Interventional Cardiac Electrophysiology
A Multidisciplinary Approach

Interventional Cardiac Electrophysiology
A Multidisciplinary Approach

EDITOR-IN-CHIEF

Sanjeev Saksena, MBBS, MD

ASSOCIATE EDITORS

Ralph J. Damiano, Jr., MD

N.A. Mark Estes III, MD

Francis E. Marchlinski, MD

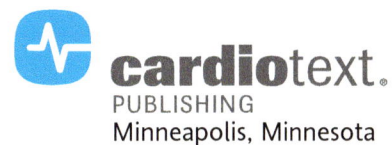

cardiotext.
PUBLISHING
Minneapolis, Minnesota

© 2015 Sanjeev Saksena

Cardiotext Publishing, LLC
3405 W. 44th Street
Minneapolis, Minnesota 55410
USA

www.cardiotextpublishing.com

Updates and disclosures for this book may be found at: www.cardiotextpublishing.com/interventional-cardiac-electrophysiology

Comments, inquiries, and requests for bulk sales can be directed to the publisher at: info@cardiotextpublishing.com.

All rights reserved. No part of this book may be reproduced in any form or by any means without the prior permission of the publisher.

All trademarks, service marks, and trade names used herein are the property of their respective owners and are used only to identify the products or services of those owners.

This book is intended for educational purposes and to further general scientific and medical knowledge, research, and understanding of the conditions and associated treatments discussed herein. This book is not intended to serve as and should not be relied upon as recommending or promoting any specific diagnosis or method of treatment for a particular condition or a particular patient. It is the reader's responsibility to determine the proper steps for diagnosis and the proper course of treatment for any condition or patient, including suitable and appropriate tests, medications or medical devices to be used for or in conjunction with any diagnosis or treatment.

Due to ongoing research, discoveries, modifications to medicines, equipment and devices, and changes in government regulations, the information contained in this book may not reflect the latest standards, developments, guidelines, regulations, products or devices in the field. Readers are responsible for keeping up to date with the latest developments and are urged to review the latest instructions and warnings for any medicine, equipment or medical device. Readers should consult with a specialist or contact the vendor of any medicine or medical device where appropriate.

Except for the publisher's website associated with this work, the publisher is not affiliated with and does not sponsor or endorse any websites, organizations or other sources of information referred to herein.

The publisher and the authors specifically disclaim any damage, liability, or loss incurred, directly or indirectly, from the use or application of any of the contents of this book.

Unless otherwise stated, all figures and tables in this book are used courtesy of the authors.

Library of Congress Control Number: 2015937687

ISBN: 978-0-9790164-8-6

Printed in the United States of America

20 19 18 17 16 15   1 2 3 4 5 6 7 8 9 10

DEDICATION

This book is dedicated to our families and our mentors, without whose unselfish and unstinting support and encouragement, we could not have made this work a reality.

CONTENTS

Contributors xiii
Preface xxv
Abbreviations xxvii

SECTION 1: Technology and Therapeutic Techniques 1

Section 1A: Electrophysiologic Techniques 1

Chapter 1: Fundamental Aspects of Electrophysiology Procedures 3
Ann C. Garlitski, N.A. Mark Estes III

Chapter 2: Electrocardiography for the Invasive Electrophysiologist 11
Christopher J. McLeod, Traci L. Buescher, Samuel J. Asirvatham

Chapter 3: Complex Catheter Recording and Mapping Techniques in the EP Lab ... 23
Andrew K. Krumerman, John D. Fisher

Chapter 4: Advances in Electroanatomic Mapping Systems 35
Brian J. Cross, Ann C. Garlitski, N.A. Mark Estes III

Chapter 5: Intraoperative Mapping for the Surgeon and Electrophysiologist 45
John M. Miller, Daniel J. Beckman, Yousuf Mahomed

Chapter 6: Special Considerations for Pediatric Electrophysiological Procedures ... 55
George F. Van Hare

Section 1B: Imaging Technology 63

Chapter 7: Fundamentals and Applications of Echocardiographic Methods and Systems in the Electrophysiology Laboratory 65
Shantanu P. Sengupta, A. Jamil Tajik, Bijoy K. Khandheria

Chapter 8: The Role of 3D Transthoracic and Transesophageal Echocardiography in Interventional Electrophysiology 71
Wael AlJaroudi, Fadi G. Hage, Navin C. Nanda

Chapter 9: Intracardiac Echocardiography 83
Susan S. Kim, Bradley P. Knight, Robert Schweikert, Sanjeev Saksena

Chapter 10: Radiological Principles of Cardiac Computed Tomography, Magnetic Resonance Imaging, and Fusion Imaging 97
Alejandro Jimenez, Timm M. Dickfeld

Chapter 11: Cardiac Computed Tomography and Magnetic Resonance Image Interpretation During Interventional Procedures 119
Saman Nazarian, Henry R. Halperin, Hugh Calkins

Chapter 12: Hybrid Operating Rooms 127
Joseph Yammine, Gregory F. Michaud, William G. Stevenson, Laurence M. Epstein

Section 1C: Device Technology 133

Chapter 13: New Developments in Lead and Introducer Systems 135
Brian J. Cross, Mark S. Link

Chapter 14: New Innovations in Implantable Pulse Generators and Heart Failure Devices 141
Helge U. Simon, Johannes Brachmann

Chapter 15: Implantable and Remote Monitoring 149
Werner Jung

Chapter 16: Percutaneous Left Atrial Appendage Occlusion 165
Heyder Omran

Chapter 17: Principles and Techniques for Lead Extraction and Device System Revision for the Surgeon and Interventionalist 171
Melanie Maytin, Laurence M. Epstein

Section 1D: Ablation Technology 185

Chapter 18: Anatomy and Histopathology of Ablation Interventions 187
S. Yen Ho

Chapter 19: Physical and Experimental Aspects of Radiofrequency Energy, Generators, and Energy Delivery Systems 205
Munther K. Homoud, Abram Mozes

Chapter 20: Cryothermal Ablation Technology and Catheter Delivery Systems 219
Rohit Bhagwandien, Paul Knops, Luc Jordaens

Chapter 21: Laser, Ultrasound, and Microwave Ablation 227
Paul J. Wang

Chapter 22: Ablation Technology for the Surgical Treatment of Atrial Fibrillation 233
Richard B. Schuessler, Ralph J. Damiano, Jr.

Chapter 23: Remote Navigation in Catheter Procedures 241
J. David Burkhardt, Luigi DiBiase, Andrea Natale

Section 1E: Drug Therapy 247

Chapter 24: How to Perform Drug Testing and Use Antiarrhythmic Drugs
in Clinical Electrophysiology 249
*Manoj N. Obeyesekere, Peter Leong-Sit, Lorne J. Gula, Raymond Yee, Allan C. Skanes,
George J. Klein, Andrew D. Krahn*

Chapter 25: Clinical Pharmacology of Anesthetic Agents and Their Application
in Cardiac Electrophysiologic Procedures 267
Jun Lin, David G. Benditt, Fei Lü

SECTION 2: Interventional Electrophysiology Procedures 281

Section 2A: Diagnostic & Mapping Techniques During Percutaneous Catheter & Surgical EP Procedures 281

Chapter 26: Sinus Node and AV Conduction System 283
Stavros E. Mountantonakis, Edward P. Gerstenfeld

Chapter 27: Paroxysmal Supraventricular Tachycardias................................. 299
Thorsten Lewalter

Chapter 28: Atrial Tachycardia and Atrial Flutter.. 315
Frederick T. Han, Nitish Badhwar

Chapter 29: Atrial Fibrillation: Clinical Electrophysiologic Evaluation 327
Rangadham Nagarakanti, Nicholas D. Skadsberg, Sanjeev Saksena

Chapter 30: Ventricular Tachycardia with Heart Disease 345
Wendy S. Tzou, Francis E. Marchlinski

Chapter 31: Idiopathic Ventricular Arrhythmias.. 355
Bruno R. Andrea, Gerhard Hindricks, Arash Arya

Chapter 32: Polymorphic Ventricular Tachycardia and Ventricular Fibrillation:
Mapping in Percutaneous Catheter and Surgical EP Procedures....... 391
*Mélèze Hocini, Ashok J. Shah, Shinsuke Miyazaki, Lena Rivard, Amir S. Jadidi, Daniel Scherr,
Stephen B. Wilton, Laurent Roten, Patrizio Pascale, Michala Pedersen, Nicolas Derval,
Sébastien Knecht, Frédéric Sacher, Pierre Jaïs, Michel Haïssaguerre*

Chapter 33: Mapping of Arrhythmias During Pediatric Electrophysiology Procedures 405
Larry A. Rhodes

Chapter 34: Intraoperative Mapping During Surgical Ablation Procedures 417
Takashi Nitta, Shun-ichiro Sakamoto

Section 2B: Catheter Ablation: Procedural Techniques and Endpoints 431

Chapter 35: Anesthesia and Airway Management for Ablation 433
Natalia S. Ivascu, Brigid C. Flynn

Chapter 36: High-Frequency Jet Ventilation in Electrophysiology 441
Jeff E. Mandel, Nabil M. Elkassabany

Chapter 37: Anesthesia for Electrophysiological Surgery and Procedures:
Quality, Safety, and Outcomes.. 451
Alfred J. Albano, Alexander G. Wolf, Michael England

Chapter 38: Atrioventricular Junction Ablation.. 463
Andrea Corrado, Antonio Rossillo, Paolo China, Antonio Raviele

Chapter 39: Sinus Node and Ablation and Atrioventricular Nodal Reentry Ablation.................. 475
Wanwarang Wongcharoen, Shih-Ann Chen

Chapter 40: Catheter Ablation of Accessory AV Pathways
(Wolff–Parkinson–White Syndrome and Variants) 489
Hiroshi Nakagawa, Warren M. Jackman

Chapter 41: Atrial Flutter: Right Atrial and Left Atrial Flutter 505
Steven M. Markowitz, Bruce B. Lerman

Chapter 42: Atrial Fibrillation.. 519

    A: Atrial Fibrillation: Linear Catheter Ablation 519
    Carlo Pappone, Vincenzo Santinelli

    B: Atrial Fibrillation: Focal and Map-guided Ablation 527
    Mauricio S. Arruda, Ashish A. Bhimani

    C: Laser and Cryothermal Balloon Ablation of Pulmonary Veins to Treat Atrial Fibrillation ... 543
    Thorsten Lewalter, Rangadham Nagarakanti, Sanjeev Saksena

Chapter 43: Ventricular Tachycardia in the Apparently Normal Heart:
Optimizing Safety and Results with Ablative Therapy 553
Amit Noheria, Mohamed Nosair, Traci L. Buescher, Christopher J. McLeod, Samuel J. Asirvatham

Chapter 44: Ventricular Tachycardia with Ischemic and Nonischemic Heart Disease 571
William W.B. Chik, Ioan Liuba, Pasquale Santangeli, Francis E. Marchlinski

Chapter 45: Epicardial Ablation.. 589
Wendy S. Tzou, Francis E. Marchlinski

Chapter 46: Ventricular Fibrillation.. 599
Ashok J. Shah, Daniel Scherr, Xingpeng Liu, Nicolas Derval, Michel Haïssaguerre

Chapter 47: Complications of Catheter Ablation and Their Management 607
Riccardo Cappato, Luigi De Ambroggi

Section 2C: Surgical Ablation.. 617

Chapter 48: Ventricular Tachycardia with Hybrid Endocardial and Epicardial Approaches............ 619
Nimesh D. Desai, Michael A. Acker

Chapter 49: Surgical Ablation for Atrial Fibrillation: Current Procedures and Clinical Outcomes 629

    A: Surgical Ablation for Atrial Fibrillation: The Cox-Maze IV Procedure 629
        Timo Weimar, Ralph J. Damiano, Jr.

    B: Surgical Ablation for Atrial Fibrillation: The Cryosurgical Cox-Maze Procedure
       Using Argon-based Cryoprobes 635
        Niv Ad

    C: Surgical Ablation for Atrial Fibrillation: Left Antral Pulmonary Vein Isolation, Ganglionic
       Plexi Ablation, and Excision of the Left Atrial Appendage 643
        Randall K. Wolf, Sandra Burgess

    D: Surgical Ablation for Atrial Fibrillation: Extended Left Atrial Lesion Set 653
        James R. Edgerton, Karen L. Roper, Stuart J. Head

    E: Surgical Ablation for Atrial Fibrillation: Ganglionic Ablation 659
        Rishi Arora, Richard Lee

    F: Surgical Ablation for Atrial Fibrillation: Hybrid Atrial Fibrillation Procedures 667
        Mark La Meir, Laurent Pison

Chapter 50: Surgical Ablation of Inappropriate Sinus Tachycardia 679
    Timo Weimar, Ralph J. Damiano, Jr.

Chapter 51: Complications of Surgical Ablation 685
    Peyman Benharash, Richard J. Shemin

Section 2D: Device Implantation: Intraoperative, Surgical, and Device Management 691

Chapter 52: Implantation Techniques for Permanent Pacemakers and Single- and
Dual-Chamber Implantable Cardioverter-defibrillator Devices 693
    Mark L. Blitzer, Mark H. Schoenfeld

Chapter 53: Surgical Considerations in Device Implantation 705
    Raj R. Kaushik, Sanjeev Saksena

Chapter 54: Ventricular and Atrial Resynchronization Devices:
Technology and Implantation Methods 717
    Robert K. Altman, Jagmeet P. Singh

Chapter 55: Organizing Best Practices in the Device Clinic 731
    Melanie Turco Gura

Chapter 56: Postoperative Management and Follow-up of Cardiac Rhythm Management Devices 753
    Bharat K. Kantharia, Arti N. Shah

Chapter 57: Optimization of Cardiac Resynchronization Therapy: Techniques and Patient Selection ... 767
    Kevin P. Jackson, Brett D. Atwater, James P. Daubert

Chapter 58: Radiologic Aspects of Cardiovascular Implantable Electronic Devices 783
    *John C. Evans, Karin Chia, Mintu P. Turakhia, Henry H. Hsia, Paul Zei,
Marco V. Perez, Paul J. Wang, Amin Al-Ahmad*

Chapter 59: Device-based Monitoring for Arrhythmias 803
Paul D. Ziegler, Douglas A. Hettrick, Rangadham Nagarakanti, Sanjeev Saksena

Chapter 60: Indications and Outcomes of Lead Extraction and Replacement Procedures
for Pacemaker and Defibrillator Systems 823
Steven P. Kutalek

SECTION 3: Clinical Indications and Evidence-based Outcomes Standards in Interventional Electrophysiology 837

Chapter 61: Catheter Ablation of AV Junction and Paroxysmal SVT 839
Sanjaya Gupta, Karl J. Ilg, Hakan Oral

Chapter 62: Catheter Ablation of Atrial Flutter and Fibrillation 847
Jasbir S. Sra, Sanjeev Saksena

Chapter 63: Ventricular Tachycardia and Ventricular Fibrillation 867
Indrajit Choudhuri, Masood Akhtar

Chapter 64: Permanent Pacing: Clinical Indications and Evidence-based
Outcomes Standards in Interventional Electrophysiology 891
Jaimie Manlucu, Bhavanesh Makanjee, Andrew D. Krahn, Raymond Yee

Chapter 65: Clinical Indications and Evidence-based Outcomes Standards in Interventional
Electrophysiology: Implantable Cardioverter-defibrillator Therapy 907
Bharat K. Kantharia, Arti N. Shah, Sanjeev Saksena

Chapter 66: Indications for Surgical Ablation of Tachyarrhythmias 921

    A: Atrial Fibrillation/Atrial Flutter 921
    David C. Kress

    B: Ventricular Tachycardia 929
    Lindsey L. Saint, Jason O. Robertson, Ralph J. Damiano, Jr.

SECTION 4: New Directions for Interventional Therapy 941

Chapter 67: Hybrid Device, Ablation, and Drug Therapy in Atrial Fibrillation 943
Sanjeev Saksena

Chapter 68: Staged Therapy Approaches in Atrial Fibrillation 967
Mario D. Gonzalez, Gerald V. Naccarelli

Chapter 69: Hybrid Device, Ablation, and Drug Therapy in Ventricular Tachyarrhythmias 981
Carlo Lavalle, Massimo Santini

Index 997

CONTRIBUTORS

Editor-in-Chief

Sanjeev Saksena, MBBS, MD, FACC, FHRS, FESC, FAHA, FRSM
Clinical Professor of Medicine, Rutgers Robert Wood Johnson Medical School; Medical Director, Electrophysiology Research Foundation, New Brunswick and Warren, New Jersey

Associate Editors

Ralph J. Damiano, Jr., MD, FACC, FACS
Evarts A. Graham Professor of Surgery; Chief, Division of Cardiothoracic Surgery; Vice-Chairman, Department of Surgery, Washington University School of Medicine, Barnes-Jewish Hospital, St. Louis, Missouri

N.A. Mark Estes III, MD, FACC, FHRS, FAHA, FESC
Professor of Medicine, Tufts University School of Medicine; Director, New England Cardiac Arrhythmia Center, Tufts Medical Center, Boston, Massachusetts

Francis E. Marchlinski, MD, FACC, FHRS, FAHA
Director Cardiac Electrophysiology, Department of Medicine, Division of Cardiovascular Medicine, University of Pennsylvania Health System; Professor of Medicine, University of Pennsylvania School of Medicine, Philadelphia, Pennsylvania

Contributors

Michael A. Acker, MD, FACC, FASA
Chief, Division of Cardiovascular Surgery; Director, Penn Medicine Heart and Vascular Center, University of Pennsylvania Health System, Philadelphia, Pennsylvania

Niv Ad, MD
Chief, Cardiac Surgery; Director, Cardiac Surgery Research; Professor of Surgery, Virginia Commonwealth University, Inova Heart and Vascular Institue, Falls Church, Virginia

Masood Akhtar, MD, FACC, MACP, FAHA, FHRS
Clinical Adjunct Professor of Medicine, University of Wisconsin School of Medicine and Public Health; Director, Electrophysiology Research and Cardiovascular Continuing Medical Education Program, Aurora Cardiovascular Services, Aurora Sinai/Aurora St. Luke's Medical Centers, Milwaukee, Wisconsin

Amin Al-Ahmad, MD, FACC, FHRS
Texas Cardiac Arrhythmia Institute, St. David's Medical Center, Austin, Texas

Alfred J. Albano, MD
Fellow, Cardiac Electrophysiology, Tufts Medical Center, Boston, Massachusetts

Wael AlJaroudi, MD, FACC, FAHA, FESC, FASE
Assistant Professor of Medicine, Division of Cardiovascular Medicine/Cardiovascular Imaging, American University of Beirut Medical Center, Beirut, Lebanon

Robert K. Altman, MD
Department of Medicine, Mount Sinai St. Luke's Roosevelt Hospital, New York, New York

Bruno R. Andrea, MD
Fellow of Rhythmology and Electrophysiology, Heart Centre Leipzig, University of Leipzig, Germany; Electrophysiology Staff and Director of the Corritmo Group, Rio de Janeiro, Brazil

Rishi Arora, MD
Associate Professor, Medicine–Cardiology, Northwestern University Feinberg School of Medicine, Chicago, Illinois

Mauricio S. Arruda, MD
Associate Professor of Medicine, Case Western Reserve University; Director, Electrophysiology and Atrial Fibrillation Center, University Hospital Harrington Heart & Vascular Institute, Cleveland, Ohio

Arash Arya, MD
Cardiologist and Interventional Electrophysiologist Senior Consultant at Heart Center University of Leipzig, Germany; Electrophysiology Fellowship Coordinator, Heart Center University of Leipzig, Germany

Samuel J. Asirvatham, MD, FACC, FHRS
Consultant, Division of Cardiovascular Diseases and Internal Medicine, Division of Pediatric Cardiology; Professor of Medicine and Pediatrics, Mayo Clinic College of Medicine; Research Translation Cardiovascular Liaison, Program Director, EP Fellowship Program, Mayo Clinic, Rochester, Minnesota

Brett D. Atwater, MD
Assistant Professor of Medicine, Division of Clinical Cardiac Electrophysiology, Duke Cardiology, Duke University Medical Center, A Division of the Department of Medicine, Durham, North Carolina

Nitish Badhwar, MBBS, MD
Associate Professor of Medicine, Cardiac Electrophysiology Fellowship Director, University of California, San Francisco, California

Daniel J. Beckman, MD, FACS
Director, Cardiovascular Critical Care, Indiana University Health Methodist, Indianapolis, Indiana

David G. Benditt, MD, FACC, FHRS, FRCPC, FESC
Cardiac Arrhythmia / Syncope Center, Cardiovascular Division, University of Minnesota Medical School, Minneapolis, Minnesota

Peyman Benharash, MD
Assistant Professor, Department of Bioengineering, UCLA Cardiothoracic Surgery, Los Angeles, California; Cardiothoracic Surgery, Ronald Reagan UCLA Medical Center, UCLA Medical Center, Santa Monica, California

Rohit Bhagwandien, MD
Cardiac Electrophysiology, Erasmus MC, Thorax Centre, Rotterdam, The Netherlands

Ashish A. Bhimani, MD
Assistant Professor of Medicine, University of Texas Medical Branch; Director, Atrial Fibrillation Program, Galveston, Texas

Mark L. Blitzer, MD
Assistant Clinical Professor of Medicine (Cardiology), Yale School of Medicine; Yale-New Haven Hospital, New Haven, Connecticut

Johannes Brachmann, MD, FACC, FHRS
Professor of Internal Medicine, Chief, Division of Internal Medicine II, Klinikum Coburg, Germany

Traci L. Buescher, RN, BSN, CEPS, FHRS
Heart Rhythm Services, Division of Cardiovascular Diseases and Internal Medicine, Mayo Clinic, Rochester, Minnesota

Sandra Burgess, BS, BA
Program Director, Hearts in Rhythm, Houston, Texas

J. David Burkhardt, MD, FACC, FHRS
Director of Research, Texas Cardiac Arrhythmia Institute, Austin, Texas; Director of Complex Arrhythmia Ablation, Scripps Clinic, La Jolla, California

Hugh Calkins, MD, FACC, FHRS, FAHA
Nicholas J. Fortuin MD Professor of Cardiology, Professor of Medicine; Director, Cardiac Arrhythmia Services; Director, Electrophysiology Laboratory, The Johns Hopkins Medical Institutions, Baltimore, Maryland

Riccardo Cappato, MD, FHRS, FESC
Director, Center of Clinical Arrhythmia and Electrophysiology, IRCCS Policlinico San Donato, San Donato Milanese (MI), Italy

Shih-Ann Chen, MD
Attending Physician, Division of Cardiology; Professor of Medicine and Director of Department of Medicine, Taipei Veterans General Hospital and National Yang-Ming University, Taipei, Taiwan

Karin K.M. Chia, MBBS, MD, PhD, FRACP, FCSANZ
Staff Cardiac Electrophysiologist, Senior Lecturer, Department of Cardiology, Royal Brisbane and Women's Hospital, University of Queensland, Brisbane, Australia

William W.B. Chik, MBBS, MD, PhD, FRACP
Clinical Cardiac Electrophysiology and Pacing Fellow, Cardiac Electrophysiology Department, Hospital of The University of Pennsylvania, Philadelphia, Pennsylvania

Paolo China, MD
Cardiovascular Department, Dell'Angelo Hospital, Mestre–Venice, Italy

Indrajit Choudhuri, MD
Clinical Adjunct Assistant Professor of Medicine, University of Wisconsin School of Medicine and Public Health; Attending, Clinical Cardiac Electrophysiology Service, Aurora Cardiovascular Services, Aurora Sinai/Aurora St. Luke's Medical Centers, Milwaukee, Wisconsin

Andrea Corrado, MD
Cardiovascular Department, Dell'Angelo Hospital, Mestre–Venice, Italy

Brian J. Cross, MD
Cardiac Electrophysiology, Regional Cardiovascular and Medical Center, Inc., Steubenville, Ohio

James P. Daubert, MD
Professor of Medicine, Duke Cardiology, A Division of the Department of Medicine, Durham, North Carolina

Luigi De Ambroggi, MD, FESC
Professor of Cardiology, University of Milan; Senior Consultant at IRCCS Policlinico San Donato, San Donato Milanese, Milan, Italy

Nicolas Derval, MD
L'Institut de Rythmologie et Modélisation Cardiaque, Institut Hospitalo-Universitaire; Hôpital haut Lévèque, Universite de Bordeaux, Bordeaux, France

Nimesh D. Desai, MD, PhD, FRCSC, FAHA
Director, Thoracic Aortic Surgery Research Program; Assistant Professor, Division of Cardiovascular Surgery, Hospital of The University of Pennsylvania, Philadelphia, Pennsylvania

Luigi Di Biase, MD, PhD, FACC, FHRS
Section Head Electrophysiology; Director of Arrhythmia Services; Associate Professor of Medicine, Department of Medicine (Cardiology), Albert Einstein College of Medicine at Montefiore Hospital, New York, New York; Senior Researcher at Texas Cardiac Arrhythmia Institute, St. David's Medical Center, Austin, Texas; Adjunct Associate Professor, Department of Biomedical Engineering, University of Texas, Austin, Texas; Assistant Professor, Section of Cardiology, University of Foggia, Foggia, Italy

Timm M. Dickfeld, MD, PhD, FACC, FHRS
Maryland Arrhythmia and Cardiology Imaging Group (MACIG), Director of Electrophysiology, VA Baltimore; Associate Professor, University of Maryland; Division of Cardiology, University of Maryland Medical Center, Baltimore, Maryland

James R. Edgerton, MD, FACC, FHRS, FACS
Surgical Director of Atrial Fibrillation Center of Innovation, Director of Education and Training, The Heart Hospital, Baylor Plano, Plano, Texas

Nabil M. Elkassabany, MD, MS
Assistant Professor of Anesthesiology and Critical Care at the Hospital of The University of Pennsylvania and the Veteran's Administration Medical Center, Departments of Anesthesiology and Critical Care, Philadelphia, Pennsylvania

Michael England, MD
Division Chief, Cardiac Anesthesiology; Assistant Professor, Tufts University School of Medicine, Boston, Massachusetts

Laurence M. Epstein, MD
Chief, Cardiac Arrhythmia Service; Director, Electrophysiology and Pacing Laboratory, Brigham and Women's Hospital; Associate Professor of Medicine, Cardiovascular Division, Harvard Medical School, Boston, Massachusetts

John C. Evans
Clinical Cardiac Electrophysiologist, Renown Institute for Heart and Vascular Health, Reno, Nevada

John D. Fisher, MD, FACP, FACC, FHRS, FAHA, FESC
Professor of Medicine, Albert Einstein College of Medicine; Program Director, CCEP, Montefiore Medical Center, Bronx, New York

Brigid C. Flynn, MD
Associate Professor, University of Kansas City Medical Center, Kansas City, Kansas

Ann C. Garlitski, MD, FACC, FHRS
Assistant Professor of Medicine, Hofstra North Shore-LIJ School of Medicine, Manhasset, New York

Edward P. Gerstenfeld, MD, FACC, FHRS
Professor of Medicine; Chief, Cardiac Electrophysiology, University of California, San Francisco, California

Mario D. Gonzalez, MD, FACC, FHRS
Professor of Medicine; Director, Clinical Electrophysiology, Penn State Heart and Vascular Institute, Milton S. Hershey Medical Center, Penn State University, Hershey, Pennsylvania

Lorne J. Gula, MD, MSc, FRCP(C)
Associate Professor of Medicine, Division of Cardiology, Western University, London, Ontario, Canada

Sanjaya Gupta, MD, FACC
Assistant Professor of Internal Medicine, University of Missouri–Kansas City, Cardiac Electrophysiologist, St. Luke's Hospital, Kansas City, Missouri

Melanie Turco Gura, MSN RN, CNS, CCDS, FHRS, FAHA, AACC
Director, Pacemaker & Arrhythmia Services, Northeast Ohio Cardiovascular Specialists, Akron, Ohio

Fadi G. Hage, MD, FACC
Assistant Professor of Medicine, University of Alabama at Birmingham; Division of Cardiovascular Disease, Birmingham Veterans Affairs Medical Center, Birmingham, Alabama

Michel Haïssaguerre, MD, FESC
Professor of Cardiology, L'Institut de Rythmologie et Modélisation Cardiaque, Institut Hospitalo-Universitaire; Hôpital haut Lévèque, Universite de Bordeaux, Bordeaux, France

Henry R. Halperin, MD, MA, FAHA, FHRS
David J. Carver Professor of Medicine; Professor of Biomedical Engineering and Radiology, Johns Hopkins University; Division of Cardiology, The Johns Hopkins Hospital, Baltimore, Maryland

Frederick T. Han, MD, FACC, FHRS
Assistant Professor of Medicine, University of Utah Health Sciences Center, Division of Cardiovascular Medicine, Section of Cardiac Electrophysiology, Salt Lake City, Utah

Stuart J. Head, MD, PhD
Department of Cardiothoracic Surgery, Erasmus University Medical Center, Rotterdam, The Netherlands

Douglas A. Hettrick, PhD
Medical Affairs Director/Technical Fellow, Coronary and Renal Denervation, Medtronic Inc., Mounds View, Minnesota

Gerhard Hindricks, MD
Professor of Medicine (Cardiology) Heart Center, University of Leipzig, Germany; Director of Department of Electrophysiology Leipzig, Germany

S. Yen Ho, PhD, FRCPath, FESC, FHEA
Head, Professor of Cardiac Morphology, Royal Brompton Hospital, London, UK

Mélèze Hocini, MD
Professor of Medicine, L'Institut de Rythmologie et Modélisation Cardiaque, Institut Hospitalo-Universitaire; Hôpital haut Lévèque, Universite de Bordeaux, Bordeaux, France

Munther K. Homoud, MD, FACC, FHRS, FACP
Associate Professor of Medicine, Tufts University School of Medicine; Co-Director, Cardiac Electrophysiology and Pacemaker Laboratory, Tufts Medical Center, Boston, Massachusetts

Henry H. Hsia, MD, FACC, FHRS
Health Science Professor of Medicine; Chief, Electrophysiology Service, VA Medical Center, University of California, San Francisco, San Francisco, California

Karl J. Ilg, MD
Cardiac Electrophysiologist, Genesys Regional Medical Center, Grand Blanc, Michigan

Natalia S. Ivascu, MD
Associate Professor of Clinical Anesthesiology; Associate Medical Director, Cardiothoracic Surgical Intensive Care Unit, New York Presbyterian Hospital–Weill Cornell Medical College, New York, New York

Warren M. Jackman, MD, FACC, FHRS
George Lynn Cross Research Professor, Senior Scientific Advisor, Heart Rhythm Institute, University of Oklahoma Health Sciences Center, Oklahoma City, Oklahoma

Kevin P. Jackson, MD
Division of Clinical Cardiac Electrophysiology, Department of Medicine, Duke University Medical Center, Durham, North Carolina

Amir S. Jadidi, MD
L'Institut de Rythmologie et Modélisation Cardiaque, Institut Hospitalo-Universitaire; Hôpital haut Lévèque, Universite de Bordeaux, Bordeaux, France

Pierre Jaïs, MD
L'Institut de Rythmologie et Modélisation Cardiaque, Institut Hospitalo-Universitaire; Hôpital haut Lévèque, Universite de Bordeaux, Bordeaux, France

Alejandro Jimenez, MD
Consultant Cardiologist/Electrophysiologist, Wellington Hospital; Senior Lecturer, University of Otago, Wellington School of Medicine, Wellington, New Zealand

Luc Jordaens, MD, PhD, FESC
Professor of Clinical and Experimental Electrophysiology, Erasmus MC, Rotterdam, The Netherlands; Professor of Cardiology, University of Ghent, Ghent Belgium

Werner Jung, MD, FESC, FHRS
Professor of Medicine-Cardiology, Head of the Department of Cardiology, Schwarzwald-Baar Klinikum, Academic Teaching Hospital of the University of Freiburg, Villingen-Schwenningen, Germany

Bharat K. Kantharia, MD, FRCP, FAHA, FACC, FESC, FHRS
Professor of Medicine; Director, Clinical Cardiac Electrophysiology Fellowship Training Program, The University of Texas Health Science Center at Houston; Director, Cardiac Electrophysiology Laboratories-Memorial Hermann Hospital, Houston, Texas

Raj R. Kaushik, MD, FACC, FACS
Chief, Cardiothoracic and Vascular Surgery, Dubois Regional Medical Center; Assistant Professor of Surgery, Columbia University College of Medicine, DuBois, Pennsylvania

Bijoy K. Khandheria, MD, FACC, FACP, FESC, FASE, FAHA
Clinical Adjunct Professor of Medicine; Director, Echocardiography Services; Director, Echocardiography Center of Innovation and Research; Aurora Sinai/Aurora St. Luke's Medical Centers; University of Wisconsin School of Medicine and Public Health, Milwaukee, Wisconsin

Susan S. Kim, MD, FACC
Assistant Professor of Medicine; Director, Cardiac Implantable Electronic Device Clinic; Cardiac Electrophysiology, Department of Medicine, Division of Cardiology, Northwestern University Feinberg School of Medicine, Chicago, Illinois

George J. Klein, MD, FRCP(C)
Professor of Medicine, Division of Cardiology, Western University, London, Ontario, Canada

Sébastien Knecht, MD, PhD
L'Institut de Rythmologie et Modélisation Cardiaque, Institut Hôspitalo-Universitaire; Hôpital haut Lévèque, Universite de Bordeaux, Bordeaux, France

Bradley P. Knight, MD, FACC, FHRS
Director of Cardiac Electrophysiology, Bluhm Cardiovascular Institute of Northwestern Memorial Hospital; Chester C. and Deborah M. Cooley Distinguished Professor of Cardiology, Feinberg School of Medicine, Northwestern University; Department of Cardiology, Chicago, Illinois

Paul Knops, Ing
Cardiac Electrophysiology, Erasmus MC, Thorax Centre, Rotterdam, The Netherlands

Andrew D. Krahn, MD
Sauder Family and Heart and Stroke Foundation Chair in Cardiology; Paul Brunes Chair in Heart Rhythm Disorders; Professor of Medicine and Chief of Cardiology, University of British Columbia, Vancouver, British Columbia, Canada

David C. Kress, MD, FACS
Chief, Department of Cardiothoracic Surgery; Director, Surgical Arrhythmia Program, Aurora Sinai/Aurora St. Luke's Medical Center, Milwaukee, Wisconsin

Andrew K. Krumerman, MD, FACC, FHRS
Associate Professor of Clinical Medicine, Division of Cardiac Electrophysiology, Albert Einstein College of Medicine; Montefiore Medical Center, Bronx, New York

Steven P. Kutalek, MD, FACC, FHRS
Associate Professor of Medicine and Pharmacology; Director, Clinical Cardiac Electrophysiology; Associate Chief, Division of Cardiology, Drexel University College of Medicine, Hahnemann University Hospital, and Medical College of Pennsylvania, Philadelphia, Pennsylvania

Mark La Meir, MD, PhD
Professor of Cardiac Surgery, Department of Cardiothoracic Surgery, University Hospital Brussels, Brussels, Belgium; Department of Cardiothoracic Surgery, Maastricht University Hospital, Maastricht, The Netherlands

Carlo Lavalle, MD
Associate Director, Cardiac Electrophysiology Laboratory, San Filippo Neri Hospital, Rome, Italy

Richard Lee, MD, MBA
Co-Director; Vice-Chair, Surgery, Center for Comprehensive Cardiovascular Care at St. Louis University Hospital, St. Louis, Missouri

Peter Leong-Sit, MD, FRCP(C)
Assistant Professor of Medicine, Division of Cardiology, Western University, London, Ontario, Canada

Bruce B. Lerman, MD
H. Altschul Master Professor of Medicine; Chief, Division of Cardiology; Director, Cardiac Electrophysiology Laboratory, Weill Cornell Medical Center, New York Presbyterian Hospital, New York, New York

Thorsten Lewalter, MD, PhD, FESC
Professor of Internal Medicine–Cardiology, University of Bonn, Bonn, Germany; Head, Department of Medicine–Cardiology and Intensive Care, Isar Heart Center Munich, Munich, Germany

Jun Lin, MD, PhD
Associate Professor, Department of Anesthesiology, Stony Brook University, Health Science Center, Stony Brook, New York

Mark S. Link, MD
Professor of Medicine, Division of Cardiology, Tufts Medical Center, Boston, Massachusetts

Xingpeng Liu, MD
Heart Center, Chao-Yang Hospital, Capital Medical University, Beijing, China; Hôpital Cardologique du Haut-Lévèque and the Universite Bordeaux II, Bordeaux, France

Ioan Liuba, MD, PhD
Cardiac Electrophysiology Fellow, Hospital of The University of Pennsylvania, Cardiac Electrophysiology Department, Philadelphia, Pennsylvania

Fei Lü, MD, PhD, FACC, FHRS
Associate Professor of Medicine, Director Cardiac Electrophysiology Laboratories, University of Minnesota Cardiology, Minneapolis, Minnesota

Yousuf Mahomed, MD, FACC, FACS
Professor of Surgery, Department of Surgery Division of Cardiothoracic Surgery, Indiana University School of Medicine, Indiana University Health, Indianapolis, Indiana

Bhavanesh Makanjee, MD, FRCP(C)
Arrhythmia Service, Division of Cardiology, Western University, London, Ontario, Canada

Jeff E. Mandel, MD, MS
Assistant Professor of Anesthesiology & Critical Care, Perelman School of Medicine at the University of Pennsylvania, Philadelphia, Pennsylvania

Jaimie Manlucu, MD, FRCP(C)
Assistant Professor of Medicine, Division of Cardiology, Western University, London, Ontario, Canada

Steven M. Markowitz, MD, FACC, FHRS
Professor of Medicine, Weill Cornell Medical College, New York, New York

Melanie Maytin, MD
Instructor of Medicine, Cardiovascular Division, Harvard Medical School, Boston, Massachusetts

Christopher J. McLeod, MBChB, PhD
Assistant Professor of Medicine, Heart Rhythm Services, Division of Cardiovascular Diseases, Mayo Clinic, Rochester, Minnesota

Gregory F. Michaud, MD, FACC, FHRS
Assistant Professor of Medicine, Harvard Medical School, Division of Cardiology, Boston, Massachusetts

John M. Miller, MD, FACC, FHRS
Professor of Medicine, Indiana University School of Medicine; Director, Clinical Cardiac Electrophysiology Service, Methodist Hospital, Indianapolis, Indiana

Shinsuke Miyazaki, MD
L'Institut de Rythmologie et Modélisation Cardiaque, Institut Hospitalo-Universitaire; Hôpital haut Lévèque, Universite de Bordeaux, Bordeaux, France

Stavros E. Mountantonakis, MD
Electrophysiologist, North Shore University Hospital; Assistant Professor of Medicine, Hofstra North Shore-LIJ School of Medicine, Hampstead, New York

Abram Mozes, MD
Cardiac Electrophysiology, Cardiology Associates of Richmond, CJW Medical Center, Richmond, Virginia

Gerald V. Naccarelli, MD
Professor of Medicine; Associate Director, Penn State Heart and Vascular Institute; Chief, Division of Cardiology, Milton S. Hershey Medical Center, Penn State University, Hershey, Pennsylvania

Rangadham Nagarakanti, MD, FACC, FHRS
Asssistant Professor of Medicine, Rutgers Robert Wood Johnson Medical School; Attending Electrophysiologist, Dvision of Cardiology, Robert Wood Johnson University Hospital, New Brunswick, New Jersey

Hiroshi Nakagawa, MD, PhD
Professor of Medicine; Director, Clinical Catheter Ablation Program; Director, Translational Electrophysiology, Heart Rhythm Institute–University of Oklahoma Health Sciences Center, Oklahoma City, Oklahoma

Navin C. Nanda, MD, FACC
Distinguished Professor of Medicine and Cardiovascular Disease, Department of Medicine, Division of Cardiovascular Disease, University of Alabama at Birmingham, Birmingham, Alabama

Andrea Natale, MD, FACC, FHRS, FESC
Executive Medical Director, Texas Cardia Arrhthmia Institute, St. David's Medical Center, Austin, Texas; Consulting Professor, Division of Cardiology, Stanford University, Palo Alto, California; Senior Medical Director, Electrophysiology and Arrhythmia Services Atrial Fibrillation and Complex Arrhythmia Program California Pacific Medical Center; Clinical Associate Professor of Medicine, Case Western Reserve University, Cleveland, Ohio; Director, Interventional Electrophysiology, SCRIPPS Clinic, La Jolla, California

Saman Nazarian, MD, PhD
Assistant Professor; Director, Ventricular Arrhythmia Ablation Service Cardiac Electrophysiology, Johns Hopkins Hospital, Baltimore, Maryland

Takashi Nitta, MD, PhD
Professor and Chairman of Cardiovascular Surgery, Nippon Medical School, Tokyo, Japan

Amit Noheria, MBBS, SM
Resident in Clinical Cardiac Electrophysiology, Mayo Clinic, Rochester, Minnesota

Mohamed Nosair, MD, FRCP(C)
Assistant Professor University of Montreal, Interventional Cardiologist, Montreal Heart Institute, Montreal, Canada

Manoj N. Obeyesekere, MBBS, MRCP, FRACP
Consultant Cardiac Electrophysiologist, Department of Cardiology/Northern Heart, Northern Health, Victoria, Australia

Professor Dr. Heyder Omran, MD
Head of Department of GFO Kliniken Bonn, St. Marien Hospital and St. Josef Hospital, Academic Hospital of the University of Bonn, Bonn, Germany

Hakan Oral, MD
Frederick G. L. Huetwell Professor of Cardiovascular Medicine; Professor of Internal Medicine; Director, Cardiac Arrhythmia Service, University of Michigan, Ann Arbor, Michigan

Carlo Pappone, MD, PhD, FACC
Professor, Department of Arrhythmology, Maria Cecilia Hospital, GVM Care & Research, Cotignola, Italy

Patrizio Pascale, MD
L'Institut de Rythmologie et Modélisation Cardiaque, Institut Hospitalo-Universitaire; Hôpital haut Lévèque, Universite de Bordeaux, Bordeaux, France

Michala Pedersen, MD
L'Institut de Rythmologie et Modélisation Cardiaque, Institut Hospitalo-Universitaire; Hôpital haut Lévèque, Universite de Bordeaux, Bordeaux, France

Marco V. Perez, MD
Assistant Professor, Stanford University, Stanford, California

Laurent Pison, MD, PhD
Department of Cardiothoracic Surgery, Maastricht University Hospital, Maastricht, The Netherlands

Antonio Raviele, MD, FESC, FHRS
Cardiovascular Department, Dell'Angelo Hospital, Mestre–Venice, Italy

Larry A. Rhodes, MD
Professor of Pediatrics, West Virginia University School of Medicine, Division Chief, Pediatric Cardiology, Morgantown, West Virginia

Lena Rivard, MD
L'Institut de Rythmologie et Modélisation Cardiaque, Institut Hospitalo-Universitaire; Hôpital haut Lévèque, Universite de Bordeaux, Bordeaux, France

Jason O. Robertson, MD, MS
Research Fellow, Division of Cardiothoracic Surgery, Washington University School of Medicine, Barnes-Jewish Hospital, St. Louis, Missouri

Karen L. Roper, PhD
Senior Research Scientist, The Cardiopulmonary Research Science and Technology Institute, Dallas, Texas

Antonio Rossillo, MD
Cardiovascular Department, Dell'Angelo Hospital, Mestre–Venice, Italy

Laurent Roten, MD
L'Institut de Rythmologie et Modélisation Cardiaque, Institut Hospitalo-Universitaire; Hôpital haut Lévèque, Universite de Bordeaux, Bordeaux, France

Frédéric Sacher, MD
L'Institut de Rythmologie et Modélisation Cardiaque, Institut Hospitalo-Universitaire; Hôpital haut Lévèque, Universite de Bordeaux, Bordeaux, France

Lindsey L. Saint, MD
Research Fellow, Division of Cardiothoracic Surgery, Washington University School of Medicine, Barnes-Jewish Hospital, St. Louis, Missouri

Shun-ichiro Sakamoto, MD, PhD
Assistant Professor, Cardiovascular Surgery, Nippon Medical School, Tokyo, Japan

Pasquale Santangeli, MD, PhD
Clinical Cardiac Electrophysiology and Pacing Fellow, Hospital of The University of Pennsylvania, Cardiac Electrophysiology Department, Philadelphia, Pennsylvania

Vincenzo Santinelli, MD
Scientific Director, Arrhythmology Department, Policlinico San Donato, University of Milan, Milan, Italy

Massimo Santini, MD, FESC, FACC
Director, Cardiovascular Department, San Filippo Neri, Rome, Italy

Daniel Scherr, MD
L'Institut de Rythmologie et Modélisation Cardiaque, Institut Hospitalo-Universitaire; Hôpital haut Lévèque, Universite de Bordeaux, Bordeaux, France

Mark H. Schoenfeld, MD, FACC, FHRS, FAHA
Clinical Professor of Medicine, Yale University School of Medicine; Director, Cardiac Electrophysiology and Pacemaker Laboratory, Yale-New Haven Hospital, Saint Raphael Campus; Past President, Heart Rhythm Society; Past Governor, Connecticut Chapter, American College of Cardiology; Fellow, Saybrook College, Yale University, New Haven, Connecticut

Richard B. Schuessler, PhD
Research Professor of Surgery and Biomedical Engineering; Director, Cardiothoracic Surgery Research Laboratory, Washington University School of Medicine, St. Louis, Missouri

Robert Schweikert, MD, FACC, FHRS
Chief of Cardiology, Akron General Medical Center; Associate Professor, Northeast Ohio Medical University, Akron, Ohio

Shantanu P. Sengupta, MD, DNB, FASE, FCCP
Director, Sengupta Cardiovascular Services, Sengupta Hospital and Research Institute, Nagpur, India

Arti N. Shah, MS, MD, FACC, FACP
Assistant Professor of Medicine, Icahn School of Medicine at Mount Sinai; Director of Electrophysiology, Elmhurst Hospital Center, Queens Hospital Center, Elmhurst, New York

Ashok J. Shah, MD
L'Institut de Rythmologie et Modélisation Cardiaque, Institut Hospitalo-Universitaire; Hôpital haut Lévèque, Universite de Bordeaux, Bordeaux, France

Richard J. Shemin, MD
Cardiothoracic Surgery, UCLA Medical Center, UCLA Medical Center, Santa Monica, California

Helge U. Simon, MD, FACC
Director, Internal Medicine Division I, Cardiology, Electrophysiology, HELIOS Frankenwaldklinik, Kronach, Germany

Jagmeet P. Singh, MD, DPhil
Professor of Medicine, Harvard Medical School; Director, Resynchronization and Advanced Cardiac Therapeutics Program, Cardiac Arrhythmia Service, Massachusetts General Hospital Heart Center, Boston, Massachusetts

Nicholas D. Skadsberg, PhD
Adjunct Assistant Professor, Department of Surgery, University of Minnesota, Minneapolis, Minnesota

Allan C. Skanes, MD, FRCP(C)
Associate Professor of Medicine, Division of Cardiology, Western University, London, Ontario, Canada

Jasbir S. Sra, MD, FACC, FAHA, FHRS
Clinical Adjunct Professor of Medicine, University of Wisconsin School of Medicine and Public Health; Vice President and Medical Director of Electrophysiology, Aurora Cardiovascular Services; Director, Clinical Electrophysiology Laboratory, Aurora St. Luke's Medical Center; Director, Electrophysiology Research Laboratory, Aurora Sinai Medical Center; Program Director, Clinical Cardiac Electrophysiology Fellowship, Aurora Health Care, Milwaukee, Wisconsin

William G. Stevenson, MD
Director, Cardiac Electrophysiology Program, Brigham and Women's Hospital; Professor of Medicine, Harvard Medical School, Boston, Massachusetts

A. Jamil Tajik, MD, FACC, FAHA
Clinical Adjunct Professor of Medicine; President, Aurora Cardiovascular Services; Director, Aurora Cardiac Specialty Centers; Aurora Sinai/Aurora St. Luke's Medical Centers, University of Wisconsin School of Medicine and Public Health, Milwaukee, Wisconsin

Mintu P. Turakhia, MD, MAS, FHRS, FAHA
Assistant Professor of Medicine and (by courtesy) of Health Research & Policy, Stanford University School of Medicine; Director of Cardiac Electrophysiology, VA Palo Alto Healthcare System, Stanford, California

Wendy S. Tzou, MD
Assistant Professor of Medicine, University of Colorado School of Medicine; Associate Laboratory Director, Cardiac Electrophysiology, University of Colorado Hospital, Aurora, Colorado

George F. Van Hare, MD
Director, Pediatric Cardiology; Louis Larrick Ward Professor of Pediatrics; Co-Director, St. Louis Children's and Washington University Heart Center, St. Louis, Missouri

Paul J. Wang, MD, FACC, FHRS
Professor of Medicine, Professor of Bioengineering (by courtesy), Stanford University School of Medicine; Cardiovascular Medicine, Department of Medicine, Stanford University Medical Center, Stanford, California

Timo Weimar, MD
Cardiac Surgeon, Sana Cardiac Surgery Stuttgart GmbH, Stuttgart, Germany

Stephen B. Wilton, MD, MSc
L'Institut de Rythmologie et Modélisation Cardiaque, Institut Hospitalo-Universitaire; Hôpital haut Lévèque, Universite de Bordeaux, Bordeaux, France

Alexander G. Wolf, MD
Instructor of Anesthesiology, Tufts University School of Medicine; Cardiothoracic Anesthesiologist, Baystate Medical Center, Springfield, Massachusetts

Randall K. Wolf, MD, FACC, FACS
Professor of Surgery; Surgical Director, AFIB Center of Excellence, University of Texas, Texas Medical Center, Memorial Hermann Hospital, Houston, Texas

Wanwarang Wongcharoen, MD
Attending Physician, Division of Cardiology, Department of Internal Medicine; Associate Professor of Medicine; Faculty of Medicine, Chiang Mai University, Chiang Mai, Thailand

Joseph Yammine, MD, FACC
Clinical Assistant Professor of Medicine, Warren Alpert Medical School of Brown University; Cardiovascular Center, Memorial Hospital of Rhode Island, Pawtucket, Rhode Island

Raymond Yee, MD, FRCP(C)
Professor of Medicine; Director, Arrhythmia Service, Division of Cardiology, Western University, London, Ontario, Canada

Paul Zei, MD
Clinical Associate Professor of Medicine; Chief, Cardiology Clinics, Cardiovascular Medicine, Stanford University Medical Center, Stanford, California

Paul D. Ziegler, MS
Senior Principal Scientist and Technical Fellow, Medtronic Diagnostics and Monitoring Research, Mounds View, Minnesota

PREFACE

True progress quietly and persistently moves along without notice.
—St. Francis of Assisi

This textbook is a serious effort to encompass the knowledge base in a new cardiovascular superspeciality that has come of age. It has a long and storied pedigree, starting with medical educational events that brought together an entire spectrum of researchers and scientists culminating in a new medical discipline, Interventional Cardiac Electrophysiology. In 1990, the first international symposium on *Interventional Cardiac Electrophysiology in the Management of Cardiac Arrhythmias* brought U.S. and European investigators together to both coin the name of and open the door to this new medical discipline. Today, the discipline is a robust, thriving field that occupies the dominant role in medical practice of cardiac electrophysiology.

Like the first meeting, this textbook ventures into new educational frontiers that define the current status and future directions of interventional cardiac electrophysiology. In this text, we have assembled a global team of experts in the field and created a comprehensive, extensively color-illustrated text complemented by an online information presentation that includes the complete text, illustrations, and additional videos for teaching procedural aspects of this specialty.

This unique text has been developed at multiple levels to make it suitable for students, current practitioners, and researchers in multiple specialties involved in the care of the arrhythmia patient. Thus, we have geared sections to cardiologists, clinical and interventional electrophysiologists, cardiac surgeons practicing arrhythmia surgery, radiologists, anesthesiologists, pharmacologists, cardiac pathologists, pediatric electrophysiologists, and allied health professionals that form the healthcare team for these patients. We have chosen an approach that combines applied science fundamental to understanding the technologic aspects of this field, with the implementation of that technology in the medical environment in current-day and future practice.

Chapters are designed to progress from fundamental understanding of the techniques and technology to advanced practice of complex interventional and surgical procedures. The importance of understanding the technology in our current practice environment is paramount. Electronic recording techniques, computer-based medical reconstruction for cardiac navigation and mapping, and medical imaging have become part of daily practice in this area. The text provides the reader with the fundamental knowledge needed for these tools for the interventional electrophysiology team.

The cardiac electrophysiology suite in the modern hospital is now a multidisciplinary operating arena. The transition of the suite into a hybrid operating facility is the trend of the future and is highlighted in this text. The interventional team has been highlighted in the multidisciplinary contributions from anesthesiologists, cardiac surgeons, allied health professionals, pharmacologists, and of course, clinical electrophysiologists. Sections and chapters directed at the entire team provide a truly 360-degree view of the current cardiac electrophysiology service at a tertiary care center.

The physiologic underpinnings of the clinical interventional procedures and cardiac mapping, which often have been less prominent in recent years, have been elegantly presented by leading authorities and translated into the clinical interventional technique and its implementation. Pharmacologic and anesthetic approaches, which are critical but often overlooked, are addressed in distinct chapters. State-of-the-art therapeutic interventions with transcatheter and surgical arrhythmia ablation techniques form the core of this multidisciplinary text. There are entire sections dedicated to mapping techniques, interventional procedures for the full array of cardiac arrhythmias as well as device therapy for bradycardias and tachycardias.

We have assembled a global team of experts to prepare information about these interventions, which is supplemented by extensive illustrations and multimedia imaging. A digital version of this text provides video files to illustrate these procedures for both the new student and advanced learner. Consistent with modern best practices, we have brought together the evidence-based clinical practice guidelines relevant to this discipline in an attempt to standardize the delivery of optimal care on a worldwide basis. This section is both a factual compendium of guidelines as well as a critical assessment by leading workers in this area. Finally, the text concludes with some potential future avenues of fruitful investigation.

Albert Einstein critically wrote in another context, *"It has become appallingly obvious that our technology has exceeded our humanity."* In this volume, I hope we have embraced both aspects, to the betterment of care for our patients. In this effort, I have been truly fortunate to enlist the superb skills and unstinting support of my associate editors, who are leaders in this arena. Drs. Damiano, Estes, and Marchlinski helped develop the concept of this text, fleshed out its content and contributors, and executed the editorial process with great commitment and extraordinary patience. We are all truly indebted to them for this final product. The fine production and editorial team at Cardiotext, particularly Ms. Caitlin Altobell and Ms. Carol Syverson, made this project a reality with their tireless efforts that have spanned several years in bringing this book to fruition. For this, I can simply only express my deepest appreciation and admiration. Finally, to the reader, I hope that our experience has led us to divine your needs in great measure, and that this effort meets your requirements to achieve a superlative standard of medical practice in this discipline.

—*Sanjeev Saksena*
Editor-in-Chief

ABBREVIATIONS

2D	two-dimensional		ATP	antitachycardia pacing/ atrial tachycardia pacing
3D	three-dimensional		A-V	atrioventricular
3DRA	3D rotational angiography		AV	arteriovenous
4D	four-dimensional; "real-time 3D"		AVB	atrioventrical block
AAD	antiarrhythmic drug		AVJ	atrioventricular junction
ABL	ablation catheter		AVN	atrioventricular node
ACC	American College of Cardiology		AVNRT	atrioventricular nodal reentry tachycardia
ACT	activated clotting time		AVRT	atrioventricular reentry tachycardia
ACT	anesthesia care team		BBB	bundle branch block
AEF	atrioesophageal fistula		BCL	basic cycle length
AF	atrial fibrillation		BiV-ICD	biventricular ICD
AFCL	AF cycle length		bpm	beats per minute
AFL	atrial flutter		BSA	body surface area
AHA	American Heart Association		BT	bypass tract
AHRE	atrial high-rate episodes		CABG	coronary artery bypass grafting
ANS	autonomic nervous system		CAD	coronary artery disease
Ao	aorta		CCM	cardiac contractility modulation
AP	accessory pathway		CEAP	clinically employed allied professional
AQI	Anesthesia Quality Institute		CFAE	complex fractionated atrial electrograms
ARVD	arrhythmogenic right ventricular dysplasia		CFE	complex fractionated electrograms
ARVD/C	arrhythmogenic right ventricular dysplasia/cardiomyopathy		CFx	polycarbon-monofluoride batteries
AS	anteroseptal		CHADS$_2$	Congestive heart failure, Hypertension, Age, Diabetes, prior Stroke
ASA	American Society of Anesthesiologists		CHF	congestive heart failure
AT	atrial tachycardia			

CICSH	cardioinhibitory carotid sinus hypersensitivity	ECI	electrical coupling index
CIED	cardiac implantable electronic devices	ECMO	extracorporeal membrane oxygenation
CL	cycle length	EF	ejection fraction
CLS	closed loop stimulation	EGM	electrogram
CMP	Cox-Maze procedure	EHRA	European Heart Rhythm Association
CMR	cardiac magnetic resonance	EMI	electromagnetic interference
CPT	current procedural terminology	EOL	end of battery life
CPVA	catheter pulmonary vein ablation	EP	electrophysiology, electrophysiologic
CPVT	catecholaminergic polymorphic ventricular tachycardia	EPL	EP laboratory
		ERI	elective replacement interval
CRM	cardiac rhythm management	ERP	effective refractory period
CRT	cardiac resynchronization therapy	ESC	European Society of Cardiology
CRT-D	CRT plus defibrillator	FAM	fast atrial mapping
CRT-P	CRT plus pacemaker	FDA	U.S. Food and Drug Administration
CS	coronary sinus	FDG	18F-fluorodeoxyglucose
CSNRT	corrected sinus node recovery time	FLE	fiducial localization error
CT	computed tomography, computed tomographic	FO	fossa ovalis
		FOV	field of view
CTA	CT angiography	FRE	fiducial registration error
CTI	cavotricuspid isthmus	FRI	functional recovery index
CVE	cardiovascular event	FT	Fourier transform
DC	direct current	GETA	general endotracheal anesthesia
DE	delayed enhancement	GP	ganglionated plexi
DEEP	dual endocardial and epicardial procedures	HB	His bundle
		HCM	hypertrophic cardiomyopathy
DFT	defibrillation threshold testing	HF	heart failure
DICOM	Digital Imaging and Communications in Medicine standard	HFJV	high-frequency jet ventilation
		HIFU	high-intensity focused ultrasound
EAD	early after-depolorization	HRA	high right atrium/atrial
EAM	electroanatomic mapping	HRS	Heart Rhythm Society
EAMS	electroanatomic mapping system(s)	HU	Hounsfield units
EBM	evidence-based medicine	IAS	intraatrial septum
ECG	electrocardiogram, electrocardiograph		

IAVA	idiopathic annular ventricular arrhythmia	LL	left lateral
ICD	implantable cardioverterdefibrillator	LMA	laryngeal mask airway
ICE	intracardiac echocardiography	LP	left posterior
ICM	ischemic cardiomyopathy	LPL	left posterolateral
IDCM	idiopathic dilated cardiomyopathy	LQTS	long QT syndrome
IEAP	industry employed allied professional	LSPV	left superior pulmonary vein
IEGM	intracardiac electrogram	LSVC	left superior vena cava
IHM	implantable hemodynamic monitor	LV	left ventricle, left ventricular
IHR	intrinsic heart rate	LVEF	left ventricular ejection fraction
IJV	internal jugular vein	LVOT	left ventricular outflow tract
ILR	implantable loop recorder	MAC	monitored anesthesia care
INR	international normalized ratio	MCV	middle cardiac vein
IR	inversion recovery	MDP	mid-diastolic potential
IST	inappropriate sinus tachycardia	MI	myocardial infarction
IV	intravenous	MIP	maximum intensity projection
IVA	idiopathic ventricular arrhythmia	MRA	magnetic resonance angiography
IVC	inferior vena cava	MRI	magnetic resonance imaging
IVCD	intraventricular conduction delay	MS	midseptal
IVS	interventricular septum	MUGA	multiple uptake gated acquisition
LA	left atrium/atrial	MV	mitral valve
LAA	left atrial appendage	MVA	mitral valve annulus
LAL	left anterolateral	NBT	nitroblue tetrazolium
LAO	left anterior oblique	NCC	noncoronary cusp
LAP	left atrial pressure	NICM	nonischemic cardiomyopathy
LBBB	left bundle branch block	NIDCM	nonischemic dilated cardiomyopathy
LCA	left coronary artery	NMR	nuclear magnetic resonance
LCC	left coronary cusp	NPO	nothing per oral
LFVT	left fascicular ventricular tachycardia	NYHA	New York Heart Association
LGE	late gadolinium enhancement	OAC	oral anticoagulation
Li	lithium	OR	operating room
LIPV	left inferior pulmonary vein	OSA	obstructive sleep apnea
		OT-VT	outflow tract ventricular tachycardia

PA	posteroanterior/pulmonary artery	RA	right anterior/right atrium
PACU	postoperative care unit	RAA	right atrial appendage
PAF	paroxysmal atrial fibrillation	RAO	right anterior oblique
PapM	papillary muscle	RBBB	right bundle branch block
PE	pericardial effusion	RCA	right coronary artery
PEA	peak endocardial acceleration	RCC	right coronary cusp
PECA	percutaneous epicardial catheter ablation	RCM	remote catheter manipulator
PET	positron emission tomography	RF	radiofrequency
PFO	patent fossa ovalis	RFA	radiofrequency ablation
PJRT	permanent junctional reciprocating tachycardia	RIP	respiratory inductance plethysmography
PLA	posterior left atrium	RIPV	right inferior pulmonary vein
PM	pacemaker	RL	right lateral
PMVT/VF	polymorphic ventricular tachycardia and ventricular fibrillation	RM	remote monitoring
		RP	refractory period/right posterior
PNP	phrenic nerve palsy	RPL	right posterolateral
PONV	postoperative nausea and vomiting	RSPV	right superior pulmonary vein
POTS	postural orthostatic tachycardia syndrome	RV	right ventricle, right ventricular
		RVA	right ventricular apex
PPI	post-pacing interval	RVOT	right ventricular outflow tract
PPM	permanent pacemaker	SA	sinoatrial
PPV	positive predictive value	SACT	sinoatrial conduction time
PSMA	posteroseptal on mitral annulus	SAR	specific absorption rate
PSTA	posteroseptal on tricuspid annulus	SCD	sudden cardiac death
PSVT	paroxysmal supraventricular tachycardia	SEC	spontaneous echocardiographic contrast
PV	pulmonary vein	SHD	structural heart disease
PVAC	pulmonary vein ablation catheter	SND	sinus node dysfunction
PVAI	PV antrum isolation	SNRT	sinus node recovery time
PVC	premature ventricular complex	SPECT	single-photon emission computed tomography
PVI	pulmonary vein isolation		
QALY	quality-adjusted life-years	SR	sinus rhythm
QoR	quality of recovery	SSD	shaded surface display

SSS	sick sinus syndrome	**TSN**	transseptal needle
ST	sinus tachycardia	**TTE**	transthoracic echocardiography
SVC	superior vena cava	**TTM**	transtelephonic monitoring
SVO	silver vanadium oxide	**ULV**	upper limit of vulnerability
SVR	surgical ventricular restoration	**VA**	ventricular arrhythmia
SVT	supraventricular tachycardia	**VF**	ventricular fibrillation
TA	tricuspid annulus	**VRP**	ventricular response pacing
TCL	tachycardia cycle length	**VSD**	ventricular septal defect
TDI	tissue Doppler imaging	**VT**	ventricular tachycardia
TEE	transesophageal echocardiography	**VTA**	ventricular tachyarrhythmia
TLE	transvenous lead extraction	**VVI**	velocity vector imaging
TRE	target registration error	**WPW**	Wolff–Parkinson–White
TSC	transseptal catheterization		

SECTION 1A

TECHNOLOGY AND THERAPEUTIC TECHNIQUES

Electrophysiologic Techniques

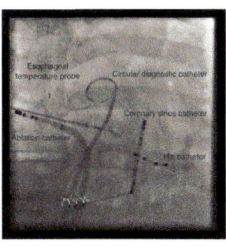 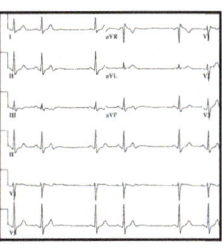 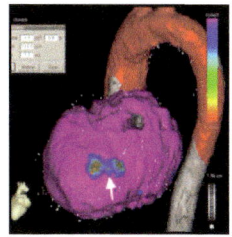 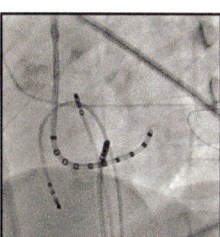

CHAPTER 1

Fundamental Aspects of Electrophysiology Procedures

Ann C. Garlitski, MD; N.A. Mark Estes III, MD

Introduction

For the first-year fellow, the electrophysiology (EP) laboratory may be an overwhelming environment with its vast array of complex procedures involving a cadre of personnel and equipment. It is important to understand the role of each individual, the placement of each catheter, the anatomic views provided by multiple imaging modalities, and the characteristics and patterns of electrograms—all of which allow for a safe and successful procedure. The goal of this chapter is to provide the novice electrophysiologist with an overview of the fundamentals of EP procedures. Armed with this foundation of knowledge, he or she will be ready to enter the complex and exciting world of the EP laboratory.

Informed Consent

Obtaining informed consent is both an ethical and a legal obligation. As with any invasive procedure, consent for an EP procedure involves an understanding of the diagnosis, the purpose of the treatment, risks and benefits, as well as alternatives. The patient should be allowed ample time to ask questions in a private setting. If the patient is deemed incompetent, then a healthcare proxy will function on the patient's behalf.

Among the risks of EP procedures are bleeding, infection, radiation exposure, cardiac perforation, heart block, stroke, and death. The likelihood of a particular complication is based on the type of procedure that is planned; therefore, consent should be tailored to the specific case. For example, a patient undergoing a diagnostic study with only right-sided catheter placement has minimal risk for major a complication such as stroke, whereas a patient undergoing ablation of a slow pathway for the treatment of atrioventricular (AV) nodal reentry tachycardia is at risk for heart block requiring pacemaker placement. On the other end of the spectrum, a life-threatening atrio-esophageal fistula, albeit rare, is a well-described complication of atrial fibrillation ablation. Although it is not possible to account for every scenario, the physician must communicate the nature of the treatment adequately to the patient.

History

Before an invasive EP study is undertaken, it is important to note certain aspects of the patient's medical and surgical history. A comprehensive assessment of the cardiac history is important, specifically the presence of congenital or acquired structural heart disease, coronary artery disease, or congestive heart failure. In the case of a patient with significant ischemia, for example, isoproterenol is avoided. In a patient with severe congestive heart failure symptoms, one may choose to avoid an irrigated catheter, which may result in the administration of a significant amount of volume during the procedure.

Other pertinent information includes a history of hematologic disorders, peripheral vascular disease, thromboembolic disease, or reaction to contrast agents. For instance, if a patient has an inferior vena cava filter, then it is reasonable to consider alternate access sites (although successful advancement of these catheters has been reported).[1] Patients who have a history of contrast allergies should be premedicated with steroids and antihistamines prior to the procedure if there is a suspicion that a vascular study will be required. Hematologic disorders or an elevated prothrombin time, partial thromboplastin time, or international normalized ratio should be addressed before the procedure so that the appropriate blood products or reversal agents are administered. Of note, progressively more data support the practice of performing device implants and atrial fibrillation ablation on patients who are therapeutically anticoagulated.[2,3] Whether anticoagulation is to be held, bridged, or continued is a decision based on the risks and benefits for that particular patient as well as the comfort level of the interventionalist.

External Defibrillators

Before performing any invasive procedure in the EP lab, electrocardiogram (ECG) electrodes must be placed on the patient in order to perform continuous cardiac monitoring. In addition, an external defibrillator should be immediately available (ie, in the room). Either self-adhesive pads or paddle electrodes may be used for cardioversion/defibrillation. In order to reduce the risk for cutaneous burns, saline-soaked gauze or conductive gel should be placed between paddles and skin. However, during an invasive study, self-adhesive pads may be favored as they may be placed on the patient at the onset of the procedure without the impediment of the fluoroscopy unit, which may impede access to the patient's chest wall. In order to improve electrode-to-skin contact and reduce transthoracic impedance, it is recommended that the patient's chest be shaved.[4,5] With regard to electrode placement, there are four pad positions (anterolateral, anteroposterior [AP], anterior–left infrascapular, and anterior–right infrascapular)[6] that are equal in their shock efficacy in treating atrial or ventricular arrhythmias.[7-9] Many studies have indicated that larger pad/paddle size (8- to 12-cm diameter) lowers transthoracic impedance.[9] It is important to note that defibrillation should not be performed directly over an implantable device.

Defibrillators deliver a shock with either a monophasic (current that flows in one direction) or biphasic (current that flows in a positive direction and then reverses) waveform, although the latter is now standard in all new devices. There are two main types of monophasic waveform: a monophasic damped sinusoidal waveform that gradually returns to zero current flow and a monophasic truncated exponential waveform that is electronically terminated before current flow reaches zero. There are two main types of biphasic waveform: the biphasic truncated exponential and rectilinear biphasic.[9] Studies have shown that lower-energy biphasic waveform shocks have equivalent, if not higher, success for termination of ventricular fibrillation than either type of monophasic waveform shock.[10,11] Of note, recommended energy levels for biphasic defibrillators vary by type of device and manufacturer.

If the manufacturer's recommended dose is not known, defibrillation at the maximal dose is reasonable.[9]

In electrical cardioversion, as opposed to defibrillation, the shock must be synchronized to the R wave (rather than with the T wave) on the ECG in order to avoid the unwanted consequence of inducing ventricular fibrillation. Ventricular fibrillation may be induced if a shock is delivered during the relative refractory portion of the cardiac cycle.

Sedation

EP procedures may be performed under local anesthesia, conscious sedation, deep sedation, or general anesthesia. Sedation may be administered under the care of an electrophysiologist with conscious sedation privileges or by an anesthesiologist. The decision to proceed with a particular form of sedation is based on several factors, including airway assessment, body habitus, length of procedure, medical comorbidities, allergies, and renal and liver function. An additional factor that may play a role in dictating the level of sedation is the mechanism of the tachycardia to be treated. Automatic tachycardias such as focal atrial tachycardias as well as right or left ventricular outflow tract tachycardias may be particularly sensitive to sedation and often require an adrenergic state in order to induce the tachycardia. The choice of sedative agents should also be planned in advance; commonly used drugs include fentanyl, midazolam, dexmedetomidine, and propofol. However, general anesthesia may be necessary for more complex cases, such as ventricular tachycardia (VT) ablation or laser lead extractions, in which hemodynamic instability may be expected.

Most importantly, communication between the cardiologist and the anesthesiologist or support staff is crucial to allow for optimal mapping conditions while maintaining patient safety. For example, certain conditions are more frequently encountered in the realm of cardiac EP, and it is important to remind colleagues and staff that QT-prolonging drugs and bradycardia should be avoided in patients with long QT syndrome and that inotropes should be avoided in patients with hypertrophic cardiomyopathy. In addition to physiologic considerations, logistical concerns such as the location of the anesthesia cart and the ventilator in relationship to the fluoroscopy unit and the availability of extension tubing for intravenous (IV) lines, oxygen, and long breathing circuits should be addressed before the procedure. Later chapters in this book will discuss sedation.

Vascular Access

The majority of EP procedures require central venous access, although some ablations such as that of left-sided VTs or left-sided accessory pathways may require arterial access for a retrograde aortic approach. In other instances, a radial or femoral arterial line may be used for more accurate hemodynamic monitoring during what may be expected to be a long or complex procedure. In the case of either venous or arterial access, the Seldinger technique, first described in 1953 by Sven Ivar Seldinger, is still the fundamental tool for obtaining vascular access.[12] A healthy respect not only for the arterial system but also for the venous system is recommended, as vascular complications are a possibility with any intervention. To avoid potential complications such as hematomas, pseudoaneurysms, aneurysms, or dissections, it is useful to be aware of a few "tricks of the trade."

A micropuncture kit is a particularly useful tool for those who have not yet honed the skill of obtaining vascular access, or even for those who are well trained but are performing a procedure on a patient who is therapeutically anticoagulated. The majority of these kits include a 21-gauge needle and a 5-Fr introducer sheath. In addition to the use of anatomic and fluoroscopic landmarks to guide the puncture, ultrasound may be used during the procedure to provide real-time localization of the relationship of the needle to the vessel.

The majority of catheters are introduced into sheaths placed via femoral venous access. Therefore, an understanding of the anatomy is critical to ensuring uncomplicated access. The superficial and deep femoral veins join to form the common femoral vein, which becomes the external iliac vein above the level of the inguinal ligament. The common femoral vein lies medial to the common femoral artery at the level of the inguinal ligament, which can be approximated by drawing an imaginary line from the anterosuperior iliac crest to the symphysis pubis. Of note, it is important not to be distracted by the inguinal fold, which does not necessarily correlate to the level of the inguinal ligament, especially in obese patients. The common femoral vein can be accessed about 0.5 cm medial to the femoral artery pulsation at the mid-inguinal ligament. Once the femoral vein is accessed, a guidewire is introduced. Under fluoroscopy, venous access can be confirmed by advancement of the guidewire on the right side of the spine along the inferior vena cava. Likewise, arterial access can be confirmed by advancement of the guidewire on the left side of the spine along the aorta. Multiple venipunctures of the femoral vein can be performed in order to advance more than one catheter.

The internal jugular vein (IJV) may also be used as an access site. The right IJV is more frequently chosen than the left as it is more convenient for a right-handed operator and is the most direct route to the superior vena cava. When preparing for IJV puncture, it is often helpful to place the patient in a Trendelenberg position if central venous pressure is suspected to be low, particularly as most patients will have been kept NPO overnight. An important anatomic landmark is the triangle formed by the two heads of the sternocleidomastoid muscle and the medial third of the clavicle. The IJV is lateral and anterior to the carotid artery. Ultrasound guidance is a useful technique that minimizes the chance of carotid artery puncture or pneumothorax.

Once the procedure is completed, the catheters and sheaths are removed, and manual compression is most commonly used to achieve hemostasis. Of course, if the patient is anticoagulated during the procedure, then an activated clotting time (ACT) test should be conducted before the sheaths are withdrawn. The definition of an acceptable ACT for sheath removal varies among laboratories as it may depend on the number and size of the sheaths as well as the patient's body habitus. The practice of using a percutaneous vascular closure device for the femoral artery has been adopted by some electrophysiologists. These devices mechanically close the puncture site using a suture, an extravascular clip, or a collagen plug.

Radiation

Radiation exposure is a consequence of the continued reliance on fluoroscopy as the fundamental imaging source in EP. Fellows who undergo formal training are more likely to be aware of safe levels of radiation exposure.[13] High cumulative radiation exposure can potentially have stochastic and deterministic effects. Stochastic effects refer to biologic effects that increase as the dose increases, but the intensity of the effect is not a function of the absorbed dose. Stochastic effects include cancer and genetic risks. Deterministic effects, such as erythema, desquamation, and cataracts, have a dose threshold, and the intensity of the effect increases with increasing dose.[14,15] Although care should be taken to minimize exposure to all patients, women of reproductive potential should all undergo a pregnancy test before the procedure in order to avoid or minimize fetal exposure.

The impact of radiation exposure affects not only the patient but also the physician and all personnel. Reductions in radiation exposure may be achieved by reducing radiation time (avoiding a "lead foot"), maintaining a safe distance from the source of radiation, and wearing barriers to radiation. The radiation beam attenuates according to the inverse square law ($1/d^2$), decreasing exponentially with distance from the radiation source. Therefore, the patient tissue receiving the greatest radiation dose is the skin area of the back at the entrance point of the x-ray beam. Of note, staff who are positioned on the same side as the x-ray tube receive a greater amount of scatter radiation. Collimation of the radiation field decreases the scattered dose. Lead aprons, thyroid collars, lead glasses, and tableside and drop-down shields are all important barriers for the physician in order to protect against scatter radiation.[14,15]

As a result of technologic advances, echocardiography, computed tomography (CT), magnetic resonance imaging (MRI), three-dimensional (3D) mapping systems, and remote navigational equipment have the potential to significantly decrease fluoroscopy times and, therefore, exposure. Today, some laboratories have gone so far as to demonstrate the feasibility of using these advanced imaging modalities to entirely replace the need for fluoroscopy.[16]

Imaging

The use of x-rays can be traced back to 1895, to Wilhem Roentgen. As noted above, single-plane or biplane fluoroscopy is still the mainstay of imaging during EP procedures. The most commonly used views are AP as well as varying degrees of left anterior oblique (LAO) and right anterior oblique (RAO). The medial-to-lateral relationship of catheters and cardiac structures can be appreciated in the LAO view, whereas the RAO view allows evaluation of the anterior-to-posterior relationship. For example, a transseptal puncture with advancement of the needle, dilator, and sheath is often performed in LAO (rather than RAO) views since the lateral border of the left atrium may be appreciated in this view. In the RAO view, the AV groove fat pad is a radiolucent area that corresponds to the tricuspid annulus and is a helpful landmark for the positioning of diagnostic catheters.

Prior to the procedure, it is valuable to consider what additional imaging tools would be useful. For instance, if an atrial fibrillation ablation or left-sided accessory pathway ablation is planned, then intracardiac echocardiography is useful for localization of the fossa ovalis during transseptal puncture. Tenting of the membrane with the needle under echocardiography can be used in conjunction with fluoroscopy to identify a safe site for puncture. For complex ablation procedures, 3D mapping may be useful to delineate anatomy, voltage, and activation patterns. Once again, it is prudent to plan ahead of time to use this equipment as these imaging systems involve patches and cables that may be challenging to place once the patient is already sedated with catheters in place.

Recordings

Recording systems utilize a process of amplification of signals as well as filtering. Band-pass filtering enables one to define a band of frequencies that are not attenuated. Low-pass filters reduce high-frequency noise (> 250 to 500 Hz), while high-pass filters reduce low-frequency noise (< 30 Hz, for example). In the EP laboratory, electrical noise can be introduced into recording systems via a common AC current. As a result, a specific use of band-pass filtering called notch filtering attenuates frequencies of 50 or 60 Hz.[17]

Catheters

There are many ways to approach a diagnostic EP study. Quadripolar catheters are typically placed in the high right atrium (HRA), the His position (His), and the right ventricular apex (RVA). The HRA catheter has a single deflection representing atrial depolarization. Occasionally, atrial and ventricular depolarization may be noted if the catheter is placed in the right atrial appendage. The His catheter reveals three deflections: electrograms from the atrium, His bundle, and ventricle. A quadripolar His catheter can be divided into three bipoles revealing three sets of electrograms: proximal His, mid His, and distal His. The catheter in the ventricle reveals a single ventricular deflection. In addition, deca- or duodecapolar catheters may be very useful as they can depict activation patterns along the length of the coronary sinus (CS). The duodecapolar catheter also displays electrograms from the cavotricuspid isthmus, which may be useful for cavotricuspid isthmus–dependent flutter or a right-sided pathway.

In addition, the CS catheter is a useful landmark for the mitral annulus, although it should be appreciated that the CS does not always run at the exact level of the annulus. These catheters may be immensely helpful because signature activation patterns, such as those of typical atrial flutter (Figure 1.1) or a left lateral accessory pathway, can be revealed at a glance. Circular diagnostic catheters are often used in atrial fibrillation ablation procedures to demonstrate isolation (or dissociation) of pulmonary vein (PV) potentials (Figures 1.2 and 1.3). Of note, the distal pole on multipolar catheters is, by convention, designated as 1.

Elements of a Comprehensive Electrophysiology Study

The birth of invasive cardiac EP dates back to the late 1960s and 1970s, when techniques to record intracardiac signals from the His bundle[18] and programmed electrical stimulation were developed to study Wolff–Parkinson–White syndrome[19] as well as VT.[20] Since that time, a standard set of variables is collected in order to assess the EP aspects of the cardiac conduction system. Baseline data should include the initial rate and rhythm, PR interval, QRS duration, and corrected QT interval. Baseline intracardiac data include AH interval (45 to 140 ms) and HV interval (35 to 55 ms). The AH interval should be measured from the His catheter at the position where the A and V electrograms are equal in size. On occasion, a split His can be noted; this denotes intra-Hisian delay. The HV interval should be measured from the His deflection to the earliest V (either on an intracardiac electrogram or the QRS deflection from the 12-lead ECG). Of note, it is normal for the V on the right ventricular apex catheter to precede the V on the His catheter. Ventricular preexcitation is denoted by an HV interval of 0 ms or a negative interval (Figure 1.4).

Different pacing maneuvers may be performed to characterize the conduction system as well as induce a tachycardia. The stimulator provides the electrophysiologist with the ability to pace from a specified bipole on a catheter. The output can be adjusted based on voltage or

Chapter 1: Fundamental Aspects of Electrophysiology Procedures • 7

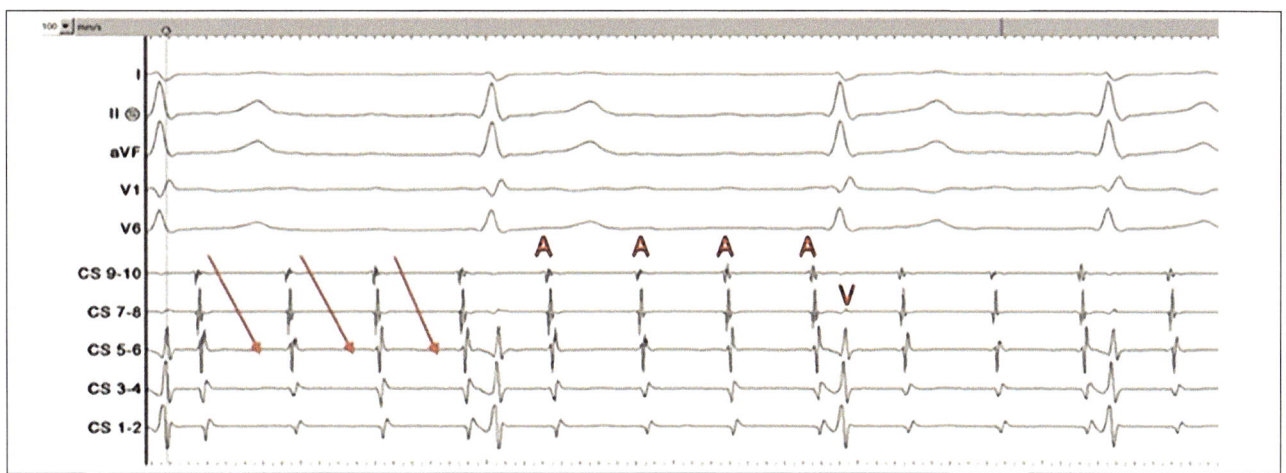

Figure 1.1 Leads I, II, aVF, V1, and V6 as well as intracardiac electrograms from the coronary sinus catheter at a sweep speed of 100 mm/second. Leads I, II, aVF, V1, and V6 are used to evaluate P-wave, QRS complex, and T-wave morphology. The CS catheter is a decapolar catheter with five bipoles. By convention, CS 1 is distal. Electrograms on the CS catheter depict left-sided atrial (**A**) and ventricular (**V**) activation. There is 4:1 atrioventricular conduction. The **arrows** depict counterclockwise activation, which is consistent with typical cavotricuspid isthmus–dependent atrial flutter.

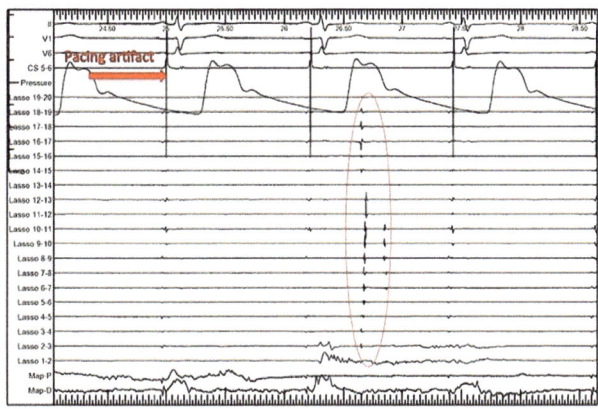

Figure 1.2 Electrograms from leads II, V1, V6, bipole 5-6 from the CS catheter, and pulmonary vein electrograms on the circular 20-pole lasso catheter, which is placed in the ostium of a pulmonary vein during atrial fibrillation ablation. The pressure waveform is obtained from an arterial line in the femoral artery. Atrial pacing is depicted by the artifact noted in the CS catheter. Pulmonary vein electrograms (**circled**) are dissociated from the atrium.

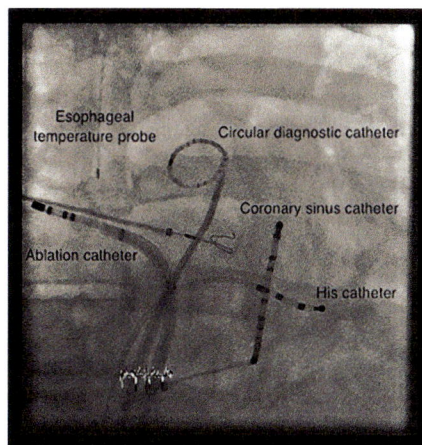

Figure 1.3 Fluoroscopic image (right anterior oblique projection) of a circular diagnostic catheter in the right superior pulmonary vein and an ablation catheter, through a sheath, in a right inferior pulmonary vein. A quadripolar diagnostic His catheter and decapolar diagnostic coronary sinus catheter are used during this procedure both as landmarks during transseptal puncture and for atrial and ventricular pacing. The esophageal temperature probe is used to monitor esophageal temperature increases when ablation is performed in the posterior aspect of the left atrium.

pulse duration. Once the threshold is determined, the output is set to twice the diastolic threshold. The operator specifies the channel from which pacing or sensing is performed. Incremental or burst pacing refers to pacing at a fixed cycle length. The extrastimulus technique refers to pacing at a fixed cycle length (by convention, a drive train of 8 beats, which are denoted as (S1) followed by a single premature beat (S2), two premature beats (S2 and S3, known as "doubles"), or three premature beats (S2, S3, and S4, known as "triples"). Antegrade (or retrograde) curves are often performed at a baseline cycle length of 600 ms, and an S2 is introduced at a decremental coupling interval of 10 ms. These interrogations of the electrical aspects of the cardiac tissue are used to define the effective refractory period of the atrium, AV node, and ventricle. The effective refractory period is defined as the longest premature coupling interval that fails to conduct.

The sinus node is evaluated by placing a catheter in the HRA and by pacing faster than the sinus rate for 60 seconds with the intention of overdrive suppressing the sinus node. A sinus node recovery time (SNRT; upper limit of 1,500 ms) and corrected SNRT (cSNRT) are obtained. The cSNRT is equal to the SNRT–BCL (basic cycle length), and the upper limit is 525 ms. There is more than one method to obtain the sinoatrial conduction time (SACT), which ranges from 45 to 125 ms.

The characteristics of the AV node are assessed by pacing the atrium and obtaining the cycle length at which

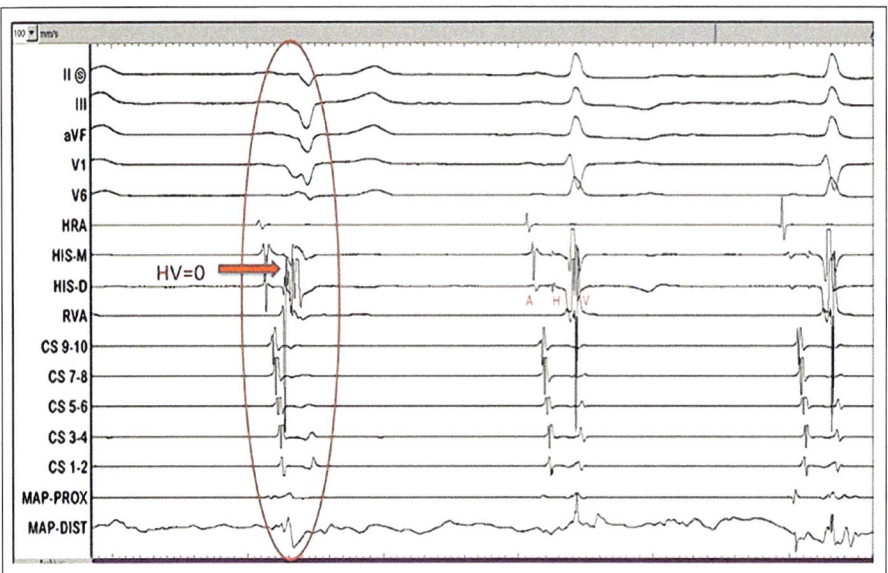

Figure 1.4 Leads II, III, aVF, V1, and V6 as well as intracardiac electrograms from the HRA catheter, His catheter (HIS-Mid, HIS-Distal), coronary sinus catheter (CS 1-10), and ablation catheter (MAP-PROX and MAP-DIST) at a sweep speed of 100 mm/second. The circled beat is preexcited as the His to earliest V interval is 0. The following two beats are a result of successful radiofrequency application resulting in antegrade conduction over the atrioventricular node such that distinct A (atrial), H (His), and V (ventricular) intracardiac signals are noted on the His catheter. The HV interval is no longer 0.

antegrade Wenckebach (Figure 1.5) and 2:1 AV block occur. When pacing the RVA, ventriculoatrial conduction should be concentric and midline (Figure 1.6). An interrogation of the retrograde characteristics of the AV node include retrograde Wenckebach and 2:1 ventriculoatrial block. AV nodal physiology will, of course, be affected by sympathetic tone as well as adrenergic agents such as isoproterenol.

Programmed atrial stimulation may be used to induce atrial fibrillation or atrial flutter. Protocols vary, particularly in the number or extrastimuli. A compilation of the reported literature reveals a sensitivity and specificity of 75% and 69%, respectively, for the induction of atrial fibrillation.[21] In atrial fibrillation ablation procedures in which the goal is to isolate the PVs, bidirectional block may be confirmed by loss of PV potentials and failure to capture the left atrium by pacing at bipolar pairs of electrodes on a circumferential catheter positioned at the entrance of the PV.[22] Of note, coronary sinus or left atrial appendage pacing may be used to distinguish far-field versus near-field signals in the PVs. Detailed protocols are addressed in later chapters of this book.

Typically, ventricular stimulation, with the intention of inducing a monomorphic VT, is performed at two or three different cycle lengths (600, 500, and/or 400 ms) at the RVA and/or right ventricular outflow tract.[23] Programmed electrical stimulation is performed with a basic drive train of eight beats immediately followed by single, double, and triple ventricular extrastimuli (known as "singles," "doubles," and "triples," respectively). With an increase in the number of extrastimuli, there is a trade-off between a higher sensitivity but a lower specificity. A positive study, in the strictest sense, results in the reproducible induction of monomorphic VT that is sustained (>15 seconds) or hemodynamically unstable requiring cardioversion.[23] In a population of patients with coronary artery disease, Hummel et al[24] showed that a stimulation protocol that uses four extrastimuli improves the specificity and efficiency of programmed ventricular stimulation without compromising the yield of monomorphic VT. There is

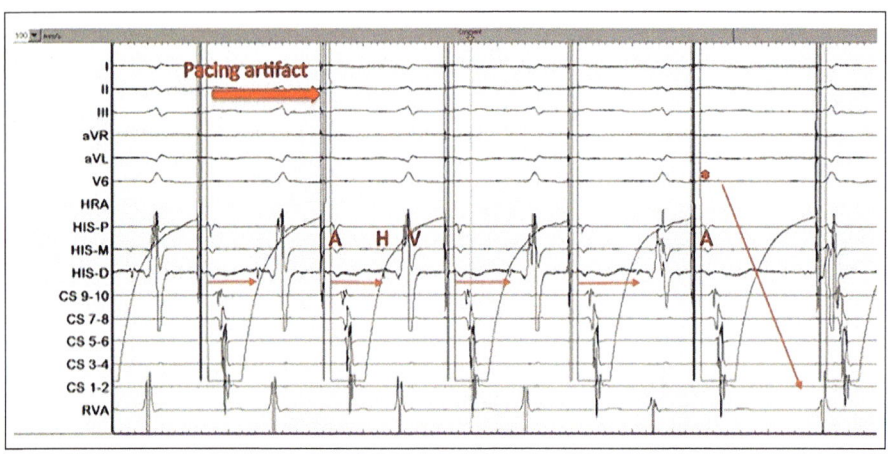

Figure 1.5 Leads I, II, III, aVR, aVL, and V6 as well as intracardiac electrograms from the HRA catheter, His catheter (HIS-Proximal, HIS-Mid, HIS-Distal), CS 1-10 catheter, and RVA catheter at a sweep speed of 100 mm/second. The artifact on the HRA catheter depicts incremental pacing in the atrium, which results in prolonged AH intervals until atrioventricular nodal Wenckebach is achieved. There is a stimulus artifact followed by atrial capture on the His and CS catheters (**asterisk**). However, there is a notable absence of His and ventricular electrograms (**long diagonal arrow**).

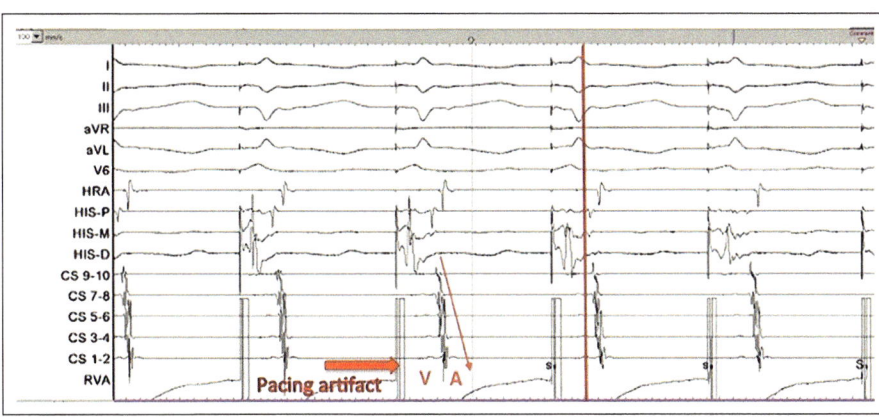

Figure 1.6 Leads I, II, III, aVR, aVL, and V6 as well as intracardiac electrograms on the HRA catheter, His catheter (HIS-Proximal, HIS-Mid, HIS-Distal), CS 1-10 catheter, and RVA catheter at a sweep speed of 100 mm/second. A stimulus artifact is noted on the RVA catheter; this denotes right ventricular pacing. Right ventricular pacing results in 1:1 ventriculoatrial conduction and a concentric activation pattern. The earliest retrograde A is in the His catheter as denoted by the diagonal line in the third beat. These findings are consistent with retrograde conduction through the atrioventricular node.

less robust data on the sensitivity and specificity of programmed electrical stimulation in patients with nonischemic cardiomyopathy. Of note, the induction of ventricular fibrillation was initially thought to be nonspecific. However, in patients who present with syncope, ventricular fibrillation and ventricular flutter induced during an EP study is an independent risk factor for arrhythmia occurrence in follow-up.[25]

Many different combinations of sensing and pacing can be used. As a result, the field of EP lends itself to creativity. Figure 1.7 demonstrates the use of sensed doubles in the atrium in order to induce AV nodal reentry tachycardia. For example, bundle branch reentry VT may require long-short ventricular sequences for induction. In addition to pacing maneuvers, the administration of a drug may be a useful tool during the EPS.

Provocative Drug Testing

Provocative drug testing in the form of IV medications can be useful in elucidating the characteristics of conduction or can assist in the induction of tachycardia. Adenosine, with a half-life of less than 10 seconds, can transiently inhibit conduction through the AV node. However, to the benefit of the electrophysiologist, it usually does not slow conduction through an accessory pathway, resulting in the unmasking of the pathway. It is used in 6-mg IV increments, followed by an IV saline bolus via a central line. IV administration of adenosine triphosphate has also been used to induce transient PV reconduction following PV isolation in patients undergoing atrial fibrillation ablation.[26,27]

Isoproterenol, which increases sinus rate and AV conduction velocity via a β1 effect, may be used to facilitate induction of both supraventricular tachycardias and VTs. Furthermore, it may be used in the dose range of approximately 1 to 20 μg/min for the assessment of inducibility of atrial fibrillation following PV isolation.[28] The β2 effect leads to peripheral vasodilation and may lead to a drop in systolic blood pressure. It is used cautiously in patients with ischemic heart disease. IV epinephrine and atropine are other options for arrhythmia induction, and the same caveat holds. A complete discussion of provocative drug testing during EP studies is provided in later chapters of this book.

Complications

Practicing invasive cardiology means being imminently aware of potential complications. The essential equipment for cardiopulmonary resuscitation should be immediately available. A crash cart with essential drugs used in advanced cardiac life support protocols should be located in the EP laboratory. Equipment required to oxygenate

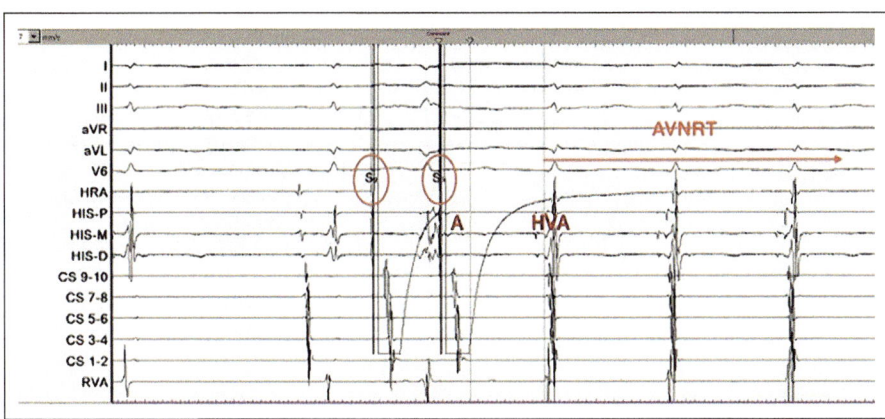

Figure 1.7 Leads I, II, III, aVR, aVL, and V6 as well as intracardiac electrograms on the HRA catheter, His catheter (HIS-Proximal, HIS-Mid, HIS-Distal), CS 1-10 catheter, and RVA catheter. Two stimulus artifacts, sensed doubles (**circled**), are noted on the HRA catheter; these denote right atrial pacing. Sensed doubles in the atrium induce typical atrioventricular nodal reentry tachycardia with antegrade slow and retrograde fast limbs.

(such as a non-rebreather mask), ventilate (such as a bag valve mask), and intubate the patient must be accessible with the ability to page respiratory therapy or anesthesia for assistance. A type and screen and/or a type and cross should be sent for procedures that are deemed high risk. A pericardiocentesis kit should be stocked in the EP laboratory, and familiarity with the technique of pericardiocentesis is necessary. In high-risk procedures, the availability of cardiothoracic surgery is required. Unfortunately, all physicians who practice invasive cardiac EP will encounter complications at one time or another. The key is to be prepared for a complication, to recognize the signs, and to have the equipment and personnel available to assist in the treatment.

Conclusion

The field of EP is an exciting area of medicine because it involves many emerging technologies and challenges us to integrate simultaneously the patient's clinical status, intracardiac electrograms, and multimodal images in order to deliver potentially curative treatments for an array of arrhythmias. The key to understanding a complex procedure is to first understand the basic concepts that have been introduced in this chapter and then to build on these fundamentals as one's experience broadens.

References

1. Sinha SK, Harnick D, Gomes JA, Mehta D. Electrophysiologic interventions in patients with inferior vena cava filters: safety and efficacy of the transfemoral approach. *Heart Rhythm*. 2005;2(1):15-18.
2. Ramirez A, Wall TS, Schmidt M, Selzman K, Daccarett M. Implantation of cardiac rhythm devices during concomitant anticoagulation or antiplatelet therapy. *Expert Review of Cardiovascular Therapy*. 2011;9(5):609-614.
3. Hakalahti A, Uusimaa P, Ylitalo K, Raatikainen MJ. Catheter ablation of atrial fibrillation in patients with therapeutic oral anticoagulation treatment. *Europace*. 2011;13(5):640-645.
4. Sado DM, Deakin CD, Petley GW, Clewlow F. Comparison of the effects of removal of chest hair with not doing so before external defibrillation on transthoracic impedance. *Am J Cardiol*. 2004;93:98-100.
5. Deakin CD, Nolan JP, Sunde K, Koster RW. European Resuscitation Council Guidelines for Resuscitation 2010 Section 3. Electrical therapies: automated external defibrillators, defibrillation, cardioversion and pacing. *Resuscitation*. 1020;81(10):1293-1304.
6. England H, Hoffman C, Hodgman T, et al. Effectiveness of automated external defibrillators in high schools in greater Boston. *Am J Cardiol*. 2005;95:1484-1486.
7. Krasteva V, Matveev M, Mudrov N, Prokopova R. Transthoracic impedance study with large self-adhesive electrodes in two conventional positions for defibrillation. *Physiol Meas*. 2006;27:1009-1022.
8. Boodhoo L, Mitchell AR, Bordoli G, Lloyd G, Patel N, Sulke N. DC cardioversion of persistent atrial fibrillation: a comparison of two protocols. *Int J Cardiol*. 2007;114:16–21.
9. Link MS, Atkins DL, Passman RS, et al. Part 6: Electrical therapies: Automated external defibrillators, defibrillation, cardioversion, and pacing: 2010 American Heart Association Guidelines for Cardiopulmonary Resuscitation and Emergency Cardiovascular Care. *Circulation*. 2010;122(18 Suppl 3):S706-S719.
10. van Alem AP, Chapman FW, Lank P, Hart AA, Koster RW. A prospective, randomised and blinded comparison of first shock success of monophasic and biphasic waveforms in out-of-hospital cardiac arrest. *Resuscitation*. 2003;58:17-24.
11. Morrison LJ, Dorian P, Long J, et al. Out-of-hospital cardiac arrest rectilinear biphasic to monophasic damped sine defibrillation waveforms with advanced life support intervention trial (ORBIT). *Resuscitation*. 2005;66:149-157.
12. Higgs ZC, Macafee DA, Braithwaite BD, Maxwell-Armstrong CA. The Seldinger technique: 50 years on. *Lancet*. 2005;366(9494):1407-1409.
13. Kim C, Vasaiwala S, Haque F, Pratap K, Vidovich MI. Radiation safety among cardiology fellows. *Am J Cardiol*. 2010;106(1):125-128.
14. Limacher MC, Douglas PS, Germano G, et al. ACC expert consensus document. Radiation safety in the practice of cardiology. American College of Cardiology. *J Am Coll Cardiol*. 1998;31(4):892-913.
15. Weiss EM, Thabit O. Clinical considerations for allied professionals: radiation safety and protection in the electrophysiology lab. *Heart Rhythm*. 2007;4(12):1583-1587.
16. Ferguson JD, Helms A, Mangrum JM, et al. Catheter ablation of atrial fibrillation without fluoroscopy using intracardiac echocardiography and electroanatomic mapping. *Circulation*. 2009;2(6):611-619.
17. Stevenson WG, Soejima K. Recording techniques for clinical electrophysiology. *J Cardiovasc Electrophysiol*. 2005;16(9):1017-1022.
18. Scherlag BJ, Lau SH, Helfant RH, Berkowitz WD, Stein E, Damato AN. Catheter technique for recording His bundle activity in man. *Circulation*. 1969;39(1):13-18.
19. Durrer D, Schoo L, Schuilenburg RM, Wellens HJ. The role of premature beats in the initiation and the termination of supraventricular tachycardia in the Wolff–Parkinson–White syndrome. *Circulation*. 1967;36(5):644-662.
20. Josephson ME, Horowitz LN, Farshidi A, Spear JF, Kastor JA, Moore EN. Recurrent sustained ventricular tachycardia. 2. Endocardial mapping. *Circulation*. 1978;57(3):440-447.
21. Krol RB, Saksena S, Prakash A, Giorgberidze I, Mathew P. Prospective clinical evaluation of a programmed atrial stimulation protocol for induction of sustained atrial fibrillation and flutter. *J Interv Card Electrophysiol*. 1999;3(1):19-25.
22. Essebag V, Baldessin F, Reynolds MR, et al. Non-inducibility post-pulmonary vein isolation achieving exit block predicts freedom from atrial fibrillation. *Eur Heart J*. 2005;26(23): 2550-2555.
23. Thomas KE, Josephson ME. The role of electrophysiology study in risk stratification of sudden cardiac death. *Prog Cardiovasc Dis*. 2008;51(2):97-105.
24. Hummel JD, Strickberger SA, Daoud E, et al. Results and efficiency of programmed ventricular stimulation with four extrastimuli compared with one, two, and three extrastimuli. *Circulation*. 1994;90:2827-2832.
25. Link MS, Saeed M, Gupta N, Homoud MK, Wang PJ, Estes NA III. Inducible ventricular flutter and fibrillation predict for arrhythmia occurrence in coronary artery disease patients presenting with syncope of unknown origin. *J Cardiovasc Electrophysiol*. 2002;13(11):1103-1108.
26. Matsuo S, Yamane T, Date T, et al. Dormant pulmonary vein conduction induced by adenosine in patients with atrial fibrillation who underwent catheter ablation. *Am Heart J*. 2011;161(1):188-196.
27. Jiang CY, Jiang RH, Matsuo S, Fu GS. ATP revealed extra pulmonary vein source of atrial fibrillation after circumferential pulmonary vein isolation. *Pacing Clin Electrophysiol*. 2010;33(2):248-251.
28. Crawford T, Chugh A, Good E, et al. Clinical value of noninducibility by high-dose isoproterenol versus rapid atrial pacing after catheter ablation of paroxysmal atrial fibrillation. *J Cardiovasc Electrophysiol*. 2010;21(1):13-20.

CHAPTER 2

Electrocardiography for the Invasive Electrophysiologist

Christopher J. McLeod, MBChB, PhD;
Traci L. Buescher, RN; Samuel J. Asirvatham, MD

Introduction

The 12-lead electrocardiogram (ECG) is, without question, both an invaluable tool for diagnosing arrhythmia mechanism and a guide for initial treatment for the patient with a cardiac rhythm disorder. However, less appreciated is the paramount importance of specific and detailed analysis of the ECG for guiding invasive electrophysiologists in planning and executing a safe and effective ablation procedure. In the early days of cardiac electrophysiology (EP), the operator was typically well versed in the nuances of ECG interpretation, and the invasive diagnostic study was readily seen as an extension of such analysis.

More recently, with anatomic and substrate-based approaches along with advances in mapping and ablation energy delivery, the correlative value of the ECG has been less appreciated.

In this chapter, we attempt to point out characteristics of the ECG relevant to invasive EP that are complementary to the analysis and understanding of the underlying anatomy and substrate for ablation. We discuss specific arrhythmias and summarize the key points that allow direct correlation between the ECG and procedural planning.

Outflow Tract Ventricular Tachycardia

The origins of the great arteries are seated in perhaps the most complex region of the heart, sharing intimate relationships with the coronary arteries, atria, and ventricular outflows. The invasive electrophysiologist should be very familiar with this anatomy but can also be guided by the ECG to identify the source of ventricular tachycardia (VT) arising in this region. The classic ECG of a patient with right ventricular outflow tract (RVOT) tachycardia shows left bundle branch block (LBBB) morphology with a strong inferior axis evidenced by tall R waves in leads II, III, and aVF and negative QS complexes in aVR and aVL. In addition, certain salient features should be distinguished from the 12-lead ECG.

Electrocardiographic Correlates

In general, mapping to identify the focal source of outflow tract tachycardia is a straightforward procedure. When difficulty occurs, however, it can often be related to an underlying failure to appreciate the complex regional anatomy and correlation with specific ECG patterns.

Importance of an R Wave in Lead V1

Lead V1 is placed anteriorly and to the right of the midline on the chest wall. The proximal infundibular portion of the outflow tract lies immediately beneath the anterior sternum, and as such, most arrhythmia originating in the RVOT present with a QS pattern in lead V1 (ie, LBBB morphology) (Figure 2.1). When an initial R wave is seen in lead V1, arrhythmia origin that is either on the left side of the body or posterior (away from the location of V1) should be suspected.

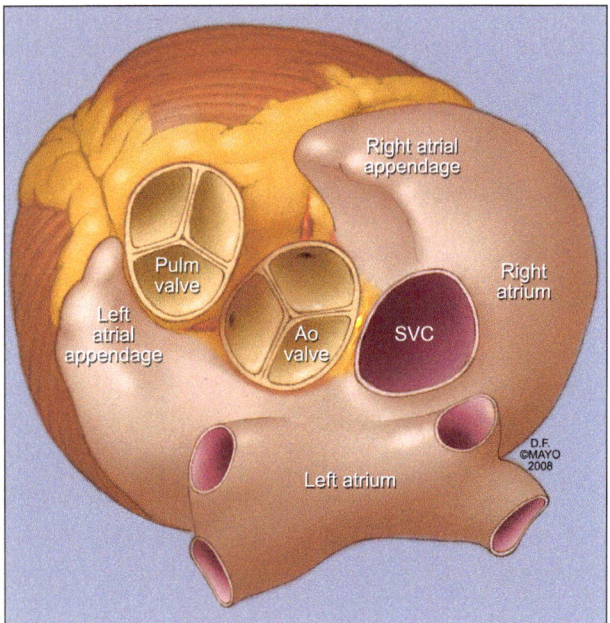

Figure 2.1 The base of the heart. Note: the pulmonic valve lies to the left of the LVOT and is contiguous with the more centrally located aortic valve. LVOT = left ventricular outflow track; Ao = aorta; SVC = superior vena cava. Source: Reproduced with permission of the Mayo Foundation for Medical Education and Research. All rights reserved.

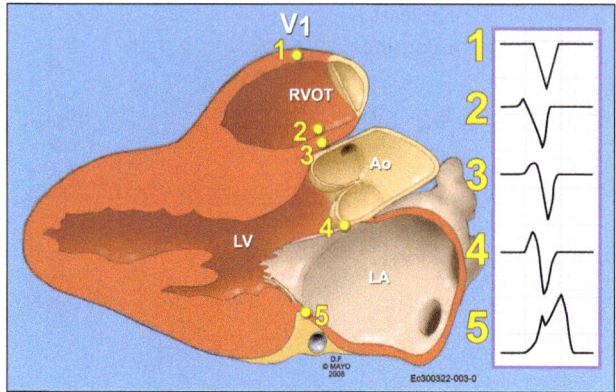

Figure 2.2 The heart is sectioned in an anteroposterior plane, and the arrhythmia origin is correlated with the characteristic ECG morphology in lead V1 (inset). Lead V1 is an anterior lead, and hence, VT arising on the anterior RVOT (1) results in a typical left bundle branch block morphology without any visible R wave in this lead. Sites 2 and 3 are contiguous between the anterior right coronary cusp of the aortic valve and the posterior RVOT. A small but variable R wave is consistently seen in lead V1. VT arising more posteriorly (4) in the region of the left coronary cusp/aortic mitral continuity/noncoronary cusp origin is characterized on the ECG with a distinct R wave in lead V1, as more of a posterior to anterior vector is provided. Ao = aorta; LA = left atrium; LV = left ventricle; RVOT = right ventricular outflow tract; VT = ventricular tachycardia. Source: Reprinted with permission of the Mayo Foundation for Medical Education and Research. All rights reserved.

The distal RVOT and pulmonary valve are on the left side of the body and located leftward of the aortic valve and distal left ventricular outflow tract (LVOT). As a result, when the RVOT focus is near or above the level of the pulmonary valve, the initial vector is from left to right and creates a small R wave in lead V1.[1,2]

When the focus of tachycardia is on the *posterior* RVOT or in the LVOT lying immediately behind the posterior RVOT, once again, a vector toward lead V1 (posterior to anterior) exists and gives rise to a small R wave in lead V1 (Figure 2.2). Further, posterior origin, such as the posterior aortic annulus or mitral annulus, gives progressively larger R waves in V1, eventually merging with a right bundle branch block (RBBB) morphology. Close analysis of lead I can help distinguish whether the cause of the small R wave in V1 is a leftward (peripulmonary valve) or posterior origin (Figure 2.3). With leftward origin, a predominant S wave (negative deflection) would be seen in lead I, whereas origin of arrhythmia in the posterior RVOT more to the right of the body would typically give rise to a prominent R wave in lead I.

Isoelectric or Positive QRS in Lead AVL

The vast majority of outflow tract VT will be negative, with QS complexes in leads aVL and aVR, as they arise from the superior portion of the heart. An isoelectric or positive QRS complex in lead aVL should immediately alert the clinician to the significance of the arrhythmia arising from the peri-His bundle origin. The peri-His bundle region lies most rightward and inferior in the RVOT, and therefore, the vector toward lead aVL (a left-sided lead) is either isoelectric or slightly positive (Figure 2.4). Recognizing the significance of an isoelectric or positive initial deflection in aVL is important when counseling patients ahead of the planned ablation procedure. The potential for His-bundle injury and

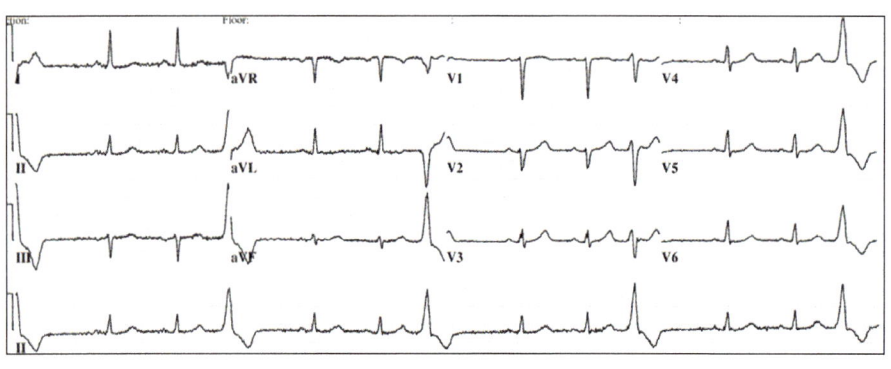

Figure 2.3 Ventricular ectopy noted to have the characteristic findings in the limb leads, suggesting an outflow tract origin. Lead V1, however, has a small R wave, which would suggest posterior RVOT at the level of the valve or the LVOT cusps. This arrhythmia was mapped to the left coronary cusp and successfully ablated. LVOT = left ventricular outflow tract; RVOT = right ventricular outflow tract.

the likelihood of at least RBBB resulting following the procedure should be considered.

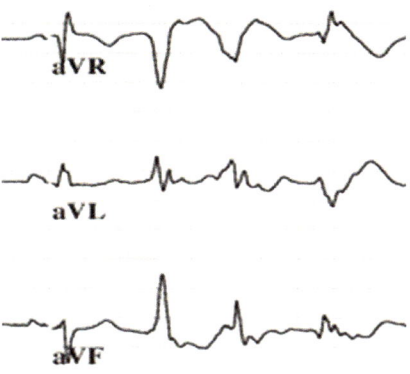

Figure 2.4 VT arising from the peri-His bundle region is typically positive or biphasic in lead aVL while remaining negative in the aVR lead and positive in the inferior leads.

Electrocardiography and Ablation—Key Correlations—Outflow Tract VT

- The RVOT lies anterior and to the *left* of the LVOT.
- An initial R wave seen in lead V1 signifies either peripulmonary valve origin or posterior origin of the outflow tract arrhythmia.
- Lead I can be helpful for distinguishing between leftward or posterior RVOT focus.
- aVR and aVL leads are simultaneously negative in the majority of outflow tract arrhythmia. When aVL is not negative, suspect a peri-Hisian source.

Fascicular Ventricular Tachycardia

VT originating in the infra-Hisian conduction system has characteristic electrocardiographic findings, which upon careful analysis can guide the ablation procedure.

The classically described Belhassen's VT exits to the ventricle in the region of the left posterior fascicle. The electrocardiographic appearance is that of typical RBBB and leftward axis (see Figure 2.5), similar to what is seen in patients with RBBB and left anterior fascicular block. The highly typical nature of the RBBB often mistakenly leads to the diagnosis of supraventricular tachycardia with bifascicular block.[3] Several specific electrocardiographic features are worth noting for the invasive electrophysiologist:

- VT origin in the posterior papillary muscle can produce an electrocardiographic vector very similar to left posterior fascicular tachycardia. At times, these two arrhythmias may be indistinguishable, but papillary muscle VT tends to be wider and has a less sharp initial deflection. Analyzing the timing for retrograde atrial activation may also be of value. Usually, fascicular-origin tachycardia has a short refractory period (RP) interval (sometimes even mistakenly leading to the diagnosis of atrioventricular [AV] node reentry). However, given the myocardial origin for papillary muscle tachycardia, the RP interval is generally longer.

- Anterior fascicular VT is seen far less frequently with this type of arrhythmia, and although it retains the characteristic right bundle configuration, the vector is directed more rightward from the anterior fascicle exit site.[4]

- Rare forms of fascicular VT may also originate above anterior and posterior fascicular branching, and hence, there is a narrow QRS due to near-simultaneous retrograde activation of the right bundle.[5]

- Moderator-band VT arises, as the name suggests, from this structure within the right ventricle. Because this structure also contains the right bundle branch itself, the arrhythmia arising from here renders a typical LBBB pattern but with a left axis[6] (Figure 2.6).

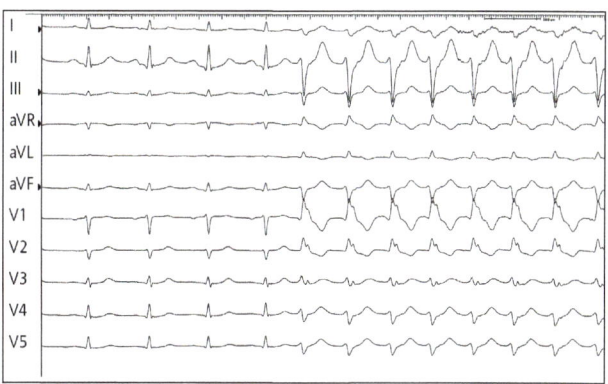

Figure 2.5 12-lead ECG from a patient with Belhassen's ventricular tachycardia, displaying the classical right bundle branch block, left axis pattern.

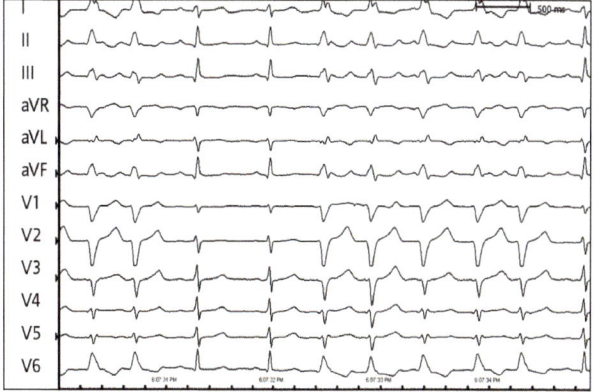

Figure 2.6 Salvos of ventricular tachycardia arising from the moderator band with two sinus beats interspersed. This arrhythmia arises close to the right bundle exit site and will inscribe a typical left bundle branch block pattern.

Ventricular Tachycardia with Structural Heart Disease

When automatic VT occurs in the structurally normal heart, electrocardiographic correlation with arrhythmia origin is relatively straightforward. The more common VT in the setting of structural heart disease (ischemic or dilated cardiomyopathy) has important differences in the principles used to correlate the electrocardiographic data in the invasive EP laboratory.

When ventricular scar or fibrosis forms, reentrant tachycardia using areas of slow conduction to perpetuate the circuit is the underlying arrhythmogenic mechanism. The electrocardiographic pattern does not necessarily relate to the area of slow conduction or diseased tissue (the true arrhythmogenic substrate) but rather to the "exit" site. The exit site usually represents the transition zone between the diseased myocardium housing the reentrant circuit and the relatively normal surrounding myocardium. As a result, analysis of the electrocardiographic vector does not usually lead to localizing the site of successful ablation (Figure 2.7). However, careful analysis of the ECG, along with knowledge of where myocardial scar, previous infarction, etc, exists, can be very useful for the ablationist when interpreting activation mapping and entrainment data.

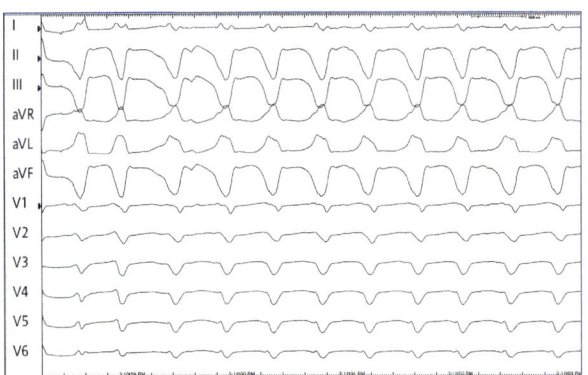

Figure 2.7 An example of ischemic VT showing a very wide left bundle branch block pattern with negative concordance across the chest leads. In this instance, successful ablation was achieved at the basal inferior left ventricle adjacent to the septum.

For example, RBBB tachycardia would typically have an exit in the left ventricle. Further, if lead I shows a QS complex, a left ventricular free-wall origin can be surmised. The analysis of leads II, III, and aVF will help define the exit site as being on either the anterior wall (tall R waves) or the inferior wall (QS complexes). Finally, further analysis of the QRS vector in lead aVR (a basal lead) and V4 (a relatively apical lead) can help define the base-to-apex orientation of the exit site. If aVR is negative and V4 positive, the exit is close to the base, whereas if V4 is negative and aVR positive, the exit is likely apical. If both aVR and V4 are positive, either the exit site is very apical (vector travels to both V4 and then to aVR) or the exit is midway between V4 and aVR. In the former case, the R wave in V4 will be less positive than a tall R wave in aVR, and leads V5 and V6 will be negative as well. Using such deductive logic, once the exit site is anticipated, one can "back into" the slow zone and diseased myocardium in the EP laboratory from knowing where low-voltage electrograms (arrhythmogenic sites and scar regions) are and based on entrainment data. (In entrainment data, postpacing interval equals tachycardia cycle length but with progressively longer stimulus to QRS delays as one goes from the exit toward the slow zone.)[7]

Although specific reentrant circuits can rarely be deduced from ECG analysis alone, some prototypical reentrant VTs do have recognizable ECG patterns. The best documented example of this situation is so-called mitral isthmus VT.[8,9] Patients usually have an inferior wall myocardial infarction with relative sparing of the myocardium between the infarct and the mitral valve. A region of slow conduction therefore exists close to the annulus. Because the exit site is near the base, the precordial leads are usually positive. Exceptions do exist, as in a large zone of slow conduction that is relatively apically displaced.

Differing but characteristic electrocardiographic patterns are manifested depending on both the exact location of the slow zone on the mitral annulus and the direction of the reentrant wave's rotation around the annulus (clockwise vs counterclockwise). If, for example, clockwise rotation with exit septal to an inferior slow zone is responsible for VT, then right ventricular myocardium and annular myocardium from anterior to posterior are activated. This activation results in LBBB morphology but with a left superior axis vector (Figure 2.8). The opposite situation holds with a right bundle but right axis deviation tachycardia, which may be seen with rotation of the circuit in the opposite direction and with the slow zone more laterally displaced.

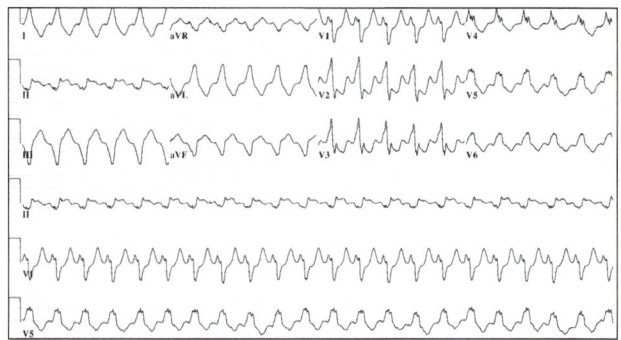

Figure 2.8 Mitral isthmus VT arising from the inferoseptal aspect of the mitral valve. The QRS vector is therefore directed toward leads I and aVL and is negative in the inferior leads.

Sinus Tachycardia and Automatic Atrial Tachycardia

Inappropriate sinus tachycardias and high right atrial "cristal" tachycardias both produce similar activation patterns on the 12-lead ECG. There is a negative P wave in lead aVR and positive deflections in leads I and II, while V1 is biphasic (positive and then negative, reflecting right atrial and subsequent left atrial activation). Using a single

ECG, differentiating between these entities can be extremely difficult, and one would rely on an abrupt initiation rather than gradual onset as a hallmark of atrial tachycardia; even so, the absence of this sign does not necessarily exclude this diagnosis.

Sinus rhythm with its characteristic initial positive P wave followed by a negative terminal P wave in lead V1 (initial activation from posterior to anterior in the right atrium, and then from right atrium to the posterior left atrium) may be indistinguishable from high crista terminalis origin because the junction of the crista terminalis and the superior vena cava (SVC) is the usual site of origin of the epicardially located sinus node. However, cristal tachycardias may occur anywhere along the crista terminalis. Lower portions of the crista terminalis arrhythmia will have a negative P wave in leads II, III, and aVF, whereas midportions may have an isoelectric P wave in lead II and isoelectric or negative P waves in lead III and aVF (Figure 2.9). For diagnosing cristal tachycardias versus sinus tachycardia, incessant tachycardia and relatively abrupt origin of tachycardia are generally clinically more useful markers than analyzing the P-wave axis alone.

- Pulmonary vein tachycardias can also be identified on the ECG, and several algorithms can be employed to aid in pinpointing the anatomic source.[10,11] A few key points are important to remember. The "true" atrial septum extends posterosuperiorly from the apex of Koch's triangle and involves the superior limbus and oval fossa (Figure 2.10). Arrhythmias originating in this region have rapid simultaneous access to both atria and hence are associated with a very narrow P wave on the surface ECG. The right-sided pulmonary veins lie in close proximity to this part of the atrial septum and can often be hallmarked by this feature (Figure 2.11). Tachycardia originating lower down on the septum, such as coronary sinus ostial tachycardia, is not originating from within the true atrial septum and does not have easily facilitated atrial activation; therefore, such tachycardia has broader P-wave inscriptions and is negative in the inferior leads (Figure 2.12). Broad-based P waves that remain positive in lead V1 can allude to left-sided pulmonary vein tachycardias because they activate from the posterior left atrium in an anterior fashion.

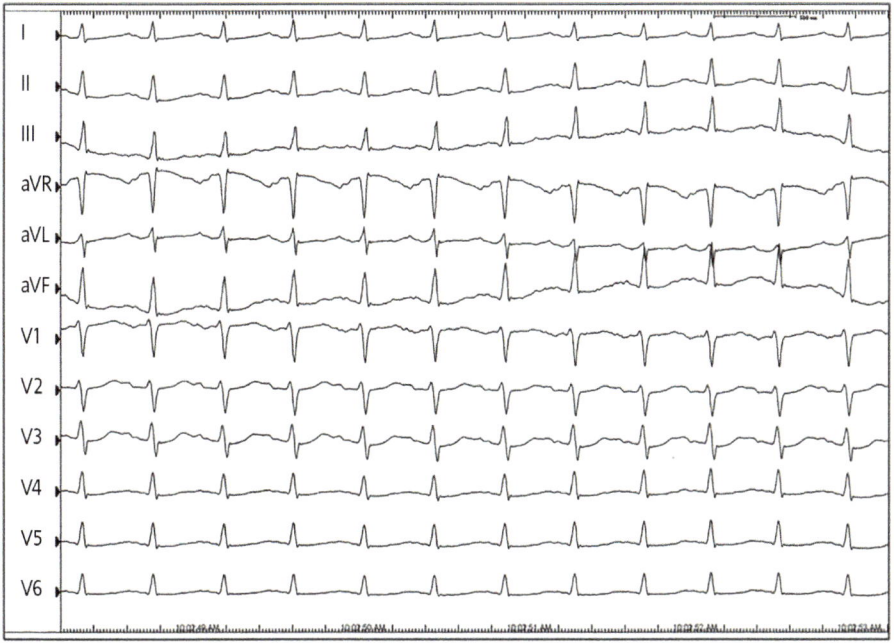

Figure 2.9 A 12-lead ECG taken during ablation of an atrial tachycardia that was arising from the mid–crista terminalis.

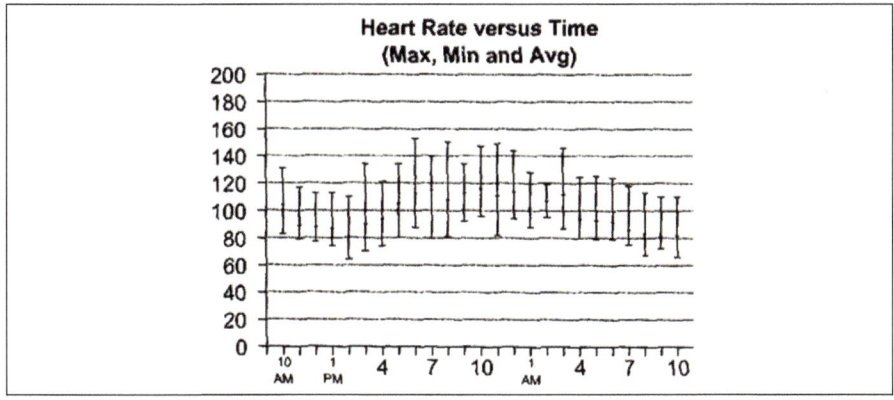

Figure 2.10 24-hour Holter monitoring taken from a 24-year-old woman with inappropriate sinus tachycardia. Note the high average heart rate, especially during waking hours (99 bpm).

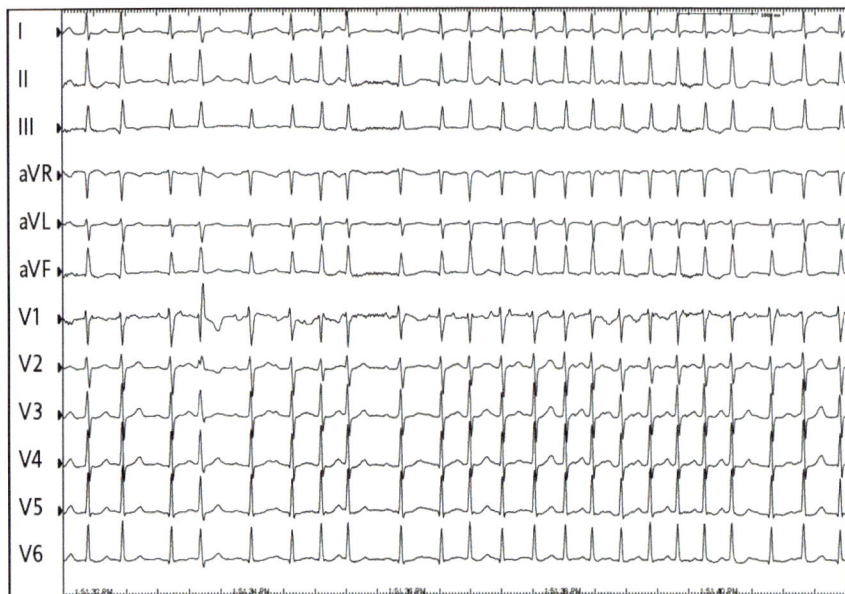

Figure 2.11 Sinus rhythm is evident in this ECG, but interspersed are salvos of atrial tachycardia that were found to be originating from the right upper pulmonary vein. This atrial activity is characterized by the narrow P-wave morphology that is positive in lead V1 but is not wide and biphasic (like sinus rhythm).

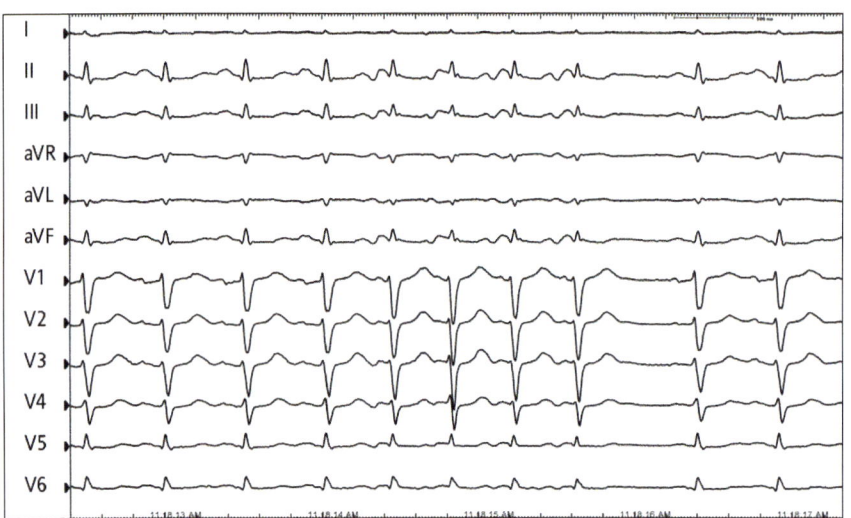

Figure 2.12 Ectopic tachycardia from the coronary sinus. The hallmark ECG's changes are evident in the inferior leads, characterized by broad negative P waves, in contrast to the sinus P wave, as evident in the last two beats of this tracing. Although a septally located structure, the coronary sinus is not part of the true septum; hence, rapid biatrial activation is not facilitated.

Electrocardiography and Ablation—Key Correlation—Automatic Atrial Tachycardia

- Analyzing the P-wave vector can be very useful in diagnosing the site of origin of ectopic atrial tachycardias.

- Sinus tachycardia and superior cristal tachycardias have a biphasic P wave with the initial component being positive and the terminal component being negative.

- A completely negative P wave in lead V1 should suggest right atrial appendage or anterior tricuspid annulus origin.

- A completely positive P wave in lead V1 should suggest left atrial and, more specifically, posterolateral left atrial origin (example, left-sided pulmonary veins).

- Coronary sinus tachycardias have a wide negative P wave in leads II, III, and aVF.

Wolff–Parkinson–White Syndrome

One can use several published algorithms to predict the location of an accessory pathway from the 12-lead ECG,[12-14] but only one of these has been prospectively validated[15] (Figures 2.13 and 2.14). This approach relies on only 5 ECG leads (I, II, III, V1, and aVF) and is highly accurate in identifying coronary sinus diverticulum/middle cardiac vein pathways as well as midseptal and anteroseptal pathways near the AV node. It is essential to recognize a few key features when using this method:

- In identifying a left-sided pathway, the ECG should show either an isoelectric *or* negative delta wave in lead I, *or* an R wave larger than S wave in lead V1. Importantly, it is necessary to fulfill only one of these criteria and not all (Figure 2.15).

- An early (initial 20 ms) negative delta wave in lead II should be seen as a hallmark of a middle cardiac vein pathway (Figure 2.16).

Chapter 2: Electrocardiography for the Invasive Electrophysiologist • 17

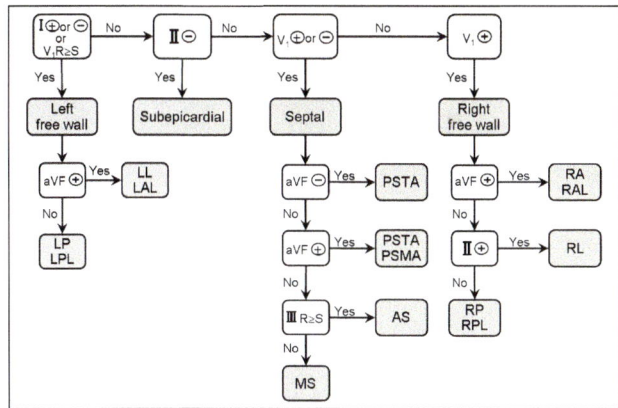

Figure 2.13 Algorithm devised by Arruda and colleagues to predict the location of an accessory pathway from a 12-lead ECG. It initially excludes left lateral pathways and subepicardial/middle cardiac vein accessory pathways before dissecting septal and right-sided ones. LL = left lateral; LAL = left anterolateral; LP = left posterior; LPL = left posterolateral; PSTA = posteroseptal on tricuspid annulus; PSMA = posteroseptal on mitral annulus; AS = anteroseptal; MS = midseptal; RA = right anterior; RL = right lateral; RP = right posterior; RPL = right posterolateral. *Source:* Reprinted with permission from Arruda MS, et al.[15]

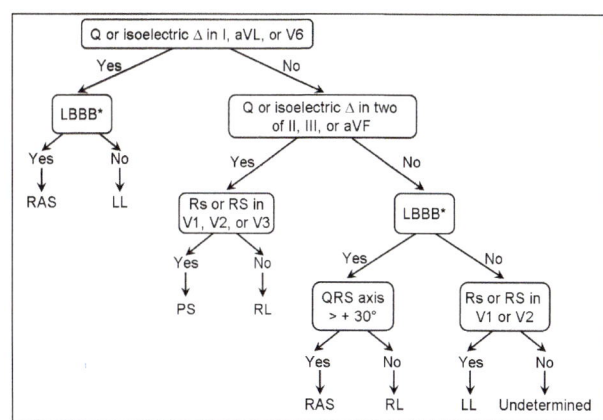

Figure 2.14 The Milstein et al algorithm considers delta wave polarity and the presence of either right or left bundle branch block QRS pattern in the right precordial electrocardiographic leads to define the location of the accessory pathway. LL = left lateral; RAS = right anteroseptal; PS = posteroseptal; RL = right lateral. *Source:* Reprinted with permission from Milstein S, et al.[14]

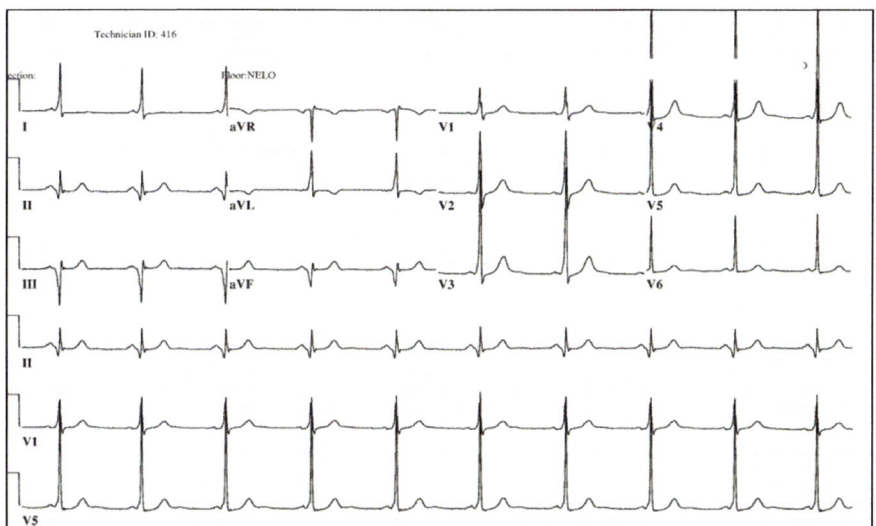

Figure 2.15 The R > S wave in lead V1 confirms a left-sided pathway despite the delta wave being negative in lead I.

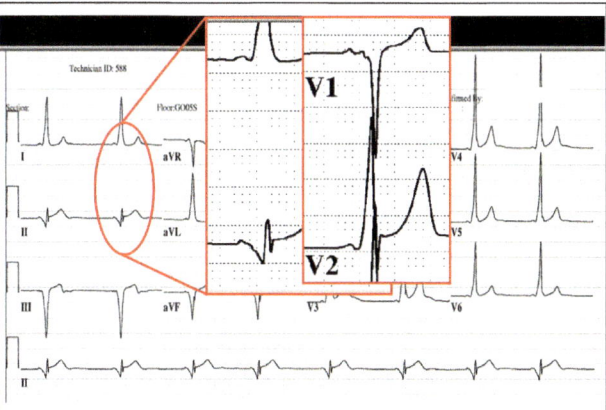

Figure 2.16 The sharply negative delta wave in lead II strongly suggests a middle cardiac vein accessory pathway. If this criteria is fulfilled, the Arruda algorithm does not require that one even view the delta wave in V1, yet its biphasic nature does suggest that the pathway is on the septum.

Electrocardiography and Ablation—Key Correlations—Accessory Pathway

- A left free-wall accessory pathway can be excluded if the delta wave is positive in lead I *and* the R wave is smaller than the S wave in lead V1.

- Septal accessory pathways have an initial negative or isoelectric delta wave in V1 that transitions to a positive delta wave in V2.

- However small, a positive delta wave in lead V1 strongly suggests pathway occurrence *off* the septum (Figure 2.17).

- An initial negative delta wave in lead II highly correlates with epicardial pathway origin in the region of the middle cardiac vein.

- Minimal preexcitation or multiple pathways are difficult to localize with the 12-lead ECG in sinus rhythm.

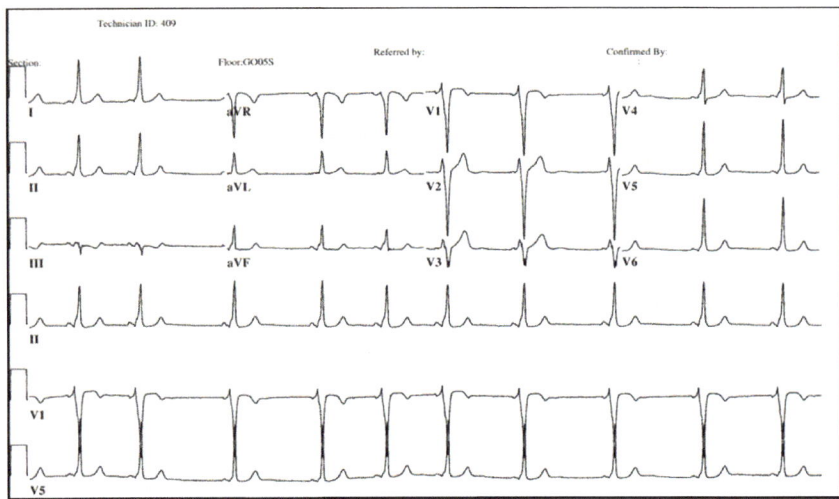

Figure 2.17 A small positive delta wave in lead V1 critically indicates that the accessory pathway is not located on the septum, and thus, inadvertent septal ablation near the AV node should be avoided.

Atrioventricular Nodal Reentry Tachycardia

As mentioned earlier, arrhythmias that originate within the true septum characteristically give narrow P waves in lieu of their facilitated access to both atria (Figure 2.18). This is also valuable in distinguishing the fast pathway exit site in typical atrioventricular nodal reentry tachycardia (AVNRT). This arrhythmia does exit low on the true septum, giving a narrow P wave that is negative in the inferior leads (as opposed to the atypical AVNRT). In this uncommon variety, atrial activation occurs via the slow pathway that is near or within the coronary sinus, inscribing wide negative P waves in the inferior leads (Figure 2.19). This is also the case for paroxysmal junctional reciprocating tachycardia and atrial tachycardias in the coronary sinus (Figure 2.20).

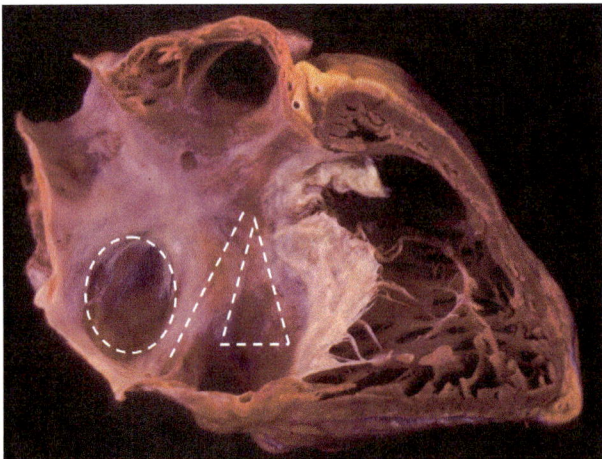

Figure 2.18 The "true" atrial septum extends posterosuperiorly from the apex of Koch's triangle and involves the superior limbus and oval fossa. Arrhythmias originating in this region have rapid simultaneous access to both atria and hence are associated with a very narrow P wave on the surface ECG. The **triangle** identifies the Koch's triangle, the **straight line** is drawn over the Tendon of Todaro, and the **circle** outlines the oval fossa.

Atrial Flutter

- The P wave in atrial flutter is inscribed on the 12-lead ECG when the electrical wavefront exits the slow zone of the circuit. Hence, in light of the fixed anatomic substrate, typical flutter is easily recognized; conversely, atypical flutters are difficult to characterize by the surface flutter waves. Typical flutter can be counterclockwise or clockwise, yet both utilize the cavotricuspid isthmus as a critical isthmus. In this setting, emergence of electrical activity thus occurs in the cavotricuspid isthmus; and, in the more common counterclockwise direction, a broad negative flutter wave is seen in the inferior leads as the vector moves away from this inferior aspect of the right atrium (Figure 2.21). Consequently, the P wave will also be positive in lead V1 as activation then moves toward this anterior lead. The reverse sequence can be expected in the clockwise direction, with negative P waves in V1 and positive P waves in the inferior leads.

Electrocardiography and Ablation— Key Correlations—Atrial Flutter

- A terminal positive flutter wave in lead V1 correlates with cavotricuspid isthmus-dependent flutter.

- Along with the pattern above, if the flutter waves appear negative in the inferior leads, counterclockwise typical flutter is likely; in contrast, positive flutter waves in the inferior leads suggest clockwise, isthmus-dependent flutter.

- All positive or all negative flutter waves in lead V1 generally exclude cavotricuspid isthmus flutter and strongly suggest another scar-related or atypical atrial flutter (Figure 2.22).

- Analyzing patterns of flutter-wave morphology in patients with a surgical maze procedure or extensive prior ablation in the left atrium can be difficult. Thus, an approach similar to that discussed for mapping the exit site of VT with structural heart disease may be utilized.

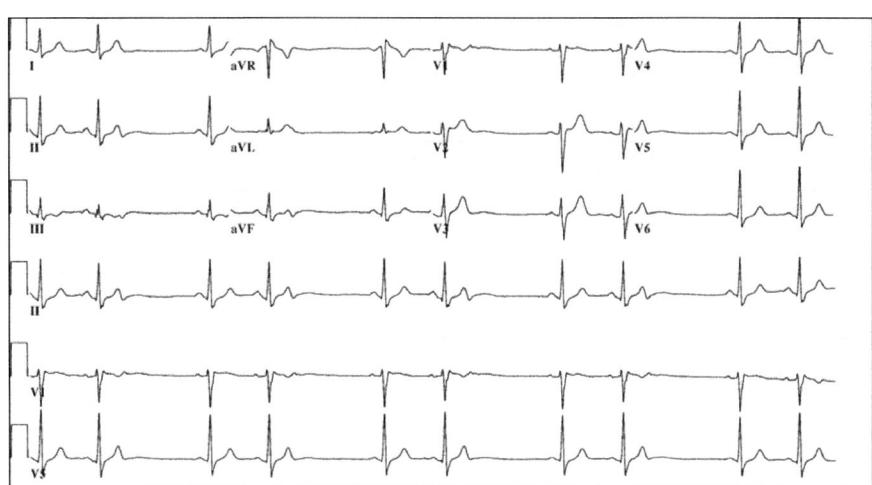

Figure 2.19 Atypical atrioventricular nodal reentry tachycardia was successfully ablated in this patient by targeting the slow pathway. The preablation ECG displays evidence of sinus rhythm with echo beats that return to the atrium via the slow pathway on every other beat, giving the impression of blocked premature beats. Most evident in the inferior leads is that, as the atrium is activated via the slow pathway/coronary sinus ostium, one can contrast the P wave during sinus rhythm with the broad negative P wave inscribed by the echo beat.

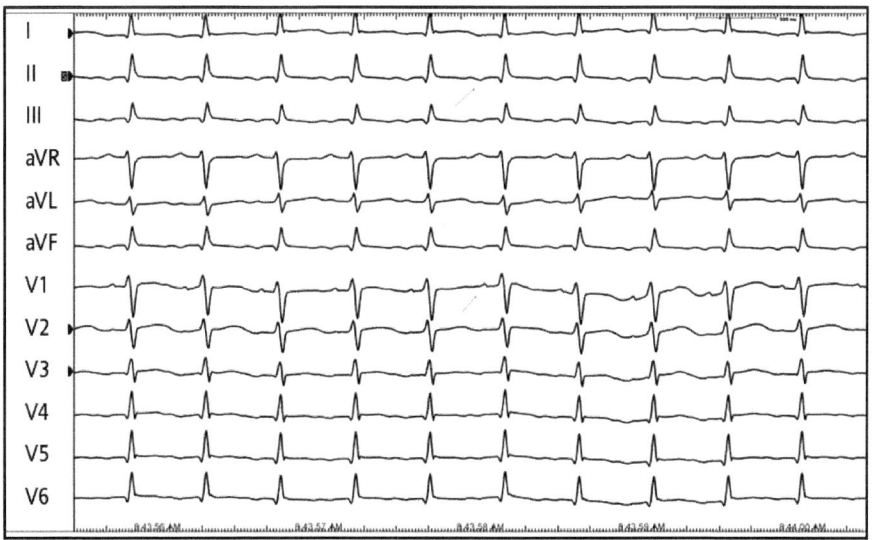

Figure 2.20 This ECG shows permanent junctional reciprocating tachycardia. It shows negative P waves in the inferior leads that are not distinctly narrow and yet are positive in the right anterior lead V1. This illustrates a long R-P tachycardia with a retrograde, decrementally conducting pathway that resides on the septum.

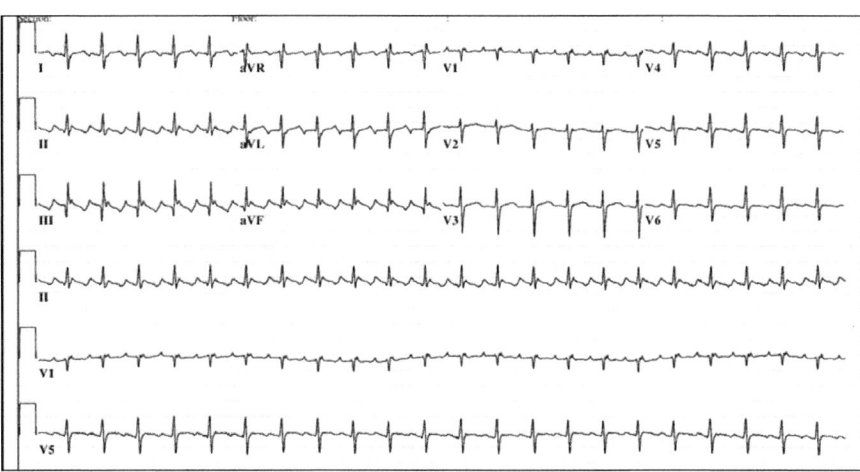

Figure 2.21 Typical cavotricuspid-dependent counterclockwise atrial flutter showing the negative P waves inferiorly and the positive P wave in lead V1.

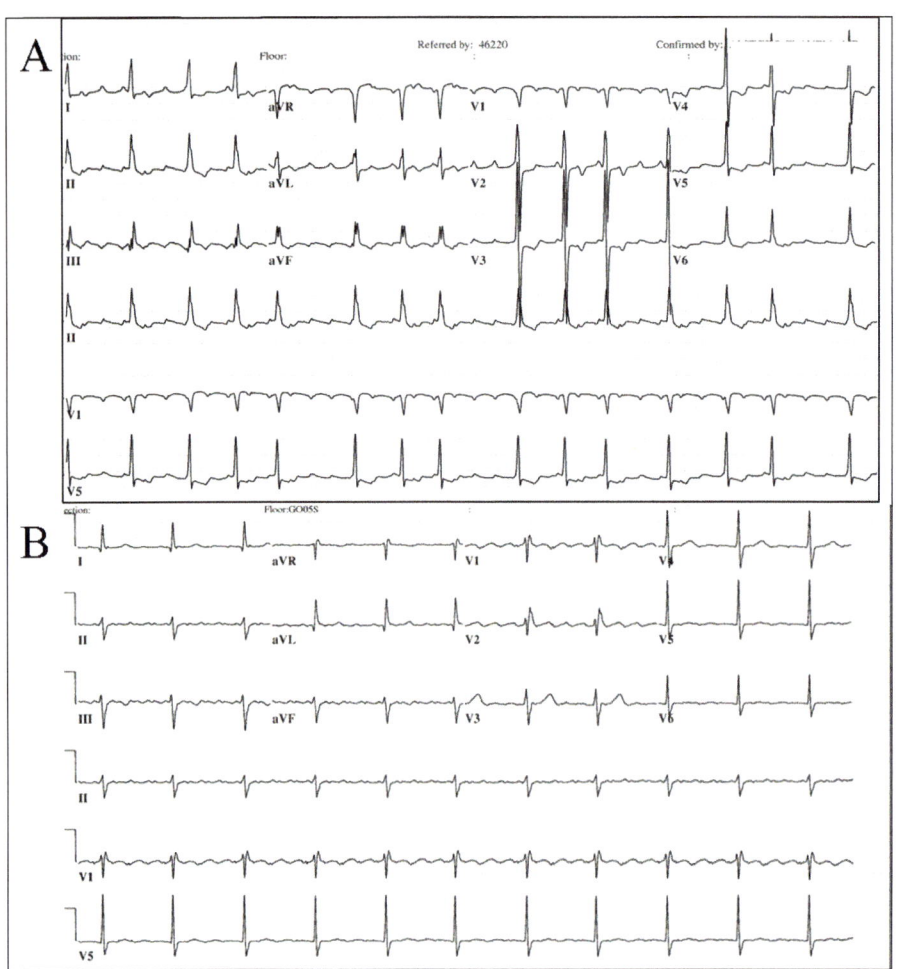

Figure 2.22 Atypical atrial flutter with a regular ventricular response.

Repolarization Abnormalities

Although current practice does not offer much opportunity for the electrophysiologist to treat these syndromes in an invasive manner, correctly identifying these diseases is critical. Early cardiac repolarization abnormalities (commonly grouped as J-wave syndromes) display unique electrocardiographic signatures based on which part of the heart is chiefly affected and which ion channel is pathological. The Epsilon wave, occurring as a discrete upward deflection immediately after the QRS, is important to recognize, given its relationship with arrhythmogenic right ventricular dysplasia (ARVD). Brugada pattern ECGs are variable but also vital to recognize. The typical coved pattern (type I) has a gradually descending ST-segment and negative T wave (Figure 2.23).

The remaining types II and III have the saddleback ST configuration and positive T wave. Based on the location of leads V1 and V2 immediately over the RVOT (which is principally affected in Brugada), these leads are characteristically most affected. A detailed description of each long QT syndrome subtype is beyond the scope of this chapter. The majority of subtypes, however, comprise long QT 1 (broad-based T wave), long QT 2 (low-amplitude, notched T wave), and long QT 3 (late-occurring T wave). Long QT 7 is also characteristic, with a prominent U wave. In these syndromes, T-wave alternans should also be sought because it can herald VT or ventricular fibrillation. Short QT syndromes are typically associated with atrial fibrillation, and the T wave can be difficult to accurately discern. Because of the high risk for sudden cardiac death from ventricular fibrillation, a QT interval less than 360 ms (and typically less than 300 ms) should alert the clinician. Given the link with ventricular fibrillation and sudden cardiac death, early repolarization syndromes are no longer considered "benign." Moreover, global early repolarization appears to be perhaps the most malignant phenotype, with inferior/inferolateral ECG changes also associated with a higher risk.[16]

Miscellaneous Arrhythmia Patterns

Premature Ventricular Complexes (PVCs) and Ventricular Fibrillation

PVCs inducing ventricular fibrillation are uncommon yet well described. They rely on the ectopic tachycardia occurring within a vulnerable repolarization window.[17] The surface ECG can help the electrophysiologist identify the source of this arrhythmia, which frequently can be

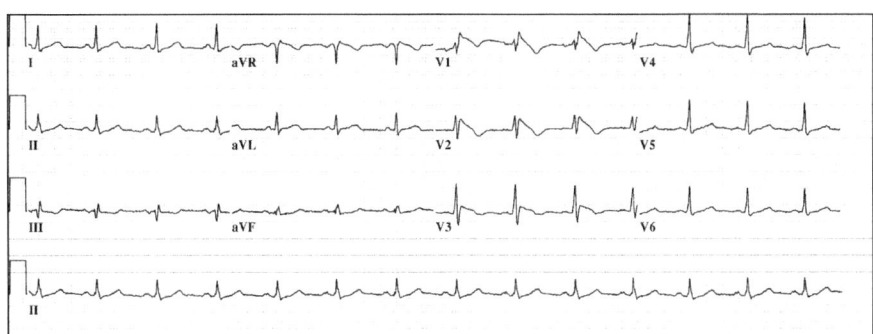

Figure 2.23 An ECG from a patient with Brugada syndrome (Type I), illustrating the typical coved ST segments, most prominently noted over the right ventricular outflow tract in leads V1 and V2.

traced to the papillary muscle or left bundle fascicle. This site of early activation within the left ventricle usually gives an RBBB morphology that is fairly narrow in QRS width based on its proximity to the Purkinje system. Papillary muscle sources often have an initial negative deflection in lead aVR because this structure is depolarized before the rest of the ventricle, and depolarization of this structure occurs before the subsequent positive R wave.

Bundle Branch Reentrant VT

In diseased hearts, a reentrant mechanism utilizing the bundle branch system and emerging at either the left or right bundle exits (rendering a typical LBBB or RBBB configuration, potentially similar to that in sinus rhythm) can occur. Reverse typical bundle branch reentry, in which the circuit ascends the right bundle and goes down the left bundle, may occur; in this instance, a relatively typical RBBB morphology VT may be seen (Figure 2.24).

Bundle branch reentrant VT may present as a relatively polymorphic tachycardia. Even though the same circuit is used, deferring exits in the region of the right bundle may create the pattern of polymorphic arrhythmia.

Hypertrophic Cardiomyopathy

Hypertrophic cardiomyopathy can present with a multitude of electrocardiographic abnormalities that can involve left atrial enlargement, depolarization, and repolarization. Perhaps the most striking features are the repolarization changes that are frequently confused with ischemia (Figure 2.25).

Digoxin Toxicity

Rarely seen these days, digoxin toxicity can be lethal, so several characteristic ECG patterns are important for the electrophysiologist to recognize. Although digoxin toxicity can result in almost any arrhythmia, bidirectional VT is a fairly unique hallmark. In addition, atrial fibrillation with complete heart block and a junctional escape should also prompt urgent therapy.

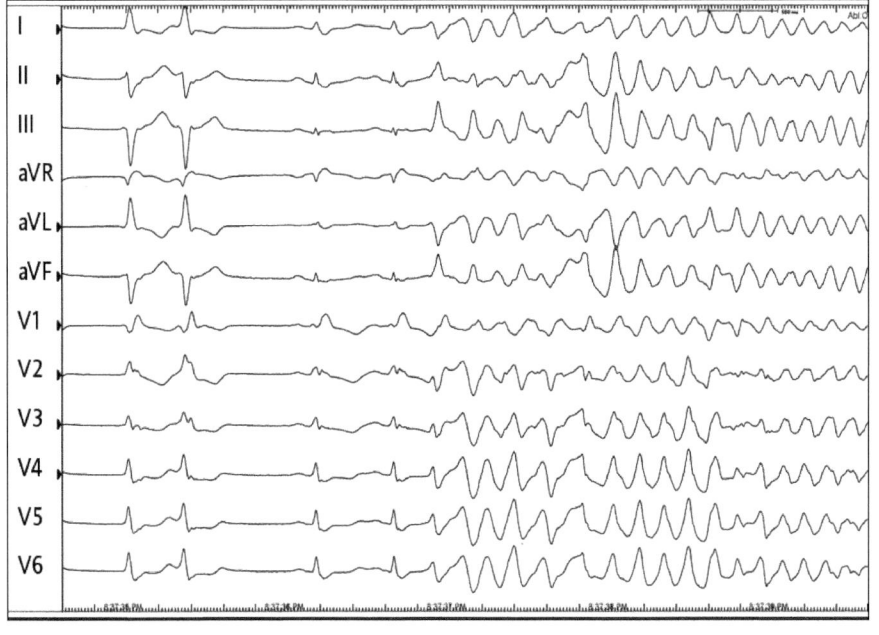

Figure 2.24 Premature ventricular complexes originating from the left posterior fascicle with a right bundle branch block configuration and a left axis. Ventricular fibrillation is precipitated.

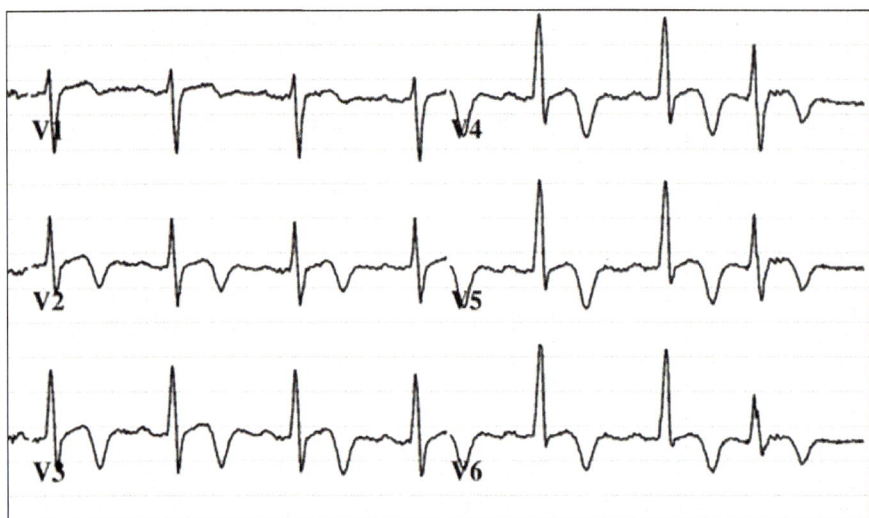

Figure 2.25 Deeply inverted T waves and prominent R-wave voltage associated with hypertrophic cardiomyopathy.

Conclusion

Even with the availability and widespread use of sophisticated mapping technology and excellent energy delivery techniques, the invasive electrophysiologist can significantly benefit from carefully analyzing the ECG before performing invasive mapping and ablation. With automatic tachycardias, the site of origin can be predicted relatively accurately, as with accessory pathway localization. With reentrant tachycardias (such as atrial flutters and VT) in the setting of ischemic or dilated cardiomyopathy, the ECG is valuable because it optimally predicts the exit site of the circuit from the diseased myocardium to relatively normal myocardium.

References

1. Asirvatham SJ. Correlative anatomy for the invasive electrophysiologist: outflow tract and supravalvar arrhythmia. *J Cardiovasc Electrophysiol*. 2009;20:955-968.
2. Gami AS, Noheria A, Lachman N, et al. Anatomical correlates relevant to ablation above the semilunar valves for the cardiac electrophysiologist: a study of 603 hearts. *J Interv Card Electrophysiol*. 30:5-15.
3. Belhassen B, Rotmensch HH, Laniado S. Response of recurrent sustained ventricular tachycardia to verapamil. *Br Heart J*. 1981;46:679-682.
4. Scheinman MM. Role of the His-Purkinje system in the genesis of cardiac arrhythmia. *Heart Rhythm*. 2009;6:1050-1058.
5. Ramprakash B, Jaishankar S, Rao HB, Narasimhan C. Catheter ablation of fascicular ventricular tachycardia. *Indian Pacing Electrophysiol J*. 2008;8:193-202.
6. Abouezzeddine O, Suleiman M, Buescher T, et al. Relevance of endocavitary structures in ablation procedures for ventricular tachycardia. *J Cardiovasc Electrophysiol*. 21:245-254.
7. Ellison KE, Friedman PL, Ganz LI, Stevenson WG. Entrainment mapping and radiofrequency catheter ablation of ventricular tachycardia in right ventricular dysplasia. *J Am Coll Cardiol*. 1998;32:724-728.
8. Kumagai K, Yamauchi Y, Takahashi A, et al. Idiopathic left ventricular tachycardia originating from the mitral annulus. *J Cardiovasc Electrophysiol*. 2005;16:1029-1036.
9. Tada H, Tadokoro K, Miyaji K, et al. Idiopathic ventricular arrhythmias arising from the pulmonary artery: prevalence, characteristics, and topography of the arrhythmia origin. *Heart Rhythm*. 2008;5:419-426.
10. Tada H, Nogami A, Naito S, et al. Simple electrocardiographic criteria for identifying the site of origin of focal right atrial tachycardia. *Pacing Clin Electrophysiol*. 1998;21:2431-2439.
11. Tang CW, Scheinman MM, Van Hare GF, et al. Use of P wave configuration during atrial tachycardia to predict site of origin. *J Am Coll Cardiol*. 1995;26:1315-1324.
12. Epstein AE, Kirklin JK, Holman WL, et al. Intermediate septal accessory pathways: electrocardiographic characteristics, electrophysiologic observations and their surgical implications. *J Am Coll Cardiol*. 1991;17:1570-1578.
13. Gallagher JJ, Sealy WC, Kasell J, Wallace AG. Multiple accessory pathways in patients with the pre-excitation syndrome. *Circulation*. 1976;54:571-591.
14. Milstein S, Sharma AD, Guiraudon GM, Klein GJ. An algorithm for the electrocardiographic localization of accessory pathways in the Wolff–Parkinson–White syndrome. *Pacing Clin Electrophysiol*. 1987;10:555-563.
15. Arruda MS, McClelland JH, Wang X, et al. Development and validation of an ECG algorithm for identifying accessory pathway ablation site in Wolff–Parkinson–White syndrome. *J Cardiovasc Electrophysiol*. 1998;9:2-12.
16. Antzelevitch C, Yan GX. J-wave syndromes. From cell to bedside. *J Electrocardiol*. 2011;44:656-661.
17. Viskin S, Lesh MD, Eldar M, et al. Mode of onset of malignant ventricular arrhythmias in idiopathic ventricular fibrillation. *J Cardiovasc Electrophysiol*. 1997;8:1115-1120.

CHAPTER 3

Complex Catheter Recording and Mapping Techniques in the EP Lab

Andrew K. Krumerman, MD; John D. Fisher, MD

Introduction

This chapter is designed to provide the reader with an understanding of mapping techniques that identify cardiac arrhythmia. It should serve as a general overview for approaching all types of arrhythmia. The chapter reviews basic catheter setup, recording systems, atrial mapping techniques, and ventricular mapping techniques.

The approach to mapping and ablation must be individualized for each patient. It is imperative to obtain electrocardiogram (ECG) tracings demonstrating arrhythmia prior to performing an electrophysiologic (EP) study. Determination of the optimal catheter choices and arrangements (rig) for performing an EP study will be based on findings gleaned from the history, physical examination, and ECG. Often a patient presents with palpitations and short runs of tachycardia recorded on a noisy transtelephonic monitor. When in doubt, the standard multipurpose rig will be sufficient for diagnosis and treatment of almost any tachyarrhythmia.

Catheter Rigs Used for Complex Mapping

Standard Multipurpose Rig

Whether one is seeking to identify the etiology of wide or narrow complex tachycardia, the standard multipurpose (four-) catheter rig will provide the tools necessary for rapid identification and treatment of cardiac arrhythmia. The most common rig used in our laboratory consists of three quadripolar catheters positioned to record electrograms (EGMs) from the high right atrium (HRA), His bundle (HIS), and right ventricular apex (RVA). If certain ablations are anticipated, the HRA catheter is likely to double as a roving probe capable of both mapping and ablation. A fourth multi-electrode catheter is inserted into the coronary sinus (CS) and records EGMs from the epicardial aspect of the left atrium and left ventricle (Figure 3.1). Recordings from all electrodes and the 12-lead ECG are analyzed using a multi-electrode recording system. A pacing stimulator connected to the recording system allows for stimulation from any catheter.

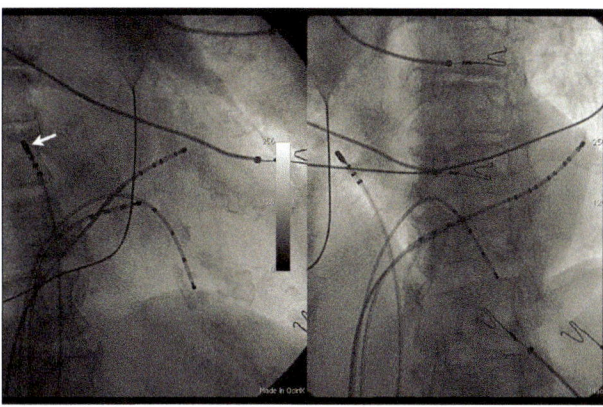

Figure 3.1 The multipurpose four-catheter rig as seen in right anterior oblique (**left**) and left anterior oblique (**right**) views. Catheters are positioned to record electrograms from the high right atrium (HRA), bundle of His, right ventricular apex, and coronary sinus. A 4-mm tip radiofrequency ablation catheter (**arrow**) is used to record and stimulate the HRA.

Alternative Rigs

Patients presenting to the EP laboratory with short RP tachycardia will likely be instrumented with a multipurpose rig as described above. However, individuals presenting with typical atrial flutter should be instrumented with a 20-pole catheter placed adjacent to the tricuspid annulus (Figure 3.2). Some operators prefer that the 20-pole catheter be placed in an inverted "U" position in the right atrium with a separate lead in the CS. Others place the distal poles of the 20-pole lead in the CS with the more proximal poles crossing the cavotricuspid isthmus (CTI) and then curving superiorly along the lateral tricuspid annulus. Recordings from the tricuspid annulus will rapidly reveal the activation sequence and facilitate pacing maneuvers that confirm its mechanism.

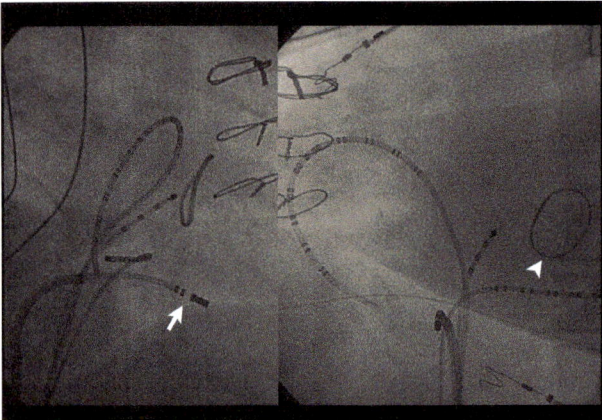

Figure 3.2 Right anterior oblique (**left**) and left anterior oblique (**right**) views of a typical rig used to map cavotricuspid isthmus (CTI)–dependent atrial flutter. A catheter with 20 electrodes is positioned adjacent to the tricuspid annulus. The distal electrode (T1) sits on the lateral CTI. A decapolar coronary sinus (CS) catheter is positioned with its distal electrode pair (CS 1, 2) in the lateral CS. A quadripolar catheter records septal activation at the bundle of His (**arrow**). An ablation catheter inserted via a long introducer is positioned in the basilar right ventricle in preparation for radiofrequency application along the CTI. A mitral valve annuloplasty ring (**arrowhead**) clearly delineates the mitral valve annulus.

Some patients presenting with one arrhythmia will have multiple arrhythmias noted during the EP study. The operator should be prepared to exchange catheters in order to facilitate rapid diagnosis and treatment. Whenever possible, an electroanatomic mapping (EAM) system should be kept on standby. Table 3.1 lists commonly used catheter rigs.

Transeptal, Transaortic, and Epicardial Approaches

The approach to left atrial and left ventricular mapping is often operator dependent. Both transseptal and transaortic (retrograde) approaches have been used successfully to map and ablate left-sided accessory pathways in patients with atrioventricular (AV) reentry tachycardia (AVRT).[1] In left atrial tachycardia, a transseptal approach is clearly advantageous as extensive mapping and ablation of the left atrium is impractical via a retrograde approach. To make things more complicated, the diagnosis of septal atrial tachycardia originating from the noncoronary aortic sinus often requires right atrial, left atrial, and transaortic mapping.[2] Left ventricular mapping and ablation may also be performed via a transseptal or transaortic approach.[3] The preferred approach depends not only on operator preference but also on a number of patient variables. The transaortic approach is contraindicated in patients with significant peripheral vascular disease, significant aortic stenosis, or mechanical aortic valve prosthesis. Figure 3.3 shows right anterior oblique and left anterior oblique views of a typical catheter rig used for left atrial and pulmonary vein mapping. EAM systems can be extremely useful when mapping left atrial tachycardia and atrial fibrillation.

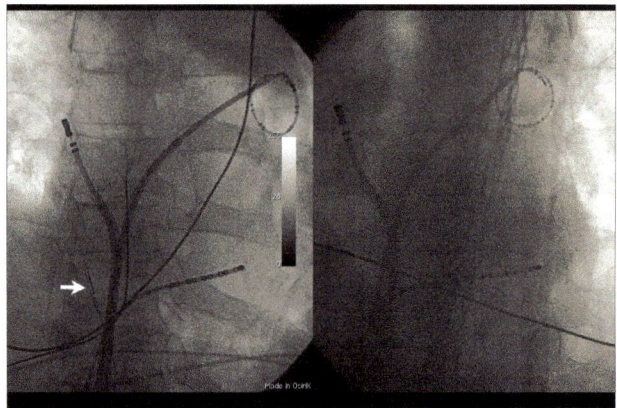

Figure 3.3 Right anterior oblique (**left**) and left anterior oblique (**right**) views showing the catheter rig used for left atrial mapping procedures. Access to the left atrium is obtained via transseptal puncture. Ablation and lasso catheters are positioned in the left atrium via long transseptal introducers. The ablation catheter is positioned inside the right superior pulmonary vein, and a 20-pole variable lasso catheter is positioned inside the left superior pulmonary vein. Intracardiac ultrasound (**arrow**) and multi-electrode coronary sinus catheters complete the rig.

The epicardial approach to mapping and ablation of ventricular tachycardia (VT) was first described in patients with cardiomyopathy secondary to Chagas disease.[4] Surface ECG recordings demonstrating a psuedo-delta wave or delayed intrinsicoid deflection time in lead V2 raise suspicion for an epicardial source of VT (Figures 3.4 and 3.5).[5,6] Epicardial mapping should always be performed in concert with endocardial mapping. Important considerations when mapping the epicardium include avoiding damage to the coronary arteries, left phrenic nerve, and lungs. A more detailed description of the approach to epicardial mapping and ablation can be found in Chapter 43.

Chapter 3: Complex Catheter Recording and Mapping Techniques in the EP Lab • 25

Table 3.1 Commonly used rigs for electrophysiologic studies

Rhythm Abnormality	Rig*
Short RP tachycardia	Standard rig: HRA/ABL, HIS, RVa (quadripolar), CS (decapolar); EAM system optional
Long RP tachycardia (atrial flutter)	ABL, 20-pole catheter along with TA, CS, RVa; EAM system optional
Atrial fibrillation (PVI)	CS (decapolar), 20-pole lasso catheter, ABL (irrigated tip), IUS, EAM system
Wide complex tachycardia (ventricular tachycardia)	Standard rig, EAM system, +/- epicardial mapping catheter

*Although the multipurpose rig used for short RP tachycardia may be useful for mapping and ablation of any arrhythmia, alternative rigs can optimize mapping and ablation of certain arrhythmia substrates. The HRA catheter is frequently used as the mapping and ablation catheter following induction of tachycardia.

ABL = ablation catheter; CS = coronary sinus catheter; EAM = electroanatomic mapping (3D systems including contact and noncontact technologies); HIS = His bundle catheter; HRA = high right atrium catheter; IUS = intracardiac ultrasound catheter; PVI = pulmonary vein isolation; RVa = right ventricular apex catheter; TA = tricuspid annulus catheter.

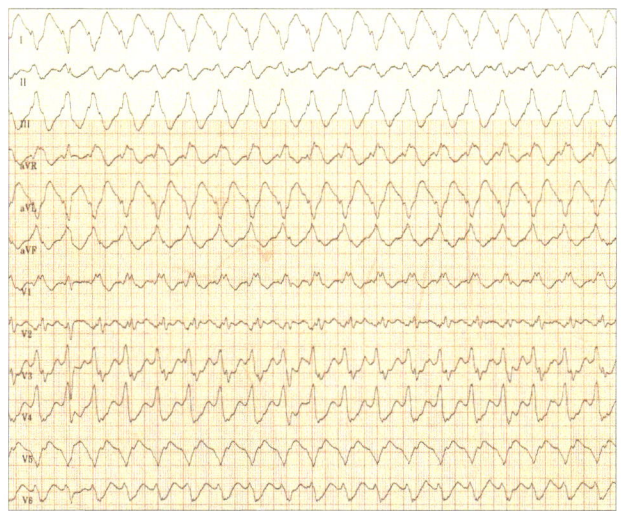

Figure 3.4 Twelve-lead ECG demonstrating ventricular tachycardia. Pseudo-delta waves measured in the precordial leads are 40 ms. The intrinsicoid deflection in lead V2 is 100 ms. See text for details. This patient had a focal ventricular tachycardia mapped to the epicardial aspect of the lateral left ventricle.

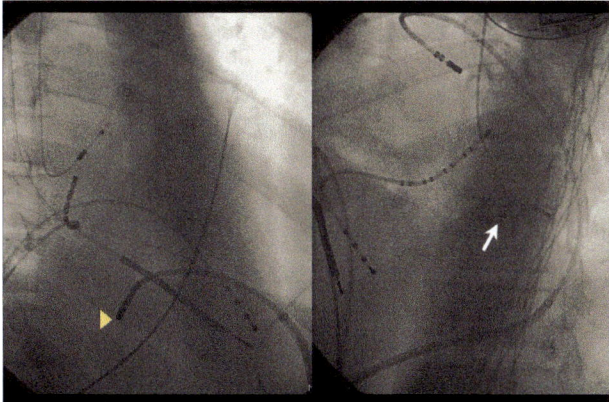

Figure 3.5 Right anterior oblique (**left**) and left anterior oblique (**right**) views of an epicardial mapping rig. Following endocardial mapping, a roving catheter (**arrowhead**) is inserted via a long introducer to map the epicardium. Multipolar catheters are observed at the right ventricular apex and coronary sinus positions. A unipolar epicardial pacing lead from a cardiac resynchronization therapy/implantable cardioverter-defibrillator system is also seen in the LAO view (**arrow**).

Recording Systems and Techniques

Signal Filtration and Inter-electrode Spacing

During EP studies, the ability to distinguish between macro and micro events is based on the effects of signal filtration and inter-electrode spacing. These variables allow simultaneous recording of a QRS complex and depolarization of the bundle of His. The QRS complex is best measured with EGMs filtered at about 0.5 to 100 Hz. Most of the electrical energy of the heartbeat occurs in these low-frequency ranges, and low-frequency signals also propagate over greater distances than high-frequency signals.

Intracardiac catheters typically record high-frequency bipolar signals from catheters with short inter-electrode spacing (2 to 2.5 mm). Lower frequencies (starting at 0.5 Hz) and relatively wide inter-electrode spacing are avoided because they maximize inclusion of "far-field" signals from parts of the heart that are not in close proximity to the recording electrodes. "Local" events, such as precise timing of a Purkinje potential, are best accomplished by filtration settings beginning at 30 or 40 Hz and going up to 500 Hz or higher. This takes advantage of the facts that higher frequencies do not propagate as well as lower frequencies and that many of the structures of interest (such as the His bundle) contain relatively few cardiac fibers and thus relatively low amounts of energy. Close inter-electrode spacing (2 to 10 mm—the latter needed with large-tip ablating catheters) together with filtering at 30 to 500 Hz combine to maximize recording of local micro signals and exclude far-field or macro signals. It is possible to focus in even more closely on local events by filtering at 100 to 1,000 Hz.

Cardiac mapping requires accurate recording of micro signals from areas of diseased myocardium. Activation and substrate mapping techniques are dependent on accurate localization of low-voltage, slowly conducting EGMs.

Timing of Electrical Events

Conduction in the heart can be measured between two electrode pairs rather easily using simple calipers or rulers. As indicated in the previous section, filtration and interelectrode distance affect the ability to record events at varying distances from a given point within the heart. All recorded signals will have characteristics such as duration and amplitude. As a general rule, if one is looking for the first evidence of an electrical event, several simultaneously recorded leads are observed for onset of a deflection that is used for the relevant measurement. The local timing of an event is important during mapping studies when one is interested in the timing of an event at the site where the mapping electrode or probe is located. Here, far-field signals are unwelcome and closely spaced electrodes filtered at 30 to 500 Hz are critical. As a wavefront approaches the electrodes from afar, there will be a progressively steeper deflection that culminates in a point. At this point, as the wavefront passes by the recording electrodes, there is a very rapid reversal in slope, making a near-vertical deflection; this deflection has the highest dV/dt of the entire EGM and is known as the intrinsic deflection.[7] It culminates in another reversal of direction as the wavefront continues to move away from the recording electrodes and inscribes a deflection that is a mirror image of the curve inscribed by the approaching wavefront.

Unipolar Recordings and Focal Tachycardias and Accessory Pathways

Several factors can alter the shape of a wavefront. If the recording electrodes are in close proximity to the initial site of ventricular repolarization (eg, near the site of initial depolarization during sinus rhythm, at the site of a tachycardia focus), the intrinsic deflection may come very early in the overall complex. This is particularly notable if unipolar recordings are made; an initial rapid negative intrinsic deflection is evidence that a recording electrode is at the initial site of depolarization. This is because unipolar recordings are made at low frequency (eg, 0.5 to 500 Hz) and compare local with very far-field (surface) potentials.

At the site of origin of a focal tachycardia, or the first site depolarized by an accessory pathway, all depolarization will be moving away from the intracardiac lead, and this will manifest as a QS complex. When recordings are made in areas that are scarred or damaged, overall signal amplitude may be low (< 1.0 mV) and there may be a series of low-amplitude deflections, none of which fulfills the criteria for local or intrinsic deflection. Usually the first of the relatively larger deflections (this can be quite subjective) is used for local timing. Low-voltage potentials are often masked by far-field signals on unipolar recordings. As a result, bipolar recordings are favored when mapping low-amplitude signals in abnormal regions of myocardium. A complete review of EP recording techniques is not within the scope of this chapter and may be found elsewhere.[8,9]

Supraventricular Tachycardia

Principles of Entrainment

The majority of supraventricular tachycardias (SVTs) are due to reentry. Entrainment mapping is the basis for defining and localizing a reentrant circuit. The concept of entrainment was initially described by Albert Waldo while treating patients with atrial flutter following coronary artery bypass graft surgery.[10] Table 3.2 lists the four entrainment characteristics of all reentrant circuits. Tachycardias due to enhanced impulse formation (abnormal automaticity or triggered activity) cannot be entrained and emanate from a focus or point source.

Table 3.2 Entrainment criteria of reentrant circuits[56]

First criterion: During tachycardia, overdrive pacing will result in constant fusion on the surface electrocardiogram (ECG), with the exception of the last beat, which will be captured but not fused.

Second criterion: During tachycardia, overdrive pacing at progressively faster rates will result in progressive degrees of fusion that is constant at any given rate.

Third criterion: Overdrive pacing that interrupts tachycardia will cause localized conduction block to a site for one beat followed by the activation of that site by the next paced beat from a different direction and with a shorter conduction time.

Fourth criterion: During tachycardia, overdrive pacing and progressively faster rates will ultimately result in progressive change in conduction time and intracardiac electrogram (EGM) activation sequence consistent with an entirely paced ECG and EGM morphology.

Intraatrial Reentry

CTI-dependent atrial flutter is the classic atrial reentrant rhythm. In atrial flutter, a macroreentrant circuit is bound between the crista terminalis and the tricuspid annulus. Atrial activation travels in a clockwise or counterclockwise direction. In order to confirm the mechanism of macroreentrant atrial flutter, one must overdrive pace 10 to 40 ms faster than the tachycardia cycle length (TCL). During overdrive pacing, an orthodromic and antidromic wave of depolarizing tissue will exit the pacing site. The orthodromic wavefront travels in the same direction and the antidromic wavefront travels in the opposite direction as the tachycardia (Figure 3.6B). The antidromic wavefront is responsible for fusion noted on the ECG or on intracardiac EGMs (also termed manifest entrainment). When pacing from a protected isthmus within a reentry circuit, such as the CTI in atrial flutter, the antidromic wavefront is blocked and does not alter the intracardiac activation sequence. As a result, fusion is not observed. This is known as concealed entrainment.

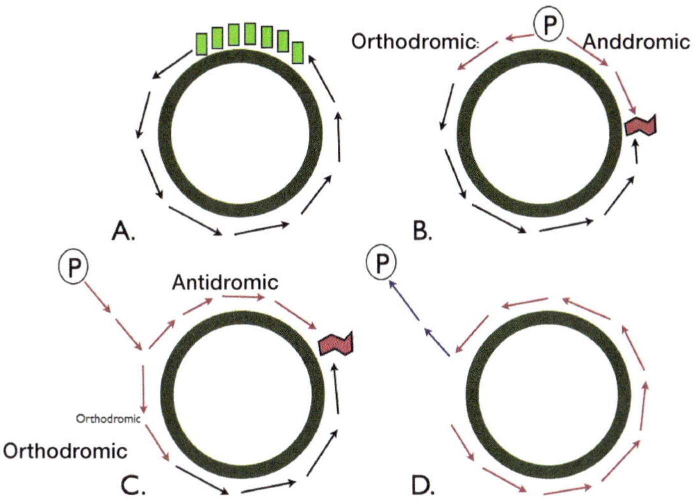

Figure 3.6 Entrainment mapping of reentrant arrhythmia. **(A)** The depolarizing wavefront of a reentrant rhythm (**black arrows**) will travel around an unexcitable barrier. The excitable gap—the area of excitable tissue denoted by **green rectangles**—separates the head and the tail of the depolarizing wavefront, allowing an arrhythmia to perpetuate. **(B)** The **large circle** represents the tricuspid annulus. A pacing catheter (P) is placed along the annulus. Overdrive pacing produces orthodromic and antidromic depolarizing wavefronts (**red arrows**). Upon termination of overdrive pacing, the last paced beat will travel once around the tricuspid annulus with a cycle length that is equal to that of the tachycardia cycle length. Because the catheter is within the reentry circuit, changes in the atrial activation sequence will not be noticeable; this is known as concealed entrainment. **(C)** Overdrive pacing remote from the reentry circuit produces depolarizing wavefronts moving toward and away from the reentry circuit, resulting in a change in the atrial activation sequence or manifest entrainment. **(D)** Upon cessation of overdrive pacing, the time it takes to travel from the pacing catheter into the reentry circuit and back to the pacing catheter is called the post-pacing interval (PPI). A prolonged PPI will be recorded when the pacing catheter is remote from the reentry circuit. See text for details.[11]

Entrainment Mapping

Entrainment can be used to localize a critical isthmus responsible for reentrant tachycardia. The post-pacing interval (PPI) can be used to locate a reentrant circuit. To determine the PPI, the tachycardia circuit should be overdrive paced at 10 to 40 ms shorter than the TCL. The PPI is defined as the interval between the stimulation artifact of the last paced beat and the next EGM measured at the pacing catheter. Thus the PPI is a measurement of the time it takes for an impulse to travel from the pacing catheter into and around the reentry circuit and back. When the PPI is within 30 ms of the TCL, then the mapping catheter is likely within the reentry circuit. When the PPI is significantly longer than the TCL (> 30 ms), the pacing catheter is remote from the tachycardia circuit (Figure 3.6D). A protected isthmus within the tachycardia circuit is identified when overdrive pacing results in concealed entrainment with a PPI that is equal to the TCL. If the protected isthmus is narrow, as in the case of the CTI, then ablation at the pacing site will result in termination of tachycardia. An example of entrainment mapping for CTI-dependent atrial flutter is shown in Figure 3.7. The pacing catheter is located on the CTI. Upon termination of pacing, the PPI is equal to the TCL. Concealed fusion is noted on both the surface ECG and intracardiac activation recordings.

Pitfalls of Entrainment Mapping

Entrainment mapping has many pitfalls. Overdrive pacing may result in termination or acceleration of tachycardia. Occasionally, arrhythmia can no longer be induced following pace termination, precluding an accurate diagnosis. Careful attention to measurement of PPIs and TCLs is imperative. If the last paced beat does not capture, the PPI will appear to be "perfect" even if the pacing catheter is far from the tachycardia circuit. Always ensure capture of the last paced beat as well as reproducibility of all findings. A complete overview of entrainment and entrainment mapping is not within the scope of this chapter and may be found elsewhere.[11-13]

Pacing Maneuvers in Supraventricular Tachycardia

SVT is probably the most common rhythm abnormality encountered in the EP laboratory. Most SVTs can be easily identified using a standard four-catheter rig in combination with the 12-lead ECG. Typical intracardiac EGM patterns noted at onset, offset, and during tachycardia are critical to the diagnosis.[14] Before performing ablation, pacing maneuvers are used to prove the diagnosis.[15-20] A series of chapters in this book describes mapping and ablation of specific tachycardias. The following should serve as a general overview.

Upon induction of SVT, a glance at the recording system will reveal a particular pattern leading to a differential diagnosis. The ventriculoatrial (VA) interval should be closely examined during tachycardia. A VA interval shorter than 70 ms has a high specificity for the diagnosis of AV node reentry tachycardia (AVNRT).[21] A series of pacing maneuvers may then performed in order to confirm the mechanism of tachycardia (Table 3.3).

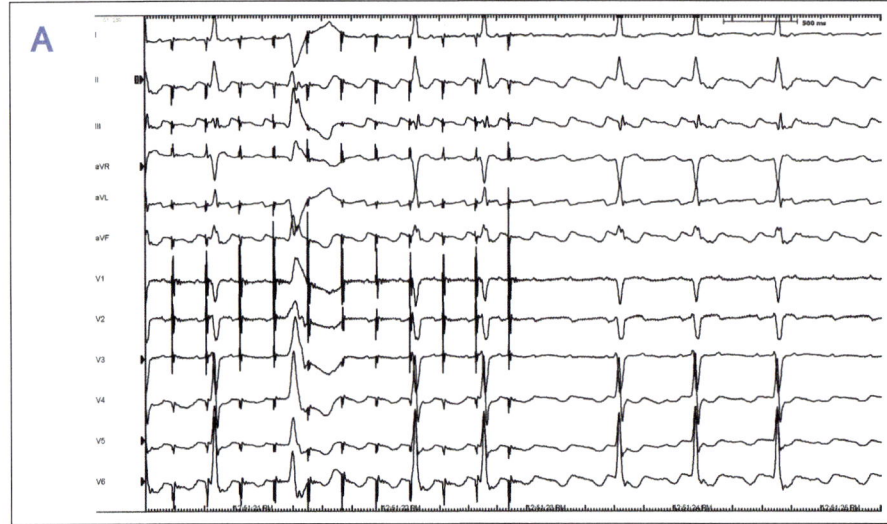
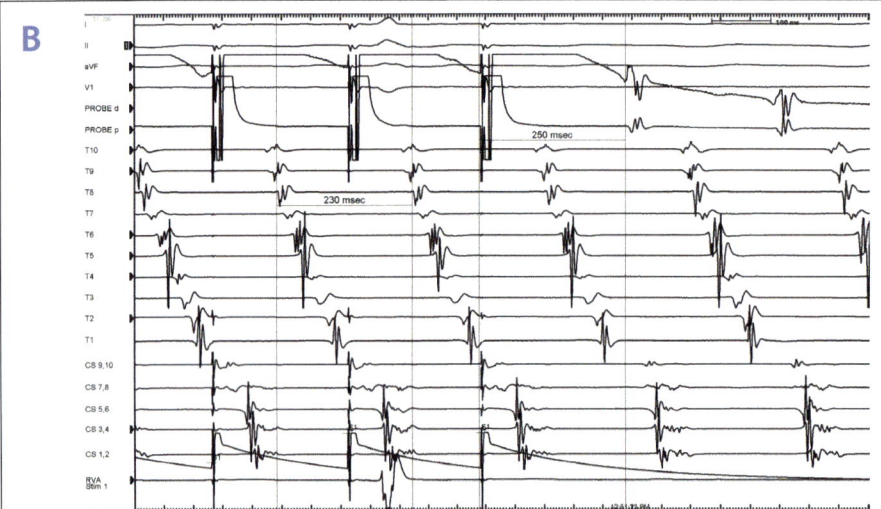

Figure 3.7 Concealed entrainment of cavotricuspid isthmus (CTI)–dependent atrial flutter. (**A**) The surface electrocardiogram (ECG) demonstrates concealed fusion during overdrive atrial pacing from the CTI. (**B**) Intracardiac electrograms (EGMs) reveal concealed fusion during overdrive pacing. The pacing catheter (Probe d) is located on the CTI. Upon termination of pacing, the post-pacing interval is 250 ms and is equal to the tachycardia cycle length. Recording system leads from top to bottom: surface ECG leads I, II, aVF, and V1; Probe D; Probe P; T10–T1 = adjacent to tricuspid annulus with T10 on septal annulus and T1 on lateral CTI isthmus; CS9,10–CS1,2 = decapolar coronary sinus catheter with CS9,10 recording from the CS os and CS1,2 from the distal CS; RVA = right ventricular apex.

Table 3.3 Pacing maneuvers used to confirm mechanisms of tachycardia[15,17,27]

Rhythm	12-Lead ECG	Intracardiac EGM	Pacing Maneuvers
AVNRT	Short RP tachycardia	VA interval < 70 ms CS concentric activation	V pacing with atrial entrainment produces V-A-V-A response
AVRT	Short RP tachycardia	VA interval > 70 ms CS eccentric activation	His-synchronous premature ventricular contraction advances atrial depolarization
Atrial tachycardia	Long RP tachycardia	CS eccentric act A > V	V pacing with atrial entrainment produces V-A-A-V Differential atrial pacing
Atrial flutter	Saw-toothed pattern	Clockwise or counterclockwise pattern of activation around tricuspid annulus	Concealed entrainment from cavotricuspid isthmus

AVNRT = atrioventricular node reentry tachycardia; AVRT = atrioventricular reentry tachycardia; CS = coronary sinus; VA = ventriculoatrial.

Ventricular Pacing Maneuvers

Ventricular pacing with 1:1 VA conduction (atrial entrainment) can help to differentiate reciprocating SVT from atrial tachycardia. Following induction of tachycardia, ventricular pacing 10 to 60 ms faster than the TCL is performed until there is 1:1 VA conduction. When pacing is discontinued, a V-A-V-A response is consistent with a diagnosis of AV node or AV reciprocating tachycardia, whereas a V-A-A-V response is consistent with a diagnosis of atrial tachycardia.[17] Careful attention to atrial entrainment is imperative to interpreting the response to pacing. Pitfalls noted with this maneuver include the inability to entrain the atrium without termination of tachycardia and a pseudo V-A-A-V response in patients with long HV intervals.[22]

Single premature ventricular complexes (PVCs) programmed during SVT can rule out atrial tachycardia and confirm the participation of an accessory pathway in AVRT. If a PVC, programmed while the His bundle is refractory, terminates tachycardia without atrial depolarization, then the diagnosis of atrial tachycardia is ruled out. The diagnosis of AVRT with retrograde conduction up an accessory pathway is confirmed when preexcitation of the atrium results following a His-synchronous PVC.[23] It is important to keep in mind that failure of PVCs to advance atrial depolarization does not rule out AVRT.[24]

When His-synchronous PVCs and the atrial activation sequence do not give the diagnosis away, ventricular pacing with entrainment of tachycardia may be useful in differentiating AVNRT from AVRT.[18-20] This maneuver is based on the fact that the ventricle is part of the reentry circuit in AVRT but not in AVNRT. Thus entrainment during V pacing should result in shorter PPIs in AVRT than in AVNRT. Sensitivity and specificity of these maneuvers are enhanced when one corrects the PPI for AV node decrement (cPPI). PPI values allowing for differentiation of AVNRT and AVRT are listed in Table 3.4.[19,25]

Table 3.4 Differentiation of AVNRT and AVRT[19,25]

Measurement	AVNRT	AVRT
cPPI-TCL	> 110 ms	< 110 ms
(S-A)-VA interval	> 80 ms	< 80 ms

CPPI = post-pacing interval corrected for AV node delay; TCL = tachycardia cycle length; S-A = ventricular pacing stimulus to atrial interval.

Atrial Pacing Maneuvers

Atrial pacing maneuvers are particularly useful for long RP tachycardias. The differential diagnosis of long RP tachycardia includes atypical (fast-slow) AVNRT, AVRT with a slowly conducting bypass tract, and atrial tachycardia. Differential atrial pacing is useful for supporting the diagnosis of atrial tachycardia.[26-28] Atrial overdrive pacing (10 to 40 ms faster than TCL) from the HRA and the proximal CS electrodes, without termination of tachycardia, is a sensitive and specific maneuver for diagnosing atrial tachycardia (Table 3.5). The retrograde limb in a reciprocating tachycardia is fixed, and little difference will be noted when comparing the return VA interval following overdrive atrial pacing. Conversely, in atrial tachycardia, the return VA interval following atrial overdrive pacing will be variable and the absolute value of the difference between the VA interval following HRA pacing and that following CS pacing will be greater than 10 ms.[27]

Table 3.5 Differential atrial pacing[27]

Measurement	AVNRT/AVRT	Atrial Tachycardia
[VA(HRA)] – [VA(CS)]	Fixed (< 10 ms)	Variable (> 10 ms)

AVNRT = atrioventricular node reentry tachycardia; AVRT = atrioventricular reentry tachycardia; VA(CS) = ventriculoatrial timing following coronary sinus overdrive pacing; VA(HRA) = ventriculoatrial timing following high right atrial overdrive pacing.

Activation Mapping for Focal Tachycardia

Focal SVT and VT may be mapped using a standard multipurpose rig. In focal atrial tachycardia, a roving (probe) catheter is maneuvered around the atrium and the activation sequence is recorded. A CS EGM is typically used for a timing reference. Unipolar EGMs and surface ECG recordings are also used in confirming areas of earliest activation prior to ablation.[29] Focal atrial tachycardia is usually mapped to characteristic anatomic regions such as the crista terminalis, the tricuspid and mitral valve annuli, and the pulmonary veins.[30] Likewise, idiopathic focal VT also originates from characteristic locations around the right and left ventricular outflow tracts, the aortomitral continuity, and the Purkinje fibers along the left ventricular septum.[31-33] Knowledge of the characteristic regions responsible for focal tachycardia will facilitate mapping and ablation.

EAM systems are instrumental in mapping focal tachycardia. These systems allow one to visualize any cardiac chamber as a three-dimensional image. Activation mapping is performed using a stable intracardiac or surface ECG reference. The EAM computer assigns colors that represent activation timing. In the Carto® System (Biosense Webster, Diamond Bar, CA), the color red represents areas of early activation. Figure 3.8 shows an EAM of the left atrium and pulmonary veins. A focal tachycardia is noted, with earliest activation mapped to the left atrial appendage. Application of radiofrequency energy to this area terminated the tachycardia. It is important to remember that EAM systems are used in concert with standard mapping techniques.

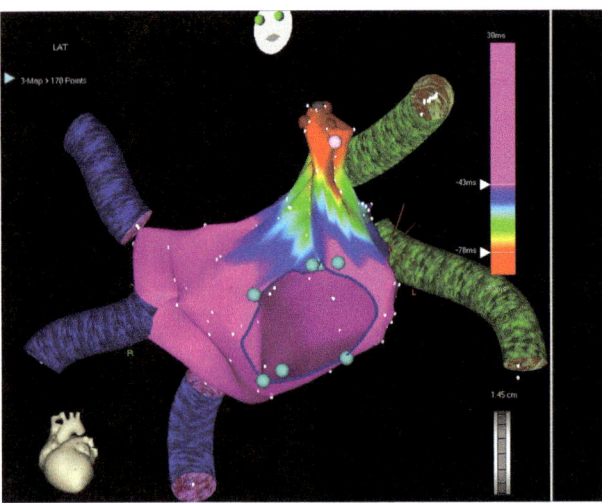

Figure 3.8 Left anterior oblique view of an electroanatomic map of the left atrium and pulmonary veins. A focal atrial tachycardia was mapped to the left atrial appendage. Activation mapping is translated into color isochrones, with red representing early activation and purple late activation. Focal atrial tachycardia was successfully eliminated by ablating within the left atrial appendage.

Ventricular Tachycardia

Mapping techniques for ventricular arrhythmia are similar to those for SVT. Idiopathic VT can be mapped to characteristic focal regions of the right and left ventricles using activation and pace mapping techniques.[31,32] Reentrant ventricular arrhythmia is often associated with chronic ischemic heart disease and concomitant LV dysfunction.[34] Activation and entrainment mapping for VT can be challenging due to hemodynamic instability, multiple VT morphologies, and acceleration of tachycardia during overdrive pacing. In cases in which VT is unmappable, substrate mapping must be used.

Substrate Mapping

Substrate mapping is used to identify narrow isthmuses of tissue that are critical to reentry circuits producing VT. In cases in which activation and entrainment mapping are not possible due to multiple reentry circuits or unstable VT, substrate mapping is required.[35-37] An EAM system is used to create a bipolar voltage map of the ventricle. Voltages are color coded and displayed on a 3D map of the ventricle. By using voltage, one can differentiate infarcted or injured areas from normal myocardium. Regions with EGMs greater than 1.5 mV are considered normal. Regions with EGMs between 0.5 and 1.5 mV are classified as border zones separating normal tissue and dense scar.[37,38] Reentry isthmuses critical for maintenance of VT are usually found along these border zones. Dense scar is defined as myocardium with EGMs measuring less than 0.5 mV. Unipolar pacing has been used to help identify areas of unexcitable scar (areas where the pacing threshold exceeds 10 mA), providing a more detailed map of potential reentry circuits.[39] After completion of voltage mapping, induction of VT with activation and entrainment mapping allows for further delineation of reentry circuits. In cases in which tachycardia is unstable, pace mapping should be utilized.

Pace Mapping

Pace mapping is used to map both reentrant and focal VT. Simply stated, pacing from a catheter placed at the exit site of a tachycardia circuit or focus should produce a QRS morphology that matches the morphology of the clinical tachycardia on a 12-lead ECG. Numerous studies have demonstrated effective localization of an idiopathic VT focus using this technique.[32,40-43] Pace mapping alone may lead to successful VT localization when tachycardia is not inducible. However, Bogun and colleagues demonstrated that pace maps have insufficient accuracy for identifying the site of VT origin in 20% of patients.[44] Thus concomitant activation mapping should be performed when feasible. Proper surface ECG lead placement is critical when using this technique. Tachycardia should be induced in the EP laboratory to ensure identical lead placement for pace mapping and recording of VT.

In patients with abnormal ventricles, pace mapping is used in conjunction with measurement of localized conduction delay to identify reentry circuits. Stevenson and colleagues demonstrated that pacing from the exit site of a reentrant circuit produces a QRS morphology similar to the morphology of the clinical VT.[45] During pace mapping, the extent of conduction delay between the pacing stimulus and the QRS complex on the surface ECG (S-QRS) should be recorded. Areas with a good pace map and a prolonged S-QRS interval (> 40 ms) are located proximal to the exit sites in isthmuses responsible for VT.[46] Isolated potentials recorded from areas of myocardial scar during sinus rhythm are also important in identifying arrhythmogenic substrate in both ischemic and nonischemic cardiomopathy. When mapping of isolated potentials is combined with pace mapping, identification of critical isthmus sites is enhanced.[47,48] Pitfalls encountered during pace mapping are due to propagation differences in diseased myocardium. Several groups have reported differing QRS morphologies when pacing from areas that are within close proximity to one another.[43,49] As a result, pace mapping should be used as one of several techniques to identify critical sites responsible for reentry tachycardia.[50]

Entrainment Mapping

In stable VT, a combination of activation and entrainment mapping may be used to define a VT reentry circuit. As most patients with structural heart disease do not tolerate long periods of VT, prior substrate mapping is recommended.[51] The principles of entrainment mapping can be found earlier in this chapter. During entrainment mapping, the PPI is used as a measure of proximity to the reentry circuit. When the mapping catheter is positioned along a protected isthmus that is part of the VT circuit, the PPI-TCL is less than 30 ms and concealed fusion is observed on the surface ECG. If the PPI-TCL is less than 30 ms but manifest fusion is noted on the surface ECG, the pacing catheter is located in an outer loop of the circuit.[13] The exit or central portions of a protected isthmus are ideal targets for ablation. As with pace mapping, the S-QRS interval is measured during entrainment mapping to further define portions of the isthmus. S-QRS intervals are recorded at sites where entrainment with concealed fusion and a short PPI are observed. Sites where the S-QRS interval is less than 70% of the TCL have the highest incidence of termination and are within the isthmus[13] (Figure 3.9). Characteristics of different reentry circuit sites determined during entrainment mapping are listed in Table 3.6.

Mid-diastolic Potentials

Bogun and colleagues demonstrated that concealed entrainment has a positive predictive value of identifying a successful ablation site only 54% of the time.[52] Mid-diastolic potentials (MDPs) recorded during VT represent narrow areas of slowly conducting myocardium critical for maintenance of a reentry circuit.[53] Entrainment mapping can determine whether an MDP is linked to the tachycardia circuit. VT termination is more likely to occur at sites demonstrating both MDPs that are linked to the reentry circuit and concealed entrainment.[53,54] Well-known pitfalls when mapping MDPs include mapping of isolated potentials that are not linked to the tachycardia and failure to recognize far-field potentials during entrainment.[55]

Ultimately, successful mapping VT requires a combination of several techniques. Several groups have demonstrated that a combination of pace, substrate, and entrainment mapping should be utilized to maximize success rates of ablation.[36,48,50] A complete overview of VT mapping and ablation can be found in Chapters 30 and 31.

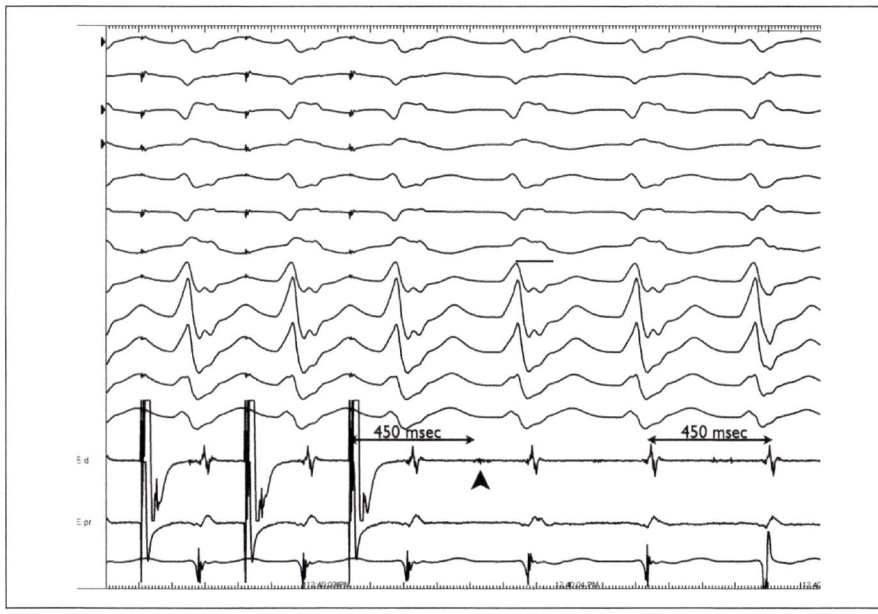

Figure 3.9 Entrainment mapping of ventricular tachycardia (VT) in a patient with structural heart disease. Overdrive pacing from the mapping catheter (Probe d) entrains VT with concealed fusion. The post-pacing interval equals the tachycardia cycle length (TCL), and the S-QRS interval is 40% of the TCL. A mid-diastolic potential is noted (**arrowhead**). Based on these characteristics, the mapping catheter is located in a protected isthmus of the reentry circuit, proximal to the exit site. Application of radiofrequency energy at this site resulted in termination of tachycardia.

Table 3.6 Entrainment mapping for ventricular tachycardia[13]

Location of Pacing Catheter	PPI-TCL	Fusion	S-QRS
Exit from protected isthmus	< 30 ms	Concealed	≤30% of TCL
Proximal isthmus	< 30 ms	Concealed	31%–70% of TCL
Outer loop	< 30 ms	Manifest	
Bystander	> 30 ms	Concealed	

PPI = post-pacing interval; S-QRS = interval between the stimulus artifact and the QRS complex during overdrive pacing of ventricular tachycardia; TCL = tachycardia cycle length.

Conclusion

The advent of catheter ablation of tachycardias has led to a revolution in electrophysiology. The desire for a purely scientific understanding of arrhythmias has been complemented and boosted by what may be called "applied electrophysiology." This term includes (1) the continuing identification of mapping and stimulation algorithms that identify specific arrhythmias, (2) the ever-broadening range of "ablatable" tachycardias, and (3) the technologic advances that have resulted in a wealth of new tools that facilitate effective ablation.

References

1. Kistler PM, Kalman JM. Locating focal atrial tachycardias from P-wave morphology. *Heart Rhythm.* 2005;2(5):561-564.
2. Ouyang F, Ma J, Ho SY, et al. Focal atrial tachycardia originating from the non-coronary aortic sinus: electrophysiological characteristics and catheter ablation. *J Am Coll Cardiol.* 2006;48(1):122-131.
3. Schwartzman D, Callans DJ, Gottlieb CD, Marchlinski FE. Catheter ablation of ventricular tachycardia associated with remote myocardial infarction: utility of the atrial transseptal approach. *J Interv Card Electrophysiol.* 1997;1(1):67-71.
4. Sosa E, Scanavacca M, D'Avila A, et al. Endocardial and epicardial ablation guided by nonsurgical transthoracic epicardial mapping to treat recurrent ventricular tachycardia. *J Cardiovasc Electrophysiol.* 1998;9(3):229-239.
5. Bazan V, Gerstenfeld EP, Garcia FC, et al. Site-specific twelve-lead ECG features to identify an epicardial origin for left ventricular tachycardia in the absence of myocardial infarction. *Heart Rhythm.* 2007;4(11):1403-1410.
6. Berruezo A, Mont L, Nava S, Chueca E, Bartholomay E, Brugada J. Electrocardiographic recognition of the epicardial origin of ventricular tachycardias. *Circulation.* 2004;109(15):1842-1847.
7. Fisher J, Baker J, Ferrick K, et al. The atrial electrogram during clinical electrophysiologic studies: onset versus the local/intrinsic deflection. *J Cardiovasc Electrophysiol.* 1991;2:398-407.
8. Fisher JD. Clinical electrophysiology techniques. In: Saksena S, Camm AJ, eds. *Electrophysiological Disorders of the Heart.* Philadelphia: Elsevier; 2005:153-174.
9. Stevenson WG, Soejima K. Recording techniques for clinical electrophysiology. *J Cardiovasc Electrophysiol.* 2005;16(9):1017-1022.
10. Waldo AL, MacLean WA, Karp RB, Kouchoukos NT, James TN. Entrainment and interruption of atrial flutter with atrial pacing: studies in man following open heart surgery. *Circulation.* 1977;56(5):737-745.
11. Waldo AL. Atrial flutter: entrainment characteristics. *J Cardiovasc Electrophysiol.* 1997;8(3):337-352.
12. Waldo AL, Wit AL. Mechanism of cardiac arrhythmias and conduction disturbances. In: Fuster V, Alexander RW, O'Rourke RA, Roberts R, King SB, Wellens HJJ, eds. *Hurst's The Heart.* 10th ed. New York: McGraw-Hill; 2001:751-796.
13. Stevenson WG, Friedman PL, Sager PT, et al. Exploring postinfarction reentrant ventricular tachycardia with entrainment mapping. *J Am Coll Cardiol.* 1997;29(6):1180-1189.
14. Josephson ME. *Clinical Cardiac Electrophysiology: Techniques and Interpretation.* 2nd ed. Philadelphia: Lea & Febiger; 1993:xi, 839.
15. Knight BP, Ebinger M, Oral H, et al. Diagnostic value of tachycardia features and pacing maneuvers during paroxysmal supraventricular tachycardia. *J Am Coll Cardiol.* 2000;36(2):574-582.
16. Knight BP, Michaud GF, Strickberger SA, Morady F. Electrocardiographic differentiation of atrial flutter from atrial fibrillation by physicians. *J Electrocardiol.* 1999;32(4):315-319.
17. Knight BP, Zivin A, Souza J, et al. A technique for the rapid diagnosis of atrial tachycardia in the electrophysiology laboratory. *J Am Coll Cardiol.* 1999;33(3):775-781.
18. Michaud GF, Tada H, Chough S, et al. Differentiation of atypical atrioventricular node re-entrant tachycardia from orthodromic reciprocating tachycardia using a septal accessory pathway by the response to ventricular pacing. *J Am Coll Cardiol.* 2001;38(4):1163-1167.
19. Gonzalez-Torrecilla E, Arenal A, Atienza F, et al. First postpacing interval after tachycardia entrainment with correction for atrioventricular node delay: a simple maneuver for differential diagnosis of atrioventricular nodal reentrant tachycardias versus orthodromic reciprocating tachycardias. *Heart Rhythm.* 2006;3(6):674-679.
20. Segal OR, Gula LJ, Skanes AC, Krahn AD, Yee R, Klein GJ. Differential ventricular entrainment: a maneuver to differentiate AV node reentrant tachycardia from orthodromic reciprocating tachycardia. *Heart Rhythm.* 2009;6(4):493-500.
21. Benditt DG, Pritchett EL, Smith WM, Gallagher JJ. Ventriculoatrial intervals: diagnostic use in paroxysmal supraventricular tachycardia. *Ann Intern Med.* 1979;91(2):161-166.
22. Vijayaraman P, Lee BP, Kalahasty G, Wood MA, Ellenbogen KA. Reanalysis of the "pseudo A-A-V" response to ventricular entrainment of supraventricular tachycardia: importance of His-bundle timing. *J Cardiovasc Electrophysiol.* 2006;17(1):25-28.
23. Sellers TD Jr, Gallagher JJ, Cope GD, Tonkin AM, Wallace AG. Retrograde atrial preexcitation following premature ventricular beats during reciprocating tachycardia in the Wolff-Parkinson-White syndrome. *Eur J Cardiol.* 1976;4(3):283-294.
24. Benditt DG, Benson DW, Jr, Dunnigan A, et al. Role of extrastimulus site and tachycardia cycle length in inducibility of atrial preexcitation by premature ventricular stimulation during reciprocating tachycardia. *Am J Cardiol.* 1987;60(10):811-819.
25. Veenhuyzen GD, Coverett K, Quinn FR, et al. Single diagnostic pacing maneuver for supraventricular tachycardia. *Heart Rhythm.* 2008;5(8):1152-1158.
26. Maruyama M, Kobayashi Y, Miyauchi Y, et al. The VA relationship after differential atrial overdrive pacing: a novel tool for the diagnosis of atrial tachycardia in the electrophysiologic laboratory. *J Cardiovasc Electrophysiol.* 2007;18(11):1127-1133.
27. Sarkozy A, Richter S, Chierchia GB, et al. A novel pacing manoeuvre to diagnose atrial tachycardia. *Europace.* 2008;10(4):459-466.
28. Man KC, Niebauer M, Daoud E, et al. Comparison of atrial-His intervals during tachycardia and atrial pacing in patients with long RP tachycardia. *J Cardiovasc Electrophysiol.* 1995;6(9):700-710.
29. Delacretaz E, Soejima K, Gottipaty VK, Brunckhorst CB, Friedman PL, Stevenson WG. Single catheter determination of local electrogram prematurity using simultaneous unipolar and bipolar recordings to replace the surface ECG as a timing reference. *Pacing Clin Electrophysiol.* 2001;24(4 Pt 1):441-449.

30. Kistler PM, Roberts-Thomson KC, Haqqani HM, et al. P-wave morphology in focal atrial tachycardia: development of an algorithm to predict the anatomic site of origin. *J Am Coll Cardiol.* 2006;48(5):1010-1017.
31. Callans DJ, Menz V, Schwartzman D, Gottlieb CD, Marchlinski FE. Repetitive monomorphic tachycardia from the left ventricular outflow tract: electrocardiographic patterns consistent with a left ventricular site of origin. *J Am Coll Cardiol.* 1997;29(5):1023-1027.
32. Movsowitz C, Schwartzman D, Callans DJ, et al. Idiopathic right ventricular outflow tract tachycardia: narrowing the anatomic location for successful ablation. *Am Heart J.* 1996;131(5):930-936.
33. Lin D, Hsia HH, Gerstenfeld EP, et al. Idiopathic fascicular left ventricular tachycardia: linear ablation lesion strategy for noninducible or nonsustained tachycardia. *Heart Rhythm.* 2005;2(9):934-939.
34. de Bakker JM, van Capelle FJ, Janse MJ, et al. Reentry as a cause of ventricular tachycardia in patients with chronic ischemic heart disease: electrophysiologic and anatomic correlation. *Circulation.* 1988;77(3):589-606.
35. Soejima K, Suzuki M, Maisel WH, et al. Catheter ablation in patients with multiple and unstable ventricular tachycardias after myocardial infarction: short ablation lines guided by reentry circuit isthmuses and sinus rhythm mapping. *Circulation.* 2001;104(6):664-669.
36. Ellison KE, Stevenson WG, Sweeney MO, Lefroy DC, Delacretaz E, Friedman PL. Catheter ablation for hemodynamically unstable monomorphic ventricular tachycardia. *J Cardiovasc Electrophysiol.* 2000;11(1):41-44.
37. Marchlinski FE, Callans DJ, Gottlieb CD, Zado E. Linear ablation lesions for control of unmappable ventricular tachycardia in patients with ischemic and nonischemic cardiomyopathy. *Circulation.* 2000;101(11):1288-1296.
38. Callans DJ, Ren JF, Michele J, Marchlinski FE, Dillon SM. Electroanatomic left ventricular mapping in the porcine model of healed anterior myocardial infarction. Correlation with intracardiac echocardiography and pathological analysis. *Circulation.* 1999;100(16):1744-1750.
39. Soejima K, Stevenson WG, Maisel WH, Sapp JL, Epstein LM. Electrically unexcitable scar mapping based on pacing threshold for identification of the reentry circuit isthmus: feasibility for guiding ventricular tachycardia ablation. *Circulation.* 2002;106(13):1678-1683.
40. Calkins H, Kalbfleisch SJ, el-Atassi R, Langberg JJ, Morady F. Relation between efficacy of radiofrequency catheter ablation and site of origin of idiopathic ventricular tachycardia. *Am J Cardiol.* 1993;71(10):827-833.
41. Rodriguez LM, Smeets JL, Timmermans C, Wellens HJ. Predictors for successful ablation of right- and left-sided idiopathic ventricular tachycardia. *Am J Cardiol.* 1997;79(3):309-314.
42. Coggins DL, Lee RJ, Sweeney J, et al. Radiofrequency catheter ablation as a cure for idiopathic tachycardia of both left and right ventricular origin. *J Am Coll Cardiol.* May 1994;23(6):1333-1341.
43. Josephson ME, Waxman HL, Cain ME, Gardner MJ, Buxton AE. Ventricular activation during ventricular endocardial pacing. II. Role of pace-mapping to localize origin of ventricular tachycardia. *Am J Cardiol.* Jul 1982;50(1):11-22.
44. Bogun F, Taj M, Ting M, et al. Spatial resolution of pace mapping of idiopathic ventricular tachycardia/ectopy originating in the right ventricular outflow tract. *Heart Rhythm.* Mar 2008;5(3):339-344.
45. Stevenson WG, Sager PT, Natterson PD, Saxon LA, Middlekauff HR, Wiener I. Relation of pace mapping QRS configuration and conduction delay to ventricular tachycardia reentry circuits in human infarct scars. *J Am Coll Cardiol.* Aug 1995;26(2):481-488.
46. Brunckhorst CB, Delacretaz E, Soejima K, Maisel WH, Friedman PL, Stevenson WG. Identification of the ventricular tachycardia isthmus after infarction by pace mapping. *Circulation.* Aug 10 2004;110(6):652-659.
47. Bogun F, Good E, Reich S, et al. Isolated potentials during sinus rhythm and pace-mapping within scars as guides for ablation of post-infarction ventricular tachycardia. *J Am Coll Cardiol.* May 16 2006;47(10):2013-2019.
48. Kuhne M, Abrams G, Sarrazin JF, et al. Isolated potentials and pace-mapping as guides for ablation of ventricular tachycardia in various types of nonischemic cardiomyopathy. *J Cardiovasc Electrophysiol.* Sep 2010;21(9):1017-1023.
49. Kadish AH, Childs K, Schmaltz S, Morady F. Differences in QRS configuration during unipolar pacing from adjacent sites: implications for the spatial resolution of pace-mapping. *J Am Coll Cardiol.* Jan 1991;17(1):143-151.
50. El-Shalakany A, Hadjis T, Papageorgiou P, Monahan K, Epstein L, Josephson ME. Entrainment/mapping criteria for the prediction of termination of ventricular tachycardia by single radiofrequency lesion in patients with coronary artery disease. *Circulation.* May 4 1999;99(17):2283-2289.
51. Raymond JM, Sacher F, Winslow R, Tedrow U, Stevenson WG. Catheter ablation for scar-related ventricular tachycardias. *Curr Probl Cardiol.* May 2009;34(5):225-270.
52. Bogun F, Bahu M, Knight BP, et al. Comparison of effective and ineffective target sites that demonstrate concealed entrainment in patients with coronary artery disease undergoing radiofrequency ablation of ventricular tachycardia. *Circulation.* Jan 7 1997;95(1):183-190.
53. Fitzgerald DM, Friday KJ, Wah JA, Lazzara R, Jackman WM. Electrogram patterns predicting successful catheter ablation of ventricular tachycardia. *Circulation.* Apr 1988;77(4):806-814.
54. Stevenson WG, Khan H, Sager P, et al. Identification of reentry circuit sites during catheter mapping and radiofrequency ablation of ventricular tachycardia late after myocardial infarction. *Circulation.* Oct 1993;88(4 Pt 1):1647-1670.
55. Tung S, Soejima K, Maisel WH, Suzuki M, Epstein L, Stevenson WG. Recognition of far-field electrograms during entrainment mapping of ventricular tachycardia. *J Am Coll Cardiol.* Jul 2 2003;42(1):110-115.
56. Waldo AL. From bedside to bench: entrainment and other stories. *Heart Rhythm.* May 2004;1(1):94-106.

CHAPTER 4

ADVANCES IN ELECTROANATOMIC MAPPING SYSTEMS

BRIAN J. CROSS, MD; ANN C. GARLITSKI, MD; N.A. MARK ESTES III, MD

Introduction

Electroanatomic mapping systems have evolved during the last decade into essential tools for catheter ablation by enabling three-dimensional (3D) nonfluoroscopic catheter navigation and reconstruction of cardiac anatomy, activation, and voltage mapping. The ability to reconstruct electrophysiological mechanisms is essential to ensure optimal ablation outcomes, particularly of complex arrhythmias.[1-11]

Current mapping systems have clinical utility for defining patient-specific cardiac anatomy as well as arrhythmia mechanisms by integrating mapping data.[1-11] These systems allow precise 3D spatial localization of the ablation and diagnostic catheters. Use of these mapping systems has been associated with a reduction in total procedure time, fluoroscopy duration, and radiofrequency energy delivery time. Owing to the elucidation of mechanisms of paroxysmal atrial fibrillation (AF) and the dramatic growth of catheter ablation in the clinic, an advanced mapping system has become the standard of care for catheter ablation of AF.[12-17] Advanced mapping systems also have clinical utility for defining optimal ablation sites for a wide range of supraventricular and ventricular arrhythmias.

Two nonfluoroscopic mapping systems are currently available for clinical use in catheter ablation. These include the CARTO System (Biosense Webster, Inc., Diamond Bar, CA) and EnSite Velocity™ Cardiac Mapping System (St. Jude Medical, Inc., St. Paul, MN).[2,4,6] The EnSite Velocity system uses impedance measurements between individual intracardiac catheter electrodes and external patches placed on the patient's chest and abdomen.[2,4,6] By contrast, the CARTO System utilizes magnetic location technology to accurately visualize magnetosensor-equipped catheter tips.[1,2,4,6,7,18] With both systems, the precise localization of the catheter tip is influenced by catheter tip stability, respiratory motion, and cardiac motion. However, magnetic location technology functions independently of patient body habitus and physiological changes that can occur during the procedure.[7] Conversely, the accuracy of impedance-based localization is sensitive to rapid transthoracic impedance changes, which may result from an uneven respiratory pattern, significant fluid shifts, and development of tissue edema.

The impedance-based system allows the operator to simultaneously visualize multiple catheters/electrodes, whereas until recently, the magnetic system could visualize only the tip of the ablation catheter. The recently released CARTO 3 System includes several enhancements to facilitate procedures that use its guidance. These include catheter location technology that combines magnetic location technology with current-based visualization data to better visualize the catheter's tip and curve. This technology allows one to simultaneously visualize multiple electrodes.

All systems can integrate with preacquired computed tomography (CT) and magnetic resonance imaging (MRI).[18,19] The CARTO 3 System also includes the ability to integrate images obtained from intracardiac echocardiography (ICE) to reconstruct cardiac anatomy.[20,21]

Carto

Carto is a 3D electroanatomic mapping system that makes use of magnetic fields to localize and visualize intracardiac catheter position. This process is driven by the placement of magnetic field–emitting coils, each of unique strength, in a pad placed posteriorly to the patient's heart on the procedure table. Equipped with proprietary localizing sensors, mapping and ablation catheters can be localized within the region of interest based on calculations of the strength and orientation of the sensed magnetic fields.[22] Significant limitations of earlier generations of the system included reliance exclusively on proprietary catheters and a time-consuming point-by-point data collection process for making high-density cardiac maps.

The most recent system, Carto 3, addresses these limitations by expanding the data collection process through a new hybrid technology that makes use of both magnetic and impedance-based localization.[5] The system uses coils to generate magnetic fields, which are sensed by proprietary catheters in the standard Carto manner. In addition, the system employs 6 electric field–emitting patches (placed in x, y, and z axes relative to the heart) that localize any catheters equipped with sensing electrodes. This system also uses the data from the magnetic-based imaging to calibrate the data from the current-based imaging, thereby increasing peripheral accuracy.[23]

Proprietary software augments electroanatomic mapping with data from separate imaging modalities. A CartoMerge™ Image Integration Software Module (Biosense Webster) imports structures identified on previously acquired CT or MRI images of the cardiac anatomy into the electroanatomic map. This can help to guide the positioning of ablation catheters with respect to anatomically significant structures, such as the left atrial appendage and the mitral valve annulus (Figure 4.1).[5]

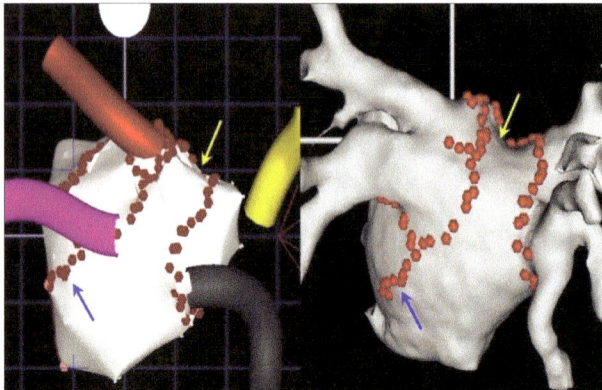

Figure 4.1 **Left panel:** Electroanatomic map of the left atrium (LA) during an atrial fibrillation ablation; **red dots** indicate sites of delivered radiofrequency lesions. **Right panel:** LA after integration with a CT image of the LA using the CartoMerge Image Integration Software Module. The **arrows** indicate corresponding anatomic sites. *Source:* Reprinted with permission from Kabra R, Singh J, their Figure 1.[5]

Integrating preacquired MRI images with electroanatomic mapping increases the accuracy of left ventricular substrate mapping.[19] This approach employs electroanatomic mapping of the ascending and proximal descending aorta, along with the left ventricle, to improve integration accuracy (Figure 4.2).[19]

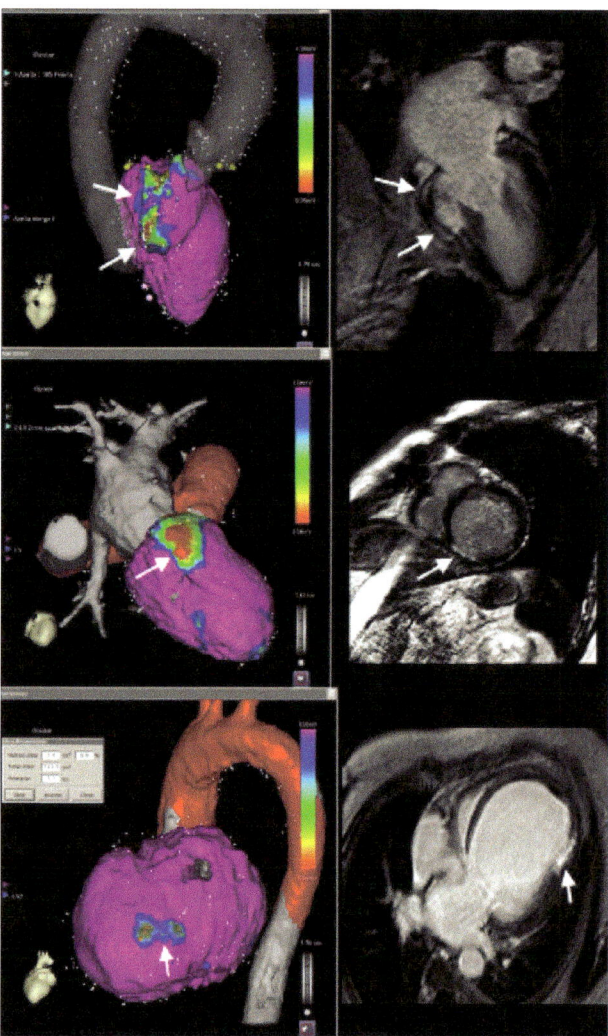

Figure 4.2 Comparison of left ventricular scar localization using either electroanatomic voltage maps generated with Carto 3 software and merged with imported MRI images (**left images**) or cardiac magnetic resonance scar imaging using delayed enhancement (**right images**). **Rows 1 and 2** depict localization of inferior-wall scar; **row 3** depicts localization of anterolateral scar. **Arrows** in all images point to the regions of scar. *Source:* Reprinted with permission from Pandozi C, et al.[19]

Images acquired by sensor-tipped ICE catheters can be integrated with the electroanatomic data using the CartoSound® module.[20,21] This integrated imaging may augment anatomic reconstruction, facilitate transseptal access, and improve endocardial tissue contact.[20,21] Left atrial (LA) anatomic mapping performed at the beginning of AF ablation procedures may be conducted by acquiring images of the LA from an ICE catheter located within the right atrium (RA).[20,21] In this manner, the creation of an anatomic map of the LA from a catheter positioned in the RA may aid in subsequent transseptal access as well as decrease the time of catheter placement within the LA.[20,21] Placement of the ICE catheter in the LA following transseptal access may help to improve registration of the Carto map with preacquired CT images of the LA[20,21] (Figures 4.3, 4.4).

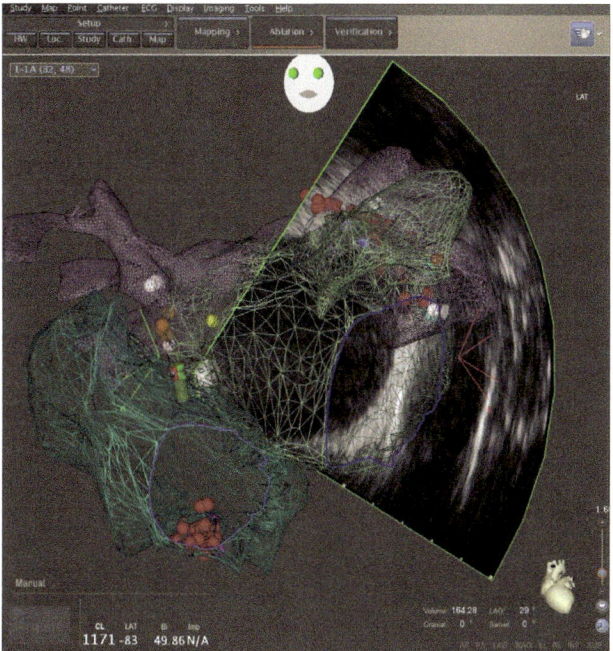

Figure 4.3 Electroanatomic map of the right atrium (RA) (**blue mesh**) and left atrium (LA) (**gray mesh**) acquired from the RA with CartoSound during a combined atrial fibrillation and typical atrial flutter ablation procedure. Ablation points can be seen around the pulmonary vein antra as well as along the cavotricuspid valve isthmus.

Anatomic renderings of cardiac anatomy generated by electroanatomic mapping are particularly helpful during anatomically driven procedures, such as catheter ablation of AF.[24] The use of cardiac mapping to augment imaging during catheter ablation of AF has been associated with improvements in procedural safety.[4] In pulmonary vein isolation procedures, decreased overall procedural time and fluoroscopy time have been demonstrated using this electroanatomic mapping technology compared with procedures that do not use 3D mapping systems.[2] Anatomic mapping can also be used to decrease fluoroscopy time in ablations of typical (cavotricuspid value isthmus–dependent) atrial flutter, in which stable ablation-catheter positioning during lesion delivery may be viewed on the anatomic map in place of a running fluoroscopic window (Figure 4.5).[11]

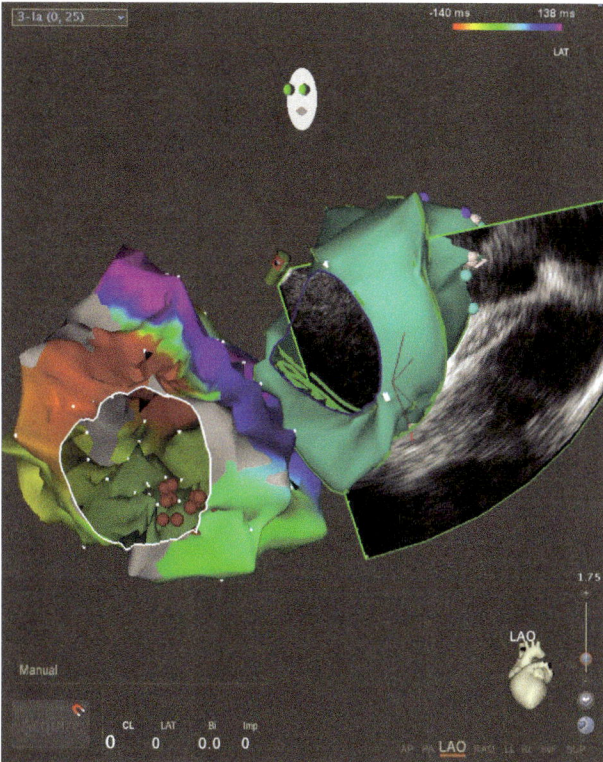

Figure 4.4 Electroanatomic activation map of the right atrium (RA) revealing a macroreentrant circuit consistent with typical atrial flutter, as well as ablation lesions along the cavotricuspid valve annulus. To the right of the RA map is a 3D reconstruction of the left atrium (LA) anatomy (without activation mapping) generated from CartoSound images of the LA acquired from an intracardiac echocardiographic catheter located in the RA.

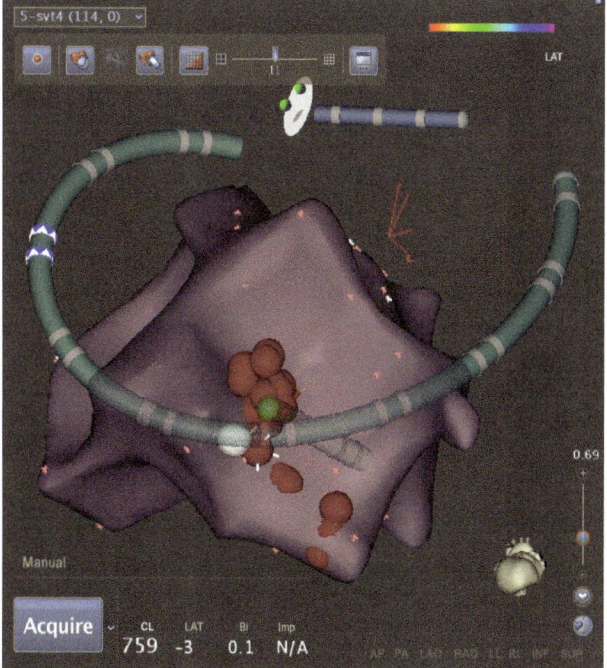

Figure 4.5 Carto 3 electroanatomic map of the right atrium showing catheter positioning and ablation lesions along the cavotricuspid valve isthmus delivered during radiofrequency ablation of typical atrial flutter.

Anatomic mapping may also help identify significant intracardiac structures during specific ablation procedures. For example, it can locate the bundle His during a slow atrioventricular (AV) nodal pathway ablation in the setting of AV nodal reentrant tachycardia.[3] In addition, fluoroscopy time during slow AV nodal pathway ablations has been reportedly lower in procedures augmented with Carto imaging than in fluoroscopy-only procedures (Figure 4.6).[3]

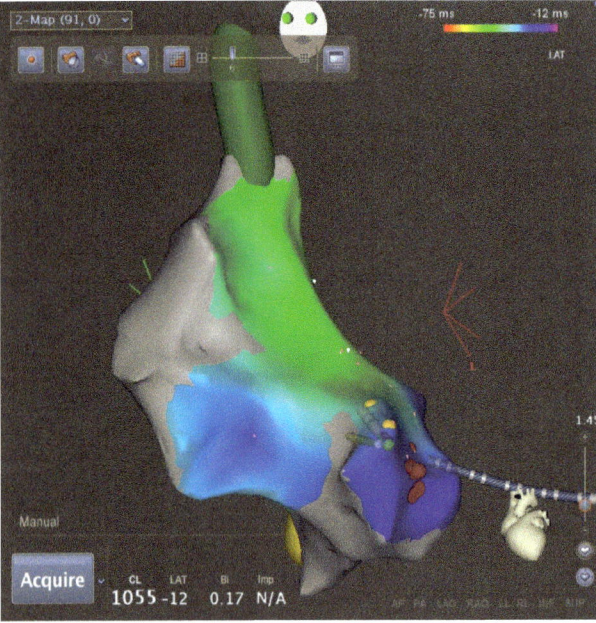

Figure 4.6 Left anterior oblique (LAO) image of the right atrium. The **yellow dots** indicate the location of the bundle of His, which was identified and marked prior to ablation of the slow atrioventricular (AV) nodal pathway (**red dots**) in a patient with typical AV nodal reentrant tachycardia.

In catheter-based ablations of monomorphic ventricular tachycardia (VT), electroanatomic mapping can be used to color-code cardiac anatomy with zones of myocardial voltage to help delineate regions of scar from healthy tissue.[10] Left ventricular voltage mapping to identify border zones between scarred and nonscarred myocardium is helpful for anatomically localizing potential sites for successful lesion delivery (Figure 4.7).[10]

Activation mapping acquired during tachycardia allows regions of cardiac depolarization to be visually depicted relative to a timing reference.[25] This technique can help to identify sites of focal activation, such as atrial tachycardias or focal VTs, in which the activation wavefront can be seen to spread from a focal site (Figure 4.8).[25] Activation wavefronts with circuitlike propagation patterns are more typical of macroreentrant arrhythmias. Ablation of reentrant cardiac arrhythmias can be guided by activation-mapping depictions of critical isthmuses (▶ Video 4.1).[26]

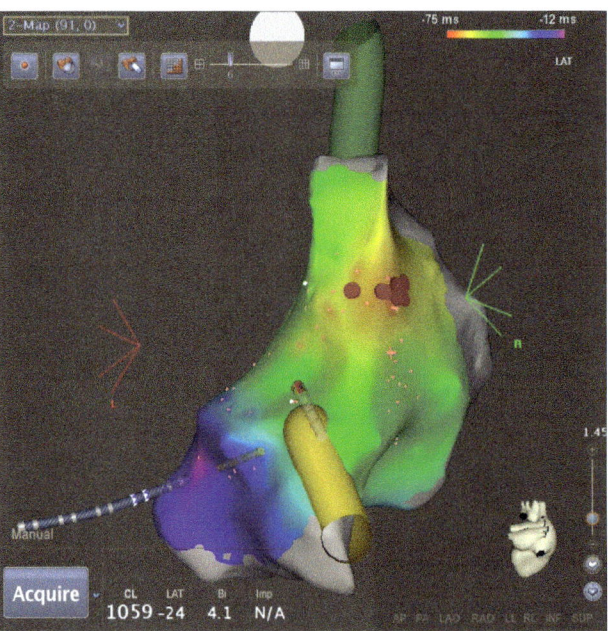

Figure 4.8 Posterior view of the right atrium during activation mapping of a supraventricular tachycardia. A focal site of activation can be seen along the posterolateral wall of the right atrium. Ablation markers overlie the earliest site of activation, where ablation lesion delivery terminated the tachycardia.

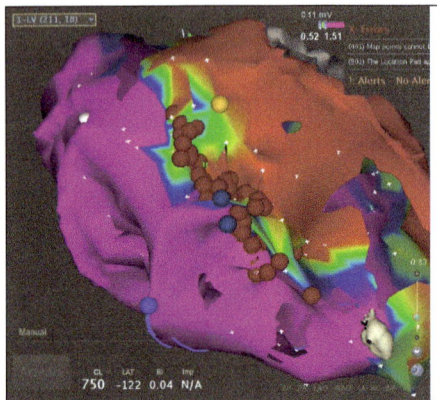 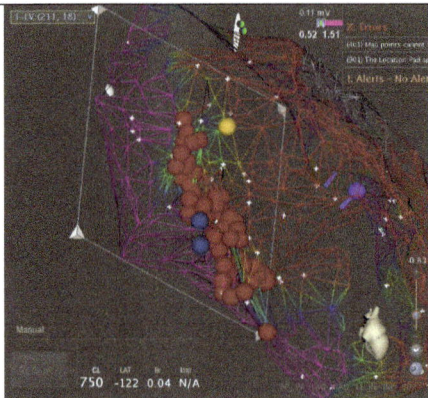

Figure 4.7 Electroanatomic voltage map of the left ventricle (LV) obtained during a radiofrequency (RF) ablation of ischemic ventricular tachycardia. **Left panel:** RF lesions that have been delivered along the scar tissue transition near the mid-LV septum, as viewed from a right lateral perspective. **Right panel:** the complete lesion set seen by "cutting out" sections of the posteroseptal LV wall.

EnSite Velocity Cardiac Mapping System

The EnSite Velocity Cardiac Mapping System uses a system of body-surface patch electrodes to create a 3D orthogonal space for mapping and catheter navigation.[2,4,6] Between patch electrode pairs, a high-frequency alternating current electrical signal (8 kHz) is delivered, and sensing electrodes on intracardiac catheters relay the relative voltages (with respect to a reference electrode) to the processing computer, which can then reconstruct electrode and catheter locations in 3D.[2,4,6] The Velocity system can operate up to 128 electrodes. Geometric data of cardiac anatomy can be collected as point clouds by sweeping catheters across the chamber walls in order to create a structural anatomic shell.[2,4,6] This mapping system now enables simultaneous, real-time acquisition and display of anatomic as well as electrophysiological data. It does this by "shrink-wrapping" a surface that follows concave and convex details, subsequently eliminating the need to segment structures such as the LA and pulmonary veins into individual surfaces. Among the features of this system is simultaneous generation of anatomic points and their corresponding surfaces while characterizing and displaying electrophysiological information collected from the same catheter electrodes. Electrogram signals that lie on or sufficiently close to the surface are automatically included in the map. Voltage mapping to identify regions of myocardial scar or other arrhythmogenic, nonmyocardial cardiac tissues may be displayed as colors coded for voltage values within a set range. Segmentation software allows for preablation cardiac CT and MRI images to be fused with the live 3D map. Including these preablation images is not only helpful for identifying pulmonary vein anatomy for AF ablation, but may also demonstrate the location of the fossa ovalis prior to transseptal puncture.[10]

The system has the added ability to create a map of complex fractionated electrograms (CFEs). These sites, presumed to be involved in the maintenance of AF, are non–pulmonary vein targets for ablation in patients with nonparoxysmal AF.[27,28] The automated CFE mapping algorithm has been validated and allows the user to define a signal width and refractory period over a given sampling period. The software then tags deflections that meet these criteria and calculates the mean interval between deflections; this value is known as the "CFE mean."[28,29] As a result, a high-density electrogram map can be rapidly and accurately created with a multipolar catheter to guide AF ablation[27-31] (Figures 4.9, 4.10).

Using this system, catheter localization can also be performed through magnetic field mapping. Transmitter coils generating magnetic fields of 10–13 kHz are mounted on the fluoroscopic image intensifier. These magnetic fields are then sensed by sensor coil–equipped catheters that encode catheter position and orientation at these sensor coils. Additionally, this technology incorporates a live catheter icon display superimposed over one or more preacquired fluoroscopy cine loops (Figure 4.11).

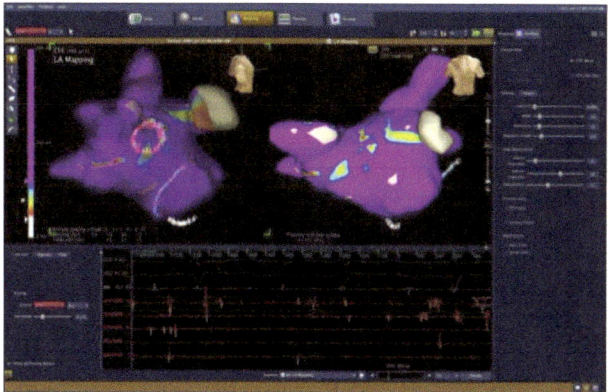

Figure 4.9 Mapping complex fractionated atrial electrical activity. The left atrial reconstructions display regions of electrical activity of a defined amplitude and fractionation, projected on a purple background. The intracardiac electrogram display at the bottom of the screen identifies these deflections with yellow markers from electrode pairs of the red circular mapping catheter.

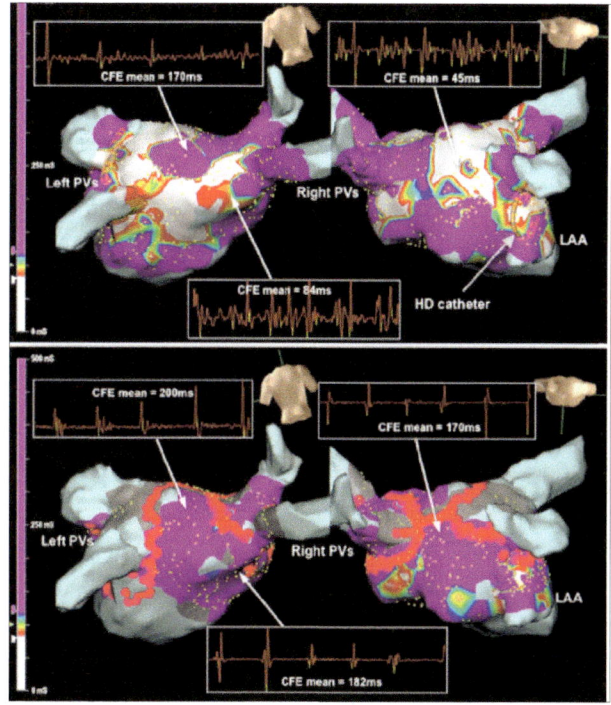

Figure 4.10 Complex fractionated electrogram map in persistent atrial fibrillation. Posterior (**left**) and anterosuperior (**right**) projections of left atrial complex fractionated electrogram (CFE) maps acquired by the high-density (HD) catheter at a preablation baseline (**upper panel**) and after pulmonary vein isolation with LA roofline of ablation (**lower panel**). This example demonstrates a significant organizational effect of pulmonary vein isolation and linear ablation with marked prolongation of local mean cycle lengths (CFE mean). PV = pulmonary vein; LAA = left atrial appendage. *Source:* Reprinted with permission from Jones DG, et al.[31]

40 • Section 1A: Electrophysiologic Techniques

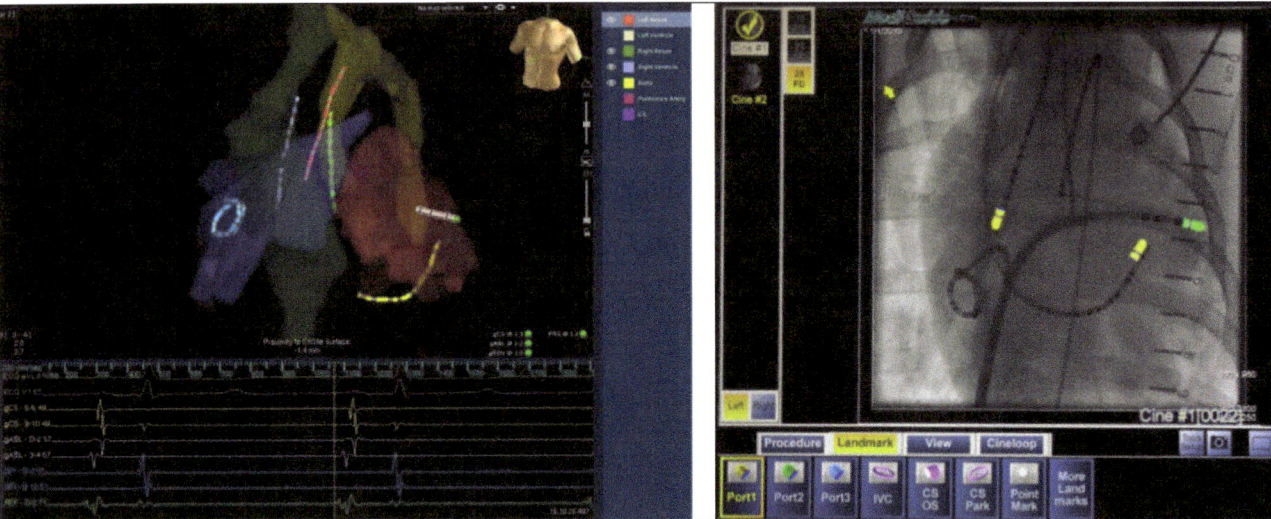

Figure 4.11 Cardiac catheter localization using MediGuide's Medical Position System (MPS) (MediGuide, Ltd., Haifa, Israel) superimposed on a fluoroscopic image (**right panel**) and simultaneously displayed on EnSite NavX™ (St. Jude Medical, St. Paul, MN) (**left panel**). Bullet-shaped MediGuide catheter tip icons (**yellow and green, right**) portray a sense of orientation in or out of the fluoroscopic image plane.

A visual metric has been designed to quantitatively display catheter contact with cardiac tissue. The EnSite Contact technology employs a tip-selective impedance signal, called electrical coupling index (ECI), which can be displayed on the mapping screen in a graphical format. Resistance and reactance values between the catheter tip and tissue are combined to calculate the ECI. The ablation catheter tip "beacon" projection changes in color and size as a qualitative display of ablation-tip radiofrequency energy coupling to the adjacent myocardium (Figure 4.12).

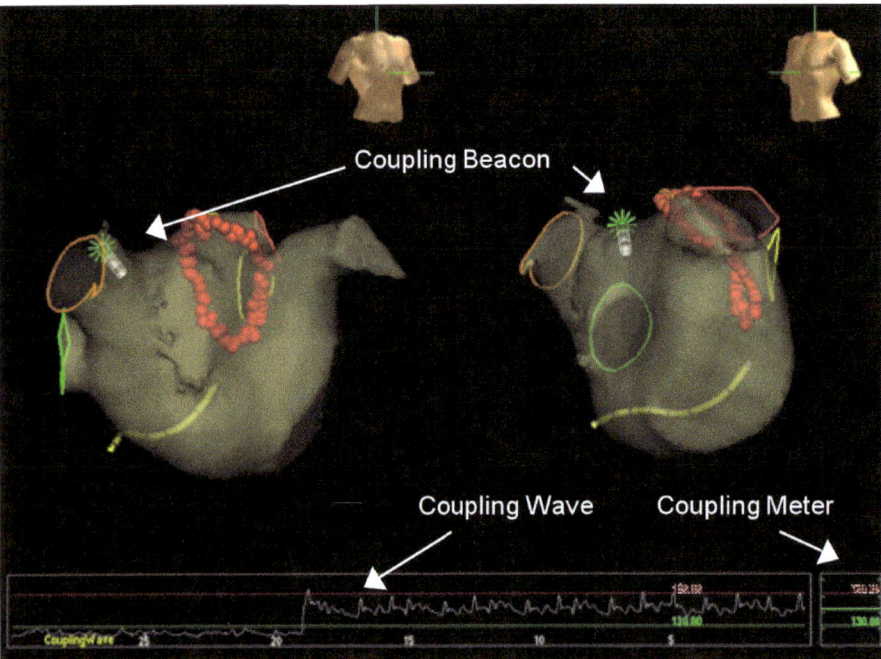

Figure 4.12 Visualization of effective electrical coupling to adjacent cardiac tissue of an ablation catheter tip electrode using EnSite Contact technology. *Source:* Dr. Gerhard Hindricks.

In addition to the use of point-to-point collection of electrical data locally at the catheter sensing electrodes, voltage and activation mapping of cardiac arrhythmias can be performed. This can be accomplished by creating virtual unipolar electrograms using a mathematical inverse solution to estimate the electrical potentials. As a result, noncontact mapping of conduction through a cardiac chamber is performed in a single cycle of the tachycardia. The noncontact catheter contains a balloon-expandable woven braid of 64 electrodes that can be used to sense more than 3,000 simultaneous far-field electrograms. This technique is most useful for mapping nonsustained or poorly tolerated, hemodynamically unstable arrhythmias for which point-by-point contact mapping is not favorable

(Figure 4.13). This noncontact mapping technology has been studied in patients with arrhythmogenic right ventricular dysplasia.[32] Using this technology, clinical VT was successfully ablated and could not be reinduced in all 15 patients[32] (Figure 4.14).

Radiation Safety

Among the advantages of the current electroanatomic mapping systems is a reduction in radiation exposure to the patient, operator, and electrophysiology lab personnel. Patients with cardiovascular conditions are increasingly being exposed to diagnostic and therapeutic procedures involving radiation, including CT, coronary angiography, and coronary intervention.[34-39] Elevated radiation exposure has been shown to increase malignancy rates and lead to other adverse outcomes.[37] Radiation protection programs and procedural measures instituted in the electrophysiology laboratory can reduce fluoroscopy radiation exposure to some extent. Even so, a considerable reduction in radiation exposure during fluoroscopy without changing the procedural technique could be beneficial.[35,39] Casella et al described 38 out of 50 cases in which EnSite mapping technology was the sole imaging mode utilized during electrophysiology study and radiofrequency ablation of supraventricular tachycardias.[33] The skin patch can be used as a positional reference in order to construct 3D venous anatomy from the femoral sheath, along the inferior vena cava, and into the cardiac chambers[33] (Figure 4.15).

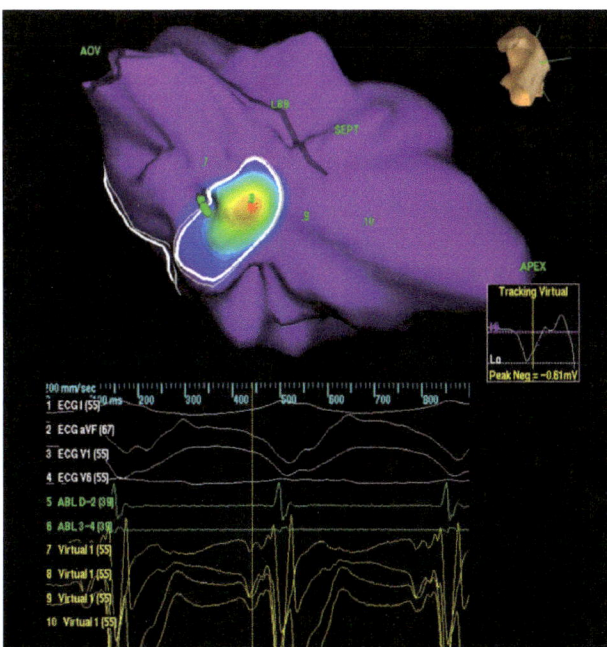

Figure 4.13 Noncontact mapping of ventricular tachycardia in the left ventricle using the EnSite Array™ Catheter illustrates localization of an early breakout before spreading to the remainder of the ventricle. Virtual unipolar electrogram signals (**yellow**) correspond to the 4 endocardial locations with **green numeric designations** at the point in the cardiac cycle denoted by the **vertical yellow line**. AOV = aortic valve; LBB = left bundle branch; SEPT = ??; ECG = electrocardiogram; ABL = ablation.

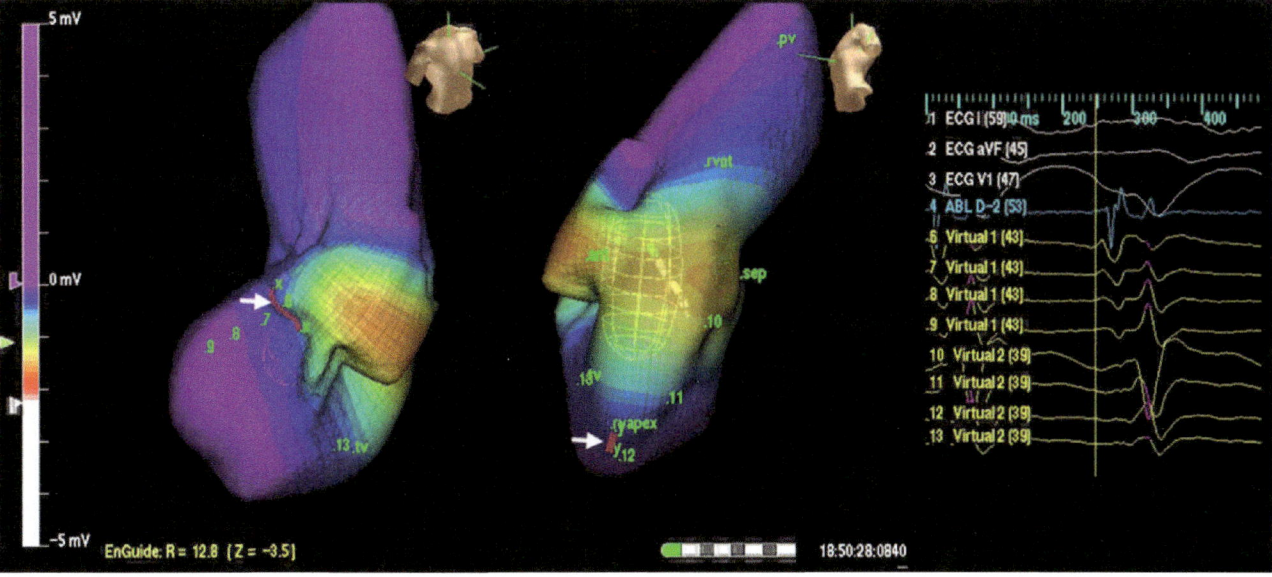

Figure 4.14 EnSite map of ventricular tachycardia (VT) in a patient with VT of multiple morphologies. All the VTs were, however, shown to turn around a single area in the right ventricle (**red line–white arrow**). Ablation along this line rendered all the VTs noninducible. ECG = electrocardiogram; ABL = ablation. *Source:* Reprinted with permission from Nair M, et al, their Figure 1.[32]

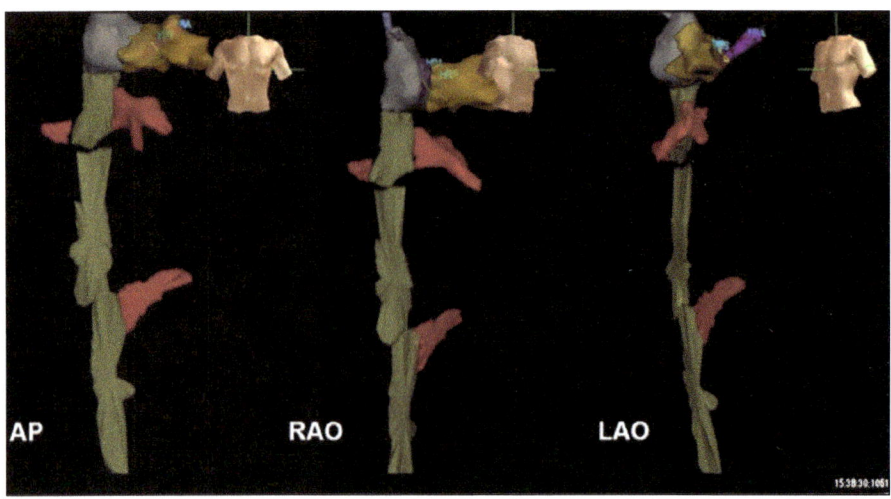

Figure 4.15 Nonfluoroscopic 3D-view reconstruction of the venous system (**olive green**) up to the right atrium (**gray**). Collateral branches (**red**) are clearly visualized. Catheter advancement is continuously monitored using 2 simultaneous views; if the catheter tip diverges from the femoral–caval axis, a collateral branch is identified, and it is possible to retract the tip to the branching point and advance it back into the correct trajectory. AP = anteroposterior; RAO = right anterior oblique; LAO = left anterior oblique. *Source:* Reprinted with permission from Casella M, et al.[33]

References

1. Shpun S, Gepstein L, Hayam G, Ben-Haim SA. Guidance of radiofrequency endocardial ablation with real-time three-dimensional magnetic navigation system. *Circulation.* 1997;96:2016-2021.
2. Khaykin Y, Oosthuizen R, Zarnett L, et al. Carto-guided vs. NavX-guided pulmonary vein antrum isolation and pulmonary vein antrum isolation performed without 3-D mapping: effect of the 3-D mapping system on procedure duration and fluoroscopy use. *J Interv Card Electrophysiol.* 2011;30:233-240.
3. Kopelman H, Prater S, Tondato F, et al. Slow pathway catheter ablation of atrioventricular nodal re-entrant tachycardia guided by electroanatomical mapping: a randomized comparison to the conventional approach. *Europace.* 2003;5:171-174.
4. Lo LW, Chen SA. Developments and recent advances in catheter ablation of paroxysmal atrial fibrillation. *Future Cardiol.* 2009;5:557-565.
5. Kabra R, Singh J. Recent trends in imaging for atrial fibrillation ablation. *Indian Pacing Electrophysiol.* 2010;10:215-227.
6. Knackstedt C, Schauerte P, Kirchhof P. Electroanatomic mapping systems in arrhythmias. *Europace.* 2008;10(Suppl 3):iii28-34.
7. Juneja R. Radiofrequency ablation for cardiac tachyarrhythmia: principles and utility of 3D mapping systems. *Current Science.* 2009;97:416-424.
8. Beinart R, Kabra R, Heist KE, et al. Respiratory compensation improves the accuracy of electroanatomic mapping (Carto) of the left atrium and pulmonary veins during atrial fibrillation ablation. *J Interv Card Electrophysiol.* 2011;32:105-110.
9. Braun MU, Knaut M, Rauwolf T, Strasser RH. Microwave ablation of an ischemic sustained ventricular tachycardia during aortocoronary bypass, mitral valve and tricuspid valve surgery guided by a three-dimensional nonfluoroscopic mapping system (Carto). *J Interv Card Electrophysiol.* 2005;13:243-247.
10. Verma A, Marrouche N, Schweikert R, et al. Relationship between successful ablation sites and the scar border zone defined by substrate mapping for ventricular tachycardia post-myocardial infarction. *J Cardiovasc Electrophysiol.* 2005;16:465-471.
11. Willems S, Weiss C, Ventura R, et al. Catheter ablation of atrial flutter guided by electroanatomic mapping (Carto): a randomized comparison to the conventional approach. *J Cardiovasc Electrophysiol.* 2000;11:1223-1230.
12. Haïssaguerre M, Jaïs P, Shah DC, et al. Spontaneous initiation of atrial fibrillation by ectopic beats originating in the pulmonary veins. *N Engl J Med.* 1998;339:659-666.
13. Haïssaguerre M, Shah DC, Jaïs P, et al. Electrophysiological breakthroughs from the left atrium to the pulmonary veins. *Circulation.* 2000;102:2463-2465.
14. Natale A, Pisano E, Shewchik J, et al. First human experience with pulmonary vein isolation using a through-the-balloon circumferential ultrasound ablation system for recurrent atrial fibrillation. *Circulation.* 2000;102:1879-1882.
15. Pappone C, Oreto G, Lamberti F, et al. Catheter ablation of paroxysmal atrial fibrillation using a 3D mapping system. *Circulation.* 1999;100:1203-1208.
16. Pappone C, Oreto G, Rosanio S, et al. Atrial electroanatomic remodeling after circumferential radiofrequency pulmonary vein ablation: efficacy of an anatomic approach in a large cohort of patients with atrial fibrillation. *Circulation.* 2001;104:2539-2544.
17. Pappone C, Rosanio S, Oreto G, et al. Circumferential radiofrequency ablation of pulmonary vein ostia: a new anatomic approach for curing atrial fibrillation. *Circulation.* 2000;102:2619-2628.
18. Piorkowski C, Hindricks G, Schreiber D, et al. Electroanatomic reconstruction of the left atrium, pulmonary veins, and esophagus compared with the "true anatomy" on multislice computed tomography in patients undergoing catheter ablation of atrial fibrillation. *Heart Rhythm.* 2006;3:317-327.
19. Pandozi C, Dottori S, Lavalle C, et al. Integration of MR images with electroanatomic maps: feasibility and utility in guiding left ventricular substrate mapping. *J Interv Card Electrophysiol.* 2010;29:157-166.
20. Schwartzmann D, Zhong H. On the use of CartoSound for left atrial navigation. *J Cardiovasc Electrophysiol.* 2010;12:656-664.
21. Singh S, Heist E, Donaldson D, et al. Image integration using intracardiac ultrasound to guide catheter ablation of atrial fibrillation. *Heart Rhythm.* 2008;5:1548-1555.
22. Gepstein L, Hayam G, Ben-Haim S. A novel method for nonfluoroscopic catheter-based electroanatomical mapping of the heart: in vivo and in vitro accuracy results. *Circulation.* 1997;95:1611-1622.

23. Sciarra L, Dottori S, De Ruvo E, et al. The new electroanatomical CARTO 3 mapping system: three-dimensional right ventricular fast anatomical map resolution in comparison to magnetic resonance image. *J Cardiovasc Med.* 2011;12:434-435.
24. Jilek C, Hessling G, Ammar S, et al. Visualization of multiple catheters in left atrial ablation procedures. *Herzschrittmacherther Elektrophysiol.* 2010;22:39-45.
25. Gonzalez-Torrecilla E, Arenal A, Quiles J, et al. Non-fluoroscopic electroanatomical mapping (CARTO system) in the ablation of atrial tachycardias. *Rev Esp Cardiol.* 2004;57:37-44.
26. Stevenson W, Delacretaz E, Friedman P, Ellison K. Identification and ablation of macroreentrant ventricular tachycardia with the CARTO electroanatomical mapping system. *Pacing Clin Electrophysiol.* 1998;21:1448-1456.
27. Nademanee K, McKenzie J, Kosar E, et al. A new approach for catheter ablation of atrial fibrillation: mapping of the electrophysiologic substrate. *J Am Coll Cardiol.* 2004;43:2044-2053.
28. Elayi CS, Verma A, Di Biase L, et al. Ablation for longstanding permanent atrial fibrillation: results from a randomized study comparing three different strategies. *Heart Rhythm.* 2008;5:1658-1664.
29. Aizer A, Holmes DS, Garlitski AC, et al. Standardization and validation of an automated algorithm to identify fractionation as a guide for atrial fibrillation ablation. *Heart Rhythm.* 2008;5:1134-1141.
30. Hunter RJ, Berriman TJ, Diab I, et al. Long-term efficacy of catheter ablation for atrial fibrillation: impact of additional targeting of fractionated electrograms. *Heart.* 2010;96:1372-1378.
31. Jones DG, McCready JW, Kaba RA, et al. A multi-purpose spiral high-density mapping catheter: initial clinical experience in complex atrial arrhythmias. *J Interv Card Electrophysiol.* 2011;31:225-235.
32. Nair M, Yaduvanshi A, Kataria V, Kumar M. Radiofrequency catheter ablation of ventricular tachycardia in arrhythmogenic right ventricular dysplasia/cardiomyopathy using non-contact electroanatomical mapping: single-center experience with follow-up up to median of 30 months. *J Interv Card Electrophysiol.* 2011;31:141-147.
33. Casella M, Pelargonio G, Dello Russo A, et al. "Near-zero" fluoroscopic exposure in supraventricular arrhythmia ablation using the EnSite NavX™ mapping system: personal experience and review of the literature. *J Interv Card Electrophysiol.* 2011;31:109-118.
34. Estner HL, Deisenhofer I, Luik A, et al. Electrical isolation of pulmonary veins in patients with atrial fibrillation: reduction of fluoroscopy exposure and procedure duration by the use of a non-fluoroscopic navigation system (NavX). *Europace.* 2006;8:583-587.
35. Lakkireddy D, Nadzam G, Verma A, et al. Impact of a comprehensive safety program on radiation exposure during catheter ablation of atrial fibrillation: a prospective study. *J Interv Card Electrophysiol.* 2009;24:105-112.
36. Rotter M, Takahashi Y, Sanders P, et al. Reduction of fluoroscopy exposure and procedure duration during ablation of atrial fibrillation using a novel anatomical navigation system. *Eur Heart J.* 2005;26:1415-1421.
37. Wagner LK, Eifel PJ, Geise RA. Potential biological effects following high x-ray dose interventional procedures. *J Vasc Interv Radiol.* 1994;5:71-84.
38. Faulkner K, Werduch A. An estimate of the collective dose to the European population from cardiac x-ray procedures. *Br J Radiol.* 2008;81:955-962.
39. Georges JL, Livarek B, Gibault-Genty G, et al. Reduction of radiation delivered to patients undergoing invasive coronary procedures. Effect of a programme for dose reduction based on radiation-protection training. *Arch Cardiovasc Dis.* 2009;102:821-827.

Video Legend

Video 4.1 Left anterior oblique projection of the right atrium with a barrel view down the tricuspid valve. Activation mapping reveals bidirectional block following cavotricupid isthmus ablation. The lesion set is depicted by three-dimensional red circles.

CHAPTER 5

Intraoperative Mapping for the Surgeon and Electrophysiologist

John M. Miller, MD; Daniel J. Beckman, MD; Yousuf Mahomed, MD

Introduction

Pharmacological agents were the first form of direct treatment for cardiac arrhythmias. These medications suppress arrhythmias or their symptoms but do not alter the underlying pathophysiology. In addition, they must be taken on a consistent basis to maintain arrhythmia control. Their use is further limited by the development of side effects as well as eventual loss of efficacy in many cases. Because of these shortcomings, starting in the 1960s, surgical therapies were sought that could confer a more lasting freedom from arrhythmia recurrence.

Fundamental tenets of surgical therapy efforts were that (1) the arrhythmia had a defined source, (2) the source could be located, and (3) the source could be safely and effectively eliminated using a surgical approach. In addition, some surgical procedures require working in the vicinity of the normal conduction system, damage to which should be avoided. The process of locating the arrhythmia source as well as the normal conduction system is known as mapping. This chapter will discuss various forms of mapping and the surgical procedures that follow from them.

Mapping

Intraoperative mapping of a variety of arrhythmias enjoyed substantial popularity in the 1980s. With the advent of the implantable cardioverter-defibrillator (ICD) and improved tools and techniques for catheter ablation of arrhythmias, the role of surgical therapy, along with its associated intraoperative mapping, has declined to a remnant of what it had been. Nonetheless, the principles of modern arrhythmia mapping remain relevant, as they were developed in the surgical environment, which afforded direct visual inspection of sites from which electrical information was being sampled and allowed for unsurpassed correlation between anatomy and pathophysiology.

Locating the tissue responsible for an arrhythmia requires an understanding of the nature of the rhythm disturbance, for which two broad categories exist: focal and macroreentrant. In *focal arrhythmias,* a cell or small group of cells fires autonomously. This focus can be identified when it is firing by sampling electrical recordings from various sites in the cardiac chambers and comparing the timing of these signals to a reference recording. The focus is that site from which the earliest electrical activation is recorded, surrounded by later recordings.

In *macroreentrant arrhythmias,* the cardiac electrical impulse propagates through a circuit, usually of several centimeters' size, that may be located in atrial or ventricular tissue. The circuit usually exists in the presence of prior damage that has replaced portions of myocardium with nonconductive scar tissue, leaving surviving strands of myocardium to form a potential circuit. Other circuits are mediated by an atrioventricular (AV) bypass tract (BT) and involve both atrium and ventricle. In these circuits, the impulse propagates through the normal AV conduction system, through the ventricles, and returns to the atria over the bypass tract that traverses the mitral or tricuspid annulus. In macroreentrant arrhythmias, mapping seeks the narrowest (thus, most vulnerable) portion of the circuit. In patients with AV BTs, this narrowest part is the pathway itself at the valve annulus.

Mapping Process

In order to locate the tissue responsible for arrhythmias, several conditions must be present:

- The heart has to be warm and electrically active (ie, not cooled or arrested with cardioplegia);
- The tissue being sought must be working (ie, the arrhythmia must be either present at the time of the mapping procedure or inducible); and
- The operator must be able to pace and record from the heart with good quality signals.

The fundamental features of most mapping studies are as follows. First, the heart is exposed after performing a median sternotomy, and cannulated for cardiopulmonary bypass if this is planned. Second, electrodes are attached to the heart for pacing as well as timing references and connected to a stimulator and amplifier/recording apparatus. From this point, there is substantial diversity of how the procedure unfolds. In all cases, however, there must be good coordination and communication between the surgeon acquiring the data and the electrophysiologist analyzing the recordings and interpreting their meaning in the context of the arrhythmia.

Different institutions have developed mapping coordinate schemes to facilitate communication and serve as a common framework for determining where the mapping electrode is at any particular time (Figure 5.1). In this context, if the electrophysiologist asks the surgeon to move the mapping electrode to a certain coordinate on their agreed-upon mapping grid, each knows what the other means.

Preparation for Intraoperative Mapping

Before taking a patient to the operating room for mapping and ablation of arrhythmias, all mapping equipment must be in good working order and additional mapping electrodes and connectors readily available in case the sterility of one is accidentally compromised. In addition, as much information as possible should be obtained for planning the procedure. This includes data on the substrate (normal heart, scar due to infarction or cardiomyopathy, prior surgery, etc) as well as mapping information derived from preoperative electrophysiologic testing. This information is valuable in two regards. Because of the time constraints of intraoperative mapping (see discussion of scar-related ventricular tachycardia, below), having ample information on the origin of the arrhythmia focus or reentrant zone helps save time as well as avoid mapping irrelevant areas.

Before effective catheter ablation techniques became available, all types of arrhythmias (eg, AV BTs, atrial tachycardias [ATs], and ventricular tachycardia [VT]) were extensively mapped preoperatively to direct the surgical team's attention to specific regions of interest during the operation. Since catheter ablation has been used and its techniques refined, it is unusual to surgically treat arrhythmias due to catheter technique failure. Indeed, if catheter ablation has failed, one could question the accuracy of the mapping information, which would then be of limited benefit during surgery. An additional benefit of mapping arrhythmias preoperatively is that, in some cases, the arrhythmia may not be inducible during surgery. If so, the surgical team may have to rely on results of preoperative mapping or ECGs of atrial or ventricular tachycardias to infer their likely origins.

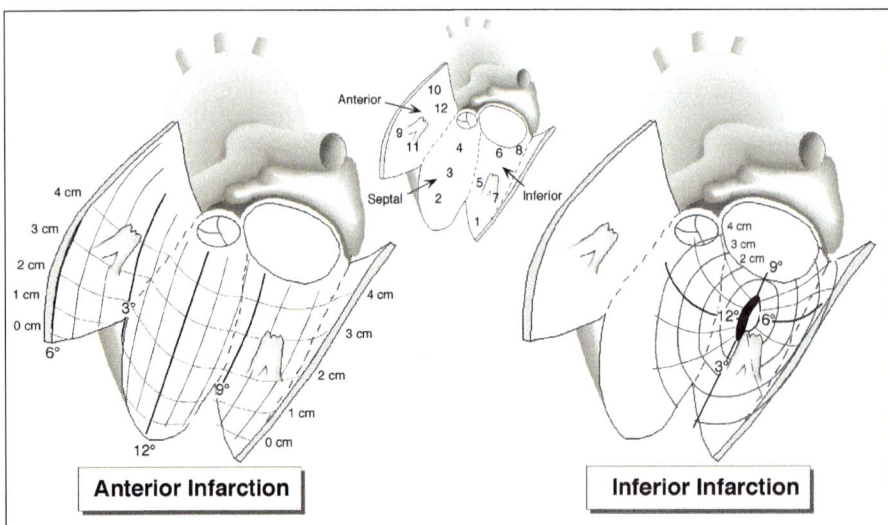

Figure 5.1 Coordinate system used during intraoperative mapping of the left ventricular (LV) endocardium. Figures show a stylized LV opened along the lateral margin, with anterior and inferior walls slightly everted. LV access was obtained by incising the infarct or aneurysm, and then mapping was begun using these grids. A clockface was used for orientation at the ventricular opening, and electrograms were sampled along this edge as well as at 1 cm concentric radii in the chamber. Using this system, the surgeon (acquiring data) and electrophysiologist (analyzing the signals) can determine where the electrode is at all times and return to areas of interest. The figure at top is for orientation and shows sites used in catheter mapping of the LV.

Atrioventricular Bypass Tracts: Wolff–Parkinson–White and Variants

The broadest initial application of successful arrhythmia surgery was for interrupting accessory AV connections or BTs responsible for rapid supraventricular tachycardias. In the early experience with AV BTs, a bipolar recording electrode was used to explore the epicardial surface of the AV rings (mitral and tricuspid); the electrode was seeking the site of earliest ventricular activation (in the case of manifest preexcitation) or earliest atrial activation during ventricular pacing (in concealed BTs). In these procedures, the heart would be exposed and a pericardial cradle created to suspend it, such that minimal manipulation of the heart would be necessary to access all relevant mapping regions, especially the posterior portion of the AV groove. Separate electrodes were affixed to atrium and ventricle for pacing and as a timing reference. When mapping during ventricular pacing, rapid rates were often necessary to minimize the degree to which atrial activation could occur over the normal AV conduction system and confuse the mapping data.

Originally, mapping consisted of moving an electrode, either in the form of a ring on the surgeon's index finger with exposed bipolar electrodes or a tube of glass with embedded electrodes exposed at one end (Figure 5.2).

The so-called roving or probe electrode was moved from site to site (≤ 1 cm at a time) along the atrial or ventricular side of the AV groove, while the electrophysiologist monitored the relative timing of activations acquired at each site. Usually, the recordings were printed on a physiological recorder, and measurements of "early" versus "late" were made by handheld calipers. Subsequently, a diagram could be constructed showing earliest activation times in anterograde or retrograde directions (Figure 5.3), but this was not available in the operating room at the time of the procedure.

In later years, a multipolar electrode array consisting of a strip in which electrodes were embedded was positioned along the epicardial aspect of the AV rings. This array afforded a comprehensive view of all the atrial or ventricular activation along this region (Figure 5.4). It could readily identify earliest atrial (during retrograde conduction) or ventricular (with anterograde conduction) breakthrough, allowing the surgeon to perform a limited epicardial dissection while the heart was warm and beating.

Rarely, the strip electrode could diagnose a second BT, indicated by a primary and secondary breakthrough during retrograde activation during tachycardia (Figure 5.5). Using this technique, successful division of the BT was readily apparent (eg, in loss of delta wave, loss of or change in pattern of retrograde conduction during ventricular pacing). So-called sock electrodes (a distensible mesh with electrodes embedded at roughly evenly spaced intervals), coupled to a computer for analysis and display, were also available for mapping. However, since the most important area in this disorder was the AV grooves, much of the information the electrodes on the sock acquired was irrelevant. (The surgical techniques for division of AV BTs are discussed in later chapters of this book.)

Following presumed BT obliteration, pacing is repeated to ensure that no residual conduction remains over any BT; on occasion, a second pathway will become evident only after eliminating the first. If BT conduction remains after attempted surgical division, the process of mapping and ablation are repeated until no evidence of BT conduction remains.

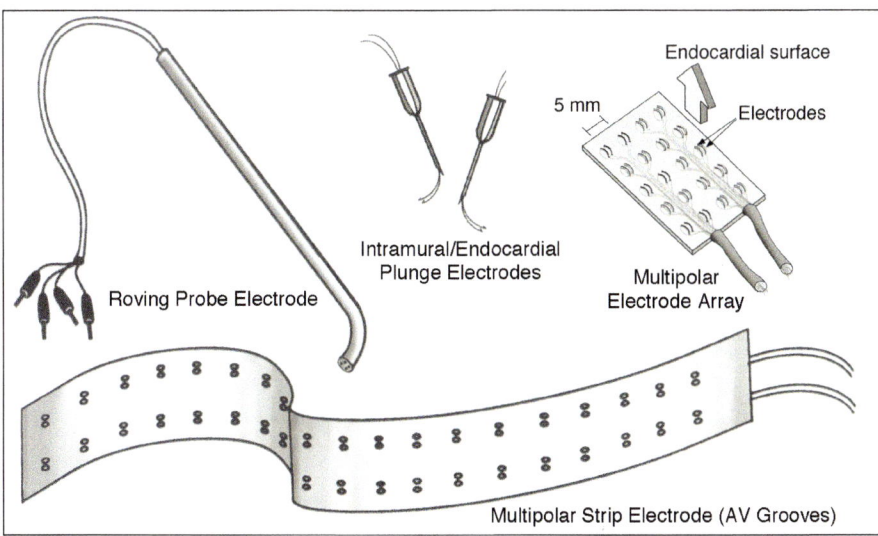

Figure 5.2 Mapping tools. Shown are the roving probe electrode (quadripolar in this illustration), needle-delivered bipolar plunge electrodes for timing reference and stimulation, a multipolar electrode array for acquiring additional detail from an endocardial site, and a multipolar strip electrode laid along the atrioventricular (AV) groove to map AV bypass tract insertions.

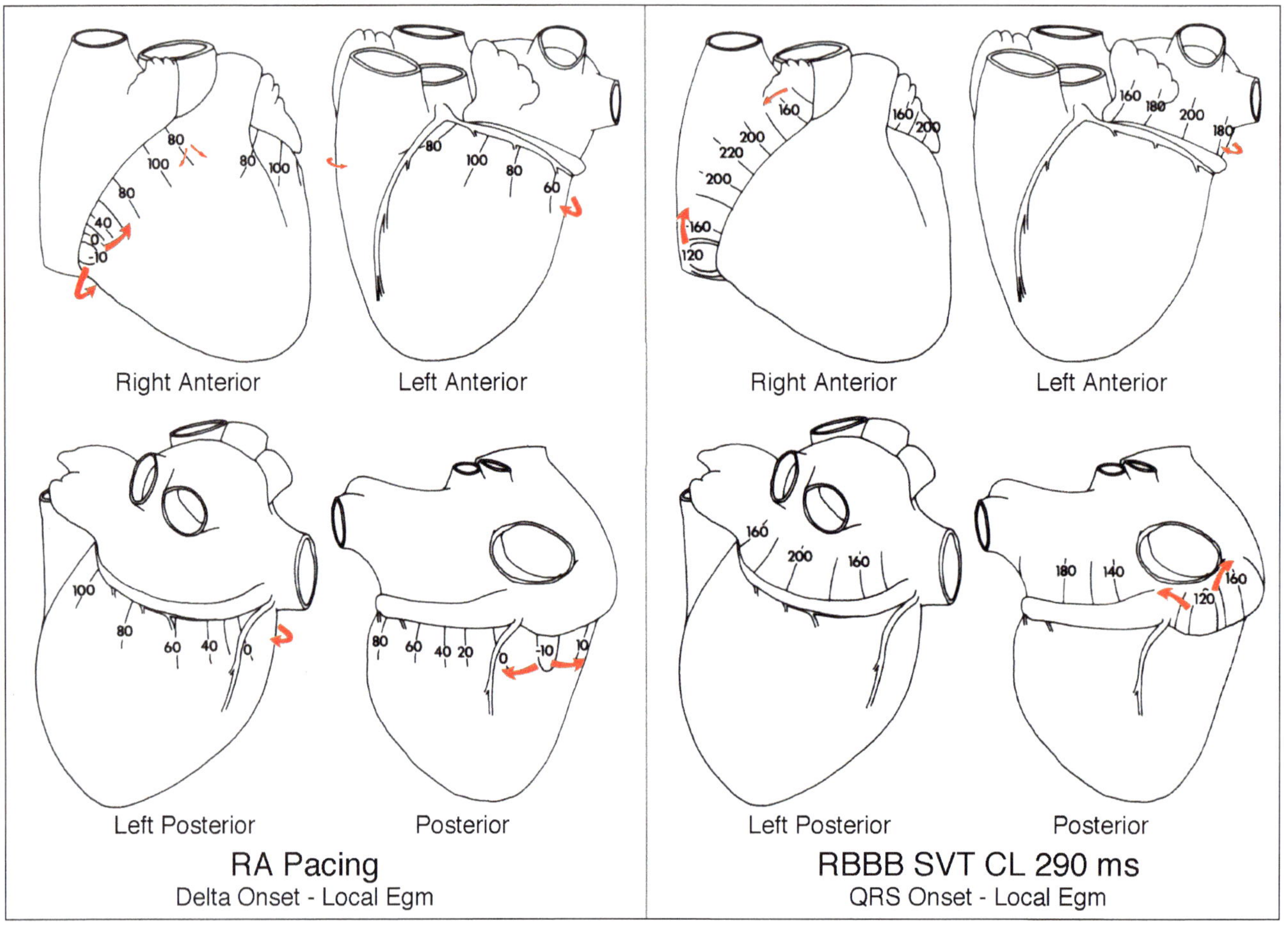

Figure 5.3 Isochronal intraoperative activation maps of anterograde ventricular activation during atrial pacing (**left set**) and retrograde atrial activation during right bundle branch block (RBBB) supraventricular tachycardia (SVT) (**right set**) in several attitudes of the heart in a patient with an atrioventricular bypass tract. **Numbers** indicate ms after the reference (surface ECG QRS onset). **Red arrows** show propagation from site of earliest activations in each instance, indicating bypass tract insertion site. Egm = electrogram.

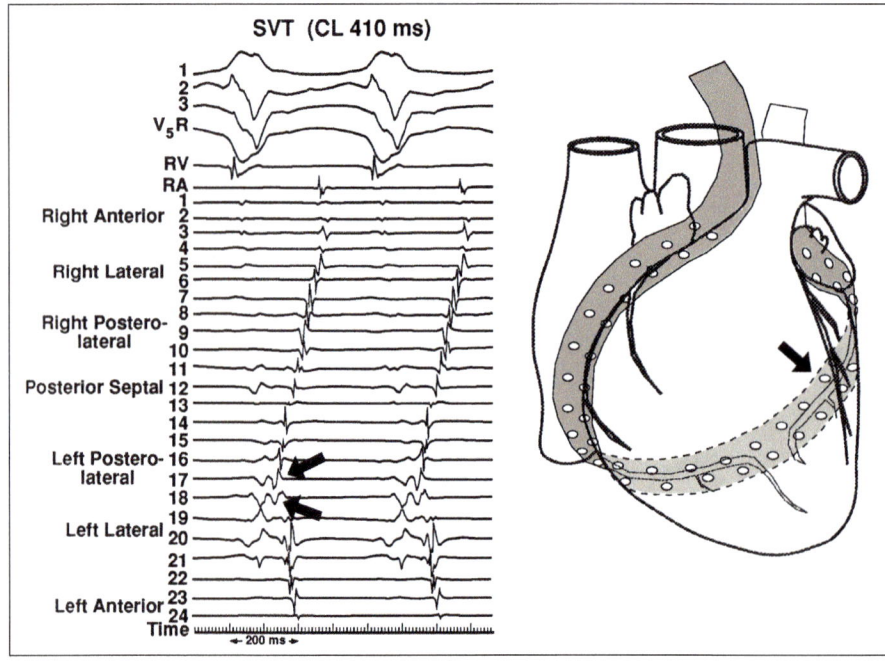

Figure 5.4 Use of a multipolar strip electrode for rapid intraoperative mapping of the atrioventricular (AV) groove in a patient with a concealed bypass tract. Mapping is performed during supraventricular tachycardia (SVT) with the strip straddling the AV groove. Earliest atrial activation, corresponding to the atrial insertion site of the bypass tract, is readily observed (**arrows on left** correspond to a particular location on the strip; **single arrow** on diagram **at right**).

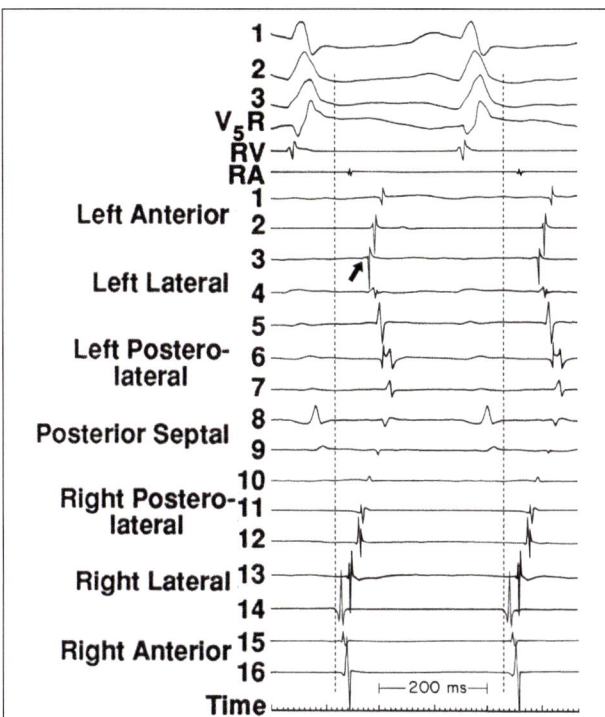

Figure 5.5 Multipolar strip electrode showing two retrogradely conducting bypass tracts (BTs). Two complexes during supraventricular tachycardia (SVT) are shown with the strip electrode around the atrial aspect of the atrioventricular groove, as in Figure 5.4 (oriented in opposite direction). **Dashed line** denotes earliest atrial activation (lateral right atrial BT); however, instead of an orderly progression of later activations from that point, a second breakthrough is noted in the lateral left atrium (**arrow**).

Ventricular Tachycardia

Scar-related Ventricular Tachycardia

Almost all surgical mapping procedures for VT have been performed in patients with prior myocardial infarction (MI) with resultant scar. Much less commonly, patients with idiopathic cardiomyopathy or arrhythmogenic right ventricular dysplasia underwent surgical mapping and ablation. The first known successful arrhythmia surgery consisted of eliminating VT after removing a left ventricular aneurysm.[1] However, this did not translate into widespread application of surgery to treat VT owing to morbidity, mortality, and poor overall results of the procedure. The procedure's limited efficacy resulted from the fact that the arrhythmia substrate is usually located at the border of scar and more normal myocardium—a region not addressed by simple aneurysmectomy.

Intraoperative mapping was introduced to delineate areas responsible for VT. Initially, epicardial mapping was performed during induced VT, but such mapping rarely revealed sites that were activated before the onset of the QRS complex, and it soon became clear that, in most cases, the responsible pathophysiology was instead on the endocardial surface. Consequently, many centers began directly with endocardial mapping.

In endocardial mapping, the heart is exposed after sternotomy, suspended in a pericardial cradle, and cannulated for cardiopulmonary bypass. Once normothermic bypass is initiated and the heart decompressed, an aneurysm or infarct is readily apparent as a "sucked-in" region (generally, its location is known prior to surgery). It is important to maintain bypass at normal or even slightly warmer body temperature because heat loss from the air-exposed endocardial surface may inhibit the induction of sustained VT. The aneurysm or infarct is opened in a line using blade or scissors, exposing the endocardial surface (Figure 5.6), which is inspected and any loose thrombus removed with forceps. The electrophysiologist then induces VT using programmed stimulation through the previously placed reference electrodes and begins the mapping process. This can either be done in a set, standardized sequence of data acquisition from all points on the coordinate scheme, or targeted if time is short and/or episodes of VT are nonsustained. Because most patients have more than one morphology of VT (generally, but not always, related to the same 5–8 cm^2 region), mapping time may have to be curtailed somewhat to fit into the roughly 45 to 60 minutes allowed for this purpose.[2] The electrophysiologist may ask the surgeon to revisit several sites of interest that were previously mapped or to apply a multipolar electrode array for higher-density data acquisition. The electrophysiologist may request that the surgeon press with the mapping probe at a certain site that, if critical to maintaining the VT, will cause the arrhythmia to slow down or cease (Figure 5.7).

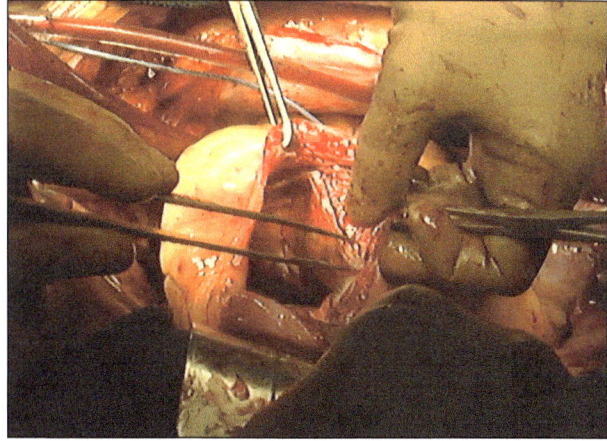

Figure 5.6 Opening an anterior left ventricular aneurysm at surgery prior to endocardial mapping. The apex is tipped slightly toward the viewer and the large opening in the aneurysm allows for visual inspection and manipulation of mapping electrodes on the endocardial surface.

Another endocardial mapping technique consists of introducing a deflated electrode-studded balloon into the closed ventricle through the mitral valve and then inflating the balloon to achieve endocardial electrode contact. VT initiation and mapping can then be performed.

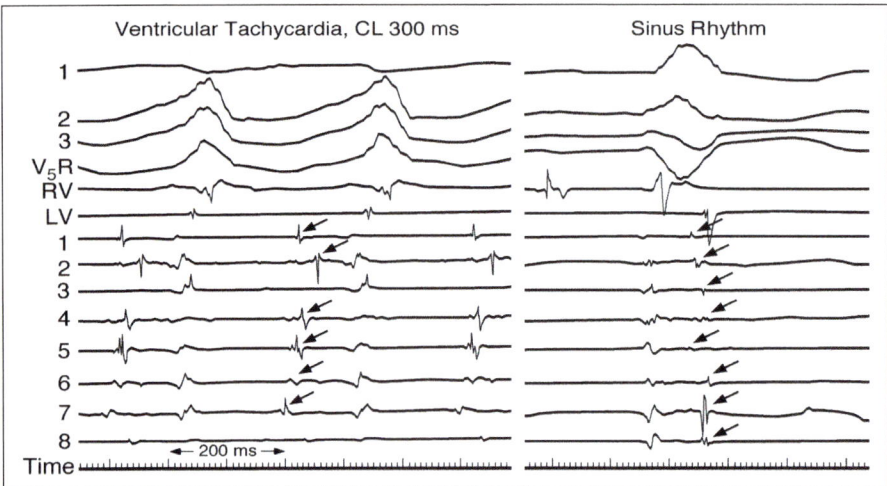

Figure 5.7 Surface ECG and intracardiac recordings using a multipolar electrode array (see Figure 5.2) during ventricular tachycardia (VT) and sinus rhythm at same location. Selected electrodes from the array are shown during VT. **Arrows** denote mid-diastolic potentials during VT that correspond to discrete split potentials during sinus rhythm. V5R = right-sided V5; RV = right ventricular plunge electrode; LV = left ventricular plunge electrode.

After endocardial mapping using one or more of these techniques is complete, a variety of surgical techniques may be applied to remove or ablate the mapping-designated arrhythmogenic regions. These include endocardial resection (to "peel" or remove the superficial 2–3 mm of endocardium in the region), encircling ventriculotomy or cryoablation (to isolate the arrhythmogenic region from the rest of the heart), and laser photoablation or cryoablation (Figure 5.8) to directly ablate the arrhythmogenic tissue without removing it. These techniques are discussed more fully in later chapters of this book. In many cases, surgical ablation is performed during normothermic bypass and, after it is finished, stimulation can be repeated. If VT can still be induced, further mapping and ablation are carried out until no further VT can be initiated.[3]

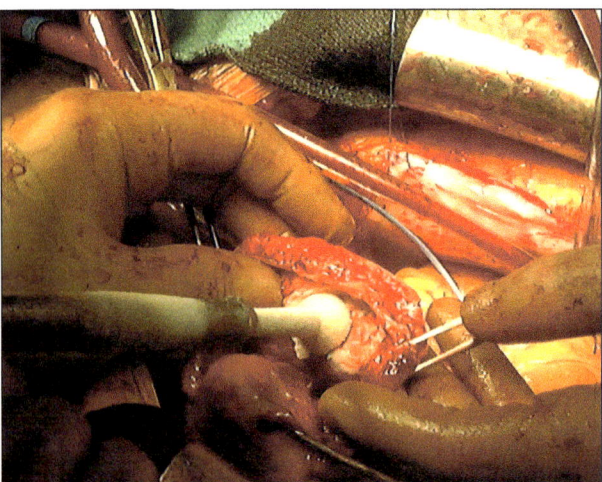

Figure 5.8 Cryoablation during intraoperative mapping. The cryoprobe tip (round white structure near center) is freezing a portion of the anterior wall after the mapping indicated a site of interest during ventricular tachycardia.

Increasingly frequently, epicardial mapping and ablation are performed in the catheterization laboratory using subxiphoid pericardial access. Most such cases are patients with various forms of cardiomyopathy, such as dilated idiopathic, arrhythmogenic ventricular dysplasia, and sarcoidosis. However, occasionally patients with postinfarct VT must be approached in this way because of either the inability to map and ablate from an endocardial approach or the presence of ventricular thrombus that could be dislodged during endocardial mapping. Although in most cases the electrophysiologist can obtain pericardial access quickly and safely, this may not be feasible in some patients, especially those with prior heart surgery in whom the pericardium may closely adhere to the epicardial surface. Adherence makes pericardial access impossible, and even if it can be obtained, the ability to manipulate the catheter in the scarred pericardial space makes extensive mapping futile. In these cases, a surgeon can obtain very good access to the pericardial space using a 3- to 5-cm subxiphoid incision through which the pericardium can be exposed and freed from the epicardial surface with blunt dissection. A mapping catheter can then be introduced into the pericardial space, and epicardial mapping can proceed. Surgical pericardioscopy can further aid catheter maneuvering if needed.

Focal Ventricular Tachycardia

Very few patients with focal VT (which generally occurs in the absence of structural heart disease) have undergone intraoperative mapping and ablation. Even so, some of the early reports of successful VT therapy described this group of patients.[4] Currently, surgical mapping and ablation for idiopathic focal VT are usually performed either following failure of catheter ablation or in patients with epicardial VT in whom the focus is too close to a proximal coronary artery to safely ablate. Preferably, epicardial mapping is performed in the operating room, since it is inadvisable to make an incision in normal ventricular muscle (doing so could result in mechanical dysfunction or serve as a barrier for subsequent reentrant VT). For epicardial mapping, the target site is identified during VT as having the earliest site of activation, preceding QRS onset by 20 to 50 ms. The electrogram at that site is often normal, but in tissue in which prior ablation has caused some damage, an abnormal, fragmented signal may be present (Figure 5.9).

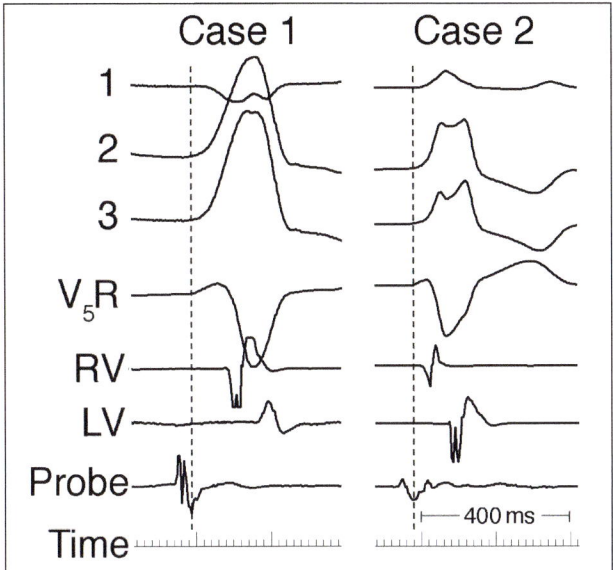

Figure 5.9 Intraoperative mapping of idiopathic focal ventricular tachycardia (VT). Single VT complexes from two different patients are shown, with respective earliest sites of activation. Case 1 had not undergone prior catheter ablation and has a normal electrogram at the "probe" site. In Case 2, prior catheter ablation had been performed; however, it was only partially successful and left a low-amplitude, fragmented electrogram at the site of earliest activation. **Dashed lines** denote QRS onset.

Cryothermy is the preferred method for ablating the focus (–70°C for 1–6 minutes, usually with multiple, closely spaced applications). This technique has the advantage of destroying the tissue without disrupting the collagenous interstitium; it leaves a homogenous, well-demarcated lesion that becomes homogeneous scar. In some focal VT cases, general anesthesia renders the focus inactive despite giving large doses of catecholamines. In our own experience, catecholamine infusion often accelerated the sinus node firing rate and, although ventricular ectopy was occasionally observed, it was overdriven by the fast sinus rates. In one case, ice was applied to the sinus node to decrease its rate, allowing the VT focus to emerge. In other cases, successful presumptive cryoablation has been performed at various sites. The cryoablation was directed by visual correlation of fluoroscopic locations obtained at the time of catheter mapping and unsuccessful ablation attempts (ie, 5 mm distal to the bifurcation of the left main coronary artery). Use of cryomapping (applying a cryoprobe cooled only to 0°C) is helpful for confirming the correct target site for ablation during an ongoing arrhythmia. This is true especially if important structures are nearby, where damage should be avoided (eg, a normal conduction system in the case of septal BTs or VTs, or VTs on the epicardial surface near a coronary artery).

Atrial Tachycardias

The principles underlying mapping focal ATs are the same as those for focal VT, and the constraints are likewise similar (eg, anesthetic agents render the AT focus quiescent). The setup for mapping focal ATs is similar to that for patients with AV BTs, except that electrodes are placed on each atrium. AT is then initiated with burst pacing or catecholamine infusion, and the atrial surface is mapped according to a predetermined grid system. The site of origin of the tachycardia is one that precedes all others and the surface P-wave onset by at least 20 ms. In many cases, the site is on the endocardial surface and epicardial mapping may not identify a pre-P-wave site. If so, the earliest site may be frozen from the epicardial surface or a small atriotomy made to further investigate its origin. Rarely, ATs arise from the atrial septum or coronary sinus musculature—areas not readily accessible to epicardial mapping. Indicators of septal origin are a very narrow P wave during AT (both atria being activated almost simultaneously) and, on epicardial mapping, several sites on the medial left and right atrium having equivalent activation times that are not pre–P wave. Ideally, preoperative catheter mapping in the electrophysiology laboratory clarifies the regionalization of tachycardia origin.

Macroreentrant Atrial Tachycardias

Less information is available on intraoperative mapping of ATs related to large circuits; these, like scar-related VT, are almost always the result of prior atrial injury. Unlike scar-related VT, however, the injury was usually incurred during repair of congenital heart disease in which one or more long atrial incisions were made. Prior procedures include atrial septal defect repair, Mustard or Senning repair of transposition of the great arteries, repair of tetralogy of Fallot through an atriotomy, and Fontan corrections of a variety of defects, to name a few. The authors have no direct experience in these cases, and there is almost no literature that reviews this area. Currently, surgical treatment is almost exclusively used on Fontan atria, and the greatly enlarged right atrium is decompressed by forming a lateral caval tunnel. During these extensive procedures, little or no mapping is performed; instead, a series of linear lesions are made, generally with radiofrequency current, in the form of a right atrial maze.

Atrial Fibrillation

One of the most complex of all arrhythmias, atrial fibrillation (AF) has posed the greatest challenges to surgical mapping and ablation. Several teams of researchers have used various arrays of electrodes to acquire activation data from one or both atria during induced AF, usually in patients undergoing surgery for Wolff–Parkinson–White syndrome.[5] In general, these studies have shown that AF is characterized by very complex activation patterns, with moving lines of block and changing patterns of activation. Multiple wavelets of reentry have been observed, as well as more organized patterns of activation, usually in the right (as opposed to the left) atrium.[6] These techniques have rarely been used to guide surgical therapy for AF. However, occasional cases have been reported during which mapping rapid discharges (resulting in fibrillatory patterns of activation) has successfully targeted areas of the heart for ablation.[7]

In recent years, it has become clear that paroxysmal AF usually originates in the pulmonary veins (PVs) or around their ostia, which are also important (though apparently less so) in the genesis of persistent AF. Thus, most catheter-based and surgical procedures now focus on electrical isolation of the PVs. With the recent widespread adoption of anatomically based surgical treatment of AF, mapping has had a very limited role to play (eg, in open-chest procedures, such as the traditional cut-and-sew maze procedure; a similar lesion set using radiofrequency, cryoablation, laser, or microwave energy; or closed-chest procedures using similar ablation energy sources). However, some surgeons have begun to use modified mapping to assess the results of ablation (eg, for confirming PV isolation). In this setting, pacing of a PV is performed using a handheld electrode. Then, to assess whether the PV has been isolated, either visual inspection for atrial contraction or recording from a separate electrode in the body of the left atrium is done (Figure 5.10).[8]

It has been known for many years that neural influences mediate some episodes of AF, especially those arising from the parasympathetic system. So-called vagally mediated AF could potentially be treated by identifying and destroying ganglionated plexi (GPs) of the parasympathetic system. GPs are present in several relatively consistent locations on the posterior aspect of the atria, medial to the ostium of each major PV. Based on this concept, the posterior left atrium is exposed (usually during mini-thoracotomy or thoracoscopy) and presumptive areas of parasympathetic ganglia are stimulated (for 1–20 sec, 5–100 V, at 20 Hz). Sites at which stimulation causes a ≥ 50% heart rate decrease (during sinus rhythm or AF) are thus identified as the location of a GP, which can then be ablated with radiofrequency or cryoenergy. Cycles of stimulation and further ablation are repeated in the region until the heart-rate depression is no longer observed. Combining this technique with standard PV antral isolation has yielded encouraging results in several small series of patients: 82% and 56% successful elimination of AF in patients with paroxysmal and persistent AF, respectively.[9] Ample evidence from other settings (eg, orthotopic heart transplantation) shows that reinnervation can occur, and thus, the permanency of these results remains to be seen.

Identifying the Normal Atrioventricular Conduction System

Equally important for locating tissue responsible for the arrhythmia(s) is identifying areas that should not be damaged, such as sinoatrial and AV nodes and the His bundle. Avoiding damage to the more distal portions of the conduction system (bundle branches and beyond) is less critical because there is more redundancy in the conduction system at these levels. Although less common nowadays, over 50 years ago, delineation of the normal conduction system was one of the original applications of intraoperative mapping.[10]

Parts of the normal conduction system and procedures that pose potential risks to these structures include the following:

1. *Sinus node.* Cardiac transplantation using atrial–atrial anastomotic techniques can damage the sinus node or its arterial supply. The bicaval technique (in which caval anastomoses are created instead of direct donor–recipient atrial apposition) largely avoids this. The sinus node is not generally mapped because it is a relatively large, diffuse structure with standard location (posterolateral right atrium, near the junction of the superior vena cava and trabeculated right atrium). Surgical repair of congenital heart disease incorporating an atriotomy can likewise damage the sinus node.

2. *AV node.* Surgical division of posterior septal and midseptal AV BTs endangers the AV node, as does repair of congenital heart defects such as ostium primum atrial septal defect (AV canal), tricuspid valve repair and replacement, and mitral valve repair or replacement. Discrete potentials from the AV node itself cannot be recorded using available

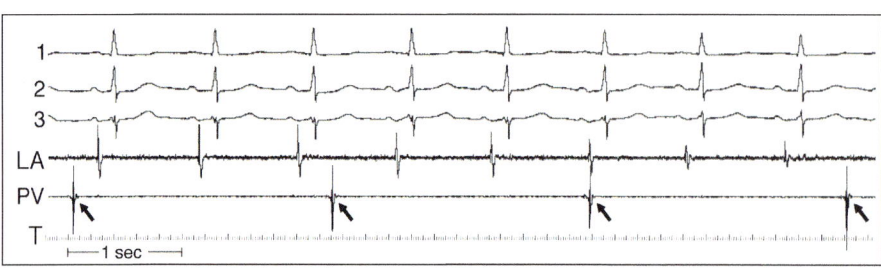

Figure 5.10 Pulmonary vein isolation. Three surface ECG leads are shown along with recordings from electrodes on the left atrium (LA) and a pulmonary vein (PV) after surgical PV isolation. **Arrows** indicate PV potentials that are slowly firing independent of sinus rhythm in the rest of the atrial mass, indicating successful entrance block into and exit block out of the PV.

technology; however, the AV node's location is relatively standard, at the apex of the triangle of Koch (formed by the tendon of Todaro, septal tricuspid annulus, and coronary sinus ostium). The location of the His bundle can be identified by its discrete deflection, derived from a narrow (1–3 mm) bipolar electrode probe. Prior to the development of catheter-based techniques that eliminate slow pathway conduction, this region had been mapped during surgical cryoablation of portions of the AV node for treating AV nodal reentrant SVT.[11]

3. *His bundle and proximal bundle branches.* The His bundle can be injured during surgical division of superoparaseptal ("anterior septal") and para-Hisian AV BTs. It is also at risk from repairs to membranous ventricular septal defects (VSDs) and aortic valve surgery (since the His bundle courses on the rightward side of the noncoronary and right coronary cusps). Among these procedures, mapping is performed prior to division of AV pathways (to locate the pathway to destroy as well as the His bundle to avoid) and occasionally during VSD closure.[12] The His bundle usually courses over the posterior aspect of a VSD. However, when the VSD occurs in the setting of L-transposition (ventricular inversion or so-called congenitally corrected transposition), the His and proximal bundle branches typically course on the anterior aspect of the VSD, and therefore mapping may be useful to delineate its course in order to avoid injury with sutures.[13] In endocardial cushion defects, the normal conduction system may be displaced posteriorly, toward the coronary sinus ostium.

Limitations of Intraoperative Mapping

Although most intraoperative mapping procedures are carried out without complications, the orderly sequence of events can be disrupted in many ways.

1. *No target.* Absence of the target arrhythmia during surgery is the most common and unsettling impediment to a smooth procedure. Fortunately, this rarely happens in cases of AV BTs.
   a. *Normal heart/focal arrhythmias.* Noninducibility is not at all unusual in patients who do not have structural heart disease and a focal mechanism of either AT or VT. This can often (but not always) be circumvented by infusing isoproterenol or epinephrine. If the heart becomes too cool, owing to heat loss from air exposure or too-cool cardiopulmonary bypass perfusate, it may be unable to support a sustained arrhythmia regardless of mechanism (focal or macroreentry). Warming the patient usually suffices in this instance.
   b. *Noninducibility of VT.* In some patients with postinfarct VT, opening the aneurysm and/or removing adherent-organized endocardial thrombus may render VT noninducible. If no previous attempt to initiate VT has been made, it raises the question of whether endocardial cooling or other factors may be responsible. However, if VT had been easily induced earlier in the procedure, or VT terminated abruptly during ventriculotomy or thrombus removal, it is likely that the circuit was critically damaged and that no further mapping may be possible (or necessary) for that morphology of VT.

2. *Polymorphic VT.* In some cases, only polymorphic VT can be initiated in patients who always had monomorphic VT previously. In this situation, rapidly infusing 1 gm procainamide may slow conduction enough during the arrhythmia to "organize" it into a monomorphic VT. Polymorphic VT may also indicate significant ongoing ischemia despite the heart being mechanically unloaded; for instance, tipping the apex upward may "kink" the left main or left anterior descending coronary artery. In such cases, one must use good judgment to decide how important it is to acquire detailed mapping data versus proceeding with coronary bypass.

3. *Equipment failure.* Time is a significant constraint during intraoperative mapping procedures. The surgeon and electrophysiologist must be able to work quickly together in a coordinated fashion to achieve optimal results within the time frame allotted. Problems such as random equipment failure or poor function (eg, an electrode not recording properly, poor contact with the stimulating electrode, empty cryotanks) must be identified and remedied as quickly as possible. Planning for such contingencies, having backup equipment, and testing equipment before attempting to initiate the arrhythmia are always helpful.

Conclusion

Although intraoperative mapping techniques are rarely used because of advances in catheter mapping and ablation of arrhythmias, they provided the foundation for understanding arrhythmia mechanisms and correlating anatomy with physiology. Understanding the pathophysiology of postinfarction VT, for instance, led to the development of catheter-based strategies for ablation of this arrhythmia that are in wide use today. Despite being limited to a minor role in AF surgery and in patients with failed catheter ablation for other arrhythmias, intraoperative mapping has had an important role in the daily practice of electrophysiology. As the importance of demonstrating exit block from PVs is more widely appreciated, it is likely that intraoperative mapping will make a comeback for the treatment of arrhythmias. Continued collaboration between the electrophysiologist and the electrophysiological surgeon will likely lead to enhanced results in the coming years.

References

1. Couch OA Jr. Cardiac aneurysm with ventricular tachycardia and subsequent excision of aneurysm; case report. *Circulation*. 1959;20(2):251-253.
2. Miller JM, Kienzle MG, Harken AH, Josephson ME. Morphologically distinct sustained ventricular tachycardias in coronary artery disease: significance and surgical results. *J Am Coll Cardiol*. 1984;4(6):1073-1079.
3. Kron IL, Lerman BB, Nolan SP, et al. Sequential endocardial resection for the surgical treatment of refractory ventricular tachycardia. *J Thorac Cardiovasc Surg*. 1987;94(6):843-847.
4. Gallagher JJ, Anderson RW, Kasell J, et al. Cryoablation of drug-resistant ventricular tachycardia in a patient with a variant of scleroderma. *Circulation*. 1978;57(1):190-197.
5. Cox JL, Canavan TE, Schuessler RB, et al. The surgical treatment of atrial fibrillation. II. Intraoperative electrophysiologic mapping and description of the electrophysiologic basis of atrial flutter and atrial fibrillation. *J Thorac Cardiovasc Surg*. 1991;101(3):406-426.
6. Konings KT, Kirchhof CJ, Smeets JR, et al. High-density mapping of electrically induced atrial fibrillation in humans. *Circulation*. 1994;89(4):1665-1680.
7. Harada A, Sugimoto T, Asano T, Yamada K. Intraoperative map-guided operation for chronic atrial fibrillation. *Ann Thorac Surg*. 1998;66(4):1401-1403.
8. Ishii Y, Nitta T, Kambe M, et al. Intraoperative verification of conduction block in atrial fibrillation surgery. *J Thorac Cardiovasc Surg*. 2008;136(4):998-1004.
9. Edgerton JR, Jackman WM, Mack MJ. Minimally invasive pulmonary vein isolation and partial autonomic denervation for surgical treatment of atrial fibrillation. *J Interv Card Electrophysiol*. 2007;20(3):89-93.
10. Stuckey JH, Hoffman BF, Amer NS, et al. Localization of the bundle of His with a surface electrode during cardiotomy. *Surg Forum*. 1960;10:551-554.
11. Cox JL, Ferguson TB Jr, Lindsay BD, Cain ME. Perinodal cryosurgery for atrioventricular node reentry tachycardia in 23 patients. *J Thorac Cardiovasc Surg*. 1990;99(3):440-449; discussion 449-450.
12. Krongrad E, Malm JR, Bowman FO Jr, et al. Electrophysiological delineation of the specialized atrioventricular conduction system in patients with congenital heart disease. I. Delineation of the His bundle proximal to the membranous septum. *J Thorac Cardiovasc Surg*. 1974;67(6):875-882.
13. Waldo AL, Pacifico AD, Bargeron LM, et al. Electrophysiological delineation of the specialized A-V conduction system in patients with corrected transposition of the great vessels and ventricular septal defect. *Circulation*. 1975;52(3):435-441.

CHAPTER 6

Special Considerations for Pediatric Electrophysiological Procedures

George F. Van Hare, MD

Introduction

The saying "children are not just small adults," while certainly a cliché, is nonetheless true. However, many aspects of pediatric electrophysiology (EP) practice are identical, or nearly so, to adult EP practice. Most of the common arrhythmia mechanisms are the same, with small differences between the adult and pediatric scenarios. Therefore, both the pediatric cardiologist who trains in an adult program and the adult electrophysiologist called to assist with pediatric cases start with a great deal of fundamental knowledge that will be essential in the enterprise.

This chapter will attempt to address the areas where pediatric and adult practice diverge, and will offer specific recommendations on how to proceed safely and effectively with pediatric EP procedures. The special considerations that will be addressed comprise development, procedure setting, sedation/anesthesia, differences in diagnoses encountered, and indications for ablation that relate to natural history, equipment, and biophysical characteristics of ablation.

Developmental and Psychosocial Considerations

One is often asked: How does one define the pediatric age-group? The question implies that there is an easy age cutoff such as 13, 18, 21, or 25. There is, of course, no such cutoff, as childhood development proceeds from fetal life through early childhood, the teenage years, and into young adulthood. Part of the mission of the pediatrician is to be well versed in all the developmental stages and to be able to provide developmentally appropriate care for patients at all stages. Certainly, as children transition from early and mid-childhood to the teenage years, they become more like adults in terms of heart size and intellectual ability. Even so, they have their own set of unique needs and issues, including the tendency to consider themselves to be "immortal."[1] Furthermore, they come with a concerned family who will have many questions. Although most teenagers are legally unable to give consent for their own procedures, it is essential that they be involved in the discussions that lead to obtaining consent, and the clinician has a duty to establish that they are themselves willing to undergo the proposed procedure. In younger children, this is less of an issue but still may be an important consideration. In young adults who are 18 and over, the mere fact that they must sign the form themselves does not mean that they are not relying on their parents' advice and judgment. Therefore, the clinician has a duty to determine, with the young adult, how involved the parents should be in the discussions.

Laboratory Setting

Of course, the EP laboratory must be properly equipped and all the staff must be fully qualified to perform the procedures planned. For patients less than 13 years of age, this almost always means that the electrophysiologist is a pediatric cardiologist with special training and experience in pediatric EP procedures. Although exceptions include adult electrophysiologists who have gained this expertise, in this case, a pediatric cardiologist is usually involved as well.[2] Likewise, the nursing and technical staff must have the appropriate level of expertise in dealing with children, including in the areas of sedation and resuscitation.

Beyond these considerations, a number of age-appropriate ancillary services must be present to do procedures safely, specifically in the under-13-year age-group. These include the following: skilled surgical backup (ideally by a pediatric cardiac surgery team) in case of perforation or cardiac tear; pediatric anesthesia services; the availability of a pediatric intensive care unit or pediatric cardiac intensive care unit as well as the ability to deploy extracorporeal membrane oxygenation (ECMO) rapidly for a child-size patient[3]; a postanesthesia care unit skilled and experienced in pediatric patients; and the availability of child life workers for patients and family education and support. Of course, all these services are likely to be readily available in a children's hospital. In other settings, in order to do procedures safely, these elements need to be assembled and available. Examples where this has been done effectively include settings in which a children's hospital adjoins an adult hospital that houses the EP laboratory, and general hospitals with pediatric units in the same building.

Sedation/Anesthesia Considerations

Pediatric EP practice has evolved over the past two decades. Early in the ablation experience, essentially from 1989 through the 1990s, pediatric procedures were often performed under conscious or deep sedation. However, currently most busy pediatric laboratories rely on anesthesia services, and procedures are done under monitored deep sedation or general anesthesia. There are a number of reasons for this, perhaps the most important of which is simply patient safety. In general, children under the age of 13 cannot be relied upon to be patient and cooperative during a long, boring, and sometimes uncomfortable procedure, so conscious sedation is not really an option. The administration of deep sedation requires a higher level of training and expertise, including the ability to effectively manage airways of various sizes.[4] In most settings, this expertise is most easily found with a pediatric anesthesia team. While some teenagers may well be capable of tolerating an ablation procedure while conscious, this is (in the author's opinion) unpredictable. Furthermore, dysphoric reactions to common conscious sedation medications such as midazolam are common in teenagers, and this leads to the need to either terminate the procedure or deepen the sedation. In general, the patient and family's experience is likely to be superior when anesthesia services are employed.

Common concerns regarding the use of anesthesia are that it may suppress certain arrhythmias, making them more difficult to initiate and map. In practice, this is not a concern for accessory pathways and atrioventricular nodal reentry tachycardia (AVNRT) (two diagnoses that make up the great majority of procedures in children)

because the effects of anesthesia in these substrates can easily be overwhelmed by the use of isoproterenol infusion[5] (Table 6.1). General anesthesia may be problematic for certain automatic focus tachycardias, such as atrial, junctional, and ventricular tachycardia, making them difficult to initiate.[6] In such cases, one often decides to defer procedures until patients are old enough, and mature enough, to undergo study with little or no sedation.

Table 6.1 Useful pharmacological agents in pediatric electrophysiology procedures

Agent	Dose	Purpose/Indication
Isoproterenol	0.025–0.05 mcg/kg/min continuous infusion	• Facilitation of inducibility of atrioventricular node reentry under anesthesia • Emergence of automatic focus tachycardias, especially junctional ectopic and atrial ectopic tachycardias
Atropine	0.01–0.03 mg/kg intravenously	• Facilitation of inducibility of atrioventricular node reentry under anesthesia
Procainamide	10–15 mg/kg intravenous bolus over 30 to 45 minutes	• Challenge test to elicit Brugada syndrome pattern on electrocardiogram • Control of atrial fibrillation with rapid conduction in Wolff–Parkinson–White syndrome
Epinephrine	0.05–0.2 mcg/kg/min, continuous infusion	Epinephrine challenge test for long QT syndrome type 17

Diagnoses and Natural History

As mentioned in the introduction to this chapter, the types of arrhythmias seen in children, adolescents, and adults, and the indications for ablation procedures, greatly overlap. It is beyond the scope of this chapter to cover the differences in detail, but several general principles can be mentioned.

First, the types of tachyarrhythmias seen differ with growth and development. In the newborn, atrial flutter is occasionally seen, and once converted to sinus, tends not to recur whether or not antiarrhythmic medications are given. The most common form of supraventricular tachycardia (SVT) is caused by accessory pathways, either manifest or concealed. Atrioventricular node reentry is thought to be rare in infants.[8] As one moves up in age to school-aged (5- to 12-year-old) children, AVNRT becomes more common, perhaps nearly as common as accessory pathways. In the teen years and on into adulthood, AVNRT becomes predominant.

Atrial flutter and atrial fibrillation are quite uncommon in children with structurally normal hearts. In fact, the occurrence of atrial fibrillation in an otherwise healthy child should prompt the search for an explanation. In some cases, it is an early manifestation of myocardial disease, such as hypertrophic or dilated cardiomyopathy. Alternatively, it can be seen in patients who have previously undiagnosed, more common forms of SVT, especially AVNRT. Finally, it is also seen in pediatric patients with Wolff–Parkinson–White (WPW) syndrome.[9]

Indications and Complications

The indications for catheter ablation in children have been published and are driven largely by safety concerns as well as natural history considerations.[2] The only form of SVT for which good data regarding natural history are available is WPW,[10] and even that is controversial.[11] Knowledge about WPW is extended to patients with concealed accessory pathways. Little is known about the natural history of AVNRT in childhood, and less is known concerning more rare substrates. However, with respect to WPW (and presumably concealed accessory pathways), infants who present in the newborn period have an excellent chance at spontaneous resolution by one year of age.[10] Interestingly, a substantial minority whose condition spontaneously resolves in the first year go on to experience relapse, often at 4 to 6 years of age. However, once established at that age, subsequent spontaneous resolution is thought to be rare, at least in childhood and most of adulthood.

Along with natural history considerations, procedural results and complication rates play an important role in informing the indications for catheter ablation. As one might expect, complication rates for catheter ablation are higher in younger and smaller children, but interestingly seem to plateau at a low incidence in children aged 4 and greater.[12] With current techniques, in skilled hands, there is no real rationale for waiting beyond age 4 for performing a clinically indicated ablation if the concern is risk. Based on natural history, there is also no rationale for delaying treatment at this age in hopes of spontaneous resolution. This is a general practice guideline that does not cover all scenarios, of course. One major exception, for some, is the situation of an anteroseptal or para-Hisian pathway, in which the electrophysiologist might prudently wait until the child is bigger, to minimize the risk of atrioventricular (AV) block as a complication of ablation.[13] It is useful to note that the increasing use of cryomapping and cryoablation has certainly influenced considerations of indications and timing in pediatric ablation. Previously, with RF ablation, the general consensus held that the risk of AV block from ablation of septal substrates would be minimized by waiting until adolescence for the procedure. Now, ablation at an earlier age is feasible for these substrates. With the opportunity to perform "test" lesions (cryomapping) to observe for the occurrence of transient AV block at a candidate site, the risk of permanent AV block can be minimized.

Several additional potential complications are specific to treating small children. While it may seem that cardiac perforation would be a bigger problem in the pediatric population than in older patients, large multiple-center studies have not identified this as a particular concern.[14] Similarly, significant damage to the cardiac valves was not observed in one large prospective study.[15] On the other hand, the small size of infants and children's hearts may put the epicardial coronary arteries at risk, particularly when performing ablation of accessory pathways. Coronary injury has been produced experimentally[16] and has been reported in a number of locations.[17] The best method for avoiding this complication is unknown, but it is reasonable to use the minimum power necessary to achieve a therapeutic ablation temperature with radiofrequency (RF). A high index of suspicion is warranted, and some clinicians advocate postablation coronary angiography following right-sided accessory-pathway RF ablation in young patients.[18] While this complication has been reported only infrequently, it is not often looked for. Thus, in young patients, the possibility of coronary injury provides a rationale for considering cryoablation for the right freewall pathway, as well as for posteroseptal pathways.[19]

The pediatric EP patient population includes a substantial number of patients who have arrhythmias following surgery for palliation or repair of congenital heart disease. It is beyond the scope of this chapter to describe the anatomy that supports these arrhythmias and the approach to ablation. However, the new onset of arrhythmias, such as atrial flutter, in a patient who has previously undergone surgery for congenital heart disease may well be the first sign of significant hemodynamic impairment. One must always consider that noninvasive diagnostic imaging and cardiac catheterization may be needed to rule out, or to treat, these factors. Such factors might include worsening ventricular function, the development of conduit stenosis, or worsening valve insufficiency. Likewise, patients who develop arrhythmias in the setting of repair for congenital heart disease may be in the situation of having frequent tachyarrhythmias that contribute to worsening ventricular function. Finally, antiarrhythmic medications proposed for treating these supervening arrhythmias may worsen ventricular function (if they are negative inotropic agents) and preexisting sinus node or AV node disease. Indications for ablation in this patient population are complex because one is often dealing simultaneously with hemodynamic and electrophysiological problems.

Access

Although it may seem a simple matter, access is often a major problem in children. In larger patients and adults, one can easily place 3 sheaths in a single femoral vein; in younger patients, this is not recommended. In the typical 4-year-old, one may place two 5-Fr sheaths in one femoral vein, and a larger sheath, for use with an ablation catheter, in the other. Some clinicians favor approaching the coronary sinus via the right internal jugular (IJ) vein (Figure 6.1), while others favor placing deflectable catheters into the coronary sinus from below (Figure 6.2). An advantage of the IJ approach is that it reduces the number of femoral lines needed.

Often, when an additional pacing or recording electrode is needed in a small patient, it is preferable to employ an esophageal lead (Figure 6.3). Commercially available 7-Fr and 10-Fr bipolar catheters are available and can be easily passed down the esophagus, to be positioned behind the left atrium.[20] The lead is positioned to obtain the maximum atrial electrogram amplitude, and one typically records a large ventricular electrogram as well. Atrial capture is facilitated by the use of a longer pulse width: ideally 15 to 20 ms, though 9.9 ms is usually adequate.[21]

In patients with unusual anatomic variants, such as interruption of the inferior vena cava or bilateral femoral venous occlusion, the transhepatic approach is available. It has the advantage of shortening the distance from the operator's hand to the tip of the catheter, fostering precise manipulation, and is quite low risk.[22]

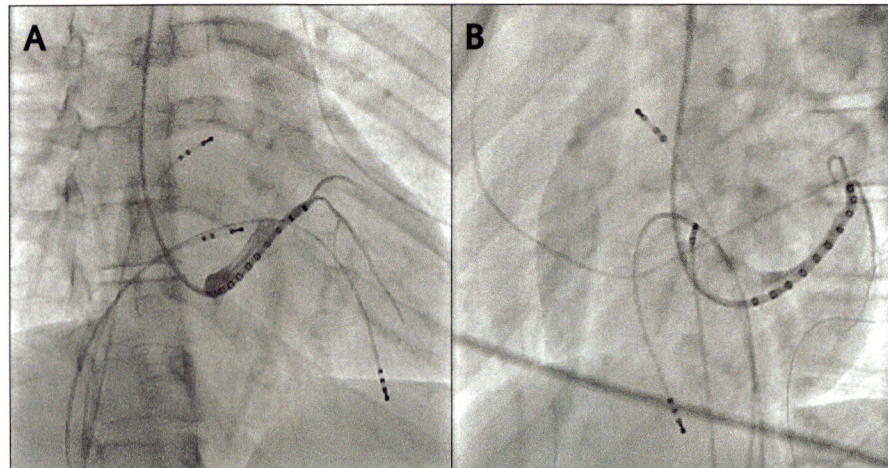

Figure 6.1 Catheter positions in a 15-year-old with Wolff–Parkinson–White syndrome. A 7-Fr nondeflectable decapolar catheter is advanced from the internal jugular vein to the coronary sinus. Through a lumen in the catheter, several milliliters of radiographic contrast is injected, outlining the coronary sinus (CS) anatomy, excluding the presence of a CS diverticulum, and identifying the relationship of the mouth of the CS to the electrode pairs.
Panel A: Right anterior oblique projection.
Panel B: Left anterior oblique projection.

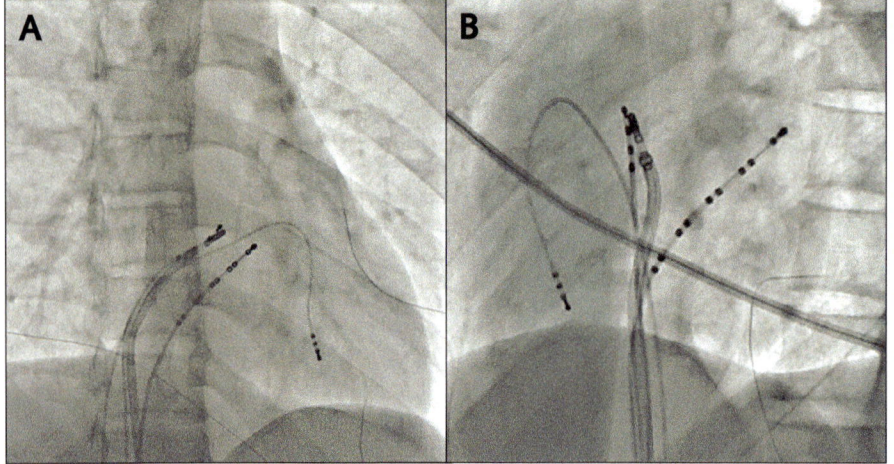

Figure 6.2 12-year-old with supraventricular tachycardia due to a concealed anteroseptal accessory pathway. A 6-Fr deflectable catheter has been advanced into the coronary sinus from below, ie, via the right femoral vein and inferior vena cava. Note also that an ablation catheter is deployed to the pathway site by the use of an 8-Fr long positioning sheath.
Panel A: Right anterior oblique projection.
Panel B: Left anterior oblique projection.

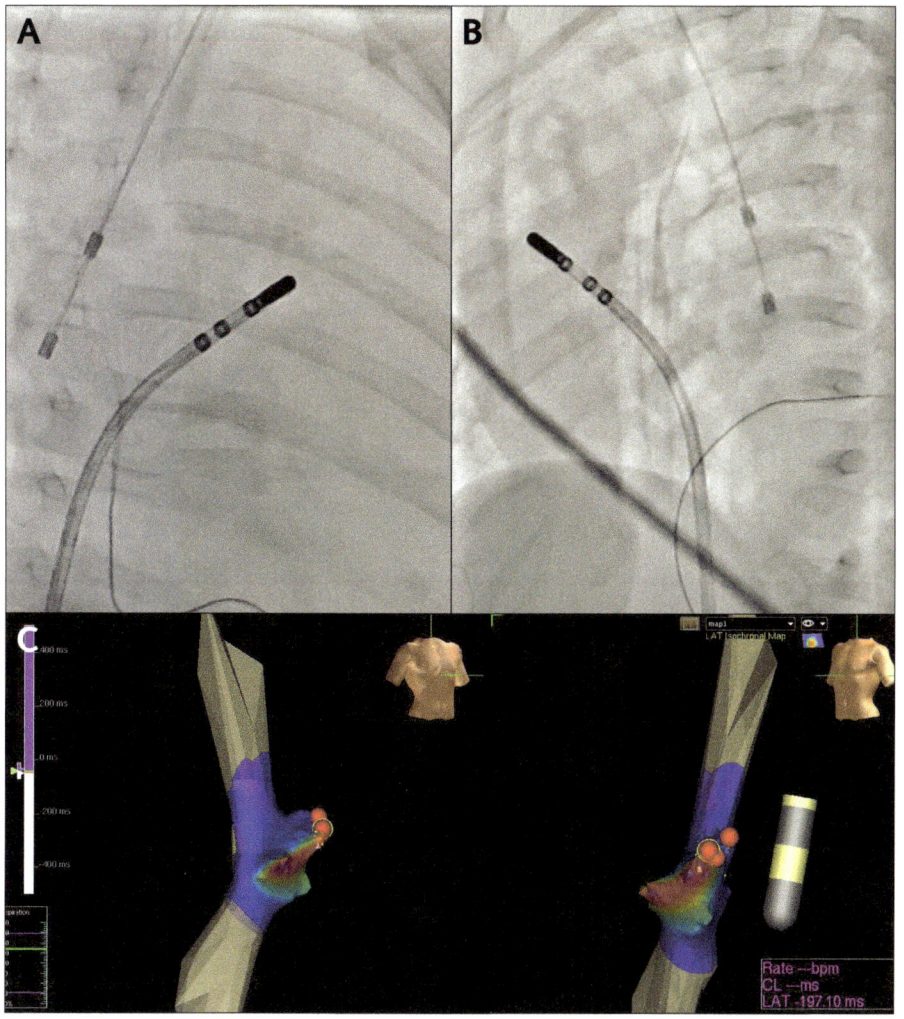

Figure 6.3 Catheter positions in a 5-month-old male infant with incessant atrial ectopic tachycardia and tachycardia-induced cardiomyopathy. Note the presence of an esophageal catheter used for timing, and a single 7-Fr mapping and ablation catheter in the right atrial appendage. **Panel A:** Right anterior oblique projection. **Panel B:** Left anterior oblique projection. **Panel C:** Electroanatomic map using the NavX system (St. Jude Medical, St. Paul, MN), generated via the single mapping catheter, and presenting electrogram timings relative to the atrial activation recorded by the esophageal bipolar catheter. bpm = beats per minute.

Equipment

Patients undergoing an EP study should always be connected to a cardiac defibrillator with adhesive defibrillator patches. Modern defibrillators generate biphasic waveforms, and the energy setting needed to defibrillate are lower than with the older, monophasic waveform devices. Studies comparing defibrillation thresholds by waveform have been done in adults but not in children; consequently, no official recommendations have been made for biphasic defibrillation dosage in children. However, in practice, doses are chosen that are about half of what was previously recommended. The rationale for limiting energy delivery in order to minimize postshock myocardial dysfunction is sound.[23]

Patch size is important for effective defibrillation. The use of patches that are too small can raise the defibrillation threshold. Most pediatric patients should have full-sized adult defibrillator patches placed, and infant patches are reserved for patients who are less than one year of age or weigh less than 10 kg.[24]

Catheters for diagnostic EP study and ablation are, for the most part, not designed for pediatric applications. Therefore, the clinician must adapt and choose from what is available to get a good fit for the particular clinical indication and heart size (Figures 6.4, 6.5, and 6.6). For standard quadripolar catheters for smaller hearts, a tighter interelectrode distance is preferable so that both the distal and proximal electrode pairs are in the same chamber (eg, a 2-5-2 configuration). Generally 4-Fr and 5-Fr catheters are small enough for even the smallest infants.

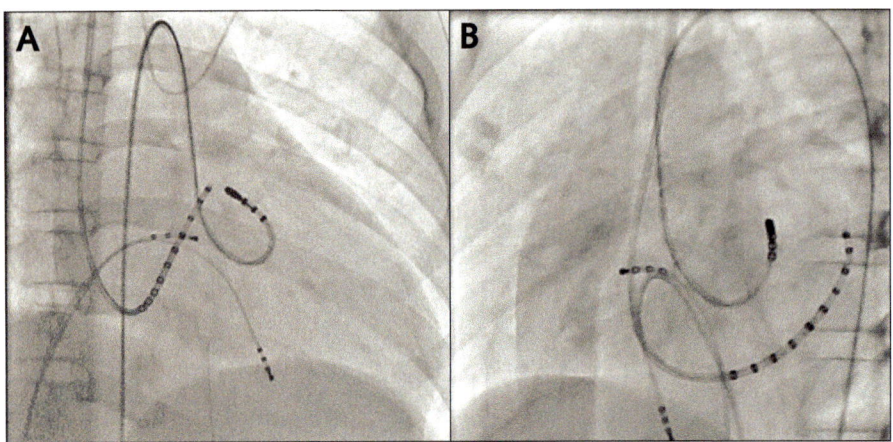

Figure 6.4 Retrograde approach. This 11-year-old girl had a single left anterolateral accessory pathway and Wolff–Parkinson–White syndrome. Note that the coronary sinus catheter is positioned from above, via the internal jugular vein. The ablation catheter has been advanced in a retrograde fashion across the aortic valve and positioned on the anterior mitral annulus under the anterior leaflet. **Panel A:** Right anterior oblique projection. **Panel B:** Left anterior oblique projection.

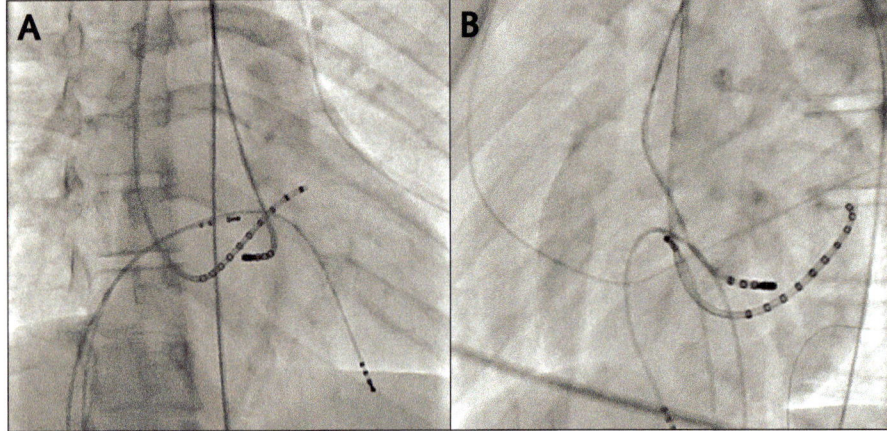

Figure 6.5 These images are from the same patient shown in Figure 6.1. The pathway was mapped to coronary sinus (CS) electrode pair 7,8, which was clearly a left-sided position based on results of CS venography. The pathway was approached in a retrograde fashion.
Panel A: Right anterior oblique projection.
Panel B: Left anterior oblique projection.

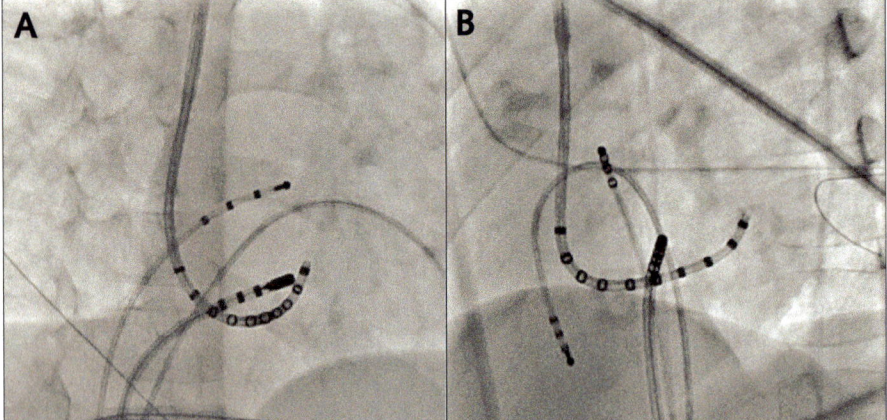

Figure 6.6 Catheter positions in a 4-year-old found to have atrioventricular node reentry. The coronary sinus (CS) catheter is positioned from above, via the internal jugular vein. The ablation catheter is positioned on the interatrial septum, just superior to the CS.
Panel A: Right anterior oblique projection.
Panel B: Left anterior oblique projection.

RF ablation catheters are available in 5-Fr, 6-Fr, and 7-Fr sizes from various manufacturers. While French size is an important factor when performing ablation in small children, curve radius, torquability, and tip softness are perhaps more important considerations.

Cryoablation is feasible in children,[25] although catheters smaller than 7 Fr are not available.

Biophysical Issues

In performing RF ablation in smaller children, one is of course dealing with a smaller heart. In practice, for most patients, settings used for RF ablation are similar to those used in older and larger patients. However, in pediatric patients, the possibility of catheter trapping is perhaps greater; that is, the catheter tip may be placed in a location that provides little or no tip cooling from blood flow. Although current ablation systems have effective control circuits to regulate power in order to achieve a set temperature, small catheter movements can lead to sudden loss of adequate tip cooling and a sudden rise in temperature. The control circuit of the RF generator may not ramp down power output quickly enough to avoid a significant temperature overshoot. In practice, when performing ablation in the smallest hearts, very low outputs are chosen initially, and of course, tip temperature is always monitored.

The total impedance seen by the RF generator also depends on other factors, such as patch size and body surface area (BSA). Interestingly, this is mainly an issue for BSA above 1.5 m², in which there is a linear relationship.[26] Below this BSA value, there is no correlation, and so standard power outputs can be utilized.

Conclusion

Basic principles of ablation are the same for patients of all ages, but pediatric patients require an organized and age-appropriate approach so that procedures are performed safely and effectively. These requirements are not limited to purely technical issues but include all elements of good pediatric care.

References

1. Bernstein D, Shelov SP. *Pediatrics for Medical Students*. Philadelphia: Lippincott Williams & Wilkins; 2012.
2. Friedman RA, Walsh EP, Silka MJ, et al. NASPE Expert Consensus Conference: Radiofrequency catheter ablation in children with and without congenital heart disease. Report of the writing committee. North American Society of Pacing and Electrophysiology. *Pacing Clin Electrophysiol*. 2002;25:1000-1017.
3. Kane DA, Thiagarajan RR, Wypij D, et al. Rapid-response extracorporeal membrane oxygenation to support cardiopulmonary resuscitation in children with cardiac disease. *Circulation*. 2010;122:S241-S248.
4. Cote CJ, Wilson S. Guidelines for monitoring and management of pediatric patients during and after sedation for diagnostic and therapeutic procedures: an update. *Pediatrics*. 2006;118:2587-2602.
5. Moore JP, Kannankeril PJ, Fish FA. Isoproterenol administration during general anesthesia for the evaluation of children with ventricular preexcitation. *Circ Arrhythm Electrophysiol*. 2011;4:73-78.
6. Lai LP, Lin JL, Wu MH, et al. Usefulness of intravenous propofol anesthesia for radiofrequency catheter ablation in patients with tachyarrhythmias: infeasibility for pediatric patients with ectopic atrial tachycardia. *Pacing Clin Electrophysiol*. 1999;22:1358-1364.
7. Vyas H, Ackerman MJ. Epinephrine QT stress testing in congenital long QT syndrome. *J Electrocardiol*. 2006;39 (4 Suppl):S107-S113.
8. Blaufox AD, Warsy I, D'Souza M, Kanter R. Transesophageal electrophysiological evaluation of children with a history of supraventricular tachycardia in infancy. *Pediatr Cardiol*. 2011;32:1110-1114.
9. Harahsheh A, Du W, Singh H, Karpawich PP. Risk factors for atrioventricular tachycardia degenerating to atrial flutter/fibrillation in the young with Wolff–Parkinson–White. *Pacing Clin Electrophysiol*. 2008;31:1307-1312.
10. Perry JC, Garson A Jr. Supraventricular tachycardia due to Wolff–Parkinson–White syndrome in children: early disappearance and late recurrence. *J Am Coll Cardiol*. 1990;16:1215-1220.
11. Santinelli V, Radinovic A, Manguso F, et al. The natural history of asymptomatic ventricular pre-excitation a long-term prospective follow-up study of 184 asymptomatic children. *J Am Coll Cardiol*. 2009;53:275-280.
12. Park JK, Halperin BD, McAnulty JH, et al. Comparison of radiofrequency catheter ablation procedures in children, adolescents, and adults and the impact of accessory pathway location. *Am J Cardiol*. 1994;74:786-789.
13. Schaffer MS, Silka MJ, Ross BA, Kugler JD. Inadvertent atrioventricular block during radiofrequency catheter ablation. Results of the Pediatric Radiofrequency Ablation Registry. Pediatric Electrophysiology Society. *Circulation*. 1996;94:3214-3220.
14. Van Hare GF, Javitz H, Carmelli D, et al. Prospective assessment after pediatric cardiac ablation: demographics, medical profiles, and initial outcomes. *J Cardiovasc Electrophysiol*. 2004;15:759-770.
15. Van Hare GF, Colan SD, Javitz H, et al. Prospective assessment after pediatric cardiac ablation: fate of intracardiac structure and function, as assessed by serial echocardiography. *Am Heart J*. 2007;153:815-820; 820.e1-6.
16. Sturm M, Hausmann D, Bokenkamp R, et al. Incidence and time course of intimal plaque formation in the right coronary artery after radiofrequency current application detected by intracoronary ultrasound. *Z Kardiol*. 2004;93:884-889.
17. Schneider HE, Kriebel T, Gravenhorst VD, Paul T. Incidence of coronary artery injury immediately after catheter ablation for supraventricular tachycardias in infants and children. *Heart Rhythm*. 2009;6:461-467.
18. Kriebel T, Kroll M, Paul T. Radiofrequency catheter ablation therapy in the young: current status. *Expert Rev Cardiovasc Ther*. 2003;1:421-437.
19. Kriebel T, Hermann HP, Schneider H, et al. Cryoablation at growing myocardium: no evidence of coronary artery obstruction or intimal plaque formation early and late after energy application. *Pacing Clin Electrophysiol*. 2009;32:1197-1202.
20. Van Hare GF, Dubin AM, Collins KK. Invasive electrophysiology in children: state of the art. *J Electrocardiol*. 2002;35 (Suppl):165-174.
21. Benson DW Jr, Sanford M, Dunnigan A, Benditt DG. Transesophageal atrial pacing threshold: role of interelectrode spacing, pulse width and catheter insertion depth. *Am J Cardiol*. 1984;53:63-67.
22. Singh SM, Neuzil P, Skoka J, et al. Percutaneous transhepatic venous access for catheter ablation procedures in patients with interruption of the inferior vena cava. *Circ Arrhythm Electrophysiol*. 2011;4:235-241.
23. Berg MD, Banville IL, Chapman FW, et al. Attenuating the defibrillation dosage decreases postresuscitation myocardial dysfunction in a swine model of pediatric ventricular fibrillation. *Pediatr Crit Care Med*. 2008;9:429-434.
24. Hazinski MF, Cummins RO, Field JM. *2000 Handbook of Emergency Cardiovascular Care for Healthcare Providers*. Dallas, TX: American Heart Association; 2000.
25. Collins KK, Schaffer MS. Use of cryoablation for treatment of tachyarrhythmias in 2010: survey of current practices of pediatric electrophysiologists. *Pacing Clin Electrophysiol*. 2011;34:304-308.
26. Park JK, Halperin BD, Kron J, et al. Analysis of body surface area as a determinant of impedance during radiofrequency catheter ablation in adults and children. *J Electrocardiol*. 1994;27:329-332.

SECTION 1B

TECHNOLOGY AND THERAPEUTIC TECHNIQUES

Imaging Technology

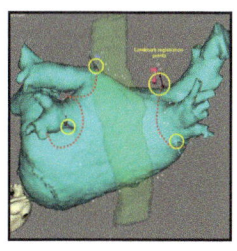 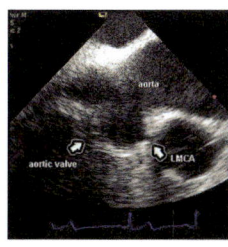 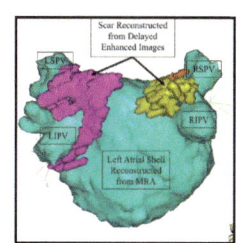 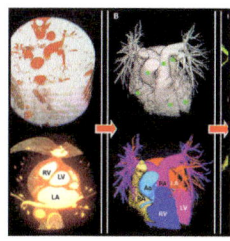

CHAPTER 7

Fundamentals and Applications of Echocardiographic Methods and Systems in the Electrophysiology Laboratory

Shantanu P. Sengupta, MD; A. Jamil Tajik, MD; Bijoy K. Khandheria, MD

Introduction

Echocardiography plays a key role in risk stratification and management of various arrhythmias. The development of newer electrophysiological (EP) mapping and ablation procedures for treating atrial fibrillation (AF), ventricular arrhythmias, and cardiac resynchronization therapy has led to the advent of new echocardiography applications. Use of echocardiography in the EP laboratory has made procedures safer for both patients and electrophysiologists and given echocardiographers an opportunity to expand their role in the field of cardiology. Both the range of indications for and the efficacy and safety of interventional EP have improved considerably. This progress is attributed to both the accumulating experience of electrophysiologists and advances in technological tools facilitating the diagnosis and treatment of cardiac arrhythmias. Three-dimensional (3D) echocardiography and intracardiac echocardiography (ICE) allow real-time visualization of cardiovascular structures during ablative procedures. This chapter will discuss the principles, approaches, and potential future applications of echocardiography in the EP laboratory.

Catheter Ablation for Arrhythmias

During the last decade, advances in the area of catheter ablation have led to a paradigm shift in interventional EP. In contrast to conventional ablation procedures, such as ablation of accessory pathways or atrioventricular (AV) nodal reentry, ablations of complex arrhythmias (eg, atrial fibrillation or postincisional tachycardias) require new definitions of ablation targets. These targets are defined not by EP assessment but by the relationship between electrograms and anatomic structures. Identification and ablation of anatomic structures necessary for arrhythmia triggering or maintenance is an important substrate of arrhythmia management.

Why Is There a Need for Echocardiography in the EP Lab?

For many decades, the main imaging modality used to guide catheter navigation in EP has been fluoroscopy. This technique has several drawbacks: It is associated with risk of radiation to patients and medical personnel, use of contrast injection, and poor resolution of soft tissue.[1] The use of computed tomography (CT) and magnetic resonance imaging (MRI) in EP procedures also has a few drawbacks: They are time-consuming and consist of pre-acquired images that often differ from electroanatomic mapping volumes owing to changes in heart rate, respiration, volume, and hemodynamic status. Being noninvasive, echocardiography provides substantial information about the structure and function of cardiac structures.

Real-time 3D transesophageal echocardiography (TEE) now helps in direct and live visualization of structures responsible for arrhythmias in the EP laboratory. In addition, real-time 3D TEE reduces the dose of radiation in the catheterization laboratory by more than 50%.[2]

Intracardiac Echocardiography

ICE provides a complete visualization of the cardiac anatomy along with hemodynamic information. This helps with live and accurate positioning of catheters and reduces the radiation exposure time of fluoroscopy. ICE's usage has increased in the last few years, mainly in ablation of AF and ventricular arrhythmias. In AF ablation, ICE helps to visualize the anatomy of the left atrium and pulmonary veins (PVs). It also helps in transseptal punctures, locating the ostium and antrum of the PVs and monitoring tissue injury during radiofrequency use.[3] ICE enables accurate localization of endocardial structures, which is important for successful catheter ablation. The images of intracardiac structures that ICE provides are superior or equivalent to those obtained with cardiac MRI.[4] ICE-guided ablation procedures are safer than those without ICE guidance, as ICE allows immediate identification of complications such as cardiac perforation, pericardial effusion, and tamponade. 3D ICE has been developed recently and is being used for catheter navigation during EP procedures.[5]

Echocardiography in Atrial Fibrillation

The most common arrhythmia in clinical practice is AF, with an overall prevalence of 0.4% in the general population.[6] Among the various diagnostic tools, echocardiography plays an important role in evaluating cardiac structure and function and stratifying risk, and is listed in the guidelines for management of patients with AF.[7] Use of ICE has allowed the real-time guidance of percutaneous interventions, including radiofrequency catheter ablation of foci in the PVs and left atrial appendage (LAA)–closure procedures for patients with AF.[8]

Assessment of Left Atrial Size and Function by Echocardiography

Two-dimensional (2D) assessment of left atrial (LA) size using M-mode echocardiography tends to underestimate LA size.[9] This is because of the asymmetrical enlargement of the left atrium, which is anteriorly guarded by the sternum and posteriorly by the thoracic spine. Hence, 2D-derived LA volume assessment using the biplane area–length or Simpson's methods gives an accurate measure of LA size.[10] Of late, 3D echocardiography for assessing LA volume has become available and demonstrated good correlation with biplane 2D measurements.[11] Assessment of LA volume helps identify patients with a high likelihood of maintaining sinus rhythm after successful AF ablation. An increased LA volume index can predict the recurrence of AF after radiofrequency ablation, and a large LA volume can predict low probability of successful cardioversion of AF.[12-14] It has been demonstrated that successful radiofrequency ablation of isolated AF can reverse morphological remodeling of LA after reverting to sinus rhythm and does not affect LA function.[15,16]

Assessment of Left Atrial Function

Echocardiography provides information about global and regional LA function and can provide in-depth insights about electromechanical remodeling in patients undergoing AF ablation. Recent developments in tissue Doppler and strain analysis allow noninvasive assessment of LA mechanics. All tissue Doppler imaging-derived parameters of the LA (including tissue velocities, strain, and strain rate) have been reported to be significantly reduced in patients with AF compared with healthy controls.[4] Documentation of LA spontaneous echo contrast or LA thrombus is also important in patients with AF. Hartono and colleagues reported that the presence of LA spontaneous echo contrast is a poorer atrial substrate.[17] Also, it is associated with less sinus rhythm post-catheter ablation and requires more antiarrhythmic drugs for longer durations.

Use of Intracardiac Echocardiography in Atrial Fibrillation Ablation

The traditional ablation of AF requires LA access through two transseptal punctures, with the patient fully anticoagulated, and a more extensive approach through multiple radiofrequency lesions. It is time-consuming and presents a higher risk for complications (eg, thromboembolism, PV stenosis, or esophageal injury).[18] ICE provides detailed anatomic information about the PVs and demonstrates the presence of anatomic variations, such as the common drainage and accessory veins.

The Heart Rhythm Society/European Heart Rhythm Association/European Cardiac Arrhythmia Society (HRS/EHRA/ECAS) Expert Consensus Statement on Catheter and Surgical Ablation of Atrial Fibrillation[19] recommends the use of ICE based on the following advantages:

1. Uses safer transseptal puncture (through the direct visualization of the interatrial septum without the need to use iodine contrast). ICE allows punctures to be performed in fully anticoagulated patients, thus decreasing the chances of thrombus formation within the left atrium and cardiac tamponade.

2. Defines the complete anatomy of PVs.

3. Allows precise positioning of circular mapping catheters in the PV ostium, helping to determine the sites where radiofrequency must be applied and preventing its use within the PVs (which increases the risk of vein stenosis).

4. Evaluates contact between the catheter and cardiac tissue, which is essential for promoting the transmurality of ablation lesions.

5. Identifies thrombus formation within the left atrium early.[20]

6. Identifies and predicts stenosis of the PVs by measuring flow velocity in the PV ostium before and after the procedure.

7. Prevents esophageal injury by identifying the esophagus and visualizing morphological changes on the posterior atrial wall adjacent to the anterior esophageal wall.

Recently, an ICE-based 3D imaging method has been developed by mounting a magnetic sensor on the tip of a 10-Fr phased-array ICE catheter (SoundStar™, Biosense Webster Inc., Diamond Bar, CA).[21] The 3D ICE-derived geometry can either be used as an imaging tool for catheter navigation or integrated with preacquired, segmented CT or MRI volume images. The use of this 3D ultrasound imaging system for guiding AF ablation proved feasible.[22] Its main advantage is the availability of conventional electroanatomic mapping with the added benefits of using ICE. These benefits include detailed delineation of peculiarities in cardiac anatomy, validation of adequate catheter contact, early recognition of collateral damage, and reduced fluoroscopic exposure. The ICE images can be integrated into the electroanatomic mapping systems (CartoSound™, Biosense Webster Inc.) to generate LA geometry. This technique may be especially helpful for preventing x-ray exposure in children, pregnant women, and obese patients undergoing LA ablation. The emerging development of 3D TEE and ICE is expected to improve the quality of real-time, echocardiography-based imaging during EP procedures.

Intracardiac Echocardiography for Ablation of Atrial Flutter

Ablation of typical atrial flutter is carried out through a cavotricuspid isthmus block line. Sometimes, anatomic differences make ablation of this isthmus difficult. ICE provides a way to directly visualize the isthmus and its variations (eg, the presence of crests, recesses, sacs, and trabeculations), thereby facilitating ablation of the isthmus flutter.[23] ICE is very useful in some congenital heart diseases, like Ebstein's anomaly, which are associated with cavotricuspid isthmus abnormalities due to apical orientation of the tricuspid valve. ICE also helps position the ablation catheter by visualizing the contact between the catheter and the tissue as well as the radiofrequency lesions in deep recesses and prominent trabeculations.

ICE also is helpful in the occlusion of the LAA by percutaneous prosthesis, which is an up-and-coming therapy being developed for patients with AF who are at high risk for embolic events. ICE facilitates the performance of the procedure by locating the LAA and guiding the position of the prosthesis, in addition to facilitating the transseptal puncture.

Real-time 3D Transesophageal Echocardiography for Arrhythmias

There is increasing interest in the utility of 2D TEE and 3D TEE for guiding EP procedures. 3D TEE allows fast sequential scanning of multiple planes by arranging thousands of new piezoelectric crystals of the phased-array transducer in multiple rows (to form a matrix-array probe) rather than one row.[5] Thus far, catheter navigation has been done using fluoroscopy. However, this technique lacks soft-tissue contrast and adequate visualization of the target region inside the heart, especially during ablation of AF in the left atrium. Real-time 3D TEE offers an *en face* view of the cardiac structures and visualizes most intracardiac catheters along their tract, clearly depicting their position in relation to surrounding structures. Owing to the esophagus's proximity to the right and left atria, real-time 3D TEE can visualize both right and left anatomic structures. Pulmonary ostia, which are often a target of ablation, can easily be visualized using real-time 3D TEE. Also, the latest real-time 3D TEE systems provide good spatial and temporal resolution, which is helpful for tracking the ablation catheter in real time.[24]

The electrophysiologist is generally not aware of the orientation of the 3D TEE images. Hence, to solve this issue, real-time 3D TEE can be obtained with images equivalent to or better than fluoroscopy projections, such as left anterior oblique (LAO) and right anterior oblique (RAO). Acquiring 3D TEE (in addition to standard 2D TEE) images may be useful before the procedure, both for its planning and during transseptal puncture. Before the procedure, 3D TEE may help one to understand the morphology of the interatrial septum and fossa ovalis. Also, 3D TEE can be extremely helpful for patients at high risk for transseptal puncture by imaging extreme rotation of the cardiac axis, repeated septal puncture, various sizes of fossa ovalis, and fossa ovalis aneurysm. During the procedure, 3D TEE may provide better guidance for the transseptal catheter (▶ Video 7.1, ▶ Video 7.2, and ▶ Video 7.3) compared with 2D TEE. The most appropriate site for the puncture is indeed usually identified after recognizing 2D TEE "tenting" of the fossa ovalis.[23] Quite often, the septal indentation is not seen on 2D TEE but can be visualized by real-time 3D TEE, owing to the 3D depth of the interatrial septum. An *en face* view can show the position and size of the fossa ovalis, and real-time 3D TEE can help directly visualize catheter-wall contact and the act of burning. Many times, it is difficult to see the tip of the catheter. During radiofrequency delivery, burning of tissue may be appreciated by the development of 3D microbubbles flowing away from the ablation catheter tip, owing to the phenomenon of cavitation caused by heating tissue. Acquiring full-volume images with real-time 3D TEE comes at lower frame rates; however, it does not impair imaging the septal structures, as the septum does not move much with every beat.

Real-time 3D TEE is also helpful in identifying the cavotricuspid isthmus and crista terminalis, both of which are structures of the right atrium and important for electrophysiologists.[25] The cavotricuspid isthmus is a well-defined anatomic area responsible for isthmus-dependent atrial flutter, while the crista terminalis is one of the most frequent sources of focal atrial arrhythmias.[25]

Real-time 3D TEE provides a unique, instantaneous assessment of the position of catheters at the level of each PV ostium. Point-by-point navigation around the PV with minimal use of fluoroscopy can be monitored continuously. This enables assessment of catheter stability and contact in challenging ablation areas such as the prominent lateral crest. For PV isolation, this region is particularly challenging because of possible suboptimal catheter contact and catheter instability. Moreover, the thickness of this area varies from patient to patient and tends to be greater with respect to LA wall thickness in other areas. Continuous real-time 3D TEE visualization of this area may ensure better catheter contact and stability while providing greater confidence in safely delivering long-lasting, high-energy radiofrequency applications until stable PV isolation is achieved.

Several challenges are involved with the use of real-time 3D TEE in EP procedures. Relatively rapid movements of the catheter can result in the need for a larger area to be scanned. Doing so requires imaging a larger volume size at a high frame rate, which in turn decreases spatial resolution. An acceptable compromise can be obtained by zooming the pyramidal data set to 60 × 60 degrees. The other problems encountered are the result of artifacts produced by highly reflective structures such as metallic catheters. These artifacts are reverberations (ie, multiple reflections between structures) and shadowing (ie, areas of dropout in the image) and can be minimized by moving the catheter more gradually during real-time 3D acquisition and keeping the probe more parallel to the catheter. Finally, catheters from different vendors have a variety of 3D imaging features owing to different acoustic impedance of the components.

Echocardiography in Ventricular Arrhythmia

The main substrates in ventricular arrhythmia are scars, ischemia, aneurysms, or nonviable myocardium. In many disease processes, this nonviable myocardium is predictive of ventricular tachycardia prevalence, mortality, or both. Transthoracic 3D echocardiography is used in EP to identify the site of origin of ventricular ectopic activity, especially in the anatomically complex region of ventricular outflow tracts.[26] Tissue-tracking imaging has helped identify the site of arrhythmia origin by detecting the earliest color-coded signal in the myocardium during ventricular premature contractions.[27] This region is then targeted by ablation.

The use of ICE in the ablation of ventricular tachycardia presents the following advantages:

1. Identification of the arrhythmogenic substrate: scars, aneurysms, akinesia, or dyskinesia.

2. Continuous monitoring of complications during the ablation: cardiac perforation and tamponade, valvular injury, and thromboembolic events.

3. Accurate localization of the catheter and its contact with the endocardium.

4. Identification of the ostia of the coronary arteries and their association with the positioning of the ablation catheter in cases of ventricular tachycardia related to the left ventricular outflow tract.[3]

5. In procedures carried out on the epicardial surface, guiding the subxiphoid pericardial puncture and visualizing puncture-related complications (ventricular perforation).

Echocardiography for Cardiac Resynchronization Therapy

A rapid development in EP has been in the treatment of cardiac resynchronization therapy (CRT). With CRT, heart failure patients have seen significant improvement in exercise-tolerance prognosis.[28-30] But CRT is not helpful in 25% of patients who are nonresponders. Hence, identifying these nonresponders is important before initiating therapy.

In this respect, echocardiography has been studied extensively. Echocardiographic assessment of left ventricular (LV) systolic performance and diastolic parameters, both before and after CRT, plays a key role in disease management in these conditions. LV diastolic function is physiologically coupled with LV systolic performance and is an important determinant of symptoms and outcomes in patients with heart failure who are undergoing CRT. The American Society of Echocardiography and European

Association of Echocardiography have published recommendations for the evaluation of LV diastolic function by echocardiography, which can be applied in depth in patients preparing for CRT.[31] This statement consists of adequately sensitive, specific, and relatively novel indices for the quantification of LV diastolic function.

Waggoner et al[32] reported an improvement in mitral E-wave velocity, E/A ratio, and estimated filling pressure after 4 months of CRT only in patients with increased LV systolic performance as assessed by echocardiography. Porciani et al[33] reported an improvement in systolic as well as diastolic function by CRT. In the presence of advanced diastolic dysfunction, evidenced by a restrictive filling pattern, CRT reverses the filling pattern. In contrast, in patients without reverse remodeling and no clinical response, LV filling pressures remained elevated. Aksoy et al[34] compared the most sensitive and specific indices of diastolic dysfunction (septal E/e′, average E/e′, lateral E/e′, mitral E/flow propagation velocity, and LA volume index). They reported that the indices of diastolic function significantly improved among responders. No significant change was seen in nonresponders. Hence, assessment of diastolic flow indices is helpful in patients undergoing CRT. Response to CRT also can be documented by assessing the LV using 2D speckle tracking. 2D speckle-tracking echocardiography is a new modality used in conjunction with 2D or 3D echocardiography for understanding the multidirectional components of LV deformation. The tracking system is based on gray-scale B-mode images and is obtained by automatically measuring the distance between two pixels of an LV segment during the cardiac cycle, independent of the angle of insonation.[35,36]

Despite much promising work, the recent multicenter Predictors of Response to Cardiac Resynchronization Therapy (PROSPECT) study reported no significant improvement in selection of CRT candidates using different tissue Doppler criteria.[37,38] To visualize the 3D morphology of the left ventricle, use of 3D echocardiography offers higher potential for identifying dyssynchrony. It helps identify the optimal pacing site that would result in resynchronization via real-time 3D echocardiography transducers with a matrix array. The 3D data sets help generate LV volumes and mass. Dyssynchrony is performed by the software provided by the respective vendors of the machine. Global and segmental functional parameters are calculated, which allows for precisely assessing the effect of CRT on LV remodeling. Color-coded display of time to maximum contraction, as represented by a bull's-eye format, helps identify the site of maximum mechanical delay and, hence, the optimal pacing site. Saksena et al[39] and Bai et al[40] each documented the advantage of ICE-based optimization for CRT patients by adjusting CRT programming in daily practice. Further advances in the field of 3D ICE for optimal treatment of dyssynchrony are in progress.

Conclusion

The need for precise information regarding cardiac structures during cardiac catheter ablation has revolutionized the use of echocardiography in the EP laboratory. Ablation targets are not defined by EP recordings but by assessing the relationship of electrograms with the anatomic structures documented by 3D echocardiography or ICE. Ongoing developments suggest that these two imaging modalities will be the future of cardiac imaging in the EP laboratory.

References

1. Gerber TC, Gibbons RJ. Weighing the risks and benefits of cardiac imaging with ionizing radiation. *JACC Cardiovasc Imaging*. 2010;3:528-535.
2. Picano E. Informed consent and communication of risk from radiological and nuclear medicine examinations: how to escape from a communication inferno. *Br Med J*. 2004;329:849-851.
3. Lamberti F, Calo L, Pandozi C, et al. Radiofrequency catheter ablation of idiopathic left ventricular outflow tract tachycardia: utility of intracardiac echocardiography. *J Cardiovasc Electrophysiol*. 2001;12:529-535.
4. Zanchetta M, Rigatelli G, Pedon L, et al. Intracardiac echocardiography: gross anatomy and magnetic resonance correlations and validations. *Int J Cardiovasc Imaging*. 2005;21:391-401.
5. Faletra F, Regoli F, Acena M, Auricchio A. Value of real-time transesophageal 3-dimensional echocardiography in guiding ablation of isthmus-dependent atrial flutter and pulmonary vein isolation. *Circ J*. 2012;76:5-14.
6. Peters NS, Schilling RJ, Kanagaratnam P, Markides V. Atrial fibrillation: strategies to control, combat, and cure. *Lancet*. 2002;359:593-603.
7. Fuster V, Rydén LE, Asinger RW, et al. ACC/AHA/ESC Guidelines for the Management of Patients With Atrial Fibrillation: Executive Summary–A Report of the American College of Cardiology/American Heart Association Task Force on Practice Guidelines and the European Society of Cardiology Committee for Practice Guidelines and Policy Conferences (Committee to Develop Guidelines for the Management of Patients With Atrial Fibrillation) Developed in Collaboration With the North American Society of Pacing and Electrophysiology. *Circulation*. 2001;104:2118-2150.
8. Haïssaguerre M, Jaïs P, Shah DC, et al. Spontaneous initiation of atrial fibrillation by ectopic beats originating in the pulmonary veins. *N Engl J Med*. 1998;339:659-666.
9. Lester SJ, Ryan EW, Schiller NB, Foster E. Best method in clinical practice and in research studies to determine left atrial size. *Am J Cardiol*. 1999;84:829-832.
10. Lang RM, Bierig M, Devereux RB, et al. Recommendations for chamber quantification: a report from the American Society of Echocardiography's Guidelines and Standards Committee and the Chamber Quantification Writing Group, developed in conjunction with the European Association of Echocardiography, a branch of the European Society of Cardiology. *J Am Soc Echocardiogr*. 2005;18:1440-1463.
11. Jenkins C, Bricknell K, Marwick TH. Use of real-time three-dimensional echocardiography to measure left atrial volume:

comparison with other echocardiographic techniques. *J Am Soc Echocardiogr.* 2005;18:991-997.
12. Brodsky MA, Allen BJ, Capparelli EV, et al. Factors determining maintenance of sinus rhythm after chronic atrial fibrillation with left atrial dilatation. *Am J Cardiol.* 1989;63:1065-1068.
13. Dittrich HC, Erickson JS, Schneiderman T, et al. Echocardiographic and clinical predictors for outcome of elective cardioversion of atrial fibrillation. *Am J Cardiol.* 1989;63:193-197.
14. Shin SH, Park MY, Oh WJ, et al. Left atrial volume is a predictor of atrial fibrillation recurrence after catheter ablation. *J Am Soc Echocardiogr.* 2008;21:697-702.
15. Reant P, Lafitte S, Jaïs P, et al. Reverse remodeling of the left cardiac chambers after catheter ablation after 1 year in a series of patients with isolated atrial fibrillation. *Circulation.* 2005;112:2896-2903.
16. Jeevanantham V, Ntim W, Navaneethan SD, et al. Meta-analysis of the effect of radiofrequency catheter ablation on left atrial size, volumes and function in patients with atrial fibrillation. *Am J Cardiol.* 2010;105:1317-1326.
17. Hartono B, Lo LW, Cheng CC, et al. A novel finding of the atrial substrate properties and long-term results of catheter ablation in chronic atrial fibrillation patients with left atrial spontaneous echo contrast. *J Cardiovasc Electrophysiol.* 2012;23:239-246.
18. Di Salvo G, Caso P, Lo Piccolo R, et al. Atrial myocardial deformation properties predict maintenance of sinus rhythm after external cardioversion of recent-onset lone atrial fibrillation: a color Doppler myocardial imaging and transthoracic and transesophageal echocardiographic study. *Circulation.* 2005;112:387-395.
19. Calkins H, Brugada J, Packer DL, et al. HRS/EHRA/ECAS expert Consensus Statement on catheter and surgical ablation of atrial fibrillation: recommendations for personnel, policy, procedures and follow-up. A report of the Heart Rhythm Society Task Force on catheter and surgical ablation of atrial fibrillation. *Heart Rhythm.* 2007;4:816-861.
20. Ren JF, Marchlinski FE, Callans DJ. Left atrial thrombus associated with ablation for atrial fibrillation: identification with intracardiac echocardiography. *J Am Coll Cardiol.* 2004;43:1861-1867.
21. Packer DL, Johnson SB, Kolasa MW, et al. New generation of electro-anatomic mapping: full intracardiac ultrasound image integration. *Europace.* 2008;10(Suppl 3):iii35-41.
22. Regoli F, Faletra FF, Nucifora G, et al. Feasibility and acute efficacy of radiofrequency ablation of cavotricuspid isthmus-dependent atrial flutter guided by real-time 3D TEE. *JACC Cardiovasc Imaging.* 2011;4:716-726.
23. Silvestry FE, Kerber RE, Brook MM, et al. Echocardiography-guided interventions. *J Am Soc Echocardiogr.* 2009;22:213-231.
24. Faletra FF, Ho SY, Auricchio A. Anatomy of right atrial structures by real-time 3D transesophageal echocardiography. *JACC Cardiovasc Imaging.* 2010;3:966-975.
25. Kalman JM, Olgin JE, Karch MR, et al. "Cristal tachycardias": origin of right atrial tachycardias from the crista terminalis identified by intracardiac echocardiography. *J Am Coll Cardiol.* 1998;31:451-459.
26. Tada H, Toide H, Naito S, et al. Tissue tracking imaging as a new modality for identifying the origin of idiopathic ventricular arrhythmias. *Am J Cardiol.* 2005;95:660-664.
27. Kautzner J, Peichl P. 3D and 4D echo—applications in EP laboratory procedures. *J Interv Card Electrophysiol.* 2008;22:139-144.
28. Abraham WT, Hayes DL. Cardiac resynchronization therapy for heart failure. *Circulation.* 2003;108:2596-2603.
29. Cleland JG, Daubert JC, Erdmann E, et al. The effect of cardiac resynchronization on morbidity and mortality in heart failure. *N Engl J Med.* 2005;352:1539-1549.
30. Bristow MR, Saxon LA, Boehmer J, et al. Cardiac-resynchronization therapy with or without an implantable defibrillator in advanced chronic heart failure. *N Engl J Med.* 2004;350:2140-2150.
31. Nagueh SF, Appleton CP, Gillebert TC, et al. Recommendations for the evaluation of left ventricular diastolic function by echocardiography. *J Am Soc Echocardiogr.* 2009;22:107-133.
32. Waggoner AD, Faddis MN, Gleva MJ, et al. Improvements in left ventricular diastolic function after cardiac resynchronization therapy are coupled to response in systolic performance. *J Am Coll Cardiol.* 2005;46:2244-2249.
33. Porciani MC, Valsecchi S, Demarchi G, et al. Evolution and prognostic significance of diastolic filling pattern in cardiac resynchronization therapy. *Int J Cardiol.* 2006;112:322-328.
34. Aksoy H, Okutucu S, Kaya EB, et al. Clinical and echocardiographic correlates of improvement in left ventricular diastolic function after cardiac resynchronization therapy. *Europace.* 2010;12:1256-1261.
35. Geyer H, Caracciolo G, Abe H, et al. Assessment of myocardial mechanics using speckle tracking echocardiography: fundamentals and clinical applications. *J Am Soc Echocardiogr.* 2010;23:351-369.
36. Arias-Godínez JA, Guadalajara-Boo JF, Patel AR, Pandian NG. Function and mechanics of the left ventricle: from tissue Doppler imaging to three dimensional speckle tracking. *Arch Cardiol Mex.* 2011;81:114-125.
37. Yu CM, Abraham WT, Bax J, et al. Predictors of response to cardiac resynchronization therapy (PROSPECT)—study design. *Am Heart J.* 2005;149:600-605.
38. Cleland JG, Abdellah AT, Khaleva O, et al. Clinical trials update from the European Society of Cardiology Congress 2007: 3CPO, ALOFT, PROSPECT and statins for heart failure. *Eur J Heart Fail.* 2007;9:1070-1073.
39. Saksena S, Simon AM, Mathew P, Nagarakanti R. Intracardiac echocardiography-guided cardiac resynchronization therapy: technique and clinical application. *Pacing Clin Electrophysiol.* 2009;32:1030-1039.
40. Bai R, Di Biase L, Mohanty P, et al. Positioning of left ventricular pacing lead guided by intracardiac echocardiography with vector velocity imaging during cardiac resynchronization therapy procedure. *J Cardiovasc Electrophysiol.* 2011;22:1034-1041.

Video Legends

Video 7.1 Bicaval view from transesophageal echocardiography showing the atrial septum.

Video 7.2 Tenting of the atrial septum seen with the transseptal needle.

Video 7.3 Real-time three-dimensional (3D) imaging is used more frequently to help guide transseptal catheter placement. This is an example of real-time 3D imaging showing the transseptal catheter in the left atrium.

CHAPTER 8

THE ROLE OF 3D TRANSTHORACIC AND TRANSESOPHAGEAL ECHOCARDIOGRAPHY IN INTERVENTIONAL ELECTROPHYSIOLOGY

Wael AlJaroudi, MD; Fadi G. Hage, MD; Navin C. Nanda, MD

Introduction

The use of echocardiography in the context of invasive electrophysiology (EP) procedures is widespread. It includes, to name a few: (1) assessing the left atrium appendage (LAA) for thrombus prior to atrial flutter/fibrillation cardioversion or ablation; (2) guiding left atrial appendage occlusion using the percutaneous closure device; (3) quantifying left ventricular ejection fraction (LVEF) before inserting an implantable cardioverter-defibrillator (ICD); (4) evaluating pacemaker or ICD leads for possible thrombus or vegetations prior to lead extractions; (5) diagnosing nonischemic cardiomyopathies, such as arrhythmogenic right ventricular dysplasia (ARVD), LV noncompaction, or hypertrophic obstructive cardiomyopathy (HCM), which might require an ICD in specified clinical scenarios; (6) evaluating LV mechanical dyssynchrony and predicting response to cardiac resynchronization therapy (CRT); and (7) diagnosing pericardial effusions and tamponade when suspected as a complication of some EP ablation procedures.

Two-dimensional transthoracic echocardiography (2D TTE) is of limited value for evaluating the atrial appendage because it often fails to visualize all the appendage lobes and can miss the presence of a thrombus.[1] The quantification of LVEF is also hindered by the 2D views and the geometric assumptions embedded in the methods used by 2D TTE.[2] As such, gated radionuclide angiography, multiple uptake gated acquisition (MUGA) scans and cardiac magnetic resonance imaging (MRI) became the gold standards (until challenged by 3D echocardiography).[3] In regards to dyssynchrony, the Predictors of Response to CRT (PROSPECT) study, a randomized, blinded study using 2D TTE, constituted the last nail in the coffin of echocardiography, mainly owing to the wide inter- and intraobserver variability and lack of reliability of the technique.[4]

However, three-dimensional transthoracic echocardiography (3D TTE), which has been in clinical use for the last few years, has emerged as a robust technique that surmounted many of 2D TTE's limitations and has gained respect and popularity. In addition, transesophageal echocardiography (TEE), although semi-invasive, is routinely used in the EP lab and offers many advantages, particularly when performed with 3D acquisition (Figure 8.1). This chapter will summarized the roles of 3D TTE and TEE in daily invasive EP practice.

3D Echocardiography: General Overview of the Technique

The evolution of echocardiography started from M-mode, progressed to B-mode, then to the addition of color Doppler, then to tissue imaging, and finally to 3D echocardiography. 3D echocardiography represents the latest development in ultrasound imaging of the heart. It is an innovative and revolutionary noninvasive imaging tool.[5-7] There have been many attempts to provide 3D echocardiographic images, including via the use of a 2D transducer probe and mechanically rotating it.[8] However,

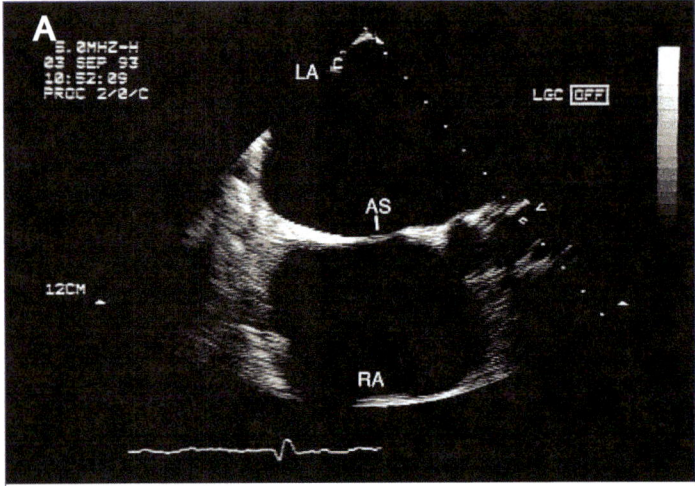
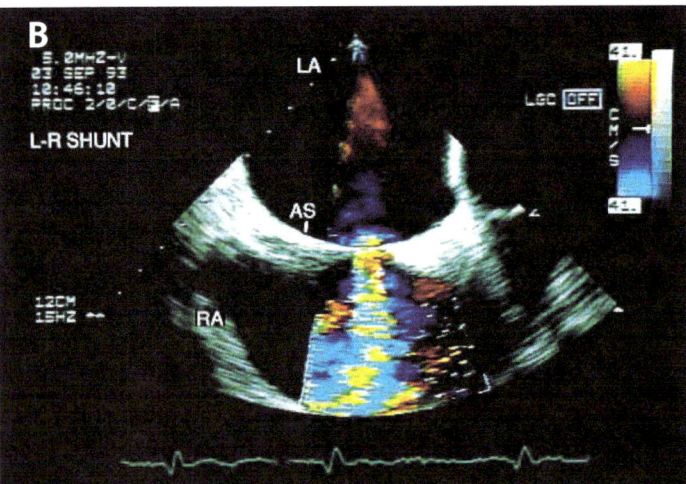
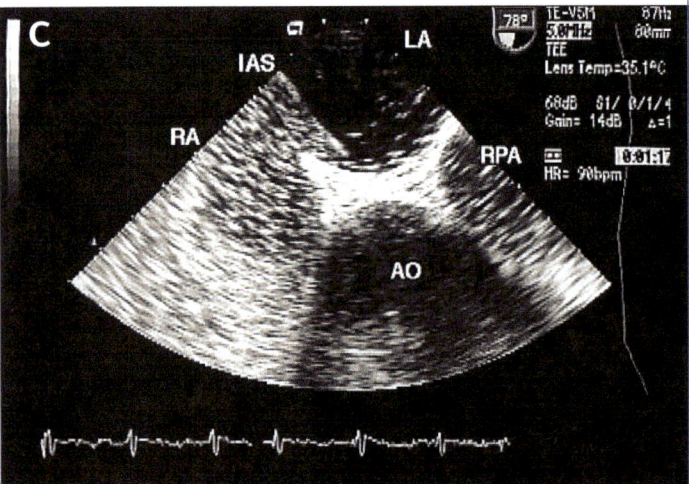

Figure 8.1 Transesophageal echocardiographic examination of the atrial septum (AS) (**Panels A–C**). Although the AS, with the fossa ovalis represented by its midportion, appears intact in **A**, color Doppler examination clearly shows shunting into the right atrium (RA) in **Panel B. Panel C:** Bubble study shows microbubbles crossing over from the RA into the left atrium (LA) through a patent foramen ovale. AO = aorta, IAS = interatrial septum; RPA = right pulmonary artery. *Source:* Reproduced with permission from Nanda NC, Domanski MJ. *Atlas of Transesophageal Echocardiography.* 2nd ed. Philadelphia, PA: Lippincott Williams & Wilkins; 2007.

the advent of a full matrix array transducer probe[9] (broadband 4 MHz × 4 phase arrays, >6,400 elements, 10,000 channels, and >150 mini-circuit boards) has permitted live or real-time 3D acquisition of a 3D volume-rendered pyramidal dataset with color Doppler, harmonic imaging, and recently, speckle tracking. The miniaturization of the probe has subsequently led to live 3D TEE.[10] The technology is now advanced so that the data can be generated in a single heartbeat. A 3D dataset is provided and can be cropped or dissected in any imaging plane, live or offline, using special software. The examination protocol is the same as in 2D TTE, with similar views (eg, left and right parasternal, apical, subcostal, and suprasternal/supraclavicular for TTE[11]; and midesophageal, gastric, and deep transgastric views for TEE) but yielding substantially more information and increased applications, as will be discussed shortly.

Atrial Appendage

Atrial arrhythmias, such as flutter and fibrillation, are commonly referred to an electrophysiologist for cardioversion or ablation. However, both conditions may be associated with left atrial appendage thrombi (right atrial appendage clots are very uncommon) that preclude such procedures because of the risk of embolization and stroke. The current guidelines recommend using 2D TEE to evaluate for the presence of left atrial thrombi in patients with atrial flutter or fibrillation before restoring sinus rhythm.[12] In fact, this is routinely done in clinical practice prior to cardioversion or ablation and is considered standard of care. 2D TEE provides high spatial resolutions of the left atrial appendage, which lies directly in front of the probe in the midesophageal view. One of the limitations of 2D TEE, however, is the inability to visualize all the side lobes of the appendage in some instances, which can lead to falsely interpreting a transverse pectinate muscle as a clot (Figure 8.2).[1] Using a TEE probe with 3D capabilities solves this problem. The disadvantage of this approach, nevertheless, is that 2D TEE is semi-invasive, thus requiring sedation and esophageal intubation, which could be associated with serious complications.[13]

In one of the largest series using 3D TTE to visualize the left atrial appendage, 92 patients had 2D TEE, 2D TTE, and 3D TTE, and the images were interpreted by a blinded observer.[1] Left atrial appendage clot was identified in the

Chapter 8: 3D Transthoracic and Transesophageal Echocardiography • 73

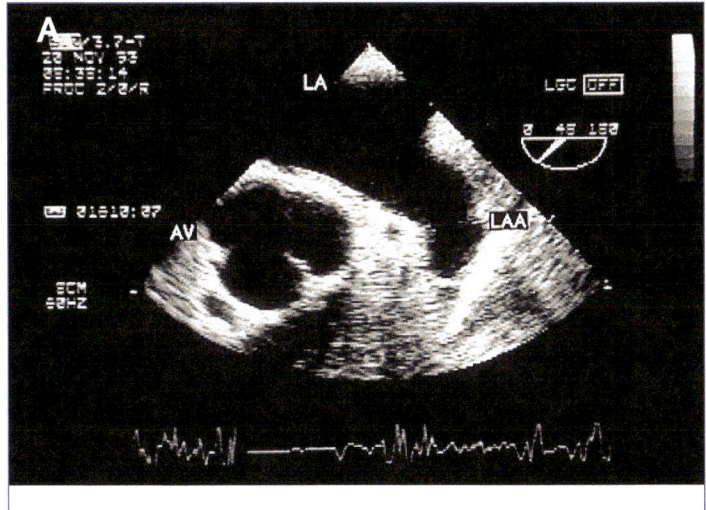

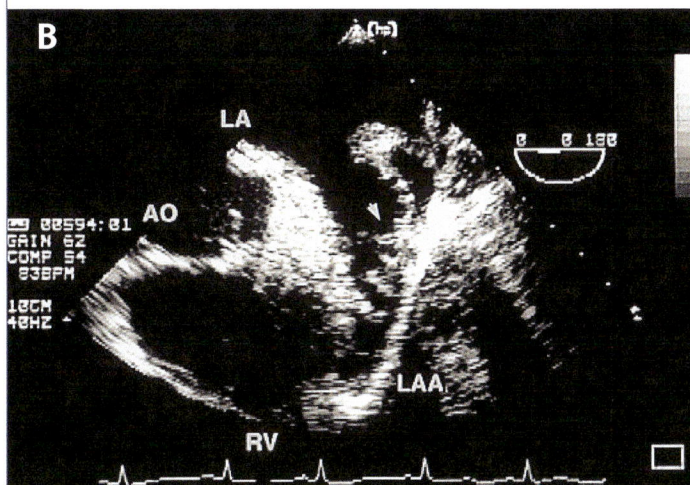

Figure 8.2 Transesophageal echocardiographic examination of the left atrial appendage (LAA) (**Panels A and B**). Aortic short axis view showing the left atrial appendage with (**A**) and without (**B**) pectinate muscles (**arrowhead**). The pectinate muscles are usually transversely oriented and should not be mistaken for clots. AO = aorta; AV = aortic valve; LA = left atrium; RV = right ventricle. Source: Reproduced with permission from Nanda NC, Domanski MJ. *Atlas of Transesophageal Echocardiography*. 2nd ed. Philadelphia, PA: Lippincott Williams & Wilkins; 2007.

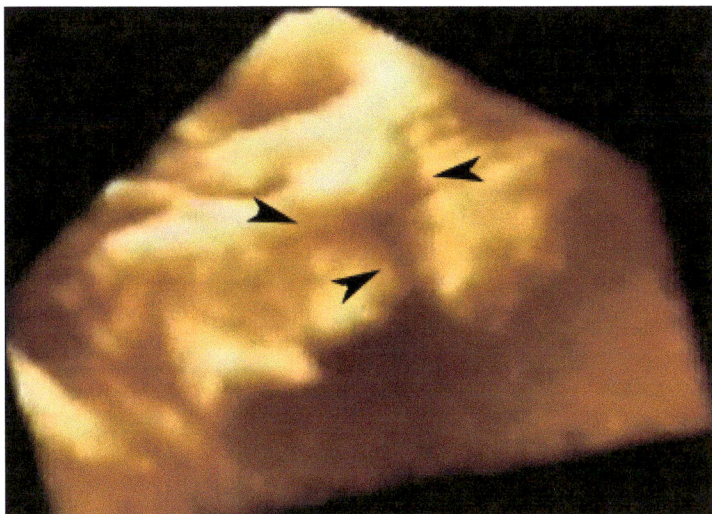

same 7 patients by both TTE studies. However, 2D TEE identified 11 other patients with "clots" that were found to be transversely oriented pectinate muscles by 3D TTE (false-positive rate of 2D TEE 11/85 = 13%). No 3D TEE was done in that study. Also, in 20 patients with atrial flutter or fibrillation in whom 2D TEE was contraindicated, 3D TTE was performed; one patient had a thrombus, while the remainder had none. All 19 patients successfully underwent successful cardioversion or ablation with no complications.[1] Of note, all patients had adequate images and the appendage was well visualized.

The main advantages of 3D TTE are as follows:

1. The ease and feasibility of performing it in a short time;
2. Lack of sedation or need for esophageal intubation;
3. Ability to visualize all lobes of the appendage and cropping them in any plane;
4. Ability to distinguish a clot from transversely oriented pectinate muscles;
5. Quantifying the thrombus size, extent, and volume; and
6. Demonstrating clot lysis by sectioning the clot and viewing echolucencies, as the clot dissolves inside to outside, and determining the time course of lysis (Figures 8.3 and 8.4, A and B).[14]

Using a TEE probe with 3D capabilities offers the same advantages as 3D TTE and with better spatial resolution; however, it requires esophageal intubation and sedation. 3D TTE can also visualize the right atrial appendage (Figure 8.5) using the right parasternal approach, and similarly, TEE can visualize it using midesophageal bicaval view.

Figure 8.3 Live/real-time 3D transthoracic echocardiographic image of left atrial appendage. The **arrowheads** point to individual lobes, as visualized by cropping a 3D dataset of the left atrial appendage. *Source:* Reproduced with permission from Karakus G, et al. *Echocardiogr.* 2008;25:918-924.[1]

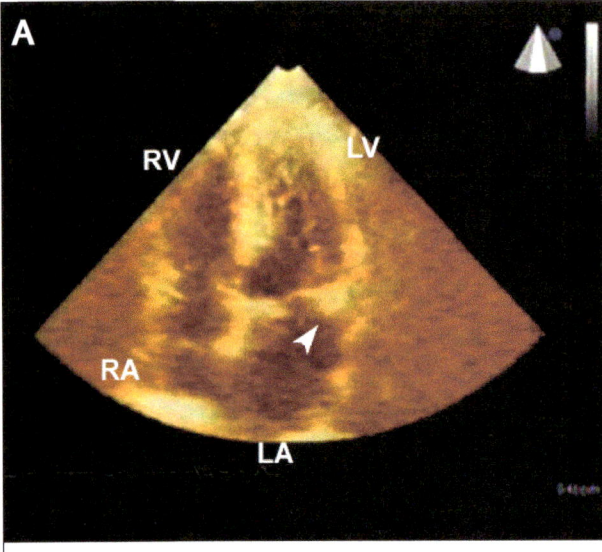

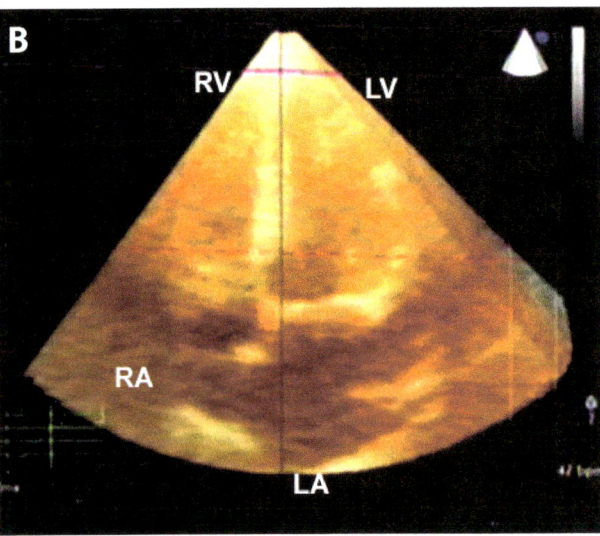

Figure 8.4 Live/real-time 3D transthoracic echocardiogram. **Panel A:** The **arrowhead** points to a thrombus in the left atrial appendage (LAA) with an echolucency in the center suggestive of clot lysis. **Panel B:** Repeat study 54 days later. LAA (magnified) is free of thrombus. LA = left atrium; LV = left ventricle; RA = right atrium; RV = right ventricle. (See Videos 8.1 and 8.2.)

▶ Video 8.1 (Figure 8.4A, Part 1) from another patient shows a thrombus (**arrowhead**) in the left atrial appendage (LAA) viewed in the 2D aortic short axis view. MPA = main pulmonary artery. A similar image is then acquired in 3 dimensions and the thrombus cropped to show absence of clot lysis. ▶ Video 8.2 (Figure 8.4A, Part 2), from a different patient shows 2 prominent linear pectinate muscles (**arrowheads**), which, when viewed in short axis, mimic clots in the LAA. Use of 3D echocardiography with cropping of datasets clarifies their true nature. AV = aortic valve. *Source:* Karakus G, et al.[1]

The current guidelines recommend TEE rather than 3D TTE to assess the left atrial appendage prior to restoring normal sinus rhythm,[12] mainly because limited studies

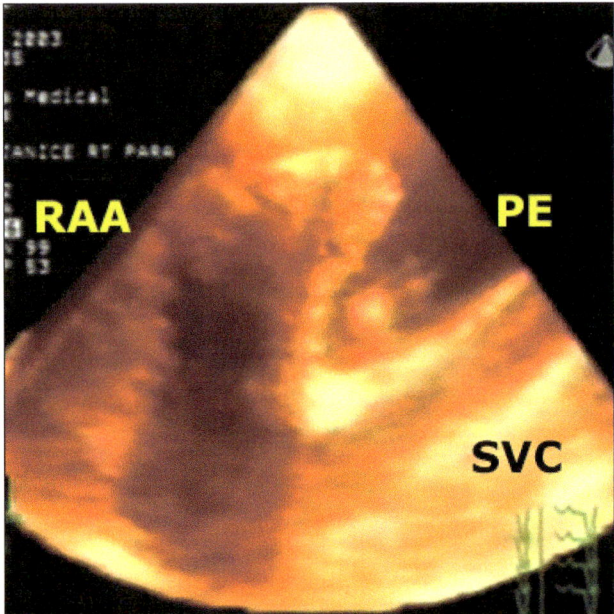

Figure 8.5 Live/real-time 3D right parasternal transthoracic echocardiographic examination of the right atrial appendage (RAA). The RAA and its relationship to superior vena cava (SVC) is demonstrated. ▶ Video 8.3 also shows the relationship of RAA to ascending aorta (AA) and pulmonary artery (PA). The bubble study shows contrast entering the RAA following an intravenous injection. The large echo-free space around the RAA represents pericardial effusion. PE = pericardial effusion. *Source:* Reproduced with permission from Patel V, et al. *Echocardiogr.* 2005;22:349-360.

have been conducted with 3D TTE. With the continuing improvement in 3D TTE acquisition, image resolution, and availability, however, further comparative studies with 2D and 3D TEE will be required to assess whether 3D TTE can be safely used as an alternative noninvasive imaging modality to rule out appendage clot.

In addition to cardioversion, electrophysiologists often perform pulmonary vein isolation and ablation. The procedure requires them to make a transseptal puncture and to guide a catheter through the small interatrial septal defect into the left atrium in order to reach the pulmonary vein ostium. TEE is often used to guide the electrophysiologist when making the transseptal puncture in order to allow direct visualization of the interatrial septum, guide the needle, and avoid aortic-root needle puncture, atrial wall puncture, and subsequent pericardial tamponade.[15]

With the increasing disease burden of atrial fibrillation and associated stroke, the percutaneous closure of the left atrial appendage emerged as a novel technique to prevent a clot from forming in the appendage and subsequently embolizing. This treatment was found to be noninferior to warfarin.[16] The current technique is being used with TEE guidance. TEE allows the operator to visualize the interatrial septum and to guide the transseptal puncture safely, with minimal risk of injuring adjacent structures, particularly the aorta, and to guide a catheter-based delivery system to seal the ostium of the left atrial appendage, and to verify adequate device size, positioning, and stability

(Figure 8.6). It also allows the assessment and early recognition of potential complications such as perforation, leak, device embolization, and pericardial effusion/tamponade.

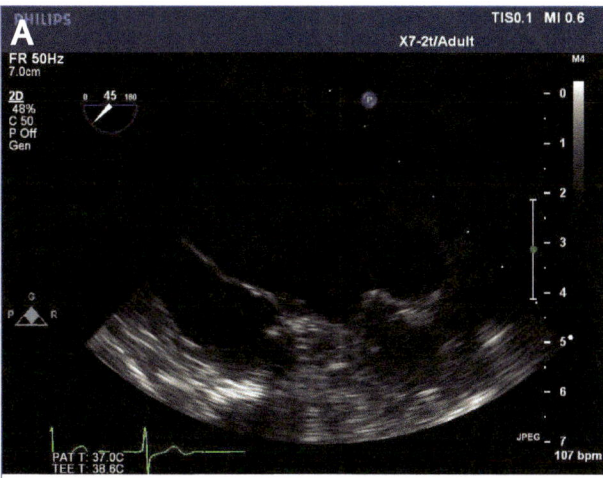
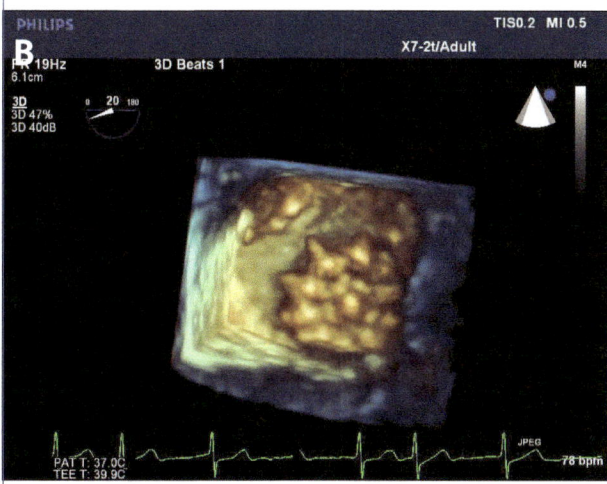
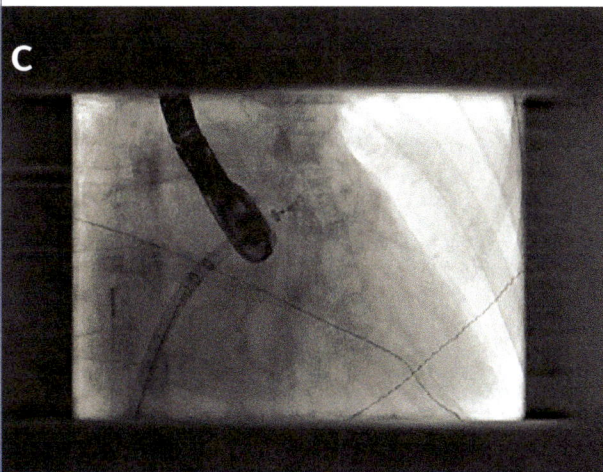

Figure 8.6 Percutaneous closure of the left atrial appendage under transesophageal echocardiography (TEE) and fluoroscopy guidance. **Panel A:** 2D TEE; **Panel B:** live 3D TEE; and **Panel C:** fluoroscopy images of the Watchman device (**arrow**) that has sealed the left atrial appendage.

Cardiomyopathies: Indications for ICD and/or CRT

Left Ventricular Ejection Fraction and Volumes

ICDs are a cornerstone of therapy in patients with cardiomyopathy.[17] The indications for implanting the device evolved from survivors of sudden cardiac death (SCD) to primary prevention in all patients with depressed LVEF.[18,19] Such devices are expensive and not without complications, but they do save lives in well-selected patients. Accurate, reproducible, and unbiased LVEF quantification is hence critical as part of the decision making for implanting an ICD.

2D TTE has several pitfalls for calculating LVEF:

1. It provides 2D views of a 3D structure;

2. LVEF is calculated based on geometrical assumptions that are often invalid; and

3. LV apical foreshortening often leads to inaccuracy.

For many years, clinicians have shifted away from 2D TTE to MUGA scans, and recently, toward cardiac MRI for taking accurate LVEF measurements. While both MUGA and MRI techniques provide robust, semiquantitative means of calculating LVEF, they are not perfect. MUGA scans necessitate the administration of radioactive tracers and are time-consuming, while MRI is contraindicated in some patients, expensive, and requires breath-holding for image acquisition. 3D TTE with live/real-time imaging, coupled with online software analysis, solves most of these problems (Figures 8.7, A and B). It provides a 3D dataset of the LV in one or few cardiac beats, avoiding arrhythmia artifact; it makes no geometrical assumptions; the machine is portable; and there is no radiation exposure or contraindication for the patient.[2,20,21]

Sugeng et al[22] compared LVEF in 31 patients using 3D TTE (Philips 7500 system, 4D-LV analysis software [TomTec Imaging system, Unterschleisheim, Germany]) with cardiac computed tomography using cardiac MRI as a gold standard. LVEF measurement by 3D TTE was accurate (+0.3%; P = 0.68) compared with MRI and underestimated LV volumes by 5 to 6 mL only. On the other hand, computed tomography significantly underestimated LVEF (−2.8%; $P < 0.05$) and overestimated LV volumes by 19 to 26 mL.

In another study, 58 patients underwent both cardiac MRI and 3D TTE (Philips iE33, offline TomTec Echoview version 5.2). LVEF, LV volumes, and LV mass measurements were found to be reproducible, with very low inter- and intraobserver variability (r = 0.95), and correlated well between both techniques ($r > 0.95$), with mild underestimation of LV volume (15 mL) and overestimation of LV mass (8 g) (Figure 8.8, A and B).[23] The main

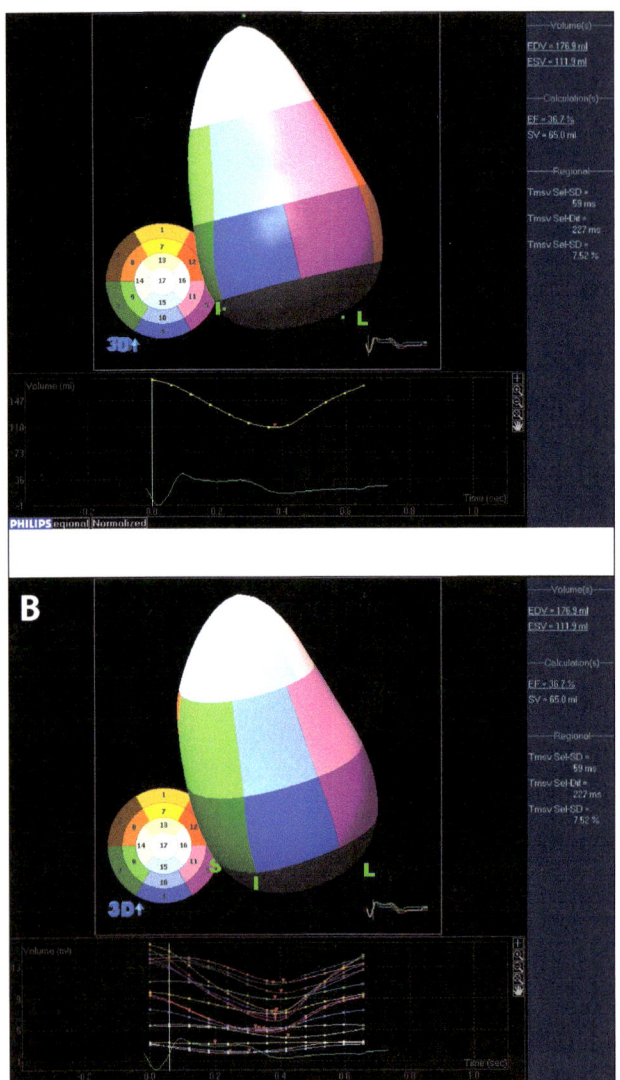

Figure 8.7 Live/real-time 3D transthoracic echocardiographic assessment of left and right ventricular function. **Panel A:** Shows global function in this patient. The LV end-diastolic volume (EDV) is 176.9 mL, end-systolic volume (ESV) is 111.9 mL, stroke volume (SV) is 65.0 mL, and ejection fraction (EF) 36.7%. **Panel B:** Shows segmental volume curves in the same patient. SD = standard deviation.
Source: Reproduced with permission from Nanda NC, et al. *Live/Real Time 3D Echocardiography.* West Sussex, UK: Wiley-Blackwell; 2010:125.

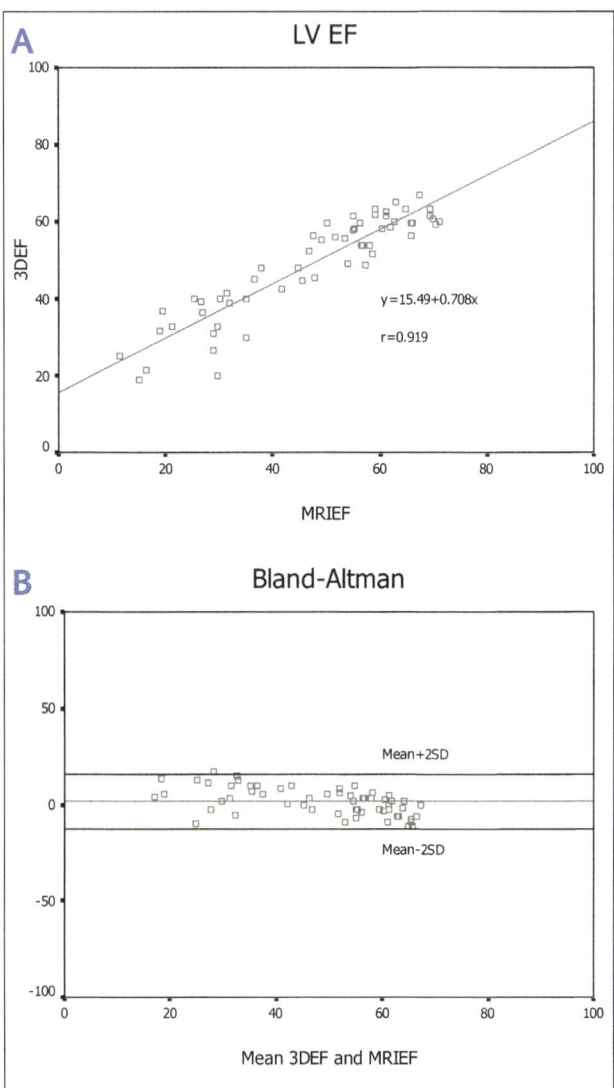

Figure 8.8 Panels A and B: Comparison of live/real-time 3D transthoracic echocardiographic (3DEF) and magnetic resonance imaging (MRI)–derived measures (MRIEF) of left ventricular ejection fraction (LVEF). *Source:* Reproduced with permission from Qi X, et al.[23]

limitation of 3D TTE remains in the setting of patients with poor acoustic windows. While 3D TEE has better spatial resolution and often overcomes a poor acoustic window, it is not routinely used to assess LV function.

Nonischemic Cardiomyopathies

Patients with certain nonischemic cardiomyopathies often benefit from an ICD implantation. These include patients with HCM, LV noncompaction, or ARVD, especially those with certain high-risk features (eg, interventricular septum > 3.0 cm in HCM, runs of ventricular tachycardia, syncope, SCD, or family history of SCD).[17] While 2D TTE often makes the diagnosis and is the current imaging modality of choice, 3D TTE can have additive value.

In patients with or suspected of having HCM, several studies have shown the incremental benefit of performing 3D TTE in order to differentiate HCM from other causes of asymmetrical ventricular-wall hypertrophy or other mimickers of the disease such as athletic heart, sigmoid septum, severe systemic hypertension, or aortic stenosis.[24-26] 2D TTE often misses the apical variant of HCM (also associated with SCD and often seen in Japan but not uncommonly in the United States), and in some cases, does so even with the intravenous administration of echo contrast. However, 3D TTE can visualize the LV apical region, which is almost obliterated in systole, and often makes the diagnosis.[27] LV outflow tract obstruction and systolic anterior motion of the mitral valve are seen in more than 25% of patients and are better defined by 3D TTE, given the live 3D realistic view of the outflow tract.[28,29] Also, the diastolic dysfunction often seen in these patients can be better assessed with 3D TTE, especially after interventions aimed at obliterating the LV outflow gradient.[30]

LV noncompaction is another form of nonischemic cardiomyopathy and is often associated with heart failure, thrombus formation, arrhythmias, and SCD.[31] LV noncompaction is thought to be a consequence of premature arrest of the compaction process during morphogenesis, which results in a thick noncompaction layer on the endothelial layer and a ratio of noncompaction to compaction of 2 or greater. The role of 3D TTE in LV noncompaction includes, to name a few: (1) accurate diagnosis of noncompaction and differentiating it from other mimickers; (2) quantifying the trabeculations; (3) diagnosing right ventricular noncompaction; and (4) identifying thrombus within the trabeculations (Figure 8.9, A and B).[32,33] From an EP perspective, an added benefit of 3D TTE is its ability to accurately diagnose the disease and identify LV clots. Identification of the latter is particularly important, especially prior to defibrillator threshold testing. When cropping the 3D dataset and looking *en face*, the LV noncompaction has a honeycomb appearance, whereas clots appear more echogenic and "gel like" owing to their hypermobility.[32]

Finally, 3D TTE might be particularly useful for diagnosing ARVD. The 3D pyramidal dataset provides a good anatomic view of the right ventricle. It also detects aneurysmal right ventricular wall-motion abnormalities and depressed right ventricular EF, which are major criteria for diagnosing ARVD.[34]

The role of TEE in diagnosing cardiomyopathies remains limited except for patients with poor acoustic windows.

The role of TEE in diagnosing cardiomyopathies remains limited except for patients with poor acoustic windows.

Left Ventricular Dyssynchrony

CRT is currently an effective option for managing certain patients with advanced heart failure that is refractory to optimal medical therapy. Randomized clinical trials have shown that it improves combined cardiovascular end points, reduces rehospitalizations, and significantly improves heart failure symptoms.[35-38] In addition to a depressed LVEF and advanced heart failure symptoms, the current guidelines require that a prospective patient show evidence of electrical dyssynchrony (ie, QRS ≥ 120 milliseconds or left bundle branch block). However, recent studies have shown that the correlation between electrical and mechanical dyssynchrony is only fair ($r = 0.4–0.5$).[39-41] In fact, up to one-third of patients who receive a biventricular-ICD (BiV-ICD) device do not benefit from it.[42,43]

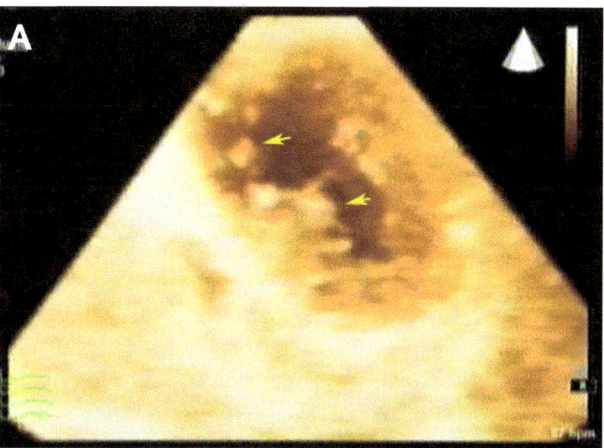

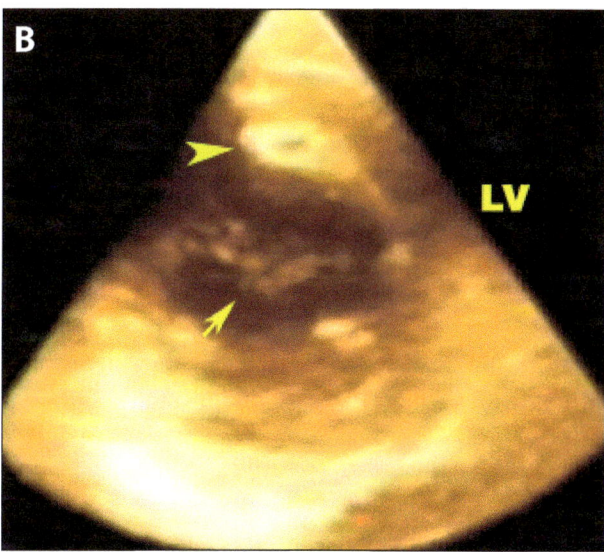

Figure 8.9 Live/real-time 3D transthoracic echocardiography. Isolated left ventricular noncompaction and thrombi in an adult patient. **Panels A and B:** The **arrows** point to multiple trabeculations in LV. In (**B**), one of the echodensities (**arrowhead**) was cropped, revealing a prominent echolucency that is typical of clot lysis. (See also ▶ Video 8.4 and ▶ Video 8.5). *Source:* Yelamanchili P, et al.[33]

Conversely, recent studies have shown that a significant number of patients who do *not* meet the published criteria for a BiV-ICD (eg, those with mild-to-moderate LV dysfunction or right ventricular–dependent pacing) have significant mechanical dyssynchrony.[44,45] In fact, a recent study by Tanaka et al[45] demonstrated that, after CRT, patients with right ventricular pacing have similar mechanical dyssynchrony to patients with left bundle branch block and similar improvement in clinical outcomes. Furthermore, mechanical dyssynchrony indices, obtained from phase analysis of gated single-photon emission computed tomography (SPECT) myocardial perfusion imaging, were recently shown to be prognostic markers in patients with cardiomyopathy.[41]

A large body of literature has assessed mechanical dyssynchrony using various imaging modalities, including echocardiography, radionuclide angiography, phase analysis of gated SPECT myocardial perfusion imaging, cardiac MRI, and cardiac CT.[43,46,47] Echocardiography has the advantage of being a portable, safe, and fast technique that does not involve radiation, especially if serial evaluation and follow-up are required. However, there are many problems with evaluating LV dyssynchrony by 2D TTE. The largest randomized clinical trial, the PROSPECT study, enrolled 498 patients who underwent 2D TTE for the evaluation of mechanical dyssynchrony.[4] Twelve echocardiographic parameters were evaluated based on conventional and tissue Doppler techniques. None of them was predictive of dyssynchrony because of poor reproducibility and wide inter- and intraobserver variability. These echocardiographic parameters were extracted from a 2D dataset and extrapolated to the whole LV, a 3D structure; also, they were influenced by tethering, wall motion, and signal dropout.[4]

The combination of 3D TTE with speckle tracking may be helpful in this regard. Tanaka et al[45] successfully measured 3D speckle radial strain as opposing wall delay on time-to-peak and its standard deviation with a 9% and 8% inter- and intraobserver variability, respectively. The more common parameter of dyssynchrony currently used is the standard deviation of time-minimal systolic volume using a 16-segment model, with 16 milliseconds being the cutoff.[48]

Another advantage of 3D TTE is that it can determine the site of latest mechanical activation (Figure 8.10). In fact, this is critical for optimizing CRT. It is important to place the LV lead at the site of latest activation in order to promote maximal synchrony and derive the maximal benefit. The LV lead is usually placed in the coronary vein at the posterior or lateral wall, wherever it is easier to place. However, in patients with left bundle branch block, the site of latest mechanical activation varies, with 14% being in the inferior wall, 49% posterior, 24% lateral, and 3% apical.[45] Placing the lead at the wrong site would produce suboptimal results and may explain the relatively large proportion of patients who are nonresponders to CRT. In fact, Deplagne et al[49] showed that individual optimization of LV lead placement during CRT under 3D TTE guidance provided an improvement in stroke volume and LVEF.

The technique and dyssynchrony analysis are easy to perform. After acquiring the 3D pyramidal volume, 3D speckle tracking software is applied and the dataset is displayed in 3 short axis views, apical 4- and 2-chamber views, and divided into a 16-segment model. The regions of interest are marked and the software generates the time-strain curves with a different color encoding for every segment. The opposing wall delay in time-to-peak radial strain and time to minimal systolic volumes are determined, along with the standard deviation. Also, the time to mechanical activation is determined for every segment and displayed on a polar map (Figure 8.11).[45]

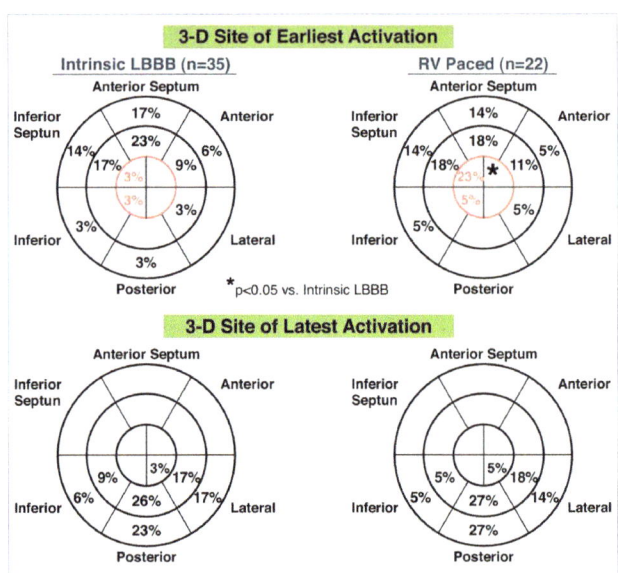

Figure 8.10 3D site of earliest and latest activation by live/real-time 3D transthoracic echocardiography with speckle tracking in patients with LBBB and RV pacing. LBBB = left bundle branch block; RV = right ventricular pacing. *Source:* Reproduced with permission from Tanaka H, et al, Figure 4.[45]

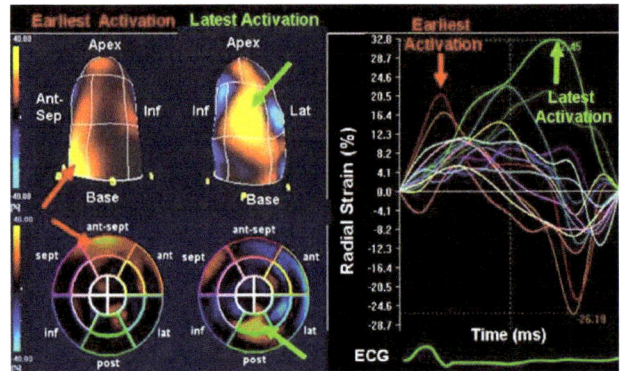

Figure 8.11 Assessment of mechanical dyssynchrony by live/real-time 3D transthoracic echocardiography. **Left panel:** Color-coded 3D strain of the left ventricle and bull's-eye plot; **right panel:** time-strain curves in a patient with left bundle branch block (LBBB). *Source:* Reproduced with permission from Tanaka H, et al, their Figure 5A.[45]

Recently, Sonne et al[46] studied 135 normal subjects using 3D TTE to establish normal values for LV mechanical synchrony and applied these results to 32 patients with dilated cardiomyopathy, half of whom had left bundle branch block and 16 of whom had normal LV function and left bundle branch block. They reported increased LV dyssynchrony in patients with cardiomyopathy, irrespective of the presence or absence of left bundle branch block. Surprisingly, 94% of cardiomyopathy patients with no left bundle branch block had LV dyssynchrony in this study, raising concern by the authors that this measurement may not be clinically useful and that it may directly correlate with LVEF rather than with true dyssynchrony. Nevertheless, the true value of 3D TTE may be in its ability to more precisely measure LVEF than 2D TTE, which serves as a current selection criterion for the placement of CRT. In addition, 3D TTE may be useful for following patients after CRT placement in order to assess their response to therapy. Currently, TEE plays a limited role in assessing dyssynchrony and planning CRT.

One of the main complications of device implantation, unfortunately, is lead infection, which often results in endocarditis and bacteremia and requires device extraction. 3D TTE evaluates the right atrial and ventricular pacemaker or defibrillator leads for thrombus or vegetations (Figure 8.12) and assesses innominate and superior vena cava veins using supraclavicular views (Figure 8.13).[50,51] Similarly, TEE is often required as an alternative imaging technique whenever the acoustic window or images are suboptimal or nondiagnostic with 3D TTE.

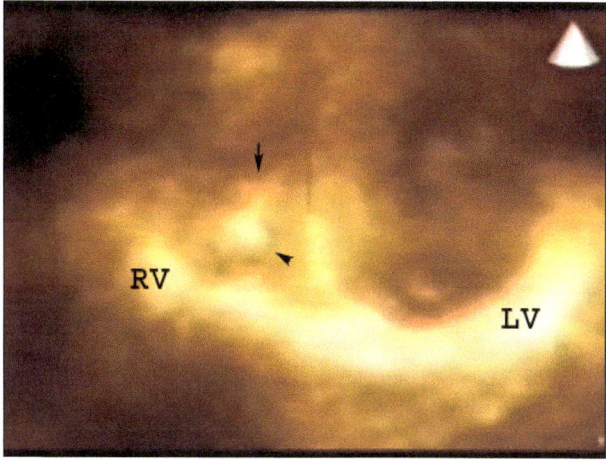

Figure 8.12 Live/real-time 3D transthoracic echocardiographic detection of a vegetation on a pacemaker/defibrillator lead. The **arrows** point to a mobile vegetation on the pacemaker/defibrillator lead in the right ventricle (RV). LV = left ventricle. Source: Reproduced with permission from Pothineni KR, et al. *Am J Geriatric Cardiology*. 2006;15:62-63.

Pericardial Effusions

Cardiac tamponade is a rare but serious complication that may occur in an EP laboratory.[52] Several events can lead to pericardial effusion and tamponade if not treated promptly. These include perforation of the right ventricular apex during ventricular lead implantation or extraction, of the coronary sinus during implantation of an LV lead for CRT, of the pulmonary veins during atrial fibrillation ablation, and of the LV myocardial wall during ventricular tachycardia or Wolff–Parkinson–White syndrome accessory pathway ablation. Although 2D TTE can detect pericardial effusion and tamponade, 3D TTE has the advantages of providing a 3D view in real time, more easily assessing fluid behind the heart, and better guiding the needle during pericardiocentesis.[53] Echogenic material, which is better seen using cropping and multiplane imaging, often indicates hematoma or fibrinous materials (Figure 8.14). This is a helpful tip for distinguishing it from regular effusion, especially in patients who have chronic effusion prior to starting the EP procedure.[53] In addition, ascites is often differentiated from pericardial effusion by the location of the falciform ligament, which is easier to identify with 3D TTE than 2D TTE. Whereas on 2D TTE it appears as a thin structure mimicking a fibrin strand, it is better delineated by 3D TTE and can be viewed *en face* as a sheet of tissue.[54]

For epicardial ventricular tachycardia ablation, a catheter is placed in the pericardial space. 3D TTE can guide the needle to access the space and to position the catheter at the site of ablation, which is easier and safer to perform using a 3D view. Furthermore, 3D TTE has the potential role of guiding the placement of the right ventricular lead at the apex and avoiding perforation in complicated cases.

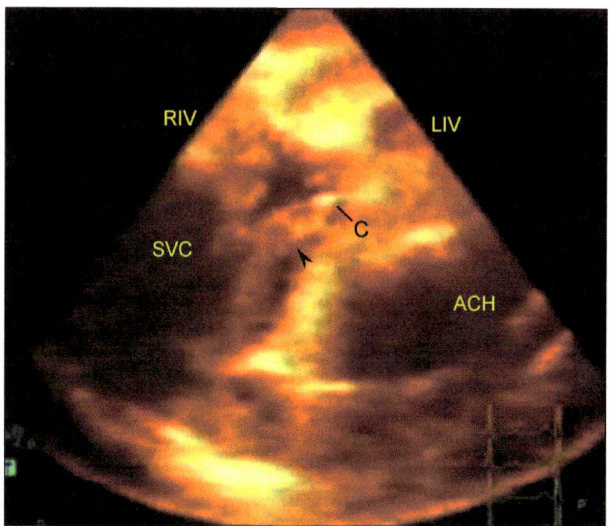

Figure 8.13 Live/real-time 3D transthoracic echocardiographic assessment of thrombus in the innominate vein and superior vena cava (SVC) utilizing supraclavicular approaches. The **arrowhead** points to a portion of the thrombus extending to involve the left innominate vein (LIV). ACH = aortic arch; C = catheter; RIV = right innominate vein. ▶ Video 8.6: The asterisk in the video clip denotes a mobile component of the thrombus, particularly prone to embolization. Source: Reproduced with permission from Upendram S, et al.[51]

Conclusions

In summary, 3D TTE and TEE play a major role in the EP laboratory and can be quite helpful as supplementary tools to 2D TTE. They provide incremental information to that derived from a routine 2D TTE study using the same machine. More recently, 3D TTE has been able to be performed with the same transducer used for 2D TTE and hence does not require switching the transducer. 3D TEE

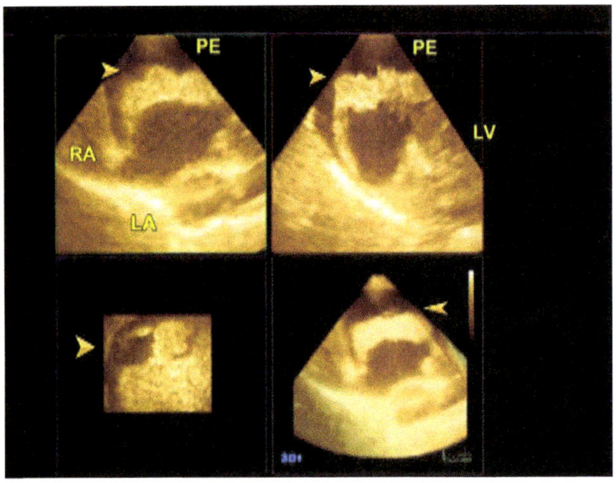

Figure 8.14 Live/real-time 3D transthoracic echocardiography of pericardial effusion in a 64-year-old female. Subcostal examination. The **arrowheads** show multiple fibrin deposits on the right atrial visceral pericardium, resulting in a rugged appearance. LA = left atrium; LV = left ventricle; PE = pericardial effusion; RA = right atrium. ▶ Video 8.7: *Source:* Reproduced with permission from Hernandez CM, et al.[53]

is performed with the same 2D TEE probe in place. They are noninvasive or semi-invasive, portable, widely available, and relatively safe techniques. In the hands of an experienced operator, they both can detect or rule out left atrial appendage thrombus and LV apical clot, and diagnose rare forms of cardiomyopathies. 3D TTE can also quantify LV ejection fraction and volumes, identify responders to CRT, optimize the placement of the LV lead to achieve better synchrony, and guide the needle during pericardiocentesis or access to the pericardial space. On its part, TEE may guide the electrophysiologist during transseptal puncture and left atrial appendage closure.

References

1. Karakus G, Kodali V, Inamdar V, et al. Comparative assessment of left atrial appendage by transesophageal and combined two and three-dimensional transthoracic echocardiography. *Echocardiogr.* 2008;25:918-924.
2. Jenkins C, Bricknell K, Hanekom L, Marwick TH. Reproducibility and accuracy of echocardiographic measurements of left ventricular parameters using real-time three-dimensional echocardiography. *J Am Coll Cardiol.* 2004;44:878-886.
3. Lang RM, Mor-Avi V, Sugeng L, et al. Three-dimensional echocardiography: the benefits of the additional dimension. *J Am Coll Cardiol.* 2006;48:2053-2069.
4. Chung ES, Leon AR, Tavazzi L, et al. Results of the Predictors of Response to CRT (PROSPECT) trial. *Circulation.* 2008;117:2608-2616.
5. Hage FG, Nanda NC. Real-time three-dimensional echocardiography: a current view of what echocardiography can provide? *Indian Heart J.* 2009;61:146-155.
6. Feigenbaum H. Evolution of echocardiography. *Circulation.* 1996;93:1321-1327.
7. Krishnamoorthy VK, Sengupta PP, Gentile F, Khandheria BK. History of echocardiography and its future applications in medicine. *Crit Care Med.* 2007;35:S309-S313.
8. Ghosh A, Nanda NC, Maurer G. Three-dimensional reconstruction of echo-cardiographic images using the rotation method. *Ultrasound Med Biol.* 1982;8:655-661.
9. Salgo I, Bianchi M. Going "live" with 3-D cardiac ultrasound. *Today in Cardiology.* 2002;5.
10. Pothineni KR, Inamdar V, Miller AP, et al. Initial experience with live/real time three-dimensional transesophageal echocardiography. *Echocardiogr.* 2007;24:1099-1104.
11. Nanda NC, Kisslo J, Lang R, et al. Examination protocol for three-dimensional echocardiography. *Echocardiogr.* 2004;21:763-768.
12. Fuster V, Ryden LE, Cannom DS, et al. ACC/AHA/ESC 2006 Guidelines for the Management of Patients with Atrial Fibrillation: a report of the American College of Cardiology/American Heart Association Task Force on Practice Guidelines and the European Society of Cardiology Committee for Practice Guidelines (Writing Committee to Revise the 2001 Guidelines for the Management of Patients With Atrial Fibrillation): developed in collaboration with the European Heart Rhythm Association and the Heart Rhythm Society. *Circulation.* 2006;114:e257-e354.
13. Ellis K, Ziada KM, Vivekananthan D, et al. Transthoracic echocardiographic predictors of left atrial appendage thrombus. *Am J Cardiol* 2006;97:421-425.
14. Duncan K, Nanda NC, Foster WA, et al. Incremental value of live/real time three-dimensional transthoracic echocardiography in the assessment of left ventricular thrombi. *Echocardiogr.* 2006;23:68-72.
15. Earley M. How to perform a transseptal puncture. *Heart.* 2009;95:85-92.
16. Holmes DR, Reddy VY, Turi ZG, et al. Percutaneous closure of the left atrial appendage versus warfarin therapy for prevention of stroke in patients with atrial fibrillation: a randomized non-inferiority trial. *Lancet.* 2009;374:534-542.
17. Epstein AE, DiMarco JP, Ellenbogen KA, et al. ACC/AHA/HRS 2008 Guidelines for Device-Based Therapy of Cardiac Rhythm Abnormalities: a report of the American College of Cardiology/American Heart Association Task Force on Practice Guidelines (Writing Committee to Revise the ACC/AHA/NASPE 2002 Guideline Update for Implantation of Cardiac Pacemakers and Antiarrhythmia Devices) developed in collaboration with the American Association for Thoracic Surgery and Society of Thoracic Surgeons. *J Am Coll Cardiol.* 2008;51:e1-e62.
18. Connolly SJ, Hallstrom AP, Cappato R, et al. Meta-analysis of the implantable cardioverter defibrillator secondary prevention trials. AVID, CASH and CIDS studies. Antiarrhythmics vs Implantable Defibrillator study. Cardiac Arrest Study Hamburg. Canadian Implantable Defibrillator Study. *Eur Heart J.* 2000;21:2071-2078.
19. Moss AJ, Zareba W, Hall WJ, et al. Prophylactic implantation of a defibrillator in patients with myocardial infarction and reduced ejection fraction. *N Engl J Med.* 2002;346:877-883.
20. Jenkins C, Chan J, Hanekom L, Marwick TH. Accuracy and feasibility of online 3-dimensional echocardiography for measurement of left ventricular parameters. *J Am Soc Echocardiogr.* 2006;19:1119-1128.
21. Jenkins C, Bricknell K, Chan J, et al. Comparison of two- and three-dimensional echocardiography with sequential magnetic resonance imaging for evaluating left ventricular volume and ejection fraction over time in patients with healed myocardial infarction. *Am J Cardiol.* 2007;99:300-306.

22. Sugeng L, Mor-Avi V, Weinert L, et al. Quantitative assessment of left ventricular size and function: side-by-side comparison of real-time three-dimensional echocardiography and computed tomography with magnetic resonance reference. *Circulation*. 2006;114:654-661.
23. Qi X, Cogar B, Hsiung MC, et al. Live/real time three-dimensional transthoracic echocardiographic assessment of left ventricular volumes, ejection fraction, and mass compared with magnetic resonance imaging. *Echocardiogr*. 2007;24:166-173.
24. Maron BJ, McKenna WJ, Danielson GK, et al. American College of Cardiology/European Society of Cardiology clinical expert consensus document on hypertrophic cardiomyopathy. A report of the American College of Cardiology Foundation Task Force on Clinical Expert Consensus Documents and the European Society of Cardiology Committee for Practice Guidelines. *J Am Coll Cardiol*. 2003;42:1687-1713.
25. Caselli S, Pelliccia A, Maron M, et al. Differentiation of hypertrophic cardiomyopathy from other forms of left ventricular hypertrophy by means of three-dimensional echocardiography. *Am J Cardiol*. 2008;102:616-620.
26. Bicudo LS, Tsutsui JM, Shiozaki A, et al. Value of real time three-dimensional echocardiography in patients with hypertrophic cardiomyopathy: comparison with two-dimensional echocardiography and magnetic resonance imaging. *Echocardiogr*. 2008;25:717-726.
27. Frans EE, Nanda NC, Patel V, et al. Live three-dimensional transthoracic contrast echocardiographic assessment of apical hypertrophic cardiomyopathy. *Echocardiogr*. 2005;22:686-689.
28. de Gregorio C, Recupero A, Grimaldi P, Coglitore S. Can transthoracic live 3-dimensional echocardiography improve the recognition of midventricular obliteration in hypertrophic obstructive cardiomyopathy? *J Am Soc Echocardiogr*. 2006;19:1190; e1191-e1194.
29. Yang HS, Lee KS, Chaliki HP, et al. Anomalous insertion of the papillary muscle causing left ventricular outflow obstruction: visualization by real-time three-dimensional echocardiography. *Eur J Echocardiogr*. 2008;9:855-860.
30. Hage FG, Karakus G, Luke WD Jr, et al. Effect of alcohol-induced septal ablation on left atrial volume and ejection fraction assessed by real time three-dimensional transthoracic echocardiography in patients with hypertrophic cardiomyopathy. *Echocardiogr*. 2008;25:784-789.
31. Engberding R, Yelbuz TM, Breithardt G. Isolated noncompaction of the left ventricular myocardium—a review of the literature two decades after the initial case description. *Clin Res Cardiol*. 2007;96:481-488.
32. Bodiwala K, Miller AP, Nanda NC, et al. Live three-dimensional transthoracic echocardiographic assessment of ventricular noncompaction. *Echocardiogr*. 2005;22:611-620.
33. Yelamanchili P, Nanda NC, Patel V, et al. Live/real time three-dimensional echocardiographic demonstration of left ventricular noncompaction and thrombi. *Echocardiogr*. 2006;23:704-706.
34. Kjaergaard J, Hastrup Svendsen J, Sogaard P, et al. Advanced quantitative echocardiography in arrhythmogenic right ventricular cardiomyopathy. *J Am Soc Echocardiogr*. 2007;20:27-35.
35. Hunt SA, Abraham WT, Chin MH, et al. 2009 focused update incorporated into the ACC/AHA 2005 Guidelines for the Diagnosis and Management of Heart Failure in Adults: a report of the American College of Cardiology Foundation/American Heart Association Task Force on Practice Guidelines: developed in collaboration with the International Society for Heart and Lung Transplantation. *Circulation*. 2009;119:e391-e479.
36. Cleland JG, Daubert JC, Erdmann E, et al. The effect of cardiac resynchronization on morbidity and mortality in heart failure. *N Engl J Med*. 2005;352:1539-1549.
37. Bristow MR, Saxon LA, Boehmer J, et al. Cardiac-resynchronization therapy with or without an implantable defibrillator in advanced chronic heart failure. *N Engl J Med*. 2004;350:2140-2150.
38. Anand IS, Carson P, Galle E, et al. Cardiac resynchronization therapy reduces the risk of hospitalizations in patients with advanced heart failure: results from the Comparison of Medical Therapy, Pacing and Defibrillation in Heart Failure (COMPANION) trial. *Circulation*. 2009;119:969-977.
39. Trimble MA, Borges-Neto S, Smallheiser S, et al. Evaluation of left ventricular mechanical dyssynchrony as determined by phase analysis of ECG-gated SPECT myocardial perfusion imaging in patients with left ventricular dysfunction and conduction disturbances. *J Nucl Cardiol*. 2007;14:298-307.
40. Trimble MA, Borges-Neto S, Honeycutt EF, et al. Evaluation of mechanical dyssynchrony and myocardial perfusion using phase analysis of gated SPECT imaging in patients with left ventricular dysfunction. *J Nucl Cardiol*. 2008;15:663-670.
41. Aljaroudi WA, Hage FG, Hermann D, et al. Relation of left-ventricular dyssynchrony by phase analysis of gated SPECT images and cardiovascular events in patients with implantable cardiac defibrillators. *J Nucl Cardiol*. 2010;17:398-404.
42. Bax JJ, Bleeker GB, Marwick TH, et al. Left ventricular dyssynchrony predicts response and prognosis after cardiac resynchronization therapy. *J Am Coll Cardiol*. 2004;44:1834-1840.
43. Bax JJ, Abraham T, Barold SS, et al. Cardiac resynchronization therapy: Part 1—issues before device implantation. *J Am Coll Cardiol*. 2005;46:2153-2167.
44. Atchley AE, Trimble MA, Samad Z, et al. Use of phase analysis of gated SPECT perfusion imaging to quantify dyssynchrony in patients with mild-to-moderate left ventricular dysfunction. *J Nucl Cardiol*. 2009;16:888-894.
45. Tanaka H, Hara H, Adelstein EC, et al. Comparative mechanical activation mapping of RV pacing to LBBB by 2D and 3D speckle tracking and association with response to resynchronization therapy. *JACC Cardiovasc Imaging*. 2010;3:461-471.
46. Sonne C, Sugeng L, Takeuchi M, et al. Real-time 3-dimensional echocardiographic assessment of left ventricular dyssynchrony: pitfalls in patients with dilated cardiomyopathy. *JACC Cardiovasc Imaging*. 2009;2:802-812.
47. Russel IK, Zwanenburg JJ, Germans T, et al. Mechanical dyssynchrony or myocardial shortening as MRI predictor of response to biventricular pacing? *J Magn Reson Imaging*. 2007;26:1452-1460.
48. Fang F, Chan JY, Yip GW, et al. Prevalence and determinants of left ventricular systolic dyssynchrony in patients with normal ejection fraction received right ventricular apical pacing: a real-time three-dimensional echocardiographic study. *Eur J Echocardiogr*. 2010;11:109-118.
49. Deplagne A, Bordachar P, Reant P, et al. Additional value of three-dimensional echocardiography in patients with cardiac resynchronization therapy. *Arch Cardiovasc Dis*. 2009;102:497-508.
50. Upendram S, Nanda NC, Mehmood F, et al. Images in geriatric cardiology: live three-dimensional transthoracic echocardiographic assessment of right atrial thrombus. *Am J Geriatr Cardiol*. 2004;13:330-331.
51. Upendram S, Nanda NC, Vengala S, et al. Live three-dimensional transthoracic echocardiographic assessment of thrombus in the innominate veins and superior vena cava utilizing right parasternal and supraclavicular approaches. *Echocardiogr*. 2005;22:445-449.

52. Kim RJ, Siouffi S, Silberstein TA, et al. Management and clinical outcomes of acute cardiac tamponade complicating electrophysiologic procedures: a single-center case series. *Pacing Clin Electrophysiol.* 2010;33:667-674.
53. Hernandez CM, Singh P, Hage FG, et al. Live/real time three-dimensional transthoracic echocardiographic assessment of pericardial disease. *Echocardiogr.* 2009;26:1250-1263.
54. Cardello FP, Yoon DH, Halligan RE Jr, Richter H. The falciform ligament in the echocardiographic diagnosis of ascites. *J Am Soc Echocardiogr.* 2006;19:1074 e1073-e1074.

Video Legends

Video 8.1 (Figure 8.4A, Part 1) Video from another patient shows a thrombus (arrowhead) in the left atrial appendage (LAA) viewed in the 2D aortic short axis view. MPA = main pulmonary artery. A similar image is then acquired in 3 dimensions and the thrombus cropped to show absence of clot lysis.

Video 8.2 (Figure 8.4A, Part 2) Video from a different patient shows 2 prominent linear pectinate muscles (**arrowheads**), which, when viewed in short axis, mimic clots in the LA appendage. Use of 3D echocardiography with cropping of datasets clarifies their true nature. AV = aortic valve. *Source:* Karakus G, et al.[1]

Video 8.3 (Figure 8.5A) Video shows the relationship of RAA to ascending aorta (AA) and pulmonary artery (PA). The bubble study shows contrast entering the RAA following an intravenous injection. The large echo-free space around the RAA represents pericardial effusion. PE = pericardial effusion. *Source:* Reproduced with permission from Patel V, et al. *Echocardiogr.* 2005;22:349-360.

Video 8.4 (Figure 8.9A) *Source:* Yelamanchili P, et al.[33]

Video 8.5 (Figure 8.9B) *Source:* Yelamanchili P, et al.[33]

Video 8.6 (Figure 8.13) The asterisk in the video clip denotes a mobile component of the thrombus, particularly prone to embolization. *Source:* Reproduced with permission from Upendram S, et al.[51]

Video 8.7 (Figure 8.14) *Source:* Reproduced with permission from Hernandez CM, et al.[53]

CHAPTER 9

Intracardiac Echocardiography

Susan S. Kim, MD; Bradley P. Knight, MD;
Robert Schweikert, MD; Sanjeev Saksena, MBBS, MD

Introduction

With the increase in the number and variety of percutaneous intracardiac procedures, as well as the advance in intracardiac echocardiography (ICE) technology, the applicability and utility of ICE are steadily growing. In this chapter, the use of ICE during cardiac electrophysiology (EP) procedures will be discussed. To start, comparison of available ICE technologies and acquisition of baseline images will be discussed. Next, the use of ICE will be discussed for the following procedures: evaluation for the presence of left atrial appendage (LAA) thrombus; placement of percutaneous LAA occlusion devices; transseptal catheterization; and catheter ablation for atrial fibrillation (AF) and ventricular tachycardia (VT). Finally, the integration of ICE imaging with other imaging modalities and with EP mapping will be described.

Currently Available ICE Technologies

Intraprocedural echocardiographic imaging can provide invaluable information during percutaneous cardiac interventions—real-time anatomic information as well as how to best position intracardiac catheters relative to cardiac structures. Given the limitations of both transthoracic and transesophageal imaging, the advent of ICE imaging has made for ready access to echocardiographic imaging during EP procedures.

The types of images available depend on the type of ICE catheter and imaging console used. There are currently three companies that provide ICE catheters (Table 9.1). These catheters can be grouped by mechanism of image acquisition. One company provides a catheter that contains a single transducer element that rotates mechanically 360° (Figure 9.1A), similar to those used in intravascular ultrasound. In this device, there is one large transducer element that emits ultrasound waves at a fixed frequency (9 Hz) and accepts the reflected ultrasound waves, which are ultimately translated into a digital image (Figure 9.1B). Based on this rotational mechanism, a 360° cross-sectional image is produced, with the transducer located in the middle of the image (Figure 9.1C).

The other two companies provide catheters that contain up to 64 transducer elements used to acquire phased-array images. In phased-array imaging, multiple rectangular blocks of ultrasonic elements (piezoelectric crystals) are lined up side by side. The crystals emit individual ultrasound pulses in a sequence that ultimately results in a summative beam whose angle can be steered electronically. This results in a searchlight-like sweep of a fixed area, producing a 90° sector-based image (Figure 9.1D).

84 • Section 1B: Imaging Technology

Table 9.1 Three commercially available ICE catheters and their characteristics

Available ICE Catheters

Ultrasound Method/ Catheter	Size (Fr)	Frequency Range (MHz)	Viewing Sector (degrees)	Depth of Field (cm)	Steering	Doppler and Color Flow?	Cost
Single-element, mechanical rotational (Boston Scientific, Natick, MA)	9	9	360	Up to 5	None	No	+
Phased-array, sector-based (St. Jude Medical, St. Paul, MN) *Viewflex Catheter Viewmate Z Machine*	9	4.5–8.5	90	Up to 21	Anterior/ posterior (120°)	Yes	+++
Phased-array, sector-based (Johnson & Johnson/ Biosense Webster, Diamond Bar, CA) (Siemens/Acuson) *AcuNav/Soundstar Catheter (Siemens or GE Machine)*	8 or 10	5.0–10.0	90	Up to 16	Anterior/ posterior (160°) Left/right	Yes	+++

Source: Adapted with permission from Kim SS, et al, their Table 2.[14]

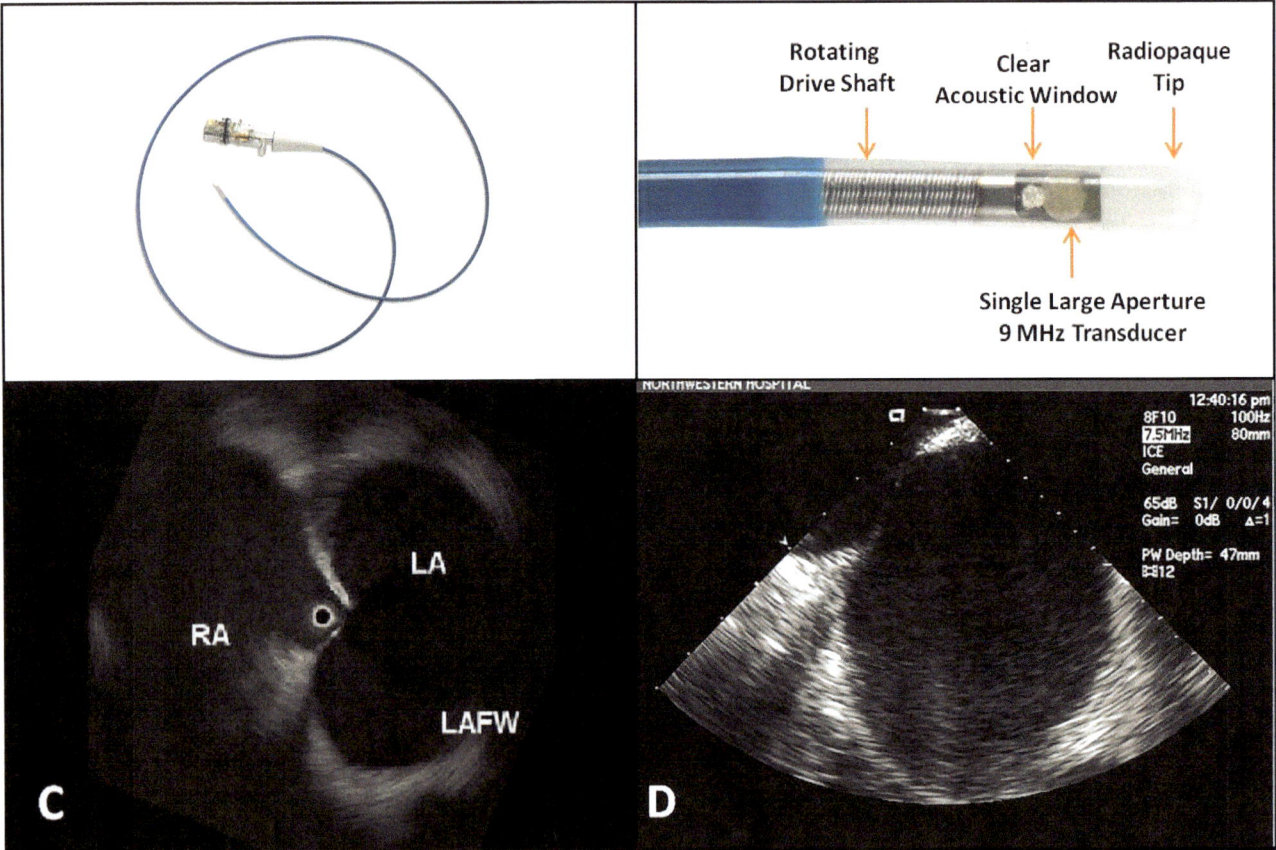

Figure 9.1 **Panel A:** Single-element, rotational intracardiac echocardiography (ICE) catheter. *Source:* Reprinted with permission from Boston Scientific Corp. **Panel B:** Close-up view of the single-element transducer seen in the rotation ICE catheter. Reprinted with permission from Boston Scientific Corp. **Panel C:** Cross-sectional 360° image produced by the rotational ICE catheter seen in panel A. Note the catheter in the center of the image abutting the interatrial septum. LA = left atrium; LAFW = left atrial free wall; RA = right atrium. **Panel D:** 90° sector-based image produced by the phased-array ICE catheter.

While the rotational catheter allows for excellent near-field imaging of the fossa ovalis (FO), which is useful for guiding transseptal catheterization, its absolute depth of field is somewhat limited at 5 cm. In addition, the rotational ICE catheter is not steerable and so requires placement through a long guide sheath. Finally, the rotational catheter does not offer Doppler and color-flow analysis. In contrast, the phased-array catheters allow for imaging up to 16 cm and 21 cm in depth and offer both Doppler and color-flow imaging. Between the two phased-array catheters, there are some differences in size and steering options.

Baseline Image Acquisition Using ICE

A wide range of clinical structures can be well imaged with the ICE catheter. Because the phased-array (as opposed to rotational) catheters are much more commonly used for percutaneous procedures, the subsequent discussion will assume the use of a phased-array ICE catheter.

For procedures to be performed in the atria, imaging can start in the right atrium in the "home" position.[1] Here, the transducer elements are pointed "up," toward the ventral aspect of the patient's body (patient's chest), with no tilt (anterior–posterior or left/right). With the ICE catheter positioned as such in the right atrium, the right atrium, tricuspid valve, and right ventricular inflow region can be well visualized. The imaging depth should be adjusted to allow for imaging to the apex of the right ventricle. This allows one to assess the pericardium at baseline (usually there is trivial to no fluid). In addition, the frequency should be adjusted to a relatively low level (4.5–5 MHz) to allow for optimal far-field imaging. For documentation of baseline anatomy, a clip may be saved of this view.

Next, the ICE catheter can be rotated clockwise 20° to 30°, which turns the plane of imaging leftward and more dorsal relative to the patient. This leads to the next standard view: right atrium, right ventricular inflow, as well as right ventricular outflow tract, and aortic valve and root. Further clockwise torque of ~30° leads to imaging of the right atrium, interatrial septum, left atrium (LA), mitral valve, LAA, left ventricle, and often, the coronary sinus (Figure 9.2, ▶ Video 9.1). In this view, the FO can be seen as a very thin, membranous portion of the interatrial septum. Applying subtle torque further clockwise (~10–15°), the left-sided pulmonary veins can be seen, often as a "pair of pants" (Figure 9.3). The left superior pulmonary vein appears just posterior (clockwise) to the atrial appendage, and care must be taken to differentiate the two. Here, flow rates and patterns in the pulmonary veins can be assessed. In the setting of mitral regurgitation, reversal of flow can be seen in the veins. In addition, baseline flow rates can be assessed and compared with future flow rates to assess for pulmonary vein stenosis. Note that visualization of actual stenosis is challenging with ICE alone and often requires venography for complete assessment.

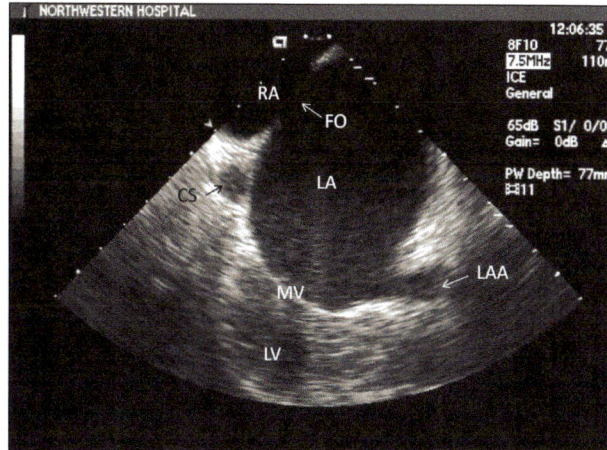

Figure 9.2 ICE image of the left atrium also showing the left ventricle and left atrial appendage. CS = coronary sinus; FO = fossa ovalis; LA = left atrium; LAA = left atrial appendage; LV = left ventricle; MV = mitral valve; RA = right atrium.

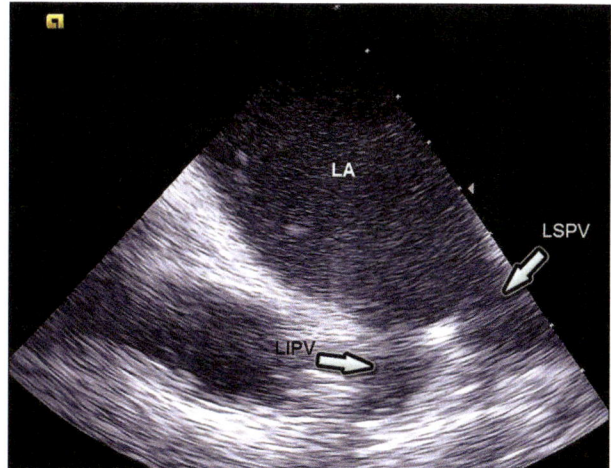

Figure 9.3 ICE image of the left atrium and left pulmonary veins. LA = left atrium; LIPV = left inferior pulmonary vein; LSPV = left superior pulmonary vein.

Torquing the ICE catheter further clockwise brings the posterior LA into view. The descending aorta will also come into view, as will the esophagus. The latter appears as a set of parallel bright stripes running just behind the LA (Figure 9.4). Further clockwise torque will now turn the imaging plane more ventral, in the rightward direction relative to the patient. This will bring the right-sided pulmonary veins into view (Figure 9.5). Finally, further clockwise torque will bring the posterior right atrium into view, followed by the crista terminalis with further clockwise torque. Further clockwise torque will return the imaging plane to the home view.

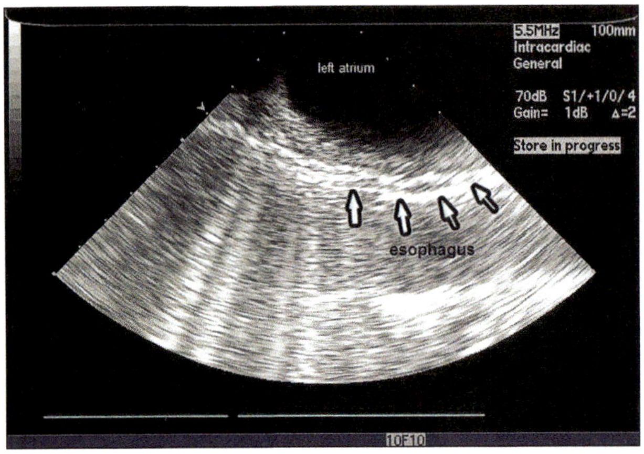

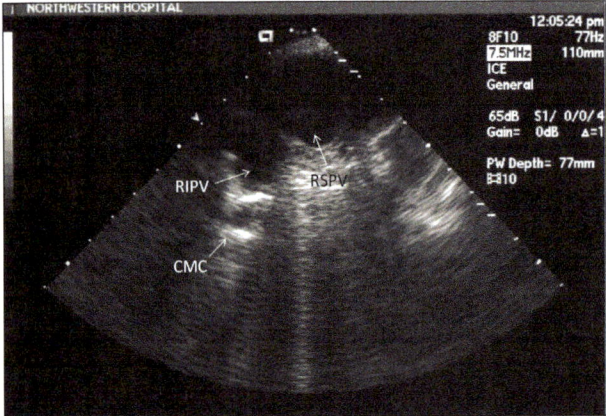

Figure 9.4 ICE image of the left atrium with adjacent esophagus (**arrows**). The esophagus has been highlighted by having the patient swallow carbonated fluid.

Figure 9.5 ICE image of the right-sided pulmonary veins. A circular mapping catheter is positioned within the right inferior pulmonary vein, past the ostium. CMC = circular mapping catheter; RIPV = right inferior pulmonary vein; RSPV = right superior pulmonary vein.

Further imaging of the LA and LAA can be achieved by placing the ICE catheter in the coronary sinus. Further imaging of the left ventricle can be achieved through the coronary sinus as well as the right ventricle.

Use of ICE to Guide Electrophysiology Procedures

Evaluation of Left Atrial Appendage for Thrombus

Before performing procedures in the left atrium (LA), assessment of the LAA for presence of thrombus can be useful. Both anatomic and functional assessment using flow measurements can be performed. For adequate imaging of the LAA, rotational ICE catheters require positioning in the LA through a transseptal puncture; in contrast, imaging of the LAA can be achieved by placing phased-array catheters in the right atrium or right ventricle. For phased-array catheters, to optimize imaging of the LAA, adjustments to depth, ultrasound frequency, and focal length may be made.

With clockwise torque of ~60° to 70° from the home position, the LA and LAA can be well visualized (Figure 9.2). The left atrial cavity is seen as an echo-free chamber with the LAA arising in the inferolateral aspect of the chamber. Because the left superior pulmonary vein often abuts the posterior aspect of the LAA, care must be taken to distinguish these two structures. In most cases, the main body of the LAA should be visualized in the same plane as the mitral valve. With further clockwise torque, the left superior and inferior pulmonary vein ostia can be visualized, oftentimes with the appearance of a "pair of pants." In addition, the LAA may demonstrate ridges of muscle and trabeculation at the base and in the main body.

When assessing the LAA, care must be taken to distinguish these muscle protrusions from actual thrombus. Note that trabeculations commonly occur at the mouth of the appendage and can mimic thrombus in this area. Thrombus is usually seen as a well-circumscribed mass, which can be either sessile and immobile or pedunculated with varying degrees of mobility. If a mass is seen in two or more views, thrombus should be strongly suspected. Examining a mass in varying views can help make the distinction between muscle and thrombus. More commonly occurring than actual thrombus is the presence of spontaneous echocardiographic contrast (SEC), which appears as areas of diffuse, echo-dense swirling within the main body of the LA. When SEC appears, systematic adjustments should be made to levels of gain in order to exclude artifact induced by excessive gain. Once artifact is ruled out, the contrast (which represents a state of low flow) can be graded as more severe (filling the entire cavity, apparent throughout the full cardiac cycle) or more mild (seen in only part of the cavity and/or appearing more intermittently).

Transesophageal echocardiography (TEE) has been the standard imaging modality for assessing LAA thrombus. One study, the Intracardiac Echocardiography Guided Cardioversion Helps Interventional Procedures (ICE-CHIP) study, compared ICE with TEE imaging of the LA.[2] In this study, LA and LAA thrombus was seen infrequently (in 6.9% of patients using TEE, and in 5.2% of patients with ICE), and concordance between ICE and TEE for the presence or absence of thrombus was high: 97% in the LA and 92% in the LAA. Similarly, detection of SEC did not differ significantly in the LA between ICE and TEE (16.9% with TEE, 12.5% with ICE), though TEE detected SEC more frequently in the LAA when compared with ICE (15.7% with TEE, 5.3%

with ICE; $P = 0.005$). Given these findings, ICE should probably be reserved as a complement to TEE for imaging the LA and LAA in order to detect thrombus. Imaging with ICE from the coronary sinus or from the LA directly may obviate the limitations of imaging the LAA from the right atrium. ICE imaging may be considered especially if cardioversion or left atrial ablation is considered.[3]

Of note, in the ICE-CHIP study, all patients with LA or LAA thrombus showed dense or moderate "smoke" in the cavity. Thus, absence of SEC is an important negative finding in assessing thrombotic risk. Low appendageal flow velocities are typically present in patients with thrombus. Thus, a Doppler flow measurement would also have value in assessing risk.

A small study by Blendea et al recently demonstrated that imaging the LAA with an ICE catheter in the LA can correlate well with measurements of the ostium and LAA depth made on computed tomography (CT) and magnetic resonance imaging (MRI).[4] This finding raises the potential for the use of ICE over the use of TEE for procedures such as placement of LAA closure devices.

Transseptal Catheterization

With the increase in the volume of left-sided EP procedures, such as catheter ablation for AF and ventricular tachycardia, transseptal catheterization (TSC) has become a commonly performed procedure. At its inception, fluoroscopy alone was used to guide TSC.[5] With the ready availability of ICE, real-time ICE imaging during TSC has become much more common.

This is not surprising, given that ICE allows for a detailed understanding of intracardiac anatomy and its relationship to catheters and the transseptal apparatus. To start, TSC allows the presence or absence of pericardial fluid to be assessed. In addition, the relationship of the FO to nearby structures, such as the aortic root and the left atrial walls, can be examined. The FO itself can also be characterized in detail in terms of length, thickness, and redundancy. This can be especially useful in the setting of repeat TSC. Also, the presence or absence of a patent foramen ovale can be assessed; its presence is suggested by redundancy in the FO and possibly confirmed with color-flow Doppler imaging.

At the time of TSC, ICE allows for a clearer understanding of the relationship between the TSC apparatus (sheath, dilator, and needle) and the FO. Optimal positioning of the tip within the middle of the FO (in both anterior–posterior and cranial–caudal aspects) can be performed. With ICE guidance, adjustments away from critical structures (eg, the aortic root anteriorly or the posterior wall of the LA) can be made. Also, more-selective positioning of the TSC apparatus (eg, more inferiorly or anteriorly) can be made. Following optimal positioning of the TSC apparatus, the needle can be advanced and "tenting" of the FO appreciated (Figure 9.6, ▶ Video 9.2). This allows for more confidence when applying pressure to the needle (or turning on radiofrequency [RF] for powered needles) for transseptal puncture (▶ Video 9.3). Resolution of tenting and visualization of contrast or saline in the LA allow confirmation of successful crossing (Figure 9.7, Video 9.3).

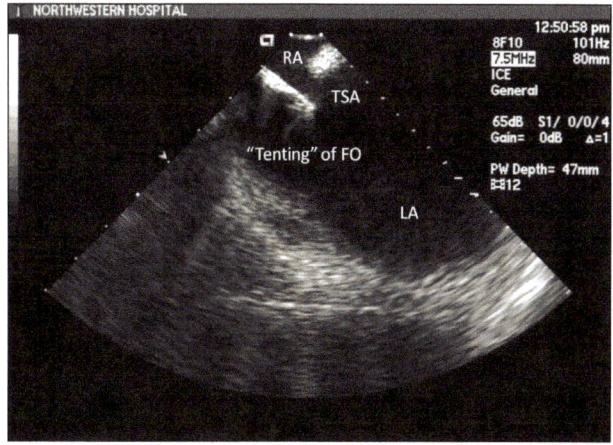

Figure 9.6 ICE image taken just prior to transseptal puncture. The tip of the transseptal apparatus is positioned in the right atrium against the fossa ovalis, resulting in "tenting" of the fossa. FO = fossa ovalis; LA = left atrium; RA = right atrium; TSA = transseptal apparatus.

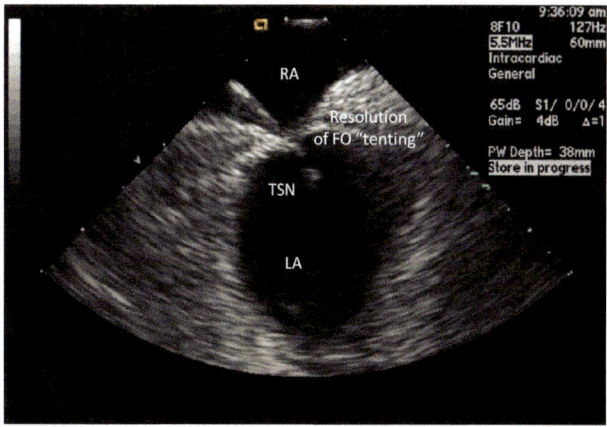

Figure 9.7 ICE image taken just after transseptal puncture. The tip of the transseptal needle is seen in the cavity of the left atrium. The "tenting" of the fossa ovalis has resolved. FO = fossa ovalis; LA = left atrium; RA = right atrium; TSN = transseptal needle.

Finally, unlike fluoroscopy alone, ICE can reveal thrombus on the catheter and sheath, which may allow for its timely removal (Figure 9.8). Clearly, fluoroscopy, angiography, and pressure monitoring remain indispensable to guide TSC; in addition to these tools, ICE has become a remarkably useful tool for guiding transseptal puncture.

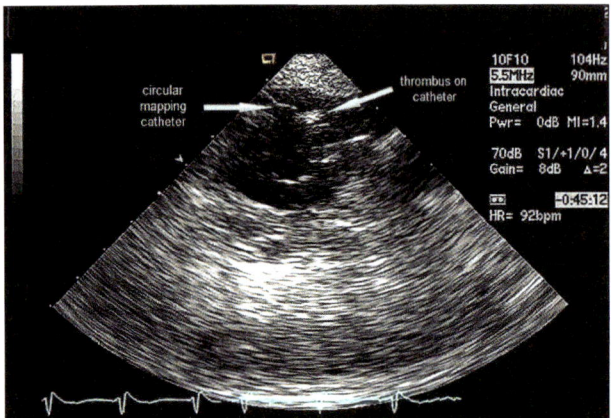

Figure 9.8 ICE image of the left atrium showing a mobile echodensity consistent with thrombus or char on the circular mapping catheter.

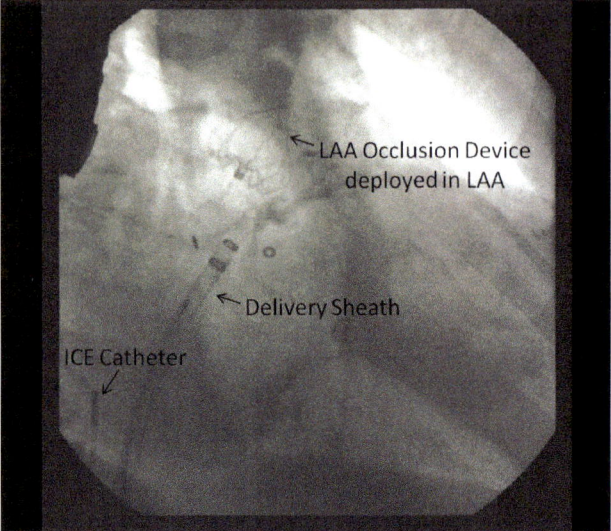

Figure 9.9 Fluoroscopic image of a left atrial appendage occlusion device having just been deployed in the left atrial appendage. The delivery sheath remains in the left atrium. The ICE catheter is seen positioned in the right atrium. ICE = intracardiac echocardiography; LAA = left atrial appendage.

Percutaneous Left Atrial Appendage Occlusion

With its tendency to cause bleeding, anticoagulation can pose an unacceptable risk for some patients with AF. However, thromboembolic risk in these patients remains. Given that about 90% or more of thrombi formed in patients with atrial fibrillation (AF) arise in the LAA, LAA occlusion devices are being investigated as possible alternatives for thromboembolic risk reduction in patients with AF.[6,7]

One device is a self-expanding nitinol frame covered with a permeable membrane designed to occlude the ostia of the LAA. The devices are inserted percutaneously through the femoral vein, across the interatrial septum via transseptal puncture, and into the LAA (Figure 9.9, ▶ Video 9.4). In addition to preoperative CT and intraprocedural fluoroscopy, angiography, and TEE, ICE can be utilized during these procedures. These modalities are used to rule out LAA thrombus and to evaluate the size, shape, and orientation of the LAA ostium (in conjunction with a preoperative CT). TEE is further utilized to guide device deployment: assessing proper positioning and orientation pre- and post-deployment as well as assessing the degree of occlusion postdeployment.

Currently, the use of ICE has been limited primarily to guiding TSC. One study, however, compared ICE with TEE in patients undergoing LAA occlusion device placements.[8] In this study, 10 patients undergoing placement of the Percutaneous Left Atrial Appendage Transcatheter Occlusion system (PLAATO) device (ev3 Inc./Covidien, Plymouth, MN) underwent imaging with both ICE and TEE during deployment. The images were found to be reasonably comparable, particularly when ICE imaging was performed closer to the LAA, either from the coronary sinus or a left-sided pulmonary artery. The presence or absence of LAA thrombus and LAA ostial dimensions were imaged comparably with ICE and TEE. A second study demonstrated a strong correlation between LAA ostial dimensions and depth with the ICE catheter placed in the LA, compared with CT and MRI.[4]

To date, the data to support the use of ICE alone, without TEE, for LAA occlusion procedures are limited. However, with the elimination of an additional two operators (the echocardiographer and anesthesiologist), the use of ICE alone could significantly streamline the procedure.

Coronary Sinus Lead Placement

ICE was initially described as an aid in gaining access to the coronary sinus.[9] More recently, it has been described as a tool with further capabilities: to guide lead placement as well as assess the impact of pacing modes and optimize atrioventricular and right–left ventricular timing delays. In addition to direct measurement of left ventricular systolic function, flow across the aortic valve has been used to quantify the response to various pacing locations and programmable pacing parameters.[10] More recently, intraprocedural quantification of left ventricular dyssynchrony with vector velocity imaging (VVI) was used to guide LV lead position and device programming.[11] In this study of 104 patients undergoing either ICE/VVI–guided versus conventional LV lead placement, ICE/VVI guidance appeared to predict response and was associated with a higher number of cardiac resynchronization device (CRT) responders.

Use of ICE During Catheter Ablation

Image Integration/ICE Fuse with Electrophysiological Mapping

With the advent of increasingly more complex ablation procedures, three-dimensional (3D) electroanatomic mapping systems (EAMSs) have become an essential tool for orientation, mapping, and lesion delivery. Initially, EAMS relied on real-time chamber reconstruction based on acquiring information from a mapping catheter. Then, software was developed to allow this real-time map to be merged with a computed tomogram or MRI obtained days prior to the procedure and imported into the EAMS. This image fusion allowed for a more detailed and nuanced map of the chamber of interest. However, because the images (real-time chamber reconstruction versus CT/MRI) were obtained at different times (and potentially, during different cardiac rhythms and hemodynamic states), there was the potential for anatomic differences between the two images and a less than ideal match. In addition, the preprocedure imaging ultimately led to increases in contrast exposure and, potentially, to increases in ionizing radiation exposure for the patient.

The next step in EAMS enhancement has been the development of ICE-based 3D chamber reconstruction. With this technique, multiple two-dimensional (2D) ICE images are acquired in multiple planes throughout the chamber of interest (eg, for the LA: mitral-valve plane with LAA, left-sided pulmonary veins, posterior LA with aorta and/or esophagus, and right-sided pulmonary veins). Images are acquired from the right atrium because acquisition from the LA has been found to be slightly less optimal.[12] Next, critical structures are outlined and labeled in each plane; the images are then combined to create a 3D chamber, with the real-time shell created using the mapping catheter or the preprocedure CT/MRI image (Figure 9.10, ◎ Video 9.5). This allows for an improved real-time understanding of the anatomy and the relationship between the catheter and the lesions delivered to the chamber of interest. Use of real-time 3D ICE imaging, merged with the image created with the mapping catheter alone, may obviate the need for a preprocedure CT/MRI, potentially decreasing contrast and radiation exposure for the patient. An ideal next step for ICE imaging would be direct, real-time 3D imaging that eliminated the need for tracing structures and acquiring multiple 2D images. This advance would significantly decrease the time required for this portion of the procedure.

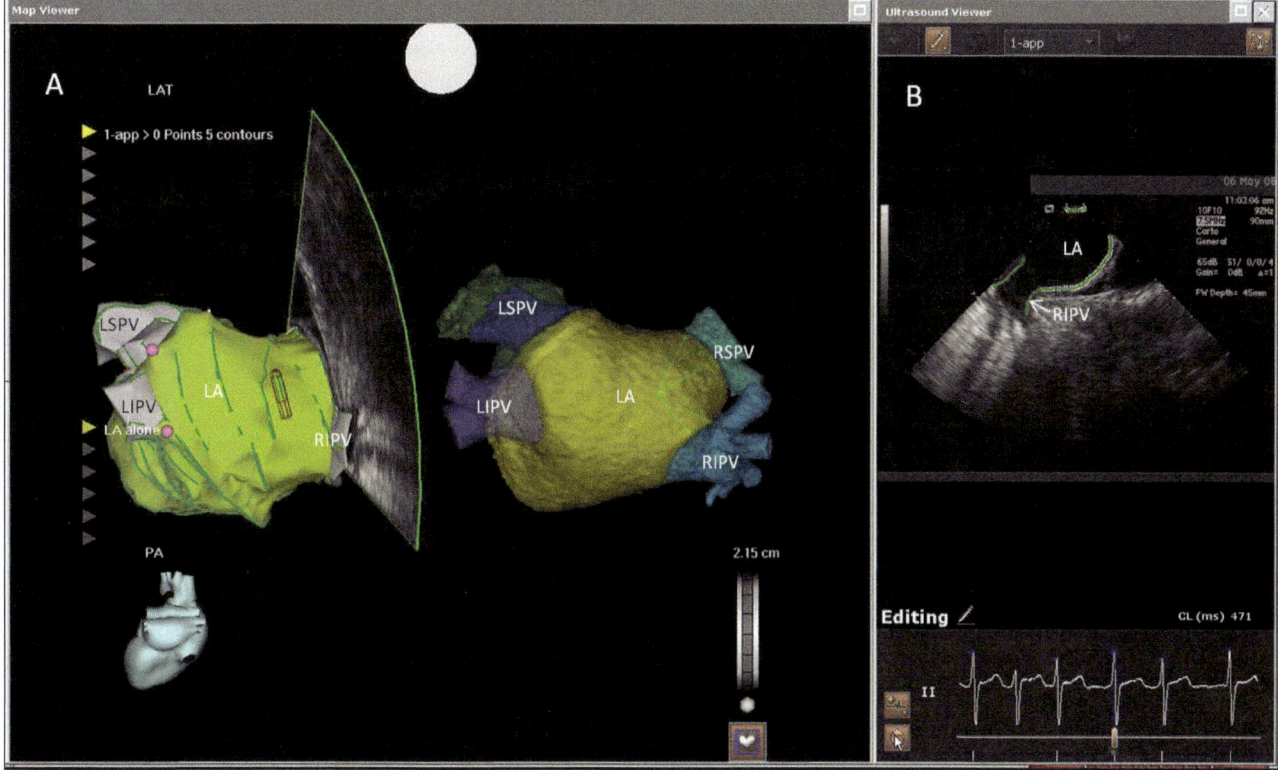

Figure 9.10 **Panel A:** The image at **left** shows the 3D composite of outlines acquired from various 2D ICE views. An example of one such ICE view is seen in **Panel B**. The image at **right** in **Panel A** shows the preprocedural computed tomogram of the LA, which can be merged with the composite ICE image (see Video 9.5). LA = left atrium; LIPV = left inferior pulmonary vein; LSPV = left superior pulmonary vein; RIPV = right inferior pulmonary vein, RSPV = right superior pulmonary vein.

Use of ICE During Catheter Ablation for Atrial Fibrillation and Ventricular Tachycardia

ICE has become an important tool for performing catheter ablation procedures in the EP laboratory. This importance reflects the emergence of anatomic and substrate-based techniques for catheter ablation of a variety of complex cardiac arrhythmias. The most common use of ICE in this regard has been with catheter ablation of AF; however, ICE has also been useful for other complex arrhythmias that are targeted anatomically, such as atypical atrial flutters and ventricular arrhythmias.[13-15] Previously, anatomic information was derived from preprocedural imaging such as cardiac CT, which did not provide real-time information. Fluoroscopy provides real-time imaging but lacks anatomic detail, and the addition of intravenous contrast for angiography is still inferior to the detail provided by ICE. Angiography does not provide ongoing real-time images and is associated with exposure to the potentially toxic effects of the intravenous contrast agent and that of the radiation. ICE lessens or potentially avoids the patient's exposure to radiation and intravenous contrast and can be used to monitor other aspects of the procedure, such as complications (eg, pericardial effusion and thrombus formation). There have been reports of using ICE for catheter ablation of AF without the need for any fluoroscopy.[16] More recently, as noted above, technology has been developed to acquire 3D ICE images and then "merge" such images with other 3D imaging, such as electroanatomical mapping systems, cardiac CT, and so forth.

ICE imaging has several potential applications within the catheter ablation of AF. In fact, some techniques for catheter ablation of AF utilize ICE imaging in a fundamental role.[17,18] Multiple aspects and stages of the AF catheter ablation procedure can be guided by ICE imaging, including the following:

- Making the transseptal puncture(s)
- Evaluating cardiac anatomy (including structure, dimensions, and function)
- Evaluating for intracardiac abnormalities (such as thrombus in the LAA)
- Monitoring locations of transseptal sheaths and catheters
- Monitoring the ablation catheter–tissue interface
- Assessing for complete pulmonary vein occlusion during cryoballoon ablation
- Visualizing adjacent extracardiac structures
- Monitoring for complications such as pericardial effusion
- Performing a color Doppler assessment of blood flow in various regions, including the pulmonary veins, cardiac valves, LAA, and across the interatrial septum.

As discussed previously in this chapter, ICE can be quite useful for guiding transseptal punctures—a potentially challenging portion of any procedure that requires LA instrumentation. The challenge can be greater for the AF patients, owing to several factors: ongoing tachycardia, the advanced age of many such patients, and the fact that many patients are undergoing a repeat procedure and the septum has become resistant to puncture on account of scar tissue from previous transseptal procedures. Moreover, many centers are performing AF catheter ablation without interrupting oral anticoagulation (eg, warfarin),[19] which lessens the tolerance for any misplaced puncture attempts. Similarly, some operators prefer to administer heparin intravenously just prior to making transseptal punctures in order to lessen the chance of thrombus formation on the transseptal sheaths once they are positioned across the septum into the LA. Under such circumstances, avoidance of puncturing the posterior wall or roof of the atrium or aorta becomes critically important.

Another advantage of ICE imaging for transseptal puncture is the ability to puncture specific regions of the septum to achieve the most advantageous point at which to cross the septum for that particular type of procedure or technique. Depending upon the tools and techniques used, decisions can be made regarding crossing points on the septum both superiorly to inferiorly and posteriorly to anteriorly. For example, some operators find it best to avoid puncturing the septum too far anteriorly, as this can make it difficult to reach the right inferior pulmonary vein. A suitably posterior puncture site is one in which the transseptal puncture site is visualized in the same imaging plane as the left pulmonary veins (Figure 9.11).

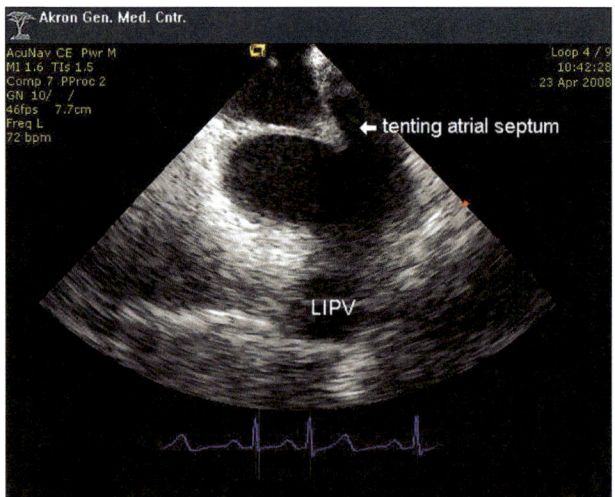

Figure 9.11 ICE image of the atrial septum, left atrium, and proximal left pulmonary veins during transseptal puncture. Note the transseptal sheath apparatus tenting the atrial septum with the left pulmonary veins in the same imaging plane to help cross the septum sufficiently posteriorly. LIPV = left inferior pulmonary vein.

Another application of ICE in the catheter ablation of AF (and perhaps, for some techniques, the most valuable) is the ability to visualize the proximal portions of the pulmonary veins, including delineation of the vestibule or so-called antrum proximal to the pulmonary vein. Regardless of the various tools and techniques used for catheter ablation of AF, uniform consensus holds that delivering ablation lesions within the pulmonary veins should be avoided owing to risk for subsequent stenosis.[20] In this regard, phased-array ICE technology provides a distinct advantage over radial imaging technology because the proximal portions of all the pulmonary veins can be readily visualized with the ICE catheter positioned only in the right atrium, not needing to be placed into the chamber of interest (Figures 9.3 and 9.12). As shown in the figures, longitudinal views of the various left and right pulmonary veins can be achieved by manipulating the phased-array ICE catheter within the right atrium. Such ICE guidance can be helpful for positioning not only a circular mapping catheter but also for balloon-based ablation systems.[21] Proper positioning of the balloon outside the tubular portion of the pulmonary vein remains important, and proper contact of the balloon can be readily assessed using ICE color Doppler imaging (Figure 9.13).

ICE imaging can be valuable for monitoring complications during interventional EP procedures, where rapid detection and treatment might be crucial. This is particularly true for catheter ablation of AF, which typically involves a high degree of anticoagulation, and for procedures done in some centers without interrupting oral anticoagulation therapy such as with warfarin. Under such circumstances, cardiac perforation leading to pericardial effusion and tamponade needs to be discovered early and treatment instituted immediately to avert a life-threatening crisis. The phased-array ICE probe can be very quickly manipulated to obtain views of the left ventricle and surrounding pericardium, thereby rapidly assessing for the presence of a pericardial effusion (Figure 9.14). This is very useful during the ablation procedure, as it is not infrequent to encounter transient hypotension (such as due to sedative or anesthetic agents), and so a quick look at the pericardial space without evidence of effusion is reassuring to everyone. On the other hand, if an effusion is present, the diagnosis has been made quickly and proper measures can be implemented immediately (Figure 9.15).

ICE imaging can also detect other complications during interventional EP procedures, such as thrombus or char formation on the catheters or intravascular sheaths[17,22] (Figure 9.8). Additionally, limited views of the esophagus can be obtained with ICE imaging (Figure 9.4), and with other measures, this could potentially be useful for avoiding ablation-related damage to this structure.[17,22,23]

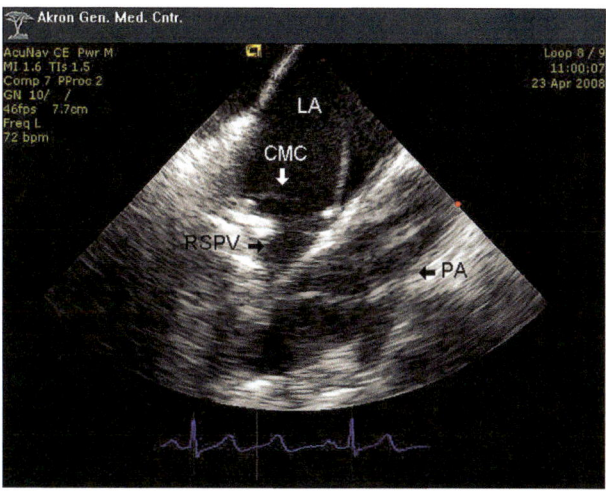

Figure 9.12 ICE image of the left atrium demonstrating the circular mapping catheter at the antrum of the right superior pulmonary vein. CMC = circular mapping catheter; LA = left atrium; PA = pulmonary artery; RSPV = right superior pulmonary vein.

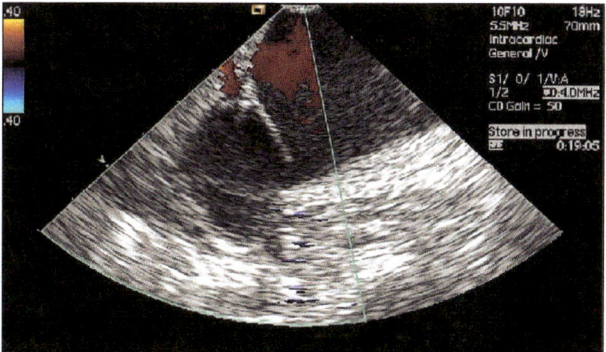

Figure 9.13 Color Doppler ICE image showing balloon-based ablation system (**light black arrows**) occluding right inferior pulmonary vein (**heavy black arrow**). LA = left atrium; RIPV = right inferior pulmonary vein.

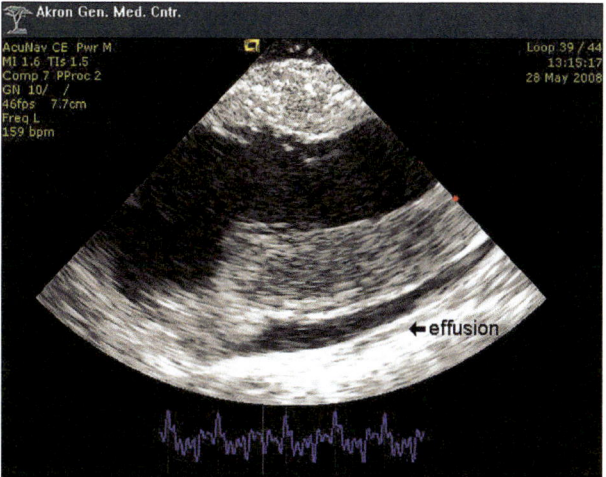

Figure 9.14 ICE image of the left ventricle in longitudinal view, demonstrating a pericardial effusion that appears as a hypoechoic region outside the ventricular myocardium (**arrow**). This image was obtained by retroflexion of the ICE catheter and positioning the catheter across the tricuspid valve and partially within the right ventricle.

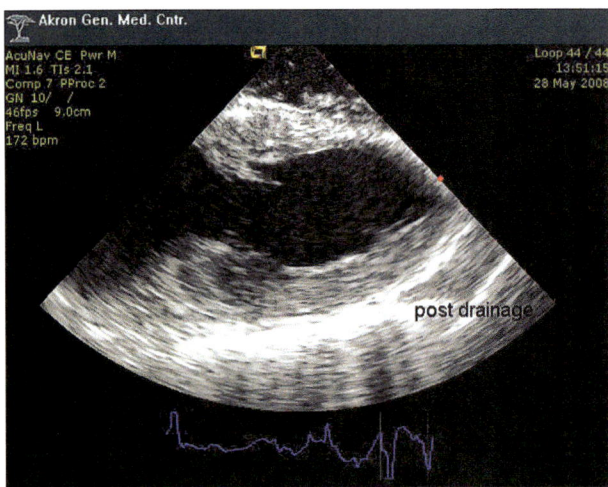

Figure 9.15 The same patient as in Figure 9.14, after percutaneous drainage of the pericardial effusion.

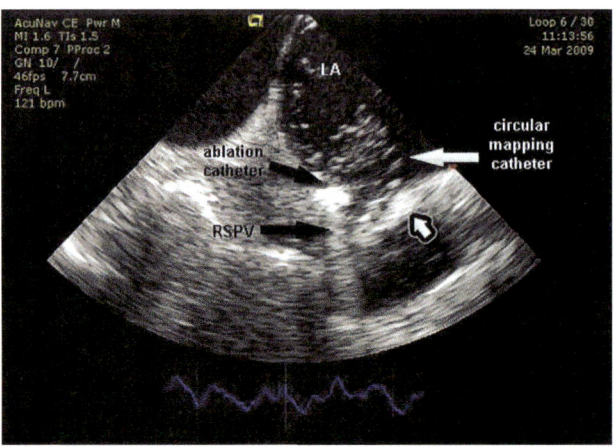

Figure 9.16 ICE image of circular mapping catheter at the right superior pulmonary vein (**large arrow**) and an open-irrigation ablation catheter delivering an ablation lesion at the inferior aspect of the vein. The tissue at the superior aspect of the vein (**small arrow**) has already been ablated with resultant increased echogenicity of the tissue. LA = left atrium; RSPV = right superior pulmonary vein.

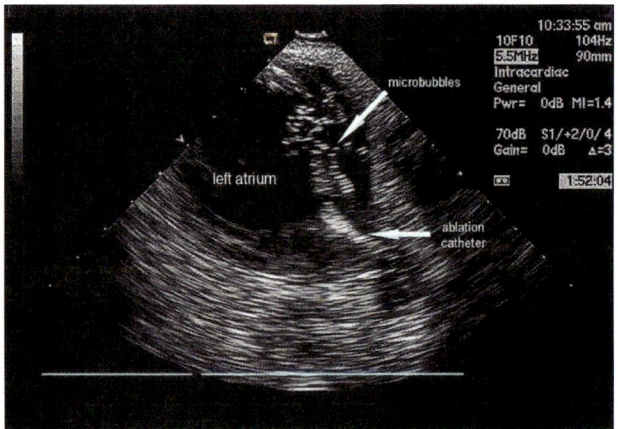

Figure 9.17 ICE image of the left atrium and left pulmonary veins with circular mapping catheter at the left superior pulmonary vein. Ablation is being performed at the left superior pulmonary vein, with formation of microbubbles indicating tissue overheating.

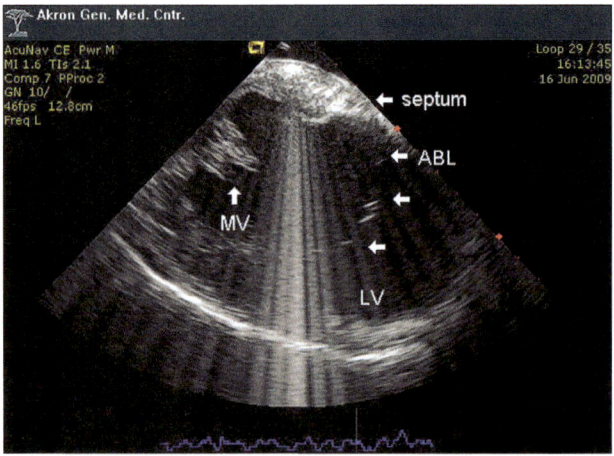

Figure 9.18 Longitudinal ICE image of the left ventricle showing myocardial scar involving the mid- to distal septum. ABL = ablation catheter; LV = left ventricle; MV = mitral valve.

ICE imaging is capable of visualizing the positions of various catheters within the chamber of interest, including the mapping/ablation catheter itself. The ablation catheter–tissue interface can be visualized, and this can be helpful for assessing catheter contact with the tissue and lesion formation within the tissue (Figure 9.16). Although not as prevalent at many centers (owing to the advent of open-irrigation ablation systems), for those operators using conventional nonirrigated or internally cooled ablation systems, monitoring the catheter–tissue interface can still be valuable. There is evidence that "microbubble" formation indicates overheating of the tissue, and such overheating can increase the risk for tissue explosion, char, and/or thrombus formation as well as damage to adjacent structures (Figure 9.17).[23-25] The use of ICE to monitor for such microbubble formation and to titrate power delivery in order to avoid it has been described and used effectively. One study demonstrated less esophageal heating with such a technique.[23]

Similarly, ICE imaging can be useful for catheter ablation of ventricular arrhythmias.[22,26–28] Many of the applications of ICE described above for the LA also apply to procedures targeting the left ventricle. This procedure can also utilize a transseptal approach, so the guidance of the transseptal puncture with ICE can be valuable, as described above. As with other ablation procedures, ICE can help visualize the catheters and the catheter–tissue interface, provide information regarding the characteristics of lesion formation, and monitor for complications, as outlined above. For left ventricular ablation procedures in particular, ICE can provide important anatomic information. ICE can identify regions of myocardial scar or aneurysm that represent the arrhythmogenic substrate (Figure 9.18). Additionally, ICE can identify the presence and location of papillary muscles, which can complicate the mapping process by mimicking inadequate tissue contact with the chamber wall (Figure 9.19).

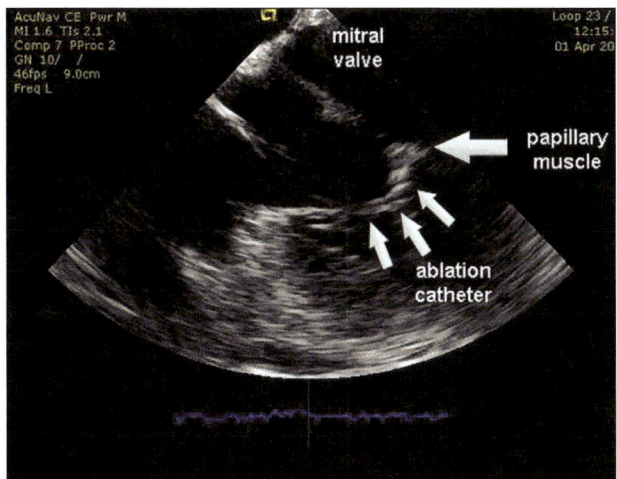

Figure 9.19 Longitudinal ICE image of the left ventricle showing the ablation catheter across the mitral valve with its tip at the papillary muscle.

ICE can also be valuable for mapping and catheter ablation of the variant of outflow tract ventricular arrhythmias that arise from the coronary cusps. Not uncommonly, mapping and ablation of such arrhythmias must be performed within the coronary cusp near the origin of the coronary arteries. ICE images can identify the coronary cusps and the origins of the coronary arteries and help guide the mapping/ablation catheter to perhaps avoid damaging such structures (Figures 9.20 and 9.21).[28] As demonstrated by the images, ICE provides the operator with excellent anatomic information regarding not only the target ablation site but also adjacent structures.

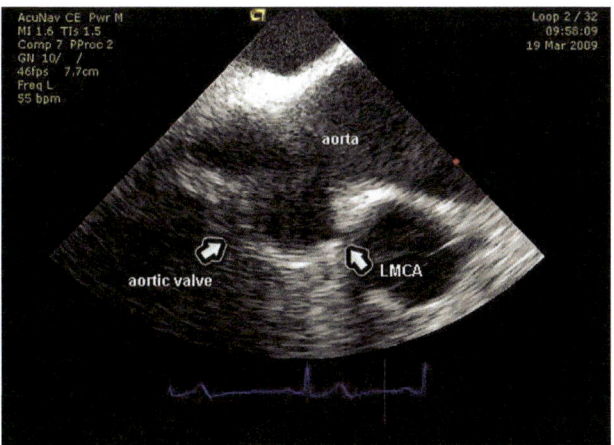

Figure 9.20 ICE image of the aortic valve and proximal aorta in longitudinal view. Note the left main coronary artery (LMCA) arising from the left coronary cusp.

More recently, further advances in ICE imaging technology have had a direct application to the performance of complex arrhythmia catheter ablation procedures. The use of 3D ICE imaging and the ability to integrate such images into other imaging modalities, such as cardiac CT and computerized EP mapping systems, have become a reality.[14,29,30] Such developments, discussed in further detail elsewhere in this chapter, will provide more powerful tools for the interventional electrophysiologist involved in complex catheter ablation procedures.

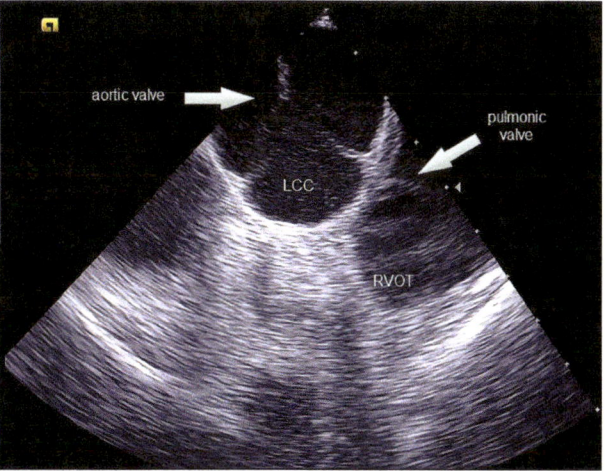

Figure 9.21 ICE image of the aortic valve in cross-sectional view. Note the close anatomic relationship of the coronary cusps, particularly the left coronary cusp (LCC), to the right ventricular outflow tract (RVOT).

Three-dimensional Imaging with ICE

While standard 2D ICE has become an invaluable tool in the EP laboratory, its use is somewhat limited. In particular, when attempting to visualize the location of a catheter tip or the position of the transseptal apparatus in relation to the FO, active rotation of the ICE catheter is required to bring the tool of interest "in plane." This can be cumbersome for a single operator or require the assistance of a second operator. In addition, fluoroscopy may be required to confirm catheter positioning.

Eventually, 3D/four-dimensional (4D or "real-time 3D imaging") may overcome these disadvantages. Challenges to developing clinically practical and useful 3D/4D ICE catheters include adequate miniaturization of components to achieve an acceptable catheter size and creation of a high-quality image with a large imaging sector. Knackstedt et al have employed a custom-made prototype stepper motor to perform automatic rotation around the longitudinal axis from 90° to 360° in 2° to 5° steps. They acquired 2D images of a complete cardiac cycle, triggered by respiration and electrocardiogram signals; next, the digitized ultrasound images underwent 3D reconstruction. Experimental validation in pigs confirmed the system's feasibility, which was tested in 6 patients during EP studies. 3D acquisition and reconstruction of both atria and ventricles, Doppler flows in great vessels, and ablation catheter locations all could be demonstrated with good image quality within 3 to 5 minutes.[31]

Lee et al[32] recently described the development of a 10-Fr ICE catheter capable of 4D ICE imaging using an integrated micromotor. Using porcine and canine models, they were able to demonstrate a marked difference between 2D and 3D images. They demonstrated that, with 2D imaging, ICE catheter rotation is required to bring mapping catheters into view. And even with rotation, only part (if any) of the catheter can be seen at one time. With volume rendering or 3D imaging, the entire mapping catheter and its distal electrodes can be seen and contact of the tip with the tissue can be confirmed—all in one view. Szili-Torok and coworkers applied this 3D ICE concept in the clinic by identifying the site of septal lead placement for Bachmann's bundle pacing in the clinical laboratory study.[33] These images demonstrate the promise of 3D/4D ICE imaging to provide clearer 3D appreciation of catheter positioning, less need for ICE catheter manipulation, and possibly less reliance on fluoroscopy in the future.

Summary

In summary, as percutaneous intracardiac procedures increase in number and type, the applicability and utility of ICE are growing, especially in cardiac EP. This chapter compared in detail ICE technologies and acquisition of baseline images. Also, it described the use of ICE during LAA evaluation for thrombus, LAA occlusion device placement, transseptal catheterization, and catheter ablation for AF and VT. It also detailed current integration of ICE with other imaging modalities and EP mapping. Future directions for ICE imaging will include the development of real-time 3D ICE imaging as well as combining ICE imaging with EP interventional tools.

References

1. Morton JB, Kalman JM. Intracardiac echocardiographic anatomy for the interventional electrophysiologist. *J Interv Card Electrophysiol*. 2005;13(Suppl 1):11-16.
2. Saksena S, Sra J, Jordaens L, et al. A prospective comparison of cardiac imaging using intracardiac echocardiography with trans esophageal echocardiography in patients with atrial fibrillation: the intra-cardiac echocardiography guided cardioversion helps interventional procedures study. *Circ Arrhythm Electrophysiol*. 2010;3:571-777.
3. Reddy VY, Neuzil P, Ruskin JN. Intracardiac echocardiographic imaging of the left atrial appendage. *Heart Rhythm*. 2005;2:1272-1273.
4. Blendea D, Heist EK, Danik SB, et al. Analysis of the left atrial appendage morphology by intracardiac echocardiography in patients with atrial fibrillation. *J Interv Card Electrophysiol*. 2011;31(3):191-196.
5. De Ponti R, Cappato R, Curnis A, et al. Trans-septal catheterization in the electrophysiology laboratory: data from a multicenter survey spanning 12 years. *J Am Coll Cardiol*. 2006;47(5):1037-1042.
6. Hanna IR, Kolm P, Martin R, et al. Left atrial structure and function after percutaneous left atrial appendage transcatheter occlusion (PLAATO): six-month echocardiographic follow-up. *J Am Coll Cardiol*. 2004;43(10):1868-1872.
7. Sick PB, Schuler G, Hauptmann KE, et al. Initial worldwide experience with the WATCHMAN left atrial appendage system for stroke prevention in atrial fibrillation. *J Am Coll Cardiol*. 2007;49(13):1490-1495.
8. Ho IC, Neuzil P, Mraz T, et al. Use of intracardiac echocardiography to guide implantation of a left atrial appendage occlusion device (PLAATO). *Heart Rhythm*. 2007;4:567-71.
9. Shalaby AA. Utilization of intracardiac echocardiography to access the coronary sinus for left ventricular lead placement. *Pacing Clin Electrophysiol*. 2005;28(6):493-497.
10. Saksena S, Simon AM, Mathew P, Nagarakanti R. Intracardiac echocardiography-guided cardiac resynchronization therapy: technique and clinical application. *Pacing Clin Electrophysiol*. 2009;32(8):1030-1039.
11. Bai R, Biase LD, Mohanty P, Hesselson AB, Ruvo ED, Gallagher PL, Elayi CS, Mohanty S, Sanchez JE, David Burkhardt J, Horton R, Joseph Gallinghouse G, Bailey SM, Zagrodzky JD, Canby R, Minati M, Price LD, Lynn Hutchins C, Muir MA, Calo' L, Natale A, Tomassoni GF. Positioning of left ventricular pacing lead guided by intracardiac echocardiography with vector velocity imaging during cardiac resynchronization therapy procedure. *J Cardiovasc Electrophysiol*. 2011;22:1034-1041.
12. Singh SM, Heist EK, Donaldson DM, Collins RM, Chevalier J, Mela T, Ruskin JN, Mansour MC. Image integration using intracardiac ultrasound to guide catheter ablation of atrial fibrillation. *Heart Rhythm*. 2008;5:1548-1555.
13. Banchs JE, Patel P, Naccarelli GV, Gonzalez MD. Intracardiac echocardiography in complex cardiac catheter ablation procedures. *J Interv Card Electrophysiol*. 2010;28:167-184.
14. Kim SS, Hijazi ZM, Lang RM, Knight BP. The use of intracardiac echocardiography and other intracardiac imaging tools to guide noncoronary cardiac interventions. *J Am Coll Cardiol*. 2009;53:2117-2128.
15. Hijazi ZM, Shivkumar K, Sahn DJ. Intracardiac echocardiography during interventional and electrophysiological cardiac catheterization. *Circulation*. 2009;119:587-596.
16. Ferguson JD, Helms A, Mangrum JM, et al. Catheter ablation of atrial fibrillation without fluoroscopy using intracardiac echocardiography and electroanatomic mapping. *Circ Arrhythm Electrophysiol*. 2009;2:611-619.
17. Saliba W, Thomas J. Intracardiac echocardiography during catheter ablation of atrial fibrillation. *Europace*. 2008;10(Suppl 3):iii42-47.
18. Callans DJ, Wood MA. How to use intracardiac echocardiography for atrial fibrillation ablation procedures. *Heart Rhythm*. 2007;4:242-245.
19. Wazni OM, Beheiry S, Fahmy T, et al. Atrial fibrillation ablation in patients with therapeutic international normalized ratio: comparison of strategies of anticoagulation management in the periprocedural period. *Circulation*. 2007;116:2531-2534.
20. Calkins H, Kuck KH, Cappato R, et al. 2012 HRS/EHRA/ECAS expert consensus statement on catheter and surgical ablation of atrial fibrillation: Recommendations for patient selection, procedural techniques, patient management and follow up, definitions, endpoints and research trial design. *Heart Rhythm*. 2012;9(4):632-696.
21. Schmidt M, Daccarett M, Marschang H, et al. Intracardiac echocardiography improves procedural efficiency during cryoballoon ablation for atrial fibrillation: a pilot study. *J Cardiovasc Electrophysiol*. 2010;21(11):1202-1207.

22. Ren JF, Marchlinski FE. Utility of intracardiac echocardiography in left heart ablation for tachyarrhythmias. *Echocardiogr.* 2007;24:533-540.
23. Cummings JE, Schweikert RA, Saliba WI, et al. Assessment of temperature, proximity, and course of the esophagus during radiofrequency ablation within the left atrium. *Circulation.* 2005;112:459-644.
24. Marrouche NF, Martin DO, Wazni O, et al. Phased-array intracardiac echocardiography monitoring during pulmonary vein isolation in patients with atrial fibrillation: impact on outcome and complications. *Circulation.* 2003;107:2710-2716.
25. Oh S, Kilicaslan F, Zhang Y, et al. Avoiding microbubbles formation during radiofrequency left atrial ablation versus continuous microbubbles formation and standard radiofrequency ablation protocols: comparison of energy profiles and chronic lesion characteristics. *J Cardiovasc Electrophysiol.* 2006;17:72-77.
26. Jongbloed MR, Bax JJ, van der Burg AE, et al. Radiofrequency catheter ablation of ventricular tachycardia guided by intracardiac echocardiography. *Eur J Echocardiogr.* 2004;5:34-40.
27. Dravid SG, Hope B, McKinnie JJ. Intracardiac echocardiography in electrophysiology: a review of current applications in practice. *Echocardiogr.* 2008;25:1172-1175.
28. Vaseghi M, Cesario DA, Mahajan A, et al. Catheter ablation of right ventricular outflow tract tachycardia: value of defining coronary anatomy. *J Cardiovasc Electrophysiol.* 2006;17:632-637.
29. Kautzner J, Peichl P. 3D and 4D echo—applications in EP laboratory procedures. *J Interv Card Electrophysiol.* 2008;22:139-144.
30. Packer DL, Johnson SB, Kolasa MW, et al. New generation of electro-anatomic mapping: full intracardiac ultrasound image integration. *Europace.* 2008;10 Suppl 3:iii35-41.
31. Knackstedt C, Franke A, Mischke K, et al. Semi-automated 3-dimensional intracardiac echocardiography: development and initial clinical experience of a new system to guide ablation procedures. *Heart Rhythm.* 2006;3(12):1453-1459.
32. Lee W, Griffin W, Wildes D, et al. A 10-Fr ultrasound catheter with integrated micromotor for 4-D intracardiac echocardiography. *IEEE T Ultrason Ferr.* Jul 2011;58(7):1478-1491.
33. Szili-Torok T, Kimman G-J P, Schoelten M, et al, Interatrial Septum Pacing Guided by Three-Dimensional Intracardiac Echocardiography. *J Am Coll Cardiol.* 2002;40:2139-2143.

Video Legends

Video 9.1 ICE video of left atrial anatomy in view of the mitral valve. At the apex of the ICE image sector, the right atrial chamber is seen. Below this appears the thin-walled fossa ovalis, below which is seen the left atrium. At 9 o'clock on the left atrium, the coronary sinus is seen in cross-section. At 5 o'clock, the left atrial appendage is seen. Between the coronary sinus and the appendage, the mitral valve is seen with the left ventricle seen below this (see also Figure 9.2).

Video 9.2 ICE video of tenting of fossa ovalis prior to transseptal puncture. The tip of the transseptal apparatus is seen abutting the fossa ovalis, which leads to "tenting" of the fossa (see also Figures 9.6 and 9.11).

Video 9.3 ICE video of transseptal puncture using a radiofrequency needle. At the apex of the ICE image sector, the right atrial chamber is seen. Below this appears the thin-walled fossa ovalis, below which is seen the left atrium. The tip of the transseptal puncture apparatus is seen "tenting" the fossa ovalis. At 00:01, artifact from the radiofrequency energy is seen, followed by successful puncture of the fossa ovalis by the needle. Contrast is seen in the left atrium following needle crossing (see also Figure 9.7).

Video 9.4 Cine angiogram of left-atrial appendage occlusion device deployment. To start, the device is still attached to the delivery catheter. At 00:08, after positioning has been optimized, the device is deployed and the delivery catheter retracted into the delivery sheath (see Figure 9.9).

Video 9.5 Animation showing merged preprocedural computed tomogram of left atrial anatomy with intraprocedurally acquired 3D composite of left atrial anatomy based on a series of 2D ICE images (see Figure 9.10).

CHAPTER 10

Radiological Principles of Cardiac Computed Tomography, Magnetic Resonance Imaging, and Fusion Imaging

Alejandro Jimenez, MD; Timm M. Dickfeld, MD, PhD

Introduction

Because of current advances in technology, cardiac imaging plays an increasingly important role in diagnosis and treatment of complex cardiac arrhythmias. Traditional imaging methods, such as x-ray fluoroscopy, allow visualization of radio-opaque structures and enable the electrophysiologist to navigate catheters within the heart and vessel contours. However, they lack the ability to display tissue characteristics and to visualize in detail specific intracardiac structures that are necessary to safely and effectively perform complex procedures such as atrial fibrillation (AF) and ventricular tachycardia (VT) ablations.

Novel three-dimensional (3D) mapping techniques using electromagnetic fields and/or electrical currents allow for creation of detailed electroanatomic maps of the heart and great vessels. These can be utilized in real time to manipulate catheters and assess electrical properties of the myocardium. However, the creation of such nonlinear 3D models is susceptible to interaction with intravascular volume changes, respiratory or positional changes, and surrounding equipment noise. All these factors can distort the electromagnetic or current field impedance and produce significant location errors, leading to inaccurate representation of the anatomy. On the other hand, linear image acquisition techniques such as computed tomography (CT) and magnetic resonance imaging (MRI) result in stable and accurate image acquisition.[1] This chapter reviews the use of cardiac CT and MRI and details their ability to offer high-resolution anatomic visualization that can be integrated into clinical 3D mapping systems to guide complex ablation procedures.

Computed Tomography Imaging Fundamentals and Technical Considerations

Imaging Process

CT is an imaging modality that employs x-ray beams, projected in fan-shaped configurations. These beams are funneled to a selected area of interest with the use of a collimator, which eliminates all x-rays not traveling in parallel to the specified direction the collimator defines. This arrangement allows for the creation of an image in a biplane coordinate system, which is referred to as the imaging plane. Although conventional planar x-ray systems can create images of high resolution, they are unable to differentiate adjacent structures within an imaging plane. The result is a superimposed image composed of multiple structures, which makes it very difficult to view separately a particular organ or structure within the projected image. By virtue of its ability to obtain specific anatomic cross-sections (hence the name transverse axial tomography), CT imaging achieves minimal superimposition of tissue and allows one to visualize contrast differences within adjacent anatomic structures.

In CT imaging systems, a filter is positioned in front of the x-ray beam. This beam filter, made of aluminum, absorbs very-low-energy x-rays that lack sufficient energy to penetrate the body tissue and thus would only increase patient exposure without contributing to the imaging process. This process is known as beam hardening and results in a more uniform average beam energy; this beam energy is clinically applicable for creating tissue images and reduces patient radiation exposure by as much as 50%.

Cardiac medical imaging is currently obtained using state-of-the-art, multislice helical CT systems. Multislice technology was developed to address slow image acquisition with early CT scanners, which required several minutes to reconstruct each slice of an imaging data set. Helical (or spiral) scanning allowed a higher image acquisition speed, which also helped reduce patient motion artifacts. Both of these advances were crucial to allow the use of CT in imaging of the heart and adjacent structures. Sixty-four-slice and higher resolution systems (currently up to 320-row detectors) have subsecond rotational speeds that enable accurate reconstruction of cardiac and coronary anatomy as well as evaluation of functional parameters (when combined with ECG gating).

Synchronizing the movements of the x-ray tube/detectors in the gantry, as well as the imaging table, is crucial in order to adequately space the images and prevent image overlapping or false-space creation. In helical CT, this is referred to as pitch, defined as the ratio of the patient's movement through the gantry during one 360° beam rotation relative to the beam collimation. Another important factor in defining image slices and their position relative to one another is the distance between the reconstructed axial slices in the z-axis. This is referred to as increment, or the distance between the slices. This distance can be adjusted to allow some overlap, which may be necessary for 3D image reconstructions and for better image resolution in specific areas.

Multislice helical CT requires continuous radiation, gantry rotation, imaging table motion, and data transfer from the detector array. Acquiring an adequate image data set mandates that a correct balance be found between scan length, collimation, increment, and number of slices generated. A current multislice helical CT system is composed of a series of conductive rings; these rings allow power and signals to be transferred to and from the rotating gantry. Digital data received from the detectors is transmitted back to the computer using high-speed radiofrequency (RF) signals. The computer then synchronizes the gantry and table motion to acquire data from known positions of the gantry rotation and the imaging table position, allowing for fast, high-speed data acquisition.[2]

Image Data Acquisition and Reconstruction

The data acquired from the helical motion of the gantry is obtained as projection data, which represent the attenuated beam of radiation from which a specific algorithm determines an attenuation coefficient at each pixel in an image matrix. Once the patient volume is scanned, the raw data obtained from the scan can be reconstructed using various parameters to obtain images of clinical diagnostic value. The beam width, as set by the detector size and collimator, determines the maximal resolution obtainable.

The helical projection data require special algorithms for adequate image reconstruction. The reconstructed segments or voxels are isotropic (ie, having the same dimensions in x, y, and z axes). The pixel values (a measure to quantify a gray-scale spectrum) assigned in the image are measured in Hounsfield units (HU) and represent the amount of x-ray attenuation. They are obtained by calculating the relative difference between the linear attenuation coefficient of tissue and water [HU = (μ_{tissue} − μ_{water})/(μ_{water} × 1000)] and are represented as 12-bit binary numbers resulting in 2^{12} (4,096) possible values. The Hounsfield scale ranges from −1,024 HU to +3,071. For example, the HU for water is zero, for air it is −1,000, and for bone (depending on its density), it can vary from 500 to 1,000. Cardiac tissue has an average HU of 10 to 60. HU are also referred to as CT numbers.

After the raw data from the scan have been acquired, several parameters must be defined before reconstructing the images. The field of view (FOV) determines the image area to be reconstructed, while the matrix determines the pixel size in each image plane. All three are closely related because pixel size = FOV/matrix. (eg, a field of view of 250 mm divided by a matrix of 512 × 512 mm² will give a pixel size of 0.49 mm). Another important parameter in image processing is the kernel reconstruction, which defines the amount of smoothing to be applied in the image reconstruction process. Multiple kernels are available, depending on the body area or clinical application. Higher kernel numbers provide sharper images, whereas lower numbers provide smoother images.

For cardiac CT imaging, ECG gating is required. To avoid respiratory motion artifacts, scanning is usually performed during held expiration. The acquired data are then synchronized with the QRS complex and used to define cardiac systole and diastole. Multiple images acquired during consecutive cardiac time intervals can be combined to obtain an image of the heart at the exact same phase of the cardiac cycle, in a prospective or retrospective fashion.

Image Display and Storage

Owing to the great variability in the HU of a given human body image (from −850 HU for lung air to 500 HU for bone), displaying CT information digitally is very challenging. Because the human eye can discern only 30 to 100 different shades of gray, and digital image size is measured in bytes (each byte made up of 8 bits), a typical gray scale for CT images comprises 256 intensity values from black to white. Thus, different tissues may be viewed using different window centerlines and widths.

CT images can be viewed as slices (traditional method) or displayed as volumetric image data sets. These 3D reconstructed images have great applicability in electrophysiology (EP) because they provide accurate anatomic reconstruction of cardiac structures and great vessels that can be integrated with electroanatomic mapping systems. These images can also be used for real-time navigation of intracardiac catheters and for delineating potential arrhythmogenic areas. The two techniques for volumetric image reconstruction are maximum intensity projection (MIP) and shaded surface display (SSD). MIP images are generated by taking a stack of image slices and projecting back the maximum intensity of the brightest pixel along that path. SSD images utilize shading and artificial light sources to create the illusion of real anatomy.

Once studies are completed and images acquired, they are stored in a proprietary format. Owing to the large size of these image data sets, the scanner information is then transferred from the scanner computer to a network server. In order to allow for seamless exchange of image information between different centers and image manufacturers, a medical image standard known as DICOM (Digital Imaging and Communications in Medicine) is used to share stored radiographic image studies worldwide.

Radiation and New Methods of Radiation Reduction

Radiation exposure during cardiac CT scanning is substantial. This has led investigators to devise new approaches in scanning protocols and hardware design modifications in order to minimize the radiation burden. Exposure during a standard cardiac CT can be as high as 10 to 12 mSv. Until recently, most cardiac CT scans used retrospective gating, a technique in which the target organ is imaged several times during the different phases of the cardiac cycle. This technique allowed for comprehensive assessment of cardiac dynamics during systole and diastole but also resulted in increased radiation exposure. To minimize radiation exposure, prospective gating can be performed, during which images are acquired only at a predefined ECG window (frequently 75%–80% of the R-R interval). Radiation exposure can be reduced to < 2 mSv using this technique.

Another approach to minimize radiation during scanning is tube current modulation, which automatically adjusts the tube current (milliamperes [mA]) according to the patient attenuation. This approach can reduce the patient's radiation exposure by more than 50%.[3]

Another technological advance is dual source scanners, which have two detector systems and can acquire a full CT slice with only half a rotation. This significantly shortens the scanning time (< 10 seconds for full-chest CT), minimizes motion artifact, and further decreases radiation exposure. With these advances, cardiac CT imaging with a radiation exposure of less than 1 mSv and an acquisition time of 0.27 seconds is now feasible.[4]

Magnetic Resonance Imaging Fundamentals and Technical Considerations

Imaging Process

Cardiac magnetic resonance (CMR) imaging makes use of nuclear magnetic resonance (NMR) to image the nuclei of atoms inside the body. NMR is based on the principles of absorption and emission of energy in the RF range of the electromagnetic spectrum. The human body is composed primarily of water and fat, both of which are made up of hydrogen ions. Therefore, RF waves in the electromagnetic spectrum excite the hydrogen nuclei (tissue magnetization), which the nuclei then decays (relaxes), releasing energy (radio waves or echoes); this energy is converted into images of radio signals (spatially resolved sinusoid waves) by Fourier transform (FT).[5] Strong magnetic field gradients cause nuclei at different locations to rotate at different speeds, and 3D spatial information can be obtained by providing gradients in each direction. The magnetic resonance scanner is composed of superconducting magnets, an RF transmitter and receiver, as well as gradient coils (solenoids) that create magnetic fields when they are subjected to high electrical pulses. The strength of these magnetic fields is graded in tesla (T) units. For CMR imaging, the usual clinical magnet strengths are 1.5 or 3 T.[6]

Images are constructed when the protons in different tissues return to their equilibrium state at different rates, and these differences are detected by the system. Five different tissue variables (spin density, T_1 and T_2 relaxation times, and flow and spectral shifts) can be employed to construct tissue images. By changing these parameters on the scanner, and adding contrast agents, one can create contrast between different types of body tissue to suit particular clinical imaging needs. The FT breaks down signals into a series of sine waves, each one with a different frequency, phase, and amplitude. The FT of the signal in the time domain can be represented in the equivalent frequency domain by a series of peaks of various amplitudes. In MRI, the signal is spatially encoded by changes in phase/frequency; the signal is then decoded by performing a 2D FT to identify pixel intensities and display the image.[7]

To create an image of the heart and blood vessels using MRI, a signal from resonating protons within the heart must be acquired. This is accomplished by applying a static magnetic field (*B0*) with the MRI scanner (ranging from 0.5 to 3 T). A static magnetic field is necessary to align randomly oriented hydrogen nuclei (protons) in the body in order to generate a net (longitudinal) magnetization and to make the protons rotate at a predefined frequency, known as the *Larmor frequency*. An RF pulse with the Larmor frequency of certain duration is applied, bringing the protons into resonance and flipping the net longitudinal magnetization from the horizontal to the transverse plane. This transverse magnetization induces a current in a receiver coil, and after switching off the RF pulse, the transverse magnetization fades out and the longitudinal magnetization progressively increases, restoring the original longitudinal magnetization.

This fading process is specific to different tissue types and allows for the generation of image contrast between different structures. The magnetic resonance signal is spatially encoded by rapidly switching three separate magnetic field gradients applied in sequence: slice-section gradient along the z-axis, phase-encoding gradient along the y-axis, and frequency-encoding gradient along the x-axis. This encoding leads to small changes in the Larmor frequency of the protons and enables identification of a proton position in a 3D plane.[8] This process defines an image slice that is perpendicular to the z-axis (transaxial plane). Other slice orientations can be obtained by reassigning each gradient to a different axis. Angled slices can therefore be obtained by combining gradients along two or more axes to perform each localization task.

In MRI, the term *relaxation* is used to describe several processes by which nuclear magnetization, prepared in a nonequilibrium state, returns to the equilibrium distribution. In simple terms, relaxation describes how fast spins "forget" the direction in which they are oriented. Different physical processes are responsible for the relaxation of the components of the nuclear spin magnetization vectors parallel and perpendicular to the external magnetic field (conventionally labeled *B0* and oriented along the z-axis). These two principal relaxation processes are termed *T1* and *T2* relaxation, respectively.

1. *T1 or longitudinal relaxation time (also known as spin-lattice relaxation)* represents the decay constant for the recovery of the Z component of the nuclear spin magnetization vector toward its thermal equilibrium value. This process involves redistributing the populations of the nuclear spin states in order to reach the thermal equilibrium distribution. A variety of relaxation mechanisms enable nuclear spins to exchange energy with their surroundings, thus allowing the spin populations to equilibrate. Rates of *T1* relaxation are strongly dependent on the magnetic resonance and vary considerably with the magnetic field strength.

2. *T2 or transverse relaxation time (also known as spin-spin relaxation)* is the decay constant for the vector component perpendicular to the external magnetic field (*B0*). It represents a complex phenomenon of disarray of the transverse nuclear spin magnetization. As a result, the initial phase coherence of the nuclear spins is lost, until eventually, the phases are disordered and there is no net x–y magnetization.

T1 relaxation represents the release of energy from the proton spin population as it returns to its equilibrium state. The rate of relaxation is related to the rate at which energy is released to the surrounding molecular structure; the latter, in turn, depends on the size of the molecule that contains the hydrogen nuclei and the rate of molecular motion, known as the *tumbling rate*. As molecules tumble, they give rise to a fluctuating magnetic field that protons in adjacent molecules experience. When this fluctuating magnetic field is close to the Larmor frequency, energy exchange is facilitated. Small lipid molecules in fat tissue have fast relaxation rates and, consequently, short *T1* relaxation time. Larger water molecules have a tumbling rate that is unfavorable to energy exchange and, therefore, tissues with a larger water content (eg, edematous tissue) have longer *T1* relaxation times.

Another important concept is the *K* space, which represents the unique relationship between the data points in an MR signal and the points in a given image. Even though a single data point in an MR signal contributes a particular attribute to the whole image, a single pixel in the image may have collected contributions from multiple MR signals. And, because each pixel occupies a unique location in an image space, each point of an MR signal echo belongs to a particular location (*K* space). As a result, the relationship between the image space and the *K* space is inversely proportional (where an *x, y* coordinate in the image plane will correspond to a 1/*x*, 1/*y* coordinate: This is known as *spatial frequency*.[9]

Image Modalities

CMR uses several different techniques within a single scan, whose combination results in a comprehensive assessment of the heart and cardiovascular system. Scar tissue or epicardial fat can be visualized without the use of a contrast agent; instead, sequences known as *spin–echo* (in which blood appears black in high-resolution still images) are used. To improve the signal-to-noise ratio of myocardial scar tissue, contrast agents (eg, gadolinium) are frequently employed. Also, special imaging sequences such as inversion recovery (IR) allow one to optimize the inversion time in order to null the myocardium and better differentiate between scar tissue and normal myocardium. A delay between contrast administration and scan acquisition allows clearance of the contrast medium from healthy myocardium but not from scar tissue, owing to the slow washout of the gadolinium chelates, which are hydrophilic, have a low molecular weight, and concentrate in extracellular space.[6,10] On the late gadolinium enhancement (LGE) images, normal heart muscle appears dark while areas of infarction appear bright white. Blood appears bright in these sequences because of its contrast properties and rapid flow.

Advantages and Limitations of Cardiac Magnetic Resonance Imaging Compared with X-ray–based Technologies

The main advantage of MRI technology is the lack of ionizing radiation. Few scan limitations exist aside from the bore diameter (limiting access in morbid obesity and claustrophobia), and even in obese individuals, images of high spatial and temporal resolution can be obtained. The use of gadolinium contrast has negligible nephrotoxicity but should be avoided in patients with creatinine clearance < 30 mL/minute (cases of nephrogenic systemic fibrosis have been described in the setting of renal insufficiency).[11] One of the main limitations of CMR imaging is its interaction with ferromagnetic material in implanted cardiac rhythm devices (eg, pacemakers and ICDs). These devices are present in many patients undergoing CMR imaging for a wide variety of clinical conditions such as heart failure, ischemic heart disease, VT, AF, and congenital heart disease. Owing to the combined effects of a pulsed RF and static and/or gradient magnetic field, multiple concerns have arisen: about adverse complications of thermal cardiac injury, arrhythmogenesis, rapid pacing, reed switch dysfunction, inappropriate detection of electromagnetic interference (EMI), device damage, software malfunction, and device movement.

1. *Static magnetic field interactions.* The static magnetic field caused by the superconductive magnet creates several potential hazards for various ICD components: mechanical forces on ferromagnetic components, unpredictable reed-switch closure, electrical device reset, inhibition of therapy delivery, and memory corruption.

2. *Pulsed RF field interactions.* RF pulses delivered on a background magnetic field at specified frequencies excite atomic nuclei (spins) in the soft tissue, which absorb and emit electromagnetic energy to generate an MR image. The specific absorption rate (SAR) quantifies RF energy exposure for a given pulse sequence. ICD patients undergoing MRI can therefore suffer thermal injury, oversensing, rapid pacing, arrhythmia induction, and electrical reset as a consequence of this RF interaction.[7]

3. *Gradient magnetic field issues.* Gradient magnetic fields can induce voltage and current changes in pacing and defibrillator leads. These can result in oversensing, rapid pacing, arrhythmia induction, battery drainage, and electrical reset of pulse generators.

4. *Mechanical effects.* ICDs and pacemakers contain ferromagnetic components that can suffer displacement in response to the strong magnetic field generated by the MRI scanner. The highest translational forces occur when the patient enters the scanner. Newer cardiac rhythm devices are smaller and contain less ferromagnetic material, which leads to minimal risk of motion during clinical scanning protocols.[12,13]

As a result of these concerns, MRI studies are still contraindicated in patients with ICDs and most pacemakers,[14] for device failure, lead heating, and unexpected reprogramming have all been described.[15] However, several recent studies have suggested that, with appropriate patient selection and pre- and postprocedural reprogramming, MRI can be performed in this population with an acceptable safety profile.[16-19] In addition, MRI-safe heart rhythm devices have recently become available for clinical use.[20]

Integrating Cardiac Computed Tomography/Magnetic Resonance Images with 3D Mapping Systems

In recent years, integrating preprocedural cardiac CT and MRI studies with intraprocedural 3D mapping systems has become increasingly common in the catheter ablation of complex arrhythmias such as AF, atrial tachycardia (AT), and VT.[21-23] Linear images of the different cardiac, vascular, and adjacent structures provide remarkable anatomic detail. When integrated with a 3D mapping system, these images enhance the accuracy of intracardiac catheter manipulation during anatomically based ablation for arrhythmias, such as AF and scar-mediated VT.

Several large prospective, randomized and nonrandomized trials have shown clinical benefits when image integration is incorporated into AF ablation procedures. Della Bella et al, in a study of 290 patients undergoing AF ablation, demonstrated an increase in AF-free survival after 14 ± 12 months in the CT image–integration group using CartoMerge (Biosense Webster, Diamond Bar, CA) compared with the conventional mapping group.[24] Caponi et al studied 299 patients undergoing AF ablation, randomized to traditional 3D mapping or image integration with preprocedural CMR. These investigators showed a reduction in fluoroscopy times in the image integration arm; procedural outcomes, length of procedure, and complication rates were similar between the two groups.[25] In the largest image integration series to date, Bertaglia et al evaluated 573 patients who underwent AF ablation with both conventional and CartoMerge image integration using preprocedural CT and CMR. Among the image integration patients, initial procedural time was shorter, and after one year of follow-up, recurrence of atrial tachyarrhythmias was significantly reduced.[26] Although one randomized controlled trial in 80 AF patients by Kistler et al did not show any difference between the standard and image integration arms,[27] the majority of studies seems to indicate some improvement in terms of procedural and outcomes data.

Basic Concepts of Image Integration

Commercially available 3D mapping systems are equipped with an image integration software module (CartoMerge and the EnSite Verismo™ (St. Jude Medical, St. Paul, MN), which allows the reconstruction and registration of preprocedural images obtained from cardiac CT or MRI studies. Newer technologies such as rotational 3D angiography have also been successfully integrated with commercially available 3D mapping systems.[28,29] The image integration process follows three main steps:

1. *Acquisition of preprocedural images.* Obtaining CT or MR images of sufficient quality is a prerequisite for a successful electroanatomic integration process that guarantees anatomically accurate images. Both CT and MRI provide images with high spatial resolution, and often, comparable quality. With the exception of some magnetic resonance angiography (MRA) sequences, images are acquired during diastole, using ECG gating; they should be available in a short time (ideally, during a single breath hold at end expiration or with respiratory gated sequences) to avoid motion artifact.

2. *Image segmentation.* After obtaining high-resolution images of the heart and adjacent anatomic structures, image segmentation allows for separation of the different structures and individual cardiac chambers from the CT and MRI sets using a 3D volume-reconstructed model obtained from the 2D CT and MRI slices. The use of contrast agents (iodine-based for CT and gadolinium-based for MRI) allows one to differentiate intravascular from intracardiac volumes (cardiac chambers and great vessels). The blood pool displays high signal intensity that differs from the lower intensities of the adjacent tissue, thereby delineating the endoluminal/endocardial contours of the different cardiac chambers and vessels. The process of segmentation is automated with vendor-specific software algorithms using signal threshold, boundary detection, and regional identification. These variables are crucial for obtaining quality segmented images; however, some degree of visual editing is always required in order to confirm that all structures have been properly delineated and that the geometry created accurately represents the true anatomy.[30]

3. *Image registration.* Registration represents the most critical step in the image integration process. It requires both an understanding of the anatomy as well as technical expertise in the manipulation of the image data sets into the 3D mapping software environment. Registration consists of superimposing the CT/MRI–derived reconstructed 3D images into the real-time electroanatomic map. This allows the intracardiac catheter(s) to navigate inside the registered 3D anatomy.

Technical Aspects of Image Segmentation

Thresholding represents a simple yet very effective method for segmentation. Pixels are combined into two main groups, based on their signal intensity in reference to a given threshold value. Pixels above or below the threshold are grouped together and exported for further processing. Using boundary extraction methods, which measure the intensity difference between adjacent pixels, the pixels are grouped into regions. During segmentation for procedures such as AF ablation, the boundary extraction method allows for chamber separation. It selects the higher pixel-signal-intensity region (in this case, the left atrium [LA] and pulmonary veins [PVs] filled with contrast) from adjacent structures (such as the lungs or esophagus) that have a lower pixel-signal intensity and are therefore grouped into a separate region.[31]

Technical Aspects of Image Registration

Cardiac registration of CT/MRI–derived reconstructed images and 3D maps is intermodal; that is, the CT/MR images and the 3D map reside in different image spaces. Registration algorithms are required for transforming one image space into another. This transformation function (T) can be either linear or nonlinear. Six parameters, or degrees of freedom (three translations and three rotations), are employed for linear transformation between two different 3D spaces. If the voxel sizes in each image differ, three additional calibration parameters are necessary to account for the discrepancy (represented by three additional degrees of freedom in the x-, y-, and z-axes, scaled in each direction) (Figures 10.1, A and B). In nonlinear transformation, multiple degrees of freedom (> 6) are required to avoid image distortion. A cost function is used to measure similarities (or discrepancies) between the reference and the transformed images.

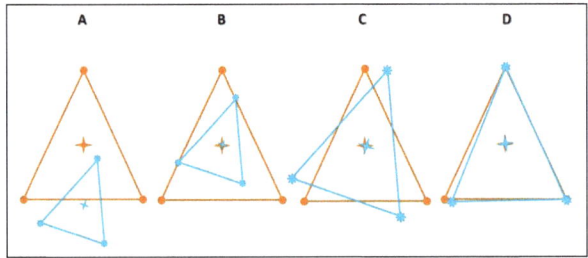

Figure 10.1A **Panel A:** Schematic representation of a geometry-based point registration process. The fiducial points are represented by **dots** for the reference image (**orange**) and **asterisks** for the CT projection (**blue**). **Panel B:** The first step in the registration process involves aligning the centroids of each image (**stars**). **Panel C:** The second step requires scaling and calibrating the images. **Panel D:** The final step consists of rotating the images to minimize fiducial registration error, or FRE.

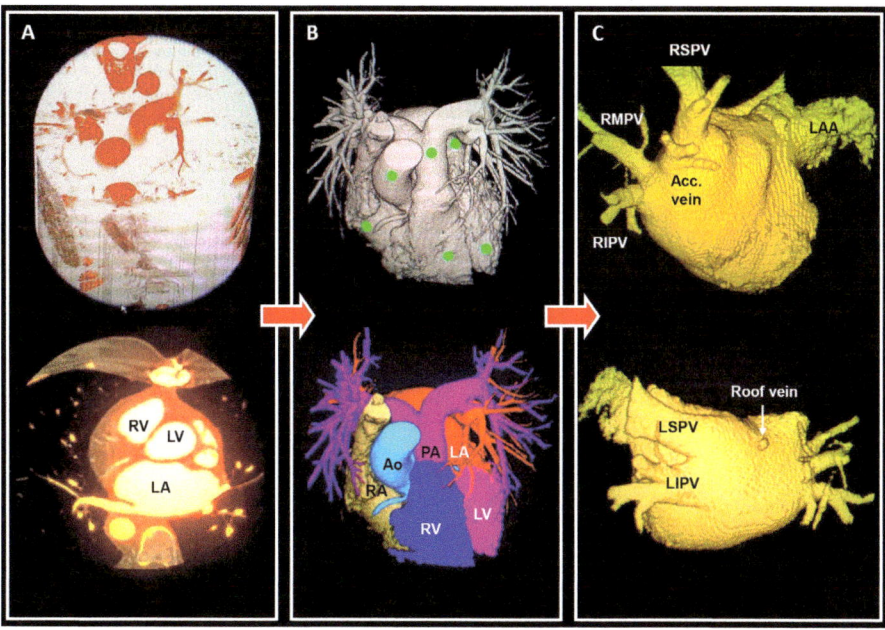

Figure 10.1B Image segmentation process for AF ablation.
Panel A: Transverse slice of the raw CT data showing the cardiac chamber of interest. By adjusting the threshold of signal intensity, the blood pool is delineated (**orange**).
Panel B: Boundaries between cardiac chambers are established using a "competitive region growth" algorithm by selecting each chamber individually (**green points, top panel**) allowing for separation of the different cardiac chambers (**color-coded 3D reconstruction, bottom panel**).
Panel C: 3D CT reconstruction of the left atrium (LA) and pulmonary veins (PVs). Note the variant anatomy of the right PVs (right middle PV [RMPV], right inferior PV [RIPV]) and a posterior roof vein. The anatomic detail provided by the 3D CT reconstruction integrated with a 3D anatomic map is very useful for accurate catheter manipulation during mapping and ablation. Ao = aorta; LAA = left atrial appendage; LV = left ventricle; PA = pulmonary artery; LIPV = left inferior pulmonary vein; LSPV = left superior pulmonary vein; RA = right atrium; RSPV = right superior pulmonary vein; RV = right ventricle.

Registration methods are divided mainly into geometry and voxel-intensity based modalities. Geometry-based methods can be further divided into point-based and surface-based registration modalities. In point-based registration, one or more sets of fiducial points in each image are registered. This is done by either aligning the two shells and using a single point pair to fuse them (frequently referred to as "visual alignment") or employing point-pair files using multiple sets (usually ≥ 5) and superimposing the correlated point-pairs (also called "landmark registration" or "fiducial point pairing"; see Figure 10.4). These fiducial points can be automatically determined, based on surface markers, but are most often manually assigned, based on anatomic landmarks. The difference between the centroids in each set of images provides an estimate of the translation required to align a given set of points. These points are consequently rotated around the new centroid until the sum of the squared distances between each corresponding point pair is minimized. The square root of the mean squared distance between point pairs is known as the *fiducial registration error* (FRE).[32]

In clinical practice, anatomically distinct endocardial areas such as the PV ostia or the atrioventricular (AV) ring are used for landmark registration.[33] As with any manual registration method, there is an inherent error associated with each registered point, which is known as the *fiducial localization error* (FLE) and represents the vector (distance) from the intended to the actual fiducial point obtained. To account for this error, the target registration error, or TRE, is computed from the FLE as a more accurate measure of registration error.

Surface-based methods for image registration are often the preferred modality for registering CT and MRI images. The surfaces represented in each of the images are delineated, registered, and transformed (*T*). The cost function provides a way to measure the distance between the different surfaces. In clinical practice, 3D CT and MRI images are registered into the 3D environment of the electroanatomic mapping system by using three translations and three rotations (assuming the internal anatomy of the patient has not changed between the time the images were obtained and the time of the actual procedure). Each device is calibrated to determine appropriate image scaling. The main limitation with surface-based methods is the assumption that the *T* function is rigid, which is not the case for cardiac registration.[34]

Registration of Computed Tomography/Magnetic Resonance Imaging Data Sets with Electroanatomic Mapping Systems

3D mapping systems spatially locate one or several catheters within the different heart chambers and great vessels. The Carto system uses ultra-low electromagnetic fields (5×10^{-5} to 5×10^{-6} T) emitted by an electromagnetic pad below the patient to assess the position of a catheter tip within the chamber of interest (defined by positioning an electromagnetic pad below the patient). The ESI NavX and Velocity (St. Jude Medical) employ voltage gradients generated by an external electrical field (generated from three patch pairs placed on the patient's skin) to localize the catheter tip. Multiple studies have validated both point and surface registration with commercially available 3D mapping systems using CT and MR images and have reported acceptable accuracy ranging from 2.9 ± 0.7 to 6.9 ± 2.2 mm for CT[35-38] and 3.8 ± 0.6 to 4.3 ± 3.2 mm for MRI.[17,39,40]

Biosense Webster's Carto XP and Carto 3 mapping systems use an image integration module known as CartoMerge. Three different types of registration algorithms can be utilized: visual alignment, landmark registration, and surface registration. All these techniques require the initial creation of landmark pairs between the two imaging data sets. If the visual alignment and surface registration algorithm are chosen for image integration, the first step involves selecting a well-defined landmark pair (eg, PV ostium or mitral valve point) and visually aligning both images. Next, 20 or ideally more surface points are acquired on the 3D electroanatomic shell throughout the chamber of interest. Finally, the surface registration algorithm is employed to align both image data sets. If one chooses a combination of landmark and surface registration to integrate the images, three or more landmark pairs must be obtained. Examples include PV ostia, antral locations, the superior vena cava–right atrial (SVC–RA) junction, and coronary sinus ostium (CS os). Surface points (>20 or more) are acquired in the same manner previously described. Whether visual alignment or landmark registration methods are used, the final step requires corroborating registration accuracy by navigating the catheter gently toward the different anatomic structures (eg, PVs, left atrial appendage [LAA]) under fluoroscopic or intracardiac ultrasound guidance. Using a canine model, the accuracy of this image registration technique was evaluated by Dong et al. Epicardial fiducial markers were placed at sites where ablation lesions were delivered. During postmortem examination, the accuracy of the integrated cardiac CT/3D map to localize the lesion sets was found to be less than 3 mm.[41]

The EnSite NavX and Velocity mapping systems use the Fusion registration module. The process consists of three main steps. First, a segmented surface rendering of a CT or MRI scan, known as the *digital image fusion*, or DIF, model is imported into the 3D mapping environment. Next, a field scaling algorithm is performed. It measures interelectrode spacing at collected geometry points in the chamber to compensate for inhomogeneities in the 3D mapping field, adjusting the volume of the 3D map to resemble the preprocedural image volume. Finally, image fusion (integration of the preprocedural CT/MR images and 3D map) is accomplished. To perform registration, the fusion module uses paired locations (fiducial points) between the mapping and the CT/MRI 3D models. A dynamic registration algorithm locally adjusts the 3D shell geometry and surface to the size and shape of the DIF model surface. Different studies have evaluated the registration accuracy of an integrated preprocedural CT image and 3D map for guiding AF ablation, using a dynamic registration module and multiple paired fiducial points. The authors described registration errors ranging from 1.9 ± 0.4 to 3.2 ± 0.9 mm and no significant difference in the PV diameters measured by CT versus the 3D map model.[42,43]

Although the same basic principles of image integration are common to both the CartoMerge and EnSite fusion systems, they differ substantially in how they accomplish the registration process. The Carto system uses a rigid registration process in which the preprocedural images can be rotated to minimize distance between the 3D map geometry and the 3D CT/MRI images, without stretching the actual 3D map. In contrast, the EnSite system uses a dynamic registration process and employs four or more fiducial points to optimize both rotation and stretching of the 3D map geometry to match the preprocedural image volume. Despite these differences in technique, clinical studies have shown comparable registration errors using both systems (Figures 10.2 and 10.3; corresponding ▶ Video 10.1 for Figure 10.3).[42,43]

Key Points to Minimize Registration Error

Because CT and MRI studies are obtained before the EP procedure, volumetric and motion-related discrepancies between the real-time electroanatomic map and the reconstructed 3D CT/MRI data sets are expected. Registration errors can be minimized by taking the following steps:

1. *Timing for preprocedural image study.* Preprocedural scans should be conducted as close to the procedure as possible (ideally ≤24 hours) to minimize variations in volume status that will affect cavity volume, particularly in the atria.

2. *Minimizing the effect of respiratory motion.* Preprocedural images are obtained mostly during the end-expiratory phase of the respiratory cycle. Respiratory gating strategies to limit respiratory motion of the catheters (which can be >10 mm) include the use of a catheter in the CS to provide a stable location reference for the 3D mapping system or limiting point acquisition to a certain phase of the respiratory cycle. New commercial solutions have been developed and are now commercially available (eg, for the Carto 3 system).

3. *Synchronization of both data sets.* The sampling of single real-time catheter mapping points is usually gated to the same cardiac phase used to reconstruct the 3D CT/MRI images (usually end diastole), thus minimizing the volume differences between the

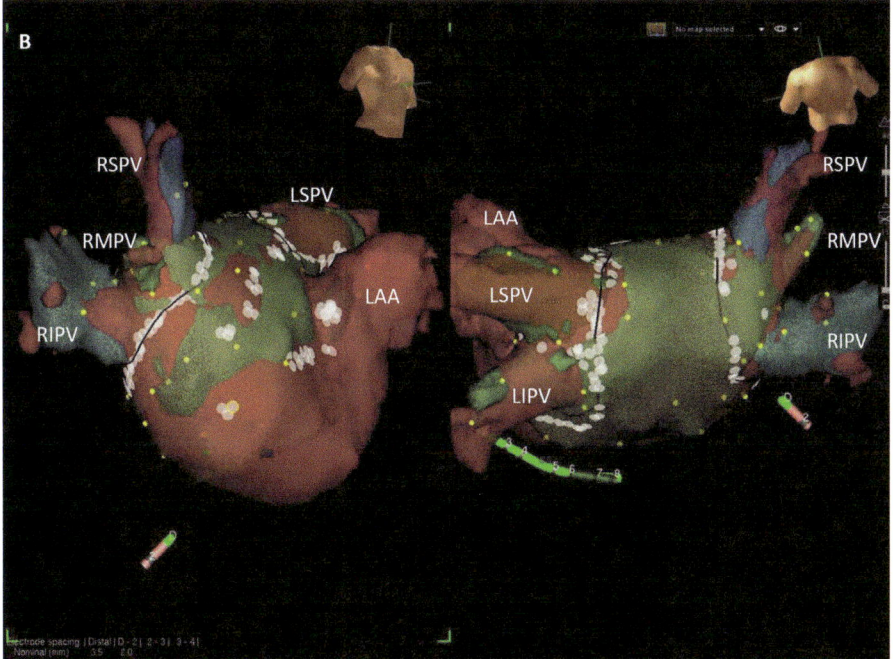

Figure 10.2 **Panel A:** Registration of left atrial images obtained with the EnSite Velocity 3D mapping system (St. Jude Medical) (**left**) and a 3D reconstruction of a cardiac CT image (**right**) using the Fusion software. The multiple fiducial points obtained from different anatomic landmarks are projected onto the surface of the images as **yellow points** and used to align both images with the help of software and visual alignment tools. **White spots** correspond to ablation points. **Panel B:** Field scaling is used to approximate the 3D map to the CT 3D volume using 4 or more fiducial points. Ablation lesions shown in **white**.

real-time catheter mapping space and the 3D surface reconstruction of the CT/MRI. However, rapid anatomic point acquisition modes (FAM mapping in the Carto 3 system and MultiPoint mapping for ESI Velocity) can acquire anatomic catheter positions without cardiac and no or limited respiratory gating. Although these mapping modes provide a quick, simple method for obtaining chamber volume and surface data, they can overestimate 3D acquisition volumes. Additionally, a change in heart rhythm between the preprocedure images and the 3D real-time electroanatomic map may affect registration accuracy; however, several studies have not substantiated significant differences in registration error indices, at least in patients with AF.[44,45]

4. *Catheter deformation.* The plasticity of the myocardial wall allows for stretching and deformation during forceful catheter manipulation, most notably in the atria; this can introduce false spacing and especially impact surface registration. During LA mapping, the areas more likely to be deformed by catheter manipulation include the roof, lateral wall, and septum. The posterior LA, on the contrary, tends to be less compliant and therefore might be more suitable for landmark/surface registration protocols.[33]

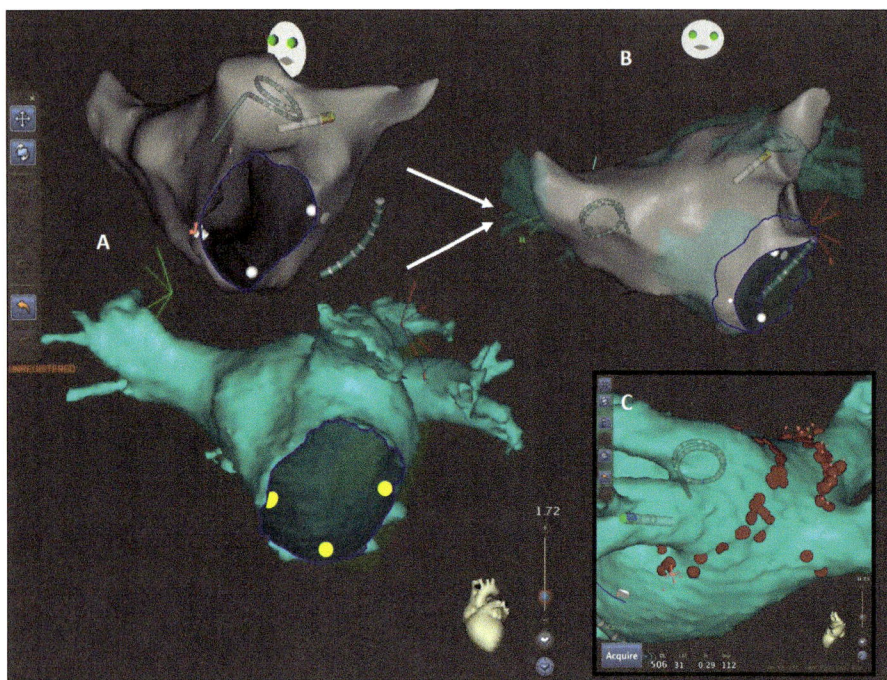

Figure 10.3 **Panel A:** Rigid registration between preprocedural 3D CT (**bottom**) reconstruction and 3D map (**top**) using the Carto 3 system and Fast Atrial Mapping (FAM) module (Biosense Webster). After landmark registration using 3 fiduciary points around the mitral annulus (**white points** on the FAM map and **blue points** on the CT), the images are fused (**Panel B**). **Panel C:** The integrated images are then used to guide real-time catheter manipulation and ablation in the left atrium (multipole circular catheter in the LSPV ostium, ablation catheter in the LIPV). Ablation lesions are shown in **red**.

Clinical Applications for Image Fusion Using Computed Tomography/Magnetic Resonance Imaging and 3D Maps

Atrial Fibrillation

Pulmonary vein isolation (PVI) remains the cornerstone of AF ablation, but this technique is not devoid of risks. Delivery of ablation lesions inside the PV ostia can lead to PV stenosis, which is associated with significant morbidity and frequently requires further interventional treatment.[46,47] In addition, the proximity of the esophagus to the posterior wall of the LA makes this organ vulnerable to injury from ablation energy sources. Sporadic cases of atrioesophageal fistula (AEF) formation post–AF ablation have been reported during recent years. A recent survey reported by Oral et al from U.S. centers performing AF ablation procedures showed an AEF incidence of 0.03% (6 out of 20,425 patients) and a mortality rate of 80% (5 out of 6 patients); the surviving patient suffered significant permanent neurological deficit.[48] Different pathological and imaging studies have shown a wide range of anatomic variability encountered in PVs; common variables include left trunk PV, right middle PV and right top PV seen in up to 38% of patients studied.[31,49] Additionally, roof pouches can be seen in 15% of AF patients, which have been implicated in occasional complications.[50] The integration of high-resolution CT and MRI images of the LA and PVs into 3D mapping systems provides a detailed display of anatomic variants and adjacent structures (eg, the esophagus) in order to minimize the risks related to this procedure (Figures 10.4 and 10.5).

Several techniques have been clinically applied to register the LA CT/MRI images with the 3D mapping system, with a registration error of 2.5 to 5 mm.[42,51-59] These methods combine visual alignment or landmark registration with surface registration of the LA and other adjacent structures, such as the descending aorta. The most common approach uses landmark registration of the junctions between the superior and inferior PVs as a reliable and reproducible method to integrate the 3D CT/MRI surface reconstruction with the catheter mapping space.[60] If an anatomic variant is present, such as middle or top PVs, their ostia can be used as additional landmark pairs.

In 30 patients undergoing AF ablation, Kistler et al evaluated the registration accuracy of a preprocedural cardiac CT integrated with a 3D map of the LA to guide PVI, using the PV origins to mark fiducial points. They achieved a registration error of 2.3 ± 0.4 mm and successful electrical PVI in 58/60 patients.[58] Tops et al assessed the accuracy of preprocedural CT/3D map integration using a combination of surface registration and fiducial point tagging (by visualizing catheter placement in the LAA under fluoroscopy and intracardiac echocardiography [ICE, also known as intracardiac ultrasound]) in 16 patients undergoing PVI for drug refractory AF. Their study showed a registration error of 2.1 ± 0.2 mm and complete PVI in all patients.[57] Machine et al used preprocedural MRA (n = 10 patients) and cardiac CT (n = 13 patients) during end inspiration and expiration to obtain fiducial points from the PV ostia and aorta in patients undergoing AF ablation. They observed significant inferior displacement of the LA relative to the aorta during end inspiration. The mean registration error using end-inspiratory data sets was 12.1 ± 11 mm, compared with 4.7 ± 0.9 for end-expiratory data sets.[56]

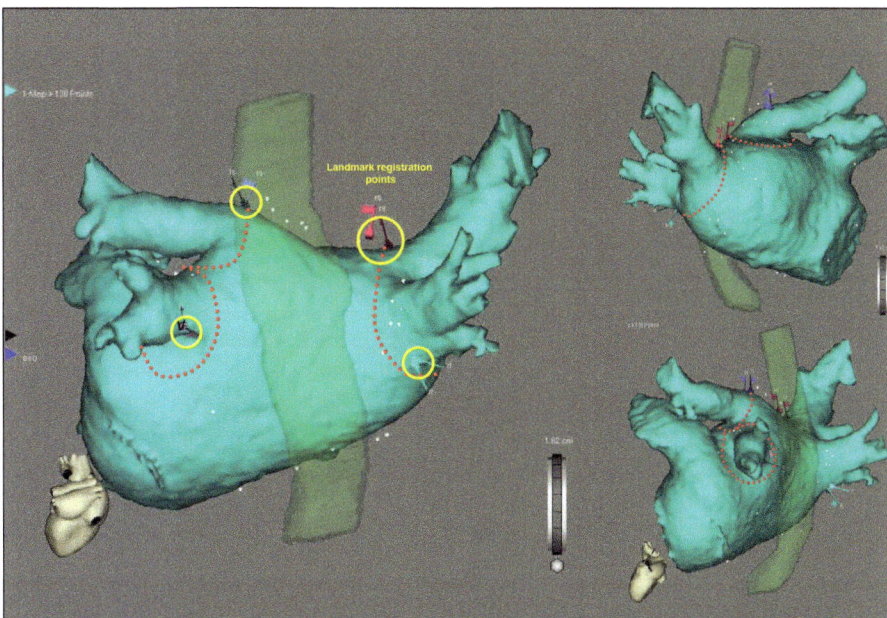

Figure 10.4 Integration of 3D CT reconstruction images of the left atrium (LA), pulmonary veins (PVs) (**blue**) and esophagus (**green**) with the Carto XP mapping system. Note the proximity of the left PVs to the esophagus, which has important implications for RF energy delivery in this region. This allows for designing lesions to isolate the veins while avoiding the areas of the LA posterior wall in closer proximity to the esophagus (**red dotted lines**). Note, however, that the exact location of the esophagus can vary significantly on account of active peristalsis, and therefore, an additional real-time indicator (eg, contrast barium or a temperature probe) is commonly used during the ablation. Landmark registration points at the PV ostium are shown as flags (**yellow circles**).

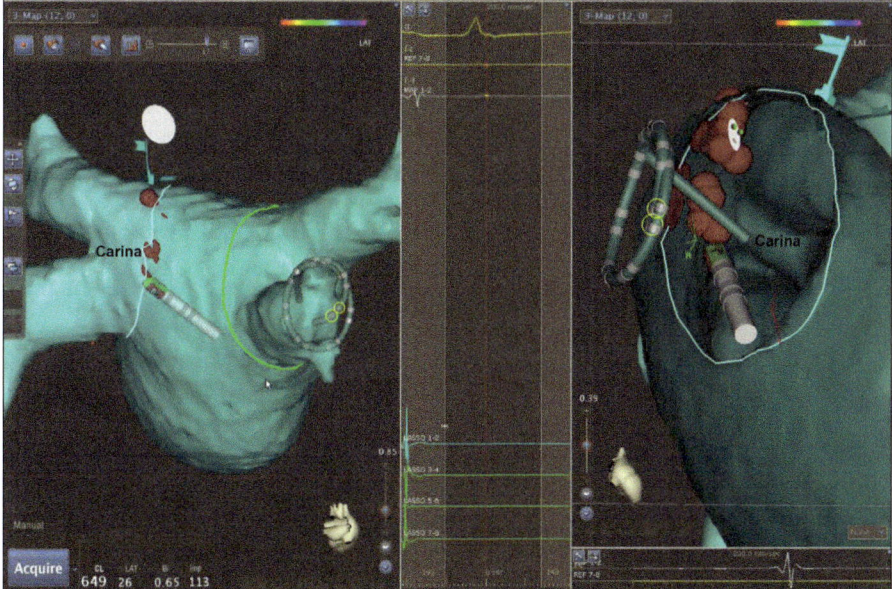

Figure 10.5 Integrated CT and Carto 3 map of the LA during AF ablation. **Left panel:** A multipole circular catheter is placed in the right inferior pulmonary vein. **Right panel:** An endoscopic view allows for visualization of the ablation catheter tip in the left carina region during ablation (**red dots**).

In a large multicenter study of 124 patients undergoing AF ablation, Fahmy et al evaluated a combination of landmark and surface registration methods between preprocedural CT and 3D electroanatomic mapping using ICE. They compared different landmark location points, such as posterior LA, PV ostia, CS, and LAA. Using landmark registration alone, the best accuracy was achieved when posterior LA points or PVs were selected (registration error: 5.6 ± 3.2), whereas landmark points taken on the anterior wall, LAA, or CS resulted in a larger registration error (9.1 ± 2.5). Although surface registration alone had an error of only 2.7 ± 1.6 mm, when this method was combined with landmark registration, it resulted in anterior shifting of the already registered landmark points, leading to a much larger registration error (from 5.6 ± 3.2 to 9.2 ± 2.1).[59] In a smaller study, Brooks et al studied 55 patients with drug-refractory AF undergoing PVI. They evaluated the accuracy of image registration between a preprocedural cardiac CT integrated with a 3D electroanatomic map; to do so, they used a combination of field scaling of the 3D map geometry with a two-step landmark point-registration method. The results showed a registration error of 1.9 ± 0.4 mm and a navigational error (defined as the distance between the catheter tip on the 3D matrix and a projected point on the 3D integrated surface) of 3.4 ± 1.6 mm.[42]

Another method of image registration integrates real-time intracardiac ultrasound imaging with acquisition of LA 3D anatomy that is incorporated into the 3D mapping system (CartoSound). Singh et al used this technique in

30 patients undergoing AF ablation and registered the ultrasound LA shell with a preprocedural CT ($n = 10$ patients) or MRI ($n = 20$ patients). Registration was achieved by visual alignment and landmark and surface registration. The registration error between the ultrasound and CT/MRI data sets was 1.83 ± 0.32 when the LA ultrasound images were obtained by advancing the probe transseptally into the LA; when the ICE probe was left in the RA and rotated to obtain LA images, the registration error was 2.52 ± 0.58.[54]

Registration accuracy can be assessed in several ways before using the fused CT/MRI images for catheter navigation. With accurate registration, the 3D electroanatomic map and the CT/MRI reconstruction can be seen alternatively overlapping the other shell, confirming that both outer boundaries are closely approximated. Further, qualitative validation can be achieved by direct visual corroboration of correct LAA and PV alignment. One can do so by gently manipulating the mapping catheter into these structures under fluoroscopic guidance and visually confirming alignment between the reconstructed 3D CT/MRI and the electroanatomic map.[30]

Some types of mapping software provide additional tools for quantifying registration error. The CartoMerge system calculates an index (the surface-to-point distance) to assess registration errors. This index represents the average distance between the real-time 3D electroanatomic map points and the registered 3D CT/MRI LA surface reconstruction. Although these measurements offer a user-independent method of quality control for the fusion process, they do not guarantee registration accuracy. Misaligned images can have a small surface-to-point distance yet lack accuracy in the registration of clinically important anatomic structures such as the PVs.[59] If the image registration is inaccurate, the process must be restarted by selecting new landmark pairs and sometimes requires sampling additional points of the LA endocardial surface, posterior wall, and PV ostia.[60]

Regardless of the technique used, factors inherent in the patient's anatomy can influence image registration accuracy. In a study by Heist et al, LA volume greater than 110 mL was associated with significant registration error between preprocedural imaging and 3D electroanatomic mapping. However, this study did not associate a significant average integration error with the presence of paroxysmal versus persistent AF, ejection fraction, days of imaging preprocedure, or preprocedural imaging technique employed (CT versus MRI).[55]

Ventricular Tachycardia

The development of electroanatomic mapping has greatly increased our understanding of and ability to treat ventricular arrhythmias. By creating accurate 3D anatomic models with endocardial and/or epicardial voltage information and electrical activation patterns, one can create highly detailed maps of complex arrhythmia circuits, including scar, border zone, and healthy tissue. These models can also differentiate and localize reentrant versus focal mechanisms of arrhythmia. The 3D environment also allows us to visualize mapping and ablation catheters to guide ablation of suitable sites for terminating arrhythmia. By incorporating preprocedural 3D reconstructed imaging data sets, the substrate can be comprehensively delineated. MRI and CT allow for a detailed evaluation of the anatomic substrate, such as wall thinning, intramural calcification, or focal aneurysms, and dynamically characterize wall-motion abnormalities using CT/MRI cine sequences. Perfusion imaging (including first-pass hypoperfusion and delayed enhancement) allows for detailed evaluation of 3D scar geometry and displays its intramural location and transmurality. The MRI- and CT-derived anatomic, dynamic, and perfusion data can be individually reconstructed to provide supplementary confirmation about location and size of the abnormal myocardial substrate.[61]

MRI and CT imaging protocols can be combined with molecular imaging techniques that use metabolically active tagged compounds, such as fluorodeoxyglucose (FDG), to simultaneously evaluate the scar substrate both anatomically and metabolically.[62-64] Preprocedural localization of scar or metabolically abnormal areas can help in planning the best approach for targeting the potential arrhythmia sources; also, it can help guide the choice of vascular access, energy delivery, and extent of endocardial versus epicardial mapping required.[39]

Several groups have demonstrated successful image fusion of preprocedural MRI, CT, and positron emission tomography (PET) data sets using 3D mapping systems for the treatment of patients with ventricular arrhythmias.[17,39,40,41,61-66] The technique for image integration and registration of ventricular chambers, outflow tract, and aorta/pulmonary artery follows the same principles as described above for the LAs and PVs. The unique shape of the right ventricle often allows acceptable registration accuracies based on its 3D form alone, especially if the pulmonary valve is included. Given the cone shape of the left ventricle, however, to minimize rotational errors, apical and mitral valve fiducial points have to be supplemented with either right ventricular or aortic mapping points. 3D substrate maps derived from contrast-enhanced MRI, CT, or PET data sets can be incorporated into the clinical mapping system after full or partial electroanatomic mapping. They can also be registered to ultrasound-created 3D chamber reconstruction in order to define substrates for VT in ischemic and nonischemic heart disease[17] (see Figure 10.5).

PET/C: The PET/CT combined imaging mode enables the metabolic-anatomic characterization of the scar substrate by evaluating myocardial viability using 18F-fluorodeoxyglucose (FDG) and perfusion with 82-rubidium chloride (Rb). A cardiac-gated multidetector

CT scanner is used to obtain chamber anatomy. Left ventricular contours and metabolic scar can then be imported and registered with the electroanatomic map. In several studies, the combination of visual alignment and surface-shell registration yielded the lowest amount of registration error (3.7±0.7; 4.34±0.6 mm),[62-64] while Fahmy et al found a surface-based registration error of 5.1±2.1 mm with this technology.[63]

Important advantages of PET are the lack of contraindications due to renal dysfunction or ICD implantation and the absence of metal artifacts. The main limitations of PET imaging are the spatial resolution of about 6 mm and poor image quality in patients with uncontrolled diabetes (Figure 10.6).

Contrast-enhanced Computer Tomography: Advances in contrast-enhanced, multidetector CT have enabled detailed characterization of the left ventricular myocardium.[61,67] Myocardial scar and border zone, as the targets of VT ablations, displays abnormal anatomic, dynamic, and perfusion characteristics during first-pass CT. In 11 patients with ischemic heart disease undergoing VT ablation, preprocedural cardiac CT integrated with 3D electroanatomic mapping had a registration accuracy of 3.31±0.52 mm. The CT 3D reconstruction predicted 82% of abnormal voltage segments, while first-pass perfusion images accurately displayed scar transmurality.[61]

Delayed-enhanced CT imaging analogous to MRI has been described in several animal models and patient series of acute or chronic infarct.[68-71] Consistent high-quality delayed-enhanced CT scar images are still challenging in chronic human infarcts, so published studies using these data for image integration is still limited. Valdigem et al used retrospective cardiac CT imaging to define cardiac anatomy, coronary arteries, and delayed-contrast enhancement in 8 patients undergoing epicardial ablation for VT in Chagasic cardiomyopathy. Registration with 3D maps rendered a positional error of 6.03±2.09 mm. Epicardial ablation was guided by combined CT-derived display of the coronary arteries but supplemented by coronary angiography. This technique led to safe energy delivery in 6 out of 8 patients[67] (see Figure 10.6).

Magnetic Resonance Imaging: With its remarkable spatial resolution, MRI technology can produce images of great anatomic detail and, with the use of LGE, accurately delineate myocardial scar tissue.[72] Using high-resolution MRI in a swine infarct model, Ashikaga et al were able to detect small, interspersed patches of fibrosis and accurately predict the activation wavefront during induced VT, based on the anatomic scar model.[73] As an additional advantage, MRI lacks the ionizing radiation to which patients are exposed during CT or PET imaging.

Prior studies have demonstrated the feasibility and clinical applicability of integrating preprocedural MRI data sets with 3D mapping systems for guiding VT ablation procedures in patients with ischemic and nonischemic cardiomyopathy. In these studies, registration accuracies ranged from 3 to 5 mm.[17,39,40,65,74] Codreanu et al studied 10 patients with ischemic cardiomyopathy prior to VT ablation. Abnormal electrogram (EGM) signals, lower voltage amplitude, and longer EGM duration were more prevalent in scar compared with healthy tissue. The best correlation between MRI and voltage-derived scar was found using a bipolar threshold of under 1.5 mV, but a scar mismatch area greater than 20% was found in 4 of 12 fibrotic areas.[74] In 14 patients with ischemic VT, Desjardins et al found that bipolar/unipolar voltages below

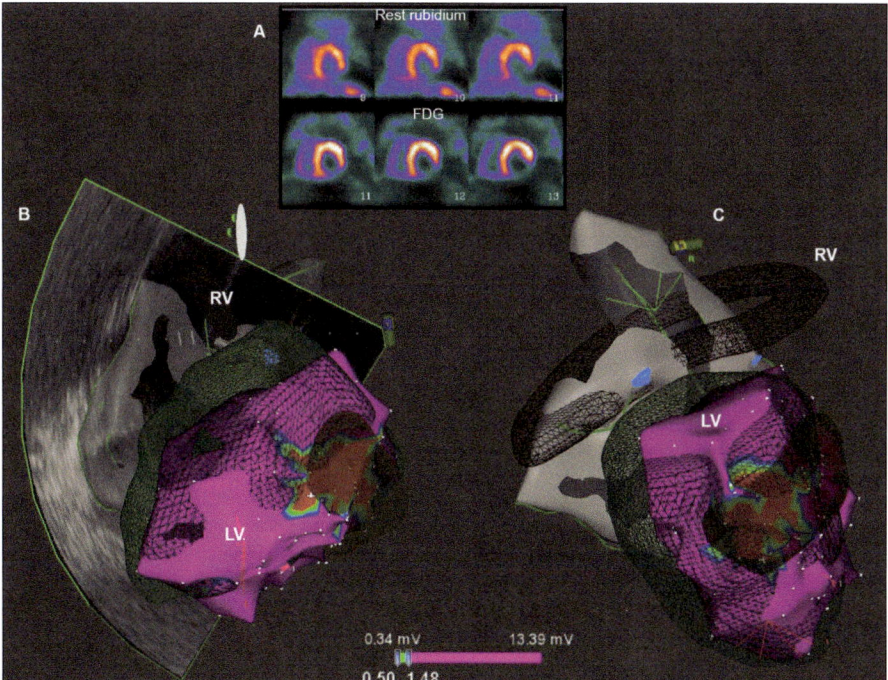

Figure 10.6 Image integration of preprocedural PET/CT with intraprocedural 3D voltage map and intracardiac ultrasound using the Carto 3 mapping system and CartoSound module for a patient with recurrent scar-mediated, monomorphic VT. A preprocedural PET (rest rubidium and FDG uptake) showed a nonviable inferolateral scar (**Panel A**). Intracardiac ultrasound and the CartoSound module allowed for quick acquisition of an RV shell in less than 5 minutes (**gray**). A 3D reconstruction of the PET CT LV (**green mesh**), RV (**brown mesh**), and LV scar (**semitransparent green**) was fused prospectively into the 3D mapping environment to guide voltage mapping to the regions of potential scar observed on the preprocedural imaging, with excellent correlation (**Panels B** and **C**). FDG = 18F-fluorodeoxyglucose.

1.0 mV and 5.8 mV, respectively, differentiated well between scar and nonfibrotic tissue. LGE was associated with isolated diastolic potentials and fractionated EGMs, and all VT and premature ventricular contractions (PVCs) originated within areas of delayed enhancement (DE). Mismatch between MRI and voltage-derived scar occurred in 18% of bipolar and 16% of unipolar voltage recordings.[40] In 5 of 14 patients with LGE and nonischemic cardiomyopathy, compared with endocardial or epicardial LGE sites, midmyocardial scar reconstructions from MRI predicted the failure of RF ablation to eliminate VT or PVCs.[65] In a study by Wijnmaalen et al, 15 patients with scar-mediated VT underwent preprocedural cardiac MRI. Three patients had only nontransmural scar and peri-infarct gray-zone areas; although these were not detected by conventional unipolar and bipolar voltage criteria, they were responsible for the VT reentrant circuits in these patients.[39]

Of special concern in MRI is the presence of ICDs in the majority of patients with structural heart disease. Although these devices are still considered a contraindication to MRI, more than 1,000 ICD patients have undergone MRI worldwide, mostly in highly experienced centers with strict inclusion and exclusion criteria. However, only limited data are available for the use of preprocedural cardiac MRI to define scar in patients with ICDs. In one study, LGE scar was successfully registered (position error: 3.9 ± 1.8 mm) in 22 ICD patients undergoing VT ablation—despite pronounced metal artifacts in LGE imaging reconstruction. Display of the registered scar was able to identify excellent pace-mapping sites. This meant forgoing complete voltage mapping in 64% of patients and identifying successful ablation sites of intramyocardial substrate despite preserved bipolar voltages (Figures 10.7 and 10.8; ▶ Video 10.2).[17]

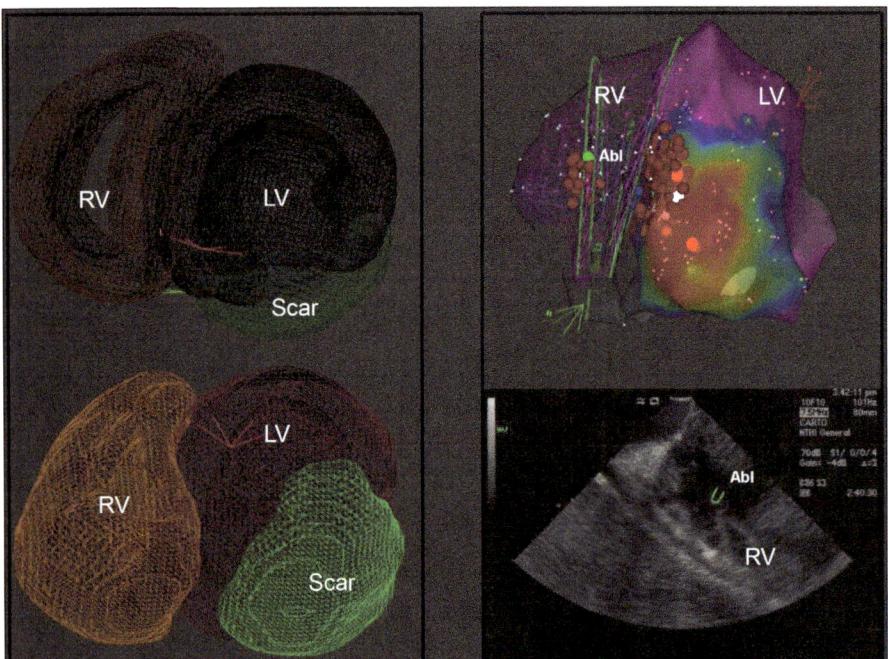

Figure 10.7 **Left panel:** 3D volume reconstruction of a preprocedural cardiac MRI showing large inferior left ventricular scar (**green mesh**). **Right panel:** Integrated voltage map and CartoSound shell (**top**) of LV showing large inferior scar (**red area** corresponding to bipolar voltage <0.5 mV). Real-time intracardiac ultrasound images (**bottom**) reveal catheter-to-tissue contact in scar areas with low voltage. Pace mapping in the septal aspect of the LV scar showed a similar pace map match for the patient's clinical VT; however, tachycardia was still inducible. Ablation (Abl) from the RV septum at a contiguous site had a near-perfect pace map match and was the successful ablation site (**green point**).

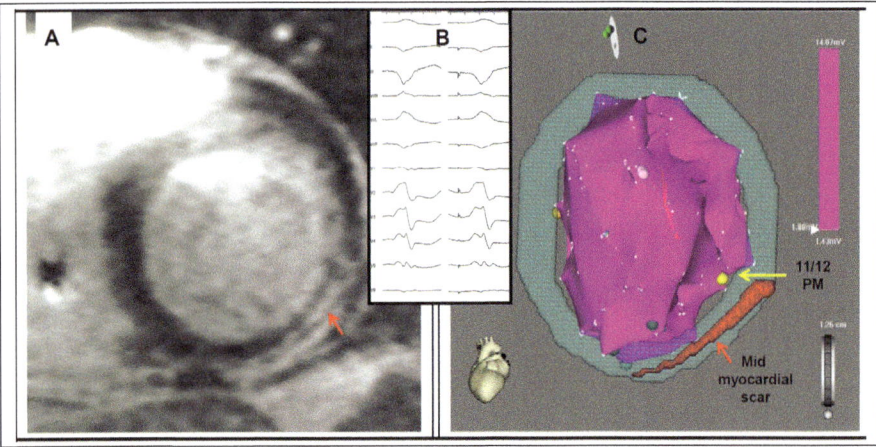

Figure 10.8 MRI-guided detection and ablation of midmyocardial scar. Normal endocardial voltage map in inferolateral wall. MR imaging plane (**Panel A, red arrow**) demonstrates an inferolateral midmyocardial scar, which was reconstructed in 3D, displaying the accurate intramyocardial location (**Panel C, red arrow**). Pace mapping at this location (**yellow dot**) resulted in a ≥11/12 pace map match (**Panel B**), and ablation eliminated the patient's clinical VT. *Source:* Adapted with permission from Dickfeld T, et al., their Figure 7B–D.[17]

Other Cardiac Arrhythmias

Given the high success rate of traditional mapping methods for AV nodal reentrant tachycardia, AV reentrant tachycardia, and typical atrial flutter, the additional cost and potential radiation exposure reserve the use of image integration techniques mostly for selected complex arrhythmias. These special situations are discussed next.

Atrial Tachycardia Occurring After Atrial Fibrillation Ablation/Surgery: Atrial tachycardia/flutter can be observed in up to 30% of patients after AF ablation and is often difficult to treat medically. In these patients, the integration of CT or MRI-derived LA and PV anatomy with 3D voltage and activation maps can help identify areas of prior intervention and possible discontinuity in the ablation lines. With the enhanced ability to visualize previous ablation lesions with MRI, the integration of postablation 3D reconstructions may enable precise catheter navigation to eliminate those gaps.[66]

Arrhythmias After Corrective and Palliative Congenital Heart Surgery: Adult congenital heart disease patients who underwent corrective or palliative surgery at a younger age for conditions such as tetralogy of Fallot, atrial and ventricular septal defect, and transposition of the great arteries can present with a wide variety of atrial and ventricular arrhythmias. These arrhythmias can be related to scar tissue from surgical incisions, patches, and/or shunts, leading to macroreentrant circuits through incision gaps, or consist of focal arrhythmias originating within or near the scar tissue. They can also derive from volume and pressure overload, leading to chamber dilatation. The supreme difficulty of navigating catheters through a distorted anatomy (eg, vessel transpositions, atrial and ventricular switches, baffle stenosis) using conventional fluoroscopy can be greatly facilitated by the use of a preprocedural contrast-enhanced CT or MRI integrated into a 3D electroanatomic map. The correlation of activation maps with detailed anatomic data is important for identifying likely reentrant pathways and arrhythmia mechanisms[75] (Figure 10.9 and corresponding ▶ Video 10.3).

Ventricular Outflow Tract Tachycardias: Traditionally, outflow tract tachycardias have been successfully mapped and ablated using fluoroscopic guidance and conventional mapping. Some areas, such as the aortic cusps and the sinuses of Valsalva, can be difficult to visualize using conventional mapping techniques. High-density electroanatomic mapping and pace mapping in the outflow tract and sub- and supravalvular regions can localize the exact site of origin and produce a successful ablation outcome. However, proximity to the coronary ostia and lack of stable contact with the aortic cusps can greatly influence the safety and efficacy of these ablations. Thus, integration of 3D reconstruction CT or MR images, including coronary artery anatomy and the addition of ICE, can help visualize the catheter tip to assess both tissue contact and distance to the coronary ostia (Figure 10.10).[76,77]

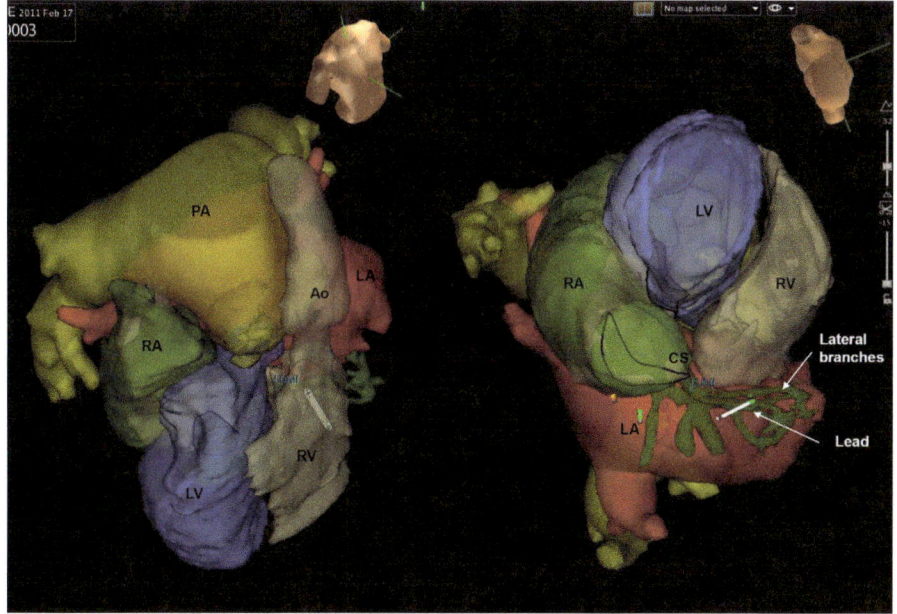

Figure 10.9 Integration of preprocedural cardiac CT with 3D electroanatomic map (EnSite Velocity) to guide systemic ventricular lead implantation in a patient with New York Heart Association (NYHA) class III heart failure due to L-transposition of the great arteries and dextrocardia. The right atrium (**green**) communicates with the morphological left ventricle (**blue**), and the left ventricular outflow tract gives rise to the pulmonary artery (**yellow**). In turn, the left atrium (**red**) empties into the morphological right ventricle, which gives rise to the ascending aorta. A 3D shell of the right atrium and coronary sinus (**green**) was fused with the cardiac CT to guide delivery of a bipolar lead (**white arrow**) into a lateral RV branch (systemic ventricle).

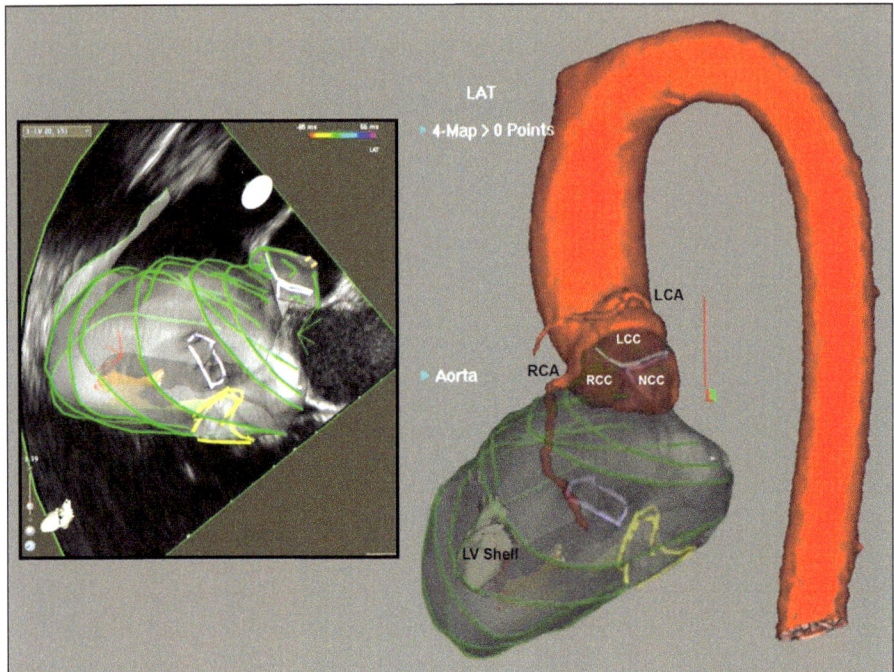

Figure 10.10 Integration of preprocedural CT with 3D reconstruction of the aortic cusps and coronary arteries (**red**) with intraprocedural intracardiac ultrasound shell of the left ventricle and aortic cusps using the CARTO 3D mapping system and the CARTOSOUND module (**left insert**). The integration of registered 3D images with real-time intracardiac ultrasound enables visualizing catheter-to-tissue contact and guiding safe energy delivery away from the coronary arteries during RF ablation. LCA = left coronary artery; LCC = left coronary cusp; NCC = noncoronary cusp; RCA = right coronary artery; RCC = right coronary cusp.

Other Imaging Modalities Used for Image Fusion with 3D Mapping Systems

Intracardiac Ultrasound and Image Fusion with 3D Mapping Systems

ICE is currently the only commercially available real-time imaging modality for detailed visualization of myocardial structures. The integration of preprocedural imaging modalities, such as cardiac CT and MRI, with a real-time imaging system offers great potential advantages for complex EP procedures. Two distinct intracardiac ICE technologies are available. One system uses a single, radial 9 MHz transducer with a field of view of 15 degrees and a rotational speed of 3,800 rpm, mounted on a 9-Fr non-steerable catheter (ClearView Cardiovascular Imaging System, Freemont, CA; Boston Scientific, San Jose, CA). The other technology uses a phased-array transducer consisting of 64 piezoelectric crystals with frequencies ranging from 5 to 10 MHz, mounted on an 8-Fr or 10-Fr catheter with 4 degrees of movement (anterior, posterior, left, and right deflections) and a 90-degree sector image (Siemens Acuson, Mountain View, CA).

The fixed catheter–radial transducer type lacks good far-field resolution and adequate imaging of intracardiac structures and requires that the catheter be positioned adjacent to such structures. The phased-array ICE catheters provides better far-field resolution (up to a depth of 15 cm) and Doppler capabilities, making it the preferred ultrasound system in many cardiac EP laboratories.[78] In addition, the phased-array ICE catheter is manufactured with an integrated magnetic location sensor (SoundStar, Siemens Acuson) and has the ability to reference the 2D ICE images to the 3D matrix of the CARTO XP or CARTO 3 mapping system (CARTOSOUND, Biosense Webster). Sequential 2D ICE images are used to build an ECG-gated, 3D geometry of the intracardiac structures and chambers, which can be fully registered with preprocedural CT, MRI, or PET images (see Figures 10.6, 10.7, and 10.10).

ICE imaging to facilitate ablation procedures has been reported for a variety of atrial and ventricular arrhythmias,[77,79,80] including fluoro-less procedures guided by ICE image fusion with preprocedural imaging.[81,82] Visualization of the ablation catheter tip *in vivo* to assess proper tissue contact can improve procedural success and facilitate safe energy delivery.[83] Combining both technologies allows for real-time confirmation that an ablation lesion has been created (ICE) in an area of registered MRI/CT scar substrate.[17]

Three-dimensional Rotational Angiography

Currently available 3D rotational angiography (3DRA) systems allow for intraprocedural rapid acquisition of angiographic images that can be fully integrated with 3D electroanatomic maps. The main advantage of 3DRA technology is eliminating the need for a preprocedural radiographic procedure altogether. Also, the acquisition of images without a significant time gap may result in fewer volumetric discrepancies and, potentially, more accurate image registration.

Contrast-enhanced cardiac fluoroscopy images are obtained using one of two commercially available 3DRA systems: Xper FD 10 system (Philips Medical Systems, Best, The Netherlands) and syngo DynaCT (Siemens, Malvern, PA) during a power injection of contrast dye through a hollow catheter. The catheter injection site is determined by the chamber of interest: the inferior vena cava–right atrial (IVC-RA) junction for right ventricular imaging; the main pulmonary trunk or selective pulmonary arteries for LA and PV imaging; and the retrograde transaortic left ventricular position for left ventricular imaging. The contrast transit time (time from injection to opacification of the chamber of interest) must be accounted for in order to appropriately time the onset of camera rotation and image acquisition. During a breath hold, the camera is rotated from 120° right anterior oblique to 120° left anterior oblique in 4 to 5 seconds, with an x-ray acquisition speed of 30 frames per second. Images are transferred to a workstation where image segmentation is conducted (in a similar fashion to conventional CT angiography [CTA] imaging). A 3D model of the heart is rendered and overlaid in the live fluoroscopy screen, and both images are registered using radio-opaque landmarks as fiduciary points, such as the carina or pacing leads. Once the 3DRA images are merged with the live fluoro images, they can be integrated with 3D electroanatomic maps using the same integration parameters described for conventional CTA.

Recent studies have validated the use of this novel image integration technique during AF and VT ablations.[84-86] The only study so far comparing 3DRA guidance with fluoroscopy and 3D electroanatomic mappings for AF ablation found no statistically significant differences in procedural time, radiation exposure, acute ablation success, or procedural outcomes.[87] Acceptable-quality images were obtained in the majority of patients studied in the different trials. Also, compared with more traditional image-integration protocols using preprocedural CT or MRI scans, researchers observed similar segmentation and registration times, x-ray exposure, and procedure duration (Table 10.1 and Figure 10.11).

Table 10.1 Studies comparing image-fusion techniques with fluoroscopy and/or 3D map–guided AF ablation procedures

Study	Pre-procedural Imaging	Groups	No. of patients	Follow up (months)	Benefits of image integration over conventional or 3D only technique
Kistler PM, et al (*J Cardiovasc Electrophysiol.* 2006)	CT	3D vs MERGE	94	6 ± 1	Reduce fluoro time; improve clinical outcomes
Kistler PM, et al (*Eur Heart J.* 2008)	CT	XP vs MERGE	80	13 ± 3	No difference between groups
Martinek M, et al (*Pacing Clin Electrophysiol.* 2007)	CT	XP vs MERGE	100	6	Reduce complications; improved clinical outcomes
Tang K, et al (*Chin Med J.* (Engl) 2008)	CT	XP vs MERGE	81	12 ± 3	Reduced fluoro and procedural time
Della Bella P, et al (*J Cardiovasc Electrophysiol.* 2009)	CT	Conventional vs MERGE	290	14 ± 12	Improved clinical outcomes, but increased fluoro and procedural time
Bertaglia E, et al (*Europace.* 2009)	CT, MRI	XP vs Conventional vs MERGE	573	11 ± 5	Reduced procedural time and improved clinical outcomes
Caponi D, et al (*Europace.* 2010)	MRI	XP vs MERGE	299	12	Reduced fluoro time
Knecht S, et al (*Heart Rhythm.* 2010)	None	XP vs 3DRA	91	10 ± 4	No difference between groups
Pratola C, et al (*Pacing Clin Electrophysiol.* 2011)	MRI	XP vs ICE vs XP + ICE	60	9 ± 2	ICE integration reduced fluoro time compared to XP or XP + ICE

3D = Carto and ESI NavX mapping systems; MERGE = Carto image integration software package; XP = Carto XP mapping system; Conventional = fluoroscopy electrogram guided PVI; 3DRA = 3D rotational angiography; ICE = intracardiac echocardiogram.

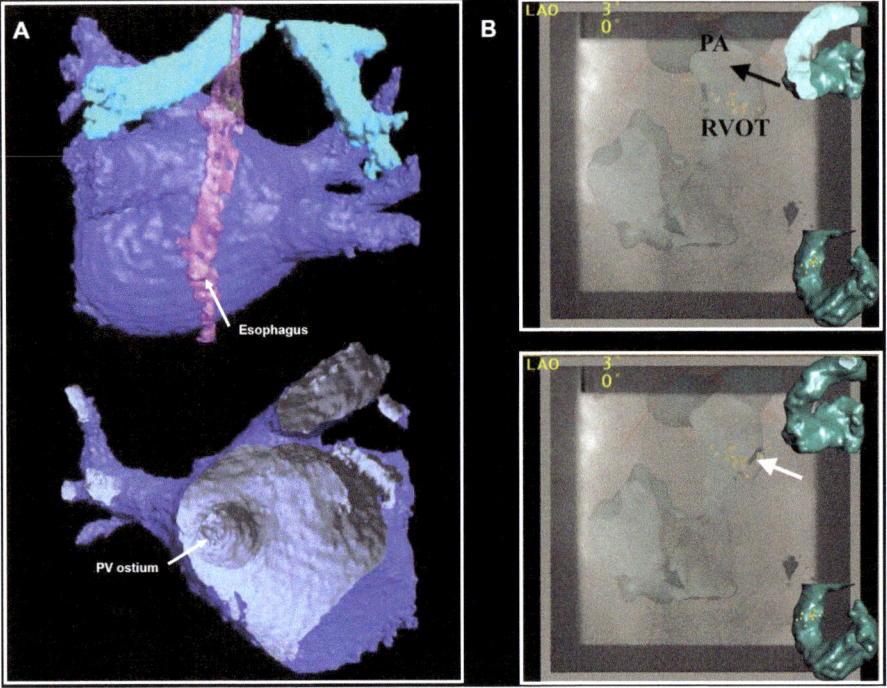

Figure 10.11 **Panel A:** Example of LA shell reconstructed from a 3D rotational angiography for an AF ablation procedure, with excellent definition of PV ostia and esophagus. **Panel B:** Anteroposterior views of image registration between a 3D rotational angiography model and live fluoroscopy during RVOT VT ablation. The bronchial carina (**light brown dot behind pulmonary artery bifurcation**) was used as a landmark for registration and visual confirmation of the catheter location in both posterior (**top**) and anterior (**bottom**) aspects of the RVOT. Ablation lesions are marked as **yellow dots**. RVOT = right ventricular outflow tract. *Source:* Panel A adapted with permission from Knecht S, et al.[87] Panel B adapted with permission from Orlov M, et al.[86]

Future Applications for Image Fusion: Real-time MRI-guided Electrophysiology Procedures, Atrial Fibrosis, and Assessment of Ablation Lesions

Future directions for image integration techniques aim to improve current technological limitations. These limitations relate to the accuracy of registration data, volumetric discrepancies between pre- and intraprocedural data sets, visualization of catheter/tissue contact, assessment of ablation lesions, and periprocedural radiation exposure. One potential modality that could overcome these limitations is real-time MRI. The basic principles of real-time cardiac MRI–guided EP studies were introduced in 2000 by Lardo et al, who demonstrated their ability to visualize intracardiac catheters and RF lesions in a canine model.[88] Subsequent studies have shown the ability of real-time cardiac MRI to monitor intraprocedural RF ablation energy delivery and assess lesion formation,[89,90] perform diagnostic EP studies[90,92] and guide interventional RF ablation.[90-92] Another possible application of real-time MRI is the use of MRI thermography to guide RF ablation and intraprocedural lesion formation. In an animal model, RF-induced lesion extent seen on thermography images correlated well with gross anatomy specimens.[93]

Significant progress has been made in cardiac MRI's ability to visualize atrial fibrosis and ablation lesions, putting this technology at the brink of clinical feasibility. Several groups have evaluated both preprocedural cardiac MRI for assessing atrial fibrosis before AF ablation to predict procedural outcomes[94,95] and postprocedural cardiac MRI for assessing lesion formation after AF ablation.[95-98] Akoum et al used DE cardiac MRI preablation to stratify 144 patients by severity of LA fibrosis and to quantify severity of LA scarring postablation. They found that, in patients with mild LA fibrosis, circumferential PV scarring was predictive of successful ablation, whereas patients with more extensive preprocedural LA fibrosis required more extensive postablation scarring to achieve procedural success.[95] In a study evaluating the LA substrate in 40 patients undergoing ablation for lone AF, Mahnkopf et al demonstrated that the degree of LA fibrosis is independent of AF type and predictive of successful outcomes postablation.[97] A study by Taclas et al compared RF ablation sites on a 3D mapping system with postprocedural DE cardiac MRI to assess scar formation in 19 patients undergoing AF ablation. They employed a rigid registration method to integrate both data sets and were able to indentify LA scar on MRI in 80% of areas postablation and to visualize gap in the intended ablation lines in up to 20% of all ablated sectors.[98] These results show that the integration of DE cardiac MRI fibrosis and scar reconstructions into 3D mapping systems may allow for a substrate-guided approach for redo AF and post-AF left and right atrial flutter ablations.

Conclusions

Image integration techniques combining pre- and postprocedural radiological studies with intraprocedural 3D electroanatomic maps can provide a detailed and comprehensive assessment of the heart. Cardiac anatomy, ventricular function, coronary perfusion, and tissue characteristics can be used to facilitate complex arrhythmia ablations by improving catheter guidance and efficient targeting of arrhythmogenic tissue. Multiple studies have demonstrated the safety and likely improved efficacy of such an approach. Paramount to the accuracy and clinical applicability of this technique is obtaining a preprocedural radiographic study of excellent quality and performing a correct image fusion process. Achieving this level of reliability requires an experienced multidisciplinary group of radiologists, electrophysiologists, and technicians. The initial role of image fusion for guiding AF ablation is expanding to other complex cardiac arrhythmias, such as VT, and has provided additional insight into disease-specific tissue characteristics and mechanisms of such complex arrhythmias. Newer imaging techniques and improvements in current MR and CT technology hold promise for further advancements in the years to come.

Acknowledgments

The authors would like to thank Howard Lowery and Thomas Severino for their assistance with some of the 3D mapping material.

References

1. Luenberger DG. *Linear and Nonlinear Programming*, 2nd ed. Reading, MA: Addison-Wesley Publishing Co.; 2005.
2. Christian PE, Waterstram-Rich, eds. *Nuclear Medicine and PET/CT: Technologies and Techniques*. 6th ed. St. Louis, MO: Mosby Elsevier; 2007.
3. Kalra MK, Maher MM, Toth TL, et al. Techniques and applications of automatic tube current modulation for CT. *Radiology*. 2004;233(3):649-657.
4. Flohr TG, Klotz E, Allmendinger T, et al. Pushing the envelope: new computed tomography techniques for cardiothoracic imaging. *J Thorac Imaging*. 2010;25(2)100-111.
5. Sra JS. Cardiac magnetic resonance imaging and computed tomography: anatomic fundamentals. *J Interv Card Electrophysiol*. 2011;31(1):39-46.
6. Hendee WR, Morgan CJ. Magnetic resonance imaging. Part I—physical principles. *West J Med*. 1984;141(4):491-500.
7. Bogaert J, Taylor AM, Van Kerkhove F, Dymarkowski S. Use of inversion recovery contrast-enhanced MRI for cardiac imaging: spectrum of applications. *AJR Am J Roentgenol*. 2004; 182(3):609-615.
8. Götte MJ, Rüssel IK, de Roest GJ, et al. Magnetic resonance imaging, pacemakers and implantable cardioverter-defibrillators: current situation and clinical perspective. *Neth Heart J*. 2010;18(1):31-37.
9. Ridgway JP. Cardiovascular magnetic resonance physics for clinicians: part I. *J Cardiovasc Magn Reson*. 2010;12:71.
10. Levine GN, Gomes AS, Arai AE, et al. Safety of magnetic resonance imaging in patients with cardiovascular devices: an American Heart Association scientific statement from the Committee on Diagnostic and Interventional Cardiac Catheterization, Council on Clinical Cardiology, and the Council on Cardiovascular Radiology and Intervention: endorsed by the American College of Cardiology Foundation, the North American Society for Cardiac Imaging, and the Society for Cardiovascular Magnetic Resonance. *Circulation*. 2007;116:2878-2891.
11. Perazella MA. Current status of gadolinium toxicity in patients with kidney disease. *Clin J Am Soc Nephrol*. 2009;4: 461-469.
12. Sommer T, Vahlhaus C, Lauck G, et al. MRI and cardiac pacemakers: in-vitro evaluation and in-vivo studies in 51 patients at 0.5 T. *Radiology*. 2000;215(3):869-879.
13. Duru F, Luechinger R, Candinas R. MRI in patients with cardiac pacemakers. *Radiology*. 2001;219:856-858.
14. Faris OP, Shein M. Food and Drug Administration perspective: magnetic resonance imaging of pacemaker and implantable cardioverter-defibrillator patients. *Circulation*. 2006;19:114(12):1232-1233.
15. Roguin A, Schwitter J, Vahlhaus C, et al. Magnetic resonance imaging in individuals with cardiovascular implantable electronic devices. *Europace*. 2008;10(3):336-346.
16. Zikria JF, Machnicki S, Rhim E, et al. MRI of patients with cardiac pacemakers: a review of the medical literature. *AJR Am J Roentgenol*. 2011;196(2):390-401.
17. Dickfeld T, Tian J, Ahmad G, et al. MRI-guided ventricular tachycardia ablation: integration of late gadolinium enhanced 3D scar in patients with ICD. *Circ Arrhythm Electrophysiol*. 2011;4(2):172-184.
18. Nazarian S, Roguin A, Zviman MM, et al. Clinical utility and safety of a protocol for noncardiac and cardiac magnetic resonance imaging of patients with permanent pacemakers and implantable-cardioverter defibrillators at 1.5 tesla. *Circulation*. 2006;114(12):1277-1284.
19. Roguin A, Zviman MM, Meininger GR, et al. Modern pacemaker and implantable cardioverter/defibrillator systems can be magnetic resonance imaging safe: in vitro and in vivo assessment of safety and function at 1.5 T. *Circulation*. 2004; 110(5):475-82.
20. Wilkoff BL, Bello D, Taborsky M, et al. Magnetic resonance imaging in patients with a pacemaker system designed for the magnetic resonance environment. *Heart Rhythm*. 2011;8(1): 65-73.
21. Dickfeld T, Calkins H, Zviman M, et al. Anatomic stereotactic catheter ablation on three-dimensional magnetic resonance images in real time. *Circulation*. 2003;108:2407-2413.
22. Richmond L, Rajappan K, Voth E, et al. Validation of computed tomography image integration into the EnSite NavX mapping system to perform catheter ablation of atrial fibrillation. *J Cardiovasc Electrophysiol*. 2008;19(8):821-827.
23. Sra J, Krum D, Hare J, et al. Feasibility and validation of registration of three-dimensional left atrial models derived from computed tomography with a noncontact cardiac mapping system. *Heart Rhythm*. 2005;2:55-63.
24. Della Bella P, Fassini G, Cireddu M, et al. Image integration guided catheter ablation of atrial fibrillation: a prospective randomized study. *J Cardiovasc Electrophysiol*. 2009;20:258-265.
25. Caponi D, Corleto A, Scaglione M, et al. Ablation of atrial fibrillation: does the addition of three-dimensional magnetic resonance imaging of the left atrium to electro-anatomic mapping improve the clinical outcome?: A randomized comparison of CartoMerge vs. Carto-XP three-dimensional mapping ablation in patients with paroxysmal and persistent atrial fibrillation. *Europace*. 2010;12:1098-1104.
26. Bertaglia E, Bella PD, Tondo C, et al. Image integration increases efficacy of paroxysmal atrial fibrillation catheter ablation: results from the CartoMerge Italian Registry. *Europace*. 2009;11:1004-1010.

27. Kistler PM, Rajappan K, Harris S, et al. The impact of image integration on catheter ablation of atrial fibrillation using electro-anatomic mapping: a prospective randomized study. *Eur Heart J.* 2008;29:3029-3036.
28. Nölker G, Asbach S, Gutleben KJ, et al. Image-integration of intraprocedural rotational angiography–based 3D reconstructions of left atrium and pulmonary veins into electro-anatomical mapping: accuracy of a novel modality in atrial fibrillation ablation. *J Cardiovasc Electrophysiol.* 2010;21(3):278-283.
29. Ejima K, Shoda M, Yagishita D, et al. Image integration of three-dimensional cone-beam computed tomography angiogram into electro-anatomical mapping system to guide catheter ablation of atrial fibrillation. *Europace.* 2010;12(1):45-51.
30. Dong J, Dickfeld T, Dalal D, et al. Initial experience in the use of integrated electro-anatomic mapping with three-dimensional MR/CT images to guide catheter ablation of atrial fibrillation. *J Cardiovasc Electrophysiol.* 2006;17(5):459-466.
31. Kato R, Lickfett L, Meininger G, et al. Pulmonary vein anatomy in patients undergoing catheter ablation of atrial fibrillation: lessons learned by use of magnetic resonance imaging. *Circulation.* 2003;107(15):2004-2010.
32. Sonka M, Fitzpatrick JM, eds. *Handbook of Medical Imaging.* Vol. 2. Bellingham, WA: SPIE Press; 2000.
33. Dong J, Dickfeld T. Image integration in electro-anatomic mapping. *Herzschrittmacherther Elektrophysiol.* 2007;18(3):122-130.
34. Sra J, Ratnakumar S. Cardiac image registration of the left atrium and pulmonary veins. *Heart Rhythm.* 2008;5(4):609-617.
35. Sra J, Krum D, Hare J, et al. Feasibility and validation of registration of three-dimensional left atrial models derived from computed tomography with a noncontact cardiac mapping system. *Heart Rhythm.* 2005;2:55-63.
36. Solomon SB, Dickfeld T, Calkins H. Real-time cardiac catheter navigation on three-dimensional CT images. *J Interv Card Electrophysiol.* 2003;8:27-36.
37. Richmond L, Rajappan K, Voth E, et al. Validation of computed tomography image integration into the EnSite NavX mapping system to perform catheter ablation of atrial fibrillation. *J Cardiovasc Electrophysiol.* 2008;19(8):821-827.
38. Kistler PM, Earley MJ, Harris S, et al. Validation of three-dimensional cardiac image integration: use of integrated CT image into electroanatomic mapping system to perform catheter ablation of atrial fibrillation. *J Cardiovasc Electrophysiol.* 2006;17(4):341-348.
39. Wijnmaalen AP, van der Geest RJ, van Huls van Taxis CF, et al. Head-to-head comparison of contrast-enhanced magnetic resonance imaging and electro-anatomical voltage mapping to assess post-infarct scar characteristics in patients with ventricular tachycardias: real-time image integration and reversed registration. *Eur Heart J.* 2011;32(1):104-114.
40. Desjardins B, Crawford T, Good E, et al. Infarct architecture and characteristics on delayed enhanced magnetic resonance imaging and electro-anatomic mapping in patients with post infarction ventricular arrhythmia. *Heart Rhythm.* 2009;6(5):644-651.
41. Dong J, Calkins H, Solomon SB, et al. Integrated electro-anatomic mapping with three-dimensional computed tomographic images for real-time guided ablations. *Circulation.* 2006;113(2):186-194.
42. Brooks AG, Wilson L, Kuklik P, et al. Image integration using NavX Fusion: initial experience and validation. *Heart Rhythm.* 2008;5(4):526-535.
43. Richmond L, Rajappan K, Voth E, et al. Validation of computed tomography image integration into the EnSite NavX mapping system to perform catheter ablation of atrial fibrillation. *J Cardiovasc Electrophysiol.* 2008;19(8):821-827.
44. Martinek M, Nesser HJ, Aichinger J, et al. Accuracy of integration of multislice computed tomography imaging into three-dimensional electro-anatomic mapping for real-time guided radiofrequency ablation of left atrial fibrillation–influence of heart rhythm and radiofrequency lesions. *J Interv Card Electrophysiol.* 2006;17(2):85-92.
45. Dong J, Dalal D, Scherr D, et al. Impact of heart rhythm status on registration accuracy of the left atrium for catheter ablation of atrial fibrillation. *J Cardiovasc Electrophysiol.* 2007;18(12):1269-1276.
46. Saad EB, Marrouche NF, Saad CP, et al. Pulmonary vein stenosis after catheter ablation of atrial fibrillation: emergence of a new clinical syndrome. *Ann Intern Med.* 2003;138(8):634-638.
47. Barrett CD, Di Biase L, Natale A. How to identify and treat patient with pulmonary vein stenosis post atrial fibrillation ablation. *Curr Opin Cardiol.* 2009;24(1):42-49.
48. Ghia KK, Chugh A, Good E, et al. A nationwide survey on the prevalence of atrioesophageal fistula after left atrial radiofrequency catheter ablation. *J Interv Card Electrophysiol.* 2009;24(1):33-36.
49. Ho SY, Sanchez-Quintana D, Cabrera JA, Anderson RH. Anatomy of the left atrium: implications for radiofrequency ablation of atrial fibrillation. *J Cardiovasc Electrophysiol.* 1999;10(11):1525-1533.
50. Wongcharoen W, Tsao HM, Wu MH, et al. Morphologic characteristics of the left atrial appendage, roof, and septum: implications for the ablation of atrial fibrillation. *J Cardiovasc Electrophysiol.* 2006;17(9):951-956.
51. Pratola C, Baldo E, Artale P, et al. Different image integration modalities to guide AF ablation: impact on procedural and fluoroscopy times. *Pacing Clin Electrophysiol.* 2011;34(4):422-430.
52. Wagner M, Butler C, Rief M, et al. Comparison of non-gated vs. electrocardiogram-gated 64-detector-row computed tomography for integrated electro-anatomic mapping in patients undergoing pulmonary vein isolation. *Europace.* 2010;12(8):1090-1097.
53. Tops LF, Schalij MJ, Bax JJ. Imaging and atrial fibrillation: the role of multimodality imaging in patient evaluation and management of atrial fibrillation. *Eur Heart J.* 2010;31(5):542-551.
54. Singh SM, Heist EK, Donaldson DM, et al. Image integration using intracardiac ultrasound to guide catheter ablation of atrial fibrillation. *Heart Rhythm.* 2008;5(11):1548-1555.
55. Heist EK, Chevalier J, Holmvang G, et al. Factors affecting error in integration of electro-anatomic mapping with CT and MR imaging during catheter ablation of atrial fibrillation. *J Interv Card Electrophysiol.* 2006;17(1):21-27.
56. Malchano ZJ, Neuzil P, Cury RC, et al. Integration of cardiac CT/MR imaging with three-dimensional electro-anatomical mapping to guide catheter manipulation in the left atrium: implications for catheter ablation of atrial fibrillation. *J Cardiovasc Electrophysiol.* 2006;17(11):1221-1229.
57. Tops LF, Bax JJ, Zeppenfeld K, et al. Fusion of multislice computed tomography imaging with three-dimensional electro-anatomic mapping to guide radiofrequency catheter ablation procedures. *Heart Rhythm.* 2005;2(10):1076-1081.
58. Kistler PM, Earley MJ, Harris S, et al. Validation of three-dimensional cardiac image integration: use of integrated CT image into electro-anatomic mapping system to perform catheter ablation of atrial fibrillation. *J Cardiovasc Electrophysiol.* 2006;17(4):341-348.
59. Fahmy TS, Mlcochova H, Wazni OM, et al. Intracardiac echo-guided image integration: optimizing strategies for registration. *J Cardiovasc Electrophysiol.* 2007;18(3):276-282.

60. Tops LF, Schalij MJ, den Uijl DW, et al. Image integration in catheter ablation of atrial fibrillation. *Europace*. 2008;10(3):iii48-iii56.
61. Tian J, Jeudy J, Smith MF, et al. Three-dimensional contrast-enhanced multidetector CT for anatomic, dynamic, and perfusion characterization of abnormal myocardium to guide ventricular tachycardia ablations. *Circ Arrhythm Electrophysiol*. 2010;3(5):496-504.
62. Dickfeld T, Lei P, Dilsizian V, et al. Integration of three-dimensional scar maps for ventricular tachycardia ablation with positron emission tomography-computed tomography. *JACC Cardiovasc Imaging*. 2008;1(1):73-82.
63. Fahmy TS, Wazni OM, Jaber WA, et al. Integration of positron emission tomography/computed tomography with electro-anatomical mapping: a novel approach for ablation of scar-related ventricular tachycardia. *Heart Rhythm*. 2008;5(11):1538-1545.
64. Tian J, Smith MF, Chinnadurai P, et al. Clinical application of PET/CT fusion imaging for three-dimensional myocardial scar and left ventricular anatomy during ventricular tachycardia ablation. *J Cardiovasc Electrophysiol*. 2008;20(6):597-604.
65. Bogun FM, Desjardins B, Good E, et al. Delayed-enhanced magnetic resonance imaging in nonischemic cardiomyopathy: utility for identifying the ventricular arrhythmia substrate. *J Am Coll Cardiol*. 2009;53:1138-1145.
66. Badger TJ, Daccarett M, Akoum NW, et al. Evaluation of left atrial lesions after initial and repeat atrial fibrillation ablation: lessons learned from delayed-enhancement MRI in repeat ablation procedures. *Circ Arrhythm Electrophysiol*. 2010;3(3):249-259.
67. Valdigem BP, da Silva NJ, Dietrich CO, et al. Accuracy of epicardial electro-anatomic mapping and ablation of sustained ventricular tachycardia merged with heart CT scan in chronic Chagasic cardiomyopathy. *J Interv Card Electrophysiol*. 2010;29(2):119-125.
68. Mahnken AH. Computed tomography imaging in myocardial infarction. *Expert Rev Cardiovasc Ther*. 2011;9(2):211-221.
69. Lautamäki R, Schuleri KH, Sasano T, et al. Integration of infarct size, tissue perfusion, and metabolism by hybrid cardiac positron emission tomography/computed tomography: evaluation in a porcine model of myocardial infarction. *Circ Cardiovasc Imaging*. 2009;2(4):299-305.
70. Gerber BL, Belge B, Legros GJ, et al. Characterization of acute and chronic myocardial infarcts by multidetector computed tomography: comparison with contrast-enhanced magnetic resonance. *Circulation*. 2006;113:823-833.
71. Lardo AC, Cordeiro MA, Silva C, et al. Contrast-enhanced multidetector computed tomography viability imaging after myocardial infarction: characterization of myocyte death, microvascular obstruction, and chronic scar. *Circulation*. 2006;113:394-404.
72. Kim RJ, Fieno DS, Parrish TB, et al. Relationship of MRI delayed contrast enhancement to irreversible injury, infarct age, and contractile function. *Circulation*. 1999;100:1992-2002.
73. Ashikaga H, Sasano T, Dong J, et al. Magnetic resonance-based anatomical analysis of scar-related ventricular tachycardia: implications for catheter ablation. *Circ Res*. 2007;101:939-947.
74. Codreanu A, Odille F, Aliot E, et al. Electroanatomic characterization of post-infarct scars comparison with 3-dimensional myocardial scar reconstruction based on magnetic resonance imaging. *J Am Coll Cardiol*. 2008;52(10):839-842.
75. Tops LF, de Groot NM, Bax JJ, Schalij MJ. Fusion of electro-anatomical activation maps and multislice computed tomography to guide ablation of a focal atrial tachycardia in a fontan patient. *J Cardiovasc Electrophysiol*. 2006;17(4): 431-434.
76. Callans DJ. Catheter ablation of idiopathic ventricular tachycardia arising from the aortic root. *J Cardiovasc Electrophysiol*. 2009;20(8):969-972.
77. Lin D, Ilkhanoff L, Gerstenfeld E, et al. Twelve-lead electrocardiographic characteristics of the aortic cusp region guided by intracardiac echocardiography and electro-anatomic mapping. *Heart Rhythm*. 2008;5(5):663-669.
78. Robinson MR, Hutchinson MD. Use of imaging techniques to guide catheter ablation procedures. *Curr Cardiol Rep*. 2010;12:374-381.
79. Verma A, Marrouche NF, Natale A. Pulmonary vein antrum isolation: intracardiac echocardiography-guided technique. *J Cardiovasc Electrophysiol*. 2004;15:1335-1340.
80. Seiler J, Lee JC, Roberts-Thomson KC, Stevenson WG. Intracardiac echocardiography guided catheter ablation of incessant ventricular tachycardia from the posterior papillary muscle causing tachycardia—mediated cardiomyopathy. *Heart Rhythm*. 2009;6:389-392.
81. Reddy VY, Morales G, Ahmed H, et al. Catheter ablation of atrial fibrillation without the use of fluoroscopy. *Heart Rhythm*. 2010;7(11):1644-1653.
82. Bunch JT, Weiss P, Crandall BG, et al. Image integration using intracardiac ultrasound and 3D reconstruction for scar mapping and ablation of ventricular tachycardia. *J Cardiovasc Electrophysiol*. 2010;21:678-684.
83. Ren JF, Marchlinski FE. Utility of intracardiac echocardiography in left heart ablation for tachyarrhythmias. *Echocardiogr*. 2007;24:533-540.
84. Orlov MV, Hoffmeister P, Chaudhry GM, et al. Three-dimensional rotational angiography of the left atrium and esophagus—a virtual computed tomography scan in the electrophysiology lab? *Heart Rhythm*. 2007;4:3-43.
85. Thiagalingam A, Manzke R, D'Avila A, et al. Intraprocedural volume imaging of the left atrium and pulmonary veins with rotational x-ray angiography: implications for catheter ablation of atrial fibrillation. *J Cardiovasc Electrophysiol*. 2008;19:293-300.
86. Orlov MV, Ansari MM, Akrivakis ST, et al. First experience with rotational angiography of the right ventricle to guide ventricular tachycardia ablation. *Heart Rhythm*. 2011;8:207-211.
87. Knecht S, Wright M, Akrivakis S, et al. Prospective randomized comparison between the conventional electro-anatomical system and three-dimensional rotational angiography during catheter ablation for atrial fibrillation. *Heart Rhythm*. 2010;7:459-465.
88. Lardo AC, McVeigh ER, Jumrussirikul P, et al. Visualization and temporal/spatial characterization of cardiac radiofrequency ablation lesions using magnetic resonance imaging. *Circulation*. 2000;102(6):698-705.
89. Dickfeld T, Kato R, Zviman M, et al. Characterization of acute and subacute radiofrequency ablation lesions with non enhanced magnetic resonance imaging. *Heart Rhythm*. 2007;4(2):208-214.
90. Kolandaivelu A, Lardo AC, Halperin HR. Cardiovascular magnetic resonance guided electrophysiology studies. *J Cardiov Magn Reson*. 2009;11:21.
91. Hoffmann BA, Koops A, Rostock T, et al. Interactive real-time mapping and catheter ablation of the cavotricuspid isthmus guided by magnetic resonance imaging in a porcine model. *Eur Heart J*. 2010;31(4):450-456.
92. Nordbeck P, Bauer WR, Fidler F, et al. Feasibility of real-time MRI with a novel carbon catheter for interventional electrophysiology. *Circ Arrhythm Electrophysiol*. 2009;2(3):258-267.
93. Kolandaivelu A, Zviman MM, Castro V, et al. Noninvasive assessment of tissue heating during cardiac radiofrequency

ablation using MRI thermography. *Circ Arrhythm Electrophysiol.* 2010;3(5):521-529.
94. Vergara GR, Marrouche NF. Tailored management of atrial fibrillation using a LGE-MRI based model: from the clinic to the electrophysiology laboratory. *J Cardiovasc Electrophysiol.* 2011;22(4):481-487.
95. Akoum N, Daccarett M, McGann C, et al. Atrial fibrosis helps select the appropriate patient and strategy in catheter ablation of atrial fibrillation: a DE-MRI guided approach. *J Cardiovasc Electrophysiol.* 2011;22(1):16-22.
96. Badger TJ, Daccarett M, Akoum NW, et al. Evaluation of left atrial lesions after initial and repeat atrial fibrillation ablation: lessons learned from delayed-enhancement MRI in repeat ablation procedures. *Circ Arrhythm Electrophysiol.* 2010;3(3):249-259.
97. Mahnkopf C, Badger TJ, Burgon NS, et al. Evaluation of the left atrial substrate in patients with lone atrial fibrillation using delayed-enhanced MRI: implications for disease progression and response to catheter ablation. *Heart Rhythm.* 2010;7(10):1475-1481.
98. Taclas JE, Nezafat R, Wylie JV, et al. Relationship between intended sites of RF ablation and post-procedural scar in AF patients, using late gadolinium enhancement cardiovascular magnetic resonance. *Heart Rhythm.* 2010;7(4):489-496.

Video Legends

Video 10.1 (Figure 10.3) Clip file during AF ablation, using a registered LA CT reconstruction fused with the 3D map. Note the position of the mapping catheter moving from the left inferior pulmonary vein (LIPV) to left superior pulmonary vein (LSPV) and the slight misregistration evidenced by the appearance of the mapping catheter tip outside of the LSPV endocardial contours.

Video 10.2 (Figure 10.7) Ablation for septal VT using an intracardiac ultrasound shell (CartoSound, **mesh**) integrated with a 3D electroanatomic map. The **colored points** represent pace-mapping sites for the clinical VT. After RF ablation in the LV septum, where good pace map matches (11/12) to the clinical VT were seen (**blue points**), the ablation catheter was positioned in the RV septum, where a perfect pace map match was seen (12/12, **green point**) and RF delivery near this site rendered the clinical VT noninducible. Live ICE images confirmed good catheter-to-tissue contact during RF ablation at this site.

Video 10.3 (Figure 10.9) 3D electroanatomic map (EnSite Velocity) fused with a CT reconstruction of the right atrium to guide systemic ventricular lead implantation in a patient with advanced heart failure with L-transposition of the great arteries and dextrocardia. As a result of the greatly distorted cardiac anatomy, a catheter with a distal bipole and a 7-Fr lumen (CPS Luminary, St. Jude Medical) was positioned in the CS ostium using the EnSite Velocity mapping system and, through this sheath, a 5-Fr lead was advanced into a ventricular lateral branch (**white/green tip**).

CHAPTER 11

CARDIAC COMPUTED TOMOGRAPHY AND MAGNETIC RESONANCE IMAGE INTERPRETATION DURING INTERVENTIONAL PROCEDURES

Saman Nazarian, MD, PhD; Henry R. Halperin, MD, MA; Hugh Calkins, MD

Introduction

Complex electrophysiology and catheter ablation procedures require the ability to interpret simultaneous, multichannel electrogram data within the context of the sampling location for each electrode pair. The ability of the electrophysiologist to process this information varies by factors including experience, patience, and computational and spatial aptitude. Fortunately for the less experienced, electroanatomic mapping systems allow for integration of preacquired computed tomography (CT) and magnetic resonance imaging (MRI) with electrogram data and greatly enhance the visual understanding of complex electroanatomic relationships. The capabilities of electroanatomic mapping systems are discussed in Chapter 4. In this chapter, we will focus on topics including the basics of cardiac CT and MRI, cardiac MRI in the setting of implanted devices, advantages of each modality in the electrophysiology laboratory, and imaging the arrhythmia substrate for interventional electrophysiology.

Basics of Cardiac Computed Tomography

Cardiac CT uses image postprocessing to generate a three-dimensional (3D) image of the heart and surrounding structures from multiple two-dimensional (2D) x-ray images taken around the CT's gantry axis of rotation. To start the CT acquisition process, typically a projection "scout" image is obtained. The scout image is essentially an anteroposterior chest x-ray view that allows one to specify the craniocaudal extent of imaging. One must pay particular attention to extend the field of view to cover the entire cardiac chamber(s) of interest in the x–y plane, with a margin of error for respiratory motion. Iodinated contrast is necessary when performing cardiac CT to illuminate cardiac chambers and vascular lumens. Adequate hydration prior to CT and the use of iso-osmolal agents may reduce the risk of contrast-induced nephropathy.[1]

The dose and duration of contrast administration may vary depending upon the primary structures of interest in addition to body mass index.[2] Additionally, the relative timing of scan acquisition from injection is critical and depends upon the structures of interest. Timing is typically determined by either the "test bolus" or the "bolus trigger" method. In the first method, sequential images of the chamber of interest are obtained in 2-second intervals after an initial 10-second delay. The optimal delay for the clinical images is then chosen based upon a qualitative review of the sequential test images. Our preferred approach is the bolus trigger method, whereby a predefined contrast threshold in the ascending aorta is used to trigger image acquisition in the chamber of interest.

Breath-holding during CT image acquisition is necessary to reduce image artifact. Image artifact is also minimized by using advanced scanners where the gantry rotates around the patient as the scanner bed advances. The "pitch" describes the ratio of distance the scanner bed travels to each rotation of the gantry; a pitch of 1 signifies one detector width advance of the scanner bed for one rotation of the gantry. The commonly utilized pitch of 0.2 allows the acquisition of overlapping data. This methodology can reduce image artifact and allows multiphase image reconstruction, albeit with increased radiation exposure.[3] Depending upon the number of detectors in a scanner, multiple heartbeats may be required to complete cardiac imaging. When images from a single phase are utilized for image reconstruction, "tube modulation" or "prospective triggering" can be used to lower or turn off the tube current (and reduce radiation exposure) during phases that are unlikely to be used for image reconstruction. Other image acquisition parameters are typically 120 kV and 600 to 900 mA, depending upon the manufacturer, but may need to be adjusted, especially in obese patients.[4]

Special attention must also be directed to postprocessing the image prior to use in the electrophysiology laboratory. Many of our patients will have ectopic beats or arrhythmias during scan acquisition. Therefore, 256-slice scanners are optimal because they enable image acquisition in a single heartbeat. If a scanner with fewer detectors is used, images acquired during ectopic beats should be excluded from the reconstruction dataset in order to minimize artifacts. Similarly, in patients with atrial fibrillation, images should be reconstructed from those acquired at a fixed interval relative to the R waves. The typical optimal phase for reconstructing the image in the electrophysiology laboratory will be end diastolic, which enables improved image registration using electroanatomic mapping systems (Figure 11.1).

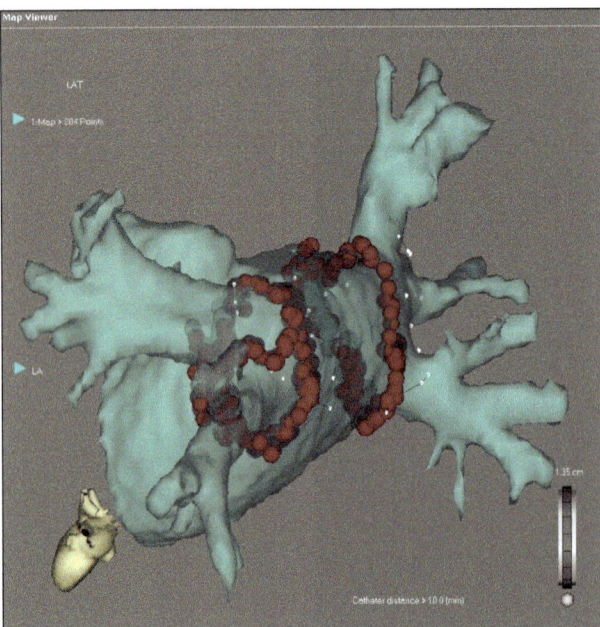

Figure 11.1 Integration of an end-diastolic CT image of the left atrium into an electroanatomic mapping system during catheter ablation of atrial fibrillation. The left atrial appendage (LAA) and posterior left atrium are visualized. Radiofrequency lesions (**red dots**) are identified encircling each pulmonary vein ostium.

Basics of Cardiac Magnetic Resonance Imaging

MRI uses high-strength magnetic and electric fields to image the body.[5-10] A strong static magnetic field orients the magnetic moments of hydrogen nuclei. Radiofrequency pulses are then used to "tip" the magnetic moments in space, by applying a resonance frequency equal to the precession frequency of the magnetic moments about the magnetic field lines. After the magnetic moment is tipped, it relaxes and emits a weak signal, which is received and used to construct the image. When performing cardiac MRI, multiple pulse sequences are available, each of which focus on particular attributes of cardiac function or structure. The availability of a multitude of pulse sequences, each with a series of programmable parameters, makes MRI a challenging test to perform requiring significant expertise for appropriate image acquisition. Cardiac MRI obtained in patients with significant arrhythmia may yield suboptimal images despite electrocardiogram (ECG) gating. In such patients, the use of single-shot images may optimize results.[11,12]

It is of paramount importance to communicate the imaging needs of the electrophysiology team to those acquiring the MRI images. If chamber volumes and valvular and contractile function are of interest, then cine imaging is required. Cine imaging is routinely performed; however, unless specifically requested, the atria may not always be completed scanned. Inversion-recovery "delayed enhancement" imaging 5 to 10 minutes after contrast administration is utilized for identifying scar tissue and is routinely performed for the ventricle.[13] This technique takes advantage of delayed washout of gadolinium contrast from scar tissue, which results in shortened T1 relaxation and hyperenhancement of scar compared with surrounding normal myocardium with rapid gadolinium washout.[14] Atrial-delayed enhancement imaging requires specialized software for respiratory gating and variations in pulse sequences to visualize the thinner muscular tissue.[15] Such a pulse sequence may not be readily available at all centers and, even when available, is not routinely performed. However, when available, such images can integrate preexisting atrial scar into the procedural space (Figure 11.2).

The potential for evaluating thrombus using delayed enhancement imaging with a long inversion time has been explored and may be useful prior to catheter ablation of atrial fibrillation or flutter. However, the accuracy of MRI for thrombus detection has not been systematically compared with transesophageal echocardiography. Importantly, based upon the most recent comparison of transesophageal echocardiography with another modality in the Intracardiac Echocardiography Guided Cardioversion Helps Interventional Procedures (ICE-CHIP) study, transesophageal echocardiography remains the most sensitive method for detecting left atrial appendage thrombus.[16]

Electrophysiologists are occasionally called upon to review cases of inflammatory myocarditis presenting with arrhythmia. Visualizing such active inflammation may change case management and can be done if T2-weighted imaging is specifically requested.[17]

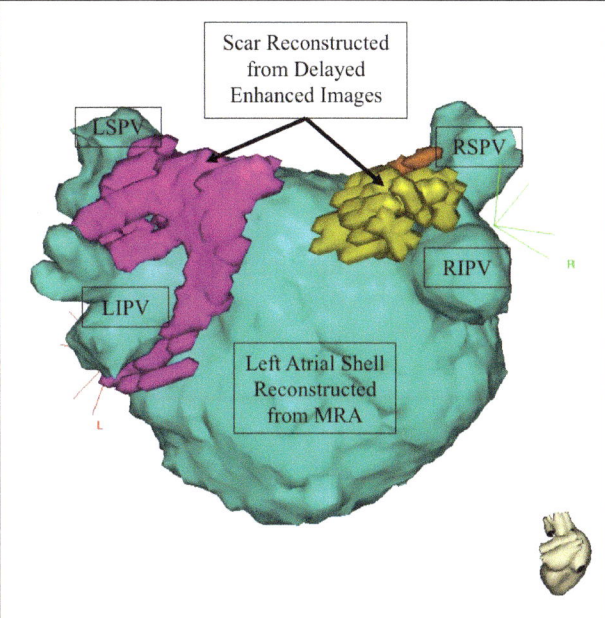

Figure 11.2 Segmentation and integration of magnetic resonance angiography (MRA) and atrial-delayed enhancement images for use during catheter ablation of atrial fibrillation. The left atrial shell and pulmonary vein ostia are visible. Scar from prior catheter ablation is highlighted in **purple**, **yellow**, and **orange**. LSPV = left superior pulmonary vein; LIPV = left inferior pulmonary vein; RSPV = right superior pulmonary vein; RIPV = right inferior pulmonary vein.

Perhaps most importantly from the electrophysiology standpoint, magnetic resonance angiography (MRA) protocols are necessary to visualize the end-diastolic dimensions of cardiac chambers and vascular structures of interest. These protocols are not routinely performed, but when MRA is requested, the chambers of interest should be specified to ensure that the field of view and scan timing relative to contrast administration are appropriately set up.

Advantages of Each Modality in the Electrophysiology Setting

One of the primary advantages of cardiac MRI compared with CT is the lack of ionizing radiation. This issue is not insubstantial, given the typical length of complex catheter ablation procedures and the potential cumulative radiation exposure to the patient. The subject deserves considerable attention—particularly in women and our young patients. The experience with and the resolution of cardiac MRI for imaging myocardial scar as a substrate for arrhythmia far surpasses that with cardiac CT. Additionally, cardiac MRI is capable of multiplanar imaging, whereas 3D reconstruction and volume rendering are necessary to visualize unconventional planes when using CT. Finally, if used in patients with glomerular filtration rate (GFR) > 30 mL/min/1.73 m^2 to avoid nephrogenic systemic fibrosis, gadolinium-based contrast agents appear to have an improved safety profile compared with iodinated contrast agents used for cardiac CT.[18] In general, patients with a variety of conditions (eg, mild renal insufficiency, history of multiple myeloma, risk for contrast-induced nephropathy, recent radioactive iodine therapy, and hyperthyroidism) are better served with cardiac MRI and gadolinium contrast versus iodinated CT contrast.[4]

On the flipside, cardiac CT has a substantially shorter acquisition time than cardiac MRI and may be the preferred alternative for a claustrophobic patient and patients who have difficulty holding their breath. Typical acquisition times for detailed CT images of the entire heart and vasculature are on the order of 15 seconds. Compare this with cardiac MRI, which requires several minute-long acquisitions that vary in length depending upon sequence settings and patient heart rate. Additionally, when evaluating chamber dimensions, pulmonary vein, coronary artery, and other vascular boundaries, cardiac CT provides superior resolution. Additionally, cardiac CT can acquire images of the esophagus and cardiac chambers in the same sequence, thereby allowing importation of both structures into the electroanatomic mapping systems without requiring "double-merge" techniques. While cardiac CT is easier to perform in the setting of permanent pacemakers and implantable cardioverter-defibrillators (ICDs), techniques for safe MR imaging in this setting are available.[19,20] Importantly, the artifact due to leads tends to be significantly smaller in cardiac MRI compared with cardiac CT.

Cardiac MRI in the Setting of Implanted Cardiac Devices

Owing to underlying structural heart disease and its accompanying conduction system disease and/or risk of ventricular arrhythmia, a significant proportion of patients referred for cardiac MRI have permanent pacemakers and ICDs.[21-25] It has been estimated that a patient with a pacemaker or ICD has a 50% to 75% likelihood of having a clinically indicated MRI during the lifetime of the device.[26] The potential for the devices' movement,[27] programming changes, asynchronous pacing, activation of tachyarrhythmia therapies, inhibition of demand pacing,[28] and induced lead currents leading to heating and cardiac stimulation[29] are all matters of concern. Device manufacturers[30-32] and MRI authorities[33-35] have addressed the performance and safety of MRI procedures in recipients of implantable cardiac devices. However, in recent years, several case series have reported the safety of

MRI in the setting of pacemakers.[36-41] A small case series has also reported neurological MRI in the setting of select ICD systems.[42] Although overall safety has been reported, acute changes in battery voltage, lead thresholds,[39] and programming[42] can occur in these devices.

At our institution, we have developed a two-pronged protocol including (1) device selection based on previous *in vitro* and *in vivo* testing[43] and (2) device programming to minimize inappropriate activation or inhibition of bradyarrhythmia/tachyarrhythmia therapies. The protocol (Figure 11.3) is unique in selecting device generators previously tested under worst-case scenario MRI conditions: ie, imaging over the region containing the generator, with a specific absorption rate of up to 3.5 W/kg.[43] The protocol also suggests steps to identify and exclude patients with leads that are more prone to movement and heating. Figure 11.3 summarizes the protocol's programming steps to reduce the risk of inappropriate pacemaker inhibition or activation, or inappropriate activation of tachyarrhythmia functions.[20,44] Using this protocol, we have safely performed more than 1,000 MRI examinations. Image quality is unaffected when the device is outside the field of view. However, thoracic images can be affected, with significant susceptibility artifacts. Artifacts can be minimized by using spin-echo sequences or shortening the echo time (Figure 11.4).[45]

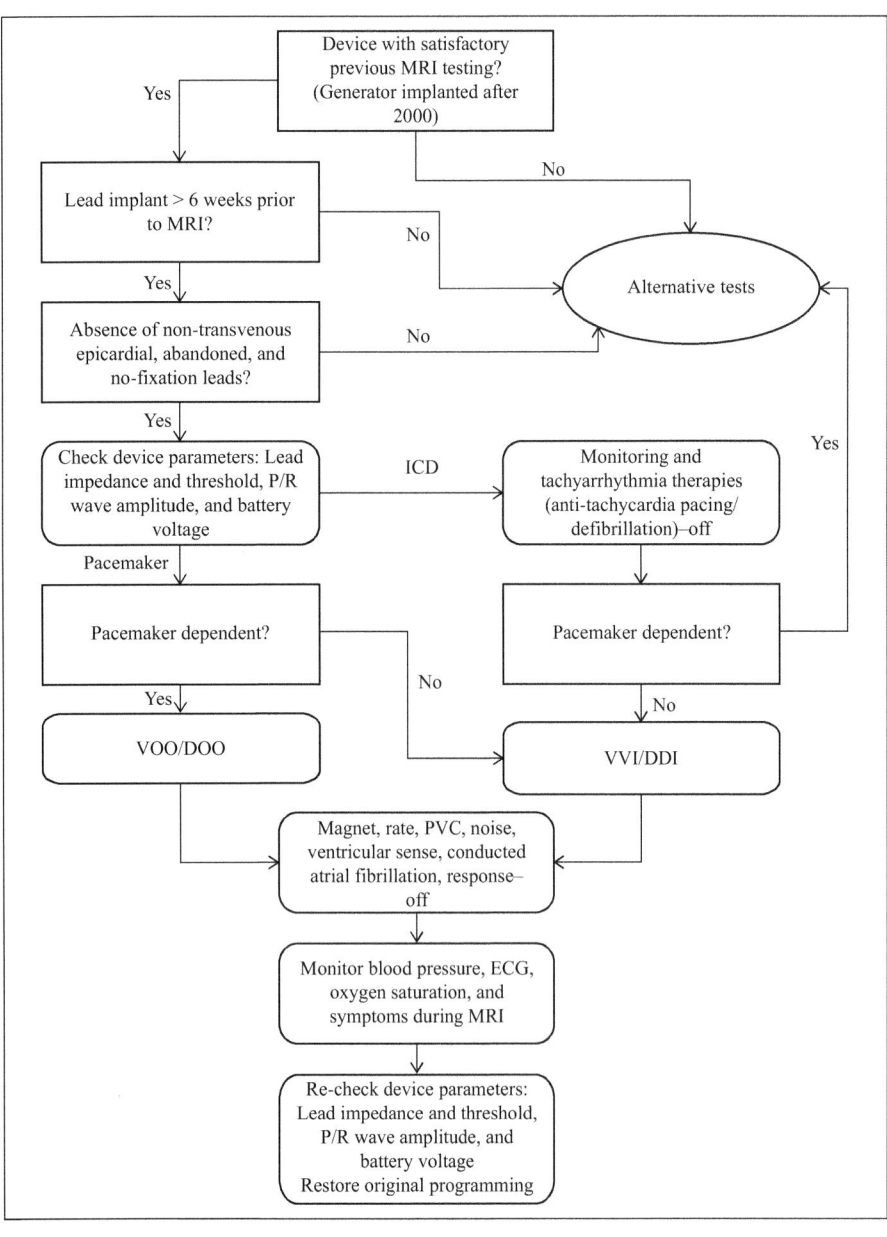

Figure 11.3 Safety protocol for MRI in the setting of implanted cardiac devices. MRI = magnetic resonance imaging; ICD = implantable cardioverter-defibrillator; PVC = premature ventricular contraction; ECG = electrocardiogram. *Source:* Modified with permission from Nazarian S, et al.[20]

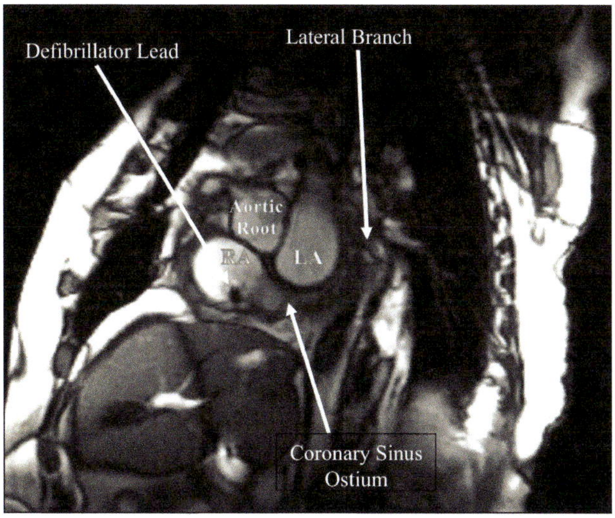

Figure 11.4 Short-axis, steady-state, free precession MRI image showing the patency of the coronary sinus and a lateral branch in the setting of an implanted cardioverter-defibrillator and postsurgical ventricular reconstruction. The aortic root, as well as left atrium (LA) and right atrium (RA) at the level of the coronary sinus ostium, are also visualized.

Imaging the Arrhythmia Substrate

Ischemic Cardiomyopathy

Patients with ischemic cardiomyopathy are at risk for ventricular arrhythmia, typically caused by reentry around the infarct scar. Cardiac magnetic resonance (CMR) techniques for visualizing infarcted myocardium rely primarily upon steady-state, free precession cine for evaluating function and delayed-enhancement CMR (DE-CMR) to assess scar burden. In pioneering work to image the substrate of ventricular tachycardia (VT), Bello et al showed that measurements of infarct surface area and mass by CMR can identify the substrate for inducible monomorphic VT.[46] Yan et al provided evidence for the relation of the scar substrate to clinical events. Their study revealed a strong association between the extent of the peri-infarct zone characterized by CMR and all-cause and cardiovascular mortality.[47] Most recently, Schmidt et al showed that increased "tissue heterogeneity" in the peri-infarct zone correlates with inducible VT at electrophysiology study.[48] Integration of 3D reconstructed CT datasets of chamber morphology and scar/border-zone substrate into electroanatomic mapping systems has been reported and will likely improve the outcome of catheter ablations in the electrophysiology laboratory.[49] Our group and others[50] are also focusing on the development of methodologies for integrating MRI scar images (in the setting of ischemic cardiomyopathy) into electroanatomic mapping systems.

Nonischemic Cardiomyopathy

Although syncope and sudden cardiac death are rarely the initial manifestations of nonischemic cardiomyopathy, nonischemic cardiomyopathy is often associated with VT. The anatomic and functional abnormalities of nonischemic cardiomyopathy are readily assessed by CMR. DE-CMR using gadolinium contrast can be used to identify scar in the evaluation of patients with nonischemic cardiomyopathy. Although absence of hyperenhancement is the most common finding in nonischemic cardiomyopathy, midwall striae or patches of enhancement can be identified in up to one third of cases. Compared with ischemic cardiomyopathy, the pattern and location of delayed enhancement in nonischemic cardiomyopathy is often atypical, making it difficult to distinguish artifact from true scar. The presence of scar should therefore be verified by using multiple planes.

Utilizing CMR to delineate scar distribution, we showed that the VT substrate in nonischemic cardiomyopathy is midwall scar involving greater than 25% of wall thickness.[51] In a recent prospective study of patients with nonischemic cardiomyopathy, Assomull et al demonstrated that this high-risk midwall fibrosis pattern predicts sudden cardiac death and spontaneous VT.[52] We have found critical sites for VT maintenance in nonischemic cardiomyopathy to correspond to scar border zones on cardiac MRI (Figure 11.5). It is likely that methodologies for integrating MRI scar images in the setting of nonischemic cardiomyopathy into electroanatomic mapping systems will improve procedural planning and efficacy.

Hypertrophic Cardiomyopathy

Patients with hypertrophic cardiomyopathy are at risk for sudden cardiac death. CMR is an appropriate adjunct or alternative to echocardiography for confirming the diagnosis or identifying atypical cases. An example of an atypical case, apical hypertrophy is presented in ▶ Video 11.1. In addition, DE-CMR can detect midwall and patchy scar in regions with hypertrophy, most commonly at the right ventricular insertion points. The degree of fibrosis measured by CMR appears to correlate with arrhythmia risk.[53]

Arrhythmogenic Right Ventricular Cardiomyopathy

Arrhythmogenic right ventricular cardiomyopathy (ARVC) commonly presents with VT and is associated with sudden cardiac death. Owing to its ability to characterize fibrofatty infiltration of the right ventricle, in experienced centers, CMR has rapidly evolved into the diagnostic standard for identifying ARVC. DE-CMR appears to predict inducibly sustained VT at electrophysiology study.[54] A caveat is that the time inversion for myocardial signal

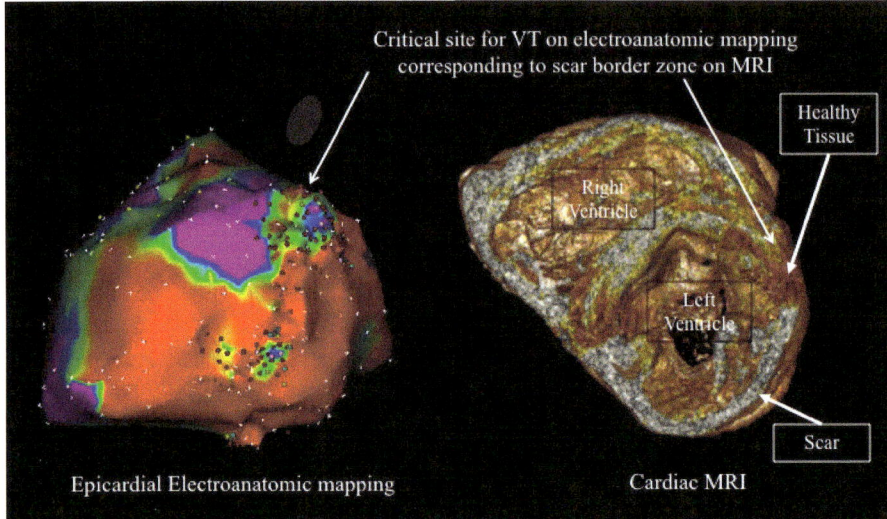

Figure 11.5 Epicardial electroanatomic mapping (**left panel**) and posttransplant ex vivo contrast-enhanced MRI in a patient with nonischemic cardiomyopathy. The scar areas appear **white** on the reconstructed cardiac MRI; healthy tissues are **brown**, and heterogeneous regions are **yellow**. Critical sites for VT maintenance corresponded to scar border zones, as identified by cardiac MRI. MRI = magnetic resonance imaging; VT = ventricular tachycardia.

suppression in DE-CMR appears to be different between the left and right ventricles and therefore must be optimized. Furthermore, substantial normal right ventricular variations (eg, reduced wall motion near the moderator band, variable trabeculation, and fat deposits surrounding the coronary vessels and epicardium) can lead to reduced specificity. Importantly, assessing right ventricular dilation and regional function on cine images is essential for establishing the correct diagnosis ▶ Video 11.2).

Sarcoidosis

Sarcoidosis with cardiac involvement is relatively uncommon (5%), but sudden cardiac death due to arrhythmia may be its initial clinical presentation. Techniques for assessing cardiac involvement, including echocardiography, scintigraphy, and myocardial biopsy, are often inadequate for stratifying arrhythmic risk. Thus, in patients with systemic sarcoidosis suspected of cardiac involvement, CMR may provide a diagnostic alternative and a method for following disease activity. The occurrence of CMR abnormalities in patients with ongoing systemic sarcoidosis has been described. However, the relation of CMR findings to either risk or the electroanatomic mapping substrate of VT in sarcoidosis has not been assessed.

Surgical Scar

Surgical scar can serve as an anatomic barrier for arrhythmic reentry. Reentrant arrhythmias observed in the postsurgical setting include VT after ventriculotomy or patch repair. CMR is capable of delineating cardiac structure and function after cardiac surgery, a setting in which echocardiography is often hindered because of chest-wall changes that diminish the acoustic window. DE-CMR has been shown to identify fibrous tissue in the postsurgical state. However, the relation of CMR findings to postsurgical risk or the electroanatomic mapping substrate of VT has not been assessed.

Chagas Disease

Chagas disease results in ventricular scar and commonly manifests with VT. Importantly, VT due to Chagas disease may develop before cardiomegaly or heart failure is detected. CMR can accurately assess morphological and functional aspects of cardiac involvement in Chagas disease. Chagas disease patients with a previously documented VT event typically have fibrosis detectable by DE-CMR.[55] The relation of CMR findings to risk or the electroanatomic mapping substrate of VT in Chagas disease has not been prospectively assessed.

Conclusion

Current electroanatomic systems are capable of integrating cardiac CT or MRI datasets into the procedural mapping space. When used as an adjunct to bipolar and unipolar local electrograms, imaging information regarding chamber dimensions, vascular proximity, and scar and border-zone characteristics can provide powerful information to aid catheter ablation procedures. Basic familiarity with the unique advantages and shortcomings of CT and MRI, image acquisition techniques, and image interpretation will be indispensable for patient management in the modern electrophysiology laboratory.

References

1. Lencioni R, Fattori R, Morana G, Stacul F. Contrast-induced nephropathy in patients undergoing computed tomography (CONNECT)—a clinical problem in daily practice? A multicenter observational study. *Acta Radiol*. 2010;51(7):741-750.
2. Bae KT, Seeck BA, Hildebolt CF, et al. Contrast enhancement in cardiovascular MDCT: effect of body weight, height, body surface area, body mass index, and obesity. *AJR Am J Roentgenol*. 2008;190(3):777-784.

3. Henzler T, Hanley M, Arnoldi E, et al. Practical strategies for low radiation dose cardiac computed tomography. *J Thorac Imaging*. 2010;25(3):213-220.
4. Moloo J, Shapiro MD, Abbara S. Cardiac computed tomography: technique and optimization of protocols. *Semin Roentgenol*. 2008;43(2):90-99.
5. Edelman RR. Basic principles of magnetic resonance angiography. *Cardiovasc Intervent Radiol*. 1992;15(1):3-13.
6. Edelman RR, Warach S. Magnetic resonance imaging (1). *N Engl J Med*. 1993;328(10):708-716.
7. Edelman RR, Warach S. Magnetic resonance imaging (2). *N Engl J Med*. 1993;328(11):785-791.
8. McVeigh ER, Henkelman RM, Bronskill MJ. Noise and filtration in magnetic resonance imaging. *Med Phys*. 1985;12(5):586-591.
9. Henkelman RM, Kucharczyk W, Bronskill MJ. Making magnetic resonance images and beyond. *Can Assoc Radiol J*. 1990;41(1):8-13.
10. Hinks RS, Bronskill MJ, Kucharczyk W, et al. MR systems for image-guided therapy. *J Magn Reson Imaging*. 1998;8(1):19-25.
11. Sievers B, Elliott MD, Hurwitz LM, et al. Rapid detection of myocardial infarction by subsecond, free-breathing delayed contrast-enhancement cardiovascular magnetic resonance. *Circulation*. 2007;115(2):236-244.
12. Kaji S, Yang PC, Kerr AB, et al. Rapid evaluation of left ventricular volume and mass without breath-holding using real-time interactive cardiac magnetic resonance imaging system. *J Am Coll Cardiol*. 2001;38(2):527-533.
13. Simonetti OP, Kim RJ, Fieno DS, et al. An improved MR imaging technique for the visualization of myocardial infarction. *Radiology*. 2001;218(1):215-223.
14. Kim HW, Farzaneh-Far A, Kim RJ. Cardiovascular magnetic resonance in patients with myocardial infarction: current and emerging applications. *J Am Coll Cardiol*. 2009;55(1):1-16.
15. Peters DC, Wylie JV, Hauser TH, et al. Detection of pulmonary vein and left atrial scar after catheter ablation with three-dimensional navigator-gated delayed enhancement MR imaging: initial experience. *Radiology*. 2007;243(3):690-695.
16. Saksena S, Sra J, Jordaens L, et al. A prospective comparison of cardiac imaging using intracardiac echocardiography with transesophageal echocardiography in patients with atrial fibrillation: the Intracardiac Echocardiography Guided Cardioversion Helps Interventional Procedures Study. *Circ Arrhythm Electrophysiol*. 2010;3(6):571-577.
17. Friedrich MG, Sechtem U, Schulz-Menger J, et al. Cardiovascular magnetic resonance in myocarditis: A JACC White Paper. *J Am Coll Cardiol*. 2009;53(17):1475-1487.
18. Martin DR, Krishnamoorthy SK, Kalb B, et al. Decreased incidence of NSF in patients on dialysis after changing gadolinium contrast-enhanced MRI protocols. *J Magn Reson Imaging*. 2010;31(2):440-446.
19. Nazarian S, Halperin HR. How to perform magnetic resonance imaging on patients with implantable cardiac arrhythmia devices. *Heart Rhythm*. 2009;6(1):138-143.
20. Nazarian S, Roguin A, Zviman MM, et al. Clinical utility and safety of a protocol for noncardiac and cardiac magnetic resonance imaging of patients with permanent pacemakers and implantable-cardioverter defibrillators at 1.5 Tesla. *Circulation*. 2006;114:1277-1284.
21. Brown DW, Croft JB, Giles WH, et al. Epidemiology of pacemaker procedures among Medicare enrollees in 1990, 1995, and 2000. *Am J Cardiol*. 2005;95(3):409-411.
22. Moss AJ, Zareba W, Hall WJ, et al. Prophylactic implantation of a defibrillator in patients with myocardial infarction and reduced ejection fraction. *N Engl J Med*. 2002;346(12):877-883.
23. Abraham WT, Fisher WG, Smith AL, et al. Cardiac resynchronization in chronic heart failure. *N Engl J Med*. 2002;346(24):1845-1853.
24. Bristow MR, Saxon LA, Boehmer J, et al. Cardiac-resynchronization therapy with or without an implantable defibrillator in advanced chronic heart failure. *N Engl J Med*. 2004;350(21):2140-2150.
25. Bardy GH, Lee KL, Mark DB, et al. Amiodarone or an implantable cardioverter-defibrillator for congestive heart failure. *N Engl J Med*. 2005;352(3):225-237.
26. Kalin R, Stanton MS. Current clinical issues for MRI scanning of pacemaker and defibrillator patients. *Pacing Clin Electrophysiol*. 2005;28(4):326-328.
27. Shellock FG, Tkach JA, Ruggieri PM, Masaryk TJ. Cardiac pacemakers, ICDs, and loop recorder: evaluation of translational attraction using conventional ("long-bore") and "short-bore" 1.5- and 3.0 Tesla MR systems. *J Cardiovasc Magn Reson*. 2003;5(2):387-397.
28. Erlebacher JA, Cahill PT, Pannizzo F, Knowles RJ. Effect of magnetic resonance imaging on DDD pacemakers. *Am J Cardiol*. 1986;57(6):437-440.
29. Hayes DL, Holmes DR Jr, Gray JE. Effect of 1.5 Tesla nuclear magnetic resonance imaging scanner on implanted permanent pacemakers. *J Am Coll Cardiol*. 1987;10(4):782-786.
30. Smith JM. Industry viewpoint: Guidant: pacemakers, ICDs, and MRI. *Pacing Clin Electrophysiol*. 2005;28(4):264.
31. Stanton MS. Industry viewpoint: Medtronic: pacemakers, ICDs, and MRI. *Pacing Clin Electrophysiol*. 2005;28(4):265.
32. Levine PA. Industry viewpoint: St. Jude Medical: pacemakers, ICDs and MRI. *Pacing Clin Electrophysiol*. 2005;28(4):266-267.
33. Shellock FG, Crues JV. MR procedures: biologic effects, safety, and patient care. *Radiology*. 2004;232(3):635-652.
34. Prasad SK, Pennell DJ. Safety of cardiovascular magnetic resonance in patients with cardiovascular implants and devices. *Heart*. 2004;90(11):1241-1244.
35. Faris OP, Shein MJ. Government viewpoint: U.S. Food & Drug Administration: pacemakers, ICDs and MRI. *Pacing Clin Electrophysiol*. 2005;28(4):268-269.
36. Gimbel JR, Johnson D, Levine PA, Wilkoff BL. Safe performance of magnetic resonance imaging on five patients with permanent cardiac pacemakers. *Pacing Clin Electrophysiol*. 1996;19(6):913-919.
37. Sommer T, Vahlhaus C, Lauck G, et al. MR imaging and cardiac pacemakers: in vitro evaluation and in vivo studies in 51 patients at 0.5 Tesla. *Radiology*. 2000;215(3):869-879.
38. Vahlhaus C, Sommer T, Lewalter T, et al. Interference with cardiac pacemakers by magnetic resonance imaging: are there irreversible changes at 0.5 Tesla? *Pacing Clin Electrophysiol*. 2001;24(4 Pt 1):489-495.
39. Martin ET, Coman JA, Shellock FG, et al. Magnetic resonance imaging and cardiac pacemaker safety at 1.5 Tesla. *J Am Coll Cardiol*. 2004;43(7):1315-1324.
40. Del Ojo JL, Moya F, Villalba J, et al. Is magnetic resonance imaging safe in cardiac pacemaker recipients? *Pacing Clin Electrophysiol*. 2005;28(4):274-278.
41. Shellock FG, Fieno DS, Thomson LJ, et al. Cardiac pacemaker: in vitro assessment at 1.5 Tesla. *Am Heart J*. 2006;151(2):436-443.
42. Gimbel JR, Kanal E, Schwartz KM, Wilkoff BL. Outcome of magnetic resonance imaging (MRI) in selected patients with implantable cardioverter defibrillators (ICDs). *Pacing Clin Electrophysiol*. 2005;28(4):270-273.
43. Roguin A, Zviman MM, Meininger GR, et al. Modern pacemaker and implantable cardioverter/defibrillator systems can be magnetic resonance imaging safe: in vitro and in vivo

assessment of safety and function at 1.5 Tesla. *Circulation.* 2004;110(5):475-482.
44. Nazarian S, Hansford R, Roguin A, et al. A prospective evaluation of a protocol for magnetic resonance imaging of patients with implanted cardiac devices. *Ann Intern Med.* 2011;155(7):415-424.
45. Sasaki T, Hansford R, Zviman MM, et al. Quantitative assessment of artifacts on cardiac magnetic resonance imaging of patients with pacemakers and implantable cardioverter-defibrillators. *Circ Cardiovasc Imaging.* 2011;4(6):662-670.
46. Bello D, Fieno DS, Kim RJ, et al. Infarct morphology identifies patients with substrate for sustained ventricular tachycardia. *J Am Coll Cardiol.* 2005;45(7):1104-1108.
47. Yan AT, Shayne AJ, Brown KA, et al. Characterization of the peri-infarct zone by contrast-enhanced cardiac magnetic resonance imaging is a powerful predictor of post-myocardial infarction mortality. *Circulation.* 2006;114(1):32-39.
48. Schmidt A, Azevedo CF, Cheng A, et al. Infarct tissue heterogeneity by magnetic resonance imaging identifies enhanced cardiac arrhythmia susceptibility in patients with left ventricular dysfunction. *Circulation.* 2007;115(15):2006-2014.
49. Tian J, Jeudy J, Smith MF, et al. Three dimensional contrast enhanced multi-detector CT for anatomic, dynamic, and perfusion characterization of abnormal myocardium to guide VT ablations. *Circ Arrhythm Electrophysiol.* 2010;3:496-504.
50. Desjardins B, Crawford T, Good E, et al. Infarct architecture and characteristics on delayed enhanced magnetic resonance imaging and electroanatomic mapping in patients with postinfarction ventricular arrhythmia. *Heart Rhythm.* 2009;6(5):644-651.
51. Nazarian S, Bluemke DA, Lardo AC, et al. Magnetic resonance assessment of the substrate for inducible ventricular tachycardia in nonischemic cardiomyopathy. *Circulation.* 2005;112(18):2821-2825.
52. Assomull RG, Prasad SK, Lyne J, et al. Cardiovascular magnetic resonance, fibrosis, and prognosis in dilated cardiomyopathy. *J Am Coll Cardiol.* 2006;48(10):1977-1985.
53. Teraoka K, Hirano M, Ookubo H, et al. Delayed contrast enhancement of MRI in hypertrophic cardiomyopathy. *Magn Reson Imaging.* 2004;22(2):155-161.
54. Corrado D, Leoni L, Link MS, et al. Implantable cardioverter-defibrillator therapy for prevention of sudden death in patients with arrhythmogenic right ventricular cardiomyopathy/dysplasia. *Circulation.* 2003;108(25):3084-3091.
55. Rochitte CE, Oliveira PF, Andrade JM, et al. Myocardial delayed enhancement by magnetic resonance imaging in patients with Chagas' disease: a marker of disease severity. *J Am Coll Cardiol.* 2005;46(8):1553-1558.

Video Legends

Video 11.1 Horizontal long-axis MRI steady-state, free precession cine sequence showing extensive apical hypertrophy.

Video 11.2 Axial MRI steady-state, free precession cine sequence showing right ventricular dilation and basal dyskinesis.

CHAPTER 12

Hybrid Operating Rooms

Joseph Yammine, MD; Gregory F. Michaud, MD;
William G. Stevenson, MD; Laurence M. Epstein, MD

Concept

Over the past decade, the evolution of cardiovascular medicine has blurred the traditional boundaries between surgical and interventional fields. The concept of "hybrid procedures," which became popular first in coronary and vascular areas, preceded the development of state-of-the-art hybrid operating rooms. One of the first reports of a hybrid procedure appeared in 2006, by Angelini and associates, who described a combined percutaneous coronary intervention with minimally invasive coronary artery bypass grafting surgery to treat multivessel coronary heart disease.[1] Lately, hybrid cases have been performed for electrophysiology (EP) and valvular procedures. Additionally, advances in imaging technologies and the importance of anatomic considerations have piqued interest in the potential use of advanced imaging tools, such as magnetic resonance imaging (MRI), during interventional or surgical procedures.

In EP, the scope of interventional procedures has exploded. These include an array of interventions: epicardial ablation via a percutaneous subxiphoid approach, left atrial ablation via a transseptal approach for atrial fibrillation, left atrial appendage occlusion using both endocardial and epicardial devices, novel hemodynamic monitoring devices implanted for heart failure management, and challenging pacing lead implants and explants. Concurrently, patients and market forces continue to push for minimally invasive surgical strategies over more traditional, open surgical approaches. However, these minimally invasive procedures may require combined expertise in percutaneous interventional and thoracotomy or thoracoscopic approaches. Early data on some minimally invasive and hybrid procedures, mainly in high-risk populations (elderly, neonates), suggest that they may decrease morbidity and mortality.[2]

A hybrid EP procedure integrates the efforts of a cardiac electrophysiologist, who may be facile with the use of advanced robotics, multiple imaging and navigation systems, and diverse percutaneous access tools, with those of a cardiac surgeon. The latter contributes cardiothoracic surgery skills and a cardiothoracic surgery team, including backup cardiac bypass resources, in the hope of ultimately providing the safest, least traumatic, and most effective arrhythmia therapies.

Hybrid Procedures

A partial list of hybrid procedures is included in Table 12.1. In cardiac EP, atrial fibrillation ablation is the most prevalent ablation procedure (see "Illustrative Example of a Hybrid Procedure," below), but hybrid approaches for this arrhythmia are only beginning to gain momentum. Surgical ablation for atrial fibrillation is most commonly combined with minimally invasive mitral valve repair and a mini coronary artery bypass grafting (CABG) procedure. Combining surgical ablation with methods to assess the electrophysiologic integrity of ablation lines is hoped to improve success rates. Doing so could make hybrid approaches that combine percutaneous endocardial with thoracoscopic epicardial ablation of great interest for treating atrial fibrillation. At our institution, ventricular tachycardia ablation is facilitated by a combined approach with a cardiac surgeon. Indications include when epicardial access is needed but is limited because of scarring from previous pericardiotomy or pericarditis, or when the ablation target is epicardial, in proximity to a coronary artery.[3] A combined approach with an interventional cardiologist is employed for transcoronary ethanol ablation of VTs that cannot be approached with catheter ablation.[4]

Table 12.1 Select cardiovascular procedures performed in hybrid operating rooms

Cardiac Electrophysiology Procedure
• Ventricular tachycardias ablation (including those requiring ablation from ventricular epicardium, the LV summit below coronary arteries, intramural sites, and the endocardium in the presence of LV thrombus)
• Atrial fibrillation ablation
• Ablation of difficult accessory pathways (Ebstein's anomaly, epicardial pathways, appendage to ventricular connections)
• Access to epicardial space for any EP procedure when subxyphoid approach is limited by pericardial scarring, as from previous surgeries
• Device implantation: CRT with epicardial pacing leads; ICD for high defibrillation threshold or cases of unsuitable vascular access for transvenous leads
• ICD/pacemaker lead extraction
Other Hybrid Cardiovascular Procedures
• Hybrid coronary revascularization, including different combinations of PCI and CABG
• Carotid artery stenting and carotid endarterectomy
• Peripheral vascular stenting
• Endovascular repair of coarctation of the thoracic aorta
• Aortic aneurysm repair and arch reconstruction
• Percutaneous and transapical aortic valve replacement
• Endovascular and transapical mitral valve repair
• Transpulmonary valve replacement
• Atrial and ventricular septal defect repair with septal occluder deployment
• Hybrid therapies for congenital heart diseases
• Endovascular leak coiling and repair

EP = electrophysiology; CRT = cardiac resynchronization therapy; ICD = implantable cardioverter-defibrillator; PCI = percutaneous coronary intervention; CABG = coronary artery bypass grafting.

Hybrid Room Design

The optimal environment for performing hybrid procedures is a hybrid suite. Such a facility is uniquely designed so that cardiac surgery can be performed safely and effectively (including the ability to implant cardiopulmonary bypass and other forms of hemodynamic support) and combined with cardiac EP procedures that incorporate sophisticated mapping and imaging. The construction of a hybrid suite requires a deep understanding of the underlying technologies and their implications for interventional (whether EP, coronary, vascular, or valvular) and surgical workflow, which can vary widely. Before planning such a project, a clear vision for its utilization should be established. The range of intended applications should determine the needed resources, including location, space, and equipment. Such a facility should be capable of accommodating these procedures with uncompromised attention to anesthesia safety and sterility measures.

Hybrid rooms are larger than cardiac catheterization and EP laboratories: between 600 and 1,500 square feet (Figures 12.1 and 12.2), with a minimum clear area of 500 square feet. Floor-to-ceiling distance should be at least 10 feet in order to accommodate floor- or ceiling-mounted C-arms capable of rotational angiography. The rooms should have an open plan for potentially adding new equipment as new cardiac technologies arise and, if they are to be used in other fields of intervention, for noncardiac instruments that support neuroradiology and oncologic surgery. Currently, even in high-volume tertiary care centers, these rooms must have efficient utilization and scheduling to achieve a sufficient caseload in order to justify the enormous resources required for construction, planning, and operating these laboratories. To that end, the allocation of equipment and human resources, the space distribution, and the procedural chronological scheduling and flow should all be well designed. They also should take into account issues of sterility, anticoagulation management, sedation and anesthesia, preoperative preparation, and postoperative recovery.[5]

Radiation Measures

Shielding of hybrid rooms or suites may be different than that required of EP/cath labs and regular surgical rooms, especially if a high load of procedures, including bradytherapy or rotational tomography, is to be performed there.[6] Lead-lined walls in the range of 2 to 3 mm in thickness may be needed, depending on state regulations. In addition, protecting the patient as well as the operating professionals from radiation during hybrid procedures can be challenging. To address this issue, innovative strategies and tools (eg, RADPAD drapes [Worldwide Innovations & Technologies, Inc., Kansas City, KS] for the patient) might be needed to achieve adequate shielding without compromising visual fields, access areas, and sterility standards.[7]

Operating Table

One or more interventional/operating table(s) could be installed in the hybrid rooms. The OR table should be preferably thin but highly stable and should provide complete clearance underneath it, to allow panning x-ray systems to be freely moved. An example is the Diethrich IC 2020 table (Special Table Concepts, Phoenix, AZ): a thin carbon-fiber table with only one pedestal support[8] (Figure 12.3).

Chapter 12: Hybrid Operating Rooms • 129

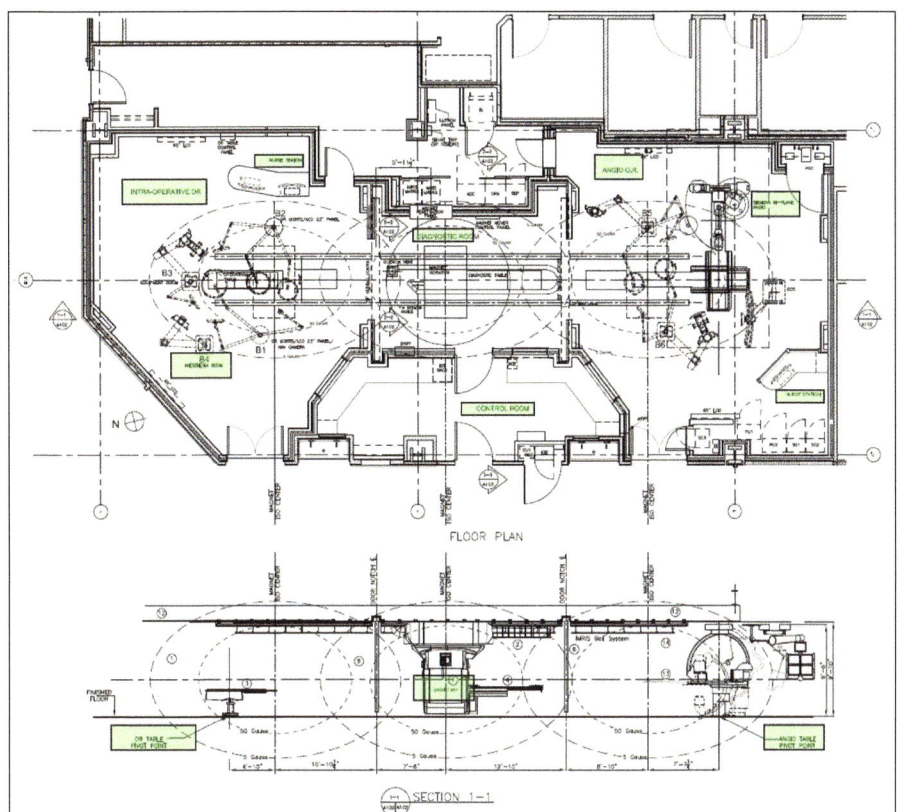

Figure 12.1 Blueprint of a hybrid operating room: the Advanced Multimodality Image Guided Operating Room. *Source:* Courtesy of IMRIS Inc., Winnipeg, Manitoba.

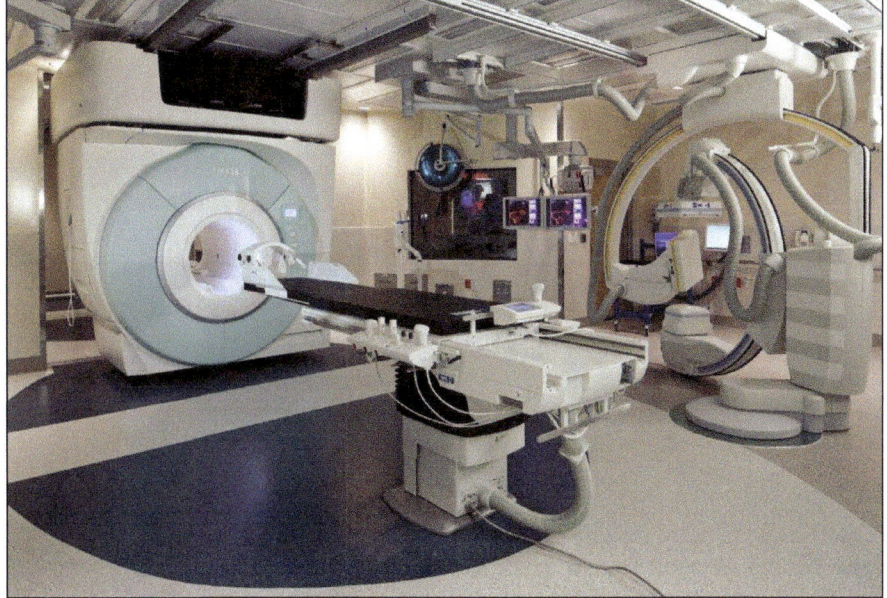

Figure 12.2 MRI section of the Advanced Multimodality Image Guided Operating Room. *Source:* Courtesy of IMRIS Inc., Winnipeg, Manitoba.

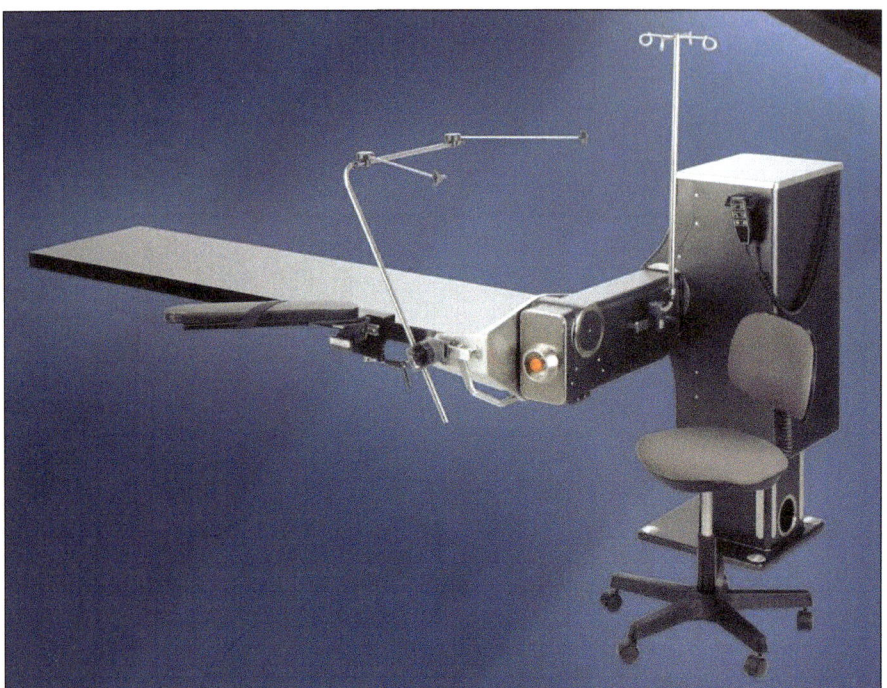

Figure 12.3 Diethrich IC 2020 surgical table: Thin, carbon fiber–made and unipedestal. *Source:* Courtesy of Special Table Concepts, Inc., Phoenix, AZ.

Imaging

In some laboratories, flat-panel detectors have replaced image intensifiers, enabling fluoroscopy to transition into three dimensions (3D) and to produce computerized tomography (CT)–like images. The contrast resolution of CT is approximately 1 Hounsfield unit (HU), whereas that of CT-like images obtained from CT fluoroscopy is around 10 HU; hence, CT fluoroscopy is not meant to replace diagnostic CT. Rotational CT angiography (CTA) is a recently developed hybrid imaging system where the C-arm swiftly revolves around the heart, obtaining serial, radially oriented images. These anatomic reconstructions can then be registered with other 2D or 3D imaging modalities (eg, electroanatomic maps, MRI, magnetic resonance angiography [MRA], positron emission tomography [PET], single-photon emission computed tomography [SPECT], or ultrasound).

Wireless Technologies

Managing the connections extending from the amplifiers and imaging equipment to the computers and monitors required is important for minimizing electrical noise and ensuring adequate functioning. Wireless technology could potentially move EP laboratories into a new era by reducing or even eliminating some of the considerable limitations and burdens of hard-wiring these environments. Such an approach could improve space utilization, opening up the room for other tools and mobile units, such as operating tables, fluoroscopy arms, cameras, and magnets to be rotated and transferred but without becoming tangled in the wired network.[9]

Equipment

A short list of the equipment commonly required in hybrid laboratories is included in Table 12.2.

Table 12.2 Partial list of cardiovascular equipment found in hybrid operating rooms

- Operating table(s)
- Electrophysiology recording systems
- Fluoroscopy units with compact, high-tube-heat capacity; semimobile, biplane capability; and flat panel monitors
- Electroanatomic mapping and navigation systems
- Ablation devices: radiofrequency energy generator, surgical and catheter cryoablation consoles, and laser energy source
- Robotic systems
- Echocardiography consoles for transthoracic, transesophageal, and intracardiac echocardiography
- Angiography and percutaneous coronary intervention equipment
- Anesthesia station(s) with related extensions and storages, gases
- Control area(s) with sufficient space to accommodate all monitors
- Nursing station(s)
- Storage facilities
- Anatomic and physiological imaging systems (MRI, CT, CTA, PET)

MRI = magnetic resonance imaging; CT = computed tomography; CTA = CT angiography; PET = positron emission tomography.

Personnel

The staff should be familiar with the different types of procedures being performed in these suites. To that end, cross-training is mandatory to build up knowledge of the different specialties involved and the multiple protocols related to sterility, catheter usage, radiation safety, equipment operation, and anesthesia.

Management

Hybrid rooms' administration, including procedural scheduling, teams' assignments, equipment traffic, inventory updating, billing, and professional development, should all be carried out through a multidisciplinary central core team. Protocols for the varied procedures should be developed and periodically revisited.

Outcomes

Individual procedural time might not be abridged, but aggregate procedural time should be reduced compared with a staged approach. In a staged approach, the patient would have to undergo different procedures in different suites on different days, with repeated preprocedural preparations and postprocedural recovery times, and with potentially recurrent anesthesia exposures, increased radiation doses, and infection risk.

The success of and complications arising from hybrid procedures should be compared against those of staged, separate procedures. At an institutional level, quality measures including efficacy and complications should be tracked. Quality assurance measures should include radiation exposure, procedural time, and postprocedure recovery. Investigational hybrid procedures should undergo evaluation and approval be obtained from the institutional review board (IRB). As the number of hybrid laboratories increases and procedures become more standardized, scientific organizations should provide guidance for performance and consider creating national data registries.

Cost

Hybrid operating rooms are more expensive to construct and to operate than conventional ones. Costs are estimated to be approximately double those of conventional operating rooms and 80% to 130% more than those of cardiac catheterization and EP laboratories. Even so, efficiencies, better outcomes, and lower complication rates have the potential to reduce overall costs for the patient populations being treated. If multiple procedures can be replaced by a single procedure, savings could be realized on recurring anesthesia costs and equipment that is otherwise redundant in EP, catheterization, and surgical rooms. Cost analyses will be required to shed more light on this question.

Education

As mentioned above, cross-training staff to work in the hybrid environment is important. In addition, training cardiology and surgery programs should incorporate more exposure to hybrid therapies for the management of cardiovascular diseases.[10] The development of educational materials for physicians and staff is likewise desirable. Regular, joint multidisciplinary conferences ("hybrid boards," similar to "tumor boards" in oncology) that review patients and outcomes may be important to both educate the team on an ongoing basis and optimize the utilization of this cost- and resource-intensive facility.

Illustrative Example of a Hybrid Procedure: Atrial Fibrillation

Catheter ablation for atrial fibrillation has a number of limitations. These probably contribute to the difficulties in achieving a high and sustainable cure rate—particularly for persistent atrial fibrillation. Incomplete, nontransmural lesions and the inability to ablate some epicardial regions are likely factors. Surgical Maze operations appear to have a very high success rate, likely because surgical atriotomy lines are usually transmural with no gaps.[11] Less invasive, surgical thoracoscopic approaches are, however, less reliable than open-heart surgical approaches, making EP assessment of completion of radiofrequency (RF) lines potentially more important. Standard surgical operating rooms, however, are not well equipped to perform electroanatomic mapping to assess the completeness of lesion lines or to map atrial tachyarrhythmias that may not be addressed in the anatomic lesion set.[12]

Combining endocardial catheter and surgical techniques is a potential approach for achieving a more durable lesion set than with catheter ablation alone, and at the same time, overcoming some of the limitations by facilitating mapping.[13] Furthermore, a surgical hybrid epicardial approach may help to avoid damaging the esophagus and the phrenic nerve. Such an approach also potentially allows for ablation of autonomic ganglia, ablation along the ligament of Marshall, and elimination of the left atrial appendage.[14] For all these reasons, a hybrid procedure performed in a hybrid environment by a multidisciplinary panel, including EP, surgery, and anesthesia teams, could address these issues (Figure 12.4).

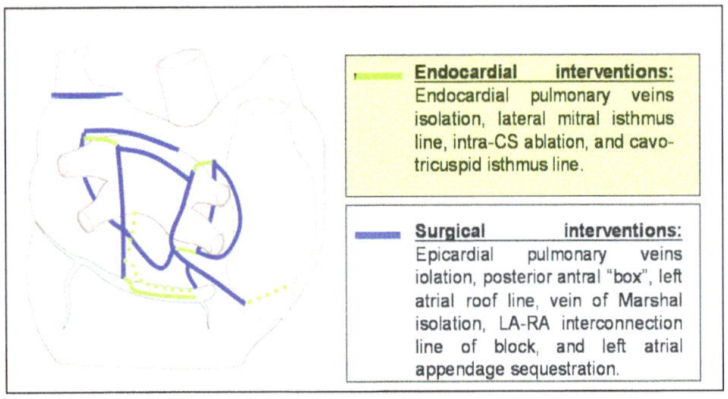

Figure 12.4 Diagram of hybrid heart procedures performed by endocardial and surgical teams in a hybrid environment. CS = coronary sinus; LA–RA = left atrium–right atrium.

Endocardial interventions: Endocardial pulmonary veins isolation, lateral mitral isthmus line, intra-CS ablation, and cavo-tricuspid isthmus line.

Surgical interventions: Epicardial pulmonary veins iolation, posterior antral "box", left atrial roof line, vein of Marshal isolation, LA-RA interconnection line of block, and left atrial appendage sequestration.

Recently, Kiser et al published the six-month results of the "convergent procedure." Their procedure combined surgical epicardial RF ablation and EP transseptal endocardial ablation to electrically isolate the 4 pulmonary veins, exclude the posterior left atrium, ablate the coronary sinus, and confirm block at the cavotricuspid isthmus. The study included patients with persistent and long-standing persistent AF, in whom an isolated endocardial ablation approach has traditionally shown a 6-month success rate of less than 50%.[15] In this study, at 6 months, 76% of patients were free from AF and antiarrhythmic drugs.[16] More data are needed to adequately compare approaches.

Periprocedural Evaluation and Care

Ideally, a multidisciplinary clinic should be designed to give the patient a chance to efficiently meet all specialists, including anesthesia personnel, involved in the procedure. This practice would extend the concept of the consolidated approach to preoperative preparations. If such a system is not in place, the multispecialty team of allied health care professionals (nurses and physician assistants) should at least coordinate the preprocedural workup and evaluation and then resume postoperative follow-up in a seamless fashion.

Conclusion

With the growing trend toward more complex cardiac procedures that combine multidisciplinary skills, we believe that the hybrid laboratory will soon become an integral part of every major cardiovascular center. Careful planning is key to the development, implementation, and ongoing optimal utilization of this complex resource.

References

1. Angelini GD, Wilde P, Salerno TA, et al. Integrated left small thoracotomy and angioplasty for multivessel coronary artery revascularization. *Lancet*. 1996;16:757-758.
2. Holzer R, Marshall A, Kreutzer J, et al. Hybrid procedures: adverse events and procedural characteristic—results of a multi-institutional registry. *Congenit Heart Dis*. 2010;5(3):233-242.
3. Soejima K, Couper G, Cooper JM, et al. Subxiphoid surgical approach for epicardial catheter-based mapping and ablation in patients with prior cardiac surgery or difficult pericardial access. *Circulation*. 2004;110(10):1197-1201.
4. Sacher F, Sobieszczyk P, Tedrow U, et al. Transcoronary ethanol ventricular tachycardia ablation in the modern electrophysiology era. *Heart Rhythm*. 2008;5(1):62-68.
5. Kpodonu J. The operating room of the future. *J Card Surg*. 2010;25:704-709.
6. National Council on Radiation Protection and Measurements. NCRP Report No. 147: *Structural shielding design for medical x-ray imaging facilities*. Bethesda, MD: National Council on Radiation Protection and Measurements; 2004.
7. Sawdy JM, Gocha MD, Olshove V, et al. Radiation protection during hybrid procedures: innovation creates new challenges. *J Invasive Cardiol*. 2009;21(9):437-440.
8. Special Table Concepts. http://www.specialtableconcepts.com.
9. Kpodonu J, Raney A. The cardiovascular hybrid room a key component for hybrid interventions and image guided surgery in the emerging specialty of cardiovascular hybrid surgery. *Interact Cardiovasc Thorac Sur*. 2009;9:688-692.
10. Hu S. One step hybrid approach for cardiovascular disease: from conception to practice. *Ann Thorac Cardiovasc Surg*. 2008;6(14):345-346.
11. Cox JL. Surgical treatment of atrial fibrillation: a review. *Europace*. 2004;5(Suppl 1):S20-S29.
12. Skanes AC, Klein GJ, Guiraudon G, et al. Hybrid approach for minimally-invasive operative therapy of arrhythmias. *J Interv Card Electrophysiol*. 2003;9:289-294.
13. Krul SPJ, Driessen AH, van Boven WJ, et al. Thoracoscopic video-assisted pulmonary vein antrum isolation, ganglionated plexus ablation and periprocedural confirmation of ablation lesions: first results of a hybrid surgical-electrophysiological approach for atrial fibrillation. *Circ Arrhythm Electrophysiol*. 2011;4(3):262-270.
14. Han FT, Kasirajan V, Kowalski M, et al. Results of a minimally invasive surgical pulmonary vein isolation and ganglionic plexi ablation for atrial fibrillation: single-center experience with 12-month follow-up. *Circ Arrhythm Electrophysiol*. 2009;2(4):370-377.
15. HRS/EHRA/ECAS. Expert Consensus Statement on catheter and surgical ablation of atrial fibrillation: recommendations for personnel, policy, procedures and follow-up. A report of the Heart Rhythm Society (HRS) Task Force on catheter and surgical ablation of atrial fibrillation. *Heart Rhythm*. 2007;4(6):816-861.
16. Kiser A, Landers M, Horton R, et al. The convergent procedure: a multidisciplinary atrial fibrillation treatment. *Heart Surg Forum*. 2010;5(13):E317-E321.

SECTION 1C

TECHNOLOGY AND THERAPEUTIC TECHNIQUES

Device Technology

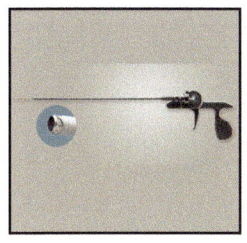 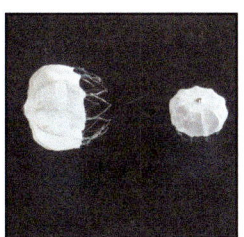 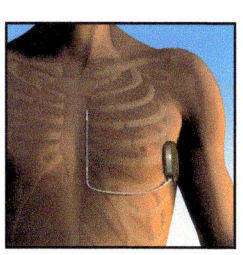 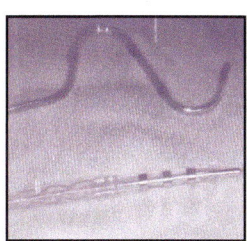

CHAPTER 13

NEW DEVELOPMENTS IN LEAD AND INTRODUCER SYSTEMS

Brian J. Cross, MD; Mark S. Link, MD

Introduction

Advances in device-based electrophysiological therapies have led to the innovations of smaller, more efficient, and more programmable implantable pacemakers and defibrillators. Importantly, concomitant technological breakthroughs in the leads and lead systems have further advanced the field of cardiac pacing and defibrillation. This chapter will provide an overview of the advances and directions in lead systems used in contemporary implantable cardioverter-defibrillator (ICD) and biventricular pacemaker implantation.

Overview of ICD Lead Developments

Following the introduction of surgically placed epicardial defibrillation pads in 1980, transvenously placed endocardial defibrillation systems were rapidly designed throughout the decade. By the mid-1990s, transvenously placed ICDs were the standard of care for primary and secondary prevention of sudden cardiac death.

Since their introduction, transvenous ICD leads have gone through several notable changes, including the advent of active fixation mechanisms and tip steroid elution, bipolar electronic design, and decreasing lead-size diameter. These improvements in lead design have helped to decrease lead-related complication rates from greater than 20% during the initial stage of ICD development to less than 10% currently.

This progress has, however, also been met with setbacks. One notable example is the Sprint Fidelis® lead, which became a commercially successful lead owing to several design advances and small 6.6 Fr caliber, with more than 268,000 leads placed worldwide. Nonetheless, despite its design advances, increased lead failure rates were encountered.[1] These manifested primarily as increased impedances and oversensing errors caused by conductor fractures at the distal ring electrode and, more proximally, near the anchoring tie-down, as well as in defibrillation failure due to fracture of the high-voltage conductor. These lead fractures have been associated with at least 13 patient deaths,[2] and in October 2007, the device's manufacturer, Medtronic, Inc. (Minneapolis, MN), pulled the lead from the market.[3] The Heart Rhythm Society Task Force on Lead Performance has responded to these examples of lead malfunction by encouraging clinicians to review the expected longevity of leads and devices with patients as a part of the informed consent process prior to implantation.[4]

Overview of Left Ventricular Leads

In select patients with left ventricular (LV) systolic dysfunction and delayed intraventricular conduction, programmed biventricular pacing to deliver cardiac resynchronization therapy (CRT) has been demonstrated to decrease heart failure symptoms and hospitalizations.[5-7] Pacing of the LV has been experimentally achieved through three mechanisms: endocardial LV pacing, pacing of the LV myocardium via surgically placed epicardial leads, and transvenous epicardial pacing via coronary venous access. Among these three, transvenous pacing has arisen as the most clinically viable method of LV pacing, because of the unreasonably high risks for systemic embolization and surgical morbidity, respectively, with the former two methods.

Within the past decade, extensive experience with transvenous epicardial LV pacing has brought it from an investigational intervention to a standard-of-care therapeutic modality for advanced heart failure worldwide. Developments of new technologies of LV lead design and techniques in lead placement have advanced concurrently with the growth in the field of CRT.

From an electrical perspective, leads used for LV pacing are similar to traditional pacing leads designed for endocardial placement in the right atrium (RA) or right ventricle (RV). Like the more traditional leads, LV leads comprise a connector pin at the proximal end and a pacing electrode at the distal end, with a flexible insulation made of polyurethane or silicone throughout the body of the lead. Also similar to their RA and RV lead counterparts, LV leads can function either as unipolar leads, with a cathodic end at the lead tip in circuit with an anodic pacing generator, or as true bipolar leads, with a cathodic tip and a proximal anodic ring. Pacing programming may make use of the various polarity settings for optimal CRT.

Unlike endocardial RA and RV leads, however, LV leads are endovascular devices and therefore have several structural aspects of lead design that are substantially unique to them. Given the endovascular nature of LV lead placement, passive fixation is (with the exception of the Medtronic Attain® StarFix unipolar lead) uniformly used. Accordingly, one of the most common adverse outcomes in a CRT system is LV lead dislodgement. To help achieve increased stability of LV leads after placement in the coronary sinus (CS) branches, the leads frequently have preshaped curves. When a stylet or guidewire is placed into such a lead, the lead becomes straighter and more rigid to lend support during lead delivery. When the stylet or guidewire is withdrawn, the lead assumes its curved shape within the target vessel. These curves help the lead to conform to the vessel wall and increase location stability.[8]

The design goal for newer generations of LV leads is to improve on lead deliverability, stability, and optimal LV pacing. Emerging design technologies aim to make LV leads smaller in caliber and tapered at the tip to allow for greater success in reaching and maintaining stable positioning in tortuous, distal CS branches. Additionally, newer-generation LV leads have been able to make use of lower-voltage bipolar pacing, which can increase battery life and decrease extracardiac stimulation. These improvements may have great importance because the presence of an LV lead in a cardiac pacing system is an independent risk factor for lead complications that subsequently require reoperation.[9]

Advances in Lead Delivery Systems

At its most basic level, an LV lead delivery system includes a subclavian venous sheath, a guide catheter designed to be seated in the proximal coronary sinus, and an LV lead with contouring and support aided by stylets, wires, and internal structural design. Together, these components of the LV lead delivery system are intended to facilitate access to the CS from a subclavian vein with optimal support and deliverability of the LV lead to the desired locations. Manufacturers of CRT devices have designed LV leads and lead delivery systems with characteristics intended to favor successful LV lead placement within the target CS branch.

St. Jude Medical Systems

The St. Jude Medical (St. Paul, MN) LV leads and delivery systems are categorized under the Cardiac Positioning System (CPS) family of devices. The CPS Direct® ST Slittable Outer Guide Catheter (Figure 13.1) can be used for initially accessing the CS ostium. From this point, LV leads can be advanced with an over-the-wire (OTW) approach to the desired location within the coronary venous system. Alternatively, inner catheters (CPS Aim™ Inner Catheters) that assist with coronary sinus cannulation and branch-vein subselection can be advanced within the lumen of the outer guide catheter to obtain more distal access within the body of the CS.

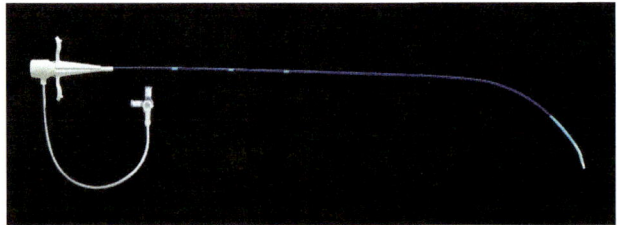

Figure 13.1A St. Jude Medical CPS Direct ST Slittable Outer Guide Catheter. *Source:* Photo courtesy of St. Jude Medical, Inc.

LV Lead Technology

St. Jude has market released the first multisite LV pacing lead, the quadripolar Quartet LV lead. This lead interfaces with a specific CRT-D device header present in the Unify-Quadra CRT-D device. Figure 13.1B shows the lead and this permits up to 10 pacing vectors shown in the table below. The lead utilizes 4 unipolar lead electrodes on a spiral S distal curve lead body. This lead permits more pacing opportunities without compromising lead stability. The options include the possibilities of more basal pacing sites. This may be associated with reverse LV remodeling and improved outcomes. It may also provide more options to manage common pacing complications, such as phrenic nerve stimulation and high pacing thresholds, resulting in less need for lead repositioning and fewer surgical revisions.

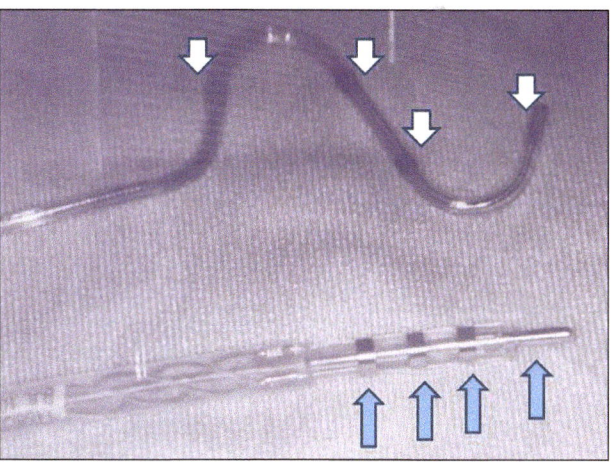

Figure 13.1B Proximal and distal ends of St. Jude Quartet LV pacing lead. The quadrupolar configuration requires a compatible header for lead electrode interface to permit multisite pacing. **White arrows** show pacing electrodes; **blue arrows** show IS-4 connector unipolar terminal pins.

Table 13.1 LV pacing lead configurations feasible using Quartet lead system

Vector	Cathode to Anode
Vector 1	Distal 1 to Mid 2
Vector 2	Distal 1 to Proximal 4
Vector 3	Distal 1 to RV Coil
Vector 4	Mid 2 to Proximal 4
Vector 5	Mid 2 to RV Coil
Vector 6	Mid 3 to Mid 2
Vector 7	Mid 3 to Proximal 4
Vector 8	Mid 3 to RV Coil
Vector 9	Proximal 4 to Mid 2
Vector 10	Proximal 4 to RV Coil

Medtronic

The Medtronic Attain Command® guide catheters (Figure 13.2) are designed to aid delivery deeply into the coronary venous system. Features designed for this purpose include a hydrophilic coating in the distal one-third of the catheter, as well as tapering, with decreases in the outer diameter from 9.0 Fr proximally to 8.5 Fr distally. The Medtronic Attain LV leads (Figure 13.3) are available in 6 Fr caliber (for medium to large veins) and 4 Fr caliber (for smaller veins with increased tortuosity). These leads may be placed using a guidewire, stylet, or both in combination. The Attain StarFix leads (Figure 13.4) have deployable lobes that are designed to increase stability of lead positioning.

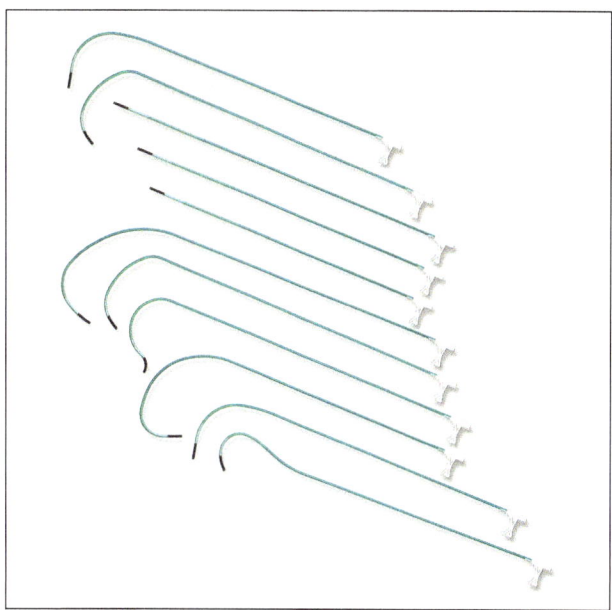

Figure 13.2 Medtronic Attain Command guide catheters, from **top to bottom:** MB2 Extra, Multipurpose Extra, Straight (57.5 cm), Straight (50 cm), Straight (45 cm), Extended Hook XL, Multipurpose, Amplatz, Extended Hook, MB2, and Multipurpose Right. *Source:* Photo courtesy of Medtronic, Inc.

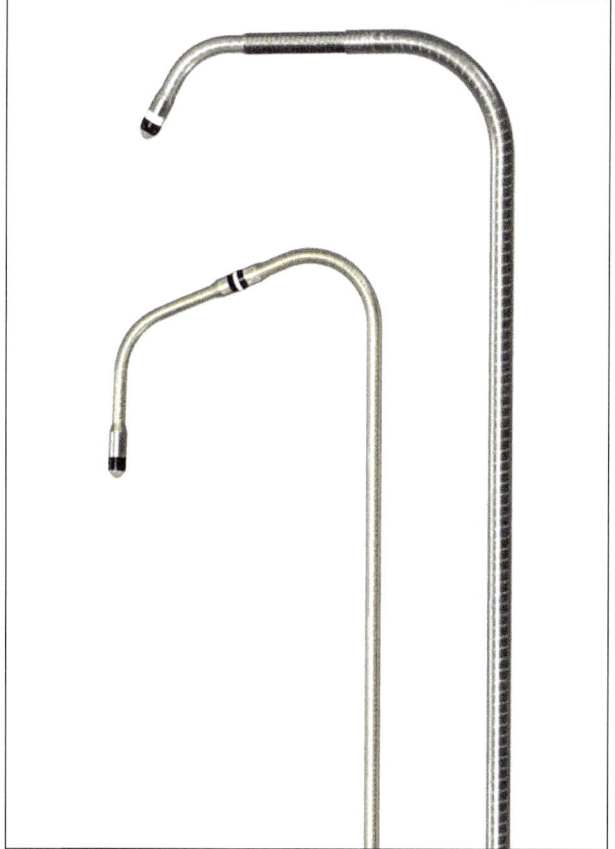

Figure 13.3 Medtronic Attain LV leads, from **left to right:** Attain Ability and Attain 4194. *Source:* Photo courtesy of Medtronic, Inc.

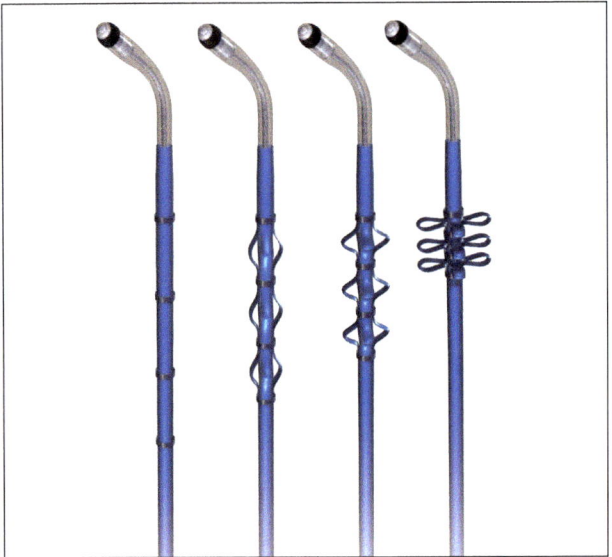

Figure 13.4 Medtronic Attain StarFix leads feature deployable lobes to increase stability of lead positioning. *Source:* Photo courtesy of Medtronic, Inc.

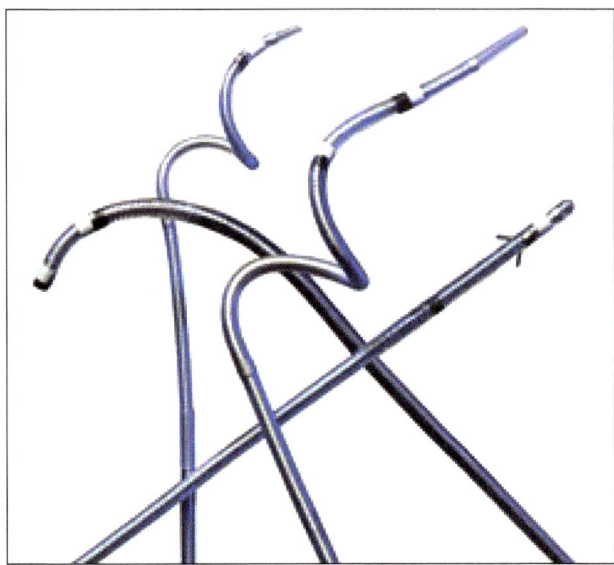

Figure 13.6 Boston Scientific LV leads, from **left to right:** ACUITY Steerable, ACUITY Spiral, EASYTRAK, and EASYTRAK 2. *Source:* Photo courtesy of Boston Scientific Corporation.

Boston Scientific

Boston Scientific (Natick, MA) LV leads (Figures 13.5 and 13.6) can be delivered within outer and inner Break-Away catheters for venous subselection. The company's LV leads are available in a range of diameter thicknesses and curve sizes to support vein stability. The smallest lead-tip profile is found in the ACUITY™ Spiral, which tapers from 4.1 Fr to 2.6 Fr, while the EASYTRAK® family of leads is better suited for larger veins. The EASYTRAK 2 and EASYTRAK 3 leads have the additional advantage of bipolar pacing, and multiple pacing polarities are available for optimal pacing without extracardiac capture.

Biotronik

The Biotronik (Berlin, Germany) Corox family of OTW LV leads, introduced through the ScoutPro catheter system (Figures 13.7, 13.8), allow for both OTW and stylet-supported lead delivery to target vessels.

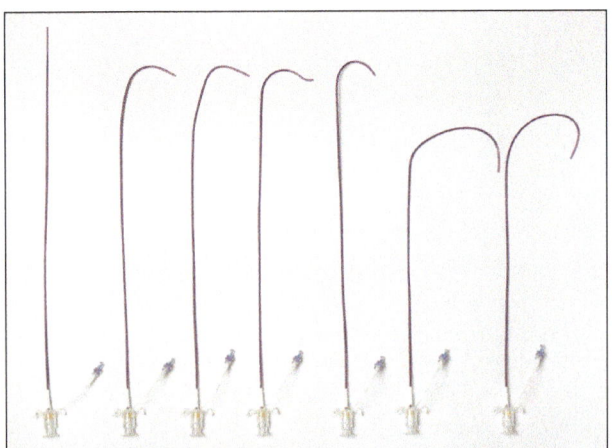

Figure 13.5 ACUITY outer catheters, from **left to right:** CS Straight, CS Hook, Multipurpose, Amplatz, Right-sided CS Hook, CS Wide, and Extended Hook. *Source:* Photo courtesy of Boston Scientific Corporation.

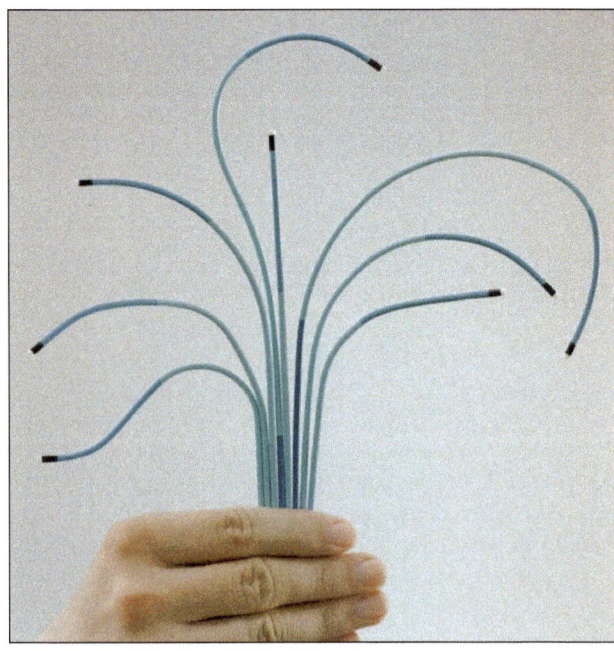

Figure 13.7 Biotronik ScoutPro ACS catheters, from **left to right:** Amplatz 6.0, Multipurpose Hook, BIO 2, Extended Hook Right, Straight, Extended Hook, Hook, and Multipurpose EP. *Source:* Photo courtesy of Biotronik, Inc.

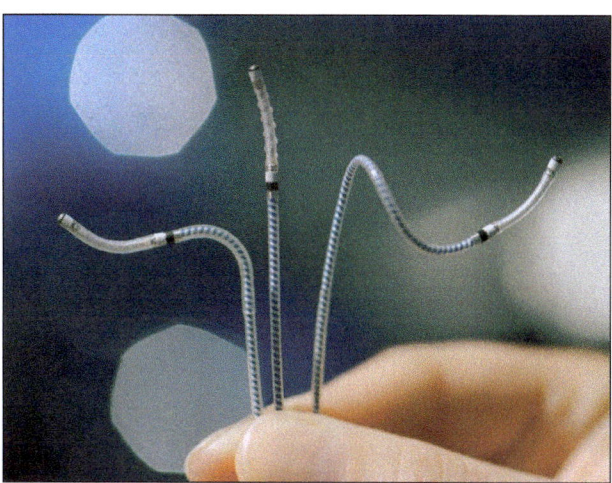

Figure 13.8 Biotronik Corox family of LV leads, from **left to right**: OTW L-BP, Corox OTW S-BP, and OTW BP. *Source:* Photo courtesy of Biotronik, Inc.

Advances in LV Pacing

Placement of an LV pacing lead can be performed from either the right or left subclavian venous system. However, the difficulty in negotiating several acute angle turns during placement from the right side often makes left-sided placement technically preferable. After successfully isolating and accessing the appropriate subclavian vein, a guide catheter is advanced into the RA. Counterclockwise torque is used to direct the guide catheter posteriorly and toward the ostium of the CS, after which careful advancement allows the catheter to engage the CS.

Once the guide catheter has engaged the CS, contrast venography is typically performed by using a balloon-tipped catheter to occlude the CS proximally while an injection of radiographic contrast opacifies the coronary venous system in a retrograde manner. The venographic images may then be used to visualize available branches of the coronary venous anatomy for LV lead placement.

Because LV leads pace the LV epicardially from their positions in the coronary venous system, locations for LV lead placement are necessarily governed by coronary venous anatomy. Technical challenges incurred by the size of a CS branch or the angle of its course may prohibit placing a lead in a desired location. Options for lead placement location may be further limited by diaphragmatic capture at a desired pacing voltage. Diaphragmatic pacing is commonly seen when LV leads are placed in inferior CS branches, but it can also occur in other branches that lie in proximity to the left phrenic nerve. Thus, the number of LV regions that are practically available for transvenous pacing lead placement is limited.

Nonetheless, as CRT use has become more widespread, the role of LV lead placement location in determining the clinical success of CRT has become increasingly evident. Early work in lead placement location associated placement of LV leads in lateral and posterolateral CS branches with desired short-term hemodynamic responses.[10] These sites have since become the most generally favored sites for lead placement, when coronary venous anatomy is favorable. However, the reported 20% to 30% clinical nonresponse rate to CRT may be at least partially the result of suboptimal lead location.

Contemporary research aiming to identify optimal anatomic sites for LV pacing has not demonstrated uniformly optimal sites for lead placement. Furthermore, this body of research has consistently shown a more patient-specific, rather than fixed-anatomic, nature of LV pacing location for CRT optimization.

As a result, subsequent research has investigated the short-term and long-term outcomes of alternative, non-anatomic criteria for site selection. Such alternative criteria have included mechanical factors (particularly, the site of latest mechanical activation, as determined by tissue Doppler imaging and speckle tracking echocardiography[11]); intracardiac electrographic assessment of LV electrical delay;[12] and real-time LV pressure/volume measurements to determine the pacing site associated with the most optimal hemodynamic effects.[13]

Intracardiac hemodynamic studies performed during LV lead placement may increase the risks and procedural time of biventricular pacemaker placement to unacceptably high levels. Therefore, future modalities to improve LV lead placement may instead use real-time electromechanical imaging to personalize LV lead placement for CRT optimization.

Magnetic Resonance Imaging of Patients with Cardiac Implantable Electronic Devices

In contemporary medical practice, magnetic resonance imaging (MRI) is an invaluable diagnostic modality that has notable prominence in cardiac applications, including for assessments of LV function, tissue viability, and structural characterization. Several studies have indicated that MRI studies can be performed safely in non–pacemaker-dependent patients with cardiac implantable electronic devices (CIEDs).[14,15] Even so, the ferromagnetic materials and electrical current–sensitive detection algorithms used in CIEDs have conventionally contraindicated most post-implant MRIs, in accordance with industry labeling as well as clinical practice guidelines.[16] In 2011, the Medtronic Revo MRI® SureScan® Pacing System and CapSureFix MRI® SureScan® pacing leads became the first CIED system designed to perform safely during postimplant MRI studies to gain approval from the U.S. Food and Drug Administration (FDA).

Despite the demonstrated safety of performing MRIs after placement of the Medtronic Revo MRI SureScan Pacing System, notable limitations and requirements apply to device placement, functioning, and programming prior to acquiring an MRI study. Specifically, the pacing system must include dual-chamber pacing with SureScan IPG pacing leads, implanted in the left or right pectoral region at least 6 weeks prior to the planned MRI study. Pacing lead impedances must be between 200 and 1,500 Ω. The leads must have capture thresholds less than or equal to 2.0 V at a pulse width of 0.4 millisecond, and in patients who will be pacing in an asynchronous mode, there must not be diaphragmatic capture at a pacing output of 5.0 V and at a pulse width of 1.0 millisecond. In addition, the imaging study must meet certain requirements to be performed. These include (but are not limited to) maximum static-field strength of 1.5 Tesla (T), patient positioning within the bore so that the MRI isocenter is superior to the C1 vertebra or inferior to the T12 vertebra, and continuous patient monitoring throughout the study with electrocardiography and plethysmography. Furthermore, health professionals performing the study must complete Medtronic SureScan® cardiology and radiology training.[17]

Conclusions

Design advances in ICD and CRT lead systems have spurred the development of smaller, more readily deliverable, and more durable leads that may improve procedural success and long-term clinical functioning. Further research into LV lead positioning will likely help to further direct the design of CRT-related devices.

References

1. Hauser RG, Hayes DL. Increasing hazard of Sprint Fidelis cardioverter-defibrillator lead failure. *Heart Rhythm*. 2009; 6(5):605-610.
2. Bloomberg News. Medtronic to settle lawsuits over devices tied to deaths. *The New York Times*. October 15, 2010:B5.
3. Medtronic, Inc. Urgent medical device information: Sprint Fidelis® lead patient management recommendations. October 15, 2007. http://www.medtronic.com/product-advisories/physician/sprint-fidelis/PROD-ADV-PHYS-OCT. Accessed January 25, 2013.
4. Maisel WH, Hauser RG, Hammill SC, et al. Recommendations from the Heart Rhythm Society Task Force on Lead Performance Policies and Guidelines: developed in collaboration with the American College of Cardiology (ACC) and the American Heart Association (AHA). *Heart Rhythm*. 2009;6(6):869-885.
5. Abraham WT, Fisher WG, Smith AL, et al. Cardiac resynchronization in chronic heart failure. *New Engl J Med*. 2002; 346(24):1845-1853.
6. Bristow MR, Saxon LA, Boehmer J, et al. Cardiac resynchronization therapy with or without an implantable defibrillator in advanced chronic heart failure. *N Engl J Med*. 2004; 350(21):2140-2150.
7. Moss AJ, Hall WJ, Cannon DS, et al. Cardiac resynchronization therapy for the prevention of heart failure events. *N Engl J Med*. 2009;361(14):1329-1338.
8. Russo A. Pacemaker and implantable cardioverter defibrillator lead design. In: Al-Ahmad A, ed. *Pacemakers and Implantable Cardioverter Defibrillators*. Minneapolis, MN: Cardiotext Publishing; 2010.
9. Kirkfeldt RE, Johansen JB, Nohr EA, et al. Risk factors for lead complications in cardiac pacing: a population-based cohort study of 28,860 Danish patients. *Heart Rhythm*. 2011;8(10):1622-1628.
10. Butter C, Auricchio A, Stellbrink C, et al. Effect of resynchronization therapy stimulation site on the systolic function of heart failure patients. *Circulation*. 2001;104(25):3026-3029.
11. Ypenburg C, van Bommel RJ, Delgado V, et al. Optimal left ventricular lead position predicts reverse remodeling and survival after cardiac resynchronization therapy. *J Am Coll Cardiol*. 2008;52(17):1402-1409.
12. Singh JP, Fan D, Heist EK, et al. Left ventricular lead electrical delay predicts response to cardiac resynchronization therapy. *Heart Rhythm*. 2006;3(11):1285-1292.
13. Derval N, Steendijk P, Gula LJ, et al. Optimizing hemodynamics in heart failure patients by systematic screening of left ventricular pacing sites: the lateral left ventricular wall and the coronary sinus are rarely the best sites. *J Am Coll Cardiol*. 2010;55(6):566-575.
14. Buendía F, Cano Ó, Sánchez-Gómez JM, et al. Cardiac magnetic resonance imaging at 1.5T in patients with cardiac rhythm devices. *Europace*. 2011;13(4):533-538.
15. Naehle CP, Strach K, Thomas D, et al. Magnetic resonance imaging at 1.5T in patients with implantable cardioverter-defibrillators. *J Am Coll Cardiol*. 2009;54(6):549-555.
16. Levine GN, Gomes AS, Arai AE, et al. Safety of magnetic resonance imaging in patients with cardiovascular devices: an American Heart Association scientific statement from the Committee on Diagnostic and Interventional Cardiac Catheterization, Council on Clinical Cardiology, and the Council on Cardiovascular Radiology and Intervention: endorsed by the American College of Cardiology Foundation, the North American Society for Cardiac Imaging, and the Society for Cardiovascular Magnetic Resonance. *Circulation*. 2007;116(24):2878-2891.
17. Medtronic, Inc. Revo MRI SureScan Pacing System: Indications, Safety, and Warnings. Minneapolis, MN: Medtronic, Inc.; February 8, 2011. http://newsroom.medtronic.com/phoenix.zhtml?c=251324&p=irol-newsArticle&ID=1771810&highlight=

CHAPTER 14

NEW INNOVATIONS IN IMPLANTABLE PULSE GENERATORS AND HEART FAILURE DEVICES

HELGE U. SIMON, MD; JOHANNES BRACHMANN, MD

New Developments and Trends in Device Therapy of Cardiac Arrhythmias

The chapter provides an overview about progress in battery technology, improved leads, and devices to reduce shocks in implantable cardioverter-defibrillator (ICD) therapy. It will discuss the approaches to avoiding lead complications altogether by use of subcutaneous leadless devices as well as new developments in cardiac resynchronization and reduced electromagnetic interference, and finally, it describes the status of the development of devices that allow patients to undergo magnetic resonance imaging (MRI).

Limitations of Current Devices

Both pacemaker and defibrillator therapy have undergone a dramatic advancement in safety, reliability, programmability, patient convenience, and affordability.

Problems remain regarding technical, battery, and electrode failures. Infections are more frequent with prolonged implantation procedures, upgrades, and battery depletion-related surgeries, often making lead extraction procedures necessary. "Leadless" device designs are being evaluated to reduce morbidity associated with intravascular permanent leads. Even so, no direct tissue injury can be demonstrated,[1] ICD shocks are associated with significant morbidity and, potentially, mortality. Therefore, sophisticated algorithms intended to reduce inappropriate shocks, as well as introduction of non-shock therapies over the last years.[2] In the field of cardiac resynchronization therapy, more reliable implant success rates have resulted from better lead placement devices, leads that are more steerable into side branches, and reduction of diaphragmatic stimulation. In particular, a new quadripolar electrode seems to improve implant success rates.[1] Other issues arise regarding interference with medical imaging such as MRI and electronic interference with devices. Finally, remote monitoring is becoming part of routine patient follow-up; this potentially leads to reduced need for face-to-face physician visits and decreases resource use while delivering faster care.

Battery Technology

Competing requirements in ICD and cardiac resynchronization therapy (CRT) devices are small battery and capacitor size, long-term physical and chemical stability of the design, short charge times of the capacitor, high energy of the delivered electric shock, and long life expectancy of the assembly.

Currently, lithium/silver vanadium oxide and polycarbon-monofluoride (CSx) batteries are benchmark technology. Silver vanadium oxide (SVO) results in consistent high-energy delivery with little increase in charge times over the battery life. Both anode-limited and cathode-limited designs are in use. *Anode-limited* refers to the fact that the anode material (lithium) depletes first, as opposed to a cathode-limited design, in which SVO content limits longevity. Cathode-limited designs reach the elective replacement interval (ERI) at lower voltage ranges (2.45–2.6 V) compared to anode-limited designs (ERI at 2.6–2.8 V). The excess lithium may serve as a cushion to prevent separator breach. Modern batteries may reach lifetimes up to 10 years in ICDs.

Polycarbon-monofluorides (CFx) have been introduced as a second cathode in modern ICDs and CRT devices to increase the energy density and discharge stability, thereby increasing battery life. Currently, these devices display longer intervals until they reach ERI, and also have a longer safety interval between ERI and end of battery life (EOL); specifically, the interval is 4.5 months in conventional lithium batteries compared to 7.5 months in Li/SVO batteries and 12.5 months in Li/SVO/CFx batteries.

To prevent erroneous information on battery longevity during device follow-up, battery voltage may not be displayed on the programmer; for example, after high-voltage charging or long episodes of radiofrequency transmission, the battery voltage may display a relaxation dip, followed by an overshoot, before returning to nominal voltage. In order to minimize erroneous data, daily battery measurements and time to ERI can be recorded, and currently some models record remaining capacity as well as battery current on their devices. Battery self-discharge is reduced from up to 5% per year in conventional designs down to 0.25% per year.

Strategies to improve battery decay (voltage delay caused by solubility of the cathode material) such as the use of phosphate oxide metal/metal phosphate battery assemblies are being explored.[3] Another promising approach in the future may be the use of body-generated energy to charge the device battery. Other strategies currently being explored to minimize battery decay are piezoelectric crystals and thermocouples. Piezoelectric crystals are being used to convert mechanical energy and thermocouples are being used to convert heat energy, both of which would provide electric current to charge a battery.[4]

Modern anodes and cathodes are separated by thin, redundant insulators that increase resistance if rapidly heated, thereby preventing internal short circuits, which could result in battery depletion. The downside of this redundant insulator design may be a slight increase in charge times over the life of the battery. Automatic adjustment of outputs according to automatically detected thresholds, requiring less than the conventionally used safety margin of twice voltage or triple impulse duration, are useful in preserving battery life, improving patient safety, and simplifying patient management and remote follow-up.[5] In clinical registries, it appears that modern devices have improved battery lives, often significantly exceeding 5 years.[6]

Lead Technology

Subcutaneous ICD

In patients without need for pacing, a new, entirely subcutaneously implanted defibrillator may avoid problems associated with endovascularly implanted leads, such as systemic infection, problems at the lead-myocardial interface resulting in loss of sensing, lead failure by long-term mechanical stress and scarring valvular insufficiency, and problems in growing patients.[7] The device is implanted in the lateral left chest with a subcutaneous lead in a parasternal position (Figure 14.1).[8] While higher shock energies are required to terminate ventricular fibrillation, this does not necessarily result in increased myocardial damage in comparison to transvenous/endocardial shock vectors, as those tend to have higher intracardiac field strengths. Problematic is the fact that the current device does not provide backup ventricular pacing after a shock. Also, in many heart failure patients, the need for atrial or biventricular pacing may arise, requiring a system change. The device size is still substantial (69 cm^3). Initial concerns of early battery depletion[9] could successfully be resolved by device reprogramming. Subcutaneous defibrillators are predominately used in young patients (children) and in cases in which no endovascular or epicardial approach to defibrillation is feasible or desired. Particularly in patients with channelopathies, who are endangered primarily by ventricular fibrillation (rather than macroreentrant ventricular tachycardia) and in whom antitachycardia pacing would be less likely effective, this device may prove beneficial.

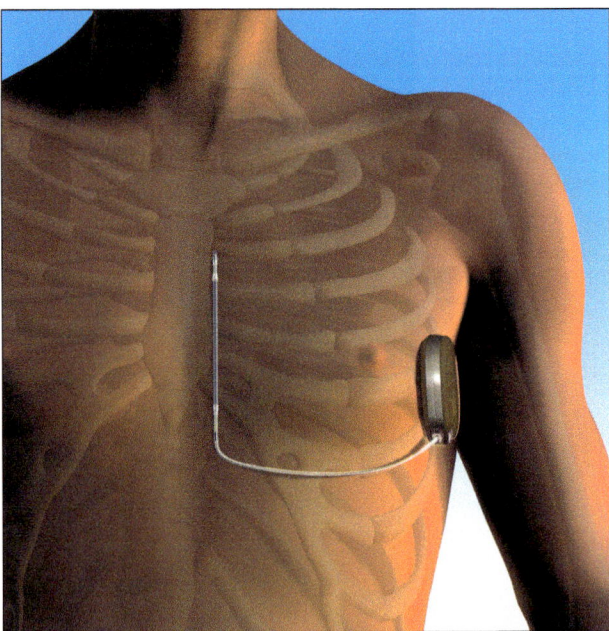

Figure 14.1 Subcutaneous ICD. *Source:* Image provided courtesy of Boston Scientific. © 2013 Boston Scientific Corporation or its affiliates. All rights reserved.

Endocardial Leads

Endocardial lead design has evolved from coaxial leads to multi-lumen leads during the last decade. This allows for smaller leads by placing multiple individually insulated conductors parallel in one lead, thereby decreasing lead size.[8] Failure rates of modern leads may vary substantially, and unanticipated high failure rates of modern design leads such as the Sprint Fidelis® (Medtronic, Minneapolis, MN) and Riata® leads (St. Jude Medical, St. Paul, MN) make surveillance of new leads and technologies such as in independently monitored registries necessary. The new DF 4 header is designed to reduce scarring and bulk of foreign body material in the pocket seen with the previously used yoke bifurcation or trifurcation, as well as potentially reducing errors by misconnection of multiple plugs and increasing convenience of the implantation procedure. Sealing rings are included in the header, consequently being replaced with each device change-out. Disadvantages may be the inability to connect pace-sense leads or additional shock coils without a special adaptor and the yet-unknown long-term reliability of the design.[9] This is being explored in ongoing trials. It is yet unknown if a design that avoids splice points outside the header (like the one used in the ENDOTAK RELIANCE® lead, Boston Scientific, Boston, MA) promises improved long-term performance.

A newly developed VDD lead with a floating atrial dipole allows for detection of atrial tachyarrhythmias to prevent inappropriate shocks. It appears to provide appropriate atrial detection;[10] however, some decay in atrial sensing was observed during follow-up. Long-term data on lead performance and avoidance of inappropriate shocks due to atrial tachyarrhythmias are needed. Timely initiation of oral anticoagulation to prevent strokes may be another benefit of the atrial sensing capability of this lead, as 13% of all patients with defibrillators demonstrate clinically otherwise undetected atrial fibrillation during device follow-up.[11]

Programming and Physiologic Stimulation

Most modern pacing devices avoid unnecessesary ventricular stimulation by maximizing atrioventricular delay in case of first-degree atrioventricular (AV) block and by switching from dual-chamber (DDD) to atrial-based pacing with monitoring of ventricular conduction in case of Wenckebach AV block, with fall back to dual-chamber pacing if two consecutive atrial events are not conducted.

Adjustment of pacing rate to a physiologic demands-rate response has conventionally been achieved by sensing respiratory rate, vibration, temperature, or a combination of these. Newer developments for more instantaneous rate adjustment involve monitoring of the QT interval and impedance changes during the cardiac cycle (closed loop stimulation, or CLS). Here, the unipolar impedance around the ventricular lead tip is measured throughout the cardiac cycle, reflecting ventricular contraction at rest. Deviation from the reference curve reflects rate demand. A more physiologic heart rate independent of comedication (like beta-blockade) and individual to the patient (reflecting increased rate response in worsening heart failure or during mental stress)[12] has been proposed. Physiologic stress (like mental stress) is reflected by a simultaneous elevation in blood pressure and heart rate and can be detected by CLS, resulting in an appropriate heart-rate increase in patients with a blunted rate response.[13] Particularly in sicker or less active patients, the rate response with CLS might reflect physiologic demands more closely than would vibration sensors.

Rate smoothing can be used in case of paroxysmal atrial tachyarrhythmias to avoid intolerable variation of intrinsically conducted ventricular cycle lengths in patients who do not tolerate those. In cases of atrial tachyarrhythmia, lock-in protection can ensure appropriate mode switching in the occasional case of atrial events that fall into the blanking period, thereby not reaching the programmed rate cutoff to adequately mode-switch.

Currently, atrial pacing can be adjusted to physiologic needs, conserving battery voltage by rate reduction at night and various atrial rate hysteresis algorhythms. Atrial antitachycardia pacing (ATP) has been proposed in selected patients to pace-terminate atrial tachyarrhythmias, yet clinical trials on this have been discouraging.[14,15] In contrast to ATP, many patients with bradycardia-related atrial tachyarrhythmias may benefit from physiologically appropriate atrial-based pacing with ventricular backup pacing only in case of ongoing AV block, which may reduce persistent atrial fibrillation by 40%.[16] Another occasionally needed feature is negative AV hysteresis to ensure ventricular pacing, if this is desired for hemodynamic reasons (eg, left ventricular stimulation or—in case of hypertrophic obstructive cardiomyopathy—right ventricular stimulation). Arrhythmia monitoring, both in the atrium and in the ventricle, can be achieved in modern pacemakers without significant effect on battery longevity. By use of frequent automatic adjustment of outputs with continuous capture control in both atrium and ventricle, device life from beginning of life (BOL) to ERI has increased to more than 10 years in some devices.

Leadless Endocardial Left Ventricular Stimulation

Conduction delay to the left ventricular lateral wall is frequently present in heart failure patients with reduced left ventricular systolic function, and CRT by epicardial pacing through a lead placed in a lateral coronary sinus branch is frequently performed. Because coronary sinus anatomy often conflicts with optimal electrical activation, conventional transvenous lead placement is not feasible, the problem being access to a suitable vein, high pacing threshold because of scarring or epicardial fat under the venous branch, unstable lead position, or phrenic nerve capture. Currently, in these cases, only surgical lead placement has been possible. A new concept for left ventricular endocardial pacing (WiseCRT) is currently under investigation. This device could allow implanting a short pacing electrode containing a piezoelectric crystal through transseptal approach into the lateral left ventricular endocardium. The piezoelectric crystal receives mechanical energy from an implanted ultrasound generator through the thoracic wall and converts it to electrical energy to pace.[17]

Alternative approaches being explored include magnetic fields to transmit energy to pace endocardially rechargeable devices.[18] These systems need to become safe during implantation and should also provide lifelong containment of the battery and circuitry. Potential problems that could arise with self-contained pacing systems include implant risks such as pneumothorax and hemopericardium in case of epicardial leads and problems with removal in case of device failure or battery depletion. Long-term exposure to transmitted energy like ultrasound needs to be safe. Also, programmability and timing of multi-chamber stimulation might become more problematic with multiple self-contained pacemakers interacting with each other.[19]

The use of a new isodiametric 5-Fr quadripolar electrode with a new, convenient IS-4 connector allows for programming of 10 different pacing vectors bipolar between the lead electrodes and using the RV shock coil electrode as anode. Initial experience demonstrated excellent thresholds and absence of phrenic nerve stimulation in 97% of patients as compared to 86% of patients using bipolar electrode configuration. In addition, the potential for improved hemodynamic response exists using this electrode, and our experience indicates successful bailouts in cases when bipolar electrodes fail (Figure 14.2).[20]

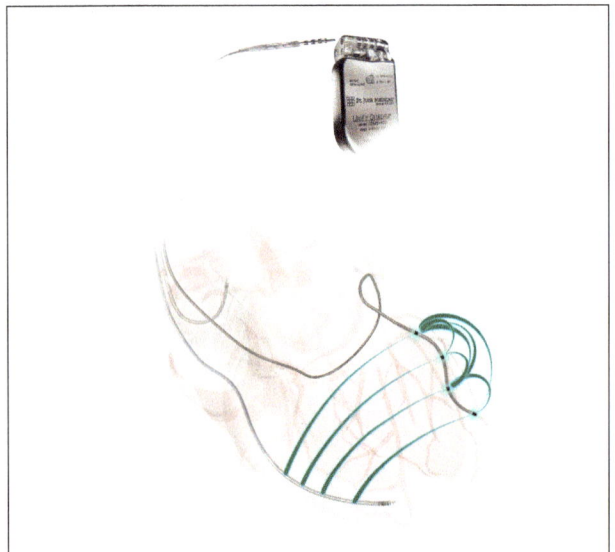

Figure 14.2 Quadripolar electrode. Ten different bipolar pacing vectors are programmable between the lead electrodes and the right ventricular shock coil. *Source:* Courtesy of St. Jude Medical, St. Paul, MN.

Cardiac Stimulation During the Refractory Period

Cardiac Contractility Modulation

Bench research has sparked interest in the effects of high-voltage impulses during the refractory period on cardiac contractility. The currently used Optimizer IV is a relatively small device shaped much like a large pacemaker. It has a battery that becomes charged by inductive charging through an external wand (Figure 14.3). One atrial and two ventricular leads are used to detect the patient's atrioventricular rhythm (either intrinsic or paced) and to set timing of the high-voltage stimulus during ventricular systole. The area of myocardium affected by the stimulus may increase over time, a phenomenon probably caused by electronic influence on myocardial membrane proteins and gap junctions.

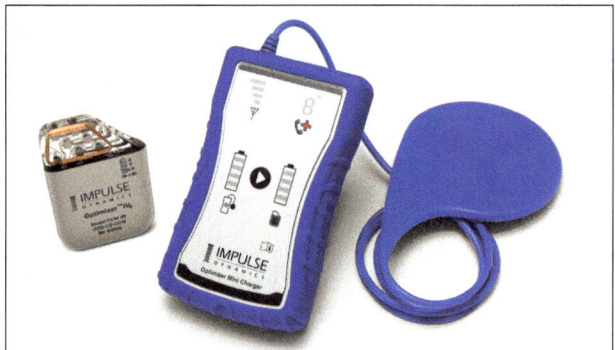

Figure 14.3 Optimizer IV system. Cardiac contractility modulation (CCM): the implantable Optimizer IV, the programmer, and the external charger. *Source:* Courtesy of Impulse Dynamics.

CCM appears to reverse pathologic ("fetal") gene expression.[21] It improves contractility without raising myocardial oxygen consumption,[22] improves peak oxygen uptake, lowers heart failure class, does not lower blood pressure, and appears to be free of proarrhythmic effects.[23] Global and regional systolic left ventricular function improves, even in myocardium remote from the stimulation lead site, reduces left ventricular end-diastolic and end-systolic volumes, thereby decreasing mitral regurgitation and improving heart failure status in a small study of 60 patients.[24] The initial promising experience with the device needs to be confirmed in large studies and registries currently under way to assess the impact of CCM on hard end points like mortality and major cardiovascular events.

Monitoring Devices/Remote Follow-up

Many implanted CRM devices are capable of monitoring battery status, lead impedances and integrity, sensing amplitude, pacing thresholds, occurrence of atrial and ventricular arrhythmias (including their intracardiac electrograms [IEGMs]), thoracic impedances as a measure of heart failure status, and patient activity. These can be radioed to a data transmitter in the patient's home, which relays the data to the follow-up clinic either by landline or mobile phone (GSM) network. Data transfer from the device to the data transmitter may take place through a wand or through wireless radiofrequency connection (which may be preferable, as it is not dependent on patient compliance). Some CRM devices may automatically adjust pacing outputs based on automatically measured pacing thresholds, and periodic transmission of all these measurements defines remote follow-up. Remote monitoring, in contrast, refers to daily device interrogation and transmission of predefined events; this follow-up pattern may reduce the number of charged (by 76%) and delivered shocks (by 52%) and reduce the number of hospitalizations due to inappropriate shocks.[25] Remote monitoring of single- and dual-chamber defibrillators results in fewer unscheduled patient visits, faster patient throughput, and less physician time required to review patient data while maintaining safety.[26] Follow-up intervals will need to be individualized based on patient status, particularly in sicker patients (like many CRT patients) and those who have had defibrillation shocks. These patients may still need to be seen in follow-up, even though follow-up often does not result in reprogramming.[27] Some remote monitoring devices may include transmission of blood pressure measurements and patient weight, thereby making remote monitoring of the patient's clinical status more reliable. Additional benefit from remote monitoring and follow-up results from the early detection of atrial fibrillation, triggering the decision to anticoagulate the patient.

Future devices may provide instant information on the hemodynamic status of the patient. This is relevant mainly for two reasons: First, in theory, a device will note a deterioration of the volume status before the patient does; moreover, the device may be more accurate in the assessment of weight measurement, thoracic impedance, and cardiac filling pressures and can transmit such data to the physician before the patient is able to call in. The benefit should be better timeliness of therapeutic decisions. Hospitalizations and other sequelae may be avoided, possibly in a cost-efficient manner. Second, according to the acute hemodynamic status of the patient, a device delivering antitachycardia therapy may help select from among several appropriate therapies (eg, antitachycardia pacing vs high-voltage shocks).

Problems of Electromechanic Interference

Magnetic Resonance Imaging (MRI) Capable Devices

The use of MRI technology has been increasing. In 2010, there were 50 million MRI scans performed worldwide, compared to 30 million MRI scans in 2006. MRI provides excellent soft tissue delineation and has become gold standard noninvasive imaging not only for many cardiac conditions, but also in particular for orthopedic and neurologic conditions.

The number of ICD implants has also been continuously increasing from about 35,000 in 1997 to almost 45,000 in 2004.[28] It is anticipated that 50%–75% of patients with CRM devices may require MRI scanning during their lifetimes.[29] Because the number of patients with CRM devices constantly increases, and the conditions assessed by MRI scan are particularly prevalent in this patient population, potential sources of interference between the physical stresses of MRI deserve attention. These are mainly the static main magnetic field, radiofrequency energy (transmitted by a variety of different coils), and gradient magnetic fields during scanning.[30]

The static magnetic field in most currently used MRI scanners ranges from 1.5 to 3 Tesla, corresponding to 40,000–60,000 times the Earth's magnetic field. It interacts with nonferromagnetic to only weakly ferromagnetic materials in most current devices. As most ex vivo investigations were performed on 1.5 T scanners, considerable concern resolves the issue of using implanted cardiac devices in scanners of higher field strength, potentially leading to projectile forces capable of injuring the patient and damaging the imaging system. It should be noted that most MR scanners are *always* exerting strong magnetic fields, even if the imaging mode is off.

The radiofrequency field pulses energy through the body, resulting in resistive heating. Energy absorption is denoted as specific absorption rate (SAR), measured in watts per kilogram (W/kg), proportional to field strength. Leads may form antennas to absorb energy, with fractured or retained leads being particularly dangerous. Local heating may result in injury or lead failure, and even late increases in thresholds have been reported. The nature of the interaction is frequency-dependent and particularly unpredictable. Blood flow at the lead tissue interface, lead geometry, position of the patient in the scanner, lead input filtering capacitance, isocenter of the scan, and imaging sequence and duration are some of the variables that can affect risk of injury.

Magnetic field gradients are induced from rapidly changing magnetic field strength and may excite peripheral nerves and potentially cardiomyocytes if transmitted through a lead. Electrocardiographic changes such as ST-segment elevations, T-wave inversions, and artifacts resembling QRS complexes have been described as a result of MRI imaging, making monitoring during scanning more problematic. Sometimes the maximal energy absorbed is distant from the site being scanned, making consultation with personnel experienced in magnetic resonance physics necessary.[30]

As a result of interference with the CRM devices, any of the following events may occur:

- pacing may be inhibited
- inadvertent reprogramming of the device may occur
- device circuitry may be damaged
- the lead-myocardial interface may become heated up, resulting in increased pacing thresholds and decreased sensing
- the battery may drain
- erroneous reed switch behavior (in up to one-third of cases)[31] may occur

Reed switch behavior is particularly unsafe in pacing-dependent patients, if electronic reset occurs at the same time. Prediction of these behaviors seems impossible, as the MRI setup, programming, coil-patient geometry, device design, and material vary substantially. Several lethal complications have been reported, and general consensus has been, that while most applications of MRI on patients with conventional pacemakers and defibrillators have been safe using precautions—such as turning tachy-therapy off, checking the device after the MR imaging, pacing asynchronous or not at all during the magnetic interference—MRI is performed only in those cases where no other reasonable imaging modality exists and the benefit clearly outweighs the risk, for example, imaging intracranial tumors of the posterior fossa.[32] An analysis of case reports and small series of MRI being performed in patients with conventional pacemakers and ICDs confirms frequent pacing-capture threshold changes, biomarker elevations, arrhythmias, and unpredictable reed switch behavior.[33] MRI is not endorsed in most circumstances in patients with conventional ICDs or in pacing-dependent patients.[30] The interaction between CRM and MRI are now being classified as safe, conditionally safe (with specification of device, patient, and MRI properties) and unsafe.[34]

MRI-compliant pacemakers and pacemaker leads are now available, and even a conditionally safe ICD has been released. A valuable tool assessing the risk of a particular device interfering with a particular MRI setup is available online.[35]

A comprehensive review of the issue has been performed by Jung et al.[36] It is important to mention that initial safety studies on these devices were performed on maximally 1.5 T scanners, had the isocenter placed far from the heart, and limited SAR to <2 W/kg. Image quality of the MRI is significantly affected by CRM leads, particularly in cardiac imaging. Initial experience suggests diagnostic imaging possible in most patients, with acceptable image quality in the inferior aspect of the heart. Even late enhancement imaging has been performed successfully.[37] It must be stated, however, that some MRI-safe devices exclude thoracic imaging in their precautions; also, data on image quality of cardiac MRI is still incomplete. In addition, various alternative diagnostic modalities such as transthoracic and transesophageal echocardiography, computed tomography, rotational angiography, cardiac catheterization, nuclear imaging, and biopsies are available.

To achieve better MRI compatibility, reed switches may be replaced with Hall sensors. Initial studies with MRI conditionally safe–rated devices are encouraging. In two larger studies with new, conditionally safe pacemakers, no significant safety issue arose, pacing thresholds remained stable during follow-up, and no resets, arrhythmia during scanning, or episodes of death or serious injury occurred.[38,39]

If performed, it is felt that MRI scanning should take place at institutions with considerable expertise in both MRI and electrophysiology. Patients need to be informed about the risk of device failure, damage to the device, arrhythmia, injury, and death. Personnel and equipment to perform advanced cardiac life support (including a defibrillator) need to be close to the patient, and the device should be interrogated and programmed before and after the procedure. The patient should be verbally monitored throughout the procedure, and electrocardiographic as well as pulse-oxymetric monitoring of heart rate should be performed. Modern devices considered conditionally safe for MRI scanning can be programmed to "MRI mode," which may involve asynchronous or switched-off pacing, maximized pacing outputs (or sensed-only mode) and adjusted sensitivity, ICD detection, and therapy disabled. After the scan, in ICD patients, defibrillation threshold testing has been advocated if the patient does not have an MRI conditionally safe device. Patients with older devices or retained leads might potentially be scanned safely in low magnetic field open MRI scanners.[40]

Acknowledgments

The authors wish to express their gratitude to Dr. Karin Simon Demel for her assistance in the preparation of this manuscript.

References

1. Toh N, Nishii N, Nakamura K, et al. Cardiac dysfunction and prolonged hemodynamic deterioration after implantable cardioverter-defibrillator shock in patients with systolic heart failure. *Circ Arrhythm Electrophysiol*. 2012;5(5):898-905.
2. Bhakta D, Foreman LD. Implantable cardioverter-defibrillator shock reduction: the new paradigm. *Heart Rhythm*. 2011;8(12):1887-1888.
3. Bock DC, Marschilok AC, Takeuchi KJ, Takeuchi ES. Batteries used to power implantable biomedical devices. *Electrochim Acta*. 2012;84:155-164.
4. Bhatia D, et al. Pacemakers charging using body energy. *J Pharm Bioallied Sci*. 2010;2(1):51-54.
5. Pierantozzi A, Landolina M, Agricola T, et al. Automatic adjustment of stimulation output in resynchronization therapy: impact and effectiveness in clinical practice. *Europace*. 2011;13(9):1311-1318.

6. Thijssen J, Borleffs CJ, van Rees JB, et al. Implantable cardioverter-defibrillator longevity under clinical circumstances: An analysis according to device type, generation, and manufacturer. *Heart Rhythm.* 2011;9(4):513-519.
7. Gradaus R, Breithardt G, Bocker D. ICD leads: design and chronic dysfunctions. *Pacing Clin Electrophysiol.* 2003;26(2 Pt 1):649-657.
8. Bardy GH, et al. An entirely subcutaneous implantable cardioverter-defibrillator. *N Engl J Med.* 2010;363(1):36-44.
9. Sticherling C, Burri H. Introduction of new industry standards for cardiac implantable electronic devices: balancing benefits and unexpected risks. *Europace.* 2012;14(8):1081-1086.
10. Safak E, Schmitz D, Konorza T, et al. Assessment of atrial sensing quality in ICD patients with a floating atrial dipole ICD lead (interim results). *Europace.* 2011;13 (suppl 3):Abstract P1027.
11. Daubert JP, Zareba W, Cannom DS, et al. Inappropriate implantable cardioverter-defibrillator shocks in MADIT II: frequency, mechanisms, predictors, and survival impact. *J Am Coll Cardiol.* 2008;51(14):1357-1365.
12. Proietti R, Manzoni G, Di Biase L, et al. Closed loop stimulation is effective in improving heart rate and blood pressure response to mental stress: report of a single-chamber pacemaker study in patients with chronotropic incompetent atrial fibrillation. *Pacing Clin Electrophysiol.* 2012;35(8):990-998.
13. Coenen M, et al. Closed loop stimulation and accelerometer-based rate adaptation: results of the PROVIDE study. *Europace.* 2008;10(3):327-333.
14. Gillis AM, et al. Impact of atrial antitachycardia pacing and atrial pace prevention therapies on atrial fibrillation burden over long-term follow-up. *Europace.* 2009;11(8):1041-1047.
15. Janko S, Hoffmann E. Atrial antitachycardia pacing: do we still need to talk about it? *Europace.* 2009;11(8):977-979.
16. Sweeney MO, et al. Minimizing ventricular pacing to reduce atrial fibrillation in sinus-node disease. *N Engl J Med.* 2007;357(10):1000-1008.
17. Lee KL, et al. First human demonstration of cardiac stimulation with transcutaneous ultrasound energy delivery: implications for wireless pacing with implantable devices. *J Am Coll Cardiol.* 2007;50(9):877-883.
18. Wieneke H, et al. Leadless pacing of the heart using induction technology: a feasibility study. *Pacing Clin Electrophysiol.* 2009;32(2):177-183.
19. Benditt DG, Goldstein M, Belalcazar, A. The leadless ultrasonic pacemaker: a sound idea? *Heart Rhythm.* 2009;6(6):749-751.
20. Simon HU, et al. Erste Erfahrungen mit einer neuen quadripolaren Stimulationselektrode zur kardialen Resynchronisationstherapie. *Clin Res Cardiol.* 2012;101(Suppl 2).
21. Butter C, et al. Cardiac contractility modulation electrical signals improve myocardial gene expression in patients with heart failure. *J Am Coll Cardiol.* 2008;51(18):1784-1789.
22. Butter C, et al. Enhanced inotropic state of the failing left ventricle by cardiac contractility modulation electrical signals is not associated with increased myocardial oxygen consumption. *J Card Fail.* 2007;13(2):137-142.
23. Borggrefe MM, et al. Randomized, double blind study of non-excitatory, cardiac contractility modulation electrical impulses for symptomatic heart failure. *Eur Heart J.* 2008;29(8):1019-1028.
24. Yu CM, et al. Impact of cardiac contractility modulation on left ventricular global and regional function and remodeling. *JACC Cardiovasc Imaging.* 2009;2(12):1341-1349.
25. Guedon-Moreau L, et al. A randomized study of remote follow-up of implantable cardioverter defibrillators: safety and efficacy report of the ECOST trial. *Eur Heart J.* 2012;34(8):605-614.
26. Varma N, et al. Efficacy and safety of automatic remote monitoring for implantable cardioverter-defibrillator follow-up: the Lumos-T Safely Reduces Routine Office Device Follow-up (TRUST) trial. *Circulation.* 2010;122(4):325-332.
27. Lunati M, et al. Follow-up of CRT-ICD: implications for the use of remote follow-up systems. Data from the InSync ICD Italian Registry. *Pacing Clin Electrophysiol.* 2008;31(1):38-46.
28. Roguin A, Schwitter J, Vahlhaus C, et al. Magnetic resonance imaging in individuals with cardiovascular implantable electronic devices. *Europace.* 2008;10(3):336-346.
29. Roguin A. Myron Prinzmetal 1908-1987: the man behind the variant angina. *Int J Cardiol.* 2008;123(2):129-130.
30. Levine GN, Gomes AS, Arai AE, et al. Safety of magnetic resonance imaging in patients with cardiovascular devices. *Circulation.* 2007;116(24):2878-2891.
31. Vahlhaus C, Sommer T, Lewalter T, Schimpf R, Schumacher B, Jung W, Lüderitz B. Interference with cardiac pacemakers by magnetic resonance imaging: are there irreversible changes at 0.5 Tesla? *Pacing Clin Electrophysiol.* 2001;24(4 Pt 1):489-495.
32. Roguin, A. Magnetic resonance imaging in patients with implantable cardioverter-defibrillators and pacemakers. *J Am Coll Cardiol.* 2009;54(6):556-557.
33. Jung W, Zvereva V, Hajredini B, Jäckle S. Safe magnetic resonance image scanning of the pacemaker patient: current technologies and future directions. *Europace.* 2012;14(5):631-637.
34. American Society for Testing and Materials (ASTM) International. ASTM F2503-05: Available at http://www.astm.org/Standards/F2503.htm. Accessed April 28, 2013: Standard Practice for Marking Medical Devices and Other Items for Safety in the Magnetic Resonance Environment. West Conshohocken, Pa: ASTM International; 2005.
35. Shellock, FG. Institute for Magnetic Resonance Safety, Education, and Research website. Available at http://www.mrisafety.com. Accessed July 31, 2013.
36. Jung W, et al. Initial experience with magnetic resonance imaging-safe pacemakers: a review. *J Interv Card Electrophysiol.* 2011;32(3):213-219.
37. Junttila MJ, Fishman JE, Lopera GA, et al. Safety of serial MRI in patients with implantable cardioverter defibrillators. *Heart.* 2011;97(22):1852-1856.
38. Forleo GB, Santini L, Della Rocca DG, et al. Safety and efficacy of a new magnetic resonance imaging-compatible pacing system: early results of a prospective comparison with conventional dual-chamber implant outcomes. *Heart Rhythm.* 2010;7(6):750-754.
39. Wilkoff BL, Bello D, Taborsky M, et al. Magnetic resonance imaging in patients with a pacemaker system designed for the magnetic resonance environment. *Heart Rhythm.* 2010;8(1):65-73.
40. Strach K, Naehle CP, Mühlsteffen A, et al. Low-field magnetic resonance imaging: increased safety for pacemaker patients? *Europace.* 2010;12(7):952-960.

CHAPTER 15

IMPLANTABLE AND REMOTE MONITORING

WERNER JUNG, MD

Introduction

The exponential growth of cardiovascular implantable electronic devices (CIEDs) necessitates novel methods of surveillance with a view toward optimizing long-term device follow-up. With increasing awareness of indications for pacemakers (PMs), and especially implantable cardioverter-defibrillators (ICDs) and cardiac resynchronization devices (CRTs), the number of patients with implantable devices has been growing steadily. According to the recent American College of Cardiology/American Heart Association/European Society of Cardiology (ACC/AHA/ESC) guidelines,[1] patients with a PM should be followed up every 3 to 12 months, and those with an ICD every 3 to 6 months (with more frequent follow-ups as the battery approaches elective replacement). This implies frequent visits for the patient and for the outpatient clinic—a significant increase in workload. In addition, the magnitude of recent PM and ICD advisories demands a further increase in follow-up visits that raises the need for accurate monitoring of the integrity of implantable devices.[2] Recent advances and innovations in telecommunications may offer an alternative to the current practice of device interrogation and alleviate the burden of pacemaker–defibrillator and CRT clinics and provide considerable convenience for patients.

Transtelephonic monitoring (TTM) was introduced in 1971 and, until recently, remained the main technology for remotely following the performance of PMs. It is aimed mostly at ascertaining the integrity of the system, especially with regard to battery performance and longevity, appropriate capture, and sensing. However, TTM entails active patient participation and raises compliance issues. In contrast to PM devices, remote monitoring (RM) of ICDs was not developed until the early 1990s. With the adoption of a specific signal transmission band and further advancement of ICD technology, sophisticated monitoring systems have been designed to accommodate the complexity of the new devices.[2] The current systems utilize a wanded or wireless transmitter to transmit signals via a wireless or digital phone line from the device to a central computer system; this transmission system renders the device information available on the Internet for analysis. The scope of this chapter is to provide the state of technology of the current RM systems and to discuss the results of the major clinical studies and registries pertaining to RM of CIEDs.

Remote Monitoring Systems

The current CIEDs being interrogated remotely include PMs, ICDs, CRTs, implantable loop recorders (ILRs), and implantable hemodynamic monitors (IHMs).[3] The advent of remote wireless communication from the CIED to a home monitor/communicator made it possible to transmit and store all data that the CIED is capable of collecting. As a result, manufacture-specific RM systems proliferated and became the new standard for remote follow-up. These systems include the Medtronic CareLink® Network (Medtronic, Minneapolis, MN); the Boston Scientific LATITUDE® Patient Management System (Boston Scientific, Natick, MA); the Biotronik Home Monitoring® (HM) system (Biotronik, Berlin, Germany); Sorin's SMARTVIEW™ Remote Monitoring (Sorin Group, Milan, Italy); and the St. Jude Merlin.net® Patient Care Network (St. Jude Medical, St. Paul, MN). The circumstances in which remote follow-up and monitoring occurs and the protocols for obtaining the information and disseminating it to the caregivers vary by manufacturer and the capabilities of each RM system.

Home transmitters that are able to interrogate the device are available from most major device companies. They work either manually, by the patient using a telemetry wand, or automatically, using wireless technology. The data downloaded from the device by the transmitter is then sent to the physician using an analog landline phone, a digital subscriber line, a device accessory phone line, or the GSM (global system for mobile communications) network. Many current PMs and ICDs are able to automatically execute the tests that are performed manually at the outpatient clinic, such as battery status, lead impedances, or sensing and capture thresholds. Data acquired automatically on a predefined periodic basis by the device can then be sent from the patient's home to the physician using the transmitter (thus avoiding an unnecessary clinic visit), hence the term "remote follow-up."[4] The physician can receive a company alert notification via pager, fax, SMS (short message service), voice message, or e-mail. Many systems require access to a dedicated (device- or company-specific) website to obtain detailed information on the interrogation. The physician can activate, either manually or automatically, message calls to patients for a variety of purposes: to remind them of upcoming remote follow-up appointments, to notify them if they miss a remote follow-up appointment, to ask them to call the clinic, to inform them that their remote transmissions have been reviewed by the clinic, and so on.

RM data can be acquired automatically on a daily basis by the device, and unscheduled transmission of predefined alerts can be sent to the physician. These alerts may involve device integrity (eg, battery status, lead impedance); programming issues (eg, disabling of ventricular fibrillation therapy, insufficient safety margins for sensing or capture); or medical data (eg, arrhythmias, indication of accumulating lung fluid). Therefore, RM has the potential to offer improved patient safety and quality of care. Comprehensive reviews of RM are available in the literature.[2-7] Recently, an expert consensus document on RM of CIEDs was published by the International Society for Holter and Noninvasive Electrocardiology (ISHNE/EHRA).[8]

Biotronik Home Monitoring System

Biotronik's HM system transmits data on a daily basis, at fixed time intervals, and immediately upon the occurrence of a clinically relevant event.[4] With the introduction of its first system in 2001, Biotronik pioneered the technology of RM, with applications in more than 50 countries. Event triggers and monitoring parameters are individually programmable online. Depending on the type of implantable device, the monitoring covers device functions and several clinical elements, including atrial fibrillation (AF), heart failure (HF), sense and pace measurements, high-definition intracardiac electrogram (IEGM), and therapies delivered. For standard monthly, quarterly, or biannual remote follow-ups, the clinician can also access the accumulated transmission files posted on a secure Internet site. This enables an expeditious offsite review of trend reports and other stored data instead of scheduling a follow-up in the outpatient clinic.

Biotronik HM technology utilizes a triple-band and a quad-band exterior wireless transmitter, the CardioMessenger®. This transmitter is connected to a cellular telephone network that provides automatic, patient-independent wireless transmission of diagnostic CIED data. The transmission utilizes encrypted technology to transfer data to a dedicated service center located in Berlin, Germany, that may alert the physician via electronic mail, facsimile, or pager. The automatic transmission of all data is an important issue today because the patient may not have a landline phone connection (owing to the increased use of cell phones); instead, they may have a digital landline connection (currently incompatible with all device systems) or a DSL/VoIP (digital subscriber line/voice over Internet protocol) connection that requires special filters and converters. Automatic transmission also means that the patient can be monitored continuously, around the clock, as the CardioMessenger has a rechargeable battery that allows it to be carried around by the patient. The novel quad-band transmitter supports all four major frequency bands in GSM and is compatible with all major GSM cellular networks worldwide, allowing freedom of travel. Parameters for the alerts can be fully configured on the secured Web page without having to bring the patient into the clinic for a manual transmission. IEGMs of 30-second duration are sent periodically that may assist with data interpretation. A callback light on the CardioMessenger can advise the patient to immediately contact the physician.

The HM system provides exceptionally fast transmission speed: less than 30 seconds for the Lumax® family of ICDs and CRT-defibrillators (CRT-Ds) (Biotronik). It also automates the transmission for all currently available devices without needing the involvement of the patient, provided that the patient is within approximately 6 feet (1.8 meters) of the portable transceiver unit. The newest family of CIED devices is capable of transmitting the equivalent of a complete in-office interrogation, including IEGMs. The wireless HM system is not susceptible to electromagnetic interference.

Currently, more than 55,000 patients worldwide are using Biotronik HM, and data on more than 24,000 Biotronik devices that use HM have been published in peer-reviewed journals. This comprises the overwhelming majority of existing data for CIED RM systems.

Medtronic CareLink Network

The Medtronic CareLink Network is a large and widely used remote follow-up and monitoring system for CIED patients. Operational in the United States since 2002 and introduced in Europe starting in 2005, more than 600,000 patients have subscribed to the service worldwide and more than 61,000 patients are registered in Europe.

The CareLink Network is designed to remotely interrogate and transmit the entire set of CIED parameters, equivalent to an in-office device interrogation. The system enables physicians or other authorized medical reviewers to remotely check the implanted device's performance. It also enables early management of cardiac status or safety issues, based on continuous monitoring of device and diagnostic variables in the CIED, and generates automatic data transmission and physician notification if any monitored parameter exceeds the predefined range.

CareLink supports and integrates onto one platform almost all existing Medtronic device models, ranging from PMs, ICDs, and CRT-Ds to insertable cardiac monitor (ICM) devices. In this way, the network makes RM available both to new patients and to those already being treated with device therapy or diagnostics. All supported CIED models can be manually interrogated by the patient and thus allow for remote device follow-up. However, ICDs, CRT-Ds, and CRT-pacemakers (CRT-Ps) with wireless telemetry provide full automatic device interrogation without patient intervention and offer event-driven RM functionality.

The CareLink Network comprises three components with which patients and clinicians interact: the Patient Monitor, the secure Data Server, and the Clinician Website. The CareLink Patient Monitor is a small, easy-to-use stationary device. It incorporates a telemetry wand that enables manual device interrogations by the patient. Monitor models for CIEDs equipped with an antenna feature automatic wireless interrogation that uses Medtronic Connexus® Wireless Telemetry. This SmartRadio™ Technology selects one of 10 channels within the Medical Implant Communication Service (MICS) frequency band (402–405 MHz). The physician can remotely initiate prescheduled automatic transmissions for remote follow-up via the CareLink website, with a minimum time interval of 21 days. Nevertheless, manual device interrogation by the patient after consultation with the follow-up clinic is feasible at any time, without limitations.

Wireless monitors are permanently connected to a power outlet and a standard analog landline, preferably (but not necessarily) at the patient's bedside to ensure highly reliable telemetry operation within the recommended distance of 3 meters (<10 feet). The monitor automatically sends the device information to the secure CareLink Data Server using a toll-free number. While a standard monitor is intended for use in the patient's country of residence, for patients who frequently travel internationally or permanently live outside their country of residence, an international monitor solution can be ordered. Moreover, for these or other patients who do not have access to a landline telephone, the M-Link™ accessory (a GPRS [general packet radio service] mobile device connectable to the CareLink Monitor) is offered as a simplified way to connect to the CareLink Network.

The patient's device data are stored long term on the secure European CareLink Data Server (United Kingdom) and can be viewed and analyzed by the medical reviewer on the password-protected clinician website. Data include entire device and diagnostic parameters, all stored electrograms (EGMs), and a 10-second real-time EGM equivalent to an in-office EGM printout. Recently manufactured Medtronic CIEDs also include the complete set of automatically performed electrode threshold tests, thus providing full device automaticity that facilitates full remote follow-up. All device and patient data can be exported as reports, either by printing them out or saving them in PDF format for further electronic data processing. Using the additional Medtronic Mainspring™ Report Export application, CareLink reports are easily and automatically moved to the clinic network to give an electronic health record or other clinic system access to imported data based on a unique file name.

The CareLink website is designed to easily navigate and tackle new patient enrollments, view and triage actual transmissions, and manage patients' follow-up schedules. The local CareLink Network structure and website can be individually customized by the administrative user to fit the clinic's needs. This includes an array of capabilities: adding users with assigned permissions within the website; customizing website content; customizing reports; configuring preferences for receiving wireless CareAlert® notifications; and setting up local CareLink Network satellite structures to share and manage CareLink device and diagnostics in collaboration with associated medical caregivers, thereby optimizing therapy management.

The RM of Medtronic CIEDs (ICDs, CRT-Ds, and CRT-Ps) is event-driven. Instead of daily monitoring, battery longevity that affects the system's transmissions is based on continuous monitoring of the device and diagnostic variables by the CIED. Thus, it immediately triggers automatic data transmission and notifies the physician only in case of a relevant event, that is, if any of the monitored parameters exceeds the predefined ranges. Thresholds for these CareAlerts can be programmed individually for each patient in the CIED for a wide range of variables that relate to system integrity and diagnostics. These include unique monitoring features of Medtronic CIEDs, such as the Lead Integrity Alert algorithm, which early detects lead failures, as well as the OptiVol® algorithm, which detects early signs of intrathoracic fluid accumulation as a proxy for worsening of HF.

The level of urgency (red and yellow alert), including the CareAlert notification type (e-mail, SMS) and notification time, can be predefined for each CareAlert setting on the CareLink website. This helps with CareAlert case management. If the CIED is unable to establish transmission operation in the first attempt, it silently repeats communication with the monitor every 3 hours for 3 days (audible alerts to the patient are the final backup system) to ensure highly reliable alert notification. CareLink combines early detection and notification of events that need medical attention with information on the entire device, including unique Medtronic Cardiac Compass® trend data (eg, variables such as heart rate, patient's daily activity, OptiVol intrathoracic detection of fluid accumulation, occurrence of arrhythmias). These data allow physicians to manage symptoms early, with the potential to improve therapy outcomes.

St. Jude Medical Merlin.net System

The Merlin Patient Care System (PCS) serves as an Internet-based repository of patients' device data. The system provides the option of transmitting wireless data between a supported device and the Merlin PCS transmitter. In addition, it enables transmission of real-time EGMs, stored EGMs, and details of delivered therapies. The Merlin PCS transmitter system sends the data to an Internet-based central computer system (Merlin.net) via a digital transtelephonic route. Remote interrogation of the patient's device may occur through either manual activation or, for the latest generation of CRT-D and ICD devices, wireless communications technology. The Merlin PCS also offers human interaction with an operator via an arrhythmia monitoring service and allows clinicians to select their alert preferences. The Merlin.net Patient Care Network allows key device data to be merged with existing patient data. This provides a single point of access for accurate, relevant patient information that may enable physicians to spot trends earlier and make decisions faster, allowing them to efficiently allocate clinic resources and improve their response to changing patient needs.

The Merlin@home® Transmitter monitors the device daily and, in case an alert has been detected, initiates a full interrogation of the device to send to Merlin.net. In addition, the physician can schedule a follow-up interrogation on Merlin.net to obtain a regular overview of the device. The physician also can upload all information from the Merlin PCS programmer to make all data available online at any time. The wireless transmitter (Merlin@home) was introduced in Europe in 2008. U.S. Food and Drug Administration (FDA) and European Conformity (CE) mark approvals were obtained in 2008 and 2009, respectively. More than 200,000 patients have been enrolled in Merlin.net worldwide, and approximately 10,000 patients enrolled in Europe.

The Merlin@home Transmitter system communicates automatically by radiofrequency with the implantable device and sends data to the physician via a landline or mobile network. Future versions of Merlin@home will also be able to send data via Wi-Fi. As with the other available systems, Merlin@home makes RM possible by sending alerts via e-mail, fax, or SMS to notify the physician of events. The Mobile DirectAlerts™ Notification feature enables physicians to access alert-initiated follow-ups directly on their smartphones. The DirectCall™ feature allows the physician to indicate alerts or reminders of scheduled in-office visits on the patient's transmitter, and to send automated phone calls to patients indicating the results of the remote follow-up (eg, that everything is normal). Wireless functionality allows clinics to benefit from efficiencies gained through wireless implants, follow-ups, and daily RM. Physicians can select which critical changes in a patient's device or disease status require immediate attention using Merlin.net PCN's DirectAlerts notifications. The DirectTrend™ viewer gathers daily device information into an interactive report, which provides enhanced visualization of disease trends and progression, thereby improving clinical insight and streamlining patient management. Device-specific alert and notification options for enhancing patient safety and ensuring therapy delivery include the following: high-voltage therapy delivered, atrial tachycardia/atrial fibrillation (AT/AF) duration, lead impedance out of range, and device at elective replacement indicator (ERI). The method of communication delivery (fax, phone, e-mail, or SMS text) and the time of notification (during or after office hours) can be chosen to best meet physician and clinic protocols.

Boston Latitude Patient Management System

The Boston Scientific Latitude Patient Management System provides remote surveillance of most models of Boston Scientific cardiac implantable devices. The latest CRT-D devices are capable of transmitting a wireless signal to the Latitude communicator at preset intervals determined by a physician. The Latitude Patient Management System transmits data to the central computer via a standard phone line. This system provides comprehensive diagnostics and IEGMs. A unique feature of this system is the possibility of connecting wireless weight scales and blood pressure cuffs to remotely monitor HF status. These data may become useful for remote HF management. The Latitude Patient Management System can also provide customized, color-coded (upon red and yellow alerts) alert notifications, according to urgency level. The interactive screen of the portable transmitter allows patients to enter information about their condition through a series of questions that appear on the transmitter screen that are also asked by the portable unit. The questions address the patient's breathing, alteration in weight, and paroxysmal nocturnal symptoms and are particularly useful in the management of patients with HF. Furthermore, the system allows customizable data to be transmitted to different physicians (eg, the general practitioner or general cardiologist in addition to the heart rhythm specialist), thereby improving the networking of HF management.

Review of Major Studies on Remote Monitoring

RM has many potential benefits for patients and their caregivers, follow-up centers, the healthcare infrastructure, and device manufacturers. Several major landmark studies have provided strong evidence for RM, in addition to a large-scale CIED registry (ALTITUDE[15]). These studies include the Remote Follow-up for ICD-Therapy in Patients Meeting MADIT II Criteria (REFORM) trial; the One Day Pacemaker Implantation Program with Home-monitoring (OEDIPE) trial; the Prospective Randomized Evaluation of a New Fabric Attenuation Device in Endovascular Interventional Radiology (PREFER) study; the Lumos-T Safely Reduces Routine Office Device Follow-up (TRUST) trial; the Clinical Evaluation of Remote Notification to Reduce Time to Clinical Decision (CONNECT) trial; and the randomized trial of long-term remote monitoring of PM recipients (COMPAS trial).[9-14]

In the very early days of RM, concern was expressed (as with most new technologies) that patients and caregivers would not be satisfied with RM because they would lose the advantage of a face-to-face visit. This was despite the fact that scheduled, routine follow-up visits have very low actionability rates in practice. Today, multiple studies have shown that patients and caregivers are satisfied with RM in terms of both ease of use and acceptability.[16,17] Researchers observed a high level of acceptance and satisfaction after one year of using remote control with Biotronik HM.[16] Clinicians were pleased with the performance of the network and the quality of the Web-accessed data, finding it comparable with in-office device interrogation.[17]

Reduction of In-office Visits and Workload

The clinical goals of remote follow-up were to obviate the need for device patients to come to the office, facilitate the follow-up of patients who live in remote areas, and improve the efficiency of device follow-up clinics. Patients require fewer overall visits to the follow-up clinic when RM is employed.

In a retrospective study by Brugada,[18] 271 patients with the Biotronik HM system were followed up for 12 months, with routine follow-up occurring every 3 months. Analysis of these data showed that as many as half of the regular scheduled visits may have been skipped, without impairing patient safety. More recently, Heidbuchel et al[19] retrospectively analyzed data from 1,739 in-clinic ICD visits in 169 patients. The authors found that only 6% of scheduled in-clinic visits resulted in device reprogramming or patient hospitalization. Thus, in 94% of all scheduled visits, remote follow-up would have sufficed. Furthermore, they estimated that ICD RM could potentially diagnose more than 99% of arrhythmia- or device-related problems if combined with clinical follow-up by the local general practitioner and/or referring cardiologist.[19]

Lazarus and colleagues[20] observed for RM a variety of benefits from the AWARE trial ("remote, wireless, ambulatory monitoring of implantable pacemakers, cardioverter defibrillators, and cardiac resynchronization therapy systems: a worldwide database"). They evaluated 3,004,763 transmissions made by 11,624 recipients of PMs (n = 4,631), defibrillators (ICDs; n = 6,548), and CRT-D systems (n = 445) worldwide. The vast majority (86%) of events were disease-related. They concluded that applying a monitoring system strongly supports the care of cardiac device recipients, enhances their safety, and optimizes the allocation of health resources.

The REFORM trial, initiated in 2004, was completed in 2008. In this analysis of a 12-month follow-up with Biotronik HM, Elsner et al[9] calculated a €71,200 savings per 100 patient-years, and 81 fewer physician hours (plus a few extra visits for alerts initiated by HM or patients) compared with a standard 3-month follow-up schedule. After subtracting a 3.9% increase in visits attributable to HM and a 7.9% increase due to patient-initiated visits, the number of visits in the HM group had been reduced by 63.2%. No significant difference was observed in rates of hospitalization and mortality between the 2 treatment assignments.[9]

In the study by Raatikainen et al,[21] physicians' and nurses' time required for an office visit was compared with a follow-up by RM. The physician time required to review the RM data (8.4 ± 4.5 min; range: 2–30 min) was significantly shorter than the time needed to complete a device follow-up visit in the clinic (25.8 ± 17.0 min; range: 5–90 min); P < 0.001. Likewise, allied professionals spent more time on an in-clinic visit compared with an RM follow-up assessment (45.3 ± 30.6 vs 9.3 ± 15.9 min; P < 0.001). Two very large trials, CONNECT[13] and TRUST,[12] demonstrated a significant reduction in the total number of in-office visits: 3.92 for RM and 6.27 in office in CONNECT; and 2.1 for RM and 3.8 in office in TRUST.

The OEDIPE trial[10] examined the safety and efficacy of an abbreviated hospitalization after implantation or replacement of a dual-chamber PM, using a telecardiology-based ambulatory surveillance program. Patients (N = 379) were randomly assigned to an active group, discharged from the hospital 24 hours after a first PM implant or 4 to 6 hours after replacement, and followed up for 4 weeks with Biotronik HM; a control group was followed up for 4 weeks according to usual medical practices. At least one treatment-related major adverse event was observed in 9.2% of patients (n = 17) assigned to the active group versus 13.3% of patients (n = 26) in the control group (P = 0.21): a 4.1% absolute risk reduction (95% CI; 22.2–10.4; P = 0.98). By study design, the mean hospitalization duration in the active group was 34% shorter than in the control group (P < 0.001), and HM facilitated the early detection of technical issues and detectable clinical anomalies. Early discharge with HM after PM implantation or replacement was found to be safe and facilitated the monitoring of patients in the month following the procedure.[10]

The first data to support the usefulness of remote follow-up were obtained in PM patients.[4] The PREFER study[11] was a prospective, randomized, parallel, unblinded, multicenter trial that compared the identification of "clinically actionable events" with inductive remote patient transmission at 3, 6, and 9 months following single- or dual-chamber PM implantation; standard 6-month in-office visits were interspersed with TTM every 2 months. An inductive transmission requires that the patient apply a wand over their device during data transfer; patients are provided with a modem that can upload the data to a central Web server for physician review. In the control group, patients with a dual-chamber PM were seen in the office at 6 months; all patients in the study were seen in the office at 12 months.

There were 866 clinical events reported in 382 patients in the study. Clinically actionable events were detected on average 2 months earlier in the RM arm. The number of events reported per patient was 0.517 in the remote arm and 0.308 in the TTM. Of note, only 3 (2%) of the 190 clinically actionable events in the TTM arm were detected during a TTM transmission; the majority of events were detected only during an in-office evaluation. In contrast, 446 (66%) of the 676 clinically actionable events in the RM arm were detected during a remote transmission. However, the most frequently detected clinically actionable event was an episode of nonsustained VT followed by AT episodes lasting 48 hours or longer.[11]

The next advance in RM came with the release of wireless devices, which do not require the patient to apply a wand over the device to initiate or maintain the data transfer. These devices automatically transmit data to a bedside communicator, which forwards the data to a central server. Transmitted data include the following: (1) programmable alerts related to device and lead function, as well as atrial and ventricular arrhythmias that are transmitted on a daily or weekly basis; (2) a real-time IEGM that is transmitted on a monthly or quarterly basis; and (3) a complete device data download that can either be initiated by a patient in response to symptoms (including an ICD discharge) or is scheduled to occur on a quarterly basis.

The clinical value of RM using wireless ICDs was evaluated recently in a randomized control trial.[12] The TRUST trial was a prospective (noninferiority) trial that compared the safety and efficacy of the Biotronik HM system with quarterly in-office evaluations in a cohort of 1,450 non–PM-dependent patients following single- or dual-chamber ICD implantation. Patients in the HM arm were seen in the office 3 months after enrollment and then a year later. In the interim, physicians were notified for the following "alert" conditions: out-of-range impedance, ERI, ventricular tachycardia/ventricular fibrillation (VT/VF) detection turned off, episodes of AF, other supraventricular tachycardia or VT/VF, delivery of an ineffective 30-J ICD shock, mode-switch duration >10% over 24 hours, and device transmission failure for more than 3 days. The primary end point of the study was the number of total in-office device evaluations in the 2 groups.

The mean number of scheduled and unscheduled visits was reduced by 45% in the remote HM arm; there was no difference in the likelihood of observing an adverse event. Additionally, HM reduced the median time from the onset of an arrhythmic event (AF, VT, or VF) to physician evaluation to 1 day as compared with 35.5 days in the conventional arm. Eighty-nine percent of the alert notifications could be managed remotely. The remaining 11% alert notifications necessitated an in-office visit; 52% of these visits resulted in a clinical intervention (device reprogramming, drug initiation, or adjustment in drug dosing). Important to note, RM increased patient compliance with their scheduled in-office visits.

The CONNECT study[13] was a multicenter, prospective, randomized evaluation involving 1,997 patients from 136 clinical sites who underwent insertion of an ICD (including CRT devices) and were followed up for 15 months. Healthcare utilization data included all cardiovascular-related hospitalizations, emergency department visits, and clinic office visits. The primary objective was to determine whether wireless RM with automatic clinician alerts, compared with patients receiving standard in-office care, reduces the time from a clinical event to a clinical decision in response to arrhythmias, cardiovascular disease progression, and device issues. A secondary objective was to compare the rates of cardiovascular healthcare utilization for patients in the remote and in-office arms.

Researchers found that the median time from clinical event to clinical decision per patient was reduced from 22 days for the in-office arm to 4.6 days in the RM arm ($P < 0.001$). The healthcare utilization data revealed a decrease in mean length of stay per cardiovascular hospitalization visit: from 4.0 days for the in-office arm to 3.3 days in the RM arm ($P = 0.002$).

The COMPAS randomized, multicenter, noninferiority trial[14] examined the safety of long-term RM of PMs. Between December 2005 and January 2008, 538 patients were randomly assigned to RM follow-up (active group) or standard care (control group). The primary objective was to confirm that the proportion of patients who experienced at least one major adverse event (including all-cause deaths and hospitalizations for device-related or cardiovascular adverse events) was not more than 7% higher in the active than in the control group. The characteristics of the study groups were similar.

Major adverse event–free survival rates and quality of life were compared in both groups. Over a follow-up of 18.3 months, 17.3% of patients in the active and 19.1% in the control group experienced at least one major adverse event ($P < 0.01$ for noninferiority). Hospitalizations for atrial arrhythmias (6 vs 18, respectively) and strokes (2 vs 8) were fewer ($P < 0.05$), and the number of interim ambulatory visits was 56% lower ($P < 0.001$) in the active group than the control group. Changes in PM programming or drug regimens were made in 62% of visits in the active versus 29% in the control group ($P < 0.001$). Quality of life remained unchanged in both groups.

The large-scale ALTITUDE study[15] provided 1- and 5-year survival outcome data in more than 194,000 recipients of implanted devices from a single manufacturer (Boston Scientific). It demonstrated that survival for these patients was equivalent to patients studied in the pivotal randomized trials. The 1- and 5-year survival rates were 92% and 68% for ICDs, respectively, and 88% and 54%, respectively, for CRT-Ds. Patients transmitting data remotely had the best survival rate, while shock therapies were associated with worsened survival rates in both ICD- and CRT-D recipients. The 1- and 5-year risks of shock were 14% and 38% for ICD recipients, respectively, and 13% and 33% for CRT-D subjects.[15] However, the lack of clinical profile data and specific knowledge of comorbid conditions in this registry limits the ability to interpret its results and to assign clinical significance to this novel observation. Thus, future studies aimed at confirming this observation are recommended.

Benefits of Remote Monitoring

RM promises three distinct advantages.[5] The first is the detection of lead malfunction and device-related issues (eg, ERI device status, inadvertent device programming that results in ventricular arrhythmia detections being turned off, and an electrical reset condition within the device). The second is the detection of asymptomatic atrial and ventricular arrhythmias. Of these, substantial interest surrounds the clinical utility of detecting atrial high-rate episodes (AHREs), given the association of AF with congestive HF and stroke. The third promise of these devices is identifying patients with an impending exacerbation of congestive HF. Because the vast majority of ICD recipients have some degree of left ventricular systolic dysfunction, these patients are at risk for HF hospitalizations, which impose an economic burden on the healthcare system.

Remote Monitoring and Implantable System Integrity

System-related short- and long-term complications in device recipients are not uncommon. A majority of these complications are related to lead failure. The estimated annual failure rate of defibrillation leads may reach 35% in 10-year-old leads.[2] Lead failure may cause inappropriate ICD therapy (due to oversensing of noise) or failure of therapy (due to undersensing of ventricular arrhythmias).

Thus, early detection of these complications is desirable to ensure a patient's safety. Lead failure may manifest as alteration in lead impedance and other parameters, such as short sensing intervals. These critical changes can be detected with RM systems earlier than with routine follow-up visits.[2] Furthermore, remote follow-up may be particularly useful for early identifying of lead failure and other potentially lethal (and asymptomatic) system problems (eg, ERI, high-voltage circuitry failure). This response will permit prompt surgical intervention (eg, for lead failure) or conservative treatment (eg, to prevent potential inappropriate ICD therapies due to AF with rapid ventricular response).

A nonsustained ventricular arrhythmia notification may be triggered by system issues such as lead electrical noise artifacts caused by fracture or nonphysiological electrical signals. Therefore, identifying patients with a high burden of these system issues may facilitate intervention to preempt premature battery depletion. Notification for disabled VF detection is also important as more patients with different comorbidities undergo procedures in different clinic departments. In PMs, lead failures such as conductor wire breaks and insulation breaches may lead to ineffective pacing and oversensing or undersensing. In ICDs, lead failures can result in inappropriate shocks, ineffective shocks, or inappropriate withholding of therapy.[6]

Small retrospective studies have found that, in patients with ICD lead failure, inappropriate shocks were experienced in only 27% of those who received HM compared with 53% of patients who had traditional follow-up.[22,23] The investigators estimated that remote follow-up identified problems 54 days earlier than traditional follow-up. In the TRUST trial,[24] RM with Biotronik HM also significantly reduced the time to detection of device and lead malfunction. Because device and lead malfunction may not be associated with patient symptoms, it may not be otherwise amenable to early detection. In the TRUST study,[24] 62 device-related events (53 for HM vs 9 in conventional monitoring) were observed in 46 patients (40 [4.4%] in HM vs 6 [1.39%] in conventional group; $P = 0.004$), 47% of which were asymptomatic. HM detected generator and lead problems earlier (a median of 1 vs 5 days for HM vs conventional; $P = 0.05$). A total of 20 device problems (eg, lead fracture, ERIs) requiring surgical revision (0.012 per patient-year) were found: 15 in the HM group and 5 in the conventional group. Other events were managed nonsurgically (eg, by reprogramming, initiation of antiarrhythmics).

The TRUST study[24] demonstrated that HM may provide a stringent method of postimplant ICD evaluation in which system components are tested daily and out-of-range values reported rapidly. Similarly, the CareLink RM system is being used to provide long-term performance data on the Medtronic Sprint Fidelis ICD lead.[5] (In 2007, Medtronic voluntarily suspended distribution of these leads, owing to their potential for lead fracture.) Immediate notification about lead failure can be life-saving in case of a Fidelis lead fracture, which may result in incessant ICD shocks.[2] Remote surveillance of device lead function can more accurately assess the risk of malfunction than traditional methods, such as analysis of returned products.

In a recent study,[25] 2,834 patients with the Sprint Fidelis advisory lead were followed using Boston Scientific LATITUDE Patient Management System for a mean duration of 17.2 months. Only 15 (0.53%) patients demonstrated increased right ventricular pacing impedance, and only one ICD therapy was adjudicated as inappropriate during this follow-up period. These results suggest that, while the risk of this lead failure is real, its incidence remains relatively low.

Remote Monitoring of Patients with Atrial Fibrillation

ICDs continually monitor heart rhythm and rate and store information on the frequency and duration of arrhythmias that can affect patient management. AHRE is the most common arrhythmia recorded by wireless devices.[5] It has previously been shown that an AHRE lasting ≥5 minutes doubles the risk of stroke or death in patients with sinus node dysfunction who undergo dual-chamber PM implantation.[26] However, certain considerations are not fully understood. The first is the precise relationship between the burden of AHRE and the risk of stroke. The TRENDS study[27] evaluated the risk of thromboembolism (ischemic stroke, transient ischemic attack, systemic embolism) in a cohort of PM, ICD, and CRT-D patients with a $CHADS_2$ score (Congestive heart failure, Hypertension, Age, Diabetes, prior Stroke) ≥1. Patients with at least one AHRE lasting more than 5.5 hours in a 30-day period had double the thromboembolic risk of patients with no AHRE and those in whom episodes lasted <5.5 hours.

The second consideration is whether detecting AHRE can aid in the management of patients. Initial studies demonstrated the efficacy of RM for the identification and management of atrial arrhythmias.[28,29] Since these devices are also capable of RM and physician notification based on prescribed criteria, they can serve as early-warning systems should an arrhythmic event be detected. In the TRUST study,[12] the time to physician evaluation for a detected AF event was reduced dramatically—from 40 to 6 days. Whether this improvement results in a favorable clinical outcome was not tested. This technology, however, could be exploited to trigger targeted anticoagulation (or antiarrhythmic therapy) if and when AF is detected in an early phase (eg, at 12 to 48 hours after onset), or even anticoagulation withdrawal when AF has subsided.

The ongoing IMPACT study (Combined Use of Biotronik HM and Predefined Anti-coagulation to Reduce Stroke Risk)[30] is seeking to clarify this issue. The IMPACT study[30] was designed to test the hypothesis that, compared with conventional clinical management, initiating and withdrawing oral anticoagulant therapy (guided by continuous ambulatory monitoring of the atrial EGM) improves clinical outcomes by reducing the combined rates of stroke, systemic embolism, and major bleeding. The study will enroll 2,718 patients with a $CHADS_2$ score ≥1 who undergo ICD or CRT-D implantation. Patients are randomized to receive remote HM or conventional in-office follow-up. In this study, the decision to initiate as well as discontinue anticoagulation is based on both the duration of an AHRE and the patient's underlying $CHADS_2$ score. The hypothesis of the study is that HM-facilitated detection of an AHRE will result in the earlier initiation of systemic anticoagulation, which will translate into a reduced risk of thromboembolism.[30] The results are increasingly important, given the recent release of a new anticoagulant with rapid offset and offset of action.

Remote Monitoring of Patients with Heart Failure

The rapidly expanding role of CIEDs in HF patients presents an opportunity to broaden the paradigm of outpatient HF monitoring. The concept of device-based monitoring and intervention represents a major opportunity for improving outcomes in chronic HF disease management. Most hospitalizations for worsening HF relate to volume overload and congestion. A large clinical trial recently demonstrated the feasibility of monitoring weight daily (with the physician alerted to a weight gain or loss of 2 pounds over 2 days or 5 pounds over a week).[31] However, indirect measures of volume overload, such as weight and symptoms, are usually insensitive and unreliable predictors of decompensated HF.

Several methods are available for diagnosing patients at high risk for HF. Commercially available methods include assessing weight as well as measuring intrathoracic impedance. Fluid accumulation in the lungs can be estimated by measuring thoracic impedance, between a lead placed within the right ventricle and a device that can be positioned in the pectoral area. Among patients hospitalized for acute decompensated HF, a strong inverse correlation has been recognized between intrathoracic impedance and pulmonary capillary wedge pressure as well as between impedance and net fluid loss.[32]

OptiVol Fluid Status Monitoring (Medtronic) uses a proprietary system that compares daily impedance measurements with a baseline reference value. The reference value is a slow-moving average of preceding impedance values. The difference in impedance between the daily measurement and the reference value is summed to generate an OptiVol fluid index whose increase corresponds to a cumulative decrease in impedance measurements, reflecting a gradual increase in pulmonary fluid content. In a small study, 33 patients were given an implantable system for measuring intrathoracic impedance to identify potential fluid overload before HF hospitalization. The authors reported that intrathoracic impedance began decreasing approximately 2 weeks before hospitalization for decompensated HF.[32]

The development of IHM technology evolved from the belief that early detection and treatment of rising intracardiac pressures could prevent decompensation and associated hospitalization. Leads and devices that use a special transducer located in the RVOT to estimate pulmonary artery pressure have been developed. In the COMPASS-HF (Chronicle Offers Management to Patients with Advanced Signs and Symptoms of Heart Failure) trial,[33] 274 patients with New York Heart Association (NYHA) class III or IV HF had a specialized device (Medtronic's Chronicle Implantable Hemodynamic Monitor) implanted. This device utilizes a lead with a pressure sensor on its tip to calculate pulmonary artery pressure. Patients were randomized to 2 groups: one in which information was available to clinicians, and the other in which the clinicians were blinded to the information.

After 6 months, a 21% decrease in the primary end point (HF-related events, including hospitalizations, emergency room visits, or unplanned clinic visits) was found, but did not meet statistical significance. Post hoc analysis suggested that active management of abnormal hemodynamic parameters was associated with a 36% decrease in the relative risk of HF-related hospitalizations. Failure to meet the primary efficacy end point may have been related to a lower-than-expected event rate in the control cohort. This finding suggests that future studies, potentially with increased statistical power, will be necessary to more clearly define the utility of IHM in this patient population.

Continuous monitoring of left atrial pressure (LAP) may provide a more robust target for implantable sensor-based strategies. The HeartPOD™ device (St. Jude Medical) is a permanently implantable LAP sensor inserted during transseptal cardiac catheterization. In an early-stage safety and efficacy observational study,[34] 40 patients with NHYA class III or IV HF were implanted with the LAP sensor and followed for a median of 25 months. LAP-guided therapy improved several important efficacy end points, including reductions in mean daily LAP, improvements in functional capacity, and higher doses of neurohormonal antagonists with reductions in daily diuretic requirements. Further studies will be necessary to validate the impact of LAP sensors on clinical outcomes.

Another emerging technology for IHM sensors is direct pulmonary pressure measurement via the CardioMEMS implantable pulmonary artery pressure transducer (CardioMEMS, Atlanta, GA). The hypothesis of the pivotal CHAMPION (CardioMEMS Heart Sensor Allows Monitoring of Pressure to Improve Outcomes in NYHA Class III HF Patients) trial[35] was that management of HF by use of pulmonary artery pressures would greatly reduce the rate of HF-related hospitalization. Patients with NYHA class III HF were randomly assigned to the use of a wireless IHM system (treatment group) or to a control group. In 6 months, 83 HF-related hospitalizations were reported in the treatment group ($n = 270$) compared with 120 in the control group ($n = 280$; rate: 0.31 vs 0.44; hazard ratio [HR] 0.70; $P < 0.0001$). During the entire follow-up (mean: 15 months), the treatment group had a 39% reduction in HF-related hospitalization compared with the control group (153 vs 253; HR 0.64; $P < 0.0001$). These results are consistent with, and extend, previous findings by definitively showing a significant and large reduction in hospitalizations for patients with NYHA class III HF who were managed with a wireless IHM system.[8]

The Remote Active Monitoring in Patients with Heart Failure (RAPID-RF) study[36] is a multicenter registry that will enroll up to 1,000 patients on the LATITUDE Patient Management System from approximately 100 centers. The study's primary objective is to examine physician responses to LATITUDE Active Monitoring data alerts by assessing alert-related medical interventions. After implant, the minimum follow-up time will be 3 months, with a maximum follow-up of 24 months. The LATITUDE Patient Management System is the first HF management tool to use wireless telemetry in a CRT-D device. The device is linked to remotely collect blood pressure and weight measures, permitting a single transmission for reporting device data. This system has several advantages, including ease of data transmission and the ability to correlate among measures of HF status, arrhythmic events, and device performance. The RAPID-RF study will provide important preliminary data on how remotely collected HF and arrhythmic surveillance data alter the management of HF patients with CRT-D devices.[36]

Device Advisory

Recent incidents pertaining to CIED reliability have shown remote surveillance from a new perspective.[1] For example, gaining immediate access to patient and device information may become critical when a safety alert is issued. Also, automatic remote surveillance of devices on advisory lists can help detect device and lead failure as early as possible. Early detection would eliminate the need to proceed with large numbers of unnecessary, premature replacements and provide patients with the highest level of reassurance.[2]

Patient Quality of Life and Acceptance

The first studies evaluating patient satisfaction by remote follow-up of ICDs were published in 2004 using the

Medtronic CareLink system[17] and the St. Jude Medical HouseCall II™.[37] Patient satisfaction with the systems was high in both studies. In an Italian study,[38] 67 patients implanted with a Medtronic CRT-D were followed remotely using the CareLink system. Remote follow-ups were preferred to in-clinic visits by 78% of the patients. Physician satisfaction was also very favorable. Likewise, in another study using the CareLink system, conducted in Finland,[21] patients' and physicians' levels of satisfaction with the RM system were high.

The aim of a recently published study was to evaluate patient acceptance and satisfaction of RM through a self-made questionnaire after 1 year of follow-up using the Biotronik HM remote control technology. Patients with an implanted device who were chronically followed up using the HM remote control system showed a high level of acceptance and satisfaction with this new technology. All investigated areas of the questionnaire had more than 90% positive responses. After 1-year follow-up, of 119 patients, only 3 refused to continue to be followed by HM. The questionnaire showed a good internal consistency.[16]

These studies demonstrate that RM is strongly supporting patients' peace of mind, psychological well-being, and safety, specifically following an advisory. Therefore, RM is seen as an important alternative to the current standard of care.

Legal Considerations

The rapid evolution and growing use of RM will likely present new legal challenges. Telemedicine and RM raise multiple legal complexities, including the following:

- Defining responsibilities (eg, what is an acceptable amount of time for notifying a patient after identifying a possible problem)
- Potential liability to health professionals (eg, whether healthcare providers are medically liable if information provided by the device is not documented)
- Maintaining patient confidentiality
- Licensing issues for physicians who are monitoring patients in states in which they are not licensed to practice[6]

At present, no guidelines or standards of practice exist for the timeliness of accessing information stored in such devices. Perhaps patient involvement in the alert process will help mitigate potential legal issues related to notification of device-generated alerts for possible problems.

Patient confidentiality is an important issue that will become more critical during the next decade. Currently, manufacturers maintain remote follow-up data repositories, and information regarding specific patients can be accessed by designated providers through a password system. Database vulnerability remains problematic and will become increasingly critical as database size increases and providers rely more heavily on database information.[6]

Legal aspects of the RM process include physician reliability, clinical practice standards, medical purposes, data protection, data ownership, and data access.[3] Sensitive data comprise data revealing or relating to racial or ethnic origin, political opinions, religious or philosophical beliefs, trade union membership, and health status or sex life. A typical example is health information about a patient processed via an RM network. Medical ethics holds that the physician has a duty to at least inform the patient of the best available treatment options. This duty supersedes other duties to society, self, practice, and insurer. In general, the physician should follow the rule: "Doing for the patient what you would do for yourself is ethical." Courts have ruled, "Should customary medical practice fail to keep pace with developments and advances in medical science, adherence to custom might constitute a failure to exercise ordinary practice." The trend in case law from a variety of jurisdictions holds as follows:

Where new technology is fairly readily available, and would have been helpful in a particular instance, plaintiff's lawyers will argue that the new technology has become the relevant standard of care. If a certain device is available and an adverse event occurs that might have been avoided through use of the technology, it is very likely that a plaintiff's attorney will attempt to establish the use of the device as the appropriate standard of care through expert testimony.[39]

Concerns over delayed review of remote data have been raised. The following aspects should be considered: (1) the concept of unreasonable burden over weekends and nights, (2) on-call issues for non-electrophysiologists/implanters, and (3) professional society guidelines, which would be very helpful. No court is *likely* to expect more than daily monitoring (weekends are a more difficult question). Instead, it is more likely that greater liability will result from not using the technology than from using it imperfectly—especially if patients are made aware of how data will be handled (and that discussion is documented).

Physician reliability includes the following aspects: (1) utilizing RM and alerts for the benefit of patients; (2) instructing patients not to send "unscheduled" transmissions without first calling; (3) signing an agreement that the RM system is *not* an emergency system; (4) checking the RM website at least once daily; and (5) having nurses on call 24-7 to deal with device issues. Patients need to be informed of the purpose and limitations of RM—for example, that it does not replace an emergency service or deal with alert events outside office hours. Before initiating RM and follow-up, the patient may be requested to sign a written informed consent form stating these points, authorizing transmission of personal data to third parties, respecting privacy, and subjecting the confidentiality of patient data collected by device companies to strict rules, as described in contracts.[39]

The transmission, storage, sharing, and interpretation of CIED diagnostics should be closely scrutinized to ensure that patients' and healthcare providers' rights are maximally protected.[8] In the United States, the Health Insurance Portability and Accountability Act of 1996 (HIPAA), the Health Information Technology for Economic and Clinical Health (HITECH) Act, and the Code of Federal Regulations (CFR) provide a general framework addressing the security and privacy of "protected health information." Healthcare providers and healthcare organizations that are involved in RM of CIEDs will typically sign a "terms of use" agreement and, when applicable, a "business associate agreement" with each CIED vendor. These legal documents outline the provisions of RM between the CIED vendor and the user.[8]

A European Directive and National Legislation on data protection has been released.[39] The principles of this European directive are summarized as follows:

1. Data must be processed fairly and lawfully.

2. Data must be obtained only for specified and lawful purposes and not further processed in any manner incompatible with those purposes.

3. Data must be adequate, relevant, and not excessive in relation to the purposes for which it is processed.

4. Data must be accurate and kept up to date.

5. Data must not be kept for longer than is necessary for that purpose.

6. Data must be processed in accordance with the rights of data subjects.

7. Appropriate technical and organizational measures must be taken to prevent unauthorized or unlawful processing of, accidental loss of, or destruction or damage to data, particularly where processing is outsourced to third parties.

8. Data must not be transferred to a country outside the EEA [European Economic Area] unless that country ensures an "adequate level of protection" for the rights of data subjects in relation to processing personal data.

The United States is *not* considered by the European Union to have an "adequate level." For that reason, European RM servers are hosted in the European Union.[39]

In order to test the vulnerability of security breaches by hackers accessing devices with wireless capability, Halperin et al[40] performed laboratory tests on a Medtronic Maximo DR ICD. After having partially reversed the ICD's communications protocol with an oscilloscope and a software radio, they performed several software radio–based attacks that were able to retrieve unencrypted personal patient data, as well as change device settings (including commanded shocks). This report triggered considerable media coverage, although it is believed that the risk of unauthorized access to an ICD is unlikely, given the considerable technical expertise required.[40] There have been no reports to date of hacking into implantable devices. Another consideration, however, is hacking into an Internet server database that stores RM information.

Reimbursement Considerations

Unfortunately, economic evaluation of remote device management has been hampered by a number of obstacles:[41] (1) There is a paucity of available data regarding clinical effectiveness, efficacy, and costs, requiring assumptions that decrease robustness of the analyses; (2) A multitude of parameters affect cost in this field, and these parameters are heterogeneous (eg, variations in distances traveled, different reimbursement policies), particularly in Europe; (3) Possible differences in performance between systems may affect the drivers of economic models; and (4) Medical devices and communication technology are constantly evolving, making it difficult to make mid- or long-term projections of cost.

The paucity of available data on economic analysis related to remote device and patient management stems from a number of factors. Until recently, no randomized controlled trials had demonstrated the effectiveness and efficacy of RM to provide robust data for performing economic analysis.[41] In most healthcare systems worldwide, despite a strong growing interest in health economics, reimbursement decisions do not require formal health economic evaluations. Indeed, reimbursement for remote patient follow-up was granted in some countries in Europe (eg, Germany) in 2008 without requiring any proof of cost-savings. Therefore, there was no need thereafter to conduct cost analysis in these countries. In Europe, reimbursement for remote follow-up is restricted to a few countries, limiting the number of patients and thus the possibility of creating large international registries. In addition, reimbursement of remote CIED follow-up varies substantially across Europe, and only a few countries define specific tariffs.[42] In turn, healthcare payers may be reluctant to reimburse remote device management owing to lack of robust economic analysis and evidence of improved patient outcomes, despite acknowledging the strategy to be safe. In the United Kingdom, Germany, and Portugal, reimbursement for RM is similar to that offered for standard follow-up visits.[42]

In the United States, since 2006, Medicare and Medicaid have expanded reimbursement for remote device monitoring for all states. Reimbursement rates vary from state to state and are, in some instances, the same as for an in-office visit without device programming. These coverage guidelines permit reimbursement on a quarterly basis for remote follow-up of PMs and ICDs. In addition, reimbursement is available to physicians for monthly remote follow-up of an ILR and "implantable cardiovascular monitor system." The latter, which can either be a stand-alone device or incorporated into a PM or ICD system, provides physiological cardiovascular data elements from internal (transthoracic impedance, heart rate variability, respiratory rate, intracardiac pressures) and external (weight and blood pressure) sensors.

The implications of remote device management for the different parties involved and analysis of costs (from the payer's perspective) have been published elsewhere.[41] The financial implications resulting from RM vary according to the perspective. For example, if RM reduces the number of hospitalizations, this is financially attractive for the payer but may result in lost income for the healthcare provider (eg, hospital or physician). However, if only duration of hospital stay is reduced, then the provider is likely to benefit financially, especially if a diagnostic-related group system is applied, because the same reimbursement will be received for less use of resources. Another example is monitoring battery status. Automatic device transmissions use additional energy that may shorten battery life (the magnitude of this impact, however, is not well defined by manufacturers); even so, this does not make it mandatory to increase the frequency of in-office visits and may allow select patients to delay the box change (eg, those who are not PM-dependent), since an alert message is sent when elective replacement is reached.[41]

Studies on Economic Evaluation of Remote Monitoring and Follow-up

Few reports have been published on economic analysis of remote cardiac device management based on prospectively collected data. Cost analyses in telemedicine have been published for a variety of other applications (such as teleconsultations and medical videoconferencing), but health and economic implications are very different in these contexts. Furthermore, many reports suffer from limitations that were addressed in a recent publication that suggested a framework for economic evaluation of telemedicine networks.[41]

In 2009, the UK National Health Service (NHS) Purchasing and Supply Agency performed an economic evaluation of remote follow-up.[41] Assuming an impact on neither clinical outcome nor quality of life with remote follow-up, and a cost of £1,000 per home transmitter (including service), it was calculated that the strategy led to reduction in costs after 6 years, if the frequency of in-office visits were reduced to once a year. However, details of the analysis (eg, travel costs, number of remote follow-ups, and their reimbursement) were not reported.

CIEDs have the potential to automatically acquire and transmit physiological information that could make follow-up more cost-effective. Several studies have attempted to evaluate the cost-effectiveness of remote follow-up.[6] At this time, there are two obvious sources for cost-savings: a decrease in patient follow-up visits and early identification of problems that could, if managed aggressively and expeditiously, lead to a reduction in hospitalizations. In one study,[21] investigators found that, compared with in-office visits, RM was associated with decreased demands on patient time (7 min vs 3 h) and physician time (8 vs 26 min, $P < 0.001$). It has also been estimated that RM could decrease the 5-year costs of standard device monitoring by $2,100 to $3,000 per patient. Data from the TRUST study[12] suggest that RM can safely reduce in-person follow-up visits by 50%. In patients with HF, more substantial cost-savings could be realized if RM were shown to reduce hospitalizations.

With RM, the intervals between in-office visits may be even extended over yearly visits (as currently recommended).[1] In the CONNECT trial,[13] ICD and CRT-D patients had in-office visits after a 14-month interval, and in the COMPAS trial[14] in PM patients, this interval was even prolonged to 18 months without increased risk. For RM to fall below NICE's generally accepted threshold of £30,000 per quality-adjusted life-year (QALY) gained, it was calculated that it requires only a 5% relative risk reduction of stroke (resulting from earlier detection of AF).[41] Assuming a 20% relative risk reduction, the incremental cost-effectiveness ratio would only be £4,069/QALY. Results from a computer-based simulation[43] showed a reduction in stroke risk by 9% to 18% with respect to standard in-person follow-up visits with intervals of 6 to 12 months comparable to the 25% rate that was reported in the COMPAS trial[14] over an 18-month follow-up. Further beneficial effects of RM, such as reduction in stroke-related deaths, HF hospitalizations, or inappropriate shocks, may lead to even more cost-effective savings.

The first studies evaluating the economic impact of remote follow-up focused on estimated savings on transportation costs.[44] In many countries, these costs are paid by the healthcare insurer. Depending on the distance to be covered, 5-year cumulative avoidable transportation costs ranged from $1,377 to $4,113 US. This savings would not only allow recovery of the technology-related costs (ie, transmitter and communication, estimated at ~$,1200 US) but also lead to substantial overall savings after a few years.[44] Other, rather small, studies have further focused on the cost effect of RM from a societal perspective (eg, of the healthcare payer). In a Finnish study,[21] savings on reimbursement for consultation, transportation (with a mean distance of 130 km), and sickness allowance led to reduced expenditures of €524/patient over the 9-month study period.

Most recent trials on RM have had safety or efficacy primary end points, but some of them have included an estimation of economic variables as a secondary outcome. Preliminary results of the REFORM trial[9] have been published, involving 115 patients with a MADIT II ICD indication randomized to 3 monthly in-hospital visits or yearly in-hospital visits (and 3-month remote follow-ups), with RM of events in both groups. Time taken for performing the visits and costs related to transportation were tracked. Researchers found that remote follow-up reduced the total number of visits by 63%. This, in turn, led to a reduction in transportation costs of €110 per patient-year. Also, the physician's time was reduced by 40% (representing about 50 min/patient-year), which translated into an estimated cost-savings to the hospital of €712/patient-year, assuming reallocation or reduction of resources. In the CONNECT trial,[13] patients in the RM arm had an 18% reduction in hospitalization duration ($P = 0.002$), which translated into an estimated savings of $1,659 US per hospitalization.

The Evolution of Management Strategies of Heart Failure Patients with Implantable Defibrillators (EVOLVO) study was a multicenter randomized trial[45] involving 200 patients. It compared RM with standard patient management consisting of scheduled visits and patient response to audible ICD alerts. The primary end point was the rate of emergency department or urgent in-office visits for HF, arrhythmias, or ICD-related events. Over 16 months, such visits were 35% less frequent in the remote arm (75 vs 117; $P = 0.005$). A 21% difference was observed in the rates of total healthcare utilization for HF, arrhythmias, or device-related events (4.40 vs 5.74 events/year; $P < 0.001$). These studies showed that RM reduced emergency department and urgent in-office visits in particular, and total health utilization in general in patients with ICD and CRT-D devices.

The ongoing EuroEco (European Health Economic Trial on Home Monitoring in ICD and CRT-D Patients) trial[46] is a prospective healthcare economics study. It will evaluate the cumulative follow-up costs for physicians and hospitals (from a provider's perspective) and for the healthcare payer (from a societal perspective). Although there is a paucity of published data on the economic aspects of remote device management, ongoing studies (most of which are being conducted in Europe) will hopefully help to assess the economic viability of this new technology.

Future Directions

With rapidly developing telecommunications technology, RM of cardiac devices may play an increased role in the care of patients with CIEDs. Also, with the latest generation of ICDs, the amount and quality of transmitted information using remote surveillance technology continue to improve and have reached the level of an in-office interrogation. However, several technical and medicolegal issues need to be resolved before these systems will replace a majority of in-office visits.

Remote follow-up has shown to be safe and is even preferred by both patients and physicians to in-office visits. It is likely to add little overall cost to follow-up and will probably be readily adopted in Europe, as it has been in the United States, although reimbursement still needs to be addressed. RM raises more complex issues, however, because the increase in workload (and possibly in costs related to alert messages) needs to be offset by improved patient outcomes. Nevertheless, because of ongoing technological progress, eventually a remote management strategy is likely to become the standard of care.

The expanding role of implantable sensors and invasive hemodynamic parameters is leading to a paradigm shift in HF management and will likely provide HF specialists with additional information. When coupled with RM, these data will allow for early intervention in these patients. RM of more sophisticated parameters that reflect additional physiological information in HF is already being evaluated in experimental settings.

References

1. Wilkoff BL, Auricchio A, Brugada J, et al. HRS/EHRA Expert Consensus on the Monitoring of Cardiovascular Implantable Electronic Devices (CIEDs): description of techniques, indications, personnel, frequency and ethical considerations: developed in partnership with the Heart Rhythm Society (HRS) and the European Heart Rhythm Association (EHRA); and in collaboration with the American College of Cardiology (ACC), the American Heart Association (AHA), the European Society of Cardiology (ESC), the Heart Failure Association of ESC (HFA), and the Heart Failure Society of America (HFSA). Endorsed by the Heart Rhythm Society, the European Heart Rhythm Association (a registered branch of the ESC), the American College of Cardiology, the American Heart Association. *Europace*. 2008;10:707-725.
2. Orlov MV, Szombathy T, Chaudry GM, Haffajee CI. Remote surveillance of implantable cardiac devices. *Pacing Clin Electrophysiol*. 2009;32:928-939.
3. Jung W, Rillig A, Birkemeyer R, et al. Advances in remote monitoring of implantable pacemakers, cardioverter defibrillators and cardiac resynchronization therapy systems. *J Interv Card Electrophysiol*. 2008;23:73-85.
4. Burri H, Senouf D. Remote monitoring and follow-up of pacemakers and implantable cardioverter defibrillators. *Europace*. 2009;11:701-709.
5. Movsowitz C, Mittal S. Remote patient management using implantable devices. *J Interv Card Electrophysiol*. 2011;31: 81-90.
6. Kusumoto F, Goldschlager N. Remote monitoring of patients with implanted cardiac devices. *Clin Cardiol*. 2010;33:10-17.
7. Sticherling C, Kühne M, Schaer B, et al. Remote monitoring of cardiovascular implantable electronic devices. Prerequisite or luxury? *Swiss Med Wkly*. 2009;139:596-601.
8. Dubner S, Auricchio A, Steinberg J, et al. ISHNE/EHRA expert consensus on remote monitoring of cardiovascular implantable electronic devices (CIEDs). *Europace*. 2012;14: 278-293.

9. Elsner C, Sommer P, Piorkowski C, et al. A prospective multicenter comparison trial of home monitoring against regular follow-up in MADIT II patients: additional visits and cost impact. *Comput Cardiol.* 2006;33:241-244.
10. Halimi F, Clémenty J, Attuel P, Dessenne X, Amara W, on behalf of the OEDIPE trial investigators. Optimized post-operative surveillance of permanent pacemakers by home monitoring: the OEDIPE trial. *Europace.* 2008;10: 1392-1399.
11. Crossley GH, Chen J, Choucair W, Cohen TJ, Gohn DC, Johnson WB, on behalf of the PREFER study investigators. Clinical benefits of remote versus transtelephonic monitoring of implanted pacemakers. *J Am Coll Cardiol.* 2009;54: 2012-2019.
12. Varma N, Epstein A, Irimpen A, et al. Efficacy and safety of automatic remote monitoring for implantable cardioverter-defibrillator follow-up. The Lumos-T Safely Reduces Routine Office Device Follow-Up (TRUST) Trial. *Circulation.* 2010;122:325-332.
13. Crossley GH, Boyle A, Vitense H, Chang Y, Mead RH, and CONNECT investigators. The CONNECT (Clinical Evaluation of Remote Notification to Reduce Time to Clinical Decision) Trial. The value of wireless remote monitoring with automatic clinician alerts. *J Am Coll Cardiol.* 2011;57:1181-1189.
14. Mabo P, Victor F, Bazin P, Ahres S, Babuty D, Da Costa A, on behalf of the COMPAS trial investigators. A randomized trial of long-term remote monitoring of pacemaker recipients (the COMPAS trial). *Europace.* 2012;33:1105-1111.
15. Saxon LA, Hayes DL, Gilliam FR, et al. Long-term outcome after ICD and CRT implantation and influence of remote device follow-up: the ALTITUDE survival study. *Circulation.* 2010;122:2359-2367.
16. Ricci RP, Morichelli L, Quart A, et al. Long-term patient acceptance of and satisfaction with implanted device remote monitoring. *Europace.* 2010;12:674-679.
17. Schoenfeld MH, Compton SJ, Mead RH, et al. Remote monitoring of implantable cardioverter defibrillators: a prospective analysis. *Pacing Clin Electrophysiol.* 2004;27(Pt I):757-763.
18. Brugada P. What evidence do we have to replace in-hospital implantable cardioverter defibrillator follow-up? *Clin Res Cardiol.* 2006;95(Suppl 3):III3-III9.
19. Heidbuchel H, Lioen P, Foulon S, et al. Potential role of remote monitoring for scheduled and unscheduled evaluations of patients with an implantable defibrillator. *Europace.* 2008;10:351-357.
20. Lazarus A. Remote, wireless, ambulatory monitoring of implantable pacemakers, cardioverter defibrillators, and cardiac resynchronization therapy systems: analysis of a worldwide database. *Pacing Clin Electrophysiol.* 2007;30(Suppl 1):S2-S12.
21. Raatikainen MJ, Uusimaa P, van Ginneken MM, et al. Remote monitoring of implantable cardioverter defibrillator patients: a safe, time-saving, and cost-effective means for follow-up. *Europace.* 2008;10:1145-1151.
22. Neuzil P, Taborsky M, Holy F, Wallbrueck K. Early automatic remote detection of combined lead insulation defect and ICD damage. *Europace.* 2008;10:556-557.
23. Spencker S, Coban N, Koch L, et al. A potential role of home monitoring to reduce inappropriate shocks in implantable cardioverter defibrillator patients due to lead failure. *Europace.* 2009;11:483-488.
24. Varma N, Michalski J, Epstein AE, Schweikert R. Automatic remote monitoring of ICD lead and generator performance: the Lumos-T Safely RedUceS RouTine Office Device Follow-Up (TRUST) trial. *Circ Arrhythm Electrophysiol.* 2010;3:428-436.
25. Saxon LA, Sharma A, Estes MNA III. Performance of the Medtronic Sprint Fidelis lead on the Latitude patient network. *Heart Rhythm.* 2008;5:S191.
26. Glotzer TV, Hellkamp AS, Zimmerman J, et al. Atrial high rate episodes detected by pacemaker diagnostics predict death and stroke. *Circulation.* 2003;107:1614-1619.
27. Glotzer TV, Daoud EG, Wyse DG, et al. The relationship between daily atrial tachyarrhythmia burden from implantable device diagnostics and stroke risk. The TRENDS Study. *Circ Arrhythm Electrophysiol.* 2009;2:474-480.
28. Varma N, Stambler B, Chun S. Detection of atrial fibrillation by implanted devices with wireless data transmission capability. *Pacing Clin Electrophysiol.* 2005;28(Suppl 1):S133-S136.
29. Ricci RP, Morichelli L, Santini M. Remote control of implanted devices through home monitoring technology improves detection and clinical management of atrial fibrillation. *Europace.* 2009;11:54-61.
30. Ip J, Waldo A, Lip GYH, et al, for the IMPACT investigators. Multicenter randomized study of anticoagulation guided by remote rhythm monitoring in patients with implantable cardioverter-defibrillator and CRT-D devices: rationale, design, and clinical characteristics of the initially enrolled cohort: The IMPACT study. *Am Heart J.* 2009;158:364-370.e1.
31. Mortara A, Pinna GD, Johnson P, et al. Home telemonitoring in heart failure patients: the HHH study (Home or Hospital in Heart Failure). *Eur Heart J.* 2009;11:312-318.
32. Yu CM, Wang L, Chau E, et al. Intrathoracic impedance monitoring in patients with heart failure: correlation with fluid status and feasibility of early warning preceding hospitalization. *Circulation.* 2005;112:841-848.
33. Bourge RC, Abraham WT, Adamson PB, et al., COMPASS-HF Study Group. Randomized controlled trial of an implantable continuous hemodynamic monitor in patients with advanced heart failure: the COMPASS-HF study. *J Am Coll Cardiol.* 2008;51:1073-1079.
34. Ritzema J, Melton IC, Richards AM, et al. Direct left atrial pressure monitoring in ambulatory heart failure patients: initial experience with a new permanent implantable device. *Circulation.* 2007;116:2952-2959.
35. Abraham WT, Adamson PB, Bourge RC, on behalf of the CHAMPION Trial Study Group. Wireless pulmonary artery haemodynamic monitoring in chronic heart failure: a randomised controlled trial. *Lancet.* 2011;377:658-666.
36. Saxon LA, Boehmer JP, Neuman S, Mullin CM. Remote Active Monitoring in Patients with Heart Failure (RAPID-RF): design and rationale. *J Cardiac Fail.* 2007;13:241-246.
37. Joseph GK, Wilkoff BL, Dresing T, et al. Remote interrogation and monitoring of implantable cardioverter defibrillators. *J Interv Card Electrophysiol.* 2004;11:161-166.
38. Marzegalli M, Lunati M, Landolina M, et al. Remote monitoring of CRT–ICD: the multicenter Italian CareLink evaluation—ease of use, acceptance, and organizational implications. *Pacing Clin Electrophysiol.* 2008;31:1259-1264.
39. Jung W. Potential medico-legal troubles and troubleshooting with remote monitoring. XIV International Symposium on Progress in Clinical Pacing. Rome, November 30–December 3, 2010.
40. Halperin D, Heydt-Benjamin TS, Ransford B, et al. Pacemakers and implantable cardiac defibrillators: software radio attacks and zero-power defenses. Proceedings of the 2008 IEEE Symposium on Security and Privacy. Oakland, CA, May 18–21, 2008;129-142.
41. Burri H, Heidbüchel H, Jung W, Brugada P. Remote monitoring: a cost or an investment? *Europace.* 2011;13:ii44-ii48.

42. Boriani G, Burri H, Mantovani L, et al. Device therapy and hospital reimbursement practices across European countries: a heterogeneous scenario. *Europace*. 2011;13:ii59-ii65.
43. Ricci RP, Morichelli L, Gargaro A, et al. Home monitoring in patients with implantable cardiac devices: is there a potential reduction of stroke risk? Results from a computer model tested through Monte Carlo simulations. *J Cardiovasc Electrophysiol*. 2009;20:1244-1251.
44. Fauchier L, Sadoul N, Kouakam C, et al. Potential cost savings by telemedicine-assisted longterm care of implantable cardioverter defibrillator recipients. *Pacing Clin Electrophysiol*. 2005;28:S255-S259.
45. Landolina M, Perego G, Lunati M, et al. Remote monitoring reduces health care use and improves quality of care in heart failure patients with implantable defibrillators: the Evolution of Management Strategies of Heart Failure Patients with Implantable Defibrillators (EVOLVO) study. *Circulation*. 2012;125:2985-2992.
46. European Health Economic Trial on Home Monitoring in ICD and CRT-D Patients (EuroEco). http://www.clinicaltrials.gov. Accessed February 13, 2013.

CHAPTER 16

PERCUTANEOUS LEFT ATRIAL APPENDAGE OCCLUSION

HEYDER OMRAN, MD

Introduction

Thromboembolism is the most feared complication in patients with permanent atrial fibrillation (AF).[1] The risk of embolism may vary from <1% to 20% depending on the underlying disease of the patient. Obviously, patients with previous strokes have the highest risk of embolism. Transesophageal echocardiography (TEE) studies show that most thrombi are located in the left atrial appendage (LAA), and only a few thrombi originate in the left atrium itself.[2,3] Although prospective, randomized studies show that oral anticoagulation (OAC) reduces the risk of thromboembolism significantly,[4] patients often may not receive OAC because of bleeding complications, increased bleeding risk, allergies to coumarin derivates, or fear of complications.[5] Occluding the LAA is another way to reduce the risk of thromboembolism. Hence, the LAA is often occluded or removed in patients undergoing cardiac surgery who have concomitant AF. Surgical obliteration of the LAA in patients at high risk for thromboembolism is a well-established procedure for eliminating the predilection of this site for developing thrombi.[6-8]

In 2001, an alternative procedure was introduced for patients with contraindications for oral anticoagulation: the interventional occlusion of the LAA.[9-11] This chapter provides information on the indications for and techniques, safety, results, imaging, and potential future applications of percutaneous LAA occlusion.

Indications

Oral anticoagulation is contraindicated for at least an estimated 30% of patients with AF. Furthermore, it has been shown that contraindications for oral anticoagulation are particularly common in elderly patients.[5] Interventional occlusion of the LAA is suggested for patients at high risk for embolism and contraindicated for oral anticoagulation. Often the so-called $CHADS_2$ score (Congestive heart failure, Hypertension, Age, Diabetes, prior Stroke 2) is used for defining the risk of embolism.

In addition to assessing the patient's individual thromboembolic risk, other factors need to be addressed:

- Life expectancy of the patient
- Procedural risk
- Technical considerations (eg, access to the LAA, anatomy of the appendage)
- Morphological features

Hence, any decision to perform an interventional occlusion of the LAA has to be an individual one; that is, it has to balance the advantages and possible disadvantages of the therapy.

Recently, the FDA's Circulatory System Devices Advisory Panel recommended the approval of the WATCHMAN® LAA Closure Technology (Atritech, Inc., Plymouth, MN), stating that it is comparable with long-term warfarin therapy for the prevention of stroke in warfarin-eligible patients with nonvalvular AF.

Devices and Implantation Techniques

The first device for the interventional occlusion of the LAA was introduced by M. Lesh and coworkers in animal studies.[9] The device was called PLAATO (Percutaneous Left Atrial Appendage Transcatheter Occlusion). It consists of a self-expanding, balloon-shaped nitinol cage with an expanded polytetrafluoroethylene (ePTFE) membrane (Figure 16.1) with three rows of anchors stabilizing the device in the appendage. The membrane covers the atrial surface of the device, whereas the opposite surface is uncovered, allowing secondary thrombosis of the lumen by the device. The morphology of the LAA was evaluated by angiography and simultaneous TEE. The maximal diameter of the LAA orifice was determined by both methods, and a mean diameter obtained. A 20% to 30% oversized occlusion device was selected. The device was introduced via a 14-Fr femoral vein sheath and advanced into the LAA after transseptal puncture of the atrial septum. Then the device was expanded and the position controlled using both angiography and TEE (Figure 16.2). The mean size of the devices used was 29 mm. After verifying the optimal position and adequate sizing of the device, it was released and the final position was assessed by repeated angiography.

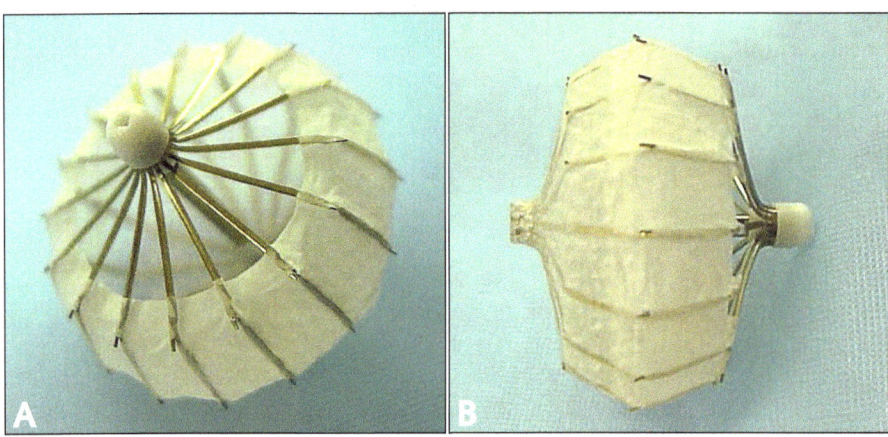

Figure 16.1 First left atrial appendage occlusion device: Percutaneous Left Atrial Appendage Transcatheter Occlusion (PLAATO) (ev3 Endovascular, Inc., Plymouth, MN). It consists of a self-expanding, balloon-shaped nitinol cage with an expanded ePTFE membrane with three rows of anchors. **Panel A:** view from the front. **Panel B:** side view showing anchors.

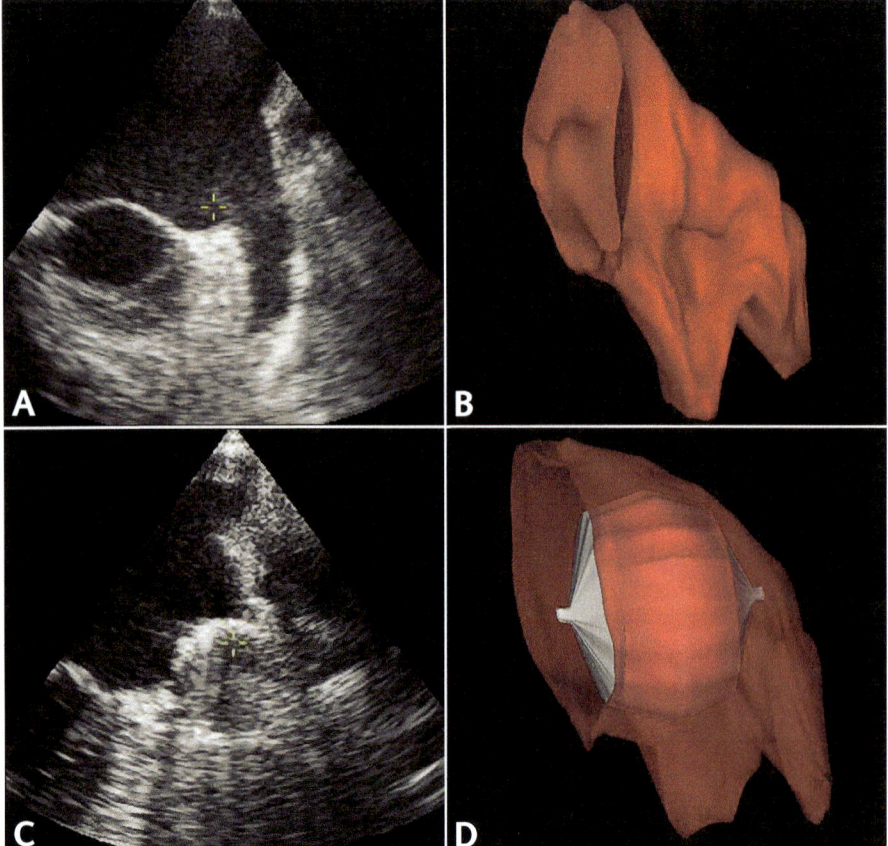

Figure 16.2 Left atrial appendage as imaged by transesophageal echocardiography (**Panel A**) and the corresponding 3D reconstruction of the left atrial appendage (**Panel B**). Left atrial appendage with occlusion device (**Panel C**) and the corresponding 3D reconstruction are shown (**Panel D**).

A similar device was introduced by Atritech, Inc. Called the WATCHMAN LAA Closure Technology device (Figure 16.3),[12] it is similar to the PLAATO device and consists of a self-expanding nickel titanium frame structure with external fixation barbs and a permeable polyester fabric cover (sizes range from 21 to 33 mm). The procedure of implanting the device resembles the implantation of the PLAATO device.

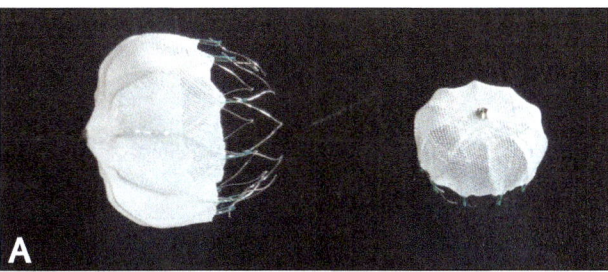

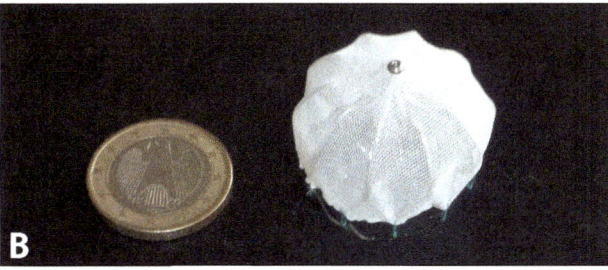

Figure 16.3 The WATCHMAN LAA Closure Technology device (Atritech, Inc., Plymouth, MN) with a self-expanding nitinol frame structure with external fixation barbs. **Panel A:** Side view and front view showing nitinol cage and covered surface. **Panel B:** Device size varies between 21 and 33 mm.

Meier and coworkers published a study on the successful occlusion of the LAA using an AMPLATZER device that was not designed uniquely for this purpose.[13] In December 2008, AGA Medical (Plymouth, MN) received the European Conformity (CE) mark of approval for an LAA occlusion device different from the previously described ones. It is called a cardiac plug and is designed to achieve optimal occlusion of the LAA; it consists of a distal lobe and disc, which is supposed to cover the orifice of the LAA (Figure 16.4). The diameter of the lobe ranges from 16 to 30 mm, and the corresponding disc diameter ranges from 20 to 36 mm.

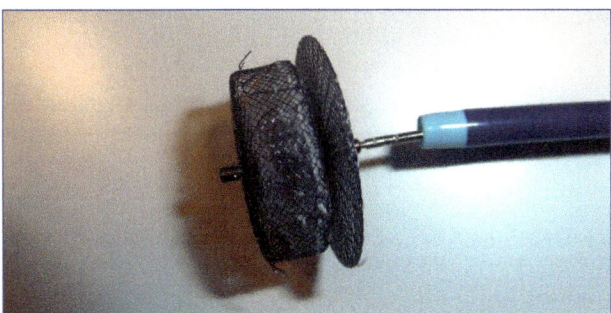

Figure 16.4 Cardiac plug LAA occlusion device (AGA Medical, Plymouth, MN) consisting of a distal lobe and a disc.

The accompanying video files provide details on the echocardiographic assessment of the LAA and major steps for implantation of an LAA occlusion device:

1. Echocardiographic exclusion of alternative cardioembolic sources (▶ Video 16.1, ▶ Video 16.2, ▶ Video 16.3, ▶ Video 16.4, ▶ Video 16.5, and ▶ Video 16.6)
2. Guidance of transseptal puncture (▶ Video 16.7.1 and ▶ Video 16.7.2)
3. Angiographic assessment of the LAA (▶ Video 16.8)
4. Wiring of the left upper pulmonary vein and introduction of the pigtail catheter (Video 16.8 and ▶ Video 16.9)
5. Introduction of the sheath (▶ Video 16.10 and ▶ Video 16.11)
6. Introduction of the device and deployment of the distal lobe (▶ Video 16.12)
7. Deployment of the proximal part of the device (▶ Video 16.13)
8. Stability test (▶ Video 16.14 and ▶ Video 16.15)
9. Release of the device (▶ Video 16.16)
10. Angiographic control (▶ Video 16.17 and ▶ Video 16.18)
11. Safety issues (▶ Video 16.19, thrombus on sheath; ▶ Video 16.20, thrombus on PLAATO device; ▶ Video 16.21, small pericardial effusion; and ▶ Video 16.22, thrombus on AGA cardiac plug device)

Safety and Results

In various studies, data about the safety and success of the LAA occlusion procedure were collected for both the PLAATO (Figure 16.5) and the WATCHMAN devices.[12,14]

The researchers evaluating the PLAATO device showed that the LAA occlusion procedure is feasible and may be performed within 2 hours.[14] Detailed results concerning 111 patients with attempted LAA occlusion were published in 2005.[14] The procedure was successful in 97% of the patients. Migration of the device or formation of mobile thrombi on the surface of the device was not observed during a follow-up 10 months later. One of the patients in the study group died owing to procedural complications. Pericardiocentesis was performed in 3 patients in response to cardiac tamponade. In addition, 1 patient developed left-sided hemothorax. Hence, relevant procedural complications were not uncommon. However, they occurred less frequently with increasing experience of the operator.

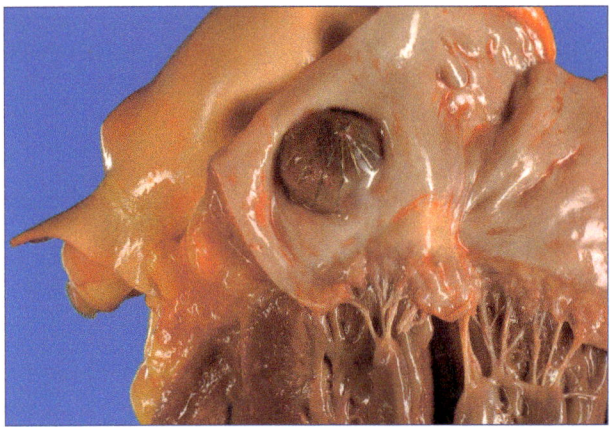

Figure 16.5 Postmortem image of PLAATO device in the left atrial appendage.

Two patients had a stroke, and two patients experienced transient ischemic attacks during the observation period. No thrombi formed on the device in any of the patients. Another study followed up the patients closely using echocardiography and showed that the implant was covered with a neointima after 6 months and that the device did not alter pulmonary vein flow.[11] Furthermore, no significant atrial septal defects were detected after the puncture of the intra-atrial septum with a 14-Fr sheath.[15] Owing to the high rate of complications, a randomized study comparing anticoagulation and device therapy was requested. Such a study has not been performed yet, and the company has since halted distribution of the device. Long-term follow-up data have not systematically been published.[16-18]

Similar experiences were reported for Atritech's Watchman device. Sick et al provided information on 75 patients who had the device implanted,[12] among whom there was a failure rate of 10%. Two patients experienced device embolization; both devices were successfully retrieved percutaneously. Two cardiac tamponades and one air embolism occurred. One device had a wire fracture and needed to be explanted surgically. In four patients, flat thrombi had formed on the atrial surface of the device by the time of the 6-month echocardiographic follow-up. Two neurological complications occurred during the follow-up period.

To assess how effectively strokes and bleeding events were reduced in patients with AF by occluding the LAA with the Watchman device, a prospective study (Watchman Left Atrial Appendage System for Embolic Protection in Patients with AF [PROTECT-AF]) was performed in patients with nonvalvular AF and a $CHADS_2$ score >1.[19] PROTECT-AF is a key study for evaluating the concept of LAA occlusion for the prevention of thromboembolism in patients with AF; hence, the study will be discussed in detail.

The trial included patients aged 18 years or older with all types of nonvalvular AF and at least one risk factor on the $CHADS_2$ scale. Patients were excluded if they had contraindications for warfarin or had comorbidities requiring the usage of chronic oral anticoagulation. In addition, patients were excluded from the study if they had an LAA thrombus, a patent foramen ovale with atrial septal aneurysm and right-to-left shunt, mobile atheroma, or symptomatic carotid artery disease. Patients were randomized in a 2:1 ratio to receive either interventional occlusion of the LAA or warfarin therapy. After implantation of the Watchman device, patients were treated for 45 days with warfarin. Thereafter, clopidogrel (75 mg) and aspirin (81–325 mg) were prescribed once daily for the remaining period, up to the 6-month follow-up visit. Then, clopidogrel was discontinued.

The primary end point of the study was to show noninferiority of the device as compared with warfarin therapy; this composite end point consisted of efficacy (ischemic and hemorrhagic stroke), cardiovascular or unexplained death, or systemic embolism. The safety end point consisted of excessive bleeding events and procedure-related complications. Patients were followed for an aggregate of 1,065 patient-years. Successful implantation was performed in 88% of patients scheduled for intervention. An international normalized ratio (INR) range of 2 to 3 was achieved in 66% of patients in the medical treatment group. The primary efficacy event rate was 3.0 per 100 patient-years in the intervention group and 4.9 in the control group. The probability of noninferiority of the intervention was 99.9%. Hemorrhagic strokes occurred in 0.1% in the intervention group and in 1.6% in the control group.

Primary safety events occurred at a significantly higher rate in the intervention group than in the control group (7.4 vs 4.4) and were associated mainly with procedural complications (ie, 22 patients had serious pericardial effusions). Device embolization was observed in 3 patients. The rate of serious pericardial effusion declined with experience of the operator.

In summary, the results of the PROTECT-AF trial demonstrated noninferiority of LAA occlusion to warfarin therapy for the primary efficacy end point. However, there was a higher initial safety event rate for device implantation.

More recently, it was demonstrated that implant success and device safety increase over time, reflecting the influence of increased operator experience. Compared with patients included in the original PROTECT-AF trial ($N = 542$), patients enrolled in the Continued Access Protocol (CAP) registry ($n = 460$) had fewer safety events (7.7% vs 3.7%). In particular, the rate of serious pericardial effusion was lower in the CAP registry (5.0% vs 2.2%).[20]

Other studies on LAA occlusion included many fewer patients. Meier et al provided information on the use of the Amplatzer device for occluding the LAA in 16 patients.[13] One patient had an embolization of the device; all other patients had no serious complications. In a larger study on LAA occlusion with the Amplatzer cardiac plug, occlusion of the appendage was successful in 96% of patients (n = 132). Serious complications (stroke, device embolization, pericardial effusions, and transient myocardial ischemia) were observed in 7% of the cases.[21]

Other devices are being assessed in animal models. Fumoto et al reported the successful implantation of a third-generation atrial exclusion device in 14 dogs.[22] Jayakar et al investigated a tissue-welding technology for obliterating the LAA.[23] However, it is important to recognize that long-term data or data from randomized, prospective trials are not available yet.

Imaging

Imaging the left atrium and its appendage is very important for planning and performing LAA occlusion. In addition, potential thrombi in the LAA need to be excluded. The anatomy of the left atrium and the LAA is complex and varies considerably, as shown by anatomic studies.[24,25] The LAA orifice is usually oval in shape and averages 17.4 (4) mm.[25] Adjacent structures are the left upper pulmonary vein (11 (4.1) mm) and the mitral valve (10.7 (2.4) mm). Histological examination of the LAA shows that the wall is very thin in places, which explains the high risk of perforation during the procedure. Hence, visual guidance of the procedure is of extreme importance.

Multiplane TEE has been shown to exclude left atrial thrombi very accurately and should be performed in all patients considered for LAA occlusion.[26-29] Both transesophageal and intracardiac echocardiography may be used to guide the procedure, as follows:[30,31]

- Guidance of transseptal puncture
- Visualization of the delivery sheath position
- Analysis of the position of the device
- Monitoring of potential complications

Furthermore, imaging is very important for the followup of the patients. All patients should be assessed for thrombus formation on the device before discontinuing the anticoagulants.

Computed tomography (CT) has been used for analyzing the size and morphology of the LAA. However, measurements vary considerably between TEE and CT.[32] Hence, further studies are needed to ascertain whether CT may be used as an alternative for device sizing prior to the procedure.

Summary

Multiple reports have shown that LAA occlusion is technically feasible. However, the procedure still carries considerable risk.[33] Potentially, increased operator experience, better patient selection, and improved technology will lead to a decrease in the complication rate. Hence, careful patient selection for the procedure is very important. Significantly, the randomized PROTECT-AF study demonstrated noninferiority of LAA occlusion with the WATCHMAN device for preventing stroke compared with treating patients with warfarin. Nevertheless, ideal candidates for LAA occlusion have contraindications for long-term oral anticoagulation therapy or refuse to take oral anticoagulants. In any case, the risk and benefits have to be carefully weighed.

Next-generation anticoagulants are being developed and tested clinically. These medications may have fewer side effects and a lower bleeding rate than current oral anticoagulants, as recently shown in the Randomized Evaluation of Long-Term Anticoagulation Therapy (RE-LY) study.[34] Therefore, the clinician is well advised to observe these developments carefully and decide accordingly.

In conclusion, LAA occlusion devices are an important alternative to oral anticoagulation in patients with AF.

References

1. Albers GW, Dalen JE, Laupacis A, et al. Antithrombotic therapy in atrial fibrillation. *Chest.* 2001;119:194S-206S.
2. Mügge A, Kühn H, Nikutta P, et al. Assessment of left atrial appendage function by biplane transesophageal echocardiography in patients with nonrheumatic atrial fibrillation: identification of a subgroup of patients at increased embolic risk. *J Am Coll Cardiol.* 1994;23:599-607.
3. Fatkin D, Kelly RP, Fenely MP. Relations between left atrial appendage blood flow velocity, spontaneous echocardiographic contrast and thromboembolic risk in vivo. *J Am Coll Cardiol.* 1994;23:961-969.
4. Stroke Prevention in Atrial Fibrillation Investigators. Adjusted-dose warfarin versus low-intensity, fixed dose warfarin plus aspirin for high-risk patients with atrial fibrillation: Stroke Prevention in Atrial Fibrillation III randomized clinical trial. *Lancet.* 1996;348:633-638.
5. Sudlow M, Thomson R, Thwaites B, et al. Prevalence of atrial fibrillation and eligibility for anticoagulants in the community. *Lancet.* 1998;352:1167-1171.
6. Johnson WD, Ganjoo AK, Stone CD, et al. The left atrial appendage: our most lethal human attachment: surgical implications. *Eur J Cardiothorac Surg.* 2000;17:718-722.
7. Blackshear JL, Odell JA. Appendage obliteration to reduce stroke in cardiac surgical patients with atrial fibrillation. *Ann Thorac Surg.* 1996;61:755-759.
8. Healey JS, Crystal E, Lamy A, et al. Left Atrial Appendage Occlusion Study (LAAOS): results of a randomized controlled pilot study of left atrial appendage occlusion during coronary bypass surgery in patients at risk for stroke. *Am Heart J.* 2005; 150(2):288-293.
9. Nakai T, Lesh MD, Gerstenfeld EP, et al. Percutaneous Left Atrial Appendage Occlusion (PLAATO) for preventing cardioembolism—first experience in canine model. *Circulation.* 2002;105:2217-2222.
10. Sievert H, Lesh MD, Trepels T, et al. Percutaneous left atrial appendage transcatheter occlusion to prevent stroke in high-risk patients with atrial fibrillation. *Circulation.* 2002;105: 1887-1889.

11. Omran H, Hardung D, Schmidt H, et al. Mechanical occlusion of the left atrial appendage. *J Cardiovasc Electrophysiol.* 2003;14(Suppl 9):S56-S59.
12. Sick PB, Schuler G, Hauptmann KE, et al. Initial worldwide experience with the WATCHMAN left atrial appendage system for stroke prevention in atrial fibrillation. *J Am Coll Cardiol.* 2007;49(13):1490-1495.
13. Meier B, Palacios I, Windecker S, et al. Transcatheter left atrial appendage occlusion with AMPLATZER devices to obviate anticoagulation in patients with atrial fibrillation. *Catheter Cardiovasc Interv.* 2003;60(3):417-422.
14. Ostermayer SH, Reisman M, Kramer PH, et al. Percutaneous Left Atrial Appendage Transcatheter Occlusion (PLAATO system) to prevent stroke in high-risk patients with non-rheumatic atrial fibrillation: results from the international multi-center feasibility trials. *J Am Coll Cardiol.* 2005;46(1):9-14.
15. Hanna IR, Kolm P, Martin R, et al. Left atrial structure and function after Percutaneous Left Atrial Appendage Transcatheter Occlusion (PLAATO): six-month echocardiographic follow-up. *J Am Coll Cardiol.* 2004;43(10):1868-1872.
16. Onalan O, Crystal E. Left atrial appendage exclusion for stroke prevention in patients with nonrheumatic atrial fibrillation. *Stroke.* 2007;38(Suppl 2):624-630.
17. Bayard YL, Ostermayer SH, Hein R, et al. Percutaneous devices for stroke prevention. *Cardiovasc Revasc Med.* 2007;8(3):216-225.
18. El-Chami MF, Grow P, Eilen D, et al. Clinical outcomes three years after PLAATO implantation. *Catheter Cardiovasc Interv.* 2007;69(5):704-707.
19. Holmes DR, Reddy VY, Tri ZG, et al. Percutaneous closure of the left atrial appendage versus warfarin therapy for prevention of stroke in patients with atrial fibrillation: a randomized non-inferiority trial. *Lancet.* 2009;374:534-542.
20. Reddy VY, Holmes D, Doshi SK, et al. Safety of percutaneous left atrial appendage closure: results from the Watchman Left Atrial Appendage System for Embolic Protection in Patients with AF (PROTECT AF) clinical trial and the Continued Access Registry. *Circulation.* 2011;123(4):417-424.
21. Park JW, Bethencourt A, Sievert H, et al. Left atrial appendage closure with AMPLATZER cardiac plug in atrial fibrillation: European experience. *Catheter Cardiovasc Interv.* 2011;77(5):700-706.
22. Fumoto H, Gillinov AM, Ootaki Y, et al. A novel device for left atrial appendage exclusion: the third-generation atrial exclusion device. *J Thorac Cardiovasc Surg.* 2008;136(4):1019-1027.
23. Jayakar D, Gozo F, Gomez E, Carlos C. Use of tissue welding technology to obliterate left atrial appendage—novel use of Ligasure. *Interact Cardiovasc Thorac Surg.* 2005;4(4):372-373.
24. Agmon Y, Khandheria BK, Gentile F, Seward JB. Echocardiographic assessment of the left atrial appendage. *J Am Coll Cardiol.* 1999;34:1867-1877.
25. Su P, McCarthy KP, Ho SY. Occluding the left atrial appendage: anatomical considerations. *Heart.* 2008;94(9):1166-1170.
26. Omran H, Jung W, Rabahieh R, et al. Imaging of thrombi and assessment of left atrial appendage function: a prospective study comparing transthoracic and transesophageal echocardiography. *Heart.* 1999;81:192-198.
27. Omran H, Jung W, Rabahieh R, et al. Echocardiographic predictors of maintenance of sinus rhythm after internal atrial defibrillation. *Am J Cardiol.* 1998;81:1446-1449.
28. Yao S, Meisner JS, Factor SM, et al. Assessment of left atrial appendage structure and function by transesophageal echocardiography: a review. *Echocardiogr.* 1998;15:243-255.
29. Mráz T, Neuzil P, Mandysová E, et al. Role of echocardiography in percutaneous occlusion of the left atrial appendage. *Echocardiogr.* 2007;24(4):401-404.
30. Jorgensen J, Palmer S, Kalogeropoulos A, et al. Implantation of left atrial appendage occlusion devices and complex appendage anatomy: the importance of transesophageal echocardiography. *Echocardiogr.* 2007;24(2):159-161.
31. Ho IC, Neuzil P, Mraz T, et al. Use of intracardiac echocardiography to guide implantation of a left atrial appendage occlusion device (PLAATO). *Heart Rhythm.* 2007;4(5):567-571.
32. Budge LP, Shaffer KM, Moorman JR, et al. Analysis of *in vivo* left atrial appendage morphology in patients with atrial fibrillation: a direct comparison of transesophageal echocardiography, planar cardiac CT, and segmented three-dimensional cardiac CT. *J Interv Card Electrophysiol.* 2008;23(2):87-93.
33. Stöllberger C, Schneider B, Finsterer J. Serious complications from dislocation of a Watchman left atrial appendage occluder. *J Cardiovasc Electrophysiol.* 2007;18(8):880-881.
34. Connolly SJ, Ezekowitz MD, Yusuf S, et al. Dabigatran versus warfarin in patients with atrial fibrillation. *N Engl J Med.* 2009;361:1139-1151.

Video Legends

Videos 16.1–16.6 Echocardiographic exclusion of alternative cardioembolic sources.

Videos 16.7.1 and 16.7.2 Guidance of transseptal puncture.

Video 16.8 Angiographic assessment of the LAA.

Videos 16.8 and 16.9 Wiring of the left upper pulmonary vein and introduction of the pigtail catheter.

Videos 16.10 and 16.11 Introduction of the sheath.

Video 16.12 Introduction of the device and deployment of the distal lobe.

Video 16.13 Deployment of the proximal part of the device.

Videos 16.14 and 16.15 Stability test.

Video 16.16 Release of the device.

Videos 16.17 and 16.18 Angiographic control.

Videos 16.19–16.22 Safety issues. Includes information on thrombus on sheath, thrombus on PLAATO device, small pericardial effusion, and thrombus on AGA cardiac plug device.

CHAPTER 17

Principles and Techniques for Lead Extraction and Device System Revision for the Surgeon and Interventionalist

Melanie Maytin, MD; Laurence M. Epstein, MD

History

The discipline of transvenous lead extraction (TLE) has evolved exponentially since its inception as a rudimentary skill with limited technology and therapeutic options. Prior to the introduction of successful intravascular countertraction techniques, options for lead extraction were limited and dedicated tools nonexistent. Early techniques involved simple manual traction that frequently proved ineffective for chronically implanted leads and carried a high risk of myocardial avulsion, tamponade, and death.[1,2] Bilgutay and colleagues attempted to improve the success rate of simple traction by creating a graded weight-and-pulley system to deliver sustained gentle traction on the externalized portion of a lead.[3] This method failed to significantly improve outcomes and suffered from similar limitations. In addition, weighted traction typically required prolonged bedrest and heightened the risk of infection. Also, the significant morbidity and mortality associated with these early extraction techniques limited their application to life-threatening situations such as infection and sepsis.

The past three decades have witnessed significant advances in lead extraction technology, resulting in safer and more efficacious techniques and tools. With the development of the field, the community of TLE experts has grown. This growth has coincided with a marked decline in the incidence of procedure-related morbidity and mortality. More recent registries at high-volume centers are reporting high success rates with exceedingly low complication rates (Figure 17.1).[4-7]

Lead–Body Interaction

The challenges and risks of TLE are principally related to the foreign-body response to the cardiovascular implantable electronic device (CIED). This response begins at implantation with thrombus development along the lead. Fibrosis of the thrombus occurs next, and near-complete encapsulation of the leads by a fibrin sheath takes place within 4 to 5 days of implant.[8,9] Robust fibrosis develops in areas of direct contact between the lead and both the vasculature and endocardium (Figures 17.2A and B). The most common adhesion sites include the venous entry site, the superior vena cava (SVC), and the electrode tip–myocardial interface; the majority of patients have multiple areas of scar tissue.[10] Calcification of the fibrotic lesions can occur over time, further cementing the adhesion site and increasing the difficulties and risks of extraction. Although predictors of severe scar formation have not been clearly identified, it appears that younger patients develop more vigorous fibrotic responses and more frequently develop progressive calcification.[11]

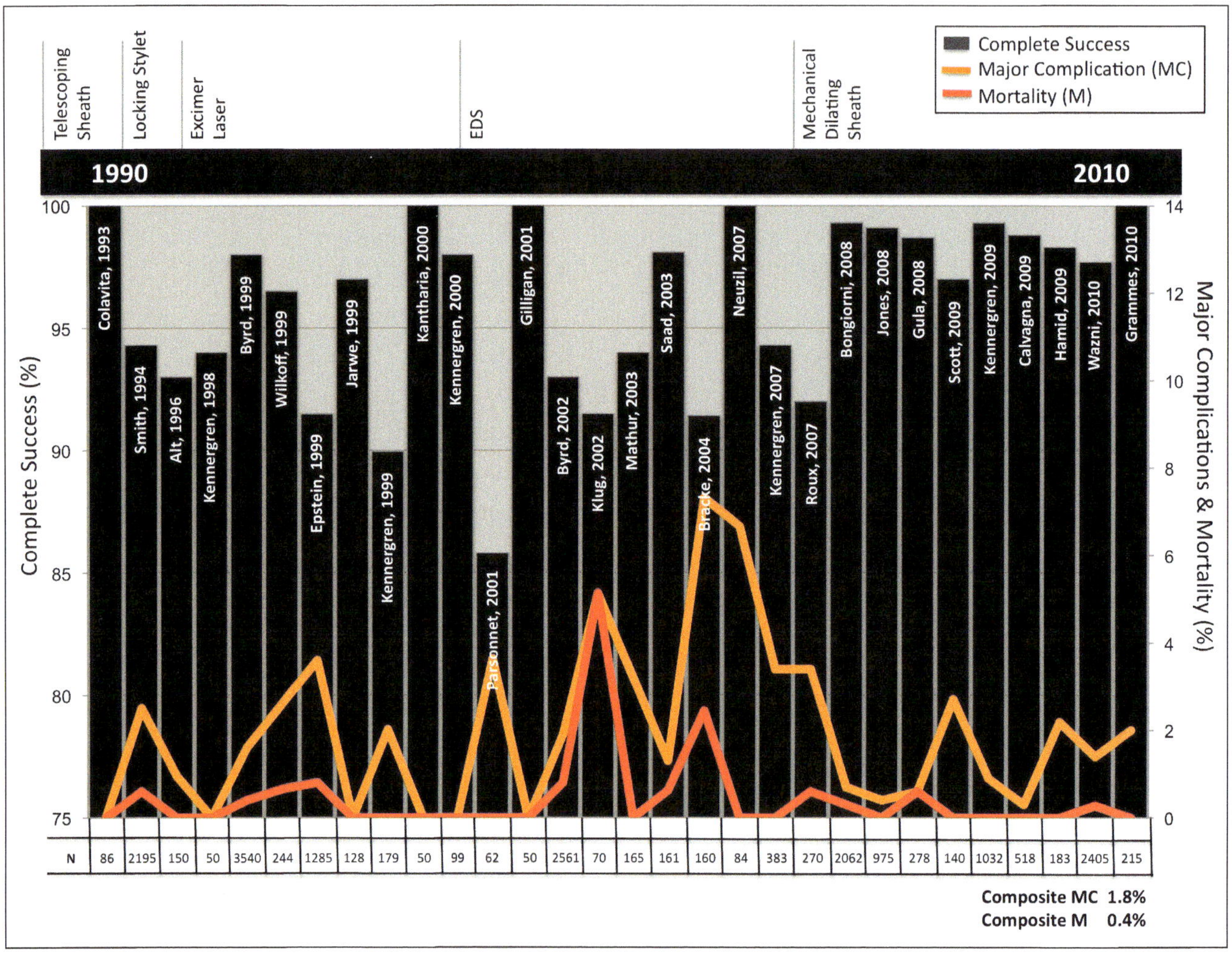

172 • Section 1C: Device Technology

Figure 17.1 Success, morbidity, and mortality of transvenous lead extraction in a series of large trials. Graphic representation of complete success as a function of time, represented by black columns. Secondary y-axis represents % morbidity (**orange**) and mortality (**red**). Timeline of extraction techniques and tools commensurate with reported trials shown at **top**. Values below the graph represent the number of leads (N) extracted in each study. Composite major complication (MC) and mortality (M) rates were calculated. Only studies with ≥50 leads extracted *and* data regarding mortality and major complications were included. EDS = electrosurgical dissection sheaths.

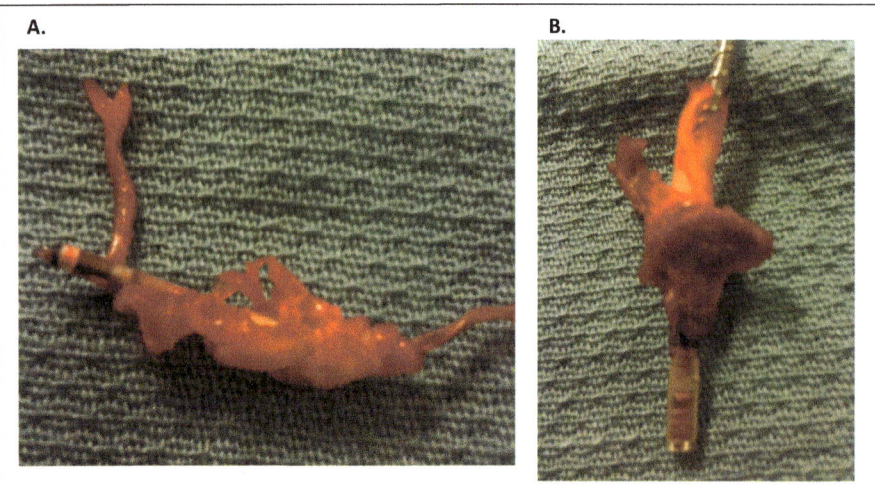

Figure 17.2 Vigorous fibrosis that developed in areas of direct contact between the lead and the vasculature and myocardium. **Panel A:** Extracted atrial lead with intense fibrosis at its distal portion. **Panel B:** Extracted defibrillator lead found to have a large amount of organized fibrosis at the electrode tip–myocardial interface.

Lead Management

CIED use has increased exponentially over the past decade,[12-14] with more than 4.5 million active devices and more than 1 million new leads implanted annually.[15,16] With expanded CIED utilization and indications for device therapy, observed complications have increased in parallel.[17-25] More frequent device system revisions for complications,[17-19] system upgrade,[26-28] and/or lead malfunction,[20-24] and longer patient life expectancies have all mandated a paradigm shift toward premeditated lead management strategies—from implant to removal or replacement. Proactive lead management requires both forethought and conscious decisions at the time of CIED implantation with respect to a variety of factors: hardware selection (eg, single-coil vs dual-coil defibrillator leads), implant vein access (ie, traditional vs nontraditional venous access), and if necessary, lead abandonment versus extraction.

Definitions

Standardized definitions are essential for ensuring uniformity of procedure classification and outcomes reporting. They are outlined in the 2009 Heart Rhythm Society (HRS) Expert Consensus Statement on Transvenous Lead Extraction.[29] The term *lead removal* is used to describe the removal of a pacing or defibrillator lead by any method and encompasses both lead explant and lead extraction. *Lead explant* refers to the removal of a pacing or defibrillator lead with simple traction (ie, without additional tools other than standard implant stylets). *Lead extraction*, in contrast, is defined as lead removal with the use of specialized tools (eg, locking stylets, countertraction sheaths) via a venous route other than the implant vein, and/or the removal of a lead(s) with implant duration(s) that exceeds one year. Similarly, standardized definitions have been created for TLE techniques and tools.

Uniformly accepted end points are crucial for the critical comparison of individual operator experience and results. *Complete procedural success* is defined as the complete removal of all leads planned for extraction in their entirety. *Clinical success* describes incomplete removal of all leads planned for extraction; only a small fragment of the lead(s) is retained, but it does not adversely affect the goal of the procedure or cause additional harm. *Failure* comprises the inability to achieve either complete procedural success or clinical success, or the occurrence of a permanent disabling complication or procedure-related death.

Complications are defined as a function of time and severity. *Intraprocedural complication* refers to a procedural complication that occurs any time between the patient entering and leaving the operating room. In contrast, a *postprocedural complication* is one that becomes evident within 30 days following the procedure. The severity of complications is divided into major and minor (Table 17.1). *Major complications* are those that threaten life, require significant surgical intervention, cause persistent or significant disability, or result in death. Complications that do not meet the major complication criteria are classified as *minor complications*.

Training

Complication rates with TLE directly parallel operator experience. Major and minor complications are reduced by approximately 50% with increased operator experience: from 20 to 120 cases to >300 cases performed.[30] Large-scale multicenter, randomized trials have confirmed the effect of experience on outcomes.[7,10,30-32] Likewise, observational registries of experienced, high-volume extractionists have consistently demonstrated even higher success rates (>99%), with exceedingly low major complication (<1.0%) and mortality rates (<0.3%).[4-6] Consequently, the 2009 HRS Expert Consensus Statement on Lead Extraction recommends that physicians being trained in TLE extract a minimum of 40 leads as the primary operator under the direct supervision of a qualified physician and extract a minimum of 20 leads annually to maintain their skills.[29] This recommendation is a minimum. The difficulty of any case can be quite variable,

Table 17.1 Potential complications of transvenous lead extraction

Major Complications	Minor Complications
• Death	• Pericardial Effusion Not Requiring Intervention
• Cardiac Avulsion Requiring Intervention (Percutaneous or Surgical)	• Hemothorax Not Requiring Intervention
• Vascular Injury Requiring Intervention (Percutaneous or Surgical)	• Pocket Hematoma Requiring Reoperation
• Pulmonary Embolism Requiring Surgical Intervention	• Upper Extremity Thrombosis Resulting in Medical Treatment
• Respiratory Arrest/Anesthesia-related Complication Prolonging Hospitalization	• Vascular Repair Near Implant Site or Venous Entry Site
	• Hemodynamically Significant Air Embolism
• Stroke	• Migrated Lead Fragment Without Sequelae
• CIED Infection at Previously Noninfected Site	• Blood Transfusion as a Result of Intraoperative Blood Loss
	• Pneumothorax Requiring a Chest Tube
	• Pulmonary Embolism Not Requiring Surgical Intervention

and future challenges will most likely not be experienced with the extraction of only 40 leads. For new extractors and programs, a conservative approach of attempting more difficult cases as experience is gained seems warranted. There is also an extraction community of experienced physicians available for consultation and advice.

Given the limited number of high-volume extraction centers, obtaining adequate training during fellowship can be difficult and the opportunity for formal training after fellowship is almost nonexistent. The challenges of obtaining sufficient training have led to the invention of alternative training tools. One such approach has been the development of computerized simulation models. While preliminary studies have demonstrated an improvement in simulated-extraction skills with practice, the correlation of these findings to clinical outcomes remains to be validated.

Indications

As advances in extraction techniques have made the procedure safer and more successful, TLE indications have expanded to include more clinical situations.[29] The recently published 2009 HRS Expert Consensus Statement on Transvenous Lead Extraction extended class I indications to include patients with CIED pocket infection, occult gram-positive infection, and functional leads that, owing to design or failure, may pose an immediate threat if left in place (Table 17.2). The class II indications for TLE were further divided into class IIa (reasonable to perform the procedure) and class IIb (may consider performing the procedure) indications. Class IIa indications for TLE include the following: CIED patients with occult gram-negative bacteremia, severe chronic pain, ipsilateral venous occlusion with contraindication to contralateral implantation, nonfunctional leads, and need for magnetic resonance imaging (MRI) with no other imaging alternatives, and in whom implantation would result in more than 4 leads on one side or more than 5 leads through the SVC. Class IIb indications for TLE include CIED patients with superfluous functional or nonfunctional leads, those with functional leads that pose a risk of device interference, or those whose device (owing to design or failure) poses a potential future risk.

In assessing an individual's indication for TLE, comparing the risks of extraction with the risks of lead abandonment is mandated (Figure 17.3). The consideration of patient and lead characteristics and, importantly, operator experience must be factored into the assessment of extraction risk. The risk assessment evaluation must pay specific attention to the number of leads, implant duration, defibrillator versus pacing electrodes, and patient age.

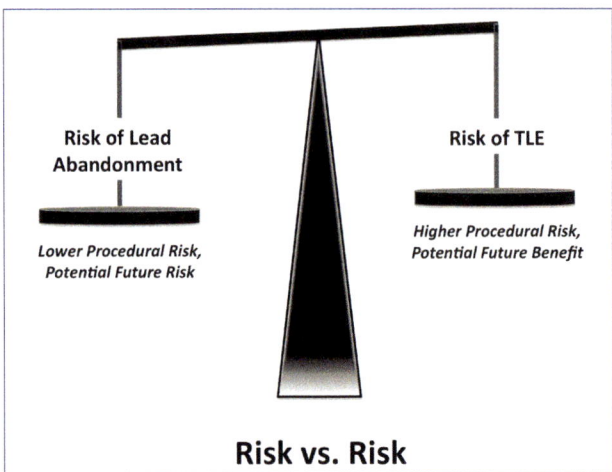

Figure 17.3 Risk of lead abandonment versus lead extraction. The decision regarding lead extraction or abandonment requires weighing the current risks of lead extraction against the future risks of both lead abandonment and potential lead extraction.

Decisions regarding lead extraction must be made on a case-by-case basis, integrating various patient and lead characteristics and operator-related variables. Lead extraction with the potential for significant morbidity and mortality may not be warranted in patients with a poor prognosis or where the risks of intervention clearly outweigh the risks of lead abandonment. Additionally, operators who are inexperienced in the procedure should not perform lead extractions, nor should those who lack the necessary tools to attain complete success or those in a practice setting not prepared and committed to the complete and safe performance of the procedure.[29]

TLE Techniques and Tools

Preoperative Planning

General: TLE, like any surgical procedure, requires a team approach that anticipates and plans for all potential situations. The required personnel of the extraction team include, at a minimum, the following: the physician performing the extraction, a cardiothoracic surgeon (if not the primary operator), anesthesia support, an x-ray technician or other person to operate the fluoroscopy, and both scrubbed and nonscrubbed assistants. Although complications will occur, the single most important factor in preventing a major complication from becoming a death is the time to intervention. Thus, the procedure location (eg, operating room or catheterization or electrophysiology lab) is less important than the immediate availability of cardiothoracic surgical intervention. This contingency mandates that a surgeon proficient in managing the potential complications be on site during the extraction procedure and that the equipment necessary for cardiopulmonary bypass be readily available.

Table 17.2 Indications for transvenous lead extraction[29]

Indication	Class I Procedure SHOULD be performed	Class IIa REASONABLE to perform procedure	Class IIb Procedure MAY BE CONSIDERED	Class III Procedure should NOT be performed
Infection	1. Definite CIED infection, eg, valvular endocarditis, DRE, or sepsis. (LOE: B) 2. CIED pocket infection, eg, abscess, erosion, or chronic draining sinus. (LOE: B) 3. Valvular endocarditis without definite lead and/or device involvement. (LOE: B) 4. Occult gram-positive bacteremia. (LOE: B)	1. Persistent occult gram-negative bacteremia. (LOE: B)		1. Superficial or incisional infection without involvement of device/leads. (LOE: C) 2. Chronic bacteremia due to a source other than CIED when long-term suppressive antibiotics are required. (LOE: C)
Thrombosis or venous stenosis	1. Clinically significant TE events associated with thrombus on lead or fragment. (LOE: C) 2. Bilateral SCV or SVC occlusion precluding implant of needed TV lead. (LOE: C) 3. Planned stent deployment in vein with TV lead already to avoid entrapment. (LOE: C) 4. Symptomatic SVC stenosis/occlusion. (LOE: C) 5. Ipsilateral venous occlusion precluding implant of additional lead when contralateral implant contraindicated (AVF, shunt, or vascular access port, mastectomy). (LOE: C)	1. Ipsilateral venous occlusion precluding ipsilateral implant of additional lead without contraindication to contralateral implant. (LOE: C)		
Functional leads	1. Life-threatening arrhythmias due to retained leads. (LOE: B) 2. Leads, due to design or failure, may pose immediate threat if left in place. (LOE: B) 3. Leads that interfere with CIED function. (LOE: B) 4. Leads that interfere with treatment of malignancy (radiation, surgery). (LOE: C)		1. Leads with potential interference with CIED function. (LOE: C) 2. Leads, due to design or failure, that pose a potential threat if left in place. (LOE: C) 3. Abandoned leads. (LOE: C) 4. Need for MRI imaging without alternative. (LOE: C) 5. Need for MRI conditional CIED system. (LOE: C)	1. Redundant leads with <1 yr life expectancy. (LOE: C) 2. Known anomalous lead placement (SCA, Ao, pleura, etc.) or through a systemic atrium or ventricle.* (LOE: C) *Can be considered with surgical backup.
Nonfunctional leads		1. Leads, due to design or failure, that pose a potential threat if left in place. (LOE: C) 2. CIED implant would yield >4 leads on 1 side or >5 leads through SVC. (LOE: C) 3. Need for MRI without alternative. (LOE: C)	1. At time of indicated CIED procedure without contraindication to TLE. (LOE: C) 2. Need for MRI conditional CIED system. (LOE: C)	1. Redundant leads with <1 yr life expectancy. (LOE: C) 2. Known anomalous lead placement (SCA, Ao, pleura, etc.) or through a systemic atrium or ventricle.* (LOE: C) *Can be considered with surgical backup.
Chronic pain		1. Severe chronic pain at device or lead insertion site with significant discomfort not manageable by medical or surgical techniques and without acceptable alternative. (LOE: C)		

CIED = cardiovascular implantable electronic device; DRE = device-related endocarditis; TE = thromboembolic; SCV = subclavian vein; SVC = superior vena cava; SCA = subclavian artery; Ao = aorta; TV = transvenous; TLE = transvenous lead extraction; LOE = level of evidence; MRI = magnetic resonance imaging. *Source:* Adapted from Wilkoff BL, et al.[29]

Additional emergency equipment should be present in the room or immediately available. This includes transthoracic and transesophageal echocardiography, a pericardiocentesis tray, vacuum containers for chest tube drainage, temporary pacing equipment, an anesthesia cart for general anesthesia, and vasopressors and other emergency medications. We have fashioned a mobile "extraction cart" that contains all the aforementioned emergency equipment in addition to extraction tools (locking stylets, nonpowered and powered sheaths, femoral workstations, extraction snares, etc) and CIED implant tools (stylets, wrenches, fixation tools, introducer sheaths, intravenous contrast, repair kits, etc).

Transvenous Lead Extraction Cart Contents
• Stylets
• Wrenches
• Fixation tools
• Introducer sheaths
• Venous access kits
• Coronary sinus sheaths (with valves and splitters)
• Intravenous contrast
• Repair kits
• IS-1 and DF-1 pins
• Locking stylets (LLD® and Liberator®)
• #5 silk
• Bulldog™ lead extenders
• Mechanical dilating sheaths
• Evolution® (11 Fr, 13 Fr) and Evolution® Shortie (9 Fr, 11 Fr) sheaths
• Laser sheaths (12 Fr, 14 Fr, 16 Fr) and outer sheaths (S, M, L)
• Byrd femoral workstations™
• Extraction snares (Needle's Eye®, Tulip, and Amplatz GooseNeck snares)
• Bioptome forceps
• Blazer radiofrequency ablation catheter (medium and large curve)
• Temporary pacing equipment
• Pericardiocenteis tray
• Vacuum containers for pericardial/chest tube drainage

Recognizing the potential need for emergent surgical intervention, our patients are prepared for the procedure so as to eliminate any delays. We prep and drape our patients to allow access for contralateral implant or emergent pericardiocentesis, thoracentesis, thoracotomy, sternotomy, or cardiopulmonary bypass. It is our practice that all patients have bilateral peripheral venous access with large bore catheters, femoral venous access, invasive hemodynamic monitoring with a radial arterial line, general endotracheal anesthesia, and 4 units of packed red blood cells immediately available.

Patient-specific: Prior to scheduling, many patient-specific factors must be considered. In addition to the usual preoperative considerations, one must also be sure of what hardware is actually implanted. Some leads require specific tools, such as stylets, to retract an active fixation screw. Registered device/lead information can be inaccurate, and abandoned leads may not be properly identified. We recommend a chest x-ray in all patients to identify what hardware is present and its anatomic location. If there is any concern that a lead may no longer be intravascular or cardiac, further imaging such as computed tomography (CT) scanning is suggested. Does the patient have a history of prior cardiac surgery? This reduces the risk of perforation but increases the difficulty of surgical intervention if required. Are you going to reimplant at the time of extraction? And, if so, what is the plan for vascular access? If the implant vein occluded, removing the lead with traction may cause you to lose access. Will the patient require temporary pacing for the procedure or for some time afterward in case of infection?

TLE Tools

There is no one "right" tool for lead extraction. Each patient presents a unique clinical scenario, so having all available tools is important to success. While many extractors have individual preferences for a given situation, all experienced extractors agree that having a full "quiver" of tools is required to achieve the highest possible success rate safely.

Locking Stylets: The ability to successfully extract a lead with traction is directly dependent upon the lead construction and its tensile strength.[11] Locking stylets were developed to reinforce the lead, transmit the extraction force to the tip of the lead, reduce the risk of lead disruption, and increase the likelihood of complete lead removal.[33-35] Several types of locking stylets have been designed. While the original locking stylets had to be sized to the luminal diameter of the conductor coil, the most commonly utilized locking stylets today are designed to accommodate a range of conductor coil diameters. The Liberator (Cook Medical, Bloomington, IN) and Lead Locking Device (LLD) EZ (Spectranetics, Colorado Springs, CO) stylets offer similar support but differ in their locking mechanism design. The locking mechanism of the Liberator is located at the distal tip of the stylet, providing focal traction at the tip of the lead, whereas the LLD EZ stylet grabs the lead in multiple areas and exerts force along the length of the lead (Figures 17.4A and B).

If a lead cannot receive a locking stylet (either because of extensive damage or a solid-core design), applying sufficient traction to it can prove challenging. The Bulldog Lead Extender (Cook Medical, Bloomington, IN) is a tool that can be useful in this situation (Figure 17.5). It consists of a wire with a threadable handle through which the lead is passed and secured, thereby locking the insulation and conductor to the extender.

The advent of locking stylets has permitted safer and more successful transvenous lead extraction via the implant vein, stimulating the development of related techniques and technologies.

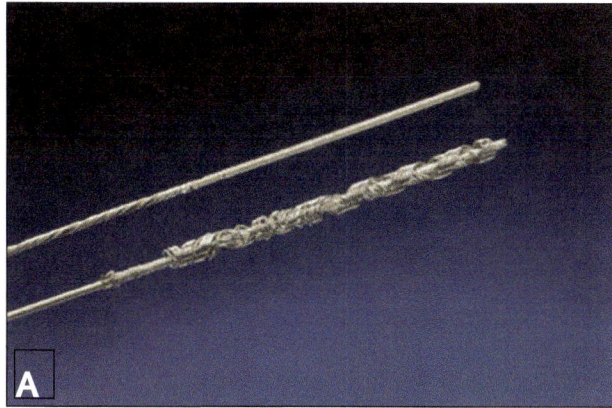

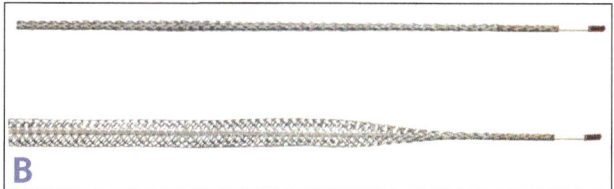

Figure 17.4 Locking stylets for transvenous lead extraction. (**A**) The Liberator Locking Stylet (Cook Medical, Bloomington, IN) fits leads with lumen diameters of 0.016 to 0.032 inches. An undeployed Liberator locking stylet is shown above a deployed Liberator locking stylet. When deployed, the wound spring at the end of the stylet opens up, locking into place. *Source:* Courtesy of Cook Medical. (**B**) The Lead Locking Device (LLD) EZ (Spectranetics, Colorado Springs, CO) has a radiopaque tip and accommodates inner coil diameters of 0.015 to 0.026 inches (undeployed stylet, **top**). In contrast to the Liberator Locking Stylet, the LLD locking stylet has a braided mesh over the entire length of a solid lead that expands when deployed (**bottom**). *Source:* Courtesy of Spectranetics.

Telescoping Sheaths: Telescoping sheaths are nonpowered sheaths available in a range of sizes from 7 Fr to 16 Fr.

They are made of different materials with varying properties, including stainless steel, Teflon®, and polypropylene (Figures 17.6A, B, C). Teflon is soft and flexible but is unable to cut through dense scar tissue; in contrast, polypropylene is stiffer and better at disrupting encapsulating scar but must be used with caution so as to avoid vascular injury. Stainless steel sheaths are employed only for disrupting dense and calcified fibrosis as the central venous circulation is entered. The inner and outer sheath pair is advanced along the lead with alternating counterclockwise and clockwise motions while applying moderate pressure. The soft inner sheath is used as a guide, while the more rigid outer sheath serves to disrupt and dilate the encapsulating fibrous tissue. Sufficient traction is essential to ensure that the sheaths track the path of the lead and remain within the confines of the vasculature under fluoroscopic guidance. Using telescoping sheaths, TLE success rates via a superior (eg, implant vein) approach range from 71% to 97%.[33,34,36,37]

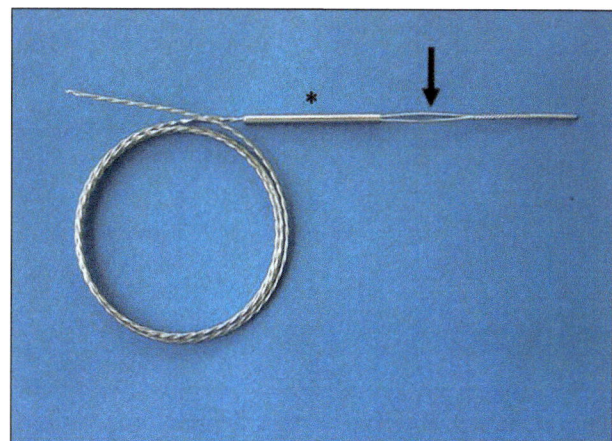

Figure 17.5 The Bulldog Lead Extender (Cook Medical, Bloomington, IN). This useful tool is meant for leads that cannot receive a locking stylet, owing to either extensive damage or a solid-core design. The exposed end of the lead is passed through the loop of the Bulldog (**arrow**), and the metal sleeve (**asterisk**) is advanced over the loop grasping the lead. *Source:* Courtesy of Cook Medical.

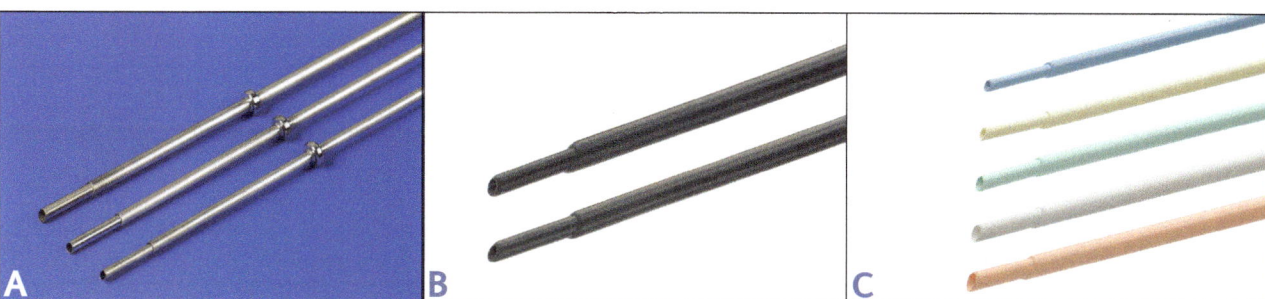

Figure 17.6 Telescoping nonpowered countertraction sheaths. Telescoping sheaths are available in a range of sizes from 7 Fr to 16 Fr and are made of different materials with varying properties, including (**A**) stainless steel, (**B**) Teflon, and (**C**) polypropylene. *Source:* Courtesy of Cook Medical.

Powered Sheaths: Powered sheaths employ a source of energy to make the dissection of encapsulating fibrous tissue easier and more efficient. They enable the advancement of the sheath along the lead with reduced countertraction and counterpressure forces.[11,38] One such powered sheath is the Excimer Laser System (Spectranetics, Colorado Springs, CO), a "cool" pulsed ultraviolet laser at a wavelength of 308 nm and available in 12, 14, and 16 Fr sizes (Figures 17.7A and B). The laser sheath applies circumferential pulses of energy from its distal end. This energy dissolves tissue that comes in contact with the tip of the sheath by photochemical destruction of molecular bonds and photothermal ablation that vaporizes water and ruptures cells with resultant photomechanical creation of kinetic energy (Figure 17.8).[39] The sheath is advanced over the lead body, utilizing the standard techniques of counterpressure and countertraction, and laser energy is delivered when encapsulating fibrous tissue halts sheath advancement. Tissue in direct contact with the sheath tip is ablated to a depth of 50 μm until the distal electrode is reached; countertraction is still necessary to dislocate the lead tip. Compared with mechanical telescoping sheaths, laser-assisted extraction resulted in more frequent complete lead removal and shortened extraction times without an increase in procedural risk.[31,32,40] The introduction of laser extraction has changed the landscape of transvenous extraction, providing a highly effective and low-morbidity technique with broad applications.[7,31,32]

The Perfecta® Electrosurgical Dissection Sheath (Cook Medical, Bloomington, IN) represents another type of powered sheath. The electrosurgical dissection sheath consists of an inner polytetrafluoroethylene (PTFE) sheath with bipolar tungsten electrodes exposed at the distal tip and an outer sheath for counterpressure and countertraction. Radiofrequency energy is delivered between the bipoles to dissect through fibrous binding sites, much like a surgical cautery tool, although the lead tip must be liberated with countertraction. In contrast to the Excimer Laser Sheath, the Electrosurgical Dissection Sheath permits localized application of radiofrequency energy with linear rather than circumferential dissection of the encapsulating fibrous tissue. The focused and steerable dissection plane offers the potential advantages of improved precision and diminished risk. The Electrosurgical Dissection Sheath offers a cost-effective alternative to the Excimer Laser System without compromising safety or efficacy.[41]

Despite the improved success rates of lead extraction with powered sheath technologies, disruption of calcified binding sites remains difficult with either system. The most recent addition to the armamentarium of lead extraction tools provides a solution. The Evolution® and Evolution® Shortie Mechanical Dilator Sheaths (Cook Medical, Bloomington, IN) are "hand-powered" mechanical sheaths that consist of a flexible, braided stainless steel sheath with a stainless steel spiral-cut dissection tip. The sheath is attached to a trigger-activation handle that rotates the sheath and allows the threaded metal end to bore through calcified and dense adhesions (Figure 17.9).[42] In our experience, we have found the Evolution® sheath quite useful for disrupting sites of calcified fibrosis, though often at the expense of functional leads that we were attempting to preserve. Regardless, this technology has provided an effective alternative for dealing with the challenges of densely scarred venous entry sites and heavily calcified adhesions.[43]

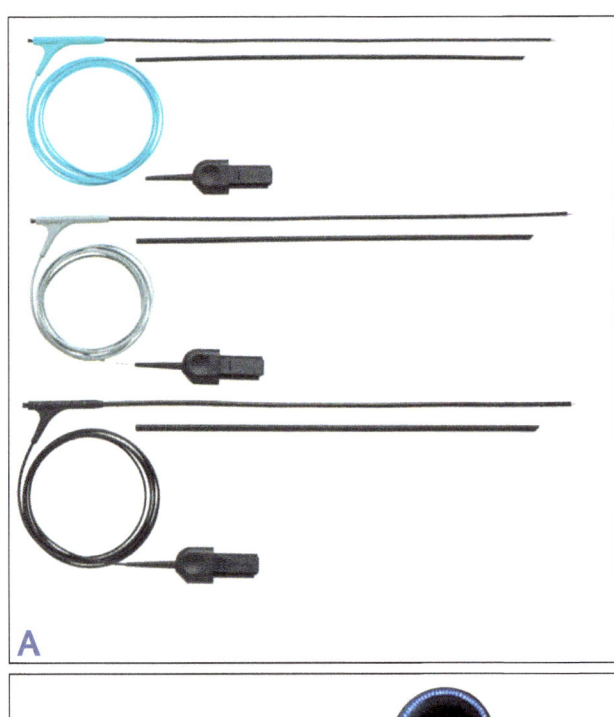

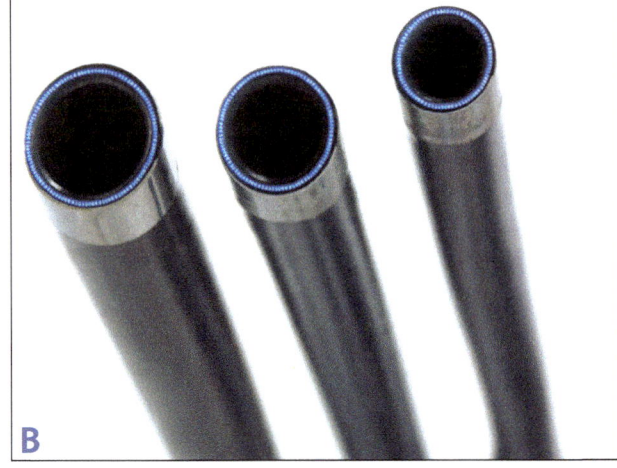

Figure 17.7 Excimer laser sheaths (Spectranetics, Colorado Springs, CO). **Panel A:** The Excimer laser sheath utilizes ultraviolet laser energy to vaporize tissue in contact with the tip of the sheath, where the optical fibers terminate. The sheath is available in a range of sizes (12 Fr, 14 Fr, and 16 Fr), displayed from top to bottom. **Panel B:** End-on view of the laser sheath showing the distal end, where the optical fibers terminate. *Source:* Courtesy of Spectranetics.

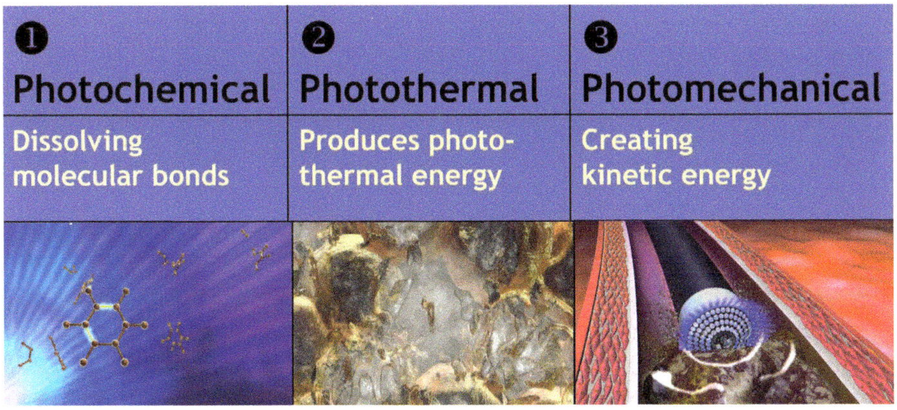

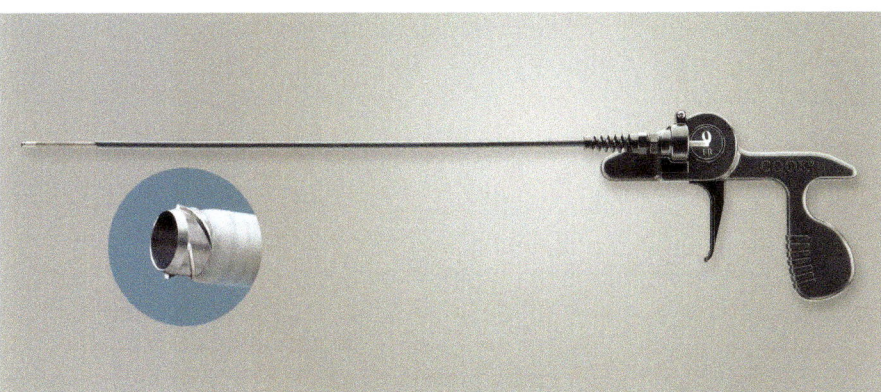

Figure 17.8 Mechanism of photoablation. The laser sheath applies circumferential pulses of energy at its distal end. The ultraviolet energy disrupts molecular bonds to a depth of 50 μm, causing cells to rupture and fibrotic tissue to dissolve, forming a vapor bubble. The vapor bubble expands and implodes, clearing debris from the distal end of the sheath. *Source:* Courtesy of Spectranetics.

Figure 17.9 The Evolution Mechanical Dilator Sheath (Cook Medical, Bloomington, IN). This "hand-powered" mechanical sheath consists of a flexible, braided stainless steel sheath with a stainless steel spiral-cut dissection tip (**inset**). The sheath is attached to a trigger handle that rotates the sheath and allows the threaded metal end to bore out the scar tissue. *Source:* Courtesy of Cook Medical.

Femoral Tools: Transfemoral lead retrieval with the Byrd Workstation™ (Cook Medical, Bloomington, IN) is a necessary skill for successful lead extraction. This is true particularly in cases where the lead is not accessible from the implant vein, as in a cut or fractured lead (Figure 17.10). The Byrd Workstation consists of a 16-Fr outer sheath with a one-way valve that is advanced over a wire into the femoral vein and a 12-Fr inner sheath through which a number of retrieval snares can be advanced. The Workstation package contains a Needle's Eye snare (although a number of other snares can be utilized, including Tulip and Amplatz GooseNeck snares). If lead retrieval with a Needle's Eye snare proves unsuccessful, we have found the combination of a gooseneck snare and bioptome forceps to be quite successful. In this situation, we preload the gooseneck snare on the bioptome, advance the two together to the lead fragment, grasp the free lead tail with the bioptome, and then advance the gooseneck snare over the bioptome to the ensnare the lead.

The challenge of femoral retrieval remains manipulating the tools and snaring the lead in three dimensions while using two-dimensional fluoroscopic imaging. The recent description of a novel technology to facilitate extraction and maintenance of vascular access proposed a hybrid superior and inferior approach. This approach, which involves femoral snaring of the lead to stabilize the lead while countertraction and counterpressure are used to free the lead, reinforces the clinical importance of femoral retrieval.[44]

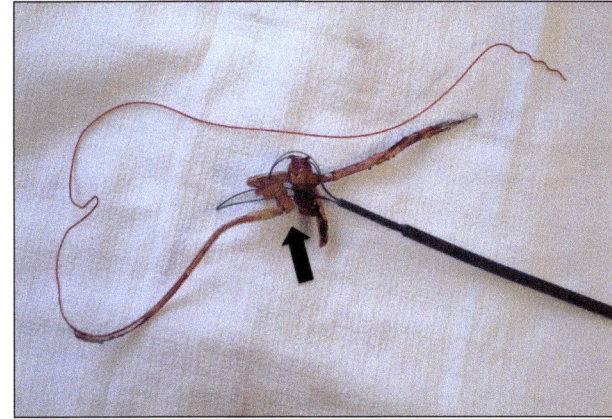

Figure 17.10 Transfemoral snaring of a lead. Transfemoral lead retrieval with the Byrd Workstation (Cook Medical, Bloomington, IN) is a necessary skill for successful lead extraction, particularly in cases where the lead is not accessible from the implant vein, as in a cut or fractured lead. Here the lead has been snared and wound up by the Needle's Eye snare (**arrow**), allowing successful removal of the lead.

TLE Techniques

In every case, we employ a stepwise approach to lead extraction with the goal of complete success utilizing the fewest tools (Figure 17.11). Because we routinely perform TLE by superior approach via the implant vein, the first step in the extraction procedure is making an appropriately positioned incision that permits easy access to the venous entry site in a plane parallel to the leads (Video 17.1). It is our practice to attempt to use the existing incision whenever possible and perform an elliptical incision excising the existing incisional scar. Occasionally, two incisions are necessary: one over the venous entry site of the leads and a second over the pocket or area of skin erosion or adherence. Once the pocket is entered, microbial cultures of pocket tissue are obtained in all cases of CIED infection. Then the device is removed and the leads are dissected free, back to their venous entry site. Dissection around the venous entry site is important because it allows for easy passage of any devices that may be necessary for lead extraction. However, aggressive dissection can result in transient problems with hemostasis secondary to back bleeding. The anchor sleeves are then removed and all extraneous material, including suture material, is eliminated from the pocket. Complete removal of infected tissue and foreign material is mandatory in cases of CIED infection. Additionally, we routinely perform a capsulectomy whenever ipsilateral reimplantation is planned.

If ipsilateral reimplantation is planned, ipsilateral venous access is attempted under fluoroscopic guidance with or without the aid of intravenous contrast. In our experience, stenotic lesions can often be crossed by using a 5 Fr dilator and Terumo Glidewire® (Terumo Interventional Systems, Somerset, NJ) (Video 17.2). If the vein is successfully cannulated and a wire can be passed into the inferior vena cava (IVC), or if ipsilateral reimplantation is not planned, lead removal with simple traction is attempted. If this proves unsuccessful, the lead is cut and a locking stylet with #5 silk is introduced and traction reattempted. The #5 silk is used to reinforce the lead and to prevent the insulation from bunching up or "snowplowing" under the force of counterpressure (Video 17.3). If lead removal still proves unsuccessful, a nonpowered or powered sheath is employed (Video 17.4). Sheath selection is determined by the clinical situation and the operator's preference and experience. If the lead is not retrievable from the implant vein or lead disruption occurs, transfemoral retrieval is performed.

Counterpressure is the force applied by the nonpowered or powered sheath as it is advanced over the lead, interrupting areas of adherent scar tissue. Sufficient traction must be applied to the lead and locking stylet so as to allow the sheath to follow the lead body and not damage the vasculature as the lead curves within the vein. Countertraction is a technique employed once the sheath has been advanced to the lead tip–myocardium interface. Applying countertraction limits the traction forces on an entrapped electrode to the circumference of the sheath at the lead tip–myocardium interface. Once the lead is released from the fibrous tissue, the myocardium falls away from the sheath, thereby reducing the risk of myocardial invagination and injury (Figure 17.12).[33,36,45]

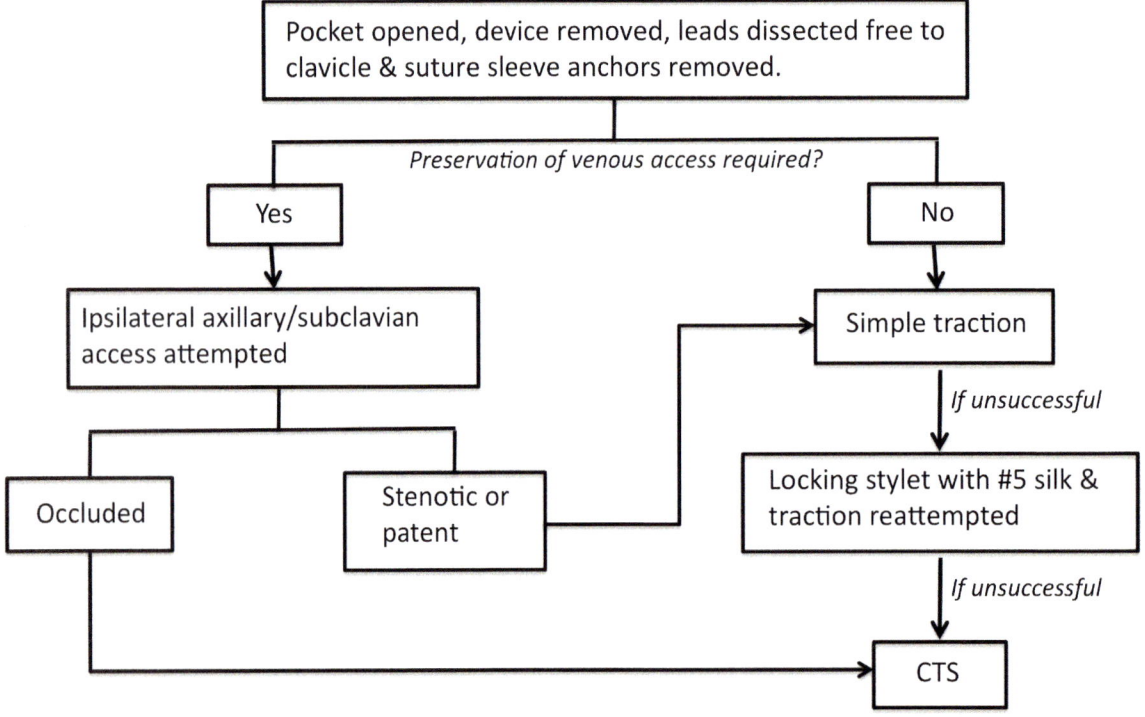

Figure 17.11 Stepwise approach to transvenous lead extraction. We routinely employ a stepwise approach to lead extraction so as to achieve the highest rate of complete success utilizing the fewest tools. CTS = countertraction sheath.

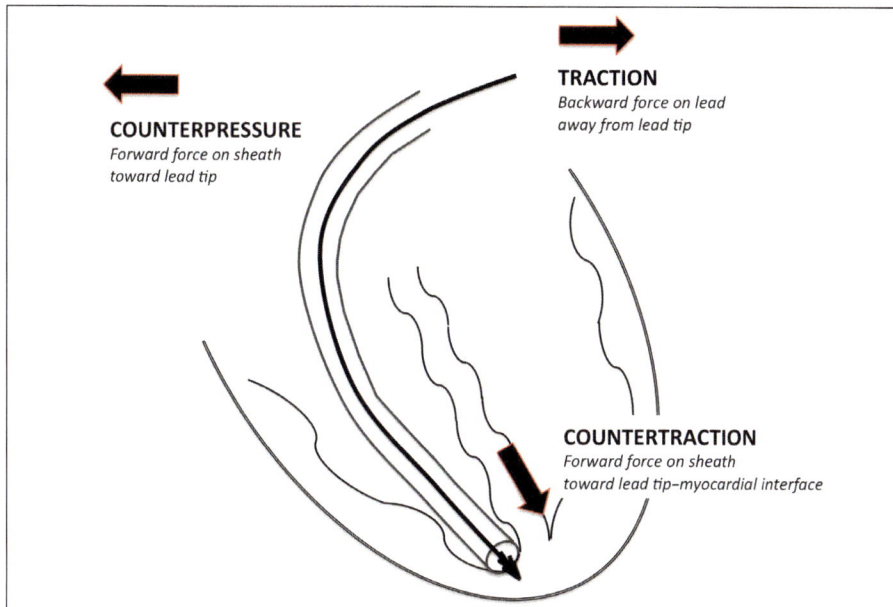

Figure 17.12 Schematic representation of the forces of counterpressure, traction, and countertraction. Counterpressure is the force applied by the nonpowered or powered sheath as it is advanced over the lead, interrupting areas of adherent scar tissue. Traction is the pulling force on the lead to provide a straight "rail" so as to allow the sheath to follow the lead. Countertraction is the forward force applied by the sheath at the myocardium to limit the traction forces on an entrapped electrode to the circumference of the sheath at the lead tip–myocardium interface. Once the lead is released from the fibrous tissue, the myocardium falls away from the sheath, thereby reducing the risk of myocardial invagination and injury.

Lead Extraction Approach

Leads are typically extracted by a superior approach via the implant vein, although alternative approaches are used in certain situations. For example, when the free lead tip cannot be reached from the implant vein, an inferior approach via the femoral vein is necessary. Occasionally, hybrid or alternative venous approaches are utilized. Bongiorni and colleagues reported on the success of a combined approach via the femoral and internal jugular veins for free-floating leads and leads with dense SVC adhesions.[6] Lead stabilization by femoral snaring via an inferior approach provides a straighter "rail" for extraction approach from the right internal jugular vein, decreasing the likelihood of SVC avulsion. Recently, Fischer et al[44] described a hybrid superior and inferior approach with femoral snaring of the lead to provide stability from below while counterpressure and traction were applied from above. They demonstrated this to be a safe and effective technique for lead extraction while maintaining venous access.

Surgical Extraction

Today, surgical lead extraction is reserved primarily for cases of incomplete or failed TLE or for individuals at excessive risk from the TLE procedure. The surgical extraction of transvenous leads can prove technically challenging and should be performed by skilled cardiac surgeons. Three surgical approaches have been described for lead extraction: open heart with cardiopulmonary bypass, right ventriculotomy, and the transatrial approach. An open-heart procedure with cardiopulmonary bypass via standard median sternotomy is a typical cardiac surgical approach and the most familiar. This approach allows for direct visualization of the transvenous leads and removal with direct traction.

Right ventriculotomy can be performed via median sternotomy or a small incision in the anterior left fifth intercostal space. In contrast to an open-heart procedure, the lead tip is identified by fluoroscopy, a purse string suture is placed around the lead tip, and the ventriculotomy performed. Lead removal is achieved by direct traction.

The transatrial approach was developed to minimize the invasive nature and postoperative morbidity of surgical lead extraction. It was first described by Byrd and colleagues in 1985[46] and remains a useful technique for lead extraction or implantation if avoiding the SVC or IVC is desired. A limited incision is made in the right anterior chest wall, and the third or fourth costal cartilage is removed to expose the right atrium. A purse string suture is placed in the atrium, and atriotomy is performed. The lead is grasped via the atriotomy and cut. The proximal portion is removed with direct traction, while the distal portion of the lead is removed with countertraction sheath assistance. If indicated, lead implantation can be performed via the atriotomy.

Venoplasty

Venoplasty is a technique that can be used in conjunction with, or as an alternative to, lead extraction. It is indicated in cases of venous obstruction among patients who require the addition of a lead or leads to the existing CIED. Spittell and colleagues first described the procedure in 1990 in two patients with pacemakers and indications for device system revision.[47] Since its inception, few studies about the use of venoplasty in the setting of lead revision had been reported until recently. Worley et al[48] described an 11-year experience of subclavian venoplasty among 373 patients with a 99.5% success rate and no complications.

Following peripheral contrast venography to identify the location of the obstruction, a 5-Fr dilator is advanced over a J-wire to the level of the obstruction and the stenosis is crossed with a Glidewire, as previously described. Once the lesion has been crossed, the Glidewire is replaced with extra-stiff wire to provide additional support. An appropriately sized peripheral balloon is advanced over the stiff wire to the area of obstruction and deployed with inflation to 15 to 30 atmospheres. Some operators employ stents to maintain venous patency. However, we feel strongly that this is never an option unless all existing transvenous leads have been removed to avoid trapping hardware between the stent and the vessel wall.

Complications can arise when the wire is unknowingly advanced into a collateral or branch vein or through fibrous tissue, resulting in venous rupture or dissection. Other potential complications include existing lead damage and contrast-induced nephropathy.

Device Reimplantation

CIED reimplantation following TLE can be ipsilateral or contralateral, immediate or delayed. The timing of reimplantation depends on the indication for extraction. Reimplantation can be performed at the time of TLE in cases of extraction for sterile indications (nonfunctional leads, superfluous functional leads, etc). However, reimplantation in cases of CIED pocket infections, bacteremia, and device-related endocarditis requires complete eradication of the active infection to reduce the chance of recurrence.

Following CIED infection, a critical appraisal of the continued need for device therapy is mandated prior to reimplant. If continued device therapy is indicated, specific recommendations regarding the timing of reimplant are available.[29,49] First, the location of CIED reimplantation should not be ipsilateral to the site of extraction. In cases of device pocket infection, positive lead-tip cultures, bacteremia, and sepsis, reimplantation can be performed after 72 hours of negative blood cultures from the time of extraction. In the case of device-related endocarditis, it is reasonable to delay reimplantation for a minimum of two weeks.

Pacemaker-dependent patients pose a particular challenge, given their continued pacing requirements during the sterilization time. Although temporary transvenous pacing is a reasonable solution, transvenous pacing catheters are frequently uncomfortable and can be unstable, as they are affected by patient position and thus necessitate bed rest. Moreover, the potential for additional complications limits the safe use of temporary transvenous pacing to several days. Alternatively, semipermanent pacing via a tunneled active transvenous pacing lead attached to an externalized, resterilized pulse generator affixed to the chest wall provides stable, long-term temporary pacing without discomfort or restrictions on mobility.[50]

Potential Complications and Management

Complications are inevitable, even among experienced extractionists. Rapidly recognizing and responding to complications are essential and represent the most important factors in preventing a major complication from becoming a death. Because different complications require different surgical approaches, rapid response requires not only the immediate availability of cardiac surgery but communication with the surgeon regarding the circumstances leading up to the complication and the believed anatomic location of the injury.

The most common causes of hypotension during TLE are vagal responses, cardiac tamponade, and hemothorax. Immediately available echocardiography (transthoracic and transesophageal) is necessary for the prompt diagnosis and treatment of cardiac tamponade. In addition, all extractionists should be capable of performing emergent pericardiocentesis. In our experience, pericardial bleeding frequently stabilizes and stops following percutaneous drainage. However, surgery should be performed in all cases of continued significant pericardial bleeding. Bleeding into the pleural space can be transiently masked by aggressive fluid resuscitation and, thus, this needs to be considered in any patient requiring significant volume resuscitation for the maintenance of blood pressure. It is not uncommon for patients to lose several liters of blood into the pleural space before the problem is diagnosed. Vascular injuries above the pericardial reflection or to the SVC require immediate surgical intervention in almost all cases. Vagal responses occur commonly in the setting of direct myocardial traction and will respond to fluid resuscitation and atropine. The majority of vagal responses are self-limiting.

Less common complications of TLE include acute tricuspid valve injury, arteriovenous fistula, and venous thrombosis. Traumatic tricuspid regurgitation can frequently be managed medically, although surgical repair is sometimes necessary in severe cases. Arteriovenous fistulae can manifest acutely at the time of the procedure or several days postprocedure, and management ranges from observation to percutaneous or open surgical correction. Venous thrombosis probably occurs more commonly than is recognized, but anticoagulation is warranted only in symptomatic cases. In cases of pocket infection, pocket hematomas are common following debridement.

Postprocedure Care

Although the overwhelming majority of complications become apparent intraoperatively, close attention should be paid to the patient's hemodynamic status in the immediate postoperative period. TLE recovery is typically rapid, and we usually obverse patients in hospital for 24 hours. Postprocedure care consists of chest radiography to exclude complications and evaluate new lead placement if applicable, periprocedural antibiotic therapy, and pain control. Postprocedure recovery from surgical lead extraction is longer as a result of pain and pericardial and pleural drainage management.

Failed Extraction

TLE can fail for various reasons—from lead construction to robust lead–body interactions and lack of operator experience. Specific predictors of failed extraction include implant duration, younger patient age, ventricular versus atrial leads, and operator inexperience. Anecdotal evidence suggests that the likelihood of complications is higher with challenging extractions that require multiple techniques and attempts. Experienced operators repeatedly reevaluate the risk-to-benefit ratio of further extraction attempts. Alternative strategies include taking a more invasive surgical approach, referring the patient to a high-volume center, or abandoning further extraction attempts.

Conclusions

TLE has evolved dramatically over the past 30 years, and exponentially throughout the past decade. Despite these advances, the basic tenets of counterpressure, traction, and countertraction remain critical to ensuring successful and safe outcomes. As indications for device therapy expand and younger patients receive devices, it is likely that the number of lead extractions performed will increase. As they do, the pressure on the field to continue to evolve not simply as a technique but as a discipline and a science will gain strength.

The 2009 HRS Expert Consensus on Transvenous Lead Extraction provides several recommendations to help the specialty of lead extraction evolve. The document creates standard definitions, recommends guidelines for safe lead extraction, identifies indications for extraction, and emphasizes the importance of reporting outcomes. As new extraction tools and novel leads designed to facilitate future extraction are introduced, standardized reporting of outcomes will be even more essential. Data collection will serve to advance our collective knowledge and allow us to draw conclusions regarding the safety of and complications resulting from these techniques. Questions regarding the benefits of lead extraction in specific situations remain, so a nationwide database of extraction outcomes and complications would allow us to critically evaluate and rigorously answer these questions. Moreover, collaboration among those performing lead extraction will be critical to building a community of lead extractors and creating a field of experts committed to quality. The future of lead extraction lies in the development of new techniques and tools, the creation of a collaborative community, and the growth of the science.

References

1. Madigan NP, Curtis JJ, Sanfelippo JF, Murphy TJ. Difficulty of extraction of chronically implanted tined ventricular endocardial leads. *J Am Coll Cardiol*. 1984;3:724-731.
2. Rettig G, Doenecke P, Sen S, et al. Complications with retained transvenous pacemaker electrodes. *Am Heart J*. 1979;98:587-594.
3. Bilgutay AM, Jensen NK, Garamella JJ, et al. Incarceration of transvenous pacemaker electrode. Removal by traction. *Minn Med*. 1968;51:489-491.
4. Kennergren C, Bjurman C, Wiklund R, Gabel J. A single-centre experience of over one thousand lead extractions. *Europace*. 2009;11:612-617.
5. Jones SO, Eckart RE, Albert CM, Epstein LM. Large, single-center, single-operator experience with transvenous lead extraction: outcomes and changing indications. *Heart Rhythm*. 2008;5:520-525.
6. Bongiorni MG, Soldati E, Zucchelli G, et al. Transvenous removal of pacing and implantable cardiac defibrillating leads using single sheath mechanical dilatation and multiple venous approaches: high success rate and safety in more than 2000 leads. *Eur Heart J*. 2008;29:2886-2893.
7. Wazni O, Epstein LM, Carrillo RG, et al. Lead extraction in the contemporary setting: the LExICon study: an observational retrospective study of consecutive laser lead extractions. *J Am Coll Cardiol*. 2010;55:579-586.
8. Robboy SJ, Harthorne JW, Leinbach RC, et al. Autopsy findings with permanent pervenous pacemakers. *Circulation*. 1969;39:495-501.
9. Huang TY, Baba N. Cardiac pathology of transvenous pacemakers. *Am Heart J*. 1972;83:469-474.
10. Smith HJ, Fearnot NE, Byrd CL, et al. Five-years experience with intravascular lead extraction. U.S. Lead Extraction Database. *Pacing Clin Electrophysiol*. 1994;17:2016-2020.
11. Smith MC, Love CJ. Extraction of transvenous pacing and ICD leads. *Pacing Clin Electrophysiol*. 2008;31:736-752.
12. Hammill SC, Kremers MS, Kadish AH, et al. Review of the ICD Registry's third year, expansion to include lead data and pediatric ICD procedures, and role for measuring performance. *Heart Rhythm*. 2009;6:1397-1401.
13. Maisel WH, Moynahan M, Zuckerman BD, et al. Pacemaker and ICD generator malfunctions: analysis of Food and Drug Administration annual reports. *JAMA*. 2006;295:1901-1906.
14. DeFrances CJ, Lucas CA, Buie VC, Golosinskiy A. 2006 National Hospital Discharge Survey. *Natl Health Stat Report*. 2008:1-20.
15. Borek PP, Wilkoff BL. Pacemaker and ICD leads: strategies for long-term management. *J Interv Card Electrophysiol*. 2008;23:59-72.
16. Agarwal SK, Kamireddy S, Nemec J, et al. Predictors of complications of endovascular chronic lead extractions from pacemakers and defibrillators: a single-operator experience. *J Cardiovasc Electrophysiol*. 2009;20:171-175.
17. Eckstein J, Koller MT, Zabel M, et al. Necessity for surgical revision of defibrillator leads implanted long-term: causes and management. *Circulation*. 2008;117:2727-2733.
18. Voigt A, Shalaby A, Saba S. Continued rise in rates of cardiovascular implantable electronic device infections in the United States: temporal trends and causative insights. *Pacing Clin Electrophysiol*. 2010;33:414-419.
19. Cabell CH, Heidenreich PA, Chu VH, et al. Increasing rates of cardiac device infections among Medicare beneficiaries: 1990-1999. *Am Heart J*. 2004;147:582-586.

20. Haqqani HM, Mond HG. The implantable cardioverter-defibrillator lead: principles, progress, and promises. *Pacing Clin Electrophysiol*. 2009;32:1336-1353.
21. Kleemann T, Becker T, Doenges K, et al. Annual rate of transvenous defibrillation lead defects in implantable cardioverter-defibrillators over a period of >10 years. *Circulation*. 2007;115:2474-2480.
22. Dorwarth U, Frey B, Dugas M, et al. Transvenous defibrillation leads: high incidence of failure during long-term follow-up. *J Cardiovasc Electrophysiol*. 2003;14:38-43.
23. Ellenbogen KA, Wood MA, Shepard RK, et al. Detection and management of an implantable cardioverter defibrillator lead failure: incidence and clinical implications. *J Am Coll Cardiol*. 2003;41:73-80.
24. Luria D, Glikson M, Brady PA, et al. Predictors and mode of detection of transvenous lead malfunction in implantable defibrillators. *Am J Cardiol*. 2001;87:901-904.
25. Pakarinen S, Oikarinen L, Toivonen L. Short-term implantation-related complications of cardiac rhythm management device therapy: a retrospective single-centre 1-year survey. *Europace*. 2010;12:103-108.
26. Vatankulu MA, Goktekin O, Kaya MG, et al. Effect of long-term resynchronization therapy on left ventricular remodeling in pacemaker patients upgraded to biventricular devices. *Am J Cardiol*. 2009;103:1280-1284.
27. Sweeney MO, Shea JB, Ellison KE. Upgrade of permanent pacemakers and single chamber implantable cardioverter defibrillators to pectoral dual chamber implantable cardioverter defibrillators: indications, surgical approach, and long-term clinical results. *Pacing Clin Electrophysiol*. 2002;25:1715-1723.
28. Foley PW, Muhyaldeen SA, Chalil S, et al. Long-term effects of upgrading from right ventricular pacing to cardiac resynchronization therapy in patients with heart failure. *Europace*. 2009;11:495-501.
29. Wilkoff BL, Love CJ, Byrd CL, et al. Transvenous lead extraction: Heart Rhythm Society expert consensus on facilities, training, indications, and patient management: this document was endorsed by the American Heart Association (AHA). *Heart Rhythm*. 2009;6:1085-1104.
30. Byrd CL, Wilkoff BL, Love CJ, et al. Intravascular extraction of problematic or infected permanent pacemaker leads: 1994-1996. U.S. Extraction Database, MED Institute. *Pacing Clin Electrophysiol*. 1999;22:1348-1357.
31. Epstein LM, Byrd CL, Wilkoff BL, et al. Initial experience with larger laser sheaths for the removal of transvenous pacemaker and implantable defibrillator leads. *Circulation*. 1999;100:516-525.
32. Wilkoff BL, Byrd CL, Love CJ, et al. Pacemaker lead extraction with the laser sheath: results of the pacing lead extraction with the excimer sheath (PLEXES) trial. *J Am Coll Cardiol*. 1999;33:1671-1676.
33. Byrd CL, Schwartz SJ. Transatrial implantation of transvenous pacing leads as an alternative to implantation of epicardial leads. *Pacing Clin Electrophysiol*. 1990;13:1856-1859.
34. Fearnot NE, Smith HJ, Goode LB, et al. Intravascular lead extraction using locking stylets, sheaths, and other techniques. *Pacing Clin Electrophysiol*. 1990;13:1864-1870.
35. Goode LB, Byrd CL, Wilkoff BL, et al. Development of a new technique for explantation of chronic transvenous pacemaker leads: five initial case studies. *Biomed Instrum Technol*. 1991;25:50-53.
36. Byrd CL, Schwartz SJ, Hedin N. Intravascular techniques for extraction of permanent pacemaker leads. *J Thorac Cardiovasc Surg*. 1991;101:989-997.
37. Brodell GK, Castle LW, Maloney JD, Wilkoff BL. Chronic transvenous pacemaker lead removal using a unique, sequential transvenous system. *Am J Cardiol*. 1990;66:964-966.
38. Bongiorni MG, Giannola G, Arena G, et al. Pacing and implantable cardioverter-defibrillator transvenous lead extraction. *Ital Heart J*. 2005;6:261-266.
39. Gijsbers GH, van den Broecke DG, Sprangers RL, van Gemert MJ. Effect of force on ablation depth for an XeCl excimer laser beam delivered by an optical fiber in contact with arterial tissue under saline. *Lasers Surg Med*. 1992;12:576-584.
40. Byrd CL, Wilkoff BL, Love CJ, et al. Clinical study of the laser sheath for lead extraction: the total experience in the United States. *Pacing Clin Electrophysiol*. 2002;25:804-808.
41. Neuzil P, Taborsky M, Rezek Z, et al. Pacemaker and ICD lead extraction with electrosurgical dissection sheaths and standard transvenous extraction systems: results of a randomized trial. *Europace*. 2007;9:98-104.
42. Dello Russo A, Biddau R, Pelargonio G, et al. Lead extraction: a new effective tool to overcome fibrous binding sites. *J Interv Card Electrophysiol*. 2009;24:147-150.
43. Hussein AA, Wilkoff BL, Martin DO, et al. Initial experience with the Evolution mechanical dilator sheath for lead extraction: safety and efficacy. *Heart Rhythm*. 2010;7:870-873.
44. Fischer A, Love B, Hansalia R, Mehta D. Transfemoral snaring and stabilization of pacemaker and defibrillator leads to maintain vascular access during lead extraction. *Pacing Clin Electrophysiol*. 2009;32:336-339.
45. Byrd CL, Schwartz SJ, Hedin N. Lead extraction. Indications and techniques. *Cardiol Clin*. 1992;10:735-748.
46. Byrd CL, Schwartz SJ, Sivina M, et al. Technique for the surgical extraction of permanent pacing leads and electrodes. *J Thorac Cardiovasc Surg*. 1985;89:142-144.
47. Spittell PC, Vlietstra RE, Hayes DL, Higano ST. Venous obstruction due to permanent transvenous pacemaker electrodes: treatment with percutaneous transluminal balloon venoplasty. *Pacing Clin Electrophysiol*. 1990;13:271-274.
48. Worley SJ, Gohn DC, Pulliam RW, et al. Subclavian venoplasty by the implanting physicians in 373 patients over 11 years. *Heart Rhythm*. 2011;8:526-533.
49. Baddour LM, Epstein AE, Erickson CC, et al. Update on cardiovascular implantable electronic device infections and their management: a scientific statement from the American Heart Association. *Circulation*. 2010;121:458-477.
50. Zei PC, Eckart RE, Epstein LM. Modified temporary cardiac pacing using transvenous active fixation leads and external re-sterilized pulse generators. *J Am Coll Cardiol*. 2006;47:1487-1489.

Video Legends

Video 17.1 Incision. One approach to skin incision is described.

Video 17.2 Crossing a venous obstruction with a 5 Fr dilator. A stenotic subclavian vein is crossed using a 5-Fr dilator and Glidewire.

Video 17.3 Lead preparation. Both an ICD and pacemaker leads are prepped for insertion of a locking stylet.

Video 17.4 Removal of an ICD lead with a laser sheath. Detailed example of extraction of an ICD lead from a dual-chamber system utilizing a laser sheath.

SECTION 1D

TECHNOLOGY AND THERAPEUTIC TECHNIQUES

Ablation Technology

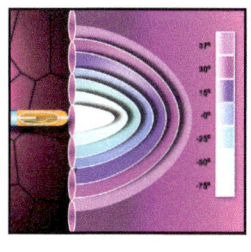
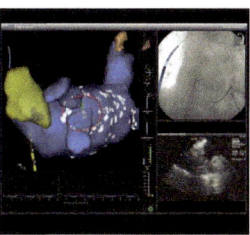
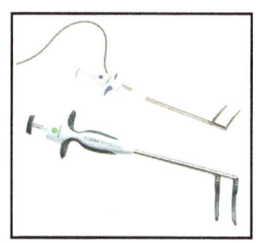
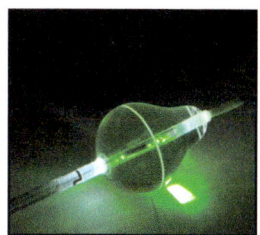

CHAPTER 18

ANATOMY AND HISTOPATHOLOGY OF ABLATION INTERVENTIONS

S. YEN HO, PHD

Introduction

For the interventional cardiac electrophysiologist, knowledge of relevant cardiac anatomy is crucial for reducing the risk of complications. Recent developments in imaging techniques can allow three-dimensional reconstructions and merging with fluoroscopy to provide the operator with better appreciation of spatial relationships of the cardiac chambers and important structures. Any information on wall thickness, architecture, and composition that can be gleaned from imaging, however, is less readily available. This chapter is illustrated with images from human heart specimens and discusses some of the important anatomic landmarks and structures. These include the cardiac conduction system, the terminal crest, Eustachian valve, cavotricuspid isthmus, left atrial ridge, pulmonary veins, the atrial septum, and ventricular outlets. Our aim is to facilitate a better understanding of cardiac anatomy relevant to catheter ablation.

Relationship of the Heart to the Thoracic Structures

To begin with, the neighborhood of the heart contains important structures that can be vulnerable to damage from ablation energies. Lying within the middle component of the mediastinum, the heart is enclosed within its fibrous pericardial sac. Accessing the heart via the pericardial space is a relatively new portal for most interventional electrophysiologists. The fibrous pericardium is continuous superiorly with the adventitia of the great vessels, like cuffs attaching to the ascending aorta and pulmonary trunk, and to the superior caval vein several centimeters above the site of the sinus node. Anteriorly, it is attached to the posterior surface of the sternum by the superior and inferior sternopericardial ligaments that are variably developed. Laterally are the pleural coverings of the mediastinal surface of the lungs. The esophagus, descending thoracic aorta, and posterior parts of the mediastinal surface of both lungs are related posteriorly. Inferiorly, the fibrous pericardium is attached to the central tendon of the diaphragm and a small muscular area to the left. The diaphragm separates the pericardium from the liver and fundus of the stomach. There is a small area behind the lower left half of the body of the sternum and the sternal ends of the left fourth and fifth costal cartilages where the fibrous pericardium is in direct contact with the thoracic wall. This area does allow the pericardial space to be accessed, but the operator should take care not to enter the right ventricle, which lies behind the space.

Immediately behind the fibrous pericardium covering the posterior wall of the left atrium runs the esophagus. Its descent in the posterior mediastinum is related variably to the middle of the posterior wall, more toward the right pulmonary veins or more toward the left pulmonary veins.[1] Indeed, this relationship can vary with peristalsis even within the individual. Just prior to its penetration through the diaphragm, the esophagus curves along the inferior wall of the left atrium to become related to the coronary sinus (Figure 18.1A). Although the course of the descending thoracic aorta is relatively distant from the atrial walls, in some cases, it can pass close to the orifices of the left pulmonary veins.

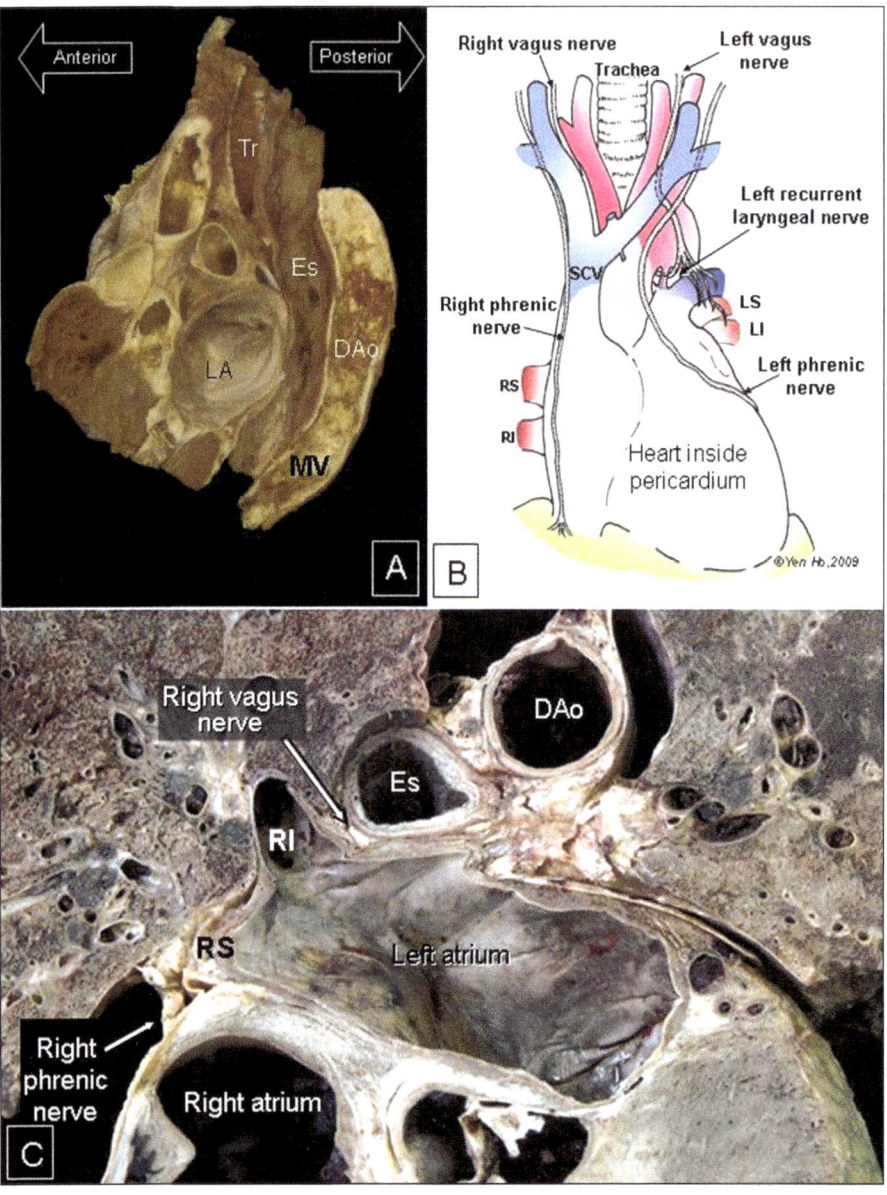

Figure 18.1 **Panel A:** Longitudinal section showing the course of the esophagus (Es) adjacent to the posterior and inferior walls of the left atrium (LA). **Panel B:** Diagram showing the courses of the vagus and phrenic nerves. **Panel C:** Transverse section showing relationship of the right phrenic nerve to the right superior pulmonary veins (RS) and the right vagus nerve anterior to the esophagus. DAo = descending thoracic aorta; LI = left inferior; LS = left superior; MV = mitral valve; RI = right inferior pulmonary vein; SCV = superior caval vein; Tr = trachea. *Source:* Photograph courtesy of Professor Damián Sanchez-Quintana, MD.

The larger nerve bundles can also be vulnerable. The importance of the phrenic nerves is often underrecognized. Accompanied by the pericardiophrenic vessels, the phrenic nerves descend bilaterally onto the fibrous pericardium (Figure 18.1B).[2,3] The right phrenic nerve descends almost vertically, initially along the right brachiocephalic vein, then along the right anterolateral surface of the superior caval vein, and continues its descent immediately in front of the right pulmonary veins in the lung hilum before reaching the diaphragm. It is intimately related to both the superior caval vein and the right pulmonary veins, running within millimeters of the lumens of these veins. The left phrenic nerve passes over the left atrial appendage in its descent and then takes an anterior course to be related to the great cardiac vein, or leftward, to overlie the obtuse marginal vein. It becomes at risk during implantation of leads into these veins or when ablating foci located epicardially in these regions.

Also important are the vagus nerves that extend on both sides directly posterior to the lung hilums to form the posterior pulmonary plexuses. From the caudal part of the left pulmonary plexus, two branches descend on the anterior surface of the esophagus, joining with a branch from the right pulmonary plexus to form the anterior esophageal plexus (Figure 18.1C). After penetrating the diaphragm, the posterior and anterior esophageal plexuses become the posterior and anterior vagal trunks that innervate the pyloric sphincter and the gastric antrum. Damage to them may account for delayed gastric emptying syndrome 3 to 48 hours after an ablation procedure.[4,5]

Relationships of the Cardiac Chambers

Walmsley[6] in 1958 commented that descriptions of cardiac anatomy disregard the cardinal principle of using terms in relation to anatomic position. He noted that many textual descriptions and figures throughout the medical literature view the heart as an isolated organ held in the hand, with the atria above the ventricles and the left and right chambers lying alongside each other in a sagittal plane—basic and false concepts that have caused untold confusion in the past. By standing the heart on its apex, it is easy to see how the anterior and posterior descending coronary arteries acquired their names. Later, MacAlpine[7] in 1975 emphasized the importance of describing the heart in its anatomic location for appropriate clinical correlations in his exquisitely illustrated atlas. He termed the orientation of the heart seen in its living condition as attitudinal. The heart positioned within the chest, in situ, has its long axis oriented from the right shoulder toward the left hypochondrium.

In the normal individual, two-thirds of the bulk of the cardiac mass is usually to the left, with one-third to the right. The so-called right heart chambers are anterior and to the right, with the right ventricle lying behind the sternum (Figure 18.2A). The right atrium is positioned anteriorly relative to its left counterpart. Being the most posterior of the cardiac chambers, the left atrium lies directly in front of the esophagus. The ventricular chambers extend anteriorly and leftward of their respective atrial chambers. The plane of the right atrioventricular junction containing the annular insertion of the tricuspid valve is oriented nearly vertically. In contrast, the plane of the pulmonary valve is nearly horizontal and located well cephalad, making the pulmonary valve the most superiorly situated of the cardiac valves. Like the tricuspid valve, the plane of the annular insertion of the mitral valve, marking the atrioventricular junction, is nearer vertical than horizontal.

The aortic root is located centrally in the heart, with the aortic valve immediately adjacent to the mitral valve. When viewed from the cardiac base, it is wedged between the tricuspid and mitral orifices (Figure 18.2B). On the epicardial side, the root of the aorta is embraced by right ventricular musculature separating the tricuspid from the pulmonary valves. Thus, the right ventricle sweeps from posterior to anterior and passes cephalad such that its outflow tract lies superior to that of the left ventricle, giving the outlets a crossover relationship.

As shown in Figure 18.2A, the main coronary arteries supplying the ventricles run on the epicardial surface and are usually covered over by fat. The right coronary artery emerges almost perpendicularly from the aortic sinus to enter the fatty tissues of the right atrioventricular groove to become sandwiched between the right atrial wall and the right ventricular wall. The tip of the right atrial appendage may overlie the proximal portion of the artery. The sinus nodal artery commonly arises from within a centimeter of the origin of the right coronary artery to enter the interatrial groove. The left coronary artery takes an acute angle after its origin to pass leftward and anteriorly before branching into the anterior descending and circumflex arteries. The left main stem and the circumflex may be overlapped by the left atrial appendage. Thus, owing to the crossover relationship of the ventricular outflow tracts, the musculature of the right ventricular outflow tract is also related to the locations of the proximal portions of the main coronary arteries.

The ascending aorta passes to the right of the pulmonary trunk and then curves left and posteriorly, continuing into the normal left aortic arch passing to the left of the trachea. The pulmonary trunk is directed cephalad and posteriorly. Its bifurcation into the right and left pulmonary arteries is close to the roof of the left atrium, allowing the right pulmonary artery to pass rightward underneath the aortic arch. The ligamentous remnant of the arterial duct usually attaches the pulmonary bifurcation to the underside of the arch in the vicinity of the recurrent left laryngeal nerve (see Figure 18.1B).

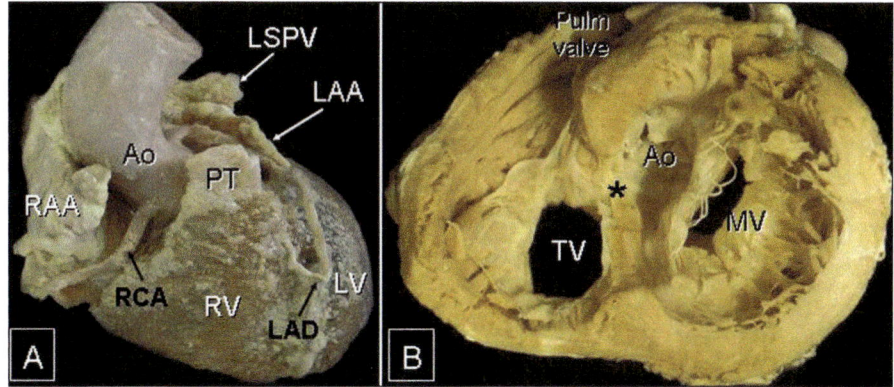

Figure 18.2 **Panel A:** Heart viewed from the front. The epicardial surface of the ventricles has been removed to display the courses of the right coronary artery (RCA) and left anterior descending coronary artery (LAD). The RCA marks the site of the right atrioventricular groove, while the LAD marks the site of the ventricular septum. **Panel B:** This transverse cut through the ventricles and viewed from the cardiac apex approximates a left anterior oblique projection. Muscle separates the pulmonary valve from the tricuspid valve, but there is fibrous continuity between the aortic and mitral valves. The **asterisk** marks the membranous septum. Ao = aorta; LAA = left atrial appendage; LSPV = left superior pulmonary vein; LV = left ventricle; MV = mitral valve; PT = pulmonary trunk; RAA = right atrial appendage; RV = right ventricle; TV = tricuspid valve.

The Atria, Septum, Conduction System, and Atrioventricular Junctions

The Right Atrium

The right atrium marks the right border of the heart. The superior and inferior caval veins enter the posterior and smooth-walled portion of the atrium, termed the *venous component*. The triangular atrial appendage occupies the anterior and lateral wall of the atrium. Its tip is superior and anterior and lies over the anterosuperior aspect of the right atrioventricular groove (Figure 18.2A). The rough wall of the appendage is characteristic, as it bears an extensive array of pectinate muscles on its endocardial surface. The areas in between the muscle bundles are paper-thin (Figure 18.3A).

The Terminal Crest

The border between the appendage and the smooth venous component is marked by the terminal crest (*crista terminalis*). Pectinate muscles arise from the crest nearly perpendicularly and fan out as they reach the smooth atrial vestibule that surrounds the orifice of the tricuspid valve. The crest itself appears like a C-shaped band extending from the septal aspect to pass in front of the orifice of the superior caval vein and then descends toward the lateral side of the orifice of the inferior caval vein. Its distal portion branches into an array of smaller muscle bundles that continue onto the inferior atrial wall, encroaching toward the orifice of the coronary sinus. The strands of myocardium making up the terminal crest run along its length.

The crest is important to interventional electrophysiologists for several reasons. First, it contains the sinus node at its junction with the superior caval vein (Figure 18.3A), and ablation of the terminal crest has been performed in patients with inappropriate sinus tachycardia.[8,9] Second, it is the origin of many focal atrial tachycardia in patients without structural heart disease.[10] Third, it is a barrier to conduction in isthmus-dependent atrial flutter.[11,12]

The Cavotricuspid Isthmus

The area of terminal ramifications of the crest is of particular significance in the setting of typical atrial flutter because it is part of the cavotricuspid isthmus. Within this

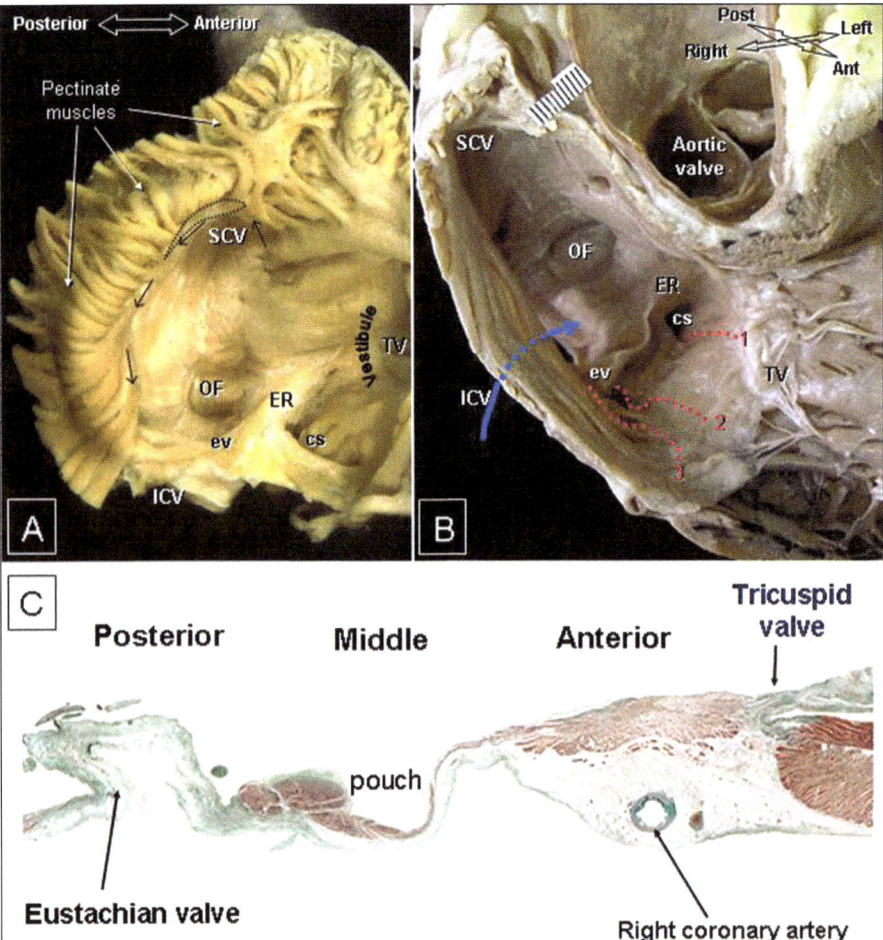

Figure 18.3 **Panel A:** The right atrium has been opened and its parietal wall deflected back to show the terminal crest (**small arrows**) and the extensive array of pectinate muscles. The terminal crest separates the rough wall of the appendage from the smooth intercaval posterior wall. The **dotted shape** marks the anticipated site of the sinus node. The Eustachian ridge (ER) extending from the Eustachian valve (ev) is fairly prominent in this heart. **Panel B:** The region of the cavotricuspid isthmus is marked by 3 **dotted lines** representing (1) the "septal" isthmus, (2) the inferior (typical flutter) isthmus, and (3) the inferolateral isthmus. The **blue arrow** indicates an inferior approach via the inferior caval vein (ICV). **Panel C:** Histological section through the inferior isthmus shows a smooth portion anteriorly, a thin-walled pouch in the middle portion, and a combination of muscle trabeculations and fibrous tissue in the posterior portion. This Masson's trichrome stain shows myocardium in **red** and fibrous tissue in **green**. cs = coronary sinus; OF = oval fossa; SCV = superior caval vein; TV = tricuspid valve.

area, bordered posteriorly by the Eustachian valve and anteriorly by the hinge line (annulus) of the tricuspid valve, three isthmuses are recognized (Figure 18.3B). The most inferiorly situated isthmus on right anterior oblique (RAO) and left anterior oblique (LAO) projections is frequently utilized to abolish common flutter. This inferior isthmus is an extensive and complex structure, possessing posterior, middle, and anterior zones. The posterior zone (closest to the inferior caval vein) is often fibrous, while the anterior zone is the vestibule (Figure 18.3C). The middle zone contains the distal branches of the terminal crest and pectinate muscles with fibrous tissue in between. Frequently, the middle zone is pouchlike and the depression is known as the sinus of Keith or sub-eustachian sinus.[13,14]

The pouch may make it more difficult to achieve a complete line of bidirectional block. In some cases, interventionists instead deploy a longer ablation line along the inferolateral isthmus (7 o'clock on LAO). The shortest of the three isthmuses is situated between the orifice of the coronary sinus and the tricuspid valve, dubbed the septal isthmus (5 o'clock on LAO). It is ablated for the "slow pathway" in atrioventricular nodal reentrant tachycardia. The so-called fast pathway, on the other hand, putatively sweeps from the anterior and superior part of the atrium to approach the apex of the triangle of Koch.[15,16] Owing to its proximity to the atrioventricular node, fast-pathway ablation is associated with a higher incidence of postprocedural heart block.[17]

The Eustachian Valve, Ridge, and Thebesian Valve

The orifice of the inferior caval vein is guarded by the Eustachian valve, while the coronary sinus is guarded by the Thebesian valve (see Figure 18.3A). Although the Eustachian valve is usually a triangular flap, in some individuals it may be more extensive, aneurysmal, or take the form of a Chiari network. These configurations can make it more challenging for the ablationist to reach the cavotricuspid isthmus. From the commissure between the Eustachian and the Thebesian valves springs a slender tendinous structure: the tendon of Todaro, which passes anterosuperiorly within the musculature of the Eustachian ridge (sinus septum) to insert into the central fibrous body. The ridge is prominent in some hearts but flat in others. The Thebesian valve is attached posteroinferiorly such that its free margin is oriented superiorly. It is usually a crescentic membrane with or without fenestrations or is represented by fibrous bands or a filigree network. The study by Hellerstein and Orbison[18] reported large flaplike valves that may present as obstacles to intubation in 25% of hearts.

The Septal Aspect

The oval-shaped depression of the oval fossa valve that is surrounded by a muscular rim (or limbus) is a characteristic feature of the right atrium, though the rim is not always prominent. Although the septal aspect appears extensive at first sight, Walmsley and Watson[19] cautioned about the importance of distinguishing between "medial wall of right atrium" and "interatrial septum." The anterior part of the "medial wall" is termed the *aortic mound* on account of its close relationship to the root of the aorta (see Figure 18.3B). Perforation of the atrial wall in this region leads to the transverse pericardial sinus and the aorta. The true extent of the atrial septum is discussed below.

The Conduction Tissues

The Location of the Sinus Node

Discovered in 1907 by Keith and Flack,[20] the sinus node in almost all individuals is positioned laterally in the terminal groove at the junction of the right atrium with the superior caval vein. The sinus node is a small, tadpole-shaped structure, approximately 15 mm long and set within the terminal groove (Figure 18.4A). Its head is immediately subepicardial, wedged between the wall of the superior caval vein and the musculature of the terminal crest. Its body and tail portions penetrate for various distances through the thickness of the crest to descend toward the orifice of the inferior caval vein.[21] It is interesting that in a study on hearts from children, we found that in one-tenth of the specimens, the node also extended in horseshoe fashion across the crest of the right atrial appendage.[22] In a subsequent study of adult human hearts, however, we did not encounter any horseshoe nodes.[21]

Although recognizable as a discrete structure, owing to its unique composition of specialized myocardial cells within a meshwork of fibrous tissue, it is important to stress that the node is not isolated from surrounding atrial myocytes (Figures 18.4B, C). Rather, there are short transitions of nodal cells with the atrial myocardium throughout the boundary between the node and the terminal crest. We have also observed prongs of nodal cells extending into the crest and the myocardial sleeve of the superior caval vein. In some cases, the tail portion is represented by fragmented islands of nodal cells.[21] It is noteworthy that, in most individuals, a prominent artery takes its course through the middle of the node, although the specific arrangement varies from heart to heart.[43] In just over half of individuals, this artery to the sinus node is an early branch of the right coronary artery; in just under half, it originates from the initial course of the circumflex artery; in rare individuals, it exhibits a lateral origin from more distal parts of the right or circumflex arteries.[22]

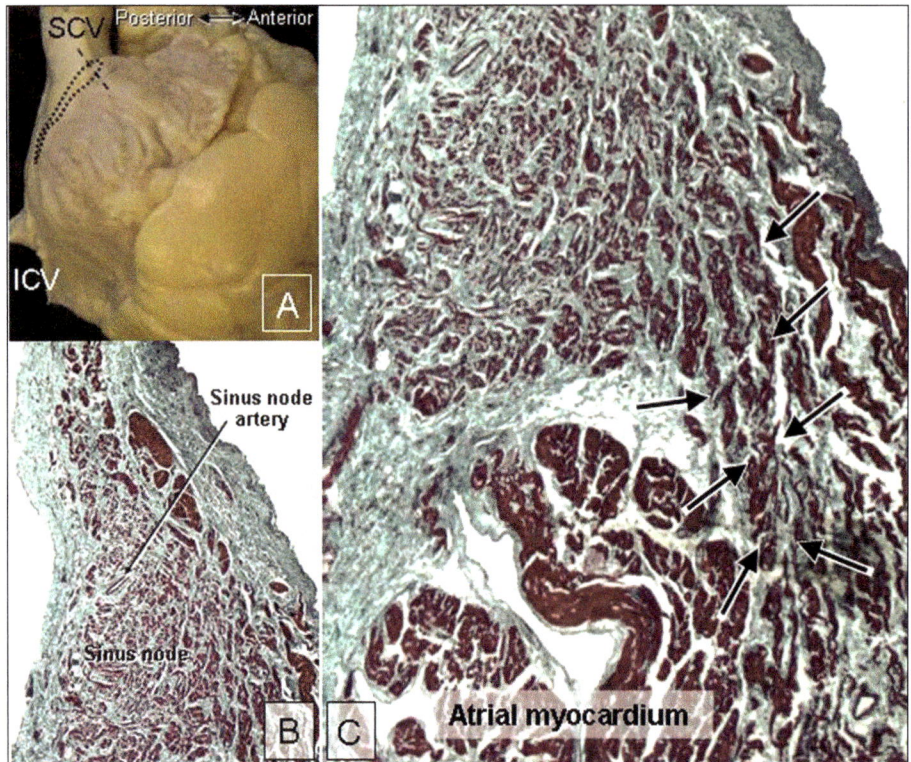

Figure 18.4 Panel A: The external aspect of the right atrium viewed from the right to show the location of the sinus node (**dot-outlined shape**) and the cutting plane for the histological sections (**broken line**). Panel B: The sinus node is recognizable as a cluster of small specialized myocytes (**red**) in a fibrous matrix (**green**) and supplied by a nodal artery. Panel C: On higher magnification of the nodal border, a prong of specialized cells (**between arrows**) can be seen extending into ordinary atrial myocardium. Masson's trichrome stain shows myocardium in **red** and fibrous tissue in **green**. ICV = inferior caval vein; SCV = superior caval vein.

The Triangle of Koch, Location of the Atrioventricular Node, and the His Bundle

The inferior paraseptal region of the right atrium contains the triangle of Koch, which is the gross anatomic landmark for the location of the atrioventricular node (Figures 18.5A, B). The compact node, along with its surrounding zones of transitional cells, is positioned at the base of the atrial septum, occupying the upper part of the triangular area. Although the triangle is a good landmark for the atrioventricular node, one should not forget that the atrioventricular node is an interatrial structure that also comes in contact with left atrial myocardium through its transitional cell zones.[23,24]

At the apex of the triangle is the atrioventricular component of the membranous septum that, in continuity with the right fibrous trigonal area of fibrous continuity between the aortic and mitral valves, forms the central fibrous body. The compact atrioventricular node, resembling a dense knot of specialized myocytes, rests against the fibrous body (Figure 18.5C). Surrounding the compact node are transitional cells interposing between the node and surrounding ordinary myocardium from both atria. The node becomes the His bundle as the conduction tissues penetrate through the central fibrous body. Indeed, the composition of the cells within the atrioventricular node and the penetrating bundle (of His) is often similar. Upon entering the fibrous body (Figure 18.5C), the His bundle is insulated from both atrial and ventricular myocardium. The anterior border of the triangle is the annular insertion of the septal leaflet of the tricuspid valve. In most hearts, the hinge line crosses the right ventricular aspect of the membranous septum, dividing it into atrioventricular and interventricular components. The more posterior border consists of the fibrous strand continuation of the valve of the inferior caval vein: the tendon of Todaro, buried within the Eustachian ridge. In 45° RAO projection, the plane of the triangle of Koch is in the plane of the image. Thus, the region of the His bundle is superior, while the coronary sinus (together with the vestibule forming the septal isthmus) marks the inferior border of the nodal triangle (Figure 18.5B). The two inferior extensions of the compact node and the inferior inputs of the transitional cell zones occupy the inferior border. While this projection displays the His bundle as coinciding with the commissure of the tricuspid valve that lies between the anterosuperior and the septal leaflets, the commissure actually veers away from the septum.

The Internodal Myocardium

The greater parts of the atrial walls are made up of ordinary working myocytes that are aggregated into myocardial strands within a supporting matrix of fibrous tissue. The parallel alignment of these strands favors preferential conduction along the direction of their long axis, and the overall arrangement is one of nonuniform anisotropy.[25] The walls of both the right and left atria can be likened to baskets with holes made by large venous orifices. Through them, conduction follows the broad bands of tissue

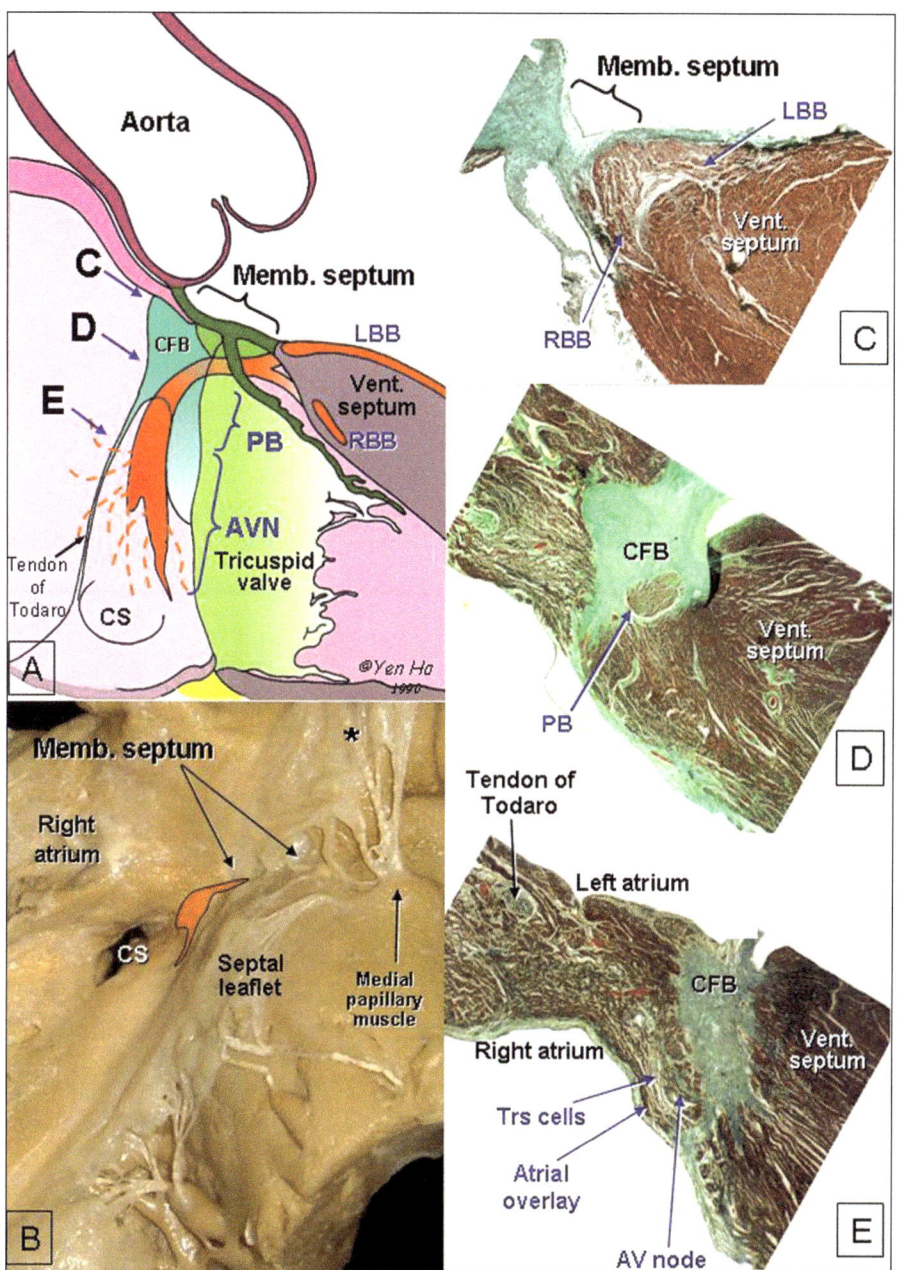

Figure 18.5 Panel A: This diagram depicts the triangle of Koch with the central fibrous body (CFB) at its apex. The **orange** areas represent the atrioventricular conduction system of the atrioventricular node (AVN), penetrating bundle (PB), and the atrioventricular conduction bundle that then branches and gives origin to the left bundle branch (LBB) and right (RBB) bundle branch. Transitional cells (**broken orange lines**) interpose between ordinary atrial myocardium and the compact atrioventricular node. **Panels C, D,** and **E** correspond to the planes of the histological sections shown on the right-hand panels. **Panel B:** The right atrium and right ventricle have been opened to show the septal leaflet of the tricuspid valve and its commissure (**asterisk**) with the anterosuperior leaflet. The latter is marked by the commissural cord extending from the medial papillary muscle. The insertion (annulus) of the septal leaflet crosses the membranous (memb) septum, dividing it into an atrioventricular portion and an interventricular portion. The **orange shape** represents the atrioventricular node and its extension into the penetrating bundle. CS = coronary sinus. **Panel C:** Surrounded by a fibrous tissue sheath, the branching bundle sits slightly to the left of the crest of the ventricular (vent) septum. The left bundle branch descends in the subendocardium, whereas the cordlike right bundle branch passes through the septal myocardium to emerge in the subendocardium on the right side. **Panel D:** The penetrating bundle is surrounded by tissues of the CFB. **Panel E:** The compact atrioventricular (AV) node leans against the central fibrous body. Transitional (Trs) cells pass between it and ordinary atrial myocardium.

continuity composed of ordinary myocytes that lack histologically specialized characteristics. Other than the cardiac nodes and their transitional cell zones, small nodelike remnants of the embryonic ring tissue show histologically specialized characteristics. They can be found within the insertions of the right atrial vestibule into the orifice of the tricuspid valve. In the normal heart, these nodal remnants (originally described by Kent in 1893[26]) make no contact with ventricular myocardium. It has been suggested that the part of the original ring in the septal isthmus forms the inferior extensions of the atrioventricular node and is the slow pathway into the atrioventricular node.[27] The nodelike structures, nonetheless, can function as part of accessory atrioventricular connections, for example, in the so-called Mahaim type of preexcitation or as an atrioventricular node in congenitally malformed hearts.[28]

The Inferior Pyramidal Space

The right atrial wall of the nodal triangle is a thin layer of myocardium. It is separated from the underlying ventricular myocardium by an extension from the fibro-fatty atrioventricular groove, which occupies the inferior pyramidal space recognized by cardiac surgeons.[29,30] The superior vertex of the pyramid is the central fibrous body, the lateral sides are the right and left atria, the anterior floor is the muscular ventricular septum with diverging left and right ventricular walls, and the coronary sinus at its base. Epicardially, the pyramidal space is traversed by the artery to the atrioventricular node (Figure 18.6A), which takes its origin from the dominant coronary artery (this being the right coronary artery in nine-tenths of the population).[30] The artery courses superiorly, entering the compact node, which is located in the union of the right and left atrial walls at the apex of the triangle.

Accessory atrioventricular pathways, referred to as septal and paraseptal pathways, traverse this region. Thus, inferior paraseptal pathways can be ablated from inside the coronary sinus or in the middle cardiac vein, which opens near the orifice of the coronary sinus. Since only a thin overlay of ordinary myocardium overlies the triangle of Koch, ablating septal and paraseptal accessory pathways from the right atrium risks inadvertent damage to the atrioventricular node.[31,32] By contrast, the central fibrous body affords the His bundle more protection from damage when ablating superficially located para-Hisian accessory pathways.

The Right Atrioventricular Groove

Containing fatty and fibrous tissues, the atrioventricular grooves provide the insulation between atrial and ventricular myocardium. When seen from the atrial aspect, the vestibular myocardium overlaps ventricular wall but is separated by epicardial tissues of the groove (Figure 18.6B). The groove contains the right coronary artery—the small cardiac vein. There are also various anterior veins draining the anterior surface of the right ventricle directly into the right atrial appendage. Very rarely, these venous walls are muscular, providing the potential for accessory atrioventricular pathways.[33]

The Left Atrium

Like the right atrium, the left atrium has smooth and rough components, but its smooth component is considerably larger. This is because the rough component is confined mainly to its appendage, which in the left atrium is characteristically small and fingerlike (Figures 18.7A, B). The appendage usually points anterosuperiorly and overlies the left atrioventricular groove. When the appendage is long, its tip can overlie the right ventricular outflow tract or pulmonary trunk. Accessory pathways can connect the left atrial appendage with the left ventricle. There is no terminal crest demarcating the border between the ostium (os) of the appendage and the body of the atrium, which is occupied mainly by the pulmonary venous component on the posterior aspect of the atrial chamber. Thus, in the vicinity of the os, it is quite usual to find pits and troughs in the atrial wall giving the impression of pectinate muscles "spilling out" of the appendage. Being mainly smooth-walled, there is no clear border between the vestibular portion and the venous portion of the left atrium. As with the right atrium, the vestibular musculature inserts into the left atrioventricular junction around the margins of the annulus of the mitral valve. The pulmonary venous component is shaped like a pillow; the pulmonary veins enter the four corners, with the left veins more superiorly located than the right veins.

Left Atrial Walls

Externally, the posterior wall is related to the esophagus and its nerves (vagal nerves) and the thoracic aorta, whereas the coronary sinus tracks along the posteroinferior part (Figure 18.7B).[1] In an anatomic study, the thickness of the posterior wall between the pulmonary vein orifices measured 2.1 to 2.9 mm, being thinner in the midportion (2.2 mm) in the hearts of patients with atrial fibrillation.[34] The superior wall, or dome, is related to the pulmonary arteries; its thickness ranges from 3.5 to 6.5 mm, with a tendency to be thinner near the left pulmonary veins. The anterior wall just behind the aorta ranges from 1.5 to 4.8 mm thick; however, there is usually a small area inferior to Bachmann's bundle that is exceptionally thin and was recognized by McAlpine as the "unprotected area."[35]

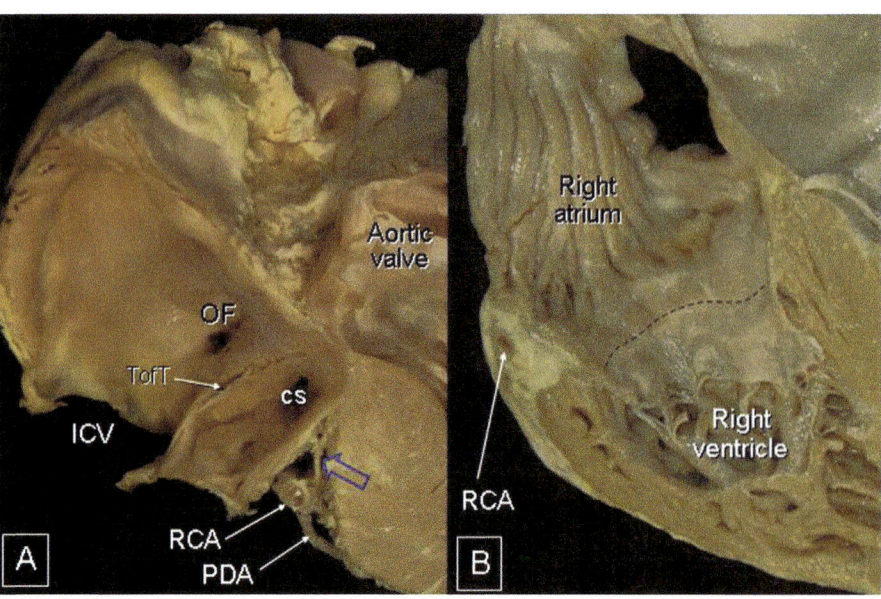

Figure 18.6 **Panel A:** This cut through the inferior pyramidal space shows the atrioventricular nodal artery (**open arrow**) originating from the right coronary artery (RCA) close to the takeoff of the posterior descending coronary artery (PDA). **Panel B:** This cut through the parietal right atrioventricular junction shows the fat-filled atrioventricular groove and the right coronary artery. There is a deep incursion of fatty tissues between atrial and ventricular walls. The **broken line** marks the level of the tricuspid annulus. cs = coronary sinus; ICV = inferior caval vein; OF = oval fossa; TofT = tendon of Todaro.

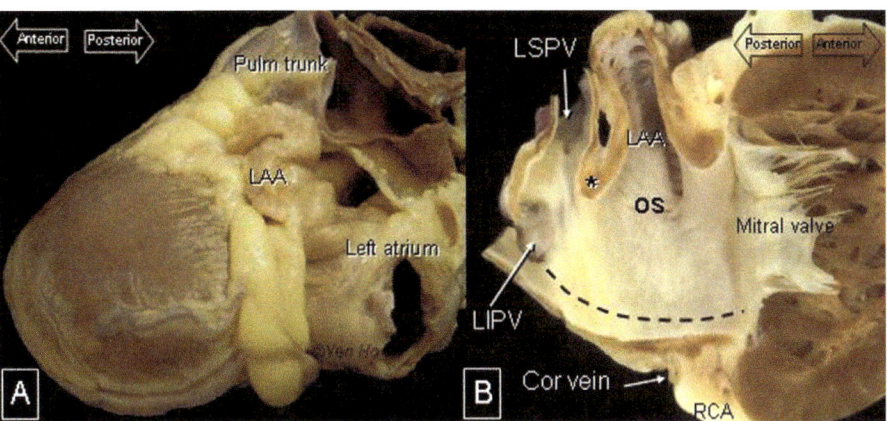

Figure 18.7 **Panel A:** This view from the left side shows the fingerlike left atrial appendage (LAA) with its tip reaching the pulmonary (pulm) trunk. **Panel B:** This longitudinal cut though the left atrium and left ventricle shows the narrow ostium (OS) to the appendage and the infolding (**asterisk**) of the atrial wall that appears like a ridge when it is viewed from inside the atrial chamber. The **broken line** represents the mitral isthmus. It transects the coronary sinus/great cardiac vein on the epicardial aspect. LIPV = left inferior pulmonary vein; RCA = right coronary artery.

Unlike the right atrium, the wall on the septal aspect of the left atrium lacks a muscular rim because this is the area of the flap-valve of the fossa. Apart from a few pits and troughs, it is relatively smooth. There is usually a reverse C-shape in the anterosuperior part, marking the edge of the foramen ovale, which is the interatrial channel in fetal life. Posterolaterally, between the os of the left atrial appendage and the left pulmonary veins, the atrial wall folds upon itself and appears like a ridge when viewed from within the chamber. The remnant of the oblique vein of the left atrium (known as the vein of Marshall), accompanied by fibro-fatty tissue and autonomic nerves, lies in this fold. The elegant histological studies by Kim et al[36] and Makino et al[37] demonstrated multiple myocardial "tracts" present within the ligament of Marshall. These tracts insert directly into the coronary sinus musculature, either near the origin of the vein of Marshall or distally, into the posterior free wall of the left atrium. This so-called ridge in the left atrium has variable widths; the narrower ridges can make it tricky to achieve a complete ablation line for encircling the left pulmonary veins.[38,39]

Left Atrial Isthmus

Electrophysiologists refer to left atrial isthmus or mitral isthmus when they draw an ablation line along the posteroinferior wall of the left atrium to connect the veno-atrial junction of the left inferior pulmonary vein to the mitral annulus. Anton Becker's anatomic study showed marked variability in the dimensions of the mitral isthmus and considerable differences in the thickness of the left atrial myocardium at various levels.[40] According to Becker's study, the wall nearest the veno-atrial junction was thickest, with a mean of 3 mm. By contrast, our study showed the thickest wall (mean: 3.8 mm) to be midway between the veno-atrial junction and the mitral annulus, with tapering at either end.[41] We found atrial arteries embedded in the wall passing closer than 5 mm from the endocardium. The isthmus is also in proximity to the circumflex artery and the coronary sinus. Depending on the precise location of the ablations, the line constructed may also transect the ligament of Marshall. Also relevant to ablation is the presence of small crevices that may entrap the tip of the catheter, thereby increasing the risk of isthmus perforation.

Pulmonary Veins

The transition between atrium and pulmonary vein is smooth. Inside the atrial chamber, it is often difficult to define entrances, or ostia, of the veins. Although commonly there are four pulmonary veins, the ipsilateral veins may coalesce into a short antrum (or vestibule) before entering the atrial chamber proper. Clinical imaging studies using magnetic resonance and multislice computed tomography have demonstrated the complex anatomy of the pulmonary veins and detailed their significant variability in dimensions, shape, and branching patterns.[42-44] Important to note, the orifices of the right pulmonary veins are directly adjacent to the plane of the atrial septum. Thus, in a postero-anterior (PA) projection, the portion of the right superior pulmonary vein closest to its orifice passes behind the posterior junction of right atrium with the superior caval vein.

The venous wall shows an innermost layer, formed by a thin endothelium overlying an irregular media of connective tissue and smooth muscle cells, and a thick outer layer comprising fibrous adventitia. At the pulmonary veno-atrial junction, the endocardium of the left atrium continues as the endothelial lining of the vein. The transition from the venous media to the left atrial wall is represented by a gradual decline in the number of smooth muscle cells, and the venous medial is overlapped on the outside by extensions of left atrial myocardium. A thin plane of fibro-fatty tissues interposes between the overlap. Thus, the muscle sleeve lies external to the venous wall and within the epicardium/adventitia. The length of muscle extension varies, with the longest sleeves usually along the upper veins.[45-47] At the venous insertions, the sleeves are thicker and tend to surround the entire epicardial aspect of the vein. The distal margins of the sleeves, however, are usually thinner and irregular as the musculature fades out.[45,46] Myocardial strands can extend between adjacent veins in various arrangements and as bridges.[38,48]

The Atrial Septum

Accessing the left atrium from the right requires an appreciation of the extent of the true atrial septum. From the right atrial aspect, the true septum is marked by the valve of the oval fossa (see Figure 18.3A). This is the area that can be perforated without risk of exiting the heart or damaging the arterial supply to the sinus node.[49-51] The muscular rim (limbus) surrounding the valve of the fossa is an infolding of the right atrial wall, whereas the fossa valve is a thin flap, 1 to 3 mm thick, on the left atrial side that closes upon the rim. The infolding contains epicardial fat and is known as the *interatrial groove* (Figures 18.8A, B). A puncture through the interatrial groove (which may be of considerable thickness) may subsequently render the catheter less maneuverable than if the puncture had been made through the thinner substance of the flap valve. Worse still, in a highly anticoagulated patient, it may result in hemopericardium. Important to note, the anteromedial wall of the right atrium appears to be "septal," but transgressing it leads to the back of the aorta (Figure 18.3B). Furthermore, the anterior rim of the oval fossa can exhibit holes or crevices. The walls are also very thin close to this point, increasing the risk of exiting the heart during attempted septal puncture.

Variability in the Fossa Ovalis

Although in RAO projection the oval fossa is usually posterior and superior relative to the orifice of the coronary sinus, the fossa rim exhibits considerable variations in location, size, and topography.[52,53] In some cases, the fossa valve is aneurysmal, herniating into the atrial chambers. Using transesophageal echocardiography, Schwinger and colleagues found abrupt change in the atrial septal plane from thick rim to thin valve in 82% of patients and gradual thinning in 18%.[53] A raised rim allows the operator to detect a change in topography when the needle descends from the rim to drop into the fossa and then tent the valve.

Probe patency of the oval fossa (PFO) is found in approximately one-fourth of the normal population in whom the C-shaped free edge of the fossa valve has not adhered completely to the muscle rim (Figure 18.9A). Through this margin, a probe or catheter can be pushed obliquely and anterosuperiorly along the fossa surface on the right side to enter the left atrium. It is worth noting that utilizing the PFO instead of making a transseptal puncture has disadvantages. Since this portal is located anterosuperiorly, the catheter emerges onto the anterior and superior walls of the left atrium where, not infrequently, there are pits with thin areas in the wall (eg, the "unprotected" area described by McAlpine, where perforations lead to the aortic root) (Figure 18.9B).[35] Also, if the PFO is small, it restricts catheter maneuverability, particularly for reaching the orifices of the right pulmonary veins.

Apart from the true septum, there are other sites of muscular interatrial connection. The most prominent interatrial bundle is Bachmann's bundle. This is a broad muscular band that runs in the subepicardium from the anterior wall of the superior caval vein into the anterior walls of both atria, crossing the interatrial groove. The muscular strands in Bachmann's bundle (as in the terminal crest) are well aligned, allowing for preferential conduction. They run in parallel with the circularly aligned left atrial myocardial strands (Figure 18.10A).[54] Bachmann's bundle is not encased by a fibrous tissue sheath; instead, at its margins, especially at its right and left atrial insertions, its myocardial strands blend into the atrial wall.[54,55]

Other interatrial muscular bridges are common (Figure 18.10B). They vary tremendously in width, number, and location. Broad bands have been seen connecting the posterior or inferior wall of the left atrium to the intercaval area of the right atrium or to the insertion of the inferior caval vein.[54,55] These provide the potential for inferior breakthrough of sinus impulse.[56] Smaller muscle bridges connecting the right pulmonary veins (or the left atrial

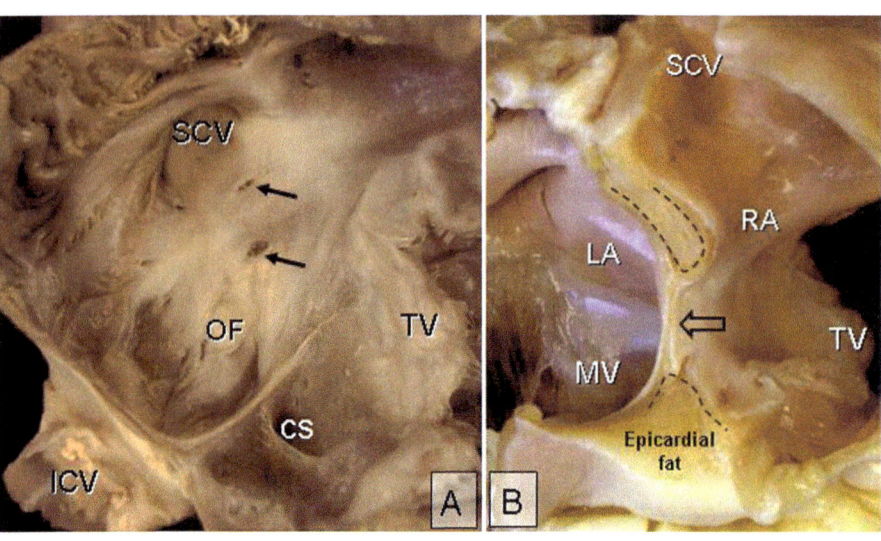

Figure 18.8 **Panel A:** The right atrium is opened to show the atrial septum *en face*. The oval fossa (OF) is not well demarcated because its muscular rim is flat. There are several pits in the wall on the septal aspect. **Panel B:** The heart is viewed from the back after removal of the posterior walls of both atria. The infolding of the muscular rim on the right atrial side is marked by the **broken lines**. The thin flap valve of the fossa (**arrow**) is on the left atrial side. CS = coronary sinus; ICV = inferior caval vein; LA = left atrium; MV = mitral valve; RA = right atrium; SCV = superior caval vein; TV = tricuspid valve.

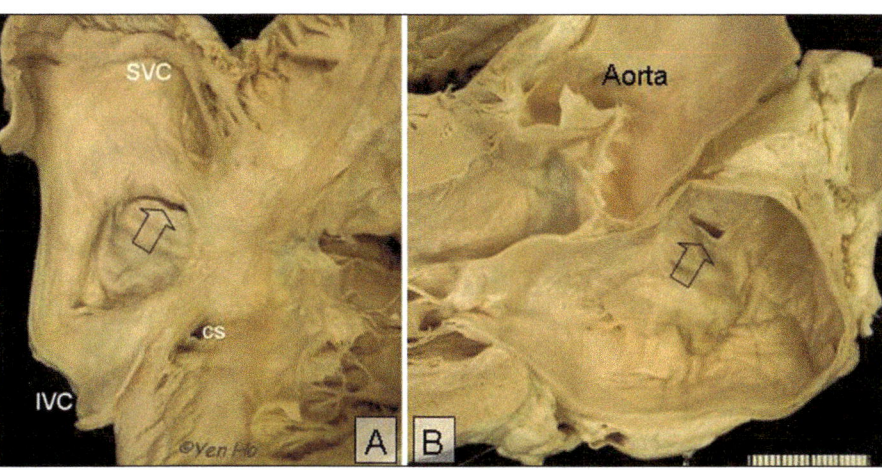

Figure 18.9 Panels A and B are right and left atrial aspects, respectively, of a probe patent oval fossa (**open arrows**) resulting from lack of adhesion between the fossa valve and its muscular rim. The fossa valve in this heart is slightly aneurysmal. CS = coronary sinus; ICV = inferior caval vein; SCV = superior caval vein.

wall between the veins) with the right atrium or the muscular sleeve of the superior caval vein have been observed.[49,54] Interatrial muscular connections may play a role in perpetuating atrial fibrillation. However, targeting these with endocardial ablation may be difficult since they are located subepicardially and cross the septal raphe some distance away from the true septum.[57,58]

Further bridges connect the musculature of the coronary sinus and vein/ligament of Marshall with the left atrium. A recent study found an association between presence of the vein of Marshall and a higher incidence of arrhythmic foci from the left superior pulmonary vein; however, vein of Marshall activity could not be confirmed.[59]

The Left Atrioventricular Junction

The left atrioventricular junction surrounds the orifice of the mitral valve, and part of it is the area of fibrous continuity between the mitral and aortic valves (see Figure 18.2B). The potential for accessory atrioventricular connections is limited mainly to the junction supporting the hinge line of the mural leaflet of the mitral valve. Accessory pathways tend to be strandlike, either single or multiple, with branching at the ventricular insertions, and run close to the annular insertions of the mitral valve.[31,60] Some run obliquely through the fibro-fatty tissue plane. When viewed in LAO projection, this is the junction that can be traced from posterosuperior to posterior and inferior (see Figure 18.2B). The inferior area harbors the coronary sinus, and its tributary, the great cardiac vein, can be seen in the parietal area. Hence, a catheter inserted in the coronary sinus and advanced into the great cardiac vein can guide the operator to the mitral annulus. The inferior paraseptal region (the so-called posterior septum) is the inferior pyramidal space that contains epicardial fibro-fatty tissues together with the artery supplying the atrioventricular node (see Figure 18.6A).[61,62]

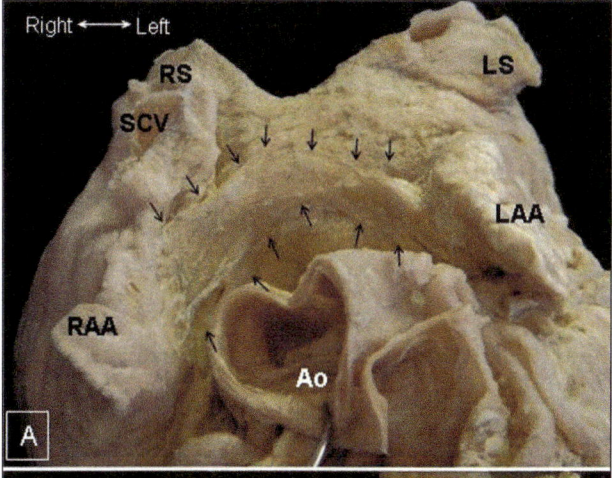
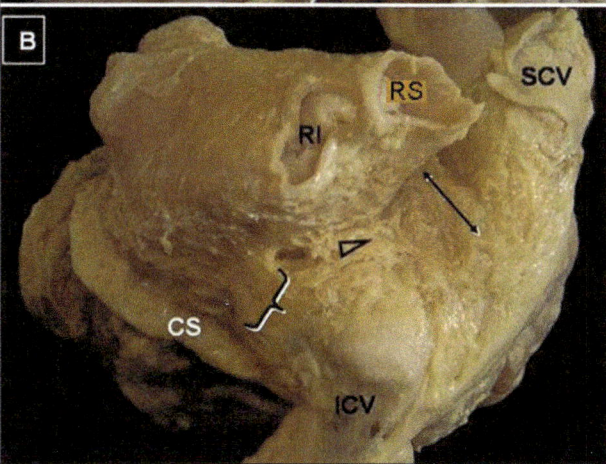

Figure 18.10 Panel A: This dissection of the anterior walls of the atria shows Bachmann's bundle (**short arrows**). The aorta (Ao) is pulled forward and the tip of the right atrial appendage (RAA) is deflected rightward. Panel B: This view of a heart from the right posterior and inferior shows a broad interatrial muscle band (}) located inferiorly and further muscle bridges (∆ and ↔) crossing the interatrial groove. CS = coronary sinus; ICV = inferior caval vein; LAA = left atrial appendage; LI = left inferior pulmonary vein; LS = left superior pulmonary vein; RI = right inferior pulmonary vein; RS = right superior pulmonary vein; SCV = superior caval vein.

The Coronary Sinus and Venous Tributaries

The venous return from the myocardium is either channeled via small Thebesian veins that open directly into the cardiac chambers or, more significantly, collected by the greater coronary venous system that drains 85% of the venous flow.[63,64] As the great cardiac vein ascends into the left atrioventricular groove, it passes close to the first division of the left coronary artery and under the cover of the left atrial appendage. Approaching the coronary sinus, the great vein is joined by tributaries from the left ventricular obtuse margin and the inferior wall, as well as veins from the left atrium (Figure 18.11). The distribution, course, and caliber of the left ventricular veins vary from individual to individual. When accessing the left ventricular veins for ablating ventricular tachycardia from a source close to the epicardium, the interventionist should be aware of the location of the phrenic nerve.[2,3] Although coronary veins are usually superficial to arteries, crossovers between arteries and veins are not uncommon.[65] Furthermore, when deploying catheters or wires in superficial veins, care should be taken since venous wall is thin and "unprotected" by muscle on the epicardial side.

The entrance of the vein or ligament of Marshall marks the venous end of the tube-shaped coronary sinus. When persistent, this is the left superior caval vein that descends along the epicardium between the left atrial appendage and the left superior pulmonary vein. In most individuals (even when a lumen is present), it is narrow, rarely exceeding 2 cm in length before tapering to a blind end. If adequately wide, this channel may be utilized for ablating the left atrial wall. In the absence of the vein of Marshall or its remnant, Vieussens' valve is taken as the anatomic landmark for the junction between the coronary sinus and the great cardiac vein. Found in 80% to 90% of hearts, this very flimsy valve has 1 to 3 leaflets that can provide some resistance to the catheter. Once past Vieussens' valve, a sharp bend in the great cardiac vein can cause further obstruction in 20% of cases.[66] Another marker for the junction between vein and coronary sinus is the end of the muscular sleeve around the sinus. However, in some cases, the sleeve may extend to 1 cm or more over the vein.[67] In many cases, bundles from the sleeve run into the left atrial wall, and in some, they also cover the outer walls of adjacent coronary arteries.[68]

The middle cardiac vein drains into the coronary sinus just within the sinus os. Occasionally, the middle vein enters the right atrium directly and opens adjacent to the os of the coronary sinus; this provides the coronary sinus catheter with an alternative, but undesired, portal. The middle vein passes just superficial to the right coronary artery at the cardiac crux. It is a useful portal for ablating accessory atrioventricular pathways located in the inferior pyramidal space.[69] Very rarely, the entrance of the middle vein is dilated and surrounded by a cuff of muscle, giving the potential for accessory atrioventricular connections.[70,71]

The small cardiac vein receives tributaries from the right atrium and the inferior wall of the right ventricle. It then courses in the right atrioventricular junction to open to the right margin of the coronary sinus orifice or into the middle cardiac vein. When joined by the acute marginal vein, or vein of Galen, the small vein enlarges. Several other veins, from the anterior surface of the right ventricle and from the acute margin, drain directly into the right atrium. In some hearts, the anterior veins merge into a venous "lake" in the right atrial wall. Again, these may be surrounded by a cuff of myocardium that gives the potential for accessory atrioventricular connection as the vein passes through the atrioventricular groove.[33,71]

The Ventricles

The ventricles make up the bulk of the muscle mass of the heart. Each ventricle has its own muscle wall, but they are conjoined at the septum and across the interventricular grooves. In the normal adult heart at autopsy, the parietal wall of the right ventricle is 3 to 5 mm thick, excluding trabeculations, and that of the left ventricle is 12 to 15 mm thick. Conventionally, these wall measurements are taken at 2 cm proximal to the pulmonary valve and 2 cm distal to the mitral valve. The ventricular septum curves as it is traced from inlet toward the outlet portions, allowing the right ventricle to curve over the left ventricle (see Figure 18.2B). Anatomically, each ventricle is described as having three portions: inlet, apical trabecular, and outlet.

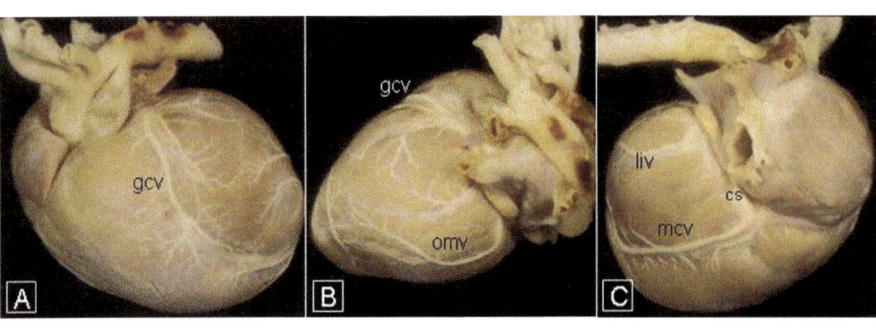

Figure 18.11 Panels A, B, and C are anterior, left, and inferior views, respectively, of a heart that has been injected to display the coronary veins on the ventricular surfaces. cs = coronary sinus; gcv = great cardiac vein; liv = left inferior vein; mcv = middle cardiac vein; omv = obtuse marginal vein.

The Right Ventricle

Apart from being the most anteriorly situated cardiac chamber, the right ventricle also marks the inferior border of the heart. The right ventricle is triangular when viewed from the front. When seen from the apex, the right edge of the right ventricle is sharp, forming the acute margin of the heart. In cross-section, the cavity appears like a crescent. In the roof of the right ventricle is the supraventricular crest (the ventriculo-infundibular fold), which separates the tricuspid valve from the pulmonary valve (Figure 18.12A).

The inlet portion of the right ventricle extends from the hinge line of the tricuspid valve to the papillary muscles that anchor the leaflets, via the tendinous cords, to the ventricular wall. The leaflets can be distinguished as septal, anterosuperior, and inferior or mural. The septal leaflet, with its cords inserting directly into the ventricular septum, is characteristic of the tricuspid valve. The medial papillary muscle (a small outbudding from the septum) supports the zone of apposition (or commissure) between the septal and anterosuperior leaflets. This muscle is a good marker for the right bundle branch, which emerges from the ventricular septum to the subendocardium at the base of this muscle (see Figures 18.5B, 18.12A). It is from here that the cordlike right bundle branch descends along the surface of the septomarginal trabeculation, taking an anterior course toward the ventricular apex. A robust muscle bundle, the moderator band, originates from the septomarginal trabeculation to insert into the parietal wall of the right ventricle. It carries within its musculature a part of the right bundle branch. The apical portion of the right ventricle is crisscrossed by coarse trabeculations and, at the very apical part, the ventricular wall tapers to 1 mm thickness (Figure 18.12A).

The outlet portion is anterior and superior in relation to the supraventricular crest and, therefore, to the bundle of His. This portion is relevant to ablations for idiopathic ventricular tachycardias that originate from this region, some forms of arrhythmogenic right ventricular cardiomyopathy, and scar-related ventricular tachycardias that develop after surgical repair of tetralogy of Fallot.

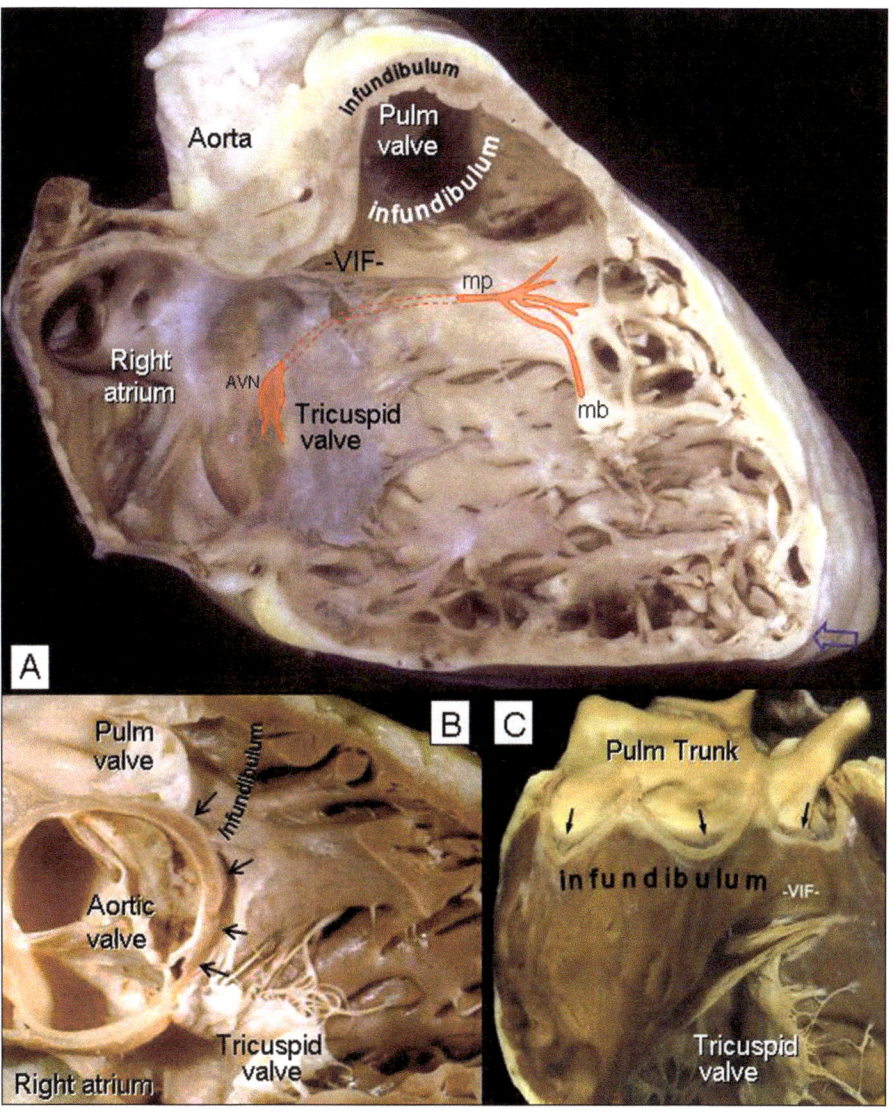

Figure 18.12 **Panel A:** The anterior walls of the heart have been removed to display the right atrium and right ventricle. The apical portion of the right ventricle is crisscrossed by thick trabeculations, and ventricular wall at the apex (**open arrow**) is very thin. The outlet is a cone of muscle (infundibulum) supporting the pulmonary (Pulm) valve. The ventriculo-infundibular fold (VIF) extends from the septum to the parietal wall, thus separating tricuspid from pulmonary valves. The **orange shape** in the right atrium represents the compact atrioventricular node; the **broken lines** represent the continuation of the atrioventricular conduction system. The cordlike right bundle branch in its initial course is intramyocardial; it emerges in the subendocardium at the base of the medial papillary muscle (mp) to descend on the septomarginal trabeculation, branching farther (**orange shape**). AVN = atrioventricular node; mb = moderator band. **Panel B:** Removal of the ventriculo-infundibular fold (**arrows**) reveals the aortic valve behind it. **Panel C:** The infundibulum is opened through a longitudinal incision. The leaflets of the pulmonary valve have been removed to show their semicircular insertion lines crossing the ventriculo-arterial junction, which is the border between darker colored myocardium and the pale wall of the pulmonary trunk. This arrangement results in segments of right ventricular myocardium at the deepest parts of the sinuses (**arrows**).

The Infundibulum: The infundibulum, or conus, describes that portion of the outflow tract that lies immediately beneath the pulmonary valves (Figures 18.12B, C). At its proximal part, it is the regular thickness of the right ventricle, but it tapers to a millimeter or so distally. Although its distal portion is well demarcated by the pulmonary valve, clear anatomic margins do not exist proximally. Its length differs from heart to heart, even if an arbitrary proximal margin can be assigned.

The distal margin of the infundibulum marks the ventriculo-arterial junction, showing a clear and circumscribed change from muscle wall to arterial wall. The semilunar attachments of the valvular leaflets crossing the ventriculo-arterial junction enclose parts of the infundibular wall (ventricular myocardium) into the pulmonary sinuses (Figure 18.12C). This region is of considerable interest to electrophysiologists who ablate within the sinuses to destroy foci of tissue responsible for some cases of ventricular tachycardia.[72,73] However, the anatomy of this region can be perplexing: The myocardium within the sinuses is considered "supravalvular" by electrophysiologists, whereas it is part and parcel of the valvular apparatus to morphologists![74-78] Describing the myocardium as supravalvular conveys an image of myocardial sleeves (akin to the sleeves around pulmonary veins) that extend several centimeters beyond the ventriculo-arterial junction. Also, by virtue of the semilunar arrangement of the hinge lines of the leaflets, three triangles of arterial walls are incorporated into the ventricles when the valve closes.

In terms of spatial relationships with adjacent cardiac chambers, the infundibulum projects anterosuperiorly, with its distal parts elevated from the ventricular septum; this makes the pulmonary valve the most superiorly situated of the cardiac valves. Two of the pulmonary sinuses are adjacent to two aortic sinuses, although the planes of the aortic and pulmonary valves are at an angle to one another (Figure 18.13A). The adjacent or "facing" aortic sinuses are those giving origin to the coronary arteries. The third pulmonary sinus is unrelated to the aorta.

The freestanding nature of the infundibulum is clearly demonstrated on cardiac sections that simulate the echocardiographic parasternal long-axis plane or the apical two-chamber plane (Figure 18.13B). This view shows the free anterior wall that blends and continues into the parietal wall of the rest of the right ventricle. Diametrically opposite to this is the posterior wall, which runs seamlessly into the ventricular septum. On the epicardial aspect, the posterior (paraseptal) wall is related to the coronary sinuses of the aortic valve and therefore to the proximal portions of the right coronary artery and the left anterior descending coronary artery (Figure 18.13A). In a heart with a longer subpulmonary infundibulum, the left main coronary artery may pass beneath the posterior wall. Any perforation in the paraseptal part is more likely to go outside the heart than into the left ventricle. The septal component is found only in the most proximal part of the infundibulum, where the supraventricular crest fuses with the septomarginal trabeculation (see Figure 18.12B).

The Left Ventricle

The left ventricle approximates a conical shape. When the heart is viewed from the front, most of the left ventricle is hidden behind the right ventricle. Its outlet overlaps its inlet. Compared with that of the tricuspid valve, the annulus of the mitral valve is very limited at the septum. A long-axis section through the four cardiac chambers shows the mitral valve's location farther away from the apex than that of the tricuspid valve (Figure 18.14A). Viewed in RAO projection, the mitral and tricuspid "rings" merge anterosuperiorly but diverge inferoposteriorly. Anatomically, this also demonstrates how the area of the triangle of Koch is in fact right atrial wall overlying epicardial tissues. These tissues, in turn, overlie the portion of the ventricular septum that was previously dubbed the atrioventricular septum (Figure 18.14B).

At the inlet portion, the two leaflets of the mitral valve are disproportionate in size. The "anterior" leaflet is deep,

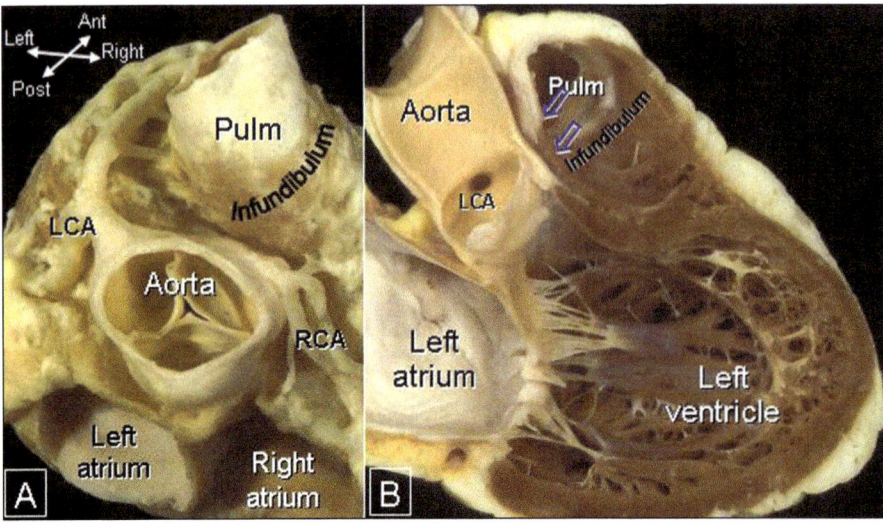

Figure 18.13 Panel A: This view shows the central location of the aortic valve and its relationship to the pulmonary valve (Pulm) and the anterior walls of both atria. The epicardium between the subpulmonary infundibulum and the aortic valve has been dissected, allowing the infundibulum to be pulled forward in order to demonstrate the higher level of the pulmonary valve relative to the plane of the aortic valve. **Panel B:** This sectional view shows infundibular muscle (**open arrow**) overlapping the sinuses of the aortic valve and the wall of the ascending aorta for some distance. Other than this overlap of muscle, no "sleeves" of muscle surround the outside of the aortic valve. LCA = left coronary artery; RCA = right coronary artery.

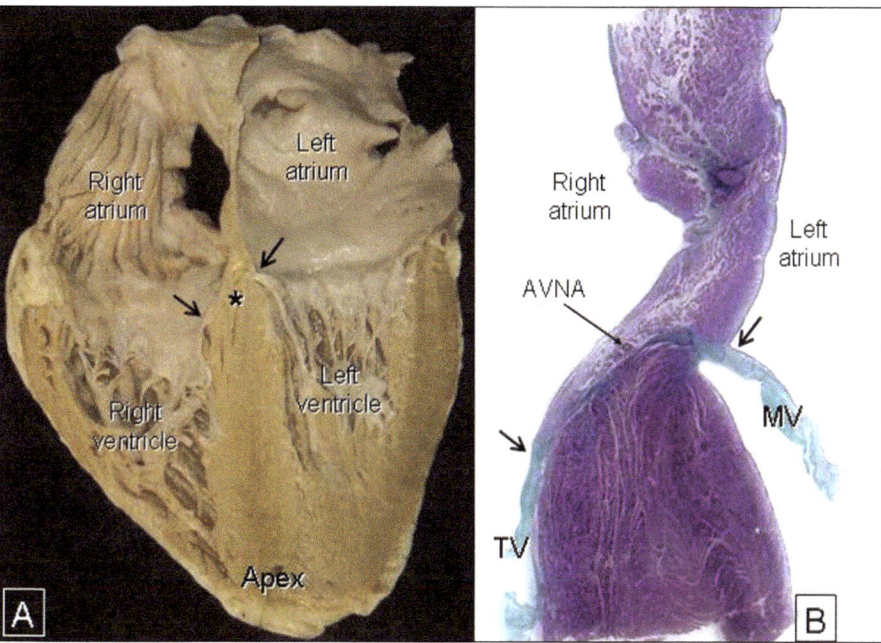

Figure 18.14 **Panel A:** A cut through the four cardiac chambers demonstrates the offset attachments (**arrows**) of the tricuspid and mitral valves at the septum, resulting in a so-called atrioventricular septum (**asterisk**). **Panel B:** This histological section shows that the area of the "atrioventricular septum" is actually a sandwich of atrial myocardium separated from ventricular myocardium by tissues from the atrioventricular groove. The artery supplying the atrioventricular node (AVNA) passes through this tissue. Masson's trichrome stain shows myocardium in **red-purple** and fibrous tissue in **blue-green**. MV = mitral valve; TV = tricuspid valve.

whereas the mural ("posterior") leaflet is shallow. The mitral leaflets are attached via tendinous cords exclusively to two groups of papillary muscles. The mural leaflet is further supported by basal cords or flaps that attach the leaflets directly to ventricular wall. At the annulus, the larger portion of the mitral valve is hinged to the parietal atrioventricular junction, whereas a third of the valve comprises the span of fibrous continuity with the aortic valve (see Figure 18.2B). At the septal end of valvular fibrous continuity is the right fibrous trigone, and at the parietal end is the left fibrous trigone. The right trigone, in continuity with the membranous septum, forms the central fibrous body.

The apical portion projects anteriorly and leftward from the level of the insertions of the papillary muscles to the ventricular apex. At the very tip, the muscular wall tapers to only 1 to 2 mm thickness (Figure 18.15A). Apical trabeculations are finer than those found in the right ventricle. Occasionally, fine muscular strands (so-called false tendons) extend between the septum and the papillary muscles or the parietal wall.[79] Often, they carry the distal ramifications of the left bundle branch; in recent years, they have been have been implicated in idiopathic left ventricular tachycardia.[24,80]

The left ventricular outlet is bordered on one side by the muscular ventricular septum curving anterosuperiorly and by the "anterior" mitral leaflet posteroinferiorly. Like the pulmonary valve, the semilunar hinge lines of the aortic valve cross the anatomic junction between ventricle and aortic wall: the ventriculo-arterial junction (Figure 18.15B). Because the outlet is bordered by muscle only on one side, only two of the aortic leaflets have muscular support. Hence, segments of ventricular myocardium can be found in the right coronary and left coronary aortic sinuses, while the noncoronary aortic sinus is in the area of aortic–mitral valvular fibrous continuity.

The two sinuses giving origin to the coronary arteries are also the sinuses nearest to the pulmonary valve (see Figures 18.13A, B, and 18.15B). Owing to this peculiar spatial relationship, the muscle of the subpulmonary infundibulum may be mistaken to be a sleeve over the aortic valve and hence a "supravalvular" muscle.[77,78] The location allows ectopic foci in the paraseptal subpulmonary infundibulum to be targeted from these aortic sinuses. Since the main coronary arteries usually arise from the upper part of the sinuses rather than deep inside them, they are not in the immediate field. Ablations within the sinuses without trauma to the coronary arteries have also been reported.[72,81] Owing to the aortic root occupying a central location in the heart, the noncoronary aortic sinus abuts the anterior walls of the atria and is close to the superior atrioventricular junction (see Figures 18.13A and 18.15B). Its position allows these areas to be mapped from this sinus and can be a portal for reaching focal atrial tachycardia in the vicinity of the His bundle.[82,83]

The upper part of the ventricular septum leading to the aortic valve is smooth; it contains the left bundle branch in its subendocardium. The left bundle branch descends from the branching atrioventricular conduction bundle. It usually branches into three main fascicles that interconnect and further divide distally into finer and finer branches as the Purkinje network, where the conduction tissues lose their fibrous sheaths.[23,24] Tracing the conduction bundle proximally, the branching atrioventricular bundle is the continuation of the common atrioventricular bundle. Whereas the branching bundle sits left of the crest of the muscular ventricular septum, the common atrioventricular conduction bundle is sandwiched between the membranous septum and the septal crest (see Figures

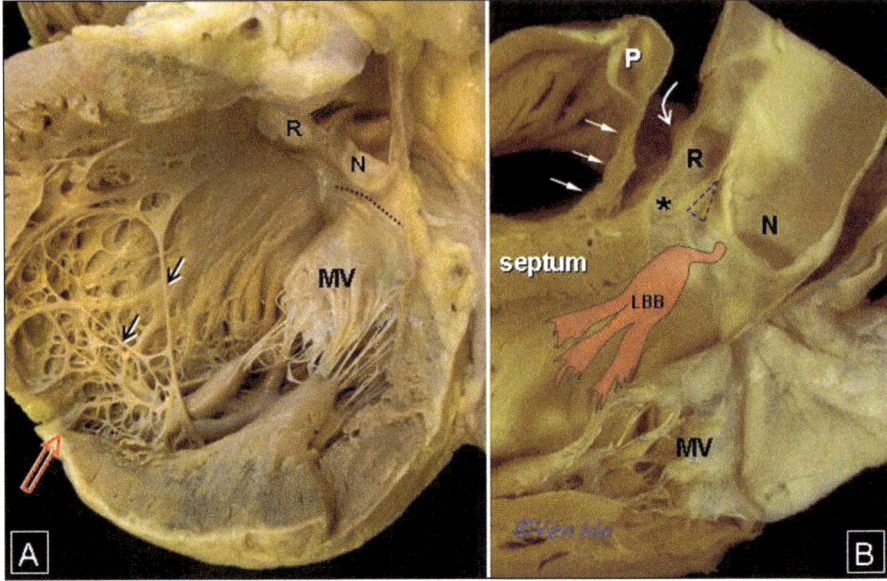

Figure 18.15 **Panel A:** The left ventricle is opened longitudinally to show the area of fibrous continuity (**dotted line**) between aortic and mitral valves. The apical trabeculations are fine, and the wall tapers to become very thin at the apex (**red arrow**). Fine muscle strands (**black arrows**) known as false tendons cross the cavity. N and R = non- and right coronary aortic leaflets, respectively. **Panel B:** This longitudinal section shows the aortic valve with its leaflets removed. There is muscle (**asterisk**) of the ventricular septum in the depth of the right coronary aortic sinus (R) but no muscle in the noncoronary aortic sinus (N). The infundibulum (**straight arrows**) with a remnant of the pulmonary valve (P) is pulled forward to show the epicardial tissue plane in front of the right aortic sinus and the origin of the right coronary artery (**curved arrow**). The interleaflet fibrous triangle (**dashed lines**) between the right and noncoronary aortic sinuses adjoins the membranous septum. The atrioventricular conduction bundle (**irregular red shape**) is sandwiched between the membranous septum and the muscular ventricular septum. From there descends the left bundle branch (LBB). MV = mitral valve.

18.5A and 18.15B). The anatomic landmark for the site where the atrioventricular conduction bundle emerges from the fibrous body is the membranous septum that adjoins the fibrous triangle between the crescentic hinge lines of the right and noncoronary leaflets of the aortic valve. In some hearts, the atrioventricular bundle itself continues beyond the bifurcation as a third bundle, termed the *dead-end tract*.[84]

Conclusions

A better understanding of detailed anatomy is essential to interventional electrophysiologists. Undeniably, the description of the heart in attitudinal orientation, as promoted in McAlpine's atlas[7] published in 1975, is crucial for understanding living cardiac anatomy. It is especially useful for grasping the spatial relationships that exist between and within cardiac chambers and important structures. This, in turn, can help avoid or minimize complications during interventional procedures, provide the anatomic background for some substrates of certain arrhythmias, and aid in the development of new approaches to electrophysiology procedures.

References

1. Sánchez-Quintana D, Cabrera JA, Climent V, et al. Anatomic relations between the esophagus and left atrium and relevance for ablation of atrial fibrillation. *Circulation*. 2005;112:1400-1405.
2. Sánchez-Quintana D, Cabrera JA, Climent V, et al. How close are the phrenic nerves to cardiac structures? Implications for cardiac interventionalists. *J Cardiovasc Electrophysiol*. 2005;16:309-313.
3. Sánchez-Quintana D, Ho SY, Climent V, et al. Anatomic evaluation of the left phrenic nerve relevant to epicardial and endocardial catheter ablation: implications for phrenic nerve injury. *Heart Rhythm*. 2009;6:764-768.
4. Shah D, Dumonceau JM, Burri H, et al. Acute pyloric spasm and gastric hypomotility: an extracardiac adverse effect of percutaneous radiofrequency ablation for atrial fibrillation. *J Am Coll Cardiol*. 2005;46:327-330.
5. Ho SY, Cabrera JA, Sánchez-Quintana D. Vagaries of the vagus nerve: relevance to ablationists. *J Cardiovasc Electrophysiol*. 2006:17;330-331.
6. Walmsley R. The orientation of the heart and the appearance of its chambers in the adult cadaver. *Br Heart J*. 1958;20:441-458.
7. McAlpine WA. *Heart and Coronary Arteries*. Berlin: Springer-Verlag; 1975:1.
8. Lee RJ, Kalman JM, Fitzpatrick AP, et al. Radiofrequency catheter modification of the sinus node for "inappropriate" sinus tachycardia. *Circulation*. 1995;92:2919-2928.
9. Boineau JP, Canavan TE, Schuessler RB, et al. Demonstration of a widely distributed atrial pacemaker complex in the human heart. *Circulation*. 1988;77:1221-1237.
10. Kalman JM, Olgin JE, Karch MR, et al. "Cristal tachycardias": Origin of right atrial tachycardias from the crista terminalis identified by intracardiac echocardiography. *J Am Coll Cardiol*. 1998;31:451-459.
11. Olgin JE, Kalman JM, Fitzpatrick AP, Lesh MD. Role of right atrial endocardial structures as barriers to conduction during human type I atrial flutter. Activation and

entrainment mapping guided by intracardiac echocardiography. *Circulation*. 1995,92:1839-1848.
12. Friedman PA, Luria D, Fenton AM, et al. Global right atrial mapping of human atrial flutter: the presence of posteromedial (sinus venosa region) functional block and double potentials: a study in biplane fluoroscopy and intracardiac echocardiography. *Circulation*. 2000;101:1568-1577.
13. Cabrera JA, Sánchez-Quintana D, Ho SY, et al. The architecture of the atrial musculature between the orifice of the inferior caval vein and the tricuspid valve: the anatomy of the isthmus. *J Cardiovasc Electrophysiol*. 1998;9:1186-1195.
14. Cabrera JA, Sánchez-Quintana D, Farre J, et al. The inferior right atrial isthmus: further architectural insights for current and coming ablation technologies. *J Cardiovasc Electrophysiol*. 2005;16:402-408.
15. Antz M, Scherlag BJ, Patterson E, et al. Electrophysiology of the right anterior approach to the atrioventricular node: studies in vivo and in the isolated perfused dog heart. *J Cardiovasc Electrophysiol* 1997;8:47-61.
16. Antz M, Scherlag BJ, Otomo K, et al. Evidence of multiple atrio-AV nodal inputs in the normal dog heart. *J Cardiovascular Electrophysiol*. 1998;9:395-408.
17. Hindricks G. Incidence of complete atrioventricular block following attempted radiofrequency catheter modification of the atrioventricular node in 880 patients. Results of the Multicenter European Radiofrequency Survey (MERFS). The Working Group on Arrhythmias of the European Society of Cardiology. *Eur Heart J*. 1996;17:82-88.
18. Hellerstein HK, Orbison JL. Anatomic variations of the orifice of the human coronary sinus. *Circulation*. 1951;3:514-523.
19. Walmsley R, Watson H. The medial wall of the right atrium. *Circulation*. 1966;34:400-411.
20. Keith A, Flack M. The form and nature of the muscular connections between the primary divisions of the vertebrate heart. *J Anat Physiol*. 1907;41:172-189.
21. Sánchez-Quintana D, Cabrera C, Farre J, et al. Sinus node revisited in the era of electroanatomical mapping and catheter ablation. *Heart*. 2005;91:189-194.
22. Anderson KR, Ho SY, Anderson RH. Location and vascular supply of sinus node in human heart. *Br Heart J*. 1979;41:28-32.
23. Tawara S. *The Conduction System of the Mammalian Heart. An Anatomico-histological Study of the Atrioventricular Bundle and the Purkinje Fibers*. Suma K, Shimada M, translators. London: Imperial College Press; 2000.
24. Ho SY, McCarthy KP, Ansari A, et al. Anatomy of the atrioventricular node and atrioventricular conduction system. *J Bifurcation & Chaos*. 2003;12:3665-3674.
25. Spach MS, Kootsey JM. The nature of electrical propagation in cardiac muscle. *Am J Physiol*. 1983;244:H3-H22.
26. Kent AFS. Researches on the structure and function of the mammalian heart. *J Physiol*. 1893;14:233-254.
27. Inoue S, Becker AE, Riccardi R, Gaita F. Interruption of the inferior extension of the compact atrioventricular node underlies successful radio frequency ablation of atrioventricular nodal reentrant tachycardia. *J Interv Card Electrophysiol*. 1999;3:273-277.
28. Anderson RH, Ho SY, Gillette PC, Becker AE. Mahaim, Kent and abnormal atrioventricular conduction. *Cardiovasc Res*. 1996;31:480-491.
29. Sealy WC, Gallagher JJ. The surgical approach to the septal area of the heart based on experiences with 45 patients with Kent bundles. *J Thorac Cardiovasc Surg*. 1980;79:542-551.
30. Sánchez-Quintana D, Ho SY, Cabrera JA, et al. Topographic anatomy of the inferior pyramidal space: relevance to radiofrequency ablation. *J Cardiovasc Electrophysiol*. 2001;12:210-217.
31. Becker AE, Anderson RH, Durrer D, Wellens HJ. The anatomical substrates of Wolff–Parkinson–White syndrome. A clinicopathologic correlation in seven patients. *Circulation*. 1978;57:870-879.
32. Kuck KH, Schluter M, Gursoy S. Preservation of atrioventricular nodal conduction during radiofrequency current catheter ablation of midseptal accessory pathways. *Circulation*. 1992;86:1743-1752.
33. Heaven DJ, Till JA, Ho SY. Sudden death in a child with an unusual accessory connection. *Europace*. 2000;2:224-227.
34. Platonov PG, Ivanov V, Ho SY, Mitrofanova L. Left atrial posterior wall thickness in patients with and without atrial fibrillation: Data from 298 consecutive autopsies. *J Cardiovasc Electrophysiol*. 2008;19:689-692.
35. McAlpine WA. *Heart and Coronary Arteries*. Berlin: Springer-Verlag; 1975:58.
36. Kim DT, Lai AC, Hwang C, et al. The ligament of Marshall: a structural analysis in human hearts with implications for atrial arrythmias. *J Am Coll Cardiol*. 2000;36:1324-1327.
37. Makino M, Inoue S, Matsuyama TA, et al. Diverse myocardial extension and autonomic innervation on ligament of Marshall in humans. *J Cardiovasc Electrophysiol*. 2006;17:594-599.
38. Kistler PM, Ho SY, Rajappan K, et al. Electrophysiologic and anatomic characterisation of sites resistant to electrical isolation during circumferential pulmonary vein ablation for atrial fibrillation: a prospective study. *J Cardiovasc Electrophysiol*. 2007;18:1282-1288.
39. Cabrera JA, Ho SY, Climent V, Sánchez-Quintana D. The architecture of the left lateral atrial wall: a particular anatomic region with implications for ablation of atrial fibrillation. *Eur Heart J*. 2008;29:356-362.
40. Becker AE. Left atrial isthmus: anatomic aspects relevant for linear catheter ablation procedures in humans. *J Cardiovasc Electrophysiol*. 2004;15:809-812.
41. Wittkampf FHM, van Oosterhout MF, Loh P, et al. Where to draw the mitral isthmus line in catheter ablation of atrial fibrillation: histological analysis. *Eur Heart J*. 2005;26:689-695.
42. Kato R, Lickfett L, Meininger G, et al. Pulmonary vein anatomy in patients undergoing catheter ablation of atrial fibrillation: lessons learned by use of magnetic resonance imaging. *Circulation*. 2003;107:2004-2010.
43. Tsao HM, Yu WC, Cheng HC et al. Pulmonary vein dilation in patients with atrial fibrillation: detection by magnetic resonance imaging. *J Cardiovasc Electrophysiol*. 2001;12:809-813.
44. Mansour M, Refaat M, Heist EK, et al. Three-dimensional anatomy of the left atrium by magnetic resonance angiography: implications for catheter ablation for atrial fibrillation. *J Cardiovasc Electrophysiol*. 2006;17:719-723.
45. Saito T, Waki K, Becker AE. Left atrial myocardial extension onto pulmonary veins in humans: anatomic observations relevant for atrial arrhythmias. *J Cardiovasc Electrophysiol*. 2000:11:888-894.
46. Ho SY, Cabrera JA, Tran VH, et al. Architecture of the pulmonary veins: relevance to radiofrequency ablation. *Heart*. 2001;86:265-270.
47. Tagawa M, Higuchi K, Chinushi M, et al. Myocardium extending from the left atrium onto the pulmonary veins: a comparison between subjects with and without atrial fibrillation. *Pacing Clin Electrophysiol*. 2001;24:1459-1463.
48. Cabrera JA, Ho SY, Climent V, et al. Morphological evidence of muscular connections between contiguous pulmonary venous orifices: relevance of the interpulmonary isthmus for catheter ablation in atrial fibrillation. *Heart Rhythm*. 2009;6(8):1192-1198.
49. Ho SY, Sánchez-Quintana D, Cabrera JA, Anderson RH. Anatomy of the left atrium: implications for radiofrequency

ablation of atrial fibrillation. *J Cardiovasc Electrophysiol.* 1999;10:1525-1533.
50. Ho SY, Anderson RH, Sánchez-Quintana D. Gross anatomy of the atriums: more than anatomical curiosity? *Pacing Clin Electrophysiol.* 2002;25:342-350.
51. Tzeis S, Andrikopoulos G, Deisenhofer I, et al. Transseptal catheterization: considerations and caveats. *Pacing Clin Electrophysiol.* 2010;33(2):231-242.
52. Hanaoka T, Suyama K, Taguchi A, et al. Shifting of puncture site in the fossa ovalis during radiofrequency catheter ablation: intracadiac echocardiography–guided transseptal left heart catheterization. *Jpn Heart J.* 2003;44:673-680.
53. Schwinger ME, Gindea AJ, Freedberg RS, Kronzon I. The anatomy of the interatrial septum: a transesophageal echocardiographic study. *Am Heart J.* 1990;119:1401-1405.
54. Ho SY, Sánchez-Quintana D. The importance of atrial structure and fibers. *Clin Anat.* 2009;22:52-63.
55. Ho SY, Anderson RH, Sánchez-Quintana D. Atrial structure and fibres: morphological basis of atrial conduction. *Cardiovasc Res.* 2002;54:325-336.
56. De Ponti R, Ho SY, Salerno-Uriarte JA, et al. Electroanatomic analysis of sinus impulse propagation in normal human atria. *J Cardiovasc Electrophysiol.* 2002;13:1-10.
57. Platonov PG, Mitrofanova LB, Chireikin LV, Olsson SB. Morphology of inter-atrial conduction routes in patients with atrial fibrillation. *Europace.* 2002;4:183-192.
58. Platonov PG, Mitrofanova L, Ivanov V, Ho SY. Substrates for intra- and interatrial conduction in the atrial septum: anatomical study on 84 human hearts. *Heart Rhythm.* 2008;5:1189-1195.
59. Kurotobi T, Ito H, Inoue K, et al. Marshall vein as arrhythmogenic source in patients with atrial fibrillation: correlation between its anatomy and electrophysiologic findings. *J Cardiovasc Electrophysiol.* 2006;17:1062-1067.
60. Basso C, Corrado D, Rossi L, Thiene G. Ventricular preexcitation in children and young adults: atrial myocarditis as a possible trigger of sudden death. *Circulation.* 2001;103:269-275.
61. Kozlowski D, Kozluk E, Adamowicz M, et al. Histological examination of the topography of the atrioventricular nodal artery within the triangle of Koch. *Pacing Clin Electrophysiol.* 1998;21:163-167.
62. Sánchez-Quintana D, Ho SY, Cabrera JA, et al. Topographic anatomy of the inferior pyramidal space: relevance to radiofrequency ablation. *J Cardiovasc Electrophysiol.* 2001;12:210-217.
63. Gensini G, Giorgi SD, Coskun O, et al. Anatomy of the coronary circulation in living man. *Circulation.* 1965;31:778-784.
64. Lüdinghausen VM, Schott C. Microanatomy of the human coronary sinus and its major tributaries. In: *Myocardial Perfusion, Reperfusion, Coronary Venous Retroperfusion.* Meerbaum S, ed. Darmstadt, Germany: Steinkopff Verlag; 1990:93-122.
65. Ho SY, Sánchez-Quintana D, Becker AE. A review of the coronary venous system: a road less travelled. *Heart Rhythm.* 2004;1:107-112.
66. Corcoran SJ, Lawrence C, McGuire MA. The valve of Vieussens: an important cause of difficulty in advancing catheter into cardiac veins. *J Cardiovasc Electrophysiol.* 1999;10:804-808.
67. Lüdinghausen VM, Ohmachi N, Boot C. Myocardial coverage of the coronary sinus and related veins. *Clin Anat.* 1992;5:1-15.
68. Chauvin M, Shah DC, Haissaguerre M, et al. The anatomic basis of connections between the coronary sinus musculature and the left atrium in humans. *Circulation.* 2000;101:647-652.
69. Kozlowski D, Kozluk E, Piatkowska A, et al. The middle cardiac vein as a key for "posteroseptal" space—a morphological point of view. *Folia Morph.* 2001;60:293-296.
70. Omran H, Pfeiffer D, Tebbenjohanns J, et al. Echocardiographic imaging of coronary sinus diverticula and middle cardiac veins in patients with preexcitation syndrome: impact on radiofrequency catheter ablation of posteroseptal accessory pathways. *Pacing Clin Electrophysiol.* 1995;18:1236-1243.
71. Ho SY, Russell G, Rowland E. Coronary venous aneurysms and accessory atrioventricular connections. *Br Heart J.* 1988;60:348-351.
72. Ouyang F, Fotuhi P, Ho SY, et al. Repetitive monomorphic ventricular tachycardia originating from the aortic sinus cusp: electrocardiographic characterization for guiding catheter ablation. *J Am Coll Cardiol.* 2002;39:500-508.
73. Vaseghi M, Cesario DA, Mahajan A, et al. Catheter ablation of right ventricular outflow tract tachycardia: value of defining coronary anatomy. *J Cardiovasc Electrophysiol.* 2006;17:632-637.
74. Hasdemir C, Aktas S, Govsa F, et al. Demonstration of ventricular myocardial extensions into the pulmonary artery and aorta beyond the ventriculo-arterial junction. *Pacing Clin Electrophysiol.* 2007;30:534-539.
75. Suleiman M, Asirvatham SJ. Ablation above the semilunar valves: when, why, and how? Part I. *Heart Rhythm.* 2008;5:1485-492.
76. Ho SY. Letter to editor re: catheter ablation of right ventricular outflow tract. *J Cardiovasc Electrophysiol.* 2006;17:E7.
77. Ho SY. Structure and anatomy of the aortic root. *Eur J Echocardiogr.* 2009;10:i3-i10.
78. Ho SY. Anatomic insights for catheter ablation of ventricular tachycardia. *Heart Rhythm.* 2009;6:S77-S80.
79. Kervancioglu M, Ozbag D, Kervancioglu P, et al. Echocardiographic and morphologic examination of left ventricular false tendons in human and animal hearts. *Clin Anat.* 2003;16(5):389-395.
80. Thakur RK, Klein GJ, Sivaram CA, et al. Anatomic substrate for idiopathic left ventricular tachycardia. *Circulation.* 1996;93:497-501.
81. Shimoike E, Ohnishi Y, Ueda N, et al. Radiofrequency catheter ablation of left ventricular outflow tract tachycardia from the coronary cusp: a new approach to the tachycardia focus. *J Cardiovasc Electrophysiol.* 1999;10:1005-1009.
82. Ouyang F, Ma J, Ho SY, et al. Focal atrial tachycardia originating from the non-coronary aortic sinus: electrophysiological characteristics and catheter ablation. *J Am Coll Cardiol.* 2006;48:122-131.
83. Liu XP, Dong JZ, Ho SY, et al. Atrial tachycardia arising adjacent to noncoronary aortic sinus distinctive atrial activation patterns and anatomic insights. *J Am Coll Cardiol.* 2010;56:796-804.
84. Kurosawa H, Becker AE. Dead-end tract of the conduction axis. *Int J Cardiol.* 1985;7:13-20.

CHAPTER 19

Physical and Experimental Aspects of Radiofrequency Energy, Generators, and Energy Delivery Systems

Munther K. Homoud, MD; Abram Mozes, MD

Introduction

The introduction and development of catheter ablation of cardiac tissue using radiofrequency (RF) energy has revolutionized the management of patients with arrhythmic disorders. Catheter ablation was first used in the early 1980s using direct current (DC) energy but was replaced by RF ablation when it became available owing to ease of use, improved control of energy delivery, and reduction in barotrauma risk.[1-3] In 1987, Huang et al introduced RF energy as a new source of energy not associated with the risks and adverse features associated with DC catheter ablation.[4]

Catheter ablation has supplanted cardiac surgery in the management of recurrent arrhythmic disorders and is used to target well-localized sources of arrhythmias, such as focal atrial tachycardias and idiopathic ventricular tachycardia (VT), or to interrupt critical pathways that support arrhythmias, such as atrial flutter, reentrant supraventricular arrhythmias, and nonidiopathic VT. While other forms of energy are being investigated, the safety and consistency of RF energy has made it the predominant source of energy used for catheter ablation, and it is expected to remain as such for the foreseeable future. This chapter aims to explain how this source of energy works, its safe application, the limitations it poses, and new developments that have been introduced to overcome these limitations. The hope is to enable operators to better understand its use in the setting of contemporary interventional electrophysiology.

The Biophysics of Radiofrequency Ablation

RF energy is an alternating current generated with a frequency of 350 to 700 kHz (usually 500 kHz on commercially available RF generators) delivered in a continuous, unmodulated sinusoidal manner to create thermal injury (Figure 19.1). The current is delivered in a unipolar manner to an indifferent, large surface (100–250 cm^2), with a patch placed against the skin. The thermal injury results from the transformation of electrical energy to thermal injury when passing through tissue with high resistance (ie, resistive heating). The indifferent patch or dispersive electrode's large surface area precludes high-current densities and the risk of developing skin burns. However, care must be taken to ensure that the indifferent patch is large enough and well coated with a conducting gel to avoid points of high-current density that may lead to skin burns.[5]

The injury created with RF energy is thermal. Tissue in immediate contact with the catheter tip is subject to *resistive heating*, resulting in coagulation necrosis. Although injury will occur with tissue temperatures greater than 50°C, to achieve irreversible injury, a catheter-tip temperature of more than 60° ± 7°C is required.[6-9] Late pathological changes after RF ablation include well-demarcated necrotic lesions with fibrosis, fatty infiltration, cartilage, granulation tissue, and chronic inflammatory cell infiltration.[10] The area surrounding the necrotic zone is characterized by contraction band necrosis.

Magnetic resonance imaging (MRI) has recently been shown to display characteristic time-dependent changes after RF lesions were applied to canine right ventricular epicardium.[11] Using nitroblue tetrazolium (NBT), ultrastructural changes were seen to extend up to 6 mm beyond the pathological lesion edge. These changes particularly affected the cell membranes and gap junctions; however, preserved myocytes within the 3- to 6-mm zone had the potential to recover.[12]

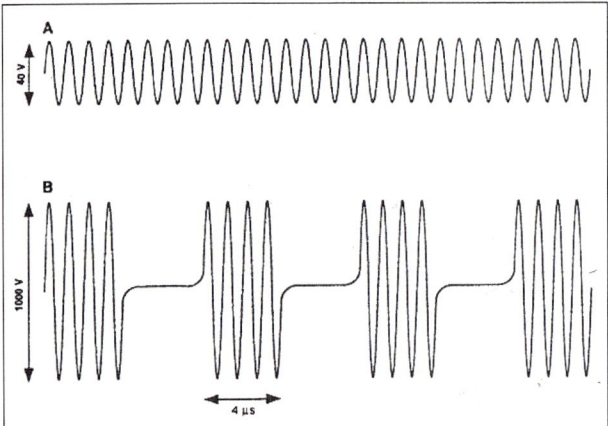

Figure 19.1 A comparison between the radiofrequency energy used in ablation, continuous (sine wave: **Panel A**) and the radiofrequency used in electrosurgery, cutting, and coagulation (intermittent and higher voltage: **Panel B**). *Source:* Reprinted with permission from Kalbfleisch SJ, Langberg JJ. Catheter ablation with radiofrequency energy: biophysical aspects and clinical applications. *J Cardiovasc Electrophysiol.* 1992;3(2):173-186. ©1992 John Wiley & Sons, Inc. All rights reserved.

The power delivered, measured in watts (W) and converted to heat, is directly proportional to the square of the current (I) and to tissue resistance (R).[13] The site of maximal endocardial temperature generation is the surface in immediate contact with the catheter tip and is directly proportional to the square of the current density at the catheter tip ($W = I^2R$).[14] Current density falls as it disperses peripherally in inverse proportion to the square of the distance from the catheter tip (current density = $1/4\pi r^2$). As tissue heating extends peripherally, thermal injury now results from *conductive heating*, with a progressive drop in temperature that is inversely proportional to the fourth power of the distance from the catheter tip. This effect explains the shallow nature (<1 mm) of the lesion created by resistive heating (heat ~ tissue resistance / $16\pi r^4$).[5,13,15] In fact, the myocardial tissue subjected to resistive heating is considerably smaller than the myocardial tissue injured by conductive heating.[5] Whereas resistive heating is immediate, conductive heating takes time; therefore, it takes 30 to 60 seconds for a mature lesion to form.[16,17] The size of the lesion depends on the catheter-tip temperature attained and the electrode radius.[5,15,18] The size of the lesion in the first 20 seconds depends on lesion duration and power delivery; beyond that, the size will depend on the amount of power delivered (Figure 19.2).[19]

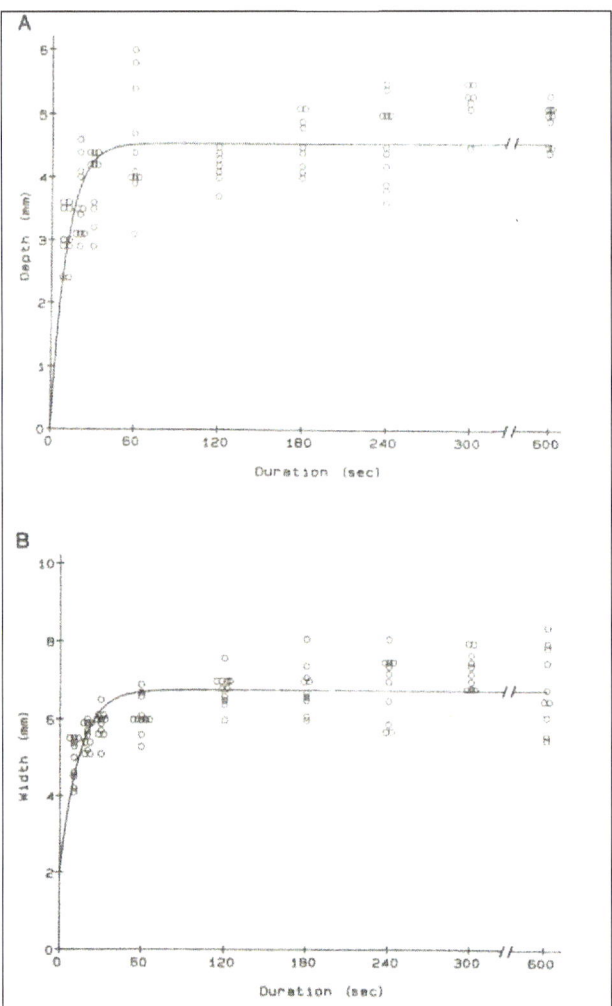

Figure 19.2 The relationship between duration of energy delivery and the depth (**Panel A**) and width (**Panel B**) of a lesion in an isolated canine right ventricular free wall. Lesion was formed using a 1.6-mm electrode with a tissue-electrode temperature of 80°C, maintained by varying the power output from the generator. Tissue heating with a fixed-temperature tip catheter displays a monoexponential curve. The lesion size approaches steady state by 40 to 50 seconds. For a catheter tip–tissue interface temperature of 80°C, thermal injury requires at least 20 seconds; to maximize the lesion size, it requires at least 40 seconds. *Source:* Reprinted with permission from Haines DE. Determinants of lesion size during radiofrequency catheter ablation: the role of electrode-tissue contact pressure and duration of energy delivery. *J Cardiovasc Electrophysiol.* 1991;2(6):509-515. ©1991 John Wiley & Sons, Inc. All rights reserved.

Heat is transferred to surrounding tissue by radial heat conduction, which establishes a gradient between the tissue in immediate contact with the catheter tip and the peripheral rim of the lesion. After energy delivery ceases, the temperatures at the catheter–tissue interface immediately drop. However, temperatures at the rim may continue to rise as a result of the heat gradient between the heat source and the rim—a phenomenon known as *thermal latency* (see Figure 19.3).[20] This explains several complications: damage to collateral structures, such as the development of atrioventricular (AV) block seconds after the cessation of energy delivery at sites close to the AV node, and the continued rise in esophageal temperatures after cessation of energy delivery at sites close to the esophagus during ablation for atrial fibrillation.

Determinants of Lesion Size

The main determinants of lesion size are twofold: the amount of power delivered to and the temperature measured at the catheter–tissue interface.[15,19] The area within the 50°C boundary (the 50°C isotherm line) is dependent on the temperature of the source.[15] However, when catheter ablation is performed in a beating cardiac chamber, other factors play a role in determining lesion size.[21] It is important to bear in mind that the temperature recorded by the catheter tip results from the transfer of heat from the tissue the catheter tip is in contact with. That is, RF energy does not directly heat the catheter tip. Thus, when the *temperature-control mode* of power delivery is employed, the cooling effect of blood flow around the catheter tip becomes an important determinant of lesion size.

In the canine thigh muscle preparation, Matsudaira et al demonstrated that lesions created by setting a low target temperature in the presence of blood flow were larger than lesions created with a higher target temperature but in the absence of surrounding flow.[22] This is similar to the findings of Eick et al, who demonstrated that lesions delivered in areas of high flow were larger than lesions delivered in areas of low or no flow, despite recording higher electrode–tissue interface temperatures in the areas of low flow.[14] Heat is lost from the electrode–tissue interface through a process of convection (convective cooling). In areas of low flow, where convective cooling is absent or minimal, high temperatures are rapidly attained at the catheter–tissue interface, reducing further delivery of power and leading to the creation of smaller lesions.

An experimental model demonstrated that the maximal temperatures achieved were inversely related to the velocity of blood flow surrounding the catheter and that the highest temperatures were recorded on the outflow side of the catheter.[23] Rapid rises in temperature with low power delivery can be seen when lesions are delivered in areas with low blood flow such as the left atrium in atrial fibrillation, the left ventricle in the setting of a cardiomyopathy, or if the catheter tip is intimately embedded within endocardial tissue or is wedged in a branch of the coronary sinus.[16] It has been observed that lesions delivered in high-flow areas result in larger lesions giving rise to the concept of cooled catheter ablation. While it is important to monitor the temperature during lesion delivery, the operator should be aware of limitations that temperature monitoring alone poses.

Lesions delivered close to blood vessels are smaller than those delivered farther away.[24] Circulating blood acts as a "heat sink," limiting the size of the ensuing lesion and protecting the surrounding vessels from thermal injury during RF catheter ablation.[24,25] This explains why vascular injury is rarely reported as a complication of catheter ablation; however, this is also one of the reasons the creation of contiguous linear lesions with RF catheter ablation is difficult.[21]

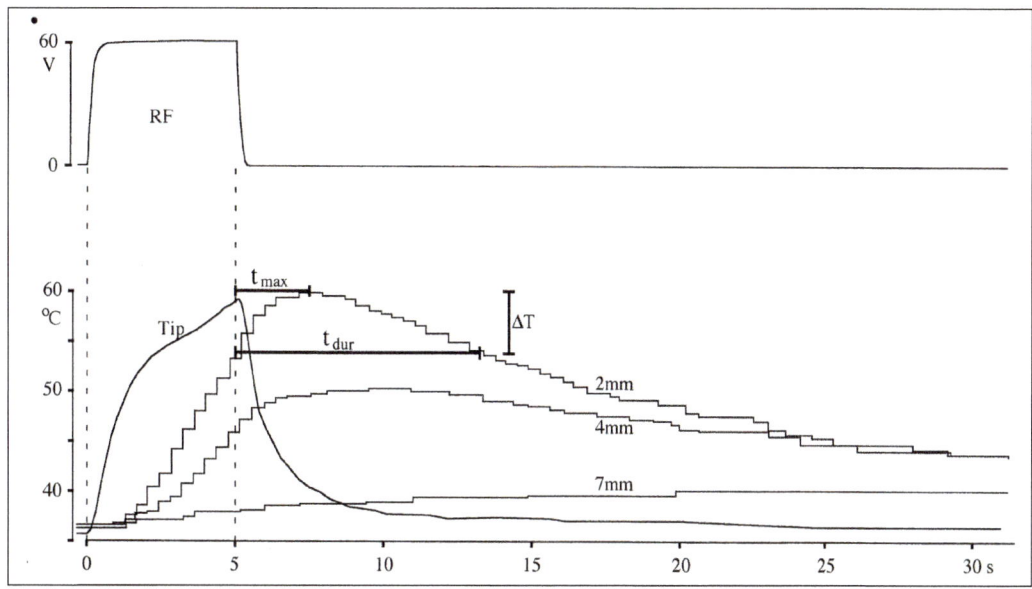

Figure 19.3 The concept of thermal latency is demonstrated in this figure plotting temperatures recorded at the tip of the catheter, 2, 4, and 7 mm after the delivery of a lesion on a thigh muscle preparation. The tip temperature falls immediately after energy delivery is terminated; however, temperatures continue to climb, reaching a peak 2.7, 5.3, and 16 seconds after termination of energy delivery at 2, 4, and 7 mm depths, respectively. t_{max} indicates the maximum temperature attained after termination of energy delivery; t_{dur} is the time it took for the temperature to return to what it was immediately before energy termination; T is the increase in tissue temperature after energy delivery termination. *Source:* Reprinted with permission from Wittkampf FH, et al, their Figure 2.[20] Copyright ©1996 American Heart Association.

Coagulum Formation

Coagulum or char formation is one factor limiting the size of the lesion created by RF current. Rapidly attaining tissue temperatures of 100°C or greater at the electrode–tissue interface during ablation can lead to tissue desiccation and protein denaturation. These, in turn, may result in coagulum, char formation, and embolization as well as limiting further delivery of energy.[26] The coagulum is not a clot in the true sense and cannot be prevented by anticoagulation with heparin.[16] Normally, the delivery of RF energy leads to a predictable fall in tissue impedance that increases current delivery and subsequent thermal injury.[5] However, the development of an insulating coagulum has the opposite effect: to impede current flow and raise impedance. This observation, in the context of lesion delivery, should lead to the immediate termination of the delivery of RF energy (Figure 19.4).[26]

This condition is more likely to be encountered in areas of low blood flow where there is inadequate catheter-tip cooling. RF delivery systems in use will automatically terminate lesion delivery when a sudden rise in impedance is encountered. This generation of ablation catheters incorporates thermocouples and thermistors into the tips that allow the monitoring of catheter tip–tissue interface temperature, thereby reducing the risk of char and coagulum formation.[27] In the *temperature-control mode,* power is delivered to achieve the desired catheter-tip temperature. This mode modifies the power output to maintain the desired catheter-tip temperature and prevent it from rising beyond the point where coagulum and char will form. More sustained, uninterrupted energy delivery would otherwise allow the formation of a larger lesion. The temperature recorded by the thermistor approximates the temperature of tissue in contact with the catheter. The recorded temperature depends on several factors: the degree of cooling from surrounding blood flow, the location of the thermistor in the catheter tip, the size of the catheter tip, and its orientation relative to the tissue surface.[28] The difference between the temperature measured by the catheter tip at the surface and the tissue temperature is greater under the following conditions: when blood flows rapidly around the catheter (convective cooling effect), when using longer tipped catheters (greater exposure to the cooling effect of blood), and when using a perpendicular or oblique orientation of the catheter tip as opposed to a parallel orientation.[28] The difference between catheter and tissue temperature is less when the catheter tip is embedded in tissue.[16]

The operator should be aware that coagulum may still form without an appreciable rise in impedance, rise in catheter temperatures, or even if the operator failed to see one on the catheter tip after its withdrawal.[16,22] The coagulum initially forms on the hotter tissue surface, and it is only when the cooler electrode tip attains higher temperatures that the impedance will rise.[16] In the canine thigh muscle preparation, Matsudaira et al demonstrated that, in the presence of blood flow, "thrombus" was detected at temperatures as low as 65°C when using a 4-mm tip catheter and 55°C when using an 8-mm tip catheter.[22] To avoid coagulum formation in high-flow areas, the temperature of a 4-mm tip catheter should not exceed 55°C, and 45°C for 8-mm tip catheters.[22]

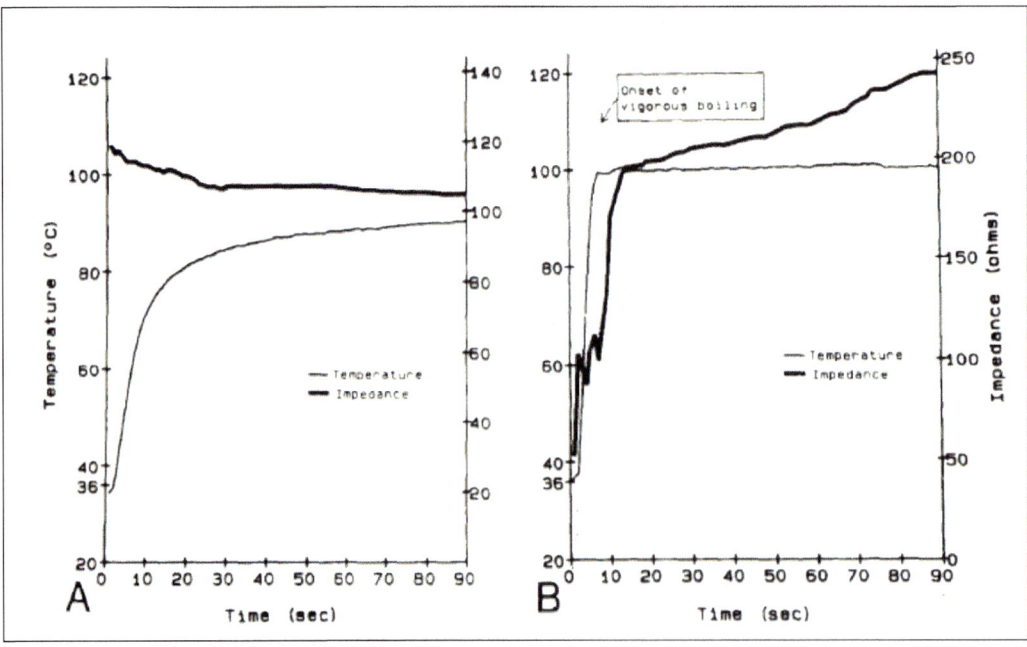

Figure 19.4 **Panel A:** The expected 5–10 Ω drop in impedance associated with a rise in catheter–tissue temperature. **Panel B:** A rise in impedance associated with a catheter–tissue temperature reaching 100°C. The resulting char and coagulum formation leads to the impedance rise, limiting the delivery of further power and the size of the lesion and creating a clot that may embolize. *Source:* Reprinted with permission from Nath S, Haines DE.[5] ©1992 Elsevier. All rights reserved.

RF Catheter Impedance for Determining the Status of the Delivered Lesion

A change in catheter impedance during power delivery has been used as an indirect surrogate for tissue heating.[7] Resistance (impedance) to current flow drops during tissue heating, a change that is attributed to an increase in ionic mobility.[29] Impedance drop is not a marker of irreversible tissue injury.[30] However, there is a good correlation between the degree of drop in lead impedance at the onset of lesion delivery and real-time tissue–electrode temperature.[29] Adequate contact and tissue heating should be signaled by a 10 ohm (Ω) drop in impedance. Ablation impedance has also been shown to correlate with contact force, which is an important determinant of both lesion size and catheter ablation–related complications.[31] A low measured impedance followed by a lack of impedance drop should suggest poor tissue contact.[30] Impedance rise can predict excessive heating at the surface or within the myocardium. Steep declines in impedance due to excessive tissue heating (>15 Ω during the first 2 seconds) can also predict an impedance rise, the development of a thrombus, or "steam pop" and should prompt the immediate discontinuation of power delivery.[30] A good way to determine the effectiveness of the delivered lesion is to observe the reduction in local EGM amplitude and the change in the slope of the distal unipolar electrogram recorded by the catheter tip.[16]

Steam Popping

Sudden rises in tissue temperature, particularly when exceeding 100°C deep in myocardial tissue, may result in deep-tissue disruption and thrombus formation at the catheter tip.[26] This is often preceded by an impedance rise and may be associated with a tactile sense of "popping." This popping results from the transformation of intramyocardial tissue water into steam and the release of the steam bubble that had formed underneath the catheter, and thus the term "steam pop." The disruption of myocardial integrity may lead to a pericardial tamponade.

Radiofrequency energy delivered in the temperature-control mode delivers power (within the limits imposed by the operator and generator) directed to achieve the desired temperature at the electrode–tissue interface. However, the electrode–tissue interface temperature is not an accurate surrogate of tissue temperature. Eick et al demonstrated in an *in vitro* porcine left ventricular model that circulating fluid flow and poor tissue contact were both associated with a higher incidence of "steam pop."[14] The lower recorded temperatures associated with higher fluid flow through convective cooling and with lower contact would propel the generator to increase the delivery of power and thus cause the intramyocardial transformation of tissue water to steam.[14]

The creation of a gaseous medium within the myocardium leads to the impedance rise often seen immediately before a steam pop and should immediately interrupt the delivery of the lesion. The patient should be evaluated for any possible consequences of myocardial tissue rupture.

Improvements in Catheter Ablation

Catheter ablation of nonidiopathic VT and atrial fibrillation requires making deeper and contiguous lesions that cannot be reliably created by standard 4-mm catheters. As attention in interventional electrophysiology has shifted to ablating scar-related tachyarrhythmias (eg, nonidiopathic VT and isolation of the pulmonary veins), the need for catheters that could create larger, contiguous, and transmural lesions has grown. The inability to create a contiguous line not only reduces the success of the procedure but may actually promote the emergence of new arrhythmias due to gaps left in the line that had been attempted to interrupt the path of the original arrhythmia.[32]

While the delivery of higher power results in larger lesions, the development of high temperatures at the electrode–tissue interface limits the amount of power that can be delivered and the depth of the lesions that can be created. Furthermore, delivering lesions in areas of low flow (such as a dilated left atrium in atrial fibrillation or a dilated hypocontractile ventricle) leads to high temperatures at the catheter–tissue interface, thus limiting the delivery of further power and precluding the creation of deeper lesions.[14] Two developments have helped overcome these limitations: larger catheter tips and catheter-tip cooling.

Large-tip Catheters

Large-tip catheters were introduced to offset the limited lesion size attained with a standard 4-mm tip catheter. To offset the lower impedance associated with large-tip catheters, generators capable of delivering greater power have to be used. Large catheter tips (5, 8, and 10 mm) result in the delivery of RF energy over larger surface areas and, in turn, create larger lesions.[33,34] The larger catheter-tip surface area also allows for greater convective cooling, higher power delivery, and larger lesion size. However, unless the large-tip catheter is coupled with a source of higher RF energy, the larger catheter-tip surface area will experience greater cooling and dissipation of energy, creating shallower lesions.[35] Compared with 4-mm tip catheters, 8-mm tip catheters result in larger lesions in part owing to increased convective cooling.[36-38]

Despite their advantages, there are several drawbacks to using large-tip catheters: (1) catheter-tip temperatures recorded from larger tips are less predictive of tissue temperature; (2) changes in catheter-tip orientation relative to the tissue surface result in significant fluctuations in delivered power; and (3) impedance changes are less predictive of tissue overheating.[16] The larger surface also reduces the fidelity of the recorded electrogram. In addition, lesions delivered by large-tip catheters lack uniformity owing to the "edge effect," in which current is concentrated at the catheter edge.[38] Also, lesions delivered by large-tip catheters with only one thermistor may result in coagulum formation at a catheter edge remote from the thermistor if the latter is located in a conventional location.[38] In fact, smaller irrigated-tip electrodes can result in deeper lesions than large-tip catheters and confer the advantage of providing sharper electrograms.[39]

A comparison between externally irrigated, internally irrigated, single-thermistor, and double-thermistor 8-mm catheters demonstrated the superiority of externally irrigated catheters to the large-tip catheters in ablating cavotricuspid isthmus–dependent atrial flutter.[40] Compared with large-tip catheters, ablation with the smaller irrigated-tip catheter was associated with shorter procedure and fluoroscopy time. Notwithstanding, large-tip catheters play an important role in ablating isthmus-dependent atrial flutter and scar-related tachyarrhythmias, such as VT. Compared with standard-tip catheters, large-tip catheters deliver energy more effectively when they are positioned parallel to the endocardial tissue, explaining their widespread use in atrial flutter ablation.

Catheter-tip Cooling

Cooling the catheter tip by using saline irrigation limits temperature rise at the electrode–tissue interface, thereby preventing the development of coagulum and char. This not only enhances the safety of power delivery but enhances the delivery of higher energies for longer periods of time that, in turn, will lead to the creation of larger lesions.[41] Petersen et al demonstrated that, for the same target temperature of 70°C, the lesion created by a temperature-controlled, irrigated catheter was larger than the lesion created with a standard catheter.[42] The larger lesions are created by expanding the size of the myocardial tissue subjected to resistive heating through the process of greater energy and longer delivery. It is important to note that irrigation alone does not lead to the formation of a larger lesion unless the power delivered is increased; otherwise, power is dissipated into the surrounding circulation.[21,43]

The seminal work by Nakagawa and his colleagues on the effect of different forms of RF ablation on the exposed canine thigh muscle demonstrates the different types of lesions created by different modes of energy delivery.[44] The smallest lesions were observed when energy was delivered at a high constant voltage, intermediate in size when variable voltage was employed to maintain a catheter–tissue interface temperature of 80° to 90°C (temperature control), and large when lesions were delivered at a high constant voltage with irrigation (see Figure 19.3). All the constant voltage applications were terminated prematurely owing to a rise in impedance secondary to high interface temperatures.

Compared with nonirrigated preparations, where the highest temperatures were recorded at the tip electrode, the highest temperatures recorded using irrigated ablation catheters were 3.5 mm below the electrode–tissue surface. Whereas the size of the lesion created with nonirrigated-tip catheters correlated with temperatures recorded by the catheter at the electrode–tissue interface, no such correlation was seen with irrigated-tip catheters. Saline cools the electrode–tissue interface, preventing temperature rises that would have otherwise limited power delivery. In part owing to the surface cooling effect and in part owing to the generation of the highest temperatures deep in the tissue, the widest part of the lesion created using an irrigated-tip catheter is below the tissue surface (Figure 19.5). Reducing the flow of irrigation reduces surface cooling that, in turn,

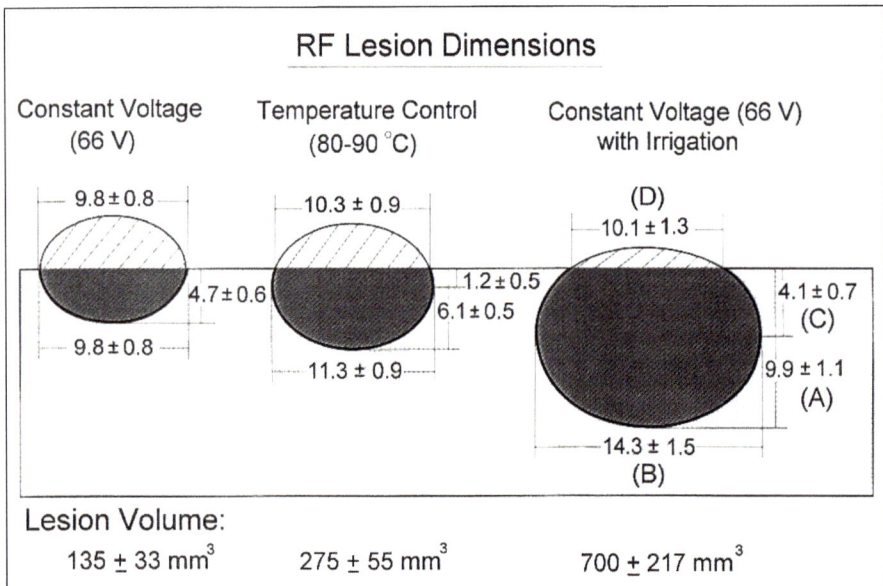

Figure 19.5 A diagram depicting the size and morphology of radiofrequency (RF) lesions. **Left to right:** RF lesions resulting from constant voltage without irrigation, temperature control, and constant voltage with irrigation. The lesion size progresses from left to right. The lesion site with the widest diameter is measured below the surface, using temperature control and the irrigated-tip catheter. *Source:* Reprinted with permission from Nakagawa H, et al, their Figure 9.[44] ©1995 American Heart Association, Inc. All rights reserved.

broadens the width of the surface lesion and allows for better tissue temperature monitoring. Conversely, increasing the rate of irrigation has been shown to reduce the surface diameter of the lesion created.[45]

The use of cooled-tip catheter technology is not free of risk. In fact, the study by Nakagawa et al showed that some of the lesions associated with irrigated-tip catheters were associated with impedance rise and "steam pop."[44] This important finding is confounded by the lack of correlation between thermistor– or electrode–tissue temperature and tissue temperature, which results in large part from saline cooling. The investigators recorded mean tip–electrode temperature as 38.4C°±5.1C°, and at no time did the temperature exceed 48°C. The investigators also observed that, 60 seconds after initiating energy delivery using the irrigated-tip catheter, a steep rise in temperature was recorded 7 mm below the surface. This finding indicates that a longer application would have led to the creation of a larger lesion.[44] This is another example of the thermal latency effect alluded to earlier and has important implications when lesions are delivered in the posterior left atrium close to the esophagus, where this type of catheter technology is often employed.

The discrepancy between catheter-tip temperature and tissue temperature was highlighted in a study by Bruce et al using an irrigated-tip catheter to ablate at the ostia of canine pulmonary vein with thermocouples attached to the atrial tissue to measure tissue temperature.[46] Energy was delivered at 5 W and uptitrated in 5 W increments to 45 W over a total of 120 seconds. Figure 19.6 shows the discrepancy between the temperature measured by the catheter tip and the tissue temperature attained with progressive increases in energy delivery.

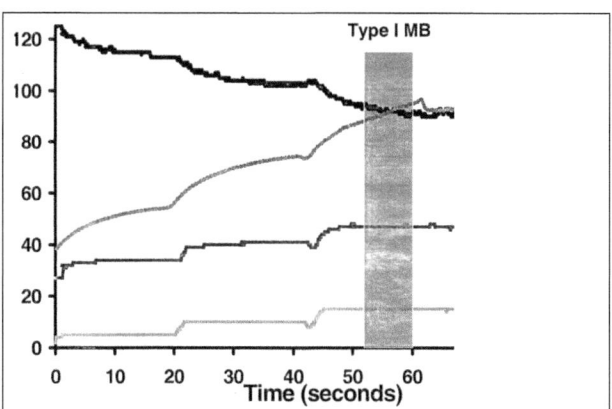

Figure 19.6 With the increase in delivery of power, both catheter-tip and tissue temperature increase. However, the discrepancy between the recorded tip temperature and the tissue temperature (which is nominally not recorded) is clearly apparent. The drop in impedance reflects tissue heating. Type I microbubbles (MB) are scattered artifacts seen on intracardiac echocardiography. They reflect tissue heating and have been proposed as a surrogate for tissue heating. *Source:* Reprinted with permission from Bruce GK, et al, their Figure 1.[46]

Dorwarth et al compared two types of irrigated-tip catheters (external and internally cooled), 8-mm, and standard 4-mm tip catheters in an *in vitro* pig left ventricle model.[43] Lesions created with the irrigated-tip and 8-mm catheters were comparable in volume and significantly larger than the lesions created with the 4-mm catheter. Cooled-tip catheters created deeper lesions than noncooled catheters, and the diameter of externally cooled catheters and 8-mm catheters was greater than the diameter of the lesions created by either the internally cooled or 4-mm catheter. Impedance rises were less likely to be seen with externally irrigated or large-tip catheters than with the internally cooled or standard-tip catheter. Impedance rises were more likely to be seen with power ≥30 W with the externally irrigated catheter compared with ≥20 W when using the internally irrigated catheter. Coagulum formation was less likely to be seen with the externally irrigated catheter.

Currently, two irrigated tip catheters are available: one with internal irrigation and the other with external irrigation. The Boston Scientific Chilli II Cooled Ablation Catheter (Boston Scientific, Natick, MA) uses a closed-loop irrigation system delivered to cool the 4-mm tip. The first cooled-tip catheter employing internal irrigation, the Boston Scientific Chilli was approved for treatment of ventricular tachycardia in 1999. It uses saline cooled to room temperature and infused at a rate of 0.6 mL/second.[47]

The NaviStar THERMOCOOL open irrigation system (Biosense Webster, Diamond Bar, CA) was approved for use by the FDA in 2009 for "type I atrial flutter in patients ≥18 years, recurrent drug/device refractory VT in post MI [myocardial infarction] patients and in drug refractory, recurrent and symptomatic paroxysmal atrial fibrillation."[48] This is a 7-Fr catheter with an 8-Fr tip containing a 3.5-mm electrode and 6 irrigation pores. During mapping, room temperature saline is irrigated at a rate of 2 mL/minute. During ablation, the irrigation rate is increased to 17 mL/minute when delivered power is less than 30 W and raised to 30 mL/minute for power higher than 30 W.

Studies have shown that the two types of cooled catheters display dissimilar properties. One study comparing large-tip catheters with internally and externally cooled catheters demonstrated that, in atrial flutter ablation, the externally cooled catheter succeeded in ablating atrial flutter with fewer applications and in less time than the internally cooled catheter.[40] Lesions delivered by both externally and internally cooled catheters were associated with steam pops. None of the patients who underwent ablation using the externally cooled catheter had recurrences compared with patients who underwent ablation using the 8 mm or the internally cooled catheter. Impedance rises interrupting the delivery of energy delivery were more frequently seen with the internally cooled catheter.

In another study, the internally cooled catheter was found to be as effective for ablating atrial flutter as an 8-mm catheter with dual sensors.[49] However, the higher incidence of impedance rise and the complexity of the internally cooled catheter rendered it less desirable than the large-tip catheter.[49] In an *in vivo* model comparing an internally irrigated catheter with an externally irrigated catheter, lesions delivered by the internally irrigated catheter were associated with a higher incidence of impedance rise and a smaller lesion size.[50]

Given the concerns about steam pop and crater formation, and owing to the lack of a reliable guide on tissue temperatures generated by irrigated-catheter ablation, the settings for energy delivery differ significantly from those used in nonirrigated catheters. As an example, in the Johns Hopkins experience using cooled catheter for ablation of atrial flutter, the limit of delivered power was 50 W with a target temperature of 45°C; in atrial fibrillation, it was 40 W and 39°C, respectively.[51] At our institution, we use the externally irrigated catheter exclusively. Ablations are not carried beyond 20 seconds at any one point before moving. A temperature limiter is set at 43°C, the initial power setting is 20 to 25 W, and careful attention is paid to the changes and in unipolar electrograms as power is being delivered. A 10 Ω change in impedance results in immediate cessation of power delivery. The power is increased only if the electrograms are not adequately attenuated.

The irrigated-tip catheter remains the most common type used in atrial fibrillation ablation.[52] Note, however, that a worldwide survey of atrial fibrillation ablation in 521 centers in 24 countries between 2003 and 2006 (albeit not a scientifically conducted study) showed that the use of an irrigated-tip catheter was not associated with a better clinical outcome than the use of a 4-mm catheter.[52] In a small study comparing the use of an irrigated-tip catheter with a 4-mm catheter for isolating the pulmonary veins in atrial fibrillation, the irrigated-tip catheter was associated with faster isolation of the pulmonary vein and a lower recurrence rate of atrial fibrillation.[53] The superiority of irrigated-tip catheter ablation has also been demonstrated in atrial flutter and intra-atrial reentrant tachycardia complicating congenital heart disease.[40,54-56]

Irrigated-tip catheters have had their largest impact on the ablation of nonidiopathic VT. Owing to the small size of lesions created by conventional catheters, the success of ablating scar-related VT had been limited by the inability to define the critical isthmus and to create a lesion large enough to incorporate the entire critical pathway.

The role of catheter ablation of ischemic VT using externally irrigated catheter ablation and electroanatomic mapping was evaluated in the Multicenter THERMOCOOL Ventricular Tachycardia Ablation Trial.[57] The patients included had a high frequency of sustained monomorphic VT despite therapy with an implantable cardioverter-defibrillator (ICD) and/or antiarrhythmic agents (an average of 11 episodes in the 6 months preceding enrollment). Patients with multiple VT morphologies, unmappable VT, or failed prior VT ablation were not excluded. The median left ventricular ejection fraction (LVEF) of the 231 patients enrolled was 25%, amiodarone had failed to control VT in 70% of patients, and 93% of patients had an ICD. After 6 months, close to half the patients were free of any VT.[57] In the epicardial space, the absence of blood flow to cool the catheter severely impairs the amount of power that can be delivered to ablate an epicardial site. Therefore, irrigated-tip catheters are the catheters of choice in the epicardial space.[58]

One of the major drawbacks of using RF energy for catheter ablation is the inability to accurately monitor tissue temperature. The introduction of catheter-tip temperature monitoring using embedded thermistors has reduced the frequency of catheter-tip "thrombus" and coagulum formation. However, the recorded temperature, particularly in irrigated catheters, is not accurate. It is important to bear in mind that the catheter tip itself does not heat up as a result of the passage of RF energy. Rather, the temperature recorded by the catheter tip is the result of passive heating from the tissue the catheter tip comes into contact with and cooled by the flow of blood around it. Thus, the temperature reading is the result of the interplay between these two factors and not the true tissue temperature.[16] For example, in an *in vitro* experiment conducted by Petersen et al, the maximum tissue temperature recorded with a standard, temperature-controlled lesion set at 70°C was 67°C (+/– 4°C).[42] When the temperature-controlled lesion was delivered using an irrigated-tip catheter, tissue temperatures were approximately 30°C higher.[42]

The efficacy and potential dangers of catheter ablation are determined by the tissue temperature attained. While externally irrigated catheters are clearly superior to internally irrigated cooled and noncooled catheters, the need to infuse saline can be a limiting factor in patients with impaired left ventricular systolic function undergoing VT ablation.[57]

Contact Force

Catheter ablation for atrial fibrillation has expanded tremendously during the last decade. However, enthusiasm for the procedure is tempered by a success rate that is lower than that for supraventricular tachycardia on the one hand, and the fear of damage to collateral structures on the other. Although the use of higher energy would decrease the likelihood of recurrence, the risk to surrounding structures would increase. As discussed earlier, the use of irrigated-tip catheters has allowed the formation of larger lesions while reducing the likelihood of thrombus and coagulum formation. Unfortunately, determining the efficacy of the lesion created has been hampered by the unreliability of recorded tip temperatures. In fact, the operator of an irrigated-tip catheter is essentially blinded to the size of the lesion being created with the power being delivered. Given the significance of contact force in determining the size of the created lesion, contact force has been introduced as a new parameter to enhance the likelihood of creating a successful lesion.

Changes in catheter–tissue contact force have been found to be as important as changes in delivered power.[31] With the catheter tip oriented perpendicularly to the tissue surface, the depth of lesions created with an irrigated-tip catheter has been found to correlate with contact force.[45] The recent development of an irrigated-tip catheter that allows measurement of contact force has allowed the evaluation of this novel parameter in order to determine lesion size and safety.[59] Contact force has been shown to correlate with lesion size, steam pops, and, in one study, thrombus formation.[31,45,59] The TactiCath® catheter (Endosense, Switzerland) (not approved in the United States) has three embedded optical sensing fibers that measure the direction and amount of applied force. In an *ex vivo* porcine model, the size of the lesions and the likelihood of a steam pop were proportional to the amount of energy delivered and the contact pressure (Figure 19.7).[31] In the United States, at the time this chapter was written, this catheter was still investigational and had been employed in the multicenter TOCCATA (TOuCh+ for CATheter Ablation) clinical trial in the United States and Europe.

The Sensei Robotic Catheter System (Hansen Medical, Mountain View, CA) employs flexible robotic technology to manipulate catheters (Figures 19.8 and 19.9).[60] The operator transmits manual instructions by manipulating an instinctive motion control device to a remote catheter manipulator (RCM) to smoothly maneuver the catheter inside the body. Tactile feedback allows the operator to determine the degree of applied force. The relationship between contact force and catheter tip–tissue contact was validated by fluoroscopy and intracardiac echocardiography in a dog model, which also demonstrated contact force to be a better predictor of lesion size than either impedance drop or voltage reduction.[61] However, the use of higher contact force was associated with significant distortion of the electroanatomical map.[61]

The use of this system in humans to perform transseptal puncture, intracardiac navigation, and atrial fibrillation and flutter ablation with results similar to conventional methods has been demonstrated.[62] However, this system requires the use of a stiff 14-Fr femoral sheath and has been associated with vascular complications and cardiac perforation.[63] One of the main advantages is lower operator exposure to radiation.

Another remotely guided ablation system uses a magnetically guided catheter (Niobe®, Stereotaxis Inc., St. Louis, MO). A weak magnetic field is created by two magnets, one on each side of the patient (Figure 19.10). A catheter with an embedded magnet in its tip is steered and moved in 1 mm increments by changing the orientation of the magnetic field without the need for direct human manipulation.[64] One of the main advantages is the ease of manipulating floppy catheters across tortuous vessels while maintaining a fixed catheter tip–endocardial contact pressure.

Clinically, the results have been mixed. In 45 consecutive patients undergoing ablation for drug-refractory atrial fibrillation, only 8% of the pulmonary veins were electrically isolated, and char was seen in 33% of the patients.[65] Using an 8-mm remote magnetic catheter navigation system, atrial flutter ablation was associated with longer ablation time and procedure duration.[66] One of the reasons proposed for the low success rate and the high incidence of char is the absence of an irrigated-tip catheter.[63] However, this experience has not been uniform. Other groups have reported better results with the remote magnetic catheter navigation system.[67,68] Although this system is very safe to use, it cannot be used in patients with implanted devices, navigation is limited to using the CARTO three-dimensional (3D) navigation system (Biosense Webster, Diamond Bar, CA), and it lacks an irrigated-tip catheter.[69] Owing to technical reasons, development of an irrigated-tip catheter for use in the magnetic navigation system was stopped in March 2008.[69]

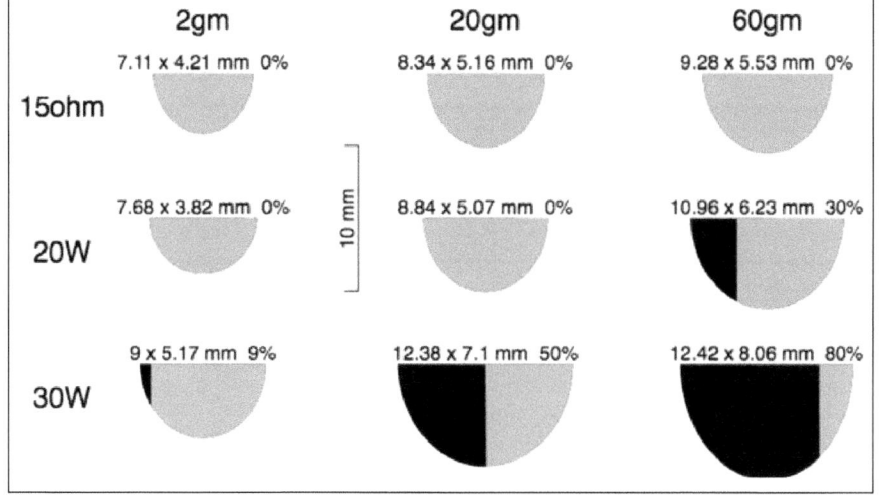

Figure 19.7 The width and depth of each lesion set created in the *ex vivo* model[34] using 3 power settings at 3 different contact pressures. In the 15 Ω power setting, variable power is delivered until the impedance drops by 15 Ω. The 20 W and 30 W power settings are fixed power settings. The size of the lesion (**gray**) increases with increasing contact pressure and power delivery. The **black** shading and the numerical representation in percentages represent the incidence of "steam pops," which also increase with greater power delivery and contact pressure. *Source:* Reprinted with permission from Thiagalingam A, et al.[31] ©2010 John Wiley & Sons, Inc. All rights reserved.

214 • *Section 1D: Ablation Technology*

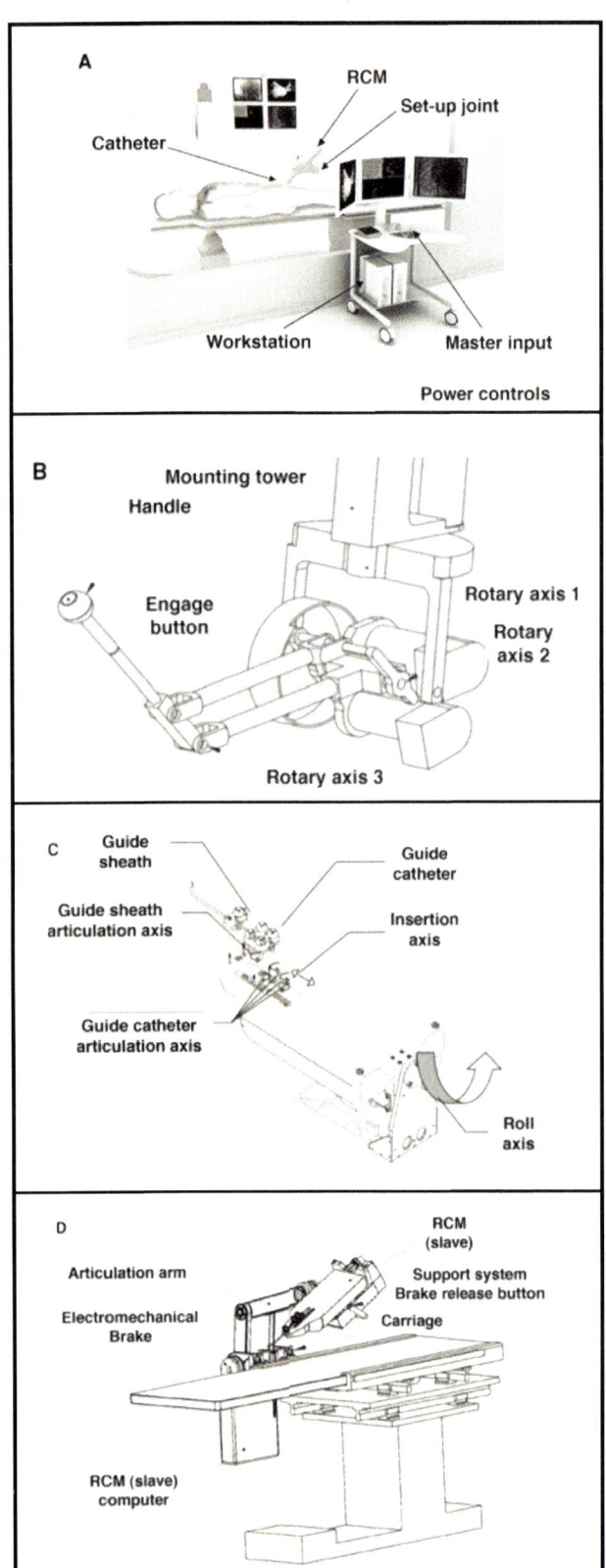

Figure 19.8 The Sensei Robotic Catheter System (Hansen Medical, Mountain View, CA). RCM = remote catheter manipulator. *Source:* Reprinted with permission from Saliba W, et al.[60] ©2006 John Wiley & Sons, Inc. All rights reserved.

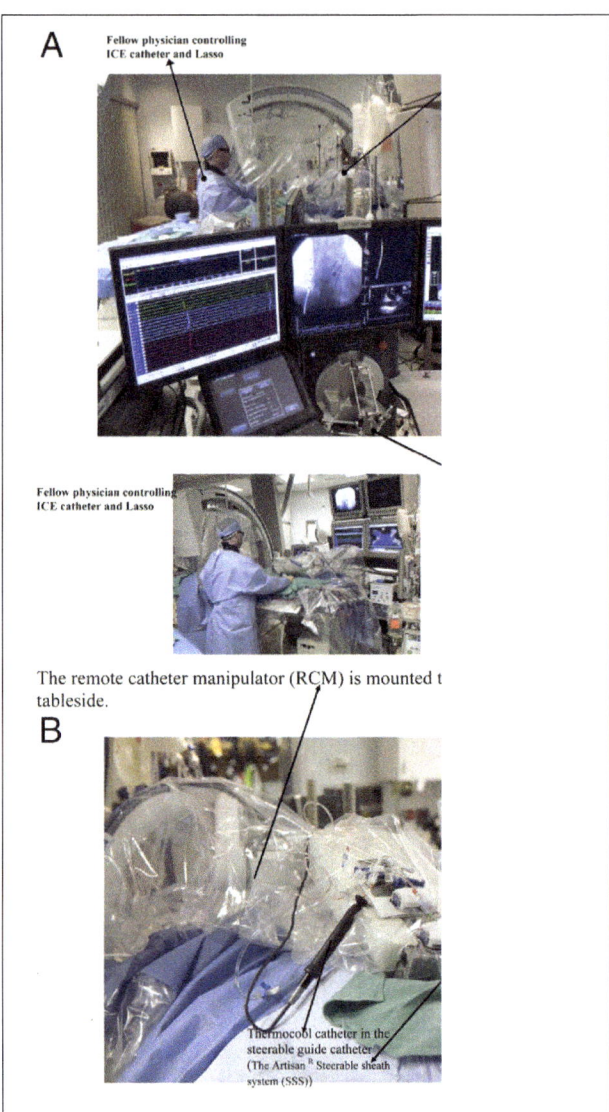

Figure 19.9 The Sensei Robotic Catheter System (Hansen Medical, Mountain View, CA). *Source:* Reprinted with permission from Saliba W, et al.[62] ©2008 Elsevier. All rights reserved.

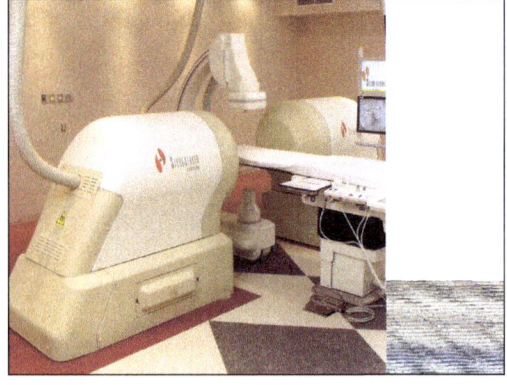

Figure 19.10 Niobe, Stereotaxis Inc., St. Louis, MO. *Source:* Reprinted with permission from Atmakuri SR, et al. Initial experience with a magnetic navigation system for percutaneous coronary intervention in complex coronary artery lesions. *J Am Coll Cardiol.* 2006;47(3):515-521. ©2006 Elsevier. All rights reserved.

Duty-cycled Phased RF Energy

To overcome the problem of lesion gaps during the creation of linear lesions, a novel multipolar catheter was developed that allows energy delivery in both the unipolar and the bipolar manner. The Pulmonary Vein Ablation Catheter® (PVAC) (Medtronic/Ablation Frontiers, Carlsbad, CA) holds ten 3 mm platinum poles, 3 mm apart, that are arranged along a 25 mm diameter array located at the end of a 9-Fr, over-the-wire catheter. The tip can be extended, giving it a spiral shape in addition to bidirectional movement of the shaft. A thermocouple is located at the anterior edge of each pole. RF energy is delivered through a dedicated duty-cycled multichannel generator (GENius™, Medtronic/Ablation Frontiers).

RF energy can be delivered in a bipolar or unipolar manner, and the power delivered is modulated to achieve a predefined target temperature. Bipolar energy is delivered between adjacent electrodes filling in linear lesions, whereas unipolar energy is delivered between the targeted pole and the dispersive pad targeting specific sites. At the time this chapter was written, this system had been approved in the United States only on an investigational basis.

The efficacy of the PVAC system was first demonstrated in 98 patients with paroxysmal or persistent atrial fibrillation.[70] All the pulmonary veins were isolated without the need to use electroanatomic mapping. There were no short-term complications, and 83% of 53 patients who were at least 6 months beyond the procedure were free of atrial fibrillation, as confirmed by a 7-day Holter monitor recording. In the first study reporting on the 1-year outcome of patients with paroxysmal atrial fibrillation undergoing pulmonary vein isolation using the PVAC system, 79.2% of patients followed for ≥12 months were free of AF.[71] Three underwent redo procedures, and no complications were reported, including the development of left atrial tachyarrhythmias.

In the first study comparing the PVAC system with point-by-point conventional circumferential isolation of the pulmonary veins with a 3D mapping system, 40 patients were randomized to each group.[72] There was no difference in the success of isolating the pulmonary vein in both groups. Both procedure time and fluoroscopy time were significantly reduced in the PVAC group. This could be attributed to the lack of need for dual transseptal or 3D mapping. One of the drawbacks was real-time interpretation of the signals from the array during lesion delivery. There was no difference in maintaining SR in both arms of this study.

Conclusions

There has been more than 20 years of experience in employing RF energy to perform catheter ablation of supraventricular and ventricular arrhythmias. The technique's safety and efficacy are well proven. The advent of irrigated-tip catheters has expanded the role of catheter ablation techniques to manage complex, scar-related arrhythmias and arrhythmias that require deep linear lesions. The major drawback of catheter ablation (particularly when using irrigated-tip catheters) is the inability to determine the extent of the lesion created. The available parameters have been arrived at through consensus and the result of animal and clinical trials. However, they should be individualized to each patient and circumstance in order to avoid the catastrophic complications that may rarely ensue. Understanding the biophysics of RF ablation allows the operator to understand the limitations of this technology and, more important, the limitations of the information that is being constantly fed back during lesion delivery. The realization that contact force is an important determinant of both efficacy and risk has led to the introduction of sensors to measure contact force and technologies that allow the operator to apply more uniform contact force (eg, remote catheter manipulation and magnetically guided catheters).

Research into other forms of energy delivery may, one day, supplant RF energy as the energy of choice for creating myocardial lesions to prevent recurrent cardiac arrhythmias. However, for the foreseeable future, RF energy will remain the preeminent choice, so fully understanding its limitations and drawbacks is imperative for any interventional electrophysiologist. In our institution, long-tip catheters (8 mm) are reserved for cavotricuspid isthmus–dependent arrhythmias, while irrigated-tip catheters are used for pulmonary vein isolation and ablation of atrial fibrillation and scar-mediated VT. The 4-mm non-irrigated catheter is used for slow pathway ablation and ablation of bypass tracts. Such a flexible approach to catheter choice is essential when dealing with an as-yet imperfect science.

References

1. Gallagher JJ, Svenson RH, Kasell JH, et al. Catheter technique for closed-chest ablation of the atrioventricular conduction system. *N Engl J Med*. 1982;306(4):194-200.
2. Scheinman MM, Morady F, Hess DS, Gonzalez R. Catheter-induced ablation of the atrioventricular junction to control refractory supraventricular arrhythmias. *JAMA*. 1982; 248(7): 851-855.
3. Evans GT Jr, Scheinman MM, Bardy G, et al. Predictors of in-hospital mortality after DC catheter ablation of atrioventricular junction. Results of a prospective, international, multicenter study. *Circulation*. 1991;84(5):1924-1937.
4. Huang SK, Graham AR, Hoyt RH, Odell RC. Transcatheter desiccation of the canine left ventricle using radiofrequency energy: a pilot study. *Am Heart J*. 1987;114(1 Pt 1):42-48.
5. Nath S, Haines DE. Biophysics and pathology of catheter energy delivery systems. *Prog Cardiovasc Dis*. 1995; 37(4):185-204.

6. Simmers TA, de Bakker JM, Wittkampf FH, Hauer RN. Effects of heating with radiofrequency power on myocardial impulse conduction: Is radiofrequency ablation exclusively thermally mediated? *J Cardiovasc Electrophysiol*. 1996;7(3): 243-247.
7. Langberg JJ, Calkins H, el-Atassi R, et al. Temperature monitoring during radiofrequency catheter ablation of accessory pathways. *Circulation*. 1992;86(5):1469-1474.
8. Nath S, DiMarco JP, Mounsey JP, et al. Correlation of temperature and pathophysiological effect during radiofrequency catheter ablation of the AV junction. *Circulation*. 1995; 92(5):1188-1192.
9. Nath S, Lynch C 3rd, Whayne JG, Haines DE. Cellular electrophysiological effects of hyperthermia on isolated guinea pig papillary muscle. Implications for catheter ablation. *Circulation*. 1993;88(4):1826-1831.
10. Huang SK, Bharati S, Lev M, Marcus FI. Electrophysiologic and histologic observations of chronic atrioventricular block induced by closed-chest catheter desiccation with radiofrequency energy. *Pacing Clin Electrophysiol*. 1987;10(4 Pt 1): 805-816.
11. Dickfeld T, Kato R, Zviman M, et al. Characterization of radiofrequency ablation lesions with gadolinium-enhanced cardiovascular magnetic resonance imaging. *J Am Coll Cardiol*. 2006;47(2):370-378.
12. Nath S, Redick JA, Whayne JG, Haines DE. Ultrastructural observations in the myocardium beyond the region of acute coagulation necrosis following radiofrequency catheter ablation. *J Cardiovasc Electrophysiol*. 1994;5(10):838-845.
13. Wagshal AB, Pires LA, Stephen SK. Management of cardiac arrhythmias with radiofrequency catheter ablation. *Arch Intern Med*. 1995;155(2):137-147.
14. Eick OJ, Gerritse B, Schumacher B. Popping phenomena in temperature-controlled radiofrequency ablation: when and why do they occur? *Pacing Clin Electrophysiol*. 2000;23(2): 253-258.
15. Haines DE, Watson DD. Tissue heating during radiofrequency catheter ablation: a thermodynamic model and observations in isolated perfused and superfused canine right ventricular free wall. *Pacing Clin Electrophysiol*. 1989;12(6): 962-976.
16. Wittkampf FH, Nakagawa H. RF catheter ablation: lessons on lesions. *Pacing Clin Electrophysiol*. 2006;29(11):1285-1297.
17. Wittkampf FH, Simmers TA, Hauer RN, et al. Myocardial temperature response during radiofrequency catheter ablation. *Pacing Clin Electrophysiol*. 1995;18(2):307-317.
18. Haines DE, Watson DD, Verow AF. Electrode radius predicts lesion radius during radiofrequency energy heating. Validation of a proposed thermodynamic model. *Circ Res*. 1990;67(1): 124-129.
19. Wittkampf FH, Hauer RN, Robles de Medina EO. Control of radiofrequency lesion size by power regulation. *Circulation*. 1989;80(4):962-968.
20. Wittkampf FH, Nakagawa H, Yamanashi WS. Thermal latency in radiofrequency ablation. *Circulation*. 1996;93(6): 1083-1086.
21. Haines D. Biophysics of ablation: application to technology. *J Cardiovasc Electrophysiol*. 2004;15(Suppl 10):S2-S11.
22. Matsudaira K, Nakagawa H, Wittkampf FH, et al. High incidence of thrombus formation without impedance rise during radiofrequency ablation using electrode temperature control. *Pacing Clin Electrophysiol*. 2003;26(5):1227-1237.
23. Jain MK, Wolf PD. A three-dimensional finite element model of radiofrequency ablation with blood flow and its experimental validation. *Ann Biomed Eng*. 2000;28(9):1075-1084.
24. Fuller IA, Wood MA. Intramural coronary vasculature prevents transmural radiofrequency lesion formation: implications for linear ablation. *Circulation*. 2003;107(13):1797-1803.
25. Simmers TA, de Bakker JM, Coronel R, et al. Effects of intracavitary blood flow and electrode-target distance on radiofrequency power required for transient conduction block in a Langendorff-perfused canine model. *J Am Coll Cardiol*. 1998;31(1):231-235.
26. Haines DE, Verow AF. Observations on electrode-tissue interface temperature and effect on electrical impedance during radiofrequency ablation of ventricular myocardium. *Circulation*. 1990;82(3):1034-1038.
27. Calkins H, Prystowsky E, Carlson M, et al. Temperature monitoring during radiofrequency catheter ablation procedures using closed loop control. Atakr Multicenter Investigators Group. *Circulation*. 1994;90(3):1279-1286.
28. Kongsgaard E, Steen T, Jensen O, et al. Temperature guided radiofrequency catheter ablation of myocardium: comparison of catheter tip and tissue temperatures *in vitro*. *Pacing Clin Electrophysiol*. 1997;20(5):1252-1260.
29. Hartung WM, Burton ME, Deam AG, et al. Estimation of temperature during radiofrequency catheter ablation using impedance measurements. *Pacing Clin Electrophysiol*. 1995; 18(11):2017-2021.
30. Thiagalingam A, D'Avila A, McPherson C, et al. Impedance and temperature monitoring improve the safety of closed-loop irrigated-tip radiofrequency ablation. *J Cardiovasc Electrophysiol*. 2007;18(3):318-325.
31. Thiagalingam A, D'Avila A, Foley L, et al. Importance of catheter contact force during irrigated radiofrequency ablation: evaluation in a porcine *ex vivo* model using a force-sensing catheter. *J Cardiovasc Electrophysiol*. 2010;21(7):806-811.
32. Perez FJ, Wood MA, Schubert CM. Effects of gap geometry on conduction through discontinuous radiofrequency lesions. *Circulation*. 2006;113(14):1723-1729.
33. Langberg JJ, Gallagher M, Strickberger SA, Amirana O. Temperature-guided radiofrequency catheter ablation with very large distal electrodes. *Circulation*. 1993;88(1):245-249.
34. Tsai CF, Tai CT, Yu WC, et al. Is 8-mm more effective than 4-mm tip electrode catheter for ablation of typical atrial flutter? *Circulation*. 1999;100(7):768-771.
35. Høgh Petersen H, Chen X, Pietersen A, et al. Lesion dimensions during temperature-controlled radiofrequency catheter ablation of left ventricular porcine myocardium: impact of ablation site, electrode size, and convective cooling. *Circulation*. 1999;99(2):319-325.
36. Otomo K, Yamanashi WS, Tondo C, et al. Why a large tip electrode makes a deeper radiofrequency lesion: effects of increase in electrode cooling and electrode-tissue interface area. *J Cardiovasc Electrophysiol*. 1998;9(1):47-54.
37. Feld G, Wharton M, Plumb V, et al. Radiofrequency catheter ablation of type 1 atrial flutter using large-tip 8- or 10-mm electrode catheters and a high-output radiofrequency energy generator: Results of a multicenter safety and efficacy study. *J Am Coll Cardiol*. 2004;43(8):1466-1472.
38. McRury ID, Panescu D, Mitchell MA, Haines DE. Nonuniform heating during radiofrequency catheter ablation with long electrodes: Monitoring the edge effect. *Circulation*. 1997;96(11):4057-4064.
39. Nakagawa H, Wittkampf FH, Yamanashi WS, et al. Inverse relationship between electrode size and lesion size during radiofrequency ablation with active electrode cooling. *Circulation*. 1998;98(5):458-465.
40. Scavée C, Jaïs P, Hsu LF, et al. Prospective randomised comparison of irrigated-tip and large-tip catheter ablation of

41. Mittleman RS, Huang SK, de Guzman WT, et al. Use of the saline infusion electrode catheter for improved energy delivery and increased lesion size in radiofrequency catheter ablation. *Pacing Clin Electrophysiol.* 1995;18(5):1022-1027.
42. Petersen HH, Chen X, Pietersen A, et al. Tissue temperatures and lesion size during irrigated tip catheter radiofrequency ablation: an *in vitro* comparison of temperature-controlled irrigated tip ablation, power-controlled irrigated tip ablation, and standard temperature-controlled ablation. *Pacing Clin Electrophysiol.* 2000;23(1):8,17.
43. Dorwarth U, Fiek M, Remp T, et al. Radiofrequency catheter ablation: different cooled and noncooled electrode systems induce specific lesion geometries and adverse effects profiles. *Pacing Clin Electrophysiol.* 2003;26(7 Part 1):1438-1445.
44. Nakagawa H, Yamanashi WS, Pitha JV, et al. Comparison of *in vivo* tissue temperature profile and lesion geometry for radiofrequency ablation with a saline-irrigated electrode versus temperature control in a canine thigh muscle preparation. *Circulation.* 1995;91(8):2264-2273.
45. Weiss C, Antz M, Eick O, et al. Radiofrequency catheter ablation using cooled electrodes: Impact of irrigation flow rate and catheter contact pressure on lesion dimensions. *Pacing Clin Electrophysiol.* 2002;25(4):463-469.
46. Bruce GK, Bunch TJ, Milton MA, et al. Discrepancies between catheter tip and tissue temperature in cooled-tip ablation: relevance to guiding left atrial ablation. *Circulation.* 2005;112(7):954-960.
47. U.S. Food and Drug Administration. Approval letter for the Chilli® Cooled Ablation System (Boston Scientific). February 2, 1999. http://www.accessdata.fda.gov/cdrh_docs/pdf/P980003a.pdf. Accessed February 6, 2013.
48. U.S. Food and Drug Administration. Approval letter for the NaviStar THERMOCOOL Catheter (Biosense Webster). February 6, 2009. http://www.accessdata.fda.gov/cdrh_docs/pdf3/P030031S011a.pdf. Accessed February 6, 2013.
49. Scavée C, Georger F, Jamart J, et al. Is a cooled tip catheter the solution for the ablation of the cavotricuspid isthmus? *Pacing Clin Electrophysiol.* 2003;26(1 Pt 2):328-331.
50. Demazumder D, Mirotznik MS, Schwartzman D. Comparison of irrigated electrode designs for radiofrequency ablation of myocardium. *J Interv Card Electrophysiol.* 2001;5(4):391-400.
51. Hugh C. Cooled ablation. *J Cardiovasc Electrophysiol.* 2004;15(Suppl 10):S12-S17.
52. Cappato R, Calkins H, Chen SA, et al. Updated worldwide survey on the methods, efficacy, and safety of catheter ablation for human atrial fibrillation. *Circ Arrhythm Electrophysiol.* 2010;3(1):32-38.
53. Pérez-Castellano N, Villacastin J, Salinas J, et al. Cooled ablation reduces pulmonary vein isolation time: results of a prospective randomised trial. *Heart.* 2009;95(3):203-209.
54. Jaïs P, Haïssaguerre M, Shah DC, et al. Successful irrigated-tip catheter ablation of atrial flutter resistant to conventional radiofrequency ablation. *Circulation.* 1998;98(9):835-838.
55. Triedman JK, Alexander ME, Love BA, et al. Influence of patient factors and ablative technologies on outcomes of radiofrequency ablation of intra-atrial re-entrant tachycardia in patients with congenital heart disease. *J Am Coll Cardiol.* 2002;39(11):1827-1835.
56. Jaïs P, Shah DC, Haïssaguerre M, et al. Prospective randomized comparison of irrigated-tip versus conventional-tip catheters for ablation of common flutter. *Circulation.* 2000;101(7):772-776.
57. Stevenson WG, Wilber DJ, Natale A, et al. Irrigated radiofrequency catheter ablation guided by electroanatomic mapping for recurrent ventricular tachycardia after myocardial infarction: the Multicenter THERMOCOOL Ventricular Tachycardia Ablation Trial. *Circulation.* 2008;118(25):2773-2782.
58. d'Avila A, Houghtaling C, Gutierrez P, et al. Catheter ablation of ventricular epicardial tissue: a comparison of standard and cooled-tip radiofrequency energy. *Circulation.* 2004;109(19):2363-2369.
59. Yokoyama K, Nakagawa H, Shah DC, et al. Novel contact force sensor incorporated in irrigated radiofrequency ablation catheter predicts lesion size and incidence of steam pop and thrombus. *Circ Arrhythm Electrophysiol.* 2008;1(5):354-362.
60. Saliba W, Cummings JE, Oh S, et al. Novel robotic catheter remote control system: feasibility and safety of transseptal puncture and endocardial catheter navigation. *J Cardiovasc Electrophysiol.* 2006;17(10):1102-1105.
61. Okumura Y, Johnson SB, Bunch TJ, et al. A systematical analysis of in vivo contact forces on virtual catheter tip/tissue surface contact during cardiac mapping and intervention. *J Cardiovasc Electrophysiol.* 2008;19(6):632-640.
62. Saliba W, Reddy VY, Wazni O, et al. Atrial fibrillation ablation using a robotic catheter remote control system: initial human experience and long-term follow-up results. *J Am Coll Cardiol.* 2008;51(25):2407-2411.
63. Burkhardt JD, Natale A. New technologies in atrial fibrillation ablation. *Circulation.* 2009;120(15):1533-1541.
64. Ernst S, Ouyang F, Linder C, et al. Initial experience with remote catheter ablation using a novel magnetic navigation system: magnetic remote catheter ablation. *Circulation.* 2004;109(12):1472-1475.
65. Di Biase L, Fahmy TS, Patel D, et al. Remote magnetic navigation: human experience in pulmonary vein ablation. *J Am Coll Cardiol.* 2007;50(9):868-874.
66. Vollmann D, Lüthje L, Seegers J, et al. Remote magnetic catheter navigation for cavotricuspid isthmus ablation in patients with common-type atrial flutter. *Circ Arrhythm Electrophysiol.* 2009;2(6):603-610.
67. Pappone C, Santinelli V. Safety and efficacy of remote magnetic ablation for atrial fibrillation. *J Am Coll Cardiol.* 2008;51(16):1614-1615.
68. Pappone C, Vicedomini G, Manguso F, et al. Robotic magnetic navigation for atrial fibrillation ablation. *J Am Coll Cardiol.* 2006;47(7):1390-1400.
69. Schmidt B, Chun KR, Tilz RR, et al. Remote navigation systems in electrophysiology. *Europace.* 2008;10(Suppl 3):iii57-iii61.
70. Boersma LVA, Wijffels MC, Oral H, et al. Pulmonary vein isolation by duty-cycled bipolar and unipolar radiofrequency energy with a multielectrode ablation catheter. *Heart Rhythm.* 2008;5(12):1635-1642.
71. Wieczorek M, Hoeltgen R, Akin E, et al. Results of short-term and long-term pulmonary vein isolation for paroxysmal atrial fibrillation using duty-cycled bipolar and unipolar radiofrequency energy. *J Cardiovasc Electrophysiol.* 2010;21(4):399-405.
72. Bittner A, Mönnig G, Zellerhoff S, et al. Randomized study comparing duty-cycled bipolar and unipolar radiofrequency with point-by-point ablation in pulmonary vein isolation. *Heart Rhythm.* 8(9):1383-1390.

CHAPTER 20

Cryothermal Ablation Technology and Catheter Delivery Systems

Rohit Bhagwandien, MD; Paul Knops, Ing; Luc Jordaens, MD, PhD

History of Cryotherapy

The use of cold to cure patients (cryotherapy) has a long history in medicine. The prefix "cryo" is derived from the Greek word "kruos," meaning cold, and "therapy" means cure. The first known application dates back to 2500 B.C.E., to the ancient Greek and Roman civilizations, when injuries and inflammation were treated with cold. During the historic retreat from Moscow, Napoleon's physician, Dominique-Jean Larrey, used cold to facilitate amputations.[1] A mixture of salt solution and crushed ice reduced both tumor size and pain in the 19th century.[2] However, the maximal freezing temperature that could be reached with this mixture was −24°C.

By the end of the 1800s and the beginning of the 1900s, new cooling gases were used. The first clinical utilization was by White, who treated diverse skin conditions with liquid air, which reached a temperature of −190°C.[3] At the beginning of the 1900s, liquid air became scarce and alternatives were being investigated. Pusey used carbon dioxide snow with a temperature of −79°C. Liquid carbon dioxide gas was supplied in pressurized steel cylinders. When the gas was allowed to escape, the loss of pressure caused the temperature fall and the formation of fine snow. The snow was transformed in various shapes for easy application.[4] In the 1920s, liquid oxygen came into clinical use. It had similar properties as liquid air, but reached −183°C. It was used to treat a variety of dermatological conditions, as was the case with liquid nitrogen, which had no explosive potential.[5,6]

The first liquid oxygen–based cryosurgical probe was developed in the 1960s (Figure 20.1) and was used to treat patients with Parkinson's disease and other movement disorders by freezing the thalamus. The probe was able to reach temperatures of −196°C.[7] Copper probes were capable of freezing tissue to depths of 7 mm.[8,9] Various other specialists, including ophthalmologists, gynecologists, urologists, thoracic surgeons, and cardiologists further refined the technique and the devices to make it more applicable in their own fields.[10,11]

The first description of cryotherapy in cardiology was in the 1950s, using carbon dioxide as refrigerant.[12,13] The essential characteristics of a lesion created by hypothermia were that it created an apparently homogenous lesion without damage to the structural integrity of the tissue, and with a sharp demarcation. In the following years, thoracic surgeons more intensively used cryotherapy. The first report of atrioventricular (AV) nodal blocks in dogs using hypothermia was by Harrison in 1977.[14] Since then, several studies have been published by thoracic surgeons describing the use of cryotherapy for ablation of the AV node, for ablation of accessory pathways, and the ablation of ventricular tachycardias.[15-19]

Transvenous catheters capable of applying cryoenergy were being developed. Gillette performed the first animal study in 1991 using a cryocatheter cooled by pressurized nitrous oxide to create total AV block in 5 miniature swine.[20] In the following years, catheters became more sophisticated. In 1998, Dubuc created lesions in dogs using a steerable cryocatheter with recording and pacing electrodes to develop the concept of cryomapping. The refrigerant used was Halocarbon 502 (Freon®).[21] Extensive animal studies helped to further elucidate the optimal freezing parameters.[21-23] One of the first multicenter prospective trials of cryothermal ablation in humans, using

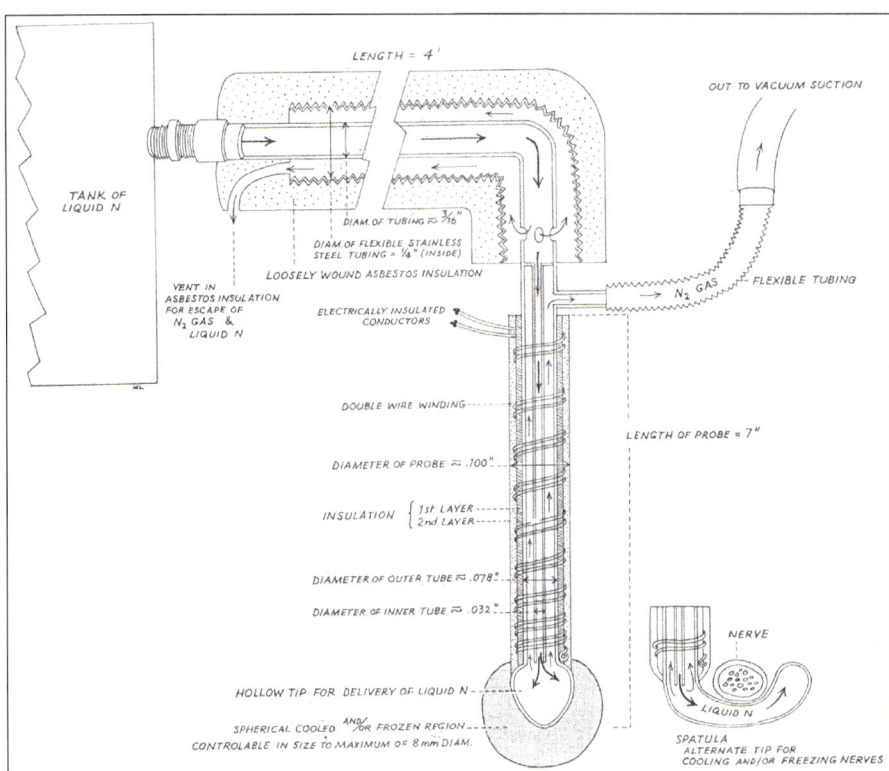

Figure 20.1 Diagrammatic illustration of mechanism of cooling cannula. *Source:* Cooper L, Lee A. Cryostatic congelation: a system for producing a limited, controlled region of cooling or freezing of biologic tissues. *J Nerv Ment Dis.* 1961;133:259-263.

the Freezor® catheter (Medtronic CryoCath Technologies, Quebec, Canada), for treatment of atrioventricular nodal reentry tachycardia (AVNRT), atrioventricular reentry tachycardia (AVRT), and atrial fibrillation (AF) was published in 2004. Cryothermal ablation proved to be a safe and effective alternative in those with AVNRT with similar success rates as patients treated with the conventional radiofrequency (RF) ablation catheters.[24]

Pathophysiology of Lesion Formation, Histological Effects, and Determinants of Lesion Size

Pathophysiology of Lesion Formation

Application of cryothermal energy with a catheter to a tissue surface results in the absorption of heat from the tissue to create a hemispherical freezing zone, or ice ball, surrounded by an outer hypothermal zone (Figure 20.2). These zones are well delineated. The cells inside the freezing zone are irreversibly damaged.[25] The lesion is formed by direct cell injury and by vascular-mediated tissue injury.[26]

Direct cell injury is caused by intracellular and extracellular ice formation. Initial mild cooling (0°C to –20°C) leads to extracellular ice formation, the extracellular space becomes hyperosmotic and water shifts from intracellular to the extracellular space. When mild cooling is applied for a short period of time (30–60 seconds), no permanent damage is inflicted; this process is reversible. However, when this period is prolonged, cellular shrinkage and subsequent cell membrane disruption occurs, ultimately leading to cell death.[27] When lower freezing temperatures are reached, subsequent intracellular ice is formed, causing irreversible damage to the intracellular organelles and the cell membranes. Intracellular ice formation can propagate though the intercellular channels, thereby influencing the lesion size. Rewarming tissue after a freezing period results in an inflammatory response; the freeze-thaw method is used to further modulate lesion size, as this results in an enhanced response.[28,29]

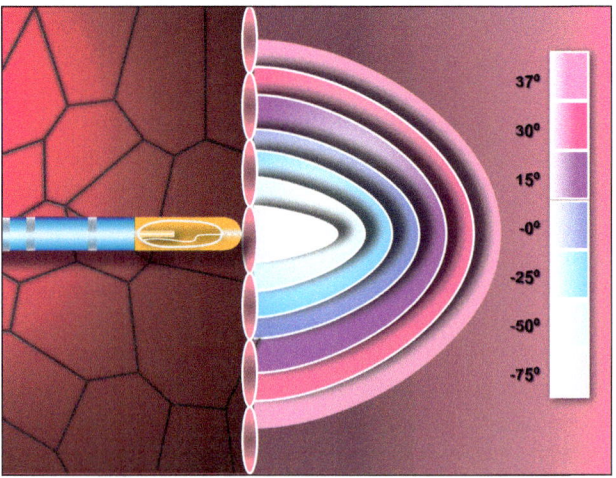

Figure 20.2 Cryocatheter applying cryothermal energy to a tissue surface creating a freezing zone (**white**) and a zone of hypothermia (**dark blue**). *Source:* Courtesy of R. Ramdan.

The second mechanism of lesion formation is by vascular-mediated tissue injury. Hypothermia causes vasoconstriction, which in turn leads to tissue hypoperfusion. During the thawing period, hyperemia results in endothelial cell damage, platelet aggregation, and microvascular obstruction.[30] These processes also result in cell necrosis.

Histological Effects on Tissue and Microcirculation

The effect on the tissue is a three-phased process. The freeze-thaw phase is mainly characterized by the intracellular and extracellular ice formation. The mechanical effect of ice formation is not clear.[25] Ice crystals do not penetrate the cell membrane, but cause irreversible damage to the organelles by damaging their membranes. The earliest changes can be seen 1 minute after thawing. They occur in the myofilaments—loss of linearity—and the mitochondria—swelling, decreased matrix density, and cristae disruption. After 10 minutes, distending vesicles appear in the sarcoplasmatic reticulum. After a few hours, all glycogen stores are depleted from skeletal muscle.[25,28] Subsequently, after approximately 48 hours, a second phase starts. This phase is characterized by hemorrhage, edema, and inflammation. In the final phase, a stable cryolesion, consisting mainly of dense collagen and fat infiltration, is formed. This takes about 2 to 4 weeks.[25]

The first effect of cryothermia on the microcirculation occurs after 30 minutes. Endothelial cells swell and protrude into the lumen. After 1 to 2 hours, the endothelial border becomes disrupted and platelets accumulate at these sites. This decreases the blood flow, eventually leading to stasis and occlusion of the vessels.[25] Although blood flow inside the lesion is decreased, blood flow in the immediate surrounding tissue is not affected.[29]

Both the effect on the tissue and microcirculation leads to formation of a sharply demarcated homogeneous lesion, while the endocardium and the fibrous stroma remain intact (Figure 20.3), possibly making lesions created with hypothermia less thrombogenic as compared to lesions created with hyperthermia.[30]

Determinants of Lesion Size

Several factors affect the lesion size. Larger probes create larger lesions, as do lower freezing temperatures. Prolonging application time also increases the lesion size, although a plateau phase is reached after 5 minutes. Repetitive freeze-thaw cycles can further enlarge lesion size. Also, increased contact pressure results in larger lesions. Lesion size is limited by convective warming due to blood flow. Lesion size is smaller in areas of high blood flow. Finally, catheter orientation influences the lesion size: horizontal orientation, parallel to the tissue, creates greater lesion depth, length, and volume.[25,31,32]

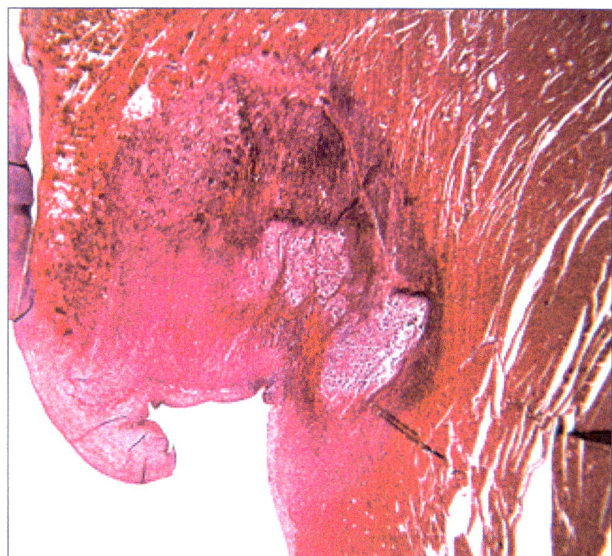

Figure 20.3 Fibroblast-rich scar tissue with inflammatory cells in a well-demarcated lesion under the mitral valve. One 240-second application at −40°C.

Advantages of Cryothermal Ablation

Cryothermal ablation has several advantages opposed to ablation using other energy sources. Cryothermal ablation is painless or at least is less associated with pain than RF ablation.[33] However, patients may experience "ice cream headache" during cryoballoon ablation in the heart, which vanishes after termination of the application. The exact mechanism is not known.

One of the properties of cryothermal ablation catheters and balloons is that they adhere to tissue during applications. This results in a stable catheter position and prevents tissue brushing.[34] Therefore, cryothermal ablation can be useful when ablating at a site where it is difficult or crucial to maintain a stable catheter position, for instance, when ablating accessory pathways, and in close proximity of critical tissue, for example, the AV node, thereby reducing the risk of an AV block. A recent meta-analysis showed that no lasting heart block has been recorded with this technique.[35] Owing to this property, cryothermal ablation during tachycardia is feasible as well. The adhesive property of the cryothermal balloon led to the development of the "pull-down" technique. If no complete occlusion of the pulmonary vein can be obtained, application is started after ensuring occlusion of the superior part of the pulmonary vein, and then, after the balloon adheres to the superior part of the pulmonary vein, the balloon is pulled down to occlude the inferior part of the vein, leading to total pulmonary vein occlusion.[36]

Cryothermal lesions are homogeneous and have, as mentioned before, sharp, well-delineated borders, making them possibly a less arrhythmogenic substrate.[34,37,38]

Because tissue architecture is maintained and no disruption of the endothelial layers occurs, cryoablation is considerably less thrombogenic as ablation using RF energy as was demonstrated in an animal study using 22 dogs.[39]

The main concern when ablating close to the coronary arteries using RF energy is that artery stenosis can occur.[40] Several pre-clinical studies have demonstrated that cryoablation near coronary arteries is safe. Furthermore, it has been shown in animal studies that ablation inside the coronary sinus is safe and feasible.[41,42] Also, a case has been described where an epicardial ventricular tachycardia is ablated by applying cryothermal energy through the anterior interventricular vein.[43] In patients with AF in whom the arrhythmogenic substrate is located at the superior vena cava (SVC) and right atrium (RA) junction, it was shown that cryoablation in the SVC can safely be performed, during continuous phrenic nerve pacing, not causing any phrenic nerve palsy even though the phrenic nerve is located in close proximity to the ablation target area.[44] This highly favorable safety profile also applies when isolating the pulmonary veins, as no pulmonary vein stenosis or atrioesophageal fistulas have been documented.

With cryoablation, temporary lesions can be created when the tissue is cooled to −20°C to −30°C. When the tissue is thawed, no permanent damage occurs to the endocardium and to the conduction tissue. So, before ablation, one can obtain a cryomap and, when the exact target site is located and no damage is done to important anatomical adjacent structures, for example, AV node, the temperature can be further lowered to create a permanent lesion.

Disadvantages of Cryothermal Ablation

Ablation has complications due to the delivery system and the type of energy delivered. Most energy types deliver thermal energy, which makes cryoablation unique. Nevertheless, both the delivery systems and the method are associated with some specific disadvantages. The balloon can mechanically damage the veins and the surrounding tissue. Tears on a frozen catheter or balloon can destroy the tissue architecture. Although cryoenergy has many advantages, there are also some concerns regarding the permanence of the lesions created. It has been shown that cryothermal energy is as effective as RF energy in ablation of AVNRT with a success rate >95%, but recurrences may occur if, for instance, the target was not in the center of the frozen area. Cryotherapy is less effective in ablating septal accessory pathways.[35,45,46] However, owing to the low risk of AV nodal block, it is still frequently used in children for perinodal arrhythmias.

Another potential disadvantage of cryoballoon ablation is that is causes reversible esophageal ulceration, not leading to any clinical manifestations. These lesions are not seen when using the cryothermal spot catheters. The lowest temperature in the esophagus is registered when ablating the inferior veins.[47]

Pulmonary vein isolation for treatment of paroxysmal AF with a cryoballoon is as effective as ablation with an RF catheter with success rates between 55% and 85%.[48-50] The main cause of reccurrence is reconduction in the veins.[51] The reconduction pattern is different from reconduction after RF.[52] This is probably due to the maintained tissue architecture without the scattered necrosis of RF. This raises the question of whether the lesions are transmural or not. Lower balloon temperature, suggesting a higher grade of occlusion of the veins, and a more complete lesion are associated with better procedural outcome.[53]

Finally, when ablating the right-sided pulmonary vein, there is a risk for phrenic nerve palsy. Fortunately, most such incidents have been transient.[48,50] This is probably not a complication attributable to the type of energy but to the location the energy is delivered, because phrenic nerve damage has been also described using RF energy.[54]

Delivery Systems

CryoCath Technologies and CryoCor developed the earliest cryoablation systems for clinical use. In 2008, CryoCath Technologies was bought by Medtronic, and CryoCor by Boston Scientific. Currently, only cryoablation catheters and balloons from CryoCath Technologies (Medtronic) are available for clinical use.

Spot/Focal Catheters

Several studies were performed with the previously available spot catheters from CryoCor. In 5 mongrel dogs, the cavotricuspid isthmus could be successfully isolated using the 6-mm tip cryocatheter. Microscopic analysis showed sharply delineated, transmural linear lesions.[51] The cryocatheter from CryoCor was also used to ablate SVTs and AF in humans.[55,56]

At present, there are 3 sizes of spot catheters available: the 4-mm (Freezor©), 6-mm (Freezor© Xtra), and 8-mm (Freezor© MAX) tip catheters (Figure 20.4). An animal study showed that lesion depth was not influenced by catheter tip size. However, lesion area and lesion volume increased with greater tip size. The tissue architecture and the endothelial cell layers are not disrupted, and the lesions were circumscribed in lesions created with either catheter. There was no difference in lowest temperature reached when comparing the 3 catheters.[56]

Linear Catheters

Linear catheter have a long linear area at the distal part of the catheter through with cryothermal energy can be delivered. In cryosurgery, linear catheters are frequently

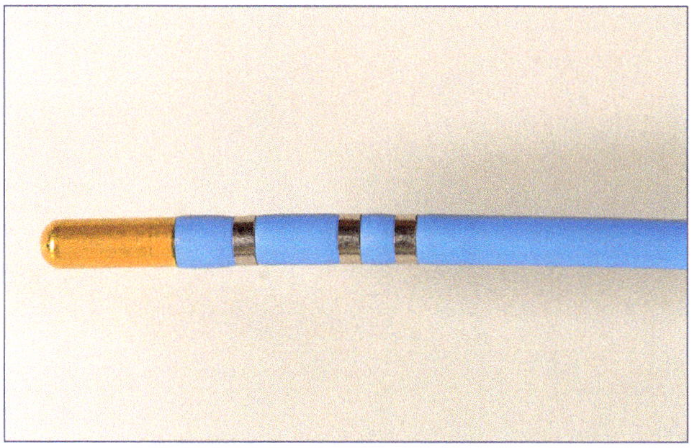

Figure 20.4 Freezor MAX spot ablation catheter. *Source:* CryoCath, Medtronic.

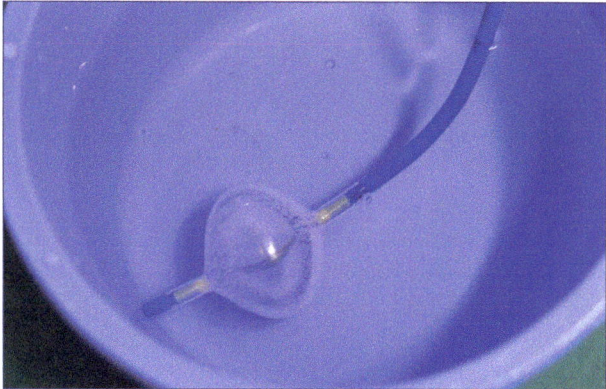

Figure 20.5 A 28-mm cryoballoon (Medtronic, Quebec, Canada) inflated.

used. The Arctic Circler™ is the only available catheter for transvenous use. There are, however, new linear catheters being developed for a variety of clinical applications.

Cryoballoon

The cryoballoon was developed to isolate the pulmonary veins to treat AF as it became apparent that the majority of the triggers in paroxysmal AF were located in the muscular sleeves inside the pulmonary veins.[59] The first experimental study using a cryoballoon was in 2004. In 13 dogs, 15-mm and 22-mm semicompliant balloons, filled with liquid nitrous oxygen, were used to isolate the pulmonary veins. Cryoballoon ablation was effective and safe regardless of the number of applications and the minimal freezing temperature reached.[58] CryoCath Technologies developed a balloon of the first generation. Finally, 23-mm and 28-mm cryoballoon became commercially available (Figure 20.5). Several studies have shown a high safety profile and similar efficacy as RF ablation for isolating the pulmonary veins. The balloon must be introduced through a 12-Fr steerable delivery sheath over the wire. Rather than a guidewire, a flexible thin lasso catheter can be used, which allows real-time recording of PV potentials.[59]

Cryosurgical Probes

Cooper Surgical manufactured the first cryosurgical probes. The probes had a curve with a 15-mm flat-face distal part. These were not disposable. Later, CryoCath Technologies developed a wide arsenal of disposable linear cryoprobes of different sizes.

Cryoconsole

Cryocatheters are controlled by a dedicated console, which contains the cylinder with pressurized liquid cooling gas as refrigerant, a computer-controlled refrigerant management system, and touch-screen interface with ablation start and stop buttons (Figure 20.6).

The system uses pressurized, liquid nitrous oxide (N_2O) as refrigerant. The desired catheter is connected to the console by an electrical connector cable and a so-called umbilical cable for delivery and aspiration of the refrigerant. Preconditioned liquid N_2O is transported to the distal tip of the focal or inflated balloon ablation catheter, where it is able to expand. This expansion causes an endothermal phase change from liquid to gas, also known as the Joule-Thomson effect. The energy needed for this process is extracted from the surrounding tissue, and results in the creation of a cryolesion.

Refrigerant flow parameters are automatically set according to the predefined parameters for the automatically detected connected catheter. The inflated Arctic Front® balloon catheter, for example, due to its larger volume and tissue contact surface, needs another amount of N_2O delivery than a focal Freezor catheter. The cryoablation catheter cooling process is managed by parameters as there are refrigerant gas flow (in square cubic centimeters, or cc^2) and gas pressure (per square inch gauge, or psig). Distal catheter temperature feedback is provided by a thermocouple. Evaporated refrigerant is evacuated from the catheter by application of a constant vacuum, and can be removed through standard hospital suction systems.

Cryosurgical Console

Epicardial or surgical cardiac cryoablation is available by Atricure (Atricure, West Chester, OH) and Medtronic (formerly CryoCath Technologies, Endocare, and ATS Medical) (Figure 20.7). The same principle as used in endocardial cryoablation systems is applied (tissue cooling by endothermal phase change of liquefied refrigerant). Atricure uses nitrous oxide as cooling gas; in contrast, Medtronic uses liquefied argon. The main different characteristic of argon is the lower temperature of $-185°C$ that can be reached at 1 atmospheric pressure level, whereas N_2O is able to reach only $-89°C$ under the same conditions. From this point of view, argon is more powerful, and can create deeper and wider lesions. The reverse: argon can reduce application time to form comparable

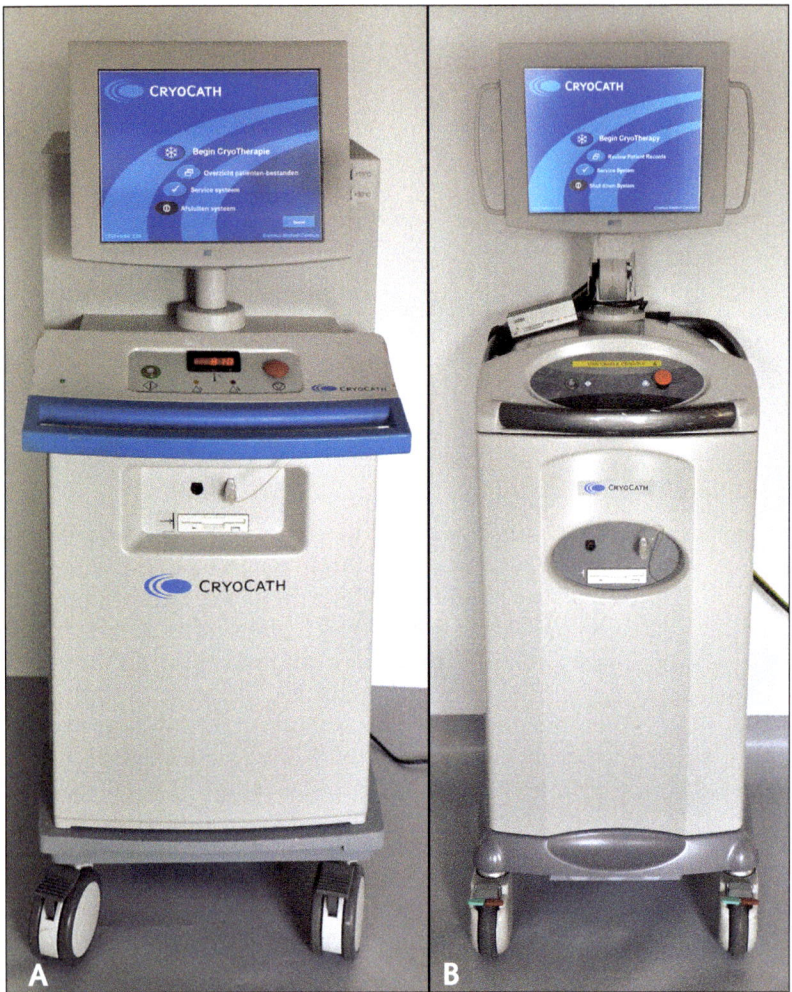

Figure 20.6 **Panel A:** First-generation cryoconsole. **Panel B:** Second-generation cryoconsole. *Source:* Medtronic, Quebec, Canada.

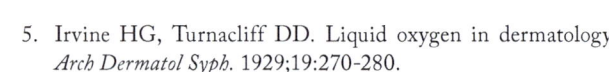

Figure 20.7 Surgical cryoconsole. *Source:* Medtronic, Quebec, Canada.

lesions. The application of the cold to the tissue is applied by either fixed, preshaped, or flexible, bendable probes.

Conclusion

The last couple of decades were witness to a fast development and improvement of cryoenergy delivery systems. However, it is clear that these can still be optimized.

References

1. Licht S. History of therapeutic heat and cold. In: Lehman JF, ed. *Therapeutic Heat and Cold*. 3rd ed. Baltimore, MD: Williams and Wilkens, 1982;1-34.
2. Arnott J. Practical illustrations of the remedial efficacy of a very low or anesthetic temperature in cancer. *Lancet*. 1850;2:257-259.
3. White AC. Liquid air: its application in medicine and surgery. *Med Rec*. 1899;56:109-112.
4. Pusey W. The use of carbon dioxide snow in the treatment of naevi and other lesions of the skin. *JAMA*. 1935;49:1354-1356.
5. Irvine HG, Turnacliff DD. Liquid oxygen in dermatology. *Arch Dermatol Syph*. 1929;19:270-280.
6. Kile RL, Welsh AL. Liquid oxygen in dermatologic practice. *Arch Dermatol Syph*. 1948;57:57-60.
7. Cooper IS. Cryogenetic surgery. A new method of destruction or extirpation of benign or malignant tissues. *N Engl J Med*. 1963;263:741-749.
8. Torre D. Alternate cryogens for cryosurgery. *J Dermatol Surg*. 1975;1:56-58.
9. Zacarian S. Cryogenics: the cryolesion and the pathogenesis of cryonecrosis. In: Zacarian SA, ed. *Cryosurgery for Skin Cancer and Cutaneous Disorders*. St. Louis, MO: Mosby, 1985;1-30.
10. Bellowes JG. *Cryotherapy of Ocular Diseases*. Philadelphia, PA: Lippincott, 1966.
11. Cahan WG. Cryosurgery of the uterus; description of technique and potential application. *Am J Obstet Gynecol*. 1964;88:410-414.
12. Hass GM. A quantitative hypothermal method for the production of local injury of tissue. *Arch Pathol*. 1948;45:563.
13. Taylor CB, Davis CB Jr, Vawter GF, Hass GM. Controlled myocardial injury produced by a hypothermal method. *Circulation*. 1951;3:239-253.
14. Harrison L, Gallagher JJ, Kasell J, Anderson RH, Mikat E, Hackel DB, Wallace AG. Cryosurgical ablation of the AV

node-His bundle: A new method for producing A-V block. *Circulation*. 1977;55:463-470.
15. Gallagher JJ, Sealy WC, Anderson RW, Kasell J, Millar R, Campbell RW, Harrison L, et al. Cryosurgical ablation of accessory atrioventricular connections: a method for correction of the preexcitation syndrome. *Circulation*. 1977;55: 471-479.
16. Guiraudon GM, Klein GJ, Gulamhusein S, Jones DL, Yee R, Perkins DG, Jarvis E. Surgical repair of Wolff–Parkinson–White syndrome: A new closed heart technique. *Ann Thorac Surg*. 1984;37:67-71.
17. Guiraudon GM, Klein GJ, Sharma AD, Milstein S, McLellan DG. Closed-heart technique for Wolff–Parkinson–White syndrome: Further experience and potential limitations. *Ann Thorac Surg*. 1986;42:651-657.
18. Lee AW, Crawford FA Jr, Gillette PC, Roble SM. Cryoablation of septal pathways in patients with supraventricular tachyarrhythmias. *Ann Thorac Surg*. 1989;47;566-568.
19. Gallagher JJ, Anderson RW, Kasell J, Rice JR, Pritchett EL, Gault HJ, Harrison L, et al. Cryoablation of drug-resistant ventricular tachycardia in a patient with a variant of scleroderma. *Circulation*. 1978;57:190-197.
20. Gillette PC, Swindle MM, Thompson RP, Case CL. Transvenous cryoablation of the bundle of His. *Pacing Clin Electrophysiol*. 1991;14:504-510.
21. Dubuc M, Roy D, Thibault B, Ducharma A, Tardif JC, Villemaire C, Leung TK, et al. Transvenous catheter ice mapping and cryoablation of the atrioventricular node in dogs. *Pacing Clin Electrophysiol*. 1999;22:1488-1498.
22. Garratt C, Camm AJ. The role of cryosurgery in the management of cardiac arrhythmias. *Clin Cardiol*. 1991;14:153-159.
23. Dubuc M, Talajic M, Roy D, Thibault B, Leung TK, Friedman PL. Feasibility of cardiac cryoablation using a transvenous steerable electrode catheter. *J Interv Card Electrophysiol*. 1998;2:285-292.
24. Friedman PL, Dubuc M, Green MS, Jackman WM, Keane DT, Marinchak RA, Nazari J, Packer DL, Skanes A, Steinberg JS, Stevenson WG, Tchou PJ, Wilber DJ, Worley SJ. Catheter cryoablation of supraventricular tachycardia: results of the multicenter prospective "frosty" trial. *Heart Rhythm*. 2004;1:129-138.
25. Lustgarten DL, Keane D, Ruskin J. Cryothermal ablation: mechanism of tissue injury and current experience in the treatment of tachyarrhythmias. *Prog Cardiovasc Dis*. 1999;41: 481-498.
26. Novak P, Dubuc M. Catheter cryoablation: biophysics and applications. In: Huang SKS, Wood MA, eds. *Catheter Ablation of Cardiac Arrhythmias*. Philadelphia, PA: W.B. Saunders; 2006:49-68.
27. Skanes AC, Klein G, Krahn A, Yee R. Cryoablation: potentials and pitfalls. *J Cardiovasc Electrophysiol*. 2004;15:S28.
28. Whittaker DK. Mechanisms of tissue destruction following cryosurgery. *Ann R Coll Surg Engl*. 1984;66:313-318.
29. Holman WL, Ikeshita M, Lease JG, et al. Cardiac cryosurgery: regional myocardial blood flow of ventricular cryolesions. *J. Surg Res*. 1986;41:524-528.
30. Khairy P, Chauvet P, Lehmann J, et al. Lower incidence of thrombus formation with cryoenergy versus radiofrequency catheter ablation. *Circulation*. 2003;42:752-758.
31. Wood MA, Parvez B, Ellebogen AL, et al. Determinants of lesion sizes and tissue temperatures during catheter cryoablation. *Pacing Clin Electrophysiol*. 2002;13:299.
32. Issa Z, Miller JM, Zipes DP. *Clinical Arrhythmology and Electrophysiology: A Companion to Braunwald's Heart Disease*. Philadelphia, PA: Saunders/Elsevier, 2009;62-91.

33. Timmermans C, Ayers GM, Crijns HJ, Rodriguez LM. Randomized study comparing radiofrequency ablation with cryoablation for the treatment of atrial flutter with emphasis on pain perception. *Circulation*. 2003;99:1250-1252.
34. Khairy P, Dubuc M. Transcatheter cryoablation part I: preclinical experience. *PACE*. 2008;31:112-120.
35. Schwagten B, Knops P, Janse P, Kimman G, Van Belle Y, Szili-Torok T. Long-term follow-up after catheter ablation for atrioventricular nodal re-entrant tachycardia: a comparison of cryothermal and radiofrequency energy in a large series of patients. *J Interv Card Electrophysiol*. 2011;30:55-61.
36. Chun KR, Schmidt B, Metzner A, Tilz R, Zerm T, Ilka Koster O, Furnkranz A, Koektuerk B, Konstantinidou M, Antz M, Ouyang F, Kuck KH. The 'single big cryoballoon' technique for acute pulmonary vein isolation in patients with paroxysmal atrial fibrillation: a prospective observational single centre study. *Eur Heart J*. 2009;30:699-709.
37. Dubuc M, Roy D, Thibault B, Ducharme A, Tardif JC, Villemaire C, Leung TK, et al. Transvenous catheter ice mapping and cryoablation of the atrioventricular node in dogs. *Pacing Clin Electrophysiol*. 1999;22:1488-1498.
38. Rodriguez LM, Leunissen J, Hoekstra A, Korteling BJ, Smeets JL, Timmermans C, Vos M, et al. Transvenous cold mapping and cryoablation of the AV node in dogs: Observations of chronic lesions and comparison to those obtained using radiofrequency ablation. *J Cardiovasc Electrophysiol*. 1998;9: 1055-1061.
39. Khairy P, Chauvet P, Lehmann J, Lambert J, Macle L, Tanguay JF, Sirios MG, et al. Lower incidence of thrombus formation with cryoenergy versus radiofrequency catheter ablation. *Circulation*. 2003;107:2045-2050.
40. Sanchez-Quintana D, Ho SY, Cabrera JA, Farre J, Anderson RH. Topographic anatomy of the inferior pyramidal space: Relevance to radiofrequency catheter ablation. *J Cardiovasc Electrophysiol*. 2001;12:210-217.
41. Skanes AC, Jones DL, Teefy P, Guiraudon C, Yee R, Krahn AD, Klein GJ. Safety and feasibility of cryothermal ablation within the mid and distal coronary sinus. *J Cardiovasc Electrophysiol*. 2004;15:1319-1323.
42. Aoyama H, Nakagawa H, Pitha JV, Khammar GS, Chandresakaran K, Matsudaira K, Yagi T, et al. Comparison of cryothermia and radiofrequency current in safety and efficacy of catheter ablation within the canine coronary sinus close to the left circumflex coronary artery. *J Cardiovasc Electrophysiol*. 2005;16:1218-1226.
43. Jordaens L, Valk S, Van Belle Y. Cardiovascular flashlight: Ablation of ventricular tachycardia in the anterior interventricular vein. *Eur Heart J*. 2009;10:1289.
44. Dib C, Kapa S, Powell BD, Packer DL, Asirvatham SJ. Successful use of "cryo-mapping" to avoid phrenic nerve damage during ostial superior vena caval ablation despite nerve proximity. *J Interv Card Electrophysiol*. 2008;22(1):23-30.
45. Kimman G, Theuns D, Szili-Torok T, Scholten M, Res J, Jordaens L. CRAVT: a prospective, randomized study comparing transvenous cryothermal and radiofrequency ablation in atrioventricular nodal re-entrant tachycardia. *Eur Heart J*. 2004;25:2232-2237.
46. Kimman G, Szili-Torok T, Theuns D, Res J, Scholten M, Jordaens L. Comparison of radiofrequency versus cryothermy catheter ablation of septal accessory pathways. *Heart*. 2003;89:1091-1092.
47. Ahmed H, Neuzil P, d'Avila A, Cha YM, Laragy M, Mares K, Brugge WR, Forcione DG, Ruskin JN, Packer DL, Reddy VY. The esophageal effects of cryoenergy during cryoablation for atrial fibrillation. *Heart Rhythm*. 2009;6:962-969.

48. Van Belle Y, Janse P, Rivero-Ayerza MJ, et al. Pulmonary vein isolation using an occluding cryoballoon for circumferential ablation: feasibility, complications, and short-term outcome. *Eur Heart J.* 2007;28:2231-2237.
49. Nault I, Miyazaki S, Forclaz A, et al. Drugs vs. ablation for the treatment of atrial fibrillation: the evidence supporting catheter ablation. *Eur Heart J.* 2010;31:1046-1054.
50. Neumann T, Vogt J, Burghard S, et al. Circumferential pulmonary vein isolation with the cryoballoon technique: results from a prospective 3-center study. *J Am Coll Cardiol.* 2008;52:273-278.
51. Furnkranz A, Chun J, Nuyens D, Metzner A, Koster I, Schmidt B, Ouyang F, Kuck KH. Characterization of conduction recovery after pulmonary veins isolation using the "single big balloon" technique. *Heart Rhythm.* 2010;7:184-190.
52. Willems S, Steven D, Servatius H, Hoffmann B, Drewitz I, Mullerleile K, Ali Aydin M, Wegscheider K, Van Salukhe T, Meinertz T, Rostock T. Persistence of pulmonary veins isolation after robotic remote-navigated ablation for atrial fibrillation and its relation to clinical outcome. *J Cardiovasc Electrophysiol.* 2010;21:1079-1084.
53. Fürnkranz A, Köster I, Chun KR, Metzner A, Mathew S, Konstantinidou M, Ouyang F, Kuck KH. Cryoballoon temperature predicts acute pulmonary vein isolation. *Heart Rhythm.* 2011;8:821-825.
54. Bai R, Datel D, Di Biase L, Fahmy TS, Kozeluhova M, Prasad S, et al. Phrenic nerve injury after catheter ablation: should we worry about this complication? *J Cardiovasc Electrophysiol.* 2006;17:944-948.
55. Tse HF, Reek S, Timmermans C, Lee KL, Geller JC, Rodriguez LM, Ghaye B, Ayers GM, Crijns HJ, Klein HU, Lau CP. Pulmonary vein isolation using transvenous catheter cryoablation for treatment of atrial fibrillation without risk of pulmonary vein stenosis. *J Am Coll Cardiol.* 2003;42:752-758.
56. Khairy P, Rivard L, Guerra P, Tanguay J, Mawad W, Roy D, et al. Morphometric ablation lesion characteristics comparing 4, 6, and 8 mm electrode-tip cryocatheters. *J Cardiovasc Electrophysiol.* 2008;19:1203-1207.
57. Haïssaguerre M, Jaïs P, Shah DC, Takashashi A, Hocini M, Quiniou G, Garrigue S, Le Mouroux A, Le Metayer P, Clementry J. Spontaneous initiation of atrial fibrillation by ectopic beats originating in the pulmonary veins. *N Engl J Med.* 1998;339:659-666.
58. Avitall B, Lafontaine D, Rozmus G, Adoni N, Le KM, Dehnee A, Urbonas A. The safety and efficacy of multiple consecutive cryo lesions in canine pulmonary veins-left atrial junction. *Heart Rhythm.* 2004:1:203-209.
59. Schwagten B, D Greef Y, Acou WJ, Stockman D. An apparent way of achieving proof of pulmonary veins disconnection during cryoballoon ablation. *Pacing Clin Electrophysiol.* 2012: 35:e337-340.

CHAPTER 21

Laser, Ultrasound, and Microwave Ablation

Paul J. Wang, MD

Introduction

Catheter ablation has become an important modality in the treatment of cardiac arrhythmias. With development of catheter ablation technologies, there has been a need to determine the optimal energy source for each application. As a result, novel energy sources such as laser, microwave, and ultrasound energy have been explored over the last two decades. Each energy source has unique characteristics and has been examined in both experimental and preclinical settings. In this chapter, we will discuss the work to date and the potential applications of these novel energy sources.

Laser Ablation

Laser energy has been used for a variety of applications including communications, information storage, and medical treatments. *Laser* comes from the phrase Light Amplification by Stimulated Emission of Radiation and provides a discrete monochromatic energy source that is coherent and collimated in its nature. Laser energy is therefore highly focused, allowing energy delivery to be precisely directed. Laser energy is created by bringing identical atoms or molecules to a particular energy state resulting in emission at a specific wavelength.[1]

Laser systems have a variety of forms and they consist of solid-state, liquid, or gas. Common gases used include argon; diode lasers use semiconductors, which emit in the near-infrared range between 700 and 1,500 nanometers. Solid-state lasers use substances such as neodymium-doped yttrium-aluminum-garnet (Nd-YAG) and holmium.[2]

The effect of laser on its target is largely due to absorption of the laser energy, resulting in vaporization and heat deposition.[3] Various tissues may become vaporized or coagulated. Energy deposition typically decreases exponentially as a function of distance, depending on the absorption characteristics of the tissue that is targeted.[4] From the area of energy deposition, there is additional thermal heating as well as laser energy scattering. Lasers are capable of producing temperatures of hundreds of degrees centigrade, although for medical uses it typically is limited to much lower temperatures. Energy transmission must be modulated to prevent excessive temperatures.

There have been several examples of the use of argon lasers for successful catheter ablation of the A-V conduction system.[5] The lesions created by this mechanism are discrete and quite localized. Argon lasers have been used intraoperatively for ventricular tachycardia ablation, as well as for ablation of accessory pathway and atrial tachycardias. In addition, argon laser has been used to create lesions in diseased human ventricles.[6,7] Histologic data demonstrate tissue vaporization as well as coagulation and necrosis, as well as some charring of tissue; moreover, heating of water within myocardial tissue, resulting in explosion, is also possible.

Nd-YAG lasers have also been used to create lesions within myocardial tissue with central vaporization. The myocardial hemoglobin content results in increased absorption.[8] The Nd-YAG laser has been used in ventricular and atrial myocardium.[9,10] Clinically, these lesions appear as transmural fibrosis. The Nd-YAG lasers have also been used epicardially in patients with monomorphic ventricular tachycardia,[11] and endocardially in patients with A-V nodal reentrant tachycardia.[12]

Diode lasers have also been demonstrated to successfully create intramyocardial lesions.[13] Diode laser technology permits wavelengths of laser to be selected, adjusting them for myocardial tissue properties. Diode lasers have been used for endocardial and epicardial applications in ventricular tachycardia.[14] Linear laser application of the diode laser has been performed in the right atrial wall in a model producing conduction block.[15]

The use of a diffusing system to permit laser energy to be used over a designated arc rather than a point source has led to new applications. Combining this approach with a balloon design has led to the greatest success clinically.[16,17] This is specifically applied to the isolation of pulmonary vein signals for the treatment of atrial fibrillation. The balloon design includes that of a balloon filled with deuterium oxide (D_2O; Figures 21.1 and 21.2). Use of deuterium oxide decreases self-heating of balloon by shifting the absorption wavelength. The ablation balloon delivers laser energy via a fiberoptic placed within the balloon and projected onto the surrounding tissue through the balloon's surface. The technology using this design has evolved from a circular target to 30° arcs. Experimental work has been successful in demonstrating the ability of this approach to create lesions in the left atrium. Gerstenfeld and Michele demonstrated in 8 swine that 10 overlapping lesions using endoscopic laser balloon ablation achieved chronic right superior pulmonary vein isolation at a mean of 28 days after ablation in 7 of 8 animals (83%). Histologically, completely transmural circumferential lesions were found in 7 of 8 animals, with 99% circumferentiality in the remaining animal.[18] This balloon system has received regulatory approval in Europe; clinical trials in the United States are currently under way. Recent multicenter data demonstrated that pulmonary veins treated using visually guided laser ablation remain isolated in 162 of 189 pulmonary veins (86%) at 3 months.[19]

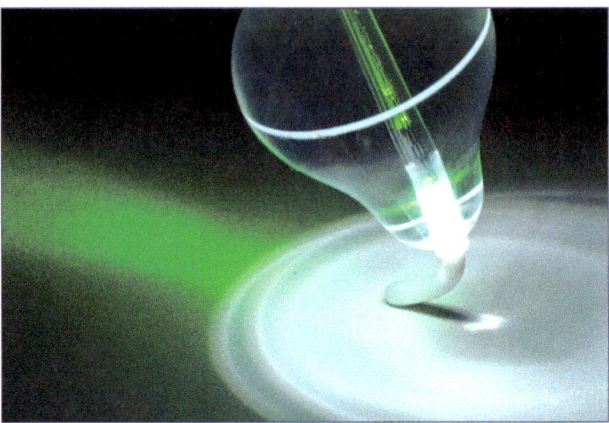

Figure 21.2 A visually guided laser ablation catheter with a flexible end-tip to permit centering of the balloon within the pulmonary vein with minimal trauma and risk of perforation. *Source:* Courtesy of Cardiofocus, Inc.

Electroanatomical mapping has revealed that isolation of the tubular portions of each pulmonary vein is at the level of the ostia, leaving the antral portions largely unablated.[20] In the first 200 patients with paroxysmal atrial fibrillation, Dukkipati et al reported freedom from atrial arrhythmias after one or two procedures in 60% of patients.[21]

Laser ablation has also been used for the surgical ablation of atrial fibrillation. Surgical atrial fibrillation ablation was performed in 16 dogs via a left atriotomy using a diode laser (980 nm) with a diffusing tip for pulmonary vein isolation. All animals had confirmed chronic isolation of the pulmonary veins, with all lesions demonstrated to be transmural with an average tissue thickness of 3.62 +/- 1.50 mm (range, 0.95–7.06 mm).[22] In epicardial experimental studies using nine different unidirectional devices (four radiofrequency, two microwave, two lasers, one cryothermic) to create continuous transmural lines of ablation from the atrial epicardium in a porcine model, Schuessler et al demonstrated that all devices except one, a radiofrequency pen, failed to penetrate 2 mm in some nontransmural sections.[23]

Ultrasound Ablation

Ultrasound ablation has been based on the ability of ultrasound to create vibration within the targeted medium. Typically, vibration frequencies of greater than 18 kHz have been used, creating a pressure wave propagated through the median and the mechanical movement of the particles. Ultrasound energy is therefore absorbed and converted to thermal energy.[24]

High-intensity focus ultrasound (HIFU) has been investigated as a noninvasive technique to apply energy from outside the structure that has been targeted.[25] HIFU energy transducers include a piezoelectric element that vibrates in the specific frequency that can be collimated to create significant depths of penetration using frequencies

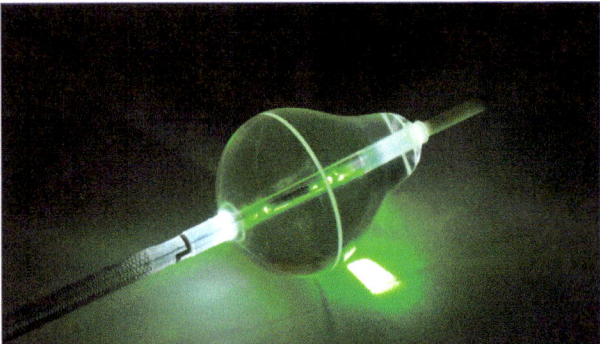

Figure 21.1 A visually guided laser ablation catheter with a compliant variable diameter balloon. The balloon is designed to be centered in the pulmonary vein so that laser energy may be delivered around the ostium at the level of the equator designated by the circumferential line. *Source:* Courtesy of Cardiofocus, Inc.

ranging from 500 kHz to 20 MHz. This energy permits oscillation and collapse of gas bubbles or microcavitation, as well as tissue absorption of the acoustic energy. Vapor cavities and bubbles may be created and result in boiling of the tissue water.[26]

Experimental studies have shown the feasibility of ultrasound for cardiac applications using energy sources from 10 to 15 MHz producing the deepest lesions.[27] Because extremely high temperatures can be created, the energy typically is modulated in order to limit the maximum temperatures below 100°C. The lesions created can be adjusted based on the target temperature. Energy transmission can be extremely rapid. This has been demonstrated in 15 seconds or less.[28] Substantial myocardial lesion depths of more than 10 millimeters have been demonstrated. The lesions are well circumscribed. In vivo extracardiac studies have been used to demonstrate the AV block. In addition, myocardial lesions can be created. In intraoperative studies, this can be accomplished at a distance of up to 6 centimeters. Koruth et al demonstrated in open-chest swine that HIFU delivered via a probe placed directly on the left anterior descending artery has the potential to create large myocardial lesions but may result in injury of the coronary artery, particularly over time.[29]

Phased-array HIFU systems use hundreds of ultrasound elements to create lesions that may be targeted up to 15 cm away. Thus, this structure may be particularly useful in the ability to achieve noninvasive energy deposition. Applications such as intrauterine fibromas have been one example.[30]

A balloon system has been designed to incorporate ultrasound energy for the treatment of atrial fibrillation. While early studies using an ultrasound system were successful experimentally, it was quickly determined that the system could not result in successful lesion formation in humans because of the variability in pulmonary vein anatomy.[31-33] A parabolic acoustic reflector was built into the back of the balloon creating a forward projecting ultrasound balloon system (Figure 21.3). Thus, the emitted sound waves traveled parallel to the axis of the transducer, which was then absorbed by the adjacent tissue.

Significant design changes were thus made in order to permit targeting of the surrounding tissue more effectively.[34] Studies have shown that significant damage can occur to adjacent structures. In a canine study using HIFU energy delivered close to the esophagus, either outside or inside the inferior pulmonary vein, endoscopy identified an esophageal ulcer immediately after ablation in 11 of 13 HIFU experiments, all with esophageal temperatures greater than or equal to 50°C. Two animals developed left atrial-esophageal fistula and died at 2 weeks.[35] Neven et al demonstrated that following pulmonary vein isolation performed using HIFU, an esophageal thermal lesion was found in 2 of 26 patients during endoscopy, and 1 patient had lethal atrial-to-esophageal fistula 31 days after ablation. In addition, 2 patients had persistent phrenic nerve palsies, 1 had ischemic stroke, 1 had pericardial effusion 48 days after ablation, and 1 patient had unexplained death 49 days after ablation.[36] Because of an excess complication rate, these studies were terminated.

HIFU has been used for the surgical ablation of atrial fibrillation. Groh et al demonstrated that in 220 patients with atrial fibrillation ultrasound surgical ablation, freedom from atrial fibrillation or left-sided atrial flutter was 86.2% at 18 months.[37] Concern of collateral damage for the epicardial HIFU ablation also exists. The epicardial delivery of HIFU may result in collateral damage of adjacent structures such as the esophagus. Prasertwitayakij

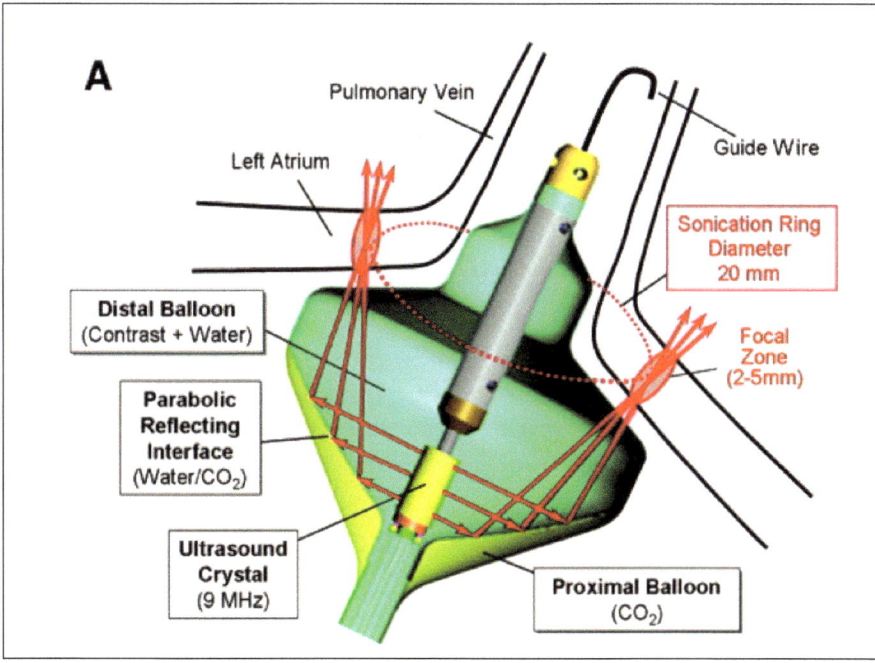

Figure 21.3 A schematic design of a parabolic ultrasound ablation catheter. The high-intensity focused ultrasound (HIFU) energy is generated by the ultrasound crystal and reflected by the parabolic reflecting interface between water and CO_2. The energy is reflected onto the left atrial surface with a focal zone of 2–5 mm and a sonication ring diameter of 20 mm. Source: Yokoyama K, Nakagawa H, Seres KA, et al.[35]

et al reported a case report of esophageal injury after atrial fibrillation ablation using an epicardial HIFU device.[38]

Microwave Ablation

Microwave energy has been shown to be able to generate energy to ablate various tissues in the body. Microwave energy requires a power source usually between 915 MHz and 2,450 MHz.[39] The energy is delivered via an antenna that is specially designed for efficient energy delivery (Figure 21.4).[40] The energy is transmitted from the power source to the antenna via a coaxial cable. There may be significant energy loss over the coaxial cable with subsequent heating, particularly when the cable diameter is small.[41]

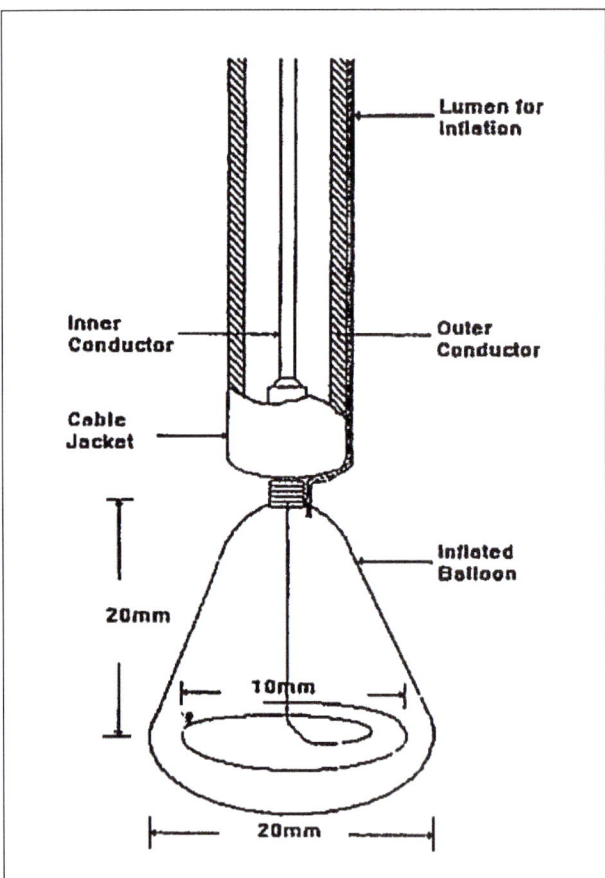

Figure 21.4 A schematic design of a microwave antenna. The antenna consists of a spiral design to direct the energy coaxially into the tissue. A coaxial cable consists of an inner and outer conductor. The spiral antenna is placed within an inflated balloon. This was tested in a porcine thigh muscle preparation. *Source:* VanderBrink BA, Gu Z, Rodriguez V, et al.[55]

For each antenna design, a specific energy distribution pattern is created.[42] The distribution is represented by a specific absorption rate pattern, which may be mapped by measuring the heating pattern in the relevant medium in three-dimensional space. There have been numerous antenna designs created for tissue ablation. The ability for microwave energy to pass through a substance is based on the dielectric properties of the substance, as assessed by the permitivity at that frequency. Energy dissipation in tissue with consequent heating is felt to be the primary mechanism for cell death and ablation.[41]

Early work demonstrated the feasibility of percutaneous microwave energy delivery for AV junction ablation.[43-44] Histopathological studies have demonstrated that ablation results in hemorrhage with coagulation necrosis. Microwave ablation has successfully resulted in atrial and ventricular myocardial ablation in experimental models.[45-50]

The clinical application for microwave energy culminated in a novel design for minimally invasive epicardial ablation for the treatment of atrial fibrillation. Using minimally invasive thoracoscopic ports, a flexible microwave device is positioned epicardially to create a "box" lesion around the four pulmonary veins. In 41 patients, the mean diameter of the left atrium was 7.19 +/− 1.44 cm and the mean follow-up time was 5.37 +/− 0.91 years; at 5 years follow-up, 39.3% of these patients (11/28) were in sinus rhythm.[51] Ahlsson et al demonstrated in 20 open-heart surgery patients with concomitant atrial fibrillation that 14 of 19 patients (74%) were in sinus rhythm with no antiarrhythmic drugs at 12 months. All patients in sinus rhythm had preserved left and right atrial filling waves, atrial wall velocities, atrial strain, and atrial strain rate.[52] Experimental studies such as those by Schuessler et al have demonstrated the inability of microwave systems to penetrate 2 mm in some sections.[53]

There have been experimental studies examining catheter ablation utilizing microwave energy. Using a swine thigh muscle preparation, Tse et al demonstrated that the independent predictors for lesion depth and microwave energy included targeted temperature ≥80°C, application duration ≥150 seconds, and use of a 20-mm antenna ($P < 0.05$).[54-56]

The development of new energy sources may provide new and improved treatments for many arrhythmias. Some catheter designs such as the HIFU balloon ablation system have been largely abandoned, while others such as the visually guided laser balloon ablation system are in the midst of clinical trials. Undoubtedly, new energy sources will find an important and sustaining role in the catheter ablation of arrhythmias in the future.

References

1. Saksena S, Gadhoke A. Laser therapy for tachyarrhythmias: A new frontier. *Pacing Clin Electrophysiol*. 1989;9:531-550.
2. Tomaru T, Geschwind HJ, Boussignac G, et al. Comparison of ablation efficacy of excimer, pulsed-dye, and holmium–YAG lasers relevant to shock waves. *Am Heart J*. 1992;123:886-895.
3. Ohtake H, Misaki T, Watanabe G, et al. Myocardial coagulation by intraoperative Nd:YAG laser ablation and its dependence on blood perfusion. *Pacing Clin Electrophysiol*. 1994;17:1627-1631.

4. Avitall B, Khan M, Krum D, et al. Physics and engineering of transcatheter cardiac tissue ablation. *J Am Coll Cardiol.* 1993;22:921-932.
5. Narula OS, Boveja BK, Cohen DM, et al. Laser catheter-induced atrioventricular nodal delays and atrioventricular block in dogs: acute and chronic observations. *J Am Coll Cardiol.* 1985;5:259-267.
6. Ciccone J, Saksena S, Pantopoulos D. Comparative efficacy of continuous and pulsed argon laser ablation of human diseased ventricle. *Pacing Clin Electrophysiol.* 1986;9:697-704.
7. Saksena S, Hussain SM, Gielchinsky I, et al. Intraoperative mapping-guided argon laser ablation of malignant ventricular tachycardia. *Am J Cardiol.* 1987;59:78-83.
8. Ohtake H, Misaki T, Watanabe G, et al. Myocardial coagulation by intraoperative Nd:YAG laser ablation and its dependence on blood perfusion. *Pacing Clin Electrophysiol.* 1994;17:1627-1631.
9. Weber HP, Enders HS, Keiditisch E. Percutaneous Nd:YAG laser coagulation of ventricular myocardium in dogs using a special laser catheter. *Pacing Clin Electrophysiol.* 1989;12:899-910.
10. Weber HP, Enders HS, Ruprecht L, et al. Catheter-directed laser coagulation of atrial myocardium in dogs. *Eur Heart J.* 1994;15:971-980.
11. Pfeiffer D, Moosdorf R, Stevenson RH, et al. Epicardial neodymium: YAG laser photocoagulation of ventricular tachycardia without ventriculotomy in patients after myocardial infarction. *Circulation.* 1996;94:3221-3225.
12. Weber HP, Kalternbrunner W, Heinze A, et al. Laser catheter coagulation of atrial myocardium for ablation of atrioventricular nodal reentrant tachycardia. *Eur Heart J.* 1997;18:487-498.
13. Ware DL, Boor P, Yang C, et al. Slow intramural heating with diffused laser light: A unique method for deep myocardial coagulation. *Circulation.* 1999;99:1630-1636.
14. d'Avila A, Splinter R, Svenson RH. New perspectives on catheter-based ablation of ventricular tachycardia complicating Chagas' disease: Experimental evidence of the efficacy of near infrared lasers for catheter ablation of Chagas' VT. *J Interv Cardiac Electrophysiol.* 2002;7:23-38.
15. Keane D, Ruskin JN: Linear atrial ablation with a diode laser and fiberoptic catheter. *Circulation.* 1999;100:e59-e60.
16. Reddy VR, Houghtaling C, Fallon J, et al. Use of a diode laser balloon catheter to generate circumferential pulmonary venous lesions in an open-thoracotomy caprine model. *Pacing Clin Electrophysiol.* 2004;27:52-57.
17. Lemery R, Vienot JP, Tang ASL, et al. Fiberoptic balloon catheter ablation of pulmonary vein ostia in pigs using photonic energy delivery with diode laser. *Pacing Clin Electrophysiol.* 2002;25:32-36.
18. Gerstenfeld EP, Michele J. Pulmonary vein isolation using a compliant endoscopic laser balloon ablation system in a swine model. *J Interv Card Electrophysiol.* 2010;29:1-9.
19. Dukkipati SR, Neuzil P, Kautzner J, et al. The durability of pulmonary vein isolation using the visually guided laser balloon catheter: Multicenter results of pulmonary vein remapping studies. *Heart Rhythm.* 2012;9:919-925.
20. Reddy VY, Neuzil P, d'Avila A, et al. Balloon catheter ablation to treat paroxysmal atrial fibrillation: what is the level of pulmonary venous isolation? *Heart Rhythm.* 2008;5:353-360.
21. Dukkipati SR, Kuck KH, Neuzil P, et al. Pulmonary vein isolation using a visually-guided laser balloon catheter: the first 200-patient multicenter clinical experience. *Circ Arrhythm Electrophysiol.* 2013;6:467-472.
22. Williams MR, Casher JM, Russo MJ, et al. Laser energy source in surgical atrial fibrillation ablation: preclinical experience. *Ann Thorac Surg.* 2006;82:2260-2264.
23. Schuessler RB, Lee AM, Melby SJ, et al. Animal studies of epicardial atrial ablation. *Heart Rhythm.* 2009;6:S41-S45.
24. He DS, Zimmer JE, Hynynen FI, et al. Application of ultrasound energy for intracardiac ablation of arrhythmias. *Eur Heart J.* 1995;16:961-966.
25. Strickberger SA, Tokano T, Kluiwstra JA, et al. Extracardiac ablation of canine antriventricular junction by use of high intensity focused ultrasound. *Circulation.* 1999;100:203-208.
26. Zimmer JE, Hynynen K, He DS, et al. The feasibility of using ultrasound for cardiac ablation. *IEEE Trans Biomed Eng.* 1995;42:891-897.
27. Zimmer JE, Hynynen K, He DS, et al. The feasibility of using ultrasound for cardiac ablation. *IEEE Trans Biomed Eng.* 1995;42:891-897.
28. He DS, Zimmer JE, Hynynen FI, et al. Application of ultrasound energy for intracardiac ablation of arrhythmias. *Eur Heart J.* 1995;16:961-966.
29. Koruth JS, Dukkipati S, Carrillo RG, et al. Safety and efficacy of high-intensity focused ultrasound atop coronary arteries during epicardial catheter ablation. *J Card Electrophysiol.* 2011;22:1274-1280.
30. Wan J, VanBaren P, Ebbini E, et al. Ultrasound surgery: comparison of strategies using phased array systems. *IEEE Trans UFFC.* 1996;43:1085-1098.
31. Lesh MD, Diederich C, Guerra G, et al. An anatomic approach to prevention of atrial fibrillation: Pulmonary vein isolation with through-the-balloon ultrasound ablation (TTB-USA). *Thorac Cardiovasc Surg.* 1999;47:347-351.
32. Natale A, Pisano E, Shewchik J, et al. First human experience with pulmonary vein isolation using a through-the-balloon circumferential ultrasound ablation system for recurrent atrial fibrillation. *Circulation.* 2000;102:1879-1882.
33. Saliba W, Wilber D, Packer D, et al. Circumferential ultrasound ablation for pulmonary vein isolation: Analysis of acute and chronic failures. *J Card Electrophysiol.* 2002;13:957-961.
34. Meininger GR, Calkins H, Lickfett L, et al. Initial experience with a novel focused ultrasound ablation system for ring ablation outside the pulmonary vein. *J Interv Card Electrophysiol.* 2003;8:141-148.
35. Yokoyama K, Nakagawa H, Seres KA, et al. Canine model of esophageal injury and atrial-esophageal fistula after applications of forward-firing high-intensity focused ultrasound and side-firing unfocused ultrasound in the left atrium and inside the pulmonary vein. *Circ Arrhythm Electrophysiol.* 2009;2:41-49.
36. Neven K, Schmidt B, Metzner A, et al. Fatal end of a safety algorithm for pulmonary vein isolation with use of high-intensity focused ultrasound. *Circ Arrhythm Electrophysiol.* 2010;3: 260-265.
37. Groh MA, Binns OA, Burton HG 3rd, et al. Ultrasonic cardiac ablation for atrial fibrillation during concomitant cardiac surgery: long-term clinical outcomes. *Ann Thorac Surg.* 2007;84:1978-1983.
38. Prasertwitayakij N, Vodnala D, Pridjian AK, et al. Esophageal injury after atrial fibrillation ablation with an epicardial high-intensity focused ultrasound device. *J Interv Card Electrophysiol.* 2011;31:243-245.
39. Whayne JG, Nath S, Haines DE. Microwave catheter ablation of myocardium in vitro: Assessment of the characteristics of tissue heating and injury. *Circulation.* 1994;89:2390-2395.
40. Vanderbrink BA, Gu Z, Rodriguez V, et al. Microwave ablation using a spiral antenna design in a porcine thigh muscle preparation: in vivo assessment of temperature profile and lesion geometry. *J Cardiovasc Electrophysiol.* 2000;11:193-198.

41. Avitall B, Khan M, Krum D, et al. Physics and engineering of transcatheter cardiac tissue ablation. *J Am Coll Cardiol.* 1993;22:921-932.
42. Nevels RD, Arndt GD, Raffoul GW, et al. Microwave catheter design. *IEEE Trans Biomed Eng.* 1998;45:885-890.
43. Langberg JJ, Wonnell T, Chin MC, et al. Catheter ablation of the atrioventricular junction using a helical microwave antenna: A novel means of coping energy to the endocardium. *Pacing Clin Electrophysiol.* 1991;14:2105-2113.
44. Yang X, Watanabe I, Kojima T, et al. Microwave ablation of the atrioventricular junction in vivo and ventricular myocardium in vitro and in vivo: Effects of varying power and duration on lesion volume. *Jpn Heart J.* 1994;35:175-191.
45. Rho TH, Ito M, Pride HP, et al. Microwave ablation of canine atrial tachycardia induced by aconitine. *Am Heart J.* 1995;129:1021-1025.
46. Liem LB, Mead RH, Shenasa M, et al. In vitro and in vivo results of transcatheter microwave ablation using forward firing tip antenna design. *Pacing Clin Electrophysiol.* 1996;19:2004-2008.
47. Liem LB, Mead RH, Shenasa M, et al. Microwave catheter ablation using a clinical prototype system with a lateral firing antenna design. *Pacing Clin Electrophysiol.* 1998;21:714-721.
48. Gu Z, Rappaport CM, Wang PJ, et al. A 2¼-turn spiral antenna for catheter cardiac ablation. *IEEE Trans Biomed Eng.* 1999;46:1480-1482.
49. Thomas SP, Clout R, Deery C, et al. Microwave ablation of myocardial tissue: the effect of element design, tissue coupling, blood flow, power, and duration of exposure on lesion size. *J Cardiovasc Electrophysiol.* 1999;10:72-78.
50. Vanderbrink BA, Gu Z, Rodriguez V, et al. Microwave ablation using a spiral antenna design in a porcine thigh muscle preparation: in vivo assessment of temperature profile and lesion geometry. *J Cardiovasc Electrophysiol.* 2000;11:193-198.
51. Vicol C, Kellerer D, Petrakopoulou P, et al. Long-term results after ablation for long-standing atrial fibrillation concomitant to surgery for organic heart disease: is microwave energy reliable? *J Thorac Cardiov Sur.* 2008;136:1156-1159.
52. Ahlsson A, Linde P, Rask P, et al. Atrial function after epicardial microwave ablation in patients with atrial fibrillation. *Scand Cardiovasc J.* 2008;42:192-201.
53. Schuessler RB, Lee AM, Melby SJ, et al. Animal studies of epicardial atrial ablation. *Heart Rhythm.* 2009;6:S41-S45.
54. Tse HF, Liao S, Siu CW, et al. Determinants of lesion dimensions during transcatheter microwave ablation. *Pacing Clin Electrophysiol.* 2009;32:201-208.
55. VanderBrink BA, Gu Z, Rodriguez V, et al. Microwave ablation using a spiral antenna design in a porcine thigh muscle preparation: in vivo assessment of temperature profile and lesion geometry. *J Cardiovasc Electrophysiol.* 2000;11:193-198.
56. VanderBrink BA, Gilbride C, Aronovitz MJ, et al. Safety and efficacy of a steerable temperature monitoring microwave catheter system for ventricular myocardial ablation. *J Cardiovasc Electrophysiol.* 2000;11:305-310.

CHAPTER 22

ABLATION TECHNOLOGY FOR THE SURGICAL TREATMENT OF ATRIAL FIBRILLATION

RICHARD B. SCHUESSLER, PhD; RALPH J. DAMIANO, JR., MD

Introduction

The Cox-Maze procedure was introduced by Dr. James Cox at Barnes-Jewish Hospital in St. Louis, MO, in 1987. The operation involved creating a number of incisions across both the right and left atria. These incisions form scar tissue, which blocks the propagation of activation. It was designed to block the multiple macroreentrant circuits that were felt at the time to be the mechanism responsible for atrial fibrillation (AF). Over the next decade, this operation became the gold standard for the surgical treatment of AF. The 10-year freedom from AF in our series has been 96%.[1] These excellent results have been reproduced by other groups around the world.[2-4] Despite its efficacy, this procedure was not widely performed because of its complexity and technical difficulty.

The introduction of ablation technology has significantly changed this attitude. To simplify the operation and make it easier to perform, the incisions of the traditional cut-and-sew Maze procedure were replaced with linear lines of ablation. Various energy sources have been used, including cryoablation, radiofrequency energy, microwave, laser, and high-frequency ultrasound. This chapter will review the present state of the art in surgical ablation therapy.

Requirements for Surgical Ablation

For ablation technology to reliably replace an incision in AF surgery, it must meet several important criteria. First, it must produce complete conduction block. This is the mechanism by which incisions prevent AF. They either block activation wavefronts or isolate trigger foci. It has been demonstrated that nontransmural lesions, which leave only a thin rim of viable tissue, can cause conduction block during AF.[5] However, our laboratory has shown that sinus rhythm and AF can conduct through even tiny gaps (≥ 1 mm) in ablation lines.[6] Since it is difficult, if not impossible, to discern the precise depth of a lesion in the operating room, the only guarantee of effectiveness is a fully transmural lesion. This always results in conduction block. Thus, a device must be able to make transmural lesions on the arrested heart from either the epicardial or endocardial surface for ablation performed during surgery. If it is used from the epicardial surface, on the beating heart, transmural lesions can be difficult because of the heat sink of the circulating intracavitary blood.[7,8]

The second important attribute of the technology is that it must be safe. This requires a precise definition of dose–response curves to limit excessive or inadequate ablation. It is also necessary to know the effects of the specific ablation technology on surrounding vital structures, such as the coronary sinus, coronary arteries, and heart valves. Third, a device should make AF surgery easier and quicker to perform. This would require features such as rapidity of lesion formation, ease of use, and adequate length and flexibility.

Finally, the device optimally should be adaptable for minimally invasive approaches. This would require the ability to insert the device through small thoracotomies or ports. It would also require the device to be capable of creating transmural epicardial lesions on the beating heart.

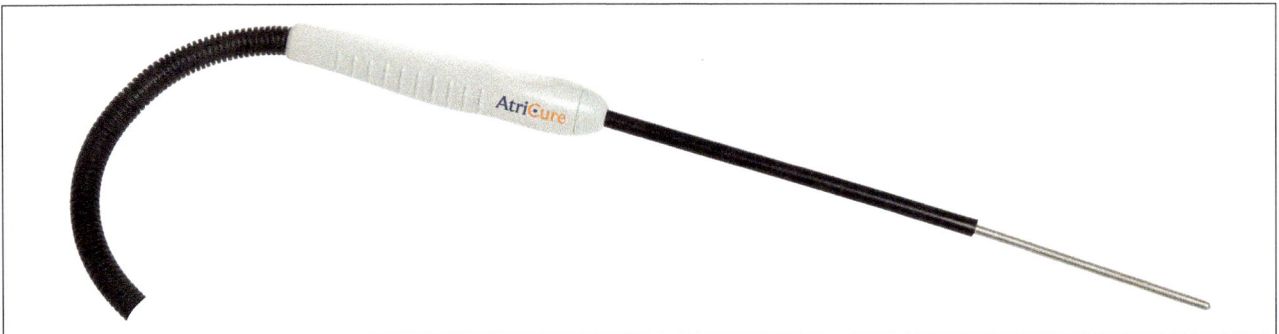

Figure 22.1 The AtriCure cryoICE™ probe. This probe is malleable. Courtesy of AtriCure.

Anatomic Considerations

It is necessary to understand the human atrial wall thickness to define the performance of any epicardial ablation device. Several studies have examined the regional wall thickness of the right atrium (RA) and left atrium (LA) of humans. In normal individuals, the atrial thickness in the posterior LA between the pulmonary veins ranged from 2.3 ± 1.0 mm between the superior veins to 2.9 ± 1.3 mm between the inferior veins.[9] In patients with a history of AF, the tissue was thinner, ranging from 2.1 ± 0.9 mm to 2.5 ± 1.3 mm. In both groups, the thickness increased moving from the superior to the inferior veins. In normal individuals, the thickness in the LA just above the coronary sinus was 6.5 ± 2.5 mm. The thickness of Bachmann's bundle, a preferential conduction pathway between the right and left atria crossing across the roof of the atria in the transverse sinus, is 4.6 ± 1.1 mm (range: 1.7–9.3 mm) in normal individuals.[10]

In patients with any cardiac disease, the mean LA thickness is 5.2 ± 1.8 (range: 3–15 mm). The crista terminalis in the RA has an average thickness of 7.7 ± 2.4 mm (range: 4.2–12.6 mm). These values include only muscle thickness and do not take into account overlying fat or underlying free-running pectinate muscles. Even in individuals who are not overweight, the fat layer at the posterior mitral annulus can be 10 mm thick. Epicardial fat is a difficult, thick barrier impeding depth of penetration for most ablation technologies.[11] In addition, in both the RA and LA, there are also free-running pectinate muscles that are not continuous with the epicardial surface. Finally, as patients grow older, their chamber size and wall thickness increase.[12] This highly variable wall thickness and anatomy provide a challenge to any unidirectional device to achieve transmural lesions.

Cryoablation

Device Characteristics

There are two commercially available sources of cryothermal energy that are being used in cardiac surgery. The older technology utilizes nitrous oxide and is manufactured by AtriCure (Cincinnati, OH). The cryoICE™ (AtriCure), uses a 10-cm malleable probe on a 20-cm shaft (Figure 22.1). Medtronic (Minneapolis, MN) has developed a device using argon. The Medtronic Cryo™ can be used in two ways: either as a malleable, single-use cryosurgical probe with adjustable insulation sleeve for varying ablation zone lengths, or as a two-in-one convertible device that incorporates a clamp and surgical probe. At one atmosphere of pressure, nitrous oxide is capable of cooling tissue to −89.5°C, while argon has a minimum temperature of −185.7°C.

Cryothermal energy is delivered to myocardial tissue by using a cryoprobe. This probe consists of a hollow shaft, an electrode tip, and an integrated thermocouple for distal temperature recording. A console houses the tank containing the liquid refrigerant. This liquid is pumped under high pressure to the electrode through an inner lumen. Once the fluid reaches the electrode, it converts from a liquid to a gas phase, absorbing energy and resulting in rapid cooling of the tissue. The gas is then aspirated by vacuum through a separate return lumen to the console. At the tissue-electrode interface, there is a well-demarcated line of frozen tissue, termed an "ice ball."

Mechanism and Histology of Tissue Injury

Cryothermal energy destroys tissue through the formation of intracellular and extracellular ice crystals. This disrupts the cell membrane and the cytoplasmic organelles. Following the cryoablation, there is development of hemorrhage, edema, and inflammation over the first 48 hours. Irreversible injury is usually evident within this early time period. There is also evidence of apoptosis, the induction of which may expand the area of initial cell death.[13]

Healing is characterized by extensive fibrosis, which begins approximately one week after lesion formation. Cryoablation is the only currently available energy source that does not alter tissue collagen; it preserves normal tissue architecture. This makes it an excellent energy source for ablation close to valvular tissue or the fibrous skeleton of the heart. Histologically, lesions exhibit dense homogenous scar formation. There is a distinct absence of cicatrization and a lack of thrombus formation over the lesions. The homogenous scar has been shown to have a low arrhythmogenic potential.[14-16] In a human study, specimens that underwent endocardial cryoablation on the arrested heart were examined. The histology revealed extensive myocellular damage and transmural lesions. Morphologic features included sarcoplasmic vacuolization, increased cell roundness with indistinct membranes, and loss of contraction bands.[17]

Ability to Create Transmural Lesions

The size and depth of cryolesions are determined by numerous factors, including probe temperature, tissue temperature, probe size, the duration and number of ablations, and the particular liquid used as the cooling agent.[16] With conventional nitrous oxide, 2- to 3-minute ablations have been shown to reliably create transmural lesions on both the right and left atrium. Because of the heat sink provided by circulating endocardial blood, epicardial cryolesions on the beating heart with nitrous oxide have not been transmural.[18]

There is an increasing number of studies investigating the use of argon cryoablation. Of three published animal studies, only one reported all samples to be transmural.[19-21] The remaining animal studies showed 25%–93% of lesions were transmural in beating heart models. Doll and colleagues examined epicardial cryoablation for 2 minutes at −160°C.[20] They were able to get transmural lesions 62% of the time around the pulmonary veins. Five of 6 lesions on the right atrial appendage were transmural, but only 2 out of 8 (25%) on the left atrial appendage were transmural. Using the cryo-clamp device epicardially on a beating heart in the canine model, 93% of lesions were transmural.[21] Thus, this device appears to be capable of creating transmural epicardial lesions. However, there has been concern regarding the use of this device on the beating heart due to fears of freezing the intracavity blood with subsequent embolization. In our laboratory, 5 of 10 pigs undergoing argon cryoablation on the beating heart showed severe signs of emboli, with necropsy confirmed pulmonary embolism in 3 animals and a large ischemic brain infarct in 1 animal.

Safety Profile

Cryoablation has the benefit of preserving the fibrous skeleton of the heart and thus is one of the safest of the technologies available. Nitrous oxide cryoablation has extensive clinical use and has had an excellent safety profile. While experience has shown that cryothermal energy appears to have no permanent effects on valvular tissue or the coronary sinus, experimental studies have shown late minimal hyperplasia of coronary arteries, and these should be avoided.[17,22-24] Esophageal injury is of concern as well. With epicardial cryoablation in a sheep model, 7 of 8 cases produced a mild or moderate esophageal lesion.[20] Additionally, a study aimed at evaluating histological changes induced on the esophagus by surgical ablation therapy reported endocardial cryoablation for 60 seconds resulted in intensive esophageal lesions in 2 of 6 sheep. Epicardial cryoablation for 120 seconds produced mainly mild alterations.[25]

There have been a number of clinical reports of argon cryoablation. The two largest studies, one with 28 patients and the other with 63 patients, reported no ablation-related complications or deaths.[26-29]

Summary

Cryoablation is unique among the presently available technologies in that it destroys tissue by freezing instead of heating. The biggest advantage of this technology is its ability to preserve tissue architecture and the collagen structure. The nitrous oxide technology reliably creates transmural lesions and generally is safe except around coronary arteries. Argon-based technology has not been studied extensively. However, it appears to be able to reliably create endocardial transmural lesions on the arrested heart. Its ability to create epicardial transmural lesions on the beating heart is unclear, but available evidence suggests that it is unreliable in this setting. Cryoablation has been shown to cause coronary injury, and its use should be avoided near the esophagus. Early clinical results have shown a good safety profile.

The potential disadvantages of cryoablation technology include the relatively long time necessary to create an ablation (2–3 minutes). There also is difficulty in creating lesions in the beating heart because of the heat sink of the circulating blood volume. The cryoclamp device may overcome this problem as early work showed 93% transmurality on the beating heart.[21] However, if blood is frozen, it coagulates, and this may be a potential risk of epicardial cryoablation on the beating heart.

Unipolar Radiofrequency Energy

Radiofrequency (RF) energy has been used for cardiac ablation for many years in the electrophysiology laboratory.[30] It was one of the first energy sources to be used in the operating room for AF ablation. RF energy can be delivered by either unipolar or bipolar electrodes.

Device Characteristics

Estech (San Ramon, CA) has two unipolar surgical probes, the COBRA™ Adhere XL Probe and the COBRA™ Cooled Surgical Probe. Both are segmented flexible and malleable devices with multiple electrodes. The cooled device has internal saline cooling. To maintain probe position during beating heart applications, the Cobra™ Adhere XL Probe (Figure 22.2) provides suction stabilization to the probe device, while the Cobra Cooled Surgical Probe does so for a minimally invasive approach.

The VisiTrax™ is available from nContact (Raleigh, NC) and is a coiled electrode that is held in place with suction and irrigated with saline for cooling. It comes in a 3- and 5-cm version. The device is designed to be used in open or closed chest procedures.

Medtronic (Minneapolis, MN) has developed different RF devices such as the Cardioblate® Standard Ablation Pen and the Cardioblate® XL Surgical Ablation Pen. These are pen-like, irrigated unipolar devices used to make ablation lesions point-by-point as well as by dragging the device across tissue to make a linear lesion. The Cardioblate® XL Pen is 20 cm in length and is designed to be used through a port or small thoracotomy.

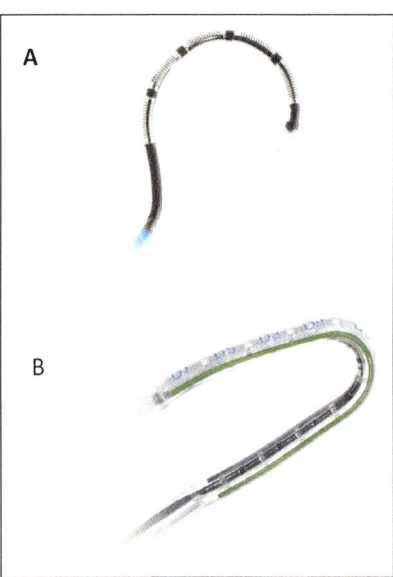

Figure 22.2 **Panel A** shows the Cobra™ Cooled Surgical Probe and **Panel B** shows the Cobra Adhere XL Probe. The Adhere uses suction to maintain contact with the atrial surface. Courtesy of Estech.

Mechanism and Histology of Tissue Injury

RF energy uses an alternating current in the range of 100–1000 kHz. This frequency is high enough to prevent rapid myocardial depolarization and the induction of ventricular fibrillation, yet low enough to prevent tissue vaporization and perforation. Resistive heating occurs only within a narrow rim of tissue in direct contact with the electrode, usually less than 1 mm. The deeper tissue heating occurs via passive conduction. With unipolar catheters, the energy is dispersed between the electrode tip and an indifferent electrode, usually the grounding pad applied to the patient.

The lesion size depends on electrode–tissue contact area, the interface temperature, the current and voltage (power), and the duration of delivery. The depth of the lesion can be limited by char formation at the tissue-electrode interface. To resolve this problem, irrigated catheters were developed; this reduces char formation by keeping temperatures cooler at the tissue interface. These irrigated catheters have been shown to create larger volume lesions than dry RF devices.[31,32] On histologic evaluation of RF lesions, a focal coagulation necrosis predominates acutely. This correlates with the irreversible nature of the injury, which occurs at high temperatures. There is destruction of myocardial/collagen matrix and replacement with fibrin and collagen in chronic studies. In chronic models, contraction and scarring occurs with large lesions. At very high temperatures (greater than 100°C), char formation predominates. Char presents as an impediment to heat transduction and has been associated with asymmetrical ablations.

Ability to Create Transmural Lesions

The dose-response curves for unipolar RF have been described.[33-35] While in animals unipolar RF has been shown to create transmural lesions on the arrested heart with sufficiently long ablation times (60–120 seconds), there have been problems in humans. After 2 minute endocardial ablations during mitral valve surgery, only 20% of the in vivo lesions were transmural.[34] Epicardial ablation has been even more difficult. Animal studies have consistently shown that unipolar RF is incapable of creating epicardial transmural lesions on the beating heart.[35,36] A recent clinical study confirmed this problem. Epicardial RF ablation in humans resulted in only 7% of lesions being transmural despite electrode temperatures of up to 90°C.[37]

Safety Profile

Because RF ablation is a well-developed technology, much is known about its safety profile. The complications of unipolar RF devices have been described after extensive clinical use and include coronary artery injuries, cerebrovascular accidents, and the devastating creation of esophageal perforation leading to atrioesophageal fistula.[25,38-41]

Summary

Unipolar RF ablation has been shown to be able to create endocardial transmural lesions most of the time, but is incapable of creating epicardial transmural lesions on the beating heart. As with all unipolar energy sources, it radiates unfocused heat, and this can cause collateral injury if not used carefully.

Bipolar Radiofrequency Energy

Device Characteristics

Bipolar technology is incorporated into devices in two ways. One means is via a clamp in which energy is applied between the two jaws of the device in which the tissue is between the two electrodes. The second is a device in which the two electrodes are side by side, and the device is applied to either the epicardial or endocardial surface.

The Isolator® Synergy™ clamp (AtriCure, Inc., Cincinnati, OH) has two electrodes embedded in each of two jaws, which are 7 cm long and in configurations of various curvatures, designed to clamp over the target atrial tissue (Figure 22.4). The device uses a continuous measurement of tissue impedance as a marker for the assessment of lesion transmurality. The conductance between the electrodes is measured 50 times per second during the ablation. When the conductance drops to a stable minimum level (high impedance), this correlates well with both experimental and clinical histology assessment of transmurality. The algorithm allows for total energy delivery to be customized to the individual tissue characteristics.

AtriCure has also developed the Isolator™ Multifunctional™ Pen (Figure 22.3) that uses bipolar energy through two side-by-side electrodes at the end of the hand-held probe. The device can be used to record electrograms or pace, in addition to using it to ablate. They also have developed the Coolrail™ Linear Pen, which is a 30 mm side-by-side electrode on a 7.5-cm shaft. The active electrode region is internally cooled with circulating saline. Both of these devices are applied for a fixed period of time. The algorithms that assess transmurality by measuring conductance between the two electrodes do not work when the electrodes are side-by-side on one surface rather than placed between the epicardial and endocardial surface.

Medtronic (Minneapolis, MN) markets two bipolar clamp devices, both with irrigated flexible jaws and an articulating head. Cardioblate® BP2 Irrigated RF Surgical Ablation System has a flexible neck and a 7-cm electrode. A similar lower-profile device is also available, the Cardioblate® LP System, for use through a small thoracotomy. They also offer a longer malleable clamp, the Cardioblate® Gemini System, which also can be used through a small lateral thoracotomy. All of the Medtronic clamps are irrigated with saline to help increase the depth of penetration.

Estech (San Ramon, CA) offers two bipolar clamps, both called the COBRA Revolution™ bipolar clamp (Figure 22.4). One utilizes disposable electrode elements with a reusable clamp. The other is a single-use system.

Mechanism and Histology of Tissue Injury

In the bipolar devices, alternating current is generated between two closely approximated electrodes. This results in a more focused ablation than with unipolar technology. Bipolar RF ablation results in discrete, transmural lesions with no evidence of contraction or scarring. Multiple chronic animal studies have revealed no evidence of thrombus or stricture formation 30 days following ablation when examining the atria, vena cava, and pulmonary veins.[42-45] By microscopic examination, 99%–100% of all lesions were transmural, continuous, and discrete with a single ablation using the conductance algorithm. Lesion width varied depending on tissue depth and the duration of ablation; the measured lesions were typically 2–3 mm

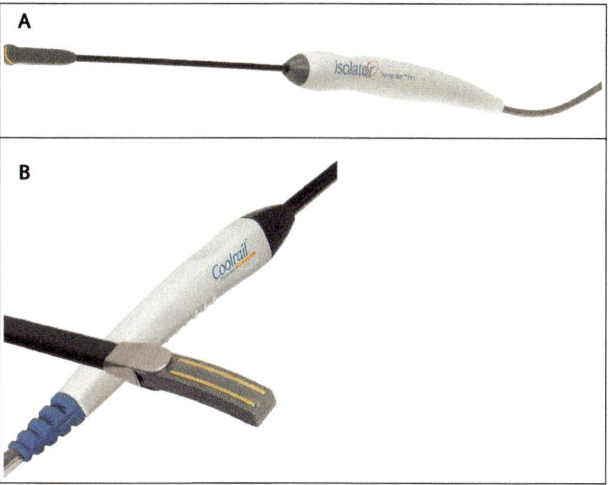

Figure 22.3 **Panel A** shows the AtriCure Isolator™ Multifunctional™ RF Pen. Courtesy of AtriCure. The Coolrail™ Linear Pen is shown in **Panel B**.

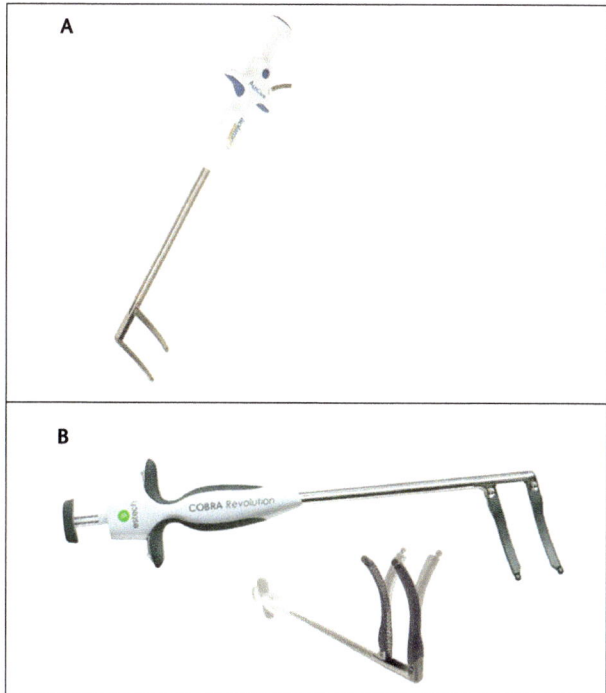

Figure 22.4 **Panel A** shows the AtriCure Isolator Synergy® clamp. Courtesy of AtriCure. **Panel B** is the Estech COBRA Revolution™ bipolar clamp. Courtesy of Estech.

but up to 5 mm in width on the thickest parts of the atrium. These studies and others have suggested that the bipolar technology produces consistent transmural lesions.

Ability to Create Transmural Lesions

Bipolar clamps are the most reliable devices for creating transmural lesions in open procedures. Bipolar RF clamp devices have been shown to be capable of creating transmural lesions without difficulty on the beating heart.[45-47] This has been shown both in animals and in humans with average ablation times between 5 and 10 seconds.[42-44,48] However, it requires that one jaw of the device is introduced into the atrium. Application in humans would have to balance the risk of introducing air into the LA. The AtriCure Isolator™ Multifunctional™ Pen has been shown to be reliable in creating transmural lesion in tissue up to 8 mm in thickness. In studies in our laboratory, the Coolrail™ Linear Pen creates transmural lesions only 80% of the time. All these data are based on a single application of the devices. Multiple applications may improve the performance. However, no animal studies have been done to determine the effects of multiple ablations at a single site. With these devices, most nontransmural lesions occur at the ends of the device. Therefore, it is important to overlap the lesions when making an extended linear lesion to ensure transmurality.

Safety Profile

Use of the bipolar RF clamp devices has eliminated most of the collateral damage that is created with the unipolar devices. The energy is focused between the two electrodes of the device, eliminating the diffuse radiation of heat. However, the devices with side-by-side bipolar electrodes have not been evaluated for safety and would have the same potential problems as unipolar devices. Application of these devices near the AV annulus increases the risk of damaging coronary arteries.

Summary

Bipolar RF ablation has the advantage of focused and discrete lesions that can be made in a fraction of the time of unipolar ablation. Moreover, by using a conductance algorithm, bipolar RF ablation is capable of creating reliable transmural lesions, both on the arrested and beating heart. Because of the focused nature of the energy, there is no chance for collateral injury.

Other Energy Sources

In the past, there have been other devices on the market based on different energy sources. These include microwave, lasers, and high-frequency ultrasound. None of these devices are presently available. Most of these devices failed to produce reliable transmural lesions. Clinical application resulted in high rates of AF recurrence.[49,50]

Conclusion

The development of ablation technology revolutionized the surgical treatment of AF. These ablation devices have taken an operation that was rarely performed and made it accessible to all cardiac surgeons. Whereas 10 years ago few patients with AF who were having cardiac surgery had a concomitant ablation procedure, at the present time, significantly more patients are undergoing AF surgery. However, a review of the Society of Thoracic Surgeons (STS) database has shown that only one-third of patients who could potentially benefit are receiving surgical treatment of their AF. These ablation technologies also have begun to allow for the development of less-invasive procedures and hold the promise of enabling a port-access, beating-heart procedure with high efficacy in the future.

Each ablation technology has its own shortcomings and complications. In the future, it will be imperative to develop a more complete understanding of the effects of surgical ablation technology on atrial hemodynamics, function, and electrophysiology. The safety of ablation depends on an intimate knowledge of the technology being used. Thus, surgeons must develop accurate dose–response curves for all new devices in clinically relevant models on both the arrested and the beating heart. While most of the devices have been shown to be reliable in the arrested heart, few have shown the capability of creating reliable transmural lesions on the beating heart. The effect of this technology on vital structures and on atrial function also must be better delineated. These devices are now being used in hybrid procedures in which a cardiac electrophysiologist records, paces, and ablates from the endocardial surface, closing gaps in nontransmural lesions. Finally, it is essential that these devices be used according to manufacturers' recommendation. For instance, the active electrode surface needs to be cleaned between ablation to remove excess blood. Desiccated blood on the active electrode surface can cause a high resistance, which can alter the energy delivery.

While this new technology has led to progress, the field is still impaired by an inadequate understanding of the mechanisms of AF. In the future, surgeons ideally will be able to design an operation based on the mechanism or substrate responsible for the arrhythmia in each patient and tailor that operation to the specific atrial geometry. In order to develop a truly minimally invasive operation, electrophysiological mapping may be necessary to confirm and guide therapy to allow for a more precise isolation or ablation of specific anatomic or electrophysiologic substrates. Finally, clinical and experimental research on the various different lesion sets that are being tried in the operating room will be essential for continuing progress.

The future presents AF surgeons with many opportunities and challenges. It is certain that the surgical treatment of AF will continue to undergo rapid evolution in the next decade, and much of this progress will be spurred by the use of new ablation technology.

Disclosure: This work was supported by NIH grants R01 HL032257 and R01 HL085113.

References

1. Prasad SM, Maniar HS, Camillo CJ, et al. The Cox-Maze III procedure for atrial fibrillation: long-term efficacy in patients undergoing lone versus concomitant procedures. *J Thorac Cardiovasc Surg.* 2003;126(6):1822-1828.
2. Raanani E, Albage A, David TE, et al. The efficacy of the Cox-Maze procedure combined with mitral valve surgery: a matched control study. *Eur J Cardiothorac Surg.* 2001;19(4):438-442.
3. Doty DB, Dilip KA, Millar RC. Mitral valve replacement with homograft and Maze III procedure. *Ann Thorac Surg.* 2000;69(3):739-742.
4. Schaff HV, Dearani JA, Daly RC, et al. Cox-Maze procedure for atrial fibrillation: Mayo Clinic experience. *Semin Thorac Cardiovasc Surg.* 2000;12(1):30-37.
5. Mitchell MA, McRury ID, Everett TH, et al. Morphological and physiological characteristics of discontinuous linear atrial ablations during atrial pacing and atrial fibrillation. *J Cardiovasc Electrophysiol.* 1999;10(3):378-386.
6. Melby SJ, Lee AM, Schuessler RB, Damiano RJ. The effect of residual gaps in ablation lines for the treatment of atrial fibrillation. *Heart Rhythm.* 2005;2(5):S15.
7. Melby S, Zierer A, Kaiser S, et al. Epicardial microwave ablation on the beating heart for atrial fibrillation: the dependency of lesion depth on cardiac output. *Ann Thorac Surg.* 2006;132:355-360.
8. Schuessler RB, Lee AM, Melby SJ, et al. Animal studies of epicardial atrial ablation. *Heart Rhythm.* 2009;6(12,S1):S41-S45.
9. Platonov PG, Ivanov V, Ho SY, Mitrofanova L. Left atrial posterior wall thickness in patients with and without atrial fibrillation: data from 298 consecutive autopsies. *J Cardiovasc Electrophysiol.* 2008;19(7):689-692.
10. Saremi F, Channual S, Krishnan S, Gurudevan SV, Narula J, Abolhoda A. Bachmann Bundle and its arterial supply: imaging with multidetector CT—implications for interatrial conduction abnormalities and arrhythmias. *Radiology.* 2008;248(2):447-457.
11. Hong KN, Russo MJ, Liberman EA, et al. Effect of epicardial fat on ablation performance: a three-energy source comparison. *J Card Surg.* 2007;22(6):521-524.
12. Pan NH, Tsao HM, Chang NC, Chen YJ, Chen SA. Aging dilates atrium and pulmonary veins: implications for the genesis of atrial fibrillation. *Chest.* 2008;133(1):190-196.
13. Steinbach JP, Weissenberger J, Aguzzi A. Distinct phases of cryogenic tissue damage in the cerebral cortex of wild-type and c-fos deficient mice. *Neuropathol Appl Neurobiol.* 1999;25(6):468-480.
14. Holman WL, Ikeshita M, Douglas JM, Jr., et al. Ventricular cryosurgery: short-term effects on intramural electrophysiology. *Ann Thorac Surg.* 1983;35(4):386-393.
15. Wetstein L, Mark R, Kaplan A, et al. Nonarrhythmogenicity of therapeutic cryothermic lesions of the myocardium. *J Surg Res.* 1985;39(6):543-554.
16. Lustgarten DL, Keane D, Ruskin J. Cryothermal ablation: mechanism of tissue injury and current experience in the treatment of tachyarrhythmias. *Prog Cardiovasc Dis.* 1999;41(6):481-498.
17. Manasse E, Colombo P, Roncalli M, Gallotti R. Myocardial acute and chronic histological modifications induced by cryoablation. *Eur J Cardiothorac Surg.* 2000;17(3):339-340.
18. Hunt GB, Chard RB, Johnson DC, Ross DL. Comparison of early and late dimensions and arrhythmogenicity of cryolesions in the normothermic canine heart. *J Thorac Cardiovasc Surg.* 1989;97(2):313-318.
19. Guiraudon GM, Jones DL, Skanes AC, et al. En bloc exclusion of the pulmonary vein region in the pig using off pump, beating, intra-cardiac surgery: a pilot study of minimally invasive surgery for atrial fibrillation. *Ann Thorac Surg.* 2005;80(4):1417-1423.
20. Doll N, Kornherr P, Aupperle H, et al. Epicardial treatment of atrial fibrillation using cryoablation in an acute off-pump sheep model. *Thorac Cardiovasc Surg.* 2003;51(5):267-273.
21. Milla F, Skubas N, Briggs WM, et al. Epicardial beating heart cryoablation using a novel argon-based cryoclamp and linear probe. *J Thorac Cardiovasc Surg.* 2006;131(2):403-411.
22. Mikat EM, Hackel DB, Harrison L, et al. Reaction of the myocardium and coronary arteries to cryosurgery. *Lab Invest.* 1977;37(6):632-641.
23. Holman WL, Ikeshita M, Ungerleider RM, et al. Cryosurgery for cardiac arrhythmias: acute and chronic effects on coronary arteries. *Am J Cardiol.* 1983;51(1):149-155.
24. Watanabe H, Hayashi J, Aizawa Y. Myocardial infarction after cryoablation surgery for Wolff–Parkinson–White syndrome. *Jpn J Thorac Cardiovasc Surg.* 2002;50(5):210-212.
25. Aupperle H, Doll N, Walther T, et al. Ablation of atrial fibrillation and esophageal injury: effects of energy source and ablation technique. *J Thorac Cardiovasc Surg.* 2005;130(6):1549-1554.
26. Mack CA, Milla F, Ko W, et al. Surgical treatment of atrial fibrillation using argon-based cryoablation during concomitant cardiac procedures. *Circulation.* 2005;112(9 Suppl):I1-I6.
27. Doll N, Kiaii BB, Fabricius AM, et al. Intraoperative left atrial ablation (for atrial fibrillation) using a new argon cryocatheter: early clinical experience. *Ann Thorac Surg.* 2003;76(5):1711-1715; discussion 1715.
28. Ad N, Henry L, Hunt S. The concomitant cryosurgical Cox-Maze procedure using Argon based cryoprobes: 12 month results. *J Cardiovasc Surg (Torino).* 2011;52(4):593-599.
29. Kim JB, Cho WC, Jung SH, Chung CH, Choo SJ, Lee JW. Alternative energy sources for surgical treatment of atrial fibrillation in patients undergoing mitral valve surgery: microwave ablation vs cryoablation. *J Korean Med Sci.* 2010;25(10):1467-1472.
30. Viola N, Williams MR, Oz MC, Ad N. The technology in use for the surgical ablation of atrial fibrillation. *Semin Thorac Cardiovasc Surg.* 2002;14(3):198-205.
31. Khargi K, Deneke T, Haardt H, et al. Saline-irrigated, cooled-tip radiofrequency ablation is an effective technique to perform the Maze procedure. *Ann Thorac Surg.* 2001;72(3):S1090-1095.
32. Nakagawa H, Wittkampf FH, Yamanashi WS, et al. Inverse relationship between electrode size and lesion size during radiofrequency ablation with active electrode cooling. *Circulation.* 1998;98(5):458-465.

33. Kress DC, Krum D, Chekanov V, et al. Validation of a left atrial lesion pattern for intraoperative ablation of atrial fibrillation. *Ann Thorac Surg.* 2002;73(4):1160-1168.
34. Santiago T, Melo JQ, Gouveia RH, Martins AP. Intra-atrial temperatures in radiofrequency endocardial ablation: histologic evaluation of lesions. *Ann Thoracic Surg.* 2003;75(5):1495.
35. Thomas SP, Guy DJ, Boyd AC, et al. Comparison of epicardial and endocardial linear ablation using handheld probes. *Ann Thorac Surg.* 2003;75(2):543-548.
36. Bugge E, Nicholson IA, Thomas SP. Comparison of bipolar and unipolar radiofrequency ablation in an in vivo experimental model. *Eur J Cardiothorac Surg.* 2005;28(1):76-80; discussion 80-82.
37. Santiago T, Melo J, Gouveia RH, et al. Epicardial radiofrequency applications: in vitro and in vivo studies on human atrial myocardium. *Eur J Cardiothorac Surg.* 2003;24(4):481-486; discussion 486.
38. Kottkamp H, Hindricks G, Autschbach R, et al. Specific linear left atrial lesions in atrial fibrillation: intraoperative radiofrequency ablation using minimally invasive surgical techniques. *J Am Coll Cardiol.* 2002;40(3):475-480.
39. Gillinov AM, Pettersson G, Rice TW. Esophageal injury during radiofrequency ablation for atrial fibrillation. *J Thorac Cardiovasc Surg.* 2001;122(6):1239-1240.
40. Laczkovics A, Khargi K, Deneke T. Esophageal perforation during left atrial radiofrequency ablation. *J Thorac Cardiovasc Surg.* 2003;126(6):2119-2120; author reply 2120.
41. Demaria RG, Page P, Leung TK, et al. Surgical radiofrequency ablation induces coronary endothelial dysfunction in porcine coronary arteries. *Eur J Cardiothorac Surg.* 2003;23(3):277-282.
42. Prasad SM, Maniar HS, Schuessler RB, Damiano RJ Jr. Chronic transmural atrial ablation by using bipolar radiofrequency energy on the beating heart. *J Thorac Cardiovasc Surg.* 2002;124(4):708-713.
43. Prasad SM, Maniar HS, Diodato MD, et al. Physiological consequences of bipolar radiofrequency energy on the atria and pulmonary veins: a chronic animal study. *Ann Thorac Surg.* 2003;76(3):836-841; discussion 841-842.
44. Gaynor SL, Ishii Y, Diodato MD, et al. Successful performance of Cox-Maze procedure on beating heart using bipolar radiofrequency ablation: a feasibility study in animals. *Ann Thorac Surg.* 2004;78(5):1671-1677.
45. Melby SJ, Gaynor SL, Lubahn JG, et al. Efficacy and safety of right and left atrial ablations on the beating heart with irrigated bipolar radiofrequency energy: a long-term animal study. *J Thorac Cardiovasc Surg.* 2006;132(4):853-860.
46. Vigilance DW, Garrido M, Williams M, et al. Off-pump epicardial atrial fibrillation surgery utilizing a novel bipolar radiofrequency system. *Heart Surg Forum.* 2006;9(5): E803-E806.
47. Voeller RK, Zierer A, Lall SC, Sakamoto S, Schuessler RB, Damiano RJ Jr. Efficacy of a novel bipolar radiofrequency ablation device on the beating heart for atrial fibrillation ablation: a long-term porcine study. *J Thorac Cardiovasc Surg.* 2010; 140(1):203-208.
48. Gaynor SL, Diodato MD, Prasad SM, et al. A prospective, single-center clinical trial of a modified Cox-Maze procedure with bipolar radiofrequency ablation. *J Thorac Cardiovasc Surg.* 2004;128(4):535-542.
49. Klinkenberg TJ, Ahmed S, Ten Hagen A, Wiesfeld AC, Tan ES, Zijlstra F, Van Gelder IC. Feasibility and outcome of epicardial pulmonary vein isolation for lone atrial fibrillation using minimal invasivesurgery and high intensity focused ultrasound. *Europace.* 2009;11(12):1624-1631.
50. Mitnovetski S, Almeida AA, Goldstein J, Pick AW, Smith JA. Epicardial high-intensity focused ultrasound cardiac ablation for surgical treatment of atrial fibrillation. *Heart Lung Circ.* 2009;18(1):28-31.

CHAPTER 23

Remote Navigation in Catheter Procedures

J. David Burkhardt, MD; Luigi Di Biase, MD, PhD; Andrea Natale, MD

Introduction

Remote navigation describes the ability to manipulate catheters from a location other than the patient's bedside. Traditionally, ablation catheters are manipulated directly at the groin of the patient when introduced through the femoral vessels. The catheter tip is guided through the chamber of interest by a combination of movements from the handle of the catheter. Completely encountering the walls of a chamber requires combinations of advance and retract, rotate and counter-rotate, and flexion and extension. Flexion of the catheter is usually performed by pull wires, which are controlled by a plunger-type mechanism. To reach a desired location, any combination of all three movements or multiple such combinations may be required. These movements are guided by fluoroscopy and electro-atomic mapping (EAM) systems. Obviously, using such complex combinations of movements requires significant dexterity, and many procedures are required to master complex ablation techniques. In addition, each of the cardiac chambers and the pericardial space are geometrically unique; the skills used for navigation in one chamber are not necessarily transferable to another chamber. In addition, the requirement that operators stand beside the fluoroscopy table exposes them to potentially harmful radiation, which is compounded by the long fluoroscopy times that many complex ablation procedures may require.

Remote navigation has been developed to attempt to reduce some of the challenges associated with manual navigation. The goals of remote navigation include making procedures less technically demanding and reducing the need for manual dexterity. Also, automation might be built into these technologies, allowing for more uniform procedures. By definition, remote navigation removes the operator from the bedside, reducing the radiation exposure to the operator. Additional benefits include potentially reducing operator fatigue, pain, and stress associated with long periods of standing while wearing leaded vests and aprons.

Currently in the United States, two types of remote navigation technologies are available: remote robotic navigation and remote magnetic navigation. Another robotic navigation device was recently approved in Europe. This robotic system manipulates standard catheter handles via preformed inserts. This allows manual type navigation from a remote location.

Remote navigation continues to mature in interventional cardiac electrophysiology. At one time, it was seen only as a toy without any meaningful clinical data to support its use; more recently, however, remote navigation has proven to be useful in ablation of simple and complex arrhythmias. Remote navigation has published results in supraventricular arrhythmias, atrial fibrillation (AF), ventricular tachycardia (VT), and epicardial procedures.

Remote Robotic Navigation

Remote robotic navigation uses a mechanical sheath that is controlled by a robotic arm to manipulate standard catheters (Hansen Medical, Mountain View, CA). The robotic sheath contains pull wires that allow the sheath itself to tightly flex. An outer sheath provides support and can also be flexed to allow a secondary curve. The robotic arm allows the inner and outer sheaths to be advanced or retracted and rotated. The entire system is controlled from a remote workstation. This uses an intuitive joystick-type device and computer console to control the movements of the sheath. The joystick is used in reference to some imaging modality such as fluoroscopy, intercardiac echocardiography (ICE), or an EAM system. If the reference image is in an anterior-posterior plane, pushing forward on the joystick advances the sheath system to the posterior of the chamber, and moving the joystick to the left moves the system to the left of the reference, and so forth. Currently, the robotic system offers integration with an EAM system (EnSite NavX, St. Jude Medical, St. Paul, MN) that allows the navigation of the robotic system from the 3D map and in any x, y, z configuration (Figure 23.1).

Other than remote navigation, the advantages of the remote robotic system include the ability to use most available radiofrequency ablation (RFA) catheters, intuitive navigation, and potentially higher stable contact forces. The inner sheath system determines the limitation of catheters that can be used with this system. In general, any ablation catheter up to 8.5 Fr in size can be used with the robotic sheaths. This size accommodates most RFA catheters but would not allow many cryoablation catheters or balloon-based ablation systems.

After set up and positioning of the system, navigation is very easy. No complex software programs or multiple mechanical devices are needed for use. The joystick control makes movement of the sheaths intuitive. Essentially, no learning curve is present for navigation alone. A person may sit down and immediately understand how the system operates. The operator sits at a control station that includes a computer console for input of data and programming of basic parameters such as response speed. Buttons allow for the movement of the outer sheath, and the joystick is positioned in the center. Three monitors are present that can display electrograms (EGMs), fluoroscopy, ICE, or the EAM system. The input to the monitors may be changed and the navigation reference may also be changed.[1,2]

Contact forces with robotic navigation appear to be higher than the average contact forces for manual ablation. This is likely due to the relative stiffness of the steel sheaths and the inability to use the flexible portion of the ablation catheter. These higher forces may improve ablation lesions but also may increase the risk of perforation.[3] Initial studies appear to show an increased rate of perforation, which may be related to these higher forces, suggesting that lower ablation power settings may be prudent.[4] A pressure sensor is available with the system that displays a numerical and graphic force indicator on the user interface. Unfortunately, this measurement appears to be inaccurate when the sheath system is not in a straight position. The development of pressure-sensing catheters may make the force sensing of the system obsolete.

The limitations of the system include the large size of the outer sheath and limited navigation outside of the left atrium. The outer sheath requires a 14-Fr introducer sheath. This is typically placed in the left femoral vein due to the proximity of the robotic arm. Initial use of the system was associated with higher rates of bleeding complications due to the size and stiffness of the sheaths. The rates of this complication waned over time with experience and with the recommendation of using a longer introducer sheath.[5]

Navigation within the left atrium is generally very easy. If the outer sheath is well seated against the septum, most positions in the left atrium are easily accessible. Unfortunately, some patients' anatomy does not allow for

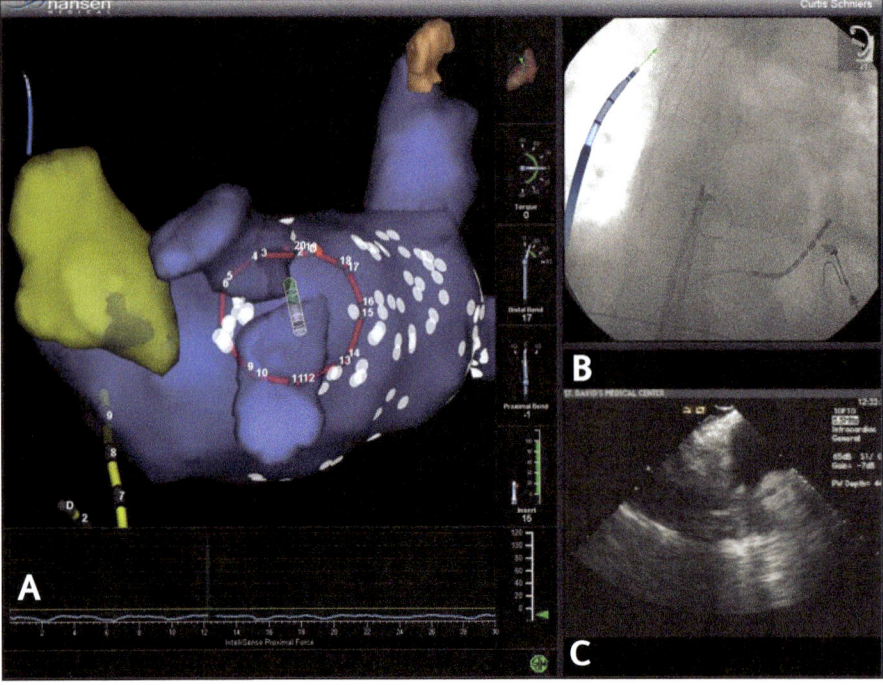

Figure 23.1 **Panel A:** Screenshot of the remote robotic navigation user interface displaying an electro-anatomic map on the left, which serves as the reference for navigation. **Panel B:** On the right side of the map screen, images portray the robotic sheath torque angle, distal and proximal bend, as well as the length of inner sheath inserted. **Panel C:** On the bottom of this screen a graphic display of contact force is shown. The upper right-hand screen displays the fluoroscopy with the circular catheter and robotic sheath in the left atrium. A virtual catheter is projected on the fluoroscopic image to show the relative curve and anterior/posterior position. The ICE image is in the lower right corner.

the outer sheath and septum to serve as a good torque point. This makes navigation analogous to manual navigation with a sheath floating in the right atrium. Also, since there is no torque point in the right atrium, navigation in the right atrium and cavotricuspid isthmus (CTI) ablation appear more difficult than left atrial navigation. The size and design of the outer sheath prohibits ablation using a retrograde aortic approach, and the reach of the inner sheath limits right and left ventricular ablation.

The majority of published experience focuses on AF ablation, although limited studies show feasibility in right ventricular outflow tract (RVOT) tachycardia and atrial flutter (AFL).[6,7] A study of the initial experience in AF ablation showed higher complication rates, including vascular access complications and cardiac perforation compared to manual ablation. Reducing ablation power, time at each ablation site, and operator experience appeared to reduce the incidence of these complications.[5] Success rates appear to mirror success rates with manual ablation. One study of 390 patients, 193 of which underwent ablation using the remote robotic system, reported a success rate of 85%. In this study of more experienced operators, complication rates were similar to manual ablation, while radiation exposure to the patient and operator were significantly reduced.[8]

The near-term future developments of remote robotic navigation are expected to address some of the limitations of the system. A robotic sheath with an extended reach may permit the system to be used for VT ablation and left ventricular mapping. Also, a proprietary ablation catheter is being developed that would allow the robotic sheaths to be downsized from its current diameter.

Remote Magnetic Navigation

Unlike robotic navigation, which uses stainless-steel, flexible sheaths to direct the shaft of an ablation catheter, remote magnetic navigation uses specially designed magnetic-tipped catheters that can be manipulated in a magnetic field. This allows the catheter tip itself to be directed. This differs from manual catheters that rely on pull wires and rotation of the shaft controlled from three feet away from the tip to direct the shaft. The magnetic ablation catheters have no pull wires and rely entirely on magnetic field changes to direct the tip in the x, y, and z axes.

The magnetic field is generated by two large, composite rare earth magnets, which are present in a housing that can be rotated to the sides of the patient. Inside this housing, the magnets are attached to a motorized system that allows them to advance, retract, rotate, and tilt (Figure 23.2). The interaction between the two large magnets creates a composite magnetic field inside the chest of the patient. The magnetic tip of the catheter aligns with this field, which can be directed in any axis. The advancing and retracting mechanism of the catheter is controlled by a separate motorized system that can be controlled by a joystick, mouse, or keyboard controls.

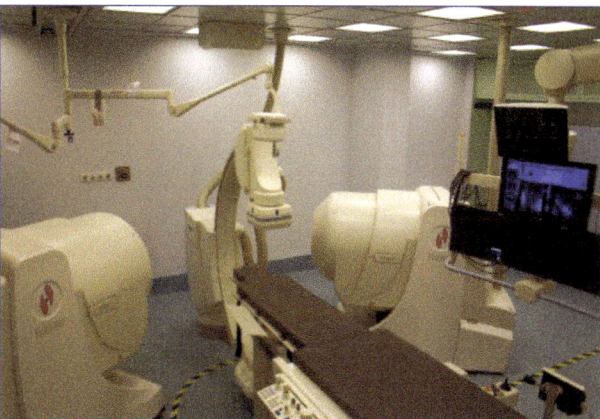

Figure 23.2 Picture showing the remote magnetic navigation system including the housing for the two large composite magnets in a semi-stowed position. The housing allows the magnets to be stored during procedures that do not require magnetic navigation.

Currently, the maximum magnetic field strength is 0.1 Tesla, significantly lower than even low-powered MRI field strengths, which are in order of 1–3 Tesla. The field strength depends on the ability to bring the magnets close to the patient. The maximum field strength may not be possible in large patients; however, most patients can achieve a field strength of 0.08 Tesla.

In addition to the magnets, catheter advancing system, and joystick, the system is computer controlled. The interactive screen can display the direction of the magnetic field in relation to a particular axis, an idealized model, displayed on a fluoroscopy screen, or on a generated EAM. The operator directs the vector, which represents the composite magnetic field, to the area of interest and magnets automatically produce this field. The catheter aligns in this field and is advanced or retracted as necessary. The magnetic navigation system is intimately linked to the Carto EAM system (Biosense Webster, Diamond Bar, CA). The systems share location information with each other, making it possible to navigate from the EAM. One can direct the catheter to a location on the map by clicking on the map itself (Figure 23.3). With this technology, it has also been possible to introduce automation. The system can reconstruct left atrial, right atrial, and RVOT anatomy without input from the operator other than starting the automation. It is also possible to direct a line of ablation automatically. Although not perfect, enhancements in automation are being developed.

Advantages of Magnetic Systems

Other than remote navigation, advantages include the ability to use the system for any cardiac chamber or even epicardially, ability to use flexible catheters, and potential

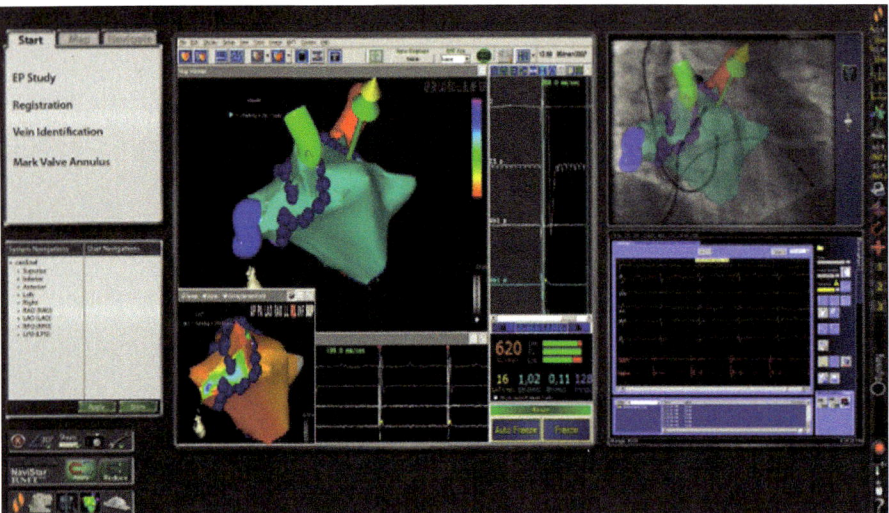

Figure 23.3 Screenshot of the remote magnetic navigation system control interface. On the left side are the system control functions. In the center, the EAM system map is displayed with the magnetic field being shown as an arrow vector. The arrow can be moved to change the magnetic field direction. On the upper right, a fluoroscopic image is displayed with the electro-anatomic map overlying the heart. On the lower right is the EGM screen.

safety. Since the magnetic system directs the tip of the catheter and does not have a major limitation on extension, it may be used in any cardiac chamber. It can navigate the entirety of the right and left atria as well as both ventricles and epicardial surface. Since it does not require specific sheaths and has the size of standard catheters, it may also be used with any approach, including retrograde aortic, transseptal, and percutaneous epicardial. Although unusual, the floppy nature of the catheter also allows its use from the internal jugular or subclavian veins with few difficulties in navigation, unlike manual catheters.[9]

Since the catheters are directed via the magnet in the tip of the catheter, the shaft does not require pull wires or have stiff characteristics. The magnetic catheters are soft and floppy, which permits the catheter to be directed in ways that manual catheters can not. They do not have a limitation on reach and can perform multiple bends to traverse tortuous anatomy. The maximum contact forces tend to be lower with magnetic catheters. In general, magnetic catheters operate at approximately 10 g of force compared to maximum forces of more than 40 g with manual catheters. Unlike manual catheters, there appears to be less variability in contact force with magnetic catheters and more constant contact. Manual catheters may actually lose contact during a cardiac cycle. Unfortunately, with solid-tipped catheters, this constant contact appears to increase the incidence of char formation. Possibly due to the constant contact, the resulting lesions from magnetic catheters tend to be larger at lower forces; however, the lesions are not as deep as the lesions that are possible with manual catheters at very high pressures.[10]

Pressure is an important factor in ablation-related steam pops and perforation; because magnetic catheters exert less force, steam pops and perforation appear to be less frequent with the magnetic system. Even initial studies with the system show a very good safety record.[11]

Limitations of Magnetic Systems

The limitations of the system include reliance on specialized catheters, requirement for specialized fluoroscopy and shielding, and size of the room required. Specialized magnetic catheters are required for use with magnetic navigation. If one prefers a particular catheter type or ablation technology, it cannot be used unless it is magnetically enabled. This is a significant limitation because most of the currently approved ablation catheters are nonmagnetic catheters. In general, the ablation technology for the magnetic system lags the standard ablation catheters. For example, an open irrigated-tip magnetic catheter was only available several years after the manual version was available. Also, due to the relatively weak magnetic field, developing technologies such as balloon-based ablation systems for magnetic use may be difficult or require large magnets for navigation.

Another major limitation is the need for a specialized room and fluoroscopy. Since the magnets are permanent, the room must be magnetically shielded and may not be near an MRI system. The magnetic housing is also large, and in general will not fit in standard EP laboratories that are being refurbished. The system is best placed in newly constructed rooms or rooms that can be enlarged into nearby space. The weight of the system also requires certain structural qualities to be present in the floor of the room(s) where it is installed.

Since x-rays are affected by magnetic fields, the system requires specially constructed fluoroscopy systems. This means that the magnetic navigation system cannot be put into existing laboratories without also replacing the fluoroscopy system. Currently, the plate size of the fluoroscopy is limited to smaller sizes due to the limitation of lateral rotation of the image intensifier by the location of the magnetic housing. Fortunately, the magnets can be stowed away from the patient, which allows the room to be used for nonmagnetic procedures, including device implants.

Use of Magnetic Systems in Treating Arrhythmias

The published experience using the magnetic navigation system is more robust. Authors have reported utilizing the system in nearly all arrhythmias, from the most simple to the most complex, including epicardial mapping and ablation. Several reports have shown utility in supraventricular tachycardia (SVTs) and potential safety in pediatric populations.[12-14] It has even been shown to be useful in arrhythmias where manual navigation would be very difficult if not impossible, including AF ablation via a retrograde aortic approach and in cases of venous anomalies.[14-16] One difficult area is in ablating typical AFL. Although some authors report high success rates, others report lower success rates and longer procedure times.[17,18]

Atrial Fibrillation

AF ablation is one of the most frequent reasons the system is utilized. Initial experience of magnetic navigation in AF ablation was particularly mixed. This appeared to be because the only catheters originally available were solid-tipped catheters. Katsiyannis reported good success rates in 20 patients while using 4-mm solid-tipped catheters, but a larger study reported that venous isolation with the catheter confirmed by circular mapping catheter was very difficult, and because of this success rates were very poor.[19] In this study, char formation was seen in nearly one-third of the cases.[20] As stated, the constant contact of the magnetic catheter with the wall of the heart may prevent the washing of the tip that occurs with loss of contact. Since the introduction of the irrigated-tip magnetic ablation catheter is relatively recent, there are limited published data on success rates using this catheter.

Ventricular Tachycardia

VT ablation can be difficult and frustrating. One area that magnetic navigation appears to shine is in the mapping and ablation of VT. Particularly, in ischemic VT, where high density maps are required, the magnetic navigation system seems to perform this mapping with less fluoroscopy and less intervening catheter induced premature beats. This combined with the improved comfort of the operator during these long cases makes the system ideal for such arrhythmias.[21]

Publications about outflow tract ventricular arrhythmias report high success rates and low complication rates. Even with the 4-mm solid-tipped ablation catheter, RVOT tachycardia success rates are greater than 80%. When using a 4-mm solid-tipped catheter, the success rates for non-outflow tract ventricular arrhythmias was dismal, but this was improved with an 8-mm solid-tipped catheter. Although the success rates were low with the 4-mm catheter, the authors reported that it enhanced the mapping portion of the procedure and ablation was carried out with a manual irrigated tip catheter.[22]

A more recent report describes the use of the irrigated-tipped magnetic catheter in ventricular arrhythmia ablation. In this case control series, 110 patients underwent mapping and ablation using this catheter, and 33% of the patients underwent epicardial mapping in addition. Thirty percent of these patients had ischemic cardiomyopathy, and 13% had NICM. Although procedure time and ablation time were longer, success rates were outstanding and compared well with manual navigation and ablation in this difficult population.[23]

Future developments in remote magnetic navigation include the introduction of a complementary robotic system to manipulate nonmagnetic catheters and allow nearly completely remote procedures and further refinement of automation. To overcome the limitation of needing another individual to move nonmagnetic catheters, a robotic system is being developed to move catheters such as a circular mapping catheter and ICE catheter. This may also be automated and allow the operator to perform complex movements of several catheters remotely. Also, the system continues to refine the automation algorithm to reduce mapping errors and improve accuracy.

Robotic Catheter Manipulation

Recently, a new robotic system that controls standard catheters using formed molds placed into a robotic controller was approved in Europe (Catheter Robotics, Budd Lake, NJ). This system has the ability to take standard catheters and manipulate in a similar mechanical manner from a remote location, without the need of a new interface. This has both potential benefits and limitations. Since the operation is familiar, the learning curve should be short. Unfortunately, since standard catheters are used, all of the limitations of standard catheters are still present. Also, the loss of tactile feedback could be a limitation.

Sparse data is available on this system. One published study described the feasibility of catheter manipulation in dogs. It reported that the system could adequately position catheters at desired locations and perform pacing. Further study will be needed to fully quantify the role of this system in ablation.[24]

Conclusion

Remote navigation has matured over the last several years. The concept of performing procedures remotely is very enticing. This would potentially allow the operator to extend his or her professional career by reducing the mechanical strain of long periods of standing with heavy lead aprons as well as lowering cumulative x-ray exposure in a field with long cases using fluoroscopy. Hopefully, the advances in technology will also improve the safety and efficacy of these procedures. In the future, these technologies may allow EP procedures to be performed in very remote locations by expert operators, expanding the availability of complex arrhythmia treatment.

References

1. Reddy VY, Neuzil P, Malchano ZJ, Vijaykumar R, Cury R, Abbara S, Weichet J, McPherson CD, Ruskin JN. View-synchronized robotic image-guided therapy for atrial fibrillation ablation: experimental validation and clinical feasibility. *Circulation.* 2007;115:2705-2714.
2. Saliba W, Cummings JE, Oh S, Zhang Y, Mazgalev TN, Schweikert RA, Burkhardt JD, Natale A. Novel robotic catheter remote control system: feasibility and safety of transseptal puncture and endocardial catheter navigation. *J Cardiovasc Electrophysiol.* 2006;17:1102-1105.
3. Di Biase L, Natale A, Barrett C, Tan C, Elayi CS, Ching CK, et al. Relationship between catheter forces, lesion characteristics, "popping," and char formation: experience with robotic navigation system. *J Cardiovasc Electrophysiol.* 2009;20:436-440.
4. Saliba W, Reddy VY, Wazni O, Cummings JE, Burkhardt JD, Haissaguerre M, et al. Atrial fibrillation ablation using a robotic catheter remote control system: initial human experience and long-term follow-up results. *J Am Coll Cardiol.* 2008;51:2407-2411.
5. Wazni OM, Barrett C, Martin DO, Shaheen M, Tarakji K, Baranowski B, et al. Experience with the hansen robotic system for atrial fibrillation ablation—lessons learned and techniques modified: Hansen in the real world. *J Cardiovasc Electrophysiol.* 2009;20:1193-1196.
6. Koa-Wing M, Linton NW, Kojodjojo P, O'Neill MD, Peters NS, Wyn Davies D, Kanagaratnam P. Robotic catheter ablation of ventricular tachycardia in a patient with congenital heart disease and Rastelli repair. *J Cardiovasc Electrophysiol.* 2009;20:1163-1166.
7. Steven D, Rostock T, Servatius H, Hoffmann B, Drewitz I, Mullerleile K, Meinertz T, Willems S. Robotic versus conventional ablation for common-type atrial flutter: a prospective randomized trial to evaluate the effectiveness of remote catheter navigation. *Heart Rhythm.* 2008;5:1556-1560.
8. Di Biase L, Wang Y, Horton R, Gallinghouse GJ, Mohanty P, Sanchez J, et al. Ablation of atrial fibrillation utilizing robotic catheter navigation in comparison to manual navigation and ablation: single-center experience. *J Cardiovasc Electrophysiol.* 2009;20:1328-1335.
9. Ernst S. Magnetic and robotic navigation for catheter ablation: "joystick ablation." *J Interv Card Electrophysiol.* 2008;23:41-44.
10. Burkhardt JD, Natale A. New technologies in atrial fibrillation ablation. *Circulation.* 2009;120:1533-1541.
11. Chun JK, Ernst S, Matthews S, Schmidt B, Bansch D, Boczor S, Ujeyl A, Antz M, Ouyang F, Kuck KH. Remote-controlled catheter ablation of accessory pathways: results from the magnetic laboratory. *Eur Heart J.* 2007;28:190-195.
12. Ricard P, Latcu DG, Yaici K, Zarqane N, Saoudi N. Slow pathway radiofrequency ablation in patients with AVNRT: junctional rhythm is less frequent during magnetic navigation ablation than with the conventional technique. *Pacing Clin Electrophysiol.* 2010;33:11-15.
13. Schwagten B, Jordaens L, Witsenburg M, Duplessis F, Thornton A, van Belle Y, Szili-Torok T. Initial experience with catheter ablation using remote magnetic navigation in adults with complex congenital heart disease and in small children. *Pacing Clin Electrophysiol.* 2009;32Suppl 1:S198-201.
14. Ernst S, Chun JK, Koektuerk B, Kuck KH. Magnetic navigation and catheter ablation of right atrial ectopic tachycardia in the presence of a hemi-azygos continuation: a magnetic navigation case using 3D electroanatomical mapping. *J Cardiovasc Electrophysiol.* 2009;20:99-102.
15. Miyazaki S, Nault I, Haissaguerre M, Hocini M. Atrial fibrillation ablation by aortic retrograde approach using a magnetic navigation system. *J Cardiovasc Electrophysiol.* 2010;21:455-457.
16. Chun JK, Schmidt B, Kuck KH, Ernst S. Remote-controlled magnetic ablation of a right anterolateral accessory pathway—the superior caval vein approach. *J Interv Card Electrophysiol.* 2006;16:65-68.
17. Arya A, Kottkamp H, Piorkowski C, Bollmann A, Gerdes-Li JH, Riahi S, Esato M, Hindricks G. Initial clinical experience with a remote magnetic catheter navigation system for ablation of cavotricuspid isthmus-dependent right atrial flutter. *Pacing Clin Electrophysiol.* 2008;31:597-603.
18. Vollmann D, Luthje L, Seegers J, Hasenfuss G, Zabel M. Remote magnetic catheter navigation for cavotricuspid isthmus ablation in patients with common-type atrial flutter. *Circ Arrhythm Electrophysiol.* 2009;2:603-610.
19. Katsiyiannis WT, Melby DP, Matelski JL, Ervin VL, Laverence KL, Gornick CC. Feasibility and safety of remote-controlled magnetic navigation for ablation of atrial fibrillation. *Am J Cardiol.* 2008;102:1674-1676.
20. Di Biase L, Fahmy TS, Patel D, Bai R, Civello K, Wazni OM, et al. Remote magnetic navigation: human experience in pulmonary vein ablation. *J Am Coll Cardiol.* 2007; 50:868-874.
21. Burkhardt JD, Saliba WI, Schweikert RA, Cummings J, Natale A. Remote magnetic navigation to map and ablate left coronary cusp ventricular tachycardia. *J Cardiovasc Electrophysiol.* 2006;17:1142-1144.
22. Di Biase L, Burkhardt JD, Lakkireddy D, Pillarisetti J, Baryun EN, Biria M, et al. Mapping and ablation of ventricular arrhythmias with magnetic navigation: comparison between 4- and 8-mm catheter tips. *J Interv Card Electrophysiol.* 2009;26:133-137.
23. Di Biase L, Santangeli P, Astudillo V, Conti S, Mohanty P, Mohanty M, et al. Endo-epicardial ablation of ventricular arrhythmias in the left ventricle with the Remote Magnetic Navigation System and the 3.5-mm open irrigated magnetic catheter: results from a large single center case-control series. *Heart Rhythm.* 2010 Aug;7(8):1029-3
24. Knight B, Ayers GM, Cohen TJ. Robotic positioning of standard electrophysiology catheters: a novel approach to catheter robotics. *J Invasive Cardiol.* 2008;20:250-253.

SECTION 1E

TECHNOLOGY AND THERAPEUTIC TECHNIQUES

Drug Therapy

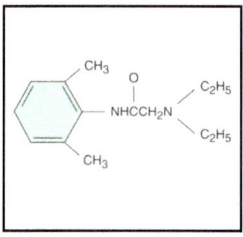 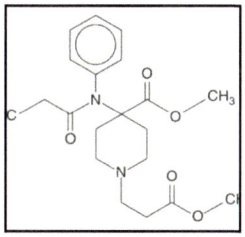 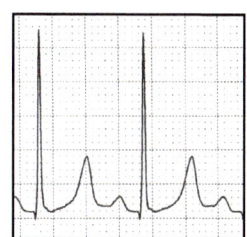 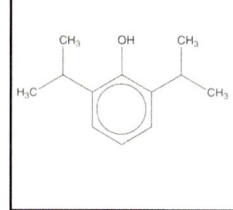

CHAPTER 24

How to Perform Drug Testing and Use Antiarrhythmic Drugs in Clinical Electrophysiology

Manoj N. Obeyesekere, MBBS; Peter Leong-Sit, MD;
Lorne J. Gula, MD, MSc; Raymond Yee, MD; Allan C. Skanes, MD;
George J. Klein, MD; Andrew D. Krahn, MD

Introduction

Historically, EP study was used to analyze the effects of antiarrhythmic drugs to select drug therapy. The evolution of effective nonpharmacological approaches to the management of VT and SVT, along with the ability to successfully use empirical antiarrhythmic drugs, has largely relegated the EP study-guided drug therapy to historical interest. Nonetheless, drugs remain a very useful adjunct for arrhythmia diagnosis in multiple contexts (eg, to unmask concealed arrhythmia substrates, to increase vulnerability to arrhythmia during EP study, for assessment of conduction in bradycardia, and following ablation).

Drug Testing in Channelopathies

Structural heart disease accounts for 90% to 95% of causes of sudden cardiac death.[1] The arrhythmogenic substrates for sudden cardiac death continue to be defined with identified channelopathies partially contributing to sudden cardiac death. Brugada syndrome, long QT syndrome (LQTS), and catecholaminergic polymorphic ventricular tachycardia (CPVT) are the most common inherited arrhythmogenic diseases predisposing to sudden cardiac death. Identification of patients requires a high level of suspicion due to the absence of structural cardiac abnormalities. Provocative testing (pharmacological and/or exercise testing) is often required due to the concealed nature of the disease.

Long QT Syndrome

LQTS is a group of genetically transmitted disorders marked by QT prolongation. It affects 1 to 2 in 5,000 individuals. LQTS patients are at increased risk of developing torsades de pointes. Episodes of torsades de pointes may present as syncope, seizures, cardiac arrest, or sudden death.[2,3] Certain triggers such as intense adrenergic or auditory stimulation appear particularly arrhythmogenic in LQTS. Swimming has been shown to trigger symptoms in nearly 15% of children and young adults with LQT1 associated with mutations in *KCNQ1*.[4] Numerous LQTS causing mutations have been identified (Table 24.1), summarized at http://www.fsm.it/cardmoc. LQT1, LQT2, and LQT3 genotypes account for an estimated 85% to 95% of LQTS.[5]

Table 24.1 Channelopathies and associated proteins and channels

Disease	Gene	Protein	Dysfunction	Frequency
LQT1	KCNQ1	Kv7.1	Loss of I_{Ks} function	~45%
LQT2	KCNH2	Kv11.1	Loss of I_{Kr} function	~30%
LQT3	SCN5A	Nav1.5	Gain of I_{Na} function	~10%
LQT4	ANK2	Ankyrin-B	Loss of $I_{Na,K}$ function	~1%
LQT5	KCNE1	Mink	Loss of I_{Ks} function	~1%
LQT6	KCNE2	MiRP1	Loss of I_{Kr} function	rare
LQT7	KCNJ2	Kir2.1	Loss I_{K1} function	rare
LQT8	CACNA1C	Cav1.2	Gain $I_{Ca,L}$ function	rare
LQT9	CAV3	Caveolin-3	Gain of I_{Na} function	rare
LQT10	SCN4B	Beta4	Gain of I_{Na} function	rare
LQT11	AKAP9	Yotiao	Loss of I_{Ks} function	rare
LQT12	SNTA1	Alpha 1 syntrophin	Gain of I_{Na} function	rare
Brugada	SCN5A	Na channel	I_{Na} loss of function	10%–30%
Brugada	GPD1-L	GPD1-L	I_{Na} loss of function	Rare
Brugada	SCN1B	β1-subunit Na channel	I_{Na} loss of function	< 1%
Brugada	SCN3B	β3-subunit Na channel	I_{Na} loss of function	< 1%
Brugada	KCNE3	β-subunit I_{to} fast	I_{to} gain of function	< 1%
Brugada	CACNA1C	α-subunit Ca channel	$I_{Ca,L}$ loss of function	< 7%
Brugada	CACNB2	β-subunit Ca channel	$I_{Ca,L}$ loss of function	< 7%
CPVT	RyR2	Ryanodine receptor	Gain of function	55%–60%
CPVT	CASQ2	Calsequestrin	Loss of function	~2%–3%
CPVT	ANK2	Ankyrin-B	Adaptor protein	rare

The longest QT intervals are generally measured in the precordial leads. The standard leads to measure the QT are V_5 and lead II. U waves should not be included in measurement. The QT interval should be measured as the time interval from the beginning of the QRS complex to the end of the T wave. The end of the T wave is defined as the intersection point between the isoelectric baseline and the tangent line representing the maximal downward or upward slope of a positive or negative T wave, respectively. In addition to measuring an absolute QT interval, a rate-corrected QT (QTc) interval should also be calculated—Bazett's formula (QT divided by the square root of the RR interval) remains widely used.[6] Intervals of 440–460 ms in men and 460–480 ms in women are considered borderline. QT and QTc measurement during AF should be averaged over 10 consecutive beats. Patients with LQT1 classically have a broad-based T wave and tend to have syncope or sudden death during physical exercise. Patients with LQT2 tend to have a notched or low-amplitude T wave, and they classically have syncope or sudden death with sudden auditory stimuli or strong emotion. Patients with LQT3 have a long, flat ST segment, a tendency toward sinus bradycardia, and a higher incidence of sudden death during sleep (Figure 24.1).

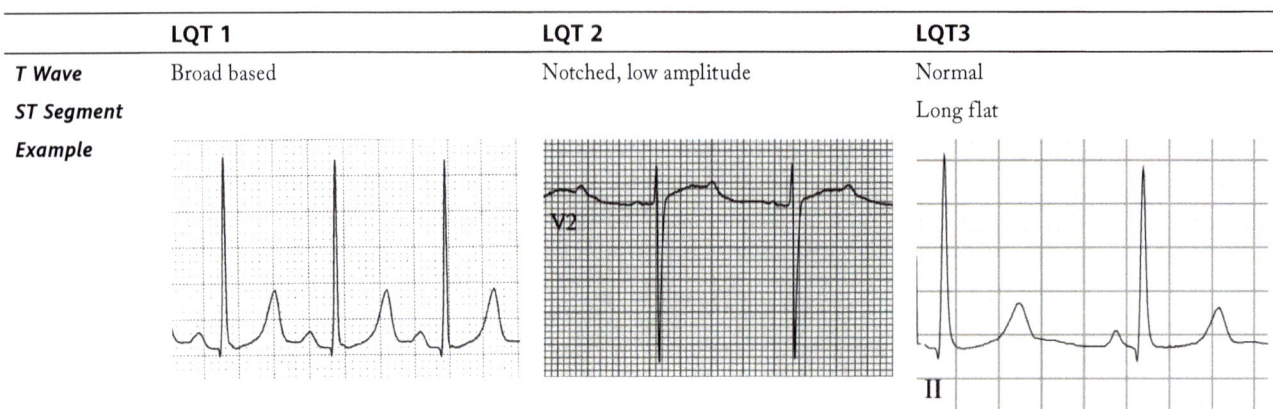

	LQT 1	LQT 2	LQT3
T Wave	Broad based	Notched, low amplitude	Normal
ST Segment			Long flat
Example			

Figure 24.1 ECG morphology in long QT syndromes 1, 2, and 3.

Mechanism of LQTS

The QT interval is the ECG manifestation of ventricular depolarization and repolarization. QT prolongation results from ion channel dysfunction that prolongs cellular repolarization.[7,8] Myocardial repolarization is primarily mediated by potassium ions. Decreased outward potassium current mediated by a loss of function mutation in I_{Ks} (slowly activating delayed rectifier potassium channel) leads to LQT1. A mutation in the *KCNQ1* that codes for the I_{Ks} channel may also disrupt other currents, including I_{Kr}, I_{Cl}, and I_{Na-Ca} that are also under sympathetic control. This leads to failure to shorten the action potential duration with adrenergic stimulation and hence the QT interval in patients with LQT1.[9] Decreased outward potassium current mediated by a loss of function mutation in I_{Kr} (rapid) leads to LQT2. I_{Kr} channels represent a smaller fraction of the potassium channels responsible for repolarization and are not as sympathetically responsive as I_{Ks} channels. I_{Kr} is activated in low adrenergic circumstances and I_{Ks} in higher adrenergic states. A gain of function mutation of I_{Na} leads to enhanced activity of inward sodium current and failed inactivation leading to LQT3. These channel dysfunctions that result in prolonged repolarization may cause EADs due to activation of inward depolarizing currents that reach threshold, causing ventricular extrasystoles. Furthermore, heterogeneity in ventricular repolarization may cause unidirectional block and cause areas of slow conduction. Although the mechanism is not fully understood, this substrate along with triggered EADs may lead to reentry and resultant torsades de pointes.

Unmasking Long QT Syndrome

Overlap of the resting QTc between unaffected people and patients with LQTS adds to the challenges of accurate diagnosis; an estimated 25%–50% of patients with LQT1, LQT2, or LQT3 display a nondiagnostic resting QTc (< 460 ms).[10] In one study,[11] the Schwartz criteria[12] iden-tified a high probability of LQTS (score > 4) with a sensitivity of 19% and specificity of 99%. The Keating criteria[13] had 36% sensitivity and 99% specificity. Alternatively, by analyzing QTc duration alone, a cutoff of 430 ms was associated with a sensitivity of 72% and specificity of 86% (area under Receiver Operator Characteristic [ROC] curve of 0.788) at identifying mutation carriers from noncarriers. Genetic testing is not universally feasible and remains expensive. Furthermore, genetic testing may identify mutations of unclear significance. This highlights the need for provocative testing to enhance diagnosis—particularly to enhance sensitivity, to guide genetic testing, and to validate genetic findings.

Since the ion channel defects (primarily I_{Ks} and to a lesser extent I_{Kr}) are stressed under sympathetic stimulation and many of the observed cardiac events are triggered by exercise, exercise stress testing and/or pharmacological adrenergic provocation have been suggested to enhance the diagnostic accuracy in LQTS.[14-17] Adrenergic provocation may reveal a paradoxical response characterized by QT lengthening rather than expected shortening that is pathognomonic for LQT1 (I_{Ks} defect). In patients with LQT2 (I_{Kr} defect), there may be a transient prolongation of the action potential duration, followed by shortening of the action potential duration due to the presence of unimpaired I_{Ks} channels.[18,19] The LQT3 phenotype is characterized by a constant reduction of the action potential duration with adrenergic stimulation due to stimulation of the intact I_{Ks} channel.[20] Thus, adrenergic provocation assesses the integrity of the I_{Ks} channel. Adrenaline-induced changes in T-wave morphology are nonspecific and may not be sensitive and should be interpreted with caution.[21]

Two major protocols have evolved for adrenaline infusion: (1) the bolus and brief infusion (Shimizu protocol)[22] and (2) the escalating dose protocol (Mayo protocol).[23] Gradually increasing the dose of adrenaline from 0.05 to 0.1, 0.2, and 0.3 mcg/kg/min in sequence can distinguish healthy controls from patients with concealed LQT1. In one study, every LQT1 patient manifested prolongation of the QT interval, whereas healthy controls and patients with LQT2 or LQT3 tended to have shortened QT intervals.[23] This study concluded that adrenergic provocation is capable of clinically evaluating the integrity of the I_{Ks} channel signaling complex in LQT1 patients.[24] In another study involving 147 genotyped patients,[10] the median change in QT interval during low-dose adrenaline infusion was −23 ms in the gene-negative group, +78 ms in LQT1, −4 ms in LQT2, and −58 ms in LQT3. The paradoxical QT response was observed in 92% of patients with LQT1 compared with 18% of gene-negative, 13% LQT2, and 0% LQT3 patients. Overall, the paradoxical QT response had a sensitivity of 92.5%, specificity of 86%, positive predictive value of 76%, and negative predictive value of 96% for LQT1 status. This study reported that patients on β-blocker therapy at the time of testing are likely to have lower diagnostic accuracy. An increase in the absolute QT by 30 ms (at 0.05 mcg/kg/min adrenaline),[23] an increase in absolute QT by 35 ms[22] or QTc prolongation by 30 ms[20] (at 0.10 mcg/kg/min adrenaline), and an increase in QTc by 65 ms[25] or to a value above 600 ms[26] during adrenaline infusion (up to 0.4 mcg/kg/min) have all been proposed as useful criteria for diagnosing LQTS that may be concealed on the resting ECG.

Graded infusions of adrenaline or isoproterenol in normal subjects is associated with QTc prolongation, which complicates interpretation; 67% to 79% of normal subjects show an abnormally prolonged QTc interval at one or more infusion levels of adrenaline or isoproterenol.[23,26] However, an absolute QT prolongation by more than 20 to 30 ms is not typically seen at any dose level of adrenaline or isoproterenol. Additionally, if catecholamine infusion is used, the need for high specificity favors use of adrenaline provocation.[27] Absolute QT interval shortening in normal individuals is greater with catecholamine infusion than with exercise.[28] Thus, false-positive results would be expected to be lower with catecholamine infusions compared to exercise testing.

Exercise stress testing has also been utilized for differentiating LQT1, LQT2, and unaffected individuals.[29] End-of-recovery QTc may have clinical use in distinguishing patients with LQTS from healthy individuals; a QTc < 445 ms at the end of recovery had a sensitivity of 92% and specificity of 88% at identifying healthy individuals. Furthermore, early-recovery QTc may be used to distinguish LQT1 from LQT2 patients;[30] early-recovery QTc < 460 ms had a sensitivity of 79% and specificity of 92% at distinguishing LQT2 patients from LQT1. Additionally, increased QT hysteresis may be a unique feature of LQT2 syndrome. QT hysteresis is calculated as the QT interval difference between exercise and 1 to 2 minutes into recovery at similar heart rates (within 10 bpm) at heart rates of approximately 100 bpm.[31] In LQT2 patients with impaired I_{Kr}, the QT fails to shorten at intermediate heart rates in early exercise. However, recruitment of I_{Ks} at higher heart rates is associated with appropriate QT shortening, which persists into the recovery phase. This consequently leads to an exaggerated QT difference between exercise and recovery, which manifests as increased QT hysteresis. QT hysteresis of > 25 ms has a sensitivity and specificity of 73% and 68%, respectively, for identifying patients with LQT2 over LQT1.[32]

Drug-induced QT prolongation is predominantly due to I_{Kr} inhibition.[33] The interval from the peak of the T wave to the end of the T wave (T_{PE}), which is thought to provide a more sensitive index of abnormal repolarization, was markedly prolonged by erythromycin (an I_{Kr} blocker) in LQT2 subjects but not in LQT1 subjects or controls.[34] A T_{PE} of > 100 ms with erythromycin infusion (1 g of erythromycin lactobionate administered intravenously over 1 hour) had a sensitivity of 80% and specificity of 75% in identifying patients with LQT2 syndrome. The small number of patients in this study precludes reaching any conclusions regarding the utility of testing with erythromycin. Thus, LQT2-specific provocative testing remains exploratory, with no clinical role that has been established.

Adenosine-induced sudden bradycardia and subsequent tachycardia has also been investigated to identify QT changes of diagnostic value in patients with LQTS. Adenosine challenge resulted in dissimilar response in LQT patients and controls in one study.[35] A QTc of > 490 ms at maximal bradycardia had a sensitivity of 94% and a specificity of 85% to detect LQTS. The small number of genotyped patients in this study series precludes reaching any conclusions regarding the utility of adenosine testing, but it is promising.

Adrenergic provocative testing may be considered to assess QT response (1) in patients with a suspicion of LQT1/2 who have not been genotyped, (2) in those with a genetic diagnosis of LQT1/2 but with a resting ECG that is normal, and (3) if the LQT1-associated mutation is novel. The test is not recommended for patients with LQT3.

These studies should be performed with appropriate medical supervision. Patients should be connected to an external cardioverter-defibrillator. The 12-lead ECG should be monitored continuously, along with frequent blood pressure monitoring. Heart rate, QT, and corrected QT interval should be measured during each stage. Recovery ECGs should also be evaluated. Both the Shimizu and Mayo protocols are well tolerated with a low incidence of adverse events. However, drugs for resuscitation, including intravenous β-blockers, should be available by the bedside (Tables 24.2, 24.3, and 24.4).

Table 24.2 Pharmacological provocation for diagnosis of channelopathies

LQTS and CPVT	Adrenaline	Infusion started at 0.05 mcg/kg/min and increased every 5 minutes to 0.1 and 0.2 mcg/kg/min for 5 minutes at each dose.
LQTS and CPVT	Isoproterenol	Infusion started at 1 mcg/min and increased every 5 minutes to a maximum of 5 mcg/min.
Brugada	Flecainide	Given intravenously at a dosage of 2 mg/kg (maximum 150 mg) over 10 minutes.
Brugada	Ajmaline	Given IV at 1 mg/kg over 10 minutes.
Brugada	Procainamide	10 mg/kg over 20–30 minutes.
Brugada	Pilsicainide	1 mg/kg over 10 minutes.

The QT interval normally shortens with appropriate sinus tachycardia and lengthens with bradycardia. Patients with LQT1 or LQT2 often display paradoxical response to exercise/adrenergic stimulation. Thus, a positive test is defined as a paradoxical response to exercise or pharmacological provocation. The test should be terminated if the test is positive or if systolic blood pressure rises above 200 mmHg, substantive increase in ventricular arrhythmia occurs, T-wave alternans develops, or the patient becomes intolerant of the infusion.

Brugada Syndrome

The incidence of Brugada ECG is estimated to be approximately 1 per 2,000.[36] The disease is more prevalent and/or more penetrant in the southeast Asian countries. Though the syndrome exhibits an autosomal dominant inheritance pattern, there is an approximately 8:1 male-to-female preponderance.

Brugada syndrome displays genetic heterogeneity, with a loss-of-function mutation in *SCN5A* gene (encoding the pore-forming subunit of voltage-gated cardiac Na channel) identified in fewer than 20% of Brugada diagnoses.[37] A loss-of-function mutation in the cardiac L-type Ca^{2+} channel has also been associated with a Brugada phenotype.[38] Additional mutations (Table 24.1) have also been identified,[39] and numerous others have been reported.[40] Reports of Brugada-like coved ST elevation in the inferior leads in association with a gene mutation in *SCN5A* may represent a variant of Brugada syndrome.[41,42]

Brugada syndrome may initially present as syncope or aborted sudden cardiac death due to polymorphic VT or VF, typically in the third or fourth decade of life. However, earlier presentations have been noted. Cardiac events typically occur at rest and may also occur during febrile illnesses[43] or with exposure to sodium channel–blocking drugs. The prevalence of cardiac arrest in Brugada individuals is reported to be 10% to 15% by the age of 60.[37] In another study, the cardiac event rate per year was 7.7% in patients with aborted sudden cardiac death, 1.9% in patients with syncope, and 0.5% in asymptomatic patients.[44] Thus, Brugada syndrome should be distinguished from Brugada pattern on ECG in asymptomatic individuals, which is a far more common presentation.

The Brugada ECG pattern is characterized by complete/incomplete RBBB with a coved morphology in the ST-segment elevation of at least 2 mm in the right precordial leads (V_1–V_3), followed by a negative T wave.[36,45] The type 2 ST-segment elevation has a saddleback appearance with a high-takeoff ST segment elevation of > 2 mm, a trough displaying > 1 mm ST elevation, and then either a positive or biphasic T wave (Figure 24.2). Type 3 has either a saddleback or coved appearance with an ST segment elevation of < 1 mm. The ECG may vary over time with change between the patterns observed in a given individual, but the type 2 and type 3 patterns in themselves are not diagnostic.

Mechanism of Brugada Syndrome

The arrhythmogenic substrate and ECG changes in Brugada syndrome are believed to be due to amplification of heterogeneities in the action potential of cells residing in epicardial and endocardial layers of the right ventricle, leading to disparity in action potential duration between these layers and, subsequently, voltage gradients.[46,47]

A reduction in the sodium current (I_{Na}) allows the transient outward (I_{to}) current to repolarize the cell in phase 1 beyond the voltage range in which L-type Ca^{+2} channels are active. Inactivity of the Ca^{+2} channel results in loss of the action potential plateau. Subendocardial cells express the I_{to} channel to a lesser extent than subepicardial cells. This results in a disparity in action potential duration between these layers and, consequently, voltage gradients.

Conduction of the action potential from sites at which it is maintained to sites at which it is lost causes local reexcitation via phase 2 reentry. This leads to development of closely coupled extrasystole capable of capturing the vulnerable window across the ventricular wall, thus triggering VT/VF.[48-50]

Unmasking Brugada Syndrome

The typical ECG pattern is often concealed or only present intermittently. In one study[51] of 176 patients in whom repetitive baseline ECGs were recorded, only 90 patients had at least one positive baseline ECG. The typical ECG features can be unmasked, however, with sodium channel blockers, including flecainide, ajmaline, procainamide, and pilsicainide.[48,52-55] Furthermore, the autonomic nervous system also modulates the ECG phenotype, with isoproterenol attenuating and acetylcholine accentuating the ECG changes in affected patients.[54] In one series, 100 of 334 patients (29.9%) could only be diagnosed with pharmacologic challenge.[56] These findings highlight the

	Type 1	Type 2	Type 3
J-wave amplitude	> 2 mm	> 2 mm	> 2 mm
T wave	negative	positive/biphasic	positive
ST morphology	coved	saddleback	either
Terminal ST portion	–	> 1 mm elevation	< 1 mm elevation
Example			

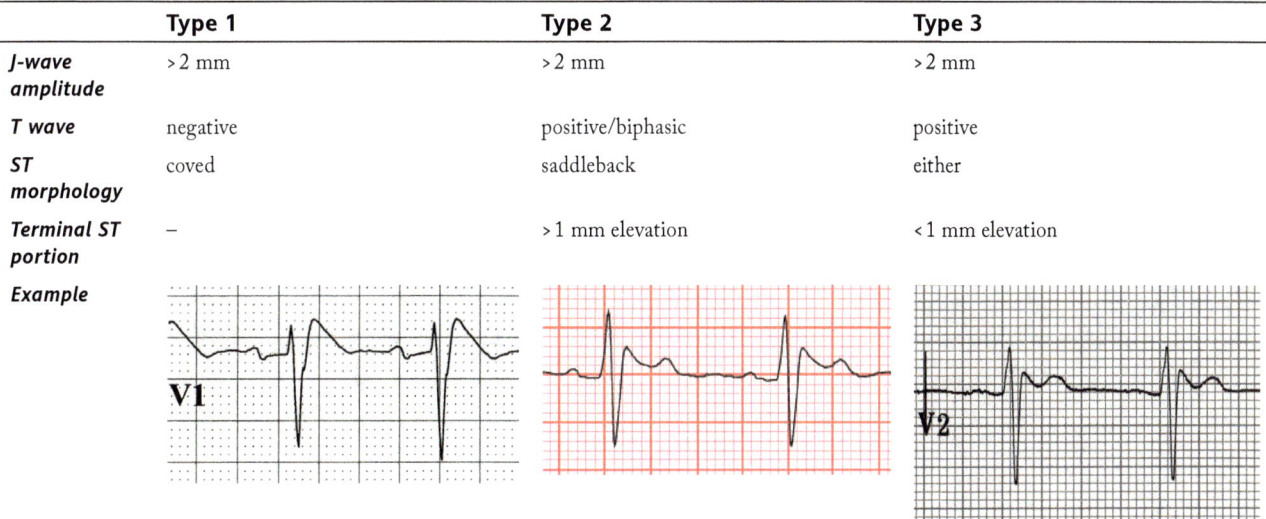

Figure 24.2 ECG morphology in Brugada syndrome.

importance of pharmacologic challenge. The highest possible sensitivity to pharmacologic challenge is warranted.[37] However, the sensitivity of provocative pharmacologic testing is still undefined, but not 100%.[37] In one study, provocative testing with flecainide had a sensitivity of 77% in the subgroup of patients carrying the *SCN5A* gene mutation.[57]

Patients with a Brugada pattern on ECG diagnosed with leads placed two intercostal spaces above the standard position may have a similar prognosis to that of individuals with a type 1 ECG recorded from the standard position[58] (Figure 24.3). The specificity of this remains to be defined.

Various drugs unmask the Brugada pattern by varied mechanisms. The varied potency of inhibiting I_{Na} and I_{to} by sodium channel blockers contributes to the varied effectiveness in unmasking the Brugada pattern. Additionally, vagotonic agents augment outward currents (I_{to}). Sodium channel blockers, cocaine, antidepressants, and antihistamines (terfenadine) reduce inward currents.[59] These drugs are summarized at www.brugadadrugs.org. With flecainide and ajmaline, I_{Na} inhibition reduces inward current and I_{to} inhibition counters this action by blocking outward current. Ajmaline and flecainide, in addition to reducing the peak amplitude of I_{to}, accelerate the decay of the current. Class IA (procainamide, disopyramide) antiarrhythmic agents that display a more rapid dissociation from the sodium channel may explain the lesser potency compared with class IC agents in unmasking the syndrome. However, in contrast to ajmaline and flecainide, procainamide produces no block of I_{to} at clinically relevant drug concentrations.[55]

One study that compared the effect of intravenous flecainide and ajmaline with respect to their ability to induce or accentuate a type 1 Brugada pattern reported disparate responses, with a failure of flecainide in 7 of 22 cases (32% vs 0% with ajmaline).[60] Greater inhibition of I_{to} by flecainide may render it less effective. In another study, pharmacological challenge with sodium channel blockers (flecainide or ajmaline) was unable to unmask most silent gene carriers (PPV, 35%).[37] Therefore, sensitivity and specificity for pharmacological provocation remains unclear. Overall, the sensitivity of the sodium channel–blocking provocative tests is estimated to be between 71% and 80%. However, this has only been evaluated in patients with an *SCN5A* mutation, which represents approximately 20% of all Brugada syndrome patients.[57,61] The single study on the sensitivity in non-*SCN5A* Brugada syndrome patients was in patients with documented but transitory type 1 ECG resuscitated from a sudden cardiac death. In this study, the sodium channel blocker test was found to be 100% sensitive.[52]

Drug challenge generally is not performed in asymptomatic patients displaying the type 1 ECG under baseline conditions because the additional diagnostic value is considered to be limited, the added prognostic value is not clear, and the test is not without risk for provoking arrhythmic events. If the ECG pattern is atypical or the extent of ST elevation is borderline, drug challenge may be warranted, including administration of isoproterenol to normalize the ST segment.

All patients should be connected to a 12-lead ECG machine. The ECG should be continuously monitored and recorded at 1-minute intervals. The author's typical adrenaline and procainamide infusion protocol is summarized in Table 24.3. After administration of the last dose (Tables 24.2, 24.3, and 24.4), the ECG should be recorded for another 10 minutes or until the ECG normalizes; plasma half-life of flecainide is 20 hours, procainamide 3–4 hours, and ajmaline is inactivated within a few minutes. Patients should be closely monitored, and resuscitation equipment should be available. Patients with conduction disease may be at increased risk of AV block (see Table 24.2 for dosing recommendations).

Testing should be terminated when a diagnostic type 1 Brugada ECG develops, premature ventricular beats or other arrhythmias develop, or the QRS widens to > 130% of baseline. A positive test is defined as a type 1 pattern occurring after sodium channel blocker administration.

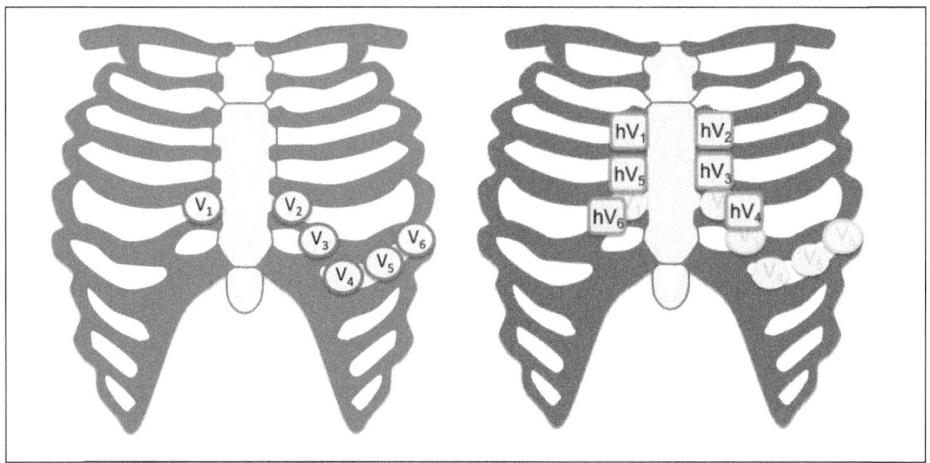

Figure 24.3 Alternative ECG lead positioning for diagnosing Brugada syndrome.

Table 24.3 Adrenaline/procainamide infusion worksheet

Progress	Time	Test	Vitals	Instructions
Adrenaline Infusion				
Baseline		ECG/Vitals		Normal placement ECG Start adrenaline 0.05 mcg/kg/min
0:05 minutes		ECG/Vitals		Increase to 0.10 mcg/kg/min Normal placement ECG
0:10 minutes		ECG/Vitals		Increase to 0.20 mcg/kg/min Normal placement ECG
0:15 minutes		ECG/Vitals		Stop adrenaline Normal placement ECG
0:25 minutes		ECG/Vitals		Normal placement ECG
0:35 minutes 20 minutes post adrenaline		ECG/Vitals		Normal placement ECG
0:45 minutes 30 minutes post adrenaline		ECG/Vitals		Normal placement ECG
Procainamide Infusion (1,000 mg over 30 minutes)				
Baseline		ECG/Vitals		ECG high alternate and normal placement Start procainamide
0:10 minutes		ECG/Vitals		Normal placement ECG
0:20 minutes		ECG/Vitals		Normal placement ECG
0:30 minutes		ECG/Vitals		Stop procainamide Normal placement ECG ECG high alternate placement
0:40 minutes 10 minutes post procainamide		ECG		ECG high alternate placement
1:00 minutes 30 minutes post procainamide		ECG/Vitals		Normal placement ECG
1:30 minutes 60 minutes post procainamide		ECG/Vitals		Normal placement ECG
If > 1 mm ST elevation in V_1 or V_2, stop procainamide and run isoproterenol 2 mcg/min.				

Table 24.4 Adrenaline infusion report

☐ Known long QT syndrome   ☐ Suspected long QT syndrome ☐ Family history of long QT syndrome   ☐ Known catecholaminergic polymorphic VT (CPVT) ☐ Suspected catecholaminergic polymorphic VT (CPVT) ☐ Family history of catecholaminergic polymorphic VT (CPVT) ☐ Suspected long QT syndrome or catecholaminergic polymorphic VT (CPVT) ☐ Previous unexplained cardiac arrest ☐ Other _____
Clinical Status ☐ Asymptomatic ☐ Symptomatic ☐ Palpitations   ☐ Syncope   ☐ Presyncope   ☐ Cardiac arrest   ☐ Other_____
Baseline ECG QT interval (ms) _____   Heart rate (bpm) _____ T-wave morphology: ☐ Normal   ☐ Borderline   ☐ Abnormal Abnormal T wave (circle any): Low amplitude   Notched   Inverted/peaked   Long isoelectric segment
The patient was on ☐ No medications ☐ Beta-blocker (details): _____ ☐ Other (list) _____
Adrenaline infusion Adrenaline was administered in doses starting at 0.05 mcg/kg/min. This was increased to 0.10 mcg/kg/min and 0.20 mcg/kg/min in 5-minute intervals. ☐ There were no side effects from the infusion. ☐ The infusion was terminated early due to side effects. Side effects were _____
Arrhythmias during infusion: ☐ No ventricular ectopy   ☐ Polymorphic/monomorphic PVCs ☐ Nonsustained monomorphic VT   ☐ Nonsustained polymorphic VT ☐ Sustained monomorphic VT   ☐ Sustained polymorphic VT or VF ☐ Other_____
QT response to infusion: ☐ No significant QT change from baseline   ☐ Borderline QT prolongation ☐ Paradoxical QT prolongation (> 30 ms absolute QT prolongation at 0.10 mcg/kg/min)

	QT	HR	QTc
Rest			
Adrenaline 0.05 mcg/kg/min			
Adrenaline 0.10 mcg/kg/min			
Adrenaline 0.20 mcg/kg/min			

Interpretation ☐ Findings do not support the diagnosis of either catecholaminergic VT or long QT syndrome. ☐ Findings support the diagnosis of long QT syndrome. ☐ Findings support the diagnosis of catecholaminergic VT. ☐ Findings support the diagnosis of both catecholaminergic VT and long QT syndrome.

Catecholaminergic Polymorphic Ventricular Tachycardia

Catecholaminergic polymorphic ventricular tachycardia (CPVT) is a rare disorder characterized by exercise- or stress-induced bidirectional and/or polymorphic ventricular tachycardia (Figure 24.3) that may lead to syncope or sudden death. The mean age at presentation is between 7 and 9 years of age, though it may present in early or mid-adulthood.[62,63] Our experience encompasses a much later age at presentation, more often in late adolescence or early adulthood. CPVT may be misdiagnosed as epilepsy or vasovagal syncope, leading to delay in accurate diagnosis. The resting ECG is usually normal with a normal or borderline QT interval, making diagnosis difficult. Mortality is high when untreated, reaching between 30% and 50% by age 30.[62,64] Although CPVT is a highly lethal condition, early diagnosis and appropriate prescription of β-blockers and exercise restriction, along with selective implantation of ICDs, can result in a favorable prognosis. Recent evidence suggests that flecainide has incremental benefit when added to β-blockers.[65]

CPVT is typically caused by mutations in the ryanodine receptor gene (*RyR2*) with autosomal dominant inheritance (chromosome 1q42–q43), or much less commonly autosomal recessive (1p31–21), caused by mutations in the cardiac calsequestrin gene (*CASQ2*). Ankyrin-B mutations have also been implicated in CPVT. Approximately 30% of the probands have a family history of sudden cardiac death before age 40. Clinical penetrance ranges from 25% to 100%, with an average of 70%–80%.

The clinical diagnosis is made based on symptoms, family history, and response to exercise and/or adrenergic stimulation. A history of exercise- or emotional stress–induced syncope or sudden death suggests a diagnosis of CPVT, similar to LQTS. A significant percentage of patients with a presumptive diagnosis of LQTS but whose genetic testing for LQT-related genes is negative have mutations associated with CPVT.[66] Swimming-triggered cardiac events should raise concern about type 1 LQTS or CPVT.[66] It is noteworthy that patients with Andersen Tawil[67] syndrome (LQT7) may also present with bidirectional VT.[68]

Mechanism of CPVT

CPVT is the result of excess intracellular calcium. The ryanodine receptor is involved in the release of calcium from the sarcoplasmic reticulum at the time of excitation-contraction coupling. *RyR2* mutations lead to a gain of function that sensitizes the *RyR2* to a premature release of calcium from the sarcoplasmic reticulum, resulting in failed reuptake of calcium into the sarcoplasmic reticulum and intracellular calcium overload.[69] Calsequestrin is a regulatory protein associated with the ryanodine receptor. Mutations in calsequestrin also contribute to abnormal regulation of cellular calcium homeostasis.[70] This abnormal calcium handling leads to calcium overload, which causes arrhythmias mediated by delayed afterdepolarizations.[71]

Unmasking CPVT

Ventricular tachyarrhythmia is induced by exercise, adrenaline, or isoproterenol infusion with ventricular ectopy, bidirectional VT, and polymorphic VT occurring in a progressively predictable order with increasing heart rate (Figure 24.4). If exercise/isoproterenol/adrenaline is continued, syncope may develop due to degeneration into sustained polymorphic VT or VF. The tachyarrhythmia resolves on discontinuation of exercise or discontinuing adrenergic stimulation. Intravenous β-blockers may be effective in terminating recurrent or sustained ventricular arrhythmia.[72] In at least 80% of CPVT patients, exercise stress test induces the appearance of premature ventricular contraction during exercise stress testing.[73] Adrenaline infusion may have incremental benefit in unmasking CPVT in patients with latent disease.[25] This may relate to a combination of sympathetic stimulation combined with vagal withdrawal during exercise that is less arrhythmogenic than a pure catecholamine trigger during adrenaline infusion in the presence of presumed normal vagal tone.

Holter monitoring is also useful in the evaluation of CPVT, demonstrating progressive arrhythmia with exercise.[63] EP studies are of limited value in the diagnostic evaluation as the tachycardia is seldom inducible by programmed stimulation.

Patients undergoing provocative adrenaline infusion should be connected to a 12-lead ECG machine during testing. The ECG should be continuously monitored and periodically recorded. After infusion (Table 24.2), the ECG should be monitored until heart rates return to baseline. Patients should be closely monitored, and resuscitation equipment should be available. Intravenous β-blocker should be on hand as a form of antidote if sustained arrhythmia is induced. Patients with conduction disease may be at increased risk of AV block. Substantive increase in ventricular arrhythmias, especially bidirectional VT and/or polymorphic VT, is considered a positive test.

Pharmacological Manipulation of Tachyarrhythmia

The electrophysiological effects of adenosine are mediated by cell surface receptors (A1 receptors) coupled to an inhibitory guanine nucleotic binding protein.[74] Stimulation of A1 receptors in the atria is accompanied by hyperpolarization of atrial myocytes and decrease in the duration of

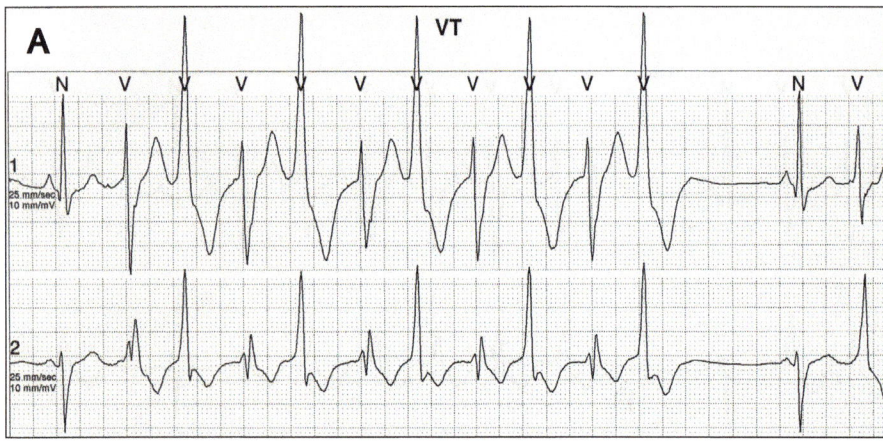
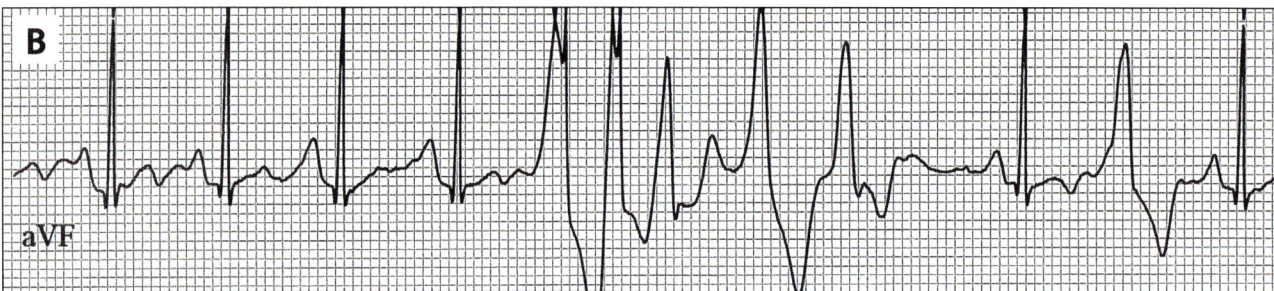

Figure 24.4 Examples of bidirectional and polymorphic VT due to CPVT with exercise/adrenergic stimulation.

atrial action potentials. Adenosine also decreases diastolic depolarization of the pacemaker cells of the SA node (negative chronotropy). The ionic mechanism of the negative dromotropic (AV block) effects of adenosine is less well known. Adenosine does, however, depress the upstroke of the action potential of the "N" cells of the AV node. This is likely to provide the basis for its AV nodal blocking action.[74] Thus, adenosine regulates atrial and ventricular rates independently of each other.

Adenosine is generally used clinically outside of the EP laboratory. However, there is also a role for adenosine in the EP lab. The patient should be continuously monitored with a 12-lead ECG and resuscitation equipment available. Doses of 6, 12, and 18 mg may be used via a large-bore IV cannula. The major advantage of adenosine is its rapid cellular metabolism, permitting rapid diagnosis with very brief side effects that are relatively benign. Induction of atrial or ventricular ectopy, AF, and aggravation of reactive airway disease may be of significant clinical concern in select patients.

Adenosine Use During Narrow-complex Tachyarrhythmia

Due to the AV nodal blocking effect of adenosine, tachycardia mechanisms that involve the AV node in their reentry circuit may be terminated by adenosine. Conduction block in the slow or fast pathway in AV node reentry and in the AV node in AVRT leads to tachycardia termination.[75] Some APs with decremental conduction properties have been shown to be sensitive to adenosine.[76] Therefore, adenosine may rarely terminate AVRT by causing conduction block in the AP rather than in just the AV node.[77]

In AV node-independent SVTs such as AFL, the primary response to adenosine is conduction block in the AV node. This decreases the ventricular rate, but the underlying tachycardia typically continues. Adenosine compounds do not typically affect AFL cycle length.[78] However, the transient AV node blocking property enables the visualization of the flutter waves on ECG clearly, which may aid in diagnosis. Occasionally, AFL may be transformed into AF by adenosine administration.[79] In these instances, AF usually is short lasting.

The effects of adenosine on focal atrial tachycardias are less predictable. Atrial tachycardia is not an AV nodal-dependent tachycardia and, therefore, atrial tachycardia will typically continue with adenosine administration despite conduction block through the AV node. Adenosine may terminate some focal atrial tachycardias that occur due to triggered activity or enhanced automaticity, and therefore, tachycardia termination with adenosine does not exclude atrial tachycardia as the diagnosis.[80] Should the atrial tachycardia continue during adenosine administration, the decreased conduction through the AV node often allows for clearer visualization of P-wave morphology, which assists in localizing focal atrial tachycardias.

In sinus tachycardia, sinus rates are transiently slowed by adenosine. In contrast, adenosine may terminate sinus node reentry tachycardia. Due to the mixed effects of adenosine, the response of a specific SVT to adenosine can only be suggestive of the diagnosis rather than being definitive.[81]

Adenosine Use in Wide-Complex Tachyarrhythmia

The administration of adenosine in patients with antidromic AVRT typically leads to tachycardia termination due to conduction block in the AV node, just as in orthodromic AVRT. Adenosine will not usually terminate reentrant tachycardia, which does not depend on the AV node, such as one that involves an AP antegradely and a second AP retrogradely, unless the AP is adenosine-sensitive. In preexcited AV node, independent tachycardia such as atrial flutter, fibrillation, or focal atrial tachycardia with antegrade conduction over a bystander AP, adenosine may have severe deleterious consequences owing to adenosine-induced AV nodal block shortening the atrial and AP refractoriness, facilitating rapid conduction solely over the AP.[82,83] This may result in AF and/or acceleration of the ventricular rate, both of which can lead to VF.[83]

Adenosine may also play a role in undifferentiated wide-complex tachycardia. Adenosine is typically well tolerated during hemodynamically stable VT episodes[84,85] and therefore may also be used to distinguish VT from SVT with aberrant conduction. In this situation, adenosine would be expected to terminate or lead to AV node conduction block in SVT with aberrancy.[84,86] However, termination of the tachycardia does not completely exclude VT because VT with a triggered mechanism may also be terminated by adenosine.[87,88] VT sensitive to adenosine usually originates in the RVOT, and is less frequently from the LVOT. No cases of adenosine-sensitive ventricular tachycardia have been documented in patients with ischemic heart disease with reentrant VT. In one study, a correct diagnosis of VT occurred more often when based on the effects of adenosine (92%) than on ECG criteria (75%).[85] However, adenosine should be used with caution in patients with structural heart disease as there are case reports of serious proarrhythmic effects in this setting.[89,90]

Adenosine Use for Intermittent, Latent, and Concealed Accessory Pathway Diagnosis

Ventricular preexcitation is often present during sinus rhythm in patients with an accessory pathway (manifest APs). However, some patients may exhibit a minor degree of preexcitation or no preexcitation despite the presence of an AP. These patients may have an intermittently conducting AP, a latent AP, or a concealed AP. Intermittently conducting APs occur in the context of a relatively long antegrade ERP. In patients with intermittent preexcitation, adenosine may transiently elicit preexcitation by shortening the action potential duration of the AP.[82] Furthermore, administration of adenosine in these circumstances may reveal preexcitation due to adenosine-related sinus bradycardia. These APs are associated with a low risk of sudden death due to the long ERP, but could be implicated in symptomatic AVRT (usually orthodromic).

Alternatively, latent APs have minimal or no preexcitation despite potentially robust antegrade conduction properties because the AV node conduction predominates in ventricular fusion. In such patients, creating transient AV nodal delay or block using adenosine results in an increase of preexcitation, which can assist in the diagnosis and ECG localization of the AP.[91]

In contrast, concealed APs by definition only conduct in the retrograde direction with no delta waves evident on the ECG due to absence of antegrade conduction. In this situation, adenosine does not help in identifying the presence of an AP on 12-lead ECG, but can play a role in identifying and localizing a concealed AP during ventricular pacing during an intracardiac EP study by transiently eliminating retrograde conduction over the AV node.

Assessing Accessory Pathway Risk for Rapid Antegrade Conduction

The mechanism of sudden death in patients with APs is usually VF due to AF conducting rapidly over the AP. Noninvasive techniques have been used to assess the antegrade refractory period of the AP and risk-stratify patients.[92,93] Intermittently conducting APs have precarious antegrade conduction, which portends a benign prognosis in the presence of AF. However, these patients may develop orthodromic AVRT. Lack of complete block in the AP with either IV procainamide[94] or ajmaline[95] has been shown to indicate a short antegrade ERP of the AP (< 270 ms). However, EP testing is the best means to determine the risk of sudden cardiac death and to evaluate for AVRT.

Diagnosing the Substrate for AV Node Reentry

Adenosine may be useful in the noninvasive diagnosis of dual AV node physiology due to differential effects of adenosine on the slow and fast pathways.[96,97] The antegrade fast pathway is more sensitive to the effects of adenosine than the antegrade slow pathway.[98] Studies have demonstrated good predictive value (PPV 72%) of adenosine in detection of dual AV node physiology compared with electrophysiological testing.[99] A sudden jump in PR interval (≥ 50 ms) was seen in 76% of patients with inducible AVNRT, but in 20 patients with undocumented tachycardia, this effect was observed in only 5% of patients without inducible AV node reentry with bedside adenosine administration.[99] Adenosine may also be of value in the noninvasive assessment following slow pathway ablation. Adenosine testing demonstrated the absence of dual AV node physiology in 96% of patients following slow pathway ablation.[97] This may potentially be utilized to predict the likelihood of recurrence of AVNRT after radiofrequency ablation in patients with ongoing symptoms.

Pharmacological Provocation in Bradycardia

Diagnostic EP testing or pharmacological provocation is not often required in the assessment of the need for permanent pacemaker implantation in suspected SA and/or AV nodal disease.[100]

Complete autonomic (sympathetic and parasympathetic) blockade of the SA node may help distinguish SA node dysfunction from sinus bradycardia due to vagal stimulation[101,102] and may also be useful in diagnosing inappropriate sinus tachycardia. Complete autonomic blockade can be achieved with a combination of β-blocker (propanolol 0.2 mg/kg) and atropine (0.04 mg/kg). The intrinsic heart rate following autonomic blockade is inversely and linearly related to a patient's age and is predicted by the following formula:[103] intrinsic heart rate = [118.1 − (0.57 × age)] ± 14% in patients < 45 years of age and ± 18% in patients > 45 years of age.

Additionally, pharmacological manipulation of the AV node can illuminate the level of AV block, especially in the context of 2:1 second-degree AV block. Conduction disease at the level of the AV node is suggested if conduction improves with atropine infusion, whereas His or infra-Hisian dysfunction is suggested by worsening conduction with atropine infusion. Block at the level of the AV node improves with atropine due to the shortening of the AV nodal ERP. Conversely, the His-Purkinje tissue ERP typically does not change with atropine, and the block at this level worsens with atropine due to a simultaneous increase in the sinus rate. For analogous reasons, vagal stimulation that improves conduction suggests infranodal dysfunction and worsening of conduction with vagal stimulation suggests AV nodal dysfunction.

Detailed and accurate assessment of sinoatrial and AV nodal function requires invasive EP study. Corrected sinus node recovery time (CSNRT) > 550 ms suggests sinoatrial nodal dysfunction, with CSNRT > 1,000 ms indicating the need for permanent pacemaker implantation. Sinoatrial conduction time > 120 ms is indicative of sinoatrial node dysfunction. An HV interval > 100 ms is an indication for permanent pacing. Some research has suggested that provocation with sodium channel blockers may be able to identify patients with SA and AV nodal disease who would benefit from permanent pacemaker implantation.[104] An increase of greater than 50% in CSNRT or sinoatrial conduction time with ajmaline (1 mg/kg) or flecainide (2 mg/kg) has been suggested to indicate sinoatrial node dysfunction.[105] The demonstration of intra- or infra-Hisian block with ajmaline may also indicate AV nodal dysfunction. These tests are now rarely used, as the indication for pacing is generally documentation of culprit arrhythmia in symptomatic patients.

Pharmacological Provocation for Interventional Procedure

Arrhythmia Induction for Tachycardia Ablation

The direct and indirect effects on vagal and sympathetic tone result in differing effects on the slow and fast AV node pathways.[106-108] Sympathomimetic and/or parasympatholytic agents can facilitate AVNRT induction during EP study. Similarly, AVRT requires differential properties of the antegrade and retrograde limbs of the circuit and is dependent on the refractoriness and conduction velocities of these two limbs.

Isoproterenol

Induction of typical (slow-fast) AV node reentry is facilitated when the antegrade refractoriness of the fast pathway is prolonged and/or antegrade conduction velocity over the slow pathway is decreased. Isoproterenol can facilitate induction of AVNRT by improving retrograde conduction of the fast pathway.[108-110] However, isoproterenol may shorten the antegrade ERP of the fast pathway so that no difference in the antegrade ERP of the fast and slow pathway could be found. This results in an inability to initiate AVNRT during atrial pacing. Isoproterenol may also facilitate antegrade[111] and retrograde AP conduction.[112]

Isoproterenol can facilitate the induction of sustained AVNRT.[110] In one study of AVNRT patients, only 64% of AVNRT was induced without isoproterenol while the remaining 36% required isoproterenol for AVNRT induction.[113] In this study, 29% of AVNRT patients demonstrated no dual AV nodal pathway physiology prior to isoproterenol induction.

Isoproterenol can be utilized to initiate and sustain ventricular tachycardias of any mechanism (automatic, triggered, or reentry mechanism). Isoproterenol has been used in patients with idiopathic ventricular tachycardias, such as RVOT, LVOT, fascicular VT, and annular VT, to facilitate mapping and ablation.[114-116] Aminophylline, calcium infusion, and atropine may also be useful to sustain tachycardia. Furthermore, macroreentrant scar-based VT (ischemic and nonischemic) can also be induced and sustained by isoproterenol. Isoproterenol has also been utilized to induce and maintain focal atrial tachycardias and junctional tachycardias.[117]

The initial dose (1 mcg/min) is gradually increased until a stable sinus rate at least 20% higher than the baseline rate is achieved. Individual isoproterenol dosage may range from 1 to 5 mcg/min.

Atropine, Calcium, and Amionophylline

Atropine may rarely be required to induce tachycardia. Atropine is a muscarinic receptor antagonist that prevents acetylcholine from binding to and activating the receptor. Thus atropine blocks the effects of vagal nerve activity on the heart, causing an increase in heart rate and conduction velocity. Atropine can improve the retrograde fast pathway conduction and thereby induce typical AVNRT.[118,119] Atropine is contraindicated in patients with glaucoma. Alternative agents for induction of SVT have also been utilized (calcium gluconate 1 g over 10 minutes, aminophylline 125–250 mg over 10 minutes), though efficacy of these agents has not been clearly defined. Aminophylline is a phosphodiesterase inhibitor that increases cAMP. It also is a nonselective adenosine receptor antagonist. Increased cAMP, through activation of cAMP-dependent protein kinases, phosphorylates target proteins including the L-type Ca^{++} channels and I_f channel. This increases inotropy, chronotropy, and conduction velocity in the heart and may assist in arrhythmia induction for EP testing.

Drug Use During Atrial Fibrillation Ablation

Adenosine

Pulmonary vein isolation (PVI) is the cornerstone for AF ablation strategies. There is, however, a significant recurrence rate after initial acute PVI, necessitating a repeat intervention to achieve long-term cure of AF. Reported success rate ranges from 50% to 80% following a single ablation procedure. The range of reported success rates is partly due to patient factors, the ablation strategy used, the technology applied, and the quality of follow-up. PV conduction recovery following the initial PVI is the main reason for recurrent AF and atrial tachyarrhythmias.[120,121] PV reconnection rates of 80% have been reported in patients undergoing repeat PVI.[122] Thus, strategies to detect and prevent PV reconnection are paramount in achieving sustained clinical freedom from AF recurrence. Studies have reported that adenosine can expose PV conduction in 25%–35% of isolated PVs.[122,123] Transient PV reconnection facilitated by adenosine may predict long-term AF recurrence.[123] Additionally, research reports show that RF applications to eliminate these transient PV reconnections induced by adenosine provocation lead to a reduction in the AF recurrences,[124,125] although further studies are required.

The mechanism by which adenosine facilitates PV reconnection continues to be investigated. Adenosine activates the outward potassium current via purinergic A1-receptor,[126] and the resulting hyperpolarization of the cell membrane and shortening of the action potential/refractory period may facilitate electrotonic conduction.[123] Finally, adenosine can also promote abnormal automatism and has been used to identify non-PV foci that may trigger AF.[127]

Isoproterenol

Though recurrence of AF following PVI is predominantly due to ectopy originating from previously isolated PVs, non-PV foci initiating AF may also play an important role. Key areas giving rise to ectopy, which can initiate AF, include the SVC, crista terminalis, coronary sinus, IAS, left atrial posterior wall, and ligament of Marshall.[128-131] Current evidence continues to shed light on the role of ablation of these non-PV foci. Non-PV foci may be observed spontaneously or with drug provocation (isoproterenol 4 to 20 mcg/min). If sustained AF occurs, the earliest ectopic site can be targeted as the initiating site. Following a sustained episode of AF (10 minutes), electrical cardioversion can be performed and the drug provocation can be repeated to ensure reproducibility. Additionally, intermittent burst atrial pacing can be undertaken to initiate AF with isoproterenol. Adenosine provocation with up to 30 mg given as a bolus may also be utilized to initiate AF. Biatrial mapping may be required with additional catheters to localize these non-PV triggers, including multielectrode basket or balloon catheters if ectopy is infrequent.

The predictive value of isoproterenol induced triggers following PVI remains to be clearly determined. In one study, inducibility of AF using isoproterenol had a sensitivity of 33%, specificity of 97%, PPV of 75%, and negative predictive value of 84% for recurrent AF post ablation.[132] Postablation response to isoproterenol has been shown to be a more accurate predictor of AF recurrence than the response to rapid atrial pacing.[132] Ablation guided exclusively by targeting induced ectopic sites has been reported,[133,134] but whether targeting these sites will result in less AF recurrence has yet to be convincingly demonstrated. A combined approach is likely to ensue if this strategy reveals further favorable results.

The mechanism by which isoproterenol induces AF may include shortening the refractory period in the PVs and atrium, facilitating calcium release from the sarcoplasmic reticulum, and promoting EADs.[133,135,136] Isoproterenol may also facilitate anisotropic reentry.[137,138] Furthermore, an increase in parasympathetic tone through isoproterenol stimulation of ganglionated plexi with the resultant shortening of atrial ERP may also contribute to promoting triggered activity.[139,140]

In summary, assessment of acute PV reconnection following PVI warrants incorporating a waiting period. Additional pharmacologic provocation with adenosine and/or isoproterenol may aid in establishing end points following PVI and may contribute to long-term AF cure.

Ibutilide

Ibutilide is a potassium channel blocker (Vaughan-Williams class III) that also enhances slow inward sodium current. Ibutilide decreases phase 3 potassium efflux and prolongs repolarization and refractory periods. Ibutilide is indicated for the conversion of AF to sinus rhythm and can be utilized in the EP lab for acute termination. Ibutilide 1 mg is administered intravenously over 10 minutes. A repeat dose may be administered once.

Ibutilide may assist in CFAE ablation that is undertaken to modify the atrial substrate in patients with persistent AF. However, the majority of CFAE may be due to passive atrial activation. Therefore, some CFAE sites may be nonspecific/noncritical targets for ablation. Ibutilide may organize areas of passive atrial activation in AF by promoting fusion of fibrillatory wave fronts and decreasing fractionated EGMs, but not affect areas critical to AF maintenance.[141] Thus, ibutilide may facilitate identification and focused ablation of critical CFAE during AF ablation. However, success with CFAE ablation has not been consistently demonstrated.

Ibutilide must be used with caution due to its effects of action potential prolongation and prolongation of the QT interval. This may cause torsades de pointes, a risk that appears to be greater in patients with severe left ventricular dysfunction and/or congestive heart failure. Cardiac monitoring for a minimum of 4 hours after administering ibutilide should be undertaken.

Conclusion

Pharmacological manipulation of arrhythmia substrate plays a crucial role in diagnosis and treatment of arrhythmia and arrhythmia substrate. A thorough understanding of normal cardiac electrophysiology, disease states, and diagnostic/therapeutic yield of pharmacological provocation is required for the safe undertaking of pharmacological provocation.

References

1. Priori SG, Aliot E, Blomstrom-Lundqvist C, et al. Task Force on Sudden Cardiac Death, European Society of Cardiology. *Europace*. 2002;4:3-18.
2. Schwartz PJ, Locati E. The idiopathic long QT syndrome: pathogenetic mechanisms and therapy. *Eur Heart J*. 1985;6 Suppl D:103-114.
3. Moss AJ, Robinson J. Clinical features of the idiopathic long QT syndrome. *Circulation*. 1992;85:I140-I144.
4. Moss AJ, Robinson JL, Gessman L, et al. Comparison of clinical and genetic variables of cardiac events associated with loud noise versus swimming among subjects with the long QT syndrome. *Am J Cardiol*. 1999;84:876-879.
5. Splawski I, Shen J, Timothy KW, et al. Spectrum of mutations in long-QT syndrome genes. KVLQT1, HERG, SCN5A, KCNE1, and KCNE2. *Circulation*. 2000;102:1178-1185.
6. Bazett HC. The time relations of the blood-pressure changes after excision of the adrenal glands, with some observations on blood volume changes. *J Physiol*. 1920;53:320-339.
7. Keating MT, Sanguinetti MC. Molecular genetic insights into cardiovascular disease. *Science*. 1996;272:681-685.
8. Chiang CE, Roden DM. The long QT syndromes: genetic basis and clinical implications. *J Am Coll Cardiol*. 2000;36:1-12.
9. Shimizu W, Antzelevitch C. Cellular basis for the ECG features of the LQT1 form of the long-QT syndrome: effects of beta-adrenergic agonists and antagonists and sodium channel blockers on transmural dispersion of repolarization and torsade de pointes. *Circulation*. 1998;98:2314-2322.
10. Vyas H, Hejlik J, Ackerman MJ. Epinephrine QT stress testing in the evaluation of congenital long-QT syndrome: diagnostic accuracy of the paradoxical QT response. *Circulation*. 2006;113:1385-1392.
11. Hofman N, Wilde AA, Kaab S, et al. Diagnostic criteria for congenital long QT syndrome in the era of molecular genetics: do we need a scoring system? *Eur Heart J*. 2007;28:575-580.
12. Schwartz PJ, Moss AJ, Vincent GM, Crampton RS. Diagnostic criteria for the long QT syndrome. An update. *Circulation*. 1993;88:782-784.
13. Keating M, Atkinson D, Dunn C, Timothy K, Vincent GM, Leppert M. Linkage of a cardiac arrhythmia, the long QT syndrome, and the Harvey ras-1 gene. *Science*. 1991;252:704-706.
14. Schwartz PJ, Priori SG, Spazzolini C, et al. Genotype-phenotype correlation in the long-QT syndrome: gene-specific triggers for life-threatening arrhythmias. *Circulation*. 2001;103:89-95.
15. Vincent GM, Jaiswal D, Timothy KW. Effects of exercise on heart rate, QT, QTc and QT/QS2 in the Romano-Ward inherited long QT syndrome. *Am J Cardiol*. 1991;68:498-503.
16. Jackman WM, Friday KJ, Anderson JL, Aliot EM, Clark M, Lazzara R. The long QT syndromes: a critical review, new clinical observations and a unifying hypothesis. *Prog Cardiovasc Dis*. 1988;31:115-172.
17. Shimizu W, Ohe T, Kurita T, Tokuda T, Shimomura K. Epinephrine-induced ventricular premature complexes due to early after-depolarizations and effects of verapamil and propranolol in a patient with congenital long QT syndrome. *J Cardiovasc Electrophysiol*. 1994;5:438-444.
18. Dumaine R, Antzelevitch C. Molecular mechanisms underlying the long QT syndrome. *Curr Opin Cardiol*. 2002;17:36-42.
19. Kass RS, Moss AJ. Long QT syndrome: novel insights into the mechanisms of cardiac arrhythmias. *J Clin Invest*. 2003;112:810-815.
20. Shimizu W, Noda T, Takaki H, et al. Epinephrine unmasks latent mutation carriers with LQT1 form of congenital long-QT syndrome. *J Am Coll Cardiol*. 2003;41:633-642.
21. Khositseth A, Hejlik J, Shen WK, Ackerman MJ. Epinephrine-induced T-wave notching in congenital long QT syndrome. *Heart Rhythm*. 2005;2:141-146.
22. Shimizu W, Noda T, Takaki H, et al. Diagnostic value of epinephrine test for genotyping LQT1, LQT2, and LQT3 forms of congenital long QT syndrome. *Heart Rhythm*. 2004;1:276-283.
23. Ackerman MJ, Khositseth A, Tester DJ, Hejlik JB, Shen WK, Porter CB. Epinephrine-induced QT interval prolongation: a gene-specific paradoxical response in congenital long QT syndrome. *Mayo Clin Proc*. 2002;77:413-421.
24. Marx SO, Kurokawa J, Reiken S, et al. Requirement of a macromolecular signaling complex for beta adrenergic receptor modulation of the KCNQ1-KCNE1 potassium channel. *Science*. 2002;295:496-499.

25. Krahn AD, Gollob M, Yee R, et al. Diagnosis of unexplained cardiac arrest: role of adrenaline and procainamide infusion. *Circulation*. 2005;112:2228-2234.
26. Kaufman ES, Gorodeski EZ, Dettmer MM, Dikshteyn M. Use of autonomic maneuvers to probe phenotype/genotype discordance in congenital long QT syndrome. *Am J Cardiol*. 2005;96:1425-1430.
27. Magnano AR, Talathoti N, Hallur R, Bloomfield DM, Garan H. Sympathomimetic infusion and cardiac repolarization: the normative effects of epinephrine and isoproterenol in healthy subjects. *J Cardiovasc Electrophysiol*. 2006;17:983-989.
28. Kawataki M, Kashima T, Toda H, Tanaka H. Relation between QT interval and heart rate: applications and limitations of Bazett's formula. *J Electrocardiol*. 1984;17:371-375.
29. Walker BD, Krahn AD, Klein GJ, Skanes AC, Yee R. Burst bicycle exercise facilitates diagnosis of latent long QT syndrome. *Am Heart J*. 2005;150:1059-1063.
30. Chattha IS, Sy RW, Yee R, et al. Utility of the recovery electrocardiogram after exercise: a novel indicator for the diagnosis and genotyping of long QT syndrome? *Heart Rhythm*. 7:906-911.
31. Krahn AD, Klein GJ, Yee R. Hysteresis of the RT interval with exercise: a new marker for the long-QT syndrome? *Circulation*. 1997;96:1551-1556.
32. Wong JA, Gula LJ, Klein GJ, Yee R, Skanes AC, Krahn AD. Utility of treadmill testing in identification and genotype prediction in long-QT syndrome. *Circ Arrhythm Electrophysiol*. 2010;3:120-125.
33. Mitcheson JS, Chen J, Lin M, Culberson C, Sanguinetti MC. A structural basis for drug-induced long QT syndrome. *Proc Natl Acad Sci USA*. 2000;97:12329-12333.
34. Jeyaraj D, Abernethy DP, Natarajan RN, et al. I(Kr) channel blockade to unmask occult congenital long QT syndrome. *Heart Rhythm*. 2008;5:2-7.
35. Viskin S, Rosso R, Rogowski O, et al. Provocation of sudden heart rate oscillation with adenosine exposes abnormal QT responses in patients with long QT syndrome: a bedside test for diagnosing long QT syndrome. *Eur Heart J*. 2006;27:469-475.
36. Antzelevitch C, Brugada P, Borggrefe M, et al. Brugada syndrome: report of the second consensus conference: endorsed by the Heart Rhythm Society and the European Heart Rhythm Association. *Circulation*. 2005;111:659-670.
37. Priori SG, Napolitano C, Gasparini M, et al. Clinical and genetic heterogeneity of right bundle branch block and ST-segment elevation syndrome: A prospective evaluation of 52 families. *Circulation*. 2000;102:2509-2515.
38. Antzelevitch C, Pollevick GD, Cordeiro JM, et al. Loss-of-function mutations in the cardiac calcium channel underlie a new clinical entity characterized by ST-segment elevation, short QT intervals, and sudden cardiac death. *Circulation*. 2007;115:442-449.
39. Frustaci A, Priori SG, Pieroni M, et al. Cardiac histological substrate in patients with clinical phenotype of Brugada syndrome. *Circulation*. 2005;112:3680-3687.
40. London B, Michalec M, Mehdi H, et al. Mutation in glycerol-3-phosphate dehydrogenase 1 like gene (GPD1-L) decreases cardiac Na+ current and causes inherited arrhythmias. *Circulation*. 2007;116:2260-2268.
41. Potet F, Mabo P, Le Coq G, et al. Novel Brugada SCN5A mutation leading to ST segment elevation in the inferior or the right precordial leads. *J Cardiovasc Electrophysiol*. 2003;14:200-203.
42. Sarkozy A, Chierchia GB, Paparella G, et al. Inferior and lateral electrocardiographic repolarization abnormalities in Brugada syndrome. *Circ Arrhythm Electrophysiol*. 2009;2:154-161.
43. Mok NS, Priori SG, Napolitano C, Chan NY, Chahine M, Baroudi G. A newly characterized SCN5A mutation underlying Brugada syndrome unmasked by hyperthermia. *J Cardiovasc Electrophysiol*. 2003;14:407-411.
44. Probst V, Veltmann C, Eckardt L, et al. Long-term prognosis of patients diagnosed with Brugada syndrome: Results from the FINGER Brugada Syndrome Registry. *Circulation*. 121:635-643.
45. Brugada P, Brugada J. Right bundle branch block, persistent ST segment elevation and sudden cardiac death: a distinct clinical and electrocardiographic syndrome. A multicenter report. *J Am Coll Cardiol*. 1992;20:1391-1396.
46. Antzelevitch C. The Brugada syndrome: ionic basis and arrhythmia mechanisms. *J Cardiovasc Electrophysiol*. 2001;12:268-272.
47. Tukkie R, Sogaard P, Vleugels J, de Groot IK, Wilde AA, Tan HL. Delay in right ventricular activation contributes to Brugada syndrome. *Circulation*. 2004;109:1272-1277.
48. Yan GX, Antzelevitch C. Cellular basis for the Brugada syndrome and other mechanisms of arrhythmogenesis associated with ST-segment elevation. *Circulation*. 1999;100:1660-1666.
49. Antzelevitch C, Brugada P, Brugada J, et al. Brugada syndrome: a decade of progress. *Circ Res*. 2002;91:1114-1118.
50. Kurita T, Shimizu W, Inagaki M, et al. The electrophysiologic mechanism of ST-segment elevation in Brugada syndrome. *J Am Coll Cardiol*. 2002;40:330-334.
51. Priori SG, Napolitano C, Gasparini M, et al. Natural history of Brugada syndrome: insights for risk stratification and management. *Circulation*. 2002;105:1342-1347.
52. Brugada R, Brugada J, Antzelevitch C, et al. Sodium channel blockers identify risk for sudden death in patients with ST-segment elevation and right bundle branch block but structurally normal hearts. *Circulation*. 2000;101:510-515.
53. Rolf S, Bruns HJ, Wichter T, et al. The ajmaline challenge in Brugada syndrome: diagnostic impact, safety, and recommended protocol. *Eur Heart J*. 2003;24:1104-1112.
54. Miyazaki T, Mitamura H, Miyoshi S, Soejima K, Aizawa Y, Ogawa S. Autonomic and antiarrhythmic drug modulation of ST segment elevation in patients with Brugada syndrome. *J Am Coll Cardiol*. 1996;27:1061-1070.
55. Shimizu W, Antzelevitch C, Suyama K, et al. Effect of sodium channel blockers on ST segment, QRS duration, and corrected QT interval in patients with Brugada syndrome. *J Cardiovasc Electrophysiol*. 2000;11:1320-1329.
56. Brugada J, Brugada R, Antzelevitch C, Towbin J, Nademanee K, Brugada P. Long-term follow-up of individuals with the electrocardiographic pattern of right bundle-branch block and ST-segment elevation in precordial leads V1 to V3. *Circulation*. 2002;105:73-78.
57. Meregalli PG, Ruijter JM, Hofman N, Bezzina CR, Wilde AA, Tan HL. Diagnostic value of flecainide testing in unmasking SCN5A-related Brugada syndrome. *J Cardiovasc Electrophysiol*. 2006;17:857-864.
58. Miyamoto K, Yokokawa M, Tanaka K, et al. Diagnostic and prognostic value of a type 1 Brugada electrocardiogram at higher (third or second) V1 to V2 recording in men with Brugada syndrome. *Am J Cardiol*. 2007;99:53-57.
59. Antzelevitch C, Brugada P, Brugada J, Brugada R, Towbin JA, Nademanee K. Brugada syndrome: 1992-2002: a historical perspective. *J Am Coll Cardiol*. 2003;41:1665-1671.
60. Wolpert C, Echternach C, Veltmann C, et al. Intravenous drug challenge using flecainide and ajmaline in patients with Brugada syndrome. *Heart Rhythm*. 2005;2:254-260.

61. Hong K, Brugada J, Oliva A, et al. Value of electrocardiographic parameters and ajmaline test in the diagnosis of Brugada syndrome caused by SCN5A mutations. *Circulation*. 2004;110: 3023-3027.
62. Priori SG, Napolitano C, Memmi M, et al. Clinical and molecular characterization of patients with catecholaminergic polymorphic ventricular tachycardia. *Circulation*. 2002; 106:69-74.
63. Leenhardt A, Lucet V, Denjoy I, Grau F, Ngoc DD, Coumel P. Catecholaminergic polymorphic ventricular tachycardia in children. A 7-year follow-up of 21 patients. *Circulation*. 1995;91:1512-1519.
64. Fisher JD, Krikler D, Hallidie-Smith KA. Familial polymorphic ventricular arrhythmias: a quarter century of successful medical treatment based on serial exercise-pharmacologic testing. *J Am Coll Cardiol*. 1999;34:2015-2022.
65. van der Werf C, Kannankeril PJ, Sacher F, et al. Flecainide therapy reduces exercise-induced ventricular arrhythmias in patients with catecholaminergic polymorphic ventricular tachycardia. *J Am Coll Cardiol*. 57:2244-2254.
66. Choi G, Kopplin LJ, Tester DJ, Will ML, Haglund CM, Ackerman MJ. Spectrum and frequency of cardiac channel defects in swimming-triggered arrhythmia syndromes. *Circulation*. 2004;110:2119-2124.
67. Andersen ED, Krasilnikoff PA, Overvad H. Intermittent muscular weakness, extrasystoles, and multiple developmental anomalies. A new syndrome? *Acta Paediatr Scand*. 1971;60:559-564.
68. Kannankeril PJ, Roden DM, Fish FA. Suppression of bidirectional ventricular tachycardia and unmasking of prolonged QT interval with verapamil in Andersen's syndrome. *J Cardiovasc Electrophysiol*. 2004;15:119.
69. Jiang D, Wang R, Xiao B, et al. Enhanced store overload-induced Ca^{2+} release and channel sensitivity to luminal Ca^{2+} activation are common defects of RyR2 mutations linked to ventricular tachycardia and sudden death. *Circ Res*. 2005;97:1173-1181.
70. Wehrens XH. The molecular basis of catecholaminergic polymorphic ventricular tachycardia: what are the different hypotheses regarding mechanisms? *Heart Rhythm*. 2007; 4:794-797.
71. Liu N, Colombi B, Memmi M, et al. Arrhythmogenesis in catecholaminergic polymorphic ventricular tachycardia: insights from a RyR2 R4496C knock-in mouse model. *Circ Res*. 2006;99:292-298.
72. Mohamed U, Gollob MH, Gow RM, Krahn AD. Sudden cardiac death despite an implantable cardioverter-defibrillator in a young female with catecholaminergic ventricular tachycardia. *Heart Rhythm*. 2006;3:1486-1489.
73. Mohamed U, Napolitano C, Priori SG. Molecular and electrophysiological bases of catecholaminergic polymorphic ventricular tachycardia. *J Cardiovasc Electrophysiol*. 2007; 18:791-797.
74. Camm AJ, Garratt CJ. Adenosine and supraventricular tachycardia. *N Engl J Med*. 1991;325:1621-1629.
75. Belhassen B, Pelleg A, Shoshani D, Geva B, Laniado S. Electrophysiologic effects of adenosine-5'-triphosphate on atrioventricular reentrant tachycardia. *Circulation*. 1983;68: 827-833.
76. Lerman BB, Greenberg M, Overholt ED, et al. Differential electrophysiologic properties of decremental retrograde pathways in long RP' tachycardia. *Circulation*. 1987;76:21-31.
77. Till J, Shinebourne EA, Rigby ML, Clarke B, Ward DE, Rowland E. Efficacy and safety of adenosine in the treatment of supraventricular tachycardia in infants and children. *Br Heart J*. 1989;62:204-211.
78. Stambler BS, Wood MA, Ellenbogen KA. Pharmacologic alterations in human type I atrial flutter cycle length and monophasic action potential duration. Evidence of a fully excitable gap in the reentrant circuit. *J Am Coll Cardiol*. 1996;27:453-461.
79. Alvarado JL, Pastelin G. Action of adenine derivatives on experimental atrial flutter in the canine heart. *Arch Med Res*. 1997;28:329-335.
80. Engelstein ED, Lippman N, Stein KM, Lerman BB. Mechanism-specific effects of adenosine on atrial tachycardia. *Circulation*. 1994;89:2645-2654.
81. Glatter KA, Cheng J, Dorostkar P, et al. Electrophysiologic effects of adenosine in patients with supraventricular tachycardia. *Circulation*. 1999;99:1034-1040.
82. Garratt CJ, Griffith MJ, O'Nunain S, Ward DE, Camm AJ. Effects of intravenous adenosine on antegrade refractoriness of accessory atrioventricular connections. *Circulation*. 1991; 84:1962-1968.
83. Rankin AC, Rae AP, Houston A. Acceleration of ventricular response to atrial flutter after intravenous adenosine. *Br Heart J*. 1993;69:263-265.
84. Sharma AD, Klein GJ, Yee R. Intravenous adenosine triphosphate during wide QRS complex tachycardia: safety, therapeutic efficacy, and diagnostic utility. *Am J Med*. 1990;88:337-343.
85. Rankin AC, Oldroyd KG, Chong E, Rae AP, Cobbe SM. Value and limitations of adenosine in the diagnosis and treatment of narrow and broad complex tachycardias. *Br Heart J*. 1989;62:195-203.
86. Griffith MJ, Linker NJ, Ward DE, Camm AJ. Adenosine in the diagnosis of broad complex tachycardia. *Lancet*. 1988; 1:672-675.
87. Lerman BB. Response of nonreentrant catecholamine-mediated ventricular tachycardia to endogenous adenosine and acetylcholine. Evidence for myocardial receptor-mediated effects. *Circulation*. 1993;87:382-390.
88. Kobayashi Y, Kikushima S, Tanno K, Kurano K, Baba T, Katagiri T. Sustained left ventricular tachycardia terminated by dipyridamole: cyclic AMP-mediated triggered activity as a possible mechanism. *Pacing Clin Electrophysiol*. 1994;17: 377-385.
89. Parham WA, Mehdirad AA, Biermann KM, Fredman CS. Case report: adenosine induced ventricular fibrillation in a patient with stable ventricular tachycardia. *J Interv Card Electrophysiol*. 2001;5:71-74.
90. Tsai CL, Chang WT. A wide QRS complex tachycardia following intravenous adenosine. *Resuscitation*. 2004;61: 240-241.
91. Garratt CJ, Antoniou A, Griffith MJ, Ward DE, Camm AJ. Use of intravenous adenosine in sinus rhythm as a diagnostic test for latent preexcitation. *Am J Cardiol*. 1990;65:868-873.
92. Wellens HJ, Bar FW, Dassen WR, Brugada P, Vanagt EJ, Farre J. Effect of drugs in the Wolff–Parkinson–White syndrome. Importance of initial length of effective refractory period of the accessory pathway. *Am J Cardiol*. 1980; 46:665-669.
93. Critelli G, Gallagher JJ, Perticone F, Coltorti F, Monda V, Condorelli M. Evaluation of noninvasive tests for identifying patients with preexcitation syndrome at risk of rapid ventricular response. *Am Heart J*. 1984;108:905-909.
94. Wellens HJ, Braat S, Brugada P, Gorgels AP, Bar FW. Use of procainamide in patients with the Wolff–Parkinson–White syndrome to disclose a short refractory period of the accessory pathway. *Am J Cardiol*. 1982;50:1087-1089.
95. Wellens HJ, Bar FW, Gorgels AP, Vanagt EJ. Use of ajmaline in patients with the Wolff–Parkinson–White syndrome to

disclose short refractory period of the accessory pathway. *Am J Cardiol*. 1980;45:130-133.
96. Belhassen B, Fish R, Glikson M, et al. Noninvasive diagnosis of dual AV node physiology in patients with AV nodal reentrant tachycardia by administration of adenosine-5'-triphosphate during sinus rhythm. *Circulation*. 1998;98:47-53.
97. Belhassen B, Fish R, Eldar M, Glick A, Glikson M, Viskin S. Simplified "ATP test" for noninvasive diagnosis of dual AV nodal physiology and assessment of results of slow pathway ablation in patients with AV nodal reentrant tachycardia. *J Cardiovasc Electrophysiol*. 2000;11:255-261.
98. Curtis AB, Belardinelli L, Woodard DA, Brown CS, Conti JB. Induction of atrioventricular node reentrant tachycardia with adenosine: differential effect of adenosine on fast and slow atrioventricular node pathways. *J Am Coll Cardiol*. 1997;30:1778-1784.
99. Tebbenjohanns J, Niehaus M, Korte T, Drexler H. Noninvasive diagnosis in patients with undocumented tachycardias: value of the adenosine test to predict AV nodal reentrant tachycardia. *J Cardiovasc Electrophysiol*. 1999;10:916-923.
100. Fujimura O, Yee R, Klein GJ, Sharma AD, Boahene KA. The diagnostic sensitivity of electrophysiologic testing in patients with syncope caused by transient bradycardia. *N Engl J Med*. 1989;321:1703-1707.
101. Szatmary LJ. Autonomic blockade and sick sinus syndrome. New concept in the interpretation of electrophysiological and Holter data. *Eur Heart J*. 1984;5:637-648.
102. Desai JM, Scheinman MM, Strauss HC, Massie B, O'Young J. Electrophysiologic effects on combined autonomic blockade in patients with sinus node disease. *Circulation*. 1981;63:953-960.
103. Jose AD, Collison D. The normal range and determinants of the intrinsic heart rate in man. *Cardiovasc Res*. 1970;4:160-167.
104. Raviele A, Di Pede F, Zanocco A, et al. [Predictive value of the ajmaline test in dysfunction of the sinus node. Prospective 4-year follow-up relative to 77 patients]. *G Ital Cardiol*. 1985;15:751-760.
105. Raviele A, Di Pede F, Callegari E, Delise P, Piccolo E. [Ajmaline test for the evaluation of sinus node function in man (author's transl)]. *G Ital Cardiol*. 1981;11:1669-1683.
106. Arnold JM, McDevitt DG. Reflex vagal withdrawal and the hemodynamic response to intravenous isoproterenol in the presence of beta-antagonists. *Clin Pharmacol Ther*. 1986;40:199-208.
107. Arnold JM, McDevitt DG. Vagal activity is increased during intravenous isoprenaline infusion in man. *Br J Clin Pharmacol*. 1984;18:311-316.
108. Hariman RJ, Gomes JA, El-Sherif N. Catecholamine-dependent atrioventricular nodal reentrant tachycardia. *Circulation*. 1983;67:681-686.
109. Hatzinikolaou H, Rodriguez LM, Smeets JL, et al. Isoprenaline and inducibility of atrioventricular nodal reentrant tachycardia. *Heart*. 1998;79:165-168.
110. Yu WC, Chen SA, Chiang CE, et al. Effects of isoproterenol in facilitating induction of slow-fast atrioventricular nodal reentrant tachycardia. *Am J Cardiol*. 1996;78:1299-1302.
111. Szabo TS, Klein GJ, Sharma AD, Yee R, Milstein S. Usefulness of isoproterenol during atrial fibrillation in evaluation of asymptomatic Wolff–Parkinson–White pattern. *Am J Cardiol*. 1989;63:187-192.
112. Yamamoto T, Yeh SJ, Lin FC, Wu DL. Effects of isoproterenol on accessory pathway conduction in intermittent or concealed Wolff–Parkinson–White syndrome. *Am J Cardiol*. 1990;65:1438-1442.
113. Charme G, Seguel M, Gonzalez R. [Clinical and electrophysiological characteristics of patients with atrioventricular nodal reentry tachycardia who underwent slow pathway ablation]. *Rev Med Chil*. 2003;131:1237-1242.
114. Doppalapudi H, Yamada T, Ramaswamy K, Ahn J, Kay GN. Idiopathic focal epicardial ventricular tachycardia originating from the crux of the heart. *Heart Rhythm*. 2009;6:44-50.
115. Mizusawa Y, Sakurada H, Nishizaki M, Ueda-Tatsumoto A, Fukamizu S, Hiraoka M. Characteristics of bundle branch reentrant ventricular tachycardia with a right bundle branch block configuration: feasibility of atrial pacing. *Europace*. 2009;11:1208-1213.
116. Yamawake N, Nishizaki M, Hayashi T, et al. Autonomic and pharmacological responses of idiopathic ventricular tachycardia arising from the left ventricular outflow tract. *J Cardiovasc Electrophysiol*. 2007;18:1161-1166.
117. Brembilla-Perrot B, Donetti J, de la Chaise AT, Sadoul N, Aliot E, Juilliere Y. Diagnostic value of ventricular stimulation in patients with idiopathic dilated cardiomyopathy. *Am Heart J*. 1991;121:1124-1131.
118. Neuss H, Schlepper M, Spies HF. Effects of heart rate and atropine on 'dual AV conduction'. *Br Heart J*. 1975;37:1216-1227.
119. Akhtar M, Damato AN, Batsford WP, et al. Induction of atrioventricular nodal reentrant tachycardia after atropine. Report of five cases. *Am J Cardiol*. 1975;36:286-291.
120. Gerstenfeld EP, Callans DJ, Dixit S, Zado E, Marchlinski FE. Incidence and location of focal atrial fibrillation triggers in patients undergoing repeat pulmonary vein isolation: implications for ablation strategies. *J Cardiovasc Electrophysiol*. 2003;14:685-690.
121. Verma A, Kilicaslan F, Pisano E, et al. Response of atrial fibrillation to pulmonary vein antrum isolation is directly related to resumption and delay of pulmonary vein conduction. *Circulation*. 2005;112:627-635.
122. Cappato R, Negroni S, Pecora D, et al. Prospective assessment of late conduction recurrence across radiofrequency lesions producing electrical disconnection at the pulmonary vein ostium in patients with atrial fibrillation. *Circulation*. 2003;108:1599-1604.
123. Arentz T, Macle L, Kalusche D, et al. "Dormant" pulmonary vein conduction revealed by adenosine after ostial radiofrequency catheter ablation. *J Cardiovasc Electrophysiol*. 2004;15:1041-1047.
124. Hachiya H, Hirao K, Takahashi A, et al. Clinical implications of reconnection between the left atrium and isolated pulmonary veins provoked by adenosine triphosphate after extensive encircling pulmonary vein isolation. *J Cardiovasc Electrophysiol*. 2007;18:392-398.
125. Matsuo S, Yamane T, Date T, et al. Reduction of AF recurrence after pulmonary vein isolation by eliminating ATP-induced transient venous re-conduction. *J Cardiovasc Electrophysiol*. 2007;18:704-708.
126. Lerman BB, Belardinelli L. Cardiac electrophysiology of adenosine. Basic and clinical concepts. *Circulation*. 1991;83:1499-1509.
127. Miyazaki S, Takahashi Y, Fujii A, Takahashi A. Adenosine triphosphate exposes multiple extra pulmonary vein foci of atrial fibrillation. *Int J Cardiol*. 2011;148(2):249-250.
128. Haïssaguerre M, Jaïs P, Shah DC, et al. Right and left atrial radiofrequency catheter therapy of paroxysmal atrial fibrillation. *J Cardiovasc Electrophysiol*. 1996;7:1132-1144.
129. Haïssaguerre M, Jaïs P, Shah DC, et al. Spontaneous initiation of atrial fibrillation by ectopic beats originating in the pulmonary veins. *N Engl J Med*. 1998;339:659-666.

130. Hwang C, Wu TJ, Doshi RN, Peter CT, Chen PS. Vein of Marshall cannulation for the analysis of electrical activity in patients with focal atrial fibrillation. *Circulation*. 2000; 101:1503-1505.
131. Lin WS, Tai CT, Hsieh MH, et al. Catheter ablation of paroxysmal atrial fibrillation initiated by non-pulmonary vein ectopy. *Circulation*. 2003;107:3176-3183.
132. Crawford T, Chugh A, Good E, et al. Clinical value of non-inducibility by high-dose isoproterenol versus rapid atrial pacing after catheter ablation of paroxysmal atrial fibrillation. *J Cardiovasc Electrophysiol*. 2009. 2010;21(1):13-20.
133. Marchlinski FE, Callans D, Dixit S, et al. Efficacy and safety of targeted focal ablation versus PV isolation assisted by magnetic electroanatomic mapping. *J Cardiovasc Electrophysiol*. 2003;14:358-365.
134. Lee SH, Tai CT, Hsieh MH, et al. Predictors of non-pulmonary vein ectopic beats initiating paroxysmal atrial fibrillation: implication for catheter ablation. *J Am Coll Cardiol*. 2005; 46:1054-1059.
135. Arora R, Verheule S, Scott L, et al. Arrhythmogenic substrate of the pulmonary veins assessed by high-resolution optical mapping. *Circulation*. 2003;107:1816-1821.
136. Van Wagoner DR, Pond AL, Lamorgese M, Rossie SS, McCarthy PM, Nerbonne JM. Atrial L-type Ca^{2+} currents and human atrial fibrillation. *Circ Res*. 1999;85:428-436.
137. Chou CC, Nihei M, Zhou S, et al. Intracellular calcium dynamics and anisotropic reentry in isolated canine pulmonary veins and left atrium. *Circulation*. 2005;111:2889-2897.
138. Chen YJ, Chen SA, Chen YC, Yeh HI, Chang MS, Lin CI. Electrophysiology of single cardiomyocytes isolated from rabbit pulmonary veins: implication in initiation of focal atrial fibrillation. *Basic Res Cardiol*. 2002;97:26-34.
139. Po SS, Scherlag BJ, Yamanashi WS, et al. Experimental model for paroxysmal atrial fibrillation arising at the pulmonary vein-atrial junctions. *Heart Rhythm*. 2006;3:201-208.
140. Scherlag BJ, Patterson E, Po SS. The neural basis of atrial fibrillation. *J Electrocardiol*. 2006;39:S180-S183.
141. Singh SM, D'Avila A, Kim SJ, Houghtaling C, Dukkipati SR, Reddy VY. Intraprocedural use of ibutilide to organize and guide ablation of complex fractionated atrial electrograms: preliminary assessment of a modified step-wise approach to ablation of persistent atrial fibrillation. *J Cardiovasc Electrophysiol*. 2009. 2010;21(6):608-616.

CHAPTER 25

Clinical Pharmacology of Anesthetic Agents and Their Application in Cardiac Electrophysiologic Procedures

Jun Lin, MD, PhD; David G. Benditt, MD; Fei Lü, MD, PhD

Introduction

Invasive cardiac electrophysiologic (EP) procedures and device implantation cause anxiety, discomfort, and pain. It is essential to perform such procedures under adequate sedation or anesthesia for patient comfort and safety. Although many procedures can be successfully performed under local anesthesia with conscious sedation, general anesthesia (defined as a reversible state of unconsciousness, amnesia, and analgesia) is often required in certain clinical settings. Typical examples of such settings include intense discomfort or pain associated with extensive surgery, very young and uncooperative patients, or prolonged procedures requiring patients to remain relatively still.

Depending on the nature of the procedure and the patient's level of cooperation, one of following anesthesia techniques, or a combination of techniques, may be used: (1) infiltration anesthesia with local anesthetics; (2) sedation at various depths with intravenous sedatives; and (3) general anesthesia with or without airway instrumentation. However, it is important to recognize that the level of sedation/anesthesia is continuous. An individual patient may have an exaggerated response to sedatives and may unexpectedly progress to the next anesthesia depth, requiring support for ventilation or airway manipulation. Therefore, it is important to monitor the patient's mental, respiratory, and hemodynamic status carefully during the procedure, and to have rescue medications, equipment, and personnel ready if needed.

The goal of clinical pharmacology in anesthesia is to offer an individualized regimen of anesthetics to achieve a desired depth of anesthesia adequate for the procedure without causing adverse effects. A thorough understanding of the pharmacology of anesthetics is essential to help prudent selection and dosing of anesthetic medications. The suggested anesthetic dosages to achieve a desired effect are usually derived from animal studies and clinical trials. Since anesthetics typically have a narrow therapeutic window, dose titration is required based upon the patient's response. The patient's sensitivity to anesthetics varies with age, body weight, composition, genetics, medical condition, and concomitant use of other medications. Unexpected sedative effect may occur at an apparently lower dose of an individual anesthetic.

Pharmacokinetic information provides guidance for selection and dosing of anesthetics. For example, the anticipated peak effect of midazolam is 9 minutes after intravenous bolus, while propofol and etomidate have peak action at approximately 2 minutes.[1] It may be prudent to bolus another dose of propofol after 3 minutes if the desired sedation is not achieved by the initial bolus. Conversely, it may not be appropriate to try to achieve the desired sedation by giving additional dose of midazolam at 3 minutes since it has not exerted its maximal effect yet; otherwise, oversedation may occur later.

Context-sensitive half-life is a useful parameter for predicting the duration of drug effects after cessation of a continuous infusion. Context-sensitive half-life is defined as the time taken for blood plasma concentration of a drug to decline by one half after an infusion designed to maintain a steady state (ie, a constant plasma concentration) has been stopped. The "context" here is referred to the duration of infusion. Context-sensitive half-life is generally a function of duration of infusion unless the drug is rapidly inactivated by metabolism. For example, remifentanil has a context-sensitive half-life of 3–4 minutes regardless of its duration of infusion.[2,3] Duration of anesthetic action following multiple small-dose boluses can also be estimated using the same concept and parameter of context-sensitive half-life.

In typical anesthetic practice, drug concentration in the blood in a particular patient is not known. A practical estimation is usually based on the typical pharmacokinetics of a given drug and its modifying factors that influence blood concentration in an individual patient. For intravenous administration, it can be considered that the drug is completely absorbed. Plasma protein binding, hepatic metabolism, and renal secretion are usually the main modifying factors. Variation of protein binding in plasma will result in alteration of available drug in the target tissue, since only the unbound drug can cross into the target tissues. Most anesthetics are metabolized in the liver and eliminated by the kidneys. The liver has a large functional reservoir for drug metabolism. However, it is difficult to evaluate the effect of liver disease on how a given drug metabolizes. If a drug is mainly metabolized and cleared by the liver, its dosage should be adjusted accordingly in the presence of significant hepatic dysfunction. Hepatic clearance capacity will be decreased when hepatic blood flow is reduced under certain circumstances, such as in congestive heart failure[4] or under inhalation agents,[5] but opioids and barbiturates do not seem to markedly affect hepatic blood flow.[6]

In patients with renal impairment, the dosing regimen also needs to be modified since intrinsic renal clearance is reduced. Endogenous creatinine clearance is commonly used to estimate renal function. Similar to the liver, reduction in renal blood flow also decreases renal clearance.[7]

Since it is rare to use only a single drug in anesthesia practice, the interactions among anesthetics need to be considered. Often, several anesthetics used in combination produce a synergistic response, which may achieve the desired state of anesthesia. Further attention also needs to be paid to the interaction between anesthetics and existing medications that the patient is taking prior to the procedure.

Local Anesthetics

Local anesthesia is frequently employed during invasive EP procedures without the need for general anesthesia. Even for patients receiving general anesthesia, local anesthesia may also be beneficial by providing postprocedure pain control. Most EP procedures can be accomplished with infiltration anesthesia using a local anesthetic combined with a desired level of sedation, that is, mild, moderate, or deep sedation. To use these local anesthetics effectively and safely, it is important to understand their pharmacological actions, pharmacokinetic properties, and toxic effects.

Classification

All the local anesthetics contain a hydrophilic domain and a hydrophobic domain. Local anesthetics are chemically divided into two categories based on the linkage between these two domains: ester and amide. Both ester and amide local anesthetics share similar mechanisms of action, pharmacological effects, and toxicity profiles. Ester linkage is hydrolyzed by serum pseudocholinesterase.[8] Patients with esterase deficiency or abnormal pseudocholinesterase will have a prolonged duration of action with ester local anesthetics and therefore be prone to local anesthetic toxicity. Paraaminobenzoic acid, a primary metabolite of procaine, has been implicated in local anesthetic allergic reaction. Metabolism of amide local anesthetics does not produce paraaminobenzoic acid. Therefore, allergies to amide local anesthetics are extremely rare.

Mechanism

Local anesthetics block the generation and propagation of nerve impulses along nerve axons, resulting in loss of sensation. The primary mechanism responsible for nerve block is intracellular blockage of voltage-gated sodium channel, preventing sodium influx during depolarization.[9,10] In addition, local anesthetics also affect other ion channels and cellular metabolism. This may account for their effects other than inhibition of nerve conductance.

Selection of Local Anesthetics

Selection of local anesthetics for infiltration anesthesia depends on onset, duration, and safety needs. The formulation suitable for injection is usually in a hydrochloride salt. Local infiltration with local anesthetics should be given in advance to allow local infiltration to take effect before incision or puncture is made. Most local anesthetics have a rapid onset for infiltrative anesthesia. Chroprocaine is probably the fastest agent, particularly when mixed with 8.4% sodium bicarbonate (10:1 volume). Lidocaine will take effect in 1 minute for local infiltration. If a large volume is needed, lidocaine can be diluted to 0.5%, which is effective for local infiltration. Sodium bicarbonate can be added to lidocaine to reduce pain associated with injection and to speed onset of action.[11] The onset of bupivacaine and ropivacaine is within 3–5 minutes. Tetracaine has the slowest onset (approximately 15 minutes) for infiltrative anesthesia. If rapid onset is desired, selection of fast-acting local anesthetic such as chloroprocaine or lidocaine is preferred. Chloroprocaine has the shortest duration of action, lasting 15–30 minutes. Lidocaine has a longer duration of action, lasting 30–90 minutes. Bupivacaine and ropivacaine last more than 2 hours.[12] The dose and potential toxicity should be monitored, and rescue equipment and medications should be readily available.

Chloroprocaine

Chloroprocaine (trade name of Nesacaine) is an ester local anesthetic. Chloroprocaine constricts blood vessels, which may be desirable for use on the surgical field to minimize bleeding. Chloroprocaine is rapidly metabolized by ester hydrolysis with a half-life of 45 seconds in the serum, and thus has low systemic toxicity.[13,14] Procaine (0.25%–0.5%) is another ester local anesthetic that was widely used in the past.

Lidocaine

Lidocaine (Figure 25.1) is an amide local anesthetic and is widely used clinically in various concentrations (0.5% to 2%) with or without epinephrine (1:50,000–1:200,000). Epinephrine delays the absorption of lidocaine, prolongs the duration of action, and potentiates the effects of lidocaine. When using the preparation containing epinephrine, its onset of action is slower because a more acidic environment is needed for the stability of epinephrine, which increases the proportion of the ionized form of lidocaine. Since systemic absorption of epinephrine can cause tachycardia and hypertension, application of epinephrine must be considered carefully in severely ill cardiac patients. Development of local anesthetic toxicity depends on not only the total dose given, but also the speed of systemic absorption and metabolism. Direct intravascular injection can be avoided by periodic aspiration during injection to ensure that the injecting needle has not entered a blood vessel. The maximum dose of lidocaine for nerve block (including local infiltration) is 4.5 mg/kg; when administered with epinephrine, it is 7 mg/kg.[13,14]

Lidocaine may also be used for intravenous administration as an antiarrhythmic agent, although this application is far less frequent than was the case 30 to 40 years ago. Furthermore, there has been a considerable interest in novel applications of lidocaine at antiarrhythmic doses for neuroprotection, anti-inflammation, and neuropathic pain.[15]

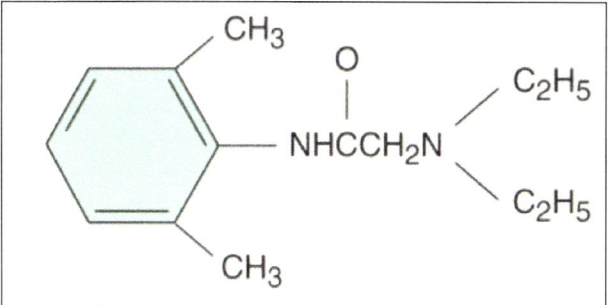

Figure 25.1 Molecular structure of lidocaine.

Lidocaine is considered safe at antiarrhythmic doses. However, overdose of lidocaine during infiltration anesthesia can occur when it is accidentally injected directly into the vascular system or by rapid injection into vessel-rich tissues, leading to systemic toxicity. Toxicities may be observed at 6 mcg/mL, but more commonly occur once levels exceed 10 mcg/mL. Lidocaine toxicity related to central nervous system dysfunction usually occurs prior to cardiovascular symptoms. Early neurological symptoms include dizziness, perioral and tongue numbness, muscle twitching, tinnitus, and blurred vision. Depression of cerebral function results in drowsiness, respiratory depression, obtundation, and coma. Blockage of selective inhibitory neurotransmission may lead to excitatory events such as agitation and seizure.[14] Convulsive activity may occur when reaching arterial blood levels of 18–21 mcg/mL. Fast-acting midazolam can be used to prevent or treat lidocaine-induced seizure since benzodiazepine increases the seizure threshold. Lidocaine-induced seizure activity can also be terminated with fast-acting barbiturate thiopental or propofol. It is vital to establish adequate oxygenation and ventilation for preventing hypoxic injury. Hemodynamic support may be needed. Lidocaine, like other local anesthetics, can depress cardiac contractility and may lead to cardiovascular collapse at high concentrations.[14]

Mepivacaine, similar to lidocaine in structure and in pharmacological properties, has a slightly faster onset and longer action duration.[16]

Bupivacaine, a long-acting amide local anesthetic, has been shown to inhibit the mitochondrial enzyme carnitine-acylcarnitine translocase and alter mitochondrial oxidative function.[17] Its high affinity to myocardium also contributes to the potential for cardiac toxicity. Intravascular injection of bupivacaine can induce severe cardiac arrhythmias, conduction block, and eventually ventricular fibrillation and asystole. Hypoxia and acidosis predispose local anesthetic toxicity and worsen resuscitation outcome.[14,18] Avoidance of intravascular injection, adherence to the maximal dose, and injection in divided doses help in prevention of local anesthetic toxicity. The maximal dose of bupivacaine is 3 mg/kg. Unlike lidocaine, bupivacaine's absorption and duration are not significantly affected by epinephrine.

Bupivacaine-induced cardiac toxicity may last for a prolonged time period. Treatment of bupivacaine cardiac toxicity may prove to be difficult. Adequate ventilation and oxygenation should be established immediately by securing the airway with tracheal intubation. Metabolic acidosis should be corrected. The cardiopulmonary bypass team should be alerted because cardiopulmonary bypass may be considered. Early application of lipid emulsion infusion in treatment of bupivacaine cardiac toxicity has been reported in multiple case studies.[19,20] Intralipid is the most commonly reported lipid emulsion, containing mostly long-chain triglycerides.[21] The regimen consists of an intravenous bolus at 1.5 mL/kg, followed by continuous infusion at 0.25 mL/kg/min for at least 10 minutes after resuming stability. Repeat bolus once or twice may be needed for persistent cardiovascular collapse. Recommended upper dose limit is approximately 10 mL/kg over the first 30 minutes. Patient's hemodynamic status should be monitored for at least 12 hours with additional lipid emulsion available.

Ropivacaine is a single (S)-stereoisomer, which is different from bupivacaine as a racemic mixture of (R)- and (S)-stereoisomers. It has the similar onset time and duration as bupivacaine. Its potency is slightly lower than bupivacaine, and it tends to have fewer motor-blocking effects. Ropivacaine has less cardiac toxicity than bupivacaine but still may cause arrhythmia at high concentrations.[14,22]

Intravenous Anesthetics

Intravenous anesthetics are used for sedation, analgesia, induction, or maintenance of general anesthesia. The goal of anesthesia is to provide a satisfactory surgical condition and patient comfort free of pain and anxiety. At times, amnesia is desired. Such a goal can be achieved by one or more intravenous anesthetics in addition to well-executed infiltration anesthesia.

Benzodiazepines

Benzodiazepines contain a benzene ring fused with a diazepine ring. The modification and substitution on these rings affect potency and duration. The effects of benzodiazepine include anxiolysis, sedation, antegrade amnesia, muscle relaxation, and anticonvulsant activity. Amnesia effects of benzodiazepines are typically more potent than their sedative effects.[23] Although analgesic effects of benzodiazepine have been reported in animals, it is generally agreed that benzodiazepines lack significant analgesic properties. However, unlike barbiturates, benzodiazepines do not induce hyperalgesia.

The pharmacological effects of benzodiazepines are mediated by potentiating the gamma aminobutyric acid (GABA) neurotransmission, the most important inhibitory system in the brain. Activation of GABA-ergic transmission results in an increase of chloride channel conductance, thus preventing the neuronal discharge evoked by excitatory stimuli. Benzodiazepines, by binding to the GABA receptors/chloride channels macro-complex, prolong the duration of chloride channel activation induced by GABA-ergic transmission.[23,24] The effect is quite specific. Without the presence of GABA receptor agonist, benzodiazepines do not have significant direct effects on chloride channel activity. Therefore, benzodiazepines are considered indirect agents and have the ceiling effect on facilitating GABA-ergic mediated functions. This might explain why benzodiazepines are safer and have higher therapeutic index, compared to other sedatives, such as barbiturates and propofol.

Midazolam (Figure 25.2A) is the most often used benzodiazepine in anesthesia practice. Midazolam is water soluble in acidic solution (pH < 4) and lipid-soluble at physiologic pH as its imidazole ring closes at physiological pH. It has a rapid onset due to its lipid solubility and reaches its peak effect 9 minutes after intravenous injection. Typically, sedation is observed within 1 minute after intravenous bolus and lasts for 15–80 minutes.[23] Termination of midazolam action follows its rapid redistribution from the central nervous system to other tissues. The initial redistribution of benzodiazepines is 3–10 minutes. The elimination half-time of midazolam is 1–4 hours, which is the shortest among the various benzodiazepines. Benzodiazepines are metabolized in the liver and their metabolites are excreted by the kidneys. Renal failure decreases elimination of pharmacological active metabolite of midazolam and prolongs the duration of sedation. The metabolism of midazolam is suppressed by erythromycin, which prolongs its duration of action.

Midazolam can be administered by oral, intranasal, buccal, sublingual, intramuscular, and intravenous routes. Typically, however, it is used as an intravenous sedative, at a dose of 0.01–0.1 mg/kg. Often, it starts at 1–2 mg bolus and titrates to desired effect by incremental bolus doses of 0.5 mg to 1 mg. In elderly and ill patients, the response to sedatives may be exaggerated. Consequently, a reduced initial dose and careful titration to desired effect is recommended.[25] It is important to keep in mind that appropriate dose and level of sedation should be maintained to avoid confusion. Disinhibition of certain brain areas by blockage of selective inhibitory neurotransmission may result in agitation, which is not uncommon and usually occurs after using midazolam for a while. Management of midazolam-induced agitation requires holding midazolam, or administrating nonbenzodiazepine sedatives (such as a small dose of propofol), or both.

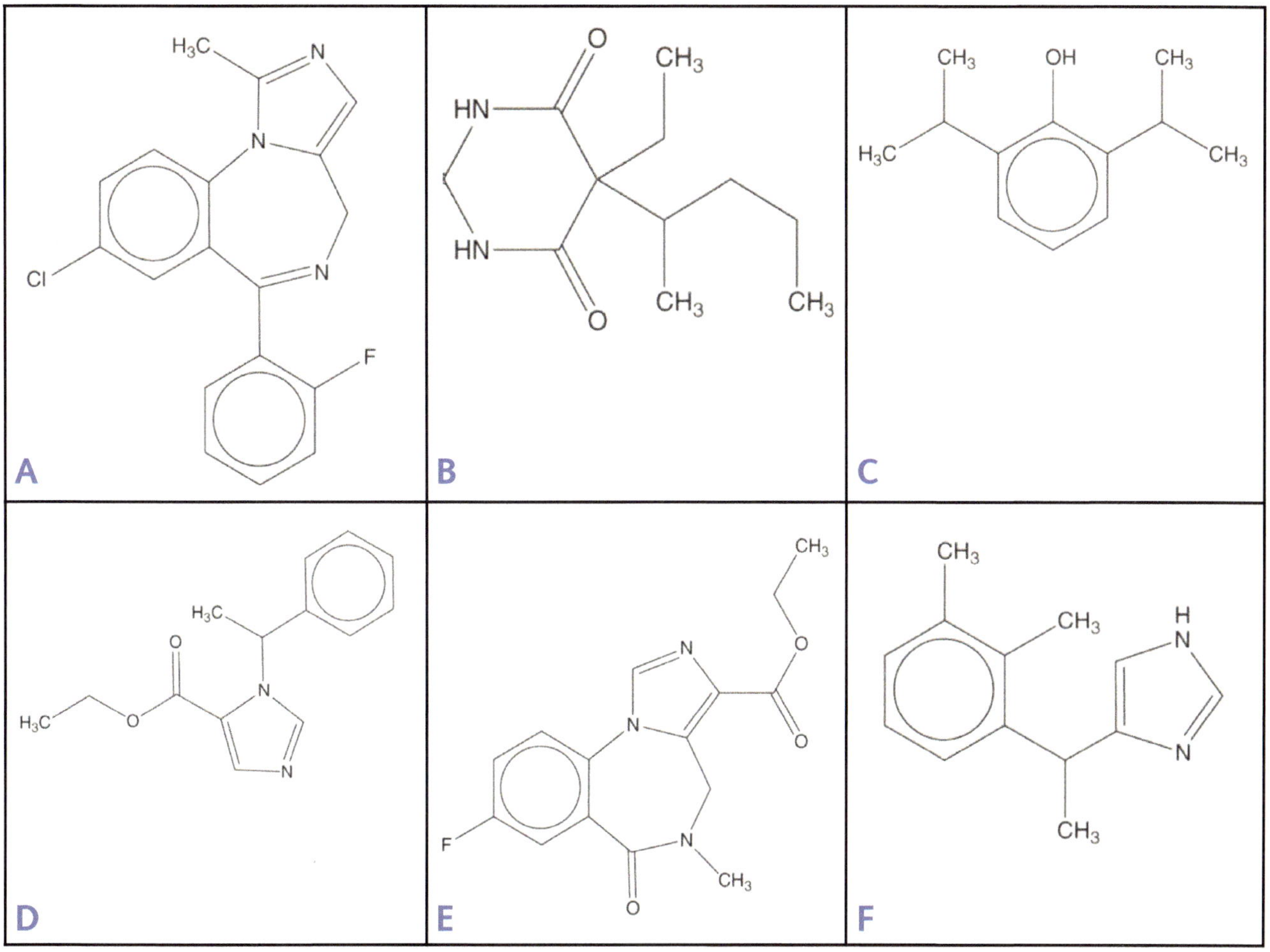

Figure 25.2 Structures of midazolam (**A**), thiopental (**B**), propofol (**C**), etomidate (**D**), ketamine (**E**), and dexmedetomidine (**F**).

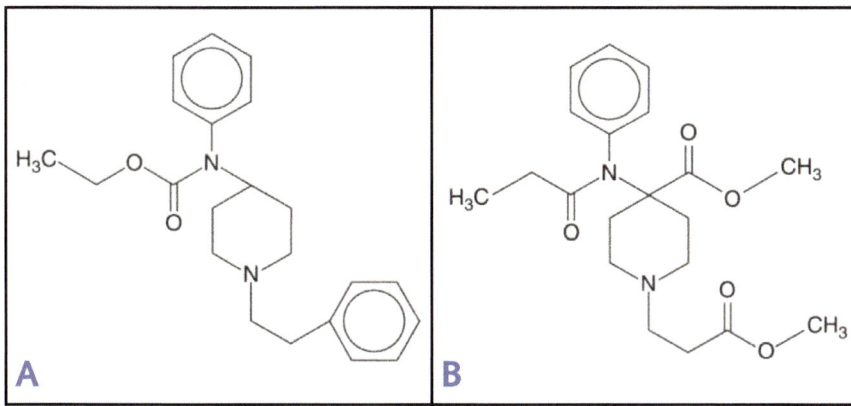

Figure 25.3 Structures of fentanyl (**A**) and remifentanyl (**B**).

Benzodiazepines have minimal effects on the cardiovascular system in therapeutic doses. Midazolam may cause vagolysis with resultant tachycardia and decrease of heart rate variability.[26] It tends to have a more profound depressing effect on cardiac output and peripheral vascular resistance than other benzodiazepines. Intravenous administration of potent benzodiazepines such as midazolam inhibits respiratory drive and may lead to apnea.

Careful monitoring of respiration and oxygenation is essential to prevent hypoxia. Benzodiazepines have synergistic effects with other sedatives and central nervous system depressants. Adjustment of dosage should be made when used in combination to avoid oversedation and respiratory arrest. Benzodiazepines potentiate the respiratory depressant effect of opioids but reduce their analgesic effects. When analgesic effect is sought, benzodiazepines should be kept to a minimal effective dose while allowing a higher dose of other anesthetic.

Diazepam is a common benzodiazepine administered orally. It is not as popular as midazolam in acute anesthesia care. Diazepam is well absorbed in the gastrointestinal tract, with peak plasma concentration in 1–2 hours. It is highly lipid-soluble and thus has a rapid onset and redistribution. After intravenous administration, the onset of sedation is usually observed in 1 minute, with the duration of 1–4 hours. Pharmacological active metabolites of diazepam are secreted in the biliary system and undergo the enterohepatic circulation, and may result in prolonged sedation. Desmethyldiazepam is a long-acting metabolite of diazepam, which may cause resedation and lead to a reduction of liver clearance of diazepam. The histamine H_2 antagonist cimetidine binds with the liver enzyme and decreases the metabolism and elimination of diazepam.[27] Diazepam has an elimination half-time of 20–35 hours. Heparin competes with plasma protein binding sites with diazepam, and increases diazepam free drug concentration.[28]

Lorazepam is a potent and long-acting benzodiazepine. Patients undergoing cardiac interventional procedure may have received lorazepam before arrival in the procedure suite. It has a slower onset and longer duration than midazolam and diazepam.[29] Lorazepam reaches its peak effect in 20–30 minutes, and duration of sedation ranges from 6 to 10 hours. After a single bolus injection of 3 mg lorazepam, it takes approximately 55 minutes to have significant sedation effect. Because of its pharmacokinetic property of slow onset and long duration, lorazepam is rarely used in the acute anesthetic care.

Benzodiazepine Antagonist

Flumazenil is a competitive benzodiazepine antagonist. It can be used to reverse the sedative or cardiac and respiratory depressing effects of benzodiazepines. Typically, it is administered as intravenous bolus at 0.2–1.0 mg, and up to 3 mg per hour. Flumazenil has rapid onset in 1–2 minutes, with peak effect in 10 minutes, and lasts 45–90 minutes. After flumazenil is metabolized to inactive products in the liver, resedation with a longer acting benzodiazepine is possible. When resedation occurs, flumazenil infusion may be required. If a patient does not respond to a total dose of 5 mg flumazenil, other causes of excessive sedation and respiratory depression must be considered and investigated.

Barbiturates

Barbiturates inhibit the neural transmission in the reticular activating system in the brain stem, which is vital for consciousness. Unlike benzodiazepine, barbiturates affect multiple neurotransmitter receptors on synapses, including GABA receptor complex, nicotinic acetylcholine receptors, adenosine receptors, α-amino-3-hydroxy-5-methyl-4-isoxazolepropionic acid (AMPA), and kainite receptors.[30,31] The relevancy of each receptor to their clinical effects is less clear. Their effects on the GABA receptor complex are both direct and indirect. At low concentrations, barbiturates enhance GABA action and increase frequency of chloride channel opening; at higher concentrations, they exert a direct effect, increasing chloride channel conductance. Their multiple involvements in the neurotransmission system probably explain why barbiturates have broader pharmacological effects and a lower therapeutic window than benzodiazepines.

Modifications of barbituric acid produce barbiturates with different lipid solubilities and pharmacological profiles. Highly lipid-soluble thiopental (Figure 25.2B) and methohexital have been used as induction agents of general anesthesia. Their onsets are within 30–60 seconds and durations are short due to rapid redistribution from the brain to other tissues in several minutes. The elimination half-life of thiopental is about 6 hours and is affected by body composition. If the peripheral tissues are saturated with thiopental, the duration of its effect will depend on the rate of elimination. The induction dose for thiopental is 2–5 mg/kg, and the sedative dose is 0.5–1.5 mg/kg.

Methohexital, metabolized 3 to 4 times faster than thiopental in the liver, is a more desired agent for sedation (0.2–0.4 mg/kg). Methohexital can be used for intravenous induction agent at 1–2 mg/kg. It can also be used for rectal induction in children. Thiopental at 50–100 mg intravenously can control most grand mal seizures.

Barbiturates typically depress respiratory drive and can cause upper airway obstruction. Apnea can be expected at induction dose. The effects of barbiturates on the cardiovascular system are dose-dependent and varying, depending on the baseline volume status, cardiac function, and sympathetic tone.[32] Typically, thiopental at induction dose results in peripheral vasodilation, decreased cardiac contractility, and inhibition of baroreceptor reflex. Tachycardia may be reflective or from a central vagolytic effect. In addition to the effects of sedatives and anesthetics, significant hypotension is usually associated with hypovolemia, significant heart disease, and beta-adrenergic blockage. Barbiturates constrict cerebral vasculature, decrease intracranial pressure, and protect the brain from transient focal ischemia episodes, possibly by reducing local metabolism.

Barbiturates do not have analgesic effect. In contrast, some can lower pain threshold. Methohexital causes involuntary muscle contraction, which may interfere with the ECG interpretation. Barbiturates are contraindicated in patients with porphyria due to its induction of the synthetic enzyme for porphyrin. Chronic use of barbiturates, as in patients with chronic seizure disorder, induces hepatic metabolic enzymes, which may affect the biotransformation of some drugs.

Propofol

Propofol (Figure 25.2C) has gained popularity in anesthesia practice and has replaced barbiturates for induction of general anesthesia and intravenous sedation. Propofol is a 2,6-diisopropylphenol compound containing a phenol ring with 2 isopropyl groups. Propofol has similar pharmacological effects with thiopental, such as sedation, hypnosis, anticonvulsion, and neuroprotection. It is also a potent respiratory and cardiovascular depressant.[33] Unlike barbiturates, it has amnesia effects at sedative dose[34] and is an antiemetic.[35] Its primary mechanism is considered by potentiating brain GABA transmission,[36] and inhibition of N-methyl-D-aspartic acid (NMDA) receptor.[37]

The most widely available propofol formulation contains soybean oil, glycerol, and egg lecithin in the aqueous solution. The egg lecithin is from egg yolk and mostly does not have an allergic cross-reaction in patients with egg albumin allergy. This formulation causes pain or burning sensation during injection, which may be ameliorated by prior lidocaine injection. The formulation of propofol supports bacterial growth. Therefore, a sterile technique should be followed and the medication should be discarded within 6 hours after the vial is opened.

Propofol is highly lipid-soluble, which accounts for its rapid onset and redistribution similar to thiopental. Clinical experience shows that awakening from propofol seems more rapid and pleasant than awakening from barbiturates. Propofol is only available for intravenous administration. It is rapidly metabolized in the liver and the lungs to inactive metabolites that are secreted by the kidneys. Moderate cirrhosis and renal failure do not seem to affect the duration of propofol action.

Induction dose is recommended at 1.5–2 mg/kg and sedation at 25–100 mcg/kg/min. Contex-sensitive half-life for propofol is duration-dependent: 15 minutes after a 2-hour infusion and 20 minutes after a 4-hour infusion. Propofol has wide interindividual variability in its pharmacological effect. In different procedures, the requirement for propofol concentration varies greatly. It should be appreciated that upper airway obstruction often occurs during sedation with propofol, requiring airway manipulation by anesthesia providers.

Inasmuch as propofol induces profound cardiovascular depression, its administration should be started at a small dose and titrated on an individual basis with careful hemodynamic monitoring. This is particularly important in elderly cardiac patients. Propofol can significantly decrease blood pressure by depressing myocardial contractility and reducing systemic vascular resistance and preload. Profound hypotension can occur after an induction dose of propofol in patients of extreme age, patients who have hypovolemia or poor ventricular function, or patients who are being treated with negative ionotropic medications or vasodilating medications, such as angiotensin converting enzyme (ACE) inhibitors.[38] Marked reduction of preload by propofol may trigger or induce vagally-mediated bradycardia, which can occasionally lead to asystole. Slow administration of small divided doses is essential to successfully use propofol for sedation or general anesthesia in critically ill patients. Patience should be exercised because the onset time is prolonged when there is a longer circulation time, such as in patients with reduced cardiac output.

Propofol may inhibit spontaneous ventricular arrhythmias. This may be undesirable when the presence of sufficient frequent ventricular arrhythmias is required for activation mapping and ablation in the EP laboratory.

Etomidate

Etomidate (Figure 25.2D) selectively enhances GABAergic neurotransmission and increases the affinity of GABA receptors.[39] It is a carboxylated imidazole compound, supplied in propylene or emulsion for intravenous use as it is unstable in water. Injection may be painful and can be ameliorated by prior lidocaine administration. It is highly lipid-soluble at physiologic pH and thus has rapid onset and redistribution. Etomidate is metabolized by the liver and the plasma esterases to inactive metabolites, which are secreted by the kidneys. Etomidate is mainly used for induction of general anesthesia (0.2–0.4 mg/kg).

Generally, etomidate has minimal effect on hemodynamics. A mild reduction in peripheral vascular resistance may occur, while myocardial performance is usually not affected. Etomidate has less depressing effect on respiratory drive than thiopental or propofol and may not induce apnea, even at induction dose. This is a favorable property when brief general anesthesia is required and airway manipulation is to be avoided, such as for cardioversion.

Like thiopental, etomidate does not have analgesic effect, and can cause nausea and vomiting which may be prevented by administration of antiemetic drugs. Etomidate has > 30% incidence of myoclonus, due to disinhibition of the extrapyramidal system. Myoclonic movements can affect recording and interpretation of ECG, which may not be desirable for cardiac EP procedures. Otherwise, etomidate is an attractive choice for general anesthesia in severely ill cardiac patients because of its minimal cardiovascular effects. Induction dose of etomidate suppresses cortisol and aldosterone synthesis for up to 5–8 hours, which probably does not have significant clinical consequence.[39] However, long-term infusion of etomidate may causes prolonged adrenal suppression and should be avoided.

Ketamine

Ketamine (Figure 25.2E) is structurally related to phencyclidine and retains phencyclidine's psychotomimetic effects with a fraction of potency. Ketamine is an NMDA receptor antagonist and suppresses brain excitatory neurotransmission in some brain areas.[40] Ketamine increases cerebral oxygen consumption, cerebral blood flow, and intracranial pressure. Its psychological effects include hallucinations, illusions, delirium, and disturbing dreams, which may be attenuated by prior administration of benzodiazepine.

Ketamine produces dissociative anesthesia: the patient may appear to be awake with eye opening, muscle movement, and swallowing, but is unable to respond to verbal or sensory stimuli. Dissociative anesthesia may be due to multiple actions. Ketamine inhibition of the communication between the thalamus and the limbic cortex is probably the main mechanism of action.

Since ketamine has an intense analgesic effect with minimal effect on ventilation, it seems to be a good choice for the invasive procedure under local or regional anesthesia without instrumentation of airway. However, ketamine stimulates centrally sympathetic discharge and inhibits reuptake of norepinephrine, results in an elevated level of available catecholamine, and consequently increases heart rate, cardiac output, blood pressure, and myocardial oxygen consumption. These are generally not desirable in the elderly cardiac patient. Because it offers analgesia, amnesia, and unconsciousness at the same time, a small dose of ketamine may be considered in the absence of severe coronary artery disease and pulmonary hypertension. If catecholamine is depleted in a severely ill patient, however, ketamine's direct cardiovascular depressant effect may be unmasked.

Ketamine can be administered as an induction agent intravenously (1–2 mg/kg) or intramuscularly (3–5 mg/kg). The onset and awakening are rapid after intravenous administration, due to its high lipid solubility and rapid redistribution. Peak plasma concentration can be expected in 10–15 minutes following intramuscular injection. Sedation can be achieved by intravenous bolus at 10–25 mg. Ketamine is taken up and metabolized in the liver, resulting in active and inactive products that are secreted by the kidneys. Its elimination half-life is approximately 2 hours.

Excessive saliva secretion induced by ketamine is disturbing and can be reduced or prevented by glycopyurrate (0.1–0.2 mg intravenously) but may result in increase of heart rate. Glycopyurrate, an anticholinergic agent, can also be used to counteract drug-induced or vagal reflexes and their associated arrhythmias (eg, bradycardia).

Dexmedetomidine

Dexmedetomidine (Figure 25.2F) is a derivative of α-methylol with high affinity for α_2 receptors in the central nervous system. Like methyldopa and clonidine, dexmedetomidine decreases central sympathetic outflow and may cause bradycardia and hypotension. However, rapid administration may cause initial paradoxical hypertension, probably due to activation of α_2 receptors in peripheral vasculature. Dexmedetomidine has sedative, anxiolytic, and analgesic effects without significant respiratory depression.[40] While this sounds attractive, and it is true that dexmedetomidine may be ideal in certain situations, it is generally not an appropriate anesthetic for cardiac EP procedures because it may interfere with the diagnostic or therapeutic intervention on cardiac rhythm due to its sympatholytic property.[41]

Opioids

Opioids refer to a group of either natural or synthetic drugs with opium-like properties. Although opioids have multiple pharmacological effects, they are primarily used as analgesics. Opioids exert their pharmacological effects by activating opioid receptors, which interact with three families of endogenous ligands: endorphins, enkephalins, and dynorphins.[42] Opioid receptors are G-protein coupled receptors, which can be classified to mu (subtypes of mu-1, mu-2), kappa, delta, and sigma. Activation of opioid receptors results in alteration of potassium and calcium channel conductance, which may account for the inhibitory effects on presynaptive release of excitatory neurotransmitters from the nociceptive neurons, and the modulatory effect on postsynaptic response. Mu receptors are associated with supraspinal analgesia (mu-1), respiratory depression and bradycardia (mu-2), and physical dependence. Kappa receptor is associated with spinal analgesia and sedation. Morphine is an agonist for mu and kappa receptors.

Opioids vary in their potency and efficacy with different subtypes of opioid receptors. Commonly used opioids in clinical anesthesia practice include morphine, meperidine, fentanyl, remifentanil, and sufentanil. In addition to analgesia and sedation, opioids have other systemic effects. A high dose of opioids, including morphine, fentanyl, alfentanil, sulfentanil, causes bradycardia, venodilation, and inhibition of sympathetic reflex. Generally speaking, however, opioids do not cause significant cardiac depression, with meperidine as an exception. Meperidine causes tachycardia due to its atropine-like activity. Meperidine is often avoided because it may induce histamine release and its active metabolite is associated with seizure activity. Morphine causes histamine release with associated hypotension and bronchospasm as well but can be attenuated by slow administration or pretreated with histamine antagonists. Morphine has a slower onset and longer duration than fentanyl.

Opioids decrease respiratory rate, increase carbon dioxide apnea threshold (so higher PCO_2 is necessary to stimulate the respiration), and inhibit hypoxic drive. Opioids cause nausea and vomiting, decrease gastrointestinal movement, and induce biliary spasm. Opioids have synergistic effect with other sedatives in sedation and respiratory and cardiovascular depression. Opioids, particularly meperidine, may interact with monoamine oxidase inhibitors, resulting in hyperpyrexia and respiratory and cardiovascular collapse.

Fentanyl (Figure 25.3A) is probably the most commonly used opioid in sedation and general anesthesia for

EP procedures. It has a rapid onset and redistribution. Initial sedation in an average adult can be achieved with intravenous 25–50 mcg of fentanyl and 1–2 mg of midazolam, followed by careful titration to desired effects. Onset of fentanyl is < 1 minute. Fentanyl has other formulations for oral, transmucosal, and transdermal administrations. Alfentanil has more rapid onset and shorter duration than fentanyl. Opioids are mainly metabolized in the liver and eliminated by the kidneys. Morphine has active metabolites that may cause prolonged sedation and respiratory depression in patients with renal failure. Remifentanil (Figure 25.3B) is unique in its metabolism. It is hydrolyzed very rapidly by nonspecific esterases in the blood and tissues. Remifentanil has an ultra-short duration of action and usually is administered as continuous infusion. Its context-sensitive half-life is approximately 3–4 minutes, independent of the duration of infusion.[2,3] The context-sensitive half-life of alfentanil after 3-hour infusion becomes steady (approximately 55 minutes). The context-sensitive half-life of fentanyl or sulfentanil is also duration-dependent. After 30 minutes of infusion, the context-sensitive half-life of fentanyl is estimated to be 25 minutes, which sharply increases as the duration of infusion increases.[2] Its context-sensitive half-life will reach 100 minutes if infusion lasts 120 minutes. Context-sensitive half-life of sulfentanil is less duration driven than fentanyl, which is estimated to be 20 minutes after 120 minutes infusion, and 30 minutes after 300 minutes infusion.[2]

Muscle Relaxants

Muscle relaxant is often given to facilitate the instrumentation of airway with general anesthesia. Muscle relaxants are divided into two categories, the depolarizing muscle relaxant and the nondepolarizing muscle relaxant.

Depolarizing Muscle Relaxants

Succinylcholine is the only clinically used depolarizing muscle relaxant. It stimulates the nicotinic acetylcholine receptors on postsynaptic membrane in the neuromuscular junction, followed by muscular relaxation. Among all current clinically available muscle relaxants, succinylcholine at induction dose (1–1.5 mg/kg) has the fastest onset (20–60 seconds) and shortest duration (< 10 minutes). This is ideal in assisting rapid control of the airway. Succinylcholine increases serum potassium by 0.5–1 mEq/L in a normal subject, which should be weighted in patients with renal failure. The effect of elevated serum potassium level on cardiac electrophysiology should be kept in mind during diagnostic and therapeutic EP procedures. Life-threatening hyperkalemia can occur in patients with myopathy, spinal cord injury, neurological diseases, massive trauma and burning, and several other conditions. Succinylcholine also induces transient increases intracranial and intraocular pressures. Succinylcholine (as well as some inhalation agents) can be a trigger for malignant hyperthermia in susceptible patients. Succinylcholine is metabolized by the serum pseudocholinesterase. In patients with atypical pseudocholinesterase, the circulating succinylcholine remains intact for hours, resulting in a remarkable prolonged duration. Because of its potential severe consequences, succinylcholine should be avoided and reserved only for the most urgent situations.

Nondepolarizing Muscle Relaxants

Nondepolarizing muscle relaxants are nicotinic receptor antagonists and do not activate the receptors like succinylcholine. Therefore, they lack the severe adverse effect of succinylcholine. However, atracurium and several other nondepolarizing muscle relaxants induce histamine release, which may cause bronchospasm and hypotension. Several long-acting nondepolarizing muscle relaxants have significant effects on the autonomic nervous system. For example, pancuronium causes tachycardia by blocking muscarinic receptors in the sinus node. Rocuronium is of choice for its fastest onset (60–90 seconds) among nondepolarizing muscle relaxants. It has intermediate duration without significant effect on the cardiaovascular system.[43]

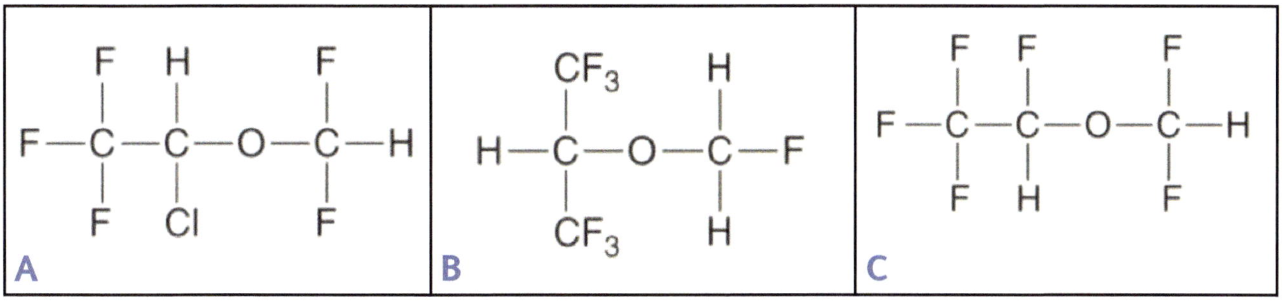

Figure 25.4   Structures of isoflurane (A), sevoflurane (B), and desflurane (C).

Inhalation Anesthetics

Inhalation anesthetic gases can be used for induction and maintenance of general anesthesia. Most commonly used inhalation gases at present are nitrous oxide and potent volatile agents, including isoflurane (Figure 25.4A), sevoflurane (Figure 25.4B), and desflurane (Figure 25.4C).

Nitrous oxide is an inorganic gas at room temperature. Its effects are a mixture of sympathetic stimulation and a direct depressing effect on the heart, such as myocardial contractility; thus, nitrous oxide often produces no significant change in cardiac output, heart rate, or blood pressure. However, the increased level of catecholamines may contribute to epinephrine-induced arrhythmia. Nitrous oxide causes pulmonary vasoconstriction and should be avoided in the patient with severe pulmonary hypertension. Nitrous oxide also mildly increases cerebral oxygen consumption and intracranial pressure.

All potent inhalation agents, more or less, depress myocardium, vascular smooth muscles, and bronchial smooth muscles, resulting in a decrease of cardiac output, vasodilation of systemic circulation, bronchodilation, and cerebral vasodilation. They also inhibit spontaneous ventilation and potentiate muscle relaxation induced by muscle relaxants.

It has been suggested that coronary artery dilation induced by isoflurane may cause coronary steal syndrome by diverting blood flow away from an obstructed artery, which may exaggerate the ischemia event.[44] Rapid increase of desflurane may result in significant sympathetic stimulation. Sevoflurane causes less change in heart rate and myocardium contractility than isoflurane and desflurane. Isoflurane, desflurane, and sevoflurane often cause QT interval prolongation with uncertain clinical significance.[45]

Interaction of Anesthetics

Generally speaking, the inhibitory effects of anesthetics on brain function, spontaneous respiration, and hemodynamic status are synergistic. When more than one anesthetic is used, adjustment of individual dose is required to avoid excessive sedation or unwanted side effects. Due to the limitation of the length of the chapter, detailed discussion of the interactions between individual anesthetics and their interactions with other medications will not be undertaken here.

Types of Anesthesia

Infiltrative Anesthesia

Local infiltration with local anesthetics is a prerequisite for invasive procedure under conscious sedation. Knowledge of sensory innervation patterns helps in achieving successful local nerve block. Dosage and toxicity of local anesthetics need to be monitored carefully. If a procedure outlasts the duration of local anesthetic, the surgical field should be reinfiltrated as needed to maintain the patient's comfort. Lidocaine is the most commonly used local anesthetic due to its fast onset of action and good cardiac safety profile. Bupivacaine is probably better avoided due to its cardiac toxicity. If used, it is prudent to have Intralipid available in enough quantity.

Conscious Sedation

Most EP procedures can be done under local infiltration with mild to moderate sedation. Synergistic effect among anesthetics should be recognized and dosing adjusted carefully. Midazolam and fentanyl are commonly used for their fast onset and titratability. It is important to maintain the patient's comfort and optimal working condition, and to avoid respiratory and hemodynamic complications by achieving an appropriate level of sedation. Communication between the anesthesiologist and the cardiologist/electrophysiologist regarding the need for the procedure and the patient's condition is essential. Propofol can be administrated for deep sedation. Propofol has very fast onset and short duration due to its rapid redistribution. Since it is a potent respiratory and cardiovascular depressant, particularly when used with other anesthetics, careful dosing and monitoring are important. A low dose of ketamine can be considered for its analgesia and minimal respiratory effect. Etomidate has a stable hemodynamic profile, but its high incidence of myoclonus and nausea make it an unpopular sedative in the EP laboratory. Providers should be trained and prepared to rescue the airway or address respiratory compromise. Emergent medications for resuscitation should be readily available when needed.

Deep Sedation

While the American Society of Anesthesiologists (ASA) defines general anesthesia as a status in which the patient is unable to make a purposeful response to an uneven, painful stimulus, deep sedation is defined as retaining the capacity to purposefully respond to painful stimulation. There is a continuum from deep sedation to general anesthesia, and the difference between them is rather vague.

A brief duration of unconsciousness can be induced by intravenous anesthetics (such as propofol) without airway intervention. For direct current (DC) cardioversion and defibrillation threshold (DFT) testing, only brief duration of unconsciousness is needed. It can be accomplished by intravenous bolus of methohexital, propofol, or etomidate. Propofol should be given at reduced and divided doses to avoid respiratory and cardiovascular compromise. The patient is given 100% oxygen before induction. Spontaneous ventilation may be maintained, but assisted or controlled ventilation by mask may be applied as indicated. Airway manipulation, such as chin lift, jaw thrust, or placement of oral or nasal airway, may be necessary to relieve airway obstruction. Endotracheal intubation and laryngeal mask airway need to be readily available to establish the airway.

General Anesthesia

When general anesthesia is required for a lengthy procedure, tracheal intubation is recommended for a secure airway. It is often difficult to access the patient's head once the procedure starts because of the draping for the procedure, resulting in a less ideal environment for intubation in the EP laboratory. Therefore, starting the case with endotracheal intubation may be a preferred choice over converting sedation to general anesthesia during the procedure. A disadvantage of laryngeal mask airway is that it is prone to be dislodged due to the frequent movement of the operating table and fluoroscope.

Before the patient is rendered unconscious by intravenous induction, he or she is asked to breathe 100% oxygen. This preoxygenation increases oxygen reserve for airway instrumentation. Tracheal intubation is then performed with a laryngoscope with a blade of choice, typically Mac #3 or 4, or Miller #2 or 3. There is an increasing trend using video laryngoscopy for tracheal intubation. Tracheal placement is confirmed by auscultation of bilateral breathing sounds and presence of end-tidal carbon dioxide. Propofol and etimidate have gained popularity as induction agents because of their rapid onset and redistribution. Fentanyl is commonly used as an adjuvant for induction. Midazolam offers anxiolytic and amnesic effect and often may be administered upon arrival in the EP laboratory. Lidocaine can be given intravenously to blunt the cardiac response to tracheal intubation. Rocuronium is a preferred muscle relaxant to facilitate the intubation though other muscle relaxants can be used. Anesthesia is usually maintained by an inhalation agent, combined with intravenous opioids such as fentanyl.

Anesthesia Considerations for EP Procedures

Prudent selection and dosing of anesthetics requires knowledge of the clinical pharmacology of anesthetics. Proper assessment and preparation of the patient before procedures, appropriate monitoring techniques, and available rescue equipment and resources are important to successfully execute anesthesia for an EP procedure. EP procedures are typically performed in an EP laboratory, outside of traditional operating rooms. A close-claim analysis suggests that procedures that take place outside operating rooms tend to deviate from the standards of anesthesia practice and guidelines, which may account for the increased incidence of adverse outcomes.[46] Therefore, the same practice standards should be emphasized and applied regardless of location of procedures. It is vital that all physicians and care providers have thorough communication and understanding regarding patient condition, procedure needs, and rescue equipment and resources.

Preoperative Preparation

Anesthesia consultation is advisable for various reasons associated with patient or procedure. Patients with history of sleep apnea, difficult airway, severe lung diseases, and other significant comorbidities require the care of an anesthesiologist.[47] A complex and lengthy procedure, such as a complex ablation procedure or a difficult implantation, may need more than mild sedation. General anesthesia or deep sedation is required for certain procedures in these patients. Appropriate laboratory tests, ECG, and other necessary tests should be ordered and results reviewed. The patient's medical condition should be optimized before planned procedures if possible.

The patient should be ordered nothing by mouth (NPO) at least 6 to 8 hours before the procedure according to the ASA guidelines.[48] For patients with gastroparesis caused by diabetes mellitus and other significant systemic diseases, or by analgesics or other medications, a stricter 8-hour NPO guideline should be required. To reduce the risk of pulmonary aspiration, 2-hour fasting is required for clear liquids and 6 hours for light meals, including nonclear beverages such as milk.

β-antagonists and $α_2$ agonists should be continued to avoid withdrawal tachycardia, hypertension, and subsequent increase of myocardium oxygen consumption unless arrhythmia induction is concerned (while on β-antagonists). For patients on analgesics, it is usually easier to manage such patients with continuation of the pain therapy before the procedure.

Monitoring During Procedure

Proper monitoring of anesthetic effects is essential for a satisfactory and safe anesthesia. Anesthetics have profound and rapid effects on the central nervous system as well as on the respiratory and cardiovascular systems. The effects are often synergistic with great variability between individuals. The individual response to anesthetics usually is not fully predictable. Nothing is more important than the vigilance of anesthesia providers as well as the team involved in the patient care. The ASA has established standards for monitoring during anesthesia, in which continuous oxygen saturation by pulse oximeter, noninvasive blood pressure measurement every 5 minutes or more frequently, and continuous ECG monitoring are considered mandatory.[49] End-tidal carbon dioxide monitoring (capnography) is very helpful in monitoring respiratory rate and pattern. However, it might be not reliable when the patient is mouth or shallow breathing. Invasive arterial pressure monitoring may be considered for patients with severely compromised cardiac function.

Anesthesia for Cardioversion

DC cardioversion can be performed in EP laboratory or at bedside. Deep sedation or general anesthesia without instrumentation of airway is often administered to avoid the pain from DC shocks. Agents with rapid onset and short duration such as propofol, etomidate, or methohexital are usually used. After standard monitoring is set up, followed by preoxygenation, a bolus of an induction agent is given. Since cardiac output is often reduced and circulation time is prolonged in this patient population, adequate time should be allowed for the administered drug to take effect before additional doses are given. After confirming unresponsiveness to voice and tactile stimulation, cardioversion can be performed. A majority of patients are able to maintain satisfactory oxygen saturation by spontaneous respiration. If needed, assisted ventilation by mask with oxygen, with or without airway manipulation, can be applied until adequate respiratory function is regained.

Vasopressor such as phenylephrine or ephedrine may be needed to treat the hypotension associated with anesthetics. If an additional cardioversion is needed, then the patient's mental status and responsiveness are assessed again and additional anesthetics can be given as needed. After cardioversion, the patient should be monitored until fully recovered from anesthesia or deep sedation.

Anesthesia for Catheter Ablation

Level of sedation varies depending upon the patient's condition and the needs of the procedure. While many ablation procedures can be performed under local infiltration anesthesia with conscious sedation, general anesthesia may be needed in certain clinical settings. For patients with sleep apnea or other significant respiratory diseases, anesthesia consultation is advised. Avoidance of coughing and partial airway obstruction will prevent patient movement, which is important for interventional procedures. Anesthetics that affect the sympathetic nervous system, such as ketamine (stimulating central sympathetic activity and inhibiting peripheral norepinephrine reuptake) and dexmedetomidine (sympatholytic), should be avoided if possible to avoid interference with arrhythmia induction or maintenance.

The anesthetic plan for a lengthy procedure needs to be individually tailored; often it must be modified or changed during the procedure when the patient's situation warrants. In principle, a decision should be made based on the patient's cooperativeness, coexisting disease, knowledge/experience of anesthetics, and availability of anesthesiologist. It has been proven to be safe and practical to keep cooperative patients oriented with anxiolytics with satisfactory local infiltration. For uncooperative patients, deeper sedation or general anesthesia is usually required.

Total intravenous anesthesia with continuous infusion of propofol has been successfully applied to catheter ablation. Continuous infusion of midazolam with or without propofol has also been used for prolonged catheter ablation. Our experience suggests that continuous infusion of midazolam alone often does not provide adequate anesthetic outcome for a prolonged procedure. Limited experience showed that continuous infusion of remifentanil may be used for catheter ablation. However, it has been reported that remifentanil may inhibit both sinus and AV node function.[50] General anesthesia is generally advised for an anticipated prolonged or complex ablation procedure because it allows the ablator to focus on ablation rather than anesthesia.

Anesthesia for Device Implantation

The implanting procedure causes significant pain or discomfort associated with venous access, creation of device pocket, and tunneling of leads. Well-performed infiltration with local anesthetics is essential for the patient's comfort, which will also reduce the requirement of systemic sedation. Sedation levels vary from mild to deep depending on patient perception and procedure duration and extent. Standard monitoring is essential. Supplemental oxygen is given via nasal cannula or face mask. Midazolam and fentanyl are commonly used to provide anxiolysis, sedation, and analgesia. Direct arterial pressure monitoring is suggested for the patient with severely compromised cardiac function. If DFT testing is required, an anesthetic agent such as propofol, etomidate, or methohexital is administered until the patient is rendered unconscious, similar to cardioversion. Synergistic effect with previously administered anesthetics should be considered and their doses should be adjusted accordingly.

Summary

Anesthesia for cardiac interventional EP procedures, cardioversion, and implantation of cardiac devices can be safely administered outside the operating room setting with proper monitoring, medications, airway management equipment, and trained personnel. Various anesthetics are available for such procedures. In addition to knowing the patient's clinical profile, a thorough understanding of the clinical pharmacology of each individual anesthetic agent is essential in order to select appropriate medications, to monitor for adverse effects, and to ensure adequate sedation and anesthesia for a comfortable, safe, and successful procedure. The commonly used anesthetics are summarized in Table 25.1 for quick reference.

Table 25.1 Common anesthetic medications and antagonists

Drug	Induction/Bolus Dose	Onset	Peak Effect (minutes)	Elimination $T_{1/2}$ (minutes)
Fentanyl	25–100 mcg IV (2–5 mcg/kg IV)	< 1 min	5–15 min	180–200 min
Morphine	2–4 mg IV (0.05–0.1 mg/kg IV)	< 1 min	10–20 min	100–120 min
Midazolam	1–2 mg IV (0.025–0.1 mg/kg IV)	< 1 min	2–5 min	60–180 min
Diazepam	0.05–0.2 mg/kg IV	1–5 min	5–10 min	>1,000 min
Sufentanil	0.2–5 mcg/kg IV	1–2 min	2–5 min	130–160 min
Remifentanil	0.025–0.2 mcg/kg/min IV	< 1 min	1–3 min	20–15 min
Thiopental	2–5 mg/kg IV	30–60 sec	5–15 min	600–700 min
Methohexital	1–2 mg/kg IV—induction 0.2–0.4 mg/kg—sedation	30–60 sec	5–15 min	180–240 min
Etomidate	0.1–0.4 mg/kg IV	30–60 sec	1–2 min	120–240 min
Ketamine	0.5–2 mg/kg IV—induction 10–25 mg IV—sedation	30–60 sec	1–5 min	120–180 min
Propofol	1.5–2 mg/kg IV—induction 25–100 mcg/kg/min—sedation	30–60 sec	1–2 min	60–90 min
(Antagonist)				
Flumazenil*	0.2–0.5 mg IV (5–20 mcg/kg IV)	1–2 min	5–10 min	30–60 min
Naloxone**	0.1–0.4 mg IV (10–50 mcg/kg IV)	1–2 min	5–10 min	60–80 min

NOTE: The information is for a healthy adult with average weight. All medications should be titrated to the desired effect. *Flumazenil is a benzodiazepine antagonist. **Naloxone is an opioid antagonist. *Source:* Loushin MK, Gold BS.[51] Modified with permission.

References

1. Johnson KB, Egan TD. Clinical pharmacokinetics and pharmacodynamics: applied pharmacology for the practitioner. In Longnecker D, Brown DC, Newman MF, Zapol W (eds): *Anesthesiology.* New York: McGraw Hill, 2008;851.
2. Egan TD, Lemmens HJ, Fiset P, et al. The pharmacokinetics of new short acting opioid remifentanyl (GI87084B) in healthy male volunteers. *Anesthesiology.* 1993;79:881-892.
3. Kapila A, Glass PS, Jacobs JR, et al. Measured context-sensitive half-times of remifentanil and alfentanyl. *Anesthesiology.* 1995;83:968-975.
4. Stenson RE, Constantino RT, Harrison DC. Interrelationships of hepatic blood flow, cardiac output, and blood levels of lidocaine in man. *Circulation.* 1971;43:205-211.
5. Gelman S, Fowler KC, Smith LR. Liver circulation and function during isoflurane and halothane anesthesia. *Anesthesiology.* 1984;61:726-730.
6. Nies AS, Shand DG, Wilkinson GR. Altered hepatic blood flow and drug disposition physiological approach to hepatic drug clearance. *Clin Pharmacokinet.* 1976;1:135-155.
7. Duchin KL, Schrier RW. Interactionship between renal haemodynamics, drug kinetics and drug action. *Clin Pharmacokinet.* 1978;3:58-71.
8. Kuhnert BR, Kuhnert RM, Philipson EH, et al. The half-life of 2-chloroprocaine. *Anesth Analg.* 1986;65:273-278.
9. Strichartz GR. The inhibition of sodium currents in myelinated nerve by quaternary derivatives of lidocaine. *J Gen Physiol.* 1973;62:37-57.
10. Courtney KR, Kendig JJ, Cohen EN. Frequency-dependent conduction block: The role of nerve impulse pattern in local anesthetic potency. *Anesthesiology.* 1978;48:111-117.
11. McKay W, Morris R, Mushlin P. Sodium bicarbonate attenuates pain on skin infiltration with lidocaine, with or without epinephrine. *Anesth Analg.* 1987;66:572-574.
12. Tucker GT. Pharmacokinetics of local anesthetics. *Br J Anaesth.* 1986;58:717-731.
13. Ritchie JM, Greene NM. Local anesthetics. In Gilman AG, Rall TW, Nies AS, et al (eds): *Goodman and Gilman's. The Pharmacological Basis of Therapeutics* (8th edition). New York: Pergamon Press, 1990;311.
14. Berde CB and Strichartz GR. *Local anesthetics.* In Miller RD, Eriksson LI, Fleisher LA, Wiener-Kronish, JP, Young WL (eds): *Miller's Anesthesia* (7th edition). Philadelphia: Churchill Livingstone, 2010;913-940.
15. Wright JL, Durieux ME and Groves DS. A brief review of innovative uses for local anesthetics. *Curr Opin Anaesthesiol.* 2008; 21:651-656.
16. Prieto-Alvarez P, Calas-Guerra A, Fuentes-Bellido J, Martínez-Verdera E, Benet-Català A, Lorenzo-Foz JP. Comparison of mepivacaine and lidocaine for intravenous regional anaesthesia: pharmacokinetic study and clinical correlation. *Br J Anaesth.* 2002;88:516-519.

17. Weinberg GL, Palmer JW, VadeBoncouer TR, et al. Bupivacaine inhibits acylcarnitine exchange in cardiac mitochondria. *Anesthesiology.* 2000;92:523-528.
18. Li Z, Xia Y, Dong X, Chen H, Xia F, et al. Lipid resuscitation of bupivacaine toxicity: long-chain triglyceride emulsion provides benefits over long- and medium-chain triglyceride emulsion. *Anesthesiology.* 2011;115:1219-1228.
19. Rosenblatt MA, Abel M, Fischer GW, et al. Successful use of 20% lipid emulsion to resuscitate a patient after a presumed bupivacaine-related cardiac arrest. *Anesthesiology.* 2006; 105:217-218.
20. Litz RJ, Roessel T, Heller AR, Stehr SN. Reversal of central nervous system and cardiac toxicity after local anesthetics intoxication by lipid emulsion injection. *Anesth Analg.* 2008; 106:1575-1577.
21. Bern S, Akpa BS, Kuo I, Weinberg G. Lipid resuscitation: A life-saving antidote for local anesthetic toxicity. *Curr Pharm Biotechnol.* 2010;12:313-319.
22. Litz RJ, Popp M, Stehr SN, et al. Successful resuscitation of a patient with ropivacaine-induced asystole after axillary plexus block using lipid infusion. *Anaesthesia.* 2006;61:800-801.
23. Reves JG, Fragen RJ, Vinik HR, et al. Midazolam: pharmacology and uses. *Anesthesiology.* 1985;62:310-324.
24. Mohler H, Richards JG. The benzodiazepine receptor: A pharmacological control element of brain function. *Eur J Anaesthesiol.* 1988;2(Suppl. 1):15-24.
25. Jacobs JR, Reves JG, Marty J, et al. Aging increases pharmacodynamic sensitivity to the hypnotic effects of midazolam. *Anesth Analg.* 1995;80:143-148.
26. Galletly DC, Williams TB, Robinson BJ. Periodic cardiovascular and ventilator activity during midazolam sedation. *Br J Anaesth.* 1996;76:503-507.
27. Greenblatt DJ, Albernaty DR, Morse DS, et al. Clinical importance of interaction of diazepam and cimetidine. *N Engl J Med.* 1984;310:1639-1643.
28. Desmond PV, Roberts RK, Wood AJ, et al. Effect of heparin administration on plasma binding of benzodiazepines. *Br J Clin Pharmacol.* 1980;9:171-175.
29. Everett E, Douglas H, Arlene N, et al. Comparative pharmacokinetics and pharmacodynamics of lorazepam, alprazolam and diazepam. *Psychopharmacology.* 1985;86:392-399.
30. Tomlin SL, Jenkins A, Lib WR, et al. Preparation of barbiturate optical isomers and their effects on GABA(A) receptors. *Anesthesiology.* 1999;90:1714-1722.
31. Judge S. Effect of general anaesthetics on synaptic ion channels. *Br J Anaesth.* 1983;55:191-200.
32. Seltzer JL, Gerson JI, Allen FB. Comparison of the cardiovascular effects of bolus vs. incremental administration of thiopentone. *Br J Anaesth.* 1980;52;527-529.
33. Angelini G, Ketzler JT, Coursin DB. Use of propofol and other nonbenzodiazepine sedatives in the intensive care unit. *Crit Care Clin.* 2001;17:863-880.
34. Veselis RA, Reinsel RA, Feshchenko VA, et al. The comparative amnestic effects of midazolam, propofol, thiopental and fentanyl at equisedative concentrations. *Anesthesiology.* 1997; 87:749-764.
35. Gan TJ, Glass PS, Howell ST, et al. Determination of plasma concentrations of propofol associated with 50% reduction in postoperative nausea. *Anestheiology.* 1997;87:779-784.
36. Sanna E, Garau F, Harris RA. Novel properties of homomeric beta 1 gamma-aminobutyric acid type A receptors: actions of the anesthetics propofol and pentobarbital. *Mol Pharmacol.* 1995;47:213-217.
37. Orser BA, Bertlik M, Wang LY, et al. Inhibition of the N-methyl-D-asparate subtype of glutamate receptor in cultured hippocampal neurons. *Br J Pharmacol.* 1995;116:1761-1768.
38. Powell CG, Unsworth DJ, McVey FK. Severe hypotension associated with angiotensin converting enzyme inhibition in anaesthesia. *Anaesth Intens Care.* 1998;26:107-109.
39. Forman SA. Clinical and molecular pharmacology of etomidate. *Anesthesiology.* 2011;114:695-707.
40. Panzer O, Moitra V, Sladen RN. Pharmacology of sedative-analgesic agents: dexmedetomidine, remifentanil, ketamine, volatile anesthetics, and the role of peripheral mu antagonists. *Anesthesiology Clin.* 2011;29:587-605.
41. Shook DC, Savage RM. Anesthesia in the cardiac catheterization laboratory and electrophysiology laboratory. *Anesthesiology Clin.* 2009;27:47-56.
42. Fukuda K. Intravenous opioid anesthetics. In Miller RD, Eriksson LI, Fleisher LA, Wiener-Kronish, JP, Young WL (eds): *Miller's Anesthesia* (7th edition). Philadelphia: Churchill Livingstone, 2010;769-824.
43. Naguib M, Lien CA. Pharmacology of muscle relaxants and their antagonists. In Miller RD, Eriksson LI, Fleisher LA, Wiener-Kronish, JP, Young WL (eds): *Miller's Anesthesia* (7th edition). Philadelphia: Churchill Livingstone, 2010;859-912.
44. Wilton NC, Knight PR, Ulrich K, et al. Transmural redistribution of myocardial blood flow during isoflurane anesthesia and its effects on regional myocardial function in a canine model of fixed coronary stenosis. *Anesthesiology.* 1993; 78:510-523.
45. Yildirim H, Adanir T, Atay A, et al. The effects of sevoflurane, isoflurane and desflurane on QT interval of the ECG. *Eur J Anaesthesiol.* 2004;21:566-570.
46. Metzner J, Posner KL, Domino KB. The risk and safety of anesthesia at remote locations: the US closed claims analysis. *Curr Opin Anaesthesiol.* 2009;22:502-508.
47. Practice Guidelines for Perioperative Management of Patients with Obstructive Sleep Apnea. A report by the American Society of Anesthesiologists task force on perioperative management of patients with obstructive sleep apnea. *Anesthesiology.* 2006;104:1081-1093.
48. Practice Guidelines for Preoperative Fasting and the Use of Pharmacologic Agents to Reduce the Risk of Pulmonary Aspiration: application to healthy patients undergoing elective procedures. A report by the American Society of Anesthesiologists task force on preoperative fasting. *Anesthesiology.* 1999;90:896-905.
49. ASA Standards, Guidelines, and Statements. Standards for basic anesthetic monitoring. October 2005.
50. Niksch A, Liberman L, Clapcich A, Schwarzenberger JC, Silver ES, Pass RH. Effects of remifentanil anesthesia on cardiac electrophysiologic properties in children undergoing catheter ablation of supraventricular tachycardia. *Pediatr Cardiol.* 2010;31:1079-1082.
51. Loushin MK, Gold BS. Anesthesia for cardioversion and device implantation. In Lü F & Benditt DG (eds): *Cardiac Pacing and Defibrillation—Principle and Practice.* Beijing, China: The People's Medical Publishing House, 2007;471.

SECTION 2A

INTERVENTIONAL ELECTROPHYSIOLOGY PROCEDURES

Diagnostic & Mapping Techniques During Percutaneous Catheter & Surgical EP Procedures

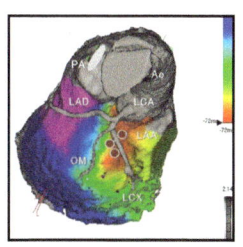
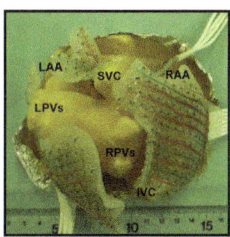
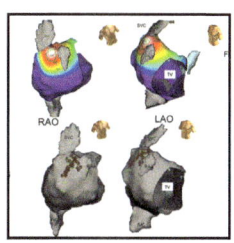
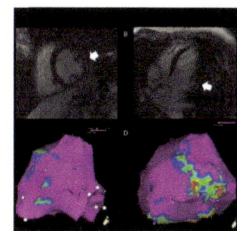

CHAPTER 26

Sinus Node and AV Conduction System

Stavros E. Mountantonakis, MD; Edward P. Gerstenfeld, MD

PART I: SINUS NODE

Anatomy and Physiology

The sinus node is a subepicardial structure localized within the sulcus terminalis of the right atrium at the junction of the SVC and RAA. It has a crescent or "comma-shaped" structure with its "head" at the SVC-atrial border and a "tail" along the crista terminalis.[1] The sinus node, as evaluated by mapping techniques, has been reported to range from 8 to 21 mm in length[2] (Figure 26.1).

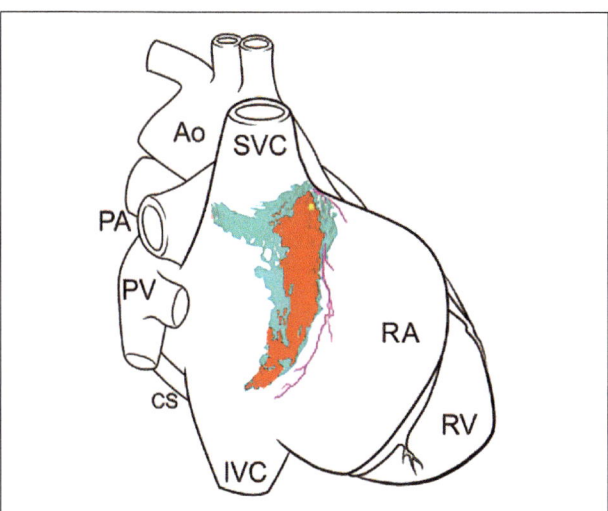

Figure 26.1 Schematic diagram of dorsal view of rabbit heart showing location and extent of central (**red**) and peripheral (**blue**) sinus node tissue. *Source:* Reproduced with permission from Dobrzynski H, Li J, Tellez J, et al. Computer three-dimensional reconstruction of the sinoatrial node. *Circulation.* 2005;111: 846-854.

However, the shape, position, and composition of the sinus node vary considerably from patient to patient.[3] Coronary perfusion to the sinus node is supplied by the sinus-node artery, which originates from the proximal right coronary artery in 65% of patients, the circumflex artery in 25%, and both in 10%. Histologically, the sinus node is composed of central smaller myocytes and an outer transitional zone of connective tissue and arteries.[3,4] Nodal cells lack myofilaments and express a set of connexins that form gap junction channels with very low conductance, which is responsible for its automatic properties.[5,6] The sinus node periphery plays a role in the functional isolation of the sinus node, allowing it to activate the atrium only through a superior, middle, or inferior exit to the atrium.[7,8]

The center of the sinus node is characterized by rich innervation with both sympathetic and parasympathetic fibers. Sensitivity to autonomic input varies, with dominance of the cranial foci during sympathetic activation and the caudal foci during increased vagal tone.[9] Due to the above arrangement, the site of impulse generation changes along the length of sinus node according to autonomic balance, with the cranial-most end being the leading site during sinus tachycardia and the caudal-most end during sinus bradycardia. Each sinus beat may also have multicentric origin, and the conduction out of the node may be variable and dependent on autonomic tone.[10]

Functionally, the sinus node is not discrete.[10] Computerized epicardial mapping system has shown that the sinus P wave arises from a wide area extending from the junction of the SVC and RAA to the IVC. This encompasses a zone of 75 × 15 mm, more than three times the size of the anatomical sinus node (Figure 26.1).[10] The presence of a functionally wide sinus area is also supported by the observation that an extensive ablation along the area of sinus node is required to achieve significant modification of the sinus rate.[11]

Electrophysiology of Sinus Node

The electrophysiology of the sinus node is complex and, despite intense investigation, remains incompletely understood. Most investigation has centered on the "funny current" (I_f), characterization of which is consistent with a major role in the spontaneous pacemaker activity of the sinus node. The resting membrane potential of normal sinoatrial cells reaches more negative values than those in the rest of the myocardium due to the presence of the small inward rectifier current, I_{K1}. When pacemaker (P) cells are maximally repolarized, activation of the hyperpolarization-cyclic-neocleotide (HCN) gated channels occurs. These channels allow the mixed Na/K+ inward current (I_f) that begins to depolarize the sinus node cells. There is a complex interaction between I_f and other currents including L-type (I_{Ca}, L) and T-type (I_{Ca}, T) calcium channels, the sodium/calcium exchanger (I_{NaCX}) sodium/potassium ATPase (I_{NaK}), and the delayed rectifier potassium current, with the balance among these currents determining the slope of diastolic depolarization and therefore the heart rate. The autonomic nervous system seems to exert its control over the sinus rate through the HCN channels. Activation of β-adrenergic receptors increases levels of cAMP, which activates the HCN channels and leads to a positive chronotropic effect. Activation of muscarinic receptors decreases cAMP levels and leads to a negative chronotropic effect.

More recent data suggest another potential contributor to sinus node depolarization. Spontaneous sarcoplasmic reticulum calcium release via ryanodine receptors, the so called "calcium clock," activates I_{NCX}, which then triggers- diastolic depolarization. It is likely that I_f and the calcium "clock" work synergistically to generate the normal heart rhythm. Inhibition of the calcium clock can lead to an inferior displacement of sinus node activity and ectopic beats from the crista terminalis in animal studies.[12]

Ivabradine is the first pharmaceutical agent to directly inhibit I_f. Ivabradine inhibits I_f in a dose-dependent manner, reducing sinus node activity and slowing the heart rate without the negative inotropic effects inherent to calcium channel and β-adrenergic antagonists. Ivabradine has been approved in Europe as a negative chronotropic agent for the treatment of refractory angina. In addition, preliminary studies suggest that it may also be useful in the treatment of inappropriate sinus tachycardia.

Sinus Node Dysfunction: Sick Sinus Syndrome and Inappropriate Sinus Tachycardia

Sick sinus syndrome (SSS) was originally described more than 4 decades ago[13] as a constellation of symptoms characterized by an inability of the sinus node to sustain adequate heart rate to meet physiological demands. The clinical manifestations may include fatigue, lightheadedness, and syncope, and the underlying rhythm can include marked sinus bradycardia, sinus pauses, sinus node exit block, or sinus arrest (Figure 26.2). SSS affects both

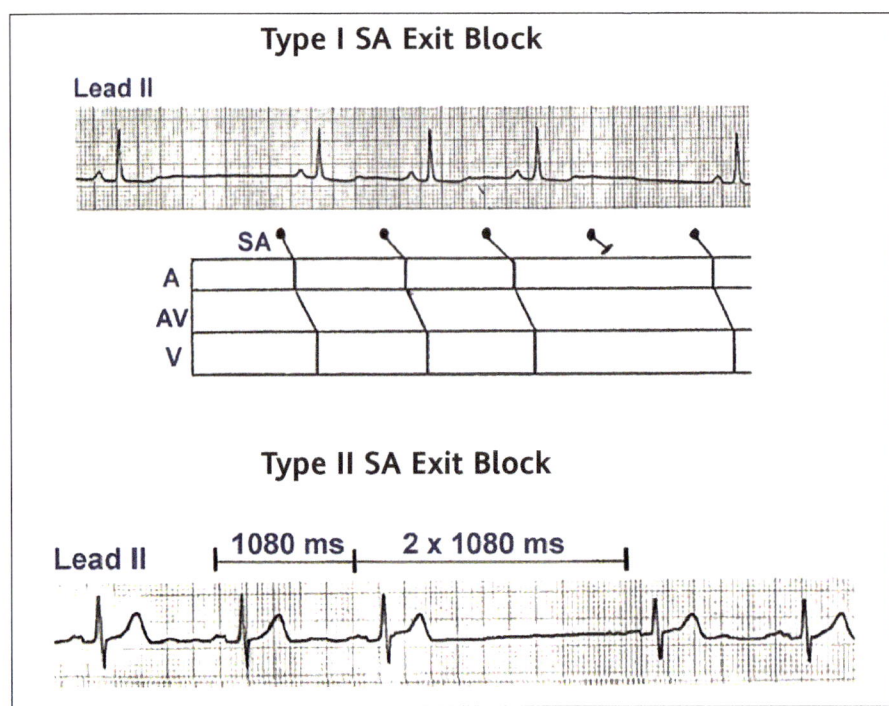

Figure 26.2 In type 1 sinoatrial block, conduction time between the sinus node and atrium progressively lengthens. The increment in conduction time decreases until the block sinus beat and therefore the PP interval of the conducted beats is decreasing. In addition, the PP interval that includes the nonconducted sinus impulse is typically less than the addition of the 2 preceding PP intervals. In type 2 sinoatrial exit block, a constant number of conducted sinus impulses occurs until one fails to conduct to the atrium. The PP of the conducted beats is constant, and the PP interval that includes the nonconducted sinus beat is twice the baseline PP interval.

genders equally, and the prevalence increases with age;[14-16] the mean age of onset is 68 years.[17] SSS is the most common indication for placement of a permanent pacemaker,[15] accounting for approximately one-half of all pacemaker implantations in the United States.[17] In addition to bradyarrhythmias, atrial tachyarrhythmias including AF have been increasingly recognized as a component of SSS. This alternation between bradyarrhythmias and tachyarrhythmias in the same patient is often described using the term "tachybrady syndrome" and tends to occur when the tachycardia converts to sinus rhythm with a pause (Figure 26.3). In the majority of cases, symptoms occur in paroxysms. Downregulation of I_f during SVT may, in part, explain the relationship between supraventricular arrhythmias and sinus node dysfunction.[18] Atrial fibrosis may also contribute to the coexistence of sinus node disease and SVTs, particularly AF.

Some patients may not exhibit evidence of sinus node dysfunction at rest; however, symptoms of fatigue or dyspnea occur reproducibly with exertion. One possible cause is chronotropic incompetence, defined as failure to increase the heart rate to >100 bpm or 70% maximum (220 − age) during a maximal exercise treadmill test (without medications that slow the sinus rate). Rate-responsive pacing may be helpful for alleviating symptoms in these patients. For patients with pure sinus node dysfunction and intact AV conduction, single-chamber atrial pacing is often sufficient.

The mechanism of SSS is considered an acceleration of the physiological sinus node aging. Causes that can accelerate this degenerative process can be intrinsic or extrinsic. In isolated sinus node dysfunction, alterations in expression of ion channels and gap connections have been described.[19] The common secondary causes of sinus node dysfunction include conditions that affect the entire right atrium[20] by increasing intra-atrial tension and promoting atrial fibrosis, such as hypertension, cardiomyopathies,[21] AF,[22] AFL,[23] atrial septal defect,[24] cardiac surgery, pericarditis, and infiltrative disorders. Coronary ischemia, especially at the right coronary distribution, has also been implicated. This is probably the mechanism involved in the high incidence of sinus node dysfunction in the donor heart post-orthotropic cardiac transplantation. The above conditions may cause a functional[23] as well structural remodeling of the sinus node, which may be reversible after the initiating condition is altered.[22] Other transient extrinsic causes of sinus-node dysfunction include the use of pharmacologic agents (eg, β-adrenergic blockers, calcium-channel blockers, digitalis, lithium, and antiarrhythmic drugs), electrolyte imbalance (hypocalcemia, hypokalemia), hypothermia, hypothyroidism, increased intracranial pressure, and excessive vagal tone. SSS occurring prematurely in the young has been associated with a mutation in the sodium (Na^+) channel *SCN5A*. This mutation results not only in reduced automaticity of the sinus node cells but also in sinoatrial exit block.[25] Regardless of etiology, a common histological finding in sinus node dysfunction is degeneration and necrosis of the sinus node cells and replacement of nodal tissue with fibrous tissue.

Inappropriate sinus tachycardia (IST) is characterized by paroxysmal or persistent sinus tachycardia disproportionate to the physiologic demand.[26] Patients typically will have a heart rate of 90–100 bpm at rest or with minimal physical exertion, and a P-wave morphology identical to sinus

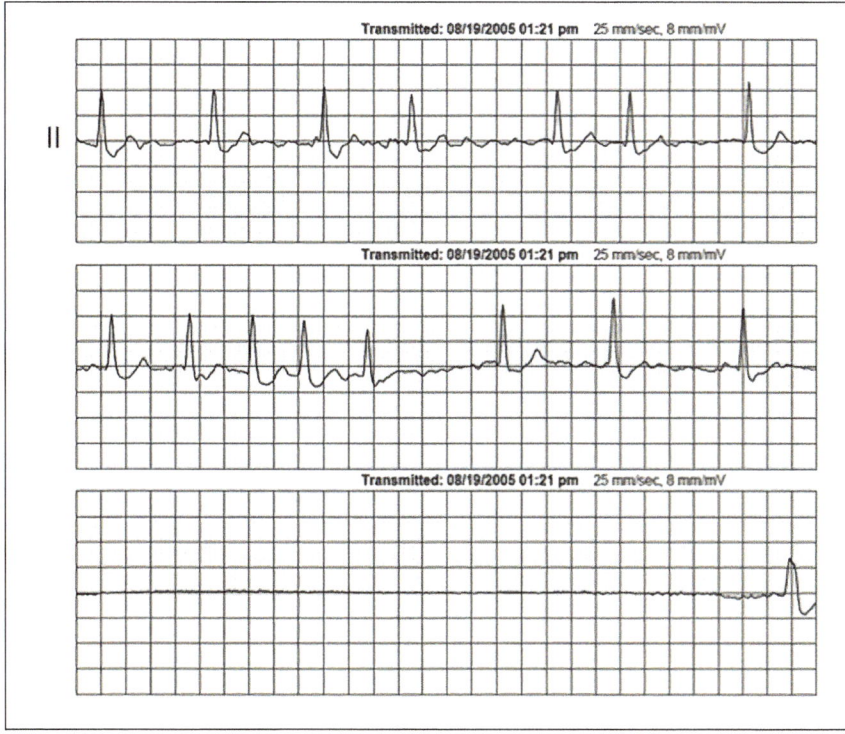

Figure 26.3 A continuous rhythm strip demonstrating a conversion pause from a patient with AF and sinus node dysfunction. These two conditions often coexist in the same patient and are referred to as tachybrady syndrome. Such pauses, if symptomatic, may require implantation of a permanent pacemaker to allow treatment with AV blocking agents.

rhythm. The condition has been reported in up to 1.2%[27] of the general population and affects predominantly females. Clinical manifestations may vary from asymptomatic tachycardia to debilitating symptoms including palpitations, shortness of breath, chest pain, dizziness, atypical precordial pain, fatigue, and syncope. Symptoms are triggered with exercise, changes in position, and physical or psychological stress, or they can occur spontaneously. Psychiatric components, including depression, stress, and anxiety, may be a part of the IST syndrome and often warrant separate evaluation.

The underlying mechanisms of IST are not well defined but can be attributed, at least in part, to autonomic dysregulation. Enhanced automaticity of the sinus node;[28,29] altered autonomic responses manifest as increased sympathetic tone, either directly or via sympathetic receptor hypersensitivity[28] or blunted parasympathetic tone; and impairment of baroreflex sensitivity are several proposed potential mechanisms.[27,30] Recently, increased levels of autoantibodies to beta-adrenergic receptors have been observed in patients with IST, suggesting an autoimmune basis.[31]

In general, IST is a diagnosis of exclusion. Secondary causes of sinus tachycardia including hyperthyroidism, pheochromocytoma, anemia, and physical deconditioning should be excluded. The differential diagnosis includes atrial tachycardia, sinus node reentry, and postural orthostatic tachycardia syndrome (POTS). The diagnosis usually can be made based on clinical symptomatology as well as ECG findings. A typical distinction between IST and POTS is the absence of hypotension during a tilt-table test.[32] Invasive EP testing or pharmacologic testing is rarely required for the establishment of diagnosis; however, treatment can be challenging.[33,34]

The mainstay of treatment of palpitations associated with IST is pharmacologic. Frequent small doses of β-blockers, that is, metoprolol 12.5 mg or pindolol 5 mg, both on a regular basis and as needed, can be effective in reducing symptoms. Giving the patient control of medication dosing, by allowing extra doses when symptoms occur, helps the patient feel empowered to manage the symptoms. It is important to explain to the patient that the treatment is not expected to completely alleviate symptoms, but render them manageable. The new I_f blocker, ivradapine, is not approved in the United States, but preliminary studies indicate that it may offer some benefit in treating IST patients. While the etiology of IST is not understood, symptomatic improvement does often occur over time, even in highly symptomatic patients, although it may take years. Weaning β-blockers may then be undertaken. In a select few patients, the symptoms are primarily related to tachycardia, and ablation or "modification" of the sinus node can be considered. This technique is described below.

Evaluation of Sinus Node Function in the EP Lab

Indications for EP Study of Sinus Node

Evaluation of sinus node function may be part of an evaluation of syncope when sinus node dysfunction is suspected. Typically, this evaluation is largely noninvasive. Careful clinical history and examination, ECG, and prolonged ambulatory ECG monitoring provide evidence of sinus node function in majority of cases. In every case, correlation of electrocardiographic findings with clinical symptoms is of the utmost importance as asymptomatic bradyarrhythmias, especially during sleep, are typically benign. Exercise testing can provide useful information on the chronotropic competence of sinus node. Carotid sinus massage is a simple maneuver that can elicit a hypersensitivity to vagal input. Sinus pauses of more than 3 seconds after 5 seconds of carotid massage are considered indicative of carotid hypersensitivity and may warrant pacemaker implantation in the appropriate clinical setting. It is important to emphasize that carotid sinus massage has low specificity and therefore should be interpreted only in correlation with clinical symptoms. Invasive electrophysiology study is often required when sinus node dysfunction is strongly suspected clinically without accompanied documentation of sinus arrhythmias.

Autonomic Testing of Sinus Node in the EP Lab

The response of sinus node to altering autonomic balance may be part of a complete sinus node evaluation, as sinus node dysfunction is often a result of exacerbated or blunted response to autonomic input. Intravenous atropine 1 mg to 3 mg can be used to assess the response of sinus node to parasympathetic tone. A normal response is considered an acceleration of the heart rate to > 90 bpm and an increase over the baseline rate of 20%–50%. A blunted response to atropine is characteristic of most patients with symptomatic sinus node dysfunction.[35]

The response of the sinus node to beta-blockade has also been evaluated. Propranolol 0.1 mg/kg typically produces a 12%–22.5% increase in sinus cycle length. However, no difference has been found in chronotropic response to propranolol between patients with or without sinus node dysfunction, suggesting that sympathetic tone is intact in patients with sinus node dysfunction.[36]

Calculation of the intrinsic heart rate (IHR) is useful to establish a diagnosis of IST and can also be useful to determine when marked sinus bradycardia is due to enhanced vagal tone. The IHR is determined during pharmacologic autonomic blockade with a combination of atropine 0.04 mg/kg and propranolol 0.2 mg/kg. The resultant heart rate can then be compared to predicted IHR as calculated by the following formula:

$$IHR = [118.1 - (0.57 \times age)] \text{ bpm}^{37}$$

An IHR higher than predicted is indicative of IST while an IHR lower than predicted is indicative of sinus node dysfunction.

EP Testing of Sinus Node Function

The amount of time required for sinus node to recover after overdriving pause is one measure of sinus node function. Like every other area with intrinsic pacemaker capability, the sinus node can be overdriven by other cells depolarizing at a faster rate. The sinus node recovery time (SNRT) is defined as the time that is required for the sinus node to depolarize after a 30- to 60-second period of atrial pacing at a cycle length shorter than the sinus rate from a site near the sinus node. Usually the maneuver is repeated more than one time starting at a cycle length just below resting sinus rate and at progressively shorter cycle lengths. The longest post-pacing pause is considered the SNRT. An important consideration in calculating SNRT is performing pacing close to sinus node in order to minimize any delay due to intra-atrial or sinoatrial conduction delay. An SNRT of >1,500 ms is considered abnormal. A limitation to SNRT is that sinus node automaticity is dependent on autonomic tone, and therefore the SNRT can vary in the same person with differing levels of autonomic tone. In order to account for this, the corrected SNRT (CSNRT) was introduced. CSNRT is calculated by subtracting the resting heart rate from the SNRT. The resting heart rate was chosen as indicative of the sympathetic input at the sinus node. CSNRT is a more reproducible measurement then the SNRT, with a CSNRT of > 550 ms considered abnormal. One of the considerations in calculating CSNRT is that the resting cycle length should be measured prior to the initiation of the pacing maneuver, as typically several seconds are required after cessation of pacing for the sinus node to resume its baseline rate. Another interval that has been used in evaluating sinus node automaticity is the total recovery time. This is the time in seconds from the point that atrial pacing is stopped until the premaneuver cycle length is reached, usually from the fourth to the sixth beat. A normal total recovery time is less than 5 seconds.

Clinical studies have shown abnormal SNRT and CSNRT in 35%–93% of patients with clinically apparent sinus node dysfunction.[36,38] The wide range of responses could be explained by different populations, inconsistency in performing the maneuvers, or a different autonomic state among the patients studied. However, despite these limitations, CSNRT remains the most widely used test to assess sinus node function. In patients with syncope, an abnormal SNRT is a reasonably specific, albeit insensitive, indicator of sinus node dysfunction.

The sinoatrial conduction time (SACT), another measure of sinus node function, evaluates conduction time through the transitional zone of connective tissue surrounding the pacing core of sinus node. Conditions that promote atrial fibrosis (eg, AF, valvular disease, ventricular cardiomyopathy) may slow or block exit and entrance of electrical conduction to the sinus node. SACT can be evaluated using two methods, Strauss[39] or Narula.[40] Using the Strauss method, late coupled atrial extrastimuli (A2) are introduced with decrementing intervals during sinus rhythm from a pacing site close to the sinus node. Assuming that A2 can penetrate to the sinus node and reset it, the duration between the last sinus beat (A1) and the first recovered (A3) will equal 2 sinus node cycle lengths (SNCLs) plus the time required for A2 to reach the sinus node and the time required for the first recovered sinus beat to exit the sinus node. Provided that the time to penetrate the sinus node equals the time required to exit it, then:

$$A2 - A3 = SNCL + 2\, SACT$$

The above method is based on several assumptions. First, it is assumed that the conduction times required to enter and exit the sinus node are the same. Experiments on animal models have shown that in fact there can be considerable difference between the conduction times in each direction. Another limitation is that the time required for A2 to reach the transitional zone is not counted. Therefore, pacing from a site away from the sinus node, or considerable intra-atrial delay, may overestimate SACT. Finally, marked sinus arrhythmia interferes with the interpretation of a post-extrastimulus pause. To overcome the difficulties of sinus rate oscillation, Narula proposed that the measurement be made after an 8-beat atrial drive at a cycle length just shorter than the underlying sinus rate. In that case, the difference between post-pacing pause and sinus cycle length should equal SACT. SACT is conceived in an effort to assess the transitional zone of sinus node and predict scenarios of sinoatrial exit. However, it is an insensitive method to identify sinus dysfunction in general, as it has been reported to be abnormal in only 40% of patients with clinical evidence of sinus dysfunction.[41] Its clinical use therefore has diminished.

Electroanatomic Mapping and Sinus Node Modification

In a select few patients with IST, the symptoms are primarily related to tachycardia, and ablation or "modification" of the sinus node can be considered if symptoms persist despite medical therapy. Early descriptions involved a primarily anatomic approach to catheter ablation using ICE to target the superior aspect of the crista terminals until there was a decrease in the resting heart rate.[42] Unfortunately, while acute improvement in the resting heart rate and heart rate response to isoproterenol has been documented, most patients developed recurrent sinus tachycardia during follow-up. Long-term symptomatic improvement was only shown in patients who underwent sufficient sinus node ablation to warrant atrial pacemaker placement. Therefore, patients are typically counseled to avoid an invasive strategy to manage this condition and reserve invasive EP study to exclude an atrial tachycardia originating near the sinus node or other SVT. However, if severe symptoms are unrelieved with medical therapy, several ablation strategies for modifying the sinus node have been described.[33,34]

During sinus node ablation, the cranial-most aspect of the sinus node, which is typically the earliest site during tachycardia, is targeted (Figure 26.4). The anatomic approach uses ICE to locate the superior aspect of the sinus node at the junction of the RAA and SVC. Traditionally, localization of sinus node was based on fluoroscopy and presence of typical sinus node EGMs along the crista terminalis. These EGMs include discrete double potentials separated by an isoelectric interval or complex fractionated activity of >50 ms duration. The location of the leading sinus node site was defined as the earliest site of activation during sinus rhythm and after a pacing train at different cycle lengths. However, the above technique was found to be inadequate for guiding sinus node modification for several reasons. First, the functional sinus node encompasses a wide area, with the earliest site changing depending on autonomic input. The sinus node is also an epicardial structure, and often the site of earliest endocardial activation in sinus rhythm represents the endocardial exit of the sinus node rather than the leading site itself. Finally, changes in the atrial electrical substrate with aging or heart disease make it difficult to identify the characteristic sinus node EGMs.

After localization of the sinus node area, multiple radiofrequency lesions are delivered at this location until sinus node slowing occurs, often with an inferiorly displaced origin of the sinus node indicated by a flat-negative P wave in lead III. The presence of an epicardial clear space, considered to represent penetration of ablation to the epicardial surface, has also been identified as a reasonable endpoint.[43] While early reports used standard 4-mm-tip ablation catheters, fewer lesions are required when irrigated-tip ablation catheters are used.[33,34]

Use of electroanatomic mapping has also gained popularity for guiding sinus node modification, as it can define the sites of earliest sinus node activation and guide a more electrically based approach. Both contact[33] and noncontact[34] mapping approaches have been used. Using a noncontact mapping approach, a multielectrode array basket catheter is first placed in the HRA and right atrial geometry is acquired. The location of the exit of sinus node depolarization is noted on the map (▶ Video 26.1) during progressive administration of isoproterenol, starting at 1 mcg/min to maximum dose of 10 mcg/min (usually in increments of 1, 2, 3, 5, and 10 mcg/min).[34] After the isoproterenol is stopped, the superior aspect of the sinus node indicated by the exit of sinus node depolarization on isoproterenol is first targeted for ablation. Ablation is continued inferiorly gradually until flattening or inversion of the P wave in lead III is noted, indicating an inferior exit of the sinus node, and rechallenge with isoproterenol (2 mcg/min) leads to a heart rate <120 bpm (Figure 26.5). Acute symptomatic relief often occurs, but the long-term recurrence rate remains unknown and multiple ablation procedures may be required. Of importance during any HRA ablation procedure is identification of phrenic course along the anterolateral border of the right atrium. Ablation in regions that exhibit phrenic capture during pacing should be avoided, as diaphragmatic paralysis may occur.

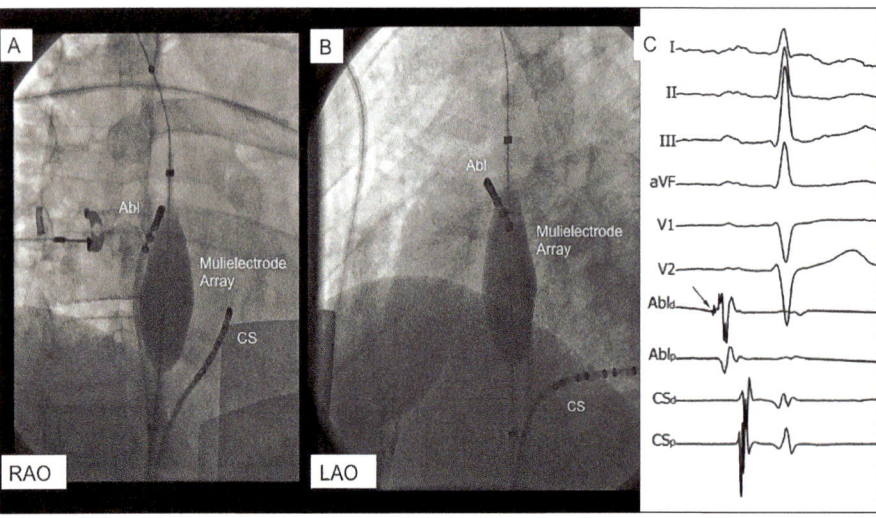

Figure 26.4 Map/ablation catheter position over the sinus node region in the RAO (**A**) and LAO (**B**) projections. At this position, an early sharp EGM that preceded the onset of a surface P wave was seen. Abl = ablation catheter; CS = coronary sinus.

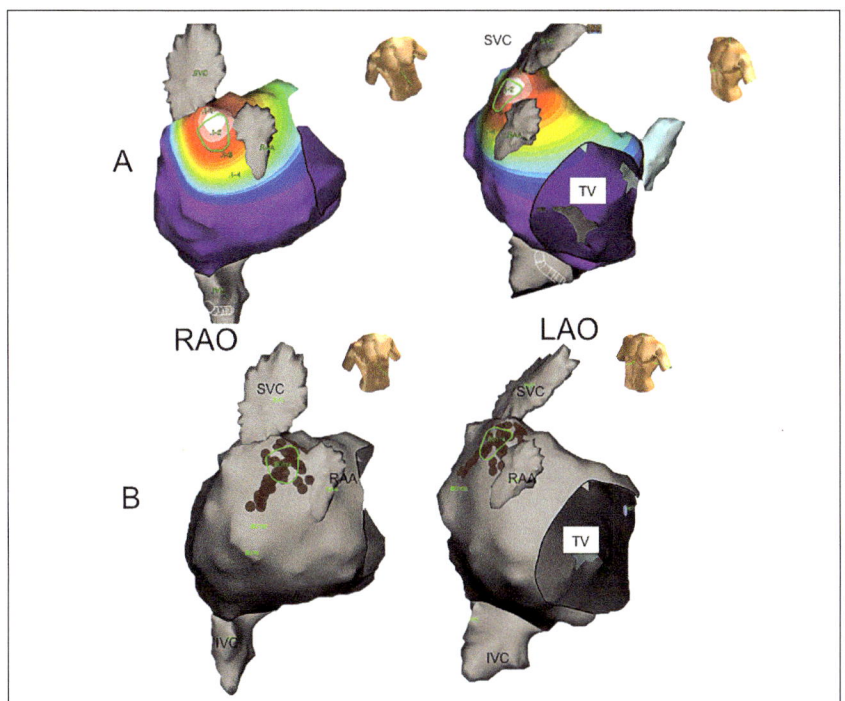

Figure 26.5 **Panel A:** Electroanatomical map with noncontact mapping of sinus rhythm during isoproterenol infusion. Notice that the earliest site of activation (**white color**) is at the most cephalad end of the right atrium at the junction of the high right atrium and the SVC. **Panel B:** Ablation lesions at the superior end of sinus node for IST. IVC = inferior vena cava; RAA = right atrial appendage; SVC = superior vena cava; TV = tricuspid valve.

One of the challenges of sinus node modification is that ablation is performed endocardially to target the sinus node, which lies subepicardially. Several authors have described an epicardial approach to sinus node modification, using percutaneous subxyphoid epicardial access.[44] This may allow a more rapid and permanent alteration of sinus node function. However, no long-term studies of this approach exist. As mentioned previously, many patients with IST are young with normal heart function. Therefore, the ablative procedures discussed above should be restricted to a select few patients with severe symptoms. Many patients, even after complete sinus node ablation and atrial pacemaker placement, can continue to feel symptoms of palpitations, fatigue, and syncope. Finally, AV junction ablation and pacemaker placement is not recommended in IST patients. These patients will continue to have sinus tachycardia in addition to problems of ventricular tracking of the atrial rate and ventricular dyssynchrony from right ventricular pacing.

PART II: ATRIOVENTRICULAR NODE

Anatomy and Histology of the Atrioventricular Node

The atrioventricular node (AVN) is a subendocardial structure located at the inferoseptal right atrium at the apex of the anatomic region called the triangle of Koch. The triangle of Koch is anatomically bounded inferiorly by the CS ostium, posteriorly by the tendon of Todaro and anteriorly by the septal leaflet of the tricuspid valve (Figure 26.6). The size and shape of the AVN varies considerably among individuals.[45] The AVN can be divided into the lower AV nodal bundle (AVNB) or bundle of His and compact node (CN).[46] The CN lies anterior to the CS os and above the insertion of the septal leaflet of the tricuspid valve. The AVNB continues from the CN more anterior and superior and penetrates the right fibrous trigone on the central fibrous body, into the lower portion of the membranous IVS. The AVNB then travels inferiorly for a few millimeters before starting to divide into two bundles in the IVS.[47] The branching variation of RBB and LBB from the AVB also shows great variation among individuals.

Two posterior extensions of the AVN have been described, which may represent the anatomic correlates of the "slow" and "fast" AV nodal pathways. The inferior or rightward extension extends posteriorly from the AVN toward the ostium of the CS.[48] The leftward nodal extension extends posteriorly from the CN superiorly to the rightward extension and is typically shorter.[48] These two extensions have differential EP properties and a different profile of connexin expression.[49] Recently, the presence of an additional extension of AV node to the left atrium has been suggested in humans. Evidence for the presence of this extension is provided mainly from cases of AVN reentrant tachycardia, where the successful site of ablation was at the inferolateral mitral annulus. The incidence of this extension is unclear and is postulated to be fewer than 1% of patients.

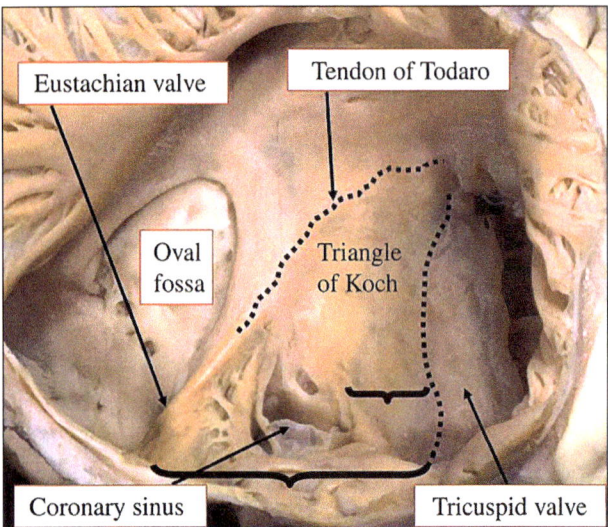

Figure 26.6 The compact AV node is located at the apex of the triangle of Koch, defined anteriorly by the septal leaflet of tricuspid valve, inferiorly by the CS os and posteriorly by the tendon of Todaro. The rightward posterior extension runs at the anterior lip of the CS node, and the leftward nodal extension extends superiorly from the compact AV node. *Source:* Reproduced with permission from Anderson RH, Cook AC. The structure and components of the atrial chambers. *Europace.* 2007:9 Suppl 6;vi3-9.

Histologically, the CN shares common characteristics to the sinus node. They both contain two distinct areas: the central CN and the transitional zone. The AVNB and bundle branches are well insulated from the rest of the myocardium by thick fibrous tissue. This ensures entrance of electrical conduction in the ventricular Purkinje network and allows rapid conduction to the ventricular myocardium. Similar to the sinus node, the AVN has rich enervation by sympathetic and parasympathetic fibers.[50] Blood supply to the AVN is from the right or left coronary artery in 73% and 19% of patients, respectively. In 8% of patients, coronary perfusion is from both right and left coronary arteries.[51] In addition, multiple anastomoses have been observed between branches of the AV nodal artery and the left anterior descending artery through septal perforators, as well as diffusion across the venous sinusoids.[52] Based on those observations, it is evident that the AV node and proximal conduction system are receiving perfusion through a complex network and are therefore well protected in case of a single coronary ischemia.

Electrophysiology of the AVN

Three main types of cells have been described in the AVN: nodal, atrionodal, and nodo-His cells. Nodal cells are structurally similar to the P cells in the sinus node. They have a relatively low resting potential and generate a small-amplitude action potential with a slow upstroke. These cells are the only cells with pacemaker activity in the AVN. The EP properties of nodal cells are based on differential expression of ion channels. Nodal cells lack Na channels; the ion currents responsible for the action potential are Ica_L and Ica_T. Because action potentials dependent on calcium channels generate a slow upstroke, AV nodal cells typically have a long refractory period and slow conduction velocity.

Another characteristic of the AV node is intrinsic automaticity. Similar to the sinus node cells, expression of the HCN channel has been documented to generate the I_f current that is responsible for spontaneous diastolic depolarization.[53] In addition, reaching the depolarization threshold in ANV cells is facilitated by their inherent lower resting membrane potential. AVN cells have a characteristic absence of I_{k1} channels. This channel is responsible for an outward potassium (K+) current that maintains a resting potential of approximately −80 mV. The absence of such current in AVN cells allows the resting potential to be closer to threshold, facilitating automaticity. Another unique attribute of the AVN is the I [ach, ado] channel. Activation of this channel in response to acetylcholine or adenosine drives the resting potential to more negative values, suppressing automaticity and prolonging conduction time. The positive chronotropic effect of the sympathetic nervous system is mainly exerted through stimulation of Ica_L current that has the opposite effect.

Atrionodal and nodo-His cells are transitional cells that have EP characteristics intermediate to those of nodal cells and surrounding tissue. They both express Na+ channels and therefore have a higher amplitude and slope of phase 0 of the action potential compared to nodal cells. Anatomically, atrionodal cells surround the CN and nodo-His occupy the transitional area between the CN and the AVNB.[54]

Gap junctions in the AVN are generally sparse with predominant Cx40 rather than Cx43.[18] The transition from expression of Cx43 to Cx40 is abrupt and correlates with the interface between the CN and the transitional zone. In general, Cx40 gap junctions conduct at a much slower velocity, and this may explain the slow conduction velocity along the AVN imparting the critical physiological AV nodal delay. In contrast, gap connections in the bundle branches are abundant and allow rapid conduction of electrical impulses.[55]

Function—Physiology

The role of AVN is multidimensional. First, it is responsible for receiving the atrial impulse and allowing its entrance to the Purkinje network and the ventricles. Normally the AVN is the only electrical connection between the atria and ventricles. The characteristic paucity of connexins among the cells of the AVN imparts the conduction delay that allows ventricular filling prior to systole. Conduction velocity and refractoriness in the AVN is primarily governed by autonomic input, rendering the AVN an important modulator of the AV conduction delay according to physiological demands. Conduction along the AVN is decremental and dependent on the interval between prior atrial impulses (AA interval). The shorter the prior AA interval, the longer the conduction time through the AVN. These conduction properties of the AVN give it the important role of protecting the ventricles in the event of rapid atrial rates, as in the cases of atrial tachycardia or AF.

Automatic activity of the AV nodal cells allows them to have the secondary role of a "rescue pacemaker" in case of sinus node failure. Typical rates of the AVN are between 30 bpm and 50 bpm and depend on autonomic input. Optical mapping studies have suggested that the leading AV nodal pacemaker is located in the CN area where P cells are more abundant and organize in clusters.[56,57] Those studies have also shown that junctional beats originating from the area of CN progress first retrograde through an anterior pathway compartment and return anterogradely through a more inferoposterior pathway before exiting to the Purkinje network.[56,58] Similar to the sinus node, a locational shift of the AVN leading pacemaker site has been shown under autonomic influence.[50]

AVN Conduction Abnormalities

Types of AVN Block

Three types of AVN conduction abnormalities have been described based on ECG characteristics. This classification has prognostic significance as has been correlated with the level of block in the conduction system, that is, whether it occurs at the AV node level or infranodal conduction system (HPS, bundle branches). First-degree AV block is more accurately referred to as delay and is characterized by stable prolongation of PR interval of more than 200 ms. Conduction delay at the level of AV block is by far the most common mechanism, whereas intra-atrial delay, especially in the setting of atrial myopathy, has also been reported. Patients with Mobitz I second-degree AV block have progressively longer PR intervals followed by a dropped ventricular beat and then resumption of AV conduction. The PP interval in Mobitz I AV block (Wenckebach) progressively shortens, and the conducted PR interval after the pause is always shorter than the last conducted PR interval. Mobitz I AV block typically occurs at the AV nodal level. Mobitz II AV block occurs when there is a P wave that occurs at the normal sinus interval and does not conduct to the ventricle without preceding PR interval prolongation. Mobitz II AV block signifies infranodal conduction disease, and typically occurs in the presence of a wide QRS complex (Figure 26.7). Complete heart block occurs when there is no evidence of AV conduction. To diagnose complete AV block, the atrial rate should be faster than the ventricular rate, and the ventricular response should be regular. Two-to-one AV block precludes differentiating Mobitz I from Mobitz II AV block because there is no opportunity to identify progressive PR prolongation. The presence of a narrow QRS and long PR interval (> 300 ms) suggests AV nodal disease, while a wide QRS or short PR interval (< 180 ms) of the conducted beats suggests infranodal conduction disease. Maneuvers can also be helpful in further identifying the level of AV block. Increasing the degree of AV block with carotid sinus massage implies that the level of block is at the AV node, while increasing AV block with exercise or adenosine suggests that the level

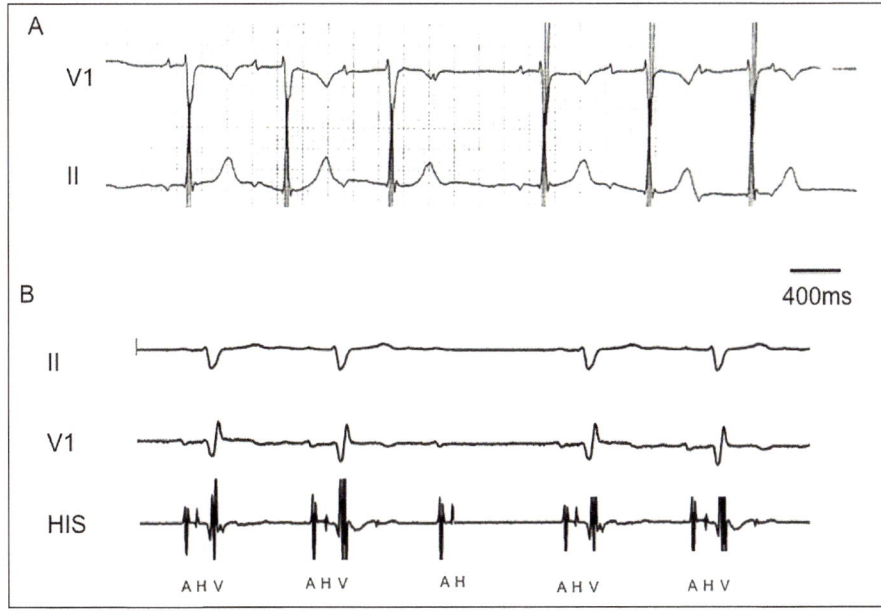

Figure 26.7 **Panel A:** Example of Mobitz I AV block with progressive PR prolongation followed by a dropped ventricular complex. **Panel B:** Example of Mobitz II AV block with a fixed PR interval and dropped QRS. Note the presence of infra-Hisian block on the His catheter recording at the bottom of Panel B.

of block is infranodal, since both these latter maneuvers result in a greater number of impulses penetrating the infranodal conduction system. Rarely, intra-His block or Wenckebach conduction can occur (Figure 26.8), which is always pathologic and should prompt pacemaker insertion. Finally, one should always be aware of the rare possibility of His extrasytoles, which may mimic intermittent AV block but has a benign prognosis. In general, block at the AV nodal level rarely requires pacemaker placement unless symptoms are present, while infranodal block implies a high likelihood of progression to complete AV block and should prompt insertion of a permanent pacemaker.

Clinical Presentation

The clinical presentation of ANV dysfunction is variable and depends largely on the level of block and the presence of escape rhythm in case of complete heart block. Patients with first-degree AV delay are typically asymptomatic. Patients with complete heart block and a stable junctional escape rhythm can be asymptomatic at rest and experience symptoms only during exercise due to inability of the heart rate to meet physiologic demands. Ventricular escape rhythms are slower and less reliable and may manifest with symptoms related to decreased cardiac output that can vary from decreased exercise intolerance and fatigue to mental status changes and syncope. Conduction delay or complete block of the AVN can occur intermittently, and therefore diagnosis of AVN block should be entertained in all patients with syncope and evidence of conduction disease on the ECG.

Common Diseases Associated with AVN Dysfunction

Congenital Complete AV Block

Neonatal lupus is the most common cause of congenital AVN block. Neonatal lupus is associated with presence of maternal autoantibodies of the Ro/La family.[59] However, the presence of those antibodies has very low specificity in predicting neonatal lupus, as only 2% of women will have a baby with complete heart block.[60] The second most common cause of congenital AV block is in the presence of congenital heart disease, with the most common disorders including congenitally corrected transposition of the great vessels and AV canal defects.[61] Isolated idiopathic congenital complete heart block can also occur and generally carries a favorable prognosis. In asymptomatic neonates and infants, prophylactic pacing is suggested in cases of marked bradycardia (< 55 bpm or < 70 bpm in the case of significant cardiac malformations). Beyond one year of age, permanent pacemaker implantation is based on the resting junctional rate (usually for a heart rate < 50 bpm) and the presence of pauses on 24-hour recordings. In adults with congenital complete heart block, the trend has been to recommend pacemaker implantation earlier than in past years. Chronic AV dysynchrony can lead to ventricular dilatation and eventually symptoms of congestive heart failure. The escape rhythm may also be unstable and lead to pauses and lightheadedness or syncope. Major indications for permanent pacing include any symptoms of presyncope or syncope, marked bradycardia (average ventricular rate < 50 bpm on 24-hour Holter or average nighttime heart rate < 45 bpm) or pauses > 3 seconds. Minor indications include the presence of complex

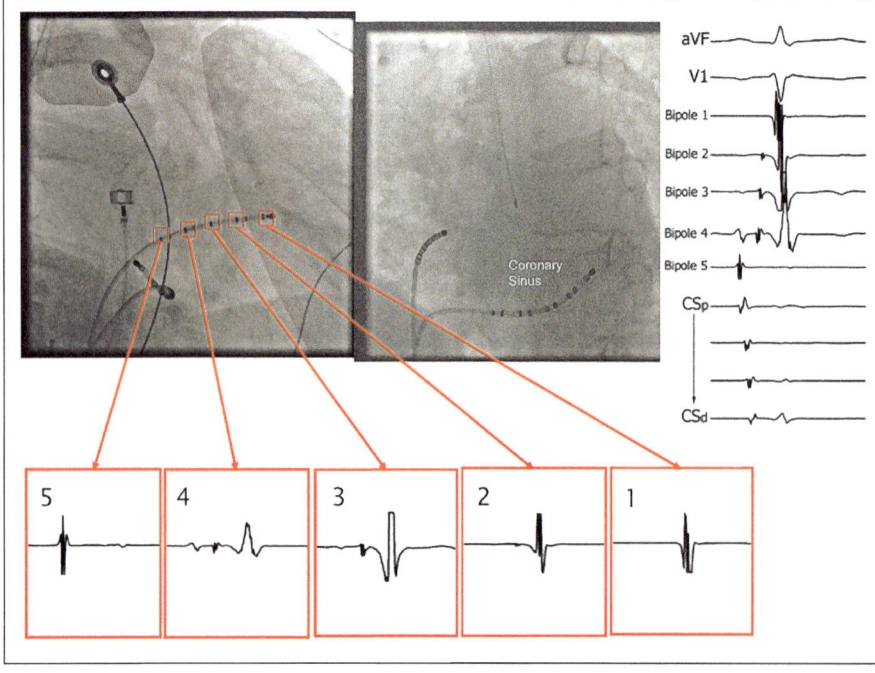

Figure 26.8 His catheter position in the right and left anterior oblique views. The distal bipole (1) records only a ventricular EGM. Bipole 2 records a right bundle potential, denoted by the absence of atrial EGM. The more proximal bipoles record a progressively sharper near-field atrial EGM and a clear His EGM.

ventricular ectopy, cardiomegaly, a wide complex escape rhythm, QT prolongation, or diminished heart rate response to exercise.

Congenital complete heart block can also rarely be due to infiltrative diseases or myocarditis.

Degenerative Diseases

Idiopathic fibrosis of the conduction system is the most common cause of acquired complete heart block, occurring in 33% of cases.[62] Fibrosis of the proximal left bundle branch and bifurcating main bundle is referred to as Lev's disease, whereas involvement of the more peripheral conduction fibers is referred to as Lenègre's disease. The etiology of either disease is unclear. Lev's disease is considered a more accelerated degenerative process of conduction system, presumably due to hypertension and atherosclerosis as it occurs in the older population. Lenègre's disease is more commonly seen in younger patients; it is has been associated with a loss-of-function mutation in the gene encoding the Na⁺ channel, *SCN5A*.[63] Prognosis of both diseases is favorable with pacemaker implantation.

Coronary Ischemia

Patients who develop permanent AVN conduction abnormalities during acute myocardial infarction have a generally worse prognosis than patients without conduction abnormalities.[64] Since blood supply to the AVN is from the right coronary artery in 73%,[51] inferior acute myocardial infarctions are more commonly associated with AVN conduction abnormalities. In addition to direct ischemia, increased vagal tone that usually accompanies inferior myocardial infarctions can contribute to the development of AV block. Despite its common occurrence, AVB in the setting of inferior myocardial infarction is usually reversible. This reversibility is due to the aforementioned rich collateral perfusion of the AVN area from septal perforators as well as direct diffusion.[52] As such, although temporary pacing may be indicated in the acute phase, a waiting period is usually suggested prior to implanting a permanent pacemaker. For those patients, prognosis is similar to the patients who did not develop AV conduction abnormalities.[64] However, AV block in setting of anterior myocardial infarction is often related to extensive necrosis of the anterior septum rather than ischemia to the AVN per se, is less likely to be reversible, and should be addressed with transvenous pacing.[64]

Systemic Inflammatory Diseases

Disruption of the normal AVN architecture can cause delay or block of AV conduction. Such disruption can occur by invasion of AVN by inflammatory cells, granulomas and fibrosis. These processes have been described in systemic inflammatory diseases (scleroderma, rheumatoid arthritis, systemic lupus erythematosus, ankylosing spondylitis, and polymyositis), infiltrative processes (amyloidosis, sarcoidosis, hemochromatosis, tuberculosis, rheumatic fever tumors), and acute and chronic infections (infective endocarditis and myocarditis, Lyme disease, Chagas' disease, measles, and mumps). Depending on the progression and stage of the disease, the AV block can be reversible with treatment of the underlying cause; however, in the majority of cases, pacemaker implantation is usually indicated due to the progressive and chronic course of these diseases.

Neuromyopathies

Neuromuscular diseases that have been associated with AV block include type 1 myotonic dystrophy, Emery-Dreifuss muscular dystrophies, and less commonly Duchenne and Becker muscular dystrophies.[65] Of importance is type I myotonic muscular dystrophy as patients with DM1 are at particular risk for sudden death due to complete heart block. Baseline ECG abnormalities and presence of atrial tachyarrhythmia were recently shown to predict sudden death.[66]

Iatrogenic Causes of AVN Conduction Block

Cardiac surgery, particularly aortic valve replacement, is often complicated by AVN conduction abnormalities. The incidence of complete heart block after cardiac surgery ranges from 3%–6% and depends on etiology of valve failure, prior cardiac operation, extent of procedure (single or dual valve, repair versus replacement), presence of preexisting conduction abnormalities, and surgical experience.[67,68] Reversible AV block due to edema rather than permanent injury is more common, and therefore, a waiting period of 7 days post–surgical procedure is usually recommended. Experience with catheter aortic valve replacement is so far limited, and different series report postprocedural heart block that varies between 5%–22%,[69,70] with the most important predictor in development of AV block being the use of a relatively large percutaneous valve.[69]

Surgical repair of congenital heart defects, especially those involving the septum and in particular ventricular septal defect, AV canal, and tetralogy of Fallot repairs, can cause reversible or irreversible heart block. They usually occur immediately after surgery or early in the postoperative period; however, they have also been reported months to years after surgery. The incidence of early AV conduction block has been reported as 0.9% and that of delayed AV conduction block as 0.3% to 0.7%.[71] Early postoperative complete heart block can be transient or permanent, with transient AV conduction block predicting risk of delayed block.[71] As in adult cardiac surgery, the duration of postoperative heart block of > 7 days is an indication for permanent pacemaker implantation. Interestingly enough, late recovery of AV conduction has been reported in up to 10% of cases, suggesting that it occurs secondary to postoperative local inflammation.[72-74]

AVN block can also occur during catheter-based procedures. Transient complete heart block is not uncommon with catheter manipulation at the right site of the septum in patients with preexistent LBBB and is due to catheter trauma of the RBB. Complete heart block following catheter alcohol ablation for hypertrophic cardiomyopathy has been reported in 8% to 14% of cases.[75,76] Female gender, extent of ablation, and presence of baseline conduction disease (especially LBBB) carry higher risk.[75] AV block can also complicate RFA close to the compact atrioventricular (AV) node or His bundle for AV nodal reentrant tachycardia or bypass tracts. It is also important to remember the risk of injury to the AVN from ablation over the coronary sinuses, especially close to the RCC.

Physiologic AV Block

AV block occurring in situations of increased vagal tone can occur in normal patients and warrants no particular intervention. Common scenarios include AV block occurring during sleep, periods of apnea, or gastrointestinal illness. Characteristically, the occurrence of AV block is preceded by slowing of the sinus rate, indicative of increased vagal stimulation.

Electrophysiology Study of AVN Function

Indications

Electrophysiological study of the AVN can be useful in cases of syncope, intermittent heart block, or investigation of SVTs. Although documentation of AV block on electrocardiogram or remote monitoring is usually sufficient in establishing the diagnosis of AV dysfunction and predicting the level of AV block, an EP study may help when such documentation is not available or in cases where the evidence is equivocal, such as in the presence of 2:1 AV block with an intermediate PR interval. In addition, the presence of dual AV nodal physiology suggests the functional substrate for development of AVNRT.

Intervals

Most information about conduction and function of the AVN and His bundle are obtained by a catheter recording the His bundle EGM (H). Usually a fixed or deflectable quadripolar catheter is passed to the right ventricle until a sharp ventricular EGM is recorded (V) (Figure 26.9). From there, the catheter is withdrawn with a clockwise torque to maintain contact against the septum. The presence of a sharp (< 30 ms) EGM before the ventricular EGM without the presence of an atrial EGM signifies the right bundle branch EGM. Withdrawing the catheter farther toward the septal tricuspid annulus where an atrial EGM (A) is seen identifies the His EGM. By convention, the ideal His EGM is the proximal-most position where a His EGM can be recorded; at this site, a large sharp atrial EGM and a smaller far-field ventricular EGM can be seen. The normal duration of a His EGM is < 30 ms. Prolonged or split His potential indicates disease in the AV bundle.

The local atrial signal (A) on the His catheter represents the timing of entrance of the atrial signal into the

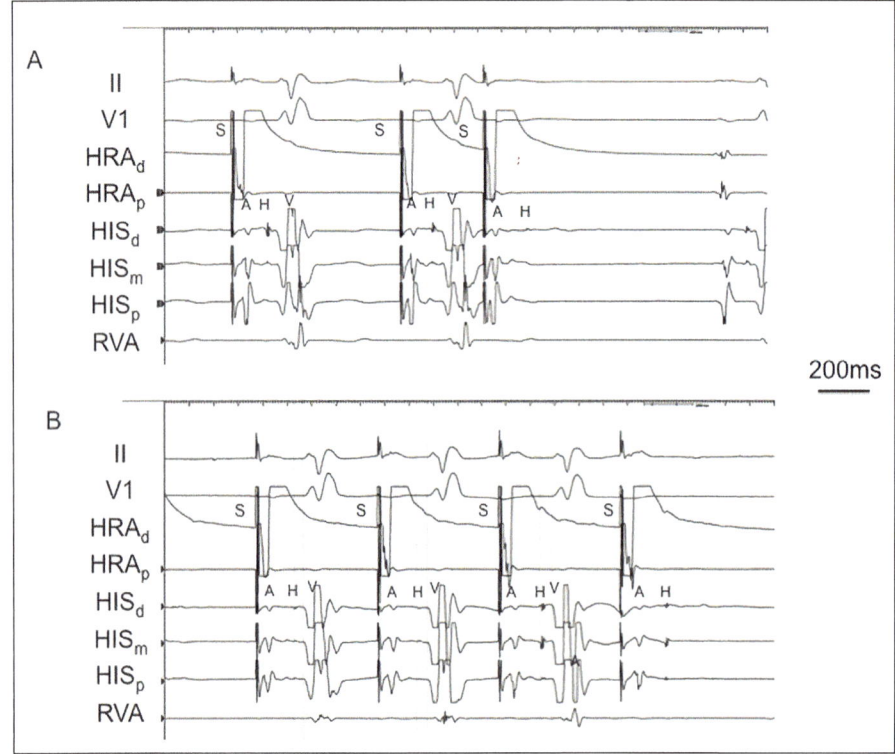

Figure 26.9 Panel A: Single atrial extrastimulus (S2) causes decremental conduction in the AV node (prolongation of AH interval) and infra-Hisian block indicated by the presence of His (H) inscription without a ventricular EGM (V). Notice the presence of bifascicular block (RBBB and left anterior hemifascicular block) on surface ECG. Infra-Hisian block with premature extrastimuli should not be considered pathologic.
Panel B: Atrial pacing at stable 400-ms cycle length causes slight prolongation of HV interval (infranodal Wenchebach) and infra-Hisian block on the last nonconducted atrial beat. This is always considered pathologic and should prompt consideration of a permanent pacemaker.

AV node. Due to slow depolarization of the AVN cells, the AVN cells do not produce a sharp EGM. Diseases at the level of the AV node affect the interval between the A and H EGM (AH interval), whereas diseases below the level of AVN prolong the delay between the H and ventricular EGM (HV interval). Therefore, recording the His bundle EGM is critical for differentiating nodal from infranodal conduction disease, the latter of which may progress to heart block and require permanent pacing. The range of normal AH conduction is 60–125 ms depending on the autonomic tone, heart rate, and the prior PP interval. The normal HV duration is 35–45 ms, and its duration is not affected by autonomic tone or heart rate. The presence of a prolonged HV interval signifies disease in the AV bundle and is almost always associated with wide QRS on surface ECG. HV interval of more than 100 ms is strongly predictive of progression to complete heart block. An HV interval < 35 ms indicates the presence of an accessory pathway with anterograde conduction between the atria and ventricles.

Decremental Conduction and Refractoriness

The refractory period of cardiac tissue is typically determined using an 8-beat drive train of pacing stimuli at constant cycle length followed by a premature extrastimulus of progressively shorter coupling interval. The Effective Refractory Period (ERP) of a structure is the longest coupling interval between extrastimuli that fails to capture that tissue. For the AVN, the ERP is defined as the longest interval between atrial extrastimuli (A1 to A2) that fails to conduct to the ventricle. However, cardiac tissue often has decremental properties that may delay arrival of a delivered extrastimulus to the more distal target. Therefore, the functional refractory period has been introduced. The functional refractory period (FRP) is the shortest coupling interval that can be elicited from a tissue by any stimulus input interval. Consequently, the AVN FRP is the shortest H1H2 interval produced by any A1A2 interval. Refractory periods depend on cycle length and autonomic input.

In response to rapid input into the AV node, the AH interval will gradually prolong until block occurs. This gradual lengthening in the AV delay followed by block, or so-called Wenckebach phenomena, limits conduction of rapid atrial rates during AF or flutter to the ventricles. Similarly, with incremental pacing, the cycle length at which AV block occurs can be documented when an atrial event is not followed by an H EGM. AVN Wenckebach will occur with rapid pacing rates in normal individuals. When it occurs with slow pacing rates (ie, less than 500 ms), it may be a sign of increased vagal tone or AV nodal conduction disease. In cases where the atrial refractory period is reached before AV nodal Wenckebach or AV nodal ERP, increasing the atrial output or performing atrial pacing from a different site usually allows determination of those parameters. Absence of a ventricular signal after the inscription of a His EGM indicates infranodal (HPS) conduction block. Infranodal block occurring with rapid pacing (< 450 ms cycle length) or during extrastimulus testing can be physiologic. However, infranodal block occurring during regular pacing at a cycle length > 450 ms is generally abnormal and evidence of infranodal conduction disease. If the presence of infranodal block cannot be determined during EP study because of a prolonged AV Wenckebach cycle length, then administration of atropine (0.5 to 1 mg IV) may improve AV nodal conduction and allow interrogation of the infranodal conduction axis.

Dual AV Nodal Physiology

The prolongation of the AH interval with atrial extrastimuli usually occurs in a gradual fashion ("decremental") until AH block occurs. An AH prolongation of more than 50 ms with an increment in the A1A2 interval of 10 ms defines the presence of "dual AV nodal physiology." Such an increase in conduction time is not expected to occur over conduction of a single nodal pathway and is indicative of transition of conduction to another pathway with different EP properties. This abrupt increase in AH interval or "jump" is suggestive of block over one AVN pathway and change to an alternate pathway, typically with slower conduction and a longer refractory period. These pathways are usually referred to as the "fast pathway" and the "slow pathway" based on the conduction velocity. During normal activation, conduction occurs over both functional pathways; however, antegrade conduction over the fast pathway reaches the AV bundle first generating a ventricular depolarization. The slow pathway therefore does not generate a ventricular depolarization unless conduction over the fast pathway is blocked. This can either occur with an atrial premature beat, provided that the refractory period of the fast pathway is longer than the slow pathway, or with a premature ventricular beat that preferentially invades the fast pathway. Evidence of multiple AVN pathways has been demonstrated with functional as well as optical mapping studies. It should be appreciated that AV nodal physiology is complex and, therefore, that the presence of two distinct AV nodal pathways is likely an oversimplification. In addition, the demonstration of functionally distinct pathways can vary in the same patient at different times and occasionally may not be apparent in patients with proven AVNRT. The EP evidence of multiple functional pathways may represent a change in AV nodal exit or the transition among multiple conducting bundles that comprise the AV node. Although there may be an anatomical basis of such differential exits, their functional significance depends on autonomic input to the AVN and therefore changes over time. The two-pathway construct, however, is useful for understanding the typical response of the AV node to extrastimuli. In addition, recent pathologic studies in humans have confirmed the presence of posterior extensions of the AV node that may correspond to the so-called "fast" and "slow" AV nodal pathways (Figure 26.10). This correlation has also been confirmed by optical mapping studies.[56,58]

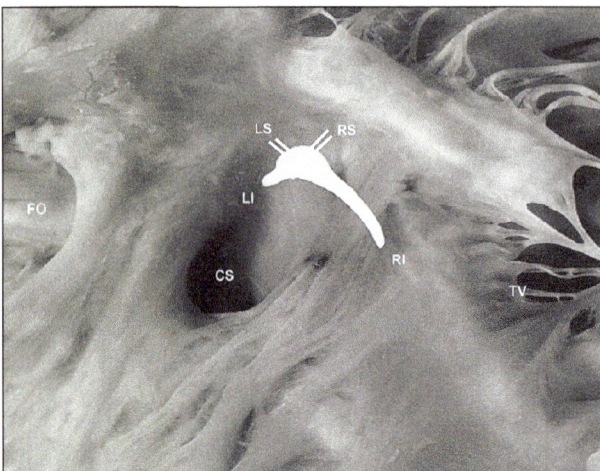

Figure 26.10 Inferior and superior atrial inputs to the AV node. One thick white line represents right or left inferior input, and two thin white lines represent right or left superior inputs. CS = coronary sinus; FO = foramen ovale; LI = left inferior input; LS = left superior input; RI = right inferior input; RS = right superior input; TV = tricuspid valve. *Source:* Figure published by Katritsis DG and Becker A. The atrioventricular nodal reentrant tachycardia circuit: a proposal. *Heart Rhythm.* 2007;4:1354-1360.

Mapping of Atrioventricular Node

Mapping the earliest atrial activation during ventricular pacing can provide information about the anatomic location of the posterior AVN extensions. At long pacing cycle lengths, retrograde conduction predominantly occurs over the fast AV nodal pathway. The location of the fast pathway is outside the triangle of Koch, just posterior to the tendon of Todaro. This region can be located by slowly withdrawing a catheter posteriorly from the His position while maintaining clockwise torque on the catheter. During ventricular pacing with retrograde conduction up the fast AV nodal pathway, earliest activation will be recorded on the His catheter followed by activation of the proximal coronary sinus.

In patients with dual AV nodal physiology, pacing at progressively shorter cycle lengths will lead to a shift in retrograde conduction to the slow pathway region. The slow pathway is located on the inferoseptal tricuspid annulus, just posterior to the CS os (Figure 26.6). A high-frequency potential may be recorded during sinus rhythm at this site representing activation through the rightward inferior AVN extension (slow pathway potential). Ablation to treat AVNRT typically targets this anatomic slow pathway region. Earlier attempts targeting the fast pathway led to a relatively high incidence of inadvertent heart block.

More recent investigations have identified the presence of left-sided extensions of the AV node. During detailed mapping of typical AVNRT in one study, the left side of the septum was activated before the right side in 53% of cases.[77] Pathologic studies have also identified the presence of left-sided AV nodal extensions.[78] The true prevalence of left-sided AV nodal extensions and how often they are involved in AVNRT is unknown.

References

1. Wiese C, Grieskamp T, Airik R, et al. Formation of the sinus node head and differentiation of sinus node myocardium are independently regulated by Tbx18 and Tbx3. *Circ Res.* 2009;104(3):388-397.
2. Sanchez-Quintana D, Cabrera JA, Farre J, Climent V, Anderson RH, Ho SY. Sinus node revisited in the era of electroanatomical mapping and catheter ablation. *Heart.* Feb 2005;91(2):189-194.
3. Chandler NJ, Greener ID, Tellez JO, et al. Molecular architecture of the human sinus node: insights into the function of the cardiac pacemaker. *Circulation.* 2009;119(12):1562-1575.
4. Boyett MR, Honjo H, Kodama I. The sinoatrial node, a heterogeneous pacemaker structure. *Cardiovasc Res.* 2000;47(4): 658-687.
5. Gros D, Theveniau-Ruissy M, Bernard M, et al. Connexin 30 is expressed in the mouse sino-atrial node and modulates heart rate. *Cardiovasc Res.* 2010;85(1):45-55.
6. Mangoni ME, Nargeot J. Genesis and regulation of the heart automaticity. *Physiol Rev.* 2008;88(3):919-982.
7. Fedorov VV, Schuessler RB, Hemphill M, et al. Structural and functional evidence for discrete exit pathways that connect the canine sinoatrial node and atria. *Circ Res.* 2009;104(7):915-923.
8. Fedorov VV, Glukhov AV, Chang R, et al. Optical mapping of the isolated coronary-perfused human sinus node. *J Am Coll Cardiol.* 2010;56(17):1386-1394.
9. Boineau JP, Schuessler RB, Roeske WR, Autry LJ, Miller CB, Wylds AC. Quantitative relation between sites of atrial impulse origin and cycle length. *Am J Physiol.* 1983;245(5 Pt 1): H781-789.
10. Boineau JP, Canavan TE, Schuessler RB, Cain ME, Corr PB, Cox JL. Demonstration of a widely distributed atrial pacemaker complex in the human heart. *Circulation.* 1988; 77(6):1221-1237.
11. Man KC, Knight B, Tse HF, et al. Radiofrequency catheter ablation of inappropriate sinus tachycardia guided by activation mapping. *J Am Coll Cardiol.* 2000;35(2):451-457.
12. Joung B, Lin SF, Chen Z, et al. Mechanisms of sinoatrial node dysfunction in a canine model of pacing-induced AF. *Heart Rhythm.* 2010;7(1):88-95.
13. Ferrer MI. The sick sinus syndrome in atrial disease. *JAMA.* 1968;206(3):645-646.
14. Kistler PM, Sanders P, Fynn SP, et al. EP and electroanatomic changes in the human atrium associated with age. *J Am Coll Cardiol.* 2004;44(1):109-116.
15. Kusumoto FM, Goldschlager N. Cardiac pacing. *N Engl J Med.* 1996;334(2):89-97.
16. Alings AM, Abbas RF, Bouman LN. Age-related changes in structure and relative collagen content of the human and feline sinoatrial node. A comparative study. *Eur Heart J.* 1995; 16(11):1655-1667.

17. Adan V, Crown LA. Diagnosis and treatment of sick sinus syndrome. *Am Fam Physician.* 2003;67(8):1725-1732.
18. Yeh YH, Burstein B, Qi XY, et al. Funny current downregulation and sinus node dysfunction associated with atrial tachyarrhythmia: a molecular basis for tachycardia-bradycardia syndrome. *Circulation.* 2009;119(12):1576-1585.
19. Dobrzynski H, Boyett MR, Anderson RH. New insights into pacemaker activity: promoting understanding of sick sinus syndrome. *Circulation.* 2007;115(14):1921-1932.
20. Sanders P, Morton JB, Kistler PM, et al. Electrophysiological and electroanatomic characterization of the atria in sinus node disease: Evidence of diffuse atrial remodeling. *Circulation.* 2004;109(12):1514-1522.
21. Sanders P, Kistler PM, Morton JB, Spence SJ, Kalman JM. Remodeling of sinus node function in patients with congestive heart failure: reduction in sinus node reserve. *Circulation.* 2004;110(8):897-903.
22. Hocini M, Sanders P, Deisenhofer I, et al. Reverse remodeling of sinus node function after catheter ablation of atrial fibrillation in patients with prolonged sinus pauses. *Circulation.* 2003;108(10):1172-1175.
23. Stiles MK, Brooks AG, Roberts-Thomson KC, et al. High-density mapping of the sinus node in humans: role of preferential pathways and the effect of remodeling. *J Cardiovasc Electrophysiol.* 2010;21(5):532-539.
24. Morton JB, Sanders P, Vohra JK, et al. Effect of chronic right atrial stretch on atrial electrical remodeling in patients with an atrial septal defect. *Circulation.* Apr 8 2003;107(13):1775-1782.
25. Benson DW, Wang DW, Dyment M, et al. Congenital sick sinus syndrome caused by recessive mutations in the cardiac sodium channel gene (SCN5A). *J Clin Invest.* 2003;112(7):1019-1028.
26. Krahn AD, Yee R, Klein GJ, Morillo C. Inappropriate sinus tachycardia: evaluation and therapy. *J Cardiovasc Electrophysiol.* 1995;6(12):1124-1128.
27. Still AM, Raatikainen P, Ylitalo A, et al. Prevalence, characteristics and natural course of "inappropriate sinus tachycardia. *Europace.* 2005;7(2):104-112.
28. Morillo CA, Klein GJ, Thakur RK, Li H, Zardini M, Yee R. Mechanism of inappropriate" sinus tachycardia. Role of sympathovagal balance. *Circulation.* 1994;90(2):873-877.
29. Bauernfeind RA, Amat-Y-Leon F, Dhingra RC, Kehoe R, Wyndham C, Rosen KM. Chronic nonparoxysmal sinus tachycardia in otherwise healthy persons. *Ann Intern Med.* 1979;91(5):702-710.
30. Still AM, Huikuri HV, Airaksinen KE, et al. Impaired negative chronotropic response to adenosine in patients with inappropriate sinus tachycardia. *J Cardiovasc Electrophysiol.* 2002;13(6):557-562.
31. Chiale PA, Garro HA, Schmidberg J, et al. Inappropriate sinus tachycardia may be related to an immunologic disorder involving cardiac beta andrenergic receptors. *Heart Rhythm.* 2006;3(10):1182-1186.
32. Deisenhofer I, Estner H, Zrenner B, et al. Left atrial tachycardia after circumferential pulmonary vein ablation for atrial fibrillation: incidence, electrophysiological characteristics, and results of radiofrequency ablation. *Europace.* 2006;8(8):573-582.
33. Marrouche NF, Beheiry S, Tomassoni G, et al. Three-dimensional nonfluoroscopic mapping and ablation of inappropriate sinus tachycardia. Procedural strategies and long-term outcome. *J Am Coll Cardiol.* 2002;39(6):1046-1054.
34. Lin D, Garcia F, Jacobson J, et al. Use of noncontact mapping and saline-cooled ablation catheter for sinus node modification in medically refractory inappropriate sinus tachycardia. *Pacing Clin Electrophysiol.* 2007;30(2):236-242.
35. Dhingra RC, Amat-Y-Leon F, Wyndham C, et al. Electrophysiologic effects of atropine on human sinus node and atrium. *Am J Cardiol.* 1976;38(4):429-434.
36. Strauss HC, Gilbert M, Svenson RH, Miller HC, Wallace AG. Electrophysiologic effects of propranolol on sinus node function in patients with sinus node dysfunction. *Circulation.* 1976;54(3):452-459.
37. Jose AD, Collison D. The normal range and determinants of the intrinsic heart rate in man. *Cardiovascular Res.* 1970;4:160-167.
38. Breithardt G, Seipel L, Loogen F. Sinus node recovery time and calculated sinoatrial conduction time in normal subjects and patients with sinus node dysfunction. *Circulation.* 1977;56(1):43-50.
39. Strauss HC, Bigger JT, Saroff AL, Giardina EG. Electrophysiologic evaluation of sinus node function in patients with sinus node dysfunction. *Circulation.* 1976;53(5):763-776.
40. Narula OS, Shantha N, Vasquez M, Towne WD, Linhart JW. A new method for measurement of sinoatrial conduction time. *Circulation.* 1978;58(4):706-714.
41. Rakovec P, Jakopin J, Rode P, Kenda MF, Horvat M. Clinical comparison of indirectly and directly determined sinoatrial conduction time. *Am Heart J.* 1981;102(2):292-294.
42. Lee RJ, Kalman JM, Fitzpatrick AP, et al. Radiofrequency catheter modification of the sinus node for "inappropriate" sinus tachycardia. *Circulation.* 1995;92(10):2919-2928.
43. Ren JF, Marchlinski FE, Callans DJ, Zado ES. Echocardiographic lesion characteristics associated with successful ablation of inappropriate sinus tachycardia. *J Cardiovasc Electrophysiol.* 2001;12(7):814-818.
44. Koplan BA, Parkash R, Couper G, Stevenson WG. Combined epicardial-endocardial approach to ablation of inappropriate sinus tachycardia. *J Cardiovasc Electrophysiol.* 2004;15(2):237-240.
45. Kawashima T, Sasaki H. Gross anatomy of the human cardiac conduction system with comparative morphological and developmental implications for human application. *Ann Anat.* 2011;20:193(1):1-12.
46. Meijler FL, Janse MJ. Morphology and electrophysiology of the mammalian atrioventricular node. *Physiol Rev.* 1988;68(2):608-647.
47. James TN. Structure and function of the sinus node, AV node and His bundle of the human heart: Part I-structure. *Prog Cardiovasc Dis.* 2002;45(3):235-267.
48. Inoue S, Becker AE. Posterior extensions of the human compact atrioventricular node: a neglected anatomic feature of potential clinical significance. *Circulation.* 1998;97(2):188-193.
49. Hucker WJ, McCain ML, Laughner JI, Iaizzo PA, Efimov IR. Connexin 43 expression delineates two discrete pathways in the human atrioventricular junction. *Anat Rec.* (Hoboken). 2008;291(2):204-215.
50. Hucker WJ, Nikolski VP, Efimov IR. Autonomic control and innervation of the atrioventricular junctional pacemaker. *Heart Rhythm.* 2007;4(10):1326-1335.
51. Futami C, Tanuma K, Tanuma Y, Saito T. The arterial blood supply of the conducting system in normal human hearts. *Surg Radiol Anat.* 2003;25(1):42-49.
52. Kennel AJ, Titus JL. The vasculature of the human atrioventricular conduction system. *Mayo Clin Proc.* 1972;47(8):562-566.
53. Yoo S, Dobrzynski H, Fedorov VV, et al. Localization of Na+ channel isoforms at the atrioventricular junction and atrioventricular node in the rat. *Circulation.* 2006;114(13):1360-1371.

54. Anderson RH, Janse MJ, van Capelle FJ, Billette J, Becker AE, Durrer D. A combined morphological and electrophysiological study of the atrioventricular node of the rabbit heart. *Circ Res.* 1974;35(6):909-922.
55. Han W, Wang Z, Nattel S. Slow delayed rectifier current and repolarization in canine cardiac Purkinje cells. *Am J Physiol Heart Circ Physiol.* 2001;280(3):H1075-H1080.
56. Hucker WJ, Fedorov VV, Foyil KV, Moazami N, Efimov IR. Images in cardiovascular medicine. Optical mapping of the human atrioventricular junction. *Circulation.* 2008;117(11):1474-1477.
57. Thibault B, de Bakker JM, Hocini M, Loh P, Wittkampf FH, Janse MJ. Origin of heat-induced accelerated junctional rhythm. *J Cardiovasc Electrophysiol.* 1998;9(6):631-641.
58. Hucker WJ, Nikolski VP, Efimov IR. Optical mapping of the atrioventricular junction. *J Electrocardiol.* 2005;38(4 Suppl):121-125.
59. Jayaprasad N, Johnson F, Venugopal K. Congenital complete heart block and maternal connective tissue disease. *Int J Cardiol.* 2006;112(2):153-158.
60. Brucato A, Frassi M, Franceschini F, et al. Risk of congenital complete heart block in newborns of mothers with anti-Ro/SSA antibodies detected by counterimmunoelectrophoresis: a prospective study of 100 women. *Arthritis Rheum.* 2001;44(8):1832-1835.
61. Walsh EP. Interventional electrophysiology in patients with congenital heart disease. *Circulation.* 2007;115(25):3224-3234.
62. Davies MJ. Pathology of chronic A-V block. *Acta Cardiol.* 1976;Suppl 21:19-30.
63. Royer A, van Veen TA, Le Bouter S, et al. Mouse model of SCN5A-linked hereditary Lenegre's disease: age-related conduction slowing and myocardial fibrosis. *Circulation.* 2005;111(14):1738-1746.
64. Simons GR, Sgarbossa E, Wagner G, Califf RM, Topol EJ, Natale A. Atrioventricular and intraventricular conduction disorders in acute myocardial infarction: a reappraisal in the thrombolytic era. *Pacing Clin Electrophysiol.* 1998;21(12):2651-2663.
65. Cox GF, Kunkel LM. Dystrophies and heart disease. *Curr Opin Cardiol.* 1997;12(3):329-343.
66. Groh WJ, Groh MR, Saha C, et al. Electrocardiographic abnormalities and sudden death in myotonic dystrophy type 1. *N Engl J Med.* 2008;358(25):2688-2697.
67. Schurr UP, Berli J, Berdajs D, et al. Incidence and risk factors for pacemaker implantation following aortic valve replacement. *Interact Cardiovasc Thorac Surg.* 2010;11(5):556-560.
68. Huynh H, Dalloul G, Ghanbari H, et al. Permanent pacemaker implantation following aortic valve replacement: current prevalence and clinical predictors. *Pacing Clin Electrophysiol.* 2009;32(12): 1520-1555.
69. Bleiziffer S, Ruge H, Horer J, et al. Predictors for new-onset complete heart block after transcatheter aortic valve implantation. *JACC Cardiovasc Interv.* 2010;3(5):524-530.
70. Dworakowski R, MacCarthy PA, Monaghan M, et al. Transcatheter aortic valve implantation for severe aortic stenosis—a new paradigm for multidisciplinary intervention: a prospective cohort study. *Am Heart J.* 2010;160(2):237-243.
71. Lin A, Mahle WT, Frias PA, et al. Early and delayed atrioventricular conduction block after routine surgery for congenital heart disease. *J Thorac Cardiovasc Surg.* 2010;140(1):158-160.
72. Batra AS, Wells WJ, Hinoki KW, Stanton RA, Silka MJ. Late recovery of atrioventricular conduction after pacemaker implantation for complete heart block associated with surgery for congenital heart disease. *J Thorac Cardiovasc Surg.* 2003;125(6):1291-1293.
73. Gross GJ, Chiu CC, Hamilton RM, Kirsh JA, Stephenson EA. Natural history of postoperative heart block in congenital heart disease: implications for pacing intervention. *Heart Rhythm.* 2006;3(5):601-604.
74. Villain E. Indications for pacing in patients with congenital heart disease. *Pacing Clin Electrophysiol.* 2008;31 Suppl 1:S17-20.
75. Chang SM, Nagueh SF, Spencer WH 3rd, Lakkis NM. Complete heart block: determinants and clinical impact in patients with hypertrophic obstructive cardiomyopathy undergoing nonsurgical septal reduction therapy. *J Am Coll Cardiol.* 2003;42(2):296-300.
76. Lawrenz T, Lieder F, Bartelsmeier M, et al. Predictors of complete heart block after transcoronary ablation of septal hypertrophy: results of a prospective electrophysiological investigation in 172 patients with hypertrophic obstructive cardiomyopathy. *J Am Coll Cardiol.* 2007;49(24):2356-2363.
77. Katritsis DG, Ellenbogen KA, Becker AE. Atrial activation during atrioventricular nodal reentrant tachycardia: studies on retrograde fast pathway conduction. *Heart Rhythm.* 2006;3:99-100.
78. Inoue S, Becker AE. Posterior extensions of the human compact atrioventricular node: a neglected anatomic feature of potential clinical significance. *Circulation.* 1998;97:188-193.

Video Legend

Video 26.1 Noncontact map.

CHAPTER 27

Paroxysmal Supraventricular Tachycardias

Thorsten Lewalter, MD, PhD

Introduction

Already in the 1900s, paroxysmal supraventricular tachycardias (PSVTs) were a well-recognized family of syndromes, becoming electrocardiographically defined arrhythmias since the early days of electrocardiography. The clinical syndrome was first described in European literature in the 19th century. In 1867, Cotton reported on an "unusually rapid action of the heart," which was further followed by additional observations made by French and German scientists.[1,2] Initially referred to as Bouveret's syndrome and later as paroxysmal atrial tachycardia, it was described classically as "a fully unprovoked tachycardia attack, lasting a few seconds or several days, in patients who as a rule have otherwise healthy hearts." It was electrocardiographically defined in the 10th Bethesda Conference on Optimal Electrocardiography as "a tachycardia usually characterized by an atrial rate of 140 to 240 beats per minute (bpm) and by an abrupt onset and termination." It may or may not be associated with intact A-V conduction. Specific electrophysiological studies may elicit specific mechanisms such as retrograde and anterograde pathways and sites of reentry.[3]

In the past 25 years, correlating and possibly due to the beginnings of radiofrequency catheter ablation, this disease has been an intensely studied arrhythmia, contributing to a current very good understanding of its genesis, presentation, subtypes, electrophysiology, and pharmacologic as well as nonpharmacologic therapy. Today we understand that this family of arrhythmias is due to either enhanced automaticity or reentry. However, while reentry tachycardias can predominate in certain populations and clinical practice, there is considerable overlap in clinical and electrocardiographic features. Automatic arrhythmias may arise from the sinoatrial region and from working atrial myocardium or the AV junction, yet reentrant rhythms may arise in these structures as well and may also involve accessory AV connections or other variants in the preexcitation syndrome. Table 27.1 provides an overview of PSVT categories by electrophysiological mechanisms and substrate.

Table 27.1 Classification of regular supraventricular tachycardias with narrow QRS complexes

Sinus Node Disorders
Paroxysmal sinus tachycardia
Nonparoxysmal sinoatrial tachycardia
AV Nodal Reentrant Tachycardias
Slow-fast
Fast-slow
Slow-slow
Reentrant and Ectopic Atrial Tachycardias
Intra-atrial reentrant tachycardia
Automatic atrial tachycardia (unifocal or multifocal)
Preexcitation Syndrome: Wolff-Parkinson-White Syndrome
Orthodromic atrioventricular reentry
Permanent junctional reciprocating tachycardia
Antidromic atrioventricular reentry
Atrial tachycardia, atrial flutter, or atrial fibrillation with or without accessory pathway conduction
Other Preexcitation Syndromes: Mahaim Conduction
Nodoventricular and nodofascicular reentry
Atrial tachycardia, AV nodal reentry, or atrial fibrillation with nodoventricular or nodofascicular bystander conduction
Atrial tachycardia, atrial flutter, or atrial fibrillation with enhanced AV nodal conduction
Automatic AV Junctional Tachycardias

AV = atrioventricular.

Diagnostic Approach to the Patient with Supraventricular Tachycardia

Investigation of supraventricular tachycardia (SVT) is based on understanding the underlying mechanism of the tachycardia and clinical context in which it occurs. A systematic approach should start with the history and physical examination, which provides two types of information: (1) the presence and type of symptoms and (2) the clinical context, particularly the existence of associated heart disease. The electrocardiographic documentation of the arrhythmia and its interpretation are essential to tachycardia management.

Differential Diagnosis of Supraventricular Tachycardias from the Surface Electrocardiogram

It is essential for the proper diagnosis and management of SVTs to obtain careful electrocardiographic documentation of the tachycardia. When the tachycardia occurs frequently or is of prolonged duration, a recording of the tachycardia episode is easily obtained. By definition, SVTs arise above the bifurcation of the His bundle, in either the atria or the AV junction and, therefore, are generally associated with narrow QRS complexes. However, SVTs can sometimes also present with wide QRS complexes, either because the patient had a pre-existing bundle branch block (BBB) or because aberrant or anomalous accessory pathway conduction is present. Differentiating SVT from ventricular tachycardia (VT) can sometimes be difficult, particularly when preexcitation is present.

Tachycardias with Narrow QRS Complexes

Most regular SVTs use the AV node either passively, such as in atrial tachycardias and atrial flutter, or as a critical component of the circuit, as in PSVT. The diagnostic approach to tachycardias with narrow QRS complexes should be undertaken in a stepwise fashion.[4-6]

As a first step, one should assess the pattern of the R–R interval. If the R–R interval is irregular, atrial fibrillation or atrial flutter should be considered the most likely diagnosis. However, when atrial fibrillation is associated with rapid ventricular response, it can also seem regular. When the R–R intervals appear regular, the next step is to look for P waves. The presence, morphology, and position of P waves in relation to the QRS complexes are important in the diagnosis of the site of origin and for the suspected mechanism of narrow QRS complex tachycardias. When the QRS complexes are preceded by P waves, which are different in configuration from the sinus P waves and conducted with a P–R interval equal or longer than the P–R interval of the sinus P waves, the most likely diagnosis is atrial tachycardia arising from an ectopic focus. The other mechanism of this type of SVT is intra-atrial or sinoatrial (SA) reentrant tachycardia, a diagnosis that requires an electrophysiological study for substantiation. If the P waves have the same configuration as the sinus P waves, the differential diagnosis includes appropriate or "inappropriate" sinus nodal tachycardia. Inappropriate sinus node tachycardia is a rare arrhythmia that has only been recognized recently. This atrial tachycardia is characterized by an inappropriate and exaggerated acceleration of heart rate during physiologic stress.[7] In the case of SVT when P waves are submerged within the QRS complex and are therefore not identifiable, the most likely diagnosis is typical AVNRT (ie, tachycardia involving the AV node and using a slow pathway in the anterograde direction and a fast pathway in the retrograde direction, resulting in a P wave within or immediately after the QRS complex).[8-9] Wellens has described an electrocardiographic sign, which is suggestive of AVNRT.[10] It consists of an incomplete BBB pattern (RSR') in lead V1 during the tachycardia that is not present in the 12-lead ECG in sinus rhythm. Di Toro and colleagues described that a notch phenomenon in lead aVL exhibits a higher sensitivity and specificity to determine the diagnosis of an AVNRT as compared to a pseudo-S wave or a pseudo-R' wave in V1.[11] However, atrial flutter with 2:1 conduction should be suspected as a differential diagnosis if the ventricular rate of the SVT with narrow QRS complexes is around 150 bpm. If P waves during SVT have been identified and follow the QRS complexes at a significant interval resulting in an R–P interval equal to or greater than the P–R interval, the most likely diagnosis is orthodromic AVRT (ie, involving the AV node in the antegrade direction and an accessory AV pathway in the retrograde direction). Other helpful electrocardiographic clues that have been reported and shed light onto the mechanism of SVT include a negative P wave in leads I and V1, due to left-to-right atrial activation in AVRT using a left-sided AV connection in its retrograde limb.[8,12] When two recordings of the tachycardia are available, one with narrow QRS complexes and the other with left BBB with a longer cycle length, a finding first described in Paris, the diagnosis of AVRT involving a left-sided accessory connection can be made.[12,13] The presence of QRS alternation is also in favor of AVRT.

The differential diagnosis between PSVT and atrial fibrillation with rapid ventricular response or atrial flutter with 1:1 conduction may at times be difficult. Vagal maneuvers, particularly carotid sinus massage and adenosine injection, may be of great help in clinical diagnosis. In AVRT or AVNRT, the arrhythmia may terminate abruptly or remain unaffected.[14] In contrast, atrial fibrillation or flutter is rarely terminated by these techniques but can be slowed in its ventricular response, thus exposing the underlying atrial flutter or fibrillation waves. PSVT and atrial flutter (AFL) may also coexist in the same patient. Adenosine administration may also be used as a diagnostic test to assess dual AV nodal pathway

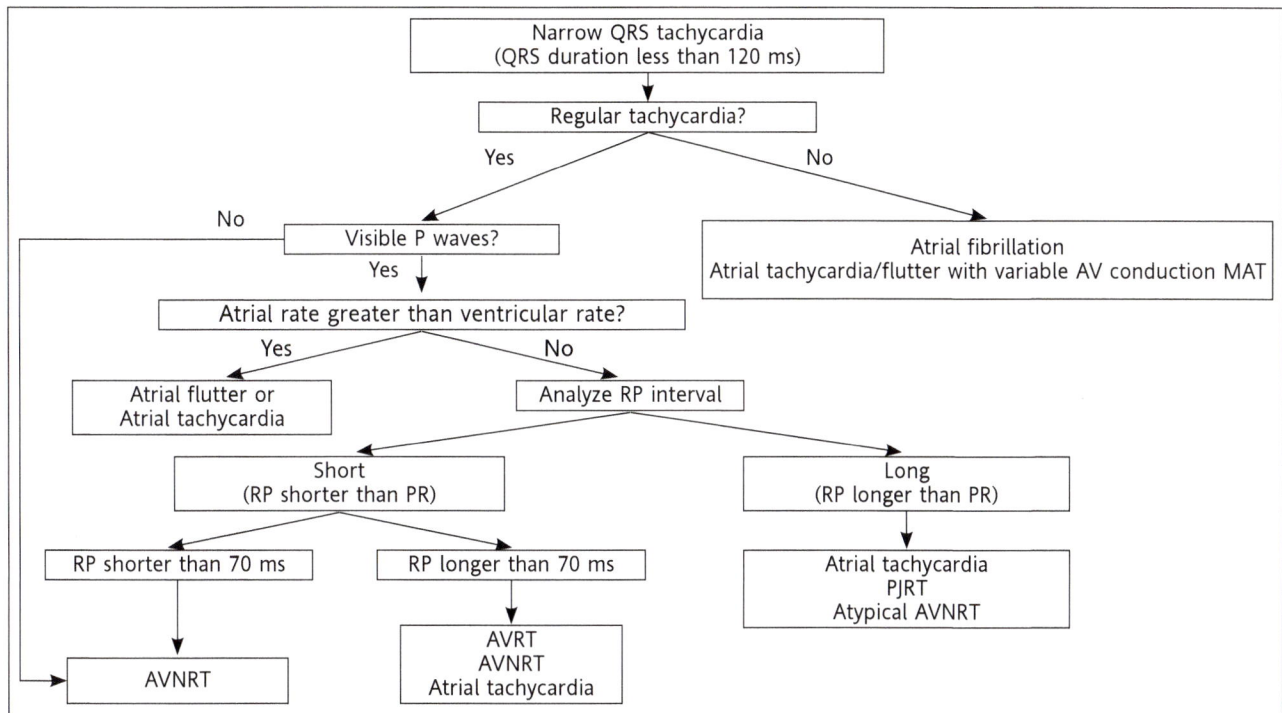

Figure 27.1 Differential diagnosis for narrow QRS tachycardia. AV = atrioventricular; AVNRT = atrioventricular nodal reentrant tachycardia; AVRT = atrioventricular tachycardia; MAT = multifocal atrial tachycardia; PJRT = permanent form of junctional reciprocating tachycardia.

conduction, efficacy of slow pathway ablation, and detection of concealed accessory pathways.[15] A unifying approach for the differential diagnosis of narrow QRS tachycardias has been proposed by the ACC/AHA/ESC guidelines and is depicted in Figure 27.1.[16]

Tachycardia with Regular Wide QRS Complex

Differentiating SVTs from VTs can be difficult since SVTs may also present with a wide (>0.12 seconds) QRS complex. In contrast to patients with VT, the vast majority of regular SVTs occur in patients without organic heart disease. The preexcitation syndrome is another etiology of wide QRS complex tachycardias. This variant may appear overt, such as in the WPW syndrome, or concealed, with the pathway only conducting in the retrograde direction, as discussed later.

Three clues may be used in the differentiation diagnosis of wide QRS tachycardias:

1. *The age of the patient.* In the child and young adult, preexcitation is more common than VT. In this instance, the ECG shows preexcitation both in sinus rhythm and during tachycardic episodes.

2. *Location of P waves during tachycardias.* The presence of AV dissociation is generally an indicator of VT. However, it is only present in about 40% of VTs. Differentiating SVT from VT may thus further require an electrophysiological study with endocavitary recordings. Wellens et al have described a number of criteria that may be of help differentiating SVT from VT.[10] Some that have proven to be particularly useful to favor a diagnosis of VT include left axis deviation (beyond –30 degrees), QRS complexes wider than 0.14 seconds, and the QRS morphology in V1 and V6 (ie, a monophasic R wave or a QR pattern in V1, or an rS or a QS pattern in V6).

3. *The presence of BBB in sinus rhythm.* An identical morphology of wide QRS complexes during the tachycardia is also suggestive of SVT. When the QRS complex is narrow in sinus rhythm but wide during SVT, aberrant conduction is also a possibility. We have found it practical to consider aberrant conduction only when the typical pattern of right or left BBB is present during tachycardia. This still does not exclude the possible diagnosis of VT. For these reasons, it is a wise rule to consider any tachycardia with wide QRS complexes as being VT unless proven otherwise. Detailed electrophysiological studies are indicated in all patients with wide QRS complex tachycardias.

Tachycardia with Preexcited QRS Complexes

When preexcited QRS complexes are present, the differential diagnosis of wide QRS complex tachycardia may be extremely difficult. Fortunately, these tachycardias represent less than 5% of all wide QRS complex tachycardias (Figure 27.2). Various mechanisms may account for a tachycardia with preexcited QRS complexes. The most common is atrial fibrillation with conduction over the

Kent bundle. In this tachycardia, the R–R interval is frequently irregular and the QRS width may be variable from one complex to another. Atrial flutter with 1:1 conduction over an accessory connection could also be present. This diagnosis should be suspected when the ventricular rate ranges from 250 to 300 bpm. Tachycardias with a left BBB and left axis deviation suggest the possibility of a Mahaim fiber, especially if the patient is young. Discerning other mechanisms may require endocavitary recordings and can thus only be ascertained through a detailed electrophysiological study.

Electrophysiological Study and Mapping of Supraventricular Tachycardia

Electrophysiological studies are nowadays routinely used for diagnostic and therapeutic purposes in patients with PSVT and other forms of arrhythmias. If SVT has not been previously recorded, it may be initiated through focal endocavitary stimulation, thus allowing ECG documentation of the tachycardia. In addition, the diagnostic procedure makes it possible to precisely define the mechanisms of the tachycardia and the critical components of its circuit. Furthermore, evaluation of the clinical symptoms during the arrhythmia can be assessed, and if indicated, radiofrequency ablation or other antiarrhythmic therapy can be administered. Since most SVTs are due to a reentrant mechanism, they may be induced in the laboratory using programmed electrical stimulation. In more than 90% of patients with AV junctional tachycardias (AVRT or AVNRT), the tachycardia can be elicited through an electrophysiological study. In patients with AVNRT, premature atrial stimulation can induce the tachycardia and reveal its mechanisms of dual AV nodal conduction. The arrhythmias associated with the WPW syndrome include reciprocating or so-called circus movement tachycardias and atrial arrhythmias. In some instances of AVNRT, there may be concomitant preexcited QRS complexes due to passive conduction over an accessory pathway, which may serve as a passive bystander. Tachycardias originating from Mahaim fibers have a particular electrocardiographic presentation that includes left BBB and left axis involvement. The ECG in sinus rhythm may show features of the WPW syndrome. The electrophysiological study will often demonstrate decremental conduction over the accessory pathway.

Atrioventricular Nodal Reentrant Tachycardia (AVNRT)

Dual Atrioventricular Nodal Pathway: During electrophysiological evaluation, typical AVNRT manifests through a characteristic dual AV nodal pathway, in which antegrade conduction occurs via a "slow" pathway and retrograde conduction via a "fast" pathway.[17,18] This dual AV nodal pathway is depicted on the ECG as a discontinuous AV node functional curve. Discontinuous AV nodal conduction is defined as a sudden increment ("jump") of 50 ms or greater in the A-H or H-A interval, with a decrement in prematurity of the extrastimulus by 10–20 ms. Typically, the jump phenomenon is followed by induction of a slow-fast AVNRT (Figure 27.3). During tachycardia of typical "slow-fast" AVNRT, one can document a long A-H combined with a short V-A interval (Figure 27.4). The earliest atrial activation (during tachycardia) can be detected by

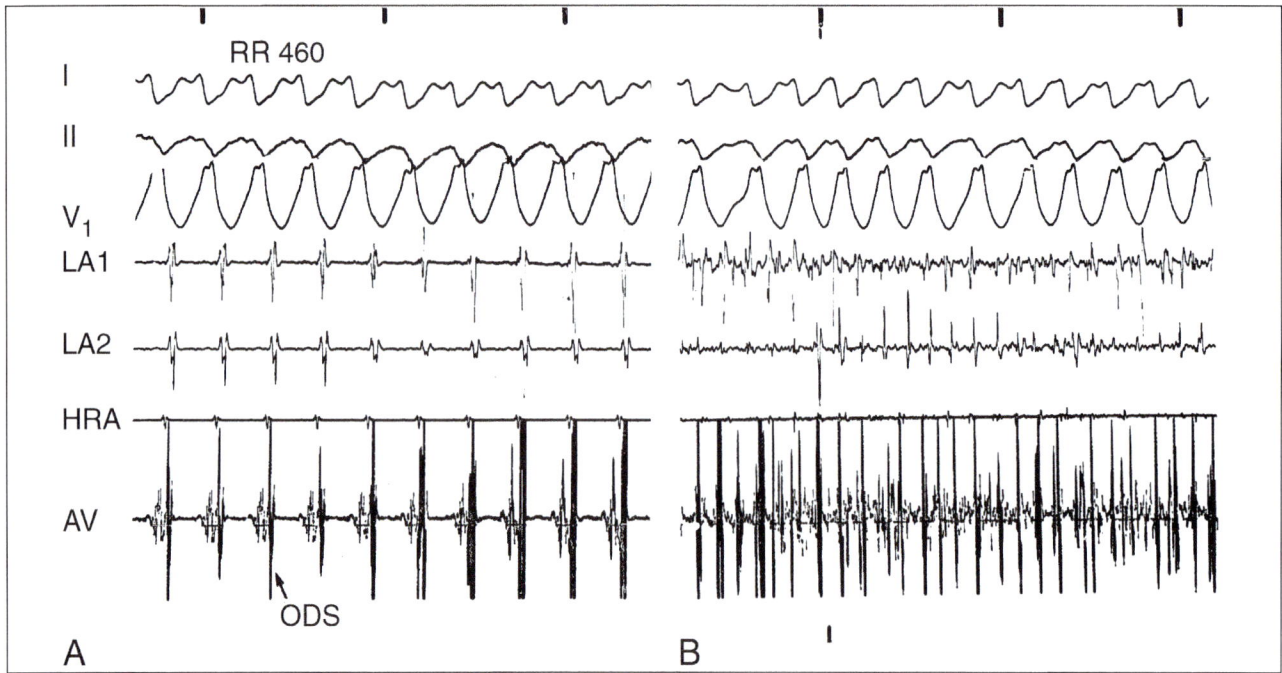

Figure 27.2 Tachycardias with preexcited QRS complexes. From top to bottom, ECG leads I, II, and V1, high right atrium (HRA), left atrium (LA1 and LA2). **Panel A** is consistent with an antidromic reciprocating tachycardia. **Panel B** shows AF conducted over a left-sided accessory AV pathway termination of SVT with vagal maneuvers.

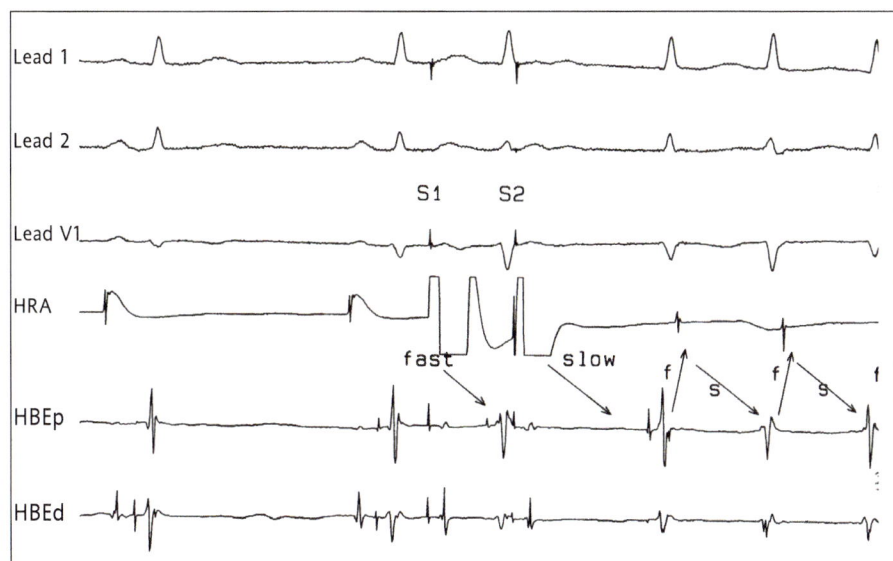

Figure 27.3 Induction AVNRT. Atrial extrastimulus pacing with an A-H jump and induction of typical slow-fast AVNRT.

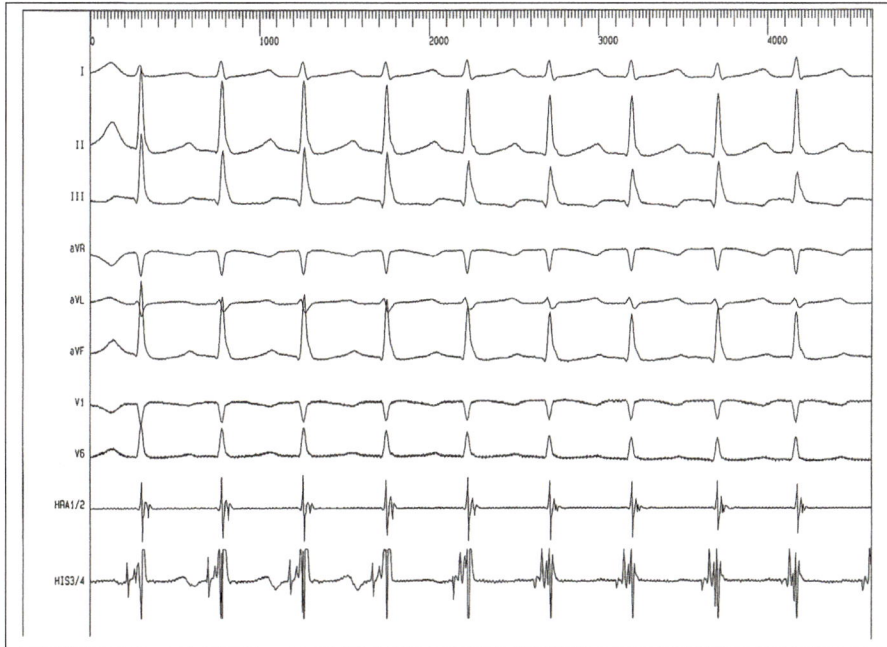

Figure 27.4 Typical slow-fast AVNRT with a short V-A interval.

endocardial mapping at the slow pathway region around the coronary sinus ostium. In contrast, atypical AVNRT has antegrade conduction through a "fast" or "slow" pathway and retrograde conduction through a "slow" pathway (Figures 27.5 and 27.6).[19,20]

To differentiate AVNRT from AVRT, the following stimulation protocols can be used:[21-23]

- V-A interval timing during tachycardia: V-A interval during "slow-fast" AVNRT is usually shorter than 50 ms, whereas during orthodromic AVRT the V-A intervals exceed 50 ms
- Miller stimulation (Figure 27.7)
- Parahisian stimulation
- Preceding stimulation (Figure 27.8)

For a long time, there has been a major question as to whether dual AV nodal pathways are fully intranodal and due to longitudinal dissociation of AV nodal tissue or extranodal involving separate atrial inputs into the AV node. This question has been illuminated by experimental (provocative) pharmacologic testing and catheter ablation in patients with AV nodal reentrant tachycardia. From clinical studies of slow pathway potentials, LH (low followed by high) frequency potentials are observed during asynchronous activation of muscle bundles above and below the coronary sinus orifice; HL (high followed by low) frequency potentials are caused by asynchronous activation of atrial cells and a band of nodal-type cells that may represent the substrate of the slow pathway.[24-27] Thus, the slow and fast pathways are likely to be atrio-nodal connections rather than discrete intranodal pathways. The results

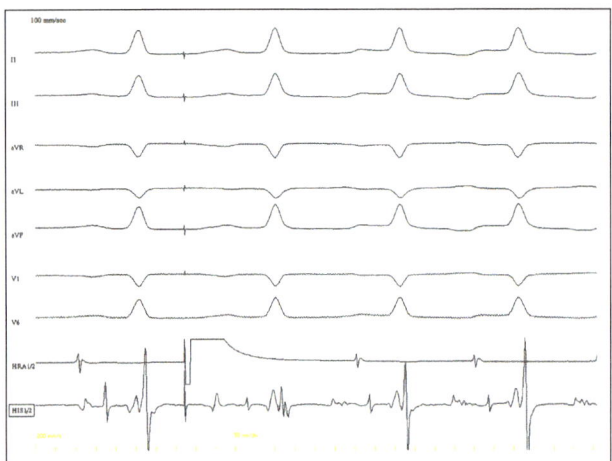

Figure 27.5 Induction of an atypical "fast-slow" AVNRT with an extrastimulus from HRA. The extrastimulus is not inducing an A-H jump because antegrade conduction is running via the fast pathway, but only a mild conduction delay in the antegrade fast pathway allowing retrograde activation of the slow pathway. From top to bottom, ECG leads II, III, aVR, aVL, aVF, V1, V6, high right atrium (HRA), and His bundle (HIS).

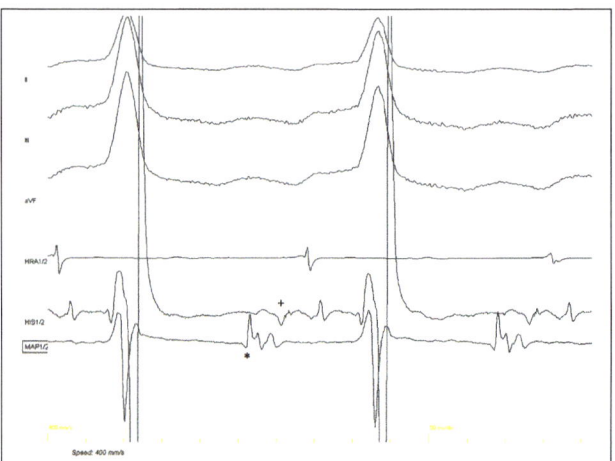

Figure 27.6 Mapping of the interatrial septum to detect earliest atrial activation during fast-slow AVNRT. During fast-slow AVNRT, the earliest atrial potential (*) can be detected at the slow pathway area (MAP-catheter); this signal is clearly earlier than the atrial deflection at the His bundle catheter (+), representing antegrade activation of the fast pathway region. From top to bottom, ECG leads II, III, aVF, high right atrium (HRA), His bundle (HIS), and (MAP) at the slow pathway region.

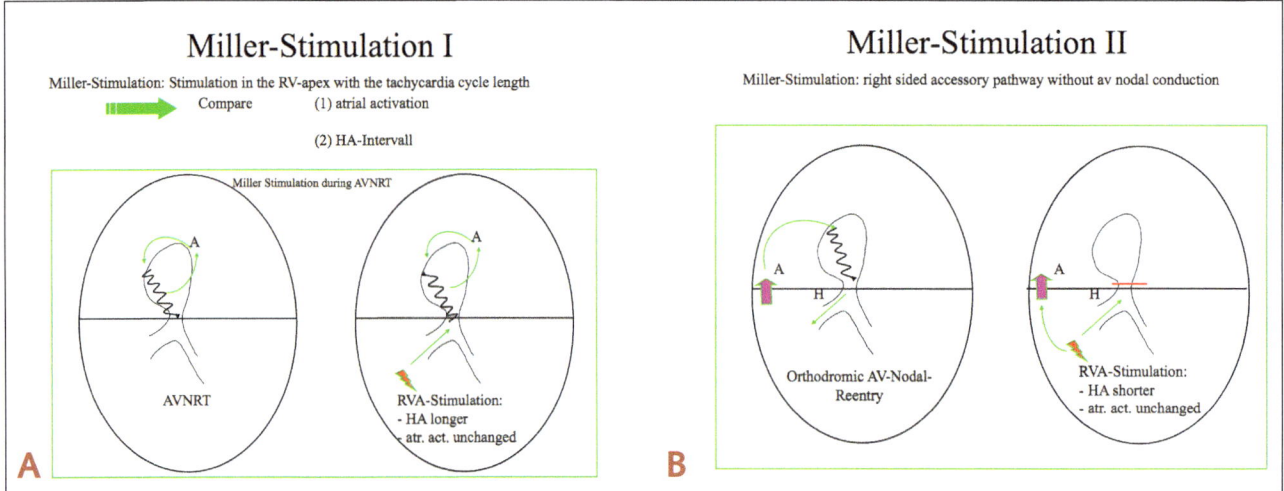

Figure 27.7 Miller stimulation.

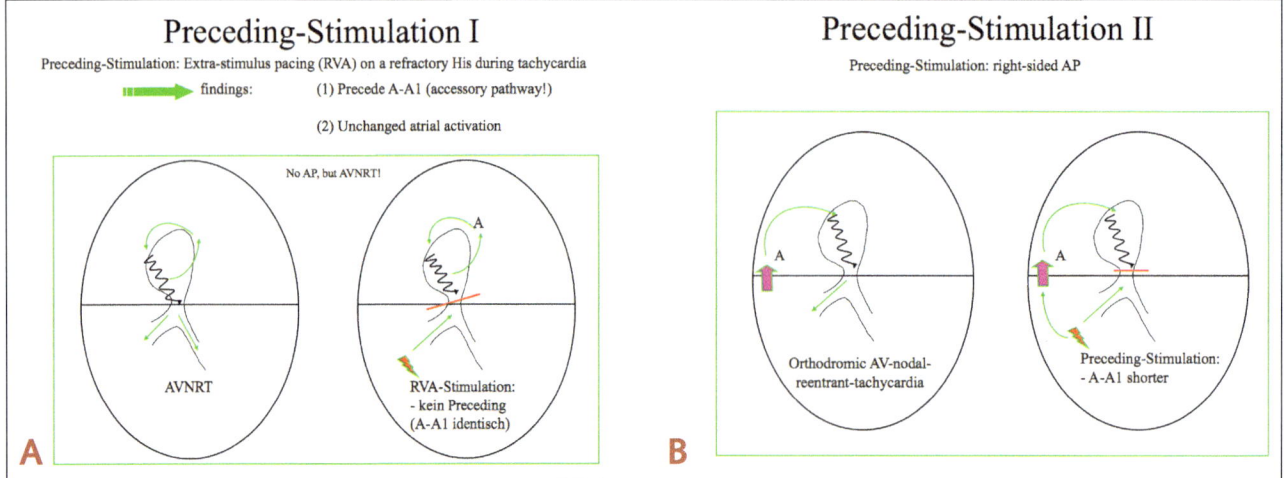

Figure 27.8 Preceding stimulation.

of catheter ablation indicate that the fast and slow pathways have their origins outside the limits of the compact AV node, and that the tissues targeted during successful ablation are composed of ordinary working atrial myocardium surrounding the AV node itself.[28-30] Furthermore, AV or VA conduction block during AVNRT favors the concept that atrial and ventricular tissue is not involved in maintenance of this tachycardia (Figures 27.9 and 27.10).[31,32]

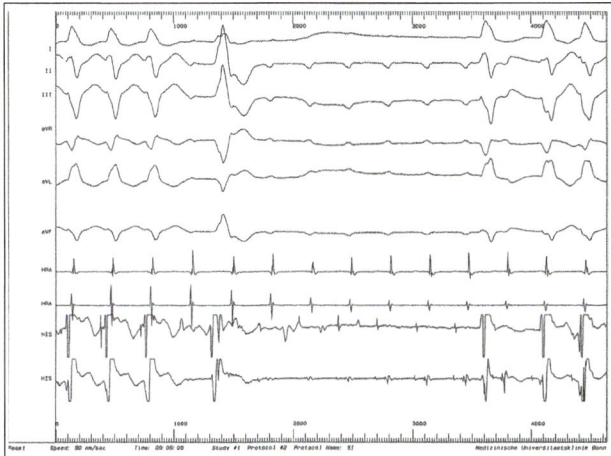

Figure 27.9 Infra-His block during typical slow-fast AVNRT. HIS = quadripolar catheter in His position; HRA = quadripolar catheter in high right atrium.

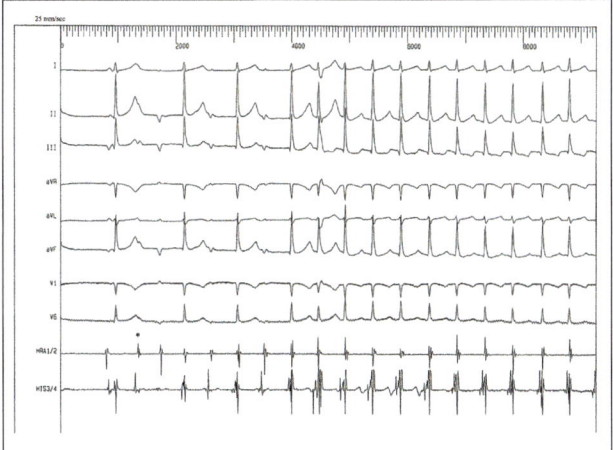

Figure 27.10 Initial 2:1 block in typical slow-fast AVNRT. Typical slow-fast AVNRT with spontaneous induction with a premature atrial complex (*) and initial 2:1 block to the ventricle; after 6 reentrant cycles with 2:1 block, 1 to 1 conduction is established.

Unusual Physiology of Dual Atrioventricular Nodal Pathways: Some patients with AVNRT have multiple antegrade and retrograde AV nodal pathways with multiple discontinuities in the AV node function curve or dual AV nodal pathways with a continuous curve during programmed electrical stimulation (Figure 27.11).[29,30] Furthermore, variant forms (slow-slow, slow-intermediate, fast-intermediate) of AVNRT have been noted (Figure 27.12).[28,33,34] Whether multiple antegrade and retrograde AV nodal pathways originate from anatomically different pathways or represent anisotropic conduction–induced functional pathways is still controversial. Several investigators have demonstrated the marked heterogeneity of the transitional cells surrounding the compact AV nodal pathway. The nonuniform properties of the AV node can produce anisotropic conduction and suggest that the antegrade and retrograde fast pathways are anatomically distant from the multiple "antegrade slow" and "retrograde slow" or intermediate pathways, respectively. Clinical studies have demonstrated that successful ablation or modification of "retrograde slow" and intermediate pathways occurs at different sites from "antegrade fast or slow" pathway, and the possibility of anatomically different antegrade or retrograde multiple pathways should be considered. Furthermore, in the patients who have successful ablation of multiple "antegrade slow" pathways or "retrograde slow" and intermediate pathways at a single site, anisotropic conduction over the low septal area of the right atrium is a possible explanation for the presence of multiple antegrade and retrograde AV nodal pathways.[29,30,35,36]

Patients with AVNRT can have continuous AV node conduction curves. These patients do not exhibit an A-H jump using 2 extrastimuli and 2 drive cycle lengths during atrial pacing from the high right atrium and coronary sinus ostium. The possible mechanisms of the continuous AV node function curves in AVNRT include: (1) the functional refractory period of the atrium limits the prematurity with which atrial premature depolarization will encounter the refractoriness in the AV node, which in turn produces inability to dissociate the fast and slow AV nodal pathways, and (2) fast and slow AV nodal pathways have similar refractory periods and conduction time.[29]

Atrioventricular Reentrant Tachycardia (AVRT)

Anatomy and Electrophysiology of Accessory Pathways: The oblique orientation of most accessory pathways has been demonstrated by detailed endocardial and epicardial mapping techniques.[34,37,38] The atrial and ventricular insertion sites of accessory pathways can be up to 2 cm disparate in location; furthermore, some accessory pathways have antegrade and retrograde conduction fibers at different locations, and this finding has been proven by different ablation sites for antegrade and retrograde conduction.[39] Thus, the anatomic and functional dissociation of the accessory pathway into atrial and ventricular insertions and antegrade and retrograde components is possible. Approximately 90% of AV accessory pathways have fast conduction properties, and the other accessory pathways (including Mahaim fibers) show decremental conduction properties during atrial or ventricular stimuli with shorter coupling intervals.[40-43] These pathways with decremental conduction may be sensitive to several antiarrhythmic drugs, including verapamil and adenosine. Accessory pathways in the right free wall and posteroseptal areas

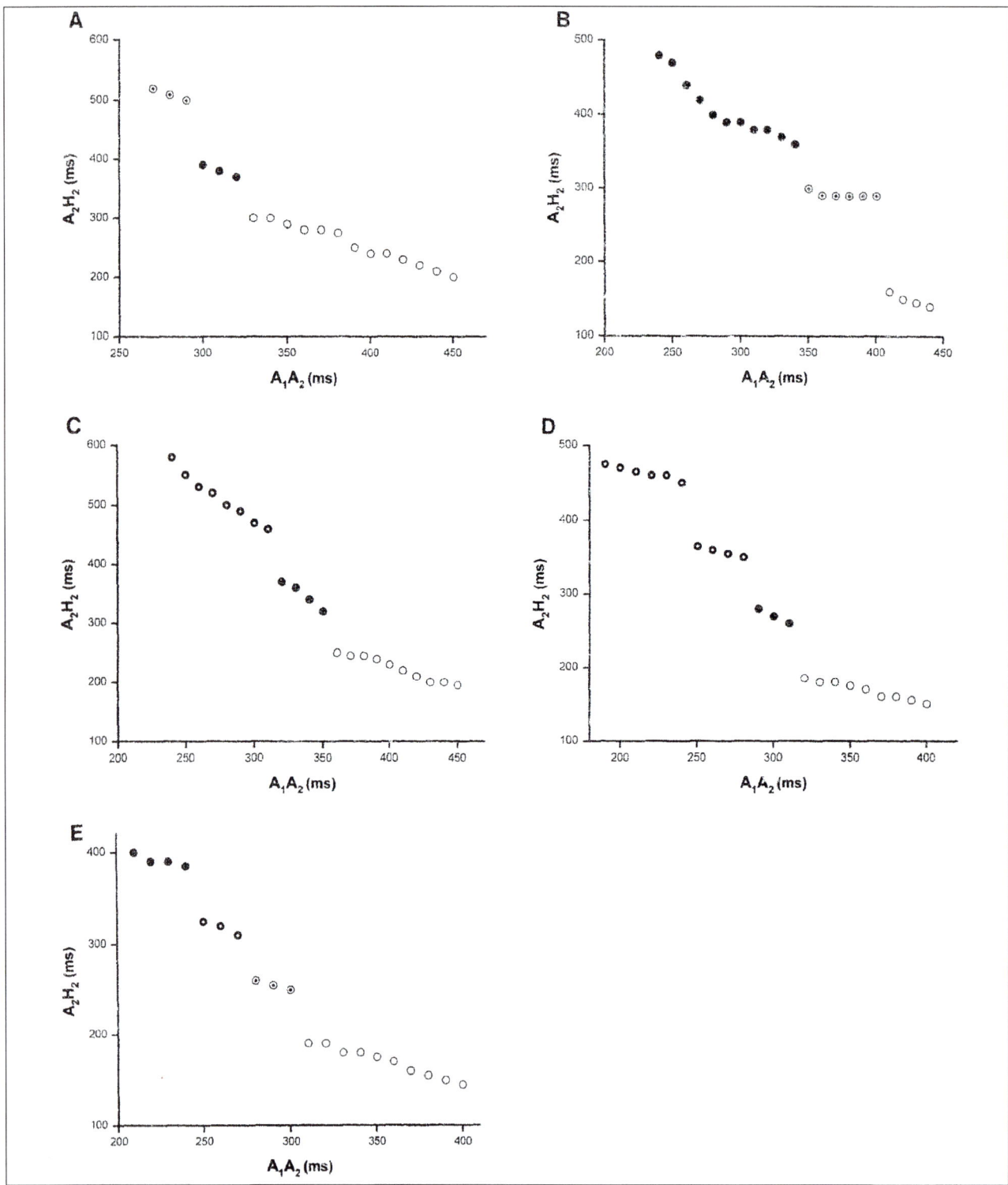

Figure 27.11 Five patterns of tachycardia (slow-fast form) induction demonstrated by atrioventricular node conduction curves (A_2H_2 vs A_1A_2). **Panel A:** Patient 17. Only the first slow pathway is used for induction and maintenance of sustained tachycardia (pattern 1). **Panel B:** Patient 20. Only the second slow pathway is used for induction and maintenance of sustained tachycardia (pattern 2). **Panel C:** Patient 12. The first slow pathway is used during sustained tachycardia; either the first or the second slow pathway is used for initiation of tachycardia (pattern 3). **Panel D:** Patient 22. The first slow pathway is used during sustained tachycardia; any of the three slow pathways is used for initiation of tachycardia (pattern 4). **Panel E:** Patient 24. The third slow pathway is used during sustained tachycardia; either the second or the third slow pathway is used for initiation of tachycardia (pattern 5). A_1A_2 = coupling interval of atrial extrastimulus; A_2H_2 = atrio-His bundle conduction interval in response to atrial extrastimulus. **Open circles** = fast pathway conduction; **circles with solid centers** = slow pathway conduction without initiation or maintenance of sustained tachycardia; **solid circles** = slow pathway conduction with initiation and maintenance of sustained tachycardia; **circles with open centers** = slow pathway conduction with initiation but without maintenance of sustained tachycardia. *Source:* From Tai CT, Chen SA, Chiang CE, et al.[29]

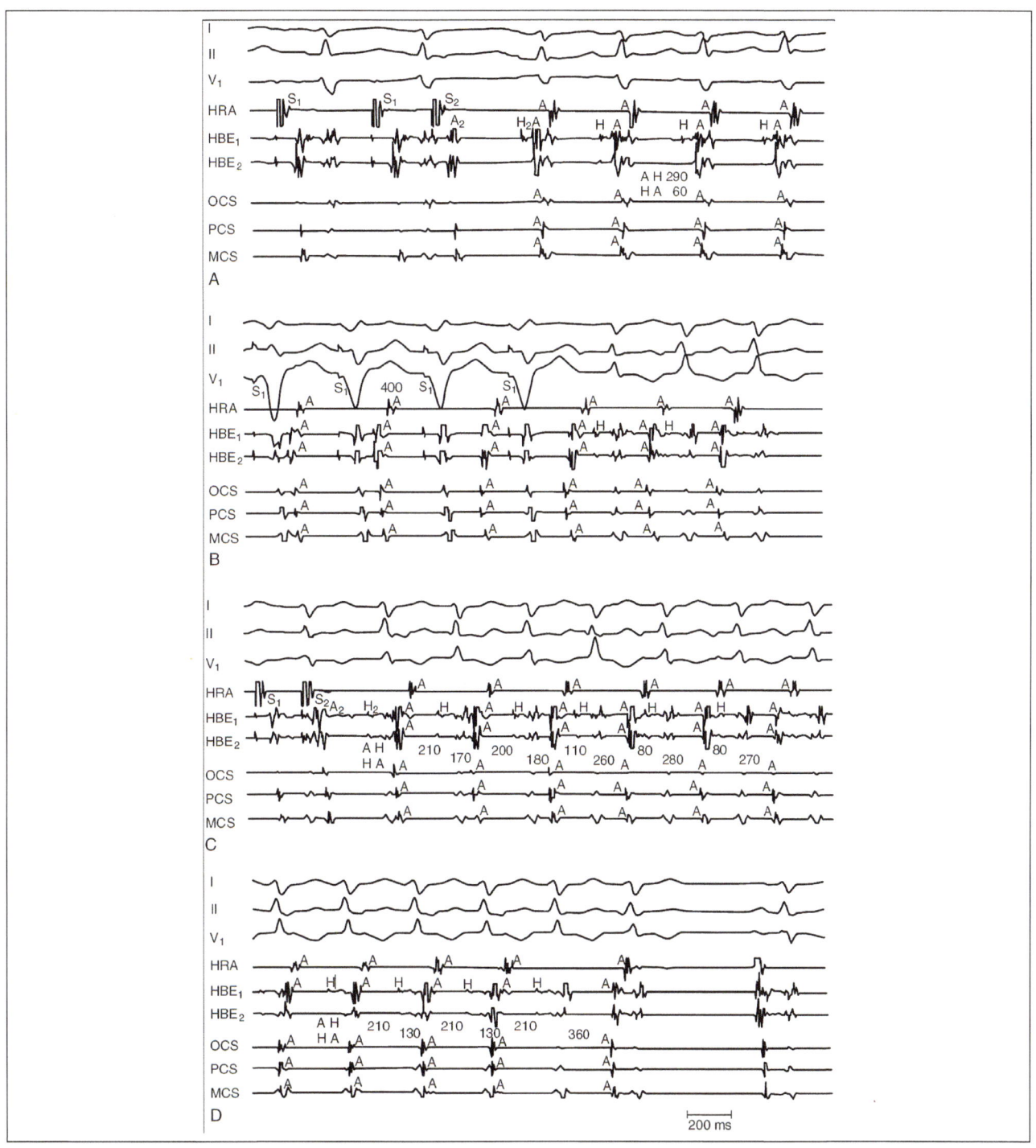

Figure 27.12 Recordings show 4 types of atrioventricular nodal reentrant tachycardia (AVNRT) and echo. **Panels A** and **B** are the baseline state. **Panels C** and **D** are intravenous infusion of isoproterenol. **Panels A:** Induction of slow-fast form of AVNRT by atrial extrastimulus, with the earliest atrial activation at the ostium of the coronary sinus (OCS). **Panel D:** A slow-slow form AVNR echo before termination of a slow-intermediate form of AVNRT. A_2 and H_2 = atrial and His bundle response to the atrial extrastimulus (S_2), respectively; HRA, HBE_1, HBE_2, PCS, and MCS = electrograms recorded from the high right atrium, the distal His bundle area, proximal His bundle area, proximal coronary sinus, and middle coronary sinus, respectively; S_1 = basic paced beats; S_2 = extrastimulus. *Source:* From Tai CT, et al.[33]

have a higher incidence of decremental conduction properties. When decremental conduction is present, the possibility of Mahaim fiber, such as atriofascicular or nodoventricular pathway, must be considered. Several studies have demonstrated that most of the ventricular insertion sites of these particular bypass tracts are close to the right bundle branch, and the typical Mahaim fiber potential can be recorded along the tricuspid annulus in patients with the atriofascicular pathways (Figure 27.13).[44-46] Accessory pathways can be located in malformation of the venous system of the heart, for example, coronary sinus diverticula (Figure 27.14).

308 • *Section 2A: Diagnostic & Mapping Techniques During Percutaneous Catheter & Surgical EP Procedures*

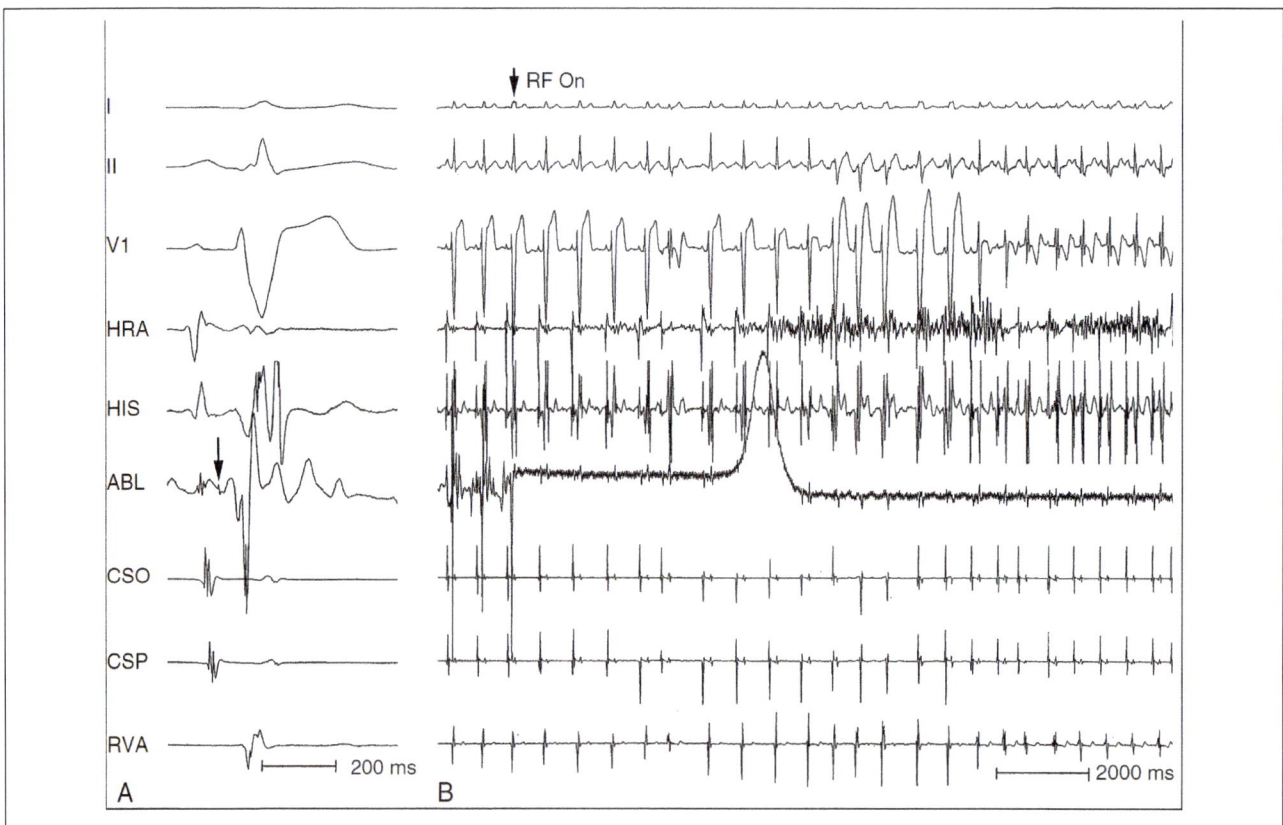

Figure 27.13 A mapping catheter along the posterolateral aspect of tricuspid annulus records the Mahaim fiber potential (**arrow in Panel A**). Application of radiofrequency energy on this point eliminates Mahaim fiber conduction with disappearance of ventricular preexcitation (**Panel B**).

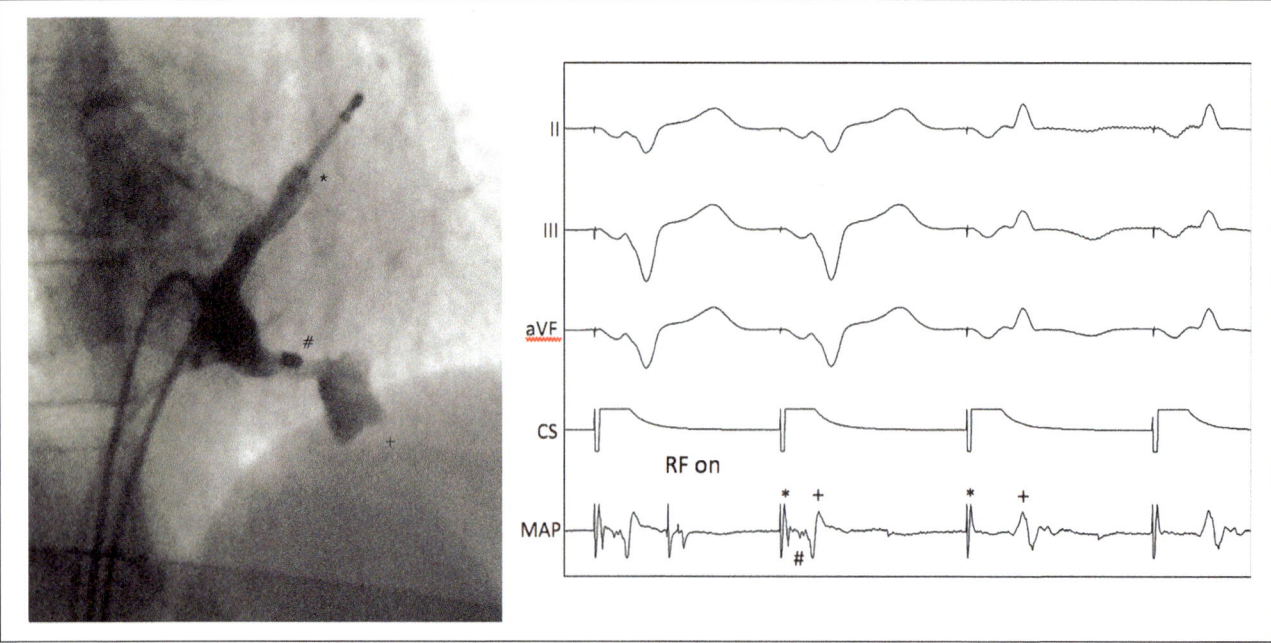

Figure 27.14 Accessory pathway catheter ablation inside the neck of a coronary sinus diverticulum. Coronary sinus (CS) phlebography was performed (★ **in left panel,** right anterior oblique view) and demonstrated a diverticulum originating from the proximal CS (+ **in left panel**). After insertion of a quadripolar ablation catheter (# **in left panel**) into the neck of the diverticulum, the ventricular signal preceded the onset of the delta wave and exhibited an AP potential (**black arrow in right panel**). During atrial pacing from the proximal CS, radiofrequency (RF) delivery (55°C, 45 W) eliminated anterograde AP conduction. The right panel (paper speed 100 mm/s) demonstrates abolition of the delta wave in ECG leads II, III, and aVF, elimination of the AP potential (# **in right panel**), and delayed ventricular activation (+) in relation to the local atrial signal (*) at the ablation catheter (MAP1/2) following conduction block in the AP. *Source:* Adapted from Lewalter T, Yang A, Schwab JO, Lüderitz B. *J Cardiovasc Electrophysiol.* 2003 Dec;14(12):1386. Used with permission.

Electrophysiological Findings in Atrioventricular Reentry Tachycardia: The manifest accessory pathway can be diagnosed from the 12-lead surface ECG with typical δ wave and is confirmed by a reduced, absent, or negative H-V interval. During electrophysiological study, recordings should be obtained from the tricuspid and mitral annulus directly or indirectly from the coronary sinus as well as the normal AV nodal His conduction system. Atrial and ventricular pacing and extrastimulation, isoproterenol provocation, and induction of atrial fibrillation to assess antegrade conduction over an accessory pathway are essential elements of electrophysiological study Ventricular pacing and extrastimulation can define retrograde conduction properties such as refractoriness and conduction time and location of the pathway. Switching of conduction between the accessory pathway and AV nodal–His axis can be demonstrated upon reaching effective refractoriness of one or the other conduction pathway. Atrial pacing or extrastimulation can accentuate antegrade preexcitation up to the refractoriness of the pathway. Tachycardia induction requires unidirectional block in one of the AV conduction pathways (AV node/His or accessory pathway) coupled with critical conduction delay in the circuit.

For the diagnosis of accessory pathway–mediated AV reentry tachycardia, a premature ventricular depolarization can be delivered during the tachycardia at a time when the His bundle is refractory and the impulse still conducts to the atrium; this indicates that retrograde propagation conducts to the atrium over a pathway other than the normal AV conduction system. The definition of AV reentry tachycardia involves reentry over one or more AV accessory pathways and the AV node, and the classic classification of AV reentry tachycardia includes orthodromic and antidromic tachycardias.[47-49] For the initiation of orthodromic tachycardia, a critical degree of AV or VA delay, which can be in the AV node or His-Purkinje system, is usually necessary. However, dual AV nodal pathway physiology, with or without AV nodal reentrant tachycardia, can be noted in some patients (Figure 27.15). Ventricular pacing from different sites can provide valuable information about retrograde conduction through the AV node or via a septal pathway (Figure 27.16). The incidence of antidromic AV reentry tachycardia is much lower than orthodromic AV reentry tachycardia (Figure 27.17). Rapid conduction in retrograde AV nodal–His axis is necessary for initiation and maintenance of antidromic tachycardia. The incidence of multiple accessory pathways is about 5%–20% and antidromic tachycardia is common in this situation where the retrograde conduction of the antidromic reentry is usually one of the retrograde conducting pathways instead of the AV node; even in PJRT, multiple slow conduction accessory pathways have been described.

The most difficult situation for differential diagnosis of AV reentry tachycardia is the so-called Mahaim tachycardia, including atriofascicular or nodofascicular (or nodoventricular) reentry tachycardia and AV nodal reentry tachycardia with innocent bystander bypass tract. These arrhythmias often appear as wide complex tachycardias with a left BBB and left axis deviation morphology. However, presence of VA dissociation favors nodofascicular tachycardia. Sternick and colleagues described a simple parameter to distinguish between decremental or rapidly conducting pathways during preexcited tachycardia: an AV interval of >150 ms during preexcited tachycardia is reliable for detecting a decrementally conducting accessory pathway.[50]

Mapping Criteria to Identify Successful Ablation Sites

Mapping Criteria for Exact Accessory Pathway Localization

The exact localization of the accessory pathway is a prerequisite for a successful catheter ablation. In *sinus rhythm* with ventricular preexcitation and delta wave indicating a rapidly conducting pathway with ventricular

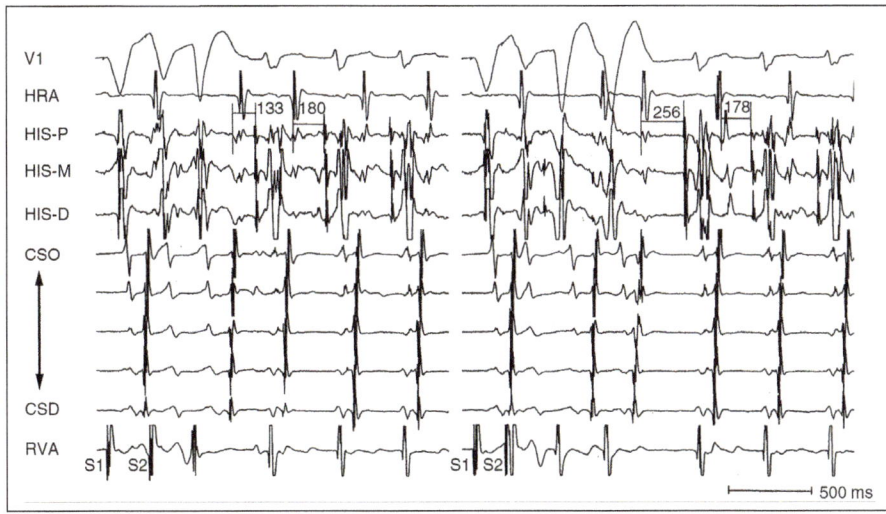

Figure 27.15 **Left** and **right panels** show right ventricular extrastimulus (S_1S_2) with V_3 phenomenon, and induces AV reentry tachycardia with retrograde conduction through the left lateral accessory pathway. In the left panel, the first and second tachycardia beats show antegrade conduction time (A-H interval) of 133 and 180 ms, respectively. In the right panel, the S_1S_2 coupling interval is shorter than the left panel, and the antegrade conduction time is much longer in the first tachycardia beat than the second tachycardia beat (256 vs 178 ms), with the difference larger than 50 ms, suggesting the possibility of antegrade conduction through the slow pathway in the first tachycardia beat.

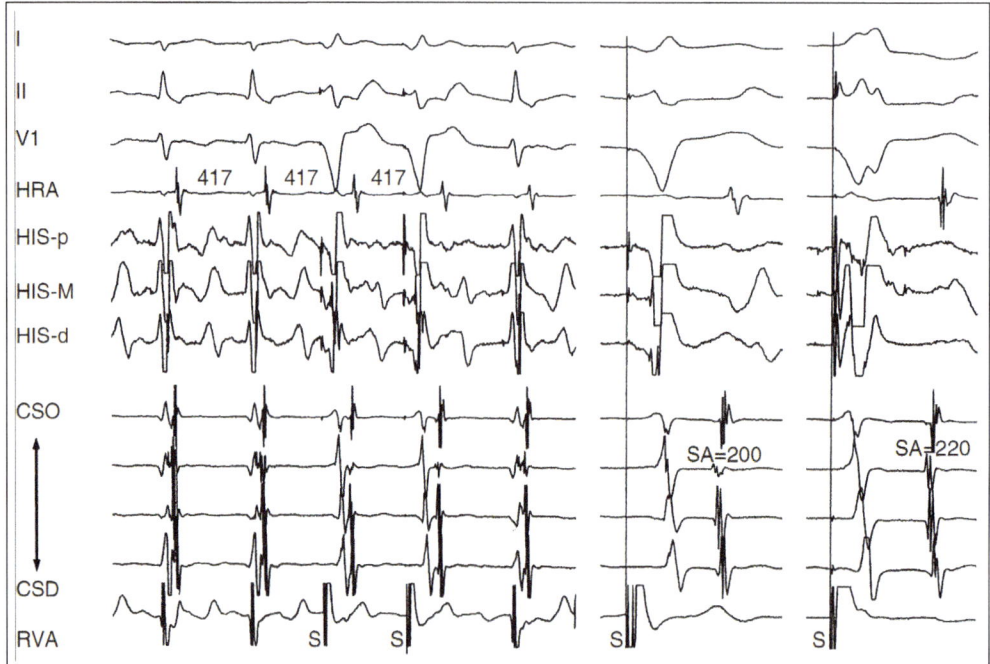

Figure 27.16 **Left panel** shows delivery of two right ventricular apex stimuli during tachycardia, without changing the tachycardia cycle length (417 ms). Furthermore, the earliest atrial activation is on the CS proximal part. The **middle panel** shows ventricular stimuli from right ventricular apex with the same pacing cycle length as tachycardia cycle length, and the interval from stimulus to atrial activation on CS is 220 ms. The **right panel** shows ventricular stimuli from the basal part of the right ventricle with the same pacing cycle length as tachycardia cycle length, and the interval from stimulus to atrial activation on CS is 220 ms. The retrograde His bundle potential is found before atrial activation. The stimulus to the A interval (220 ms) is much longer than the QRS–A interval during tachycardia. These findings suggest atrioventricular nodal reentrant tachycardia (AVNRT) with demonstration of lower common pathway during ventricular pacing and exclude the possibility of retrograde accessory pathway in the posteroseptal area.

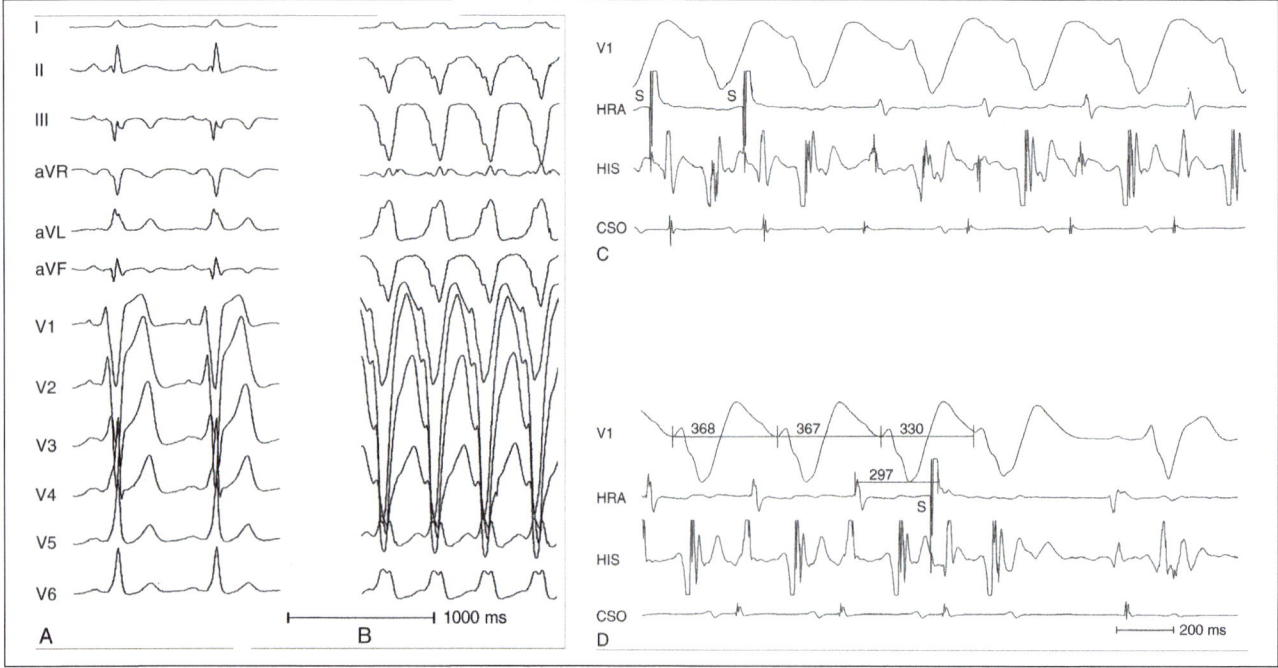

Figure 27.17 **Panel A:** A 12-lead ECG during sinus rhythm. **Panel B:** Surface 12-lead ECG of antidromic tachycardia. **Panel C:** Rapid atrial pacing (S) induces antidromic atrioventricular (AV) reentry tachycardia with antegrade conduction through right free wall accessory pathway and retrograde conduction through slow AV nodal pathway (earliest retrograde atrial activation in the CS ostium). **Panel D:** One atrial premature beat preexcites the ventricle through the accessory pathway; however, this atrial premature beat (S) also collides with retrograde atrial activation, and AV reentry tachycardia is terminated.

preexcitation, the following criteria indicate that the mapping catheter is at the accessory pathway location:

1. Earliest V-signal in relation to delta wave onset (Figure 27.18)

2. Electrical continuity or fusion between the A-signal and the V-signal ("W sign")[53] (Figure 27.18)

3. Presence of an accessory pathway potential ("Kent fiber potential") (Figure 27.19)

4. QS morphology in the unipolar recording

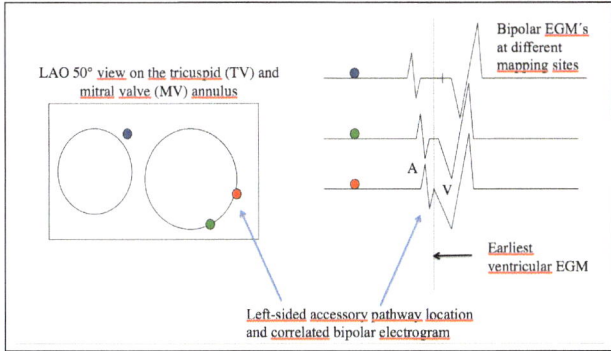

Figure 27.18 This graph illustrates the correlation of accessory pathway location to different mapping sites in terms of "earliness" of the local bipolar ventricular electrogram (EGM). In addition, the local EGM at the accessory pathway location display a "W sign."

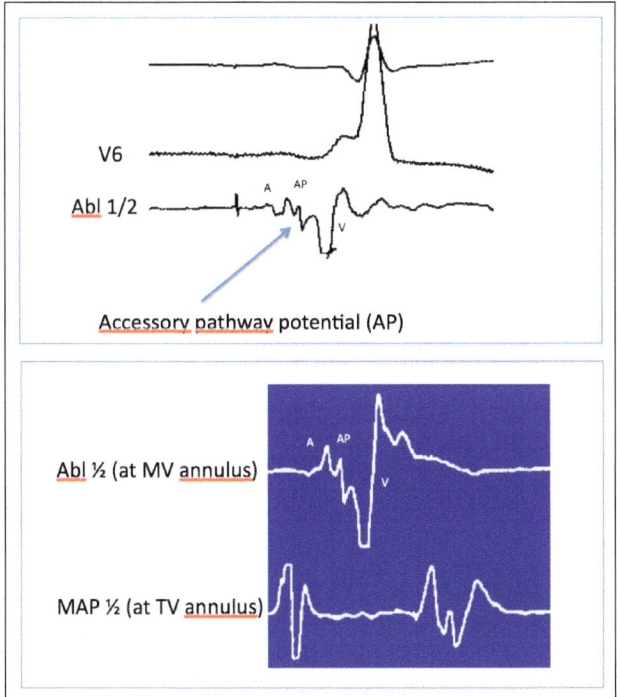

Figure 27.19 Two examples for accessory pathway potentials as an indicator for a successful ablation site. MV = mitral valve; TV = tricuspid valve.

As described in several studies, the timing of the local ventricular electrogram in relation to the preexcited QRS complex and the presence of a Kent fiber potential were the most powerful predictors for a successful ablation site.[51,52] A specific morphology of the bipolar local electrogram indicating electrical continuity between atrial and ventricular myocardium ("W sign") was described by Manolis and colleagues.[53]

During *antidromic tachycardia,* mapping criteria remain the same, whereas during *orthodromic antriventricular tachycardia,* the mapping catheter has now to detect the earliest site of retrograde atrial activation again with electrical continuity between the ventricle and the atrium. The following criteria indicate that the mapping catheter is at the accessory pathway location during atrioventricular tachycardia:

1. Earliest A-signal in relation to the retrograde P wave or any other endocardial atrial signal

2. Electrical continuity between the V-signal and the A-signal

3. Presence of an accessory pathway potential representing retrograde accessory pathway conduction

Mapping Criteria for Slow Pathway Identification

Jackman et al reported spike potentials following atrial electrograms as potentials of the slow pathway; targeting those potentials with RF energy, they obtained a good rate of success with ablation therapy.[25] Haïssaguerre, however, reported rather hump-shaped slow pathway potentials, which he could record in Koch's triangle. Those potentials were described as discrete and low-amplitude deflections with a slow rate of rise occupying the interval between the atrial and ventricular potentials.[26] For further details and description of the current ablation approach using both electrophysiological criteria to identify the slow pathway location and anatomical criteria, see chapter 39.

Cryomapping

Cryoenergy is more frequently in clinical use, either for pulmonary vein ablation or for ablation in high-risk cases like parahisian pathways or AVNRT in children. The reason for using it in such high-risk cases is that cryoenergy allows the performance of cryomapping, which makes it possible to assess the functional effect of ablation at a particular site in a reversible mode before generating a permanent lesion.[54] In clinical practice, cryomapping is carried out at a cryocatheter tip temperature of −30°C for a maximal duration of 60 seconds.[55] In case of an ineffective result (eg, no conduction block in an accessory pathway) or development of an AV block (while ablating close to the AV node), cryomapping is stopped and repeated at a new target site. If the desired effect is observed, (1) block of the accessory pathway, (2) no development of an AV block targeting for the slow pathway, or (3) abolition of nodal conduction jump or AV nodal refractory period prolongation,[55] direct freezing and cryoablation is initiated. As a limitation of cryomapping, it has to be mentioned that adverse effects on AV conduction may be observed during cryoablation despite no previous deleterious effect during cryomapping.[56] This is probably related to the fact that the cryolesion created with cryoablation is larger than suggested by cryomapping.

Drug Testing in Paroxysmal Supraventricular Tachycardia

Cardiac electrophysiology studies use intracardiac recording and programmed stimulation to define the mechanisms and most appropriate therapy for supraventricular and ventricular arrhythmias. Using these techniques, the majority of clinical tachycardias can be reproducibly initiated and terminated in the electrophysiology laboratory. With this approach, antiarrhythmic agents can be tested in a systematic, serialized fashion for efficacy, safety, and patient tolerance.[57] Suppression of arrhythmia induction is a marker for freedom from recurrence, whereas inducibility carries a higher risk of recurrence or need for alternative therapies. Nagi and colleagues, for example, could identify by electrophysiological testing an acutely effective drug in patients with an accessory pathway; those findings were highly predictive for their long-term clinical outcome.[58] In parallel to the reduced overall relevance of drug therapy in SVT, the use of drug testing, especially serial electrophysiological drug testing, has been mainly abandoned.

References

1. Bouveret, quoted by Froment R: Precis de Cardiologie Clinique. *Masson et Cie.* 1962:238-242.
2. Cotton R. Notes and observations of unusually rapid action of the heart. *BMJ.* 1867;I(629).
3. Surawicz B, Saito S. Exercise testing for detection of myocardial ischemia in patients with abnormal electrocardiograms at rest. *Am J Cardiol.* 1978;41(5):943-951.
4. Marriot H. Systematic approach to diagnosis of arrhythmias. *Practical Electrocardiography.* 7th ed. Baltimore: William & Wilkins; 1984.
5. Davies DTW. *Diagnosis of cardiac arrhythmias from the surface electrocardigram.* London: Kluwer Academic; 1988.
6. Levy S. Diagnostic approach to cardiac arrhythmias. *J Cardiovasc Pharmacol.* 1991;17(suppl 6):524-531.
7. Morillo CA, Klein GJ, Thakur RK, Li H, Zardini M, Yee R. Mechanism of "inappropriate" sinus tachycardia. Role of sympathovagal balance. *Circulation.* 1994;90(2):873-877.
8. Farre JWH. *The value of the electrocardiogram in diagnosing the site of origin and mechanisms of supraventricular tachycardia.* The Hague: Martinus Nijhoff; 1981.
9. Akhtar M, Jazayeri MR, Sra J, Blanck Z, Deshpande S, Dhala A. Atrioventricular nodal reentry. Clinical, electrophysiological, and therapeutic considerations. *Circulation.* 1993;88(1):282-295.
10. Wellens HJ, Bar FW, Vanagt E. *The differentiation between ventricular tachycardia and supraventricular tachycardia with aberrant conduction: the value of the 12-lead electrocardiogram.* The Hague: Martinus Nijhoff; 1981.
11. Di Toro D, Hadid C, Lopez C, Fuselli J, Luis V, Labadet C. Utility of the aVL lead in the electrocardiographic diagnosis of atrioventricular node re-entrant tachycardia. *Europace.* 2009;11(7):944-948.
12. Coumel P, Gourgon R, Fabiato A, Laurent D, Bouvrain Y. [Studies of assisted circulation. I. Methods of repetitive provoked extrasystole and slowing of effective heart rate]. *Arch Mal Coeur Vaiss.* 1967;60(1):67-88.
13. Slama M, Coumel P, Bouvrain Y. Tachycardies paroxystiques liees a un syndrome de Wolff-Parkinson-White inapparent. *Arch Mal Coeur Vaiss.* 1973;66:639-653.
14. Riccardi A, Arboscello E, Ghinatti M, Minuto P, Lerza R. Adenosine in the treatment of supraventricular tachycardia: 5 years of experience (2002–2006). *Am J Emerg Med.* 2008;26(8):879-882.
15. Viskin S, Fish R, Glick A, Glikson M, Eldar M, Belhassen B. The adenosine triphosphate test: a bedside diagnostic tool for identifying the mechanism of supraventricular tachycardia in patients with palpitations. *J Am Coll Cardiol.* 2001;38(1):173-177.
16. Blomström-Lundqvist C, Scheinman MM, Aliot EM, Alpert JS, Calkins H, Camm AJ, et al. ACC/AHA/ESC Guidelines for the Management of Patients With Supraventricular Arrhythmias—Executive Summary: A Report of the American College of Cardiology/American Heart Association Task Force on Practice Guidelines and the European Society of Cardiology Committee for Practice Guidelines. *Circulation.* 2003;108:1871-1909.
17. Denes P, Wu D, Dhingra RC, Chuquimia R, Rosen KM. Demonstration of dual A-V nodal pathways in patients with paroxysmal supraventricular tachycardia. *Circulation.* 1973;48(3):549-555.
18. Sung RJ, Styperek JL, Myerburg RJ, Castellanos A. Initiation of two distinct forms of atrioventricular nodal reentrant tachycardia during programmed ventricular stimulation in man. *Am J Cardiol.* 1978;42(3):404-415.
19. Wu D, Denes P, Amat YLF, Wyndham CR, Dhingra R, Rosen KM. An unusual variety of atrioventricular nodal re-entry due to retrograde dual atrioventricular nodal pathways. *Circulation.* 1977;56(1):50-59.
20. Sung RJ, Waxman HL, Saksena S, Juma Z. Sequence of retrograde atrial activation in patients with dual atrioventricular nodal pathways. *Circulation.* 1981;64(5):1059-1067.
21. Miller JM, Rosenthal ME, Gottlieb CD, Vassallo JA, Josephson ME. Usefulness of the delta HA interval to accurately distinguish atrioventricular nodal reentry from orthodromic septal bypass tract tachycardias. *Am J Cardiol.* 1991;68(10):1037-1044.
22. Chien WW, Wang YS, Epstein LM, et al. Ventricular septal summit stimulation in atrioventricular nodal reentrant tachycardia. *Am J Cardiol.* 1993;72(17):1268-1273.
23. Goldberger J, Wang Y, Scheinman M. Stimulation of the summit of the right ventricular aspect of the ventricular septum during orthodromic atrioventricular reentrant tachycardia. *Am J Cardiol.* 1992;70(1):78-85.
24. Ross DL, Johnson DC, Denniss AR, Cooper MJ, Richards DA, Uther JB. Curative surgery for atrioventricular junctional

("AV nodal") reentrant tachycardia. *J Am Coll Cardiol.* 1985;6(6):1383-1392.

25. Jackman WM, Beckman KJ, McClelland JH, et al. Treatment of supraventricular tachycardia due to atrioventricular nodal reentry, by radiofrequency catheter ablation of slow-pathway conduction. *N Engl J Med.* 1992;327(5):313-318.
26. Haïssaguerre M, Gaita F, Fischer B, et al. Elimination of atrioventricular nodal reentrant tachycardia using discrete slow potentials to guide application of radiofrequency energy. *Circulation.* 1992;85(6):2162-2175.
27. McGuire MA, Lau KC, Johnson DC, Richards DA, Uther JB, Ross DL. Patients with two types of atrioventricular junctional (AV nodal) reentrant tachycardia. Evidence that a common pathway of nodal tissue is not present above the reentrant circuit. *Circulation.* 1991;83(4):1232-1246.
28. Yeh SJ, Wang CC, Wen MS, Lin FC, Chen IC, Wu D. Radiofrequency ablation therapy in atypical or multiple atrioventricular node reentry tachycardias. *Am Heart J.* 1994;128(4):742-758.
29. Tai CT, Chen SA, Chiang CE, et al. Complex electrophysiological characteristics in atrioventricular nodal reentrant tachycardia with continuous atrioventricular node function curves. *Circulation.* 1997;95(11):2541-2547.
30. Tai CT, Chen SA, Chiang CE, et al. Multiple anterograde atrioventricular node pathways in patients with atrioventricular node reentrant tachycardia. *J Am Coll Cardiol.* 1996;28(3):725-731.
31. Wellens HJ, Wesdorp JC, Duren DR, Lie KI. Second degree block during reciprocal atrioventricular nodal tachycardia. *Circulation.* 1976;53(4):595-599.
32. Lee SH, Chen SA, Tai CT, et al. Electrophysiologic characteristics and radiofrequency catheter ablation in atrioventricular node reentrant tachycardia with second-degree atrioventricular block. *J Cardiovasc Electrophysiol.* 1997;8(5):502-511.
33. Tai CT, Chen SA, Chiang CE, et al. Electrophysiologic characteristics and radiofrequency catheter ablation in patients with multiple atrioventricular nodal reentry tachycardias. *Am J Cardiol.* 1996;77(1):52-58.
34. Tai CT, Chen SA, Chiang CE, et al. Identification of fiber orientation in left free-wall accessory pathways: implication for radiofrequency ablation. *J Interv Card Electrophysiol.* 1997;1(3):235-241.
35. Yeh SJ, Wang CC, Wen MS, et al. Characteristics and radio-frequency ablation therapy of intermediate septal accessory pathway. *Am J Cardiol.* 1994;73(1):50-56.
36. Tai CT, Chen SA, Chiang CE, Lee SH, Chang MS. Electrocardiographic and electrophysiologic characteristics of anteroseptal, midseptal, and para-Hisian accessory pathways. Implication for radiofrequency catheter ablation. *Chest.* 1996;109(3):730-740.
37. Gallagher JJ, Sealy WC. The permanent form of junctional reciprocating tachycardia: further elucidation of the underlying mechanism. *Eur J Cardiol.* 1978;8(4-5):413-430.
38. Jackman WM, Friday KJ, Yeung-Lai-Wah JA, et al. New catheter technique for recording left free-wall accessory atrioventricular pathway activation. Identification of pathway fiber orientation. *Circulation.* 1988;78(3):598-611.
39. Chen SA, Tai CT, Lee SH, et al. Electrophysiologic characteristics and anatomical complexities of accessory atrioventricular pathways with successful ablation of anterograde and retrograde conduction at different sites. *J Cardiovasc Electrophysiol.* 1996;7(10):907-915.
40. Gallagher JJ, Kasell J, Sealy WC, Pritchett EL, Wallace AG. Epicardial mapping in the Wolff-Parkinson-White syndrome. *Circulation.* 1978;57(5):854-866.
41. Farre J, Ross D, Wiener I, Bar FW, Vanagt EJ, Wellens HJ. Reciprocal tachycardias using accessory pathways with long conduction times. *Am J Cardiol.* 1979;44(6):1099-1109.
42. Tchou P, Lehmann MH, Jazayeri M, Akhtar M. Atriofascicular connection or a nodoventricular Mahaim fiber? Electrophysiologic elucidation of the pathway and associated reentrant circuit. *Circulation.* 1988;77(4):837-848.
43. Chen SA, Tai CT, Chiang CE, et al. Electrophysiologic characteristics, electropharmacologic responses and radio-frequency ablation in patients with decremental accessory pathway. *J Am Coll Cardiol.* 1996;28(3):732-737.
44. Klein LS, Hackett FK, Zipes DP, Miles WM. Radiofrequency catheter ablation of Mahaim fibers at the tricuspid annulus. *Circulation.* 1993;87(3):738-747.
45. McClelland JH, Wang X, Beckman KJ, et al. Radiofrequency catheter ablation of right atriofascicular (Mahaim) accessory pathways guided by accessory pathway activation potentials. *Circulation.* 1994;89(6):2655-2666.
46. Cappato R, Schluter M, Weiss C, et al. Catheter-induced mechanical conduction block of right-sided accessory fibers with Mahaim-type preexcitation to guide radiofrequency ablation. *Circulation.* 1994;90(1):282-290.
47. Selle JG, Sealy WC, Gallagher JJ, Fedor JM, Svenson RH, Zimmern SH. Technical considerations in the surgical approach to multiple accessory pathways in the Wolff-Parkinson-White syndrome. *Ann Thorac Surg.* 1987;43(6):579-584.
48. Yeh SJ, Wang CC, Wen MS. Catheter ablation using radio-frequency current in Wolff-Parkinson-White syndrome with multiple accessory pathways. *Am J Cardiol.* 1992;(71):1174-1180.
49. Huang JL, Chen SA, Tai CT, et al. Long-term results of radiofrequency catheter ablation in patients with multiple accessory pathways. *Am J Cardiol.* 1996;78(12):1375-1379.
50. Sternick EB, Lokhandwala Y, Timmermans C, et al. The atrioventricular interval during pre-excited tachycardia: a simple way to distinguish between decrementally or rapidly conducting accessory pathways. *Heart Rhythm.* 2009;6(9):1351-1358.
51. Calkins H, Kim YN, Schmaltz S, et al. Electrogram criteria for identification of appropriate target sites for radiofrequency catheter ablation of accessory atrioventricular connections. *Circulation.* 1992;85:565-573.
52. Hindricks G, Kottkamp H, Chen XU, et al. Localisation and radiofrequency catheter ablation of left-sided accessory pathways during atrial fibrillation. *JACC.* 1995;2:444-451.
53. Manolis AS, Wang PJ, Estes M. Radiofrequency ablation of atrial insertion of left-sided accessory pathways guided by the "W sign." *J Cardiovasc Electrophysiol.* 1995;6:1068-1076.
54. Skanes AC, Dubuc M, Klein GJ, Thibault B, Leung TK, Friedman PL. Cryothermal ablation of the slow pathway for the elimination of atrioventricular nodal reentrant tachycardia. *Circulation.* 2000;102:2856-2860.
55. De Sisti A, Tonet J. Cryoablation of atrioventricular nodal reentrant tachycardia: a clinical review. *PACE.* 2012;35:233-240.
56. Fischbach PS, Saarel EV, Dick M. Transient atrioventricular conduction block with cryoablation following normal cryomapping. *Heart Rhythm.* 2004;1:554-557.
57. Naccarelli G, Dougherty A, Berns E, Rinkenberger R. Assessment of antiarrhythmic drug efficacy in the treatment of supraventricular arrhythmias. *Am J Cardiol.* 1986;58:31C-36C.
58. Nagi H, Pinski S, Mokhtar S, Saad Y, Maloney J. Serial electrophysiological testing of drug therapy in supraventricular tachycardia related to accessory pathway. *Clev Clin J Medicine.* 1990;57:622-626.

CHAPTER 28

Atrial Tachycardia and Atrial Flutter

Frederick T. Han, MD; Nitish Badhwar, MBBS, MD

Characteristics

Atrial tachycardias (ATs) are regular atrial rhythms occurring at a constant rate greater than or equal to 100 beats per minute.[1] Focal ATs are characterized by an origin of activation from a small area (focus) outside the sinus node with centrifugal activation to both atria. Although the mechanism of a focal AT can vary among abnormal automaticity, triggered activity, and microreentry, they all share the characteristic of centrifugal endocardial activation to both atria from a focal origin. Consistent with its focal origin, significant portions of the cycle length are devoid of electrical activation during intracardiac mapping. Focal ATs arise from localized areas within the right and left atria, allowing an AT to persist independently of the AV junction and APs, which are not essential structures for maintenance of the tachycardia.[2] Focal ATs are most commonly mapped to the crista terminalis,[3] the tricuspid annulus,[4] and the pulmonary veins.[5] Less frequently, they can be found to originate from the perinodal (para-Hisian) region,[6] the CS musculature,[7] the CS ostium,[8] the IAS,[9,10] the aortic cusps,[11-14] the atrial appendages,[15,16] and the mitral annulus.[17]

Macroreentrant ATs (atrial flutter or AFL) also do not utilize the AV junction or accessory pathways as part of their mechanism and can sustain themselves in the absence of conduction through these structures. In contrast, macroreentrant ATs utilize a central conduction barrier (arbitrarily defined as > 3 cm in diameter)[1] and/or a zone of slow conduction that allows for sustained reentry. The central conduction barrier can be a fixed anatomical scar or a functional obstacle that serves as the substrate for the tachycardia. Due to the size of the central obstacle, macroreentrant ATs demonstrate an atrial activation map that spans the cycle length of the tachycardia.

Pathophysiology

Focal ATs have no specific gender or age predilection and should remain in the differential diagnosis of any patient presenting for evaluation of an SVT. As noted above, most ATs are mapped to the RA, but sites such as the IAS, the posterior RA (with its close relationship to the RSPV), and the CS musculature often require left atrial access and mapping in order to exclude a left atrial focus.[5,7,9,10] Although focal ATs are mapped to discrete foci within the atria, that does not preclude the existence of multiple foci in patients who present with an AT. In their cohort, Chen and colleagues found that 17.5% of their patients presented with more than 1 atrial focus; these patients had a higher incidence of left atrial foci and cardiovascular comorbidities as well as a shorter tachycardia cycle length (TCL). Whether these patients with multiple AT foci have the same basic mechanism underlying their arrhythmias remains to be determined.

Although the exact mechanism of focal ATs cannot be determined in every patient, identifying features consistent with an automatic, triggered, or microreentrant mechanism may help to dictate the diagnostic and therapeutic approach with the individual patient.[18,19] However, strict application of these mechanisms may be plagued by inconsistencies, so we find that a flexible application and understanding of these mechanisms holds the greatest utility.

Abnormal automaticity, defined as a net cation influx causing phase 4 depolarization, is believed to be the most common mechanism for focal ATs. Clinically, automatic tachycardias manifest a sudden onset with a "warm-up" period facilitated by increased adrenergic activity and exogenous catecholamines. Vagal stimulation, β-blockers, and calcium channel blockers may suppress automatic ATs, while adenosine may transiently suppress or slow the tachycardia.[20] Programmed electrical stimulation fails to reproducibly initiate or terminate automatic ATs, while overdrive pacing suppresses these tachycardias.

Triggered activity occurs when cells at the abnormal foci are depolarized by afterpotentials. Delayed afterpotentials occur after cellular repolarization and are of sufficient amplitude to depolarize the cell membrane to the depolarization threshold. The subsequent triggered activation of inward ionic current initiates cellular depolarization and AT initiation. Defining the prevalence of triggered activity in focal ATs has been limited to cellular electrophysiology investigations and evidence of triggered activity with digitalis toxicity.[21] Triggered activity ATs also demonstrate a warm-up period facilitated by high adrenergic output, but are differentiated by their induction with programmed electrical stimulation and burst pacing. Whereas overdrive pacing may suppress automatic ATs, overdrive pacing may accelerate ATs due to triggered activity. Triggered activity ATs may be terminated with vagal maneuvers, calcium channel blockers, β-blockers, and adenosine.[20,22]

With focal ATs, a discrete circuit (< 3 cm in diameter) creates a microreentrant circuit. The size of the circuit allows microreentrant ATs to be successfully ablated with a single ablation lesion, whereas a macroreentrant AT usually requires a series of linear ablation lesions. Focal ATs demonstrate a discrete origin with a centrifugal pattern of atrial activation, but are characterized by their initiation/termination with programmed atrial extrastimuli as well as their ability to be entrained with a postpacing interval approximating the TCL. Adenosine insensitivity and the presence of low-amplitude, fractionated EGMs at the site of origin of these ATs also support a microreentrant mechanism.[23]

A macroreentrant AT, as noted above, requires a central obstacle. There is no single focus of activation, and atrial myocardium outside the circuit is activated from various parts of the circuit. Defining the circuit requires defining the atrial anatomy in order to define the boundaries of the circuit and a potential critical isthmus that serves as a zone of slow conduction and target of ablation. Knowledge of preexisting anatomical variations, previous cardiac surgeries, and areas of atrial scar is helpful in planning for potential mapping and ablation of the AT.

Differential Diagnosis of Focal Atrial Tachycardia

As most patients with an AT present with a diagnosis of an SVT, examination of the R-P relationship on the 12-lead ECG or telemetry tracings provides early clues for the diagnosis.[24] AT typically presents as a long-RP SVT, whereas AVNRT and AVRT are usually short-RP tachycardias. Rare variants of AT, AVNRT, and AVRT can affect the expected RP relationship of SVT, as in the case of an AT with prolonged AV conduction producing a short-RP tachycardia and an atypical AVNRT or AVRT utilizing a slowly conducting AP manifesting as a long-RP tachycardia. Analysis of intracardiac EGMs during tachycardia as well as the tachycardia response to pharmacologic manipulation, pacing, and programmed electrical stimulation allows one to differentiate AT from AVNRT or AVRT. A summary of the diagnostic criteria for a focal AT is listed in Table 28.1. Spontaneous termination of the tachycardia with an atrial depolarization without a ventricular depolarization makes an AT extremely unlikely, as one would have to postulate that the AT terminated simultaneously with AV conduction block. Variable VA intervals with fixed TCL strongly favor a diagnosis of AT (Figure 28.1). Variable AV conduction with more atrial than ventricular signals excludes an AV reciprocating tachycardia and strongly suggests an AT, given the rarity of AVNRT with lower common

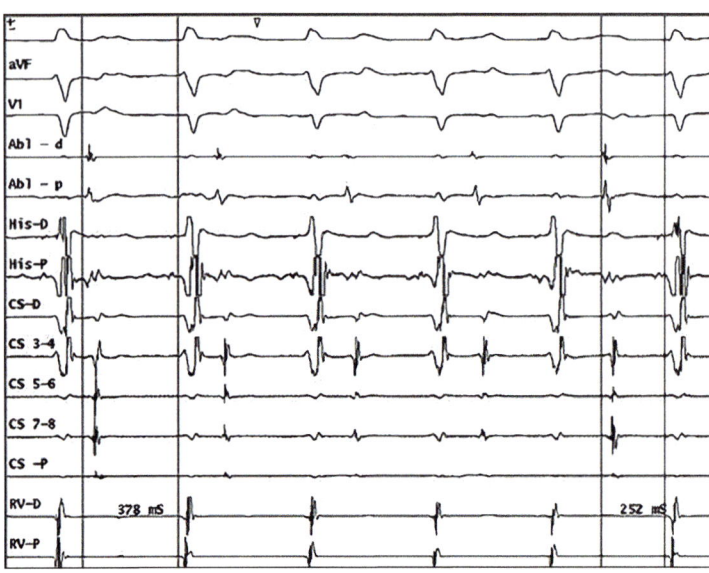

Figure 28.1 Supraventricular tachycardia (SVT) that shows variable VA relationship with a fixed TCL that favors a diagnosis of AT. The variation is mainly due to a jump in the AH interval from a slow pathway to a fast pathway. In this figure, SVT occurs with earliest atrial activation at the His position that is consistent with a diagnosis of para-Hisian AT.

pathway block.[25] Analysis of the atrial activation sequence during tachycardia also can be very helpful for differentiation of an AT from an AVNRT or AVRT. Focal ATs with an origin apart from the AV valve annuli or CS ostium are inconsistent with an AVNRT or AVRT; further support for a diagnosis of AT is obtained by proving that changes in the TCL are driven by changes in the earliest atrial cycle length. However, if the tachycardia demonstrates 1:1 AV conduction and the atrial activation sequence suggests an annular location, pharmacologic and EP maneuvers must be employed to determine whether the AV node is a critical part of the tachycardia circuit.

Table 28.1 Diagnostic criteria for focal atrial tachycardia

- Overdrive pacing of tachycardia with ventricular pacing results in a V-A-A-V response (exclude pseudo V-A-A-V response)
- Delta AH interval < 20 ms (Delta AH = AH interval during atrial pacing at TCL − AH interval during tachycardia)
- Variable VA intervals (lack of VA linking) during sustained tachycardia or after overdrive atrial pacing from different sites suggest AT
- Dissociation of the ventricle from the tachycardia highly suggestive of AT
- Ventricular pacing that reproducibly terminates the tachycardia without conduction to the atrium excludes AT
- Spontaneous termination of tachycardia with an atrial activation highly unlikely for an AT
- Macroreentrant AT has been excluded (atrial activation over < 50% of TCL)

Ventricular pacing during SVT can provide critical diagnostic information in differentiating AT from AVNRT and AVRT. If burst pacing in the right ventricle at a rate slightly faster than the tachycardia rate dissociates the ventricle from the tachycardia, AVRT has been excluded by proving that the ventricle is not part of the tachycardia circuit. Conversely, if ventricular pacing terminates the tachycardia without conduction to the atrium, AT is excluded (Figure 28.2). If burst pacing in the ventricle entrains the atrium and there is a V-A-A-V response to the last paced beat, AT is the diagnosis, as the tachycardia must respond to entrainment with an initial beat from the AT focus (Figure 28.3A). Careful analysis of the last entrained atrial beat in response to ventricular pacing will allow successful differentiation of a true V-A-A-V response from a pseudo V-A-A-V response that results from a long VA conduction time (Figure 28.3B). A V-A-V response provides proof of a reentrant circuit (AVRT or AVNRT) and excludes an AT (Figure 28.3C).[26]

Atrial pacing during tachycardia also provides useful diagnostic information. Overdrive atrial pacing allows for assessment of "VA linking"—if the VA interval of the return cycle length after pacing is within 10 ms of the VA interval during tachycardia, VA linking is present and AVNRT or AVRT are the most likely diagnoses. In contrast, if the VA interval is variable (VA linking does not exist), AT is the diagnosis.[27] Analysis of the AH intervals during atrial pacing versus the AH intervals during tachycardia can also be used to identify the mechanism of a long RP tachycardia.[28] If the delta AH (AH during atrial pacing—AH interval during tachycardia) is < 20 ms, then the SVT is an AT. A delta AH between 20 and 40 ms supports the diagnosis of an AVRT, and a delta AH > 40 ms is likely an AVNRT.

As noted above, observing AV dissociation during tachycardia with persistence of the SVT is diagnostic of an AT. This can be induced pharmacologically with adenosine or by stimulation of vagal tone with carotid sinus massage. Since some ATs are adenosine-sensitive,[29] exhausting the maneuvers above or applying carotid sinus massage prior to adenosine administration may be helpful, especially if the SVT is difficult to induce.

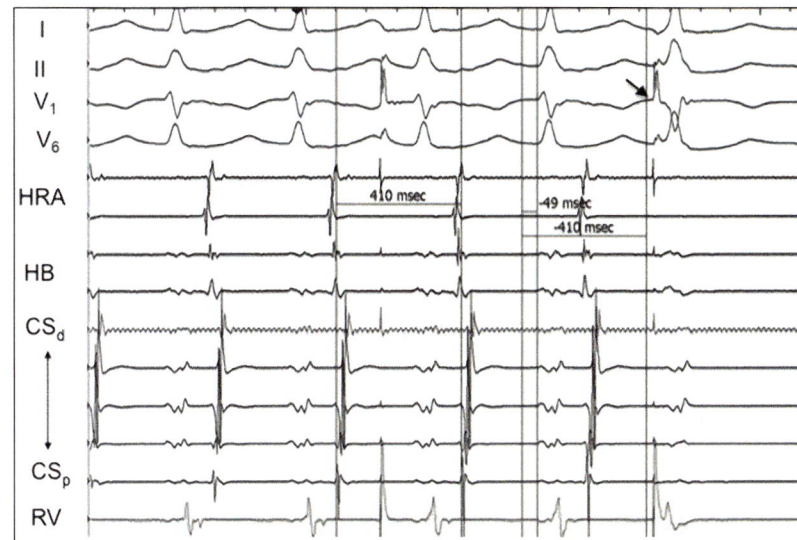

Figure 28.2 Reproducible termination of SVT by ventricular stimulation that does not conduct to the atrium excludes an AT. In this figure, SVT occurs with earliest atrial activation in the His position. A premature ventricular stimulus (fused paced QRS) is delivered after the timing of His activation (**arrow**) followed by termination of the SVT. This finding was reproducible and the patient underwent successful ablation of a right septal AP. CS_p = proximal coronary sinus; CS_d = distal coronary sinus; HB = His bundle; RA = septal right atrium; surface ECG leads I, II, V_1, V_6.

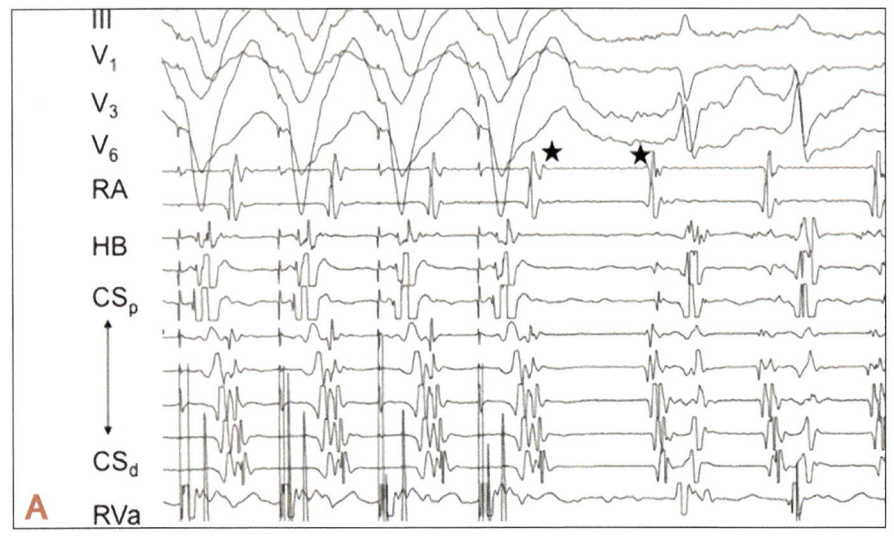
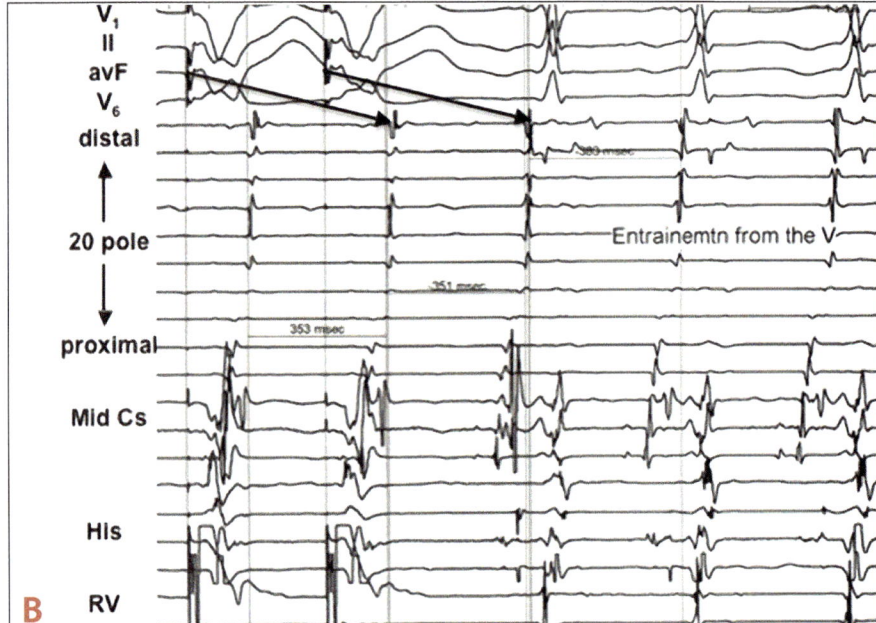
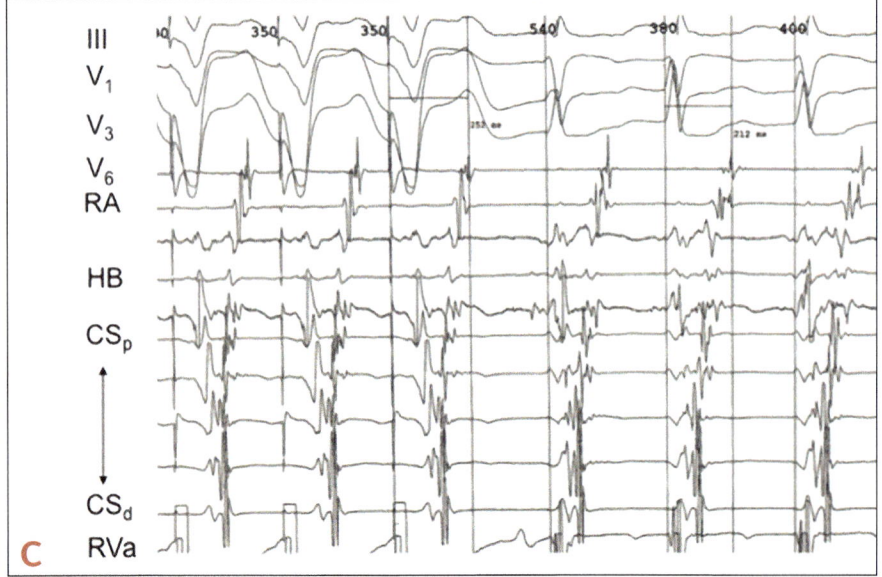

Figure 28.3 **Panel A:** V-A-A-V response after overdrive ventricular pacing (VOD) during the SVT is diagnostic of an AT. There is acceleration of the atrial rate to the ventricular rate during ventricular pacing with requirement of another atrial depolarization from the AT focus to continue SVT after pacing. The interval between the first two As (★) after VOD is similar to SVT cycle length and different from ventricular pacing cycle length. **Panel B:** Pseudo V-A-A-V response after overdrive ventricular pacing during the SVT. The interval between the first two As (★) after VOD is the same as the ventricular pacing cycle length (**arrows**). Hence the second "A" of the pseudo V-A-A-V response is caused by the last ventricular paced beat with a long VA conduction time (**arrows**). Thus, the pseudo V-A-A-V response to ventricular entrainment during tachycardia cannot be used to diagnose AT, and the response to entrainment is consistent with an atypical form of AVNRT. **Panel C:** V-A-V response after VOD of a left-sided AP-mediated AVRT. *Source:* From Kistler PM, Roberts-Thompson KC, Haqqani HM, et al[31] with permission from Elsevier.

Focal Atrial Tachycardia Localization

Once the diagnosis of AT has been established, P-wave morphology and vector analysis on the 12-lead ECG provides a useful, noninvasive method of localizing the tachycardia focus (Figure 28.4). Lead V_1 is the most useful lead in distinguishing between left and right atrial origin.[30] In developing an algorithm for AT localization, Kistler and colleagues found that a negative or biphasic (with a negative terminal portion) P wave had a sensitivity of 100% for a right atrial focus, whereas a positive or biphasic (with a positive terminal portion) P wave had a 100% sensitivity for a left atrial focus.[31]

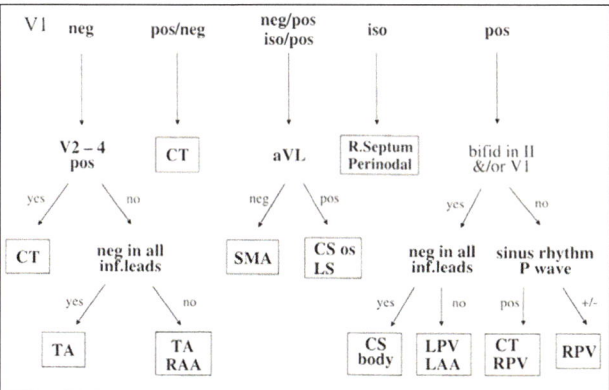

Figure 28.4 Algorithm for localization of AT origin based on surface ECG. CS = coronary sinus; CT = crista terminalis; iso = isoelectric P wave; LAA = left atrial appendage; LPV = left pulmonary vein; LS = left septum; neg = inverted P wave; pos = upright P wave; R = right; RAA = right atrial appendage; RPV = right pulmonary vein; SMA = superior mitral annulus; TA = tricuspid annulus. *Source:* From Kistler PM, Roberts-Thompson KC, Haqqani HM, et al. P-wave morphology in focal atrial tachycardia: development of an algorithm to predict the anatomic site of origin. *J Am Coll Cardiol.* 2006;48(5):1010-1017.

Since the RSPV and posterior high RA are both posterior midline structures, there is a subtle difference for focal ATs originating from these sites. Tang and colleagues[30] found that posterior high right ATs demonstrate the same P-wave morphology in V_1 during both sinus rhythm (SR) and tachycardia, whereas RSPV ATs change from a biphasic P wave during SR to an upright P wave in V_1 during tachycardia.[30] Leads II, III, and aVF are useful for differentiating a superior atrial focus (positive P wave) from an inferior origin (negative P wave). A negative P wave in lead aVR has a 95% sensitivity and 93% specificity for a lateral right atrial origin in the crista terminalis.[31] Conversely, a negative P wave in any of the inferior leads with a negative P wave in V_5 and V_6 demonstrated a 92% sensitivity and 100% specificity for an inferomedial right atrial focus.[32] The finding of narrow P waves in AT as compared to sinus rhythm with biphasic P wave in V_1 and early precordial transition is consistent with a para-Hisian origin (perinodal—at the apex of the triangle of Koch)[6] (Figure 28.5). The P waves in the inferior leads are usually negative; however, they could be positive depending on the activation sequence of the LA. Focal ATs with an apparent right atrial septal location by ECG can also be mapped to the noncoronary cusp because of the contiguous anatomy between these two sites. Noncoronary cusp ATs are characterized by narrow P waves that are positive in V_1 and positive or isoelectric P wave in the inferior leads; because of their proximity to the His bundle, these ATs may also manifest a short PR interval.[6,33] Focal ATs from the CS ostium are characterized by deeply negative P waves in the inferior leads (with a greater negative amplitude in II and III versus aVF), an isoelectric (iso) P wave in lead 1, positive P waves in aVL and aVR, and a biphasic P wave (iso/+ or −/+ pattern) in V_1.[8] RAA tachycardias have a negative P wave in V_1–V_2, positive P waves in inferior leads, and a variable transition across the precordial leads.[15,34] By specifying a P-wave transition after lead V_2, Brugada and colleagues demonstrated 100% sensitivity and 98% specificity for a RAA focus based on P-wave morphology.[34]

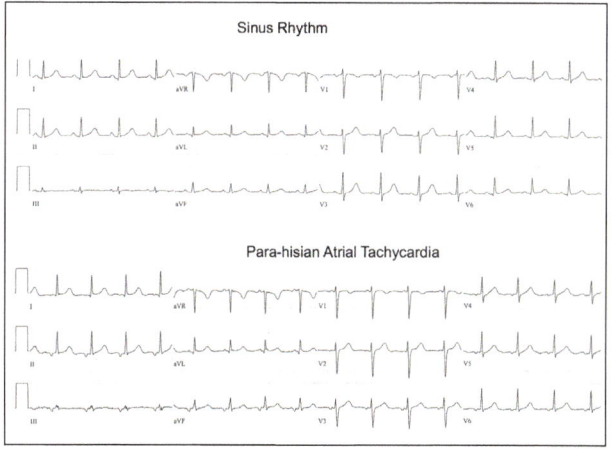

Figure 28.5 12-lead ECG during para-Hisian AT shows narrower P waves as compared to P waves during sinus rhythm. The P waves are negative in inferior leads, biphasic in V_1 with transition in V_2.

In addition to the positive P wave in V_1 indicative of a left atrial origin, pulmonary vein tachycardias demonstrate a characteristic positive P wave across the precordial leads, negative P wave in aVR and aVL (the exception being an RSPV tachycardia, which may demonstrate a positive P wave in aVL).[5] The left pulmonary vein (PV) tachycardias are characterized by notched and wider P waves with a lead III/II amplitude ratio > 0.8, while the right PV tachycardias have a positive P wave in lead 1. Left CS musculature ATs have positive P waves in aVR and V_1 with a transition to negative P waves in V_3–V_4, negative P waves in the inferior leads, and a biphasic pattern (+/− or +/iso) in aVL[7] (Figure 28.6A). Mitral annular tachycardias tend to cluster at the superior aspect of the aortomitral continuity with biphasic (−/+) P waves in V_1, negative or isoelectric P waves in I and aVL, and low-amplitude positive or isoelectric P waves in the inferior leads.[17] Consistent with its location posterior, lateral and superior to the mitral annulus, LAA tachycardias have broad, positive P waves in the precordial leads, deeply negative P waves in I and aVL, and positive P waves in the inferior leads.[16]

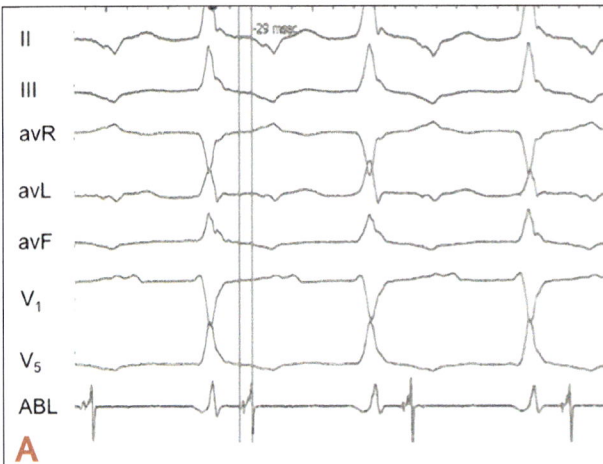

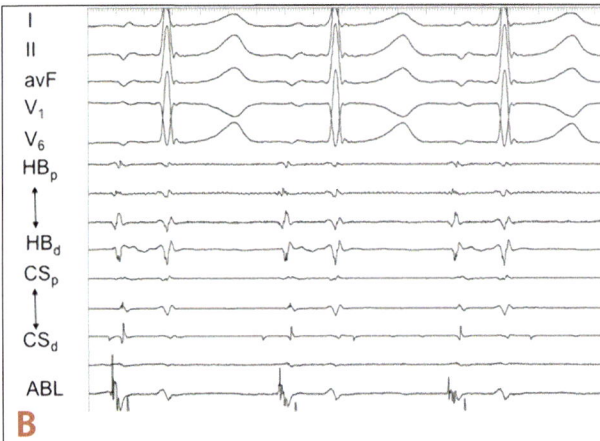

Figure 28.6 EGM targets for AT ablation. **Panel A:** Successful ablation site in a patient with AT originating from the CS musculature. ECG shows deep negative P waves in II, III (more than avF) with positive P wave in V$_1$ and negative in avL. The ablation catheter distal bipolar recording (ABL) shows fractionated EGM with local activation 29 ms before surface P-wave onset (**vertical line**). **Panel B:** Successful ablation site in a patient with para-Hisian AT showing fractionated EGM that preceded the P wave by 35 ms. The ECG shows narrow P waves that are negative in inferior leads and biphasic in V$_1$.

Although P-wave vector and morphologic analysis can be very useful for the diagnosis of a focal AT, the presence of 1:1 AV conduction can distort the P waves with the superimposed QRS complex or T waves. In this situation, pharmacologic/vagal-induced AV block or ventricular pacing can be used to unmask the P wave for analysis. It has been shown that the P-wave morphology is largely determined by the direction of septal and left atrial activation;[35] hence, the morphology may vary among patients with the same AT depending on the dominant route of LA activation. In addition, the spatial resolution of P-wave morphology on ECG is limited by the inability to detect morphologic changes at sites up to 17 mm apart.[36] As mentioned previously, differentiating a posterior right AT from an RSPV origin may be difficult by ECG analysis. ICE can be helpful to identify the anatomic relationship between these two structures.

Mapping of Focal Atrial Tachycardia

Given its focal origin and centrifugal atrial activation, successful ablation of a focal AT requires precise mapping of the tachycardia origin. Activation mapping, in which the earliest local activation is compared with the onset of the tachycardia, P wave is the most common technique for mapping and has been used with good success. Analyzing the activation sequence with multielectrode catheters in combination with the atrial activation of the His catheter can provide clues to the AT focus. Goal ablation targets should demonstrate local activation preceding P-wave onset by 15 to 60 ms. The ideal target with activation mapping should produce a QS complex during tachycardia on the unipolar atrial EGM of the mapping catheter. The atrial EGM at the target ablation site is usually characterized by a low-amplitude fractionated signal (Figure 28.6A, B).

The inability to localize an ideal early activation site should suggest the possibility of an AT arising from an unusual site. In addition to being rare, ATs from the CS musculature are characterized by the unique activation pattern of the CS in relation to the atrial myocardium.[7] The ligament of Marshall is another rare source of ATs that may not be readily apparent without careful mapping due to its epicardial location between the LAA and the LSPV. ATs with earliest activation mapped to the posterior RA should initiate mapping of the RSPV as well, given their anatomic proximity.

ATs mapped to the atrial septum present a unique challenge as the actual AT origin may lie on the left septum[9,10] or in the aortic cusp.[11] Careful mapping of these areas prior to ablation increases the chance of a successful ablation, while also avoiding potential complete heart block. With its anatomic relationship to the IAS, the aortic cusps must also be considered an atypical location for ATs (Figure 28.7). The NCC is the most frequent site of aortic sinus ATs. The IAS lies immediately posterior to the NCC and serves as a marker for the midline portion of this cusp. Mapping the right half of the NCC produces large atrial EGMs during sinus rhythm. Mapping progressively anterior along the NCC to the RCC elicits a His EGM at the commissure between the two cusps with the appearance of a large ventricular EGM confirming the location of the catheter tip in the RCC.[33] Due to its close relationship with the RAA, an atrial EGM from the RAA may be mapped to the posterior aspect of the RCC. The left aspect of the NCC and the posterior aspect of the LCC border the LA. However, these regions are rarely implicated as the site of origin for a focal AT because of the aorto-mitral continuity and the left fibrous trigone, which serve to electrically isolate the NCC and LCC from the LA. However, ATs likely originating from the LA behind the aortic wall at the level of the NCC, the posterior portion of the LCC, and the aorto-mitral continuity have been successfully mapped/ablated with a transseptal approach for the LA as well as via a retrograde approach for mapping/ablation in the LCC.[12,37]

If an AT is not sustained or is difficult to induce, pace mapping can be useful for guiding ablation. It can also serve as an adjunct to activation mapping. Pace mapping must be performed at the lowest capture threshold possible in order to avoid distortion of the P wave and also requires a "naked" P wave on 12-lead ECG for comparison. Utilizing a template of intracardiac activation during tachycardia in combination with pace mapping can also be used to help map nonsustained or quiescent ATs.[38]

Three-dimensional (3D) electroanatomic mapping systems have emerged as a useful tool for mapping ATs. A 3D geometry of the chamber(s) of interest generated during activation mapping enables precise localization of an AT focus. Points of interest can be analyzed in real time to concentrate high-density activation mapping at specific anatomic sites prior to ablation; in addition, potential candidate sites for ablation can be tagged on the 3D geometry prior to further mapping/ablation. Marking points of interest such as the His bundle can be helpful, especially with para-Hisian AT. Additionally, the ability to incorporate image integration from computed tomography or magnetic resonance angiography can facilitate mapping of multiple structures such as the LA, the IAS, and the coronary cusps. This facilitates a comparison of various sites in different chambers as well as the ability to return to a particular site for an ablation. Finally, visualization of the catheter tip in real time during mapping helps to reduce fluoroscopic exposure.

Activation mapping with a 3D mapping system can also be useful in distinguishing a focal AT from a macroreentrant AT. A macroreentrant AT will produce an activation map that spans the entire TCL with a point of earliest activation meeting the point of latest activation, whereas a focal AT will produce an activation map that spans < 50% of the TCL and a centrifugal pattern of atrial activation.

Simultaneous voltage mapping with a 3D mapping system can also be used to identify areas of scar with low-amplitude EGMs. Multielectrode arrays (EnSite array—St. Jude Medical, St. Paul, MN) can be useful for

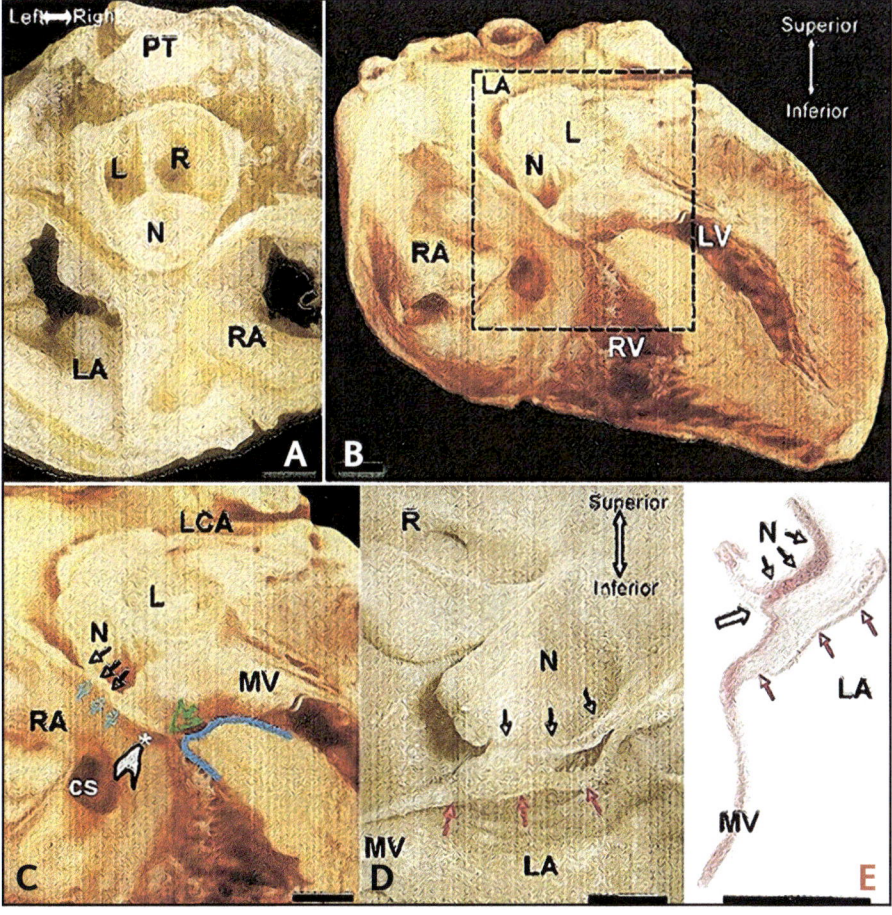

Figure 28.7 **Panel A:** This view of the cardiac base shows the central location of the aortic valve and the relationship of the NCC to the IAS and the left and right atria. **Panels B and C:** An oblique coronal section of the heart shows the relationship of the right half of the NCC (**black arrows**) to the right atrial wall (**blue arrows**). The AV node is indicated by the white shape anterior to the CS ostium, and the His bundle is marked by the asterisk. The green arrow indicates the membranous septum with the branches of the conduction system indicated by the blue line. **Panel D:** A parasternal long-axis section of the aortic valve shows the relationship of the left half of the noncoronary cusp (**black arrows**) to the left atrial wall (**red arrows**). **Panel E:** A histologic section of the aortic valve shown in panel D stained with van Gieson stain shows the extension of the fibrous continuity (open arrow) between the aortic and mitral valves on the ventricular aspect of the valves. The fibrous continuity insulates the LA from the noncoronary cusp. Gaps in the fibrous continuity may play a role in cases of left AT successfully ablated from the left half of the NCC. CS = coronary sinus; L = left coronary cusp; LA = left atrium; LCA = left coronary artery; LV = left ventricle; MV = mitral valve; N = noncoronary cusp; PT = pulmonary trunk; R = right coronary cusp; RA = right atrium; RV = right ventricle. *Source:* From Ouyang F, Ma J, Ho SY, et al[11] with permission from Elsevier.

mapping nonsustained arrhythmias. The EnSite array uses a 64-pole array mounted on a 10-cc balloon catheter. After the anatomic information of the chamber of interest has been obtained, the system utilizes a mathematical algorithm to superimpose the activation data of up to 3,200 EGMs on a 3D geometry to create an isopotential map. While providing the ability to quickly map an AT and its origin, the disadvantage of this system is a loss of spatial resolution with a very large atrium.

Ablation of Focal Atrial Tachycardias

Despite the various mechanisms of AT (abnormal automaticity, triggered activity, or microreentry), the precise mechanism does not affect the mapping strategies or success rate of ablation.

Once an ablation target has been identified, we use a standard 4 mm-tip RFA catheter in the temperature control mode (temperature limit 55°C). Depending on the location, 25 to 50 W is delivered for 30 to 60 seconds. Large-tip catheters, high-energy generators, or irrigated ablation systems are rarely required except in areas where the tissue is very thick or has pectinate muscles (appendage, crista terminalis) that prevent delivery of energy with standard RF catheter. Acceleration of the tachycardia during RF and termination within 10 seconds of ablation usually predict a successful lesion. After ablation, pacing and programmed electrical stimulation with/without isoproterenol are performed in order to attempt tachycardia reinduction before declaring acute success.

For para-Hisian ATs, use of a 3D mapping system to create a His cloud helps to identify areas to avoid during ablation. Starting the ablation with a lower energy and temperature setting and careful observation and termination of ablation for A-H prolongation help to avoid permanent damage to the conduction system.

For focal ATs originating from the CS or the pulmonary veins, lower energy and temperature settings are used to reduce the risk of perforation, thrombosis, and coagulum formation. Coronary angiography prior to and after ablation in the CS is useful to reduce the risk of ablation-associated coronary stenosis/myocardial infarction. Irrigated RF catheters (20 to 30 W for temperature limit of 50°C) can be useful if ablation with a standard RF catheter is limited by excessive impedance rises. Cautious use of irrigated catheters in the CS is recommended as the deeper lesions achieved with irrigated catheters may increase the risk of myocardial infarction. Cryoablation with the ability to perform cryomapping can be a useful tool for ATs localized to the CS or the perinodal region, especially for reducing the incidence of complete heart block in the latter situation.[39] Cryomapping refers to the technique of "chilling" the tissue to −30°C and observing for AH prolongation or AV block. If no effect is seen, then completing the cryoablation with a goal temp of ≤−70°C can be safely pursued.[40] Cryoablation can also be useful for an AT arising from the lateral RA in order to reduce the risk of phrenic nerve paralysis. Prior to ablation in the lateral RA, pacing at high output (10 mA or greater) from the ablation catheter can be used to check for phrenic nerve stimulation on fluoroscopy. If phrenic nerve stimulation is noted, cryoablation with mapping of an alternative site or displacement of the phrenic nerve away from the atrium using an intra-pericardial balloon may be necessary.[41]

ICE can be a useful tool by helping to localize anatomic structures, aiding catheter positioning and catheter tip contact, and confirming lesion size and location.[42] As noted above, using ICE to guide catheter manipulation between the right posterior atrial wall and the superior crista terminalis can help to differentiate between an AT from the crista and an AT from the RSPV (Figure 28.2). ICE can also be used to guide transseptal puncture, to help recognize early complications (perforations and clot formation), and to reduce fluoroscopy time.

Ablation of ATs localized to the aortic cusps can be undertaken with irrigated or nonirrigated catheters. We prefer the use of irrigated catheters to reduce the risk of thromboembolic complications and coagulum formation. In addition, ICE, aortography, and/or coronary angiography should be used to confirm catheter positioning away from the coronary artery ostia.

Diagnosis and Mapping of Macroreentrant Atrial Tachycardias

Macroreentrant ATs and AFLs exhibit a distinctly different pattern of atrial activation in comparison to a focal tachycardia. Continuous reentrant activation of the atrium is diagnostic of a macroreentrant tachycardia. Endocardial atrial activation is recorded continuously through the AT cycle length and the diastolic interval on the surface ECG (Figure 28.8). Consistent with a continuous reentrant circuit, there is no clear point of earliest activation during tachycardia.

Defining an obstacle for a macroreentrant circuit requires mapping of a critical slow conduction zone or line of block. Regardless of whether this obstacle is functional (crista terminalis[43]) or fixed (atriotomy, Eustachian ridge[44-46]), a line of block is characterized by the presence of double potentials indicating sequential activation of the atrium on both sides of the line of block. In order to confirm that the line of block is critical to the AT, evaluating the activation sequence and the response to entrainment of these potentials establishes whether that obstacle is a crucial part of the AT circuit. Entrainment of the double potentials and advancing their activation during pacing verifies its participation in the circuit, whereas spontaneous block of the double potentials rules out its participation in the tachycardia. Fractionated EGMs may represent slow

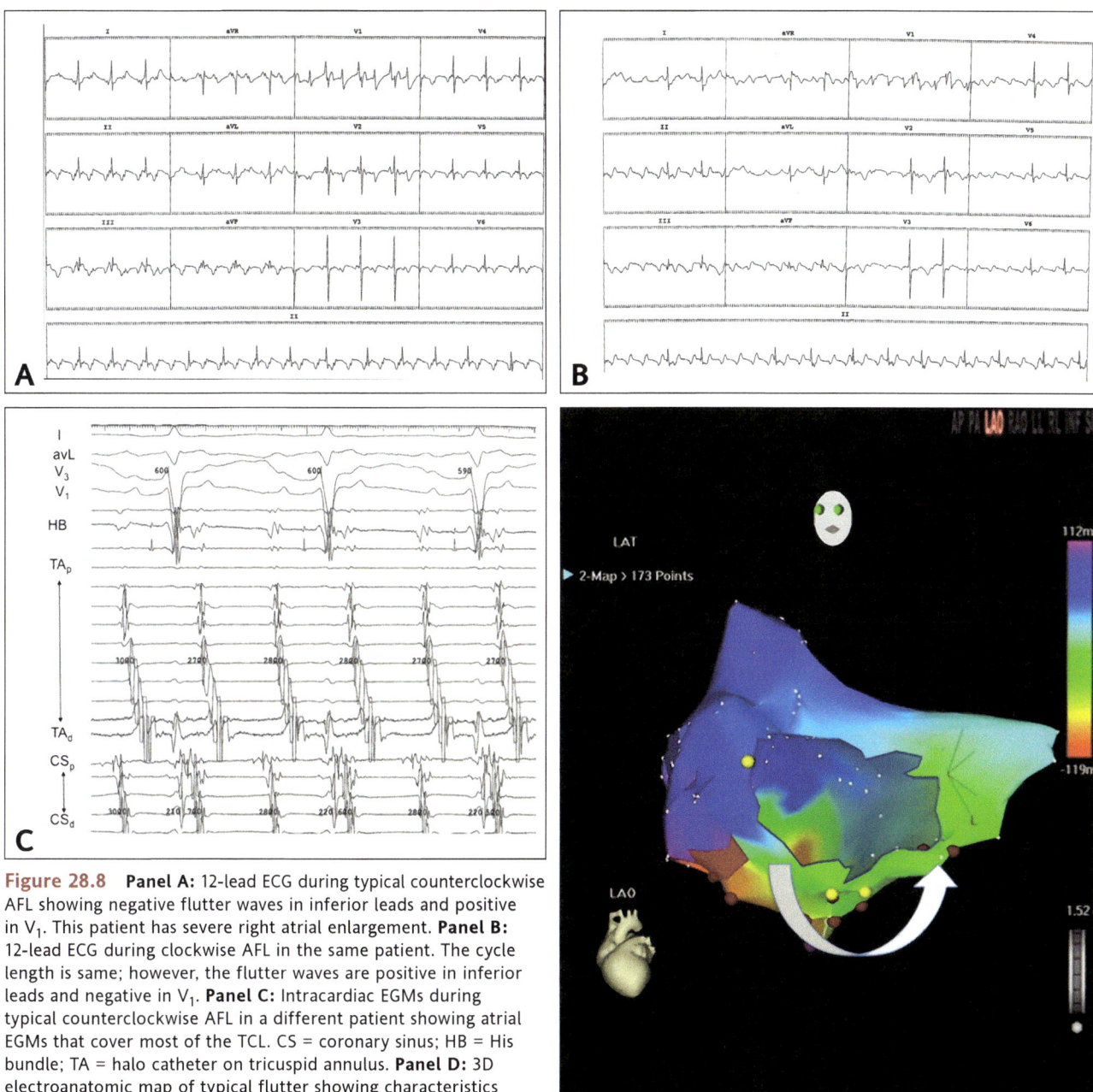

Figure 28.8 **Panel A:** 12-lead ECG during typical counterclockwise AFL showing negative flutter waves in inferior leads and positive in V_1. This patient has severe right atrial enlargement. **Panel B:** 12-lead ECG during clockwise AFL in the same patient. The cycle length is same; however, the flutter waves are positive in inferior leads and negative in V_1. **Panel C:** Intracardiac EGMs during typical counterclockwise AFL in a different patient showing atrial EGMs that cover most of the TCL. CS = coronary sinus; HB = His bundle; TA = halo catheter on tricuspid annulus. **Panel D:** 3D electroanatomic map of typical flutter showing characteristics of macroreentrant arrhythmia (atrial activation includes 90% of the cycle length and early meets late on the lateral aspect of the tricuspid annulus. The arrow illustrates counterclockwise activation of the flutter around the tricuspid annulus.

conduction zones critical to the circuit of the tachycardia. Candidate sites with an anatomic barrier serving as a conduction obstacle can be correlated with intracardiac echocardiography and a 3D electroanatomic mapping system in order to define a propagation map during tachycardia. This can be especially useful for patients with postsurgical AT.

The most common form of a macroreentrant AT is typical AFL. In typical AFL, there is a macroreentrant circuit marked by a counterclockwise circuit around the tricuspid annulus (viewed from a left anterior oblique projection). The counterclockwise pattern of activation is characterized by the presence of a "sawtooth" pattern of flutter waves in leads II, III, and aVF (Figure 28.8). The flutter waves are marked by an initial downward deflection, followed by a sharper negative deflection, and finally a sharp positive deflection, prior to the downslope of the following flutter wave (F wave). Lead V_1 demonstrates a positive deflection with an intervening isoelectric segment. In contrast, reverse typical AFL utilizes the same tachycardia circuit but with the opposite endocardial activation pattern—clockwise reentry. Consistent with this pattern of endocardial activation, the surface ECG manifests upward deflections in leads II, III, and aVF and a negative deflection in V_1 (Figure 28.8). The boundaries of the circuit are marked by the tricuspid valve anteriorly, with the crista terminalis, the Eustachian ridge, and the SVC and IVC posteriorly.[45] The CTI serves as the zone of slow conduction critical to the maintenance of tachycardia with typical AFL.

Although the diagnosis of AFL may be apparent on the surface electrocardiogram, an electrophysiology study with induction, mapping, and entrainment of the tachycardia is necessary to verify the mechanism of the tachycardia. For an EP study of a suspected right AFL, we prefer to use a duodecapolar catheter around the tricuspid annulus (Halo catheter), a quadripolar catheter in the His position, and a decapolar catheter in the CS with the proximal pair positioned at the ostium of the CS. If patients present in sinus rhythm, AFL is induced with a combination of burst atrial pacing and programmed single and double atrial extrastimuli at the CS ostium and the low lateral RA. Typical AFL (counterclockwise reentry–CCW) is more commonly initiated with pacing and programmed atrial extrastimuli from the CS ostium, while reverse typical AFL (clockwise reentry–CW) is usually initiated with pacing and programmed atrial extrastimuli from the low lateral RA.[45]

After induction of tachycardia, most macroreentrant ATs can be entrained successfully. Pacing as close as possible to the TCL helps to prevent inadvertent termination or conversion to atrial fibrillation.[47] In order to confirm successful entrainment of AFL, several criteria must be satisfied. Depending on the site of pacing, concealed entrainment or manifest entrainment may be observed. During *concealed entrainment* (achieved by pacing within the CTI), there is (1) acceleration of the tachycardia to the pacing cycle length without a change in the flutter wave (F wave) pattern on the surface ECG or the endocardial atrial activation pattern and EGM morphology; (2) immediate return of the tachycardia at the original cycle length upon termination of pacing, (3) the stimulus–F wave or stimulus–reference EGM interval equal to the local EGM–F wave or local EGM–reference EGM interval. Manifest entrainment with constant and progressive fusion of the F wave and endocardial atrial activation is observed when pacing at sites outside the CTI. Once the above criteria are satisfied, analysis of the return cycle (postpacing interval) in relation to the TCL can be performed; a postpacing interval equal to or within 20 ms of the TCL at the site of pacing for at least 2 different sites at least 2 cm apart verifies (1) the existence of a macroreentrant circuit and (2) that these sites lie within the circuit.[48] The presence of concealed entrainment with a postpacing interval ≤20 ms of the TCL indicates that entrainment has been performed from the critical isthmus of the macroreentrant AT.

Although not necessary, 3D mapping systems can be useful for defining an activation and voltage map of macroreentrant ATs, especially in the setting of scar-related ATs or variants of AFL such as upper loop reentry, lower loop reentry, or septal isthmus short circuit.[49] Since the possibility of multiple AFLs exists, especially when there are documented variations in flutter wave morphology and cycle length, 3D mapping systems can facilitate more rapid definition of these tachycardia circuits with less fluoroscopic exposure. ICE can also be useful for defining the cavotricuspid anatomy, such as a long CTI, the presence of a deep sub-Eustachian pouch, or a large Eustachian ridge.

Ablation of Macroreentrant AT

For the ablation of typical AFL and reverse typical AFL targeting the CTI, we favor the use of an 8-mm electrode-tip or irrigated-tip ablation catheter with a large curve (EP Technologies, San Jose, CA; THERMOCOOL, Biosense Webster, Diamond Bar, CA). The use of a long sheath with a fixed distal curve (SR0, RAMP™ sheath, Flutter sheath–Daig, Minnetonka, MN) improves catheter reach, stability, and tissue contact during ablation. The ablation catheter tip is advanced from the RA to the ventricular aspect of the CTI in the fluoroscopic RAO view until a 1:4 A:V ratio is achieved. After this has been achieved, the catheter is adjusted such that the catheter tip is at 6 o'clock on the LAO view. Using generator settings of 60 to 70 W for target temperatures of 50 to 70°C with an 8-mm tip catheter and 35 to 45 W for target temperatures of 40 to 45°C with an open-irrigated tip catheter, RF energy is delivered to each ablation target for up to 60 seconds. The catheter is then withdrawn several millimeters at a time, creating a line of lesions until the IVC has been reached. At the IVC, there will be no EGMs recorded on the distal tip of the ablation catheter and/or the ablation electrode will have been noted to drop off the Eustachian ridge into the IVC on fluoroscopy. Due to variations of the CTI anatomy and the presence of pectinate muscles and pouches within the central portion of the CTI, repeating the ablation line may be necessary to achieve bidirectional block across the CTI. Sometimes a lateral line along the CTI (7 o'clock) may be required in order to avoid a deep sub-Eustachian pouch that impedes the delivery of effective power (indicated by high distal tip temperatures and low power). Effective power delivery at a lateral line may be impeded by the presence of terminal pectinate muscles limiting power delivery or catheter stability. In this case, a medial ablation line (5 o'clock) across the CTI can be performed. Ablation along this line may be limited by the RCA with patient discomfort or AV nodal extensions and the small increased chance of heart block.

Conclusions

Catheter ablation for focal and macroreentrant ATs has been proven as a safe and effective therapy with success rates varying from 77 to 100%.[3,7,11,30,50,51] Catheter ablation of ATs has also been demonstrated to improve quality of life scores.[52] Fortunately, complications are rare and are usually related to vascular access or intracardiac catheter manipulation. Ablation-specific complications by location include complete heart block (near the AV node and His bundle) and phrenic nerve palsy (lateral RA). Therefore, we reserve ablation for those patients who have persistent symptoms despite medical therapy, have intolerable side effects with medical therapy, or are not willing to undergo medical therapy.

References

1. Saoudi N, Cosio F, Waldo A, et al. A classification of atrial flutter and regular atrial tachycardia according to electrophysiological mechanisms and anatomical bases; a statement from a Joint Expert Group from the working Group of Arrhythmias of the European Society of Cardiology and the North American Society of Pacing and Electrophysiology. *Eur Heart J.* 2001;22(14):1162-1182.
2. Scheinman MM, Basu D, Hollenberg M. Electrophysiologic studies in patients with persistent atrial tachycardia. *Circulation.* 1974;50(2):266-273.
3. Kalman JM, Olgin JE, Karch MR, Hamdan M, Lee RJ, Lesh MD. "Cristal tachycardias": origin of right atrial tachycardias from the crista terminalis identified by intracardiac echocardiography. *J Am Coll Cardiol.* 1998;31(2):451-459.
4. Morton JB, Sanders P, Das A, Vohra JK, Sparks PB, Kalman JM. Focal atrial tachycardia arising from the tricuspid annulus: electrophysiologic and electrocardiographic characteristics. *J Cardiovasc Electrophysiol.* 2001;12(6):653-659.
5. Kistler PM, Sanders P, Fynn SP, et al. Electrophysiological and electrocardiographic characteristics of focal atrial tachycardia originating from the pulmonary veins: acute and long-term outcomes of radiofrequency ablation. *Circulation.* 2003;108(16):1968-1975.
6. Iwai S, Badhwar N, Markowitz SM, et al. Electrophysiologic properties of para-Hisian atrial tachycardia. *Heart Rhythm.* 2011;8(8):1245-1253.
7. Badhwar N, Kalman JM, Sparks PB, et al. Atrial tachycardia arising from the coronary sinus musculature: electrophysiological characteristics and long-term outcomes of radiofrequency ablation. *J Am Coll Cardiol.* 2005;46(10):1921-1930.
8. Kistler PM, Fynn SP, Haqqani H, et al. Focal atrial tachycardia from the ostium of the coronary sinus: electrocardiographic and electrophysiological characterization and radiofrequency ablation. *J Am Coll Cardiol.* 2005;45(9):1488-1493.
9. Frey B, Kreiner G, Gwechenberger M, Gossinger HD. Ablation of atrial tachycardia originating from the vicinity of the atrioventricular node: significance of mapping both sides of the interatrial septum. *J Am Coll Cardiol.* 2001;38(2):394-400.
10. Marrouche NF, SippensGroenewegen A, Yang Y, Dibs S, Scheinman MM. Clinical and electrophysiologic characteristics of left septal atrial tachycardia. *J Am Coll Cardiol.* 2002;40(6):1133-1139.
11. Ouyang F, Ma J, Ho SY, et al. Focal atrial tachycardia originating from the non-coronary aortic sinus: electrophysiological characteristics and catheter ablation. *J Am Coll Cardiol.* 2006;48(1):122-131.
12. Shehata M, Liu T, Joshi N, Chugh SS, Wang X. Atrial tachycardia originating from the left coronary cusp near the aorto-mitral junction: anatomic considerations. *Heart Rhythm.* 2010;7(7):987-991.
13. Yamada T, Huizar JF, McElderry HT, Kay GN. Atrial tachycardia originating from the noncoronary aortic cusp and musculature connection with the atria: relevance for catheter ablation. *Heart Rhythm.* 2006;3(12):1494-1496.
14. Gami AS, Venkatachalam KL, Friedman PA, Asirvatham SJ. Successful ablation of atrial tachycardia in the right coronary cusp of the aortic valve in a patient with atrial fibrillation: what is the substrate? *J Cardiovasc Electrophysiol.* 2008;19(9):982-986.
15. Roberts-Thomson KC, Kistler PM, Haqqani HM, et al. Focal atrial tachycardias arising from the right atrial appendage: electrocardiographic and electrophysiologic characteristics and radiofrequency ablation. *J Cardiovasc Electrophysiol.* 2007;18(4):367-372.
16. Yamada T, Murakami Y, Yoshida Y, et al. Electrophysiologic and electrocardiographic characteristics and radiofrequency catheter ablation of focal atrial tachycardia originating from the left atrial appendage. *Heart Rhythm.* 2007;4(10):1284-1291.
17. Kistler PM, Sanders P, Hussin A, et al. Focal atrial tachycardia arising from the mitral annulus: electrocardiographic and electrophysiologic characterization. *J Am Coll Cardiol.* 2003;41(12):2212-2219.
18. Callans DJ, Schwartzman D, Gottlieb CD, Marchlinski FE. Insights into the electrophysiology of atrial arrhythmias gained by the catheter ablation experience: "learning while burning, Part II." *J Cardiovasc Electrophysiol.* 1995;6(3):229-243.
19. Steinbeck G, Hoffmann E. "True" atrial tachycardia. *Eur Heart J.* 1998;19 Suppl E:E10-12, E48-49.
20. Engelstein ED, Lippman N, Stein KM, Lerman BB. Mechanism-specific effects of adenosine on atrial tachycardia. *Circulation.* 1994;89(6):2645-2654.
21. Rosen MR. Cellular electrophysiology of digitalis toxicity. *J Am Coll Cardiol.* 1985;5(5 Suppl A):22A-34A.
22. Iwai S, Markowitz SM, Stein KM, et al. Response to adenosine differentiates focal from macroreentrant atrial tachycardia: validation using three-dimensional electroanatomic mapping. *Circulation.* 2002;106(22):2793-2799.
23. Markowitz SM, Nemirovksy D, Stein KM, et al. Adenosine-insensitive focal atrial tachycardia: evidence for de novo micro-re-entry in the human atrium. *J Am Coll Cardiol.* 2007;49(12):1324-1333.
24. Kalbfleisch SJ, el-Atassi R, Calkins H, Langberg JJ, Morady F. Differentiation of paroxysmal narrow QRS complex tachycardias using the 12-lead electrocardiogram. *J Am Coll Cardiol.* 1993;21(1):85-89.
25. Miller JM, Rosenthal ME, Vassallo JA, Josephson ME. Atrioventricular nodal reentrant tachycardia: studies on upper and lower "common pathways." *Circulation.* 1987;75(5):930-940.
26. Knight BP, Ebinger M, Oral H, et al. Diagnostic value of tachycardia features and pacing maneuvers during paroxysmal supraventricular tachycardia. *J Am Coll Cardiol.* 2000;36(2):574-582.
27. Sarkozy A, Richter S, Chierchia GB, et al. A novel pacing manoeuvre to diagnose atrial tachycardia. *Europace.* 2008;10(4):459-466.
28. Man KC, Niebauer M, Daoud E, et al. Comparison of atrial-His intervals during tachycardia and atrial pacing in patients with long RP tachycardia. *J Cardiovasc Electrophysiol.* 1995;6(9):700-710.
29. Glatter KA, Cheng J, Dorostkar P, et al. Electrophysiologic effects of adenosine in patients with supraventricular tachycardia. *Circulation.* 1999;99(8):1034-1040.

30. Tang CW, Scheinman MM, Van Hare GF, et al. Use of P wave configuration during atrial tachycardia to predict site of origin. *J Am Coll Cardiol*. 1995;26(5):1315-1324.
31. Kistler PM, Roberts-Thomson KC, Haqqani HM, et al. P-wave morphology in focal atrial tachycardia: development of an algorithm to predict the anatomic site of origin. *J Am Coll Cardiol*. 2006;48(5):1010-1017.
32. Tada H, Nogami A, Naito S, et al. Simple electrocardiographic criteria for identifying the site of origin of focal right atrial tachycardia. *Pacing Clin Electrophysiol*. 1998;21(11 Pt 2):2431-2439.
33. Suleiman M, Asirvatham SJ. Ablation above the semilunar valves: when, why, and how? Part II. *Heart Rhythm*. 2008;5(11):1625-1630.
34. Freixa X, Berruezo A, Mont L, et al. Characterization of focal right atrial appendage tachycardia. *Europace*. 2008;10(1):105-109.
35. Okumura K, Plumb VJ, Page PL, Waldo AL. Atrial activation sequence during atrial flutter in the canine pericarditis model and its effects on the polarity of the flutter wave in the electrocardiogram. *J Am Coll Cardiol*. 1991;17(2):509-518.
36. Man KC, Chan KK, Kovack P, et al. Spatial resolution of atrial pace mapping as determined by unipolar atrial pacing at adjacent sites. *Circulation*. 1996;94(6):1357-1363.
37. Gonzalez MD, Contreras LJ, Jongbloed MR, et al. Left atrial tachycardia originating from the mitral annulus-aorta junction. *Circulation*. 2004;110(20):3187-3192.
38. Tracy CM, Swartz JF, Fletcher RD, et al. Radiofrequency catheter ablation of ectopic atrial tachycardia using paced activation sequence mapping. *J Am Coll Cardiol*. 1993;21(4):910-917.
39. Bastani H, Insulander P, Schwieler J, et al. Safety and efficacy of cryoablation of atrial tachycardia with high risk of ablation-related injuries. *Europace*. 2009;11(5):625-629.
40. Wong T, Markides V, Peters NS, Davies DW. Clinical usefulness of cryomapping for ablation of tachycardias involving perinodal tissue. *J Interv Card Electrophysiol*. 2004;10(2):153-158.
41. Lee JC, Steven D, Roberts-Thomson KC, Raymond JM, Stevenson WG, Tedrow UB. Atrial tachycardias adjacent to the phrenic nerve: recognition, potential problems, and solutions. *Heart Rhythm*. 2009;6(8):1186-1191.
42. Chu E, Kalman JM, Kwasman MA, et al. Intracardiac echocardiography during radiofrequency catheter ablation of cardiac arrhythmias in humans. *J Am Coll Cardiol*. 1994;24(5):1351-1357.
43. Olshansky B, Okumura K, Hess PG, Waldo AL. Demonstration of an area of slow conduction in human atrial flutter. *J Am Coll Cardiol*. 1990;16(7):1639-1648.
44. Lesh MD, Van Hare GF, Epstein LM, et al. Radiofrequency catheter ablation of atrial arrhythmias. Results and mechanisms. *Circulation*. 1994;89(3):1074-1089.
45. Olgin JE, Kalman JM, Fitzpatrick AP, Lesh MD. Role of right atrial endocardial structures as barriers to conduction during human type I atrial flutter. Activation and entrainment mapping guided by intracardiac echocardiography. *Circulation*. 1995;92(7):1839-1848.
46. Nakagawa H, Lazzara R, Khastgir T, et al. Role of the tricuspid annulus and the eustachian valve/ridge on atrial flutter. Relevance to catheter ablation of the septal isthmus and a new technique for rapid identification of ablation success. *Circulation*. 1996;94(3):407-424.
47. Waldo AL. Atrial flutter: entrainment characteristics. *J Cardiovasc Electrophysiol*. 1997;8(3):337-352.
48. Stevenson WG, Nademanee K, Weiss JN, et al. Programmed electrical stimulation at potential ventricular reentry circuit sites. Comparison of observations in humans with predictions from computer simulations. *Circulation*. 1989;80(4):793-806.
49. Yang Y, Cheng J, Bochoeyer A, et al. Atypical right atrial flutter patterns. *Circulation*. 2001;103(25):3092-3098.
50. Chen SA, Tai CT, Chiang CE, Ding YA, Chang MS. Focal atrial tachycardia: reanalysis of the clinical and electrophysiologic characteristics and prediction of successful radiofrequency ablation. *J Cardiovasc Electrophysiol*. 1998;9(4):355-365.
51. Kay GN, Chong F, Epstein AE, Dailey SM, Plumb VJ. Radiofrequency ablation for treatment of primary atrial tachycardias. *J Am Coll Cardiol*. 1993;21(4):901-909.
52. Feld GK. Catheter ablation for the treatment of atrial tachycardia. *Prog Cardiovasc Dis*. 1995;37(4):205-224.

CHAPTER 29

Atrial Fibrillation: Clinical Electrophysiologic Evaluation

Rangadham Nagarakanti, MD; Nicholas D. Skadsberg, PhD; Sanjeev Saksena, MBBS, MD

Introduction

Atrial fibrillation (AF) was one of the earliest cardiac arrhythmias to be characterized; described initially in the 17th century, it was later recorded at the turn of the 19th century.[1] It is also the most common arrhythmia, with a current prevalence estimated to be in excess of 2.5 million patients in the United States alone and with a projected potential to increase to 15 million patients by 2050.[2,3]

Atrial fibrillation is associated with adverse clinical outcomes, including an increased risk of stroke, cardiovascular hospitalizations, and mortality. Many disease states are associated with AF. Hypertension is currently the most common cardiovascular disease in the Western Hemisphere, followed by coronary artery disease, valvular heart disease, and cardiomyopathy, with other diseases such as rheumatic and valvular heart disease being the major disease states in Asia and Africa.

The clinical electrophysiology (EP) laboratory is assuming an increasingly important role in the evaluation and management of the AF patient. Electrophysiological characteristics of AF may differ between different disease states, but this has been poorly characterized. While our understanding of the AF disease state and its mechanisms has progressed significantly in the last decade, limitations of current therapeutic efforts to restore rhythm control in AF have highlighted the need for further knowledge of the arrhythmia and the disease state underlying the condition. This chapter will describe observations made in the context of AF populations with mostly nonvalvular AF in the Western world, which therefore should not be extrapolated to valvular and rheumatic heart disease.

Atrial Fibrillation Definition and Clinical Classification

The clinical definition of AF must be confirmed by an electrocardiographic (ECG) recording, as relying on the arterial pulse or heart sounds alone can be misleading. On the surface ECG, AF is characterized by the absence of P waves and the presence of small, irregular oscillations (fibrillatory or F waves). Fibrillation has been defined as either fine or coarse, based on the ability to discern well-defined organized atrial activity in the surface ECG. It is generally associated with irregularly irregular RR intervals, in the absence of complete atrioventricular (AV) block. An arrhythmia with the ECG characteristics of AF that lasts at least 30 seconds on an ECG recording should be considered a sustained AF episode. Careful evaluation of ECGs, preferably with high gain or body surface mapping, can also be performed.[4] ECG recordings may also reveal evidence of varying F wave morphology and periods of atrial flutter or atrial tachycardia (Figure 29.1).[5,6]

AF patients are currently clinically classified as having either new onset AF (defined as newly discovered or first diagnosed) or recurrent AF (≥ 2 episodes), with the latter having three types of clinical presentation.[7-9] Any patient who presents to medical attention with AF for the first time is considered to have newly diagnosed AF. ECG documentation of AF is strongly recommended. Paroxysmal AF is defined as recurrent (2 or more episodes) AF that terminates spontaneously within 7 days, while persistent AF is defined as recurrent AF that is

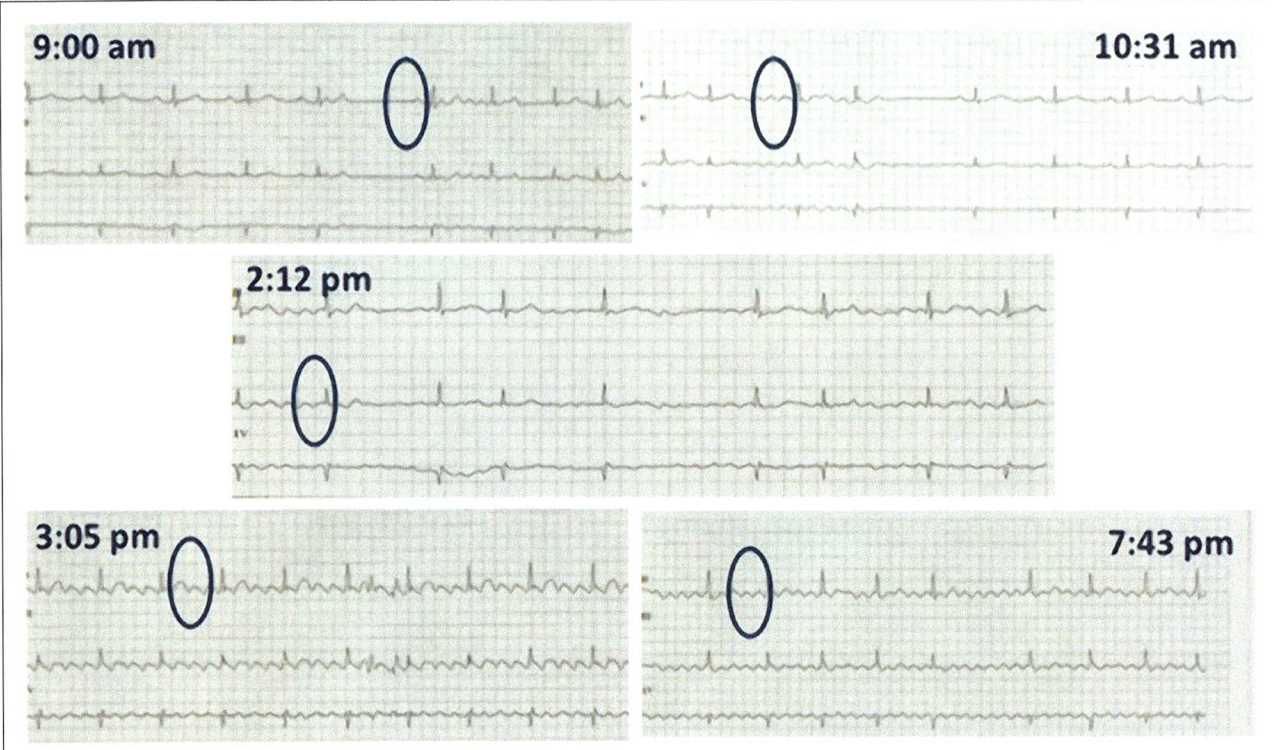

Figure 29.1 Electrocardiographic rhythm strips of recurrent paroxysms of AF in a single patient during the course of a single day demonstrating varying F wave morphology. **Top left:** Onset of spontaneous AF episode at 9:00 am triggered by premature beats with large atrial signals consistent with an ectopic focus, typically seen with focal initiation of pulmonary vein (PV) tachycardia. **Top right:** Termination of the episode at 10:30 am showing reorganization of fine fibrillation seen on the first two beats into coarse, larger F waves before termination. **Middle:** Periods of coarse and fine fibrillatory activity with and without clearly discernible F waves during a sustained AF episode. **Bottom left:** Organized atrial activity consistent with typical atrial flutter with a rate of 250 beats/min during a subsequent event. **Bottom right:** Organized atrial tachyarrhythmia with a faster cycle length consistent with atypical flutter with a rate of 300 beats/min later in the same day.

sustained beyond 7 days or requires cardioversion (drug or electrical) for termination. More recently, the 2012 ablation guidelines suggest that most paroxysmal episodes terminate within 48 hours, and termination with an intervention in this window still maintains their classification.[9] Thus, patients with AF who undergo cardioversion should be classified as having paroxysmal AF if the cardioversion is performed within 48 hours of AF onset, and persistent AF if the cardioversion is performed more than 48 hours after AF onset. A third category of AF is "long-standing, persistent AF," which is defined as continuous AF of greater than 1 year's duration.

The primary difference between the clinical AF presentations lies in the probability of AF termination in a defined time period, which in turn may be based on the complexity of the AF mechanisms initiating or maintaining AF. When cardioversion fails repeatedly (≥ 3 attempts at maximum energy) or is not attempted based on a clinical decision, the patient has been defined as having permanent AF. More recently, aggressive cardioversion using repeated high-energy shocks or intracardiac shocks has demonstrated effective termination of even so-called permanent AF, leading to a decrease in the proportion of these patients. It is recognized that a patient with persistent AF can have episodes that fall into the paroxysmal category. The relationship of the clinical categorization of AF to EP findings in each class becomes important for assessment of AF progression and its management.

Pathophysiology of Atrial Fibrillation

The pathophysiology of AF is complex, integrating electrical, mechanical, structural, and signaling processes that can evolve in the presence or absence of structural heart disease. The onset and maintenance of AF, irrespective of the underlying mechanism, requires both a triggering event that initiates the arrhythmia and the presence of a predisposing substrate that perpetuates it. The former may occur due to atrial premature beats or other atrial tachyarrhythmias, most commonly atrial tachycardias (ATs) or atrial flutter.[10] Specific triggering ATs have been described from the pulmonary and other great veins. AV reentrant tachycardias and AV nodal reentrant tachycardias may also initiate AF.[11] There is a strong association between atrial flutter and the development of AF or coexistence with AF.

The substrate is a key element in the progression of paroxysmal AF to persistent AF. This progression is more rapid in the presence of cardiovascular disease. The development of atrial fibrosis, which can occur as a result of aging, chamber dilatation (leading to transatrial force and stretch distribution changes), and inflammation can have significant role in the development of a substrate that can maintain persistent and permanent AF. Recent data suggest that both resident cardiac cells and infiltrating leukocytes can generate matrix metalloproteinases, the latter via activation of myeloperoxidase, that are key to development of fibrosis. Intracellular signaling cascades are initiated that result in deposition of atrial collagen.[12] Imaging studies show a progressive relationship between the atrial fibrosis burden and the development of more advanced forms of AF. Akoum and coworkers have described a classification on gadolinium-enhanced magnetic resonance imaging (MRI) scans to assess AF scar burden with levels 1 to 4.[13] Left atrial fibrosis involving ≥35% of the entire atrium is generally associated with persistent AF. Experimental studies have shown that ATs can initiate a tachycardia-induced remodeling cascade with changes in ionic currents and signaling proteins.[14] This can promote fibroblastic conversion of myocytes in the atrium, often within one week.[14-16] This conversion can be independent of high ventricular rates.[16]

Uncommonly, a genetic role for AF can be uncovered.[17,18] The genetic mechanisms in this AF subgroup are still being defined. Variants in *SCN5A* that encodes the alpha subunit of the sodium channel have been associated with lone and familial AF.[19,20] Mutations in atrial natriuretic peptide have been noted in familial AF. Mutations in *KCNQ1* (encoding the alpha-subunit of slow delayed rectifier potassium current (IKs) and, separately, in natriuretic peptide precursor A (NPPA) were identified, resulting in a gain of function in IKs.[21] Recent observations suggest that increased IKs due to the *KCNQ1* S140G mutation shortens atrial refractoriness and alters atrial conduction velocity, which can facilitate reentry.[22] For a more detailed description, the reader is referred to a review on the subject.[17]

Electrophysiological Mechanisms

The EP mechanisms of AF have been widely debated and have been studied extensively in several experimental models. The demonstration of critical mass phenomenon for maintenance of a fibrillatory process was initially demonstrated in the ventricle by Garry.[23] Considerable progress has been made since then in defining the specific mechanisms of initiation and perpetuation of AF, with attention focused on the triggers that induce the arrhythmia and the substrate that sustains it. Experimental mechanisms of AF have focused on two theories: "focal" initiation and "reentry" as mechanisms initiating and maintaining AF. The "reentry" hypothesis for a tachyarrhythmia was initially proposed by Mines using a fixed anatomic obstacle, around which the reentrant excitation wavefront could circulate and perpetuate the rhythm.[24] The wavelength was determined by the anatomic pathway characteristics. Moe et al[25,26] later proposed the "multiple wavelet theory" based on computer modeling and suggested that AF is the result of multiple, independent reentrant circuits that exist simultaneously and lead to chaotic activation of the atrium. Several alternate multiple reentry theories have been proposed, in the atrium or ventricle, that are based on the functional and/or anatomic characteristics of normal or diseased myocardial tissue. They suggest that initiation of reentry is dependent on transient local conditions rather than typical reentry around predetermined anatomic or functional barriers.

- *Leading circle model.*[27] Allessie et al suggested that in the absence of an anatomic obstacle, a functional reentry loop can propagate and reenter in a relative refractory tissue without a "full excitable gap," with the wavelength of the circuit being determined by the functional properties of the circuit. This type of reentry is commonly observed in normal cardiac tissue.

- *Anisotropic reentry.*[28] This macroreentrant activation and propagation is dependent on the orientation of the myocardial fibers and the direction of the propagation wavefront. The propagation velocity is many times faster along the longitudinal axis of cells compared to transverse propagation. This phenomenon is believed to be determined by connections between individual cells in the cardiac fibers and their distribution (eg, gap junctions).

- *Figure-of-8 reentry.*[29] Two macroreentrant, counter-rotating circuits coexist around two separate anatomical or functional barriers with a common pathway/isthmus. Understanding the characteristics and propagation properties of the common pathway is of great practical importance, as this could serve as a strategic region to target for surgical or catheter ablation.

- *Spiral wave reentry.*[30] According to this model of reentry, a spiral wave develops and determines the size and shape of the region or "core" around which a functional reentrant wavefront rotates. Spiral wave reentry circuits could be formed even in cardiac muscle, which is completely homogenous in its functional properties. Recent clinical data from the CONFIRM trial suggest that this may be seen in clinical reentrant rotor activity during simultaneous left and right atrial mapping using basket catheters. These circuits appear to be relatively small, according to the authors.[31]

- *Automaticity.* The primary hypothesis currently suggests that AF is due to areas of ectopic automaticity producing rapid focal electrical discharges.[32] The presence of sleeves of cardiac tissue that extend onto the pulmonary veins (PVs) was first noted by Nathan et al.[33] There is now general agreement that myocardial muscle fibers extend from the left atrium into all the PVs as well as other great veins for 1–3 cm; the thickness of the muscular sleeve is highest at the proximal ends (1–1.5 mm), and then gradually decreases distally.[34,35] The reduced action potential duration and slow conduction in proximal portion of PVs facilitate and initiate rapid reentrant circuits in the PVs.[36]

- *Electrical and structural remodeling.* Maintenance and persistence of AF may result from electrical and structural remodeling, characterized by atrial dilatation and shortening of the atrial ERP. This combination, along with other remodeling changes, facilitates the appearance of multiple reentrant atrial tachyarrhythmias that result in perpetuation of AF.

A recent expert consensus statement has discussed the key structures and the potential experimental mechanisms into a proposed overall mechanistic basis for clinical AF and its major types (Figure 29.2).[9] Atrial fibrillation onset and maintenance, irrespective of the mechanism, require a trigger that initiates the arrhythmia and the presence of substrate that perpetuates it. Additional factors (eg, neural influences, tissue factors, inflammation, or autonomic tone) may also facilitate initiation or maintenance of AF. Clinical investigations, therefore, focus on understanding these mechanisms of clinical AF in an individual patient.

The clinical EP study remains the gold standard for the investigation and evaluation of human AF.

Electrophysiological Studies for the Evaluation of Atrial Fibrillation

The clinical EP study in an AF patient should consist of a systematic approach for the analysis of arrhythmias by recording and measuring a variety of EP parameters and events with the patient in sinus rhythm and/or AF and by evaluating their response to programmed electrical stimulation and/or to a variety of interventions.

Clinical Electrophysiological Techniques

Clinical EP studies in a patient with AF should consist of a systematic approach to the analysis of arrhythmias by recording and measuring a variety of EP parameters and events with the patient in sinus rhythm, AF, or both, and by evaluating his or her response to programmed electrical stimulation. The study begins with the recording of a surface ECG, which is necessary to diagnose AF. It is recommended that the physician evaluate the electrical rhythm with a high-gain 12-lead ECG at higher paper speeds (50–100 mm/sec) to accurately assess P-wave duration and morphology (Figure 29.5B). Correlation of the P wave with intracardiac signals is valuable and should be systematically performed (Figure 29.5B). Following the

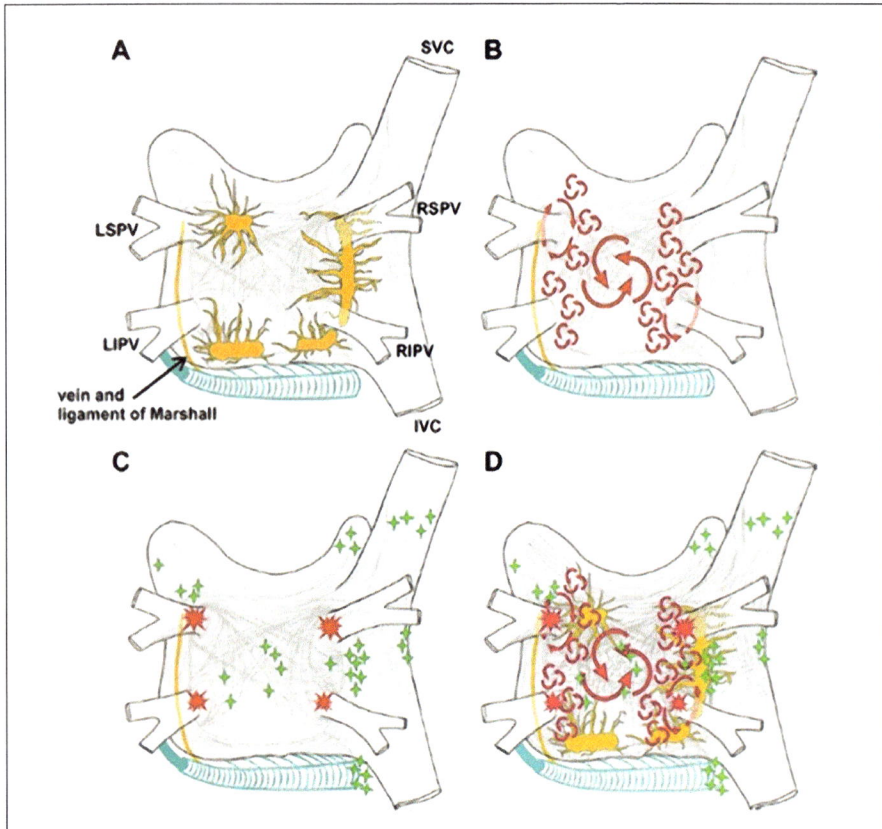

Figure 29.2 Structure and mechanisms of atrial fibrillation. *Source:* Reproduced with permission from JICE. **Panel A:** Schematic drawing of the left and right atria (as viewed from the posterior). The extension of muscular fibers onto the PVs can be appreciated. Shown in **yellow** are the five major left atrial autonomic ganglionic plexi (GP) and axons (superior left GP, inferior left GP, anterior right GP, inferior right GP, and ligament of Marshall). Shown in **blue** is the coronary sinus, which is enveloped by muscular fibers that have connections to the atria. Also shown in **blue** is the vein and ligament of Marshall, which travel from the coronary sinus to the region between the left superior PV and the left atrial appendage. **Panel B:** Large and small reentrant wavelets that play a role in initiating and sustaining AF. **Panel C:** Common locations of PV triggers (**red**) and sites of origin of non-PV triggers (shown in **green**). **Panel D:** Composite of the anatomic and arrhythmic mechanisms of AF. *Source:* Calkins H, Kuck KH, Cappato R, et al.[9] Used with permission.

assessment of the patient's ECG, the EP study includes the measurement of baseline intracardiac conduction intervals and assessment of sinus node, atrial, AV node, His-Purkinje system conduction, and refractoriness. These are described elsewhere in this text.

There have been several techniques reported for the regional catheter mapping of discrete focal sources of AF in specific atrial regions. At a minimum, this is accomplished with placement of 2 to 4 multipolar catheters in the high right atrium and/or the mid-right atrium, His bundle region, right ventricular apex, and the coronary sinus to record left atrial electrograms and activation (Figure 29.3). Right atrial recordings can be obtained from the free wall, septum, and the tricuspid isthmus for regional right atrial activation patterns. A duodecapolar catheter is widely used for this purpose in our laboratory. Unlike mapping of common flutter, we typically place this catheter with its distal electrode in the low lateral right atrial free wall with the proximal set of electrodes lying along the interatrial septum (Figure 29.4). Electrograms are recorded at paper speeds of 100 to 200 mm/sec. Intra-atrial conduction in the right atrium is best reflected by measurement of the P-A interval (from onset of P wave to the onset of atrial activation in the His bundle electrogram), and right-to-left atrial conduction is measured from the onset of the P wave to the latest atrial electrogram recorded. This is commonly found between the middle and distal coronary sinus leads and should not exceed 130 ms.

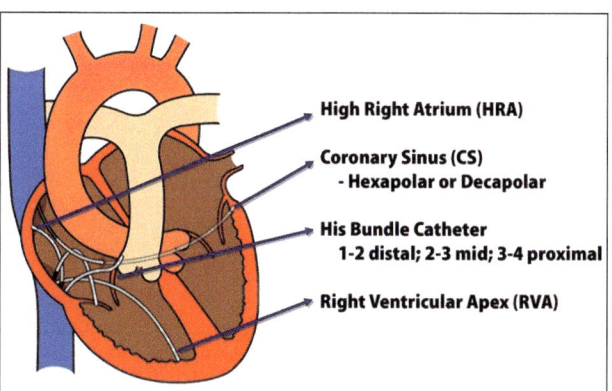

Figure 29.3 Typical right atrial diagnostic catheter placements to measure baseline conduction intervals and assessment of the conduction system for an EP evaluation in patients with AF. A total of 2 to 4 multipolar catheters are placed at the high right atrium, coronary sinus (CS), His bundle region, and the right ventricular apex.

The routes of interatrial conduction are complex and have been studied by using detailed atrial mapping with noncontact and contact approaches. Anatomic studies have recognized an interatrial connection in the anterosuperior interatrial septum referred to as Bachmann's bundle. The contributions of left and right atrial musculature to the interatrial septum have been well described, but EP studies have also noted preferential conduction along the coronary sinus now ascribed to a spiral muscle band.

Lemery and colleagues performed right and left atrial noncontact mapping during sinus rhythm and atrial pacing and demonstrated interatrial conduction over two distinct regions via Bachmann's bundle and the coronary sinus.[37]

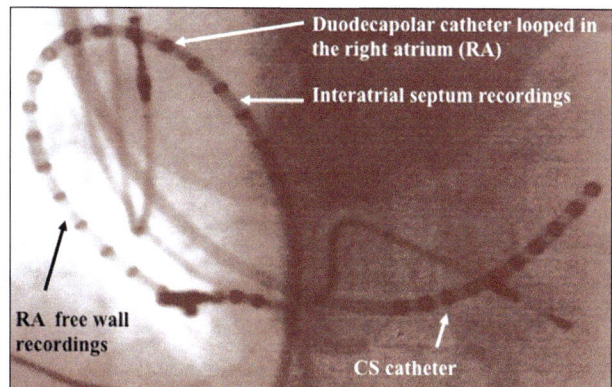

Figure 29.4 Fluoroscopic image demonstrating how right atrial recordings can be obtained from the free wall, septum, and the tricuspid isthmus for regional right atrium activation patterns. A duodecapolar catheter can be placed with its distal electrode in the low lateral right atrial free wall with the proximal set of electrodes lying along the interatrial septum.

Left atrial recordings can be indirectly obtained epicardially from the coronary sinus and the left pulmonary artery. A decapolar catheter is placed in the left pulmonary artery in a branch typically encircling the left atrial appendage (Figure 29.5A). In this fashion, recordings from the left atrial lateral wall, left superior PV, roof of the left atrium and LIPV, and RSPV can be indirectly obtained to evaluate conduction in the superior left atrium (Figure 29.5B).[38]

Direct left atrial access can be achieved with a transseptal puncture, which requires puncture at the fossa ovalis using a Brockenborough needle mounted within a transseptal sheath and dilator assembly, usually guided by intracardiac echocardiography (ICE). With the transseptal approach, the distal electrode can be placed in the left superior PV, across the left atrial roof, and in the fossa ovalis. Several variants of fossa anatomy, including lipomatous hypertrophy, fibrosis (which is noted in repeat transseptal procedures), and interatrial septal aneurysms can make transseptal puncture challenging. These anatomic variants are instantly recognizable on ICE, so this imaging modality can facilitate safe transseptal puncture. In cases of difficult transseptal puncture, an FDA-approved radiofrequency-powered transseptal needle (Baylis NRG, Montreal, Quebec, Canada) can be used to cross the interatrial septum.[39] After transseptal puncture is accomplished, specifically designed catheters can be used to map the atrium or PVs. With the transseptal approach, the distal electrode can be placed in the left superior PV, across the left atrial roof, in the left atrial appendage, and along the mitral valve isthmus. The catheter can also be manipulated into each of the PVs for

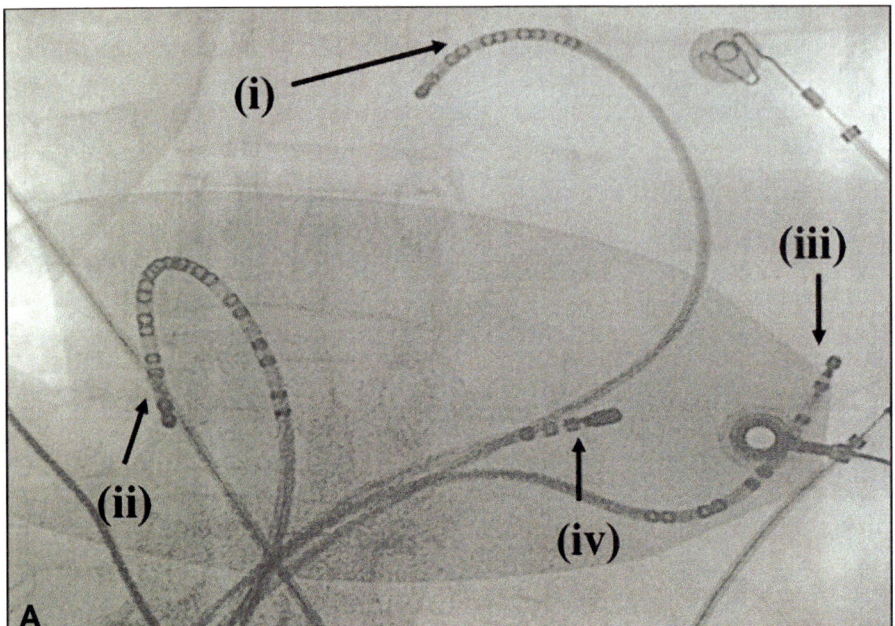
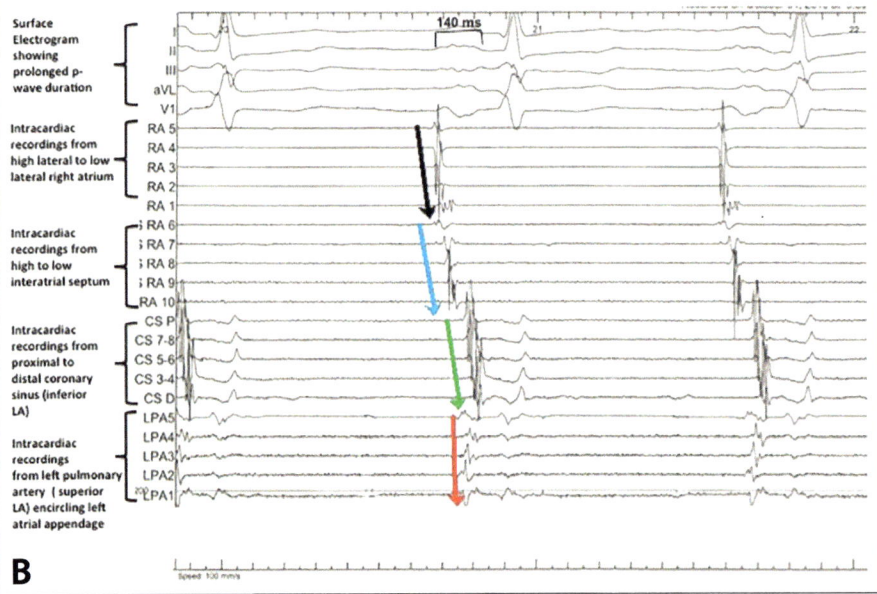

Figure 29.5 Panel A: Fluoroscopic image demonstrating the positioning of a (i) decapolar catheter in the left lower pulmonary artery in a branch typically encircling the left atrial appendage (LAA) to indirectly record electrical activity from the left atrial lateral wall, left superior pulmonary vein (PV), roof of the left atrium, and the right superior PV; (ii) duodecapolar catheter looped in the right atrium to record free wall, roof, and septal electrograms; (iii) decapolar catheter in the coronary sinus; and (iv) catheter to record His bundle signals.
Panel B: Demonstration of surface ECG (note prolonged and notched P-waves) and intracadiac electrograms in sinus rhythm with catheters positioned in the lateral right atrium, interatrial septum, coronary sinus, and left atrial intracardiac recordings with a decapolar catheter in the left lower pulmonary artery during sinus rhythm. RA = right atrium; CS = coronary sinus; LPA = left pulmonary artery recordings from superior left atrium.

mapping. Alternatively, preformed electrode catheters can be used to map the atrium or PVs. A circular preformed multielectrode catheter (eg, Lasso® catheter, Biosense Webster, Diamond Bar, CA) or small linear catheters (eg, Cardima Pathfinder®, Cardima Inc., Fremont, CA) can also be used for mapping within tubular structures such as the PVs, superior or inferior vena cava, coronary sinus, or atrial appendages (or at their ostia in the atria). The Lasso catheter comes in different configurations (10 or 20 electrode poles) and variable spacing (8 mm, 2-6-2 mm) and with fixed 15, 20, and 25 mm and variable curve diameters (Figure 29.6). It allows for circular mapping at the PV antrum, which can have varying anatomic configurations (usually 5–10 mm outside the PV ostium and in the atrium) and within the veins for segmental mapping. The Pathfinder catheter permits placement well inside the vein and its branches, to map the main vein or its secondary branches. However, as ablation within the PV is progressively undertaken with lesser frequency, this catheter is most useful in careful assessment of gaps in ablation lines. Using such technology, activation within the veins during sinus rhythm, paced atrial stimuli, and spontaneous premature atrial beats can be recorded and localized. The HD Mesh Ablator catheter (Bard, Lowell, MA) integrates high-density simultaneous multielectrode curvilinear mapping and radiofrequency energy delivery in a single device. For additional information relative to left atrial recordings, please see Chapter 3. The Mesh has been used in a recent clinical trial for mapping and ablation of spontaneous AF.[31]

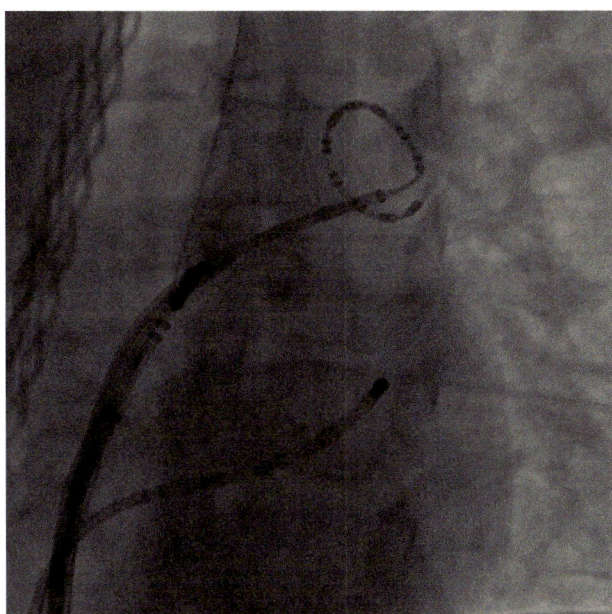

Figure 29.6 Positioning of a preformed Lasso circular catheter (Biosense Webster) in the left superior PV of the left atrium; 10 electrode poles, 8 mm spacing, 25 mm diameter. The Lasso catheter is typically used for circular mapping at the PV antrum and within the veins for segmental mapping.

Programmed Stimulation During Electrophysiological Evaluation

An important goal of EP evaluation of the AF patients is to elicit an AF episode to permit careful study of its mode of initiation, location of onset, evolution, maintenance, and termination. Ideally, a spontaneous AF event occurring during the EP study would allow for such analyses. Often, this does not occur, and we utilize programmed atrial stimulation to provoke AF during EP studies. There are several methods for induction of AF using programmed stimulation including the single and multiple extrastimuli during regular drive trains, long–short sequences, and rapid burst pacing techniques. This can be performed before and after a variety of pharmacologic provocative maneuvers that are described later.

Atrial refractoriness is assessed using programmed atrial stimulation using an extrastimulus pacing technique. In this method, a single atrial extrastimulus (S2) is delivered with progressively shorter coupling intervals in 10–20 ms decrements after an 8- to 10-beat regular drive train (S1–S1 of usually 600 ms and 400 ms). Stimulus amplitude is typically 2 to 4 times the atrial pacing threshold. The evoked atrial potentials are measured and A1–A2 interval can be measured as a function of the S1–S2 coupling interval. The longest coupling interval at which the extrastimulus fails to capture the atrium is defined as the atrial effective refractory period. In contrast, the absolute atrial effective refractory period is the longest S1–S2 interval at any S2 stimulus amplitude that fails to capture the atrium. The shortest A1–A2 interval elicited on this curve is referred to as the functional atrial refractory period. AV nodal conduction and conduction in the His-Purkinje system can be assessed using H1–H2 and H2–V2 interval measurements with corresponding effective and functional refractory periods. Additional extrastimuli (two or three) and long–short drive trains are used to elicit atrial tachyarrhythmias and AF (Figure 29.7, Panel A). Rapid atrial pacing can also be used to induce AF (Figure 29.7, Panel B). Because morphologic analysis on the surface ECG is limited, sensitivity and specificity of these methods to induce AF require consideration.

Krol and colleagues[40] employed a programmed stimulation protocol at two different atrial sites (high right atrium and coronary sinus ostium) using two drive trains (600 ms and 500 ms) of 8 beats followed by a single, double, or triple extrastimuli. These were delivered at 50 ms above the atrial refractory period followed by 10 ms decrements until atrial capture was lost. This protocol induced either AF or atrial flutter in 89% of patients with spontaneous AF events, compared to only 7% induction of arrhythmia in the control group without atrial arrhythmias. The sensitivity and specificity of this programmed stimulation protocol for induction of AF were 89% and 92%, respectively. Mapping of induced AF by the same group showed that while initial onset tachycardia cycles were in the vicinity of the pacing site, established AF could be maintained by disparate locations and tachycardias. This could be more akin to the spontaneous arrhythmia.

Spontaneous Atrial Fibrillation Induction

Spontaneous AF events sometimes may occur during an EP study (Figure 29.7C). These should be analyzed from their onset to the maintenance phase. Triggering APB locations can be identified, and the onset tachycardia can be analyzed. After onset, evolution of new tachycardias can be seen; these may involve disparate locations and even disparate atria. This is discussed further in a subsequent section in this chapter.

Isoproterenol is commonly used to elicit such events by increasing trigger activity, particularly from the PVs. Isoproterenol has been used at moderate to high doses (4–20 mcg/min) to initiate spontaneous AF.[41] Consideration of concomitant comorbid conditions—for example, the presence of ischemia or heart failure—should guide its use. Hemodynamic monitoring is desirable in this instance. Adenosine or vagomimetic drugs have also been used to induce AF. Adenosine, methacholine, and even alcohol infusions have been used to elicit AF in the laboratory.[42] They are also used to assess the efficacy of PV isolation.[43]

Alternatively, we have found that cardioversion of a sustained AF episode can allow emergence of spontaneous APBs and AF events after cardioversion. Figure 29.7, Panel D shows combined biatrial and noncontact mapping showing an early recurrence of AF with triggering APBs

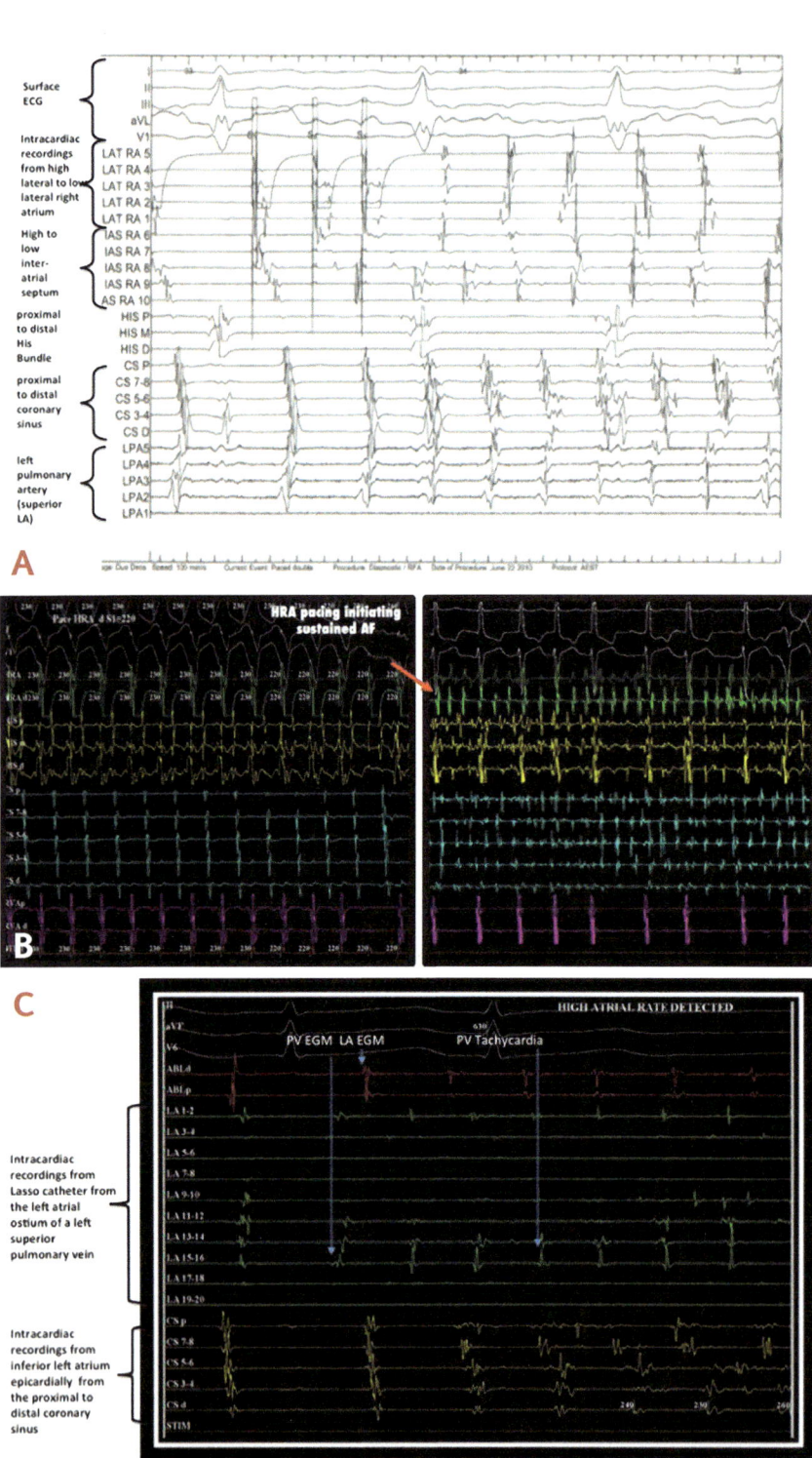

Figure 29.7 Panel A: Induction of atrial fibrillation by programmed electrical stimulation using two extrastimuli during a drive train. Surface ECG recordings and intracardiac recordings from both atrial regions are shown. The initial induced atrial cycle arises in the lateral right atrium near the pacing site, but subsequent cycles show development of a rapid atrial tachyarrhythmia in the left atrium, as seen in the coronary sinus and left pulmonary artery recordings, which is dissociated from the right atrial tachycardia and in the last cycle penetrates the septum and right atrium. **Panel B:** Induction of sustained AF with rapid atrial pacing. Surface ECG recordings and intracardiac recordings from both atrial regions are shown. **Panel C:** Spontaneous AF onset recording using a Lasso catheter at the ostium of a PV with an ablation catheter in the left atrium and another electrode catheter in the coronary sinus. A triggering premature beat (second cycle) initiates a run of atrial tachycardia arising in the PV. Earliest activation at Lasso electrodes 15–16 suggests a focal onset of the tachycardia from this region in the PV. **Panel D:** Biatrial and noncontact right atrial mapping of spontaneous onset of an AF episode following cardioversion due to early recurrence of AF. Triggering atrial premature beats (APBs; shown by **arrow**) initiating atrial tachycardia are seen. The triggering beat is recorded first in the left pulmonary artery recordings and is consistent with a superior left PV trigger and PV tachycardia. Delayed activation of the right atrium with no wavefront at onset of the premature beat is noted. Activation at Bachmann's bundle shown by the **red asterisk** confirms the bystander role of the right atrium at onset of AF in an AF patient. CS = coronary sinus; EGM = electrogram; HB = His bundle; HRA = high right atrium; IAS = interatrial septum; LA = left atrium; LPA = left pulmonary artery; PV = pulmonary vein; RA = right atrium; RV = right ventricle. Source: Saksena S, Skadsberg ND, Rao HB, Filipecki A.[38] Used with permission.

most likely arising in the PVs followed by spontaneous onset of an AF episode. Such early recurrences of AF have, in our experience, been similar to spontaneous AF events in terms of origin and propagation. Cardioversion of induced AF can also evoke spontaneous AF events and is utilized routinely in our EP studies.

Clinical Electrophysiological Findings in Atrial Fibrillation

Periods of organized f waves can often be correlated with organized tachyarrhythmias on intracardiac recordings. Any arrhythmia that has the ECG characteristics of AF and lasts sufficiently long for a 12-lead ECG to be recorded, or at least 30 seconds on a rhythm strip, should be considered an AF episode. Patients with AF generally have ECG evidence of delayed intra-atrial conduction, and this is manifested on the surface ECG as prolonged and/or notched P waves in sinus rhythm. This intra-atrial conduction defect (IACD) can result in virtual segmentation of the P wave, with three levels of intra-atrial conduction block being described based on P-wave morphology.[44] Increasing P-wave duration during sinus rhythm is associated with more advanced forms of AF, such as persistent or long-standing persistent AF, as well as with frequent relapses after AF therapy.[45,46] Prolongation of P-wave duration may also be related to temporal dissociation of right and left atrial activation, slowing of conduction, or fragmentation of atrial potentials often seen as late potentials on a P-wave signal-averaged ECG.

A high incidence of intra- and interatrial conduction abnormalities (eg, P-to-mid-distal coronary sinus duration ≥ 130 ms) and reentrant behavior has been demonstrated in patients with AF or flutter (see Table 29.1).[46] The interatrial conduction delay is especially pronounced using single extrastimulus technique, performed at < 50% of drive train, eg, 600 ms.[47] Regional intracardiac atrial electrogram recordings show a propensity for split potentials in certain locations (eg, crista terminalis, coronary sinus, Eustachian ridge at the cavotricuspid isthmus, posterior left atrium, etc), suggesting that an anatomic structure or obstacle can alter atrial electrical wavefront propagation with splitting and delayed conduction. A thorough abbreviation of atrial effective and functional refractory periods during programmed atrial stimulation is also seen in patients with AF, with concomitant loss of rate adaptation of atrial refractoriness. In addition, there is increased dispersion of atrial refractoriness in the atria in AF patients compared to controls.[48] This can promote reentry.

Our group has previously analyzed the electrophysiologic characteristics and patterns of atrial activation in patients with inducible atrial fibrillation.[49] After a drive train (8–10 beats at 600 ms and 500 ms), extrastimuli were delivered in a decremental fashion. There was an increase in intra-atrial conduction delay (stimulus S2 to local atrial electrogram A2) for the right atrial premature beats, and an increasing delay with increasing prematurity of the last extrastimulus. Maximal intra-atrial conduction delay was noted at the coronary sinus ostium, His bundle region, or interatrial septum.[49] The earliest atrial activation site of induced AF was noted at the crista terminalis or interatrial septum on the right side. This may be related to site of stimulation as the activation sequence and EP behavior of the first induced AF cycle was consistent with local reentry as a trigger mechanism of AF. This would suggest that local reentrant excitation in proximity to a triggering premature beat can be an early phenomenon in AF initiation. In a later section, spontaneous APB behavior will be discussed.

Table 29.1 Comparison of typical EP intervals and refractory periods in normal patients and patients with AF and atrial flutter

Electrophysiologic Findings	Normal	Atrial Fibrillation	P-value
P-wave duration	117 ± 11 ms	127 ± 16 ms	<0.05
RA conduction time (Onset of P wave to the onset of atrial activation in the His bundle electrogram)	35 ± 21 ms	64 ± 18 ms	<0.005
Interatrial conduction time (Onset of P wave to the onset of atrial activation in the mid and distal coronary sinus)	36 ± 16 ms	76 ± 19 ms	<0.001
Atrial effective refractory period (at drive cycle length of 600 ms from high right atrium)	233 ± 28 ms	206 ± 24 ms	0.02

Sources: Josephson ME. *Clinical Cardiac Electrophysiology Text Book,* 4th ed. Philadelphia, PA: Lippincott Williams & Wilkins; 1988, and Cosio FG, Palacios J, Vidal JM, Cocina EG, Gómez-Sánchez MA, Tamargo L. Electrophysiologic studies in atrial fibrillation: slow conduction of premature impulses: a possible manifestation of the background for reentry. *Am J Cardiol.* 1983;51:122-130.

PV Ectopy and Tachycardia

Recent reports of EP evaluation of AF have focused on the mapping of induced and spontaneous AF as well as detailed 3-dimensional (3D) or catheter activation mapping of the right and left atria for triggers, organized tachycardias, and/or identification of an abnormal atrial substrate. Focal triggers are diverse and may be facilitated by sympathetic or parasympathetic stimulation or bradycardia and atrial stretch. Atrial ectopic activity often arises from the extension of atrial myocardial "sleeves" into the PVs or vena caval junctions.

PV premature beats or tachycardia constitute PV triggers and are frequently responsible for initiation of paroxysmal AF events, in patients both with and without structural heart disease. PV triggers can be induced with catecholamines such as isoproterenol. The electrograms originating from the PVs have some distinct properties allowing them to be distinguished from atrial electrograms.[50] Pulmonary veins that trigger electrograms typically are local, high-frequency signals. They can be easily identified by the reversal of conduction pattern from PV to left atrium rather than from left atrium to PV. It is important to distinguish this from far-field activity from the adjacent PVs, the left atrium, the left atrial appendage, the superior vena cava, or the vein of Marshall. This can be accomplished by differential pacing maneuvers.[51] Pacing from different atrial locations may move the relative timing of non-PV potentials, helping to distinguish the true PV potentials.[51]

The rapid rate of PV tachycardia can cause functional block in surrounding atrial tissue, preventing it from following in 1:1 fashion. Therefore, a shorter cycle length within the PV than in the left atrium proper can help identify spontaneous PV tachycardia. Drugs such as adenosine can activate dormant conduction in ostial tissue and are used to assess the durability of ablation lesions for PV isolation.[43]

The finding of PV triggers initiating the majority of paroxysmal AF led to development of ablation strategies designed to electrically isolate the PVs from the left atrium.[52] These include segmental PV isolation and circumferential PV antral isolation approaches.[53] Single procedure success is modest, and repeated procedures are often necessary even in paroxysmal AF.[54] Reconnection of previously ablated regions for PV isolation is one major reason for recurrence in paroxysmal AF. However, recent studies have shown limited long-term success with PV isolation alone in persistent AF patients and in patients with structural heart disease and enlarged atria.[54,55]

It is now believed that identification and ablation of non-PV triggers and functional/anatomical areas of slow conduction are also necessary in 20% to 30% of all patients. In our biatrial mapping data, an average of 3 triggering APB locations can be identified in a given patient. This would suggest that non-PV triggers are more frequently identified with global mapping techniques.

Non-PV Triggers

Non-PV triggers initiating AF can be identified in up to one-third of patients referred for catheter ablation for paroxysmal AF.[56] In patients with persistent AF, extrapulmonary APBs and triggering tachycardias are more frequent than in paroxysmal AF. The superior vena cava is a common site of non-PV triggers, followed by crista terminalis; ligament of Marshall, coronary sinus, persistent left superior vena cava, inferior vena cava, and the left atrial appendage also have all been reported to demonstrate triggering premature atrial beats.[57] Provocative maneuvers such as the administration of isoproterenol in incremental doses of up to 20 mcg/min and/or cardioversion of induced and spontaneous AF can aid in the identification of non-PV triggers. They were detected in 16.5% of patients in one report.[58] In such patients, these triggers can be isolated, eg, in the superior vena cava, by interrupting conduction between the right atrium and superior vena cava or directly ablating ectopic sites in the right atrial free wall or crista terminalis. In our studies using simultaneous biatrial and 3D mapping, the presence of multiple APB sites of origin (usually three or more) in both atria was the rule rather than the exception. This is probably related to performance of global biatrial mapping and simultaneous recording of both atria. It would suggest that triggering APBs are underestimated and undermapped in routine EP studies. Supraventricular tachycardias such as AV nodal reentry or accessory pathway-mediated atrioventricular reciprocating tachycardia may also be identified in up to 4% of unselected patients referred for AF ablation and may serve as a triggering mechanism for AF. Additionally, reentrant circuits maintaining AF may be located across the right and left atria.

Complex Fractionated Atrial Electrograms (CFAEs)

Mapping of human AF has identified CFAEs in both atria. In our early studies, sites of conduction delay were identified in the crista terminalis, interatrial septum, and coronary sinus during atrial extrastimulation.[49] Jaïs et al showed regional disparities in paroxysmal AF.[59] CFAEs are defined as atrial electrograms with low voltage (≤ 0.15 mV) that have fractionated electrograms composed of two or more deflections and/or have a short cycle length (≤ 120 ms) in their maximal form giving continuous electrical activity. CFAEs identify sites of slow conduction or functional block in the atria, which can act as pivotal points for reentry circuits and have been thought to be potential key locations for maintenance of AF.[60] Some of them also demonstrate a dominant high-frequency spectral component (DF) during sinus rhythm. These may have been considered important target sites for AF ablation.[61] The CFAE region may play an important role in the perpetuation of AF based on a higher number of focal discharges, frequency of wave breaks and wave fusions, and slower conduction being recorded than in non-CFAE regions.[62] In humans, high-density mapping during AF demonstrated that the formation of CFAE was preceded in 91% of mapped sites by shortening of the atrial cycle length, which further supports the key role that cycle length plays in the generation of CFAE.[63] The primary endpoints during RF ablation targeting CFAE sites are either complete elimination of the areas with CFAE, conversion of AF to sinus rhythm, and/or noninducibility of AF. The outcomes of CFAE ablation have been mixed, raising questions about the extent of ablation as well as the endpoints. When employing the targeting of CFAE in the right atrium, Oral et al reported that CFAE ablation showed no improvement in outcomes in persistent AF patients.[64] More recently, a single-center comparative study did not show better outcomes when CFAE ablation was added to PV isolation and/or linear ablation.[65]

Atrial Fibrillation Nests (See Chapter 42B)

Real-time spectral mapping using fast Fourier transform (FFT) in sinus rhythm has identified unfiltered, bipolar atrial electrograms containing unusually high frequencies, the so-called "AF nest" (Figure 42B.13). These AF nests are thought to play a role in perpetuation of AF. Therefore, the purpose of DF mapping is to identify sites of maximal DF during AF, as it is believed that ablation at such sites results in slowing and termination in a significant proportion of paroxysmal AF patients, and may further improve outcomes when coupled with PV isolation ablation.[66,67] In AF due to multiple unstable reentry circuits, FFT generally demonstrates multiple and broad frequency peaks in both atria.[68] For more details, refer to Chapter 42B in this text.

Periatrial Ganglionic Plexi Mapping and Ablation

The autonomic nervous system, especially the parasympathetic periatrial ganglionic plexi (GP) were shown to initiate spontaneous AF in an open-chest canine model.[69] Evidence suggests that the intrinsic cardiac autonomic nervous system initiates or facilitates AF by triggered firing of the PVs and by altering the atrial refractoriness.[70,71] The majority and large GP are located at the LA–PV junctions between the bilateral superior and inferior PVs. GP are mapped by applying high-frequency stimuli (cycle length 50 ms, 12 V, 1–10 ms pulse width) at the LA–PV junction, which results in marked slowing of ventricular rate (>50%) during AF. Ablation at these sites in paroxysmal AF were initially reported to have very high success rates (90%) during a short 6-month follow-up period.[72,73] However, later reports showed highly variable success rates ranging from 25% to 75% after >1 year follow-up.[74-76] Another study demonstrated that despite successful endocardial GP ablation, there was a very high rate of acute reinduction of AF with high-frequency atrial stimulation (17/18 patients).[77] Approaches of hybrid endocardial and epicardial GP ablation and electrical stimulation of the vagoparasympathetic ganglia is currently being evaluated.

3D Electrophysiologic Mapping Techniques

Mapping Technology

It is common today to use 3D mapping systems to conduct EP mapping and subsequent ablation of AF. Today's systems allow for nonfluoroscopic catheter navigation, activation and voltage mapping, and precise identification and tagging of ablation sites. 3D mapping systems incorporate electrical data recorded from the electrode catheters in real space with structural data from MRI or computed tomography (CT). The use of these 3D mapping systems has demonstrated the ability to significantly reduce fluoroscopy exposure duration for operators.

The two most widely used systems are the Carto™ (Biosense Webster, Diamond Bar, CA) and the EnSite™ NavX™ systems (St. Jude Medical, St. Paul, MN). The Carto mapping system utilizes ultralow magnetic field technology to reconstruct 3D maps and activation sequences. With this approach, the patient is positioned over a patch that emits 3 electromagnetic waves at unique frequencies. Each signal is registered by one of 3 specifically tuned coils embedded in the mapping catheter tip to specify location in 3D space, with reference to a second catheter that is typically positioned in the coronary sinus. Electrograms and the direction of the catheter tip also create an orientation vector that can be displayed on the workstation. Sequential collection of local tissue activation at each recording site generates activation maps within the framework of the previously acquired surrogate geometry. In addition, this system records and stores both unipolar and bipolar signals, to give a snapshot view of global and local voltage at each of the individual recording sites.

The EnSite NavX system is capable of simultaneously displaying 3D positions of multiple catheters with the chamber's electrophysiological activation. This is achieved by applying a low-level 5.6 kHz current through orthogonally located skin patches. The recorded voltage and impedance at each of the catheter's 64 electrodes generated from this current allows measuring their distance from each skin patch and, ultimately, their location in space, to be triangulated with the help of a reference electrode located within the chamber of interest. The EnSite system's multielectrode array mapping balloon catheter can be employed to create dynamic EP activation sequence maps of the chamber's endocardial surface on the order of only 1 to 2 cardiac cycles. To create the endocardial geometry, we typically use identifiable landmarks, eg, for right atrium mapping, crista terminalis in the lateral right atrium, the orifices of the great veins, the entire tricuspid annulus, coronary sinus ostium, tricuspid valve-inferior vena cava isthmus, and the interatrial septum at multiple sites along a craniocaudal axis. Figure 29.8 shows a fluoroscopic image of the multielectrode mapping array balloon in the right atrium. Similar approaches are used in the left atrium. Once the 3D contour of the chamber of interest is completed, the system is ready for acquisition and analysis of different rhythms. This approach permits beat-to-beat real-time activation mapping of AF from onset to termination.

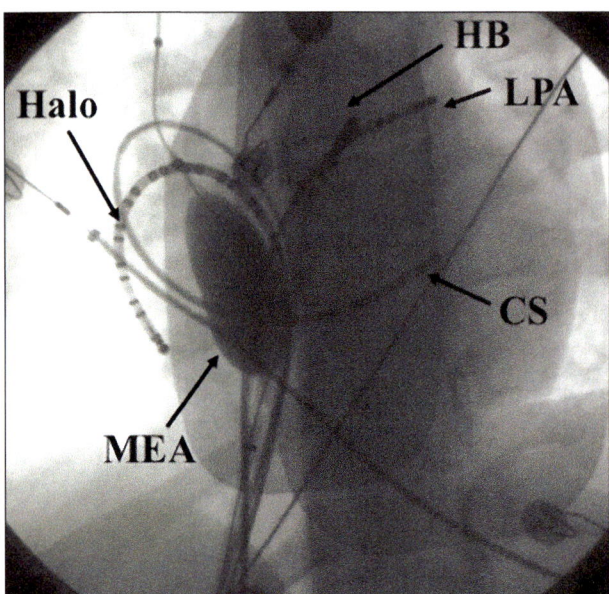

Figure 29.8 Fluoroscopic image showing positioning of the multielectrode balloon array catheter in the right atrium and biatrial contact catheters in a left anterior oblique view. CS = coronary sinus; HB = His bundle; LPA = left pulmonary artery; MEA = multielectrode array.

Electrophysiological Findings Employing 3D Mapping

Using 3D mapping, we have the unique ability to study sinus rhythm propagation, extrastimulus behavior, and induced or spontaneous arrhythmia initiation either on sequential mapping or on beat-by-beat imaging (EnSite balloon) and perform detailed 3D analysis. During sustained tachyarrhythmias, whether induced or spontaneous, we can correlate the arrhythmia propagation with specific anatomic locations. 3D mapping can also be employed to allow for automatic detection and characterization of CFAEs ranging from virtual unipolar signals (EnSite) to the FFT (Bard EP, Lowell, MA) of signals from the tip of the ablation catheter up to tiny electrodes on a specialized multipolar catheter (PentaRay®, Biosense Webster).

Insights into AF Mechanisms from Biatrial and 3D Mapping

Our studies in patients with paroxysmal and persistent AF with combined contact biatrial and noncontact 3D mapping have allowed analyses of the regional origin of APBs and atrial tachyarrhythmias during spontaneous AF.[38,49] Evolution into sustained AF and its maintenance have been examined. On simultaneous biatrial mapping over a few hours, APBs are noted to be multifocal, and often biatrial in origin in both paroxysmal and persistent AF patients. One or more APBs can trigger spontaneous AF events in a single patient (Figure 29.9). APBs triggering spontaneous AF demonstrate a wider distribution of origin in persistent AF with the highest frequency arising from the superior left atrium and septum (Figure 29.10). The onset of sustained AT may commence at a location distant from the APB origin (eg, type 1 flutter in the right atrium), or in proximity to the trigger (eg, PV trigger initiating reentrant tachycardia in the posterior left atrium). Organized ATs are seen in both paroxysmal and persistent AF, and at least two ATs, most commonly PV tachycardia and common right atrial flutter, are seen in paroxysmal AF patients (Figure 29.11). A wider spectrum of ATs can be seen, particularly in persistent AF. This includes focal PV tachycardia, left atrial flutter with macroreentry including mitral isthmus flutter, type 1 isthmus-dependent or type 2 nonisthmus-dependent right atrial flutter, upper or lower loop flutter, and/or focal atrial tachycardia. Organized AT distribution in persistent AF (right or left atrial flutter) or tachycardia demonstrated a wider biatrial origin than paroxysmal AF. Furthermore, mitral isthmus-dependent left atrial flutter was more prevalent in persistent AF patients, while isthmus- or nonisthmus-dependent right atrial flutter was comparable in prevalence in both types of AF. Therefore, AF progression is most likely related to the development of a biatrial substrate for the arrhythmia and proliferation of these ATs, which results in persistence of an individual AF event. These findings bridge the divide between observations obtained with regional catheter recordings and intraoperative findings in humans.

Simultaneous global atrial mapping has also been performed using basket catheters in the right and left atria (Figure 29.12). Narayan and colleagues have reported small reentrant circuits with areas of curvature mimicking animal models of spiral waves. These are reported to be often a few millimeters to centimeter size. Ablation at these sites has been reported to improve outcomes in the short term in one trial.[31]

Postablation Mapping

EP mapping is performed after catheter ablation to assess adequacy of ablation. Focal ablation of PV triggers is assessed by elimination of PV potentials, while PV isolation procedures require demonstration of entrance and exit block in the PV (Figure 29.13, Panel A). Entrance block evaluation requires sinus rhythm (see arrows in Figure 29.13, Panel B), coronary sinus, or left atrial appendage pacing with PV recordings. Exit block evaluation requires PV pacing and capture with left atrium recordings from sites on the opposing aspect of the isolation lesions to demonstrate linear lesion integrity (Figure 29.13, Panel C). Intravenous adenosine (12 mg) is used by some centers to assess recovery of conduction into the PVs immediately after PV isolation.[78] Recurrences of AF after PV isolation or ablation procedures have been most often ascribed to reconnection of the PV to the left atrium.

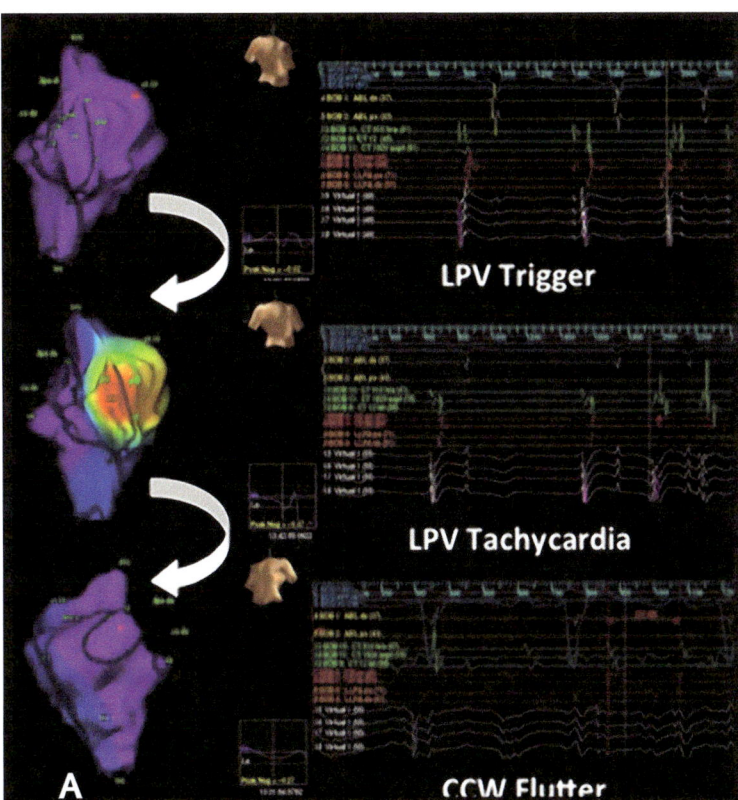

Figure 29.9 **Panel A:** Simultaneous biatrial noncontact mapping (NCM) of a spontaneous AF episode on a beat-to-beat sequence showing a triggering atrial premature beat (APB) from the superior left atrium (**top panel**) initiating a left atrial tachycardia arising in the superior left atrium in the vicinity of the PVs with breakthrough in the bystander right atrium (**middle panel**). The final panel shows the onset of a counterclockwise right atrial flutter within 5 minutes, which is tracked through the entire macroreentrant pathway on the NCM map.

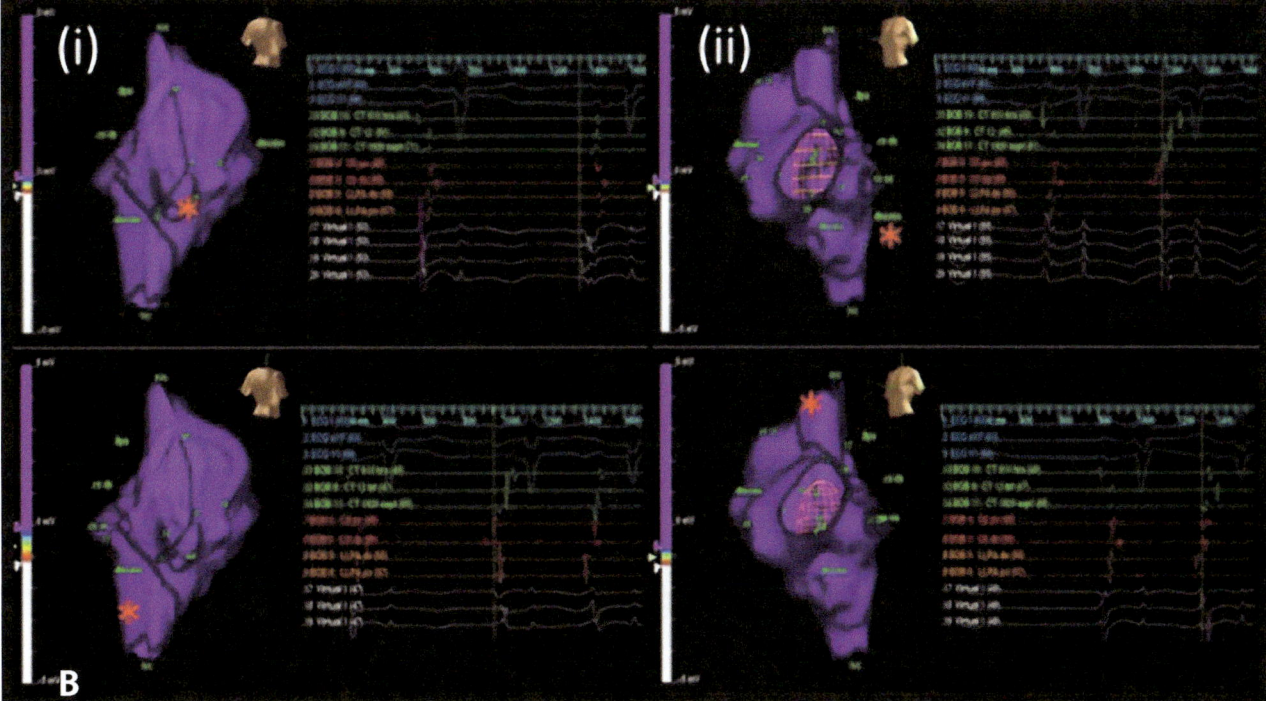

Panel B: Simultaneous biatrial and NCM identifies differing sites of origin of 4 APBs recorded in a single patient in rapid sequence in a single procedure. The right atrium 3D NCM contour is shown with the body torso orientation on the **top of each panel** and selected ECG recordings, electrograms from the biatrial contact catheter map, and virtual recordings from the NCM are shown on the **right of each panel**. The site of origin of the APB is shown with a **red asterisk** and can be spatially related using the body torso orientation. (i) APBs arising in the right atrium at two differing locations. (ii) Left atrial onset of two different APBs with widely disparate right atrial breakthrough locations and activation patterns. 3D contour locations at recording sites are marked in following locations: SVC = superior vena cava; IVC = inferior vena cava; CT 1-8 = lateral right atrium; HLRA, MLRA, LLRA = high, middle, and low lateral right atrium, respectively; HCT = high lateral CT; LCT = low lateral CT; HIAS = high interatrial septum; CT 11-20 = septal locations; CSpx = coronary sinus ostium; CS dis = coronary sinus distal; LLPA and LPA = left pulmonary artery. The numbers represent virtual electrogram recording sites. *Source:* Modified from Saksena S, Skadsberg ND, Rao HB, Filipecki A.[38] Used with permission.

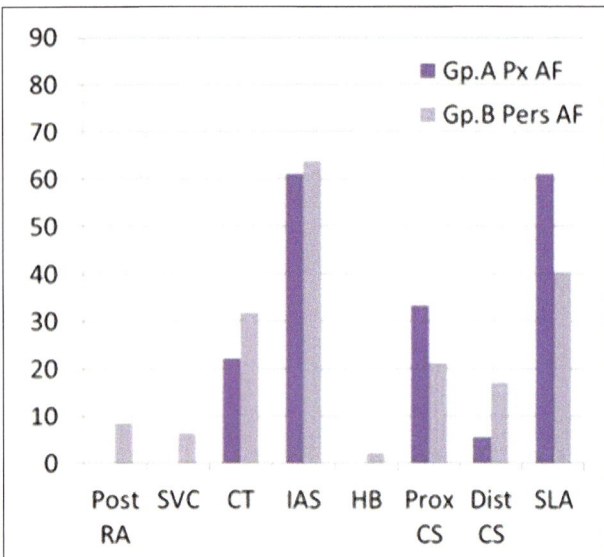

Figure 29.10 Regional distribution of atrial premature beat (APB) origin in paroxysmal AF patients (Gp.A) compared with long-standing persistent AF patients (Gp.B). Post RA = posterior right atrium; SVC = superior vena cava; CT = lateral right atrium; IAS = interatrial septum; HB = His bundle; Prox CS = proximal coronary sinus; Dist CS = distal coronary sinus; SLA = superior LA.

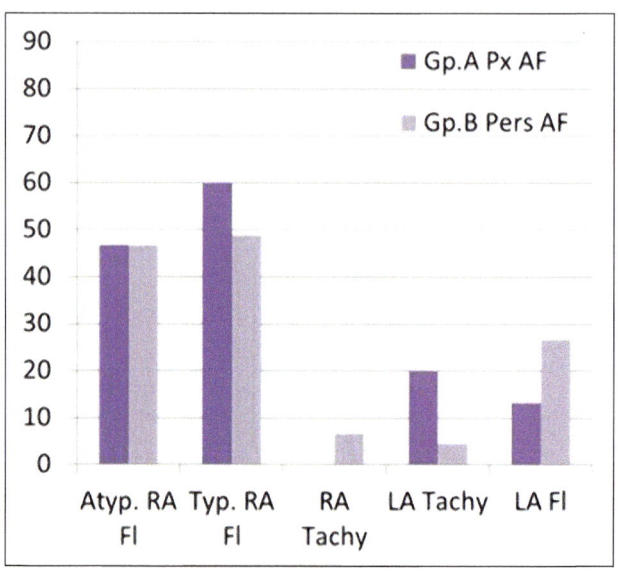

Figure 29.11 Summary of the distribution of atrial tachyarrhythmias (ATs) during spontaneous atrial fibrillation (AF) in paroxysmal AF patients (Gp.A) compared with long-standing persistent AF patients (Gp.B). Atyp RA Fl = atypical right atrial flutter; Typ RA Fl = typical (isthmus-dependent) right atrial flutter; RA Tachy = right atrial tachycardia; LA Tachy = left atrial tachycardia; LA Fl = left atrial flutter. *Source:* Narayan SM, Krummen DE, Shivkumar K, Clopton P, Rappel W, Miller JM.[31] Used with permission.

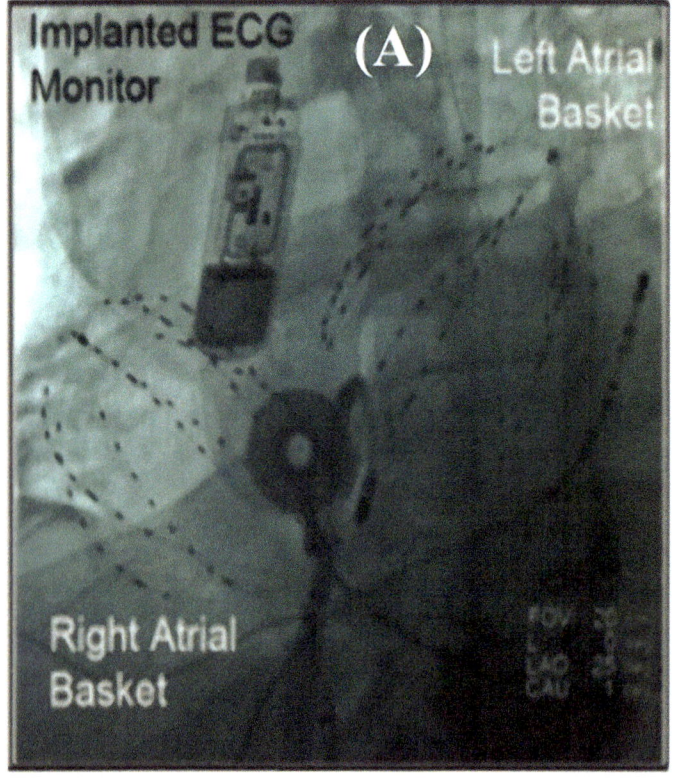

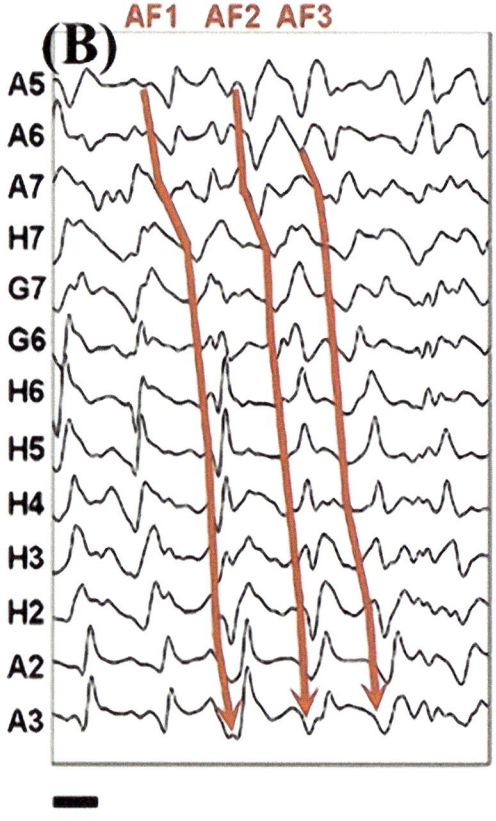

Figure 29.12 **Panel A:** Fluoroscopy shows a 64-pole catheter in each atrium. An implanted continuous ECG monitor, diagnostic catheters in the coronary sinus and left atrium, and an esophageal temperature probe are also seen. **Panel B:** Computationally processed and filtered intracardiac recordings show sequential activation over the rotor path for different AF cycles (AF1 to AF3) (**arrows**).

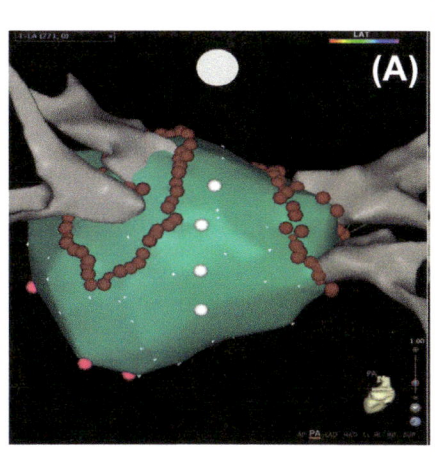
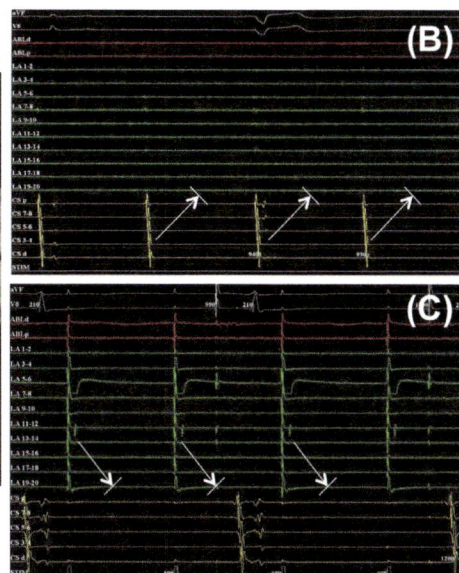

Figure 29.13 **Panel A:** Electroanatomic 3D map of the left atrium from a posterior view demonstrating wide area circumferential ablation and isolation of the bilateral pulmonary veins (PVs). **Panel B:** Electrograms demonstrating entrance block into the PVs following PV isolation. **Panel C:** Electrograms demonstrating PV capture with pacing within the PVs with exit block following PV isolation. CS = coronary sinus; EGM = electrogram; LA = left atrium; PV = pulmonary vein.

In persistent AF patients and patients with structural heart disease, substrate modification is usually performed by ablating sites of CFAEs or AF nests and by performing linear ablation lines (usually at the mitral annulus or roof of the left atrium). Endpoints of CFAE ablation are complete elimination of the areas with CFAEs, conversion of AF to sinus rhythm, and/or noninducibility of AF. Linear ablation line block is confirmed by presence of widely separated double potentials along the length of the ablation line and change in activation sequence (as the pacing site is moved away from the ablation line, the distance to the opposite side of the line decreases, and the interelectrogram interval shortens accordingly). This can also be confirmed by 3D activation mapping (early activation meets late activation or a "head to tail" relationship is demonstrated by the reentrant wavefront). Gaps in different lines can be identified by activation mapping and can be addressed intraoperatively. Figure 29.14 shows gaps in linear lesions in the left atrium (arrows) in the roof line and lateral mitral isthmus line.

Conclusions

EP studies using intracardiac recordings and advanced mapping techniques have documented triggering APBs, multiple organized ATs including PV tachycardias, and typical and atypical atrial flutters in patients with AF.[38,79] Patients with AF also generally have ECG and EP evidence of delays in intra-atrial and interatrial conduction, creating a critical functional substrate for initiation and maintenance of multiple reentrant circuits in AF patients. Electrophysiologic evaluation is critical in the evaluation of AF and permits understanding of AF mechanisms and the influence of comorbidities, and helps identify targets for non-pharmacologic interventions and the development of therapeutic strategies for the management of AF.

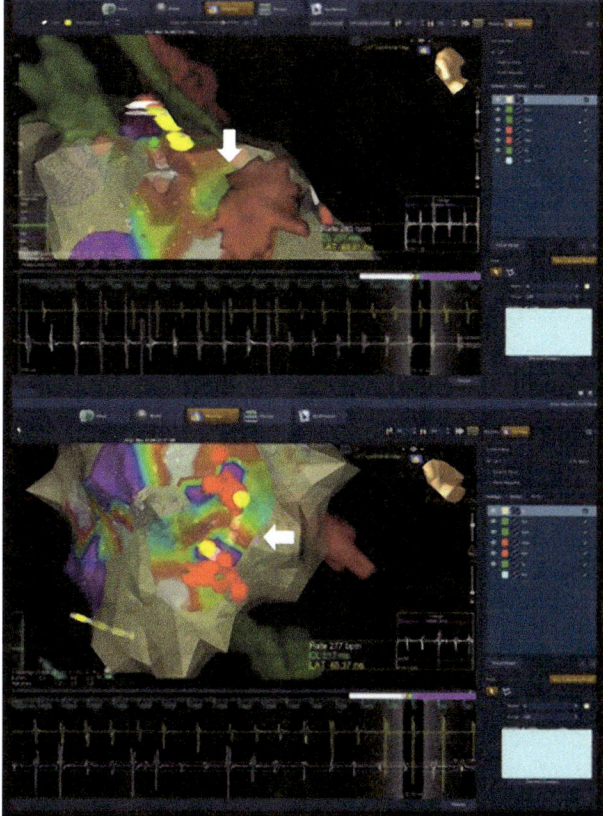

Figure 29.14 Intraoperative left atrial mapping during catheter ablation using the EnSite NavX system. The left atrium is seen in a left lateral caudal view. A sustained atrial tachyarrhythmia is in progress as seen in the electrogram recordings, and is mapped. Linear lesions are being developed, and mapping shows conduction at gaps in the linear lesions. The **top panel** shows conduction through a roof line that is incomplete and requires extension to close the gap. The **bottom panel** shows a gap in a lateral left atrial mitral isthmus line.

References

1. Einthoven W. Le telecardiogramme. *Arch Int de Physiol.* 1906;4:132-164.
2. Go AS, Hylek EM, Phillips KA, et al. Prevalence of diagnosed atrial fibrillation in adults: national implications for rhythm management and stroke prevention: the AnTicoagulation and Risk Factors in Atrial Fibrillation (ATRIA) study. *JAMA.* 2001;285:2370-2375.
3. Miyasaka Y, Barnes ME, Gersh BJ, et al. Secular trends in incidence of atrial fibrillation in Olmsted County, Minnesota, 1980 to 2000, and implications on the projections for future prevalence. *Circulation.* 2006;114:119-125.
4. Rudy Y. Noninvasive electrocardiographic imaging in humans. *J Electrocardiol.* 2005;38(4 Suppl):138-139.
5. Nault I, Lellouche N, Matsuo S, et al. Clinical value of fibrillatory wave amplitude on surface ECG in patients with persistent atrial fibrillation. *J Interv Card Electrophysiol.* 2009;26(1):11-19.
6. Cuculich PS, Wang Y, Lindsay BD, et al. Noninvasive characterization of epicardial activation in humans with diverse atrial fibrillation patterns. *Circulation.* 2010;122(14):1364-1372.
7. Fuster V, Ryden LE, Cannom DS, et al. ACC/AHA/ESC 2006 guidelines for the management of patients with atrial fibrillation—a report of the American College of Cardiology/American Heart Association Task Force on Practice Guidelines and the European Society of Cardiology Committee for Practice Guidelines (Writing Committee to Revise the 2001 Guidelines for the Management of Patients with Atrial Fibrillation). *J Am Coll Cardiol.* 2006;48:e149-e246.
8. European Heart Rhythm Association; European Association for Cardio-Thoracic Surgery, Camm AJ, Kirchhof P, Lip GY, et al. Guidelines for the management of atrial fibrillation: the Task Force for the Management of Atrial Fibrillation of the European Society of Cardiology (ESC). *Eur Heart J.* 2010;31(19):2369-2429.
9. Calkins H, Kuck KH, Cappato R, Brugada J, Camm AJ, Chen SA. 2012 HRS/EHRA/ECAS expert consensus statement on catheter and surgical ablation of atrial fibrillation: recommendations for patient selection, procedural techniques, patient management and follow-up, definitions, endpoints, and research trial design. *J Interv Card Electrophysiol.* 2012;33(2):171-257.
10. Knight BP, Michaud GF, Strickberger SA, et al. Electrocardiographic differentiation of atrial flutter from atrial fibrillation by physicians. *J Electrocardiol.* 1999;32:315-319.
11. Sauer WH, Alonso C, Zado E, et al. Atrioventricular nodal reentrant tachycardia in patients referred for atrial fibrillation ablation: response to ablation that incorporates slow pathway modification. *Circulation.* 2006;114:191-195.
12. Friedrichs K, Baldus S, Klinke A. Fibrosis in atrial fibrillation—role of reactive species and MPO. *Front Physiol.* 2012;3:214.
13. Akoum N, Daccarett M, McGann C, et al. Atrial fibrosis helps select the appropriate patient and strategy in catheter ablation of atrial fibrillation: a DE-MRI guided approach. *J Cardiovasc Electrophysiol.* 2011;22:16-22.
14. Nattel S, Shiroshita-Takeshita A, Brundel BJ, Rivard L. Mechanisms of atrial fibrillation: lessons from animal models. *Prog Cardiovasc Dis.* 2005;48:9-28.
15. Allessie M, Ausma J, Schotten U. Electrical, contractile and structural remodeling during atrial fibrillation. *Cardiovasc Res.* 2002;54:230-246.
16. Avitall B, Bi J, Mykytsey A, Chicos A. Atrial and ventricular fibrosis induced by atrial fibrillation: evidence to support early rhythm control. *Heart Rhythm.* 2008;5:839-845.
17. Campuzano O, Brugada R. Genetics of familial atrial fibrillation. *Europace.* 2009;11:1267-1271.
18. Gollob MH, Jones DL, Krahn AD, et al. Somatic mutations in the connexin 40 gene (GJA5) in atrial fibrillation. *N Engl J Med.* 2006;354:2677-2688.
19. Olson TM, Michels VV, Ballew JD, et al. Sodium channel mutations and susceptibility to heart failure and atrial fibrillation. *JAMA.* 2005;293:447-454.
20. Darbar D, Kannankeril PJ, Donahue BS, et al. Cardiac sodium channel (SCN5A) variants associated with atrial fibrillation. *Circulation.* 2008;117:1927-1935.
21. Yang Y, Xia M, Jin Q, et al. Identification of a KCNE2 gain-of-function mutation in patients with familial atrial fibrillation. *Am J Hum Genet.* 2004;75:899-905.
22. Kharche S, Adeniran I, Stott J, et al. Pro-arrhythmogenic effects of the S140G KCNQ1 mutation in human atrial fibrillation—insights from modelling. *J Physiol.* 2012;590(Pt 18):4501-4514.
23. Garry W. The nature of fibrillary contraction of the heart—its relation to tissue mass and form. *Am J Physiol.* 1913;46:349-382.
24. Mines GR. On circulating excitations in heart muscle and their possible relation to tachycardia and fibrillation. *Trans R Soc Can.* 1914;4:43-52.
25. Moe GK, Abildskov JA. Atrial fibrillation as a self-sustaining arrhythmia independent of focal discharge. *Am Heart J.* 1959;58:59-70.
26. Moe GK, et al. Multiple wavelet hypothesis of atrial fibrillation. *Arch Int Pharmacodyn Ther.* 1962;140:183.
27. Allessie MA, Bonke FI, Schopman FJ. Circus movement in rabbit atrial muscle as a mechanism of tachycardia. III. The "leading circle" concept: a new model of circus movement in cardiac tissue without the involvement of an anatomical obstacle. *Circulation.* 1977;41(1):9-18.
28. Spach MS, Dolber PC, Heidlage JF. Influence of the passive anisotropic properties on directional differences in propagation following modification of the sodium conductance in human atrial muscle. A model of reentry based on anisotropic discontinuous propagation. *Circulation.* 1988;62(4):811-832.
29. El Sherif N, Restivo M, Gough WB. The figure of eight model of reentrant ventricular rhythms in the subacute phase of myocardial infarction. In: Shenasa M, Borggrefe M, Breithardt G, eds. *Cardiac Mapping.* Mount Kisco, NY: Futura Publishing Co; 1993:159-182.
30. Pertsov AM, Davidenko JM, Salomonsz R, Baxter WT, Jalife J. Spiral waves of excitation underlie reentrant activity in isolated cardiac muscle. *Circ Res.* 1993;72:631-650.
31. Narayan SM, Krummen DE, Shivkumar K, Clopton P, Rappel W, Miller JM. Treatment of atrial fibrillation by the ablation of localized sources: CONFIRM (Conventional Ablation for Atrial Fibrillation with or without Focal Impulse and Rotor Modulation) Trial. *J Am Coll Cardiol.* 2012;60(7):628-636.
32. Scherf D, Romano FJ, Terranova R. Experimental studies on auricular flutter and auricular fibrillation. *Am Heart J.* 1948;36:241-251.
33. Nathan H, Eliakim M. The junction between the left atrium and the pulmonary veins. An anatomic study of human hearts. *Circulation.* 1966;34:412-422.
34. Ho SY, Sanchez-Quintana D, Cabrera JA, Anderson RH. Anatomy of the left atrium: implications for radiofrequency ablation of atrial fibrillation. *J Cardiovasc Electrophysiol.* 1999;10:1525-1533.

35. Weiss C, Gocht A, Willems S, Hoffmann M, Risius T, Meinertz T. Impact of the distribution and structure of myocardium in the pulmonary veins for radiofrequency ablation of atrial fibrillation. *Pacing Clin Electrophysiol.* 2002:1352-1356.
36. Arora R, Verheule S, Scott L, Navarrete A, et al. Arrhythmogenic substrate of the pulmonary veins assessed by high-resolution optical mapping. *Circulation.* 2003;107:1816-1821.
37. Lemery R, Soucie L, Martin B, Tang AS, Green M, Healey J. Human study of biatrial electrical coupling: determinants of endocardial septal activation and conduction over interatrial connections. *Circulation.* 2004;110(15):2083-2089.
38. Saksena S, Skadsberg ND, Rao HB, Filipecki A. Biatrial and three-dimensional mapping of spontaneous atrial arrhythmias in patients with refractory atrial fibrillation. *J Cardiovasc Electrophysiol.* 2005;16(5):494-504.
39. Shah DP, Knight BP. Transseptal catheterization using a powered radiofrequency transseptal needle. *J Interv Card Electrophysiol.* 2010;27(1):15-16.
40. Krol RB, Saksena S, Prakash A, Giorgberidze I, Matthew P. Prospective clinical evaluation of a programmed atrial stimulation protocol for induction of sustained atrial fibrillation and flutter. *J Interv Card Electrophysiol.* 1999;3:19-25.
41. Oral H, Crawford T, Frederick M, et al. Inducibility of paroxysmal atrial fibrillation by isoproterenol and its relation to the mode of onset of atrial fibrillation. *J Cardiovasc Electrophysiol.* 2008;19:466-470.
42. Strickberger SA, Man KC, Daoud EG, et al. Adenosine-induced atrial arrhythmia: a prospective analysis. *Ann Intern Med.* 1997;127:417-422.
43. Gula LJ, Massel D, Leong-Sit P, et al. Does adenosine response predict clinical recurrence of atrial fibrillation after pulmonary vein isolation? *J Cardiovasc Electrophysiol.* 2011;22:982-986.
44. Bayes de Luna A, Cladellas M, Cafferas F, et al. Interatrial blocks: their relationship with atrial tachyarrhythmias. In: Levy S, ed. *Cardiac Arrhythmias.* New York: Futura Company, Inc; 1984;217-229.
45. De Sisti A, Leclercq JF, Stiubei M, Fiorello P, Halimi F, Attuel P. P-wave duration and morphology predict atrial fibrillation recurrence in patients with sinus node dysfunction and atrial-based pacemaker. *Pacing Clin Electrophysiol.* 2002;25(11):1546-1554.
46. Xia Y, Hertervig E, Kongstad O, et al. Deterioration of interatrial conduction in patients with paroxysmal atrial fibrillation: electroanatomic mapping of the right atrium and coronary sinus. *Heart Rhythm.* 2004;1:548-553.
47. Buxton AE, Waxman HL, Marchlinski FE, Josephson ME. Atrial conduction: effects of extrastimuli with and without atrial dysrhythmias. *Am J Cardiol.* 1984 Oct 1;54(7):755-761.
48. Attuel P, Childers R, Cauchemez B, Poveda J, Mugica J, Coumel P. Failure in the rate adaptation of the atrial refractory period: its relationship to vulnerability. *Int J Cardiol.* 1982;2(2):179-197.
49. Saksena S, Giorgberidze I, Mehra R, et al. Electrophysiology and endocardial mapping of induced atrial fibrillation in patients with spontaneous atrial fibrillation. *Am J Cardiol.* 1999;83:187-193.
50. Takahashi Y, O'Neill M D, Jonsson A, et al. How to interpret and identify pulmonary vein recordings with the lasso catheter. *Heart Rhythm.* 2006;3(6):748-750.
51. Asirvatham SJ. Pulmonary vein-related maneuvers: part I. *Heart Rhythm.* 2007;4(4):538-544.
52. Haïssaguerre M, Shah DC, Jaïs P, et al. Mapping-guided ablation of pulmonary veins to cure atrial fibrillation. *Am J Cardiol.* 2000;86(9A):9K-19K.
53. Haïssaguerre M, Jaïs P, Shah DC, et al. Electrophysiological end point for catheter ablation of atrial fibrillation initiated from multiple pulmonary venous foci. *Circulation.* 2000; 101:1409-1417.
54. Weerasooriya R, Khairy P, Litalien J, et al. Catheter ablation for atrial fibrillation: are results maintained at 5 years of follow-up? *J Am Coll Cardiol.* 2011;57(2):160-166.
55. Haïssaguerre M, Sanders P, Hocini M, et al. Catheter ablation of long-lasting persistent atrial fibrillation: critical structures for termination. *J Cardiovasc Electrophysiol.* 2005; 11:1125-1137.
56. Lee SH, Tai CT, Hsieh MH, et al. Predictors of non-pulmonary vein ectopic beats initiating paroxysmal atrial fibrillation: implication for catheter ablation. *J Am Coll Cardiol.* 2005; 46:1054-1059.
57. Arruda M, Natale A. The adjunctive role of nonpulmonary venous ablation in the cure of atrial fibrillation. *J Cardiovasc Electrophysiol.* 2006;17:S37-S43.
58. Chen SA, Tai CT. Catheter ablation of atrial fibrillation originating from non-pulmonary vein foci. *J Cardiovasc Electrophysiol.* 2005;16:229-232.
59. Jaïs P, Haïssaguerre M, Shah DC, Chouairi S, Clementy J. Regional disparities of endocardial atrial activation in paroxysmal atrial fibrillation. *Pacing Clin Electrophysiol* 1996;19: 1998-2003.
60. Konings KT, Smeets JL, Penn OC, Wellens HJ, Allessie MA. Configuration of unipolar atrial electrograms during electrically induced atrial fibrillation in humans. *Circulation.* 1997;95(5):1231-1241.
61. Nademanee K, McKenzie J, Kosar E, et al. A new approach for catheter ablation of atrial fibrillation: mapping of the electrophysiologic substrate. *J Am Coll Cardiol.* 2004;43: 2044-2053.
62. Yamabe H, Morihisa K, Tanaka Y, et al. Mechanisms of the maintenance of atrial fibrillation: role of the complex fractionated atrial electrogram assessed by noncontact mapping. *Heart Rhythm.* 2009;6:1120-1128.
63. Rostock T, Rotter M, Sanders P, et al. High-density activation mapping of fractionated electrograms in the atria of patients with paroxysmal atrial fibrillation. *Heart Rhythm.* 2006;3:27-34.
64. Oral H, Chugh A, Good E, et al. A randomized evaluation of right atrial ablation after left atrial ablation of complex fractionated atrial electrograms for chronic atrial fibrillation. *Circ Arrhythm Electrophysiol.* 2008;1:6-13.
65. Dixit S, Marchlinski FE, Lin D, et al. Randomized ablation strategies for the treatment of persistent atrial fibrillation: RASTA study. *Circulation.* 2012;5:287-294.
66. Arruda M, Natale A. Ablation of permanent AF: adjunctive strategies to pulmonary vein isolation: targeting AF NEST in sinus rhythm and CFAE in AF. *J Interv Card Electrophysiol.* 2008;23:51-57.
67. Pachon MJ, Pachon ME, Pachon MJ, et al. A new treatment for atrial fibrillation based on spectral analysis to guide the catheter RF ablation *Europace.* 2004;6:590-601.
68. Ryu K, Sahadevan J, Khrestian CM, Stambler BS, Waldo AL. Use of Fast Fourier transform analysis of atrial electrograms for rapid characterization of atrial activation—implication for delineating possible mechanisms of atrial tachyarrhythmias. *J Cardiovasc Electrophysiol.* 2006;17:198-206.
69. Sharifov OF, Fedorov VV, Beloshapko GG, Glukhov AV, Yushmanova AV, Rosenshtraukh LV. Roles of adrenergic and cholinergic stimulation in spontaneous atrial fibrillation in dogs. *J Am Coll Cardiol.* 2004;43:483-490.

70. Patterson E, Po SS, Scherlag BJ, Lazzara R. Triggered firing in pulmonary veins initiated by in vitro autonomic nerve stimulation. *Heart Rhythm*. 2005;2:624-631.
71. Zhou J, Scherlag B, Edwards J, Jackman W, Lazarra R, Po S. Gradient of atrial refractoriness and inducibility of atrial fibrillation due to stimulation of ganglionated plexi. *J Cardiovasc Electrophysiol*. 2007;18:83-90.
72. Pappone C, Santinelli V, Manguso F et al. Pulmonary vein denervation enhances long-term benefit after circumferential ablation for paroxysmal atrial fibrillation. *Circulation*. 2004;109:327-334.
73. Platt M, Mandapati R, Scherlag BJ, et al. Limiting the number and extent of radiofrequency applications to terminate atrial fibrillation and subsequently prevent its inducibility. *Heart Rhythm*. 2004;1:S11.
74. Katritsis D, Giazitzoglou E, Sougiannis D, Goumas N, Paxinos G, Camm AJ. Anatomic approach for ganglionic plexi ablation in patients with paroxysmal atrial fibrillation. *Am J Cardiol*. 2008;102:330-334.
75. Pokushalov E, Romanov A, Shugayev P, et al. Selective ganglionated plexi ablation for paroxysmal atrial fibrillation. *Heart Rhythm*. 2009;6:1257-1264.
76. Mikhaylov D, Kanidieva A, Sviridova N, et al. Outcome of anatomic ganglionated plexi ablation to treat paroxysmal atrial fibrillation: a 3-year follow-up study. *Europace*. 2011;13: 362-370.
77. Danik S, Neuzil P, d'Avila A, et al. Evaluation of catheter ablation of periatrial ganglionic plexi in patients with atrial fibrillation. *Am J Cardiol*. 2008;102:578-583.
78. Hachiya H, Hirao K, Takahashi A, et al. Clinical implications of reconnection between the left atrium and isolated pulmonary veins provoked by adenosine triphosphate after extensive encircling pulmonary vein isolation. *J Cardiovasc Electrophysiol*. 2007;18:392-398.
79. Scheussler RB, Kawamoto T, Hand DE, et al. Simultaneous epicardial and endocardial activation sequence mapping in the isolated canine right atrium. *Circulation*. 1993;88:250-263.

CHAPTER 30

Ventricular Tachycardia with Heart Disease

Wendy S. Tzou, MD; Francis E. Marchlinski, MD

Introduction

In the setting of structural heart disease, the primary reason for developing ventricular tachycardia (VT) is the presence of scar.[1] It is well understood that patients with prior myocardial infarction (MI) and marked left ventricular (LV) systolic dysfunction are at high risk for developing not only monomorphic VT but VT that can degenerate into ventricular fibrillation (VF) and sudden cardiac death.[1-3] However, it has also become apparent that arrhythmogenic scar is present in individuals with nonischemic heart disease, including idiopathic cardiomyopathy and arrhythmogenic right ventricular cardiomyopathy/dysplasia (ARVC/D).[4,5] In these patients, the predominant mechanism for VT is reentry. To be clear, it is not the scar that is arrhythmogenic but the presence of living tissue intermixed within the scar. The latter provides the ideal milieu for reentrant circuits to initiate and propagate areas with (1) fixed or functional unidirectional block and (2) relatively slow conduction that permits recovery of previously depolarized tissue.

An estimated 40% of individuals who have an implantable cardioverter-defibrillator (ICD) placed for an index event of sustained VT will have recurrent VT.[6] This VT often necessitates the initiation of antiarrhythmic drugs to suppress additional VT episodes and prevent recurrent shocks. Unfortunately, the long-term success of these drugs for preventing recurrent arrhythmias or sudden death is limited,[7-10] and long-term use is often hindered by intolerance owing to side effects or drug toxicity.[7] With catheter mapping, however, critical components of the VT circuit can often be identified and targeted successfully with ablation. This chapter will delineate the approach to percutaneous mapping of VT in acquired structural heart disease.

Preparing for the Procedure

Much information can be gleaned noninvasively when evaluating sustained VT. Thus, before the ablation procedure, efforts should be initially directed toward optimizing the use of available tools and data.

Surface Electrocardiogram

The baseline electrocardiogram (ECG) can be very helpful in the initial assessment of confirmed VT. In sinus rhythm, the presence of Q waves in contiguous leads or ST segment elevations (in the absence of acute MI) can indicate prior MI location and potential site of VT origin. Evidence for abnormal right ventricular (RV) conduction, with QRS prolongation and/or T-wave inversions in the right-sided precordial or inferior limb leads (particularly if associated with post-QRS epsilon waves), should raise suspicion for ARVC/D if this diagnosis has not already been established. Presence of a widened QRS at baseline, which is a marker of His-Purkinje disease, suggests a predisposition for bundle branch reentrant or fascicular VT.[11] Finally, in patients with nonischemic cardiomyopathy (NICM), a sinus rhythm ECG showing a more pronounced R wave in V1 (> 0.15 mV) along with a larger S wave in V6 (> 0.15 mV) in the absence of prior infarction suggests the presence of basal–lateral scar.[12]

A 12-lead ECG obtained during VT, when available, assists greatly in preparing for mapping and ablation. It greatly helps to devise pace-mapping strategies in the setting of poorly hemodynamically tolerated or noninducible VTs and substrate-based ablation (see chapters 3 and 46). Knowing which of many potentially inducible VTs during electrophysiology (EP) study are pertinent or "clinical" also will ensure that those VTs are targeted during the ablation procedure. Finally, a 12-lead ECG obtained during VT can often determine a likely site of origin, or at least close approximation, of the VT exit from a larger macroreentrant circuit (Figure 30.1).[13]

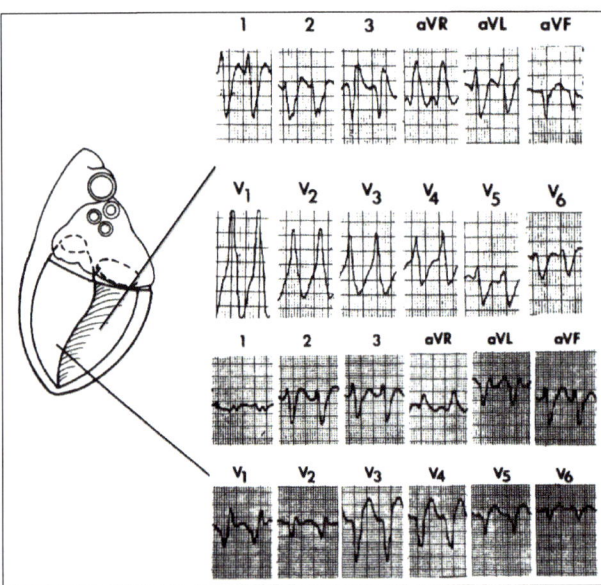

Figure 30.1 A schematic of the heart is displayed in left lateral oblique view, with the anterior and lateral left ventricular walls cut away, displaying endocardial septal and inferior wall segments. Two different ventricular tachycardias (VTs) are depicted, with corresponding sites of origin indicated (**lines**). See text for details. Source: Adapted with permission from Josephson ME, et al,[13] their Figure 2. Circulation. 1981;64:261.

A left bundle branch block (LBBB) pattern, defined by a predominantly negative QRS complex in lead V1, indicates either RV or septal LV origin. A right bundle branch block (RBBB) pattern, defined by the presence of a terminal R in V1, almost uniformly indicates LV origin, and the frontal plane axis should then be examined. In the inferior leads, a positive QRS axis will indicate a superior (thus inferiorly directed) VT exit, and a negative axis will indicate an inferior (thus superiorly directed) exit. Transition in the precordial leads, defined by the first precordial lead where R > S, if an LBBB pattern, or S > R, if an RBBB pattern, indicates how basal (transition ≤ lead V2) or apical (transition ≥ V5) the VT circuit exit or focus is located.[13] This localization strategy, coupled with intracardiac mapping (described below), works well in almost all cases except for VT occurring in the presence of a large apical infarction, in which it is difficult to distinguish septal from lateral exits.[14] Taking a recording from the RV apex either from an ICD lead or from an electrode catheter placed at the time of initiating VT in the EP laboratory can also help to define an apical septal versus a lateral exit. A delay in the time to activate the RV apex of greater than 100 ms from the onset of the QRS during VT will define an apical lateral exit for the VT circuit.[15]

The above localization strategy was developed in patients with reentrant VT due to chronic coronary artery disease (CAD) and prior infarction but can be applied to other forms of VT as well. Here, clinical history and pattern recognition can be additionally helpful. A young, athletic person with several LBBB premature ventricular contraction (PVC) or VT morphologies should raise suspicion of ARVC/D, particularly when signs of abnormal RV depolarization and repolarization on the sinus rhythm ECG are present (as discussed above). Of note, reentrant VT associated with nonischemic cardiomyopathy typically originates near the peripulmonic, aortic, and/or superior mitral valves and can mimic right/left ventricular outflow tract (RVOT/LVOT) morphology.[11]

Imaging

Noninvasive imaging is often much more sensitive than the surface ECG for assessing the presence of structural heart disease and, in particular, scar or ischemia. Such an assessment can usually be easily accomplished by traditional methods of echocardiography or nuclear scintigraphy. Magnetic resonance imaging (MRI) is a generally less accessible but often more sensitive tool for detecting both LV and RV abnormalities.[16-19] In terms of guiding mapping and ablation, it is critical to identify abnormalities that are not transmural or that are primarily epicardial or midmyocardial. The presence of an ICD or pacemaker has long been viewed as a contraindication for performing an MRI, but experiences at several centers, including our own, have shown that it can be done safely.[20,21] Recent developments have also made contrast-enhanced computed tomography (CT) potentially helpful for identifying scar and potential VT substrate.[22] Furthermore, both MRI and CT images can be integrated with real-time electroanatomic mapping to help characterize and target arrhythmogenic substrate (Figure 30.2) and define large-vessel coronary anatomy.[22,23] Also, given the high risk for thromboembolism and stroke, the presence of sessile intracardiac thrombus should be ruled out before attempting any invasive evaluation or intervention in the presence of significant structural heart disease.

ICD Electrograms

For patients with an ICD, the VT information stored on the device should be carefully reviewed. The number of events (both nonsustained and those resulting in therapy) reflects the arrhythmia burden. Such data should guide the urgency with which subsequent medical care is

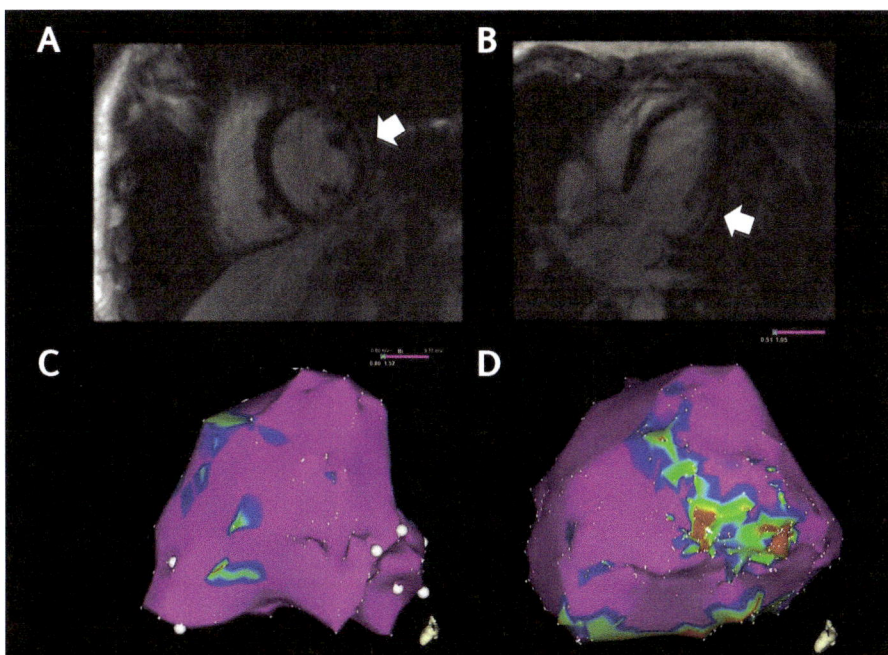

Figure 30.2 Gadolinium-enhanced cardiac magnetic resonance images from a patient with nonischemic cardiomyopathy and ventricular tachycardia (VT) are shown in short axis (**Panel A**) and 4-chamber long-axis (**Panel B**) views. The **white arrows** in **A** and **B** point to an area of epicardial delayed enhancement along the lateral–basal left ventricle. These findings were corroborated on subsequent bipolar endocardial (**Panel C**) and epicardial (**Panel D**) voltage maps during VT ablation.

executed, including initiation of antiarrhythmic therapy and catheter ablation.[1] Device-recorded intracardiac electrograms (EGMs) may be especially helpful for determining whether catheter ablation therapy is potentially useful and, if pursued, to help target ablation when a surface 12-lead ECG of the clinical VT is not available. For instance, events dominated by polymorphic VT may be less amenable to ablation, unless a reproducible PVC trigger is evident that may be targeted. A reproducible triggering event can be confirmed by analyzing EGMs at the onset of VT associated with stored arrhythmia events (Figure 30.3). Depending on patient stability, one could consider noninvasive programmed stimulation (NIPS) testing through the device. NIPS enables one to potentially identify a 12-lead ECG for a clinically occurring VT by matching the intracardiac EGM from any induced VT to those stored from spontaneous clinical events.

Before pursuing more invasive evaluation with EP study and possible ablation, it is important to have a recent evaluation of the presence and status of CAD and determination of LV function and reserve, either noninvasively (as described above) or via cardiac catheterization. Deaths related to the procedure are often caused by underestimation of the importance of ischemic burden prior to and volume overload during the procedure. Therefore, it is crucial to document the patient's anticoagulation status and, as indicated, to exclude an unstable LV thrombus. Identifying vascular access problems before the procedure will facilitate its success and safety. Severe arterial disease or the presence of aortic stenosis will require taking a transseptal LV approach to LV mapping.

Knowing the details of the patient's present and past antiarrhythmic therapy is also important. Ideally, any ongoing therapy should be discontinued for at least five half-lives before undertaking EP study and ablation (however, because of the unstable nature of many patients' conditions, this is often not possible). Many patients will have been treated with amiodarone. Its long half-life and storage in body fat will mean that amiodarone will be present even if stopped several days before the procedure. The results of programmed stimulation and subsequent ablation should be interpreted with this knowledge.

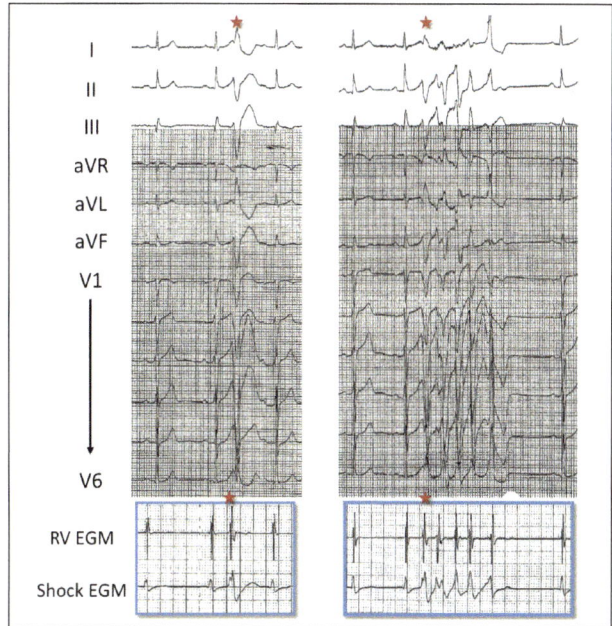

Figure 30.3 Surface 12-lead ECGs (**top rows**) and corresponding ICD electrograms (**bottom rows**) are depicted from a patient with polymorphic ventricular tachycardia and ventricular fibrillation triggered by a recurrent and monomorphic premature ventricular contraction (PVC) (**red star**). Note the signature morphology of the PVC on both the surface and intracardiac recordings. EGM = electrogram; RV = right ventricle.

Initiating VT

A hallmark of reentrant VT is its ability to be induced and terminated by ventricular programmed electric stimulation (PES) in the EP laboratory. Thus, a critical basic pacing rate in PES is often needed to initiate a reentrant tachycardia in a given patient, and several different basic pacing drive-cycle lengths with extrastimuli should be used to try to induce it.[24] Other hallmarks of reentrant VT are as follows:

- An inverse relationship between the coupling interval of the ventricular extrastimulus and the return cycle length of the tachycardia;

- The ability to entrain the VT with progressive fusion using shorter pacing cycle lengths; and

- The ability to demonstrate entrainment with concealed fusion at isthmus sites.[25]

Notably, triggered VTs also can be initiated with ventricular PES; thus, induction with PES does not exclude the latter as a mechanism for VT.[26,27] However, the other features associated with reentry described above are not characteristic of triggered VTs.

When trying to induce VT with PES, it is advisable to attempt stimulation from other ventricular sites than the right ventricular apex. In 10% to 20% of patients in whom stimulation from the RV apex is ineffective, additional stimulation from sites such as the RVOT or LV may be required to initiate a monomorphic, sustained VT. Frequently, VT with an RBBB pattern will best be initiated by stimulating from the lateral LV. Facilitating VT initiation by stimulation from the lateral LV can occasionally be observed as a proarrhythmic effect of LV pacing during biventricular pacing.[28]

Methods for PES vary significantly. Pacing for 8 beats with basic drive-cycle lengths of 600 and 400 ms, followed by the introduction of 1 to 4 extrastimuli, is generally the most accepted protocol. The ability to induce sustained monomorphic VT (MMVT) increases successively with the number of extrastimuli, up to 3. MMVT can be induced in 96% of patients with sustained clinical VT and in 75% of those who have survived sudden arrhythmic cardiac death.[26] Beyond 3 extrastimuli, there is little additional yield; sensitivity and inducibility increase marginally but with a significant decrease in specificity, as less stable and more nonclinical and/or polymorphic VTs (PMVTs) are induced.[27] The majority (80%–85%) of patients with clinical VT can be induced in this fashion; however, occasionally, induction is more effective when the basic "drive" is provided by sinus rhythm and the extrastimuli is introduced via pacing. If a specific VT is identified, then additional extrastimuli may be introduced for induction, recognizing the potential for inducing less clinically relevant arrhythmias. On occasion, a short–long–short stimulation sequence may be helpful. This stimulation has been described for the induction of bundle branch reentry, but it also can be used for inducing other VTs associated with structural heart disease that cannot be induced using a standard stimulation protocol.

Mappable VT

A small minority of reentrant VT consists of hemodynamically stable, slow VT that is easily inducible and stable in response to pacing. However, when it is present, detailed activation and entrainment mapping can be performed (Figure 30.4). The goal of activation and entrainment mapping is to identify critical elements of the reentrant circuit that are protected by anatomic or functional boundaries (eg, dense scar or valvular structures) that would therefore be easiest to successfully target with ablation. The surface ECG recording of VT typically represents the wavefront as it exits the scarred area and begins to depolarize healthy myocardium. The "exit" is frequently located at the end of the most critical portion (isthmus) of the circuit, at the border of a scar. However, it is possible for the isthmus to be situated quite a distance from the edge of the scar and the wavefront to activate diseased myocardium for several centimeters before engaging normal myocardium. Once the wavefront encounters normal myocardium, it then propagates away from this site to depolarize the rest of the ventricles; it also completes the depolarization of other portions of the circuit, including the outer scar border (outer loop) and the "entrance" to the isthmus region. Occasionally, the wavefront may propagate through a path within the scar or area of functional block (inner loop) that is not critical to maintaining the circuit.[29]

One goal during activation mapping is to identify areas with middiastolic potentials or abnormal, low-amplitude signals recorded during electrical diastole (see Figure 30.4). These recordings are believed to represent depolarization of the aforementioned important portions of the reentrant circuit, including the most critical (isthmus).[30-32] Isolated potentials recorded during VT have been found in about half of isthmus sites and represent areas at which radiofrequency energy application may be most effective in terminating VT.[30] However, the isthmus width can range from 6 to 26 mm,[33] and the presence of a broad isthmus may make activation data more difficult to interpret. Significantly, isolated diastolic potentials also have been found at bystander sites that are near to but not participating in the VT circuit; alternatively, they can even represent far-field activation of tissue remote from the mapping site. Sites critical to the reentrant circuit can sometimes be better characterized using entrainment mapping (described below) or pacing from a remote site to dissociate the potential from the VT. The presence of bystander sites, as well as the presence of multiple loops of reentry, can often confound analysis.

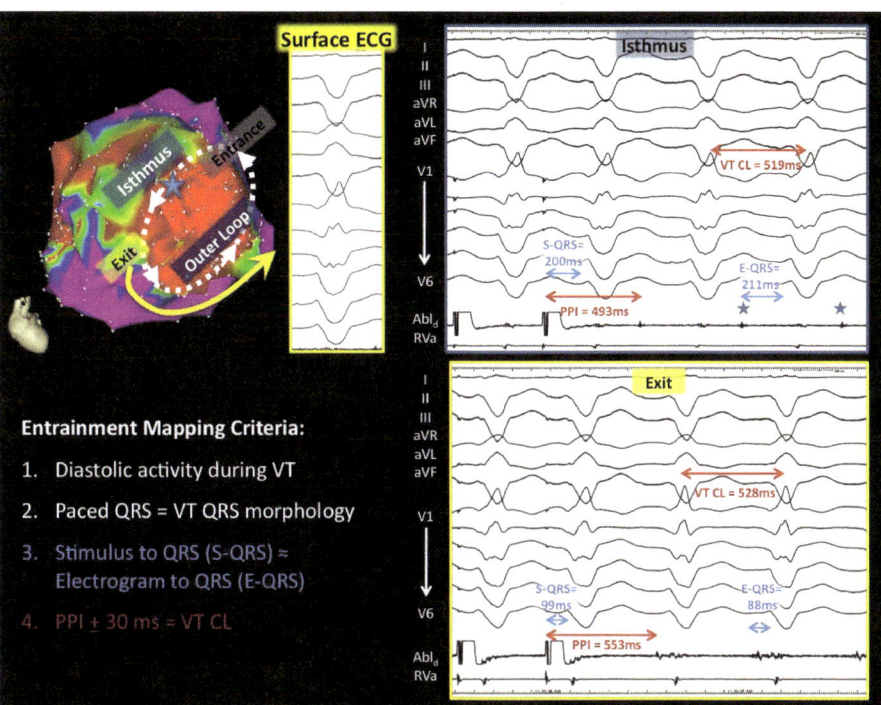

Figure 30.4 An example of hemodynamically tolerated and mappable ventricular tachycardia (VT) is demonstrated in a patient with prior anterior–apical myocardial infarction. The electroanatomic left ventricular voltage map (in anterior–posterior projection) is shown in the **top left panel**, with the presumed VT circuit and components marked, as determined by entrainment mapping, around the apical scar. The **blue star** marks the location on the voltage map where middiastolic potentials were recorded from the isthmus site during VT (**top right panel**). Entrainment results for isthmus and exit sites are also shown (**right panels**). See text for details. CL = cycle length; PPI = postpacing interval.

Entrainment mapping can be performed in hemodynamically tolerated VT that remains stable in response to pacing. Pacing slightly faster than the VT will cause continuous resetting of the reentry circuit. Sites within the circuit will have a postpacing interval (PPI), or time to return to the site of pacing, within 30 ms of the tachycardia cycle length (TCL) (Figure 30.4). Thus, the farther away from the circuit that entrainment is attempted, the larger the difference between the PPI and TCL. It should be ensured that the EGM selected for measuring PPI represents local depolarization. The latter can be very difficult to identify when multiple signals are present (as is common in scar) or when local potentials directly depolarized by pacing are obscured by the pacing artifact. Other major assumptions when interpreting the response to entrainment are that (1) pacing does not alter the path of the circuit or initiate another VT; and (2) conduction time through the circuit is unchanged with entrainment compared with VT. Care should therefore be made to pace only slightly faster than the TCL, because faster pacing has been shown to alter the VT circuit. Additionally, the presence of antiarrhythmia medications may further decrease conduction velocities during pacing and potentially confound analysis—particularly when pacing at even modestly faster rates.[29]

Assuming the above conditions are met, entrainment mapping can be very helpful in identifying reentrant circuit components. Entrainment from all isthmus sites will demonstrate concealed fusion with entrainment, or demonstrate capture with pacing, but without a change in QRS morphology of the paced beats compared with VT. At isthmus exit sites, the pacing stimulus to the QRS interval (S-QRS, which represents the conduction time from the pacing site to the reentry circuit) should be short: 30% or less of the TCL. At central isthmus sites, the S-QRS should be intermediate: 31% to 50% of the TCL. At isthmus entrance sites, the S-QRS should be longer: 51% to 70% of the TCL. At all these sites, the S-QRS time should also equal the EGM-to-QRS time during the VT (see Figure 30.4). Termination with catheter pressure can occur when mapping in this region; this suggests a narrow isthmus predisposed to block with the slightest perturbations.[29] The presence of inner-loop or adjacent bystander sites can be confusing because entrainment also will demonstrate concealed fusion when stimulation is performed at these sites. For the former, the S-QRS will be very long (usually > 70% of TCL); for the latter, the PPI will not be similar to the TCL, and the S-QRS and EGM-QRS will not be equal. At outer-loop sites, there will be manifest QRS fusion with entrainment owing to propagation of stimulated antidromic wavefronts, both away from the scar border and within the VT circuit. The fact that the site lies within the VT circuit is evident because the PPI will approximate the TCL. If the scar border along this portion of the circuit is contiguous with healthier myocardium, the width of this circuit portion may be quite broad; thus, termination with either focal ablation or catheter trauma succeeds less often (< 10%) at these sites.

Even after detailed mapping, it may not be possible to delineate the entire circuit. Parts of the reentry circuit may not be confined to the endocardium but also may course through the midmyocardium or epicardium.

Unmappable VT

The vast majority of clinical VTs either will not be hemodynamically tolerated, will be difficult to induce at the time of EP study, or will be unable to be fully characterized using the above-mentioned strategies. As a result, the sinus rhythm substrate is now characterized as part of the routine procedure for all patients being considered for VT ablation. Other ablation approaches for VT will be detailed in later chapters.

Sinus Rhythm Voltage Map

A detailed substrate and voltage map should be made, and efforts should initially focus on areas of known infarction or areas that are scar-based on prior imaging. The endocardial extent of anatomic abnormalities has been well characterized using bipolar voltage criteria of < 1.5 to 2.0 mV. In this way, normal signal amplitude recorded from the LV endocardium has been identified using a commercially available electroanatomic mapping system (Carto™, Biosense Webster, Diamond Bar, CA) with a 4 mm electrode-tip mapping catheter.[34,35] For most patients with sustained VT, low-voltage areas of endocardium typically represent arrhythmia substrate. Thus, a color range corresponding to endocardial bipolar voltages of 0.5 to 1.5 mV will highlight areas of densely scarred myocardium or aneurysm (< 0.5 mV), border zone of scar (0.5 to < 1.5 mV), and healthy myocardium (> 1.5 mV) (Figure 30.5). It is important to note that in patients with extensive septal involvement, the extent of endocardial scar identified on voltage mapping often will exceed that observed on thallium imaging. This difference may result from lower sensitivity of the latter in identifying subendocardial versus transmural infarction. Similarly, regions of scar identified on either MRI or CT have correlated well with low-voltage areas on electroanatomic mapping, and therefore, integrated systems may provide incremental utility in VT mapping and ablation.[22,23]

Late-potential Mapping and Ablation

Frequently, split and/or late potentials during sinus rhythm can be observed on bipolar recordings within or at the borders of scar that has been delineated by voltage mapping. Late potentials are distinct bipolar ECMs that are inscribed after the end of the surface QRS complex and separated from the major initial component of the local ventricular EGM, often (but not always) by an isoelectric interval (Figures 30.5 and 30.6). Split and/or late potentials are believed to represent delayed activation in the diseased myocardium and have frequently been found at critical sites in reentrant VT circuits.[36,37]

These potentials are found in 89% of isthmus sites, 57% of entrance sites, and 20% of exit sites.[37] This localization strategy, combined with voltage mapping, identifies appropriate ablation targets and provides a more refined substrate-based approach for VT ablation.

Pace Mapping

In conjunction with a detailed voltage map and available 12-lead surface ECG or ICD EGM VT morphologies, pace mapping is used to approximate the VT exit site for VT that cannot be characterized by activation or entrainment mapping owing to hemodynamic instability.[35,38] The procedure involves pacing at different ventricular sites along the border of the dense scar (0.5–1.0 mV) during sinus rhythm to identify site(s) at which the paced QRS morphology mimics that observed during VT (see Figure 30.5). There are important limitations to recognize when using pace mapping to localize the VT exit site. The paced QRS morphology may not accurately reflect the site of origin of the VT and may not identify an appropriate site for VT ablation. Bidirectional conduction from

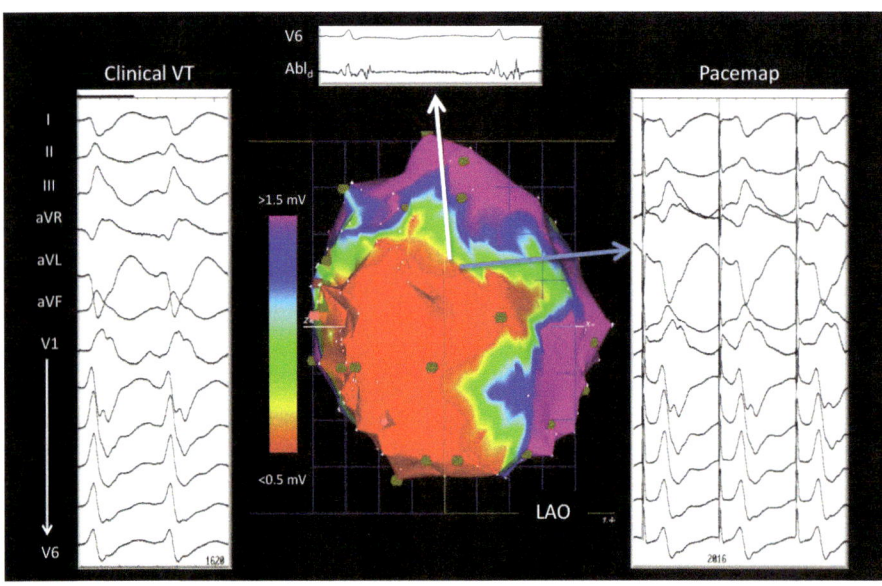

Figure 30.5 The endocardial left ventricular voltage map from a patient with prior anterior myocardial infarction and ventricular tachycardia (VT) is shown in the **middle panel** (left anterior oblique [LAO] projection), with a range of 0.5 to 1.5 mV, highlighting areas of dense scar, border zone, and healthy myocardium. The 12-lead ECG of the clinical VT is in the **left panel**. An example of late potentials is shown in the anterior–lateral scar border zone (**center white arrow**), where a VT exit might be predicted based on VT morphology and known scar distribution. Indeed, pace map (**right panel**) from the region of suspected exit (**blue arrow**) is a perfect match for the clinical VT.

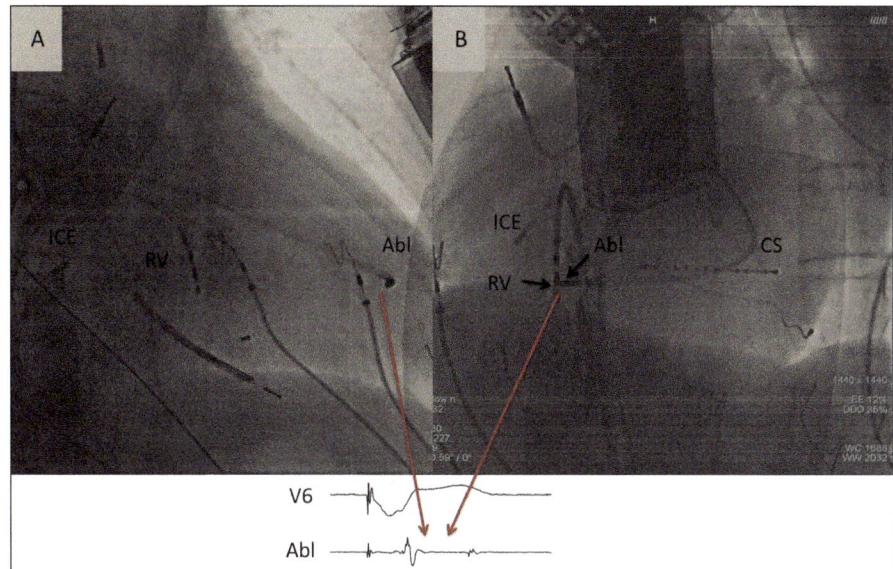

Figure 30.6 Right anterior (**Panel A**) and left anterior (**Panel B**) oblique fluoroscopic images obtained during a typical ischemic VT mapping and ablation procedure. The patient has a biventricular implantable cardioverter-defibrillator. **Black arrows** depict the distal ends of the quadripolar catheter in the right ventricle (RV) and the ablation catheter (Abl) on the left ventricular septum. Intracardiac recordings obtained at the site of the Abl (**red arrows; bottom tracings**) show late potentials in the region of scar. CS = coronary sinus catheter; ICE = intracardiac echocardiography catheter.

the pacing site may not mimic the unidirectional wavefront of activation associated with the VT circuit. Furthermore, the output used to capture with pacing, especially if high, can influence the pattern of ventricular activation. Even when pacing in a critical site of the VT circuit, the output can produce a different QRS morphology in sinus rhythm because of an increase in the size of the virtual electrode, which will differ from that during VT. Despite its drawbacks, pace mapping can approximate the exit site of the VT circuit in most patients and is a generally accepted method for mapping when more detailed options are limited because of poor hemodynamic intolerance or noninducibility of VT.

Conducting Channels

Many slower, more mappable VTs demonstrate conduction through densely infarcted myocardium (< 0.5 mV). In these cases, viable channels of conducting myocardium may be identified by decreasing the color range so that narrow channels of larger voltage surrounded by areas of extremely low voltage can be visualized (Figure 30.7).[39] Such channels can also be identified during RV pacing in the absence of ongoing VT.[40] Fractionated EGMs, with isolated delayed and/or multiple components, are often seen at isthmus sites; however, these low-amplitude signals may be obscured in sinus rhythm because of depolarization of the surrounding larger mass of more normal myocardium. As a result, changing the direction of depolarization compared with sinus rhythm (eg, with pacing) has been observed to better elucidate these signals and potential channels of conduction. RV apical pacing has been used for this purpose. Channels can also be defined by identifying viable myocardium between areas of inexcitability, defined as having a threshold >2 ms, 10 mA. While identifying conducting channels can be

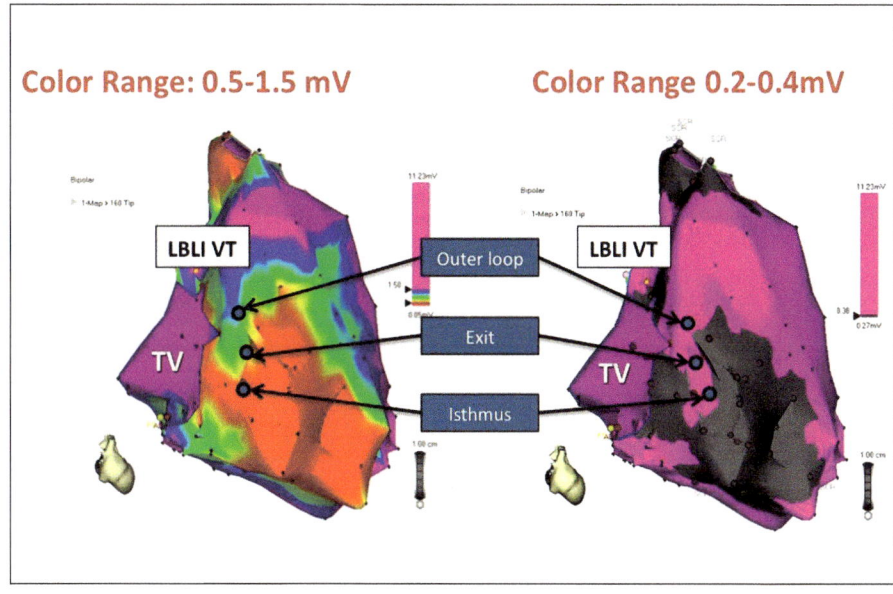

Figure 30.7 Right anterior oblique projections of bipolar endocardial right ventricular voltage maps are shown from a patient with right ventricular cardiomyopathy and left bundle, left axis, and inferiorly directed ventricular tachycardia (LBLI VT). **Left panel:** Entrainment maneuvers identifying VT outer loop, exit, and isthmus sites are shown on the voltage map with standard bipolar color range cutoffs intended to display scar border zone (0.5–1.5 mV). **Right panel:** After adjusting the voltage color range to better contrast relatively preserved voltage areas against more densely scarred areas, a channel of conduction corresponding to the sites of critical VT circuit elements is identified. TV = tricuspid valve. *Source:* Adapted with permission from Hsia HH, et al.[39] *Heart Rhythm.* 2006;3:503-512. © 2006 Elsevier. All rights reserved.

useful when used in conjunction with other methods, it is often not specific enough to be the sole mapping guide.[35,40]

Noncontact Mapping

A final approach to mapping poorly tolerated or otherwise unmappable VT is via noncontact mapping using a multielectrode system. One currently available system comprises a woven braid of 64 0.003 in diameter wires mounted on a 7.6 mL balloon on a 9 Fr catheter. Each wire has a 0.025 inch break in insulation, producing noncontact unipolar electrodes whose recorded signals are processed and displayed via a proprietary amplifier system and software (Endocardial Solutions, Inc., St. Paul, MN). This system allows for display of more than 3,300 unipolar ECGs derived from the inverse solution to Laplace's equation.[41]

Good correlation has been observed between ECMs computed using the noncontact balloon and those obtained simultaneously by direct catheter contact, and reasonably positive results have been reported in limited clinical experiences to date.[41,42] However, the system is currently a bit cumbersome to use, requiring a customized amplifier system and Silicon Graphics workstation (SGI, Inc., Fremont, CA) to run system software. Other limitations include the following: (1) potential need for contact mapping of areas that are inaccessible by the balloon system because of low-amplitude signals or excessive (> 34 mm) distance from the balloon to endocardial surface; and (2) instability of balloon position, particularly in the recommended retrograde aortic placement in patients with normal LV function.

Epicardial VT Mapping

Features that may call for epicardial mapping and ablation can be apparent on the surface 12-lead ECG recorded during VT.[43-45] These include the presence of a particularly wide QRS VT with a slurred initial aspect of the QRS complex. In patients with nonischemic cardiomyopathy, a Q wave in lead I is a particularly sensitive marker for identifying an epicardial VT site of origin. If it is present (and there is an absence of Q waves in the inferior leads), a basal–superior lateral epicardial focus is suggested. Epicardial mapping and ablation are discussed in more detail in chapter 45.

Mapping Prior to Surgical Ablation

In patients with NICM who are not amenable to catheter ablation, we have used catheter-based recordings made during endocardial and epicardial mapping to help guide more extensive surgical cryoablation. In the absence of direct intraoperative recordings, a detailed bipolar voltage map made with catheter recordings, coupled with a definition of coronary anatomy and anatomic definition of scar with MRI imaging, can be used to guide the surgical procedure.[46]

Summary

In the setting of structural heart disease, comprehensive EP evaluation of VT should incorporate details from the patient's clinical history and noninvasive data to tailor the approach for the mapping procedure and potential ablation. In addition to the patient history, surface 12-lead ECGs of the VT and cardiac imaging studies often provide insight into VT mechanism and site of origin. The majority of VTs in the setting of structural heart disease are the result of reentry, and most can be initiated with programmed stimulation, allowing for confirmation of ECG diagnosis and further evaluation. Effective mapping and ablation strategies for both hemodynamically tolerated and nontolerated VTs have been developed that allow for VT control.

References

1. Zipes D, Camm A, Borggrefe M, et al. ACC/AHA/ESC 2006 guidelines for management of patients with ventricular arrhythmias and the prevention of sudden cardiac death: a report of the American College of Cardiology/American Heart Association Task Force and the European Society of Cardiology Committee for Practice Guidelines (Writing Committee to Develop Guidelines for Management of Patients with Ventricular Arrhythmias and the Prevention of Sudden Cardiac Death). *J Am Coll Cardiol*. 2006;48:e247-e346.
2. Henkel DM, Witt BJ, Gersh BJ, et al. Ventricular arrhythmias after acute myocardial infarction: a 20-year community study. *Am J Cardiol*. 2006;151:806-812.
3. Kempf FC Jr, Josephson ME. Cardiac arrest recorded on ambulatory electrocardiograms. *Am J Cardiol*. 1984;53:1577-1582.
4. Hsia HH, Callans DJ, Marchlinski FE. Characterization of endocardial electrophysiological substrate in patients with nonischemic cardiomyopathy and monomorphic ventricular tachycardia. *Circulation*. 2003;108:704-710.
5. Marchlinski FE, Zado E, Dixit S, et al. Electroanatomic substrate and outcome of catheter ablative therapy for ventricular tachycardia in setting of right ventricular cardiomyopathy. *Circulation*. 2004;110:2293-2298.
6. Moss AJ, Greenberg H, Case RB, et al. Long-term clinical course of patients after termination of ventricular tachyarrhythmia by an implanted defibrillator. *Circulation*. 2004;110:3760-3765.
7. Randomized antiarrhythmic drug therapy in survivors of cardiac arrest (the CASCADE Study). The CASCADE Investigators. *Am J Cardiol*. 1993;72:280-287.
8. Connolly SJ, Hallstrom AP, Cappato R, et al. Meta-analysis of the implantable cardioverter defibrillator secondary prevention trials. *Eur Heart J*. 2000;21:2071-2078.
9. Mason JW. A comparison of seven antiarrhythmic drugs in patients with ventricular tachyarrhythmias. *N Engl J Med*. 1993;329:452-458.
10. Connolly SJ, Dorian P, Roberts RS, et al. Comparison of β-blockers, amiodarone plus β-blockers, or sotalol for prevention of shocks from implantable cardioverter defibrillators: The OPTIC study: a randomized trial. *JAMA*. 2006;295:165-171.
11. Riley MP, Marchlinski FE. ECG clues for diagnosing ventricular tachycardia mechanism. *J Cardiovasc Electrophysiol*. 2008;19:224-229.
12. Tzou WS, Zado ES, Lin D, et al. Sinus rhythm ECG criteria associated with basal-lateral ventricular tachycardia substrate

in patients with nonischemic cardiomyopathy. *J Cardiovasc Electrophysiol*. 2011;22:1351-1358.
13. Josephson ME, Horowitz LN, Waxman HL, et al. Sustained ventricular tachycardia: role of the 12-lead electrocardiogram in localizing site of origin. *Circulation*. 1981;64:257-272.
14. Miller JM, Marchlinski FE, Buxton AE, Josephson ME. Relationship between the 12-lead electrocardiogram during ventricular tachycardia and endocardial site of origin in patients with coronary artery disease. *Circulation*. 1988;77:759-766.
15. Patel VV, Rho RW, Gerstenfeld EP, et al. Right bundle branch block ventricular tachycardias: septal versus lateral ventricular origin based on activation time to the right ventricular apex. *Circulation*. 2004;110:2582-2587.
16. Jerosch-Herold M, Kwong RY. Optimal imaging strategies to assess coronary blood flow and risk for patients with coronary artery disease. *Curr Opin Cardiol*. 2008;23:599-606.
17. Ashikaga H, Sasano T, Dong J, et al. Magnetic resonance based anatomical analysis of scar-related ventricular tachycardia: implications for catheter ablation. *Circ Res*. 2007;101:939-947.
18. Bogun FM, Desjardins B, Good E, et al. Delayed-enhanced magnetic resonance imaging in nonischemic cardiomyopathy: utility for identifying the ventricular arrhythmia substrate. *J Am Coll Cardiol*. 2009;53:1138-1145.
19. Yokokawa M, Tada H, Koyama K, et al. The characteristics and distribution of the scar tissue predict ventricular tachycardia in patients with advanced heart failure. *Pacing Clin Electrophysiol*. 2009;32:314-322.
20. Nazarian S, Roguin A, Zviman MM, et al. Clinical utility and safety of a protocol for noncardiac and cardiac magnetic resonance imaging of patients with permanent pacemakers and implantable-cardioverter defibrillators at 1.5 Tesla. *Circulation*. 2006;114:1277-1284.
21. Naehle CP, Strach K, Thomas D, et al. Magnetic resonance imaging at 1.5-T in patients with implantable cardioverter-defibrillators. *J Am Coll Cardiol*. 2009;54:549-555.
22. Tian J, Jeudy J, Smith MF, et al. Three-dimensional contrast-enhanced multidetector CT for anatomic, dynamic, and perfusion characterization of abnormal myocardium to guide ventricular tachycardia ablations. *Circ Arrhythm Electrophysiol*. 2010;3:496-504.
23. Wijnmaalen AP, van der Geest RJ, van Huls van Taxis CF, et al. Head-to-head comparison of contrast-enhanced magnetic resonance imaging and electroanatomic voltage mapping to assess post-infarct scar characteristics in patients with ventricular tachycardias: real-time image integration and reversed registration. *Eur Heart J*. 2011;32:104-114.
24. Wellens HJ, Bar FW, Lie KI. The value of the electrocardiogram in the differential diagnosis of a tachycardia with a widened QRS complex. *Am J Med*. 1978;64:27-33.
25. Marchlinski FE. Ventricular tachycardia: clinical presentation, course, and therapy. In: Zipes D, Jalife J, eds. *Cardiac Electrophysiology: From Cell to Bedside*. Philadelphia, PA: W.B. Saunders and Co.; 1995:756-777.
26. Buxton AE, Waxman HL, Marchlinski FE, et al. Role of triple extrastimuli during electrophysiologic study of patients with documented sustained ventricular arrhythmias. *Circulation*. 1984;69:532-540.
27. Josephson ME. *Clinical Cardiac Electrophysiology: Techniques and Interpretations*. 4th ed. Philadelphia, PA: Lippincott Williams & Wilkins; 2008.
28. Nayak HM, Verdino RJ, Russo AM, et al. Ventricular tachycardia storm after initiation of biventricular pacing: incidence, clinical characteristics, management, and outcome. *J Cardiovasc Electrophysiol*. 2008;19:708-715.
29. Stevenson WG, Friedman PL, Sager PT, et al. Exploring postinfarction reentrant tachycardia with entrainment mapping. *J Am Coll Cardiol*. 1997;29:1180-1189.
30. Kocovic DZ, Harada T, Friedman PL, Stevenson WG. Characteristics of electrograms recorded at reentry circuit sites and bystanders during ventricular tachycardia after myocardial infarction. *J Am Coll Cardiol*. 1999;34:381-388.
31. El-Shalakany A, Hadjis T, Papageorgiou P, et al. Entrainment/mapping criteria for the prediction of termination of ventricular tachycardia by single radiofrequency lesion in patients with coronary artery disease. *Circulation*. 1999;99:2283-2289.
32. Soejima K, Suzuki M, Maisel WH, et al. Catheter ablation in patients with multiple and unstable ventricular tachycardias after myocardial infarction: short ablation lines guided by reentry circuit isthmuses and sinus rhythm mapping. *Circulation*. 2001;104:664-669.
33. de Chillou C, Lacroix D, Klug D, et al. Isthmus characteristics of reentrant ventricular tachycardia after myocardial infarction. *Circulation*. 2002;105:726-731.
34. Cassidy DM, Vassallo JA, Marchlinski FE, et al. Endocardial mapping in humans in sinus rhythm with normal left ventricles: activation patterns and characteristics of electrograms. *Circulation*. 1984;70:37-42.
35. Marchlinski FE, Garcia F, Siadatan A, et al. Ventricular tachycardia/ventricular fibrillation in the setting of ischemic heart disease. *J Cardiovasc Electrophysiol*. 2005;16(Suppl 51):S59-S70.
36. Miller JM, Tyson GS, Hargrove WC, et al. Effect of subendocardial resection on sinus rhythm endocardial electrogram abnormalities. *Circulation*. 1995;91:2385-2391.
37. Hsia HH, Lin D, Sauer WH, et al. Relationship of late potentials to the ventricular tachycardia circuit defined by entrainment. *J Interv Card Electrophysiol*. 2009;26:21-29.
38. Brunckhorst CB, Delacretaz E, Soejima K, et al. Identification of the ventricular tachycardia isthmus after infarction by pace mapping. *Circulation*. 2004;110:652-659.
39. Hsia HH, Lin D, Sauer WH, et al. Anatomic characterization of endocardial substrate for hemodynamically stable reentrant ventricular tachycardia: identification of endocardial conducting channels. *Heart Rhythm*. 2006;3:503-512.
40. Arenal A, del Castillo S, Gonzalez-Torrecilla E, et al. Tachycardia-related channel in the scar tissue in patients with sustained monomorphic ventricular tachycardias: influence of the voltage scar definition. *Circulation*. 2004;110:2568-2574.
41. Rajappan K, Schilling RJ. Non-contact mapping in the treatment of ventricular tachycardia after myocardial infarction. *J Interv Card Electrophysiol*. 2007;19:9-18.
42. Strickberger SA, Knight BP, Michaud GF, et al. Mapping and ablation of ventricular tachycardia guided by virtual electrograms using a noncontact, computerized mapping system. *J Am Coll Cardiol*. 2000;35:414-421.
43. Bazan V, Gerstenfeld EP, Garcia F, et al. Site-specific twelve-lead ECG features to identify an epicardial origin for left ventricular tachycardia in the absence of myocardial infarction. *Heart Rhythm*. 2007;4:1403-1410.
44. Bazan V, Bala R, Garcia F, et al. Twelve-lead ECG features to identify ventricular tachycardia arising from the epicardial right ventricle. *Heart Rhythm*. 2006;3:1132-1139.
45. Garcia F, Bazan V, Zado ES, et al. Epicardial substrate and outcome with epicardial ablation of ventricular tachycardia in arrhythmogenic right ventricular cardiomyopathy/dysplasia. *Circulation*. 2009;120:366-375.
46. Anter E, Hutchinson MD, Deo R, et al. Surgical ablation of refractory ventricular tachycardia in patients with nonischemic cardiomyopathy. *Circ Arrhythm Electrophysiol*. 2011;4:494-500.

CHAPTER 31

Idiopathic Ventricular Arrhythmias

Bruno R. Andrea, MD; Gerhard Hindricks, MD; Arash Arya, MD

Introduction

At the beginning of the 20th century, ventricular tachycardias (VTs) were observed in patients with severe heart disease and correlated mainly with coronary artery disease. Thus, these arrhythmias were considered lethally dangerous. Crawford et al observed VTs in young patients without evident structural heart disease in the early 1950s[1] and reported the term "idiopathic ventricular tachycardias." More recently, with advanced medicine and diagnostic tools, idiopathic VTs are commonly seen in practice and usually have a benign prognosis.[2] This entity accounts for 10%–20% of all VTs referred for catheter ablation.[3] The term "arrhythmias" instead of "tachycardias" might be more suitable because a great number of patients present with extrasystoles.

Idiopathic ventricular arrhythmias (IVAs) are classified in a variety of ways: by (1) the site of origin, (2) response to pharmacologic agents, (3) morphologic characteristics on surface electrocardiogram (ECG), and (4) electrophysiological mechanism (Table 31.1). Recently, several groups have adopted the classification based on the arrhythmia location, as follows:

- Outflow tract VTs (right or left);[4,5]
- Fascicular or verapamil-sensitive left VTs;[6,7]
- Left papillary muscle VTs;[8,9]
- Inflow mitral and tricuspid tract VTs;[10] and
- Epicardial VT arising close to the coronary venous system, including the anterior interventricular vein, the distal great cardiac vein, and the anterior interventricular vein–great cardiac vein junction.[11]

In patients without any heart disease, VT arises most frequently at the right ventricular outflow tract (RVOT).[2,3,10,12,13] However, some series have reported different localizations with peculiar electrophysiological and electrocardiographic characteristics, which include pulmonary artery (above pulmonary valve) and left ventricular outflow tract, underneath or above the aortic valve plane.[14,15] The reason these arrhythmias come most frequently from the RVOT is still unclear.

The main pathophysiology is widely considered to be *triggered activity* due to cyclic AMP-mediated calcium-dependent delayed afterdepolarizations (DADs) or catecholamine-dependent abnormal automaticity.[10,16] Compared with outflow VT, idiopathic VT from the mitral and tricuspid valve annulus, the papillary muscles, and the coronary sinus system are rare in prevalence. The underlying electrophysiologic mechanism appears to be the same as outflow VT.[10]

After outflow tract arrhythmias, fascicular VTs or verapamil-sensitive left VT are the most frequent and are normally presented in a younger population as compared to outflow tract VT and to papillary muscle VT.[9] The mechanism is well demonstrated to be macroreentry involving the left posteroinferior fascicle and Purkinje fibers (most common form) with an estimated distance of approximately 2 cm between its entrance and exit. VTs arising from the left anterior fascicle are uncommon (right bundle branch block morphology and right-axis deviation).

Clinical presentation is variable among those arrhythmias, and medical therapy has positive responses in 50% of the cases. Catheter ablation is feasible, safe, and has a high rate of success (Figure 31.1).[3,10,12,13,17] Treatment is normally indicated in presence of related symptoms, signs of heart failure ("arrhythmia-related" cardiomyopathy), or drug therapy failure.[2,12]

Table 31.1 Classification of idiopathic ventricular arrhythmias according to the electrophysiological mechanism

Classification	Triggered Activity (Adenosine-sensitive)	Fascicular Reentry (Verapamil-sensitive)	Automatic Focus (β-blocker-sensitive)
Clinical aspect	Exercise-induced; monomorphic and repetitive VT	Stress-induced or spontaneous	Exercise-induced; incessant
Mechanism	cAMP-mediated	Macro- or microreentry	Enhanced automaticity
Morphology	LBBB or RBBB; inferior axis	RBBB; left-superior or right-inferior axis; intrinsicoid deflection < 100 msec	RBBB; LBBB; polymorphic
Induction	PES from atrium or ventricle with/without catecholamines; bradycardia induced (sedation or BB)	PES from atrium or ventricle with/without catecholamines	Catecholamines
Origin	Right/left outflow tract	Left posterior or anterosuperior fascicle	Right or left ventricles (mitral/tricuspid annulus, other locations)
Pacing maneuvers	None	Reset/entrainment	None
Response to medications	BB (eg, Propranolol); Adenosine; Verapamil	Verapamil	BB (eg, Propranolol); Adenosine

BB = β-blockers; cAMP = cyclic adenosine monophosphate; LBBB = left bundle branch block; PES = programmed electrical stimulation; RBBB = right bundle branch block; VT = ventricular tachycardias. *Source:* Modified from Zipes DP, Jalife J.[17]

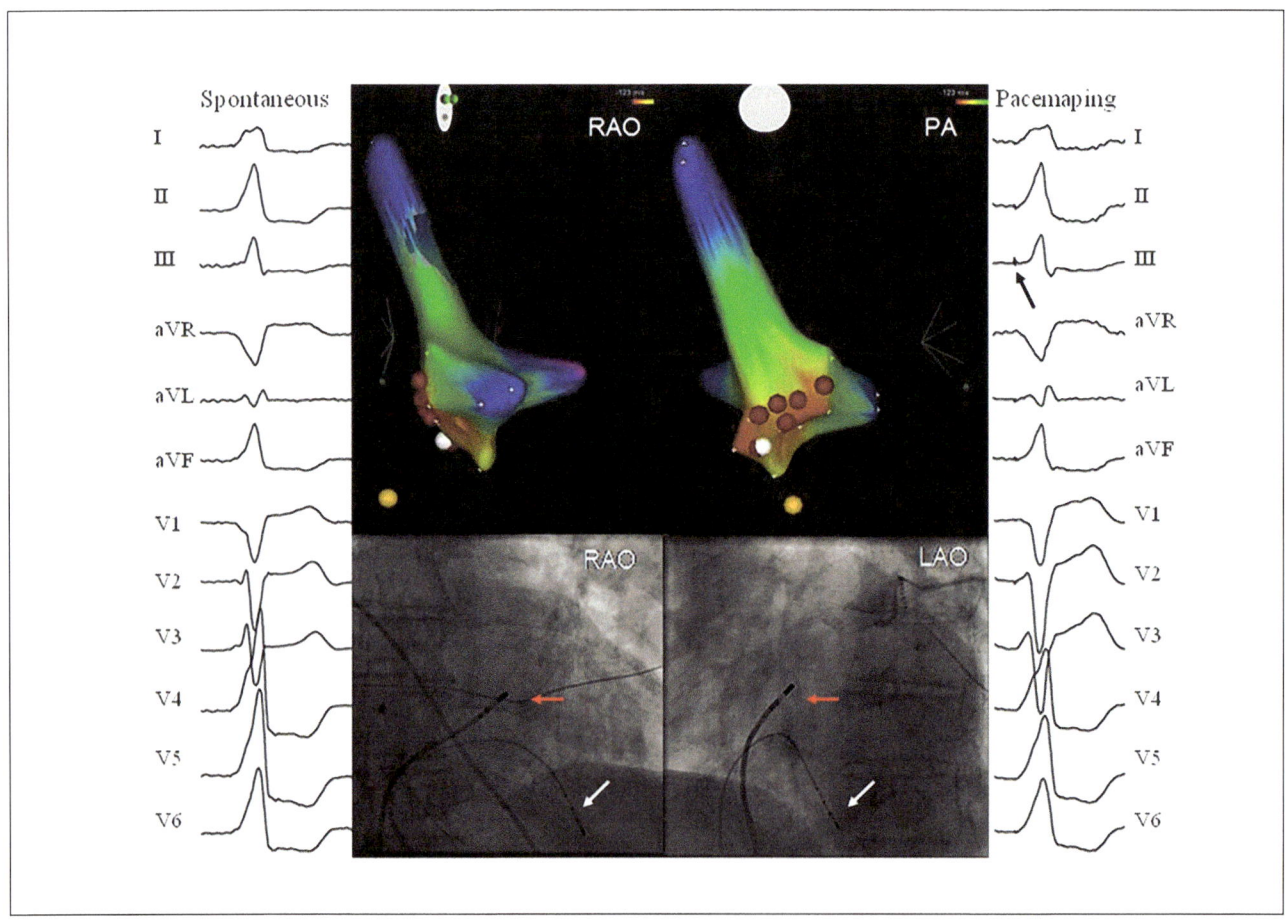

Figure 31.1 Example of a 35-year-old male patient with idiopathic and drug refractory RVOT-PVC who underwent successful catheter ablation. **Left** and **right** panels show the 12-lead ECG from the spontaneous (**left**) and the stimulus-artifact marked pace map (**right**) morphologies on the successful site of ablation, respectively. **Top center panel:** the color-coded activation map from the RVOT showing the PVC earliest activity (**red color**) and the tagged points: **white** – the best pace map; **yellow** – His bundle. On the middle inferior, the fluoroscopic views showing the successful site of ablation. Note the standard position of electrode catheter in right ventricular apex (**white arrows**) and ablation catheter in the RVOT (**red arrows**). PVC = premature ventricular contraction; RVOT = right ventricular outflow tract.

PART I: THE OUTFLOW TRACT VENTRICULAR TACHYCARDIAS

Introduction

Outflow tract ventricular tachycardias (OT-VT) are the most common form of idiopathic VT, accounting for nearly 20% of all patients referred for evaluation of VT.[18-20] In more than 80% of OT-VT cases, VT originates from the RVOT. Nevertheless, other IVA foci have been described, including the interventricular septum, left ventricular outflow tract (LVOT), pulmonary artery, aortic Valsalva sinus, the region close to the His bundle (known as para-Hisian), mitral and tricuspid valves annuli, and the epicardial surface of the ventricles.[5,21-28] Although OT-VT usually occurs in patients with no concomitant structural heart disease,[29] recent studies have debated this issue.[30-32]

Pathophysiology and Anatomy Considerations

Outflow VT is characterized by spontaneous and/or exercise-induced monomorphic VT. The basic electrophysiologic mechanism, as mentioned before, is widely accepted to be triggered activity by calcium-dependent DADs mediated by cyclic adenosine monophosphate (cAMP) overactivity or catecholamine-dependent abnormal automaticity, which explains the sensibility to adenosine and β-blockers. The literature normally suggests that the exact origin of outflow VT is determined by the successful ablation site.

Although the majority of studies on OT-VT mechanism are focused on right OT-VT, recent publications have suggested that right and left OT-VT actually share a common mechanism.[18,33] The OT-VT usually terminates in response to adenosine, β-blockers, calcium channel blockers, and Valsalva maneuvers. β-blockers and calcium channel blockers can be effective in certain forms of VT due to reentry and abnormal automaticity; however, termination of OT-VT by adenosine is pathognomonic for VT caused by cAMP-mediated DADs. There are several clues in this regard: (1) adenosine has no direct effect on the myocardium and Purkinje fibers, but only reverses the cAMP-mediated DADs; (2) adenosine has no effect on digitalis-induced VTs, developed by either early and/or delayed afterdepolarizations, which are mediated by inhibition of Na/K-ATPase with intracellular calcium overload; (3) adenosine terminates VT caused by triggered activity but can only transiently suppresses catecholamine-induced automaticity; and (4) adenosine has no effect on reentrant VT caused by structural heart disease, including catecholamine-facilitated VTs.[29,34,35]

Understanding the anatomy of the outflow tracts is crucial to comprehend this entity. Briefly, the RVOT is an infundibular structure characterized by a smooth surface when compared to the overall right ventricle chamber. Normally there is no trabecular tissue. On the other hand, the LVOT is almost indistinguishable from the rest of the left ventricle and has trabecular tissue until one reaches the aortic valve. At this juncture, it is called the aortic Valsalva sinus. The RVOT crosses superior, anteroposterior, and with a right-to-left direction to reach the atrioventricular orifice and the pulmonary valve (Figure 31.2). The muscle within the wall of the RVOT is substituted by fibrous and elastic tissue when it merges with the fibrous annulus of the pulmonary valve.

There is a close relationship between the RVOT and LVOT. The RVOT is located basally anterior and crosses the LVOT superiorly from the anterior to the posterior aspect of the heart outflow tract, slightly from left to right orientation (Figure 31.2). The septal aspect of the ROVT

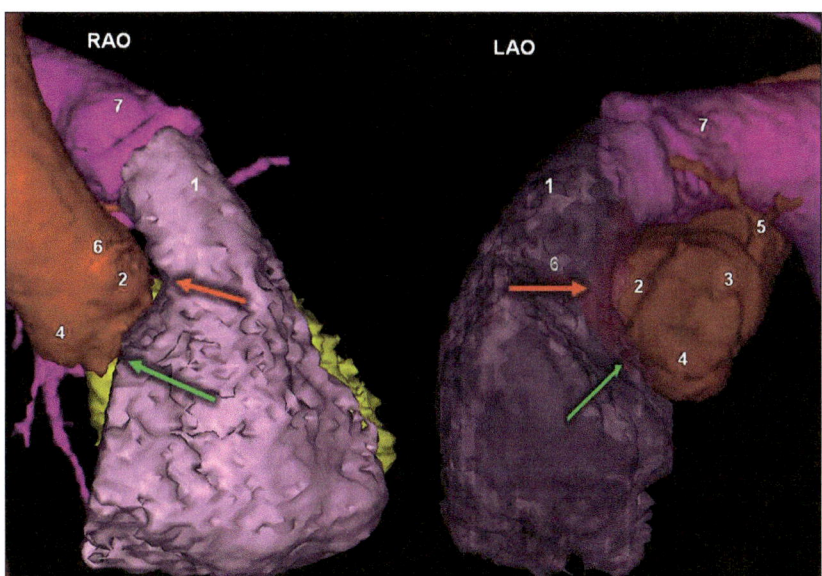

Figure 31.2 Computed tomography from the heart showing the outflow tract (in RAO and LAO views, respectively) and the relationship between RVOT and LVOT. The RVOT crosses above the LVOT/aortic Valsalva sinus with an anteroposterior orientation slightly from left to right. Notice the relationship from the septal aspect of the RVOT with the right coronary cusp (**red arrows**) and posterior aspect with the noncoronary cusp (**green arrows**). Structures presented: 1. RVOT; 2. Right coronary cusp; 3. Left coronary cusp; 4. Noncoronary cusp; 5. Left coronary artery; 6. Right coronary artery; 7. Pulmonary valve and artery. LVOT = left ventricular outflow tract; RVOT = right ventricular outflow tract.

, makes a direct contact with the septal aspect of the LVOT and the right coronary cusp. Its posterior aspect has a relationship with the noncoronary cusp. In the LVOT, one should take note of the segment comprising the area of fibrous continuity between the aortic valve and the anterior leaflet of the mitral valve, known as *the mitral-aortic continuity* (Figure 31.3). In our experience, around 20% of the LVOT-VTs arise in this area.

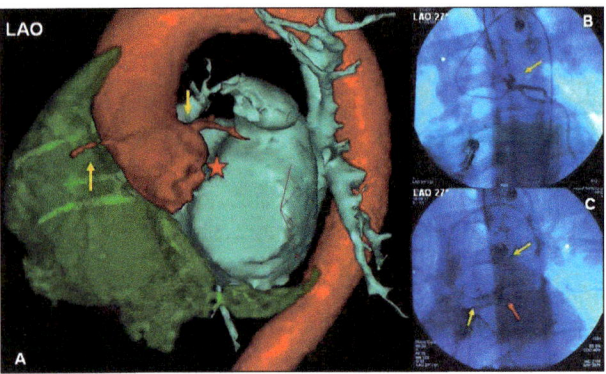

Figure 31.3 Location and anatomic correlation of the LVOT/mitral-aortic continuity. **Panel A:** Computed tomography image in LAO view showing the right atrium with CSO (**green**), the right ventricle and RVOT with transparency (**gray**), aortic valve and root with coronary arteries ostia (**red**), and left atrium with the mitral annulus. **Panel B:** Fluoroscopic image (LAO 27° projection) locating the left coronary ostium with coronariography before ablation of a LVOT-PVC. **Panel C:** Same projection in B with a mark at the monitor from the coronary arteries ostia by pen, indicated by the **yellow arrows** (same correspondence in A and B). Ablation catheter is placed within the mitral-aortic continuity (**red arrow corresponding to the red star in A**), where the PVC was successfully ablated. CSO = coronary sinus ostium; LVOT = left ventricular outflow tract; PVC = premature ventricular contraction.

Fluoroscopic images are shown in Figure 31.1. This relationship between RVOT and LVOT explains the phenomenon of shifting VT "exits" from the right ventricle to the LVOT and vice versa, spontaneously when 2 different morphologies of OT-VT are documented or during catheter ablation (Figure 31.4).[36]

This knowledge also has importance when counseling patients for catheter ablation once one knows the possibility to approach the arrhythmia from the LVOT or epicardially, within the coronary sinus or through a subxyphoidal puncture, respectively.

Clinical Aspects and Clinical Management

Diagnosis of OT-VT is based on the surface 12-lead ECG morphology and absent evidence of structural heart disease (Figure 31.1).

One important cause of RVOT-VT that must be excluded is arrhythmogenic right ventricular cardiomyopathy/dysplasia (ARVC/D). A recent review concerning the diagnostic criteria of ARVC/D has been published, which adds more definitive characteristics for making a diagnosis of this complex disease in contrast to former guidelines.[37]

Around 80% of OT-VTs come from the RVOT.[18-20] OT-VTs are more frequently found in women[38] and symptoms usually occur between the ages of 20 and 50 years.[19] Patients can refer to be asymptomatic, to have palpitations or tachycardias, or even dizziness and syncope in some cases. In this situation, patients must be carefully screened of structural or genetic heart diseases, because OT-VT might be a trigger of other malignant arrhythmias (eg, long QT syndrome, Brugada syndrome, ARVC/D in very early stages, etc). Symptoms mostly relate to physiological effort or emotional stress, meaning enhanced sympathetic tonus, which increases the burden of VTs. Some cases might show Gallavardin phenomenon (Figure 31.5). Another group of patients presents with arrhythmias in rest or during sleep. Both groups are characterized by adenosine sensitivity.

Exercise testing can induce clinical arrhythmia in 25%–50% of the patients; however, in those with

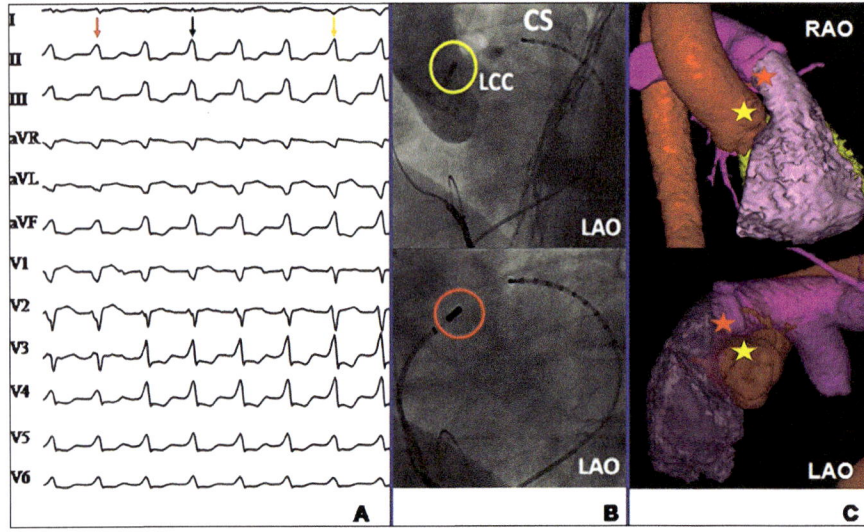

Figure 31.4 Case of a 62-year-old male patient with idiopathic RVOT-VT undergoing catheter ablation. **Panel A:** During ablation at the site of earliest activation in the RVOT. The QRS morphology changed due to the shift of the VT exit from the RVOT (**red arrow**) to the LVOT (**yellow arrow**). In between, an intermediate morphology was observed (**black arrow**). **Panel B:** Fluoroscopic images in LAO views showing the successful ablation site first at the RVOT (**lower panel**) and after at the LVOT within the Valsalva sinus above the left coronary cusp (**upper panel**); **Panel C:** Computed tomography reconstruction of the outflow tracts showing the spots of successful ablation. (RVOT—**red mark**; LVOT sinus of Valsalva from the left coronary cusp—**yellow star**). LVOT = left ventricular outflow tract; RVOT = right ventricular outflow tract; VT = ventricular tachycardia.

repetitive monomorphic VT, the exercise test often suppresses the arrhythmia. OT-VT can happen during either the exercise or recovery phases of the stress test.[39] Limited studies on heart rate variability in patients with OT-VT suggest that activation of sympathetic tone plays an important role in VT genesis.[40,41]

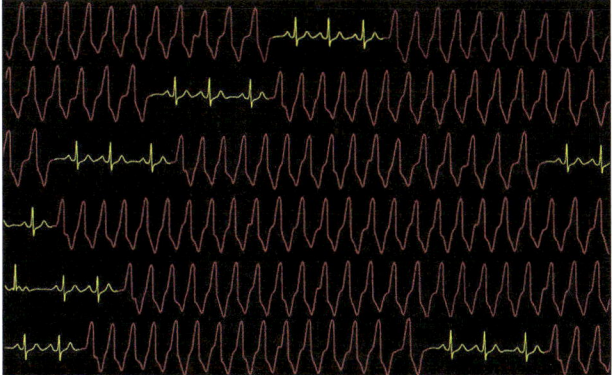

Figure 31.5 The Gallavardin phenomenon characterized by short and frequent burden of outflow tract tachycardia with the behavior of "warming up" and "cooling down" that belongs to triggered activity. Source: Courtesy of Dr. Eduardo M. Andrea, Cardioritmo group, Rio de Janeiro, Brazil.

Treatment is usually guided by the symptoms, and the first, most popular approach is pharmacological. Several medications are used, such as β-blockers, calcium-channel blockers,[42] and class I (eg, quinidin, flecainide, and propafenon)[43] and class III antiarrhythmics (eg, amiodarone and sotalol). Pharmacological treatment has limited efficacy and various side effects. Considering the fact that the patients are young and previously healthy, therapy compliance is also a limitation of this strategy. Some patients can even feel a worsening of the symptoms after starting bradycardia medication with an increase in the VT burden.

In cases of therapy failure, electrophysiology study (EPS) with catheter ablation should be indicated as class IC recommendation.[2] EPS is also indicated as class IIA in suspected cases of RVOT.[2]

The general prognosis of OT-VT is benign once structural heart diseases, especially ARVC/D, are excluded. In general, the benign form of premature ventricular contractions (PVC) have a long coupling interval,[44,45] indicating less risk for the development of primary ventricular fibrillation (VF), which may happen in short-coupled PVCs. In some cases, the frequent burden of PVCs or incessant VT can develop cardiomyopathy, a condition generally named tachycardiomyopathy or arrhythmia-related cardiomyopathy.

RVOT-VT[5]/PVC[6] are also a cause of VF in patients with genetic diseases such as Brugada syndrome, long QT syndrome, catecholaminergic polymorphic VT, and idiopathic VF.[46,47] Normally the "malignant" group presents with syncope or cardiac arrest and often polymorphic PVCs with a short coupling interval occurring on the peak of the T wave (vulnerable refractory period).[45] Therefore, radiofrequency ablation should be strongly considered for the following patients with potentially malignant forms of OT-VT: (1) history of syncope or cardiac arrest; (2) very fast VT (ventricular rates > 230 beats/minute, which can be associated with polymorphic VT); and (3) ventricular premature beats with short coupling interval and/or polymorphic OT-VT.

Primary arrhythmias originating from the LVOT (Figures 31.3 and 31.6) represent nearly 20% of all OT-VT and usually have the same clinical presentation as RVOT. Facing a middle-aged patient (40–60 years old)

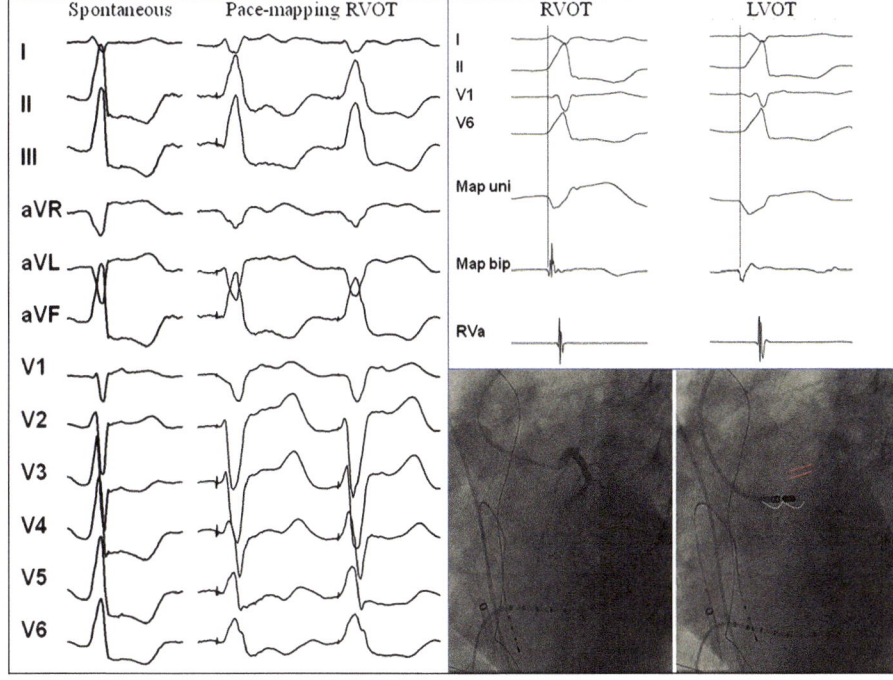

Figure 31.6 Case of a 52-year-old female with highly symptomatic outflow tract PVC sent for catheter ablation. RVOT origin was suspected; however, during the RVOT mapping, no good local EGM (early to the QRS onset or fragmented signals) were found neither a good pace mapping match morphology. Notice the late QRS transition in precordial leads during pace mapping at the RVOT compared to the clinical PVC morphology (**ECG at the left side of the panel**). Retrograde transaortic LVOT mapping revealed the successful site of ablation at the valsalva sinus above the left coronary cusp (**fluoroscopic image at the right inferior panel**) with local EGM 25 ms before QRS complex onset. The unipolar EGM reveals a total negative curve (**right superior panel**). EGM = electrogram; LVOT = left ventricular outflow tract; PVC = premature ventricular contractions; RV = right ventricle; RVOT = right ventricular outflow tract.

with new-onset LVOT-VT/PVC, structural heart abnormalities, especially from the valve leaflets, should be well investigated (eg, ischemic heart disease, aortic or mitral valve calcification). At this point, the arrhythmias should not be considered as idiopathic; however, no consensus is reached in the literature. This topic is discussed later in this chapter.

Approach in the Electrophysiology Laboratory

Electrocardiogram Analysis and Considerations

The ECG analysis must involve the characterization of VT morphology as well as the intrinsic QRS. A standard position for placement of ECG leads is especially important because it (1) will definitely help detecting the probable focus location, ie, whether the origin is within the right or left outflow tract and also endo- or epicardial, (2) aid in guiding the EP laboratory team regarding the process of setting up equipment, and (3) minimize the possibilities of lead misplacement. Unfortunately, conditions such as cardiac hypertrophies and rotations may lead to misinterpretations of a patient's ECG.

The importance of standard placement of the ECG leads for the diagnosis and treatment of patients with OT-VT has been recently reported.[48] The ECG leads placed in a standard and modified position were compared in 20 consecutive patients undergoing catheter ablation of OT-VT. This slight deviation of the limb electrodes affected limb lead vectors and therefore the accuracy of the 12-lead ECG, especially in leads I and aVR.[48]

ECG during sinus rhythm is usually normal in patients with OT-VT; however, nearly 10% of patients with OT-VT show complete or incomplete right bundle branch block.[39]

The QRS morphology during OT-VT is usually left bundle branch block configuration with an inferior axis (Figures 31.1 and 31.7).[13] The QRS duration is usually < 140 ms if it originates from the RVOT septal region.[39] QRS morphology can vary slightly during tachycardia, which is usually associated with minor variations in local EGMs near the site of origin of the tachycardia. Multiple distinct VTs are very rare and should raise the suspicion of an underlying structural heart disease.[49] The QRS morphology of the VT is the first clue to the possible successful site of ablation. There have been several reports on the application of 12-lead ECG findings for localization of OT-VT, which are summarized in Table 31.2.[22,50-55] One recent work reported good accuracy in differentiating RVOT from LVOT with the V_2 transition ratio.[55] Briefly, the V_2 or V_3 transition ratios were calculated by the percentage R wave (R/R+S) from the QRS of the VT and divided by the same ratio from the QRS in sinus rhythm. The measurement should be from the lead that shows the precordial transition of VT. Forty patients with outflow tract premature ventricular contractions (OT-PVC) were retrospectively analyzed, and the transition ratio was significantly greater for VT/PVC originated from the LVOT then from the RVOT (1.27 ± 0.60 vs 0.23 ± 0.16; $P < 0.001$, respectively). In 21 prospectively analyzed patients, a V_2 ratio > 0.6 predicted an LVOT origin with 91% accuracy.[55] Using a ratio that compares with patients' His-Purkinje QRS is also interesting because it "corrects" for physiological electric rotations and deviations.

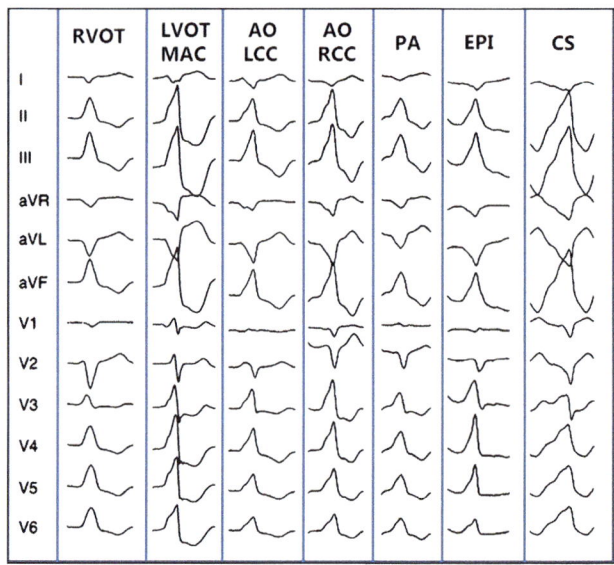

Figure 31.7 Twelve-lead electrocardiograms (ECGs) from seven different patients with idiopathic ventricular tachycardia. Note that all ECG present with a left bundle branch block morphology, inferior axis, R/S transitional zone in lead V_3, and negative QRS complex in lead I. Notice that a slurring beginning of QRS morphology is mostly observed at EPI, coronary sinus, AO LCC, and AO RCC, that is, places where epicardium is thought to be the spot of origin. AO = aortic sinus of Valsalva; CS = coronary sinus; EPI = epicardial surface (through subxyphoid puncture); LCC = left coronary cusp; LVOT MAC = left ventricular outflow tract mitral-aortic continuity; PA = pulmonary artery; RCC = right coronary cusp; RVOT = right ventricular outflow tract.

Ainsworth has recently proposed an ECG algorithm for differentiating idiopathic OT-VT from ARVC/D. The authors showed that QRS duration ≥ 120 ms in lead I had a sensitivity of 100%, specificity 46%, positive predictive value 61%, and negative predictive value 100% for ARVC/D. The addition of R < S in lead III to the above criterion increased specificity for ARVC/D to 100%.[56]

Analyzing the precordial leads, VT/PVC morphologies can be separated in definitely right-sided, intermediate, or definitely left-sided. The first situation normally shows in precordial leads the QRS transition pattern (from negative to positive) between or after V_3 and V_4. Intermediate morphology may have the transition at V_2 or V_3. Definitely left-side origin shows a positive or isodiphasic morphology in V_1. A nice example of transition changes is demonstrated in Figure 31.4. Ablation within the RVOT is performed

Table 31.2 Localization of the site of origin of OT-VT based on 12-lead ECG

Study	Finding
Hachiya[22]	• LVOT-VT suspected: S wave in lead I and an R/S ratio greater than 1 in lead V_1 or V_2. • Coronary cusp location if there is no S wave in leads V_5 and V_6.
Ouyang[50]	• The R-wave duration index (dividing the QRS complex duration by the longer R-wave duration in lead V_1 or V_2) ≥ 50% and for an R/S-wave amplitude index (in leads V_1 and V_2) ≥ 30% strongly suggest the aortic sinus cusp origin.
Hachiya[51]	• R/S transitional zone in V_1 and V_2 (suggesting LVOT-VT): S wave in lead I, tall R wave on leads II, III, and aVF, and no S wave on either lead V_5 or V_6 suggests the aortic sinus cusp origin.
Miles[52]	• Patients with LVOT-VT display significantly earlier precordial transition and more commonly have R waves in V_1 compared to patients with RVOT-VT.
Ito[53]	• S wave > 0.1 mV in lead V_6: Origin is the left ventricle endocardium. • Precordial transitional zone ≥ V_4 or lack of S in lead I: Origin in RVOT. In this case, R or RR' in lead I suggests right ventricular septum. • Transitional zone < V_4: R-duration index < 0.5 and R/S amplitude index < 0.3 suggests RVOT. • Transitional zone < V_4 (for LVOT-VT): Q wave aVL/aVR > 1.4 or V_1 S > 1.2 mV (suggests epicardial origin of the VT).
Tanner[54]	• Transitional zone V_3 alone cannot differentiate RVOT versus LVOT-VT. In this case, stepwise endocardial and epicardial mapping would help to find the site of origin of the OT-VT.
Lerman[39]	• Early precordial transition (V_1-V_2) suggests LVOT-VT. • Transition zone V_2 in patients with RVOT-VT suggests origin immediately below the pulmonary valve. • RBBB in V_1 and broad monophasic R in precordial leads suggests aorto-mitral continuity. • In RVOT-VT: aVL(QS) > aVR(QS) suggests upper left region and vice versa.
Betensky[55]	• In 40 retrospective OT-VT patients with R/S transition in leads V_2-V_3 (V_2 transition ratio) LVOT: 1.27 ± 0.60 vs RVOT: 0.23 ± 0.16; P < 0.001. • In 21 prospective patients, V(2) transition ratio ≥ 0.60 predicted an LVOT origin with 91% accuracy. • PVC precordial transition later than in sinus rhythm excluded LVOT origin (100% accuracy).

Source: Modified from Arya et al.[13]

during VT (with QRS transition between V_3 and V_4) and its morphology changes to an intermediate morphology (with QRS transition between V_2 and V_3) indicating VT exit shift to the left side (Valsalva sinus, above the left coronary cusp).[36] In our practice, when we face a definitely right-sided or intermediate VT/PVC morphology, RVOT mapping and ablation is always attempted first. In definitely left-sided morphology, this strategy is skipped; we move directly to LVOT mapping and ablation.

Finally, the QRS morphology at leads I/aVL can estimate where the VT arises within the RVOT. If both are positive, it most likely comes from the posterior or anterior free wall; if both are negative, there is a greater chance that it comes from the anteroseptal portion. When lead I is positive and aVL is negative, the focus is possibly located intermediately within the posterior or posteroseptal aspect. Figure 31.1 shows that the morphology is almost intermediate at leads I (positive) and aVL (isodiphasic). The VT was successfully ablated at the posterior aspect of the RVOT.

In summary, our stepwise routine of ECG analysis for OT-VT is the following:

1. QRS axis and V_1 pattern (LBBB or RBBB);
2. If inferior axis and RBBB pattern, definitely LVOT-VT is considered;
3. If inferior axis and LBBB pattern—QRS transition (early: V_1-V_2, intermediate: V_2-V_3 or V_3-V_4, late: V_4-V_6);
   - Early QRS transition, highly suspected LVOT-VT is considered;
   - Intermediate QRS transition, we perform V_2 or V_3 transition ratio; and
   - Late QRS transition, definitely RVOT-VT is considered.
4. QRS analysis in leads I and aVL.

Workflow in the Electrophysiology Laboratory

The workflow in the electrophysiology laboratory (EP-Lab) initiates with ECG analysis, as previously described. Suspecting its origin will help to counsel patients about the procedure, to plan the choice of vascular accesses and catheter types, to prepare the team in the EP-Lab for the intervention, to infer procedure time, and raise possible complications. The setup process involves: (1) configuration of EP-systems, radiofrequency generators, fluoroscopy, and, eventually, 3D mapping systems; (2) election of vascular access, introducers, and catheters; and (3) the strategy itself.

Our preference is to use only femoral access instead of associated subclavian or jugular vein access for electrode catheters (eg, placement within coronary sinus) because of comfort for patients and operators, less vascular complication risks, and convenience for vascular compression.

VT/PVC QRS morphologies at the ECG (see the earlier mention of this in "Electrocardiogram Analysis and Considerations") can be didactically divided in morphology as definitely right-sided, intermediate, or left-sided, and this differentiation guides for distinct strategies.

QRS Morphology Definitely from the Right Side

Study Catheters: Usually a standard 4-pole study catheter (4-, 5-, or 6-Fr) with fixed curve in the right ventricle apex (RVa) position is enough to help the procedure. During the procedure, especially if the VT is not evident, right ventricular pacing is important for VT induction and control after radiofrequency ablation. One suggestion would be the election of a soft and malleable catheter to avoid a forced position against the right ventricle wall or damage any structure like papillary muscles or chordae tendineae. RVa position is the most desirable because it normally does not interfere during mapping and the catheter stays stable. The stability is important to ensure a fixed EGM, which can serve as stable reference for 3D mapping systems. However, in practice, any position would be acceptable except the RVOT, which interferes with mapping (provoking undesirable VTs and sometimes leading to ECG misinterpretations) and ablation (difficulty for ablation catheter maneuvering) (Figure 31.1).

Ablation Catheter: In theory, ablation catheters with 4 mm, 8 mm, and open-irrigated tip can be chosen. The use of 8 mm tip surely lacks mapping precision; however, radiofrequency can be applied in a more extended area.[57] We routinely use irrigated-tip catheters for a more consistent lesion not losing mapping precision. Preferences of catheters and curves vary according to operators' experiences. The RVOT is a relatively small chamber; therefore, we recommend catheters with small curves. To carefully place the catheter within the RVOT, one should first reach His bundle position and register its EGM (see also "Intracardiac Registration and Stimulation"). Then slightly bend and advance with a 90° to 180° clockwise turn, bypassing the tricuspid valve, until good contact with the high septum is achieved. Attention should be given to the right anteroseptal papillary muscle where the catheter can get entrapped. Large moves should not be performed in order to avoid heart damages or catheter curve defects. Small moves to advance and retract repetitively can help to accommodate it within the RVOT (Figure 31.8). Sometimes the clockwise turn is not helpful to advance the catheter to the RVOT due to the position of chordae tendinae and trabeculation from the anteroseptal papillary muscle. In this situation, one can slightly retract the catheter to the level of the His bundle and do a counter-clockwise turn up to 180°.

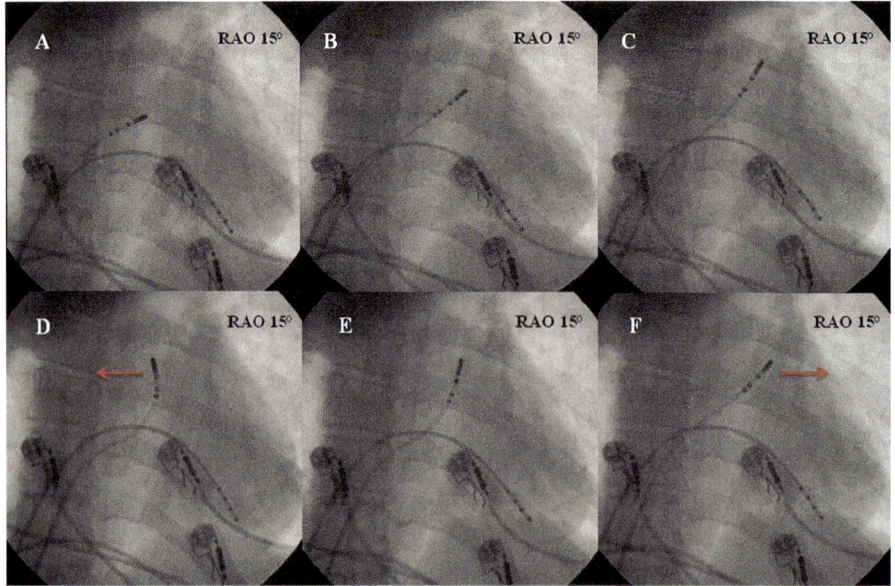

Figure 31.8 Example of 26-year-old female patient who underwent successful ablation of symptomatic RVOT-PVC. Notice the regular catheter placement within the RVOT (ablation catheter 8 mm tip) and at the right ventricular apex (fixed curve 4-electrode study catheter). **Panel A:** Ablation catheter close to His bundle position. The ablation catheter is slightly banded. **Panel B:** The operator gently advances the ablation catheter with a clockwise turn (around 90° to 180°) without releasing the curve. **Panel C:** Ablation catheter is advanced until the level underneath pulmonary valve. **Panel D:** Banding the ablation catheter makes a movement toward the posterior aspect of RVOT. **Panel E:** Middle position within the RVOT during curve release. **Panel F:** Complete release of catheter's curve moves the tip toward the anteroseptal aspect of RVOT. In addition, with this approach within the RVOT, clockwise turn should move the catheter toward posterior and free-wall regions, and counterclockwise turn moves it directing to anterior and anteroseptal aspect.

Once in the RVOT, the initial position of ablation catheter for mapping should be at the pulmonary valve level, then slightly withdraw it until achieving a good EGM. Bending the curve should lead the catheter posterior and, releasing it, the catheter lays anterior toward the septum. Achieving free-wall or septal positions can be easily managed with slightly clockwise and counterclockwise turns, respectively. Normally, movements within the RVOT can be done safely without any important restriction (Figure 31.8).

Radiofrequency Energy Settings: There are no fixed recommended protocols for power (W), temperature (°C), and time (seconds) settings in radiofrequency generators. There are variations among electrophysiology groups.[12,13,20,27] In practice, suggestions of radiofrequency settings are given as following:

- For 4 mm–tip ablation catheter: 30–50W / 40–60°C.
- For 8 mm–tip ablation catheter: 30–50W / 40–60°C.
- For 4 mm irrigated-tip ablation catheter: 20–40W / 40–48°C.
- Time of radiofrequency application: 60 or 90 seconds each pulse.

Logically these values can be modified according to the patient (eg, small size RVOT where it is desirable to give less energy) and the situation (eg, need to titrate up power).

Our standard initial approach is 40 W/50°C for 8 mm–tip ablation catheter, and 30 W/48°C for an irrigated 4 mm tip. In our experience, using 4 mm nonirrigated-tip catheters increases procedure time, increases number of radiofrequency lesions to reach success, and provides lower success rates compared to irrigated-tip catheters. Application time setting for each radiofrequency pulse is usually 90 seconds. However, when suppression is not reached, we interrupt application after 30 seconds and perform further mapping. We routinely use irrigated-tip ablation catheters.

The RVOT is a region with smooth tissue and relatively thin wall; thus, high power and temperature levels should be avoided due to the risk of "stem-POP" and cardiac tamponade.[57] Therefore, when the temperature of the irrigated-tip ablation catheter increases above 42°C in a certain spot, we avoid long application times (eg, more than 20 seconds at that place) and/or reduce power during ablation, or even slightly change position or release contact pressure, in order to increase catheter tip contact with blood and/or irrigation fluid itself.

Intracardiac Registration and Stimulation: The setup process of EP systems should be done according to operators' preferences and should have specific technical support. Of interest, the main control monitor should have 12-lead ECG, bipolar EGM from the right ventricular catheter, bipolar, and unipolar EGM from the ablation catheter.

Before they start mapping the RVOT, operators must be aware about the location of the His bundle, with or without mapping systems.

Registration of signals during mapping of OT-VT/PVC (focal arrhythmogenic activity), independently on the origin, should focus on local bipolar and unipolar signals at the tip of the ablation catheter. But why both signals? Bipolar signals have more accurate morphology to detect local voltage amplitudes and fragmentations, and unipolar signals reflect the proximity of the ablation catheter tip with the focus. Nevertheless, both signals reflect precocity in comparison to QRS onset of VT/PVC. In practice, the bipolar signal registers the local morphology and is more reliable to measure earliness of the EGM (Figures 31.6 and 31.9), and the unipolar signal (earliness and morphology) shows proximity with the focus. If a unipolar signal shows a positive deflection at its initial portion, known widely as "R wave," it means that the impulse from the arrhythmogenic area is coming toward the catheter tip producing a positive deflection, though indicating lack of proximity to the focus. A totally negative unipolar signal morphology, especially when there is a steep initial descending slope, indicates that ectopic activation begins at that spot and moves away, pinpointing the exact location of the focus. Figure 31.6 shows an example of a VT arising from the LVOT. The ECG morphology was doubtful whether right or left OT. Mapping the RVOT revealed no good earliness in both signals, despite a local negative unipolar EGM. Once performing left-side mapping (aortic Valsalva sinus), the EGMs showed a better precocity and a slightly steeper negative unipolar. Ablation was successful at the left side.

Programmed ventricular stimulation is often required to induce the clinical VT and to be a control parameter after ablation. It is not uncommon for these arrhythmias, especially PVCs, to disappear during the procedure (after sedation or even before catheter ablation). Therefore, inducing maneuvers should be done with ventricular programmed stimulation and/or pharmacological stimulation (eg, orciprenalin, isoproterenol, or dobutamine) to initially reach a heart rate between 100 and 120 bpm. Rarely increased sinus rate can inhibit the VT/PVC focus (Figure 31.10).

Stimulation protocols vary among groups and should be individualized for each patient. Protocols are not fixed for idiopathic OT-VT and are usually adapted from the ones previously described for ischemic cardiomyopathy.[2,3,10] Normally these patients are young and have no structural heart disease; therefore these maneuvers are clinically well tolerated. We usually use the following protocol:

Programmed Ventricle Stimulation: (from right ventricular apex and OT)

- Coupling cycles of 500, 430, 370, and 330 ms with 2 extrastimuli (Cycle + S3). Maximum: 500 ms + S4. Pauses from 2 to 5 seconds between cycles.

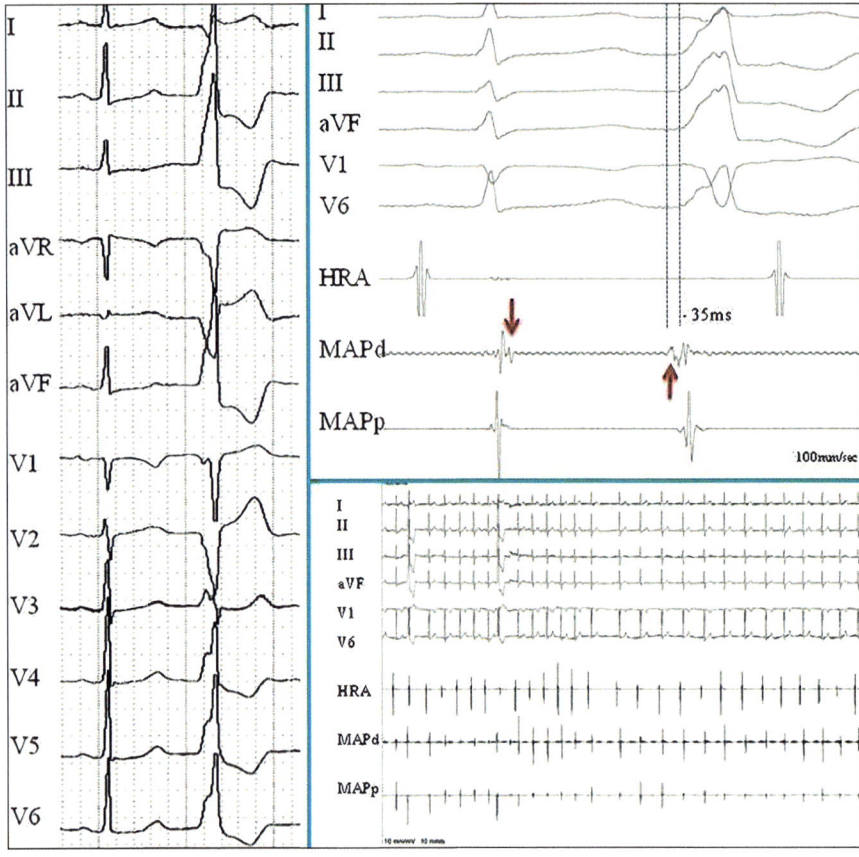

Figure 31.9 Same patient from Figure 31.8. **Left panel:** 12-lead ECG from a normal QRS and the one from the RVOT-PVC. Note the late QRS transition (V_3-V_4) itself and comparing to the normal QRS (V_2-V_3) suggesting a right ventricle origin rather than left ventricle. However, the slurring beginning of the PVC-QRS complex could suggest an epicardial origin. **Upper right panel:** EGM from the 8 mm–tip ablation catheter (MAP distal and proximal) showing the earliest spot compared to the QRS onset. In this moment the right ventricular catheter was placed at the high right atrium to avoid difficulties on moving ablation catheters as well as PVCs provoked by this (operator's preference). Notice the fragmented portion at the end of the EGM in the sinus beat (**upper red arrow**) that comes earlier, before the onset of the PVC, indicating a good spot for ablation. **Lower right panel:** The two first beats from left to right correspond to the beats seen above (upper right panel). First ablation attempt began at that moment and a few seconds later, the PVC was abolished. Time of appliance – 60 seconds, power 40 W, temperature 50°C (see text for details). The successful ablation site was found at the anteroseptal aspect, at the area shown in Figure 31.8F. EGM = electrogram; PVC = premature ventricular contractions; RVOT = right ventricular outflow tract.

- Fixed stimulation with 500, 430, 370, and 330 ms for 5 to 10 seconds. Pauses from 2 to 5 seconds between cycles.

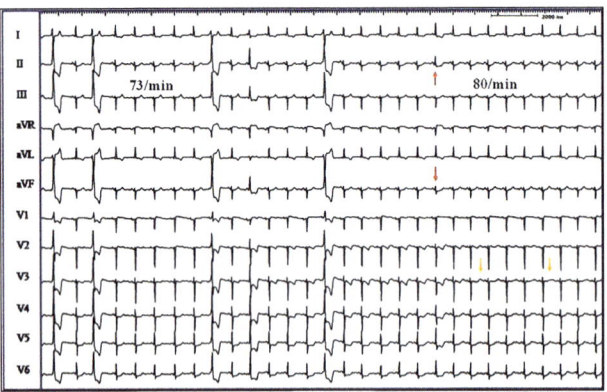

Figure 31.10 Young (32-year-old) female patient undergoing catheter ablation for idiopathic LVOT-PVC. After orciprenalin, the heart rate increased from 73 bpm to 80 bpm and inhibited the PVC focus. And before inhibition, some fusion beats could be seen (**red arrows**). Interestingly, T-wave changes could also be observed (**yellow arrows**). (ECG speed 10 mm/sec.) OT = outflow tract; PVC = premature ventricular contractions.

Mapping and Ablation Strategies: After going through all steps mentioned before—analyzing the ECG correctly, setting up the EP system and/or mapping systems, placing catheters, and inducing the arrhythmia—it is time to start mapping the right outflow tract.

The most common technique used is location of the earliest local activation compared with the VT-QRS onset. First, the ECG can give a good estimation whether the focus can be located at the anteroseptal, posterior, or free-wall aspects of the RVOT as mentioned before. In sequence, the ablation catheter can be carefully placed close to the area of interest. Mapping that area should be performed with maximum attention. It is not rare that local pressure of the catheter tip can suppress the arrhythmia ("touch-mapping").

Searching for the earliest activation place should take the QRS onset as a reference of measurement. The QRS onset is the most reliable parameter of the clinical arrhythmia. During mapping, every single beat should be analyzed individually and compared with the initial clinical arrhythmia morphology, owing to the fact that the catheter can mechanically induce VT or PVC. Figure 31.9 shows an example of a young woman with symptomatic RVOT PVCs. The earliest local EGM showed precocity of −35 ms in comparison to the QRS onset. That was the successful ablation site (anteroseptal aspect of the RVOT).

Pace mapping maneuvers are easily performed and effective to confirm the VT/PVC exit point.[10,12,13] Once the earliest spot is found or suspected, pace mapping should always be performed. The QRS morphology is then compared with the clinical VT morphology. A perfect 12-lead ECG pace mapping match (called "12/12 pace mapping match") translates the place of VT/PVC exit and a good target for radiofrequency ablation (Figure 31.1). We suggest usage of different output voltages during pacing with the following strategy: (1) Increasingly higher output voltages in order to obtain local capture once good contact is confirmed and a good ablation target is suspected (eg, earliest spot), or (2) Increasingly lower output once a good target and catheter contact are confirmed, and the PM match is not 12/12. In this last situation, higher outputs may capture a broader area of tissue, adjacent to the VT/PVC focus, disturbing QRS morphology. In practice, this might partially explain successful ablation in areas where PM match is 11/12 or even 10/12.

Three-dimensional mapping systems can be used and show feasibility and efficacy.[58,59] Systems are more frequently required for VT ablation in patients with structural heart disease.[60] One advantage is the capability to mark and define spots with great precision, and also mark places where ablation has been attempted. The mapping technique normally employed is the activation map, which shows the earliest activation area. Voltage mapping is usually required for patients with structural disease, where areas of low voltage and electric scars must be defined.[60]

Precautions: Some situations deserve specific attention as follows:

- ECG leads should be correctly placed. Misinterpretation of 12-lead ECG can compromise the whole procedure.

- Deep sedation may suppress this arrhythmia. Sometimes it is necessary to suspend sedation and wake the patient during the procedure.

- Groin punctures must be done with extra care. Punctures performed very close to one another might trouble catheter guidance and movements.

- High power and temperature settings should be avoided.

- Avoid large and strong moves to access and within the RVOT, in order to prevent lesions in structures like tricuspid valve, chordae tendineae, right ventricular papillary muscles, and AV node. This precaution is especially important to avoid suppressing VT with catheter movement or mechanically inducing other morphologies rather than the clinical one.

- After successful ablation, routine EPS should be performed in order to confirm success, analyze the physiology of cardiac electrical system, and exclude associated arrhythmias.

Intermediate VT Morphology

The VT-QRS transition within V_2 and/or V_3 may be the most common presentation of OT-VT in practice. Various studies analyzed ECG features of such VTs (Table 31.2). The recently reported V_2 transition ratio seems to have good accuracy to detect or exclude a left-sided VT.[55] In our practice, even though this ratio indicates a left ventricle VT, we usually start mapping the RVOT.

Study Catheters: Catheters that help in this case are one in the right ventricular apex and another one, deflectable, deep within the coronary sinus, trying to reach the great cardiac vein (Figure 31.11—right panel).[61] EGM registration within the coronary sinus (close to the left ventricle summit) helps comparing precocities and predicts left-side or epicardial origin.[55]

Ablation Catheter: The choice here can be the same as for the RVOT-VT; however, once intermediate morphologies may rise from the left side, catheters with irrigated tips should be preferable to conventional 4 mm or 8 mm tip. Advantages favoring irrigated-tip catheters might be: (1) deeper lesions rather than extended; (2) capacity of delivering more power with less temperature increase; and (3) maintenance of an accurate mapping capability (conventional or with 3D mapping systems), therefore increasing ablation success.

The choice of types of catheter curves depends on the operator's experience and the patient's anatomy. Fluoroscopic placement of study catheters helps knowing the anatomy. A deeply placed coronary sinus catheter contours mitral annulus and infers the position of aortic annulus. Mapping both areas, RVOT and left Valsalva sinus, normally requires a small or middle curve catheter, especially with retrograde transaortic approach. For femoral artery puncture, a 7-Fr short sheath is enough.

Radiofrequency Settings, Mapping, and Ablation Strategy: Recommended radiofrequency settings are the same as for RVOT-VT. In our experience, however, slightly higher power settings may be safely used for ablation within the left side with irrigated-tip ablation catheter. Power and temperature settings may be 30–45W / 40–48°C, titrating up to 50–55W within the mitral-aortic continuity.

Strategy for mapping and ablation is basically the same used for RVOT-VT. The difference is accessing, mapping, and ablating the left side. In this case, retrograde transaortic approach or transseptal puncture is necessary. Retrograde access is preferable because it easily reaches Valsalva sinus and obviously presents no complications related to transseptal puncture. Trespassing aortic valve can be done with the catheter already curved from the aortic root or at the aortic valve plan (Figure 31.12). Nevertheless, cardiac catheterization should be performed during the procedure in order to locate coronary vessels ostia (Figures 31.3 and 31.6).[62] Applying radiofrequency energy within or close to these ostia may lead to catastrophic consequences.

Signals interpretation should be the same for RVOT-VT with greater attention for fragmented and/or small amplitude signals, especially within the Valsalva sinus, where such signals are more frequently found compared to places under the aortic valve (Figures 31.6 and 31.11).

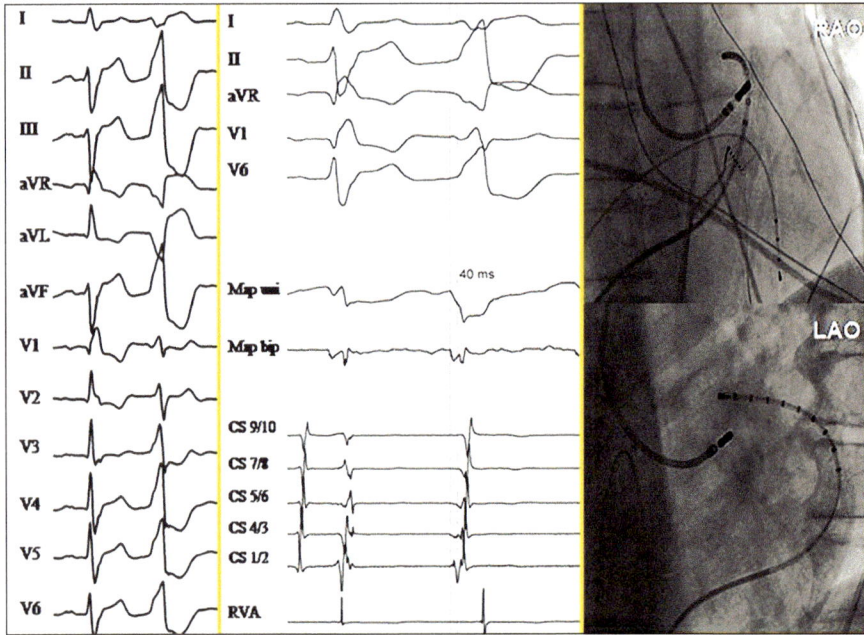

Figure 31.11 Case of a 65-year-old male patient who developed symptomatic LVOT PVC. At baseline ECG, notice the presence of LAH and RBBB. He had no detectable structural heart disease. **Left panel:** 12-lead ECG showing the baseline and the PVC-QRS morphologies. **Middle panel:** EGM showing the signals at the spot of earliest activation (40 ms before the QRS onset), which is even earlier than the distal coronary sinus catheter electrode. **Right panel:** Fluoroscopic image in RAO and LAO views showing the successful ablation site at the mitral-aortic continuity. Although no structural heart disease was found, age-related calcifications at the mitral-aortic fibrous ring could be responsible for the late development of these PVCs. CS = coronary sinus; EGM = electrogram; LAH = left anterior hemiblock; LVOT = left ventricular outflow tract; PVC = premature ventricular contraction; RBBB = right bundle branch block.

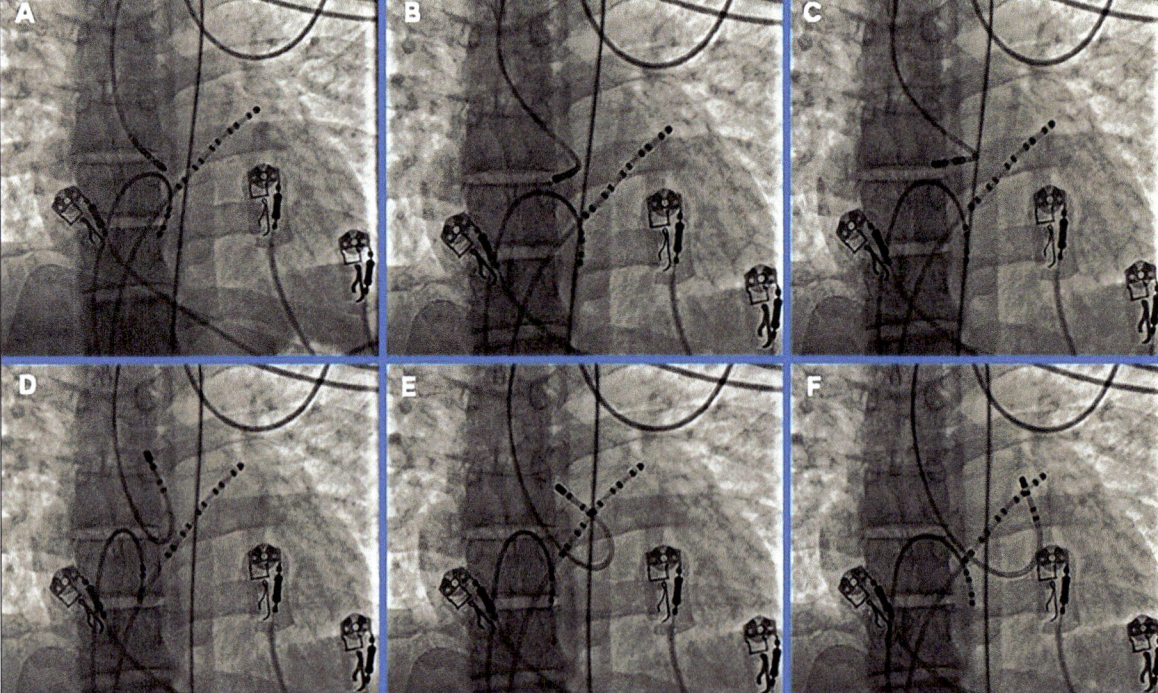

Figure 31.12 Fluoroscopy sequence showing the movement of trespassing the aortic valve with the ablation catheter. The sequence was made in AP projection, and there was one 4-electrode catheter in right ventricle, one 10-electrode catheter within the coronary sinus, and the ablation catheter executing the movement. **Panel A:** The operator advances the catheter until it reaches the aortic valve. The coronary sinus catheter is used as a landmark to distinguish the aortic valve plan, which stays around 0.5 to 1 cm above the coronary sinus level (mitral annulus). The coronary arteries' ostia lie around 2 to 3 cm above the coronary sinus level. **Panels B to D:** After recognizing the aortic valve (visually and tactile feedback of resistance), the operator advances the catheter without curve to favor a natural curve at the Valsalva sinus to the position observed in D. **Panel E:** The catheter is advanced still without curve. Notice the convexity of the curve pointing to the apex and moving below the coronary sinus catheter level. **Panel F:** Catheter finally inside the left ventricle (still without catheter curve) and the tip directs toward the mitral annulus.

Precautions: Same precautions should be taken as for RVOT-VT with the following additions:

1. Patients must receive heparin and should have the activation clotting time between 250 and 350 seconds with individualization in each case.

2. Careful groin punctures especially predicting the usage of an arterial access. A reasonable distance between the punctures' incisions helps maneuvering catheters and groin compression after the procedure. This care also avoids crossing punctures through veins and arteries, thus risk of complications.

3. Passing carefully through the aortic valve to avoid lesions, with special attention to the coronary ostia.

4. Awareness of the His bundle position from the left side is extremely important, and it should be always marked, especially with 3D mapping systems, before ablation.

ECG Morphology Definitely from the Left Side

Normally, a positive QRS pattern in V_1 during VT excludes right-side origin. In practice, the arrhythmias are more commonly associated with structural heart disease. In this scenario, the same recommendations and precautions listed before may be applied here, with the same settings for the left ventricle chamber.

To our knowledge, there is no publication of a pure idiopathic outflow ventricular tachycardia with a totally positive QRS pattern in lead V_1. These VTs are grouped into the hall of idiopathic left fascicular ventricular tachycardias and are discussed later in this chapter.

Other arrhythmias such as atrioventricular nodal reentry tachycardia (AVNRT), either spontaneous or induced, can be present in 25% of patients with idiopathic outflow tract ventricular arrhythmias undergoing catheter ablation.[63] However, it is still unclear whether ablation is necessary in the induced group.[63]

Follow-up and Prognosis

Prognosis will certainly depend on the clinical status of the patient and how your approach was successful, whether clinical or interventional.

Around 5% of patients undergoing successful ablation have recurrent VT, especially within the first year.[42] Significant predictors of recurrence following initially successful ablation were later activation at the target site, poor pace mapping matches (ECG morphology <12/12 leads), and reliance exclusively on pace mapping.[64] Serious complications occur in approximately 1% of patients, usually related to cardiac perforation.

Patients treated pharmacologically experience recurrent symptoms and/or VT in 30%–40% of the cases during long-term follow-up.[65]

Generally, OT-VT has a benign prognosis, especially when successfully treated in the first ablation procedure, and usually a second intervention is not necessary.

PART II: IDIOPATHIC LEFT FASCICULAR VENTRICULAR TACHYCARDIAS

Introduction

Idiopathic left fascicular ventricular tachycardias (LFVTs) are the second most common idiopathic ventricular tachycardia, accounting for nearly 10%–15% of all idiopathic VT. It occurs typically in young patients without any structural heart disease with the first episode often in adolescence.[66] This arrhythmia was first reported in 1979 by Zipes et al, who highlighted the inducibility after atrium pacing and its relatively narrow QRS.[67] These findings were related to the proximity to the left posteroinferior fascicle. Furthermore, in the early 1980s, Belhassen et al[67,68] described an electrophysiologic entity that was sensitive to verapamil.

Commonly named fascicular tachycardia, verapamil-sensitive VT, or Belhassen VT, is characterized by a right bundle branch block pattern and left axis deviation. The LFVTs have benign prognosis, and intravenous verapamil is highly effective in terminating VT. Other uncommon locations were described at the left ventricle anterosuperior fascicle[66] and the left superior septum.[69] Patients presenting recurrent episodes of VT may be referred for radiofrequency catheter ablation.

Anatomy and Pathophysiology

The left bundle of the cardiac conducting system is the continuation of conducting fibers from the His bundle. After leaving the membranous septum and diving into the subendocardial layer of the muscular septum, the left main branch divides into two, or sometimes three, broad groups of fibers: (1) the anterosuperior (LAS) fascicle or hemibundle, which supplies the anterior papillary muscle and the Purkinje network of the anterior and superior surfaces of the left ventricle; (2) the posteroinferior (LPI) fascicle or hemibundle supplying the posterior papillary muscle and Purkinje network of the inferior and posterior surfaces of the left ventricle. The third fascicle would be a midseptal (MS) branch that can originate independently or as a ramification of the LPI (more common) or LAS fascicles. Anatomical studies of the left conduction system by Demoulin and Kulbertus in the early 1970s showed a considerable variability in its anatomy and, in fact, in most of the cases a distinct third division of the left bundle branch was evident at the midseptal area.[70] The initial contact between Purkinje fibers and contractile myocytes permits the first contraction within the papillary muscles. After emerging at apical regions, functional contacts are made in a continuous manner within the subendocardial layer toward the base of the left ventricle. This physiological distribution means that the tension within the papillary muscles increases before ventricular contraction, which happens from the endocardium to the epicardium and from the apex toward the basis of the left ventricle. The left bundle branch cells are rapidly conducting Purkinje myocytes displaying automatic properties.

Several studies have proved that the LFVT electrophysiological mechanism is calcium-dependent reentry[71-75] and depends on the effects of the slow calcium current in partially depolarized Purkinje fibers, contrasting with other idiopathic VTs, which are triggered activity by cAMP.[76] The most common type is the one originating within the LPI-fascicle (LPI-VT) and the reentrant circuit locates at the inferior left ventricle septum extending from its basal aspect to the mid-apical region. The entrance of the circuit is located in the basal aspect of the septum and the wave front runs antegrade to the apical septum by the LPI-fascicle (antegrade arm). At the distal portion of the septum, the circuit changes its meaning with the retrograde conduction along the LPI-fascicle (retrograde arm) and antegrade conduction distally to the corresponding myocardium. This circuit can be defined as intra-fascicular (Figure 31.13A). The retrograde arm through the LAS-fascicle, known as inter-fascicular circuit, is also possible (Figure 31.13B and case mentioned in Figure 31.14A–E; see further explanation in Part IV). The anatomical substrate is not completely understood. It is widely accepted that the posterior fascicle constitutes the retrograde arm of the circuit. One hypothesis to explain the antegrade arm suggests that a longitudinal dissociation of the affected fascicle and/or even ventricular myocardium might be responsible for this reentry fashion.[77]

Clinical Aspects and Management

LFVTs normally occur in young patients (15–40 years), mainly males (60%–80%).[78,79] It frequently presents with paroxysmal episodes of tachycardic palpitations, dizziness, fatigue, shortness of breath, and, less frequently, syncope. The attacks are hemodynamically stable and may be precipitated by exercise, excitement, emotional stress, and infection. Although uncommon, persistent and incessant tachycardia can lead to tachycardiomyopathy (in around 6% of cases) and is usually reversible after ablation.[79]

In patients presenting with a hemodynamically stable tachycardia, administration of intravenous verapamil 5 or 10 mg over 2 minutes normally interrupts the tachycardia (Figure 31.15). Electrical cardioversion is mandatory in case of instability. Verapamil should be given only in patients without moderate to severe heart failure and structural disease due to the risk of hemodynamic collapse. LFVT usually does not respond to vagal maneuvers, β-blockers, or adenosine; however, patients in whom the tachycardia initiates by catecholaminergic stimulus may be responsive to acute adenosine infusion. This sensitivity is explained by the fact that cAMP can positively modulate the cellular calcium influx.[80]

Long-term treatment strategies will depend on the severity of symptoms. Verapamil can be given chronically and is helpful in patients with mild symptoms. In case of severe symptoms, refractoriness, or intolerance to pharmacologic treatment, catheter ablation is recommended.[2,67] Catheter ablation is highly successful (85%–95%) with low rate of recurrences (5%–10%), especially in those with typical LPI-VT.

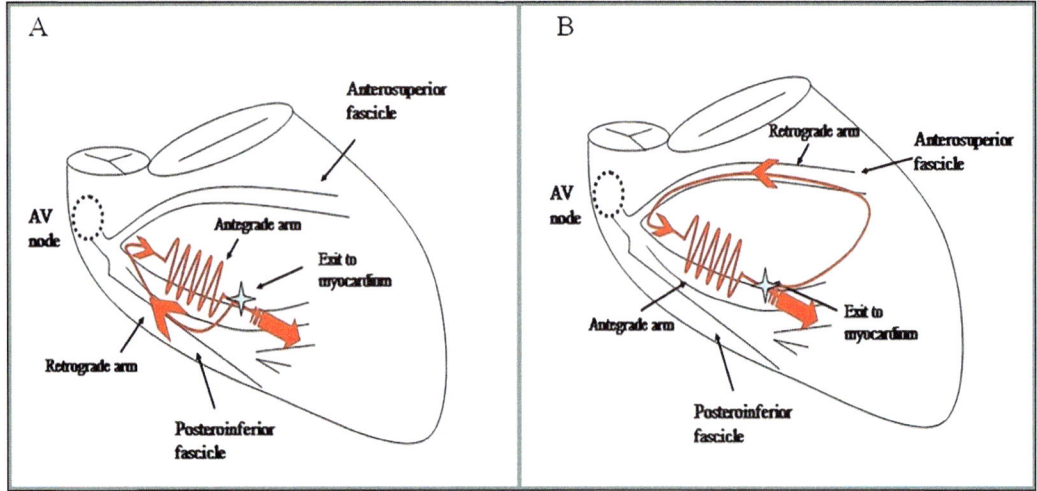

Figure 31.13 Schemes showing the mechanisms of typical left fascicular tachycardias. **Panel A:** Intra-fascicular reentry. **Panel B:** Inter-fascicular reentry.

Chapter 31: Idiopathic Ventricular Arrhythmias • 369

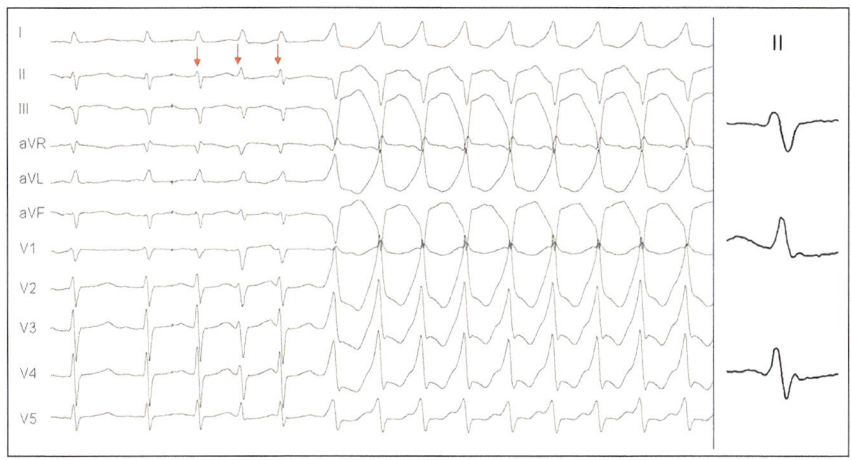

Figure 31.14A Male 60-year-old patient with an idiopathic wide complex tachycardia, which was inducible from the ventricle and easily from the atrium. **Left panel:** After 2 coupled atrium extrabeats, the baseline QRS morphology changes from LAH (**left red arrow**) to a "normal" morphology (**middle red arrow**), then to an "incomplete LAH" (**right red arrow**) and the tachycardia starts with the supposed origin at the inferobasal aspect of the left ventricle septum (based on QRS morphology). **Right panel:** Detailed QRS morphology in lead II; from up to down following the **red arrows** sequence at the right panel from left to right. LAH = left anterior hemiblock; LV = left ventricle (see text for further explanation) (ECG speed 50 mm/sec).

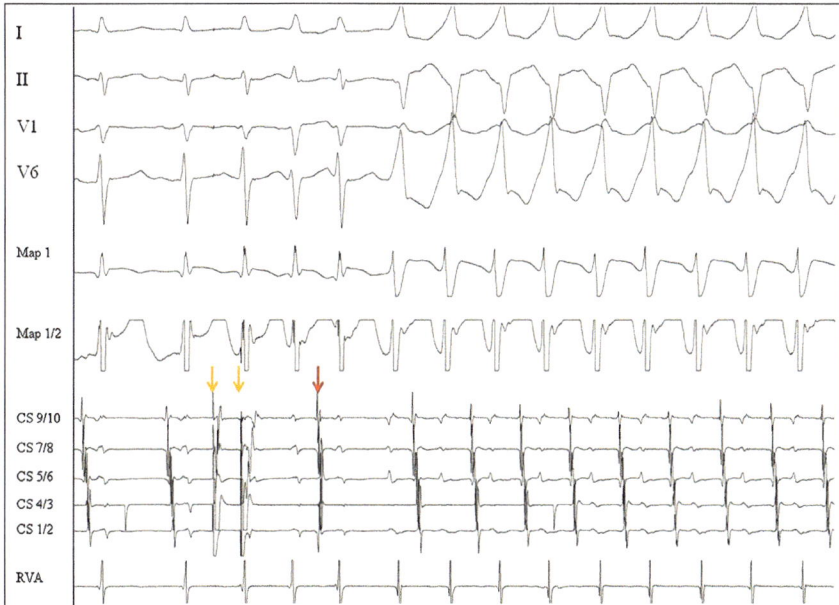

Figure 31.14B Same patient cited in Figure 31.14A with intracardiac signals. The ablation catheter (Map) was placed in the left ventricle. Description from left to right: two sinus beats; two extrastimuli from the distal coronary sinus (CS 1/2) conducting to the ventricle with the baseline QRS (LAH) and without LAH, respectively; one spontaneous PAC conducting with an incomplete LAH; tachycardia induction after QRS deflagrated by the PAC. Notice that the VT starts after a small QRS complex (**red arrow**) and there is decremental VA conduction. Wenckebach VA block follows the sequence of the tracing (not shown). LAH = left anterior hemiblock; LV = left ventricle; PAC = premature atrial contraction (see text for further explanation) (ECG speed 50 mm/sec).

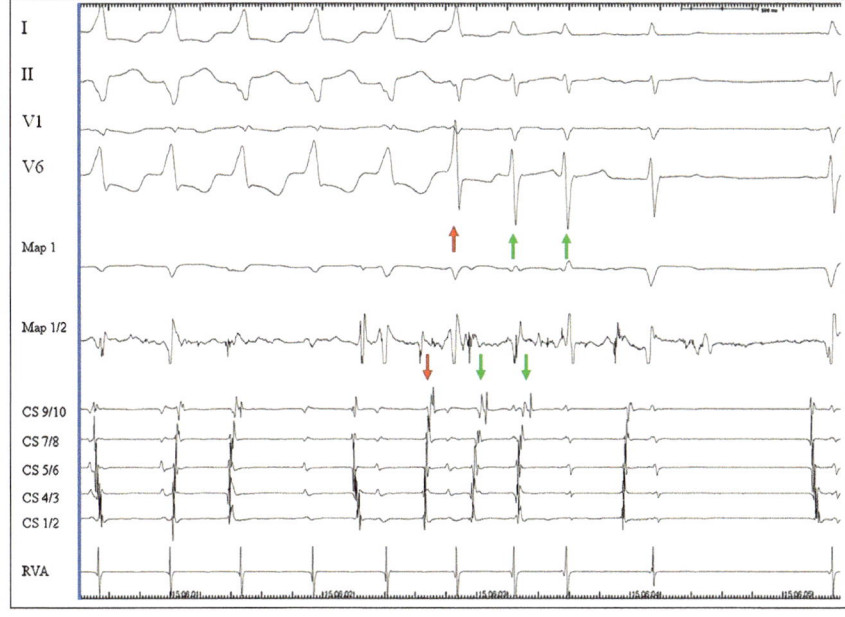

Figure 31.14C Same patient from Figure 31.14A. Tracing showing VT termination with 3 spontaneous PACs. The first PAC (**red arrow**) conducts through His-Purkinje and deflagrates a ventricular fusion beat with the VT QRS complex (**red arrow**). The second and third PACs (**green arrows**) conduct through His-Purkinje as well, fully capturing the ventricle and conducting a narrow QRS complex and terminating the VT. Notice that the termination of VT is preceded by QRS complexes with the same morphology as the basal one, ie, LAH. LAH = left anterior hemiblock; LV = left ventricle; PAC = premature atrial contraction; VT = ventricular tachycardia.

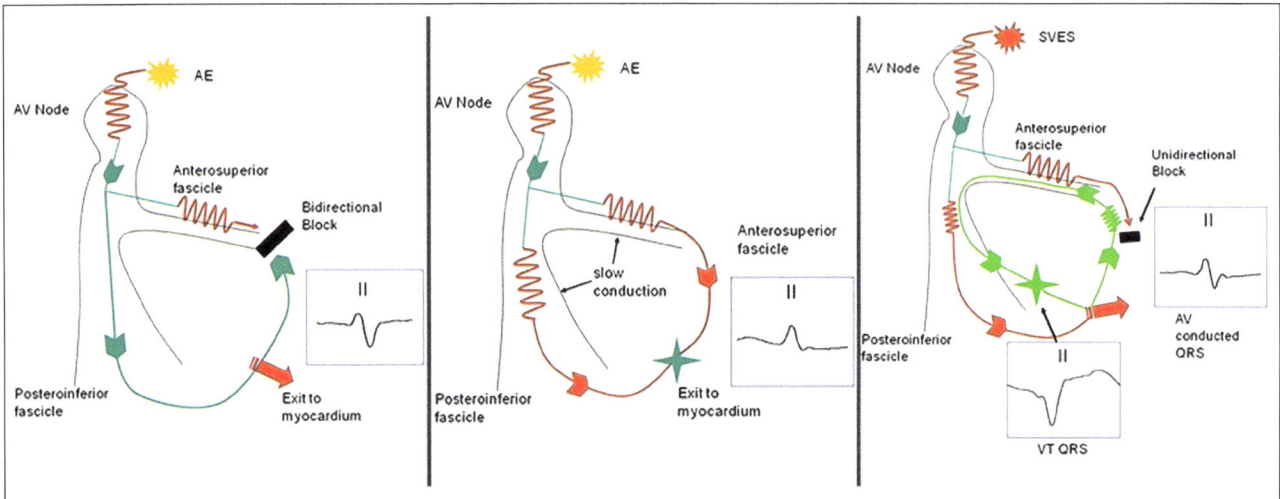

Figure 31.14D Same patient from Figure 31.14A. Scheme illustrating the suggested mechanism of inter-fascicular reentry. **Left panel:** First AE conducting to the ventricle with LAH (**left yellow arrow in Figure 31.14B**). The wavefront interferes with the conduction of the LAS, which has a fixed refractory time. **Middle panel:** Second AE conducting with delay through both fascicles due to relative refractoriness at the LPI-fascicle permitting the conduction through the LAS which and a small QRS complex appears (without the LAH morphology) (**right yellow arrow in Figure 31.14B**). **Right panel:** Spontaneous SVES (**red arrow in Figure 31.14B**) conducting with less delay through the LPI (partially recovered) raising an intermediate QRS morphology (incomplete LAH) in a first moment, then the wavefront retrogradely penetrates in the LAS (retrograde arm of the circuit—**green marker pointing retrogradely against the LAS**) to further run through the antegrade arm within the LPI (**green marker now pointing antegradely toward the LPI**) and perpetuate the VT. The QRS morphology is wide, which suggests an exit point within the adjacent ventricular myocardium. The VT has at this moment VA conduction 1:1 with coronary sinus concentric activation and slightly decremental. AE = atrium extrastimulus; LAH = left anterior hemiblock; LAS = left anterosuperior fascicle; LPI = left posteroinferior fascicle; SVES = supraventricular extrasystole; VT = ventricular tachycardia.

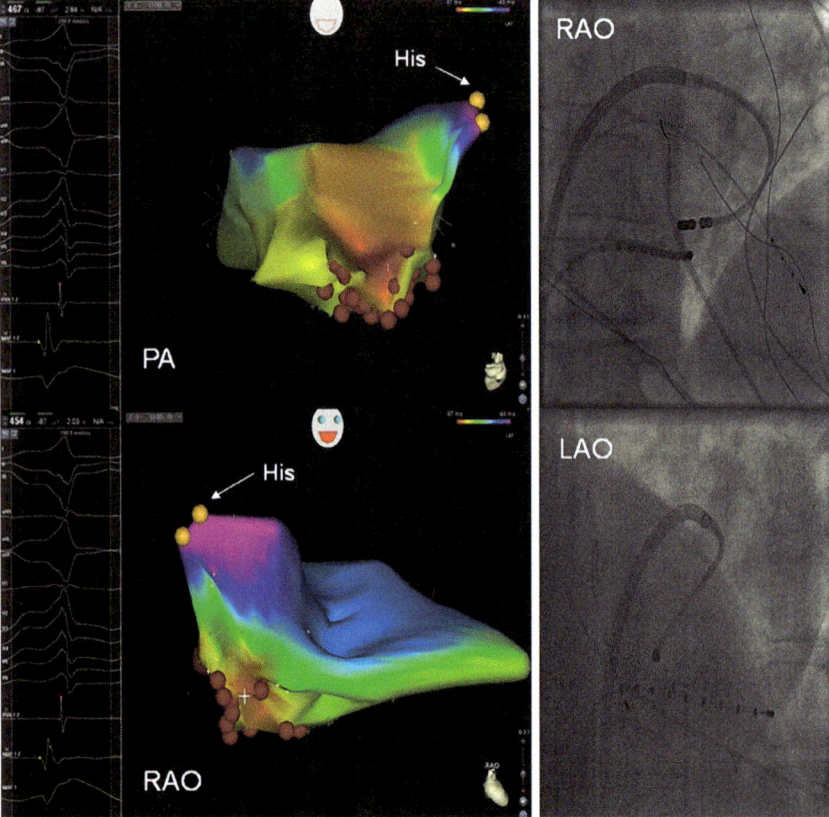

Figure 31.14E Left panel: Electroanatomical mapping (upper part in PA and inferior part in RAO views) of the earliest VT activation at the middle part of the left ventricle inferoseptal area (area of interest). The VT QRS morphology is also shown at the left side and the **yellow tagged points** mark the His bundle position as indicated. **Right panel:** Fluoroscopic images of the successful site of ablation (upper part in RAO and inferior part in LAO views).

Practice in the Electrophysiology Laboratory

The Electrocardiogram

The baseline ECG is normal in most patients; however, sometimes it may present T-wave inversion, especially after a tachycardia episode corresponding to cardiac memory. The LFVT usually shows a relatively narrow QRS complex (<150 ms) and a fast intrinsic deflection (RS interval of 60–80 ms in precordial leads). These features can lead to misdiagnosis of supraventricular tachycardia with aberrant AV conduction. The ventriculoatrial (VA) nodal conduction can either be blocked, translated by P-wave dissociation (Figure 31.15), or presented in a 1:1 fashion (Figure 31.16) or even in a Wenckebach block fashion (Figure 31.17A). The VT morphology varies depending on the site of origin of the tachycardia (exit point). As a rule, all the VTs show RBBB:

- Left posteroinferior fascicular ventricular tachycardia (LPI-VT): It accounts for around 90% of cases. The ECG exhibits an RBBB morphology and left superior axis suggesting that the exit of the circuit is located in the inferoposterior septum. Another feature, which also helps differentiating fascicular versus papillary muscle VT/PVC, is the presence of the first inferoseptal vector, translating a small Q wave in lead I and small first R wave in inferior leads (Figures 31.15A and 31.17A–D).

- Left anterosuperior fascicular ventricular tachycardia (LAS-VT): It is the second most common variant. The ECG pattern shows RBBB morphology and right inferior axis. The VT exit is found in the left ventricle anterolateral wall (Figure 31.16).[81]

- Upper septal fascicular ventricular tachycardia: This presentation corresponds to the location of the midseptal fascicle and is rare (Figure 31.18). The QRS is narrow and has a normal frontal axis. It presents generally with RBBB morphology; however, few cases with LBBB pattern have been described with a precordial R-wave transition between V_3 and V_4.[69]

Some patients with frequent symptoms and recurrent VT may present with repolarization disturbances with negative T waves corresponding to cardiac memory phenomenon.

Electrocardiographic differential diagnosis with papillary muscle arrhythmias might be a challenge and should be made before the procedure in order to plan mapping and ablation approaches. This point is discussed in Part III, Papillary Muscle Arrhythmias.

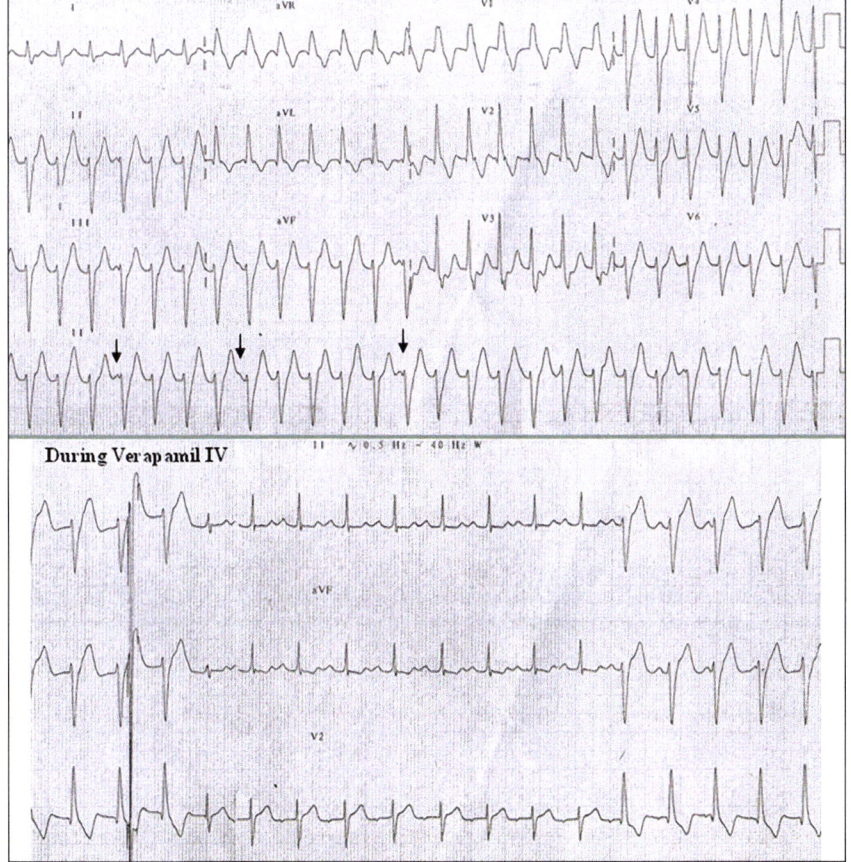

Figure 31.15 Young female patient (27 years old) presenting to the emergency room with a hemodynamically stable fascicular ventricular tachycardia due to her own interruption of verapamil intake. **Panel A:** Ventricular tachycardia. Note the dissociated sinus P waves (**arrows**). **Panel B:** Continuous tracing during slow infusion of 10 mg verapamil. Note the fusion QRS complexes (**arrows**) and after for short time when the VT slows down and is inhibited by sinus tachycardia conducting with short QRS. VT = ventricular tachycardia (ECG speed 25 mm/sec).

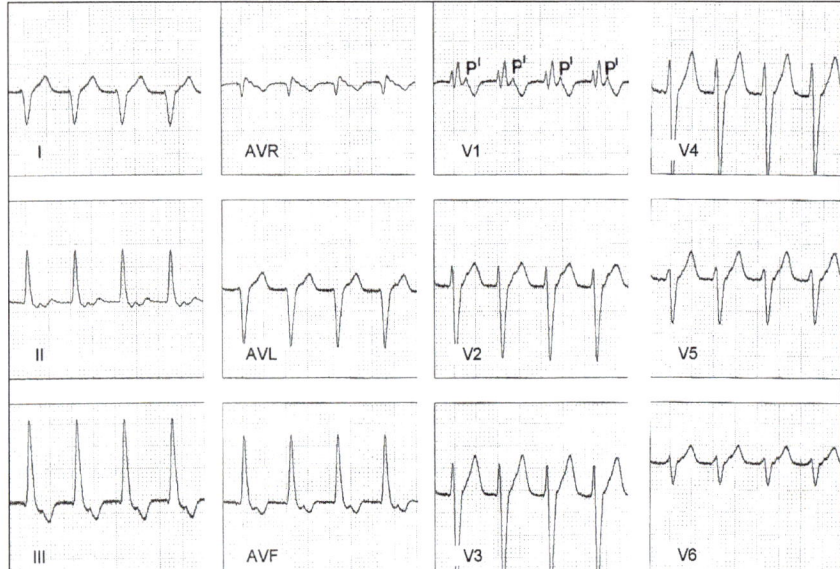

Figure 31.16 Young male patient (22 years old) without structural heart disease brought to the chest pain unit with long history of paroxysmal tachycardia. Ventricular tachycardia with RBBB morphology and inferior right-sided axis. Notice the ventriculoatrial 1:1 conduction (indicated in V_1 – P'). The patient is on verapamil and is asymptomatic. *Source:* Courtesy of Dr. Jacob Atié, Cardioritmo group, Rio de Janeiro, Brazil.

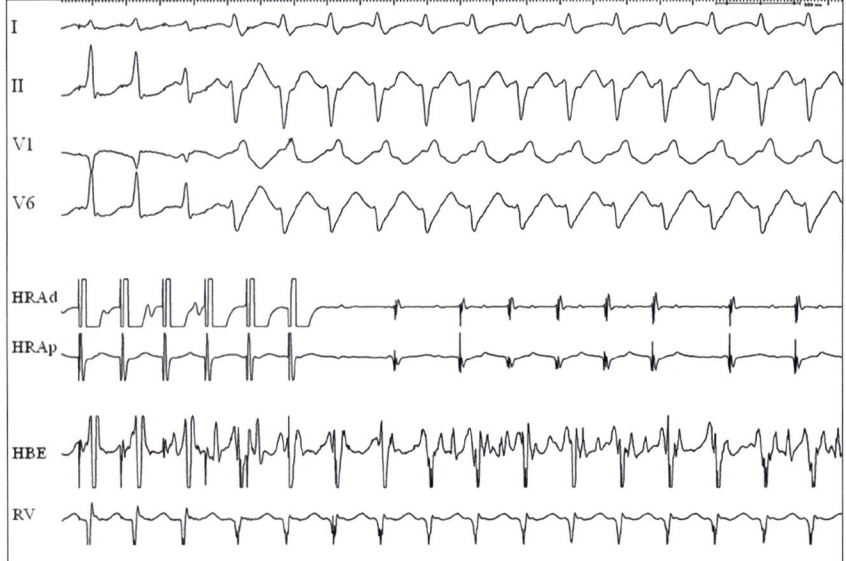

Figure 31.17A Young female (35 years old) patient undergoing catheter ablation for fascicular VT. Induction with fast atrium pacing after orciprenalin infusion. Notice ventriculoatrial conduction with Wenckebach block (tracing speed 50 mm/sec). Intracardiac signals from top to bottom: Four surface ECG leads, 2 high atrial electrograms distal and proximal (HRAd/p), His bundle recording (HBE), and right ventricle electrogram (RV). VT = ventricular tachycardia.

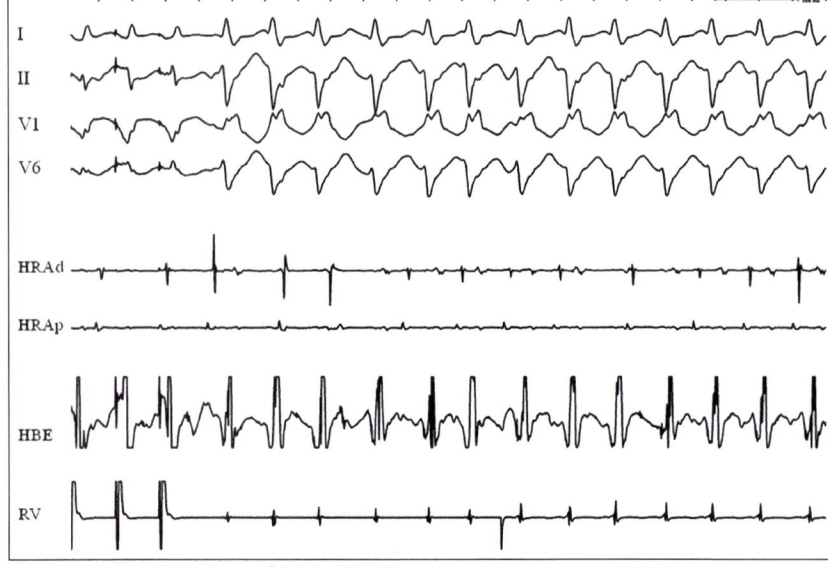

Figure 31.17B Same patient in Figure 31.17A. Tachycardia induction with ventricular fast stimulation (tracing speed 50 mm/sec).

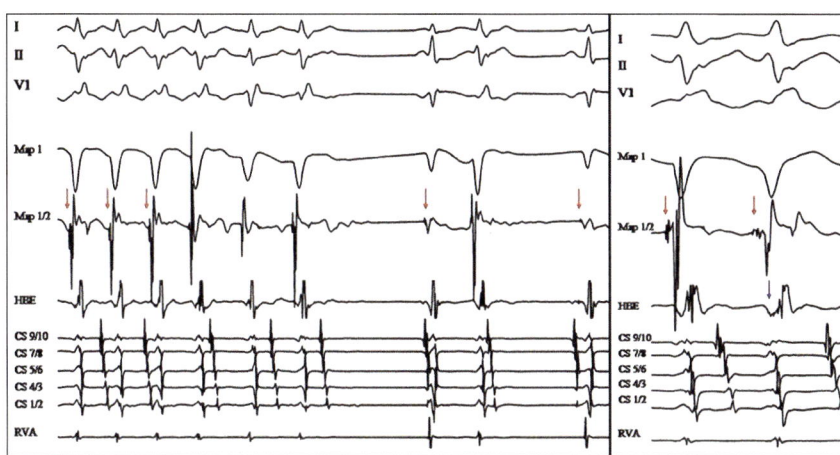

Figure 31.17C Same patient in Figure 31.17A. During mapping of the inferior midseptal area of the left ventricle during tachycardia. **Left panel** (tracing speed 50 mm/sec): Purkinje earliest activation (**red arrows**) and mechanical termination of the tachycardia. Note Purkinje potential at the ablation catheter in sinus rhythm. **Right panel** (tracing speed 100 mm/sec): Close look at the Purkinje potential (**red arrows**) and a small His bundle recording (**blue arrow**), which is also seen in the left panel after tachycardia termination.

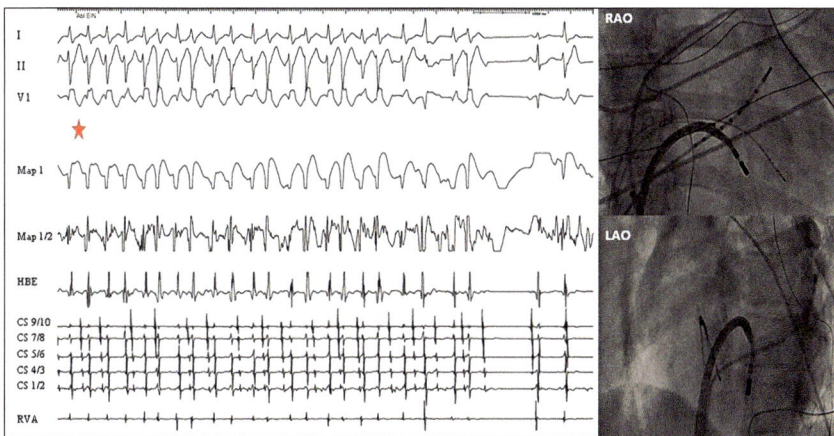

Figure 31.17D Same patient in Figure 31.17A. Successful ablation (beginning of ablation—**red star, left panel**) at the inferobasal area of the left septum (**right panel**) with the tachycardia termination. Note that after the fifth beat, the tachycardia shows a "regular" irregularity that might be related to a Wenckebach conduction block at the level of the VT circuit or exit. This phenomenon can be often observed but is poorly reported.

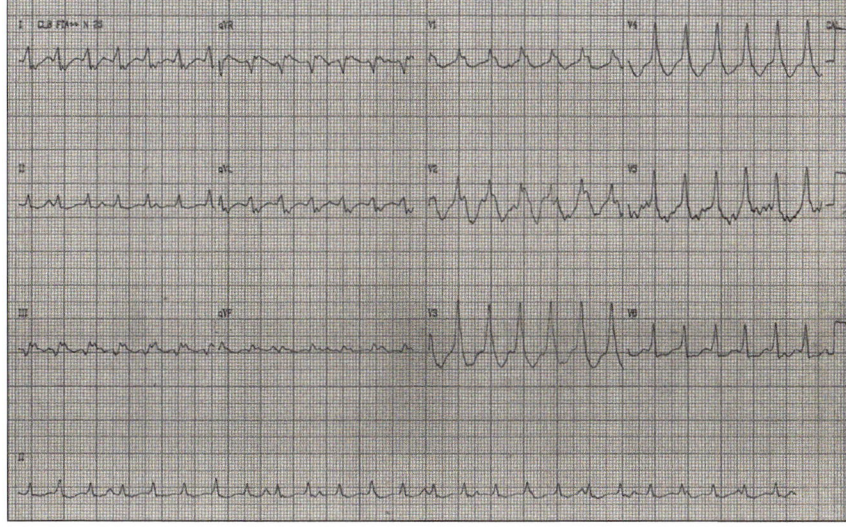

Figure 31.18 Female patient (35 years old) came to the emergency room feeling strong palpitations. Had a history of paroxysmal tachycardia since 20 years of age. Ventricular tachycardia with RBBB morphology and an axis of 0°. Notice AV dissociation. The VT exit point suggests to be midseptal at the basal portion. No structural heart disease was detected. VT = ventricular tachycardia.

Workflow in the Electrophysiology Laboratory

Following the rationale for OT-VTs, the workflow in the EP-Lab initiates with ECG analysis.

Methodology here is the same as described for OT-VTs with some particularities, including: (1) election of vascular access (depends on operators' experience to access the left ventricle, either transaortic retrograde or transseptal puncture); (2) need of anticoagulation (heparin) during the procedure; and (3) the strategy itself.

LFVTs are also didactically divided according to ECG morphology as explained before, ie, LPI-VT, LAS-VT, and MS-VT. For all three entities, means and methods for ablation share the same concepts, which are addressed stepwise as following:

Study Catheters: Standard placement of a 4-pole fixed curve study catheter in the RVa and a 10-pole deflectable catheter in the coronary sinus is of great value because:

- RVa catheter:
  - VT induction and control after radiofrequency ablation;
  - Backup ventricular pacing (eg, termination of VT);
  - Reference for mapping systems (considering in a stable position);
  - Anatomic reference at fluoroscopy.

- Coronary sinus catheter:
  - Ventricular EGM comparison whether the VT is closer to proximal or distal coronary sinus poles;
  - Back up atrial pacing (eg, eventual VT induction; atrial pacing for catheter stability);
  - Anatomic reference at fluoroscopy, especially for transseptal puncture;
  - Helps operators to infer patient's anatomy, especially left ventricle transversal size and position (horizontal or vertical hearts) according to mitral annulus position.

Ablation Catheter: In the left ventricle, where myocardium is the most robust, the use of irrigated-tip catheters is preferable because they accomplish more consistent and deeper lesions with mapping precision in comparison to 4 mm or 8 mm tips.[57] Preferences of catheters' characteristics vary among operators; however, some particularities must be addressed. Normally these patients are young with small hearts; therefore, we generally recommend catheters with small curves. However, this choice is made by evidence of other exams like echocardiography, MRI, or CT and the fluoroscopic operator's impression of the anatomy.

In our experience, once accessing retrograde through the aorta, a small or middle curve is recommended to reach the areas of LPI or LAS fascicles, respectively. Transseptal approach may lead to the opposite choice, ie, small curve to LAS area and middle to LPI area. Sometimes it is necessary to use a large curve in order to reach more easily the apical portion of the septum.

Radiofrequency Settings: Settings for radiofrequency may vary among groups.[71,80,81] Considering standard usage of irrigated-tip ablation catheter, power and temperature settings should be higher than for OT-VTs because ablation is performed in a thick myocardium (left ventricle). Suggestions would be for 40 to 50W / 40–48°C, respectively. Rarely, titration of power up to 55 or 60W is needed. Time of radiofrequency application may be the same for OT-VT (ie, 60 or 90 seconds each pulse).

Using external irrigated-tip catheters within the left ventricle chamber involves less risk for catheter thrombus, thus "stem-POP," when compared to 8 mm–tip catheters.[57] "Stem-POPs" happen not rarely within the left ventricle and show to be less harmful as within RVOT, probably because of left ventricle thickness.

Stimulation and Ablation Strategies: After all initial steps of monitoring the patient, setting up systems, sedation, groin punctures, and catheter placement, it is time to induce the clinical arrhythmia. Usually these patients already have an ECG of the clinical VT, thus stimulation maneuvers should target induction of this one. Frequently, other arrhythmias are induced, which may disturb the VT ablation, like nodal reentry tachycardia or atrial fibrillation.

Induction can be accomplished with programmed ventricular or atrial stimulation (Figure 31.17A and B). Like other arrhythmias, stimulation maneuvers are also control parameters for ablation success. Protocols vary widely (suggestion, see Parr I or OT-VT); however, importantly, refractory periods from His-Purkinje and ventricles should be reached and measured until VT induction. This parameter is the essence of VT reentry mechanism and serves as a control value as well. Sometimes pharmacological stress (eg, orciprenalin, isoproterenol, or dobutamine) must be associated with programmed stimulations to induce VT.

During VT, resetting and entrainment maneuvers from atrium or ventricle can confirm the reentrant characteristic by entrainment reproducibility and same return cycle or postpacing interval (PPI).

Next step is accessing the left ventricle, either retrograde transaortic approach or transseptal puncture. ECG morphology from VT should guide the ablation catheter placement, ie, superior axis = inferior region (LPI); inferior axis = anterior region (LAS).

A stepwise mapping process follows:

1. VT induction and left ventricle assessment;
2. Mapping VT earliest local activation;
3. Local entrainment and PPI–tachycardia cycle length (TCL) measurement;
4. Detecting diastolic Purkinje potentials during VT.

Early local activation is important to reach proximity with VT exit spot; however, evidence of early local Purkinje signal before the ventricular EGM and QRS onset indicates an excellent target for ablation because left ventricle fascicles make part of VT circuit and constitute critical arms for reentry[69,80] (Figure 31.17C and D). Purkinje signals can be seen in a "local middle diastolic" (closer to basal portion of left ventricle septum) or "presystolic" (closer to apical portion of left ventricle septum) position as seen in Figure 31.17C. Personally we prefer to ablate at a spot with "presystolic" Purkinje EGM, which may correspond to the terminal portion of reentry circuit within the fascicle or fascicle-ventricle tissue.

In practical terms, ablation is usually attempted at the inferoseptal aspect of left ventricle (in case of LPI-VT typical form), more distally as possible, ie, closer to left ventricle apex. However, sometimes it must be extended to more inferobasal areas to accomplish success.

Entrainment maneuver within the left ventricle and measurement of the returning cycle (PPI-TCL) at ablation catheter, as previously described, confirm catheter position within the circuit, ie, values between 0 and 20 ms.

Pace mapping can also be done as an adjunctive maneuver to locate VT exit, especially when VT is nonsustained. Here we also suggest usage of different output voltages because local capture may be wide and include muscle tissue rather than just Purkinje fibers. Three-dimensional mapping systems may help, especially in locating structures such as mitral annulus, papillary muscles, His bundle and fascicles, and places previously ablated.

After successful ablation, changes in the baseline QRS complex can be observed as right axis deviation with increased S waves in lead I and aVL, and increased R waves and/or qR morphology in inferior leads, meaning partial ablation of the LPI-fascicle (Figure 31.19). This sign is a good indicator of noninducibility and procedural success.[80]

One interesting case is presented in Figure 31.14, A–E. As discussed before, the LAS-fascicle could play a role in the tachycardia as being the retrograde arm of the circuit. This patient without any structural heart disease presents a VT that could be reproducibly induced from the atrium with the same behavior. The patient presented a baseline LAH, and 2 atrial extrastimuli were sufficient to make the LPI also relatively refractory, which could delay the wavefront at a critical time to enable a "pseudo-normal" intraventricular conduction, suggested by the normal QRS morphology after the second extrastimulus. This phenomenon indicates that the LAS-fascicle had no complete block but a delayed conduction. Coincidentally in this tracing, a spontaneous atrium extrasystole conducts to the ventricle with an incomplete block at the LAS-fascicle (intermediate QRS morphology) showing that the LPI-fascicle is slightly less refractory. At this moment, the wavefront reaches the distal portion of the LAS-fascicle, which permits retrograde conduction and subsequently antegrade activation of the "now recovered" LPI-fascicle with the induction and perpetuation of the VT (Figure 31.14D). Despite the broad QRS, this VT was considered to be fascicular because: (1) the patient had no structural heart abnormalities; (2) the VT could be reproducibly induced (Figure 31.14A and B) and terminated (Figure 31.14C) from the atrium; (3) the VT could be entrained from the ventricle; and (4) it was successfully ablated at the inferobasal portion of the left interventricular septum (Figure 31.14E).

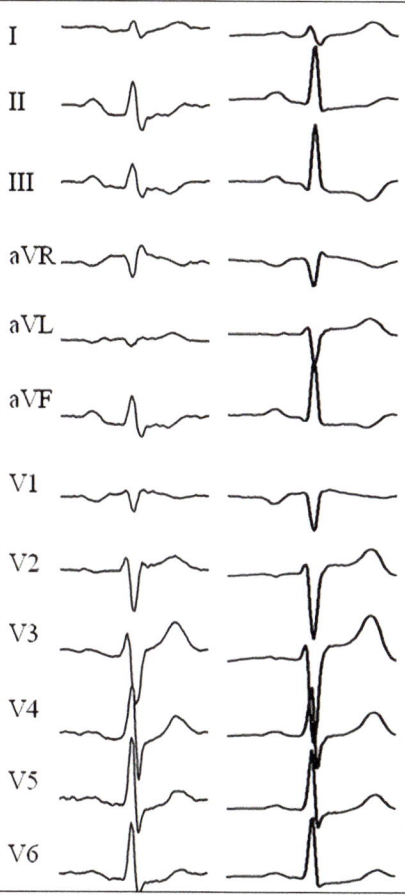

Figure 31.19 Case of the patient presented in Figure 31.14A-D. Baseline QRS morphology before (**left panel**) and after (**right panel**) ablation. Note a slight change in the QRS duration and axis with an increased S wave in I and aVL indicating partial damage of the LPI. This is one of the criteria of ablation success (see text for explanations).

Precautions:

- Careful groin punctures, especially arterial access;
- Intravenous heparin is necessary to keep an activation clotting time usually ≥ 270 seconds;
- Precautions related to transseptal punctures and/or passing through aortic valve;
- Locate His bundle during mapping and avoid ablating at its proximity;
- Careful moves within the left ventricle to avoid mechanical lesions in structures such as tendineae chordae or papillary muscles.

Follow-up and Prognosis

LFVTs are known to have an excellent prognosis but in some cases (eg, concomitant genetic syndromes) can induce other malignant arrhythmias. Patients under clinical treatment with verapamil rarely have tachycardia recurrences. In case of recurrences, changes in verapamil dosage or catheter ablation should be performed. Verapamil may be helpful in patients with mild symptoms. When symptoms are severe and pharmacologic treatment is not effective or is poorly tolerated, catheter ablation is recommended and might be the first therapy line in selected cases.[2,67] Ablation success rates as reported in various series vary between 85% and 95% and are generally higher in those patients with posterior LPI-VT with variable recurrence rates (5% vs 12.5%).[2] Procedural complications are rare, and the most common is the development of left bundle branch or atrioventricular block. Damage of the aortic valve when retrograde aortic approach is performed or complications related to transseptal puncture can also occur. LFVTs are considered benign with good prognosis and rare incidence of syncope and sudden death.

PART III: PAPILLARY MUSCLE ARRHYTHMIAS

Introduction

Since the early 1960s, several studies have sought to evaluate the anatomy and physiology of the papillary muscles (PapM), especially concerning mitral valve function in humans and animals.[82,83] Arrhythmias originating at the level of the PapM are normally linked to structural heart disease as ischemic cardiomyopathy.[84] Nevertheless, very recently these arrhythmias have been recognized as a distinct entity in patients without structural heart abnormalities.[85] These arrhythmias can arise most frequently from the left posterior (posteroseptal) papillary muscle (LP-PapM)[86,87] or from the left anterior (anterolateral) papillary muscle (LA-PapM)[86] and from the right ventricle papillary muscles (RV-PapM).[87,88] In the absence of structural heart disease, VT/PVCs originating from the RV-PapM are more uncommon and seem to have a benign prognosis.[87]

Understanding the anatomy is a key determinant for diagnosis based on the surface ECG and for the therapeutic strategy. Although this group of arrhythmias does not share the same pathophysiological mechanisms of the outflow tract VT or fascicular VT, clinical presentations may have some common features.

The decision to treat is based on symptoms or development of dilated cardiomyopathy, and catheter ablation is a feasible and efficient therapeutic method[85-87] as further detailed.

Anatomy and Pathophysiology

There are a total of five PapM in the heart—three in the right ventricle and two in the left ventricle. The anterior (free wall), inferoseptal, and midseptal PapM of the right ventricle attach to each tricuspid leaflet of the tricuspid valve via chordae tendineae and the anterior and posterior PapM of the left ventricle attach to the mitral valve. A rare third group of left accessories PapM was also described, located posterobasally.[89] There are different anatomical classifications to describe the left PapM. Some authors use a surgical classification in respect to the orthogonal plan of the heart in the thorax.[90] Analyzing the transversal view of the left ventricle, the PapM located at the free wall is posterior or lateral and superior, and the one closer to the septal aspect is anterior or septal and inferior (Figure 31.20A).[9] We use the traditional nomenclature in this chapter (Figure 31.20B).

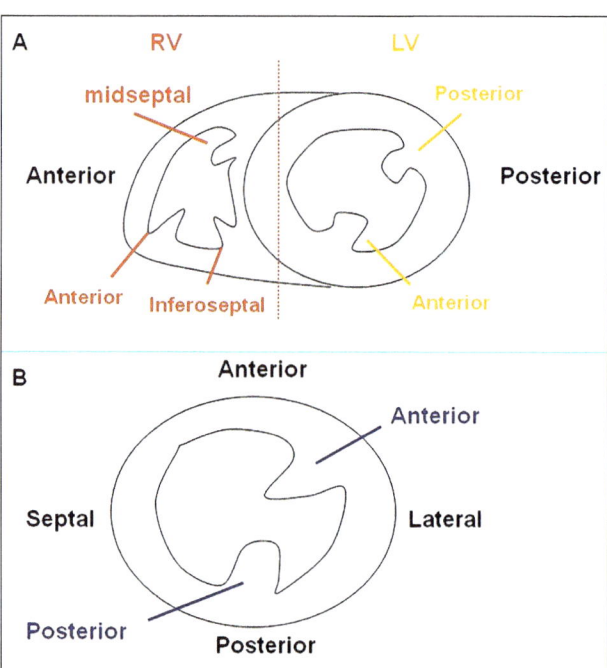

Figure 31.20 Scheme demonstrating the usual anatomy of all five papillary muscles in transversal view. **Panel A:** Spatial classification. **Panel B:** Traditional classification at the left ventricle.

The pathophysiological mechanisms of idiopathic arrhythmias originating at the PM are not completely understood. The arrhythmias are often induced by exercise and infusion of isoproterenol or epinephrine.[91]

Evidence suggests a focal mechanism instead of reentry because (1) they cannot be entrained; (2) they have a relatively late diastolic activation time at the site of ablation; (3) the local activation sequence of the first beat of the VT is the same as the subsequent beats; and (4) there has been an observed absence of fractionated potentials at the ablation site.[91] The incidence and prevalence of this arrhythmia is higher in older patients in comparison to fascicular VTs[9] and might be related to microcalcifications around and within the PapM related to aging—a phenomenon often seen within the mitral-aortic fibrous apparatus. In some cases of PapM-PVCs, the observation of a fixed coupling interval suggests a microreentry mechanism. Good et al[9] showed that 2 of 7 patients with PapM-VTs who underwent cardiac MRI had delayed enhancement within the arrhythmogenic PapM. Similar results were found in 3 of 35 patients reported by Yokokawa et al.[92]

Clinical Aspects and Clinical Management

This subtype of idiopathic ventricular arrhythmia is very uncommon in clinical practice and corresponds to 3% to 10% of all idiopathic arrhythmias referred to specialized centers for catheter ablation[9,91] and around 1% of all ventricular arrhythmias referred for catheter ablation.[93]

The mean prevalence according to age group is largely variable compared to outflow tract or fascicular VT/PVC. The mean age of first symptoms and diagnosis is between 40 and 60 years old in patients who are referred to specialized centers.[9,85,91] It is usually more prevalent in male patients, and around 50% of episodes are induced by exercise.[91]

The most common clinical presentation is in the form of PVCs, and nonsustained VT (NSVT) accounts for 75% of cases. The duration of symptoms can vary from 1 month up to 10 years.[9,85,91]

In comparison to other idiopathic ventricular arrhythmias, patients presenting with PapM arrhythmias should be screened for the presence of any heart structural disorder, which is sometimes evident with detailed cardiac imaging. Good et al[9] showed in their series that 4 of 9 patients had dilative cardiomyopathy and all presented PVCs instead of VT. Another study, a retrospective analysis of 40 cases with PapM arrhythmias by Yokokawa and colleagues, reported ischemic and dilative cardiomyopathy in 10 and 9 patients, respectively.[92]

Practice in the Electrophysiology Laboratory

The Electrocardiogram

The ECG in sinus rhythm is usually normal; however, some patients can present negative T waves following the VT/PVC axis corresponding to a cardiac memory phenomenon.

The QRS morphology during PapM-VT/PVC exhibits a right bundle branch block with a superior axis configuration in around 80% of the cases corresponding to an origin at the LP-PapM (Figure 31.21).[85,86,91]

In comparison with the fascicular VTs, the QRS duration in patients with PapM-VTs is usually wider (usually above 140 ms) (Figure 31.22). In these patients, structural heart disease and different VT/PVC morphologies (pleomorphic) are more often encountered.[9]

One diagnostic criteria of PapM-VT/PVC at surface ECG is a QRS morphology that resembles a left bundle anterior hemiblock without the first activation vector at peripheral leads (Figure 31.22). The differential diagnosis can be challenging in some cases, especially in young patients, leading to different therapeutic strategies. One must be aware of normal heart rotations that could lead to difficulties in ECG interpretations, so baseline QRS should be also carefully analyzed. This again shows the importance of standardized and correct placement of surface–ECG electrodes.[48-53]

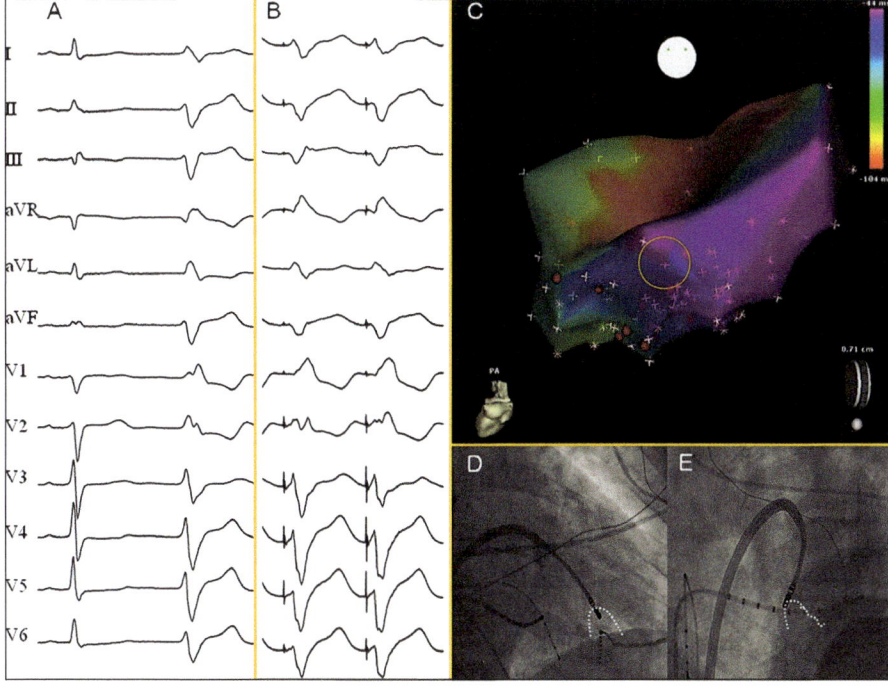

Figure 31.21 Example of a 54-year-old male patient with symptomatic PVCs refractory to β-blockers. **Panel A:** 12 lead-ECG from the normal and PVC QRS complexes, respectively. **Panel B:** Pace mapping at the successful ablation site. **Panel C:** Electroanatomical color-coded activation map showing the earliest activation at a "floating" spot corresponding to the medial aspect of the inferior PM body. Notice the high number of points around the basis of this PM. **Panels D and E:** RAO and LAO fluoroscopic projections, respectively, at the successful ablation spot. Notice in LAO that the catheter is pointing slightly inferoseptal, showing that the catheter contact, with the medial aspect of the inferolateral PM body, had been done with the lateral part of the tip. At that moment in LAO, the catheter was moving from posterior to anterior with the cycle diastole to systole, respectively, despite good contact with the PM.
PM = papillary muscle; PVC = premature ventricular contraction.

Workflow in the Electrophysiology Laboratory

As mentioned before, the recognition of the VT/PVC morphology at the surface 12-lead ECG is fundamental for the diagnosis, presumable location, and orientation for cardiac mapping and treatment (see "The Electrocardiogram" in Part IV).

The methodology of setup of all equipment, catheter selection and placement, radiofrequency settings, and vascular accesses is the same for left fascicular VT.

Stimulation and ablation strategies share the same principles for OT-VT and LFVT. QRS morphologies of PapM-VT/PVC usually have a superior axis, thus the placement of a catheter deep in coronary sinus around mitral annulus is not necessary. First, PM are complex structures with large and trabecular base and punctiform top where the chordae tendineae inserts. Arrhythmia may originate everywhere along this structure, so mapping and ablation may be more difficult and take more time compared to LFVT, especially if VT/PVC originates at the body of PapM (Figure 31.13). VT arising from the bottom or basis of PapM may show different areas of same precocities. This aspect implies that the focus might originate exactly under the PapM body, deep within the myocardium, consequently reducing efficacy of radiofrequency ablation.

Mapping techniques here should focus on EGM precocity rather than finding reentrant circuits due to the nature of electrophysiologic mechanisms discussed previously. In around one-third of cases, a Purkinje potential can be found at the successful site of ablation.[9,92] Pace mapping may be used to confirm a good target for ablation, especially if EGM precocity shows no optimal value. In summary, a place with the earliest EGM with the closest pace mapping match (higher than 10/12 leads) should be one ablation target (Figure 31.21).

Left ventricle access depends on operators' experience. In our experience, left ventricle access through transseptal puncture with a deflectable long sheath (placed at the level of mitral annulus) facilitates catheter movements around papillary muscles during mapping and ablation.

Three-dimensional mapping systems may have more advantages when used in PapM-VT compared with OT-VT and LFVT because: (1) they locate and mark more precisely His bundle and fascicles, especially LPI; (2) PapM anatomy might be more difficult to define with just fluoroscopic information; (3) trabecular tissue surrounding the PMs makes it difficult to place ablation catheter in the same position repeatedly; (4) they aid in defining areas where ablation attempts were performed with or without success; and (5) these arrhythmias can change the exit if the focus is located deep within the basis of the PapM, thus discrete changes in QRS morphology may happen during ablation. Figure 31.21 exemplifies the importance of 3D cardiac mapping for the management of PapM arrhythmias.[94]

Successful ablation is indicated mainly by termination of VT/PVC and noninducibility.

Follow-up and Prognosis

Several studies showed that the idiopathic form of PapM-VT/PVC appears to have a benign prognosis, especially after successful ablation,[9,85,91] and even after arrhythmia recurrence.[85]

In some cases of arrhythmia-associated cardiomyopathy, successful ablation can reverse ventricular dysfunction,[9] so it should be strongly considered in this situation. It is

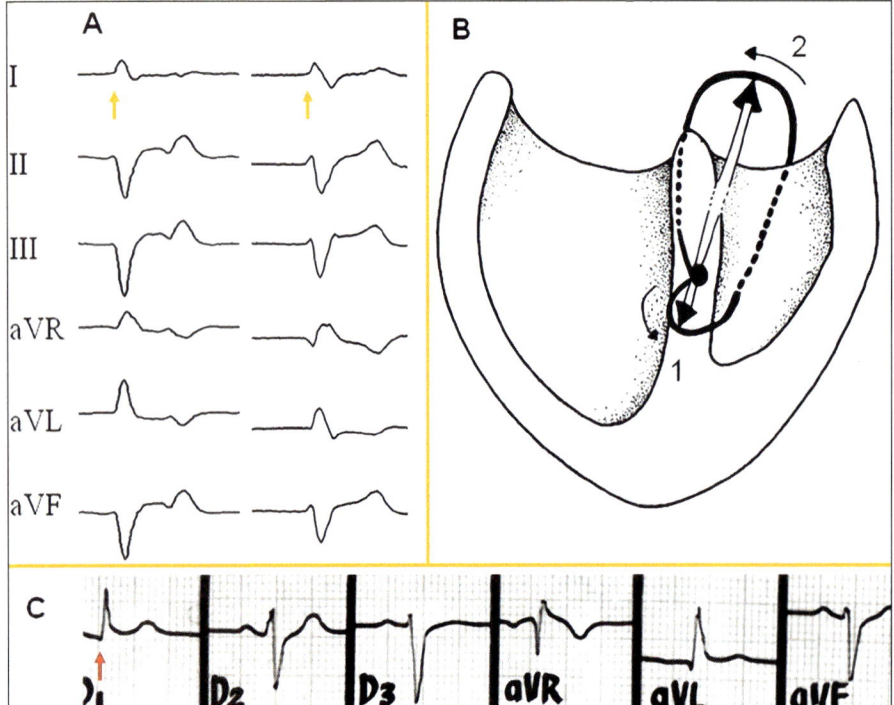

Figure 31.22 Example showing 2 different PM-PVC morphologies from 2 distinct patients at the peripheral leads (**Panel A**). **Panels B and C**: A scheme and an ECG (**peripheral leads**) of a left anterosuperior hemiblock, respectively. Notice the presence of the vector 1 (**red arrow in Panel C**) indicated by the q wave in lead I and aVL. There are no q waves in leads I and aVL from the PM-PVC QRS complexes (**indicated by the yellow arrows**). PM = papillary muscle; PVC = premature ventricular contraction.

important to investigate patients with these arrhythmias for structural heart diseases, because myocardial infarction/ischemia can be presented and carries a poor prognosis.[95] Catheter ablation must be considered in symptomatic patients in whom pharmacological approach failed or is contraindicated, or even in some cases as the first-line therapy due to high success rates, including patients with ischemic heart disease.[95]

PART IV: VENTRICULAR ARRHYTHMIAS FROM THE VALVE ANNULI

Introduction

Ventricular arrhythmias arising from the valve annuli, also sometimes known as idiopathic annular ventricular arrhythmias (IAVA), have been recognized as an independent group of idiopathic arrhythmias accounting for around 3%–15% of cases referred for catheter ablation,[96-98] thus not so uncommon. These arrhythmias manifest most frequently as isolated PVCs and originate around the rings of the tricuspid and mitral annulus, frequently within the anteroseptal area close to the His bundle.[97-99] Arrhythmias in this portion are often called para-Hisian VT/PVCs.

Treatment strategies are basically the same as those used for outflow tract arrhythmias, evolving pharmacological, and/or invasive catheter ablation approach. The latest seems to have good results with rare complications[97-100] except the para-Hisian variant, which leads to lower success rates.[97]

These arrhythmias have a benign behavior with a good prognosis; nevertheless, patients presenting such arrhythmias should be screened for structural heart disease.

Pathophysiology

The electrophysiologic mechanism of this subtype of idiopathic ventricular arrhythmia is still unclear. Some studies suggest that they could share the same mechanisms as the outflow tract tachycardias, ie, cAMP-dependent automaticity and/or microreentry within slow conduction areas, as those originating from the cusps, indicated by fractionated signals found at the successful ablation site.[50] Wu and colleagues reported that in 5 of 16 patients with IAVA referred for catheter ablation, spike early potentials were found at the successful ablation sites, which could indicate the association with remnants of Purkinje fibers.[100] However, Tada et al report no preceding Purkinje-like potentials at the successful ablation spots in 31 patients undergoing catheter ablation for arrhythmias arising at the tricuspid annulus.[97]

Both mechanisms of automaticity and reentry may be involved, with or without registration of Purkinje potentials, and might be supported by the fact that the IAVA often present a fixed coupled interval and can be induced by programmed stimulation and/or sympathomimetic medication infusion.[97]

Clinical Aspects and Management

Idiopathic arrhythmias arising from the atrioventricular annuli are uncommon, and there are just few reports in literature, so it is difficult to describe epidemiology. IAVA are often detected in older patients more than RVOT or fascicular arrhythmias. Tada et al[97] report mean age of overall incidence of 61 years old and greater frequency in male patients (3:2) in their series of tricuspid annulus arrhythmias; however, the para-Hisian variant could also occur in younger patients.[101]

IAVA manifest mostly at the form of PVCs than VTs[97,99,100] and seem to occur more within the mitral than tricuspid annulus.[100]

Patients may be asymptomatic or may develop cardiomyopathy.[96] Treatment should be considered in symptomatic patients and in those who develop or are progressively developing cardiomyopathy. This group may not be compliant to the treatment due to absence of symptoms; therefore, they should be correctly informed about the disease and its possible consequences. It is important that patients be evaluated for structural or genetic heart disorders. A detailed anamnesis, physical examination, ECG, thorax radioscopy, and echocardiography are enough for the first screening.

Practice in the Electrophysiology Laboratory

The Electrocardiogram

According to anatomy, it is logical that ECG patterns are different regarding the origin within the tricuspid or mitral annulus, following the same rationale as for accessory pathway algorithms. Wu et al[100] have compared patients with annular VT/PVCs and the corresponding ECG pattern in patients with WPW syndrome. The correlation would be quite precise except for the fact that the spontaneous preexcitation in WPW patients is rarely maximal. Moreover, the authors suggest that algorithms used to locate WPW accessory pathways could give a good clue to locate the origin of annular VT/PVCs.[102,103] In this chapter, the ECG morphologies should be divided into tricuspid annulus, mitral annulus, and para-Hisian region (Figure 31.23).

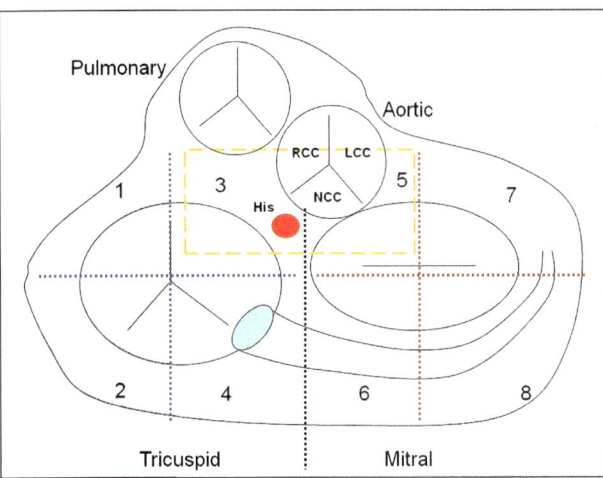

Figure 31.23 Schematic view (from the apex of the heart) of the atrioventricular septum (valves plan) and schematic division into regions. Tricuspid annulus (**blue lines**): 1 – anterolateral right; 2 – inferolateral right; 3 – anteroseptal right (para-Hisian); 4 – inferoseptal right or posteroseptal right; mitralannulus (**red lines**): 5 – anterosuperior left (mitral-aortic continuity); 6 – posteroseptal left; 7 – anterolateral left; 8 – posterolateral left. The regions 3 and 5 are close to the His bundle; however, the closest is the 3. Anatomy of the aortic cusps is also indicated: notice the relationship of the right and noncoronary cusps with the RVOT and the left and noncoronary cusps with the LVOT (basically mitral valve and mitral-aortic continuity). LVOT = left ventricular outflow tract; RVOT = right ventricular outflow tract.

Tricuspid Annulus

Arrhythmias arising from tricuspid annulus demonstrate left bundle branch block (LBBB) QRS morphology and positive QRS pattern in left leads: I, V_5, and V_6. Usually the QRS complex in lead I exhibits a complete positive pattern independently on the site of origin (sites 1 to 4 in Figure 31.23). The inferior leads (II, III, and aVF) show an inferior axis when the origin is superior or anterior (Figure 31.23, sites 1 and 3), or superior axis when the origin is inferior or posterior (Figure 31.23, sites 2 and 4). The recognition of the QRS morphology in inferior leads is very useful to distinguish between septal and lateral origins. Basically, arrhythmias coming from the regions 1 and 4 show major amplitude of the activation vector in lead II, and from regions 2 and 3, in lead III. Detailed descriptions of the possible morphologies have been recently published.[97,99]

In precordial leads, the QRS complex presents in V_1 a QS or rS pattern, and in V_6 an R pattern. The transitional zone varies and generally relies between V_3 and V_4 (Figure 31.24).[97,99]

Some authors consider the para-Hisian region as a part of the tricuspid annulus mainly due to the anatomical aspect; however, this area has distinct electrophysiological properties, and catheter ablation has a lower success rate.[97]

Yue-Chun et al[99] reported a series of 35 patients undergoing ablation of VT/PVCs arising from the vicinity of tricuspid annulus, and ECG showed some distinctive characteristics:

- rS pattern in lead V_1 most frequently from the free wall than from the septal aspect (93.1% vs 16.7%);
- Precordial late R-wave transition (beyond V_3) of VT/PVC from the free wall rather than earlier when it came from the septal portion of the TA;
- All patients had an R-wave pattern in leads I, V_5, and V_6;
- All patients had a QS pattern in aVR.

Mitral Annulus

These arrhythmias, as opposed to those from the tricuspid annulus, typically show a QRS complex with a right bundle branch block (RBBB) pattern with a pure R wave in V_1,[104,105] except when it is coming from the posteroseptal aspect of the mitral annulus, which can present a Q-wave component.[105]

Peripheral leads play a major role in locating the origin of the foci. Coming from anterior and/or anterolateral portions (regions 5 and 7 from Figure 31.23), leads I and aVL exhibit a major negative QRS complex with QS or rS pattern. The inferior leads show a positive pattern usually with a pure R wave; however, in some cases a qR or Rs morphology can be present.[105] In case of origin from the lateral or posterior region (regions 7 and 9 from Figure 31.23), leads I and aVL can show a QS or rS pattern, and inferior leads exhibit a positive polarity[104] usually with an R-wave morphology. In this situation, Kumagai et al also reported different patterns in V_6 translated in RS, rS, or Rs.[104] Once arising from the posteroseptal region (region 6 from Figure 31.23), I and aVL have a positive pattern with a monophasic R wave and the inferior leads showing the opposite with a QS or rS complex.[104,105]

As V_1 usually shows a complete positive pattern, there is no classical transitional zone unless it presents with biphasic morphology. In this situation, the transitional zone occurs very early (V_1 or V_2).[104,105]

Of interest is a report by Tada et al that a terminal S wave in lead I could help differentiate anterior and anterolateral and posterior morphologies from a posteroseptal origin. Furthermore, they observed a late-phase "notching" of the QRS complex in inferior leads in cases of anterolateral and posterior origin.[105] This finding may result from phased excitation from the left ventricle free wall to the right ventricle. We also believe that there might be a relative "slow" conduction time or a "breakthrough" conduction delay within the interventricular septum, which could also explain this "notching." In their series, the QRS duration was longer in cases of anterolateral and posterior foci (>140 ms) than in the posteroseptal origin.[105]

Mitral annulus VTs could be also compared with WPW and cusp-VT patients.[104] Kumagai et al compared the mitral annulus arrhythmias with 22 matched WPW patients, and the arrhythmias coming from the corresponding segment with maximal preexcitation showed good concordance at the surface ECG, which suggests a deep subendocardial origin (also reflected by the finding of something like a delta wave in some cases). On the other hand, when compared with VTs arising from the aortic cusps, the only important difference was a longer intrinsic deflection time of the annular VT.[105] One case is illustrated in Figure 31.25.

Para-Hisian Region

This group of IAVA presents some peculiar characteristics at the surface ECG, as follows (Figure 31.26):

- A tall monophasic R wave in lead I and aVL (this last can present also as Rs);
- A relatively narrow QRS in the inferior leads;
- Inferior axis with a R wave in lead II > III;
- LBBB morphology with a QS or Qr pattern in lead V_1;
- Early precordial transitional zone (leads V_2-V_3);
- Relatively tall R wave in V_5 and V_6.

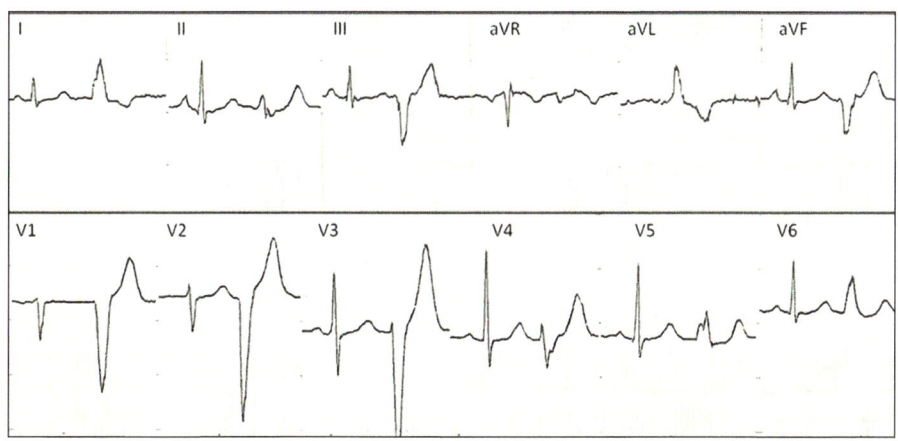

Figure 31.24 Case of a 23-year-old female patient with constant palpitations without any structural heart disease. The QRS morphology is an example of PVC coming from posterolateral aspect of tricuspid annulus.

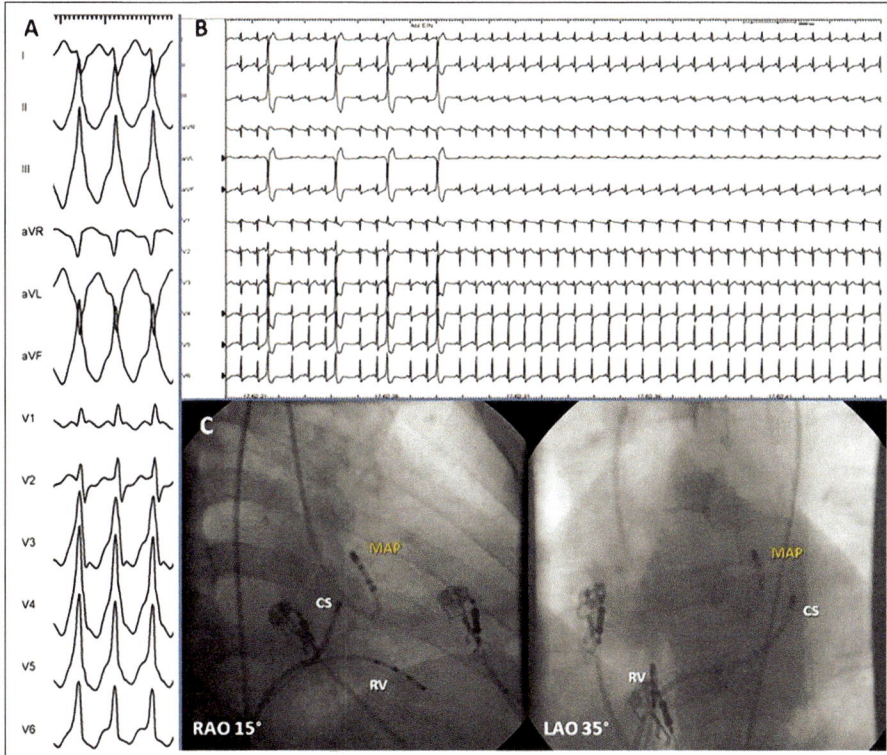

Figure 31.25 Case of a 39-year-old male patient with symptomatic VT and PVC undergoing catheter ablation. Transaortic approach was done. **Panel A:** Induced VT. **Panel B:** Spontaneous PVC. At the moment ablation began, the arrhythmia disappeared. **Panel C:** Fluoroscopy images (from left to right, RAO 15° and LAO 35°) showing the area of ablation (between regions 5 and 7 from Figure 31.23). Position of the coronary sinus (CS), right ventricle (RV), and mapping (MAP) catheters are indicated. PVC = premature ventricular contraction; VT = ventricular tachycardia.

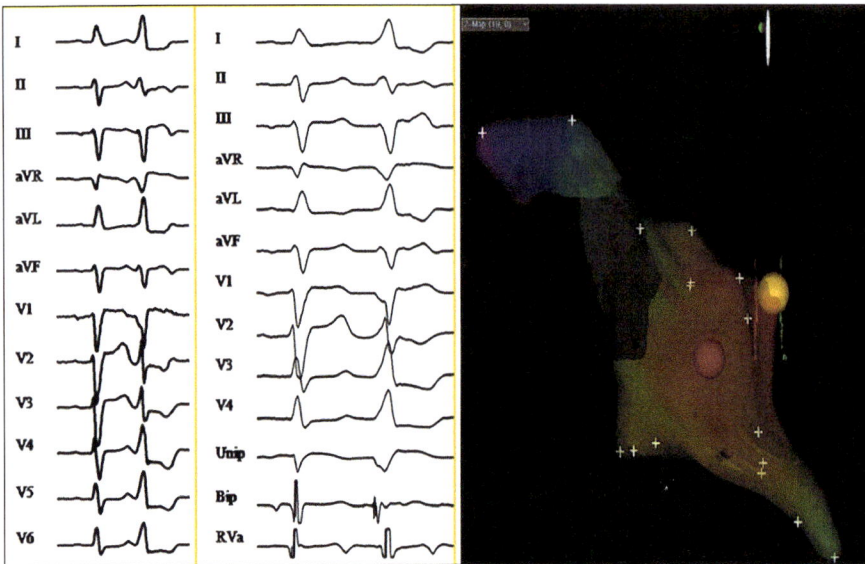

Figure 31.26 Example of a 55-year-old male patient with symptomatic extrasystoles. **Panel A:** 12-lead ECG in 25 mm/sec of the sinus rhythm QRS complex presenting a left anterior hemiblock and the QRS complex of the ventricular extrasystole. Note the monophasic R wave in lead I and aVL, QS in V_1, and early precordial transition (V_1-V_2). **Panel B:** EGM of the successful ablation site—**top to botton:** ECG leads from I to V_4, unipolar (Unip) and bipolar (Bip) EGM from the ablation catheter tip, and EGM from a catheter in RVa (speed 50 mm/sec). Notice the absence of the His signal in sinus rhythm and a spike EGM at the Bip signal from the ablation catheter. **Panel C:** Electroanatomical color-coded map of the septal aspect of the tricuspid annulus in a left lateral view (from the ventricular septum). Note the His bundle (**yellow point**) and successful ablation site (**earliest activation region in red area**), approximately 5 mm from the His bundle (**red point**). This patient had transient complete AV block during ablation. EGM = electrogram; RVa = right ventricle apex.

An interesting study comparing the electrocardiographic characteristics of patients with para-Hisian ($n = 10$) versus RVOT arrhythmias ($n = 80$) significantly showed that para-Hisian arrhythmias presented mainly with monophasic and higher R waves in lead I (100% vs 53%) and QS pattern in lead V_1 (80% vs 17%).[98] In this study, Yamauchi and colleagues suggest that a combination of these parameters strongly predicts arrhythmias originating close to the His bundle.

Workflow in the Electrophysiology Laboratory

The procedure should follow the same steps used for the other idiopathic ventricular arrhythmias regarding the site of origin, ie, right or left annulus. Careful analysis of the ECG not just from the QRS pattern of the arrhythmia but also from the His-Purkinje QRS must be the first step.

The same workflow routine used for RVOT or LVOT is applied here, obviously depending on QRS morphology. When septal or para-Hisian VT/PVC is suspected, mapping should routinely start from the right side. Patients must be well informed about risks of AV block development.

In all cases, a study electrode catheter should be placed within the right ventricle apex. An electrode catheter at His bundle position is needed for tricuspid annulus VT/PVC, and one within coronary sinus is important for mitral annulus VT/PVC.

Similar to other arrhythmias, mapping techniques rely on precocity with QRS onset and pace mapping. Precocity of EGM and QS pattern in the unipolar signal from ablation catheter is determinant for a successful ablation. In case of para-Hisian arrhythmia, recording and pace mapping from an electrode catheter at His bundle position facilitate mapping and radiofrequency ablation.[98] Pace mapping should be performed in all cases to ensure a good position.

In case of retrograde mapping of the mitral annulus, one must be aware about the subvalvar apparatus, which complicates catheter moves (Figure 31.25). A good tip is to release the curve for every change of position. So, a stepwise approach for this issue with the ablation catheter at the ZERO position (straight without curve) would be:

- to reach more lateral aspects of mitral annulus: slightly curve deflection > clockwise turn > advance the catheter while deflecting and turning (or not) more clockwise as wished.

- to reach more septal aspect of mitral annulus: counterclockwise turn > slowly advance the catheter while deflecting and turning (or not) more counterclockwise as wished.

Kumagai and colleagues report a frequent finding of spike pre-potential signals in the local EGM at the effective ablation site and suggest it could be an indicator of ablation success.[104]

In some places around the tricuspid annuli, stability of the ablation catheter can be difficult, and long sheaths, especially steerable, may be used.

Facing a para-Hisian VT/PVC when the EGM of earliest activation stays exactly at the His bundle and there is a clear indication for ablation, radiofrequency should be applied first in regions around this spot and/or with a His deflection less than 0.1 mV.[98,106] Radiofrequency energy should be delivered with less power than recommended for RVOT-VT. We usually start with 10 W/40°C and titrate up the power according to the balance between disappearance of VT/PVC versus appearance of junctional rhythm. In such cases, cryoablation might be safer than radiofrequency energy in order to avoid damaging the His bundle.

Radiofrequency catheter ablation can achieve successful elimination of VT/PVCs arising from the tricuspid[97,99] and mitral annulus[104,105] with results reaching up to 100%.[105] However, Tada et al reported success of 57% for VT/PVCs arising close to the His bundle due to an insufficient energy delivery because of the appearance of junctional rhythm and risk or AV block.[9] As exposed before, radiofrequency delivery should be done with titration of power with careful monitoring of AV and/or VA conduction.[101,107]

Follow-up and Prognosis

Clinical prognosis is usually benign and a therapeutic strategy is often not necessary. Previous studies showed high success rates of catheter ablation for VT/PVCs originating at the tricuspid and mitral annulus[97,99,104,105] except for the para-Hisian variant.[97] Tada et al report a success rate of 100% in 19 patients presenting arrhythmias coming from the mitral annulus.[105] Recurrence rates of para-Hisian VT/PVCs are much higher than those originating at the RVOT.[27,108] Some investigators further suggest that para-Hisian VT/PVCs mimicking those originating from the RVOT are not so uncommon and tend to be more resistant to radiofrequency ablation.[27,109]

Catheter ablation has proven efficacy and safety and therefore should be recommended for this group of patients, especially those refractory or noncompliant to medical treatment. Selected patients could highly profit from catheter ablation as the first-line treatment.

PART V: IDIOPATHIC EPICARDIAL VENTRICULAR ARRHYTHMIAS

Introduction

Idiopathic outflow tract VTs usually arise within the endocardial surface of the right ventricle and/or left ventricle outflow tracts.[15] However, in around 15% to 20% of cases the arrhythmias can present a deep intramyocardial or epicardial origin.[23,110] Idiopathic epicardial ventricular arrhythmias (EpiVA) have been reported to originate in different locations including the anterior interventricular vein, the distal great cardiac vein,[111] the anterior interventricular vein–great cardiac vein junction,[110] sinus of Valsalva,[11] crux of the heart near the junction of the middle cardiac vein with the coronary sinus,[112] and the left ventricular summit up to the great cardiac veins.[113]

Therapeutic catheter ablation has been recognized as a safe and effective approach, especially patients refractory to medical treatment. Success can be achieved rather percutaneously through a subxyphoid puncture[114] or with a direct surgical exposure of the pericardial space.[115]

On this issue, some important considerations for the daily electrophysiological practice will be discussed in further detail.

Anatomy, Mechanism, and Clinical Considerations

The outflow tract region is basically composed by the endocardial surface of the RVOT and its respective segments, ie, lateral or "free wall," posterior, and anteroseptal (see outflow tract tachycardias) with intimate contact with the LVOT at the level of and slightly above the aortic valve. This relationship is made by an anteroposterior orientation of the RVOT overlapping superiorly the LVOT, which has a left-to-right orientation. In between rises the main left coronary artery and its bifurcation into left anterior descendent (LAD), running anterior to the apex along the epicardial surface parallel with the distal portion of the great cardiac vein (GCV) and left circumflex artery (LCx) passing posterolaterally along the left atrioventricular sulcus in close relationship with the proximal segment of the GCV.[110] This arc, composed by the LAD, before the first septal branch, to the LCx, in close proximity to the coronary venous system, has been characterized as the left ventricle summit.[113]

Some idiopathic VTs arise from the deep myocardium or subepicardial surface of the outflow tract, which often cannot be ablated from the endocardium. This group has been defined as epicardial VT, which can originate from either the coronary venous system, the epicardial surface itself, and/or deep within the coronary sinus of Valsalva.[110] Baman and colleagues report 14% of consecutive cases of idiopathic ventricular arrhythmias had epicardial origin, identified within the coronary venous system, most often from the GCV.[110]

Another region for anatomical consideration is the epicardial surface at the inferobasal aspect, called the crux of the heart, composed by the proximal portion of the middle cardiac vein (MCV) and its intersection with the coronary sinus and the corresponding posterior descending coronary artery. Doppalapudi et al recently reported this rare subtype of idiopathic arrhythmia accounting for around 1% of their series of 340 patients referred for catheter ablation.[112]

EpiVAs share the same mechanisms purposed for outflow VTs, ie, triggered automaticity due to cAMP-dependent DADs and/or catecholamine-dependent abnormal automaticity suggested in several studies that performed arrhythmia induction in the same way with pharmacological catecholamine stimulation.[11,111-113] Moreover, patients present with similar symptoms and conditions, eg, frequent symptoms during exercise and/or emotional stress.

Clinical treatment is basically the same as that used for outflow tract tachycardias. β-blockers, calcium channel blockers, and class I or class III antiarrhythmics can be used with limited efficacy to control arrhythmia burden.

Practice in the Electrophysiology Laboratory

The Electrocardiogram

The QRS morphology will certainly depend on the site of origin, ie, from areas close to the outflow tract showing an inferior axis (Figure 31.7) or inferior regions showing a superior axis, respectively. In several studies, the inferior axis pattern is the most common variant,[110,116] probably owing to the close anatomical relationship of the outflow tracts. However, superior axis is also described.[110,112,117]

Once arising within the GCV, the VT/PVC QRS morphology exhibits similarities with arrhythmias originating from the aortic cusp (Figure 31.6).[23,25,51] Obel et al[110] defined similar characteristics in 5 patients undergoing successful ablation within the GCV. In all patients, the QRS complex in lead I showed an rS or Rs morphology. Four of 5 patients presented with RBBB morphology (R or Rs QRS complex in V_1) and 1 had early R-wave transition with a descending notching in the S wave in V_1/V_2 (example in Figure 31.4). All had a degree of slurring beginning at the QRS complex in precordial leads and in 4 cases had no S wave in V_6 (Figure 31.27). They attribute those similarities to the close anatomical relationship of these segments. Daniels et al reported that a maximum deflection index (time to maximum deflection/QRS duration) ≥0.55 in precordial leads, which translates to a delayed QRS activation, could identify an idiopathic epicardial left ventricle–VT origin located close to the aortic root and left anterior descending coronary artery, and to the posterior left ventricle septum.[11]

Broad R or r waves in lead V_1 or a slurring beginning in V_1/V_2 with an S wave descending notching in patients with an LBBB morphology may indicate an epicardial origin (Figure 31.28). Baman et al reported broader R waves in lead V_1 (≥75 ms) in 12 or 16 patients with an epicardial origin and LBBB morphology in comparison with 1 out of 17 in the control group (endocardial origin).[110] They have also reported narrower S waves in V_1 and V_2 in the epicardial group (40–50 ms vs 80 ms). When compared with VT successfully ablated at the aortic cusps, epicardial arrhythmias exhibited wider R waves in V_1 (85 ms vs 35 ms); however, there is no difference in the maximum deflection index (0.65 vs 0.69).[110]

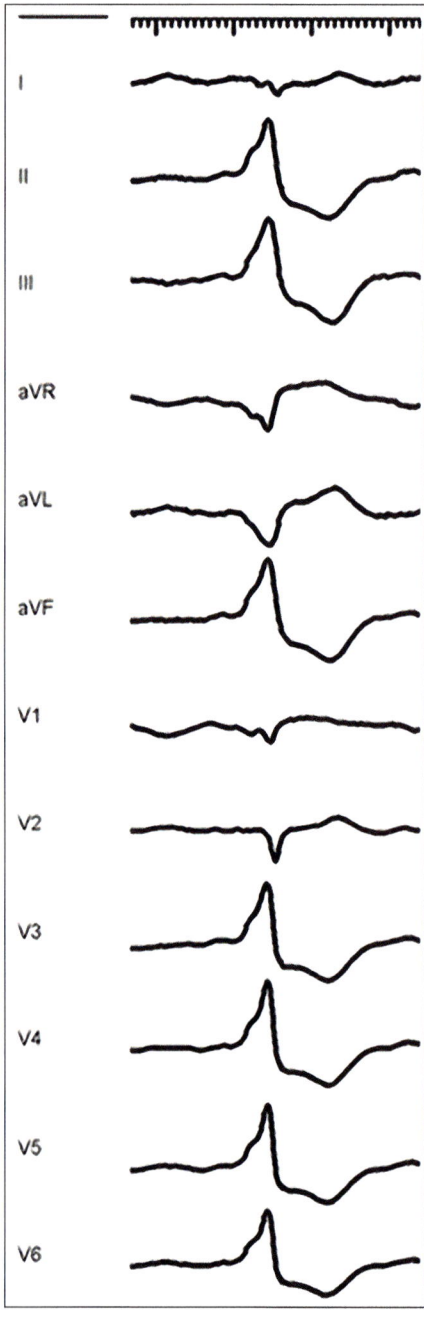

Figure 31.27 ECG morphology of a PVC coming from the vicinity of the GCV. Note the slurring at the beginning of the QRS complex and QS complex in V_1 and V_2 with notches at its beginning. Successful place of ablation was within the coronary sinus at the GCV level. CS = coronary sinus; GCV = great cardiac vein; PVC = premature ventricular contraction.

The ECG criteria generally used to identify an epicardial origin of VTs[118] can be applied with good accuracy and might be more valuable for idiopathic VTs, once these arrhythmias are focal and usually located close to the exit (QRS complex). The criteria usually used when analyzing the QRS complex of the VT/PVC are: [119] (1) time to earliest rapid deflection in precordial leads (pseudo-delta wave) ≥ 34 ms, (2) interval to peak of R wave in lead V_2 (intrinsic deflection time) ≥ 85 ms, and (3) time to earliest QRS nadir in precordial leads (shortest RS complex) ≥ 121 ms. Patients with structural heart diseases and myocardial scars often present more challenging arrhythmias originating and perpetuating within complex substrates and circuits. QRS morphology plays a role only in indicating places of VT exit. In such cases, extensive ablation lesions and lines with substrate modification are often required.

Workflow in the Electrophysiology Laboratory

Workflow with the setup process should follow the same routine as for OT-VT. After recognition of 12-lead ECG and suspecting an epicardial origin, the first step should be placement of electrode catheters in the right ventricle apex and one deep within the coronary sinus to reach the GCV (once inferior axis is presented). This standard approach is generally used for the OT-VT, especially in patients with intermediate QRS morphology. Local ventricle EGM from distal coronary sinus catheter serves as a comparable reference for endocardial mapping. RVOT should be routinely the first chamber for mapping and, sometimes, for the first ablation attempts.

In practice, if the patient undergoes the first ablation procedure, endocardial RVOT mapping should be performed first and ablation attempts should be tried when early bipolar signals (before the onset of the QRS) and/or very negative and steep unipolar signals are detected. If there is early precordial R-wave transition at the surface ECG (within V_1/V_2), mapping the LVOT may be performed directly.

In fact, patients considered to have VT/PVCs from the RVOT who undergo unsuccessful ablation might have arrhythmias originating deeper within this segment or even epicardially. Lokhandwala et al studied 40 patients with OT-VT and reported unsuccessful endocardial ablation in those who presented wide and slurred QRS complexes during VT, which might indicate a deeper intramyocardial or epicardial site of origin.[120]

Idiopathic EpiVA from the left Valsalva sinus is normally approached retrogradely from the aortic root. After detection of the earliest local activation, especially when the local potential precedes the onset of the QRS and ≥11/12 (surface ECG) morphology reproducibility during pace mapping is achieved, ablation should be attempted. In addition, Oyuang et al[50] and Tada et al[116] report in some cases the presence of a double and/or fragmented potential at that area, which could be a potential target for ablation.

In some cases, ablation can be performed inside the coronary sinus with variable success rates.[11,111,112] Baman et al report 74% of success from their series of 27 patients in whom an origin within the coronary sinus system was diagnosed.[110] The failure was attributed to an impossibility of catheter advancement in 4 patients, inadequate power delivery in 1, proximity to the phrenic nerve in 1, and to a major coronary artery in 1. In 2 cases, a transcutaneous access was needed through a subxyphoid puncture.[110]

Originally described for patients with Chagas cardiomyopathy and epicardial ventricular tachycardias, the transcutaneous access through a subxyphoid puncture[114] has been increasingly and safely used for idiopathic EpiVA.[11,110,112,117] Normally, one puncture and a nonsteerable sheath is enough to successfully guide the ablation catheter; nevertheless, in our experience, a steerable sheath can be safely used for more stability and helps reach more remote and difficult places, due to the presence of two more curves from the sheath (bidirectional) in addition to the one of the ablation catheter.

Once performing epicardial ablation through a subxyphoid puncture, extra care must be taken with important adjacent structures such as coronary arteries and the phrenic nerve. Therefore, after defining the area of interest to be ablated, coronary angiography and pacing maneuvers with high output from the ablation catheter tip should be performed.

Three-dimensional mapping systems have been constantly used in such procedures and have become fundamental tools for the success of ablation. They have capital importance in locating and marking, with acceptable accuracy, important structures such as the phrenic nerve, and defining areas with previous attempts and places where radiofrequency application achieved transitory inhibition of the arrhythmia. That area should be marked, and more attempts should be performed.

One concern about epicardial mapping is the capability of differentiating myocardium and fat, commonly found at this space, that can be confounded with areas of low voltages.

Relevant precautions are: (1) related to epicardial puncture itself; (2) invasive arterial monitoring; (3) the periodical drainage of fluid between ablation pulses once using irrigated-tip catheters; (4) location of coronary arteries and phrenic nerve before ablation (as mentioned before); (5) echocardiography control for pericardial effusion; and (6) after ablation, the pericardic introducer should be withdrawn about 2 hours after the last epicardial drainage and echocardiography control.

Epicardial punctures and mapping must be undertaken only by operators and centers with experience and cardiac surgery available.

Follow-up and Prognosis

The prognosis is generally favorable, and patients often do not need a specific treatment. For those who are symptomatic or who have a decrease of cardiac performance and pump function, clinical treatment with β-blockers or calcium-channel blockers may control arrhythmia, albeit with limited efficacy.

Several studies reported high rates of success of catheter ablation of idiopathic EpiVAs.[11,110-113,115,117] Whether performed from the Valsalva sinus, within the coronary sinus system or through a subxyphoid access, the procedure has a safe profile with low complication rates and must be performed from an experienced service where backup cardiac surgery is available.

References

1. Crawford T. Idiopathic paroxysmal ventricular tachycardia. *Memphis Med J.* 1947;22(12):202-204.
2. Zipes DP, Camm AJ, Borggrefe M, et al. ACC/AHA/ESC 2006 guidelines for management of patients with ventricular arrhythmias and the prevention of sudden cardiac death: a report of the American College of Cardiology/American Heart Association Task Force and the European Society of Cardiology Committee for Practice Guidelines (Writing Committee to Develop Guidelines for Management of Patients with Ventricular Arrhythmias and the Prevention of Sudden Cardiac Death). *J Am Coll Cardiol.* 2006;48: e247-e346.
3. Sacher F, Tedrow UB, Field ME, et al. Ventricular tachycardia ablation: evolution of patients and procedures over 8 years. *Circ Arrhythm Electrophysiol.* 2008;1(3):153-161.
4. Lerman BB, Stein K, Engelstein ED, et al. Mechanism of repetitive monomorphic ventricular tachycardia. *Circulation.* 1995;92:421-429.
5. Van Herendael H, Garcia F, Lin D, et al. Idiopathic right ventricular arrhythmias not arising from the outflow tract: prevalence, electrocardiographic characteristics, and outcome of catheter ablation. *Heart Rhythm.* 2011;8(4):511-518.
6. Maruyama M, Tadera T, Miyamoto S, Ino T. Demonstration of the reentry circuit of verapamil-sensitive idiopathic left ventricular tachycardia: direct evidence for macroreentry as the underlying mechanism. *J Cardiovasc Electrophysiol.* 2001;12:968-972.
7. Emmel M, Sreeram N, Khalil M, Adelmann R, Brockmeier K. Ablation strategies in a patient with Belhassen tachycardia. *J Electrocardiol.* 2011;44(6):802-805.
8. Abouezzeddine O, Suleiman M, Buescher T, et al. Relevance of endocavitary structures in ablation procedures for ventricular tachycardia. *J Cardiovasc Electrophysiol.* 2010;21: 245-254.
9. Good E, Oral H, Morady F, et al. Ventricular arrhythmias origination from a papillary muscle in patients without prior infarction: a comparison with fasicular arrhythmias. *Heart Rhythm.* 2008;5:1530-1537.
10. Natale A, Raviele A, Brugada J, et al. Venice chart international consensus document on ventricular tachycardia/ventricular fibrillation ablation. *J Cardiovasc Electrophysiol.* 2010;21:339-379.
11. Daniels DV, Lu YY, Morton JB, et al. Idiopathic epicardial left ventricular tachycardia originating remote from the sinus of Valsalva: electrophysiological characteristics, catheter ablation, and identification from 12-lead electrogram. *Circulation.* 2006;113:1659-1666.
12. Morady F, Kadish AH, DiCarlo L, et al. Long-term results of catheter ablation of idiopathic right ventricular tachycardia. *Circulation.* 1990;82:2093-2099.
13. Arya A, Piorkowski C, Sommer P, Gerds-Li JH, Kottkamp H, Hindricks G. Idiopathic outflow tract tachycardias: current perspectives. *Herz.* 2007;32(3):218-225.
14. Lin D, Ilkhanoff L, Callans D, et al. Twelve-lead electrocardiographic characteristics of the aortic cusp region guided by intracardiac echocardiography and electroanatomic mapping. *Heart Rhythm.* 2008;5:663-669.
15. Callans DJ, Menz V, Schwartzman D, et al. Repetitive monomorphic tachycardia from the left ventricular outflow tract: electrocardiographic patterns consistent with a left ventricular site of origin. *J Am Coll Cardiol.* 1997;29:1023-1027.
16. Lerman BB, Belardinelli L, West GA, et al. Adenosine-sensitive ventricular tachycardia: evidence suggesting cyclic AMP-mediated triggered activity. *Circulation.* 1986; 74:270-280.
17. Zipes DP, Jalife J. *Cardiac Electrophysiology: From Cell to Bedside*, 4th ed. Philadelphia: W.B. Saunders, 2004.
18. Bunch TJ, Day JD. Right meets left: a common mechanism underlying right and left ventricular outflow tract tachycardias. *J Cardiovasc Electrophysiol.* 2006;17:1059-1061.
19. Joshi S, Wilber DJ. Ablation of idiopathic right ventricular outflow tract tachycardia: current perspectives. *J Cardiovasc Electrophysiol.* 2005;16 Suppl 1:S52-S58.
20. Miller JM, Pezeshkian NG, Yadav AV. Catheter mapping and ablation of right ventricular outflow tract ventricular tachycardia. *J Cardiovasc Electrophysiol.* 2006;17:800-802.
21. Azegami K, Wilber DJ, Arruda M, LinAC, Denman RA. Spatial resolution of pacemapping and activation mapping in patients with idiopathic right ventricular outflow tract tachycardia. *J Cardiovasc Electrophysiol.* 2005;16:823-829.
22. Hachiya H, Aonuma K, Yamauchi Y, et al. Electrocardiographic characteristics of left ventricular outflow tract tachycardia. *Pacing Clin Electrophysiol.* 2000;23:1930-1934.
23. Kanagaratnam L, Tomassoni G, Schweikert R, et al. Ventricular tachycardias arising from the aortic sinus of Valsalva: an underrecognized variant of left outflow tract ventricular tachycardia. *J Am Coll Cardiol.* 2001;37:1408-1414.
24. Yamauchi Y, Aonuma K, Takahashi A, et al. Electrocardiographic characteristics of repetitive monomorphic right ventricular tachycardia originating near the His-bundle. *J Cardiovasc Electrophysiol.* 2005;16:1041-1048.
25. Tada H, Tadokoro K, Miyaji K, et al. Idiopathic ventricular arrhythmias arising from the pulmonary artery: prevalence, characteristics, and topography of the arrhythmia origin. *Heart Rhythm.* 2008;5(3):419-426.
26. Sekiguchi Y, Aonuma K, Takahashi A, et al. Electrocardiographic and electrophysiologic characteristics of ventricular tachycardia originating within the pulmonary artery. *J Am Coll Cardiol.* 2005;45:887-895.
27. Coggins DL, Lee RJ, Sweeney J, et al. Radiofrequency catheter ablation as a cure for idiopathic tachycardia of both left and right ventricular origin. *J Am Coll Cardiol.* 1994;23:1333-1341.
28. Timmermans C, Rodriguez LM, Crijns HJ, Moorman AF, Wellens HJ. Idiopathic left bundle-branch block-shaped ventricular tachycardia may originate above the pulmonary valve. *Circulation.* 2003;108:1960-1967.
29. Farzaneh-Far A, Lerman BB. Idiopathic ventricular outflow tract tachycardia. *Heart.* 2005;91:136-138.

30. Sinha S, Calkins H. Idiopathic right ventricular outflow tract tachycardia: no longer idiopathic? *J Cardiovasc Electrophysiol.* 2006;17:776.
31. Proclemer A, Basadonna PT, Slavich GA, Miani D, Fresco C, Fioretti PM. Cardiac magnetic resonance imaging findings in patients with right ventricular outflow tract premature contractions. *Eur Heart J.* 1997;18:2002-2010.
32. Globits S, Kreiner G, Frank H, et al. Significance of morphological abnormalities detected by MRI in patients undergoing successful ablation of right ventricular outflow tract tachycardia. *Circulation.* 1997;96:2633-2640.
33. Iwai S, Cantillon DJ, Kim RJ, et al. Right and left ventricular outflow tract tachycardias: evidence for a common electrophysiologic mechanism. *J Cardiovasc Electrophysiol.* 2006;17:1052-1058.
34. Lerman BB, Stein KM, Markowitz SM, Mittal S, Slotwiner D. Catecholamine facilitated reentrant ventricular tachycardia: uncoupling of adenosine's antiadrenergic effects. *J Cardiovasc Electrophysiol.* 1999;10:17-26.
35. Lerman BB, Stein KM, Markowitz SM. Adenosine sensitive ventricular tachycardia. A conceptual approach. *J Cardiovasc Electrophysiol.* 1996;7:559-569.
36. Andrea B, Richter S, Sommer P, Arya A. Changing QRS morphology during catheter ablation of outflow tract ventricular tachycardia: what is the mechanism? *Europace.* 2011;13(3):444-446.
37. Marcus FL, et al. ARVC up to date reviewed task force criteria. *Circulation.* 2010;121:1533-1541.
38. Nakagawa M, Takahashi N, Nobe S, et al. Gender differences in various types of idiopathic ventricular tachycardia. *J Cardiovasc Electrophysiol.* 2002;13:633-638.
39. Lerman BB, Stein KM, Markowitz SM, Mittal S, Iwai S. Ventricular tachycardia in patients with structurally normal hearts. In: Zipes DP, Jalife J (eds.), *Cardiac Electrophysiology from Cell to Bedside.* Philadelphia, PA: W.B. Saunders, 2004; 668-682.
40. Shimoike E, Ueda N, Maruyama T, et al. Heart rate variability analysis of patients with idiopathic left ventricular outflow tract tachycardia: role of triggered activity. *Jpn Circ J.* 1999; 63:629-635.
41. Yoshida A, Inoue T, Ohnishi Y, Yokoyama M. Heart rate variability before spontaneous episodes of ventricular tachycardia originating from right ventricular outflow tract in patients without organic heart disease. *Jpn Circ J.* 1998;62:745-749.
42. Gill JS, Blaszyk K, Ward DE, et al. Verapamil for the suppression of idiopathic ventricular tachycardia of left bundle branch block-like morphology. *Am Heart J.* 1993;126:1126-1133.
43. Buxton AE, Waxman HL, Marchlinski FE, et al. Right ventricular tachycardia: clinical and electrophysiologic characteristics. *Circulation.* 1983;68:917-927.
44. Viskin S, Rosso R, Rogowski O, Belhassen B. The short-coupled variant of right ventricular outflow ventricular tachycardia. A not so benign form of benign ventricular tachycardia. *J Cardiovasc Electrophysiol.* 2005;16:912-916.
45. Belhassen B, Viskin S. Idiopathic ventricular tachycardia and fibrillation. *J Cardiovasc Electrophysiol.* 1993;4:356-368.
46. Viskin S, Antzelevitch C. The cardiologists' worst nightmare: sudden death from "benign" ventricular arrhythmias. *J Am Coll Cardiol.* 2005;46:1295-1297.
47. Noda T, Shimizu W, Taguchi A, et al. Malignant entity of idiopathic ventricular fibrillation and polymorphic ventricular tachycardia initiated by premature extrasystoles originating from right ventricular outflow tract. *J Am Coll Cardiol.* 2005;46:1288-1294.
48. Arya A, Huo Y, Frogner F, et al. Effect of limb lead electrodes location on ECG and localization of idiopathic outflow tract tachycardia: a prospective study. *J Cardiovasc Electrophysiol.* 2011;22(8):886-891.
49. Chinushi M, Aizawa Y, Takahashi K, Kitazawa H, Shibata A. Radiofrequency catheter ablation for idiopathic right ventricular tachycardia with special reference to morphological variation and long term outcome. *Heart.* 1997;78:255-261.
50. Ouyang F, Fotuhi P, Ho SY, et al. Repetitive monomorphic ventricular tachycardia originating from the aortic sinus cusp. Electrocardiographic characterization for guiding catheter ablation. *J Am Coll Cardiol.* 2002;39:500-508.
51. Hachiya H, Aonuma K, Yamauchi Y, Igawa M, Nogami A, Iesaka Y. How to diagnose, locate, and ablate coronary cusp ventricular tachycardia. *J Cardiovasc Electrophysiol.* 2002;13:551-556.
52. Miles WM. Idiopathic ventricular outflow tract tachycardia. Where does it originate? *J Cardiovasc Electrophysiol.* 2001; 12:536-537.
53. Ito S, Tada H, Naito S, et al. Development and validation of an ECG algorithm for identifying the optimal ablation site for idiopathic ventricular outflow tract tachycardia. *J Cardiovasc Electrophysiol.* 2003;14:1280-1286.
54. Tanner H, Hindricks G, Schirdewahn P, et al. Outflow tract tachycardia with R/S transition in lead V3: six different anatomic approaches for successful ablation. *J Am Coll Cardiol.* 2005;45:418-423.
55. Betensky BP, Park RE, Marchlinski FE, et al. The V(2) transition ratio: a new electrocardiographic criterion for distinguishing left from right ventricular outflow tract tachycardia origin. *J Am Coll Cardiol.* 2011;57(22):2255-2262.
56. Ainsworth CD, Skanes AC, Klein GJ, Gula LJ, Yee R, Krahn AD. Differentiating arrhythmogenic right ventricular cardiomyopathy from right ventricular outflow tract ventricular tachycardia using multi lead QRS duration and axis. *Heart Rhythm.* 2006;3:416-423.
57. Wittkampf FH, Nakagawa H. RF catheter ablation: Lessons on lesions. *Pacing Clin Electrophysiol.* 2006;29(11):1285-1297.
58. Saleem MA, Burkett S, Passman R, et al. New simplified technique for 3D mapping and ablation of right ventricular outflow tract tachycardia. *Pacing Clin Electrophysiol.* 2005;28:397-403.
59. Friedman PA, Asirvatham SJ, Grice S, et al. Noncontact mapping to guide ablation of right ventricular outflow tract tachycardia. *J Am Coll Cardiol.* 2002;39:1808-1812.
60. Wijnmaalen AP, Zeppenfeld K. Ventricular tachycardia ablation: indications and techniques. *Minerva Cardioangiol.* 2011;59(2):149-169.
61. Arya A, Haghjoo M, Emkanjoo Z, Sadr-Ameli MA. Coronary sinus mapping to differentiate left versus right ventricular outflow tract tachycardias. *Europace.* 2005;7:428-432.
62. Vaseghi M, Cesario DA, Mahajan A, et al. Catheter ablation of right ventricular outflow tract tachycardia: value of defining coronary anatomy. *J Cardiovasc Electrophysiol.* 2006;17: 632-637.
63. Topilski I, Glick A, Viskin S, Belhassen B. Frequency of spontaneous and inducible atrioventricular nodal reentry tachycardia in patients with idiopathic outflow tract ventricular arrhythmias. *Pacing Clin Electrophysiol.* 2006;29:21-28.
64. Wen MS, Taniguchi Y, Yeh SJ, Wang CC, Lin FC, Wu D. Determinants of tachycardia recurrences after radiofrequency ablation of idiopathic ventricular tachycardia. *Am J Cardiol.* 1998;81:500-503.
65. Gill JS, Mehta D, Ward D, Camm AJ. Efficacy of flecainide, sotalol, and verapamil in the treatment of right ventricular

tachycardia in patients without overt cardiac abnormality. *Br Heart J.* 1992;68:392-397.
66. Ohe T, Shimomura K, Aihara N, et al. Idiopathic sustained left ventricular tachycardia: clinical and electrophysiologic characteristics. *Circulation.* 1988;77:560-568.
67. Zipes D, Douglas PR, Troup PJ, et al. Atrial induction of ventricular tachycardia: reentry versus triggered automaticity. *Am J Cardiol.* 1979;44:1-8.
68. Belhassen B, Rotmensch HH, Laniado S. Response of recurrent sustained ventricular tachycardia to verapamil. *Br Heart J.* 1981;46:679-682.
69. Shimoike E, Ueda N, Maruyama T, et al. Radiofrequency catheter ablation of upper septal idiopathic left ventricular tachycardia exhibiting left bundle branch block morphology. *J Cardiovasc Electrophysiol.* 2000;11:203-207.
70. Demoulin JC, Kulbertus HE. Histopathological examination of concept of left hemiblock. *Br Heart J.* 1972;34:807-814.
71. Nakagawa H, Beckman KJ, McClelland JH, et al. Radiofrequency catheter ablation of idiopathic left ventricular tachycardia guided by a Purkinje potential. *Circulation.* 1993;88:2607-2617.
72. Okumura K, Yamabe H, Tsuchiya T, et al. Characteristics of slow conduction zone demonstrated during entrainment of idiopathic ventricular tachycardia of left ventricular origin. *Am J Cardiol.* 1996;77:379-383.
73. Nogami A, Naito S, Tada H, et al. Demonstration of diastolic and presystolic Purkinje potentials as critical potentials in a macroreentry circuit of verapamil-sensitive idiopathic left ventricular tachycardia. *J Am Coll Cardiol.* 2000;36:811-823.
74. Aiba T, Suyama K, Aihara N, et al. The role of Purkinje and pre-Purkinje potentials in the reentrant circuit of verapamil-sensitive idiopathic LV tachycardia. *PACE.* 2001;24:333-344.
75. Tsuchiya T, Okumura K, Honda T, et al. Effects of verapamil and lidocaine on two components of the reentry circuit of verapamil-senstive idiopathic left ventricular tachycardia. *Am J Cardiol.* 2001;37:1415-1421.
76. Lerman BB. Response of nonreentrant catecholamine mediated ventricular tachycardia to endogenous adenosine and acetylcholine: evidence for myocardial receptor-mediated effects: *Circulation.* 1993;87:382-390.
77. Lin FC, Wen MS, Wang CC, et al. Left ventricular fibromuscular band is not a specific substrate for idiopathic left ventricular tachycardia. *Circulation.* 1996;93:525-528.
78. Gaita F, Giusteto C, Leclerc JF, et al. Idiopathic verapamil-responsive left ventricular tachycardia: clinical characteristics and long-term follow-up of 33 patients. *Eur Heart J.* 1994;15:1252-1260.
79. Ohe T, Aihara N, Kamakura S, et al. Long-term outcome of verapamil-sensitive sustained left ventricular tachycardia in patients without structural heart disease. *J Am Coll Cardiol.* 1995;25:54.
80. Arya A, Haghjoo M, Emkanjoo Z, et al. Comparison of presystolic Purkinje and late diastolic potentials for selection of ablation site in idiopathic verapamil sensitive left ventricular tachycardia. *J Interv Card Electrophysiol.* 2004;11:135-141.
81. Nogami A, Naito S, Tada H, et al. Verapamil-sensitive left anterior fascicular ventricular tachycardia: results of radiofrequency ablation in six patients. *J Cardiovasc Electrophysiol.* 1998;9:1269-1278.
82. Phillips JH, Burch GE, De Pasquale NP. The syndrome of papillary muscle dysfunction. *Ann Intern Med.* 1963;59: 508-520.
83. Marzilli M, Sabbah HN, Stein PD. Mitral regurgitation in ventricular premature contractions. The role of the papillary muscle. *Chest.* 1980;77(6):736-740. (http://chestjournal.chestpubs.org/content/77/6/736.long)
84. Sarrazin JF, Good E, Kuhne M, et al. Mapping and ablation of frequent post-infarction premature ventricular complexes. *J Cardiovasc Electrophysiol.* 2010;21(9):1002-1008.
85. Doppalapudi H, Yamada T, McElderry HT, Plumb VJ, Epstein AE, Kay GN. Ventricular tachycardia originating from the posterior papillary muscle in the left ventricle: a distinct clinical syndrome. *Circ Arrhythm Electrophysiol.* 2008;1(1):23-29. (http://circep.ahajournals.org/content/1/1/23.long)
86. Yamada T, Doppalapudi H, McElderry HT, et al. Idiopathic ventricular arrhythmias originating from the papillary muscles in the left ventricle: prevalence, electrocardiographic and electrophysiological characteristics, and results of the radiofrequency catheter ablation. *J Cardiovasc Electrophysiol.* 2010;21(1):62-69.
87. Lazzari JO, Fachinat A, Tambussi A. Clinical assessment of the right ventricle anterior papillary muscle extrasystoles with Holter recordings. *Pacing Clin Electrophysiol.* 1990;13(3): 275-284.
88. Crawford T, Mueller G, Good E, et al. Ventricular arrhythmias originating from papillary muscles in the right ventricle. *Heart Rhythm.* 2010;7(6):725-730.
89. Rusted IE, Scheifley CH, Edwards JE. Studies of the mitral valve. I. Anatomic features of the normal mitral valve and associated structures. *Circulation.* 1952;6(6):825-831.
90. Anderson RH, Frater RWM. Editorial: how can we best describe the components of the mitral valve? *J Heart Valve Dis.* 2006;15:736-739.
91. Yamada T, Doppalapudi H, McElderry HT, et al. Ventricle: relevance for catheter ablation ventricular arrhythmias originating from the papillary muscles in the left electrocardiographic and electrophysiological characteristics in idiopathic. *Circ Arrhythm Electrophysiol.* 2010;3:324-331.
92. Yokokawa M, Good E, Desjardins B, et al. Predictors of successful catheter ablation of ventricular arrhythmias arising from the papillary muscles. *Heart Rhythm.* 2010;7(11):1654-1659.
93. Sacher F, Tedrow UB, Field ME, et al. Ventricular tachycardia ablation: evolution of patients and procedures over 8 years. *Circ Arrhythm Electrophysiol.* 2008;1;153-161.
94. Shenasa M, Hindricks G, Borggrefe M, Breithardt G. *Cardiac Mapping*, 3rd ed. Wiley-Blackwell, 2009.
95. Bogun F, Desjardins B, Crawford T, et al. Post-infarction ventricular arrhythmias originating in papillary muscles. *J Am Coll Cardiol.* 2008;51(18):1794-1802.
96. Yokokawa M, Kim HM, Good E, et al. Relation of symptoms and symptom duration to premature ventricular complex-induced cardiomyopathy. *Heart Rhythm.* 2012;9(1): 92-95.
97. Tada H, Tadokoro K, Ito S, et al. Idiopathic ventricular arrhythmias originating from the tricuspid annulus: prevalence, electrocardiographic characteristics, and results of radiofrequency catheter ablation. *Heart Rhythm.* 2007;4:7-16.
98. Yamauchi Y, Aonuma K, Takahashi A, et al. Electrocardiographic characteristics of repetitive monomorphic right ventricular tachycardia originating near the His bundle. *J Cardiovasc Electrophysiol.* 2005;16:1041-1048.
99. Yue-Chun L, Wen-Wu Z, Na-Dan Z, et al. Idiopathic premature ventricular contractions and ventricular tachycardias originating from the vicinity of tricuspid annulus: results of radiofrequency catheter ablation in thirty-five patients. *BMC Cardiovasc Disord.* 2012;12(1):32.
100. Xiao-yu W, Zhao-guang L, Zhen T, Hong-yue G, Shu Z, Wei-min L. Radiofrequency catheter ablation of idiopathic ventricular tachycardia and symptomatic premature ventricular contraction originating from valve annulus. *Chin Med J.* 2008;121(22):2241-2245.

101. Ashikaga K, Tsuchiya T, Nakashima A, Hayashida K. Catheter ablation of premature ventricular contractions originating from the His bundle region. *Europace*. 2007;9,781-784.
102. Arruda MS, McClelland JH, Wang X, et al. Development and validation of an ECG algorithm for identifying accessory pathway ablation site in Wolff-Parkinson-White syndrome. *J Cardiovasc Electrophysiol*. 1998;9:2-12.
103. Atié I, Maciel W, Andréa E, et al. Wolff-Parkinson-White syndrome and other atrioventricular accessory pathways in 1,465 patients undergoing radiofrequency ablation. *Rev SOCERJ*. 2008;21(6):387-392.
104. Kumagai K, Yamauchi Y, Takahashi A, et al. Idiopathic left ventricular tachycardia originating from the mitral annulus. *J Cardiovasc Electrophysiol*. 2005;16:1029-1036.
105. Tada H, Ito S, Naito S, et al. Idiopathic ventricular arrhythmia arising from the mitral annulus: a distinct subgroup of idiopathic ventricular arrhythmias. *J Am Coll Cardiol*. 2005;45:877-886.
106. Shimoike E, Ohba Y, Yanagi N, et al. Radiofrequency catheter ablation of idiopathic right ventricular tachycardia near the His bundle. *Fukuoka Igaku Zasshi*. 1999;90:132-139.
107. Haïssaguerre M, Marcus F, Poquet F, Gencel L, Le Metayer P, Clementy J. Electrocardiographic characteristics and catheter ablation of para-Hisian accessory pathways. *Circulation*. 1994;90:1124-1128.
108. Aizawa Y, Chinushi M, Naitoh N, et al. Catheter ablation of ventricular tachycardia with radiofrequency currents, with special reference to the termination and minor morphologic change of reinduced ventricular tachycardia. *Am J Cardiol*. 1995;76:574-579.
109. Zhu DW, Maloney JD, Simmons TW, et al. Radiofrequency catheter ablation for management of symptomatic ventricular ectopic activity. *J Am Coll Cardiol*. 1995;26:843-849.
110. Baman TS. Mapping and ablation of epicardial idiopathic ventricular arrhythmias from within the coronary venous system. *Circ Arrhythm Electrophysiol*. 2010;3:274-279.
111. Obel O, d'Avila A, Neuzil P, Saad E, Ruskin J, Reddy V. Ablation of left ventricular epicardial outflow tract tachycardia from the distal great cardiac vein. *J Am Coll Cardiol*. 2006;48:1813-1817.
112. Doppalapudi H, Yamada T, Ramaswamy K, Ahn J, Neal G. Idiopathic focal epicardial ventricular tachycardia originating from the crux of the heart. *Heart Rhythm*. 2009;6:44-650.
113. Yamada T, McElderry HT, Doppalapudi H, et al. Idiopathic ventricular arrhythmias originating from the left ventricular summit: anatomic concepts relevant to ablation. *Circ Arrhythm Electrophysiol*. 2010;3(6):616-623.
114. Sosa E, Scanavacca M, d'Avila A, Pilleggi F. A new technique to perform epicardial mapping in the electrophysiology laboratory. *J Cardiovasc Electrophysiol*. 1996;7:531-536.
115. Soejima K, Couper G, Cooper JM, Sapp JL, Epstein LM, Stevenson WG. Subxyphoid surgical approach for epicardial catheter-based mapping and ablation in patients with prior cardiac surgery or difficult pericardial access. *Circulation*. 2004;110:1197-1201.
116. Tada H, Naito S, Ito S, et al. Significance of two potentials for predicting successful catheter ablation from the left sinus of Valsalva for left ventricular epicardial tachycardia. *Pacing Clin Electrophysiol*. 2004;27(8):1053-1059.
117. Villacastín J, Castellano NP, Moreno J, Álvarez L, Moreno M, Quintana J. Percutaneous epicardial radiofrequency ablation of idiopathic ventricular tachycardia. *Rev Esp Cardiol*. 2005;58(1):100-104.
118. Bazan V, Gerstenfeld EP, Garcia FC, et al. Site-specific twelve-lead ECG features to identify an epicardial origin for left ventricular tachycardia in the absence of myocardial infarction. *Heart Rhythm*. 2007;4(11):1403-1410.
119. Berruezo A, Mont L, Nava S, Chueca E, Bartholomay E, Brugada J. Electrocardiographic recognition of the epicardial origin of ventricular tachycardias. *Circulation*. 2004;109: 1842-1847.
120. Lokhandwala YY, et al. Idiopathic ventricular tachycardia–characterisation and radiofrequency ablation. *Indian Heart J*. 1994;46(6):281-285.

# CHAPTER 32

Polymorphic Ventricular Tachycardia and Ventricular Fibrillation: Mapping in Percutaneous Catheter and Surgical EP Procedures

Mélèze Hocini, MD; Ashok J. Shah, MD; Shinsuke Miyazaki, MD; Lena Rivard, MD; Amir S. Jadidi, MD; Daniel Scherr, MD; Stephen B. Wilton, MD, MSc; Laurent Roten, MD; Patrizio Pascale, MD; Michala Pedersen, MD; Nicolas Derval, MD; Sébastien Knecht, MD, PhD; Frédéric Sacher, MD; Pierre Jaïs, MD; Michel Haïssaguerre, MD

Introduction

Polymorphic ventricular tachycardia (PMVT) and ventricular fibrillation (VF) are the most life-threatening complex cardiac rhythm disorders. Ventricular fibrillation and tachycardias are responsible for 80% of the 350,000 sudden cardiac deaths (SCDs) occurring each year in Europe and the United States (20% are caused by primary arrest of cardiac activity).[1] SCD remains the single most common mode of death due to medical causes in the United States today (World Health Organization report, 2008). Every year, 350,000 sudden deaths occur in Europe. The majority of SCD events (90%) are associated with structurally diseased heart due to coronary arterial abnormalities, dilated and hypertrophic cardiomyopathies, acquired infiltrative disorders, and valvular or congenital cardiac disorder. Ten percent of SCDs can be attributed to primary electrophysiological (EP) disorders (having no identifiable structural cardiac problem) with either known ion channel abnormalities (long QT syndrome, Brugada syndrome, catecholaminergic PMVT, short QT syndrome) or unknown ion channel abnormalities (early repolarization syndrome, idiopathic VF).[2,3]

Owing to strikingly lethal characteristics and momentary presence, these arrhythmias have been mapped and studied, by and large, in animal hearts or models. Moreover, PMVT and VF are mechanistically varied and more complex in comparison with the sustained monomorphic reentrant ventricular arrhythmias.

The recently described role of the Purkinje conducting system in triggering these arrhythmias in both structurally normal and diseased hearts provides new insight into their mechanisms and potential therapy.[4,5] The role that ventricular myocardium plays in maintaining the arrhythmia employs several mechanisms: reentry involving the substrate and the Purkinje–myocardium junction, and the migratory propagation of vortices.

Initiation and Maintenance of PMVT/VF: Insights from Animal/Experimental and Clinical Studies

Role of His–Purkinje Arborization as Triggers of VF

Animal and Experimental Studies

In vitro studies have shown that the Purkinje conducting system is able to generate or maintain arrhythmias through a variety of means. These include automaticity, reentry, or triggered activity during electrolyte imbalance; catecholamine or other drug exposure; and myocardial ischemia during which Purkinje fibers can survive within the necrotic muscle.[6-8]

Wilson et al[9] first studied experimentally produced myocardial infarction in animals by recording epicardial electrograms. They then correlated changes in the local electrogram with changes in the electrocardiogram (ECG). Later, Moe et al[10] studied the initiation of VF in noninfarcted canine hearts. They found that fibrillation began locally at the stimulated site and spread therefrom to invade the rest of the ventricle.

Hoffman[6] described the role of subendocardial Purkinje fibers that survive after extensive myocardial infarction in the genesis of cardiac arrhythmias. She emphasized the important role of subendocardial layers harboring the Purkinje network. Friedman et al[7,8] described the role of surviving subendocardial distal Purkinje fibers in infarcted canine hearts. Oxygenation of this subendocardial conduction system network that comes directly from the ventricular cavity may provide survival advantage during an ischemic insult. Compared with normal subendocardial Purkinje fibers, surviving Purkinje fibers demonstrated a reduction in maximum diastolic potentials, maximum depolarization amplitudes and velocities, and prolonged action potential durations. The survivors also demonstrated spontaneous diastolic depolarization, indicating that these fibers may participate in the genesis of ventricular arrhythmias associated with myocardial infarction.

In concurrence with the previous description of Myerburg et al[11] other researchers observed distinct Purkinje activity as a rapid deflection. This activity occurs before inscription of the Q wave of the surface ECG in sinus rhythm, and often much earlier than the QRS deflection, during spontaneous ventricular ectopic beats initiating fibrillation. In an experimental model, Berenfeld et al[12] simulated the evolution of reentrant activity at the Purkinje–muscle junction and provided a mechanism for rapid focal Purkinje discharges. Thus, they were able to show that focus itself was a reentrant circuit.[13] Earlier, Overholt et al[14] had demonstrated the existence of unidirectional block between Purkinje network and ventricular layers of papillary muscles and established their added role as a substrate for ventricular arrhythmias. Later, Berenfeld et al[12] and Pak et al[15] demonstrated active involvement of both Purkinje fiber and ventricular muscle in the reentrant mechanism of polymorphic ventricular arrhythmias, thereby elucidating a vital role for Purkinje fibers in arrhythmia maintenance besides initiation. Tabereaux et al[16] highlighted the activation patterns of Purkinje fiber activation during long-duration VF and reaffirmed the role of the Purkinje network in maintaining VF. In their study, the Purkinje network was activated in more than 84% of activation wavefronts during 10 minutes of VF.

Since isolation of single Purkinje fibers is difficult, especially in small-animal research, investigation into the effects of abolition of individual Purkinje cells is likewise problematic.[17] However, to highlight the active role of the Purkinje network in VF, Damiano et al[18] applied Lugol's solution to ablate the superficial ventricular endocardium and Purkinje fibers in a dog's heart. As a consequence, a profound increase in the VF threshold was observed but without damage to the underlying myocardium. Dosdall et al[19] extended the experiment and demonstrated that chemical ablation of the Purkinje system caused early termination and activation rate-slowing of long-duration VF. In these studies, Purkinje fibers were experimentally demonstrated to play an active role in initiating and maintaining PMVT/VF.

Clinical Studies

Ashida et al[20] first performed activation and pace mapping of monomorphic right ventricular outflow tract (RVOT) ectopic beats by initiating torsades de pointes in an 18-year-old woman with recurrent syncope. The authors ablated the focal source of ectopy, which resulted in abolition of the torsades de pointes without disappearance of isolated ectopies or changes in the coupling interval. These results led them to propose that ablation had modified the substrate for rapid reentry, which was considered to be the mechanism for maintaining PMVT initiated by focal source ectopy.

In the early 2000s, Kusano et al,[21] Takatsuki et al,[22] and Saliba et al[23] reported successful abolition of focal ectopic source triggering VF in individual case reports. Using activation mapping of the ectopy initiating VF, Haïssaguerre et al[4,5] first elucidated the role of His–Purkinje triggers in initiating VF and PMVT. They did so in a series of patients with recurrent episodes, frequent premature beats, and seemingly normal heart.

In the period that followed, Purkinje arborization was also described to have multiple roles. For instance, it was discovered to play a role in the initiation of ventricular fibrillation and PMVT/VF associated with long QT, Brugada, and early repolarization syndromes.[24,25] It also helped initiate VF/electrical storm in a series of patients with myocardial infarction,[26-28] nonischemic dilated cardiomyopathy,[29] cardiac amyloidosis,[30] valvular heart disease, and infective myocarditis.[31] During the past decade, several sporadic case reports also reinforced the concept of focal onset of VF from the Purkinje/myocardial source.[23,31-49]

Invasive Mapping

Because of the rapidly lethal nature of these arrhythmias, substrate mapping remains largely restricted to *in vitro* experiments and heart models. Their focus is on the mechanisms of maintenance of cardiac fibrillation and polymorphic ventricular arrhythmias.[12,50,51] For the same reason, it is also very difficult to invasively map these arrhythmias' initiation during ongoing arrhythmia.

However, during periods of arrhythmia, isolated or repetitive ventricular premature beats (whose morphology is identical or similar to those preceding runs of VF) allow activation mapping of the culprit ectopy. The ectopies are usually more profound 2 to 3 days following the VF episodes or electrical storm.

It is crucial to record the 12-lead ECG continuously to identify ectopies prior to invasive mapping. At our center, we subject the patients to continuous 12-lead ECG during the preprocedural hospitalization. We carefully mark the position of electrodes on the patient so as to perfectly reproduce the same ECG pattern in the laboratory during mapping (Figure 32.1). Based on available evidence, the majority of such initiating ventricular complexes can be mapped to various locations in the His–Purkinje tree. This pattern is indicated by sharp potentials preceding local muscle electrogram during sinus rhythm as well as during ectopy (Figure 32.2). If the site of origin of the ectopic beat is not preceded by sharp potential during sinus rhythm, the trigger source is considered to be the local myocardium (although the ectopic beat may be preceded by sharp potential). Next, we will describe invasive mapping of triggers in difficult-to-map cardiac arrhythmias that arise in normal hearts and in patients with a wide range of electrostructural abnormalities.

Mapping Triggers of PMVT/VF in Structurally Normal Hearts: Electrophysiological Study

For sick patients experiencing recurrent episodes of VF, electrical storms, and multiple shocks from the defibrillator, a comprehensive procedure includes an EP study and radiofrequency ablation. To safely conduct these procedures, it is important to have the necessary therapeutic or prophylactic circulatory support in place (eg, extracorporeal membrane oxygenator, cardiac assist device). In relatively unstable, potentially dying patients, speed and accuracy are necessary to combat lethal arrhythmias. For this population, specialized catheters have been developed to facilitate and expedite the mapping process over a wide area of ventricular muscle. One such catheter is the PENTARAY (Flower™, Biosense Webster, Diamond Bar, CA). This deflectable-tip 7-Fr catheter provides high-density contact ventricular mapping. It comprises 30 platinum electrodes (1 mm each), precisely spaced (2-8-2 mm) along 5 soft and flexible splines (2 or 3 pairs of electrodes per spline) that radiate from the deflectable-tip span over a wide area of >60 cm^2.

In a multicenter study on mapping of VF in structurally normal hearts,[4,5,24,25,52] an EP study was undertaken either during the storm or during spontaneous or induced ventricular ectopies. Two to 4 multielectrode catheters were introduced percutaneously through the femoral vessels, including a 4 mm–tip ablation catheter (Biosense Webster, Diamond Bar, CA). Then, surface ECG leads and bipolar intracardiac electrograms (filtered at 30 to 500 Hz) were recorded simultaneously with a polygraph (model Lab system or Midas, 1–4 kHz and 10 kHz sampling rate, respectively; or Bard Electrophysiology, Lowell, MA) for offline analysis. When left ventricular access was required, it was obtained by the transseptal or retrograde aortic method. After obtaining transseptal access, a single bolus of heparin (30 IU/kg) was administered.

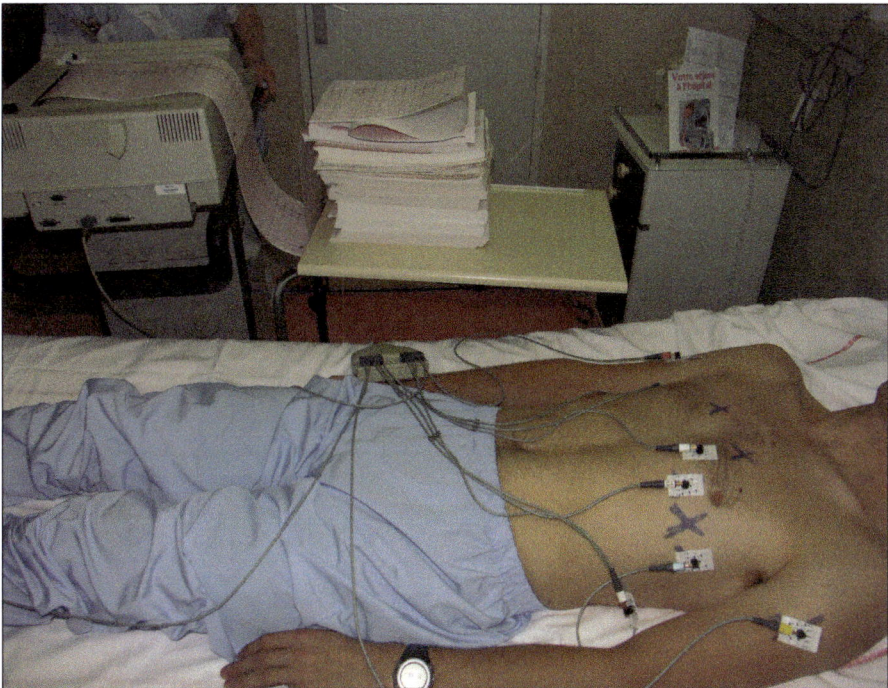

Figure 32.1 The patient is subjected to continuous 12-lead ECG during the preprocedural hospitalization. The positions of electrodes on the patient are marked so as to perfectly reproduce the ECG pattern in the laboratory during mapping.

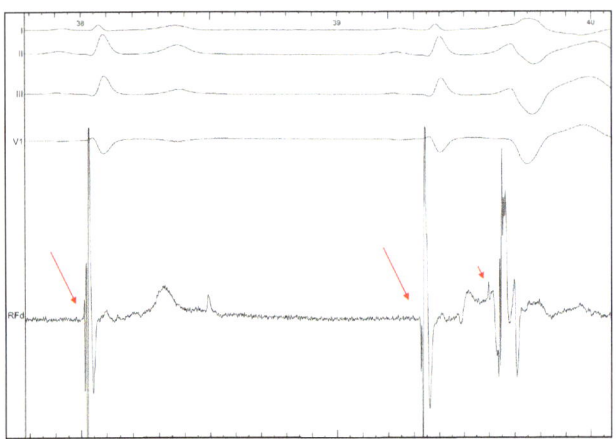

Figure 32.2 Intracardiac electrogram recorded on the ablation catheter shows distal Purkinje potential (**red arrows**) preceding the local muscle electrogram in sinus rhythm and ectopy.

Mapping the Arrhythmogenic Triggers

In the reports described by Haïssaguerre et al[4,5,24,25] and Knecht et al,[52] the clinically observed ventricular ectopies were localized by endocardial mapping of the earliest electrogram relative to the onset of the ectopic QRS complex. During sinus rhythm, the location of the mapping catheter on the distal Purkinje network was indicated by sharp potentials (<10 ms in duration) preceding the onset of QRS complex by ≤15 ms. During ectopic activity, such electrograms were distinctly earlier (≥15 ms) before the onset of ectopic QRS; this is suggestive of initiation of ectopy from the distal Purkinje arborization (Figure 32.3). The absence of Purkinje potential at the site of earliest ectopic beat during sinus rhythm indicated ventricular myocardium as the source of the culprit ectopy. Wherever required, ectopies were induced by the use of pacing maneuvers (during transient pause postburst pacing in the ventricles) and/or, rarely, with isoproterenol (1–4 mcg/kg/min) or ajmaline (1 mg/kg) by intravenous infusion. If these measures were ineffective, Purkinje mapping at the likely site of origin of ectopy was used to identify the site of origin of clinical ectopy.

Idiopathic PMVT/VF

Patient Population

The largest experience of mapping primary idiopathic VF involved 38 consecutive patients (21 men), aged 42 ± 13 years, from 6 centers across Europe.[52] Excluded were patients with structural or ischemic heart disease, ventricular tachycardia degenerating into fibrillation, long QT and Brugada syndromes, catecholaminergic polymorphic ventricular arrhythmia, and right ventricular dysplasia. Physical examination; ECG (sinus rate, 68 ± 10 bpm; PR interval, 164 ± 24 ms; QRS duration, 92 ± 15 ms; QTc interval, 398 ± 25 ms); echocardiography (left ventricular end-diastolic dimension, 42 ± 10 mm); and left ventricular ejection fraction (67 ± 9%) were normal in all the patients.[53] Patients recruited for the study experienced a median of 4 significant events (either syncope, electrical storm, documented VF, or aborted SCD) with documented ventricular ectopy–triggered VF on 12-lead ECG despite continued antiarrhythmic drug use (median 2); 87% patients had at least 2 events in the year before ablation.

Results of Trigger-mapping

Thirty patients out of 38 (81%) had clinical ectopy at the time of the procedure, whereas 8 patients (19%) did not. Clinical ectopies triggering VF arose from the right Purkinje system in 16 patients, the left Purkinje in 14 patients, in both the left and right Purkinje systems in 3 patients, and in the myocardium in 5 patients (including the RVOT in 4 patients). The coupling interval of ectopies originating from the RVOT was longer when compared with those from the Purkinje system (355 ± 23 ms vs 276 ± 22 ms; $P < 0.001$). A mean of 1.7 ± 2.0 morphologically distinct ectopies were targeted per patient. The ectopy arising from the left Purkinje system had higher morphological variation than that arising from the right Purkinje network. The latter often had more subtle changes. This difference can be explained by smaller arborial mass of the right Purkinje network compared with that of the left (anterior, septal, and intermediate) (Figure 32.4). In this series, there were only 2 patients with single morphology of ectopy from the left Purkinje tree.

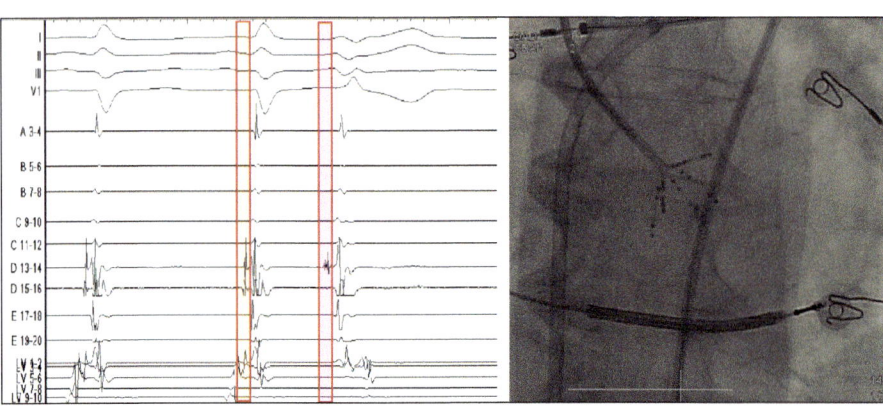

Figure 32.3 Intracardiac recording on a multipolar (PENTARAY™ [Biosense Webster]) mapping catheter (**right**). Proximal Purkinje potential is seen preceding local (**red triangles**) ventricular electrogram during sinus rhythm and ectopy (**left**).

The QRS duration of ectopies was shorter when originating from the left than the right Purkinje system (130 ± 24 ms vs 162 ± 19 ms; P < 0.002), but the QRS duration was not significantly different between the ectopies originating from the left Purkinje system and the myocardium (130 ± 24 ms vs 150 ± 16 ms, respectively; P < 0.11). During premature beat, the earliest Purkinje potential preceded the local muscle activation by a conduction interval of 38 ± 28 ms, with a greater precocity in the left than in the right ventricle (46 ± 29 vs 19 ± 10 ms; P = 0.04) (Figure 32.5).

At the same site, varying conduction times were associated with varying morphologies, suggesting either changes in ventricular activation route or origin from another part of Purkinje system. In 10 patients, 2, 3, or 4 repetitive beats were recorded, with each complex being preceded by a Purkinje potential with a variable delay ranging from 15 to 120 ms. Conduction block between Purkinje and ventricular muscle was also observed in 3 patients (Figure 32.6). Catheter manipulation produced transient bundle branch block in 4 patients (right in 3, left in 1); as a result, peripheral Purkinje potentials no longer preceded the local ventricular activation in sinus rhythm, although activation during ectopy remained unchanged (Figure 32.7).

PMVT/VF in Long QT and Brugada Syndromes

Patient Population

Seven patients with long QT syndrome diagnosed with established criteria (2 men and 2 women, aged 37 ± 8 years; QTc >460 ms) or genetically proven Brugada syndrome (2 men and 1 woman, aged 39 ± 7 years) underwent mapping of triggers inducing 1 to 21 episodes of PMVT or VF (family history positive in 3).[24] The ventricular ectopy burden was 11,559 ± 13,111/24 hours within 2 weeks of the arrhythmia episode. Clinical ectopy in the long QT syndrome had a coupling interval of 503 ± 29 ms; they were monomorphic in 2 patients and polymorphic and repetitive (sometimes bidirectional) in the other 2. In contrast, clinical ectopies were monomorphic in all the patients with Brugada syndrome; left bundle branch block–inferior axis morphology was suggestive of RVOT origin in 2 patients, and left bundle branch block–superior axis was suggestive of it in the remaining 1 patient. Coupling intervals were shorter than in the patients with long QT syndrome. Except for 2 patients with Brugada syndrome, all the other patients were on antiarrhythmic drug therapy, including quinidine.

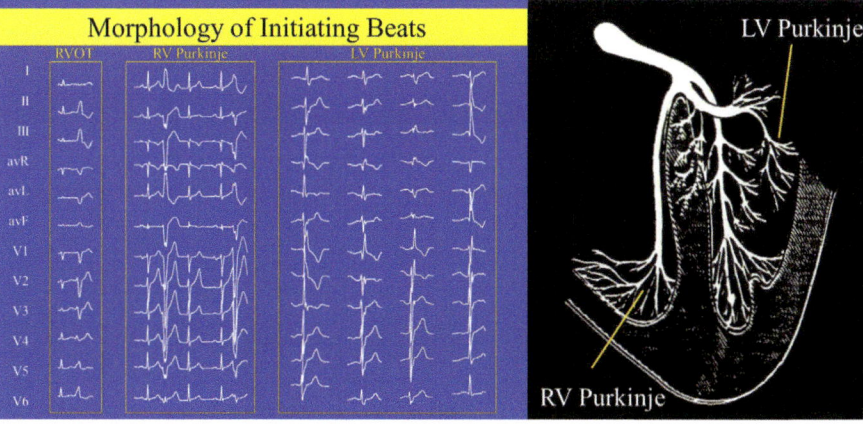

Figure 32.4 There is a higher morphological variation in the ectopies originating from the left ventricular (LV) Purkinje network when compared with those originating from the right ventricular (RV) Purkinje network or right ventricular outflow tract (RVOT) muscle. The LV Purkinje network is more arborized than the RV Purkinje network.

Ectopic Source	V1	Ectopic Duration (ms)	Earliest Potential (ms)
RVOT	-ve	130–160	32 ± 15
RV Purkinje	-ve	140–150	19 ± 10
LV Purkinje	+ve	90–120	46 ± 29

Figure 32.5 The characteristics of right and left Purkinje and right ventricular outflow tract–triggered ectopy. LV = left ventricular; OT = outflow tract; RV = right ventricular.

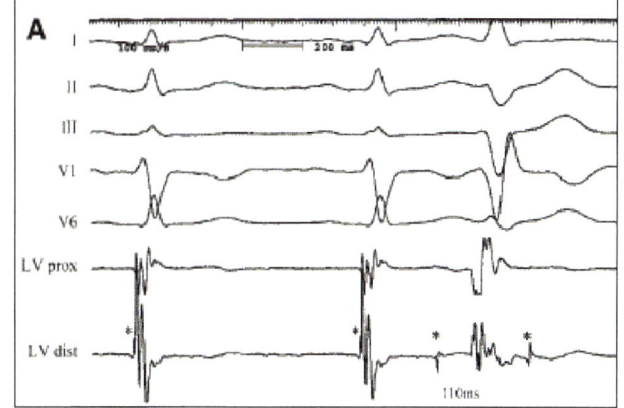

Figure 32.6 Purkinje potentials (**asterisks**) precede the local ventricular electrogram in sinus rhythm and ectopy. Blocked Purkinje potential is marked by an **asterisk** on last electrogram.

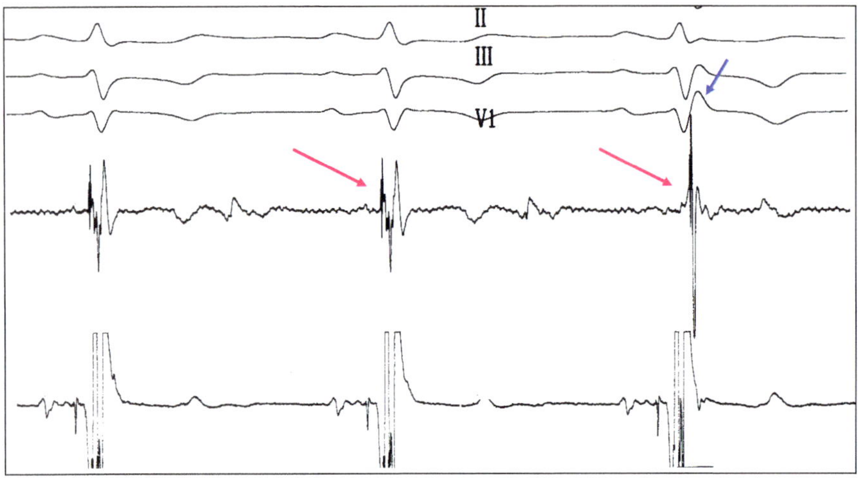

Figure 32.7 Right Purkinje potential (**red arrows**) is recorded in sinus rhythm. During mechanical right bundle branch block (**blue arrow**), the Purkinje potential is hidden within the local ventricular electrogram.

Results of Trigger-mapping

Long QT Syndrome: Purkinje arborization was triggering ectopies in 3/4 patients. In the remainder, monomorphic ectopy originated from the RVOT myocardium. Polymorphic bidirectional runs of ectopy originated from either the distal ramifications of the anterior and posterior fascicle or the intervening region, explaining the observed morphological variation. In one patient with monomorphic ectopy, the latter originated from the posterior fascicle. During monomorphic ectopy, the earliest Purkinje potential preceded the local muscle electrogram by 34 ± 17 ms. All the repetitive beats were also preceded by Purkinje activity, with a variable delay ranging from 20 to 110 ms.

Brugada Syndrome: Triggers were mapped to the muscle in the RVOT in 4 out of 5 patients and to anterior right ventricular distal Purkinje arborization in the remaining one. The myocardial trigger potential preceded the onset of ectopic QRS by 25 and 40 ms, respectively. VF was reproducibly induced from the right ventricular apex with 2 extrastimuli (S1500, S2240, and S3220 ms) in both patients with outflow-tract triggers before ablation. In one of these patients, no clinical recurrence of VF took place during a follow-up of just under 7 years (based on clinical and defibrillator logs). Furthermore, the ECG pattern of Brugada syndrome was abolished immediately after ablation of the substrate surrounding the trigger in the anteroseptal and lateral RVOT. The ECG showed no reappearance of a Brugada pattern over long-term follow-up, suggestive of a potential role for ablation in curing this primary electrical disorder[54] (Figure 32.8).

PMVT/VF in Early Repolarization Syndrome

Patient Population

In a multicenter, case-control study, 206 patients (123 men; mean age 36 ± 11 years) who had been resuscitated after cardiac arrest with idiopathic VF were assessed for early repolarization.[25] Compared with the control group, early repolarization was significantly more frequent in the patients who had been resuscitated from VF (31% vs 5%). Within the study group of patients with early

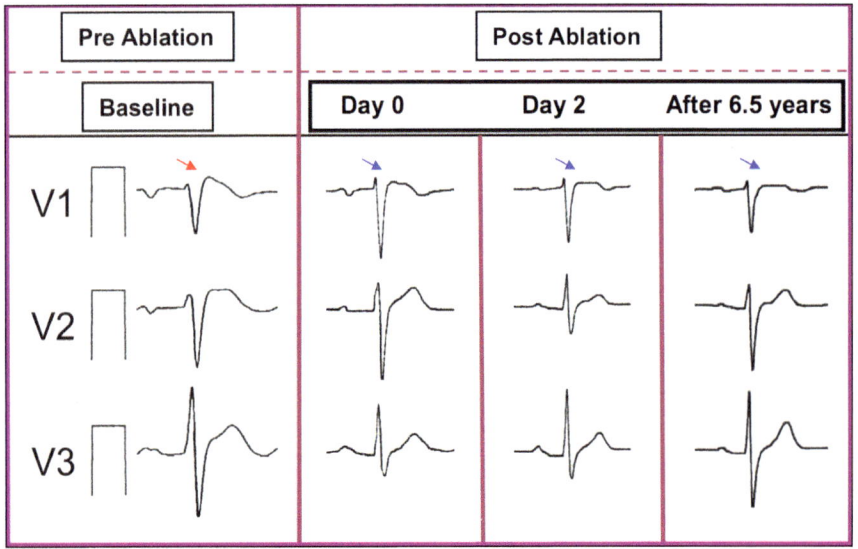

Figure 32.8 Abolition of Brugada syndrome by regional ablation, as shown on ECG. (**Arrows** represent ST elevation.)

repolarization, 8 patients with recurrent VF were subjected to catheter mapping of the triggering ectopy, which originated from the Purkinje arborization or myocardial source. (These patients' VF recurred despite being administered a wide range of antiarrhythmic drugs, including β-blockers, amiodarone, flecainide, cifenline, pilsicainide, quinidine, disopyramide, verapamil, and mexiletine.)

Results of Trigger-mapping

A total of 26 ectopic patterns were mapped either to the ventricular myocardium (16 patterns) or to Purkinje tissue (10 patterns) in 8 patients. In 6 subjects with early repolarization recorded only in inferior leads, all ectopy originated from the inferior ventricular wall. In 2 subjects with widespread early repolarization (as recorded by both inferior and lateral leads), ectopy originated from multiple regions (Figure 32.9).

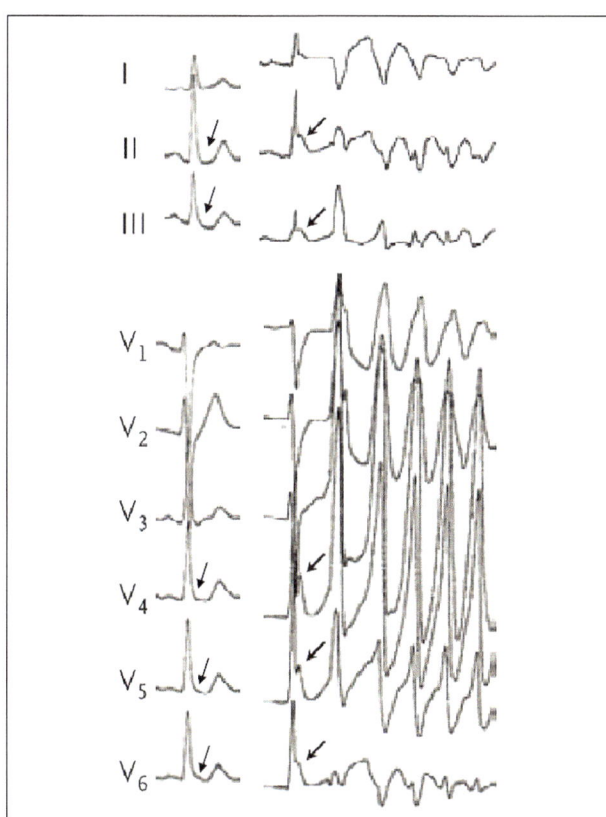

Figure 32.9 Exacerbation of early repolarization pattern (**arrows**) before the initiation of ventricular fibrillation, as seen on ECG.

Mapping Triggers of PMVT/VF in Ischemic Heart Disease

Several centers have reported their experience in ablation of triggers of VF arising in the setting of acute, subacute, and remote myocardial infarction.[26-28,55] Next, we will discuss invasive mapping in PMVT/VF occuring during the acute phase of myocardial infarction (< 1 week), or delayed (>1 week), and remotely (> 6 months)

Arrhythmia Onset Less Than One Week after Acute Myocardial Infarction

EP Study and Mapping the Arrhythmogenic Triggers

In the report by Bansch et al[26] on mapping VF storm within 1 week of acute myocardial infarction, multipolar catheters were positioned from the femoral veins into the right atrium and at the His bundle. Left ventricular mapping was performed with a 7-Fr, 4 mm–tip electrode (Biosense Webster) via a retrograde approach, with or without anterograde transseptal approach. (The latter was preferred if catheter manipulation was difficult retrogradely.) Bipolar electrograms were recorded at a filter setting of 30 to 400 Hz. Pace mapping was attempted in all patients in order to identify the origin of the ectopies in the left ventricle. In addition, earliest endocardial activation of ectopic beats was used as a target for radiofrequency ablation.

Patient Population

The study reported on 4 patients experiencing drug-refractory electrical storm within a mean of 4 ± 3 days after acute myocardial infarction (2 anterior, 1 inferior, and 1 inferior with old anterior). They had undergone successful revascularization and for severely impaired left ventricular ejection fraction (32 ± 5%) and underwent invasive EP study for mapping and ablation of frequent monomorphic ventricular ectopies triggering the storm. The site of origin of the ectopies on 12-lead ECG was concordant with the site of myocardial infarction or coronary artery stenosis. The coupling interval was 270 to 400 ms. In one patient who received intravenous phenytoin for convulsions, ectopies were suppressed and not observed during the mapping procedure. All patients were sedated with midazolam and fentanyl, mechanically ventilated, and received hemodynamic support, if required.

Results of Trigger-mapping

Mapping the culprit clinical ectopies was carried out in 3 out of 4 patients. Short-coupled, high-frequency, low-amplitude potentials (surviving Purkinje cells) preceded each extrasystole by a maximum of 126 to 160 ms and the sinus QRS by 23 to 26 ms at the local site. The activation times between these potentials and the extrasystole varied from beat to beat, with exit block in one patient. Before initiating VF, local potentials preceded ventricular activation for the first few tachycardia beats and then followed the ventricular activation in a random order. The QRS morphology during the first few tachycardia beats also resembled the initiating ectopy. This pattern favors the

Step 1

AIM: Appropriate patient selection

Multiple episodes of PMVT/VF or frequent ICD shocks unresponsive to maximum medical management or device reprogramming

Step 2

AIM: Identification and reproducible bedside documentation of one or more PMVT/VF-triggering ventricular ectopic beat(s)

Continuous 12-lead ECG recording around the period of storm

Ink-marking the precordial sites of the application of the chest electrodes

Step 3

AIM: Focus of mapping – RV vs LV and Purkinje vs myocardium of the outflow tracts

Based on the ECG information and clinical setting, the source of triggers may be localized to outflow tract areas where the Purkinje network is absent

Step 4

AIM: Facilitation of distal His–Purkinje conduction

Avoid inadvertent mechanical trauma to proximal His–Purkinje system (bundle branches) during mapping-related catheter manipulation

Step 5

AIM: Recognition of distal Purkinje as a source of clinical ectopy

Electrogram characteristics of distal Purkinje site triggering the culprit ectopy:

1. Sharp electrogram
2. <10 ms duration
3. <15 ms precocity to local V in sinus rhythm

In the absence of Purkinje potential, myocardium becomes the source of the culprit ectopy

Step 6

AIM: Ablation endpoints

Complete elimination of the arrhythmia-triggering ventricular ectopy

Complete elimination of the trigger source (Purkinje potential) responsible for generating the culprit ectopy

Consolidate lesion into ≈2 cm^2 of surrounding substrate

Step 7

AIM: Ablation strategy for absent or infrequent clinical ectopy

Frequent target ectopies are necessary for clinical success. Induction of clinical ectopy can be attempted, if required:

1. Drug provocation (eg, isoproterenol infusion or withdrawal)
2. Single-ventricular, extrastimulus-induced pause may provoke clinical ectopy from the triggering source

ECG = electrocardiogram; ICD = implantable cardioverter-defilbrillator; PMVT/VF = polymorphic ventricular tachycardia/ventricular fibrillation.

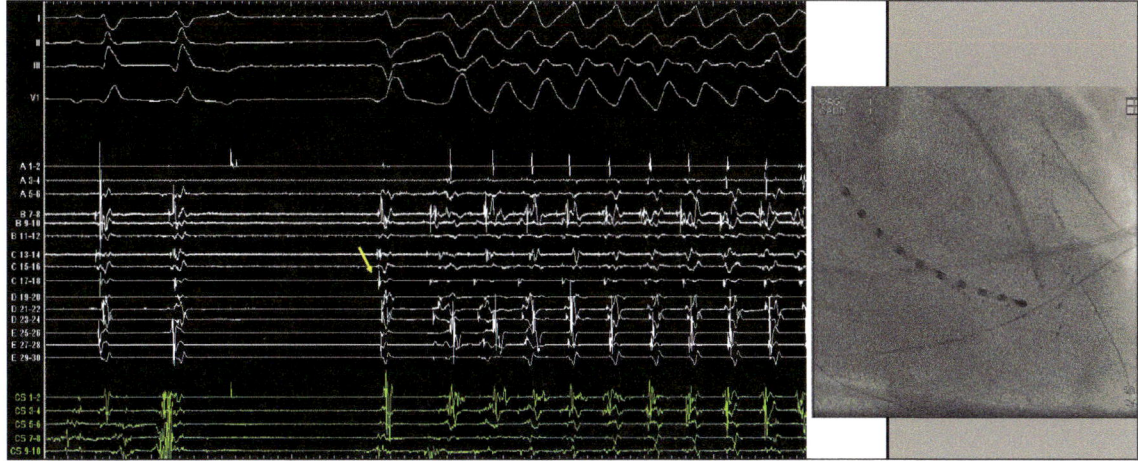

Figure 32.10 Initiation of ventricular fibrillation (VF) by clinical ectopy. **Left panel:** Purkinje potentials are seen in sinus rhythm and during VF spanning a large part of the arrhythmia cycle. (**Yellow arrow** shows Purkinje potential initiating VF.) **Right panel:** Fluroscopic image of the catheters.

role of Purkinje in initiating and maintaining VF during the first few beats, as shown in Figure 32.10.

Pace mapping at sites with QRS morphology similar to the extrasystoles showed a stimulus-to-ventricular activation interval of 0 to 50 ms. A high pacing output was necessary for capturing local myocardium. The stimulus-to-QRS time was shorter than the triggering Purkinje potential–to-QRS time; this indicated that separate capture of the triggering Purkinje network was not possible. Only pace mapping was attempted and compared with previously documented 12-lead ECGs of the extrasystoles in one patient. Areas with Purkinje potentials during sinus rhythm and pace mapping similar to the ectopy were identified and used as targets for radiofrequency ablation.

Arrhythmia Onset More Than One Week after Acute Myocardial Infarction

EP Study and Mapping the Arrhythmogenic Triggers

Szumowski et al (manuscript in preparation) studied long-term follow-up of ablation of Purkinje-triggered PMVT or VF in 14 patients. They undertook an EP study either during the storm or during frequent ventricular ectopies and supplied adequate ventilatory and circulatory support whenever necessary. One or two multielectrode catheters were introduced through the femoral vessels, including an 8 mm–tip or irrigated-tip, quadripolar roving ablation catheter (NaviStar™, Biosense Webster). The latter was introduced into the left ventricle by retrograde aortic catheterization. Surface ECG and bipolar endocardial electrograms were monitored and stored on a polygraph for offline analysis (Bard Electrophysiology, Lowell, MA; or EP-WorkMate™, St. Jude Medical, St. Paul, MN). Intracardiac electrograms were filtered at 30 to 500 Hz and measured with computer-assisted calipers at a sweep speed of 200 mm/second. Electroanatomic maps were performed using the Carto™ System (Biosense Webster; Johnson & Johnson). The border zone of the myocardial infarction was defined as the region demonstrating bipolar voltage amplitudes of 0.5 to 1.5 mV.

Activation mapping of the ectopies with preceding Purkinje potential was verified by pace mapping. Purkinje potential was defined as described above.

Patient Population

Fourteen consecutive patients (12 men; aged 63 ± 10 years) who had undergone successful revascularization were invasively studied with ventilatory support (n = 7). They had drug-refractory PMVT or VF after a mean of 10 days of an acute anterior myocardial infarction, and their mean left ventricular ejection fraction was 30% ± 9%.

Results of Trigger-mapping

All patients demonstrated frequent right bundle branch block–morphology ventricular extrasystoles (coupling interval = 390–550 ms) that initiated PMVT. The variable-morphology Purkinje potential preceded the onset of ectopies QRS by 20 to 220 ms. Repetitive Purkinje activity was documented during PMVT. The splitting of Purkinje activity and Purkinje-to-muscle conduction block was also observed.

Arrhythmia Onset More Than Six Months after Acute Myocardial Infarction

Electrophysiological Study and Mapping the Arrhythmogenic Triggers

Marrouche et al[27] reported on ablation of the triggers initiating drug-refractory VF storms in patients with at least 6-month-old myocardial infarction. Multipolar catheters were positioned from the femoral veins into the right ventricular apex and/or right atrium. Access to the left ventricle was obtained via retrograde aortic approach.

The left ventricle was mapped using a 7-Fr, 4 mm–tip catheter (NaviStar). Surface ECG leads and bipolar intracardiac electrograms were recorded and filtered at 30 to 400 Hz Prucka Cardiolab system (Prucka Inc., Milwaukee, WI). Patients were heparinized to maintain an activated clotting time of 300 to 400 seconds during left-sided mapping.

In patients with frequent ectopies resembling the clinical ectopy that initiated their electrical storm, 3D activation mapping of the ectopy was performed using Carto. If no spontaneous ectopies were detected, an isoproterenol infusion (up to 6 mcg/minute) was used. Voltage mapping was used to identify infarct-related scar and to define the scar border zone. Scar tissue was defined as a local voltage of <0.5 mV and normal tissue as >1.5 mV. In patients in whom ectopies could not be detected in sufficient quantity to permit trigger mapping, sinus rhythm substrate mapping was performed using Carto. Careful mapping along the border zone was performed to identify low-amplitude, high-frequency Purkinje-like potentials preceding the sinus QRS. Ablation targeted the site of such potentials, and the endpoint was ablation of ectopies or these potentials.

Patient Population

Out of 29 total patients having electrical storm, 8 patients (6 men; aged 65 ± 8 years) with medically refractory electrical storm were studied. The 8 patients who had undergone ablation experienced 52 ± 25 refractory episodes of VF storm despite attempted antiarrhythmic therapy with amiodarone, mexilitine, and procainamide. One patient required left ventricular assist device. These 8 patients had mean 11 ± 5-month-old myocardial infarction with an average ejection fraction of 15% ± 4%. None of the patients had acute ischemic ECG changes, significant elevations in cardiac enzymes, or new severe coronary artery lesions. Among the 29 patients, VF storm was initiated with monomorphic right bundle branch block morphology (inferior axis in 24 and superior axis in 5), ventricular ectopy with a mean QRS duration of 178 ± 25 ms, and a mean coupling interval of 195 ± 45 ms.

Results of Trigger-mapping

Spontaneous ($n = 4$) and isoproterenol-induced ($n = 1$) monomorphic ectopies triggering storm were mapped. In all 5 cases, the clinical ectopy was preceded by a low-amplitude, high-frequency potential by 68 ± 20 ms recorded from the scar border zone. The local site demonstrated Purkinje-like potential preceding QRS complex in sinus rhythm. Three patients underwent substrate-based mapping in sinus rhythm. Low-amplitude, high-frequency potentials similar to those preceding target ectopies were observed during sinus rhythm along the scar border zone. These potentials were targeted during ablation.

Mapping Triggers of PMVT/VF in Amyloid Heart Disease

EP Study and Mapping the Arrhythmogenic Triggers

Two cases of VF storm in amyloid hearts were reported by Mlcochova et al.[30] One quadripolar and one mapping/ablation catheter (NaviStar, Biosense Webster) were used via transvenous and retrograde aortic routes, respectively. The surface ECG and intracardiac electrogram were displayed on a recording system (Prucka, Inc.). The Carto System was used to localize the focal origin of ventricular ectopy using an activation map.

Patient Population

Both patients were female (aged 60 and 52 years, respectively), and cardiac amyloidosis was diagnosed on biopsy immediately after successful ablation of ventricular arrhythmias. The first patient had severe ischemic left ventricular dysfunction and developed incessant episodes of nonsustained PMVT with underlying atrial fibrillation after repeat aortocoronary bypass surgery and mitral valve replacement. The arrhythmia, unresponsive to medical treatment, worsened 3 weeks later and developed into electrical storm. The second patient had normal echocardiography and coronary arterial tree, old occipital hemorrhage, and pulmonary lobectomy; symptomatic bigeminy was her presenting feature. After having a transient response to β-blockers, bigeminy rapidly increased to PMVT, which degenerated into VF despite ongoing medical treatment. The arrhythmia transiently responded to high-dose intravenous verapamil, which resulted in complete heart block and a narrow complex, junctional escape rhythm. Prophylactic mechanical ventilation was undertaken before catheter ablation. In both cases, monomorphic right bundle branch block morphology ectopies (160 ms and 130 ms wide, respectively) with superior axis initiated the arrhythmia at coupling intervals of 370 ms and 400 ms, respectively.

Results of Trigger-mapping

In the first patient, ectopic beat was preceded by 65 ms by a low-voltage, high-frequency potential that had not been observed during sinus rhythm, suggesting a myocardial source. The site of earliest activation was detected in the healthy, normal-voltage, inferolateral apical region of the left ventricular free wall. In the second patient, the ectopic origin could be localized to the area of the proximal posterior fascicle of the left bundle, marked by fascicular potential preceding the QRS during sinus rhythm and ectopy.

Mapping Triggers of PMVT/VF in Nonischemic Dilated Cardiomyopathy

EP Study and Mapping the Arrhythmogenic Triggers

Sinha et al[29] reported on trigger-mapping and ablation of VF in 5 patients with nonischemic dilated cardiomyopathy. An EP study was conducted under conscious sedation and local anesthesia. Multipolar catheters were positioned at the right ventricular apex and/or right atrium using a femoral approach. The left ventricle was accessed retrogradely via the aorta. Left ventricular mapping was performed using a 7-Fr, 3.5 mm–tip catheter (NaviStar THERMOCOOL, Biosense Webster). Surface and bipolar intracardiac electrograms were recorded and filtered using a 30 to 400 Hz Prucka Cardiolab system (Prucka Inc.). During the procedure, patients were heparinized to maintain an activated clotting time of 300 to 400 seconds. Three-dimensional voltage mapping was performed using CARTO during sinus rhythm, with sequential mapping of repetitive extrasystoles and/or ventricular arrhythmias if they occurred. For the CARTO map, scar tissue was defined as a local voltage of <0.5 mV, and normal tissue was defined as having voltage >1.5 mV. Areas with intermediate local voltage (0.5–1.5 mV) were defined as scar border zone. Careful mapping along the scar and the border zone was performed in order to identify low-amplitude, high-frequency Purkinje-like potentials. Isoproterenol infusion (up to 10 mcg/minute) was administered if no spontaneous extrasystoles were detected.

Patient Population

Five patients with dilated nonischemic cardiomyopathy (3 men; mean age: 61 ± 13 years) and left ventricular ejection fraction of 35% ± 16% continued to suffer ongoing defibrillator discharges with VF (mean episodes: 6 ± 2) despite optimum medical treatment including antiarrhythmic drugs (β-blockers and amiodarone). None of the patients showed frequent extrasystoles or VF during sinus rhythm. Two patients also suffered from monomorphic ventricular tachycardia. At our center, we successfully mapped and ablated one patient with aortic valve replacement who presented with storm of VF on day 9 postsurgery (Figure 32.11).

Results of Trigger-mapping

At baseline sinus rhythm, none of the patients presented with frequent ventricular ectopy or VF. In 4 patients, electroanatomic mapping identified the scar along the posterior mitral annulus in the left ventricular basal myocardial region. Programmed ventricular stimulation with isoproterenol triggered ectopy in 1 patient and VF in 3 others. In the patient with sustained ectopies, the arrhythmia for a patient with nonischemic cardiomyopathy was mapped to the distal posterior Purkinje tree (precocity of 70 ms to surface QRS of the ectopic beat) in the scar border zone. In the remaining 3 patients without ectopies but with inducible fibrillatory rhythm, Purkinje-like potentials were mapped to the region of scar border zone in sinus rhythm and targeted for ablation. In 1 patient (who also had no scar), no arrhythmia was inducible and no mapping or ablation was performed.

Conclusions

PMVT and VF, the unmappable arrhythmias, are triggered by ventricular ectopies frequently arising in the His–Purkinje network in structurally normal and diseased hearts (in >80% cases) and of predominantly myocardial origin (RVOT) in Brugada syndrome. Invasive mapping helps to identify these triggers and provides

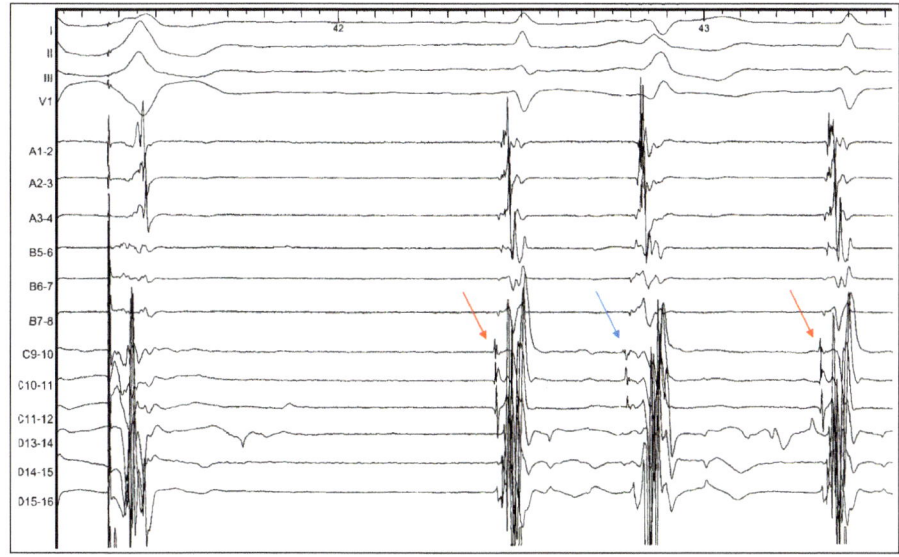

Figure 32.11 Distal Purkinje potentials are seen preceding the local ventricular electrogram during sinus rhythm (**red arrows**) and ectopy (**blue arrow**) in a patient who underwent high-density mapping of the Purkinje network after aortic valve replacement.

targets for ablation of these potentially lethal arrhythmias. Going forward, clinical knowledge about the crucial role that triggers play will promote more fundamental studies into the clinical anatomy, gross and microscopic structure, EP properties, and dynamics of the arrhythmogenic transformation of these triggers.

References

1. Wever EFD, Hauer RNW, Oomen A, et al. Unfavorable outcome in patients with primary electrical disease who survived an episode of ventricular fibrillation. *Circulation*. 1993; 88:1021-1029.
2. Wever EF, Robles de Medina EO. Sudden death in patients without structural heart disease. *J Am Coll Cardiol*. 2004;43(7): 1137-1144.
3. Huikuri HV, Castellanos A, Myerburg RJ. Sudden death due to cardiac arrhythmias. *N Engl J Med*. 2001;345:1473-1482.
4. Haïssaguerre M, Shah DC, Jaïs P, et al. Role of Purkinje conducting system in triggering idiopathic sudden cardiac death. *Lancet*. 2002;359:677-678.
5. Haïssaguerre M, Shoda M, Jaïs P, et al. Mapping and ablation of idiopathic ventricular fibrillation. *Circulation*. 2002; 106:962-967.
6. Hoffman BF. Genesis of cardiac arrhythmias. *Prog Cardiovasc Dis*. 1966;8:219-229.
7. Friedman PL, Stewart JR, Fenoglio JJ Jr, Wit AL. Survival of subendocardial Purkinje fibers after extensive myocardial infarction in dogs. *Circ Res*. 1973;33(5):597-611.
8. Friedman PL, Stewart JR, Wit AL. Spontaneous and induced cardiac arrhythmias in subendocardial Purkinje fibers surviving extensive myocardial infarction in dogs. *Circ Res*. 1973;33:612-626.
9. Johnson FD, Hill IGW, Wilson FN. The form of the electrocardiogram in experimental myocardial infarction: II. The early effects produced by ligation of the anterior descending branch of the left coronary artery. *Am Heart J*. 1935;10:889.
10. Moe GK, Harris AS, Wiggers CJ. Analysis of the initiation of fibrillation by electrographic studies. *Am J Physiol*. 1941;134:473-492.
11. Myerburg RJ, Stewart JW, Hoffman BF. Electrophysiological properties of the canine peripheral conducting system. *Circ Res*. 1970;26:361-372.
12. Berenfeld O, Jalife J. Purkinje-muscle reentry as a mechanism of polymorphic ventricular arrhythmias in a 3-dimensional model of the ventricles. *Circ Res*. 1998;82:1063-1077.
13. Janse MJ. Focus, reentry, or "focal" reentry? *Am J Physiol Heart Circ Physiol*. 2007;292:2561-2562.
14. Overholt ED, Joyner RW, Veenstra RD, et al. Unidirectional block between Purkinje and ventricular layers of papillary muscles. *Am J Physiol*. 1984;247:H584-H595.
15. Pak HN, Kim YH, Lim HE, et al. Role of the posterior papillary muscle and Purkinje potentials in the mechanism of ventricular fibrillation in open chest dogs and swine: effects of catheter ablation. *J Cardiovasc Electrophysiol*. 2006;17:777-783.
16. Tabereaux PB, Walcott GP, Rogers JM, et al. Activation patterns of Purkinje fibers during long-duration ventricular fibrillation in an isolated canine heart model. *Circulation*. 2007;116(10):1113-1119.
17. Dun W, Boyden PA. The Purkinje cell; 2008 style. *J Mol Cell Cardiol*. 2008;45(5):617-624.
18. Damiano RJ Jr, Smith PK, Tripp HF Jr, et al. The effect of chemical ablation of the endocardium on ventricular fibrillation threshold. *Circulation*. 1986;74:645-652.
19. Dosdall DJ, Tabereaux PB, Kim JJ, et al. Chemical ablation of the Purkinje system causes early termination and activation rate slowing of long-duration ventricular fibrillation in dogs. *Am J Physiol Heart Circ Physiol*. 2008;295(2):H883-H889.
20. Ashida K, Kaji Y, Sasaki Y. Abolition of torsade de pointes after radiofrequency catheter ablation at right ventricular outflow tract. *Int J Cardiol*. 1997;59(2):171-175.
21. Kusano KF, Yamamoto M, Emori T, et al. Successful catheter ablation in a patient with polymorphic ventricular tachycardia. *J Cardiovasc Electrophysiol*. 2000;11:682-685.
22. Takatsuki S, Mitamura H, Ogawa S. Catheter ablation of a monofocal premature ventricular complex triggering idiopathic ventricular fibrillation. *Heart*. 2001;86:E3.
23. Saliba W, Abul Karim A, Tchou P, Natale A. Ventricular fibrillation: ablation of a trigger? *J Cardiovasc Electrophysiol*. 2002;13;1296-1299.
24. Haïssaguerre M, Extramiana F, Hocini M, et al. Mapping and ablation of ventricular fibrillation associated with long-QT and Brugada syndromes. *Circulation*. 2003;108:925-928.
25. Haïssaguerre M, Derval N, Sacher F, et al. Sudden cardiac arrest associated with early repolarization. *N Engl J Med*. 2008;358:2016-2023.
26. Bansch D, Oyang F, Antz M, et al. Successful catheter ablation of electrical storm after myocardial infarction. *Circulation*. 2003;108:3011-3016.
27. Marrouche NF, Verma A, Wazni O, et al. Mode of initiation and ablation of ventricular fibrillation storms in patients with ischemic cardiomyopathy. *J Am Coll Cardiol*. 2004;43(9): 1715-1720.
28. Peichl P, Cihák R, Kozeluhová M, et al. Catheter ablation of arrhythmic storm triggered by monomorphic ectopic beats in patients with coronary artery disease. *J Interv Card Electrophysiol*. 2010;27(1):51-59.
29. Sinha AM, Schmidt M, Marschang H, et al. Role of left ventricular scar and Purkinje-like potentials during mapping and ablation of ventricular fibrillation in dilated cardiomyopathy. *Pacing Clin Electrophysiol*. 2009;32(3):286-290.
30. Mlcochova H, Saliba WI, Burkhardt DJ, et al. Catheter ablation of ventricular fibrillation storm in patients with infiltrative amyloidosis of the heart. *J Cardiovasc Electrophysiol*. 2006; 17(4):426-430.
31. Bode K, Hindricks G, Piorkowski C, et al. Ablation of polymorphic ventricular tachycardias in patients with structural heart disease. *Pacing Clin Electrophysiol*. 2008;31(12): 1585-1591.
32. Li YG, Gronefeld G, Israel C, Hohnloser SH. Catheter ablation of frequently recurring ventricular fibrillation in a patient after aortic valve repair. *J Cardiovasc Electrophysiol*. 2004; 15:90-93.
33. Pasquié JL, Sanders P, Hocini M, et al. Fever as a precipitant of idiopathic ventricular fibrillation in patients with normal hearts. *J Cardiovasc Electrophysiol*. 2004;15(11):1271-1276.
34. Betts TR, Yue A, Roberts PR, Morgan JM. Radiofrequency ablation of idiopathic ventricular fibrillation guided by noncontact mapping. *J Cardiovasc Electrophysiol*. 2004;15:957-959.
35. Darmon JP, Bettouche S, Deswardt P, et al. Radiofrequency ablation of ventricular fibrillation and multiple right and left atrial tachycardia in a patient with Brugada syndrome. *J Interv Card Electrophysiol*. 2004;11:205-209.
36. Nogami A, Sugiyasu A, Kubota S, Kato K. Mapping and ablation of idiopathic ventricular fibrillation from the Purkinje system. *Heart Rhythm*. 2005;2:646-649.

37. Enjoji Y, Mizobuchi M, Shibata K, et al. Catheter ablation for an incessant form of antiarrhythmic drug-resistant ventricular fibrillation after acute coronary syndrome. *Pacing Clin Electrophysiol.* 2006;29(1):102-105.
38. Yu CC, Tsai CT, Lai LP, Lin JL. Successful radiofrequency catheter ablation of idiopathic ventricular fibrillation presented as recurrent syncope and diagnosed by an implanted loop recorder. *Int J Cardiol.* 2006;110(1):112-113.
39. Kohsaka S, Razavi M, Massumi A. Idiopathic ventricular fibrillation successfully terminated by radiofrequency ablation of the distal Purkinje fibers. *Pacing Clin Electrophysiol.* 2007;30:701-704.
40. Okada T, Yamada T, Murakami Y, et al. Mapping and ablation of trigger premature ventricular contractions in a case of electrical storm associated with ischemic cardiomyopathy. *Pacing Clin Electrophysiol.* 2007;30:440-443.
41. Srivathsan K, Gami AS, Ackerman MJ, Asirvatham SJ. Treatment of ventricular fibrillation in a patient with prior diagnosis of long QT syndrome: importance of precise electrophysiologic diagnosis to successfully ablate the trigger. *Heart Rhythm.* 2007;4:1090-1093.
42. Naik N, Juneja R, Sharma G, et al. Malignant idiopathic ventricular fibrillation "cured" by radiofrequency ablation. *J Interv Card Electrophysiol.* 2008;23(2):143-148.
43. Takahashi Y, Takahashi A, Isobe M. Ventricular fibrillation initiated by premature beats from the ventricular myocardium not associated with the Purkinje system after myocardial infarction. *Heart Rhythm.* 2008;5:1458-1460.
44. Kataoka M, Takatsuki S, Tanimoto K, et al. A case of vagally mediated idiopathic ventricular fibrillation. *Nat Clin Pract Cardiovasc Med.* 2008;5:111-115.
45. Nakagawa E, Takagi M, Tatsumi H, Yoshiyama M. Successful radiofrequency catheter ablation for electrical storm of ventricular fibrillation in a patient with Brugada syndrome. *Circ J.* 2008;72(6):1025-1029.
46. Uemura T, Yamabe H, Tanaka Y, et al. Catheter ablation of a polymorphic ventricular tachycardia inducing monofocal premature ventricular complex. *Intern Med.* 2008;47(20):1799-1802.
47. Nogami A, Kubota S, Adachi M, Igawa O. Electrophysiologic and histopathologic findings of the ablation sites for ventricular fibrillation in a patient with ischemic cardiomyopathy. *J Interv Card Electrophysiol.* 2009;24(2):133-137.
48. Suh WM, Fowler SJ, Yeh T, Krishnan SC. Successful catheter ablation of focal ventricular fibrillation originating from the right ventricle. *J Interv Card Electrophysiol.* 2009;26(2):139-142.
49. Kirubakaran S, Gill J, Rinaldi CA. Successful catheter ablation of focal ventricular fibrillation in a patient with nonischemic dilated cardiomyopathy. *Pacing Clin Electrophysiol.* 2011;34(4):e38-e42.
50. Gray RA, Jalife J, Panfilov AV, et al. Mechanism of cardiac fibrillation. *Science.* 1996;270:1223-1225.
51. Kim Y-H, Xie F, Yashima M, et al. Role of papillary muscle in the generation and maintenance of reentry during ventricular tachycardia and fibrillation in isolated swine right ventricle. *Circulation.* 1999;100:1450-1459.
52. Knecht S, Sacher F, Wright M, et al. Long-term follow-up of idiopathic ventricular fibrillation ablation: a multicenter study. *J Am Coll Cardiol.* 2009;54(6):522-528.
53. Zipes DP, Camm AJ, Borggrefe M, et al. ACC/AHA/ESC 2006 guidelines for management of patients with ventricular arrhythmias and the prevention of sudden cardiac death: a report of the American College of Cardiology/American Heart Association Task Force and the European Society of Cardiology Committee for Practice Guidelines (Writing Committee to Develop Guidelines for Management of Patients With Ventricular Arrhythmias and the Prevention of Sudden Cardiac Death). *J Am Coll Cardiol.* 2006;48:e247-346.
54. Shah AJ, Hocini M, Lamaison D, et al. Regional substrate ablation abolishes Brugada syndrome. *J Cardiovasc Electrophysiol.* 2011;22(11):1290-1291.
55. Szumowski L, Sanders P, Walczak F, et al. Mapping and ablation of polymorphic ventricular tachycardia after myocardial infarction. *J Am Coll Cardiol.* 2004;44(8):1700-1706.

CHAPTER 33

Mapping of Arrhythmias During Pediatric Electrophysiology Procedures

Larry A. Rhodes, MD

Introduction

The use of radiofrequency ablation for the treatment of arrhythmias in children began in 1991.[1] In many ways, it has paralleled that of adults, although when newer mapping and ablation techniques have been introduced, they are often delayed in their use in pediatrics. The pediatric population offers challenges related not only to the patient's size but also to the long-term effects of lesions in a growing child. Particular interest has focused on several risks: the potential for damage to cardiac valves and coronary arteries in the growing and developing heart, radiation exposure, and potential damage to vessels used for vascular access. Potential obstacles to successful ablations exist in patients with congenital heart disease relative to anatomy, vascular access, and arrhythmia substrate. This chapter will focus on these and other issues related to catheter ablation in children.

Patient Safety

Prior to discussing technical issues related to mapping and ablation in children, it is important to review issues relative to both acute and chronic safety in this population. Shortly after the first reports of the use of radiofrequency catheter ablation in children, the Pediatric Electrophysiology Society established a national registry to follow the results in terms of safety and success.[2] A follow-up study in 2004[3] evaluated the use of radiofrequency ablation in 2,761 pediatric patients between 0 and 16 years with supraventricular tachycardia. This study looked at complications and initial success rates in children who did not have significant congenital heart disease.

This well-designed study evaluated subjects divided into 3 groups to eliminate bias based on recruitment. Group I consisted of 481 subjects followed prospectively; Group II was made up of 504 subjects who fulfilled entry criteria but were not enrolled in the prospective study; and Group III contained 1,776 subjects who did not qualify for the prospective study but were in the registry. Complications were evaluated relative to whether the subject had undergone an electrophysiology study alone or the addition of radiofrequency ablation.

The incidence of complications in the electrophysiology group ranged from 2.9% to 4.2%, with the most common complication being a hematoma at catheter entry (1.4%). In the radiofrequency ablation group, the incidence of complications ranged from 2.6% to 4%. Atrioventricular block was seen in 1.2%, most frequently in patients with atrial ventricular nodal reentry tachycardia. Overall successful ablation of supraventricular tachycardia was noted in 95.7% of the patients. This was an improvement on the initial rates of 83% reported in 1994[4] and 92% in 1997[2] and similar to that reported in an adult series in 2000.[5] The authors commented in this report that if success was not achieved after 50 minutes of fluoroscopy time, there continued to be an 81% chance of success if one persists. However, they stressed that the clinician should weigh the risks of additional fluoroscopy exposure against the possible benefits of eventual success.[3] There were no deaths in this study. In the original registry report by Kugler et al,[2] there were a total of 4 (0.097%) procedure-related deaths in 4,135 children from 1991 to 1996. The results of this study quickly became the benchmark for expected results in the pediatric population, in terms of both acute and long-term success as well as in the occurrence of complications.

A follow-up study in 2007 evaluated the short- and long-term outcomes of the 481 patients followed prospectively in the above publication. In addition to success rates, the patients were evaluated for any acute or long-term complications. Patients ranged from 0 to 16 years of age, having supraventricular tachycardia without congenital heart disease. The mean procedure time was 206.7 minutes, with a mean of 7.6 radiofrequency lesions.

There were 406 subjects with both pre- and postprocedure echocardiograms available for review. Mild insufficiency in at least one atrioventricular or semilunar valve was present in both preablation (42.43%) and postablation (40.49%) studies.[6] Changes in valvular insufficiency were graded numerically; a change of 1 degree (none to mild) was scored as 1, and a change of 2 (none to moderate) was scored as 2. This system was applied in the opposite direction if the insufficiency improved. In this group, 1 subject was judged to have changed by 2 points toward less severity, and none were judged to have changed by >2 points toward greater severity. In 10.26% of subjects, valvular insufficiency improved, and in 9.42%, it worsened by 1 point. The greatest percentage of worsening valvular insufficiency was noted for the tricuspid valve in left free-wall pathways addressed by a retrograde approach (26.32%), left septal pathways (25%), and right free-wall pathways (20.59%).[6]

The authors also evaluated whether a particular catheter approach had put specific valves at risk. They evaluated differences in retrograde versus transseptal approaches to left-sided pathways and the effect on the mitral and aortic valves. Tricuspid regurgitation was analyzed relative to ablation of atrioventricular nodal reentry tachycardia (AVNRT), right free-wall, and right septal pathways. They uncovered no difference based on the approach to left-sided pathways. However, they did find statistically significant differences in the degree of tricuspid valve insufficiency in patients who had ablation of AVNRT and of a right free-wall pathway.[6]

There were no thrombi noted in cardiac chambers following radiofrequency ablation. Dyskinesis was noted on echocardiography at baseline and 2 months after ablation but was slightly more frequent after ablation than before (0.66% vs 1.64%). Although this study found no clear effect of radiofrequency ablation on cardiac wall motion or left ventricular function, the authors stated that the detection of coronary artery injury cannot be ruled out by echocardiography. They suggested that assessing the impact of radiofrequency ablation on coronary artery damage would require selective angiography or cardiac perfusion studies.[6]

This study failed to identify significant injury to cardiac valves or an adverse effect of radiofrequency ablation on cardiac function. This finding contrasted with an earlier study by Minich et al, which reported on 44 pediatric patients who had serial echocardiograms prior to and following radiofrequency ablation. Their study noted a 12% increase of mitral regurgitation and a 30% increase in the incidence of aortic regurgitation following ablation of left-sided accessory pathways via a retrograde approach.[7] These differences most likely represent a learning curve effect over a 15-year period as well as advances in technology.

Patient Size

During the past two decades, experience, expertise, and technology have improved significantly in radiofrequency ablation. These factors have led to a desire to expand the application of this technique to younger and smaller patients. However, significant concerns have been raised about the impact that patient size may have on acute and long-term safety in children undergoing radiofrequency catheter ablation. For instance, the size of mapping and radiofrequency catheters relative to the size of the patient's heart and blood vessels can lead to significant morbidity based solely on size and limited mobility. This, in addition to the proximity of critical structures (such as the atrioventricular node and coronary arteries to the arrhythmia substrate) as well as the possibility of lesion growth as the heart grows, makes it easy to understand the concerns.

The largest body of experience concerning radiofrequency ablation in children was gathered in the Pediatric Radiofrequency Ablation Registry.[2] In 1997, this registry reported patient weight less than 15 kg as an independent risk factor for procedure-related complications, including an increased risk for heart block,[8] injury to blood vessels used for access, and injury to the heart itself.[9] A recent retrospective study[10] reported from the University of Michigan and the University of Utah reviewed all registry patients weighing ≤20 kg who had a radiofrequency ablation for supraventricular tachycardia between January 1994 and January 2003. They divided subjects into 2 groups: Group 1 (≤15 kg) and Group 2 (>15 kg and ≤20 kg). Group 1 had 25 procedures in 23 patients, and Group 2 had 44 procedures in 40 patients. Group 1 had a statistically greater incidence of structural heart disease than Group 2. There was no significant difference between the groups in short- or long-term success.

Overall, the rate of major complications was 4.3%. Major complications included 2 atrial perforations in Group 1: one occurring during a transseptal puncture and the other noted during recovery. Both patients required pericardiocentesis. There was also 1 patient in Group 2 with complex cyanotic congenital heart disease who developed depressed function following radiofrequency ablation but without evidence of coronary compromise, based on resting electrocardiogram or cardiac catheterization.

This study stressed the fact that, frequently, one needs to proceed with radiofrequency ablation in children who have structural heart defects at a younger age and a smaller size. This is secondary to the fact that their baseline hemodynamics may not allow them to tolerate the insult of a tachyarrhythmia or medical therapy as well as a child without a congenital defect.

The authors of this study stated that certain techniques should be employed during electrophysiology studies and radiofrequency ablation in small patients to maximize procedural safety (Table 33.1). A summary of their recommendations include the following:

- General anesthesia and held ventilation while applying radiofrequency energy to improve catheter stability;
- An esophageal electrode lead as a substitute for a right atrial catheter;
- A multipole catheter to record the bundle of His and the right ventricular apex (as well as pacing);[11]
- Smaller (5 and 6 Fr) mapping and ablation catheters;
- The delivery of few or no "test" or "insurance" lesions;
- Lower maximal temperatures (50°–55°C); and
- Shorter application cycles of energy.[10]

Table 33.1 Modifications for performing radiofrequency catheter ablation in children weighing < 20 kg

Sedation
• General anesthesia
• Supervised conscious sedation
• Precatheterization use of topical anesthetic
Catheters
• Recording and stimulation
– Esophageal lead (behind left atrium)
– Single 4-Fr or 5-Fr multipolar lead to record His and right ventricular apex
• Ablation
– 5 Fr or 6 Fr with 4 mm tip
• Transseptal
– 5 Fr
Vessel Entry
• Placement of no more than two 5-Fr sheaths in femoral vein
• Placement of multicatheter sheath
Special Techniques
• Coronary mapping
• Cryomapping
• Few to no insurance burns
• Careful monitoring of fluoroscopic times

Radiation Exposure

Another major concern when performing radiofrequency ablation in growing children is the effect of radiation, both acutely and during a lifetime of follow-up. These include malignancies, skin lesions, cataracts, and birth defects in the patients' future children.[12-14] A large subset of children undergoing ablation procedures also have congenital heart disease and have already had significant exposure to radiation related to their anatomy and palliative procedures. In studies of diagnostic and therapeutic pediatric and adult catheterization and ablation procedures, the lifetime risk of developing malignancies has been estimated at 0.08% to 0.1%.[15-18]

In addition to radiation exposure to the child, one needs to be cognizant of the cumulative exposure to staff and other laboratory personnel. This is especially important in an electrophysiology lab, where cases are frequently measured in hours, not minutes. This concern has led to a significant interest in decreasing radiation exposure, and a number of centers are moving toward nonfluoroscopic imaging.

Tuzcu published a report in 2007[19] of 26 consecutive electrophysiology studies and 24 of 28 consecutive right-sided ablations in patients performed without fluoroscopy. Patients ranged in age from 6 months to 38 years. There were 2 patients with mild Ebstein's malformation; all others had structurally normal hearts. Twenty-three of the 24 ablations were performed with cryoablation. In the electrophysiology study group, the mean procedure time was 98.7 ± 49.7 minutes with no additional fluoroscopic guidance. The mean procedure time in those undergoing ablation was 193.5 ± 80 minutes. Of those undergoing ablation procedures, 4 required additional fluoroscopic guidance. There were no complications.

These ablation data were compared with those of a control group of 19 patients who had right-side ablations prior to three-dimensional (3D) mapping. In comparing these groups, no significant differences were found between procedure time and age of patients who underwent ablation with or without fluoroscopic guidance. Overall success rates did not differ between the 2 groups.

The author stated that having 3D images of the right atrium allowed the operator to analyze the catheters from many angles, helping to achieve fast and safe placement of catheters in the heart. Another perceived advantage to this type of mapping was the ability to map the coronary sinus without the need to maintain a coronary sinus catheter throughout the case; this decreased by one the total number of catheters required in these smaller patients.

A similar retrospective study from Akron Children's Hospital in 2007[20] reported on 30 patients who underwent ablation with 3D mapping and 30 age-matched controls. In this study, as in the one above, there was a high procedural success rate (30 of 30) and a low mean fluoroscopy time of 1.05 ± 2.9 minutes, in contrast to 21.4 ± 18.3 minutes for the control group. Six of 30 patients in the 3D group required the use of fluoroscopy. There was no significant difference in procedure times between the 2 groups. Complications included transient atrioventricular block in 10 patients during applications of cryotherapy, all of which resolved by the end of the case. At a mean follow-up of 3 months (range: 1–6 months), recurrence was noted in 13% in the 3D group and 10.3% in the control group.

These authors stated that, in addition to the decreased radiation exposure, 3D mapping offers other potential benefits. These include eliminating the need to wear lead garments during procedures as well as portability, making it feasible to do an ablation in the intensive care unit rather than needing to transport a sick patient to the laboratory. They also pointed out that this type of mapping affords one the opportunity of doing ablations at times otherwise not possible, such as during pregnancy.[20]

A study from Athens in 2006[21] had similar findings. It retrospectively compared 40 consecutive pediatric patients who had undergone ablation with a nonfluoroscopic navigation system with 40 consecutive patients with similar diagnoses who had undergone radiofrequency ablation with fluoroscopic guidance. They too found shorter procedural times, similar success rates, and no significant difference in recurrence rates.

As the above studies report, there is a significant interest in decreasing radiation exposure to both the patient and healthcare providers during ablation procedures. Technology is advancing at a rate that will, in all likelihood, lead to a nonradiological electrophysiology laboratory.

Technical Issues Relative to Patient Size

In the past two decades, a number of catheter techniques have been developed to aid in the mapping and ablation in patients whose body surface area frequently is less than half an adult's. Many of these techniques have emerged through the efforts of industry in providing smaller electrophysiology catheters and sheaths for easier vascular access and less vascular trauma. Other creative innovations have been developed by practitioners that enable procedures to be performed with less vascular access. These include esophageal pacing and sensing,[10] using single catheters to record the bundle of His and the right ventricular apex, and the novel use of catheter placement in nonstandard locations to help with mapping. (See Figure 33.1.) Electrophysiologists who have attempted ablations in children have found that failed procedures are frequently the result of difficulty with catheter position and stabilization, epicardial accessory pathway location, and associated congenital heart defects leading to mapping errors.[22]

As many experienced pediatric and adult electrophysiologists know, right-sided, nonseptal pathways are frequently very difficult to map and ablate. A recent report from Turkey[23] described the placement of mapping catheters in coronary arteries to improve localization of accessory pathways along the left and right atrioventricular grooves.

The authors reported the use of microcatheter-assisted mapping during ablation procedures in 7 children with a mean age of 15.3 ± 1.6 years and a mean weight of 52.6 ± 6.5 kg. This technique took advantage of the fact that the right coronary artery is in the right epicardial atrioventricular groove and has a constant relation to the annulus.[23]

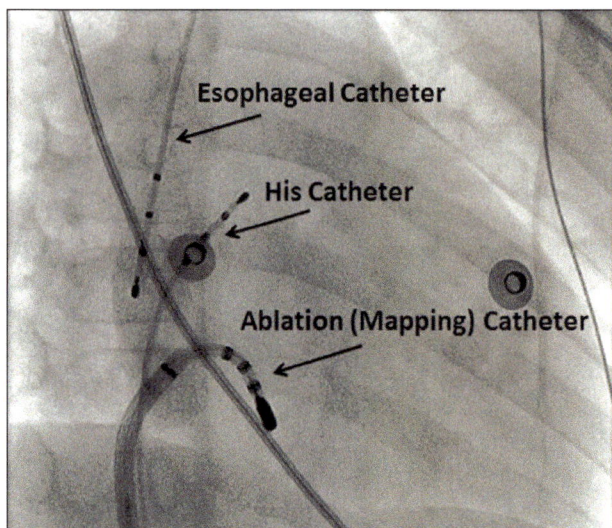

Figure 33.1 Ablation in a 4-year-old with ectopic atrial tachycardia performed with 2 intracardiac and esophageal catheters. The His catheter is used to record the bundle on the proximal electrodes and to record or pace the right ventricle on the distal pair. The esophageal catheter is used as a reference for timing atrial activity or atrial pacing if needed.

The technique included coronary arteriography in a right anterior oblique and left anterior oblique view to determine right coronary artery size. A 6-Fr right Judkins guiding catheter was placed in the right coronary artery and connected to a rotating hemostatic valve. Following this, a 2.3-Fr octapolar microcatheter (Cardima Inc., Fresno, CA) was placed in the right coronary artery. Once the microcatheter was placed, the patients underwent standard mapping and ablation procedures. Operators ablated 8 accessory pathways in 7 patients (3 with congenital heart disease), and there were no cardiac or neurological complications during the procedure or follow-up. They also performed this technique in left-sided pathways in patients with abnormalities of the coronary sinus.

The authors suggested that these techniques be employed in special circumstances: in patients with structurally normal hearts in which there is difficulty in localizing the atrioventricular groove and in complex congenital heart diseases. This technique has been particularly helpful in those patients with Ebstein's anomaly of the tricuspid valve, not only for anatomic guidance but also for sorting out the complex signals in the arrhythmias seen in these patients.

There are circumstances in children (especially those who are very small or have significant structural heart disease) that lead the provider to develop techniques to help determine the mechanism and location of an abnormal rhythm substrate. A recent example of this innovation is seen in a publication describing cryomapping in a small child with complex congenital heart disease with supraventricular tachycardia who was to undergo a significant surgical palliation and had failed numerous medications.[24]

In this report, the patient underwent a standard electrophysiology stimulation protocol with induction of supraventricular tachycardia. Mapping in supraventricular tachycardia suggested atrioventricular reentrant supraventricular tachycardia via a para-Hisian accessory pathway or AVNRT. In an attempt to determine whether the mechanism was AVNRT, cryomapping was performed during supraventricular tachycardia in areas where electrograms resembled those seen in AVNRT in structurally normal hearts. Cryomapping was performed for 30 seconds at −25°C until supraventricular tachycardia was terminated. Standard electrophysiology recordings and techniques suggested that this was typical AVNRT and not a para-Hisian pathway. This (in addition to having achieved termination of the tachycardia in the region of the slow pathway) allowed the team to proceed to cryoablation for 240 seconds at −80°C. Although the supraventricular tachycardia remained, inducibility was much more difficult, requiring double atrial extrastimuli and isoproterenol infusion. A total of 44 cryomapping applications were made during the procedure without damage to the atrioventricular node.

These authors pointed out that cryomapping offers a significant safety advantage for patients with a supraventricular tachycardia mechanism that requires ablation near the atrioventricular node. This need is more pronounced in patients with complex congenital heart disease in whom the location of the atrioventricular node and His–Purkinje system may be different from that in the normal heart.[24]

There are rare, but not insignificant, occasions in both children and adults when one is required (or at least tempted) to deliver an ablation lesion in the coronary sinus. This is generally related to a left-side epicardial accessory pathway. However, radiofrequency energy has the potential to perforate the coronary sinus, lead to thrombus formation, or damage the circumflex coronary artery—concerns that are compounded in small children. There is also the problem of delivering significant energy for an effective lesion secondary to the relative low-flow state in the coronary sinus that is partially occluded by a catheter.

A multicenter study[25] presented experiences in using cryoablation technology in the coronary sinus of 21 patients with a median age of 13.0 years and a median weight of 51 kg. They reported an initial success rate of 71% with 2 complications (a femoral arterial hematoma and transient atrioventricular block) and noted no ST segment elevations. There were 6 recurrences in a median follow-up of 257 days. The authors concluded that cryoablation of accessory pathways within the coronary sinus in children and patients with congenital heart disease has a reasonable acute success rate.

Arrhythmias in Children and Adults with Congenital Heart Disease

General Concepts

Patients with congenital heart disease frequently have rhythm disturbances related to their underlying hemodynamics, naturally occurring conduction obstacles, or those created following surgical intervention. Before entering the laboratory for an electrophysiology study and ablation, one needs to be significantly prepared. This preparation begins with a thorough understanding of the patient's underlying congenital heart disease in terms of anatomy and physiology. A careful and thorough review of all prior interventions (both catheter and surgical) is required. As part of this review, one should consider the options for vascular access. Many of these patients may have lost common sites of access either secondary to prior interventions or because of anatomy that does not allow entry to the heart (Table 33.2).

Hemodynamic insults considered trivial in patients with normal anatomy and physiology, such as sedation or prolonged tachycardia, can lead to significant morbidity in this patient population. The type of sedation to be employed during the procedure needs to be planned before entering the catheterization laboratory. In general, this patient population appears to benefit from the use of general anesthesia when delivered by an anesthesiologist who understands the patient's underlying congenital heart disease. This professional brings additional expertise to the sedation and allows the electrophysiologist to focus on the task at hand. Before beginning the procedure, it is important that there be an idea of the maximum length of time the patient can safely be in the laboratory. During a long procedure, procedure-related morbidities can result, such as respiratory problems related to prolonged supine positioning or intubation, and the potential for fluid overloading or dehydration. These cases are very intense, and so the electrophysiologist may frequently lose sight of time in pursuit of a "cure."

During the procedure, patients with congenital heart disease require meticulous monitoring of hemodynamics, including vital signs, central venous pressure, and frequent blood gas measurements. It is helpful to have a Foley catheter in place to monitor urine output and ensure patient comfort. Frequently, it is prudent to obtain baseline hemodynamic measurements, including filling pressures and mixed systemic venous saturation. Angiograms may help delineate the anatomy prior to beginning the electrophysiology study. It occasionally becomes necessary for patients to recover in an intensive care unit following the procedure.

Tools of the Trade

Many new imaging devices and mapping technologies are available to the electrophysiologist performing ablation procedures in children and adults with congenital heart disease. These devices range from those as simple as handheld ultrasound to help locate vessels for vascular access to intracardiac echocardiography to help identify intracardiac landmarks such as the origin of the atrial appendages or the limbus of the atrial septum for transeptal procedures. Although intracardiac echocardiography would appear to be especially helpful in patients with congenital heart disease, there are frequent limitations on its use relative to vascular access. In cases where ultrasound guidance is sought but intracardiac echocardiography is not feasible, transesophageal echocardiography can be very helpful.

Electroanatomic Mapping Systems

The use of electroanatomic mapping systems is not unique to the patient with congenital heart disease. However, it has been tremendously beneficial for differentiating and mapping the frequently difficult tachycardia circuits associated with abnormal cardiac anatomy. As discussed in previous chapters, much of the recent success in ablation in these patients is related to this new technology.

The balloon-mounted EnGuide system (St. Jude Medical, St. Paul, MN) generates an endocardial surface voltage map from unipolar electrograms recorded from the chamber of interest. The greatest advantage of this system is its ability to generate a map from the recording of a single beat of tachycardia. There are practical disadvantages to this system, however, because the size of the balloon can impede blood flow in relative small chambers and lead to unwanted hemodynamic changes. There are also size-related difficulties with vascular access.

Navigation and Visualization Technology

A relatively new technology borrowed from the adult experience in the ablation of atrial fibrillation is the use of CARTO or NavX Navigation and Visualization Technology, St. Jude Medical). These systems obtain anatomic reconstructions and endocardial electrograms displayed with previously obtained computed tomography (CT) or magnetic resonance imaging (MRI)–generated anatomy. Such technology allows one to have a true 3D sense of the position of the mapping catheter and the area of interest relative to the surrounding anatomy.

Voltage Mapping

Voltage mapping is becoming a significant tool for mapping and ablation of arrhythmias in patients with congenital heart disease. This technology is based on the fact that the amplitude of unipolar and bipolar electrograms are determined by the electrophysiological and structural characteristics of the myocardial tissue involved. Thus, it is very helpful for treating patients with reentry circuits involving diseased or damaged tissue. This mapping technique was well summarized in a study by De Groot et al, who described the use of voltage mapping in patients with congenital heart disease.[26] The authors demonstrated that,

Table 33.2 Congenital heart defects

Defect	Potential Arrhythmia	Arrhythmia Substrate	Operation	Barriers
Single ventricle (MA, AA, HLHS, TA, PA)	Atrial tachycardia	Atriotomy and baffle suture lines Atrial hypertension Crista terminalis	Fontan	Baffle prevents contact with atrial tissue; limited access from SVC
TGA	Atrial tachycardia	Atriotomy and baffle suture lines	Mustard Senning	Need to ablate CTI from both sides
ASD	Atrial tachycardia	Atriotomy and patch suture lines	Patch closure	
Ebstein's anomaly	Atrial tachycardia AV reentry (WPW)			Difficulty in defining annulus
TOF	Atrial tachycardia	Atriotomy and patch suture lines Atrial hypertension	Patch closure of ASD	
	Ventricular tachycardia	VSD patch, RVOT suture lines RV dilation	Patch closure of VSD Opening of RVOT	
Heterotaxy	Atrial tachycardia			Interrupted IVC

AA = aortic atresia; ASD = atrial septal defect; AV = atrioventricular; CTI = cavotricuspid isthmus; HLHS = hypoplastic left heart syndrome; IVC = inferior vena cava; MA = mitral atresia; PA = pulmonary atresia; RV = right ventricle; RVOT = right ventricular outflow tract; SVC = superior vena cava; TA = tricuspid atresia; TGA = transposition of great arteries; TOF = tetralogy of Fallot; VSD = ventricular septal defect; WPW = Wolff-Parkinson-White syndrome.

in patients with normal heart anatomy, the signal amplitudes were significantly larger than those recorded in patients with congenital heart disease. In healthy atrial tissue with normal conduction properties, large areas will be activated simultaneously and the amplitude of the signals will be relatively large. In abnormal myocardium, in contrast, fibers become separated and conduction will decrease, leading to asynchronous contraction of fibers[27,28] and smaller amplitude signals. The authors stressed the need to evaluate both unipolar and bipolar recordings because they offer complementary information. They recommended that these recordings be used in combination during voltage and activation mapping, with unipolar recordings providing information about the direction of propagation and bipolar signals giving information on voltage-based scar tissue delineation.[26]

Rhythm Disturbances: Atrial

A significant number of patients who have undergone palliation of congenital heart disease have atrial arrhythmias. These can be automatic, macro-, or microreentry tachycardias related directly to the underlying congenital heart disease or to sequelae of surgical interventions. It is well known that the Mustard and Senning procedures for transposition of the great arteries and the Fontan procedure for single-ventricle physiology leave significant intra-atrial suture lines and scarring, creating a substrate for reentry circuits (Figure 33.1). It may not be as obvious that other procedures (eg, atrial septal defect or ventricular septal defect closure) frequently use atriotomies to access the lesion. These incisions lead to scarring in the wall of the atrium. Direct cannulation of the right atrium for procedures requiring cardiac bypass also lead to scar formation. As this patient population has continued to grow in both age and numbers, the subset with rhythm disturbances requiring electrophysiology interventions has significantly increased. The majority of electrophysiologists attempting radiofrequency ablation in this population often find it to be technically demanding and, at times, very frustrating.

A number of difficulties have been identified in patients with surgically corrected congenital heart disease and atrial reentrant arrhythmias, making these procedures challenging with multiple entrance and exit sites. These circuits are frequently related to, or surrounded by, scars.[29] In order to have a reasonable chance of success in ablating these rhythm disturbances, the practitioner must thoroughly understand the patient's underlying cardiac anatomy, all prior palliative procedures, and cannulation and atriotomy sites. The surgical and catheterization records should be reviewed prior to entering the electrophysiology laboratory.

Before we discuss the techniques and results of ablation of atrial tachyarrhythmias in patients with congenital heart disease, we must first review the Fontan, Mustard, and Senning procedures.

Fontan Procedure

The Fontan procedure is a palliation for patients with one functional ventricle. It takes advantage of the concept that, in "ideal" situations, systemic venous blood can flow to the lungs passively (ie, without the use of ventricular propulsion). This palliation involves routing systemic venous blood from the inferior vena cava and superior vena cava directly to the lungs.

There have been a number of modifications made to the connections during the past quarter century (Figure 33.2). With the exception of an extracardiac conduit, all modifications have involved right atrial tissue, in part or in whole. The portion of the right atrium involved in the circuit is under increased pressure to drive blood flow through the lungs. This, in addition to atrial suture lines, becomes a significant nidus for the development of atrial arrhythmias. Most modifications of the Fontan operation have been made in an effort to decrease the incidence of atrial arrhythmias in this population. These changes in surgical technique have been met with limited success, however. An unintentional effect of these modifications has been to limit the ability to place catheters in direct contact with the atrial tissue.

The original Fontan palliation was an atriopulmonary connection, frequently an anastomosis of the right atrial appendage to the pulmonary artery (Figure 33.2A). This palliation placed the entire atrium under increased pressure, leading to both dilation and hypertrophy. The majority of adults undergoing a Fontan operation prior to the mid-1980s had this type of palliation. The advantage to the electrophysiologist is that the entire atrium can be entered and mapped. The disadvantage is that it is very difficult to map secondary to its size. The tachycardia circuits frequently involve the anastomosis site, the atriotomy site (usually low anterolateral atrium), and the crista terminalis. A number of variations on this type of palliation were performed that involved oversewing the atrioventricular valves and patching atrial septal defects, each of which have suture line–induced scars producing other potential arrhythmia substrates.

A modification of the Fontan procedure in the late 1980s involved the lateral tunnel, which consisted of an intracardiac baffle of the inferior vena cava blood flow to the pulmonary artery or the superior vena cava that was connected to the pulmonary arteries (Figure 33.2B). There are variations in the anastomosis of the superior vena cava to the pulmonary artery (end-to-side or side-to-side). These variations can lead to difficulties in venous access from the subclavian and internal jugular veins, as well as potential damage to the sinus node blood supply. The baffle separates the lateral wall of the right atrium from the remainder of the atrium. When attempting radiofrequency ablation from a venous approach, the circuit can be mapped and treated only inside the baffle, with its

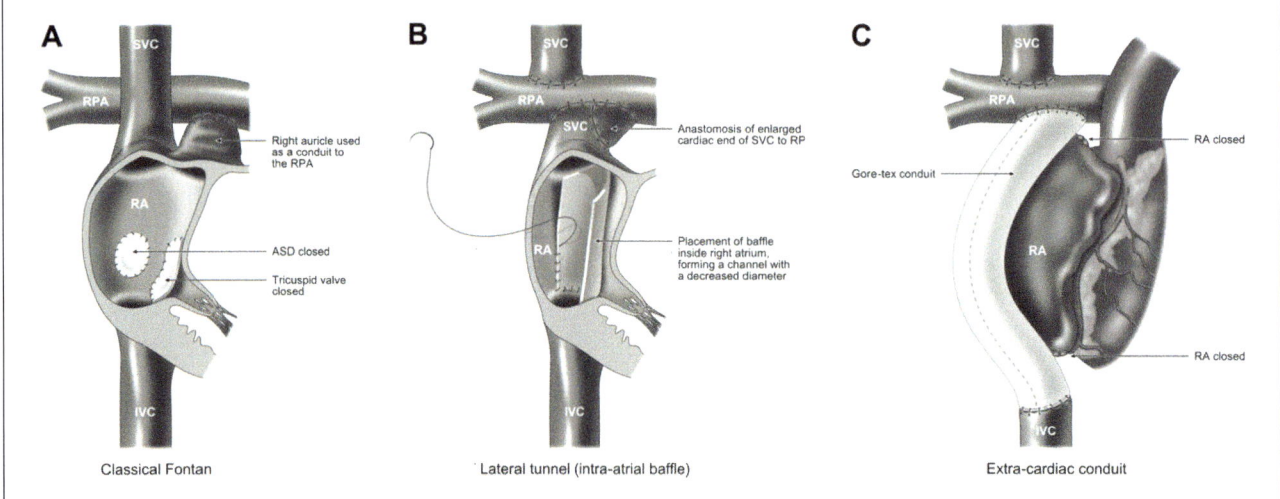

Figure 33.2 Modifications of the Fontan procedure for single ventricle anatomy and physiology. ASD = atrial septal defect; IVC = inferior vena cava; RA = right atrium; RPA = right pulmonary artery; SVC = superior vena cava. *Source:* d'Udekem Y, et al, their Figure 1. The Fontan procedure: contemporary techniques have improved long-term outcomes. *Circulation.* 2007;116(Suppl 11):I157-I164. Reprinted with permission from Wolters Kluwer Health.

relatively small area of atrial tissue. The remaining atrium can be entered retrograde from an aortic approach, either across the atrioventricular valve or by a trans-baffle puncture. The tachycardia circuits in this modification are similar to those of a classic Fontan procedure but with the addition of suture lines involving the baffle.

In a further attempt to decrease the right atrial tissue exposed to hypertension and suture lines, the extracardiac Fontan procedure was embraced in the 1990s (Figure 33.2C). In this operation, a conduit is placed connecting the inferior vena cava to the pulmonary artery or the superior vena cava but without entering the heart. Although there has been somewhat limited follow-up, it seems that this approach has not eliminated atrial tachycardia in this population but has significantly limited access to the substrate.

In the classic and lateral tunnel Fontan procedures, atrial tissue is exposed to elevated intracavitary pressures and will frequently hypertrophy to thicknesses of 1 cm or greater. This leads to later difficulty in delivering effective lesions with standard catheters. Subsequently, larger catheter tip sizes and irrigated-tip catheters were developed to deliver larger and more effective lesions.

Mustard and Senning Operations

Atrial arrhythmias seen in patients with scar-related circuits due to the Fontan procedure also occur in patients who underwent an atrial switch (ie, Mustard or Senning) procedure for transposition of the great arteries. In addition, the latter may develop cavotricuspid isthmus reentry atrial tachycardia. Although these reentry circuits mimic those seen in structurally normal hearts, several anatomic circumstances warrant further discussion. Prior to the mid-1980s, the palliation for transposition of the great arteries consisted of a Mustard or Senning procedure.

These procedures baffled the systemic and pulmonary venous return to the subpulmonic ventricle (left) and subsystemic ventricle (right), respectively, to allow oxygenated blood to reach the systemic circulation. These baffles are made of either artificial material or pericardium, as in the Mustard procedure, or right atrial free wall, as in the Senning. The location of suture lines and the coronary sinus ostium varies between the two procedures. This, in turn, impacts the site for later modification of a cavotricuspid isthmus reentry tachycardia.

The ablation of these circuits is very well summarized by Kanter et al,[30] who described how cavotricuspid isthmus–dependent atrial tachycardia frequently requires placing lesions on both sides of the baffle. Access to the tricuspid valve annulus and pulmonary venous atrium may be achieved by a transseptal approach, using a perforation of the interatrial baffle from the systemic venous atrium, or by a retrograde aortic approach. The transseptal procedure differs from that used in a "native" atrial septum. In these patients, the transseptal needle must be aimed anteriorly and slightly rightward (this can be helped by ultrasound guidance). Many who have found this technique to be challenging and nerve-wracking opt to take a retrograde approach. However, a disadvantage to the retrograde approach is the potential for damaging two cardiac valves and the difficulty of moving the catheter tip through the chordae of the tricuspid valve.

Ablation of Atrial Arrhythmias in Congenital Heart Disease

A relatively early study from Children's Hospital in Boston (2002)[31] reported acute and intermediate results from a large, single-center series of patients with congenital heart disease who had undergone radiofrequency ablation for intra-atrial reentry tachycardia. This study evaluated a number of clinical and procedural variables and their effect on clinical outcomes. They looked at 134 patients ranging in age from 1 month to 62 years with variants of single-ventricle physiology, tetralogy of Fallot, ventricular septal defect, and transposition of the great arteries. Fontan procedures were the most common surgical intervention.

In this study, standard ablation was performed using a variety of power- and temperature-controlled catheters. This was one of the first groups to use an irrigated ablation catheter in patients who had failed standard radiofrequency ablation. As previously mentioned, there are times when the practitioner must develop techniques to help these procedures succeed. So the authors used external sheath irrigation (this was prior to the availability of internally irrigated catheters) by placing a 7-Fr standard ablation catheter at the ablation site and advancing an 8-Fr-long sheath to the distal-tip electrode. There was a slow infusion of saline delivered in the sheath during the radiofrequency application, permitting higher power but without raising impedance. Once available, they used an internally irrigated catheter with a closed coolant system (Chilli®, Cardiac Pathways, Inc., Sunnyvale, CA).

In these 134 patients, a total of 369 distinct intra-atrial reentry tachycardia circuits were identified, and ablation was attempted in 268. The authors defined success as limited if one or more targeted circuits were ablated and complete if all targeted circuits were ablated. Limited procedural success was reported in 79% and complete success in 66%. Procedural success was defined as termination of the tachycardia during a radiofrequency lesion, which subsequently could not be induced by programmed stimulation. Complications were noted in 22 patients, 9 related to transient femoral vascular access issues. A pacemaker lead was damaged in 3 cases. There were transient phrenic nerve palsies in 2 cases. (There is an increased potential for this complication in patients with previous palliation of congenital heart disease, in that the phrenic nerve may be "stuck" to the heart following manipulation of the pericardium.) Transient ischemic events or atrial/superior vena caval thrombi were observed in 2 cases as well. There was a single periprocedural death in a 45-year-old patient who had palliated tricuspid atresia with incessant atrial tachycardias and severe congestive heart failure.

There were 156 procedures with sufficient follow-up for analysis. Fifty-four were classified as long-term unfavorable outcomes and 52 as long-term favorable outcomes. In these cases, univariate predictors of a favorable outcome included a higher level of right atrial saturation and complete procedural success. Predictors of unfavorable outcomes included a diagnosis of single ventricle, an older variant of the Fontan procedure, a history of atrial fibrillation, and higher numbers of intra-atrial reentry tachycardia circuits mapped and ablated.[31] Multivariate analysis showed that predictors of long-term success included the ablation of all targeted arrhythmias, the use of electroanatomic mapping to guide ablation, and a higher degree of right atrial saturation. The only negative predictor was mapping a larger number of intra-atrial reentry tachycardia circuits during the procedure. The authors stressed that, although many patients have their tachycardia recur, significant palliation of clinical symptoms can be achieved with these procedures.[31]

Although patch closure of an atrial septal defect is a relatively simple procedure when compared with a Fontan, Mustard, or Senning, it can lead to clinically significant atrial arrhythmias. Atrial septal defects are seen more frequently than transposition of the great arteries or single ventricles and lead to a larger number of potential patients with these arrhythmias. In 2005, a publication from France looked at the mechanisms of atrial tachycardia occurring after surgical repair of atrial septal defect in 22 patients. In this study, a 3D mapping system (CARTO, Biosense Webster) was used in addition to conventional mapping with entrainment to determine the mechanism of the tachycardia. Entrainment was used only in the first 4 cases because it would frequently terminate the tachycardia or induce a second, possibly nonclinical arrhythmia. In all patients, the mechanism was determined to be an intra-atrial reentry dependent on at least one critical isthmus. The authors noted that if a line of double potentials were identified in the right atrial free wall, a double-loop figure-8 reentrant circuit could be identified. If no line of double potentials were identified, a single-loop macroreentrant circuit could be identified with a peritricuspid circuit. This is similar to findings by Shah et al, who presented 5 patients with double-loop reentry circuits who had undergone prior closure of a secundum atrial septal defect.[32]

A critical isthmus was identified, bound by 2 conduction barriers consisting of a line of double potentials, the tricuspid annulus, a surgical scar, or the intercaval line.[33] This isthmus was relatively narrow. These circuits were successfully ablated by targeting the narrowest portion of the isthmus. It was deemed necessary to do a cavotricuspid isthmus ablation in all the patients, as reported by Chan et al.[34] All inducible circuits could be treated by ablation of the cavotricuspid isthmus alone in 7 of 22 patients (27%); in the remaining cases, the tachycardia was dependent on a second isthmus. With this protocol, they obtained freedom from recurrence at a mean follow-up of 25 ± 16 months.

This was the first description of a tachycardia circuit rotating around the atrial septal defect patch and the coronary sinus. The authors described a double-loop circuit involving a counterclockwise activation around the atrial septal defect patch and a clockwise activation around the coronary sinus. They also documented abrupt termination of the tachycardia during lesions delivered close to the roof of the coronary sinus, at the narrow isthmus bounded by the coronary sinus and the patch.

The authors summarized their findings by stating that atrial tachycardias following surgical repair of an atrial septal defect were frequently the macroreentry type. The cavotricuspid isthmus was not the only circuit noted in these patients, but it was critical to the circuit and therefore should be ablated in patients presenting with reentry tachycardia following atrial septal defect repair. The other tachycardias were related to the crista terminalis, surgical incisions, or cannulation sites.[33]

Not all atrial arrhythmias seen in patients with congenital heart disease are reentry circuits. A significant number of patients have focal tachycardias that can be seen in either atrium. These rhythm disturbances can be seen in the early postoperative period as well as in mid- to-late follow-up. The majority of these foci are thought to be automatic in nature, but a study by Seslar reported on the ablation of nonautomatic focal tachycardias in this population.[35] The authors used standard criteria for inducibility and termination of the arrhythmia by programmed stimulation to differentiate automatic from nonautomatic foci. In this study, they noted that 17 of 216 patients with a diagnosis of atrial tachycardia undergoing an electrophysiology study also fulfilled criteria for nonautomatic focal atrial tachycardia. Fourteen of the 17 had congenital heart disease, and 13 had postsurgical intervention status. Before an electrophysiology study, 11 of these patients were thought to have atrial flutter.

The authors emphasized that no clinical or electrocardiographic features of this arrhythmia differentiated it from ectopic atrial tachycardia or intra-atrial reentry tachycardia. Rather, in this study, the foci were found in the right atrium and were relatively easily ablated.

These varied reports reinforce the need to approach an attempted radiofrequency ablation in this population with an open mind. They also demonstrate the importance of performing a comprehensive electrophysiological evaluation prior to proceeding to an ablation in this complex cohort of patients.

Rhythm Disturbances: Ventricular Tachycardia

Prior to considering an ablation in a child with ventricular tachycardia, one should attempt to understand the mechanism, potential hemodynamic consequences, and natural history of the arrhythmia. There are children with structurally normal hearts who develop ventricular tachycardia but who have a significant potential to outgrow the rhythm disturbance. Ventricular tachycardia in children can present in the fetus, potentially leading to hydrops fetalis, or have no obvious hemodynamic consequences. Presentation during infancy is frequently found to be benign and self-limiting.[36] Toddlers and school-age children rarely present with ventricular tachycardia. There is also a presentation peak noted during puberty. Ventricular tachycardia seen in children without structural heart disease is similar to that seen in adults, and may be related to channelopathies such as long QT or Brugada syndrome.

They can also be the sequelae of myocarditis, cardiomyopathy, metabolic abnormalities, or toxic ingestions.

The highest prevalence of ventricular tachycardia in children is seen in those who have structural congenital heart disease both prior to and following palliation. Although tetralogy of Fallot is the most studied defect, both in and out of the electrophysiology laboratory, ventricular tachycardia is also seen in patients who have undergone almost every type of palliation for congenital heart disease. These include ventricular septal defect closure, left-side obstruction relief, and procedures that require the right ventricle to become the systemic ventricle (eg, atrial-level switches such as the Mustard or Senning procedure) or procedures for single-ventricle physiology (eg, the Fontan). In the majority of these cases, the ventricular tachycardia circuit involves scarring in the ventricle, related to incisions to enter the ventricle or suture lines involving patches or baffles.

Tetralogy of Fallot

The most common ventricular tachycardia in patients with congenital heart disease is seen in patients with tetralogy of Fallot. Palliation of the patient with tetralogy of Fallot results in a substrate with conduction barriers, leading to reentry circuits. Such palliative procedures involve the closure of the anterior malaligned ventricular septal defect and any other ventricular septal defects. The ventricular septal defect can be approached via the tricuspid valve or through a ventriculotomy, which leads to a scar in the ventricular muscle. In tetralogy of Fallot, there is also a need to relieve the right ventricular outflow tract obstruction. This may entail pulmonary valvuloplasty with or without resection of the subpulmonary obstruction, a transvalvular outflow patch, or a right ventricle–to–pulmonary artery conduit. These variations should be reviewed before proceeding to the electrophysiology laboratory because they may change the substrate for ablating the ventricular tachycardia.

Mapping and Ablation of Ventricular Arrhythmias in Tetralogy of Fallot

Before attempting ablation of ventricular tachycardia in a patient with tetralogy of Fallot or any other palliated congenital heart disease, one must perform a complete electrophysiology study with programmed stimulation in the atrium and ventricle. Although ventricular tachycardia is commonly seen in patients with tetralogy of Fallot, the clinical arrhythmia may be a supraventricular tachycardia involving an accessory pathway, AVNRT, or a primary atrial tachycardia such as atrial flutter or atrial fibrillation. Patients with palliated tetralogy of Fallot frequently have diastolic dysfunction relative to long-standing pulmonary insufficiency, and this leads to high atrial filling pressures. Diastolic dysfunction, along with atrial scars from atriotomies, atrial septal defect closure, or cannulation sites, serves as a substrate for primary atrial tachycardias. The combination of poor ventricular function and rapidly conducting atrial tachycardia can have the same degree of morbidity as ventricular tachycardia in patients with tetralogy of Fallot.

The most frequently encountered ventricular tachycardia in patients following palliation of tetralogy of Fallot is a macroreentrant right ventricular circuit. This ventricular tachycardia typically has a left bundle branch block QRS morphology and normal (inferior) frontal plane axis. As mentioned in the discussion of radiofrequency ablation in patients with atrial tachycardia, the walls of these chambers are frequently much thicker than those found in patients without structural heart disease. Thus, ablation in these patients often requires the use of large-tip or irrigated catheters.

The tachycardia rate or poor underlying hemodynamics may result in ventricular tachycardia not being well tolerated. In these cases, noncontact mapping of the tachycardia may be useful using the EnGuide system (Endocardial Solutions/St. Jude Medical) by creating a virtual map based on a single beat or short salvo. These circuits may also be determined by employing voltage mapping during sinus rhythm.

A landmark paper by Zeppenfeld et al in 2007 identified 4 discrete anatomic isthmuses that serve as substrates for ventricular tachycardia in patients with tetralogy of Fallot repair. The most common lies between the superior aspect of the tricuspid valve annulus and the incision or patch in the right ventricular outflow tract. A second isthmus is found between the pulmonary valve annulus and the right ventricular free-wall scar. Another is located between the ventricular septal defect patch and the pulmonary annulus, and the final one is found between the ventricular septal defect patch and the tricuspid annulus. The authors demonstrated that once an isthmus was shown to be in the circuit (either by entrainment or pace mapping), lesions placed to transect it would frequently lead to noninducibility (or arrhythmia termination if done during tachycardia).[37]

In this report, 11 patients (9 with tetralogy of Fallot) with recurrent symptomatic ventricular tachycardia after palliation of congenital heart disease were referred for catheter ablation. They had right ventricular mapping performed during sinus rhythm to construct a 3D voltage map using an electroanatomic mapping system (Carto, Biosense Webster). Electrograms <1.5 mV were defined as low voltage, and those <0.5 mV as very low voltage, on the basis of previously reported mapping data obtained in patients without structural heart disease.[38] In areas of low amplitude, unipolar pacing was performed with 10 mA at a 2 ms pulse width. Sites where there was failure to capture were marked as electrically unexcitable scar.

Once the voltage mapping was complete, ventricular tachycardia was induced. When possible, based on the patients' ability to tolerate the ventricular tachycardia, activation and entrainment mapping was performed. In those who could not tolerate the ventricular tachycardia, circuit isthmuses were defined by pace mapping where the QRS morphology matched the ventricular tachycardia in ≤ 10 of 12 leads, with an S-QRS delay of > 40 ms.[37] Once the mapping was completed, the subjects underwent radiofrequency ablation with a saline-irrigated catheter or an 8 mm–tip catheter. When possible, the ablation was performed during ventricular tachycardia. Anatomic boundaries were connected with additional lesions once the ventricular tachycardia was terminated. Lesions were placed during sinus rhythm until unipolar pacing failed to capture.[37]

The authors concluded that, after repair of congenital heart disease, ventricular tachycardia circuits are located in anatomically defined isthmuses bordered by unexcitable tissue that can be identified by 3D mapping during sinus rhythm. Radiofrequency ablation of these isthmuses during sinus rhythm can lead to successful treatment of these patients. These finding can also applied during surgical ablation as well as during catheter procedures.[37]

Summary

The use of ablation, radiofrequency, or cryoablation in the pediatric population is now the standard of care for treating arrhythmias. During the past 20 years, experience and technology have evolved to the point that these procedures are now offered to children as small as 15 kg without causing significant morbidity. This advance has had a significant impact on the quality of life of these young patients and their families. While these procedures serve as useful therapeutic tools to those with normal hearts, they have had a far greater impact on those with structural heart disease. However, these procedures remain challenging and their success rates are somewhat lower than in patients with normal anatomy. Even so, they afford these patients an opportunity to have rhythm control without resorting to medications that may have a negative effect on their hemodynamics.

References

1. Van Hare GT, Lesh MD, Scheinman M, et al. Percutaneous radiofrequency catheter ablation for supraventricular arrhythmias in children. *J Am Coll Cardiol*. 1991;17(7):1613-1620.
2. Kugler JD, Danford DA, Houston K, et al. Radiofrequency catheter ablation for paroxysmal supraventricular tachycardia in children and adolescents without structural heart disease. *Am J Cardiol*. 1997;80:1438-1443.
3. Van Hare GF, Javitz H, Carmelli D, et al. Prospective assessment after pediatric cardiac ablation: demographics, medical profiles, and initial outcomes. *J Cardiol Electrophysiol*. 2004;15(7):759-770.

4. Kugler JD, Danford DA, Deal BJ, et al. Radiofrequency catheter ablation for tachyarrhythmias in children and adolescents. *N Engl J Med.* 1994;330:1481-1487.
5. Scheinman MM, Huang S. The 1998 NASPE prospective catheter ablation registry. *Pacing Clin Electrophysiol.* 2000;23:1020-1028.
6. Van Hare GF, Colan SD, Javitz H, et al. Prospective assessment after pediatric cardiac ablation: fate of intracardiac structure and function, as assessed by serial echocardiography. *Am Heart J.* 2007;153(5):815-820.
7. Minich LL, Snider AR, Dick II M. Doppler detection of valvular regurgitation after radiofrequency ablation of accessory connections. *Am J Cardiol.* 1992;70:116-117.
8. Price IF, Kertesz NT, Snyder CS, et al. Flecainide and sotalol: a new combination therapy for refractory supraventricular tachycardia in children < 1 year of age. *J Am Coll Cardiol.* 2002;39:517-520.
9. Bokenkamp R, Wibbelt G, Sturm M, et al. Effects of intracardiac radiofrequency current application on coronary artery vessels in young pigs. *J Cardiovasc Electrophysiol.* 2000;11:565-571.
10. Aiyagari R, Saarel EV, Etheridge SP, et al. Radiofrequency ablation for supraventricular tachycardia in children ≤15 kg is safe and effective. *Pediatr Cardiol.* 2005;26(5):622-626.
11. Dick M 2nd, Law IH, Dorostkar PC, et al. Use of the His/RVA electrode catheter in children. *J Electrocardiol.* 1996;29:227-233.
12. Park T, Eichling J, Schechtman K, et al. Risk of radiation induced skin injuries from arrhythmia ablation procedures. *Pacing Clin Electrophysiol.* 1996;19:1363-1369.
13. Rosenthal L, Beck T, Williams J, et al. Acute radiation dermatitis following radiofrequency catheter ablation of atrioventricular nodal reentrant tachycardia. *Pacing Clin Electrophysiol.* 1997;20:1834-1839.
14. Lindsay B, Eichling J, Ambos H, et al. Radiation exposure to patients and medical personnel during radiofrequency catheter ablation for supraventricular tachycardia. *Am J Cardiol.* 1992;70:218-223.
15. McFadden, SL, Mooney RB, Shepherd PH. X-ray dose and associated risks from radiofrequency catheter ablation procedures. *Br J Radiol.* 2002;75:253-265.
16. Kovoor P, Ricciardello M, Collins L, et al. Risk to patients from radiation associated with radiofrequency ablation for supraventricular tachycardia. *Circulation.* 1998;98:1534-1540.
17. Calkins H, Niklason L, Sousa J, et al. Radiation exposure during radiofrequency catheter ablation of accessory atrioventricular connections. *Circulation.* 1991;84:2376-2382.
18. Bacher K, Bogaert E, Lapere R, et al. Patient-specific dose and radiation risk estimation in pediatric cardiac catheterization. *Circulation.* 2005;111:83-89.
19. Tuzcu V. A nonfluoroscopic approach for electrophysiology and catheter ablation procedures using a three-dimensional navigation system. *Pacing Clin Electrophysiol.* 2007;30:519-525.
20. Smith G, Clark J. Elimination of fluoroscopy use in a pediatric electrophysiology laboratory utilizing three-dimensional mapping. *Pacing Clin Electrophysiol.* 2007;30:510-518.
21. Papagiannia J, Tsoutsinos A, Kirvassilis G, et al. Nonfluoroscopic catheter navigation for radiofrequency catheter ablation of supraventricular tachycardia in children. *Pacing Clin Electrophysiol.* 2006;29:971-978.
22. Anderson RH, Ho SY. Anatomy of the atrioventricular junctions with regard to ventricular preexcitation. *Pacing Clin Electrophysiol.* 1997;20:2072-2076.
23. Olgun H, Karagoz T, Celiker A. Coronary microcatheter mapping of coronary arteries during radiofrequency ablation in children. *J Interv Card Electrophysiol.* 2010;27:75-79.
24. Tuzcu V, Gonzalez MB, Gonzalez Y. Diagnosis of tachycardia mechanism with cryomapping in a toddler with complex congenital heart disease. *J Interv Card Electrophysiol.* 2006;16:59-64.
25. Collins KK, Rhee EK, Kirsh JA. Cryoablation of accessory pathways in the coronary sinus in young patients: a multicenter study from the Pediatric and Congenital Electrophysiology Society's Working Group on Cryoablation. *J Cardio Electrophysiol.* 2007;18(6):592-597.
26. De Groot NMS, Schalij MJ, Zeppenfield K. Voltage and activation mapping: how the recording technique affects the outcome of catheter ablation procedures in patients with congenital heart disease. *Circulation.* 2003;108:2099-2106.
27. Spach MS, Dolber PC. Relating extracellular potentials and their derivatives to anisotropic propagation at a microscopic level in human cardiac muscle: evidence for electrical uncoupling of side to side fiber connections with increasing age. *Circ Res.* 1986;58:356-371.
28. Roberts DE, Scher AM. Effect of tissue anisotropy on extracellular potential fields in canine myocardium in situ. *Circ Res.* 1982;50:342-351.
29. Lesh MD, Van Hare GF, Epstein LM, et al. Radiofrequency catheter ablation of atrial arrhythmias: results and mechanisms. *Circulation.* 1994;89:1074-1089.
30. Kanter RJ. Pearls for ablation in congenital heart disease. *J Cardiovasc Electrophysiol.* 2010;21(2):223-230.
31. Triedman JK, Alexander ME, Love BA. Influence of patient factors and ablative technologies on outcomes of radiofrequency ablation of intra-atrial re-entrant tachycardia in patients with congenital heart disease. *J Am Coll Cardiol.* 2002;39(11):1827-1835.
32. Shah D, Jaïs P, Takahashi A, et al. Dual-loop intra-atrial reentry in humans. *Circulation.* 2000;101:631-639.
33. Magnin-Poull I, De Chillou C, Miljoen H, et al. Mechanisms of right atrial tachycardia occurring late after surgical closure of atrial septal defects. *J Cardiovasc Electrophysiol.* 2005;16(7):681-687.
34. Chan DP, Van Hare GF, Mackall JA, et al. Importance of atrial flutter isthmus in postoperative intra-atrial reentrant tachycardia. *Circulation.* 2000;102:1283-1289.
35. Seslar SP, Alexander ME, Berul CI, et al. Ablation of nonautomatic focal atrial tachycardia in children and adults with congenital heart disease. *J Cardiovasc Electrophysiol.* 2006;17(4):359-365.
36. Levin MD, Stephen P, Tanel RE, et al. Ventricular tachycardia in infants with structurally normal heart: a benign disorder. *Cardiol Young.* 2010;20(6):641-647.
37. Zeppenfeld K, Schalij MJ, Bartelings MM, et al. Catheter ablation of ventricular tachycardia after repair of congenital heart disease: electroanatomic identification of the critical right ventricular isthmus. *Circulation.* 2007;116(20):2241-2252.
38. Marchlinski FE, Callans DJ, Gottlieb CD, et al. Linear ablation lesions for control of unmappable ventricular tachycardia in patients with ischemic and nonischemic cardiomyopathy. *Circulation.* 2000;101:1288-1296.

CHAPTER 34

Intraoperative Mapping During Surgical Ablation Procedures

Takashi Nitta, MD, PhD; Shun-ichiro Sakamoto, MD, PhD

Introduction

Intraoperative mapping has guided surgeons in performing accurate procedures for treating arrhythmia. It has also contributed to the understanding of the mechanism of the various arrhythmias and the development of other non-pharmacological treatments, such as catheter ablation.

It was back in the 1960s when Durrer and colleagues[1] first studied intramural ventricular activation in isolated and perfused normal human hearts taken from 7 individuals who had died from various cerebral conditions but without any history of cardiac disease. They used plunge-needle electrodes to record 870 intramural sites and constructed a two- and three-dimensional (2D and 3D) isochronic presentation of the ventricular activation of a human heart. They further studied epicardial ventricular activation in a patient with Wolff–Parkinson–White (WPW) syndrome who underwent a surgery for an atrial septal defect. They demonstrated preexcitation in the anterolateral part of the right ventricle close to the tricuspid annulus, suggesting an accessory pathway connecting the atrium and ventricle in patients with WPW syndrome.[2]

During the past half century, combined with the development of pulse stimulators, electrodes, signal digitizers, and computers and software for data acquisition and analysis, the technique and quality of intraoperative mapping has dramatically improved. Intraoperative mapping techniques have provided direct information on the various types of atrial and ventricular arrhythmias. And, since the substrates of cardiac arrhythmias are usually invisible, surgical procedures can be directed by the findings of the mapping data. The spatial accuracy of the mapping data directly contributes to the outcome of map-directed arrhythmia surgery. This chapter describes the fundamental methodology, techniques, and specific considerations for treating each type of arrhythmia.

Electrodes for Mapping

Bipolar and Unipolar Electrodes

Both unipolar and bipolar electrodes are used in intraoperative mapping. Unipolar electrograms show the voltage change at the electrode location relative to an extracardiac reference electrode, whereas bipolar electrograms display the voltage difference between the dipoles. Unipolar electrograms may contain remote activation, such as ventricular activation in an atrial electrogram. In general, unipolar electrograms are more sensitive to noise and artifact than bipolar ones. The unipolar electrogram accurately determines local activation time by intrinsic deflection, defined as the time of the maximum negative derivative. The unipolar recording from multiple sites provides a potential distribution at an instant in time.

In bipolar electrograms recorded with two closely spaced poles, far-field effects induce similar potentials at both poles, and thus, the remote effects will be canceled. To cancel the repolarization waveforms, the high-pass filter is usually set at 10 to 50 Hz in the bipolar recording. As a result, the recording allows one to clearly identify the potentials separated by a flat baseline. Because the bipolar signals are determined by the voltage difference between the dipoles, the amplitude of the bipolar electrogram is influenced by the direction of the activation propagation and the layout of the dipole. The activation that propagates perpendicular to the dipole may not form a bipolar electrogram with a large amplitude, whereas the activation propagating parallel to the dipole may form a large electrogram.

To avoid variable amplitude typically found in the bipolar electrogram, we use a target-oriented electrode in which a cathode is surrounded by a ring-shaped anode. In the bipolar electrogram, the time of local activation is defined as the onset of the electrogram in the catheter-based electrophysiological study. However, in intraoperative mapping using a computer, the time of absolute maximum amplitude is frequently considered to be the local activation time because it is a more definitive criterion for computers to determine time than onset of the electrogram.

Various Other Types

From the beginning of the intraoperative mapping era, single-point mapping has used a pen-type handheld electrode (Figure 34.1). A variety of rhythms may be mapped with the single-point mapping technique: sinus rhythm, tachycardias with a stable cycle length (such as atrial flutter or atrioventricular reciprocating tachycardia), and hemodynamically tolerable ventricular tachycardia (VT) with stable cycle length. More recently, the single-point mapping technique has been combined with electromagnetic navigation technology into the electroanatomic mapping system. This system is used in catheter-based electrophysiological studies and ablation as well as in the operating room.

The location and size of the reentrant circuit can change as the tachycardia becomes sustained; some tachycardias may not sustain long enough for data acquisition during surgery under general anesthesia. Therefore, simultaneous recording of the electrograms from multiple sites is required for most sustained and nonsustained tachycardias in order to acquire accurate information. To accomplish this, multiple electrodes are applied on the epicardium or endocardium in various forms, as follows.

A card-type electrode patch (Figure 34.2), in which multiple electrodes are mounted on a square silicon plate, is used for mapping a limited region in the atria or ventricles. The card-type electrode patch can be used for mapping of the patients with WPW syndrome. The mapping for WPW is performed during normal rhythm for locating the abnormal pathway. In most patients with WPW syndrome, the locations of the accessory pathways have already been roughly extrapolated by the polarities of the delta waves in the electrocardiogram or the preoperative electrophysiological study. Using the card-type electrode patch, intraoperative mapping is performed on both the atrial and the ventricular epicardium across the atrioventricular groove during pacing or atrioventricular reentrant tachycardia. The intraoperative mapping helps determine the precise location of the accessory pathways and makes a spatial correlation with anatomic references.

In mapping atrial fibrillation (AF), one must especially consider temporal and spatial accuracy. AF is a variable arrhythmia in which the number and location of the activation wavefronts continue to change from moment to moment, resulting in multiple wavelets at any point of time. Hundreds of electrodes would need to be distributed over the entire atria in order to document all the activation wavefronts. Moreover, the configuration of the atrial epicardium and endocardium is 3D and complex. We use template-type electrode patches (Figure 34.3) and fit them snugly to the entire atrial epicardium during intraoperative mapping of AF. The activation maps are then displayed in a dynamic mode as a movie on 3D-constructed atrial models to keep atrial activation correlated with anatomic landmarks (Figure 34.3).

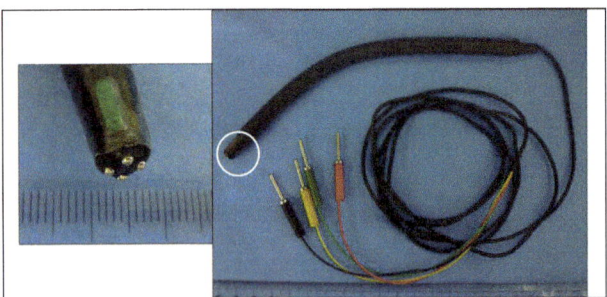

Figure 34.1 A pen-type handheld electrode. The shaft is flexible and has four electrodes on the tip. The electrode can be used for stimulation and for recording electrograms.

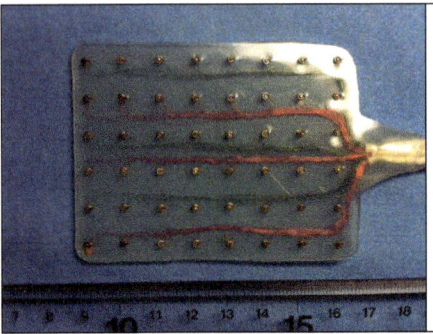
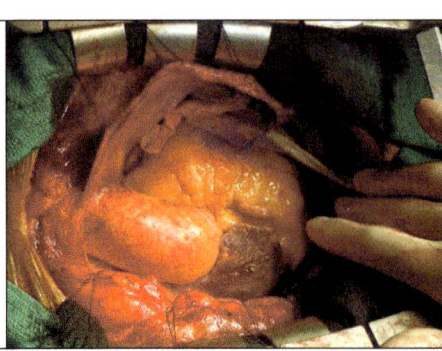

Figure 34.2 Card-type electrode patch with 48 bipolar electrodes arranged on a square silicon plate. The card-type electrode patch is placed on the anterolateral left ventricle of a patient with nonischemic ventricular tachycardia. The bipolar electrodes are target-oriented electrodes whose interelectrode distance is 10 mm.

Signal Processing and Analysis

The signals recorded by the electrodes are processed for displaying the electrograms and maps, storing data, and analyzing the maps. First of all, the signals are amplified and filtered. The high-pass filter is usually set at 10 to 50 Hz for the bipolar electrograms (for reasons described above) and at 0.05 Hz for the unipolar electrograms. The most common source of noise in the operating room is the alternating current for the power supply, which has a frequency of 50 or 60 Hz. Because this frequency band of noise may not be eliminated by the usual filter setting, grounding all the electrical equipment is extremely important when performing intraoperative mapping. The low-pass filter is usually set at 500 to 1,000 Hz for both bipolar and unipolar electrograms.

The signals are then digitized by an analog-to-digital converter and stored in the memory of a computer. The sampling rate of 1,000 Hz (which gives 1 ms temporal accuracy) is usually enough to analyze most clinical arrhythmias. A higher sampling rate may be used for research purposes. The higher the sampling rate, the higher the temporal resolution, but also the greater the memory and time required for saving and displaying the data. Use of a circular buffer as a memory device allows one to continuously record the signals by deleting the previously saved data simultaneously. The signals are also continuously displayed as electrograms, along with selected leads of the electrocardiograms on a display. Signals that have been temporarily stored in the memory are saved on a hard disk for data storage and later offline analysis.

The electrograms are analyzed by various methods according to the purpose, such as activation time mapping, potential distribution mapping, voltage mapping, frequency analysis, and others. The analyzed data are displayed as a map. A simple 2D sheet may be used for displaying maps for card-type electrodes. Since the spatial correlation between the electrophysiological data and anatomic landmarks is critical in arrhythmia surgery, a 3D display of the maps is more ideal in intraoperative mapping. The epicardium, endocardium, or both for the atria, ventricles, or whole heart can be displayed as a 3D figure on a computer.

We use a custom-made system developed by the Cardiothoracic Surgery Research Laboratory (Washington University in St. Louis, MO). The system is capable of displaying 3D figures of the epicardial and endocardial surfaces of the atria and ventricles; these figures are reconstructed from 2D images from magnetic resonance imaging (MRI) of the human heart. The figures can be rotated in 3D and seen from any direction (▶ Video 34.1). In most analyses, the analyzed data are time-domain data and are displayed on the figures as contours of time with or without a color code.

Displaying maps on the 3D figures facilitates the anatomic understanding of the electrophysiological data.

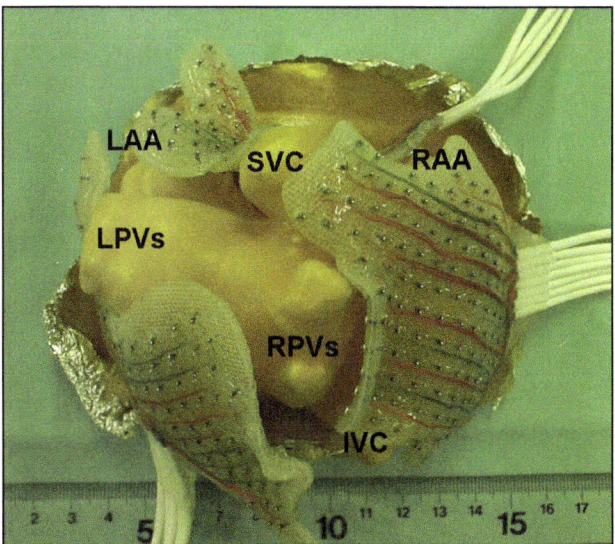

Figure 34.3 Template-type electrodes for the atria. The curvature of the atrial epicardium was copied from a mold of a cadaver heart onto 3 silicone sheets: the right atrial free wall, the left atrial free wall (including the posterior left atrium between the pulmonary veins), and the anterior atrium behind the great arteries. A total of 253 unipolar electrodes were distributed over the sheets with interelectrode distances of 5 to 7 mm. IVC = inferior vena cava; LAA = left atrial appendage; LPVs = left pulmonary veins; RAA = right atrial appendage; RPVs = right pulmonary veins; SVC = superior vena cava.

In mapping the ventricles, a card-type electrode patch may be used to map a limited area (see Figure 34.2). However, in order to map the entire surface of the ventricles, sock- or net-type electrodes (Figure 34.4) are ideal. Electrodes placed on hard templates, such as silicon plates, may not steadily record the electrograms because of the dynamic motion of the ventricular contraction. Endocardial mapping of the left ventricle through a ventriculotomy or across the mitral valve is possible with an inflatable balloon electrode array.

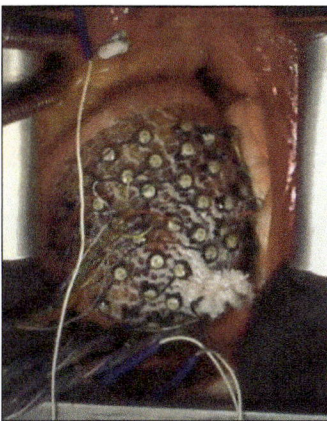

Figure 34.4 Net-type electrodes for the ventricles. A total of 64 unipolar electrodes are mounted on the stretchable net. The epicardial electrograms are stably recorded during an entire cardiac cycle of ventricular tachycardia or other cardiac rhythms. Three white cables are connected to subcutaneous tissue and provide for indifferent electrodes for recording unipolar electrograms.

However, the spatial accuracy of the maps depends on the consistency of the electrode location, on both the maps and the actual location on the heart in each patient. The size and figure of the atria or ventricles can vary among patients, and as a result, the location of each electrode may also vary, even if the electrode templates are made for individual patients based on the actual size and figure of the patient's heart.

The recently introduced electroanatomic mapping system uses an electromagnetic navigation technology, albeit for single-point mapping. This system constructs a 3D structure of the heart and draws an activation map on the figure simultaneously, allowing for a consistent spatial correlation between the electrode location on the maps and the actual location on the heart in each patient. This mapping modality more precisely localizes a tachycardia's focus or reentrant circuit for arrhythmia surgery.

Activation Time Mapping

The most popular analysis in intraoperative mapping is activation time mapping. In unipolar electrograms, the time of local activation is determined as the time of steepest downward slope, which can be determined by the maximum negative derivative of the electrogram. In bipolar electrograms, the time of local activation is usually determined to be the absolute maximum amplitude rather than the onset of the electrogram; this consistency better enables the computer to determine the time.

The underlying mechanism for surgically curing arrhythmias consists of excision or ablation of the focus of a tachycardia or interruption of the reentrant circuit by making a line of conduction block. The focus of a tachycardia can be located by finding the earliest activation time in the activation time maps. The accuracy of locating the focus of the tachycardia depends on the spatial resolution of the mapping, which is determined by the interelectrode distance of the mapping electrodes. The focus of a VT may be located in the endocardium or intramural myocardium; thus, endocardial mapping combined with epicardial mapping may precisely locate the focus. In addition to consulting the findings of the epicardial mapping, referring to the preoperative endocardial mapping data is important in the intraoperative mapping of VT.

Activation maps are usually displayed as static maps in which the local activation time is calculated as the time difference from the activation time at the reference electrode. The activation time can be sorted as the time from earliest activation site (as zero time), and each area with an activation time range is color coded. The static activation map clearly demonstrates the earliest activation site and the atrial or ventricular activation patterns that follow in a regular rhythm, eg, sinus rhythm, supraventricular tachycardia, or VT. However, in irregular arrhythmias, particularly in AF, displaying the activation sequence as a static map is not appropriate. Because in AF the atrial activation is continuous and the pattern of activation varies beat by beat, the activation maps should be displayed in a dynamic mode as a movie.

In surgery for reentrant tachycardias, such as atrial flutter or VT, it is important to localize the reentrant circuit and interrupt it. The earliest activation site the activation map locates is an epicardial or endocardial breakthrough from the reentrant circuit; therefore, this site may not be the ideal for making a lesion for ablation. Most reentrant tachycardias have an isthmus or central common pathway in their circuits.[3] The activation in the isthmus is confined within a small and narrow area of myocardium. Also, the conduction is usually slow, providing enough time for the atrial or ventricular tissue to recover from the refractory period and for sustaining the reentrant activation. In atrial flutter and incisional atrial reentry, respectively, the isthmus consists of the atrial tissue between the inferior vena cava and the tricuspid valve annulus (cavotricuspid isthmus) and the gap between the incision and the venous cannula insertion site. In reentrant VT that occurs after a myocardial infarction, the surviving myocardium surrounded by fibrous scar tissue may act as the central common pathway of the reentrant circuit.

The electrograms in the central common pathway should be recorded as diastolic potentials or as continuous activity during the time between the QRS waves of VT. Because the electrograms in the central common pathway are low amplitude and fragmented, the activation may not form a significant wave on the surface electrocardiogram. Even with hundreds of electrodes covering the entire epicardium, these electrograms are not necessarily recorded using intraoperative mapping because the pathway can be located endocardially or intramurally. Meanwhile, the diastolic potentials can be recorded from bystander or inner-loop pathways in the reentrant circuit.

Entrainment of the tachycardia and measurement of the postpacing interval are helpful for determining whether the potentials are recorded from the central common pathway—the critical lesion for sustaining reentrant VT and the target for ablation. During entrainment of the tachycardia at the central common pathway, the QRS morphologies of the electrocardiograms should be the same as the VT (concealed entrainment). The postpacing interval should be close to the tachycardia cycle length because the last paced activation is the same as the activation of the tachycardia.[4] Mapping the return cycle, which is the time interval between the first and second activations after entrainment, has been shown able to locate the central common pathway without pacing the pathway. The contours of the return cycle, equal to the tachycardia cycle length, converge on the central common pathway.[5]

Voltage Mapping

The requirement for reentrant activation is the slow conduction and dispersion of refractoriness. These conditions are frequently associated with surviving myocardium surrounded by fibrosis or scar that has been complicated by myocardial infarction or cardiomyopathy. Under these conditions, the electrograms recorded at lesions are low voltage and fragmented. Voltage mapping measures the amplitude of the local electrograms during sinus rhythm or pacing and displays the distribution of the amplitude.[6] Because, with low-voltage electrograms, the area frequently coincides with the lesion having the critical area for the VT, resection or ablation of such an area may terminate the VT. More important, ablation of the low-voltage area not only terminates the clinical VT but also potentially prevents nonclinical arrhythmias, which may not be induced or mapped during surgery or an electrophysiological study.

Potential Distribution Mapping

Potential distribution mapping is a different modality of intraoperative mapping. Instead, it is constructed from unipolar electrograms and the distribution of the potential fields. A potential minimum is developed in the potential distribution map at the earliest activation site of a VT.[7] This type of mapping has several advantages over activation time mapping—particularly when it is demonstrated in a dynamic mode as a movie. It requires less editing to construct the isopotential maps. Also, once the reference baseline for the potential maps is determined, no additional analysis is required and multiple runs of VT can be displayed.[8] Because unipolar potentials reflect distant activity, a VT's intramural sites of origin may be detected using the epicardial or endocardial electrogram recordings.

Various Types of Arrhythmias

Wolff-Parkinson-White (WPW) and Other Preexcitation Syndromes

These days, it has become infrequent to perform surgery for WPW syndrome because catheter ablation of the accessory pathways has led to satisfactory results with less invasiveness. The opportunities for surgical ablation in WPW patients are limited to patients with recurrent tachyarrhythmias after several sessions of catheter ablation and those undergoing cardiac surgeries for structural heart disease. More recently, the latter cases are usually being treated by catheter ablation prior to the surgery. Therefore, patients who require surgical ablation may have special reasons for having undergone multiple sessions of unsuccessful catheter ablation, such as an epicardial location or oblique course of the accessory pathway across the atrioventricular groove.

The purpose of intraoperative mapping in patients with WPW syndrome is to localize the accessory pathway.[9] This pathway can be localized via activation mapping of the atrioventricular groove. The ventricular end of the pathway can be localized as the earliest activation during sinus rhythm or atrial pacing, and the atrial end can be localized as the earliest activation during ventricular pacing or reciprocating tachycardia. The electrograms can be recorded using a card-type electrode patch with multiple electrodes (see Figure 34.2). The atrioventricular groove is usually covered by fatty tissue that precludes a clear recording of the electrograms close to the atrioventricular junction. Thus, additional precise mapping is recommended after dissecting the fat tissue and exposing the myocardium. The electroanatomic mapping technique enables one to precisely localize the accessory pathway (Figure 34.5).

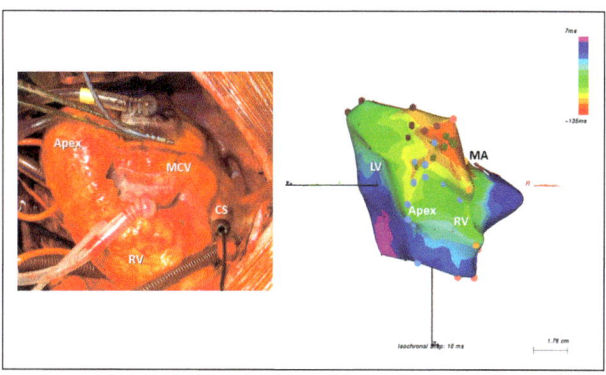

Figure 34.5 Electroanatomic mapping for Wolff–Parkinson–White syndrome with an accessory pathway connected to the middle cardiac vein. After multiple sessions of catheter ablation, the patient had conduction recur over a posterior septal atrioventricular accessory pathway. Intraoperative mapping was performed with the aid of cardiopulmonary bypass and a Tentacles® Heart Positioner (Sumitomo Bakelite, Tokyo). This setup provided sufficient exposure of the posterior aspect of the heart while maintaining stable hemodynamics and ensuring the geometric accuracy of the data. **Left panel:** Electrograms were recorded from the ventricular epicardium, along with the 3D locations by manipulating the NaviStar catheter (Biosense Webster/Johnson & Johnson, Diamond Bar, CA). **Right panel:** Activation map of the ventricles during sinus rhythm. The ventricles are seen from the apex and the isochronal contours are color coded, as shown in the scale. The earliest activation occurs at the proximal midcardiac vein that courses along the posterior septum. The **blue tags** indicate the septum between the right and left ventricles, and the **ocher tags** indicate the midcardiac vein. CS = coronary sinus; LV = left ventricle; MA = mitral annulus; MCV = midcardiac vein; RV = right ventricle.

Special attention is needed for mapping arrythmias in patients with multiple accessory pathways. In these patients, the conduction of an accessory pathway can be masked by the earlier activation of the atria or ventricles that have been preexcited by the other accessory pathways. Performing activation mapping during extrastimulation is helpful for unmasking the conduction of the second accessory pathway. In this way, the conduction of an accessory pathway with a longer refractory period is blocked or slowed during an extrastimulated cycle, and the conduction of the other accessory pathway is unveiled.

Extrastimulation is also useful for determining successful division or ablation of the accessory pathway in patients who have retrograde conduction over the atrioventricular node. Retrograde atrial activation with a constant ventriculoatrial conduction time during extrastimulation indicates residual conduction across the accessory pathway; in contrast, retrograde atrial activation with a decremental conduction indicates retrograde conduction over the atrioventricular node and successful ablation of the accessory pathway.

Atrial Tachycardia

Atrial tachycardia (AT) is defined as a supraventricular tachycardia that is initiated and maintained only with atrial myocardium. Symptomatic and medically refractory patients with AT are indicated for radiofrequency catheter ablation, which has a high success rate and a low AT recurrence rate.[10] Surgery is indicated in patients with recurrent AT after failed catheter ablation and in those who undergo (usually a redo) surgery for congenital or valvular heart disease.

Intraoperative Mapping of Atrial Tachycardia: From the perspective of intraoperative mapping, AT may be classified into two categories: focal AT and reentrant AT. Focal ATs arise from a localized area in the atria, such as the crista terminalis, pulmonary veins, ostium of the coronary sinus, or interatrial septum. Focal ATs can be induced by programmed stimulation, commonly with the aid of isoproterenol infusion. Not infrequently, some patients with focal AT continuously experience tachycardia for several years. The pattern of atrial activation is focal; in it, the atrial activation occurs at a localized atrial region (focus) and spreads toward the boundaries of the atrium with the atrioventricular annuli or connecting vessels. The latest activation usually occurs at boundaries that are remote from the focus.

Reentrant ATs most commonly occur in patients after surgery for congenital or valvular heart disease. The incisions or scars caused by a previous surgery pose obstacles, along with slow conduction at the atrial tissues around the atrioventricular annuli or the edge of the incisions or scars. This sets up perfect conditions for sustained macroreentrant activation.

Prior to surgery, obtaining sufficient precise electrophysiological data of either focal or reentrant AT is strongly recommended. This is because some focal ATs are catecholamine-sensitive and may not be inducible during surgery under general anesthesia, making intraoperative mapping impossible. In addition, patients with reentrant ATs associated with previous cardiac procedures frequently have dense adhesion with the pericardium or other surrounding tissue; these can result in incomplete recording of the epicardial electrograms.

Because precisely localizing the earliest activation is crucial for mapping focal AT, and given that most focal ATs are regular and stable, electroanatomic mapping should be an ideal modality for intraoperative mapping (▶ Video 34.2). Once the focus of the AT is determined, it can be excised, ablated, or isolated.

Template-type electrode patches that cover the entire atrial epicardium can be used in patients with reentrant AT to determine the reentrant circuit of the AT. However, intraoperative mapping of reentrant AT in patients with previous cardiac procedures may not be so straightforward. Potentially, it could fail to provide sufficient data to determine the reentrant circuit. In these patients, surgical incisions or ablation lines should be designed based on preoperative electrophysiological data; alternatively, the maze procedure should be performed in order to block all possible macroreentrant circuits.[11]

Atrial Fibrillation

Until recently, the role of intraoperative mapping had been limited to an investigation of the electrophysiological mechanism in human AF.[12,13] Although it is still a challenging modality in AF surgery, the map-guided procedure is the ideal approach to take in arrhythmia surgery. Intraoperative verification of a line of conduction block created by radiofrequency ablation also has been widely applied during surgery for AF. More recently, mapping and ablation of active ganglionated plexi (GP) have been examined to see whether they affect the sustainability of AF.

Intraoperative Mapping: Few mapping studies have been performed in patients with AF because mapping of AF carries several difficulties.[12-15] For example, analyzing the atrial activation using the usual static and 2D maps is sometimes an intricate process because of coexisting multiple wavelets during AF and the complex, 3D-structure of the atria. Therefore, simultaneously mapping the entire atria with multiple electrodes is required to analyze the coexisting multiple wavelets. The maps should be displayed in dynamic mode as a movie in 3D-constructed atrial models. This view will keep the atrial activation correlated with the anatomic landmarks, such as the atrioventricular annuli, great vessels, and pulmonary vein orifices. These technical advantages allow for a precise, accurate analysis of multiple concurrent wavelets in the atria.[15]

Intraoperative studies on the atrial activation of the entire atria[12] or lateral right atrium[13] during pacing-induced AF syndrome were undertaken in patients with WPW. They demonstrated unstable reentrant circuits of a very short cycle length in the right atrium. Harada and colleagues[14] intraoperatively mapped the right and left atria separately in patients with mitral valve disease and permanent AF. They observed regular, repetitive activations originating from the left atrium and complex, chaotic activation in the right atrium. As a result, they proposed that the left atrium acts as an electrical chamber for AF in patients with mitral valve disease.

We used 253 electrodes to map the entire atrial epicardium simultaneously in patients with permanent AF associated with mitral valve disease. We then analyzed the atrial activation on 3D-constructed atrial models in a dynamic mode[15] (Video 34.3). In this subset of patients, concurrent multiple focal activations arising from the pulmonary veins combined with fibrillatory conduction and right atrial focal or reentrant activations were the mechanism underlying multiple coexisting wavelets. A progressive conduction delay or block in the pathway from the pulmonary vein focus to the right atrium, and in the lateral right atrium, caused an irregular and complex right atrial activation that was desynchronized with the left atrium (Figure 34.6, Video 34.4). In addition to passive activation, focal activation and reentrant activation were observed in the lateral right atrium (Figure 34.7, Video 34.5). All these complex, desynchronized activations of the right and left atria formed multiple wavelets in the atrial activation and fibrillatory waves on the electrocardiograms.

Map-guided Surgery: Few attempts at map-guided surgery have been made for AF. Among these, Yamauchi and colleagues[16] performed map-guided surgery with a card-type electrode patch, carrying 60 unipolar electrodes, in 40 patients with AF associated with valvular or congenital heart disease. None of the patients had any reentrant movement or repetitive activation in the right atrium. Foci or reentry circuits located in the left atrium were clearly identified in 11 patients, and in 9 of those, sinus rhythm was resumed by placing cryoablation lesions at these sites. The exact site was not identified in the 29 remaining patients. They concluded that intraoperative mapping was

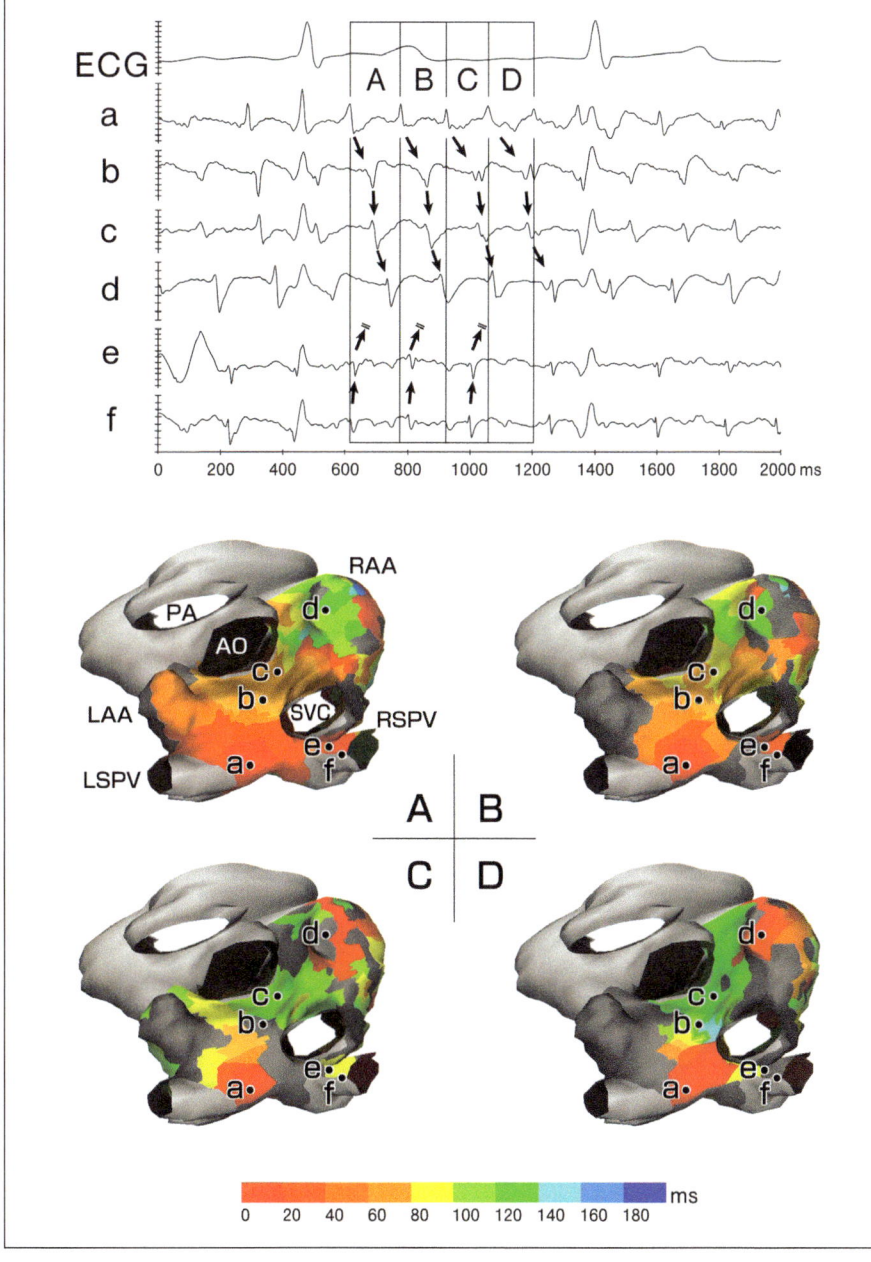

Figure 34.6 Repetitive activations arising in the pulmonary veins and fibrillatory conduction to the right atrium. Atrial activation maps constructed in a 55-year-old male patient with permanent AF associated with aortic and mitral valve disease. The maps are shown along with an electrocardiogram and selected electrograms. The maps represent a superior view of the atria, as if being observed cranially. The location of the selected electrodes (**a–f**) is indicated in the maps. The activation maps during the time windows from **A** to **D** are shown. The duration of each time window (the cycle length of the activation recorded from electrode a) is 164, 144, 140, and 141 ms, respectively. Atrial activation is shown with color coding at 20 ms increments. The **gray** represents regions where no activation is seen during the time window. See the text for an explanation. AO = aorta; ECG = electrocardiogram; LAA = left atrial appendage; LSPV = left superior pulmonary vein; PA = pulmonary artery; RAA = right atrial appendage; RSPV = right superior pulmonary vein; SVC = superior vena cava. *Source:* Nitta T, et al.[15] ©2004 The American Association for Thoracic Surgery and Elsevier Inc. All rights reserved.

useful for distinguishing the mechanism of AF and facilitating the optimal placement of the cryolesions.

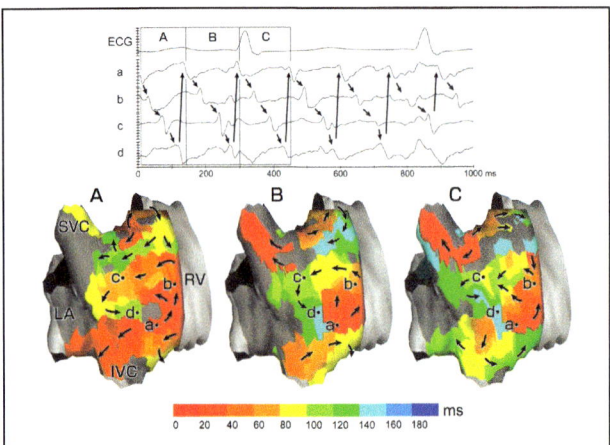

Figure 34.7 Reentrant activations in the lateral right atrium. Right atrial activation maps constructed in a 70-year-old female patient with permanent AF associated with mitral valve stenosis. The maps represent the lateral aspect of the right atrium and are shown along with an electrocardiogram and selected electrograms. The location of those electrodes (**a–d**) is indicated in the maps. The activation maps during the time windows from **A** to **C** are shown. The duration of each time window (the cycle length of the activation recorded from electrode a) is 132, 155, and 155 ms, respectively. The **arrows** indicate the activation sequence. Note the reentrant activation in the right atrium. *Source:* Nitta T, et al.[15] ©2004 The American Association for Thoracic Surgery and Elsevier Inc. All rights reserved.

Our group performed map-guided surgery in 46 patients with AF. We used a 256-channel 3D dynamic mapping system with custom-made epicardial patch electrodes in order to examine atrial activation during AF and to determine the optimal procedure.[17] The atrial electrograms had a low voltage over a broad area, and surgical intervention for AF was not indicated in 3 patients. Concurrent, multiple, and repetitive activations arising from the pulmonary veins or left atrial appendage were observed in all the other patients. Pulmonary vein isolation and left atrial incisions without any right atrial incisions were performed in 8 patients in whom the right atrial activation was passive, and all were cured of AF. The radial procedure, which consisted of biatrial incisions and pulmonary vein isolation, was performed in the remaining 35 patients, and 31 (89%) of the patients were cured of AF. These results indicate that intraoperative mapping helps determine the optimal procedure for AF in each patient.

Although these studies indicate that intraoperative mapping is useful for AF surgery, the technique has several limitations. For one, the current technique of activation mapping for AF is time-consuming because the atrial electrograms can be fragmented and have a low voltage in these patients. Thus, an analysis of the electrograms to determine the local activation time at hundreds of points frequently requires extensive editing. Either the mapping technique needs to be improved or a different modality, capable of characterizing the atrial activation during AF within a minute, needs to be developed. In addition, the interatrial septum and the coronary sinus should be mapped. That is because macroreentry conduction through the interatrial septum and interatrial electrical connections that go through the coronary sinus musculature or the septum can be mechanisms of AF.

Intraoperative Verification of Conduction Block: Creating a conduction block is the rationale behind the surgical treatment of AF. Recently, radiofrequency ablation has been widely used to create a conduction block in surgery for AF. However, radiofrequency ablation does not necessarily guarantee transmural and continuous necrosis because of the thermal sink effect, thick atrial tissue, or technical reasons. Incomplete creation of the conduction block between the pulmonary veins and left atrium may result in recurrence of AF. A conduction gap within a line of conduction block created on the atrial wall can result in reentrant AT postoperatively.

The electrical isolation of the pulmonary veins from the left atrium can be verified by demonstrating the absence of atrial activation during pacing at the pulmonary veins (Figure 34.8, ▶ Video 34.6). Verification of a complete conduction block of the linear ablation on the

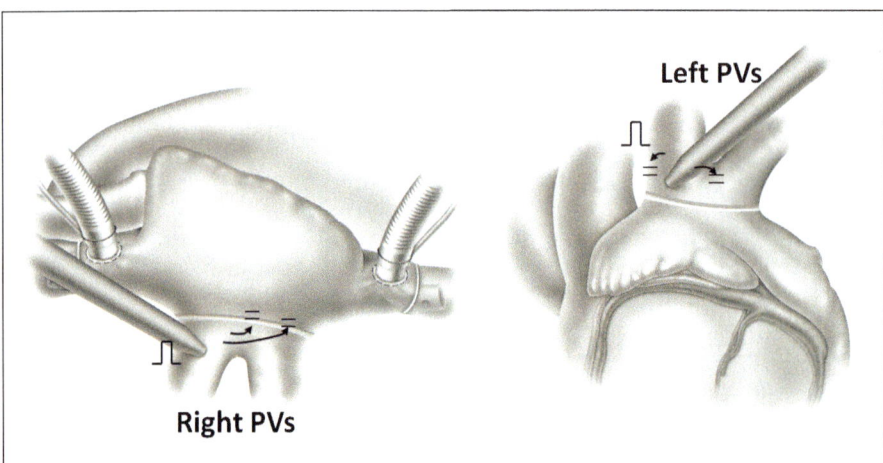

Figure 34.8 Verification of complete electrical isolation of the pulmonary veins (PVs) from the left atrium. After PV ablation, each of the 4 PVs is paced using a bipolar electrode. Conduction block between the PVs and left atrium is determined by failure of atrial capture despite maximum output from the PV pacing stimuli. If any residual conduction is demonstrated between any of the PVs and the left atrium, repeat ablation is performed until a complete conduction block is confirmed. Pacing sites indicated by **open rectangles**. *Source:* Ishii Y, et al.[20] ©2008 The American Association for Thoracic Surgery and Elsevier Inc. All rights reserved.

atrial wall *requires* atrial mapping and analysis of activation across the line of ablation. Many studies have demonstrated that incomplete ablation of the coronary sinus is the most common cause of postoperative AT.[18,19] Conduction block in the coronary sinus can be tested by analyzing the activation sequence in the coronary sinus during pacing by placing an electrode catheter in the coronary sinus[20] (Figure 34.9).

the superior aspect of the interatrial groove and the ligament of Marshall. Combined with the pulmonary vein isolation or maze procedure, ablation of active GPs has been shown to improve the short-term outcome for AF. An experimental study demonstrated that restoration of vagal effects 4 weeks after GP ablation suggests early atrial reinnervation.[24]

Ventricular Tachycardia

VT is classified into ischemic and nonischemic VTs. Ischemic VT is associated with coronary artery disease and is usually seen in patients with a prior myocardial infarction. The majority of these patients have an associated aneurysm or dyskinesis of the left ventricle. Nonischemic VT is associated with a variety of structural heart diseases, including hypertrophic or dilated cardiomyopathy, myocarditis, arrhythmogenic right ventricular cardiomyopathy,[25] cardiac tumors, and postoperative status of congenital heart disease.[26] Idiopathic VT without any structural heart disease is also seen in relatively young patients.

Implantable cardioverter-defibrillators (ICDs) have been demonstrated to prevent sudden cardiac death due to VTs. As a result, they are designated as first-line therapy in VT patients who are at high risk for sudden cardiac death. Since the ICD does not prevent the occurrence of VTs, the patients are still prone to experiencing them. A prospective study has shown that the mortality rate is higher in ICD patients who have frequent appropriate or inappropriate discharges of their ICDs. Although radiofrequency catheter ablation is initially indicated in patients with medically refractory VTs, surgical therapy is indicated in patients who have recurrent and incessant VTs, left ventricular dysfunction, or intramural VT foci in the hypertrophic myocardium.

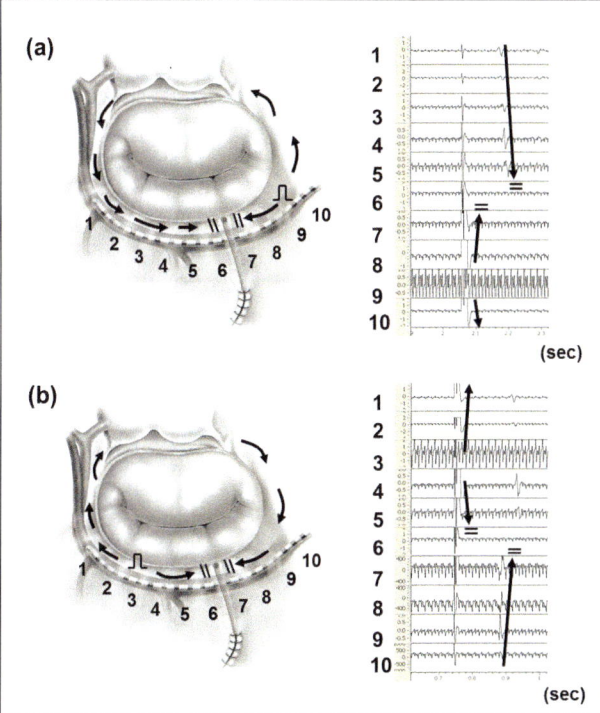

Figure 34.9 Verification of conduction block in the coronary sinus (CS). Typical activation sequence around the mitral valve after a complete CS ablation. The paced activation from the proximal (electrode No. 9) or distal (electrode No. 3) electrode (**open rectangles**) to the CS ablation lesion is completely blocked at the ablation lesion. The activation is propagated around the mitral valve in a counterclockwise (**a**) or clockwise (**b**) fashion from the pacing site to the opposite side across the ablation lesion. **Right panel:** The activation sequence is shown. Propagation of the conduction (**arrows**); conduction block (**double bars**). *Source:* Ishii Y, et al.[20] ©2008 The American Association for Thoracic Surgery and Elsevier Inc. All rights reserved.

Mapping and Ablation of Ganglionated Plexi: Increased autonomic nervous activity has been known to play a role in the initiation and maintenance of AF. Recently, identification of GP and their ablation has been expected to reduce the vagal activity that may facilitate the triggered activity in the pulmonary veins and prevent the recurrence of AF after surgical treatment of AF.[21-23] High-frequency stimulation at a rate of 1,000/minute is delivered to the fat pad beside the pulmonary veins and atrial tissue. Then, a specific area with a vagal reflex (reduction in heart rate) during stimulation is defined as an active GP (▶ Video 34.7). More than half the GPs were found in the area of

Intraoperative Mapping of Ischemic VT: From the late 1970s to the early 1980s, when Dr. Harken[27-28] first performed a surgery for ischemic VT, Drs. Josephson and Horowitz[29-30] performed an extensive mapping study of ischemic VT. They mapped both the epicardial and endocardial surfaces during VT using bipolar electrodes mounted in a ring worn on the surgeon's finger. The electrograms were recorded from 50 to 100 epicardial and 30 to 90 endocardial preselected sites. They were recorded on paper as well as on a computer for postoperative offline analyses. The local activation times were determined as the time difference from the reference electrogram, and the activation maps were drawn on schemas of the ventricular epicardium and endocardium.

Their analysis of 67 VT morphologies found that the earliest activation occurred on the endocardial surface 2 to 79 ms before the onset of the QRS complex and was followed by the epicardial breakthrough. The location of earliest activation was along the endocardial margin of the left ventricular aneurysm or healed myocardial infarction, within 2 cm inside or outside the border between the infarcted tissue and viable myocardium.

Based on their experience with intraoperative mapping, they addressed some technical problems and considerations as follows.[30] Fragmented and low-amplitude electrograms are frequently recorded near the site of origin of VT, which makes determining local activation times difficult. Motion artifact caused by ventricular contractions may produce artifact deflections on the recordings and confusion during data analysis. The other problems are related to the inducibility and reproducibility of the clinical VTs during surgery. Clinically documented VTs are not necessarily induced in the operating room, and nonclinical VTs are induced in some patients. General anesthesia, hypothermia, electrolyte variations, withdrawal or maintenance of antiarrhythmic drugs, and other factors may affect the inducibility of VTs in the operating room. Moreover, polymorphic VTs and ultrafast VTs are not possible to map using a single-point mapping technique.

Many of these problems were solved during the following two decades. Ideker and colleagues[31,32] developed a computerized method of multichannel mapping that was capable of recording multiple electrograms simultaneously and analyzing and displaying the activation maps with a combination of electrode arrays. Mickleborough and colleagues[33] used a multiballoon electrode array and a computer-generated flashing light display to obtain extensive mapping data and demonstrate the endocardial activation sequence in a relatively short period of time. They observed three basic patterns of endocardial activation: monoregional (focal), figure-8, and circular patterns. Pagé[34] also introduced an inflatable balloon electrode array into both left and right ventricular chambers through the atriotomies across the atrioventricular valves. They found that, in many patients, the localization of the earliest epicardial and endocardial activations was anatomically consistent, suggesting that epicardial mapping could locate the site of origin in free-wall VTs. They also demonstrated that the epicardial and left ventricular endocardial relation is more complex in VTs with a septal origin, which occurred in 76% of their patients. For these VTs, potential distribution mapping has been shown to precisely localize the site of origin in the interventricular septum[35] (Figure 34.10).

Because reentry is the underlying mechanism in most cases of ischemic VTs in humans, the critical region for sustaining VT is the central common pathway or the slow conduction zone of the reentrant circuit; there, the activation wavefronts are confined to a narrow isthmus. Although high-resolution mapping with hundreds of electrodes can record potentials from the critical region and localize the region, the potentials at the critical region are frequently low voltage and fractionated, as described above; thus, constructing activation maps of the reentrant circuit requires careful analysis and extensive editing. Entrainment has been widely used in localizing the critical region during catheter ablation. Demonstration of concealed entrainment and the postpacing interval close to the tachycardia cycle length suggests that the VT is paced from the central common pathway of the reentrant circuit.

Return-cycle mapping is a unique method for localizing the central common pathway. It employs fewer electrodes and does not require pacing the common pathway and analyzing the complex electrograms at the pathway. The return cycle is the time interval between the first and second activations after cessation of entrainment. Thus, the mapping method is based on the phenomenon that, irrespective of the stimulation site, the isochrones of the return cycle equaling the cycle length of the VT converge on the lines of block connected to the central common pathway[36] (Figure 34.11).

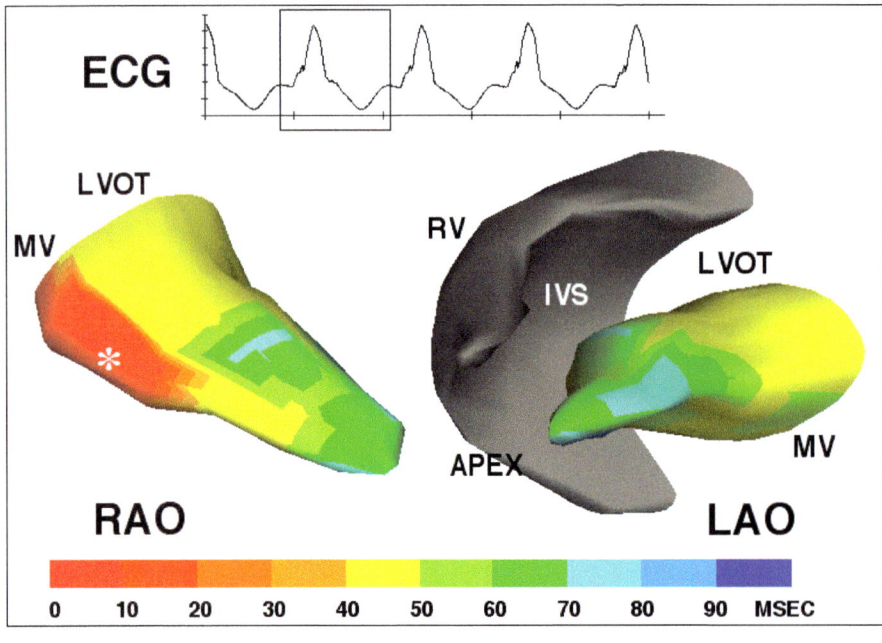

Figure 34.10 Endocardial mapping of the left ventricle (LV). In a patient with a history of inferior myocardial infarction, the LV endocardium was mapped using form-fitted sponge-made electrodes inserted from the left atrium across the mitral valve while the heart was beating. The maps represent the activation sequence of the LV endocardium during the VT. The isochronal contours are color coded, and the **asterisk** indicates the earliest activation site. The VT originated from the inferior septum of the LV endocardium. ECG = electrocardiogram; IVS = interventricular septum; LAO = left anterior oblique; LVOT = left ventricular outflow tract; MV = mitral valve; RAO = right anterior oblique; RV = right ventricle.

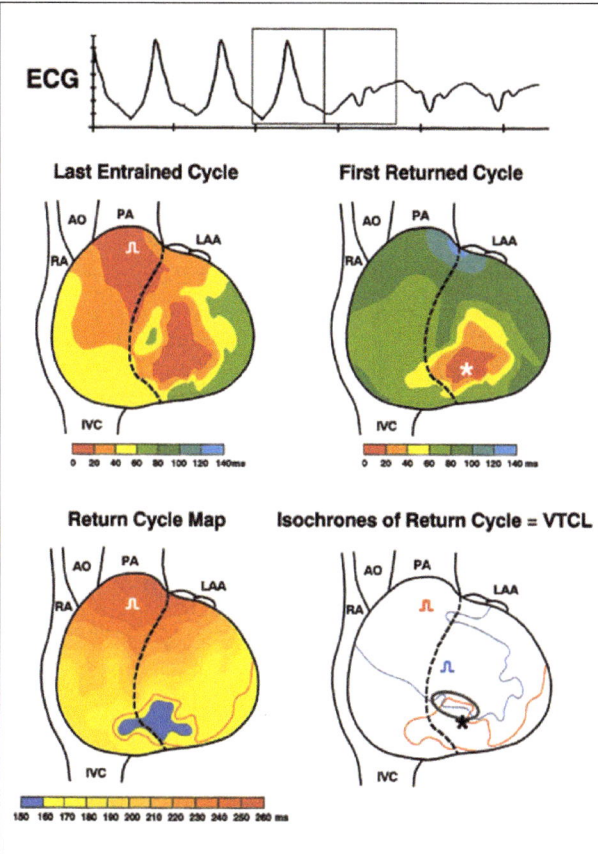

Figure 34.11 Return-cycle mapping. **Upper panel:** Electrocardiogram (ECG) during cessation of entrainment of a VT induced in a 4-day-old canine infarct. **Middle panels:** The activation maps during the first and second activation after cessation of entrainment. **Boxed areas** on the ECG at top comprise the data window analyzed to construct the activation maps. The VT was entrained from the right ventricular outflow tract (**open rectangles denote the pacing site**) at a pacing cycle length of 160 ms. After cessation of pacing, the VT resumed at a cycle length of 168 ms with the earliest activation site (EAS) located at the inferior left ventricle near the apex (**asterisk**). The activation times are represented as color codes with 20 ms increments. **Lower left panel:** Return-cycle map constructed from these activation maps by subtracting the first activation time from the second activation time after cessation pacing. The return cycle is represented as color codes with 10 ms increments. The return cycle was longest at the region around the pacing site and shorter at the region near the earliest activation site. The **blue** indicates the region where the return cycle equaled the pacing cycle length, suggesting orthodromic activation by the preceding stimulus. The **red line** indicates the return cycle isochrone equal to the VTCL. **Right lower panel:** As we changed the pacing site from the **red** to the **blue open rectangle**, this isochrone shifted from the **red line** to the **blue line**. These lines converged on a region 20 mm away from the earliest activation site and formed intersections. The VT was terminated by applying cryothermia to the region between the intersections. AO = aorta; IVC = inferior vena cava; LAA = left atrial appendage; PA = pulmonary artery; RA = right atrium; VTCL = ventricular tachycardia cycle length. Source: Nitta T, et al.[36] ©2001 The American Association for Thoracic Surgery and Elsevier Inc. All rights reserved.

Based on findings from the mapping studies, the surgical procedure for ischemic VT has been proposed. It involves resection of the fibrous scar tissue of the endocardium, combined with encircling cryoablation at the border of the endocardial resection, and followed by a surgical ventricular reconstruction. This procedure has been shown to prevent ischemic VT. However, many ischemic VT patients present with multiple VT morphologies. So not only is precisely mapping each VT morphology time-consuming, but nonclinical VT may occur even after resection of only the endocardium of induced and mapped VTs. Even so, in most patients, combining an extensive endocardial resection with encircling cryothermia (even if it is not guided by intraoperative mapping) has been shown to control VTs.[37]

Intraoperative Mapping in Nonischemic VT: In the 1980s, when Drs. Fontaine,[38] Iwa,[39] and others[40] first performed surgery for nonischemic VTs, handheld or sock-type electrodes were used to construct activation maps during sinus rhythm and VT. The findings of this initial intraoperative mapping varied according to the underlying heart disease. In arrhythmogenic right ventricular dysplasia (cardiomyopathy), for example, delayed activation was demonstrated during sinus rhythm on the right ventricle. Epicardial mapping performed during VT was able to localize the emergence of the abnormal activation and direct the surgical procedure. In idiopathic left ventricular aneurysms, postexcitation potentials were recorded during sinus rhythm around the aneurysm, and the epicardial breakthrough of the VT was localized at the border of the aneurysm. In patients with VT after repair of a tetralogy of Fallot, macroreentrant activation around the ventricular incision was observed at the right ventricular outflow tract.

Currently, most VT patients undergo one or more sessions of endocardial and/or epicardial catheter ablation. Each VT's site of origin will have been determined in the limited region of the ventricles before the patient is referred to surgery. Therefore, the intraoperative mapping should concentrate on more precisely localizing the focus or reentrant circuit of the VTs. Simultaneous multisite mapping with high-density electrodes may be used for this purpose. More recently, an electroanatomic mapping system has been used for intraoperative mapping. This system provides a consistent spatial correlation between the electrode location on the maps and the actual location on the heart; this correlation allows for precise localization of the focus or reentrant circuit of the VT in each patient[41] (Figure 34.12).

In patients with hypertrophic cardiomyopathy, radiofrequency catheter ablation frequently fails. This is because of a possible nontransmural ablation due to an epicardial or intramural activation focus or to hypertrophic myocardium. Epicardial mapping alone, or combined with endocardial mapping, may not precisely localize the intramural focus. In such patients, a plunge needle with closely separated electrodes may be useful for locating the intramural focus.

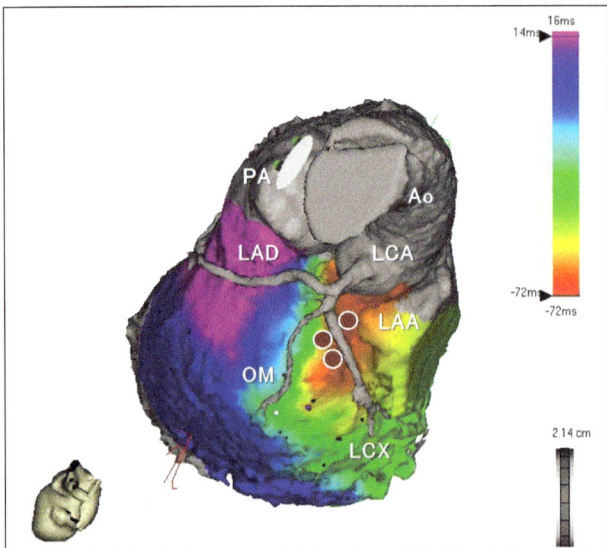

Figure 34.12 Epicardial mapping of nonischemic VT using the electroanatomic mapping system. Left anterosuperior oblique aspect of the left ventricle. The epicardial activation sequence during VT is presented as a color code. **Three red circles** denote the site of epicardial cryoablation. Ao = aorta; LAA = left atrial appendage; LAD = left anterior descending coronary artery; LCA = left coronary artery; LCX = left circumflex coronary artery; OM = obtuse marginal artery; PA = pulmonary artery.

Future Perspectives

Even with so much progress made in the past half century, limitations and problems in the intraoperative mapping of human arrhythmias remain. Cardiac mapping of human AF carries several problems. Multiple pathological and electrophysiological mechanism may participate in initiating and sustaining AF. Furthermore, the type or combination of these mechanisms varies among patients and can change from moment to moment. The complex anatomy of the atria, including the presence of the interatrial septum and complex and nonuniform trabeculae, makes atrial activation during AF extremely intricate. In addition, intraoperative activation mapping during AF is difficult and time-consuming because of fractionated, unsteady, and ambiguous electrograms caused by the underlying conditions described above.

In order to direct the optimal surgical procedures for AF in each patient, intraoperative mapping could instead focus on selected information, such as the location of the foci of an abnormal rapid activation, pattern of the atrial activation, and so on. Frequency mapping is a relatively new method in which the electrograms are analyzed in a frequency domain by calculating the power spectrum using a fast Fourier transform. Schuessler et al[42] showed that in the majority of patients with AF, a distinct region of dominant frequencies could be demonstrated during the recording period. The location of the dominant frequency was in either the right or left atrium and changed over time in half of the patients. The dominant frequency was highest in patients with chronic AF as compared with those with paroxysmal AF. Frequency mapping has an advantage over activation mapping because it is able to rapidly localize the source of AF.

Intraoperative mapping has focused on localizing the earliest tachycardia activation. This is a rational approach if the tachycardia has an automaticity or microreentry mechanism. However, it is irrational and inappropriate for treating reentrant tachycardias that have an extent of reentrant circuit, such as in ischemic VT or AF. In these reentrant tachycardias, localizing the substrate that leads to the reentry would be more useful and curative. Fractionated electrograms, continuous activity, or delayed activations have all been used as indicators of the substrate. Distribution mapping of the dispersion of the conduction and refractoriness may be able to localize the regions of the substrate.

References

1. Durrer D, van Dam RT, Freud GE, et al. Total excitation of the isolated human heart. *Circulation.* 1970;41:899-912.
2. Durrer D, Roos JP. Epicardial excitation of the ventricles in a patient with WPW syndrome. *Circulation.* 1967;35:15-21.
3. El-Sherif N, Yin H, Caref EB, Restivo M. Electrophysiological mechanisms of spontaneous termination of sustained monomorphic reentrant ventricular tachycardia in the canine postinfarction heart. *Circulation.* 1996;93:1567-1578.
4. Almendral JM, Gottlieb CD, Rosenthal ME, et al. Entrainment of ventricular tachycardia: explanation for surface electrocardiographic phenomena by analysis of electrograms recorded within the tachycardia circuit. *Circulation.* 1988;77:569-580.
5. Nitta T, Schuessler RB, Mitsuno M, et al. Return cycle mapping after entrainment of ventricular tachycardia. *Circulation.* 1998;97:1164-1175.
6. Stevenson WG, Delacretaz E, Friedman PL, Ellison KE. Identification and ablation of macroreentrant ventricular tachycardia with the CARTO electroanatomical mapping system. *Pacing Clin Electrophysiol.* 1998;21:1448-1456.
7. Harada A, D'Agostino HJ Jr, Schuessler RB, et al. Potential distribution mapping. New method for precise localization of intramural septal origin of ventricular tachycardia. *Circulation.* 1988;78(5 Pt 2):III137-III147.
8. Harada A, Tweddell JS, Schuessler RB, et al. Computerized potential distribution mapping: a new intraoperative mapping technique for ventricular tachycardia surgery. *Ann Thorac Surg.* 1990;49(4):649-655.
9. Gallagher JJ, Kasell J, Sealy WC, et al. Epicardial mapping in the Wolff-Parkinson-White syndrome. *Circulation.* 1978;57: 854-866.
10. Blomström-Lundqvist C, Scheinman MM, Aliot EM, et al. ACC/AHA/ESC guidelines for the management of patients with supraventricular arrhythmias—executive summary. A report of the American College of Cardiology/American Heart Association Task Force on Practice Guidelines and the European Society of Cardiology Committee for Practice Guidelines (writing committee to develop guidelines for the management of patients with supraventricular arrhythmias)

developed in collaboration with NASPE-Heart Rhythm Society. *J Am Coll Cardiol.* 2003;42:1493-1531.
11. Mavroudis C, Backer CL, Deal BJ, et al. Total cavopulmonary conversion and maze procedure for patients with failure of the Fontan operation. *J Thorac Cardiovasc Surg.* 2001;122:863-871.
12. Cox JL, Canavan TE, Schuessler RB, et al. The surgical treatment of atrial fibrillation. II. Intraoperative electrophysiologic mapping and description of the electrophysiologic basis of atrial flutter and atrial fibrillation. *J Thorac Cardiovasc Surg.* 1991;101:406-426.
13. Konings KT, Kirchhof CJ, Smeets JR, et al. High-density mapping of electrically induced atrial fibrillation in humans. *Circulation.* 1994;89:1665-1680.
14. Harada A, Sasaki K, Fukushima T, et al. Atrial activation during chronic atrial fibrillation in patients with isolated mitral valve disease. *Ann Thorac Surg.* 1996;61:104-111.
15. Nitta T, Ishii Y, Miyagi Y, et al. Concurrent multiple left atrial focal activations with fibrillatory conduction and right atrial focal or reentrant activation as the mechanism in atrial fibrillation. *J Thorac Cardiovasc Surg.* 2004;127:770-778.
16. Yamauchi S, Ogasawara H, Saji Y, et al. Efficacy of intraoperative mapping to optimize the surgical ablation of atrial fibrillation in cardiac surgery. *Ann Thorac Surg.* 2002;74:450-457.
17. Nitta T, Ohmori H, Sakamoto S, et al. Map-guided surgery for atrial fibrillation. *J Thorac Cardiovasc Surg.* 2005;129:291-299.
18. McCarthy PM, Kruse J, Shalli S, et al. Where does atrial fibrillation surgery fail? Implications for increasing effectiveness of ablation. *J Thorac Cardiovasc Surg.* 2010;139:860-867.
19. Henry L, Durrani S, Hunt S, et al. Percutaneous catheter ablation treatment of recurring atrial arrhythmias after surgical ablation. *Ann Thorac Surg.* 2010;89:1227-1231.
20. Ishii Y, Nitta T, Kambe M, et al. Intraoperative verification of conduction block in atrial fibrillation surgery. *J Thorac Cardiovasc Surg.* 2008;136:998-1004.
21. Mehall JR, Kohut RM Jr, Schneeberger EW, et al. Intraoperative epicardial electrophysiologic mapping and isolation of autonomic ganglionic plexi. *Ann Thorac Surg.* 2007;83:538-541.
22. McClelland J, Duke D, Reddy R. Preliminary results of a limited thoracotomy: new approach to treat atrial fibrillation. *J Cardiovasc Electrophysiol.* 2007;18:1289-1295.
23. Onorati F, Curcio A, Santarpino G, et al. Routine ganglionic plexi ablation during Maze procedure improves hospital and early follow-up results of mitral surgery. *J Thorac Cardiovasc Surg.* 2008;136:408-418.
24. Sakamoto S, Schuessler RB, Lee AM, et al. Vagal denervation and reinnervation after ablation of ganglionated plexi. *J Thorac Cardiovasc Surg.* 2010;139:444-452.
25. Misaki T, Watanabe G, Iwa T, et al. Surgical treatment of arrhythmogenic right ventricular dysplasia: long-term outcome. *Ann Thorac Surg.* 1994;58:1380-1385.
26. Misaki T, Tsubota M, Watanabe G, et al. Surgical treatment of ventricular tachycardia after surgical repair of tetralogy of Fallot. Relation between intraoperative mapping and histological findings. *Circulation.* 1994;90:264-271.
27. Harken AH, Josephson ME, Horowitz LN. Surgical endocardial resection for the treatment of malignant ventricular tachycardia. *Ann Surg.* 1979;190:456-460.
28. Horowitz LN, Harken AH, Kastor JA, Josephson ME. Ventricular resection guided by epicardial and endocardial mapping for treatment of recurrent ventricular tachycardia. *N Engl J Med.* 1980;302:589-593.
29. Josephson ME, Harken AH, Horowitz LN. Endocardial excision: a new surgical technique for the treatment of recurrent ventricular tachycardia. *Circulation.* 1979;60:1430-1439.
30. Horowitz LN, Josephson ME, Harken AH. Epicardial and endocardial activation during sustained ventricular tachycardia in man. *Circulation.* 1980;61:1227-1238.
31. Ideker RE, Smith WM, Wallace AG, et al. A computerized method for the rapid display of ventricular activation during the intraoperative study of arrhythmias. *Circulation.* 1979;59:449-458.
32. Klein GJ, Ideker RE, Smith WM, et al. Epicardial mapping of the onset of ventricular tachycardia initiated by programmed stimulation in the canine heart with chronic infarction. *Circulation.* 1979;60:1375-1384.
33. Mickleborough LL, Harris L, Downar E, et al. A new intraoperative approach for endocardial mapping of ventricular tachycardia. *J Thorac Cardiovasc Surg.* 1988;95:271-280.
34. Kawamura Y, Pagé PL, Cardinal R, et al. Mapping of septal ventricular tachycardia: clinical and experimental correlations. *J Thorac Cardiovasc Surg.* 1996;112:914-925.
35. Rokkas CK, Nitta T, Schuessler RB, et al. Human ventricular tachycardia: precise intraoperative localization with potential distribution mapping. *Ann Thorac Surg.* 1994;57:1628-1635.
36. Nitta T, Mitsuno M, Rokkas CK, et al. Cryoablation of ventricular tachycardia guided by return cycle mapping after entrainment. *J Thorac Cardiovasc Surg.* 2001;121:249-258.
37. Moran JM, Kehoe RF, Loeb JM, et al. Extended endocardial resection for the treatment of ventricular tachycardia and ventricular fibrillation. *Ann Thorac Surg.* 1982;34:538-552.
38. Fontaine G, Guiraudon G, Frank R, et al. Surgical management of ventricular tachycardia unrelated to myocardial ischemia or infarction. *Am J Cardiol.* 1982;49:397-410.
39. Iwa T, Misaki T, Kawasuji M, et al. Long-term results of surgery for non-ischemic ventricular tachycardia. *Eur J Cardiothorac Surg.* 1991;5:191-197.
40. Frank G, Lowes D, Baumgart D, et al. Surgical alternatives in the treatment of life-threatening ventricular arrhythmias. *Eur J Cardiothorac Surg.* 1988;2:207-216.
41. Nitta T, Kurita J, Murata H, et al. Intraoperative electroanatomical mapping. *Ann Thorac Surg.* 2012;93:1285-1288.
42. Schuessler RB, Kay MW, Melby SJ, et al. Spatial and temporal stability of the dominant frequency of activation in human atrial fibrillation. *J Electrocardiol.* 2006;39:S7-S12.

Video Legends

Video 34.1 Three-dimensional (3D) atrial figure. The figure was constructed from two-dimensional (2D) cross-sectional images of the atria, imported from magnetic resonance imaging (MRI) images of the human heart. The epicardial and endocardial surfaces were plotted on the MRI images, and the 3D images of the epicardial and endocardial features were reconstructed on a computer. The ventricles are cut from the figure, and the atria are seen from the back. The figure can be rotated in 3D and can be seen from any direction.

Video 34.2 Intraoperative mapping of atrial tachycardia (AT) using an electroanatomical mapping system (CARTO, Biosense Webster/Johnson & Johnson, Diamond Bar, CA). The patient was a 33-year-old female who had been suffering from a persistent AT from the age of 5 years old. Three sessions of catheter ablation were performed in multiple hospitals, but all failed to cure the tachycardia. The patient was in AT at 120 beats per minute during the surgery. The lateral right atrium (RA) was mapped with the NaviStar (Biosense Webster) catheter electrode through a small thoracotomy guided by a thoracoscopic view. The acinus diverticulum was located in the RA appendage and extended inferiorly down to the middle of the lateral RA. The computer simultaneously constructed a 3D structure of the RA and an activation map. The surface of the diverticulum was more closely mapped. The dynamic activation map revealed a focal activation arising medial to the diverticulum. The patient was cured of AT after excision of the diverticulum on the RA appendage.

Video 34.3 Intraoperative mapping of atrial fibrillation (AF) using template-type electrodes. Three silicone templates carrying a total of 253 electrodes were placed onto the posterolateral left atrium (LA), superior LA, and lateral right atrium (RA). The curved surfaces of the atria were copied to the templates in order to fit those snugly to the atrial epicardium. Burst pacing was applied to the RA appendage using a pen-type electrode to induce AF.

Video 34.4 Atrial activation during atrial fibrillation (AF): repetitive activations arising from the pulmonary veins (PVs) and fibrillatory conduction to the right atrium (RA). The atria are seen from the superior aspect, as if being observed cranially. Repetitive activations arise from 2 different left atrial (LA) regions adjacent to the right and left superior PVs. The activation arising from the left superior pulmonary vein (LSPV) was rapid and relatively regular, and the cycle length ranged from 132 to 160 ms. In the meantime, the activation arising from the right superior pulmonary vein (RSPV) was slower and irregular, and the cycle length varied from 185 to 257 ms. Because the activation arising from the LSPV was faster than that from the RSPV, only the activation from the LSPV conducted to Bachmann's bundle, and the activation arising from the RSPV was confined to a small LA region around the vein. Left-to-right interatrial conduction with a progressive conduction delay via Bachmann's bundle was also demonstrated. AO = aorta; SVC = superior vena cava.

Video 34.5 Atrial activation during atrial fibrillation (AF): reentrant activations in the lateral right atrium (RA). The map represents the lateral aspect of the RA. There were at least 2 reentrant circuits in the lateral RA. One was in the middle of the lateral RA and the other in the RA appendage. These reentrant circuits changed their location and configuration cycle by cycle. This activation pattern in the RA is sometimes seen in patients with chronic AF.

Video 34.6 Verification of a conduction block. After the left atrial (LA) antrum was circumferentially ablated bilaterally to isolate the right and left pulmonary veins (PVs) from the LA by means of a bipolar radiofrequency ablation device, atrial fibrillation was defibrillated if needed, and the conduction block across the ablation lines was tested by pacing each PV. The pacing was performed by a pen-type handheld electrode with a maximum output of 10 V at a pacing rate of 10 to 20 beats faster than the heart rate. Failure to pace the atrium despite maximum output of the stimulation suggests electrical isolation of the PV from the LA. Meanwhile, ability to pace the atrium by the PV stimulation indicates residual electrical connection between the PV and LA as a result of incomplete ablation, indicating an additional ablation of the LA antrum.

Video 34.7 Mapping and ablation of active ganglionated plexi (GP). High-frequency stimulation is delivered onto the anatomic GP location to determine the active GP. Active GP is defined as the GP site with a significant vagal reflex, such as temporary asystole or a decrease of 50% in heart rate during stimulation. After ablation of the active GP, the ablation site is restimulated to confirm that the vagal reflex has been completely eliminated.

Video 34.8 Intraoperative use of the electroanatomical mapping system. The ventricular epicardium is mapped by roving the NaviStar catheter electrode directly around on the epicardium to simultaneously record the local electrograms and location of the electrode. Ventricular tachycardia (VT) is induced by programmed electrical stimulation using the implanted defibrillator. Before inducing VT, the patients are cannulated and undergo cardiopulmonary bypass to support any hemodynamic instability during the VT and mapping.

SECTION 2B

INTERVENTIONAL ELECTROPHYSIOLOGY PROCEDURES

Catheter Ablation: Procedural Techniques and Endpoints

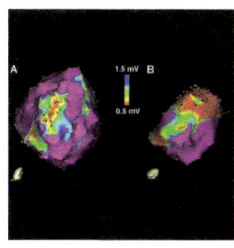 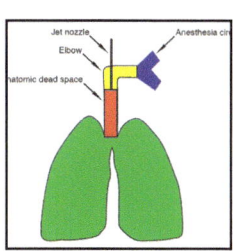 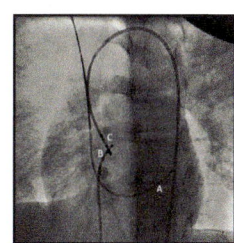 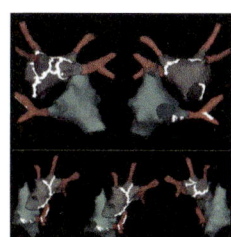

CHAPTER 35

Anesthesia and Airway Management for Ablation

Natalia S. Ivascu, MD; Brigid C. Flynn, MD

Introduction

Catheter ablations have transformed the management of cardiac dysrhythmias. Since the late 1980s, radiofrequency energy has been used to heat myocardium and produce ablative lesions. The target areas have been clarified over the years, and mapping technology has refined the procedure. Ablation procedures are a common occurrence in electrophysiology (EP) labs around the world for indications including accessory pathways, ventricular dysrhythmias, scar foci, and supraventricular tachycardias. Atrial fibrillation, the most common cardiac dysrhythmia, affects up to 5 million people in the United States. As the population ages, that number will continue to grow.

In the United States alone, tens of thousands of ablations are performed annually.[1] In an international survey of 162 centers, more than 45,000 catheter ablations were performed for atrial fibrillation alone.[2] The technology for ablations continues to advance. Some predict that the repertoire of ablation catheters and mapping devices will expand exponentially and, by 2014, may reach up to 200,000 procedures per year.[3]

Goals of Anesthesia

The goals of anesthesia for ablation procedures in the EP laboratory (EPL) are many, and can be challenging to attain (Figure 35.1). First, it is important that patients remain comfortable and immobile for lengthy procedures. Although intracardiac mapping techniques have become less sensitive to patient movement, it is critical that patients do not substantially change position. Sudden patient movement could also lead to cardiac perforation, femoral vessel damage, or falling off the operating table. Also, patient safety concerning respiratory function (with or without a controlled airway), hemodynamic perturbations, and patient positioning must be astutely monitored. Lastly, the choice of medications to be administered may affect the efficiency of the ablation and should be thoughtfully chosen. Achieving all these anesthetic goals may require utilizing various anesthetic depths, ranging from minimal sedation to general anesthesia.

Administering Anesthesia

The anesthetic process begins with anxiolysis. Patients frequently present to the EP laboratory with a variety of fears, such as what they will hear or see during the procedure or the pain they will experience. This anxiety may be worsened by the need to lie flat for several hours. Analgesia is another important consideration. There is discomfort associated with femoral catheter placement that is often not completely blocked by local anesthesia. During the periods of direct myocardial ablation, patients will also experience chest pain associated with local tissue destruction. The pain associated with being positioned on a hard, flat table may be exacerbated in older patients or in patients with chronic pain conditions.

The Continuum of Anesthetic Depth

The term "MAC," or monitored anesthesia care, has been interchangeably used to describe sedation without endotracheal intubation. The American Society of Anesthesiology has clarified that MAC should indicate only "a specific anesthesia service in which an anesthesiologist has been requested to participate in the care of a patient undergoing a diagnostic or therapeutic procedure." The continuum of sedation depth is defined in Table 35.1.

Continuum of Depth of Sedation: Definition of General Anesthesia and Levels of Sedation/Analgesia

In most instances, mild-to-moderate sedation and analgesia will be adequate for performing ablation procedures. Such sedation is frequently given at the direction of the operative electrophysiologist. There are, however, certain circumstances in which specialized anesthetic care is required.

Preprocedure Evaluation

When assessing a patient who is to undergo any sort of sedation, an airway evaluation is paramount. The Mallampati classification is often used as a cursory airway examination. The purpose of the Mallampati score is to determine size of the tongue relative to total mouth size. Class I indicates an ability to visualize the soft palate, anterior and posterior tonsillar pillars, and uvula. Class II implies a view of tonsillar pillars, but the base of uvula is hidden by the base of the tongue. A view of only the soft palate constitutes a class III view. Finally, class IV implies that the soft palate is not visible (Figure 35.2). A high Mallampati class is an indication, among others, that endotracheal intubation may be difficult. The presence of a large tongue also predicts difficulty with applying mask ventilation and an increased likelihood of airway obstruction, requiring intervention during moderate sedation.

The preprocedure evaluation should identify patients who may be more complicated to sedate. Evaluation by an anesthesiologist should also be prompted by a history of

Table 35.1 Continuum of anesthesia

	Minimal Sedation/ Anxiolysis	Moderate Sedation/ Analgesia "Conscious Sedation"	Deep Sedation/ Analgesia	General Anesthesia
Responsiveness	Normal response to verbal stimulation	Purposeful response to verbal or tactile stimulation	Purposeful response following repeated or painful stimulation	Unarousable even with painful stimulus
Airway	Unaffected	No intervention	Intervention may be required	Intervention often required
Spontaneous ventilation	Unaffected	Adequate	May be inadequate	Frequently inadequate

Source: Approved by the American Society of Anesthesiology (ASA) House of Delegates on October 27, 2004, and amended on October 21, 2009. Reprinted with permission from the ASA, 520 N. Northwest Highway, Park Ridge, IL.

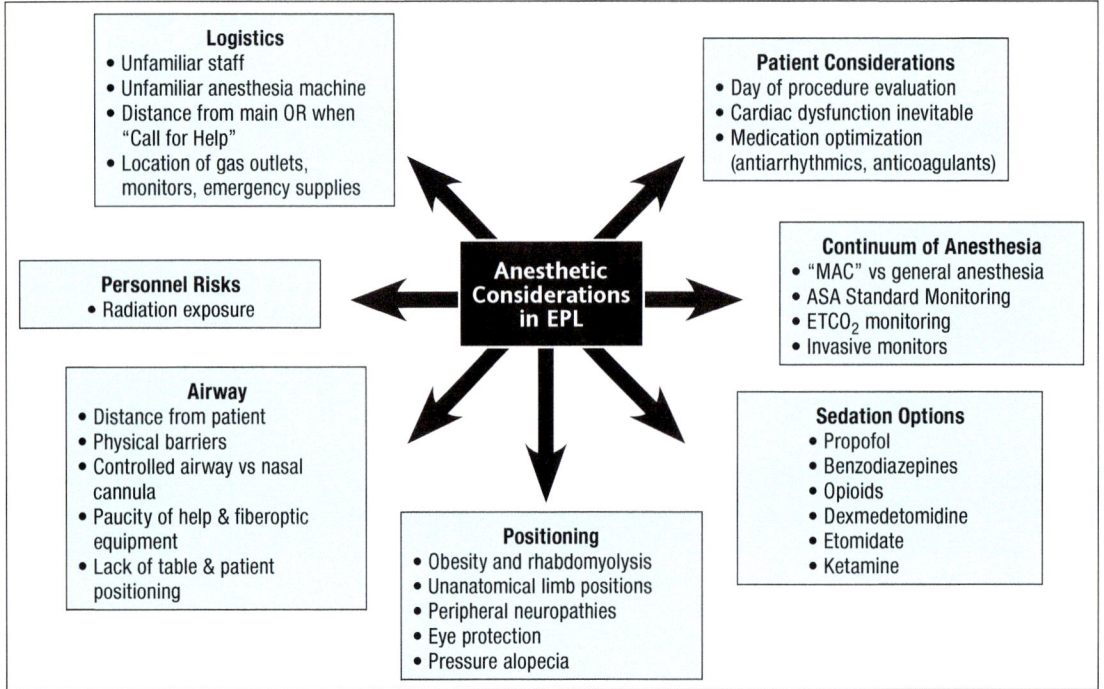

Figure 35.1 Anesthetic considerations in the electrophysiology lab.

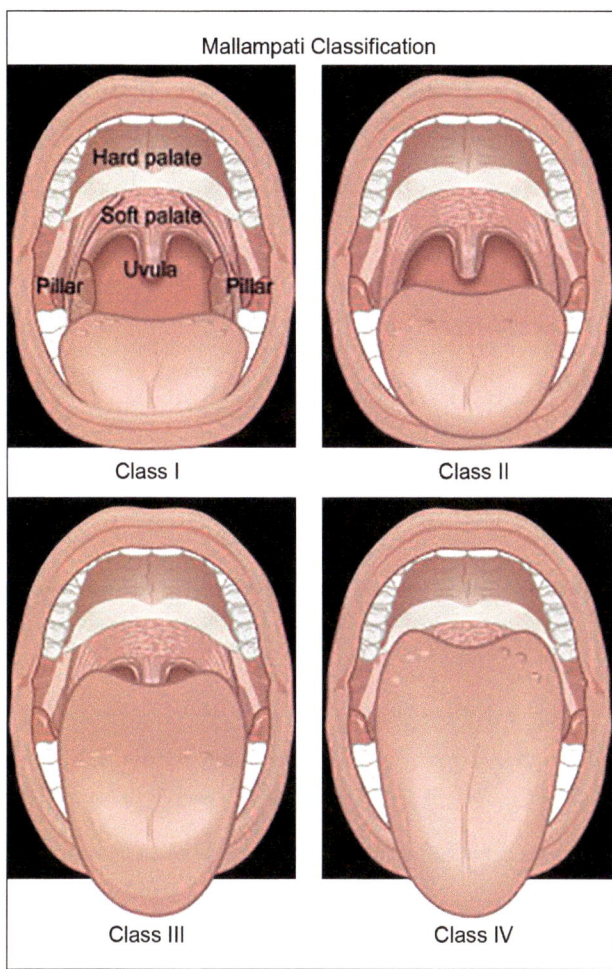

Figure 35.2 Mallampati classification system. Graphic illustraion of the four Mallampati airway classes. *Source:* Reprinted with permission from Mace SE. Challenges and advances in intubation: airway evaluation and controversies with intubation. *Emerg Med Clin North Am.* 2008;26(4):977-1000. © 2008 Elsevier Ltd. All rights reserved.

difficult intubation, obstructive sleep apnea, morbid obesity, or inability to lie flat. In addition, patients with emotional or psychiatric disorders, those taking medications that may affect the metabolism of anesthetic drugs, or those with a history of difficulty during sedation should have an anesthetic consultation.[4] It is not uncommon for a patient to have a transesophageal echocardiogram before an ablation to exclude the presence of an atrial clot. If so, the patient may arrive at the EP suite already sedated. Preanesthesia evaluations should be coordinated in order to interview the patient before sedatives are administered. Also, preoperative medications should be taken into account when determining anesthetic dosage for the ablation procedure.

Finally, one must review the patient's full medical history. Previous cardiac procedures, cardiac evaluations (such as echocardiogram and electrocardiogram), and other comorbid conditions should be elicited. An ablation is almost always an elective procedure and, as such, all other medical conditions should be optimized first. Special attention should be paid to pulmonary disease in order to anticipate respiratory complications. Patients with diabetes will need a plan to monitor blood glucose levels. Renal and hepatic function must be known to facilitate making appropriate anesthetic medication choices.

Monitoring

Adequate cardiopulmonary monitoring is essential no matter the depth of sedation. Pulse oximetry, end-tidal CO_2 monitoring, electrocardiogram, and blood pressure monitors must be employed. End-tidal CO_2 monitoring allows the anesthesiologist to monitor respiratory patterns from a greater distance, where it may not be possible to see ventilation. This is important because not only can the fluoroscopy equipment physically hinder the patient, but it also creates a radiation hazard from which the anesthesiologist should be shielded. Invasive blood pressure monitoring is preferred in ablation procedures because noninvasive blood pressure measurement is neither fast nor accurate enough during periods of dysrhythmia. Central venous access is not typically needed. In an emergency, the venous introducers placed by the electrophysiologist can be used for administering vasoactive medications or intravenous fluids.

The room temperature in the EP lab is notoriously cold to prevent overheating of the sensitive radiological machinery. The patient's temperature should be continually monitored, and underbody forced-air heating devices should be used as necessary to maintain normothermia. Finally, bladder catheterization is usually advised because, in prolonged procedures, the patient may experience tremendous discomfort associated with a full bladder. Even judicious fluid administration cannot prevent bladder distention after many hours.

Airway Management

Preanesthesia Evaluation

The most important step in airway management is a thorough preanesthesia evaluation. The unanticipated difficult airway can create a catastrophic situation in remote medical facilities such as the EP laboratory. Thus, it is paramount to attempt to identify these patients prior to sedation. The markers of difficult intubation or ventilation include Mallampati class III–IV, micrognathia, prominent incisors, presence of a beard, obstructive sleep apnea, or history of difficult intubation.[5] The presence of these factors, or a combination thereof, should prompt consideration of securing the airway at the start of the case. If the patient becomes overly sedated or otherwise unstable during the procedure, it will be far more complicated to intubate the difficult airway under duress, in a remote location with physical barriers such as fluoroscopy and other ablation equipment. Additionally, it is important that oxygenation and normocarbia be maintained because these can affect arrhythmogenicity. Avoiding airway obstruction will also prevent large changes in intrathoracic pressure, which create disruptive cardiac motion during mapping and ablation.

Nasal Cannulae

In patients with normal anatomy, most ablations will proceed with moderate conscious sedation and require only nasal cannula oxygen and end-tidal CO_2 monitoring. However, should the patient become more deeply sedated and experience upper airway obstruction, a nasal airway ("nasal trumpet") may be used to keep the oropharynx patent. If the patient is anticoagulated, great care and plentiful lubrication should be used to avoid epistaxis. In one study, up to 40% of patients under the care of an anesthesiologist needed some sort of airway intervention, ranging from nasal airway to orotracheal intubation.[6]

Laryngeal Mask Airway

Another option for airway intervention is the laryngeal mask airway (LMA). The LMA is a supraglottic device that allows for either spontaneous ventilation or positive pressure ventilation without endotracheal intubation. The depth of anesthesia needed to tolerate an LMA is consistent with general anesthesia. An LMA can be easily placed even with suboptimal patient positioning. If a favorable seal is achieved, patients can be effectively ventilated with positive pressure. It is impossible to ensure a perfect seal, and therefore, it poses a risk of insufflation of the stomach, passive regurgitation, and aspiration. In addition, spontaneous ventilation during general anesthesia for an extended period of time can lead to significant atelectasis, hypercapnia, and even respiratory failure.

Endotracheal Intubation

Endotracheal intubation is the most reliable airway during any anesthesia. The downside of intubation includes the need for a deeper level of general anesthesia to enable tolerance of the stimulus in the trachea in addition to the procedure. This level of anesthesia can blunt the autonomic responses and make certain arrhythmias more difficult to elicit. Furthermore, it may not be possible to arrange the anesthesia machine in a convenient location, making ventilation awkward. In the event of a difficult airway, additional anesthesia personnel or equipment may be very far away. Every effort should be made to anticipate these situations ahead of time and to ask for help as soon as difficulty is encountered. Endotracheal intubation is also required for high-frequency jet ventilation (HFJV), which will be discussed below.

A major advantage of endotracheal intubation is the consistency of thoracic movement that it enables. Catheter ablation techniques depend on catheter stability for accurate and effective treatment. A randomized controlled trial of more than 250 patients comparing conscious sedation with general endotracheal anesthesia (GETA) found that, while all patients achieved successful acute treatment of atrial arrhythmias, the GETA patients had significantly shorter procedure and fluoroscopy times. In addition, at 1.5- to 2-year follow-up, 88% of the GETA patients were free of arrhythmias and off antiarrhythmic drugs, compared with only 69% of the sedation group. These findings may indicate that GETA has advantages beyond airway safety that are yet to be elucidated.[7]

Anesthetic Agents

Benzodiazepines

Benzodiazepines are a common choice for light-to-moderate sedation. Anxiolysis is a key contribution these drugs make to sedation, but this class of drugs also has hypnotic, amnestic, anticonvulsant, and centrally mediated muscle relaxant properties.[8] In general, benzodiazepines do not cause significant respiratory depression; however, their synergistic effect with narcotics can produce apnea. In older patients, these drugs have been associated with postoperative delirium, which can be of particular concern for ambulatory patients.[9]

Midazolam

Midazolam is the most common benzodiazepine choice for ablation procedures owing to its shorter duration of action compared with lorazepam or diazepam. Midazolam is metabolized in the liver to form a weakly active metabolite (α-hydroxymidazolam), which is excreted in the urine. Higher doses of midazolam should be avoided in renal-insufficient patients because accumulating levels of metabolites can lead to prolonged duration of action.[10]

Lorazepam

Lorazepam is an intermediate-acting benzodiazepine. Lorazepam is metabolized in the liver to form 5 inactive metabolites. The elimination half-life of lorazepam is 5 to 10 times longer than that of midazolam. As such, this drug is not often used for moderate sedation or ambulatory patients.[11]

Opioids

Opioids are another important component of an anesthetic regimen. They are used to treat the pain associated with cannula placement, cardiac tissue ablation, and lying on a hard, flat table for a prolonged time. Opioids have a significant depressive effect on respiration. These drugs act directly on the brain stem's respiratory centers and decrease the autonomic response to increased CO_2. Opioids are effective at decreasing the heart rate response to noxious stimuli.[12] Opioid-induced bradycardia may be more pronounced in patients concurrently taking β-blockers and calcium-channel blockers.

Fentanyl

Fentanyl is a common choice of opioid owing to its quick onset, relatively short duration of action, and mild side-effect profile, which includes allergic reaction, nausea, or dysphoria. Fentanyl is approximately 100 times more potent than morphine. Boluses of fentanyl reach their peak effect within several minutes of administration. The drug is metabolized in the liver, by the cytochrome P450 pathway.[12] Fentanyl is extremely lipophilic and redistributes to adipose tissue. Increasing age contributes to prolonged elimination half-times. Although small doses are rapidly metabolized, large doses or prolonged infusions may result in elimination half-times greater than 6 hours.[12]

Remifentanil

Remifentanil is a synthetic opioid with rapid onset and ultrashort duration of action. Unlike other opioids, remifentanil is metabolized by nonspecific plasma and tissue esterases. Its context-sensitive half-time is short no matter the duration of infusion: about 4 minutes. Remifentanil should be administered as an intravenous infusion. Usual infusion rates are 0.05 to 0.2 mcg/kg/min. There is little or no postprocedure pain associated with ablation, so additional narcotics are not needed when remifentanil is discontinued.

Sedative-hypnotics

Propofol

Propofol is a sedative-hypnotic used for moderate sedation through general anesthesia (Table 35.2). Propofol causes profound respiratory depression and can easily produce apnea, especially combined with other sedatives or narcotics. The American Society of Anesthesiology recommends that propofol administration be limited to anesthesia personnel. Propofol also has significant hemodynamic effects, including hypotension, bradycardia, and myocardial depression, all of which are dose-dependent. It exerts no direct effect on the sinoatrial node, normal atrioventricular conduction, or accessory pathway conduction.[13]

Dexmedetomidine

Dexmedetomidine is an alpha-2 agonist that provides sedation while causing minimal respiratory depression. Dexmedetomidine decreases sympathetic tone and reduces narcotic requirements. This reduction in sympathetic activity may produce hypotension or bradycardia in some patients. This drug is associated with a reduction in postoperative delirium and may be a superior choice in the aged population. It is often combined with lower dosages or benzodiazepines and narcotics for a balanced approach. Loading doses or very-high-dose infusions of dexmedetomidine may be less desirable in ablation procedures because they may depress inducible dysrhythmias secondary to suppression of sinus and atrioventricular node function. Metabolism of dexmedetomidine is mostly hepatic and works via biotransformation, involving both direct glucuronidation as well as cytochrome P450–mediated metabolism. In patients with renal failure, the pharmacokinetic profile of dexmedetomidine is very similar to that in control patients.[14,15]

Etomidate

Etomidate is less frequently chosen for ablation procedures. Etomidate has several attributes that make it a less desirable sedative. First, it is associated with adrenal insufficiency even after one dose. Continuous infusion has been questioned for this reason. In addition, etomidate has a painful injection, frequently causes myoclonic jerks during induction, and has a high incidence of postoperative nausea and vomiting. One possible use for etomidate is for inducing anesthesia in a patient with poor heart function, as etomidate has little effect on the myocardial contractility or blood pressure.[11]

Table 35.2 Hemodynamic effects of common sedatives[8]

	Propofol	Midazolam	Dexmedetomidine	Etomidate	Ketamine
Heart rate	↓10 ± 10%	↓14 ± 12%	↓ 1%–27%	↓5 ± 10%	↑0–59%
Mean blood pressure	↓10–10%	↓12–26%	↓15% (indirectly) or ↑ with IV bolus	↑0–17%	↑0 ± 40%
Systemic vascular resistance	↓15–25%	↑0–20%	↓	↓10 ± 14%	↑0 ± 33%
Cardiac index	↓10–30%	↑0–25%	↓ (indirectly)	↓20 ± 14%	↑0 ± 42%
Stroke volume	↓10–25%	↑0–18%		↑0–20%	↑0 ± 21%
Left ventricular stroke work	↓10–20%	↓28–42%		↑0–33%	↑0 ± 27%

Ketamine

Ketamine causes a dissociative state consisting of analgesia and amnesia while maintaining protective reflexes and consciousness. Ketamine is known for its hallucinatory effects and is almost always given with a benzodiazepine or propofol to prevent unpleasant experiences.[11] Ketamine significantly stimulates the sympathetic nervous system. Consequently, it is unlikely to be chosen as a primary sedative for patients with cardiovascular disease.

Inhalational Anesthetics

A general anesthetic is often maintained with inhalational gases, the most common of which are isoflurane, desflurane, and sevoflurane. All these drugs are inhaled as vapor in a closed-circuit system. All 3 anesthetics cause a dose-dependent reduction in blood pressure, although desflurane is known to cause an increase in sympathetic output in higher doses. There is conflict as to whether modern inhalational agents interfere with normal cardiac conduction. Also, general anesthesia is less often used for ablation secondary to other patient safety concerns. However, when general anesthesia is required to maintain a patient airway, volatile anesthetics may be used in conjunction with opioids.

Patient Positioning

Patients under general anesthesia, or sedated to the point of minimal movement, are at increased risk for injuries caused by positioning. Ablation procedures can be very lengthy; therefore, a consistent positioning strategy should be employed.

In the supine position, the arms may be tucked under or on arm boards at the patient's sides. The ulnar nerve is at risk for pressure-related injuries, so arms and elbows must be placed in the neutral position and padded well to avoid this complication.[14]

Pressure alopecia can occur when the full weight of the head rests in one position for a long period of time. Placing monitoring cords or other objects behind the head, thereby causing focal points of pressure, can exacerbate this problem. The head should be well padded. It is also recommended that the head be rotated periodically throughout long procedures.

In extreme cases, lengthy procedures can cause rhabdomyolysis. The large gluteal muscles can develop necrosis when the patient remains immobile for a long duration. Obese patients are most at risk for this rare complication.[15] Protracted periods in the supine position may injure tissue in the sacral area. In elderly and very thin patients, limited subcutaneous fat may pose an increased risk for such damage. In the susceptible patient, this can lead to pressure ulcers. Again, appropriate padding is crucial for preventing such complications.

Finally, temperature homeostasis should be maintained. EP labs are kept notoriously cold in order to maintain the integrity of the sensitive fluoroscopy equipment. So the patient's body temperature can be monitored at a variety of sites, including the skin, axilla, and tympanic membrane. Although most of the patient's body is draped, heat loss still does occur. In a general anesthesia regime, additional heat is lost due to inspiration of cold gases. A heat-and-moisture exchanger should be used for patients on a ventilator. An underbody forced air-warming device is also very useful, especially for low-body-weight patients who may become hypothermic quickly. Temperature is best monitored using an esophageal temperature probe. The esophageal temperature will rise as the myocardial temperature rises during ablation periods, owing to the approximate positions of the esophagus and the left atrial and pulmonary vein where ablation typically occurs. Any rapid increases in this temperature should be noted and communicated to the electrophysiologist in order avoid severe myocardial or esophageal burn injury.

Patient Safety Concerns

Emergency Management

Intraoperative complications are uncommon during ablation procedures but can be rapidly lethal. Malignant dysrhythmias may require defibrillation, so pads should be placed before draping the patient. Cardioversion may also be needed during a procedure. Generally, a small dose of propofol is adequate to deepen the plane of anesthesia beyond conscious sedation for a short duration and to ensure amnesia.

Intraoperative death is extremely rare, but the most frequent cause is tamponade secondary to cardiac perforation. Tamponade is most frequently associated with ablations for atrial fibrillation and caused by perforation of the left atrium. The incidence is estimated to be 2% to 6% of cases.[16] The first sign of tamponade may be a sudden drop in blood pressure. Intracardiac ultrasound, transthoracic ultrasound, and, to a lesser extent, fluoroscopy may help make the diagnosis. Early intubation and ventilation with 100% oxygen should be accomplished as soon as personnel detect tamponade with cardiac compromise. Emergent pericardiocentesis and reversal of heparin with protamine are often sufficient to regain hemodynamic stability. In the case of continued drainage from the pericardial catheter, surgical exploration may be necessary.

Esophageal Thermal Injury

Although it is a rare complication, radiofrequency ablation for atrial fibrillation can lead to thermal injury of the esophagus. As stated above, not only is the myocardium at risk for burn injury, but the esophageal tissue is also at risk. Left atrial and pulmonary vein isolation produces high tissue temperatures in the approximate portion of the esophagus. In one small study, capsule endoscopy demonstrated postprocedure evidence of esophageal injury in up to 48% of patients. Furthermore, there was a 10-fold higher incidence when patients were under general anesthesia as opposed to conscious sedation. The reason for this increase is theorized to be a reactive peristalsis secondary to pain generated by the radiofrequency impulse. Such a reaction may lead to cooling or distribution of heat transfer.[17] Although monitoring esophageal temperature may be helpful for preventing this complication, intraluminal temperature may not reflect esophageal wall temperature. In addition, it may be difficult to use esophageal temperature probes in moderately sedated patients.

Other Techniques

High-frequency Jet Ventilation

Ablation of atrial fibrillation often requires targeting the posterior left atrial area. This location is particularly susceptible to movement associated with spontaneous or controlled ventilation. One technique to minimize thoracic movement is ventilation by HFJV, which requires endotracheal intubation and neuromuscular relaxation. A larger endotracheal tube is often chosen to provide minimal resistance to exhalation. During periods of ablation, HFJV is provided via a specialized ventilator. A ventilation rate of approximately 100 cycles/minute is generally chosen. Although exhalation is passive, normocapnia can usually be achieved, which is important for dysrhythmogenicity purposes. Arterial blood gases should be measured at least every 30 minutes to verify adequate ventilation. Because there is no practical way to deliver inhalational anesthetics while using HFJV, a total intravenous anesthetic (TIVA) is used.[18] A common combination for TIVA is infusion of propofol and remifentanil along with neuromuscular blockade.

The purported advantage of HFJV over intermittent positive pressure ventilation is decreased thoracic movement and increased catheter stability. This advantage must be weighed against the potential risks of HFJV, including lung injury, upper airway injury, and atelectasis. The experience and comfort of an individual center with these techniques best dictates choice of ventilation method.[19]

References

1. Scheinman MM. NASPE survey on catheter ablation. *Pacing Clin Electrophysiol*. 1995;18(8):1474-1478.
2. Cappato R, Calkins H, Chen SA, et al. Prevalence and causes of fatal outcome in catheter ablation of atrial fibrillation. *J Am Coll Cardiol*. 2009;53(19):1798-1803.
3. Pechisker A, Zamanian K. Diagnostic EP catheters, ablation devices see strong industry growth. Diagnostic and Interventional Cardiology. November 10, 2009. http://www.dicardiology.com/article/diagnostic-ep-catheters-ablation-devices-see-strong-industry-growth. Accessed January 31, 2013.
4. Shook DC, Savage RM. Anesthesia in the cardiac catheterization laboratory and electrophysiology laboratory. *Anesthesiol Clin*. 2009;27(1):47-56.
5. Langeron O, Masso E, Huraux C, et al. Prediction of difficult mask ventilation. *Anesthesiology*. 2000;92(5):1229-1236.
6. Trentman TL, Fassett SL, Mueller JT, Altemose GT. Airway interventions in the cardiac electrophysiology laboratory: a retrospective review. *J Cardiothorac Vasc Anesth*. 2009;23(6):841-845.
7. Di Biase L, Conti S, Mohanty P, et al. General anesthesia reduces the prevalence of pulmonary vein reconnection during repeat ablation when compared with conscious sedation: results from a randomized study. *Heart Rhythm*. 2011;8(3):368-372.
8. Reves JG, Glass P, Lubarsky DA, et al. Intravenous anesthetics. In: Miller RD, Eriksson LI, Fleisher LE, et al, eds. *Anesthesia*. 7th ed. Philadelphia, PA: Churchill Livingstone; 2010:719.
9. Parikh SS, Chung F. Postoperative delirium in the elderly. *Anesth Analg*. 1995;80(6):1223-1232.
10. Bauer TM, Ritz R, Haberthür C, et al. Prolonged sedation due to accumulation of conjugated metabolites of midazolam. *Lancet*. 1995;346(8968):145-147.
11. White PF, Eng MR. Intravenous anesthetics. In: Barash PG, Cullen BF, Stoelting RK, et al, eds. *Clinical Anesthesia*. 6th ed. Philadelphia, PA: Lippincott Williams & Wilkins; 2009:453-454.
12. Coda B. Opioids. In: Barash PG, Cullen BF, Stoelting RK, et al, eds. *Clinical Anesthesia*. 6th ed. Philadelphia, PA: Lippincott Williams & Wilkins; 2009:465-497.
13. Sharpe MD, Dobkowski WB, Murkin JM, et al. Propofol has no direct effect on sinoatrial node function or on normal atrioventricular and accessory pathway conduction in Wolff-Parkinson-White syndrome during alfentanil/midazolam anesthesia. *Anesthesiology*. 1995;82(4):888-895.
14. Practice advisory for the prevention of perioperative peripheral neuropathies: a report by the American Society of Anesthesiologists Task Force on Prevention of Perioperative Peripheral Neuropathies. *Anesthesiology*. 2000;92(4):1168-1182.
15. Bostanjian D, Anthone GJ, Hamoui N, et al. Rhabdomyolysis of gluteal muscles leading to renal failure: a potentially fatal complication of surgery in the morbidly obese. *Obes Surg*. 2003;3(2):302-305.
16. Darge A, Reynolds MR, Germano JJ. Advances in atrial fibrillation ablation. *J Invasive Cardiol*. 2009;21(5):247-254.
17. Di Biase L, Saenz LC, Burkhardt DJ, et al. Esophageal capsule endoscopy after radiofrequency catheter ablation for atrial fibrillation: documented higher risk of luminal esophageal damage with general anesthesia as compared with conscious sedation. *Circ Arrhythm Electrophysiol*. 2009;2(2):108-112.
18. Goode JS Jr, Taylor RL, Buffington CW, et al. High-frequency jet ventilation: utility in posterior left atrial catheter ablation. *Heart Rhythm*. 2006;3(1):13-19.
19. Di Biase L, Walton D, Santangeli P, Natale A. Reply to the editor—general anesthesia and catheter ablation for atrial fibrillation. *Heart Rhythm*. 2011;8(8):e1-e2.

CHAPTER 36

HIGH-FREQUENCY JET VENTILATION IN ELECTROPHYSIOLOGY

Jeff E. Mandel, MD, MS; Nabil M. Elkassabany, MD, MS

Rationale for High-frequency Jet Ventilation

Respiratory activity is associated with motion of the pulmonary vein (PV) ostia that may affect catheter stability during PV isolation. Ector and colleagues,[1] in a study of 16 patients referred for pulmonary vein isolation (PVI), tracked movement in expiration versus held inspiration. PV ostia moved 19.1 ± 8.6 mm, with a "moderate-to-strong" correlation between diaphragmatic and ostial motion. Multiple patterns of respiratory movement were seen, and this was in nonsedated patients undergoing voluntary breath holds. In patients breathing spontaneously with sedation and intermittent obstructed breathing, these effects can be considerably greater.

The use of high-frequency jet ventilation (HFJV) in PVI was first described by Goode et al,[2] who retrospectively compared 36 patients receiving HFJV with 36 patients undergoing conventional mechanical ventilation. Less motion of the posterior left atrial (LA) wall was observed with HFJV, resulting in better ablation catheter wall contact and shorter overall ablation time. More constant PV blood flow velocity was observed, and fluctuations in electrode impedance and temperature were lower, suggesting a more stable biophysical environment for ablation. Our experience, which compares HFJV with conscious sedation, supports the observation of better catheter stability, as will be discussed later. Videos illustrating the impact of various ventilation modes on catheter stability are included in the supplementary material.

Physics and Physiology of Jet Ventilation

What Is High-frequency Ventilation?

Ventilation at rates greater than 60 breaths per minute (BPM) is generally considered high-frequency ventilation.[3] Several variants of high-frequency ventilation have been described, including HFJV,[4] high-frequency oscillation (HFO),[5] superimposed high-frequency jet ventilation (SHFJV),[6] and high-frequency percussive ventilation (HFPV).[7] The latter two are of limited interest for PVI, as they superimpose high-frequency ventilation on low-frequency ventilation to improve the efficiency of CO_2 elimination and alveolar recruitment; these excursions would defeat the purpose of high-frequency ventilation for reducing respiratory motion. HFJV has been used more extensively for reducing respiratory motion than HFO, although examples of HFO can be found.[8] HFJV is more commonly used in the OR, finding major utility in laryngotracheal procedures, while HFO is used almost exclusively in critical care, particularly for neonatal use. The only devices suitable for adult use available to practitioners in the United States are the Monsoon Universal Jet Ventilator (Acutronic Medical Systems, Hirzel, Switzerland) and the SensorMedics 3100B High-Frequency Oscillator (CareFusion, San Diego, CA), although other units are available in Europe and Asia.

From a practical standpoint, HFJV is more widely used because anesthesiologists are more likely to have experience providing anesthesia with the Monsoon ventilator and to have access to it. In our institution, experience with several hundred laryngeal surgical cases predated the first application of HFJV in electrophysiology.

Breath Stacking and Auto-PEEP

During phasic ventilation, the lungs expand in inspiration and relax in expiration. Expiration is typically passive, with an exponential decay of pressure determined by the compliance of the lung and the resistance to outflow. The amount of gas leaving the lungs can be reduced by valves that produce positive end-expiratory pressure (PEEP). If the duration of expiration is long, the flow will approach zero, but typically, inspiration begins before the lung is completely relaxed. This process determines the functional residual capacity (FRC). When the ventilatory rate increases, the FRC will increase over ensuing breaths until the expiratory flow matches the inspiratory flow. This process is referred to as *breath stacking*, and the result is termed *auto-PEEP*. As lung compliance, airway resistance, and inspiratory to expiratory (I:E) ratio increase, the ventilatory rate at which significant breath stacking occurs decreases. Breath stacking can be observed both in conventional positive pressure ventilation and in high-frequency ventilation[9] but is often associated with HFJV owing to the use of this modality in patients with tracheal stenosis. It should be noted that with HFJV, it is often difficult to measure this phenomenon in vivo, and much of our understanding comes from physical analogs, which may not reflect all the nuances of a live patient.

The most significant factor causing breath stacking is airway diameter. As this diminishes to a critical value (typically 4.0–4.5 mm), the expiratory time constant increases and breath stacking increases.[10] Thus, having an endotracheal tube of 7 mm or larger is optimal. Sampling lines placed within the lumen of the endotracheal tube will decrease the effective cross-sectional area. Deflating the cuff of the endotracheal tube will provide an additional path for gas to escape, decreasing the potential for significant breath stacking. The larger diameter of a laryngeal mask airway (LMA) will also diminish breath stacking.

Another factor in the development of breath stacking is high lung compliance, which also increases the expiratory time constant. In patients with inhomogeneous lungs, regions of gas trapping may coexist with normally aerated lungs. Much of the initial experience with HFJV was obtained in critical care, and in patients with acute respiratory distress syndrome (ARDS), attempts to utilize auto-PEEP to expand an atelectatic lung could result in barotrauma to a more compliant lung. Patients undergoing PVI do not typically present with ARDS, and thus, barotrauma due to breath stacking is less likely. With appropriate settings, HFJV has been demonstrated as safe in patients with emphysema,[11] but caution should be observed in these patients.

The location of the jet nozzle in the airway has an effect on breath stacking largely because of its effect on entrainment, as will be discussed later. At frequencies of 120 to 150 BPM, the proximal location is associated with approximately twice as much auto-PEEP as the distal location.[12] Paradoxically, when HFJV is applied proximally to an area of stenosis, a distal position is associated with significantly greater auto-PEEP than it is in a more proximal location.[13]

It should be noted that, with driving pressures (DPs) less than 30 lbs/inch^2 (PSI), a lung of normal compliance and with less than 60% stenosis should develop less than 6 cm H_2O of auto-PEEP. This is rarely problematic, and for patients undergoing HFJV for PVI, this level of auto-PEEP is useful for preventing atelectasis. In our experience with more than 1,000 cases, we have not identified barotrauma in a single patient. Additionally, we find that it is difficult to recruit atelectasis when DPs are below 30 PSI. Thus, while an understanding of breath stacking is essential to safely use HFJV, it is unlikely to be manifest during PVI.

Monitoring Airway Pressure

During HFJV, monitoring airway pressure is mandatory to avoid barotrauma. Measuring auto-PEEP is not practical, however, because the pressure in the alveolus is the result of a gradient across the small peripheral airways, and the end-expiratory pressure in the central airway will underestimate this. Pressure in the central airway varies somewhat according to the location of the pressure monitoring line,[14] but there is little reason to choose a distal location over a proximal one.

The Acutronic Monsoon Universal Jet Ventilator has the capability of measuring pressure in two ways. The first uses a second hose (the red connector), which measures the pressure throughout the respiratory cycle, permitting assessment of peak inspiratory pressure (PIP). The second measures the pressure in the ventilation hose (the blue connector) during the pause between breaths (PP). The compliance of the hose is low, and typically the resistance to flow is low, so the pressure in the hose will decay rapidly, typically in less than 100 ms.[15] At high respiratory rates (RRs), the difference between PIP and PP is small, reflecting the fact that delivered tidal volumes are on the order of 100 mL; this makes monitoring PP simple and convenient. Neither form of monitoring can accurately assess auto-PEEP; this would require cessation of HFJV while clamping the endotracheal tube to determine the pressure under conditions of zero flow. Doing so is not practical in routine clinical care, and thus, the true incidence of significant breath stacking during HFJV in patients with normal lungs is unknown.

One approach to assessing high-frequency ventilation is respiratory inductance plethysmography (RIP).[16] RIP employs bands placed around the chest and abdomen that measure the change in cross-sectional area, permitting an estimate of the magnitude of breath stacking, as illustrated in Figure 36.1.

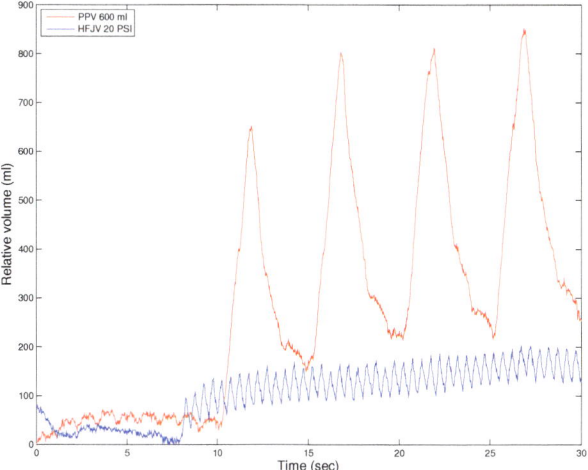 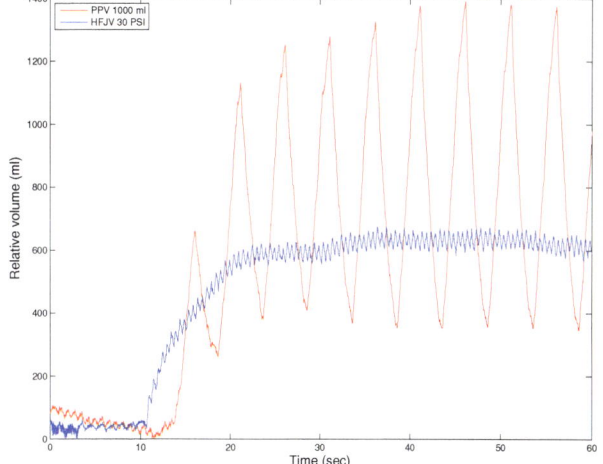

Figure 36.1 Respiratory inductance plethysmography during conventional and high-frequency jet ventilation (HFJV). **Left panel:** A patient with normal airway anatomy is ventilated with conventional mechanical ventilation (**red**) and HFJV (**blue**) initiated from apnea. Breath stacking achieves 200 mL and 100 mL, respectively, of auto-PEEP. **Right panel:** A patient with significant tracheal stenosis is ventilated with these 2 modalities, and a larger effect is seen: 400 mL and 600 mL, respectively. PPV = positive pressure ventilation; PSI = pounds per square inch.

Various approaches to external spirometry have been described,[17-19] but all require calibration to yield estimates of the volume change associated with auto-PEEP. As a result, they have not been embraced in clinical practice.

Entrainment of Gas

During HFJV, gas surrounding the nozzle is entrained into the jet stream by frictional forces. This process is erroneously referred to as the Venturi effect.[20] The magnitude of this effect is highly dependent of the geometry of the system and the hydraulic load of the patient. As the jet nozzle is progressively moved distal to the inlet to the endotracheal tube, entrainment diminishes.[21] (This effect is demonstrated in the supplementary material.) As airway resistance increases and chest wall compliance decreases, entrainment decreases.[22] Measurement of entrained volume has been described[23] but has not been employed in routine clinical care. Entrainment increases the effective minute ventilation during HFJV, though this effect can vary over time. Thus, arterial or end-tidal CO_2 must be intermittently monitored even in the absence of changes in ventilator settings, as pressure on the chest or abdomen, bronchoconstriction, and saturation of heat and moisture exchange filters can alter the entrainment ratio.

Although it is theoretically possible to entrain volatile anesthetic agents into the jet stream, it is not practical, as entrainment ratios are typically 10% to 20%, and minute ventilation is typically 10 to 15 liters per minute (LPM), which would produce an effective fresh gas flow of 100 to 300 LPM, consuming 0.5 to 1.5 mL/min/% volatile agent. Gravenstein and colleagues, working with a simple mechanical model, estimated that, at a 5 LPM fresh gas flow rate, the delivered agent concentration was 25% of the vaporizer setting.[24] Given that the agent delivery could be changing moment to moment and that end-tidal monitoring would be intermittent, the practice hardly seems worth the expense, as was borne out by the senior author's (JEM) experience in the era prior to propofol.

Open Versus Semiclosed Systems

When providing HFJV in intubated patients, the circuit can be open or semiclosed. Open systems may be configured to administer supplemental oxygen or to be open to room air. Semiclosed systems utilize valved circle systems and simplify the administration of supplemental oxygen and conversion to conventional mechanical ventilation. An illustration and photo of an open system are presented in Figures 36.2 and 36.3, respectively.

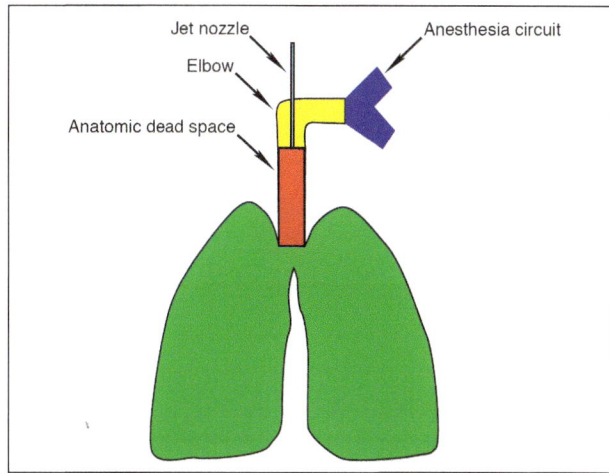

Figure 36.2 High-frequency jet ventilation via an open system. The jet nozzle is passed through a T connector, and the segments depicted in **red** and **yellow** always act as dead space. Auxiliary gas flow is delivered into the right arm of the T connector. The segment in **blue** will also act as dead space if this flow is zero, but as the flow increases, the effective dead space falls to zero.

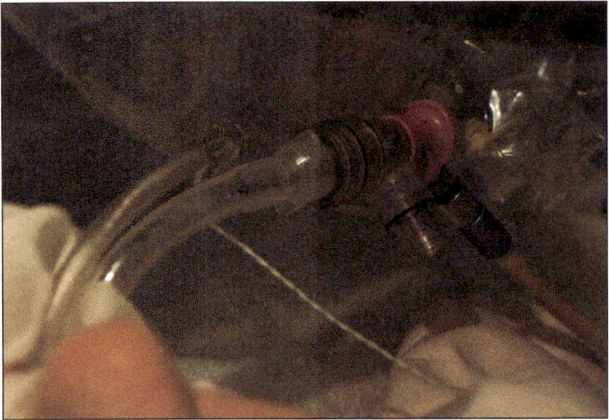

Figure 36.3 High-frequency jet ventilation via an open system.

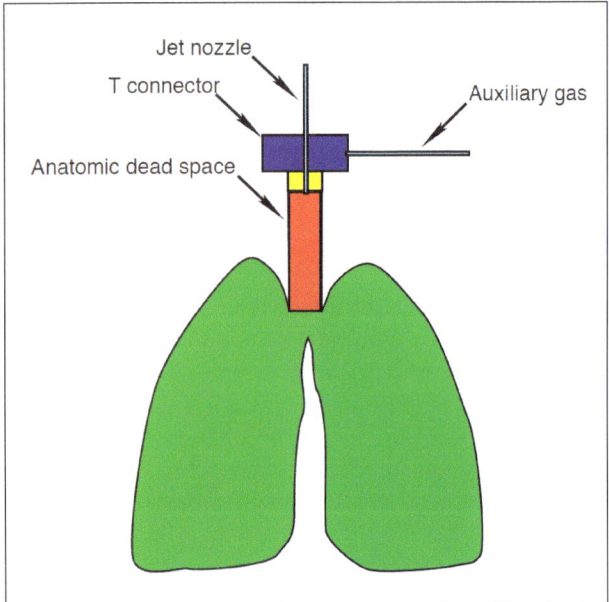

Figure 36.4 High-frequency jet ventilation via a semiclosed system. The **yellow** and **red** segments comprise the dead space. The anesthesia circuit (**blue**) may also be dead space.

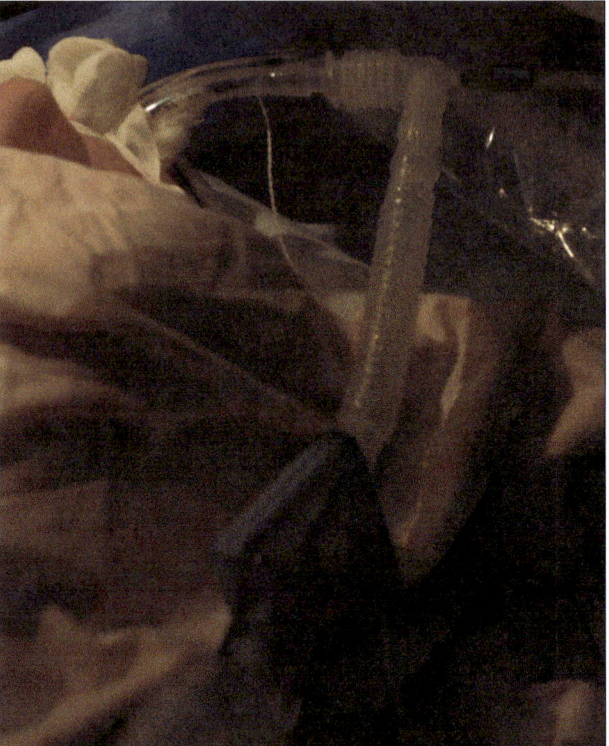

Figure 36.5 High-frequency jet ventilation via a semiclosed system.

A semiclosed system is depicted in Figure 36.4. Here, again, the yellow and red segments comprise the dead space. However, the anesthesia circuit (blue) may also be dead space, as the volume of gas moving in and out for each breath is small, and the pressure in the inspiratory and expiratory limbs of the circuit may not seat the valves of the circle system. A photograph of a semiclosed system is found in Figure 36.5.

Although open systems may have slight advantages in terms of efficient CO_2 elimination, these effects are typically small, and the practical advantage of being able to switch to conventional mechanical ventilation (CMV) without changing circuits may be more compelling. Additionally, the use of a semiclosed system permits one to add small amounts of PEEP, which may be useful when the amount of auto-PEEP is insufficient to avoid atelectasis.

Humidification

Owing to the lower efficiency in CO_2 elimination, higher minute ventilation is employed during HFJV. All the gas delivered comes from the wall source, and thus is dry. Evaporative losses can be significant, and HFJV without some form of humidification for durations exceeding 30 minutes is not recommended, as pathological changes can be observed after 4 hours without humidification. Several approaches to humidification have been described,[25-27] but the principal choices are nebulization of fluid into the jet stream and humidification of entrained gas.

The Acutronic Monsoon 2 Universal Jet Ventilator employs nebulization of sterile water, and this should be employed when using open systems. When using a semiclosed system that includes a heat and moisture exchange (HME) filter, nebulized water will quickly clog the filter, causing an increase in expiratory resistance and breath stacking. Although the humidity achieved with an HME filter is significantly less than that obtained with nebulization, it may be acceptable for several hours.

Hemodynamic Effects

The effect of HFJV on cardiac function has been studied extensively in critically ill patients, particularly those with ARDS. In these patients, the difference between HFJV and controlled mechanical ventilation (CMV) may be more significant because high peak inflating pressures are typically employed in these patients. However, when comparing the effects of HFJV in the patient population undergoing PVI, the effects are less impressive. High mean airway pressures, whether from CMV or HFJV, will increase pulmonary vascular resistance and decrease left ventricular filling, with predictable consequences. The principal benefit of HFJV is the ability to maintain the same FRC at lower mean airway pressure, leading to lower pulmonary vascular resistance.[28]

CO_2 Elimination

During CMV, convective flow of gas from the alveolus is responsible for the majority of CO_2 elimination. In high-frequency ventilation, by contrast, tidal volumes are typically less than the physiologic dead space, and elimination of CO_2 occurs by several mechanisms in addition to convective flow.[5] A variety of effects come into play: Pendeluft (convection between adjacent lung units of different time constants), Taylor dispersion, diffusion, and turbulence. These effects are influenced by the geometry of the airway and the forces applied, and the efficiency of CO_2 elimination can differ from patient to patient, and from time to time in a given patient. Monitoring CO_2 is not continuous, as there is no end-tidal plateau to observe, and interrupting HFJV to give tidal breaths affects the ablation procedure, and thus must be coordinated with the electrophysiologist.

On the Monsoon ventilator, the settings that are available to modify include the DP, I:E ratio, and RR. When I:E ratio and DP are held constant, increasing the RR above 100 will generally increase $PaCO_2$, whereas decreasing I:E ratio will decrease $PaCO_2$.[29] An increase in DP will produce a decrease in $PaCO_2$, but the relationship between DP and tidal volume varies, and it is not possible to predict the $PaCO_2$ for a given patient for any DP.[30] There does seem to be a correlation between the peak-to-PEEP pressure difference and the tidal volume and $PaCO_2$[14] even when PEEP is increased by closing the adjustable pressure limit (APL) valve in a semiclosed system. When altering these settings, it should be noted that increasing RR, DP, and I:E ratio will all increase breath stacking, which may be either useful for reducing atelectasis or deleterious in decreasing cardiac output, depending on the circumstances.

Although hypercarbia is associated with increased pulmonary vascular resistance in awake patients, remifentanil has been shown to have vasodilator properties in the pulmonary vascular bed.[31] In our experience with over 600 cases, we have never discovered hypercarbia by echocardiographic evidence of pulmonary hypertension, tachycardia, or hypertension; rather, it has been initially detected during blood gas analysis. Efforts to reduce the CO_2 levels have often resulted in hypotension due to increased auto-PEEP. Thus, alterations in ventilator settings should aim to improve the clinical situation rather than merely chasing a number.

Monitoring CO_2

During HFJV, alveolar gas is mixed with fresh gas; thus, the ability to continuously estimate arterial CO_2 from gas analysis is lost. However, it is easy enough to periodically suspend HFJV and deliver 3 to 6 tidal breaths to detect end-tidal CO_2, and this has been demonstrated to correlate with arterial CO_2. Transcutaneous measurement of CO_2 is also possible, although the correlation is not quite as reliable.[32] Newer devices permit lower sensor temperatures, and thus are more practical for extended monitoring.[33]

The Physiology of Apnea

Respiratory motion clearly can be eliminated with neuromuscular blocking agents. However, producing stable apnea without these agents requires multiple factors. While high-frequency ventilation is effective for lowering CO_2, this alone is not typically sufficient to produce prolonged apnea (although our group has reported the use of HFJV to permit brief apnea to facilitate CT angiography).[34] George[35] demonstrated that HFO could lower spontaneous minute ventilation by 19% to 46% in normocarbic volunteers, although these patients still exhibited spontaneous breathing. England found that apnea could be obtained in dogs using high-frequency ventilation during quiet wakefulness, quiet sleep, and tonic rapid eye movement (REM) sleep but not during phasic REM sleep.[61] The apneic threshold for CO_2 can be easily demonstrated in non–rapid eye movement (NREM) sleep, but volitional drives to breathe interfere with production of stable apnea in awake humans.[36] Narcotics significantly raise the apneic threshold during NREM sleep and anesthesia.

Producing NREM sleep or general anesthesia during HFJV does not guarantee apnea. van Vught and colleagues found that the CO_2 tension required to suppress breathing against the ventilator in HFJV was dependent on both PEEP and RR.[37,38] Thompson-Gorman described an interaction of CO_2, tidal volume, and mean airway pressure influencing the probability of apnea.[62] Fortunately, obtaining these conditions with HFJV is the norm, particularly when significant doses of narcotic are employed.

Implementation: Anesthetic Considerations for Pulmonary Vein Isolation

Anesthetic Goals

Like many procedures performed with catheters placed through the groin, pulmonary vein isolation is not profoundly stimulating once vascular access has been obtained, with the exception of cardioversion. The purpose of anesthesia is to render patients comfortable and motionless throughout a lengthy procedure while producing minimal interference with mapping of atrial triggers and generating AF. Finally, the anesthetic should minimize the impact of ventilatory movement on the stability of the ablation catheter.

Pressure transmitted to the pulmonary circulation during respiration results in movement, leading to dislodgement of the ablation catheter from its contact point. In a spontaneously breathing patient, airway obstruction and deep, slow breathing in response to sedatives and narcotics often accentuate this phenomenon. General anesthesia offers the advantage of a more comfortable patient and a secured upper airway. General anesthesia is associated with a higher AF cure rate, when compared with conscious sedation, and may be associated with a lower prevalence of PV reconnection at the time of repeat ablation procedures.[39]

The ablation catheter may still move throughout the respiratory cycle, especially when higher tidal volumes are used during conventional intermittent positive pressure ventilation (IPPV). HFJV has been recently introduced as a modality for ventilation in the electrophysiology laboratory in patients undergoing ablation treatment under general anesthesia. The principal benefit of HFJV in PVI is minimizing the ablation catheter's movement from its contact site in the LA during the ventilatory cycle.[40] Goode et al[2] compared ablation time during HFJV with IPPV. They concluded that ablation time, number of radiofrequency applications, and total laboratory time were significantly shorter in the HFJV group when compared with the IPPV group. The study also found that HFJV was associated with less fluctuation in LA volume and pressure, PV blood-flow velocity, and posterior LA motility—all of which suggest a more stable LA environment that may facilitate the ablation procedure. Prolonged ablation time and total procedure time may result in less efficient utilization of electrophysiology suites. Frequent dislodgement of the ablation catheter from its contact site can lead to incomplete electrical isolation of the PVs from the rest of the LA or the frequently observed PV reconnection and recurrent AF. HFJV was rapidly endorsed by the electrophysiologists in the authors' institution and was one of several technical improvements that improved ablation catheter stability, resulting in greater freedom from AF at one year despite an increase in BMI, atrial size, and the number of patients with persistent AF in our cohort.[60] This shift in the composition of the cohort is not the result of the epidemic of obesity, but rather a change in the perception of the electrophysiologists, who previously avoided PVI in such patients.

Anesthetic Management

As previously discussed, volatile anesthetic agents are not practical during HFJV, and thus, total intravenous anesthesia is typically employed. The goal of the anesthetic regimen is to permit the patient to be rendered apneic in response to minimal stimulation. We achieve this with infusions of propofol and remifentanil, relatively modest levels of which typically suffice. Normal patients will be adequately anesthetized with 50 mcg/kg/min propofol and 0.1 mcg/kg/min remifentanil. This corresponds to effect-site targets slightly greater than 2 mcg/mL propofol and 2 ng/mL remifentanil, lower than those reported by Nora and colleagues.[41] Over 95% of our patients require a phenylephrine infusion to maintain mean arterial pressure above 80 mmHg.

Anesthesia is typically induced using intravenous agents such as propofol, or in cases with poor cardiac function, etomidate. Our experience does not suggest differences in outcome between these agents, and with appropriate titration of propofol and remifentanil, hemodynamic stability is rarely problematic in this patient population.

We employ muscle relaxants sparingly. During induction, about 50% of patients receive muscle relaxants; the remainder are intubated with only propofol and remifentanil. Using propofol and boluses of remifentanil without muscle relaxants has been reported in the literature to have variable degrees of success.[42-44] We avoid muscle relaxants during maintenance to facilitate identification of the phrenic nerve with high-output pacing,[45] although other authors have utilized these agents.[2,39]

Airway Management

We typically perform these procedures with endotracheal anesthesia, although we have utilized LMAs on occasion. When employing an LMA, the LMA ProSeal (LMA North America, San Diego, CA) device may be preferable because we typically monitor esophageal temperature during ablation in the vicinity of the esophagus. Although strong evidence supports curtailing ablation to limit esophageal temperature increases,[46,47] recent evidence suggests that interaction between the radiofrequency field and the esophageal temperature probe may be a cause of injury.[48]

Proper timing for induction of general anesthesia is controversial. In some cases, we delay induction until after the ablation catheter has been inserted through the interatrial septum to permit neurological examination to rule out an embolic stroke and facilitate identification of atrial triggers with isoproterenol administration. However, induction of general anesthesia from the outset renders the patient more comfortable, secures the patient's airway under optimal conditions, and avoids issues related to sedation of a cohort with a high prevalence of obstructive sleep apnea (OSA). Although isoproterenol infusion during general anesthesia is associated with a greater need for hemodynamic support, we find an equal rate of success in completing the stimulation protocol compared with patients undergoing sedation. Inducing general anesthesia after the ablation catheter has been inserted through the interatrial septum necessitates instrumentation of the airway of a fully anticoagulated patient with an activated clotting time (ACT) exceeding 300 seconds. This may lead to an increased incidence of airway trauma and bleeding. The available physical space for the anesthesia team is reduced by the fluoroscopy units; also, measures routinely employed to provide optimal intubating conditions, such as placing the patient on a ramp, may be impractical. In these cases, we routinely employ intubation devices such as the GlideScope (Verathon, Inc., Bothell, WA), which have dramatically lowered the rate of airway injuries in our practice.

At the conclusion of the case, early extubation is favored to permit neurological assessment. In patients with morbid obesity and OSA, the need to have patients recumbent with groin pressure to avoid hematomas may preclude safe extubation. In such circumstances, a limited neurological examination may be obtained by discontinuing propofol and maintaining remifentanil at 0.05 to 0.1 mcg/kg/min to permit the patient to tolerate the endotracheal tube. Continuous positive airway pressure (CPAP) should be applied as deemed appropriate by the postoperative care team, and continuous monitoring of ventilation should be employed in patients who are extubated.

Ventilator Settings

We utilize the Monsoon 2 Universal Jet Ventilator, whose initial manufacturer-recommended settings are satisfactory for many patients. We set the RR to 120 BPM, and there is little reason to change this. The I:E ratio of 0.4 is usually adequate, although it can be decreased to improve CO_2 elimination or increased to raise auto-PEEP. We set PP to alarm at 20 cm H_2O. An initial DP of 18 PSI is typical. Note that the Monsoon 2 has been replaced by the Monsoon 3, which has additional features but basic settings are identical.

We employ both open and semiclosed circuits. Semiclosed circuits are somewhat preferred because conversion from HFJV to CMV and back does not require connecting and disconnecting the circuit. We have had several patients (typically those with smoking history) who have experienced inspissated secretions, and thus, we are increasingly employing open systems with humidity set to 70 to 80. Conversely, in obese patients, the ability to increase lung volume without increasing DP by applying 5 to 10 cm H_2O PEEP with the APL valve is sometimes useful.

Complications

Most of our knowledge about complications of HFJV comes from applying the technique in tracheal surgery. Obstruction of outflow leading to incomplete exhalation of gas is the main mechanism of the HFJV-induced auto-PEEP effect. This effect depends on RR, I:E ratio, and DP, and it may be responsible for some of the side effects. Special care therefore must be taken to ensure conditions that allow an adequate exhaust of expired gas to prevent generation of inadvertently high airway pressures. Numerous case reports have described barotrauma associated with jet ventilation, ranging from uncomplicated cervical emphysema to tension pneumothorax and subsequent heart failure.[49-53] Pneumoperitoneum, gastric distention, and gastric rupture due to misdirected or dislodged catheters have also been reported with the use of HFJV.[54] Bourgain and colleagues[55] reported their experience with transtracheal jet ventilation in 643 cases and noted a high incidence of subcutaneous emphysema (8.4%) and pneumomediastinum (2.5%). In contrast, pneumothoraces rarely occurred (1%), and no tension pneumothorax was reported. In another series of 734 cases,[56] the incidence of pneumothorax was 0.27%. In this series, a higher American Society of Anesthesiologists (ASA) physical status classification significantly correlated with an increased risk for complications during jet ventilation. (It should be noted that these reports included a large number of cases utilizing transtracheal ventilation, which is associated with a higher rate of complications than would be expected with ventilation through endotracheal tubes.)

Recent progress in transcutaneous CO_2[32] and inspiratory pressure[57] monitoring has not appreciably reduced the rate of complications associated with HFJV. The vigilance of the anesthesia provider still remains the best safeguard for preventing barotrauma.

Prolonged use of high oxygen concentrations, inadequate humidification, and warming of inspiratory gases can lead to a variety of complications: eg, mucosal edema, postoperative atelectasis, ventilation perfusion mismatching, hypoxia, and hypercarbia.[54] HFJV can cause tracheal and main bronchi damage in the form of mucosal edema and congestion, epithelial erosion, and hemorrhagic necrosis. Scanning electron microscopy after short-term HFJV has revealed flattening and histological changes in epithelial cells in piglets.[58] The relevance of these findings to adults undergoing PVI is unclear.

Both high body mass index (BMI) and OSA are independent risk factors for the development of AF. A recent study suggested that a BMI above 26 was a risk factor for CO_2 retention during suspension laryngoscopy using HFJV,[59] although in our experience, BMI is not a predictor of hypercarbia.

Conclusions

HFJV is a relatively new modality in the electrophysiology suite, and the anesthetic management of patients in this locale has evolved at a rapid pace. Early reports and anecdotal experience suggest that HFJV reduces ablation time and improves outcomes; as a result, anesthesia providers will increasingly be asked to provide this service. Modern equipment and anesthetic techniques permit the safe application of this method, but a thorough understanding of the technique's physics and physiology and vigilance to maintain patient safety are required to avoid complications.

References

1. Ector J, De Buck S, Loeckx D, et al. Changes in left atrial anatomy due to respiration: impact on three-dimensional image integration during atrial fibrillation ablation. *J Cardiovasc Electrophysiol*. 2008;19:828-834.
2. Goode JS Jr, Taylor RL, Buffington CW, et al. High-frequency jet ventilation: utility in posterior left atrial catheter ablation. *Heart Rhythm*. 2006;3:13-19.
3. Sjöstrand UH, Smith RB. Overview of high-frequency ventilation. *Int Anesthesiol Clin*. 1983;21:1-10.
4. Smith RB, Babinski MF. Clinical high-frequency jet ventilation. *Int Anesthesiol Clin*. 1983;21:89-97.
5. Bouchut JC, Godard J, Claris O. High-frequency oscillatory ventilation. *Anesthesiology*. 2004;100:1007-1012.
6. Rezaie-Majd A, Bigenzahn W, Denk DM, et al. Superimposed high-frequency jet ventilation (SHFJV) for endoscopic laryngotracheal surgery in more than 1,500 patients. *Br J Anaesth*. 2006;96:650-659.
7. Allan PF, Osborn EC, Chung KK, Wanek SM. High-frequency percussive ventilation revisited. *J Burn Care Res*. 2010;31:510.
8. Beck SM, Finley DS, Box GN, et al. High-frequency oscillatory ventilatory support during CT-guided percutaneous cryotherapy of renal masses. *J Endourology*. 2008;22:923-926.
9. Beamer WC, Prough DS, Royster RL, et al. High-frequency jet ventilation produces auto-PEEP. *Crit Care Med*. 1984;12:734-737.
10. Dworkin R, Benumof JL, Benumof R, Karagianes TG. The effective tracheal diameter that causes air trapping during jet ventilation. *J Cardiothorac Anesth*. 1990;4:731-736.
11. Conti G, Bufi M, Rocco M, et al. Auto-PEEP and dynamic hyperinflation in COPD patients during controlled mechanical ventilation and high-frequency jet ventilation. *Intensive Care Med*. 1990;16:81-84.
12. Spackman DR, Kellow N, White SA, et al. High-frequency jet ventilation and gas trapping. *Br J Anaesth*. 1999;83:708-714.
13. Ihra GC, Heid A, Pernerstorfer T. Airway stenosis-related increase of pulmonary pressure during high-frequency jet ventilation depends on injector's position. *Anesth Analg*. 2009;109:461.
14. Waterson CK, Militzer HW, Quan SF, Calkins JM. Airway pressure as a measure of gas exchange during high-frequency jet ventilation. *Crit Care Med*. 1984;12:742-746.
15. Bourgain JL, Desruennes E, Cosset MF, et al. Measurement of end-expiratory pressure during transtracheal high-frequency jet ventilation for laryngoscopy. *Br J Anaesth*. 1990;65:737-743.
16. Atkins JH, Mandel JE, Weinstein GS, Mirza N. A pilot study of respiratory inductance plethysmography as a safe, noninvasive detector of jet ventilation under general anesthesia. *Anesth Analg*. 2010;111:1168-1175.
17. Beydon L, Bourgain JL, Benlabed M, Bourgain L. Pulmonary volume measurements during high-frequency jet ventilation in anesthetized man. *Crit Care Med*. 1990;18:1102-1106.
18. Pittet JF, Morel DR, Bachmann M, et al. Predictive value of FRC and respiratory compliance on pulmonary gas exchange induced by high-frequency jet ventilation in humans. *Br J Anaesth*. 1990;64:460-468.
19. Rouby JJ, Simonneau G, Benhamou D, et al. Factors influencing pulmonary volumes and CO_2 elimination during high-frequency jet ventilation. *Anesthesiology*. 1985;63:473-482.
20. Ihra G, Aloy A. On the use of Venturi's principle to describe entrainment during jet ventilation. *J Clin Anesth*. 2000;12:417-419.
21. Benhamou D, Ecoffey C, Rouby JJ, et al. High-frequency jet ventilation: the influence of different methods of injection on respiratory parameters. *Br J Anaesth*. 1987;59:1257-1264.
22. Berdine GG, Strollo PJ. Effect of mechanical load on tidal volume during high-frequency jet ventilation. *J Appl Physiol*. 1988;64:1217-1222.
23. Jones MJ, Mottram SD, Lin ES, Smith G. Measurement of entrainment ratio during high-frequency jet ventilation. *Br J Anaesth*. 1990;65:197-203.
24. Gravenstein N, Weber W, Banner MJ. Entrainment of anesthetic agents from the circle system during high-frequency jet ventilation and anesthesia. *Anesthesiology*. 1986;65:A148.
25. Kraincuk P, Kepka A, Ihra G, et al. A new prototype of an electronic jet-ventilator and its humidification system. *Crit Care*. 1999;3:101-110.
26. Kan AF, Gin T, Lin ES, Oh TE. Factors influencing humidification in high-frequency jet ventilation. *Crit Care Med*. 1990;18:537-539.
27. Zandstra DF, Stoutenbeek CP, Miranda DR. Efficacy of a heat and moisture exchange device during high-frequency jet ventilation. *Intensive Care Med*. 1987;13:355-357.
28. Kawahito S, Kitahata H, Tanaka K, et al. Transesophageal echocardiographic assessment of pulmonary arterial and venous flow during high-frequency jet ventilation. *J Clin Anesth*. 2000;12:308-314.
29. Calkins JM, Waterson CK, Quan SF, et al. Effect of alterations in frequency, inspiratory time, and airway pressure on gas exchange during high-frequency jet ventilation in dogs with normal lungs. *Resuscitation*. 1987;15:87-96.
30. Bayly R, Sladen A, Tyler IL, et al. Driving pressure and arterial carbon dioxide tension during high-frequency jet ventilation in postoperative patients. *Crit Care Med*. 1988;16:58-61.
31. Kaye AD, Baluch A, Phelps J, et al. An analysis of remifentanil in the pulmonary vascular bed of the cat. *Anesth Analg*. 2006;102:118-123.
32. Simon M, Gottschall R, Gugel M, et al. Comparison of transcutaneous and endtidal CO_2 monitoring for rigid bronchoscopy during high-frequency jet ventilation. *Acta Anaesthesiol Scand*. 2003;47:861-867.
33. Eberhard P. The design, use, and results of transcutaneous carbon dioxide analysis: current and future directions. *Anesth Analg*. 2007;105:S48-S52.
34. Mandel JE, Perry I, Boonn WW, Litt H. Use of high-frequency jet ventilation for respiratory immobilization during coronary artery CT angiography. *J Clin Anesth*. 2009;21:599-601.
35. George RJ, Winter RJ, Johnson MA, et al. Effect of oral high-frequency ventilation by jet or oscillator on minute ventilation in normal subjects. *Thorax*. 1985;40:749-755.

36. Dempsey JA. Crossing the apnoeic threshold: causes and consequences. *Exp Physiol.* 2005;90:13-24.
37. van Vught AJ, Versprille A, Jansen JR. Suppression of spontaneous breathing during high-frequency jet ventilation. Influence of dynamic changes and static levels of lung stretch. *Intensive Care Med.* 1986;12:26-32.
38. van Vught AJ, Versprille A, Jansen JR. Suppression of spontaneous breathing during high-frequency jet ventilation. Separate effects of lung volume and jet frequency. *Intensive Care Med.* 1987;13:315-322.
39. Di Biase L, Conti S, Mohanty P, et al. General anesthesia reduces the prevalence of pulmonary vein reconnection during repeat ablation when compared with conscious sedation: results from a randomized study. *Heart Rhythm.* 2011;8:368-372.
40. Jaïs P, Weerasooriya R, Shah DC, et al. Ablation therapy for atrial fibrillation (AF): past, present and future. *Cardiovasc Res.* 2002;54:337-346.
41. Nora FS, Pimentel M, Zimerman LI, Saad EB. Total intravenous anesthesia with target-controlled infusion of remifentanil and propofol for ablation of atrial fibrillation. *Rev Bras Anestesiol.* 2009;59:735-740.
42. Schlaich N, Mertzlufft F, Soltész S, Fuchs-Buder T. Remifentanil and propofol without muscle relaxants or with different doses of rocuronium for tracheal intubation in outpatient anaesthesia. *Acta Anaesthesiol Scand.* 2000;44:720-726.
43. Klemola UM, Mennander S, Saarnivaara L. Tracheal intubation without the use of muscle relaxants: remifentanil or alfentanil in combination with propofol. *Acta Anaesthesiol Scand.* 2000;44:465-469.
44. Erhan E, Ugur G, Alper I, et al. Tracheal intubation without muscle relaxants: remifentanil or alfentanil in combination with propofol. *Eur J Anaesthesiol.* 2003;20:37-43.
45. Fan R, Cano O, Ho SY, et al. Characterization of the phrenic nerve course within the epicardial substrate of patients with nonischemic cardiomyopathy and ventricular tachycardia. *Heart Rhythm.* 2009;6:59-64.
46. Halm U, Gaspar T, Zachäus M, et al. Thermal esophageal lesions after radiofrequency catheter ablation of left atrial arrhythmias. *Am J Gastroenterol.* 2010;105:551-556.
47. Redfearn DP, Trim GM, Skanes AC, et al. Esophageal temperature monitoring during radiofrequency ablation of atrial fibrillation. *J Cardiovasc Electrophysiol.* 2005;16:589-593.
48. Deneke T, Bünz K, Bastian A, et al. Utility of esophageal temperature monitoring during pulmonary vein isolation for atrial fibrillation using duty-cycled phased radiofrequency ablation. *J Cardiovasc Electrophysiol.* 2011;22:255-261.
49. Hardy MJ, Huard C, Lundblad TC. Bilateral tension pneumothorax during jet ventilation: a case report. *AANA J.* 2000;68:241-244.
50. Chang JL, Bleyaert A, Bedger R. Unilateral pneumothorax following jet ventilation during general anesthesia. *Anesthesiology.* 1980;53:244-246.
51. O'Sullivan TJ, Healy GB. Complications of Venturi jet ventilation during microlaryngeal surgery. *Arch Otolaryngol.* 1985;111:127-131.
52. Braverman I, Sichel JY, Halimi P, et al. Complication of jet ventilation during microlaryngeal surgery. *Ann Otol Rhinol Laryngol.* 1994;103:624-627.
53. Crockett DM, Scamman FL, McCabe BF, et al. Venturi jet ventilation for microlaryngoscopy: technique, complications, pitfalls. *Laryngoscope.* 1987;97:1326-1330.
54. Ihra G, Gockner G, Kashanipour A, Aloy A. High-frequency jet ventilation in European and North American institutions: developments and clinical practice. *Eur J Anaesthesiol.* 2000;17:418-430.
55. Bourgain JL, Desruennes E, Fischler M, Ravussin P. Transtracheal high-frequency jet ventilation for endoscopic airway surgery: a multicentre study. *Br J Anaesth.* 2001;87:870-875.
56. Jaquet Y, Monnier P, Van Melle G, et al. Complications of different ventilation strategies in endoscopic laryngeal surgery: a 10-year review. *Anesthesiology.* 2006;104:52-59.
57. Baer GA. Prevention of barotrauma during intratracheal jet ventilation. *Anaesthesia.* 1993;48:544-545.
58. Davis JM, Metlay LA, Dickerson B, et al. Early pulmonary changes associated with high-frequency jet ventilation in newborn piglets. *Pediatr Res.* 1990;27:460-465.
59. Tang F, Li SQ, Chen LH, Miao CH. The comparison of various ventilation modes and the association of risk factors with CO_2 retention during suspension laryngoscopy. *Laryngoscope.* 2011;121:503-508.
60. Hutchinson MD, Garcia FC, Mandel JE, et al. Efforts to enhance catheter stability improve atrial fibrillation ablation outcome. *Heart Rhythm.* 2012;10:347-353.
61. England SJ, Sullivan C, Bowes G, Onayemi A, Bryan AC. State-related incidence of spontaneous breathing during high-frequency ventilation. *Respir Physiol.* 1985;60:357-364.
62. Thompson-Gorman SL, Fitzgerald RS, Mitzner W. Chemical and mechanical determinants of apnea during high-frequency ventilation. *J Appl Physiol.* 1988;65:179-186.

CHAPTER 37

Anesthesia for Electrophysiological Surgery and Procedures: Quality, Safety, and Outcomes

Alfred J. Albano, MD; Alexander G. Wolf, MD; Michael England, MD

Quality, Safety, and Outcomes

Clinical electrophysiology has undergone a dramatic transformation over the past several decades. Once limited to simple diagnostic procedures, the electrophysiology lab (EPL) has evolved into a complex interventional suite where intricate, life-saving therapies are delivered on a daily basis. The patient population frequently includes patients with severe coronary artery disease, hypertrophic cardiomyopathy, biventricular heart failure, and hemodynamic instability stemming from recurrent and potentially lethal dysrhythmias. These patients often have multiple comorbidities complicating their anesthesia management. To meet the clinical demands of these higher-acuity patients while ensuring safe and successful outcomes, the need for anesthesiology expertise in the EPL is steadily growing.

Throughout the field of medicine, there has been a recent focus on the quality, safety, and outcomes of clinical care. In the United States, recognizing suboptimal medical care has prompted professional societies to develop metrics and benchmarks to assess quality; their expectation is that such monitoring and reporting will lead to improved outcomes. The field of cardiovascular medicine, bolstered by a strong foundation of evidence-based guidelines, has taken a leadership role in the development of performance measures.[1-5] As pay for performance continues to evolve and the concept of "global payments" supplants traditional fee-for-service payment methods, having a comprehensive system in place that is capable of measuring and analyzing clinically important quality metrics will be critical.[6]

The field of anesthesiology has taken its own steps to advance quality improvement. In December 2008, the Anesthesia Quality Institute (AQI) was chartered by the American Society of Anesthesiologists (ASA) to serve as a primary regulator of quality management and to collect and synthesize data from its members. Currently, the AQI is gathering data from 700 facilities with 4,300 providers and more than 1,250,000 cases into a National Anesthesia Clinical Outcomes Registry (NACOR).[7] A recent in-depth systematic review identified key quality and safety metrics in anesthesia, although many are based on expert opinion rather than evidenced-based practice.[8] This highlights the need for more data-driven analyses within the field.

Although the field of quality improvement and outcomes research remains in its infancy, this chapter is devoted to summarizing published current best practices (as well as our own suggestions for quality care) in the delivery of sedation and analgesia to patients undergoing electrophysiology procedures. This is an exciting time in electrophysiology, and as quality improvement initiatives make strides, we will begin to see better results and outcomes for our patients.

Preanesthesia Evaluation

Patient History

A standard set of information should be collected and documented during the preanesthesia evaluation (Table 37.1). This initial evaluation should always begin with a comprehensive history and physical examination. A current and detailed note, including the indication for the procedure, should be completed by the electrophysiology team and made available at the time of evaluation by the anesthesia care team (ACT). The history-taking process should be devoted to eliciting a complete past medical history, obtaining an accurate medication list (including medications taken and not to be taken the day of procedure), and confirming allergies (including latex or heparin) and NPO (nothing by mouth) status. Patients should also be asked about prior personal or family history of adverse anesthesia experiences and/or difficulties with intubation or malignant hyperthermia. A history of postoperative nausea and vomiting (PONV) should routinely be elicited so that consideration can be given to prophylactic antiemetics.

Table 37.1 Preanesthesia evaluation: ASA guidelines for documentation of care

Patient History
- Patient and procedure identification
- Verification of admission status
- Medical history
- Anesthetic history
- Medical/allergy history
- NPO status

Physical Exam
- Vital signs
- Airway evaluation

Objective Data
- Laboratories
- Chest radiograph
- 12-lead electrocardiogram
- Echocardiogram

Formulation of Anesthetic Plan
- Documentation of risks
- Informed consent
- Documentation of anesthetic technique

Premedication
- Prophylactic antibiotics
- Venous thromboembolism prophylaxis
- Prophylactic antiemetics

A comprehensive understanding of patients' comorbidities is critical to ensure appropriate periprocedural management and minimize complications. In the unusual circumstance that objective data on cardiac function are unavailable, cardiac function can be grossly assessed by inquiring about functional capacity. The ability to climb a flight of stairs without dyspnea corresponds to approximately 4 METs (metabolic equivalents). Patients who smoke or have pulmonary disease (including obstructive sleep apnea [OSA]) are at higher risk for respiratory complications. The STOP questionnaire (loud *s*noring, *t*iredness during the daytime, *o*bserved apneas, and high blood *p*ressure) is a simple tool that can be used to quickly assess underlying OSA.[9] Those patients with renal or hepatic dysfunction may have elevated anesthetic risk and require medication dosage adjustments or be precluded from receiving certain medications. Diabetic patients should be counseled not to take their morning insulin or oral hypoglycemic agents on the day of the procedure and will need to have their glucose monitored and controlled with short-acting insulin during and after the procedure. In patients with poor dentition (including loose, decayed teeth or evidence of severe periodontal disease), a formal evaluation by a dental professional should be performed before implanting a device that may have the potential to become infected after a major oral surgery procedure. Medical consultations may be necessary to assist in the risk stratification and medical optimization of particularly challenging patients with multiple comorbidities. Subspecialty consultants should help assess whether the patient's comorbidities are well managed and recommend specific therapies to decrease the risk of periprocedural complications. This should be done well in advance to minimize the need to cancel and reschedule the procedure.

Physical Examination

In addition to the patient history, a thorough physical examination should be performed, noting vital signs (including bilateral upper extremity blood pressures) and evaluating the airway. Height, weight, and body mass index (BMI) should be documented. The Mallampati classification system is commonly used among anesthesiologists to predict the ease of intubation. This was originally described in 1985 as a three-class system but was then modified by Samsoon and Young in 1987 to include four anatomic landmarks: the soft palate, fauces, uvula, and pillars (Figure 37.1). A patient with a class I oropharynx has all four landmarks visible. In class II, the soft palate, fauces, and uvula are visible. In class III, only the soft palate and base of the uvula can be seen, whereas in class IV the entire soft palate is not visible.[10,11] A favorable modified Mallampati class (class I) does not always predict an easy intubation, however, nor is an unfavorable modified Mallampati class (class IV) always predictive of difficulty. In fact, a recent meta-analysis determined that the Mallampati test itself had poor-to-moderate discriminative power when used alone in this regard.[12] However, this method of airway evaluation is commonly and widely used as an initial tool in alerting the ACT that there might be an airway issue.

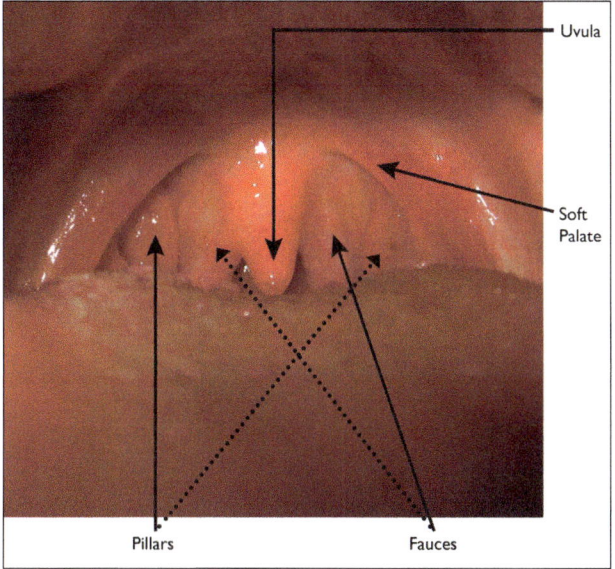

Figure 37.1 Oropharyngeal anatomy.

The value of the Mallampati score can be improved by considering it in conjunction with other predictors of difficult intubation. These factors include small mouth opening (a narrow inter-incisor distance), restricted jaw mobility (an inability to push the lower jaw forward over the upper jaw), limited head extension, and a thyromental distance of less than 7 cm.[13] Poor dentition can be a risk factor for dental damage during laryngoscopy, and certain patterns of dentition (such as overhanging central incisors) can make intubation challenging. It is suggested that additional caregivers skilled in airway management be present while attempting to intubate a patient identified in advance as having a "difficult airway." This is especially important if the location of the procedure is "off site," since there may be a delay in getting assistance in a timely fashion. The ASA has standardized the algorithm for managing anticipated and unanticipated difficult airways.[14]

The risk factors that predict difficult intubation are different from those that predict difficult ventilation with a face mask. Predictors of difficult mask ventilation include obesity, increased neck circumference, advanced age, upper airway obstruction (as in OSA), limited mandibular protrusion, and the presence of facial hair. A laryngeal mask airway (LMA) is an invaluable tool in the anesthesiologist's airway armamentarium for both elective and rescue use in a situation where the patient cannot be intubated or ventilated. Aids to intubation should be readily available and close at hand during any induction of anesthesia so that the anesthesiologist may be prepared for any complications that may ensue. In addition to an LMA (including an intubating LMA), a variety of devices may prove invaluable in the setting of a difficult airway. These include an oropharyngeal or nasopharyngeal airway, a flexible fiberoptic bronchoscope, or a video laryngoscope—either disposable units made by Airtraq and King Systems (Noblesville, IN) or reusable devices such as the GlideScope (Verathon, Bothell, WA), McGrath® (Aircraft Medical, Edinburgh, UK), and C-MAC ® (Karl Storz, Tuttlingen, Germany) (Figure 37.2). Being forewarned and forearmed is the key to avoiding an airway disaster.

An important part of the preanesthesia evaluation is determining the ASA physical status. The ASA Physical Status Classification System was introduced in 1940 as a global assessment of the patient's state of health (Table 37.2). The values range from 1 to 6, with 1 denoting a healthy patient and 6 indicating a brain-dead organ donor. Importantly, an ASA class of 5 describes a moribund patient who is not expected to survive with or without the procedure. The utility of the ASA physical status is that it clearly communicates an anesthesiologist's prediction of morbidity and mortality based on a comprehensive evaluation of the patient's current condition. This classification can also be used to stratify patients for outcomes-related data analyses.

Table 37.2 American Society of Anesthesiology Classification System of Physical Status

Physical Status	Description
1	Normal, healthy patient
2	Mild systemic disease without functional limitation
3	Severe systemic disease functional limitation
4	Life-threatening severe systemic disease
5	Moribund, not expected to survive operation
6	Brain-dead organ donor
E	Emergency operation

Review of Diagnostic Studies

Objective laboratory data, radiographic studies, prior cardiac testing, previous electrophysiology procedures, and prior surgeries (noting any previous difficulty by a former ACT) should also be carefully reviewed. A baseline 12-lead ECG should be performed on all patients, with particular emphasis on the presence of conduction system disease, ST-T wave abnormalities, and QTc prolongation. A chest radiograph should be obtained to assess for occult pulmonary disease or cardiac failure, evaluate the positioning of any devices, and establish a baseline measurement for the cardiac silhouette for postprocedure comparison (to help assess for the presence of a pericardial effusion). When a patient's (cardiac) functional capacity is ambiguous, a direct assessment of left ventricular (LV)

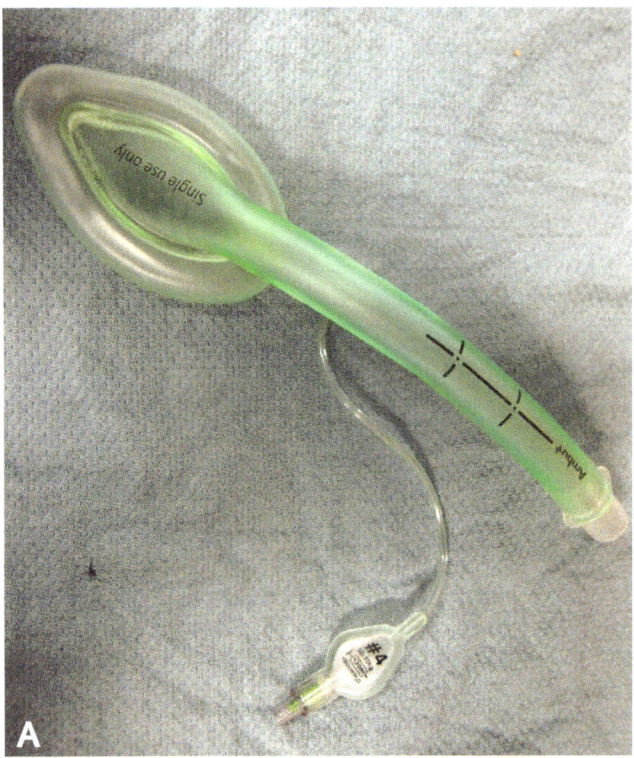
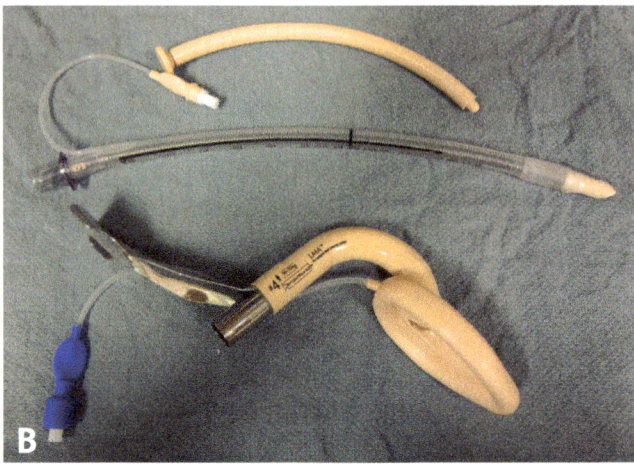
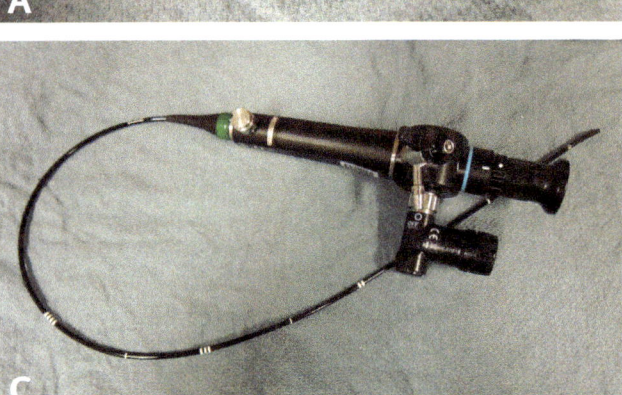
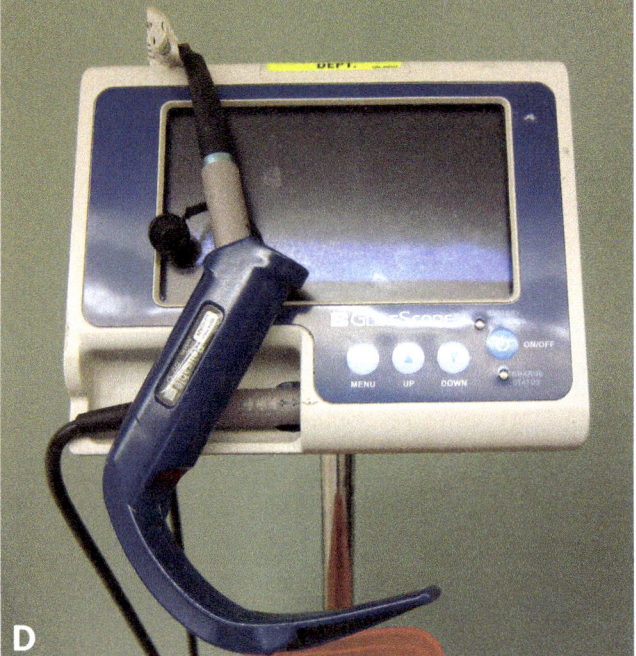

Figure 37.2 Intubation aids for patients with challenging airways. **Panel A:** Laryngeal mask airway (LMA). This supraglottic device is inserted blindly. The cuff is then inflated to provide a seal for spontaneous or positive-pressure ventilation. **Panel B:** Intubating LMA. The LMA (**bottom**) is inserted using the standard technique. The endotracheal tube (**middle**) is then pushed through the LMA into the trachea with the pink tube pusher (**top**). The LMA is then removed, leaving the endotracheal tube in place. **Panel C:** Flexible fiberoptic bronchoscope. An endotracheal tube can be threaded onto the bronchoscope. The bronchoscope is then navigated into the trachea and the tube is advanced off the device. **Panel D:** Video laryngoscope. The video screen displays an image from the fiber-optic camera at the tip of the blue plastic blade, allowing excellent visualization of airway anatomy.

function using transthoracic or transesophageal echocardiography (TEE) should be performed.

Formulating the Anesthesia Plan

The goal of anesthesia is to maintain patient comfort and a quiet surgical field through a combination of agents producing anxiolysis, amnesia, and analgesia. The extent of the procedure and the physical status of the patient should always be taken into consideration when formulating the anesthesia plan. The depth of anesthesia required for EPL procedures may vary widely, ranging from minimal sedation to general anesthesia (Table 37.3). Most procedures may be performed under minimal or moderate sedation. At our institution, the administration of this level of sedation has been successfully performed by a highly qualified nursing service. A "cocktail" of midazolam and fentanyl in small doses is very popular and successful if the procedure is short (≤4 hours). However, using this cocktail beyond the first few hours may put the patient in an uncooperative state as a result of the escalating doses of sedative required.

If the procedure is predicted to be long, and if deep sedation or general anesthesia is likely to be required, then an ACT should be scheduled in advance. It is important to note that, even though Table 37.3 defines distinct levels

Table 37.3 Distinct levels of sedation

	Minimal Sedation (Anxiolysis)	Moderate Sedation (Analgesia)	Deep Sedation (Analgesia)	General Anesthesia
Responsiveness	Normal response to verbal stimulation	Purposeful response to verbal or tactile stimulation	Purposeful response following repeated or painful stimulation	Unarousable even with painful stimulus
Airway	Unaffected	No intervention required	Intervention may be required	Intervention often required
Spontaneous ventilation	Unaffected	Adequate	May be inadequate	Frequently inadequate
Cardiovascular function	Unaffected	Usually maintained	Usually maintained	May be impaired

of sedation, they are on a continuum, so inadvertent administration of excessive analgesic and sedative agents may risk airway compromise. Thus, any plan to sedate a patient should include contingencies for immediate advanced airway management should deeper levels of sedation be achieved.

The North American Society of Pacing and Electrophysiology consensus document states that anesthesia personnel should be involved in all cases in the EPL requiring the use of deep sedation or general anesthesia with or without an artificial airway.[15] According to the ASA guidelines, nonanesthesia practitioners who administer deep sedation must be trained in appropriate rescue airway techniques.[16] The use of deep sedation in some EPLs without the oversight of an ACT is an ongoing safety concern. The incidence of such events should be an indicator of an EPL that requires a formal safety evaluation. In a survey of 95 academic electrophysiology programs in the United States, 1 of 3 different models of care for anesthesia providers was reported: 16% of labs used exclusively anesthesia professionals, 13% used exclusively nonanesthesia professionals (RNs with sedation training), and 71% used a combined model.[17] In the labs that did not use anesthesia professionals, difficulty with scheduling and lack of anesthesia availability were the two most common reasons for not employing their services.[17] A summary of recommended personnel who should be present in the EPL for an array of different procedures is summarized in Table 37.4.

In general, EPL procedures can be divided into two broad categories: device implantation and arrhythmia-based procedures. Multiple studies have demonstrated safe and successful placement of pacemakers and implantable cardioverter-defibrillators (ICDs) using only mild or minimal sedation and analgesia combined with a good local anesthetic field block. In this way, the need for an ACT may be obviated.[18-21] Patients undergoing biventricular ICD placement typically have more extensive comorbidities and require a more prolonged and technically challenging procedure; the support of an ACT should usually be requested for such patients. Despite the excellent safety record of using local anesthesia and mild conscious sedation during device implantation, in a recent study of 500 consecutive device implants, 11% of patients experienced discomfort with the procedure.[22] This may result from a lack of understanding about how much local

Table 37.4 Recommended anesthesia personnel by procedure

		Personnel				
		Staff Anesthesiologist	CRNA or Anesthesia Fellow	EP Lab RN	EP Attending	EP Fellow
Procedure	EP study			X	X	X
	Right-sided radiofrequency ablation			X	X	X
	Left-sided radiofrequency ablation	X	X	X	X	X
	Pacemaker, ICD, and CRT device implantation			X	X	X
	DFT testing	X	X	X	X	X
	Lead extraction	X	X	X	X	X
	Endocardial or epicardial VT ablation	X	X	X	X	X
	Cardioversion	X		X		X

CRNA = certified registered nurse anesthetist; CRT = cardiac resynchronization therapy; DFT = defibrillation threshold; EP = electrophysiology; ICD = implantable cardioverter-defibrillator; VT = ventricular tachycardia.

anesthetic can safely be used without causing high systemic blood levels of a local anesthetic (in a 70 kg man, ≤ 31.5 mL of 1% lidocaine, or 4.5 mg/kg subcutaneously). An inadequate field block is not easily compensated with intravenous analgesics and sedatives. It is also important to remember that bicarbonate added to local anesthetics may reduce the amount of pain on injection and make this initial step more tolerable for patients.[23]

Our institutional experience is that patients tolerate device implantation with improved comfort and less agitation with the use of dexmedetomidine (Hospira's Precedex™) rather than intermittent dosing of fentanyl and midazolam. This is especially true for longer procedures, including biventricular ICD device placement or an electrophysiology study for a challenging arrhythmia. The unique sedative, analgesic, and anxiolytic properties of dexmedetomidine and its lack of effect on respiratory drive have made it an ideal agent for use in the EPL.[24] In our informal institutional experience since the introduction of dexmedetomidine in 2004, we have not encountered any major respiratory or cardiovascular complications with the use of this drug in over 1,500 cases.

Dexmedetomidine is a highly selective alpha-2 agonist whose administration results in a reduction of sympathetic outflow. Hypotension (and, less commonly, bradycardia) occurs in a distinct minority of cases and can be readily managed with dosage titration, given the short half-life of the agent (the α half-life is 6 minutes). A minimal infusion of phenylephrine (10 mg in 250 mL of normal saline) can also be used to stabilize blood pressure when necessary. Dosing consists of a 0.4 to 1 mcg/kg bolus over 15 minutes followed by an infusion of 0.2 to 1 mcg/kg/hour. Transient hypertension may occur with more rapid bolus administration. Downward adjustments to the loading dose (or elimination of the loading dose) should be based on the presence of a low ventricular ejection fraction (LVEF < 30%) or low systolic blood pressure (< 90 mmHg).

As mentioned previously, the anesthetic properties of fentanyl and midazolam are also ideally suited for short procedures in the EPL. Fentanyl is a potent synthetic opioid with a rapid onset and short duration of action. Peak effect is reached in 3 to 5 minutes, and the duration of action is less than 20 minutes with analgesic doses of 25 to 100 mcg IV. The effects of fentanyl are terminated by redistribution rather than by metabolism; however, with repeated doses or infusions, the drug may accumulate, resulting in a prolonged duration of action. The primary adverse effects of fentanyl are dose-dependent respiratory depression and muscle rigidity with large boluses. In patients with underlying hemodynamic compromise, fentanyl can cause significant hypotension.

Midazolam is a short-acting benzodiazepine with an extremely rapid onset. Like fentanyl, its effects are terminated primarily by redistribution over 7 to 10 minutes. At a dosing range of 0.5 to 5 mg IV, midazolam provides sedation and anterograde amnesia. Although it is not a potent respiratory depressant when used in isolation, midazolam can have synergistic respiratory depressant effects when combined with an opioid. These effects are more severe in patients with OSA or other causes of upper airway obstruction. Midazolam is similar to other benzodiazepines in its lack of analgesic effect.

Prevention and management of the adverse effects of sedatives and opioids begin by using appropriate, small doses titrated to achieve the desired effect. Loss of upper airway tone and reflexes may require ventilatory support, beginning with noninvasive maneuvers (such as chin lift or jaw thrust) and proceeding to more invasive forms of management, up to and including endotracheal intubation. Hypotension induced by sedatives or opioids can be treated with intravenous fluid and vasopressors such as phenylephrine (10–60 mcg/min IV) or ephedrine (5 mg IV bolus). Benzodiazepines and opioids both have specific reversal agents that can be used to emergently terminate their effects: flumazenil antagonizes benzodiazepines at the GABA receptor, and naloxone competes with opioids at opiate receptors.

Simple arrhythmia-based procedures such as diagnostic electrophysiology studies and right-sided radiofrequency ablations (RFAs) typically require only mild-to-moderate sedation. However, more involved procedures (including left-sided procedures such as AF and VT ablations) necessitate at least deep sedation, and often, general anesthesia. Monitored anesthesia care (MAC), defined as the formal participation of an ACT in the care of the patient undergoing the procedure, should be universally employed for these complicated left-sided ablation procedures. Deep sedation is usually necessary to maintain patient comfort and allow for precise positioning of the ablation catheter. The delivery of radiofrequency energy to the endocardium frequently causes chest pain in the lightly sedated patient. Similar to device implantations, our institutional experience is that patients undergoing right-sided ablation procedures experience improved comfort and sedation with the use of dexmedetomidine. Compared with the use of fentanyl and midazolam alone, dexmedetomidine patients are more comfortable and may be at a much lower risk of developing delirium and agitation, especially during longer procedures. A criticism of dexmedetomidine is that it causes sympatholysis and could theoretically make it more challenging to induce culprit arrhythmias.[24] This has not been our institutional experience, nor has this effect been reported in the literature.

The most common agents used for sedation and/or general anesthesia in the EPL include fentanyl, midazolam, propofol, dexmedetomidine, isoflurane, and sevoflurane. The electrophysiological effects of these agents on the heart are not well studied, but in our institutional experience, difficulties inducing arrhythmia have not been observed with any of these agents.

A few small studies have evaluated the effects of fentanyl and midazolam on cardiac conduction and the inducibility of arrhythmias in the EPL and have found no difference when these agents are compared with placebo.[25-26] In another small study of children undergoing RFA, randomization to propofol or isoflurane anesthesia had no effect on cardiac conduction or the ability to induce the culprit tachyarrhythmia.[27] The effects of dexmedetomidine on the cardiac conduction system was studied in 12 children undergoing an RFA for supraventricular tachycardia by comparing electrophysiological measurements at baseline with those obtained on dexmedetomidine.[28] With dexmedetomidine, an increase in sinus cycle length, PR interval, QTc interval, sinus node recovery time, AV nodal block cycle length, and AV nodal effective refractory period was observed. No patient developed clinically significant bradycardia, and there was no effect on the inducibility of the culprit tachyarrhythmia.

There is no particular anesthetic of choice in the EPL that has demonstrated greater efficacy than others. Ultimately, the anesthetic used should be the most appropriate for the patient. In patients in whom there is a concern for the development of bradycardia (heart rate < 40 beats per minute), dexmedetomidine should generally be avoided. For pediatric patients in whom placement of a peripheral intravenous line may be both physically and emotionally challenging, a mask induction of general anesthesia may be commenced using sevoflurane, since this agent is potent with rapid induction and rarely causes airway reactions or coughing. The induction may even be performed while the patient is being held by a parent! An alternative in pediatric patients with a history of complex congenital heart disease who might not tolerate unpredictable changes in blood pressure with a mask inhalational induction would be the use of oral midazolam (0.5–1.0 mg/kg) given in advance of the procedure. Clearly, a pediatric anesthesiologist should be involved with the management of such patients.

As with all patients undergoing induction of general anesthesia, careful attention to airway management and vital signs is crucial. Following the blood pressure and heart rate in order to avoid excessive changes is the goal here. Placing an endotracheal tube (or LMA) may be very stimulating, so providing an adequate level of sedation and analgesia is vital to prevent large changes in vital signs. Once intubation has occurred, most EPL procedures are not particularly painful, so large doses of narcotics are not needed, except to help the patient tolerate the artificial airway.

If the procedure is short, as with cardioversion or defibrillation threshold (DFT) testing, then small doses of propofol may be all that is needed. The object is to carefully titrate the drug to produce unconsciousness while maintaining spontaneous ventilation with supplemental oxygen. Even patients with a depressed LVEF will tolerate a slow titration of propofol. It is important to keep in mind that, owing to the prolonged circulation time in these patients, the sedating effects may not be evident immediately and so the caregiver must be patient and resist further drug administration. Aggressive administration of propofol in a patient with heart failure can result in apnea and the need for an advanced airway.

Although device implantation is commonly performed in the EPL, removal of device leads that are infected or malfunctioning is more safely undertaken in the operating room. Device removal is routinely performed with a laser lead extraction system. The potential complications of this procedure include injury to the heart and great vessels as well as pericardial tamponade with immediate hemodynamic collapse. Therefore, a "double setup" (lead extraction and cardiac surgery) is suggested so that, if needed, the patient can be placed on cardiac bypass without delay. Therefore, general anesthesia and invasive monitoring are recommended, in addition to the immediate availability of packed red blood cells. The ability of TEE to evaluate for pericardial effusion and tamponade make it a valuable tool in this setting.

Once an anesthetic strategy is selected, it is important to document this information in the patient chart (see Table 37.1). Informed consent for the administration of anesthesia or sedation should be obtained from the patient following a detailed explanation of the benefits and risks, including, but not limited to, those discussed.

Procedural Anesthesia

Upon arrival in the EPL, an immediate review of the patient chart and a brief evaluation of the patient should be performed. Reverification of the patient, procedure, surgical site, and NPO status is a critical safety step. All equipment and drugs should also be properly labeled and inspected prior to patient arrival. When appropriate, antibiotic and deep-vein thrombosis prophylaxis should be given within one hour prior to incision. The use of a first-generation cephalosporin for device implantation is strongly supported by the American Heart Association.[29] The above verifications and checks should be made part of a standardized checklist or "ticket to safety." The ACT, nursing staff, and electrophysiologist are jointly responsible for completing the checklist. In our institution, a checklist is completed both preoperatively and after the patient is draped for the procedure. The Surgical Care Improvement Project (SCIP) was created to reduce perioperative complications and track such quality markers as timing of the last β-blocker dose, thromboembolic prophylaxis, and antibiotic administration.[30,31] The Centers for Medicare and Medicaid Services (CMS) estimates a reduction in more than 270,000 complications if the SCIP measures are followed for all surgeries performed annually in the United States.

During the procedure, the ACT maintains a time-based anesthesia record with specific documentation requirements outlined by the ASA (Table 37.5). These include vital signs, intravenous fluids and blood products, doses of drugs and agents used, and placement of intravascular catheters as well as attesting to sterile technique and notation of any access complications. Vascular catheters should be placed in the internal jugular vein with ultrasound guidance, and this technique should be noted in the medical record (including a picture of the catheter in the vein). With the digitization of medicine, more procedural suites and operating rooms will have the benefit of electronic record management systems. These systems will not only eliminate the tedious and very inaccurate record-keeping process but also lead to improvements in quality of care through the use of smart alarms, dosing recommendations, medication interaction alerts, and pop-up messages displaying differential diagnoses and suggestions for therapies during periods of patient decompensation.[32] Electronic systems also provide the ability to construct large, searchable patient databases that can be used to better assess outcomes.

Table 37.5 Procedural anesthesia: ASA guidelines for documentation of care

Patient Monitoring and Documentation
• Vital signs
• Doses of drugs, agents used, adverse reactions
• IV fluids, blood products given
• Techniques used
• Patient position
• Intravascular lines, technique, and location
• Airway devices, technique, and location
• Unusual events
• Patient status at conclusion of anesthesia

Patient Positioning

Proper patient positioning in the EPL is necessary to avoid potential iatrogenic injury due to prolonged immobility. Some procedures, especially biventricular device placement and AF/VT ablations, may require up to 4 to 6 hours of procedure time. This places the patient at risk for positioning complications, including pressure alopecia, peripheral (most commonly ulnar) nerve palsies, and even stage I pressure ulcerations. As a result, arms, elbows, sacrum, and occiput should be placed in a neutral position and padded to avoid compressive injury.[33] The AQI tracks the incidence of postprocedure peripheral neurological deficits in its NACOR database, which highlights the importance of these procedure-related complications (Table 37.6).

Table 37.6 AQI recommended quality indicators

Business Indicators
• Number of cases
• Number of providers
• Total minutes billed
• Top 10 cases performed, average duration
Process Indicators
• On-time starting percentage
• Cancellation rate
• Physician Quality Reporting Initiative (PQRI) measure compliance
• Documentation compliance
• Number of patient complaints
Clinical Outcome Indicators
• Death
• Cardiac arrest
• Perioperative MI
• Anaphylaxis
• Malignant hyperthermia
• New cerebrovascular accident
• Visual loss
• Incorrect surgical site
• Incorrect patient
• Medication error
• Unplanned admission
• Unplanned difficult airway/reintubation
• Dental trauma
• Vascular access complication
• Pneumothorax
• Peripheral neurologic deficit
Patient Experience Indicators
• Overall patient satisfaction
• Rate of postoperative nausea/vomiting
• Adequacy of pain management in postoperative care unit (PACU)
• Patient complaints

Airway and Esophageal Instrumentation

In patients requiring placement of an endotracheal tube, special care must be taken to avoid injury. Endotracheal intubation carries the risk of dental, oropharyngeal, and vocal cord trauma. Inadvertent or unrecognized esophageal intubation is a major cause of morbidity and mortality, making it especially important to identify difficult airways during the preanesthesia assessment. If necessary, the airway may need to be "secured" while the patient is awake and spontaneously breathing. It is beyond the scope of this chapter to describe this technique in detail. However, dexmedetomidine has been FDA approved for use as a sedation platform for this procedure.

Placement of TEE probes and esophageal temperature probes is commonly performed in the EPL. Complications are infrequent but may be fatal. In one large series of consecutive patients undergoing TEE, upper gastrointestinal (GI) hemorrhage occurred in 0.03% of patients.[33] This complication can result in progressive hypopharyngeal tear, leading to hematoma formation, acute upper airway obstruction, and fatal septic shock.[34-36] In addition, although many patients who require TEE and transesophageal temperature monitoring remain on therapeutic anticoagulation, the risk of GI-related injury does not appear to be increased in this well-studied patient population.[37-39] When one is placing a TEE probe in an intubated patient, care should be taken not to induce injury, since this is often done in a "blinded" fashion. Careful elevation of the mandible to create a space behind the pharynx for placing the probe is often necessary and will reduce trauma to the area. If there is any resistance to the blind passage of the probe, it is important to avoid forcing the probe. Consideration can be given to the use of a laryngoscope for better visualization. It may be necessary to reduce the volume of air in the cuff of the endotracheal balloon or to use a pediatric TEE probe.

Airway Management and Monitoring with Conscious and Deep Sedation

Close patient monitoring and continuous airway management are essential to ensuring a successful outcome in patients undergoing EPL procedures. Although most patients are initially maintained in a state of mild-to-moderate sedation in which low-flow oxygen delivered via nasal cannula is sufficient, airway compromise may occur frequently. A recent study demonstrated that up to 40% of patients may descend into a state of deep sedation requiring an airway intervention, including placement of an oropharyngeal or nasopharyngeal airway, and potentially requiring conversion to general anesthesia.[40]

The ASA Standards for Basic Anesthetic Monitoring are designed to ensure adequacy of heart rhythm, oxygenation, ventilation, circulation, and temperature. Basic monitoring includes measuring inspired oxygen concentration to prevent inadvertent delivery of a hypoxic gas mixture. Pulse oximetry has largely supplanted direct observation of patients' skin color to detect arterial hypoxemia; however, adequate illumination of the patient is still included in the ASA guidelines. Monitoring the adequacy of circulation is essential to any anesthesia procedure. Circulation may be assessed either by noninvasive blood pressure measurements taken at least every five minutes or directly, with an intra-arterial catheter.

In most EPLs, ventilation is not quantitatively assessed during routine procedures with MAC, but is as important as oxygenation. The ASA basic standards require continual monitoring for the presence of carbon dioxide in exhaled gases for all patients who receive sedative medication during a procedure. Although qualitative measures (eg, observing chest excursion and auscultation of breath sounds) or impedance plethysmography are useful, they are no replacement for the continuous measurement of end-tidal carbon dioxide ($ETCO_2$).[41-42] Apnea and airway obstruction are common during MAC, and if ventilation is not quantitatively assessed, hypoventilation may be missed. In one study, 10 (26%) of 39 patients undergoing MAC with midazolam were found to have at least one 20-second episode of apnea as measured by an O_2/CO_2 oral nasal cannula.[43] None of the 10 episodes of apnea was detected by the anesthesia provider. Capnography (the monitoring of the concentration of CO_2 in respiratory gases) enables early detection and treatment of ventilation problems. Patients who require an advanced airway intervention that culminates in an unplanned difficult airway are tracked by the AQI (see Table 37.5). All procedural cases done in our EPL that utilize any form of sedation employ $ETCO_2$ monitoring.

Normothermia should be maintained through routine temperature monitoring. This is best accomplished using an esophageal temperature probe if the patient is under general anesthesia. Otherwise, temperature probes on the skin, axilla, tympanic membrane, or within the bladder should be used. Hypothermia is commonly experienced in the EPL as a result of the cooler temperatures used to maintain fluoroscopy equipment and patient inhalation of cold gases during general anesthesia. Successful achievement of normothermia within one hour of arrival to the postoperative care unit (PACU) is a routinely employed quality metric. A forced-air warming blanket is often used for this purpose. For left-sided ablation procedures, the use of esophageal temperature monitoring is particularly helpful for reducing esophageal injury that can occur with delivery of high concentrations of radiofrequency energy to the posterior wall of the left atrium.[44]

Skin Preparation

Skin preparation and sterilization have received much media attention lately, owing to an increase in intraoperative fires following a nationwide transition to alcohol-based antiseptic solutions.[45] The use of alcohol-based chlorhexidine has rapidly escalated in response to both the 2003 recommendation by the Centers for Disease Control and Prevention (CDC) to transition to alcohol-based chlorhexidine for skin antisepsis and a randomized clinical trial in 2010 that demonstrated chlorhexidine's superiority over povidone-iodine in reducing surgical site infections.[46] However, because these solutions typically contain 70% isopropyl alcohol (which can also be found in alcohol-based preparations of povidone-iodine), they are flammable. Recognition of this rare but catastrophic complication requires training and methods to increase awareness among all EPL staff. The overwhelming majority of surgical device implants in the EPL are performed in the upper chest using cautery in proximity to an unregulated oxygen source, such as a facemask or nasal cannula. The potential for fire is further increased when alcohol-based solutions are allowed to pool on the skin or wick into hair or linens, or vapors become trapped under sterile drapes because too little time is allowed for them to evaporate. If alcohol-based antiseptic solutions are to be used, adequate drying time and minimal supplemental oxygen should be delivered. Given the severe consequences of an EPL fire, our institution has continued to use nonalcohol-based povidone-iodine solution.

Pain Control

During any procedure or surgery, pain control is a component of overall quality and will significantly influence patient satisfaction. Pain management is rarely challenging during an EPL procedure, but even so, nurses should be formally trained in acute pain management and follow established acute pain protocols. Multiple professional societies have proposed severe respiratory depression or severe hypotension that develops during pain management as a quality indicator.[8]

Postprocedure

In the Postoperative Care Unit

At the conclusion of the procedure, the patient is awakened and extubated in the procedure room and then transferred to the PACU to recover. The ACT should continue to monitor and document the same information being collected during the procedure (see Table 37.4), concluding only when the patient is stable and fully under the care of the PACU team. Transport monitors should be utilized for this transition of care. Pain management and assessment of postoperative nausea and vomiting should continue in the PACU. Vascular complications (including hematoma formation) are also common quality indicators, and routine groin checks and assessment for bleeding should be performed postprocedure. Following discharge, a personalized telephone call to the patient within 24 to 48 hours of leaving the hospital is another best practice to assist in the early identification of periprocedural complications or issues.

Recovery from Anesthesia

Several standardized scoring systems can be employed to help clinicians objectively determine postprocedural recovery from anesthesia. For example, the patient's ability to resume normal activities is an important indicator of a successful procedure and a key measure of quality. The Quality of Recovery (QoR) 9 Score is the most commonly employed instrument used to objectively gauge recovery after ambulatory surgery and anesthesia.[47] The QoR9 is a 9-item questionnaire specifically designed as a patient-centered tool to be completed by patients at various intervals throughout their treatment (preoperative baseline, on discharge from recovery room, 4 hours postoperatively, postoperative days 1–6, and postoperative weeks 1–6). The score was tested and validated in a cohort of patients undergoing primarily minor and major general surgical procedures. No specific guidelines have been written as to how to administer the questionnaire for EPL procedures, but using an abridged schedule is reasonable. Documenting the scores in the patient's chart and in a centralized database allows for periodic quality review and process improvement.

The 14-item Functional Recovery Index (FRI) is another recently developed tool that can be used to measure functional recovery after ambulatory surgery.[48] This scoring system measures three main components of recovery: pain and social activity, lower limb activity, and general physical activity. The questionnaire is designed to be performed as a daily telephone interview conducted at baseline (preprocedural) and on postprocedure days 1, 3, 5, and 7. Patients rate each of the 14 items using a 10-point scale to indicate whether the activity (such as returning to work or climbing stairs) can be performed without any difficulty (0 points) or with extreme difficulty (10 points). Because the FRI was specifically designed to evaluate patients recovering from ambulatory surgery, it is more applicable to EPL procedures than the QoR.

Conclusion

As the United States forges ahead with the most expensive healthcare system in the world, we anticipate an era of increased efficiency, cost-containment, and improved patient outcomes. This chapter offers a glimpse into how quality improvement initiatives directed at anesthesia care in the EPL may lead to improvements in patient safety, better outcomes, and reduced overall cost. The central role of practitioner education, collaboration, and data assessment should be emphasized as we continue to develop more sophisticated registries and use them to improve our practices.

References

1. Spertus JA, Eagle KA, Krumholz HM, et al. American College of Cardiology/American Heart Association Task Force on Performance Measures. American College of Cardiology and American Heart Association methodology for the selection and creation of performance measures for quantifying the quality of cardiovascular care. *J Am Coll Cardiol*. 2005;45:1147-1156.
2. Bonow RO, Masoudi FA, Rumsfeld JS, et al. ACC/AHA classification of care metrics: performance measures and quality metrics: a report of the American College of Cardiology/

American Heart Association Task Force on Performance Measures. American College of Cardiology/American Heart Association Task Force on Performance Measures. *Circulation.* 2008;118:2662-2666.
3. Estes NA III, Halperin JL, Calkins H, et al. ACC/AHA/Physician Consortium 2008 clinical performance measures for adults with nonvalvular atrial fibrillation or atrial flutter: a report of the American College of Cardiology/American Heart Association Task Force on Performance Measures and the Physician Consortium for Performance Improvement (Writing Committee to Develop Clinical Performance Measures for Atrial Fibrillation). Developed in collaboration with the Heart Rhythm Society. American College of Cardiology; American Heart Association Task Force on Performance Measures; Physician Consortium for Performance Improvement. *J Am Coll Cardiol.* 2008;51:865-884.
4. Califf RM, Peterson ED, Gibbons RJ, et al. Integrating quality into the cycle of therapeutic development. *J Am Coll Cardiol.* 2002;40:1895-1901.
5. Califf R. The benefits of moving quality to a national level. *Am Heart J.* 2008;156:1019-1022.
6. Lindenauer PK, Remus D, Roman S, et al. Public reporting and pay for performance in hospital quality improvement. *N Engl J Med.* 2007;356:486-496.
7. Anesthesia Quality Institute: Home of the National Anesthesia Clinical Outcomes Registry (NACOR). aqihq.org. Accessed February 26, 2013.
8. Haller G, Stoelwinder J, Myles PS, McNeil J. Quality and safety indicators in anesthesia: a systematic review. *Anesthesiology.* 2009;110:1158-1175.
9. Chung F, Yegneswaran B, Liao P, et al. STOP questionnaire: a tool to screen patients for obstructive sleep apnea. *Anesthesiology.* 2008;108(5):812-821.
10. Mallampati SR, Gatt SP, Gugino LD, et al. A clinical sign to predict difficult tracheal intubation: a prospective study. *Can Anaesth Soc J.* 1985;32:429-434.
11. Samsoon GLT, Young JRB. Difficult tracheal intubation: a retrospective study. *Anaesthesia.* 1987;42:487-490.
12. Lee A, Fan LTY, Gin T, et al. A systematic review of the accuracy of the Mallampati tests to predict the difficult airway. *Anesth Analg.* 2006;102:1867-1878.
13. Frerk CM. Predicting difficult intubation. *Anaesthesia.* 1991;46:1005-1008.
14. American Society of Anesthesiologists Task Force on Management of the Difficult Airway. Practice guidelines for management of difficult airway. *Anesthesiology.* 2003;98:1269-1277.
15. Bubien RS, Fisher JD, Gentzel JA, et al. NASPE expert consensus document: use of IV (conscious) sedation/analgesia by nonanesthesia personnel in patients undergoing arrhythmia specific diagnostic, therapeutic, and surgical procedures. *Pacing Clin Electrophysiol.* 1998;21:375-385.
16. American Society of Anesthesiologists Task Force on Sedation and Analgesia by Non-Anesthesiologists. Practice guidelines for sedation and analgesia by nonanesthesiologists. *Anesthesiology.* 2002;96:1004-1017.
17. Gaitan BD, Trentman TL, Fassett SL, et al. Sedation and analgesia in the cardiac electrophysiology laboratory: a national survey of electrophysiologists investigating the who, how, and why? *J Cardiothorac Vasc Anesth.* 2011;25:647-659.
18. Pacifico A, Cedillo-Salazar FR, Nasir N, et al. Conscious sedation with combined hypnotic agents for implantation of cardioverter-defibrillators. *J Am Coll Cardiol.* 1997;30:769-773.
19. Tung RT, Bajaj AK. Safety of implantation of a cardioverter-defibrillator without general anesthesia in an electrophysiology laboratory. *Am J Cardiol.* 1995;75:908-912.
20. van Rugge FP, Savalle LH, Schalij MJ. Subcutaneous single-incision implantation of cardioverter-defibrillators under local anesthesia by electrophysiologists in the electrophysiology laboratory. *Am J Cardiol.* 1999;81:302-305.
21. Pachulski RT, Adkins DC, Mirza H. Conscious sedation with intermittent midazolam and fentanyl in electrophysiology procedures. *J Interv Cardiol.* 2001;14:143-146.
22. Fox DJ, Davidson NC, Bennett DH, et al. Safety and acceptability of implantation of internal cardioverter-defibrillators under local anesthetic and conscious sedation. *Pacing Clin Electrophysiol.* 2007;30:992-997.
23. McKay W, Morris R, Mushlin P. Sodium bicarbonate attenuates pain on skin infiltration with lidocaine, with or without epinephrine. *Anesth Analg.* 1987;66:572-574.
24. Paris A, Tonner PH. Dexmedetomidine in anesthesia. *Curr Opin Anaesthesiol.* 2005;18:412-418.
25. Yip ASB, McGuire M, Davis L, et al. Lack of effect of midazolam on inducibility of arrhythmias at electrophysiologic study. *Am J Cardiol.* 1992;70:593-597.
26. Lau W, Kovoor P, Ross D. Cardiac electrophysiologic effects of midazolam combined with fentanyl. *Am J Cardiol.* 1993;72:177-182.
27. Lavoie J, Walsh EP, Burrows FA, et al. Effects of propofol or isoflurane anesthesia on cardiac conduction in children undergoing radiofrequency catheter ablation for tachydysrhythmias. *Anesthesiology.* 1995;82:884-887.
28. Hammer GR, Drover DR, Cao H, et al. The effects of dexmedetomidine on cardiac electrophysiology in children. *Anesth Analg.* 2008;106:79-83.
29. Cesar de Oliveira J, Martinelli M. Efficacy of antibiotic prophylaxis before the implantation of pacemakers and cardioverter-defibrillators. *Circ Arrhythm Electrophysiol.* 2009;2:29-34.
30. Clancy CM. SCIP: making complications of surgery the exception rather than the rule. *AORN J.* 2008;87:621-624.
31. Beya SC. Surgical care improvement project—an important initiative. *AORN J.* 2006;83:1371-1375.
32. Kheterpal S. The intra-operative anesthesia record. *Anesthesia Patient Safety Foundation Newsletter.* Summer 2001;16(2). http://apsf.org/newsletters/html/2001/summer/07record.htm. Accessed February 26, 2013.
33. Practice advisory for the prevention of perioperative peripheral neuropathies: a report by the American Society of Anesthesiologists Task Force on Prevention of Perioperative Peripheral Neuropathies. *Anesthesiology.* 2000;92:1168-1182.
34. Kallmeyer IJ, Collard CD, Fox JA, et al. The safety of intraoperative transesophageal echocardiography: a case series of 7200 cardiac surgical patients. *Anesth Analg.* 2001;92:1126-1130.
35. Saphir JR, Cooper JA, Kerbavez RJ, et al. Upper airway obstruction after transesophageal echocardiography. *J Am Soc Echocardiogr.* 1997;10:977-978.
36. Savioo JS, Hanson CW, Bigelow DC, et al. Oropharyngeal injury after transesophageal echocardiography. *J Cardiothorac Vasc Anesth.* 1994;8:76-78.
37. Klein AL, Grimm RA, Murray RD, et al. Use of transesophageal echocardiography to guide cardioversion in patients with atrial fibrillation. *N Engl J Med.* 2001;344:1411-1420.
38. Silverman DI, Manning WJ. Role of echocardiography in patients undergoing elective cardioversion of atrial fibrillation. *Circulation.* 1998;98:479-486.
39. Manning WJ, Silverman DI, Gordon SPF. Cardioversion from atrial fibrillation without prolonged anticoagulation with use of transesophageal echocardiography to exclude the presence of atrial thrombi. *N Engl J Med.* 1993;328:750-755.
40. Trentman TL, Fassett SL, Mueller JT, Altemose GT. Airway interventions in the cardiac electrophysiology

laboratory: a retrospective review. *J Cardiothorac Vasc Anesth.* 2009;23:841-845.
41. Whitaker DK. Time for capnography—everywhere. *Anaesthesia.* 2011;66:539-549.
42. Berry NH, Smith MG. Capnography during sedation. *Anaesthesia.* 2007;62:755.
43. Soto RG, Fu ES, Vila H Jr, Miguel RV. Capnography accurately detects apnea during monitored anesthesia care. *Anesth Analg.* 2004;99:379-382.
44. Singh SM, d'Avila A, Doshi SK, et al. Esophageal injury and temperature monitoring during atrial fibrillation ablation. *Circulation.* 2008;1:162-168.
45. Prasad R, Quezado Z, St Andre A, O'Grady NP. Fires in the operating room and intensive care unit. *Anesth Analg.* 2006;102:172-174.
46. Darouiche RO, Wall MJ, Itani KMF, et al. Chlorhexidine-alcohol versus povidone-iodine for surgical site antisepsis. *N Engl J Med.* 2010;362:18-26.
47. Myles PS, Hunt JO, Nightingale CE, et al. Development and psychometric testing of a quality of recovery score after general anesthesia and surgery in adults. *Anesth Analg.* 1999;88:83-90.
48. Wong J, Tong D, De Silva Y, et al. Development of the functional recovery index for ambulatory surgery and anesthesia. *Anesthesiology.* 2009;110:596-602.

CHAPTER 38

ATRIOVENTRICULAR JUNCTION ABLATION

Andrea Corrado, MD; Antonio Rossillo, MD;
Paolo China, MD; Antonio Raviele, MD

Introduction

In patients with atrial fibrillation (AF), the primary endpoint should be the maintenance of sinus rhythm with antiarrhythmic drugs or, when possible, with pulmonary vein isolation, as suggested by prominent guidelines and working groups. However, in some patients, these strategies are not effective or not indicated. Thus, rate control is considered a reasonable alternative.[1,4]

However, pharmacological rate control is never easy to achieve and/or is associated with side effects, leading to poor patient compliance as well as inadequate decrease of ventricular rate. As such, atrioventricular junction (AVJ) ablation (producing atrioventricular [AV] block), followed by implantation of a pacemaker, is a well-established, widely accepted alternative in selected patients. In these patients, evidence exists that, compared with conventional drug therapy, ablation and pacing treatment is able to reduce the specific symptoms of arrhythmia and to improve overall quality of life.

Note, however, that AVJ ablation has several limitations. In contrast with pulmonary vein isolation (in which ablation can be considered curative), AVJ ablation therapy is unable to eliminate the triggers or electrophysiological substrate of the arrhythmias and works only indirectly, by controlling a fast, irregular ventricular rate. Moreover, the procedure is necessarily associated with pacemaker implantation and a small but definite risk of short- and long-term complications. In addition, few data are available on the long-term effects of this treatment on cardiac performance, morbidity, and survival. Finally, a high rate of progression of paroxysmal to permanent AF following ablation and pacing (22% at 1 year, 40% at 2 years) has been described. For these reasons, the clinical benefit of this powerful therapy must be weighed against the risk of complications and side effects, and a careful risk-benefit evaluation must be performed for each patient who is considered for this procedure, which at present should be a last resort.

The first ablation strategy used for creating an AV block consisted of high-energy direct current (DC) shocks. DC ablation required general anesthesia and was associated with a high incidence of morbidity and mortality. The major advantage of the introduction of radiofrequency (RF) energy is the ability to precisely block the AV node and leave a junctional escape pacemaker (Figure 38.1A and B). Although this does not obviate the need for permanent pacing, it provides reassurance in case of pacemaker failure.

Some investigators have shown interest in the use of intracoronary-delivered ethanol to produce AV block within the AV node. The long-term safety of this procedure is unknown and, moreover, the resumption of AV conduction in 30% of patients has been reported. At this date, we do not believe that catheterization of the AV nodal artery and delivery of ethanol are warranted, because complete AV block can be achieved using RF delivery in almost 100% of patients. In order to avoid permanent pacemaker implantation, attempts have been made to control the heart rate by modifying the properties of the AV node by means of RF but without inducing block (through AV junction modulation). Although initial noncontrolled studies yielded encouraging results, two randomized, controlled clinical studies compared "ablate and pace" with heart rate modulation in patients with congestive heart failure and paroxysmal or permanent AF. Researchers found that ablate and pace was more efficacious than AV node modulation for improving cardiac performance and alleviating symptoms.

464 • Section 2B: Catheter Ablation: Procedural Techniques and Endpoints

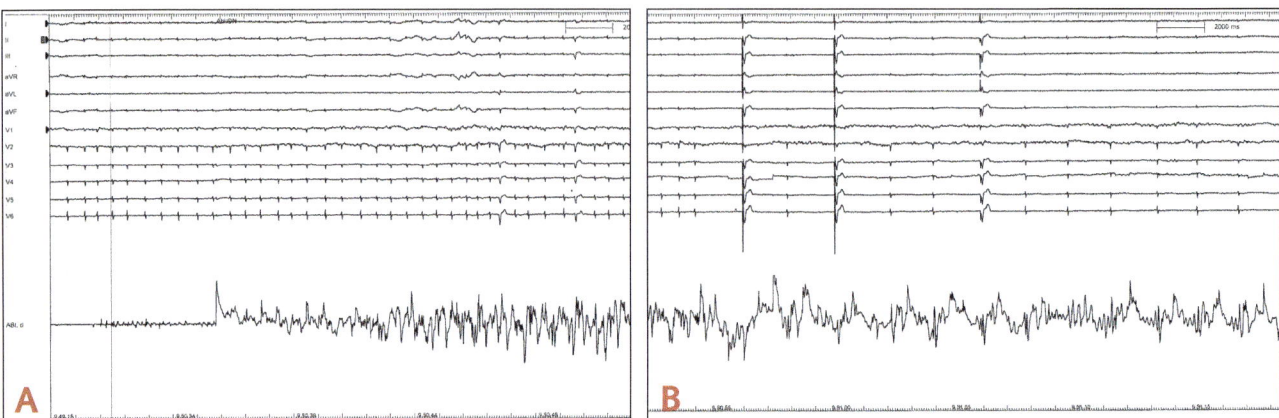

Figure 38.1 Atrioventricular junctional ablation. **Panels A** and **B, top:** the surface ECG; **bottom:** the timeline and the intracardiac signal of the ablator tip, marked with the starting energy delivery (Abl:ON) and artifacts created. **Panel A:** At the beginning of the trace, patient has atrial fibrillation with narrow QRS at ~100 to 110 beats per minute (bpm). **Panel B:** a few seconds after first energy delivery on the AV node appears an AV block with junctional escape rhythm of 36 bpm and fixed RR interval; also notable are some paced beats (programmed at the lower rate of 30 bpm).

To avoid ablation of the AV junction, pacemakers have been developed that are endowed with special algorithms designed to regularize heart rate (ventricular response pacing [VRP]) with a view to reducing symptoms and improving cardiac performance. While this modality has proved effective for regularizing heart rate in controlled studies, it has not yielded satisfactory results in terms of improving quality of life or functional capacity. Thus, both pacemaker implantation and AVJ ablation seem to be necessary in order to obtain a clinical benefit.

Indications

The definition of drug-refractory AF requires individually assessing a patient's symptoms in terms of severity and frequency. "Drug refractoriness" implies that symptoms remain uncontrolled and unacceptable to the patient, even if ventricular rate is within the normal range but remains irregular. AF can be highly symptomatic and may lead to cardiac dysfunction. However, it is important to remember that AVJ ablation is an irreversible process and results in lifelong pacemaker dependence for patients. Table 38.1 summarizes different professional groups' recommendations on AVJ ablation, based on class of recommendation and level of scientific evidence.

Methodology

Patients should be fully clinically assessed and appropriate tests performed before an AVJ ablation procedure. All efforts should be made to stabilize the patient before the intervention. Operators should be experienced in right- and left-sided heart catheterization, and the procedure should be performed in an adequately equipped and staffed cardiac electrophysiology laboratory.

In those patients who have a permanent pacemaker implanted already, this can be used for backup pacing, as long as it is understood that RF energy may inhibit or reprogram the pacemaker. The appropriate programmer should be in the room, and equipment should be set up so that emergency pacing can be commenced through the ablation catheter in the right or left ventricle.

It may be helpful to convert the patient's heart to sinus rhythm before or during the procedure. However, the procedure can be successful in most patients during AF. Choice of catheter and tip design are considered to be personal choices and reflect local practice. AVJ ablation can be accomplished by means of a right- or left-sided approach. The greater experience available with the right-sided approach and the higher prevalence of complications from left-sided catheterization make the right-sided approach the preferred choice. When the right-sided approach fails, however, left-sided ablation can be performed during the same session (the so-called sequential approach) or at another session. Left-sided ablation may be easier to perform and requires fewer RF applications, but it requires arterial catheterization. If AVJ ablation is not achieved after a total of 10 applications of RF energy at the indicated site, right-sided ablation can be considered to have failed and left-sided ablation should be attempted. Ablation can be performed sequentially first in the right and then the left side of the heart if the pacemaker is already implanted. If the pacemaker has not been implanted, and heparin infusion is given for a left-sided ablation, pacemaker implantation will normally be postponed.

Right-sided Approach

The ablation catheter is inserted via the femoral vein and positioned on the AVJ. A two-catheter approach is usually sufficient (one for the right ventricle [RV] to pace the ventricle and one to deliver RF energy), but many

Table 38.1 Comparison of recommendations on AVJ ablation therapy from professional group guidelines

Class of Recommendation	ACC/AHA/ESC 2006[2]	ESC 2010[1]
Class IIa	It is reasonable to use ablation of the AV node or accessory pathway to control heart rate when pharmacological therapy is insufficient or associated with side effects (LOE B).	Ablation of the AV node to control heart rate should be considered when the rate cannot be controlled with pharmacological agents and when AF cannot be prevented by antiarrhythmic therapy or is associated with intolerable side effects, and direct catheter-based or surgical ablation of AF is not indicated, has failed, or is rejected (LOE B).
		Ablation of the AV node should be considered for patients with permanent AF and an indication for CRT (NYHA functional class III or ambulatory class IV symptoms despite optimal medical therapy, LVEF ≤35%, QRS width ≥130 ms) (LOE B).
		Ablation of the AV node should be considered for CRT nonresponders in whom AF prevents effective biventricular stimulation and amiodarone is ineffective or contraindicated (LOE C).
		In patients with any type of AF and severely depressed LV function (LVEF ≤35%) and severe heart failure symptoms (NYHA III or IV), CRT should be considered after AV node ablation (LOE C).
Class IIb	When the rate cannot be controlled with pharmacological agents or tachycardia-mediated cardiomyopathy is suspected, catheter-directed ablation of the AV node may be considered in patients with AF to control the heart rate (LOE C).	Ablation of the AV node to control heart rate may be considered when tachycardia-mediated cardiomyopathy is suspected and the rate cannot be controlled with pharmacological agents, and direct ablation of AF is not indicated, has failed, or is rejected (LOE C).
		Ablation of the AV node with consecutive implantation of a CRT device may be considered in patients with permanent AF, LVEF ≤35%, and NYHA functional class I or II symptoms on optimal medical therapy to control heart rate when pharmacological therapy is insufficient or associated with side effects (LOE C).
Class III	Catheter ablation of the AV node should not be attempted without a prior trial of medication to control the ventricular rate in patients with AF (LOE C).	Catheter ablation of the AV node should not be attempted without a prior trial of medication, or catheter ablation for AF, to control the AF and/or ventricular rate in patients with AF (LOE C).

ACC/AHA/ESC = American College of Cardiology/American Heart Association/European Society of Cardiology; AF = atrial fibrillation; AV = atrioventricular; CRT = cardiac resynchronization therapy; LOE = level of evidence; LV = left ventricular; LVEF = left ventricular ejection fraction; NYHA = New York Heart Association; RV = right ventricular.

prefer placing an additional catheter in the His bundle position (Figure 38.2A). A stable RV position (preferably in the apex) is required, with acceptable pacing thresholds. The goal of the procedure is to ablate the compact AV node rather than interrupt the bundle of His. The compact node lies on the atrial aspect of the tricuspid annulus, just inferior and posterior to the His bundle. The ideal signal has an atrial-to-ventricular ratio greater than or equal to one, with an early and stable His deflection. The most practical technique consists of looking for the largest His potential, then moving the tip of the steerable catheter a few millimeters into the atrium toward the compact AV node until a large A wave is obtained, having a small or absent His potential (Figure 38.2B). During AF, a smaller atrial signal is acceptable and the His potential is more difficult to identify. In case of failure, successive energy applications are delivered close to this site by moving the tip a few millimeters in different directions. A different catheter curve should be considered if there are difficulties in obtaining stable or adequate signals.

Left-sided Approach

In left-sided AVJ ablation, in the absence of a permanent pacemaker, it is mandatory to place a temporary pacing catheter in the RV, as for a right-sided approach. The ablation catheter is inserted into the femoral artery and positioned through the aortic valve into the left ventricle (Figure 38.3A). The catheter is withdrawn so that the tip lies against the membranous septum a few millimeters below the aortic valve at the point of recording the largest His deflection with a small A wave (Figure 38.3B). Often, no atrial electrogram may be seen, and in this situation, the best His signal should be sought. The presence of a large A wave suggests that the tip of catheter is close to the left atrium above the aortic valve; ablation must not be attempted at this site. A good radiological reference for the left-sided catheter tip is a right-sided recording catheter placed in a conventional manner over the His bundle.

Left-sided ablation with a retrograde approach is contraindicated if there is an aortic mechanical prosthesis. Complications and technical problems are more common

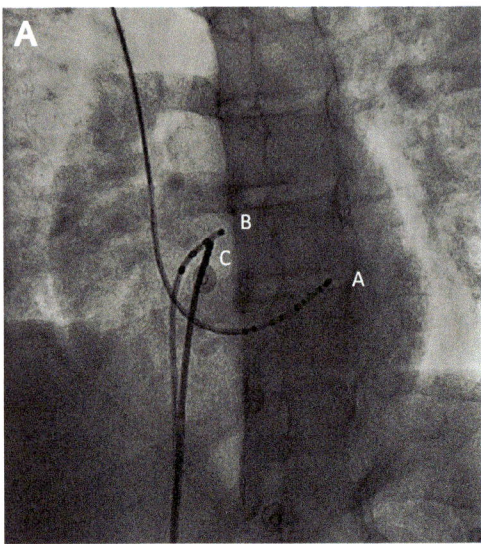
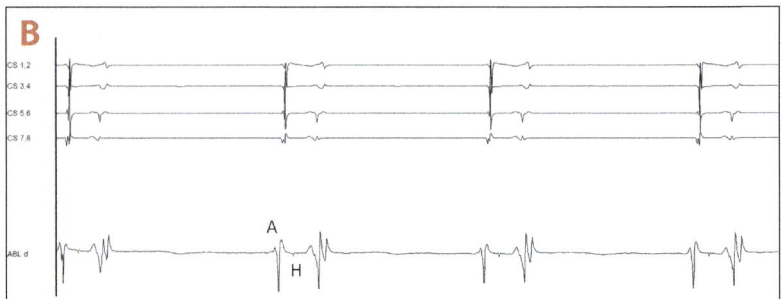

Figure 38.2 **Panel A:** Left anterior oblique projection showing the right-sided approach for atrioventricular junctional (AVJ) ablation. (**A**) Catheter in coronary sinus, (**B**) catheter in the His bundle position, and (**C**) ablator catheter positioned a few millimeters toward the atrium on the compact AV node. **Panel B:** Intracardiac signal recorded by ablator catheter (ABL d) in the site of AVF ablation by the right-sided approach, showing a large A wave (**A**) with a small or absent His potential (**H**).

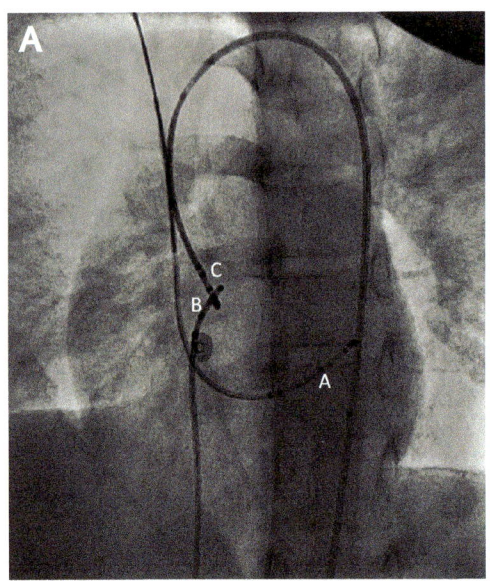
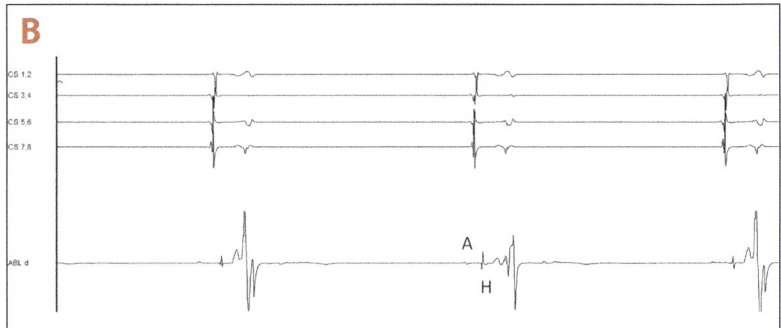

Figure 38.3 **Panel A:** Left anterior oblique projection showing the left-sided approach for atrioventricular junctional (AVJ) ablation. (**A**) Catheter in coronary sinus, (**B**) catheter in the His bundle position, and (**C**) ablator catheter positioned against the membranous septum a few millimeters below the aortic valve. **Panel B:** Intracardiac signal recorded by ablator catheter (ABL d) in the site of AVJ ablation by the left-sided approach, showing a large His deflection (**H**) with a small/absent A wave (**A**).

in the presence of disease of the aorta or aortic valve, if the patient is older, or if the patient has peripheral or coronary artery disease. In this circumstance, a further attempt should be considered from the right side on another occasion. The danger of inadvertent placement of the ablation catheter in the coronary artery and the potential for damaging the aortic valve during a left-sided approach should be recognized.

Energy

Temperature-controlled ablation is preferred, for which a temperature of 60° to 70°C should be set, with a maximum power output of 40 to 50W. Energy is applied for 10 to 30 seconds. When AV block or accelerated junctional rhythm occurs, energy delivery may be continued for a further 30 seconds, up to a total of 60 seconds.

Confirmation of AV Block

After successful ablation, temporary pacing must be commenced immediately if the escape rhythm is unstable or absent, or if there is a hemodynamic compromise. The regularity and width of the escape rhythm (if present) should be recorded by reducing the rate of pacing at regular intervals during the observation period. The target of ablation is a stable, third-degree AV block for at least 10 minutes despite giving 1 mg intravenous atropine.

Heparin Infusion During the Ablation Procedure

No controlled studies have demonstrated the efficacy of heparin infusion in preventing thromboembolic complications of AVJ ablation. However, the majority of operators give intravenous heparin for left-sided (but not for right-sided) ablation of the AVJ.

Pacemaker Implantation and Postimplantation Monitoring

There are four strategies for AVJ ablation and pacing:

1. A single procedure in which ablation of the AV junction is followed by pacemaker implantation.

2. If the right-sided ablation fails, then the pacemaker is implanted at the session and the patient returns at a later date for a left-sided approach to AVJ ablation.

3. The pacemaker is implanted initially and the patient is then readmitted approximately 1 to 3 months later (ie, when the pacemaker system is considered stable and wounds have healed) in order to review the need to proceed to AVJ ablation, with sequential right-sided and then left-sided approaches as necessary.

4. As for point 1, but with delay between ablation and permanent pacing of up to 24 hours. This is the least favored approach and should be performed only when local factors demand it. The patient must be carefully monitored during the intervening period owing to dependency on the temporary pacemaker.

Due to some malignant arrhythmias (polymorphic VT, torsade de pointes, and VF) and QT interval modifications observed immediately after AVJ ablation (with probably different mechanisms: bradycardia and sympathetic tone increase) is important to reduce this risk by routinely reprogramming the pacemaker to pace at 80-90 bpm for some weeks after the procedure. After this first period is safe, slowly reduce the lower pacing rate.

Results and Complications of Ablation

As discussed, ablation of the AVJ is easy to perform and can be carried out through either a right-sided or left-sided approach.[5] Extensive experience of ablation through the right-sided approach and the higher complication rates associated with left-sided catheterization make the right-sided approach preferable. If this fails, the left-sided approach can be undertaken during the same procedure; while this requires fewer RF deliveries, it involves arterial catheterization. Complete AV block is achieved by means of such a sequential approach in more than 95% of cases; late regression of AV block occurs in 0% to 7% of cases. Periprocedural complications are < 2% and procedure-related mortality is 0.1%, almost exclusively involving patients with severe heart failure.[5]

Clinical Efficacy

In view of the results of open studies, meta-analyses, and randomized controlled trials, the clinical efficacy of "ablate and pace" can be regarded as well established (Table 38.2).

Paroxysmal AF

One noncontrolled study[6] and two randomized controlled trials[9,17] demonstrated that ablate and pace was superior to drug therapy for improving the quality of life of patients with drug-refractory, symptomatic paroxysmal AF. After ablation, palpitations were eliminated in 80% of patients, and specific symptom scores (effort dyspnea, effort intolerance, easy tiring) improved by 30% to 80%.

Permanent AF

Observational studies comparing designated patient endpoints with baseline measures[7,14] have suggested that ablation is effective for improving quality of life during long-term follow-up. In comparison with preablation baseline values, quality of life and exercise capacity increased by 30% to 60% (although in one controlled study,[18] about 40% of this improvement was attributed to the placebo effect). These results were partially confirmed by two randomized controlled trials[19] in which ablate and pace was compared with drug treatment during long-term follow-up. Ablate and pace proved more effective for controlling specific symptoms; however, it was less effective than observed in the intrapatient comparisons. Moreover, symptoms improved to a greater degree than quality-of-life indexes (Minnesota Living with Heart Failure Questionnaire [LHFQ], NYHA class, and activity scale).

In noncontrolled studies, ablation has been seen to reduce left ventricular diameters, as measured by echocardiography. It did so especially in patients with depressed functional capacity, leading to an improvement in indexes of systolic function, ie, ejection fraction and fractional shortening.[7,8,18,20,21] Exercise capacity was also reported to improve after ablation.[6,18,21] In one randomized controlled parallel study, however, no substantial changes in echocardiographic parameters or exercise capacity were observed.[19]

Pacing Mode

The aim of permanent cardiac pacing is to restore AV synchrony during sinus rhythm and to provide an adequate increase in heart rate in response to physical activity during AF. These criteria are met by pacing in the DDDR mode. The VVIR mode, which is adequate during AF, is inadequate during sinus rhythm because it does not maintain AV synchrony and may cause pacemaker syndrome.[5] Therefore, the VVIR mode is preferred in patients with permanent AF or with persistent AF who are at high risk for progressing to permanent AF after AVJ ablation (ie, patients aged > 75 years or those who have previously undergone electrical cardioversion).[22,23]

Table 38.2 Most recent and important trials and meta-analysis on ablate and pace strategy

Study author	Year	Study type	Nr patients	AF type	Average follow-up
Kay[6]	1988	Prospective, not controlled	12 AVJAP	Paroxysmal	8 ± 2 months
Rosenqvist[7]	1990	Observational prospective single center	47 AVJAP	59% AF/AFL, 26% AVNRT, 12.5% AVRT, 2.5% AT	41 ± 23 months
Rodriguez[8]	1993	Observational retrospective	30 AVJAP : group I LVEF ≤ 50% (N=12), group II LVEF >50% (N=18)	Lone AF: 90% Paroxysmal	14 ± 20 months
Marshall[9]	1999	Prospective single-center, randomized controlled trial	37 AVJAP (DDDR/MS pacing mode with slow-or fast-switch algorithm or VVIR); 19 drugs	Paroxysmal	18 weeks
Brignole[5]	1999	Controlled prospective multicenter randomized trial in severely symptomatic patients	22 AVJAP; 21 drugs	Paroxysmal	6 months
Wood[10]	2000	Meta-analysis of all published outcome studies	1,181 patients (21 studies)	97% AF: Paroxysmal and Permanent	—
Ozcan[11]	2001	Observational retrospective case-control study	350 AVJAP; 229 drugs	45% paroxysmal 50% chronic 5% AFL (7% lone AF)	36 ± 26 months
Ozcan[12]	2003	Retrospective case-control comparison between pt with EF> or <40%	56 AVJAP; 56 controls	Paroxysmal and permanent	40 ± 23 months
Weerasooriya[13]	2003	Controlled prospective randomized multicentre trial	59 AVJAP; 50 controls	Permanent	12 months
Brignole[14]	2005	Prospective randomized, single-blind, 3-month crossover comparison between RV vs LV pacing and RV vs BiV pacing	56 AVJAP (3 different pacing modalities (RV/LV/BiV)	Permanent	12 months (6-month phase 1; 6-month phase 2)
Gasparini[15]	2008	Observational multicentre longitudinal on patients undergoing CRT	118 AVJAP (CRT); 125 drugs + CRT	Permanent	34 (10–40) months
Dong[16]	2010	Observational single-center study on patients undergoing CRT	49 AVJAP (CRT); 109 drugs + CRT	88% Permanent	2.1 (1.4–3.0) years

AF = ATRIAL fibrillation; AFL = atrial flutter; AT = atrial tachycardia; AVJAP = atrioventricular junction ablation and pacing; AVN = atrioventricular node; AVNRT = atrioventricular nodal reentrant tachycardia; AVRT = atrioventricular reciprocating tachycardia; BiV = Bi-ventricular; CHF = congestive heart failure; CRT = cardiac resynchronization therapy; FU= follow-up; CHF = congestive heart failure; LA = left atrial; LBBB = left bundle branch block; LV = left ventricular; LVEDV = left ventricular end-diastolic volume; LVEF = left ventricular ejection fraction; LVESV = left ventricular end-systolic volume; MS=mode switch; NYHA = New York Heart Association; QoL = quality of life; RV = right ventricular; SHD = structural heart disease.

Endpoints	Results	Comments
QoL and exercise capacity before and 6 weeks after ablation	Ablate and pace significantly improved QoL and exercise capacity.	
Early complication and long-term outcome	4 early complications and 1 sudden death at 2 weeks.	Direct current ablation technique.
	Improved activity level in 83% of patients with successful ablation. Significant decreased hospital admissions/year. Most patients with low LVEF showed a significant increase. New onset of CHF occurred after ablation in 4 patients (2 without SHD). Total mortality rate 17%, higher among patients with underlying SHD.	
Left heart chambers dimension and function	LVEF increased significantly and LVESV, LVEDV and LA dimensions decreased in group I.	Group I had a longer history of AF (deterioration of LV function, maybe related to duration).
	No changes in group II.	
Primary: QoL and symptoms		Exercise tolerance and LV systolic function were not significantly affected by ablation and pacing or medical therapy.
Secondary: (1) comparison of QoL intrapatient and intergroups (2) exercise capacity and LVEF		
(3) complications, development of permanent AF		
Primary: QoL and specific symptoms.	Ablate and pace is highly effective and superior to drug therapy for controlling symptoms and improving QoL.	
Secondary:(1) intrapatient comparison of QoL and specific symptoms (2) major clinical events (complications, development of permanent AF, number of hospitalizations and/or CVE)		
QoL, cardiac function, exercise duration, healthcare use	Ablate and pace significantly reduces symptoms and healthcare use and improves exercise duration and cardiac function (except fractional shortening).	
	1-year total mortality 6.3%; sudden death mortality 2.0%.	
Long-term survival	Similar survival for patients with AF, whether they received ablation or drug therapy. AVJAP did not adversely affect long-term survival.	IMA, history of CHF, and treatment with cardiac drugs after ablation-independent predictors of death.
Long-term survival in patients with EF < 40%	End FU: Mortality: 41%, 61% for cardiac causes. Normal survival in patients with reversible LV dysfunction. Poor survival in patients with persistent LV dysfunction.	LVEF increase in 68%; normalization of LVEF occurred in 29% of patients.
Primary: cardiac function (echocardiographic data and exercise tolerance).	No significant difference in LVEF or exercise duration. Peak ventricular rate lower in the AVJAP group during exercise and activities of daily life. Better QoL and symptoms in the AVJAP group.	
Secondary: ventricular rate control and QoL		
Primary: QoL and exercise capacity.	QoL and exercise capacity improved little with LV and BiV versus RV pacing.	
Secondary: effect of AVJAP on QoL and exercise capacity in subgroups: (1) patients with ≤ 40% and LBBB or not and (2) different pacing modalities	BiV pacing, but not LV pacing, was slightly better than RV in patients with LVEF > 40% and no LBBB. Compared with preablation baseline, clinically significant improvement in all pacing modalities (better in BiV group).	
Overall, cardiac, and HF survival	Total mortality 4.6%/ year; cardiac mortality 4.1%/year.	
	AVJAP group had less overall and cardiac mortality and HF.	
Clinical and survival outcomes in AF and heart failure population	AVJAP and CRT provides greater improvement in NYHA class and survival benefit (96.0% vs 76.5%).	

Long-term Follow-up

Some data on the long-term effects of ablation suggest that initially paroxysmal or persistent forms of AF frequently progress to permanent AF following ablate and pace therapy (approximately 20% per year).[24] However, to date, ablate and pace does not seem to increase thromboembolic risk in patients with AF.[25] Anticoagulant therapy should therefore be prescribed in accordance with the current guidelines. Finally, the results of randomized controlled studies[7,9,17] do not indicate an increased risk of death. Indeed, a meta-analysis carried out on 1,073 patients from 16 peer-reviewed studies revealed a one-year total mortality rate of 6.3% (95% CI; 5.5%–7.2%) and a one-year sudden death rate of 2% (95% CI; 1.5%–2.6%). These figures are very similar to the 6.7% total mortality rate and the 2.4% sudden death rate observed in 1,330 AF patients followed up for 1.3 years in the Stroke Prevention in Atrial Fibrillation Trial.[11] Thus, it is more likely that the long-term outcome is attributable to the natural course of the underlying disease than to an adverse effect of ablate and pace.

Ozcan et al[11] concluded that (1) in the absence of heart disease, survival among AF patients after undergoing ablate and pace is similar to that of the general population; (2) long-term survival is similar both in patients who undergo ablation and in those on drug therapy; and (3) ablate and pace does not impact long-term mortality. A recent subanalysis was conducted of the Atrial Fibrillation Follow-Up Investigation of Rhythm Management (AFFIRM) trial. In it, the authors showed how nonpharmacological therapy, even in more symptomatic patients with more frequent AF and faster ventricular rates during AF, led to increased time to cardiovascular hospitalization and reduced total length of stay compared with drug therapy.[26]

In contrast with its usually excellent results, ablate and pace is ineffective in a minority of patients. With regard to paroxysmal AF, inefficacy was reported in 14% of patients in a study by Rosenqvist et al[7] and in 7% of patients in a study by Kamalvand et al.[27] There are various possible explanations for this. Careful analysis of the follow-up of these patients has suggested that AF relapses were only partly responsible for their symptoms. Indeed, it is possible that their symptoms were linked to any of several factors: from DDDR pacing, to inappropriate programming, to the unfavorable hemodynamic effect of electrical stimulation from the RV apex. Moreover, Weber et al[28] found that palpitations are caused by a psychiatric illness in almost one-third of all patients. In patients with congestive heart failure, early hemodynamic deterioration was observed by Vanderheiden[29] in 7% of cases and by Twidale[30] in (9%) of cases; mitral regurgitation and a very low ejection fraction were predictors of this adverse event. Although a randomized study[19] did not confirm this result, other studies have found that pacing from the RV apex is not optimal because it determines a nonphysiological asynchronous contraction.[31]

AVJ Ablation and Cardiac Resynchronization Therapy

We now consider two other clinical situations: cardiac resynchronization therapy (CRT) in patients who are candidates for AVJ ablation, and AVJ ablation in patients who are candidates for CRT.

Cardiac Resynchronization Therapy in Candidates for AVJ Ablation

In patients who require ventricular response control through AVJ ablation (see previous section), adding CRT ("upstream") is justified by the fact that the hemodynamic benefits of regularizing cardiac rhythm may be partially offset by the adverse effects of nonphysiological stimulation of the right ventricle.[19,32] Indeed, during RV stimulation, the ventricular activation sequence resembles that of left bundle branch block, ie, the RV is activated before the left ventricle (so-called interventricular dyssynchrony) and the interventricular septum is activated before the free wall of the left ventricle (intraventricular dyssynchrony). Studies of both acute[33] (immediately after implantation) and chronic[34] (after months/years) pacing therapy have shown that stimulating the RV induces dyssynchrony of the left ventricle in about 50% of cases. Moreover, some small studies[22,35] have suggested that biventricular pacing can exert a beneficial hemodynamic effect additive to that of regularizing the ventricular rhythm by means of AVJ ablation. In sum, the abovementioned studies reveal that AVJ ablation associated with RV pacing is able to increase ejection fraction and reduce mitral regurgitation, and that biventricular pacing is able to double these effects.

Three randomized studies,[14,36,37] involving a total of 347 patients, compared the short-term clinical results of biventricular pacing with those of RV pacing. Individually, these trials were unable to demonstrate a statistically significant improvement in terms of survival, stroke, hospitalizations, or cost reduction. In two of the studies, biventricular pacing achieved a significant improvement in ejection fraction and exercise capacity. On the other hand, in noncontrolled observational studies,[38,39] upgrading to biventricular pacing in patients who developed heart failure months or years after AVJ ablation and RV pacing was seen to produce a great clinical benefit. For example, in 20 patients who had become severely symptomatic 17 months after AVJ ablation, Leon et al[38] added biventricular pacing; this led to a 29% improvement in NYHA class, a 33% improvement in Minnesota LHFQ scores, and an 81% reduction in hospitalizations. Similar results were obtained by Valls-Bertault et al.[39] In sum, the available data do not enable us to draw any definitive conclusions; therefore, larger clinical trials with long periods of follow-up are needed.

AVJ Ablation in Candidates for CRT

In patients with heart failure in whom CRT is indicated, regularizing the ventricular rhythm by means of AVJ ablation enables biventricular pacing to be optimized.

The large trials conducted on CRT have not included patients with AF. A possible explanation for this omission lies in the fact that AF potentially reduces the advantages offered by CRT. First of all, the possibility of AV resynchronization is lost, and with it, the benefits that can be obtained from lengthening the phase of diastolic filling (since only intra- and interventricular dyssynchrony can be corrected). Second, the efficacy of CRT may be impaired by the presence of a high intrinsic heart rate that renders biventricular pacing incomplete. In a small Holter-controlled study,[40] only 47% of patients had complete biventricular pacing in more than 90% of beats, while the others had fusion beats (60% of beats) and pseudo-fusion beats (24% of beats); the patients with complete capture displayed a better clinical response to CRT (responders: 86% vs 67%; P = 0.03). AV node ablation is the best way of completely controlling the heart rate and, at the same time, obtaining a regular ventricular rhythm. Moreover, this procedure offers the even greater advantage of ensuring effective CRT by means of constant biventricular pacing.

Gasparini et al[41] compared the efficacy of biventricular pacing in 48 patients with permanent AF who had not undergone AVJ ablation because their ventricular rate was apparently well controlled by drug treatment (> 85% of beats were placed in the biventricular mode) and 114 patients who had undergone biventricular pacing after AVJ ablation. During 4 years of follow-up, they observed an improvement in ejection fraction, inverse ventricular remodeling, and an increase in exercise capacity only in those patients who had undergone ablation. The improvement observed was of similar magnitude to that seen in patients in sinus rhythm. Similarly, in a study by Ferreira et al,[42] the percentage of responders (52%) was significantly lower in AF patients who had not undergone AVJ ablation than in those who had (85%) or in those in sinus rhythm (79%). Indeed, Koplan et al[43] demonstrated that the clinical efficacy of CRT is proportional to the percentage of biventricular pacing achieved; in patients who had 93% to 100% of their beats paced in the biventricular mode, the risk of events during follow-up was 44% lower than in patients who had 0% to 92% of biventricular pacing (P < 0.001). Patients with a history of tachyarrhythmia were more likely to have had fewer than 92% of their beats paced in the biventricular mode.

In some studies, however, the favorable effects of CRT have been documented even in the absence of AVJ ablation. Some authors[44,45] have reported similar results in terms of mortality and functional capacity in AF patients and patients in sinus rhythm who have not undergone AVJ ablation. In one multicenter study,[46] no differences in functional capacity or ventricular remodeling emerged between patients who had undergone AVJ ablation during CRT and those who had not.

Summary

Despite the lack of conclusive controlled studies, physiopathological assumptions, and clinical results suggest that AVJ ablation contributes to achieving good clinical results in all cases in which the intrinsic heart rate hinders constant biventricular pacing.

References

1. Camm AJ, Kirchhof P, Lip GY, et al. Guidelines for the management of atrial fibrillation: the Task Force for the Management of Atrial Fibrillation of the European Society of Cardiology (ESC). *Eur Heart J*. 2010;31:2369-2429.
2. Fuster V, Rydén LE, Cannom DS, et al. ACC/AHA/ESC 2006 Guidelines for the Management of Patients with Atrial Fibrillation: a report of the American College of Cardiology/American Heart Association Task Force on Practice Guidelines and the European Society of Cardiology Committee for Practice Guidelines (Writing Committee to Revise the 2001 Guidelines for the Management of Patients with Atrial Fibrillation): developed in collaboration with the European Heart Rhythm Association and the Heart Rhythm Society. *Circulation*. 2006;114:e257-e354.
3. Wann LS, Curtis AB, January CT, et al. 2011 ACCF/AHA/HRS focused update on the management of patients with atrial fibrillation (updating the 2006 guideline): a report of the American College of Cardiology Foundation/American Heart Association Task Force on Practice Guidelines. *J Am Coll Cardiol*. 2011;57:223-242.
4. Natale A, Raviele A, Arentz T, et al. Venice chart international consensus document on atrial fibrillation ablation. *J Cardiovasc Electrophysiol*. 2007;18:560-580.
5. Brignole M, Gammage M, Jordaens L, et al. Report of a study group on ablate and pace therapy for paroxysmal atrial fibrillation. *Europace*. 1999,1:15-19.
6. Kay GN, Bubien RS, Epstein AE, et al. Effect of catheter ablation of the atrioventricular junction on quality of life and exercise tolerance in paroxysmal atrial fibrillation. *Am J Cardiol*. 1988;62:741-744.
7. Rosenqvist M, Lee M, Mouliner L, et al. Long-term follow-up of patients after transcatheter direct current ablation of the atrioventricular junction. *J Am Coll Cardiol*. 1990;16:1467-1474.
8. Rodriguez LM, Smeets J, Xie B, et al. Improvement in left ventricular function by ablation of atrioventricular nodal conduction in selected patients with lone atrial fibrillation. *Am J Cardiol*. 1993;72:1137-1141.
9. Marshall H, Harris Z, Griffith M, et al. Prospective randomized study of ablation and pacing versus medical therapy for paroxysmal atrial fibrillation. Effects of pacing mode and mode-switch algorithm. *Circulation*. 1999;99:1587-1592.

10. Wood MA, Brown-Mahoney C, Kay GN, et al. Clinical outcomes after ablation and pacing therapy for atrial fibrillation: a meta-analysis. *Circulation.* 2000;101:1138-1144.
11. Ozcan C, Jahangir A, Friedman PA, et al. Long-term survival after ablation of the atrioventricular node and implantation of a permanent pacemaker in patients with atrial fibrillation. *N Engl J Med.* 2001;344:1043-1051.
12. Ozcan C, Jahangir A, Friedman PA et al. Significant effects of atrioventricular node ablation and pacemaker implantation on left ventricular function and long-term survival in patients with atrial fibrillation and left ventricular dysfunction. *Am J Cardiol.* 2003;92:33-37.
13. Weerasooriya R, Davis M, Powell A, et al. The Australian Intervention Randomized Control of Rate in Atrial Fibrillation Trial (AIRCRAFT). *J Am Coll Cardiol.* 2003;41:1697-1702.
14. Brignole M, Gammage M, Puggioni E, et al. Comparative assessment of right, left, and biventricular pacing in patients with permanent atrial fibrillation. *Eur Heart J.* 2005;26:712-722.
15. Gasparini M, Auricchio A, Metra M, et al. Long-term survival in patients undergoing cardiac resynchronization therapy: the importance of performing atrioventricular junction ablation in patients with permanent atrial fibrillation. *Eur Heart J.* 2008;29:1644-1652.
16. Dong K, Shen WK, Powell BD, et al. Atrioventricular nodal ablation predicts survival benefit in patients with atrial fibrillation receiving cardiac resynchronization therapy. *Heart Rhythm.* 2010;7(9):1240-1245.
17. Brignole M, Gianfranchi L, Menozzi C, et al. An assessment of atrioventricular junction ablation and DDDR mode-switching pacemaker versus pharmacological treatment in patients with severely symptomatic paroxysmal atrial fibrillation. A randomized controlled study. *Circulation.* 1997;96:2617-2624.
18. Brignole M, Gianfranchi L, Menozzi C, et al. Influence of atrioventricular junction radiofrequency ablation in patients with chronic atrial fibrillation and flutter on quality of life and cardiac performance. *Am J Cardiol.* 1994;74:242-246.
19. Brignole M, Menozzi C, Gianfranchi L, et al. Assessment of atrioventricular junction ablation and VVIR pacemaker versus pharmacological treatment in patients with heart failure and chronic atrial fibrillation. A randomized controlled study. *Circulation.* 1998;98:953-960.
20. Heinz G, Siostrozonek P, Kreiner G, et al. Improvement in left ventricular systolic function after successful radiofrequency His bundle ablation for drug refractory, chronic atrial fibrillation and recurrent atrial flutter. *Am J Cardiol.* 1992;69:489-492.
21. Twidale N, Sutton K, Bartlett L, et al. Effects on cardiac performance of atrioventricular node catheter ablation using radiofrequency current for drug-refractory atrial arrhythmias. *Pacing Clin Electrophysiol.* 1993;16:1275-1284.
22. Puggioni E, Brignole M, Gammage M, et al. Acute comparative effect of right and left ventricular pacing in patients with permanent atrial fibrillation. *J Am Coll Cardiol.* 2004;43:234-238.
23. Gianfranchi L, Brignole M, Menozzi C, et al. Progression of permanent atrial fibrillation after atrioventricular junction ablation and dual-chamber pacemaker implantation in patients with paroxysmal atrial tachyarrhythmias. *Am J Cardiol.* 1998;81:351-354.
24. Olgin J, Scheinman M. Comparison of high energy direct current and radiofrequency catheter ablation of the atrioventricular junction. *J Am Coll Cardiol.* 1993;21:557-564.
25. Gasparini M, Mantica M, Brignole M, et al. Thromboembolism after atrioventricular node ablation and pacing: long-term follow-up. *Heart.* 1999;82:494-498.
26. Saksena S, Slee A, Liu T, et al. Impact of non-pharmacologic therapies on clinical outcomes of a rate control strategy: an AFFIRM analysis. *J Am Coll Cardiol.* 2011;57:E128.
27. Kamalvand K, Tan K, Kotsakis A, et al. Is mode switching beneficial? A randomized study in patients with paroxysmal atrial tachyarrhythmias. *J Am Coll Cardiol.* 1997;30:496-504.
28. Weber BE, Kapoor WN. Evaluation and outcome of patients with palpitations. *Am J Med.* 1996;100:138-148.
29. Vanderheiden M, Goethals M, Anguera I, et al. Hemodynamic deterioration following radiofrequency ablation of the atrioventricular conduction system. *Pacing Clin Electrophysiol.* 1997;20:2422-2438.
30. Twidale N, Manda V, Nave K, et al. Predictors of outcome after radiofrequency catheter ablation of the atrioventricular node for atrial fibrillation and congestive heart failure. *Am Heart J.* 1998;136:647-657.
31. Ausubel K, Furman S. The pacemaker syndrome. *Ann Intern Med.* 1985;103:420-429.
32. Vernooy K, Dijkman B, Cheriex EC, et al. Ventricular remodeling during long-term right ventricular pacing following His bundle ablation. *Am J Cardiol.* 2006;97:1223-1227.
33. Lupi G, Sassone B, Badano L, et al. Effects of right ventricular pacing on intra-left ventricular electromechanical activation in patients with native narrow QRS. *Am J Cardiol.* 2006;98:219-222.
34. Tops LF, Schalij MJ, Holman ER, et al. Right ventricular pacing can induce ventricular dyssynchrony in patients with atrial fibrillation after atrioventricular node ablation. *J Am Coll Cardiol.* 2006;48:1642-1648.
35. Brignole M, Menozzi C, Botto GL, et al. Usefulness of echo-guided cardiac resynchronization pacing in patients undergoing 'ablate and pace' therapy for permanent atrial fibrillation and effects of heart rate regularization and left ventricular resynchronization. *Am J Cardiol.* 2008;102:854-860.
36. Leclercq C, Walker S, Linde C, et al. Comparative effects of permanent biventricular and right-univentricular pacing in heart failure patients with chronic atrial fibrillation. *Eur Heart J.* 2002;23:1780-1787.
37. Doshi RN, Daoud EG, Fellows C, et al. Left ventricular-based cardiac stimulation post AV nodal ablation evaluation (the PAVE study). *J Cardiovasc Electrophysiol.* 2005;16:1160-1165.
38. Leon AR, Greenberg JM, Kanuru N, et al. Cardiac resynchronization in patients with congestive heart failure and chronic atrial fibrillation: effect of upgrading to biventricular pacing after chronic right ventricular pacing. *J Am Coll Cardiol.* 2002;39:1258-1263.
39. Valls-Bertault V, Fatemi M, Gilard M, et al. Assessment of upgrading to biventricular pacing in patients with right ventricular pacing and congestive heart failure after atrioventricular junctional ablation for chronic atrial fibrillation. *Europace.* 2004;6:438-443.
40. Kamath GS, Cotiga D, Koneru JN, et al. The utility of 12-lead Holter monitoring in patients with permanent atrial fibrillation for the identification of nonresponders after cardiac resynchronization therapy. *J Am Coll Cardiol.* 2009;53:1050-1055.
41. Gasparini M, Auricchio A, Regoli F, et al. Four-year efficacy of cardiac resynchronization therapy on exercise tolerance and disease progression: the importance of performing atrioventricular junction ablation in patients with atrial fibrillation. *J Am Coll Cardiol.* 2006;48:734-743.

42. Ferreira AM, Adragão P, Cavaco DM, et al. Benefit of cardiac resynchronization therapy in atrial fibrillation patients vs. patients in sinus rhythm: the role of atrioventricular junction ablation. *Europace.* 2008;10:809-815.
43. Koplan BA, Kaplan AJ, Weiner S, et al. Heart failure decompensation and all-cause mortality in relation to percent biventricular pacing in patients with heart failure: is a goal of 100% biventricular pacing necessary? *J Am Coll Cardiol.* 2009;53:355-360.
44. Khadjooi K, Foley PW, Chalil S, et al. Long-term effects of cardiac resynchronisation therapy in patients with atrial fibrillation. *Heart.* 2008;94:879-883.
45. Delnoy PP, Ottervanger JP, Luttikhuis H, et al. Comparison of usefulness of cardiac resynchronization therapy in patients with atrial fibrillation and heart failure versus patients with sinus rhythm and heart failure. *Am J Cardiol.* 2007;99:1252-1257.
46. Tolosana JM, Hernandez Madrid A, Brugada J, et al. Comparison of benefits and mortality in cardiac resynchronization therapy in patients with atrial fibrillation versus patients in sinus rhythm (Results of the Spanish Atrial Fibrillation and Resynchronization [SPARE] Study). *Am J Cardiol.* 2008;102:444-449.

CHAPTER 39

Sinus Node Ablation and Atrioventricular Nodal Reentry Ablation

Wanwarang Wongcharoen, MD; Shih-Ann Chen, MD

Introduction

Supraventricular tachyarrhythmias (SVTs) are commonly encountered in clinical practice. Currently, catheter ablation has been accepted to be the curative therapy for most patients with SVTs. In this chapter, we focus on the catheter ablation of SVTs involving sinus node and atrioventricular nodal reentrant tachycardia (AVNRT).

Sinus Node Ablation

SVTs that involve sinus node and can be treated by catheter ablation include inappropriate sinus tachycardia and sinus nodal reentrant tachycardia. The electrocardiograms (ECGs) during those SVTs are identical to that of normal sinus tachycardia owing to their similar origins within the sinus node. As a result, these two conditions are frequently misdiagnosed and are often attributed to an anxiety disorder. Normal sinus tachycardia is an appropriate increase in sinus rate to more than 100 beats per minute (bpm) in response to a variety of physiological, pathological, and/or pharmacological stimuli; elimination of the underlying cause is the main treatment.[1] On the contrary, catheter ablation is generally accepted as the treatment of choice for patients with symptomatic inappropriate sinus tachycardia or sinus nodal reentrant tachycardia that is refractory to medical therapy.

Anatomy of the Sinus Node

The sinus node represents the cardiac pacemaker, which initiates each cardiac cycle. The origin of the dominant sinus pacemaker group in humans may occur over a widely distributed area: as far cranially as the right atrial–superior vena caval junction or as far caudally as the right atrial–inferior vena caval junction.

Sympathetic activation causes a cranial shift in the pacemaker location, whereas vagal stimulation results in a caudal shift along the crista terminalis.[2-4] The morphology of sinus node is crescent-like. The long axis of the nodal body is parallel to the terminal groove, with the head and tail penetrating intramyocardially toward the subendocardium.[5] The nodal length was reported to be 8 to 21.5 mm and was found to be longer than 16 mm in 50% of the studied hearts. Owing to the thickness of the crista terminalis, a large mass of the nodal tissue can be relatively distant from the endocardium. In half of the hearts, the distance from the most caudal boundaries of the nodal body to the endocardium was more than 3.5 mm. The body of the node is constantly penetrated by the sinus node artery, which in most hearts occupies a central position throughout the length of the node. Previous reporting has shown that the sinus node artery does not branch in the nodal tissue and that the main blood supply of this tissue is secured by the peripheral nodal networks.[6]

Inappropriate Sinus Tachycardia

Inappropriate sinus tachycardia is defined as a persistent increase in resting heart rate to more than 100 bpm, which is out of proportion to physiological need.[7,8] On 24-hour Holter monitoring, either the mean heart rate exceeds 95 bpm, daytime resting heart rate exceeds 95 bpm, or sinus rate from supine to upright position increases more than 25 to 30 bpm in a persistent manner.[9] Typically, the heart rate normalizes nocturnally. Because of the similarities of ECGs between normal sinus tachycardia and inappropriate sinus tachycardia, the primary underlying cause of normal sinus tachycardia (eg, hypovolemia, anemia, thyroid disease, infection, or other systemic illness) must be excluded before the diagnosis of inappropriate sinus tachycardia can be made.

The primary alteration in sinus node automaticity, coupled with sympathovagal balance, is speculated as the mechanism of inappropriate sinus tachycardia.[10] Previous studies have reported inappropriate sinus tachycardia as a complication that occurs after ablation of SVTs, for which a change of autonomic tone is the postulated explanation.[11-13]

The initial therapy for inappropriate sinus tachycardia is medical treatment with β-blockers. However, in patients with symptomatic inappropriate sinus tachycardia that is refractory to medical therapy, radiofrequency modification or ablation of the sinus node is the preferred option. As mentioned above, the sinus node is not focal but rather regional. Previous studies have shown that a change in heart rate correlates with a change in the site of origin of atrial depolarization; that is, the faster rates originate from superior pacemaker cells and slower rates from more inferiorly situated cells. Accordingly, the change in P-wave morphology is observed at different atrial rates.[14] In this regard, it is possible to guide catheter ablation to eliminate only a portion of the sinus node, specifically, that portion with the faster pacemaker cells.

Electrophysiology of Inappropriate Sinus Tachycardia

The diagnostic electrophysiological study of inappropriate sinus tachycardia includes the following feature: The P-wave morphology is indistinguishable from normal sinus rhythm. The earliest endocardial activation occurs near the sinus node area along the crista terminalis and is estimated from fluoroscopic images, intracardiac ultrasonography, or advanced three-dimensional (3D) electroanatomic techniques. The atrial depolarization sequence is usually craniocaudal, along the crista terminalis.[14] The tachycardia cannot be induced or terminated using standard programmed stimulation. Rather, a gradual increase (warm-up) and decrease (cool-down) in heart rate (spontaneously or during initiation and termination of isoproterenol infusion) are observed that are consistent with an automatic mechanism of sinus node function.[8,14]

Catheter Ablation for Inappropriate Sinus Tachycardia

Earlier experience with total ablation of the sinus node frequently resulted in the requirement for implantation of permanent pacemakers.[15] Therefore, sinus node modification (compared with more extensive ablation procedures) is preferred because it targets ablation lesions to the more superior location within the sinus node. In doing so, it can preserve the dominance of the sinus node and achieve heart rate control but without producing significant pauses and without the need for permanent pacemaker implantation.[15,16]

Several strategies have been used to target the appropriate site. These include the following: conventional activation mapping by locating the earliest atrial activation site (usually 25–50 ms preceding onset of the P wave during tachycardia); and the anatomic approach, directing lesion sites to the crista terminalis guided by the use of intracardiac echocardiography and the use of 3D electroanatomic mapping, which allows for rapid identification of the activation origin and assessment of anticipated shift in earliest activation during sinus node ablation (Figure 39.1).[8,14-19]

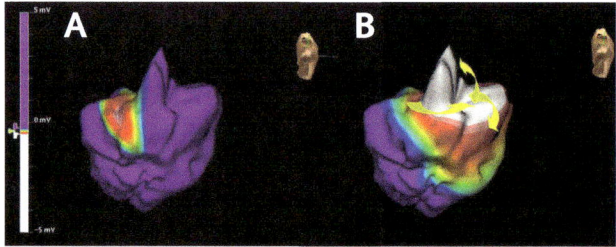

Figure 39.1 A 3D noncontact mapping system applied during inappropriate sinus tachycardia. The isopotential map shows the origin (**Panel A**) and breakout site (**Panel B**) of the earliest activation at the superior vena cava–right atrium junction.

Responses to radiofrequency catheter application on the sinus node have been reported.[15,17-19] In most of the cases, there was a migration of the site of earliest atrial activation in a cranial–caudal direction along the lateral right atrial wall. This effect was associated with flattening of the P wave in the inferior lead and, occasionally, with a slightly negative initial component of the P wave in the same ECG recordings.[18,19] In the remaining patients, the sinus rate decreased abruptly in the absence of any gradual migration of the site of earliest endocardial activation. This effect may indicate that, in these patients, inappropriate sinus tachycardia had been generated by a single pacemaker site within or adjacent to the sinus node.[18]

Although short-term success rates of catheter ablation were favorable (range: 76%–100%), it has limited long-term effects.[20] Several factors related to the anatomy of the sinus node may explain the high arrhythmia recurrence rates. The density of the matrix of connective tissue surrounding the specialized sinoatrial cells, the predominantly epicardial location of the sinus node, and the potential cooling effects of the nodal artery each may prevent delivery of effective lesions.[5,21,22] Recent reports have shown that the use of noncontact mapping with saline-irrigated ablation[23] and combined epicardial–endocardial catheter ablation may help improve the outcome.[24] Nevertheless, Shen and colleagues have shown that some patients still had symptoms despite successfully achieving a slower heart rate after sinus node modification.[20] Autonomic dysregulation was proposed to underlie the clinical symptoms in this particular group of patients. Therefore, sinus node modification is not recommended in patients with inappropriate sinus tachycardia who show evidence of autonomic abnormalities without persistent tachycardia.[14]

Procedural complications also have been reported, including the need for a permanent pacemaker,[15] superior vena cava occlusion,[15,25] and phrenic nerve paralysis.[26,27] In order to prevent phrenic nerve injury, high-output pacing should be performed before each radiofrequency delivery in order to assess diaphragmatic stimulation. In situations where the critical area of ablation has phrenic nerve capture with pacing, protecting the phrenic nerve by placing a balloon in the epicardial space has been previously reported.[28]

Sinus Nodal Reentrant Tachycardia

Sinus nodal reentrant tachycardia is a rare disorder whose incidence ranges between 1.8% and 16.9% of patients undergoing diagnostic electrophysiological study.[29] The underlying mechanism is reentry; however, the exact site of reentry (whether in the sinus node, the perinodal area, or the adjacent atrial tissue) has not been elucidated.[30]

The architecture of the sinus node potentially provides a substrate for sinus nodal reentrant tachycardia. The increase in the uncoupling of intercellular transmissions (owing to the presence of the dense matrix of connective tissue separating the nodal cells) may facilitate slow conduction.[31,32] In addition, lack of an insulating connective tissue sheath surrounding the sinus node along with the presence of nodal radiations interweaving with the working atrial myocardium mean that there are multiple potential sites of entry and exit for an excitatory wavefront. Altogether, these unique structures of the sinus node make an ideal substrate for reentry.

Electrophysiology of Sinus Nodal Reentrant Tachycardia

The ECG for sinus nodal reentrant tachycardia is similar to that of inappropriate sinus tachycardia. However, inappropriate sinus tachycardia has a nonparoxysmal character, which is opposite to the paroxysmal nature of sinus nodal reentrant tachycardia. The diagnostic electrophysiological study for sinus nodal reentrant tachycardia is characterized by high-to-low and right-to-left atrial activation during tachycardia. The activation sequence is similar to that for sinus rhythm, and the induction in the electrophysiology laboratory uses programmed stimulation with premature atrial stimuli or burst atrial pacing. The termination employs appropriately timed atrial premature stimuli, and the termination has vagal maneuvers. The induction of the arrhythmia takes place independently of atrial or atrioventricular (AV) nodal refractory periods or conduction time. In addition, there is no abnormality in sinus node function, as assessed by sinus node recovery time and sinoatrial conduction time. In contrast to inappropriate sinus tachycardia, β-blockers have little effect in terminating sinus nodal reentrant tachycardia.[33] Furthermore, adenosine has been shown to be effective for terminating episodes of sinus nodal reentrant tachycardia but not inappropriate sinus tachycardia.[34]

Catheter Ablation of Sinus Nodal Reentrant Tachycardia

Sinus nodal reentrant tachycardia does not respond well to β-blockers. Therefore, digoxin, calcium-channel blockers, and amiodarone are preferred drugs of choice.[33] In patients who remain refractory to medical therapy, radiofrequency catheter ablation has become an effective alternative for managing sinus nodal reentrant tachycardia.

Because of this arrhythmia's reentrant mechanism, the ablation of sinus nodal reentrant tachycardia requires making a focal lesion. The target ablation sites are identified by activation mapping, in which a local electrogram on the ablation catheter occurs more than 35 ms before the onset of the surface P wave during tachycardia. The intracardiac electrograms at these locations show evidence of slowed conduction (a prerequisite for reentry) exemplified by a prolonged, fractionated, and multicomponent electrogram.

Previous small studies have shown excellent outcomes for eradicating sinus nodal reentrant tachycardia with radiofrequency catheter ablation.[35-37] The 2 largest series of radiofrequency catheter ablations for sinus nodal reentrant tachycardia consisted of 10 patients each. They reported a 100% success rate in eliminating the tachycardia.[37,38]

Atrioventricular Nodal Reentrant Tachycardia Ablation

AVNRT is the most common arrhythmia in patients with regular supraventricular tachycardia. It is well established that the AV node is the underlying substrate of AVNRT, and the AV junctional region is the target of AVNRT ablation. Therefore, a comprehensive understanding of the anatomy and electrophysiology of the AV node, including different types of AVNRT, is needed in order to achieve successful ablation and minimize procedural-related complications.

Anatomy of the Atrioventricular Node

The compact AV node is situated in the triangle of Koch. This feature is delineated by the membranous septum at its apex, the inferior border at the attachment of the septal tricuspid leaflet, and the superior border at a strand of fibrous tissue extending from the central fibrous body to the sinus septum above the ostium of the coronary sinus (CS), known as the tendon of Todaro.[39] The compact AV node is around 5 to 7 mm in length and 2 to 5 mm in width.[40,41] At the apex of the triangle of Koch, the compact AV node is set against the central fibrous body, the point at which the conduction axis becomes surrounded by fibrous tissue and the compact AV node becomes the bundle of His.

The distance between the CS ostium and the His bundle recording site has been frequently used to define the dimensions Koch's triangle.[42,43] Previous studies have demonstrated mean distances from the His bundle electrogram recording site to the upper and lower lips of the CS ostium of 10 mm (range: 0–23 mm) and 20 to 25 mm (range: 9–46 mm), respectively.[44,45] However, the variability in the dimensions and morphology of Koch's triangle also has been described. In patients with a normal Koch's triangle, the AV node's position is usually in the superior third portion of the triangle. However, in 13% of patients who have a small triangle, the AV node is located in a lower position, which leads to a higher risk for heart block during application of radiofrequency energy (Figure 39.2). Therefore, in those who have a small or horizontal triangle of Koch, radiofrequency energy should be applied in the medial region of Koch's triangle (in which is found an area of subnodal tissue) in order to prevent inadvertent AV block during ablation.

Coronary Sinus Size and Morphology

The base of Koch's triangle is positioned inferiorly and is occupied by the CS. Several studies have demonstrated that the dimension of the CS diameter in patients with AVNRT is larger than that of control subjects and that there is a more windsock morphology in patients with AVNRT (Figure 39.3).[46-48] It has been suggested that the CS size and morphology may determine the presence of dual-AV nodal physiology and influence the ablation procedure in patients with AVNRT. Therefore, in particular patients who cannot achieve a successful ablation even after targeting the usual locations, a CS angiogram may be necessary.

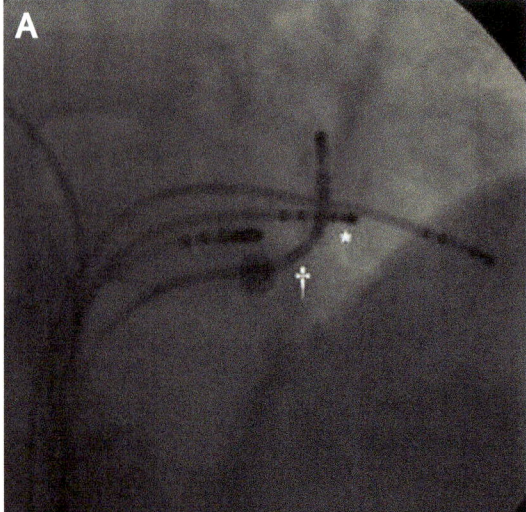 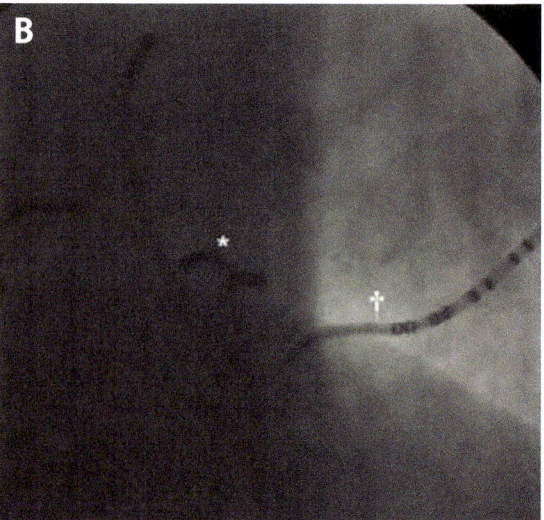

Figure 39.2 The horizontal contour of Koch's triangle in a patient with AVNRT. Notice the flattened and horizontal contour of Koch's triangle in these right anterior oblique (**Panel A**) and left anterior oblique (**Panel B**) fluoroscopic views. (The **asterisks** indicate the His bundle; the **daggers** mark the coronary sinus ostium.) Source: Adapted with permission from Lee PC, et al.[122]

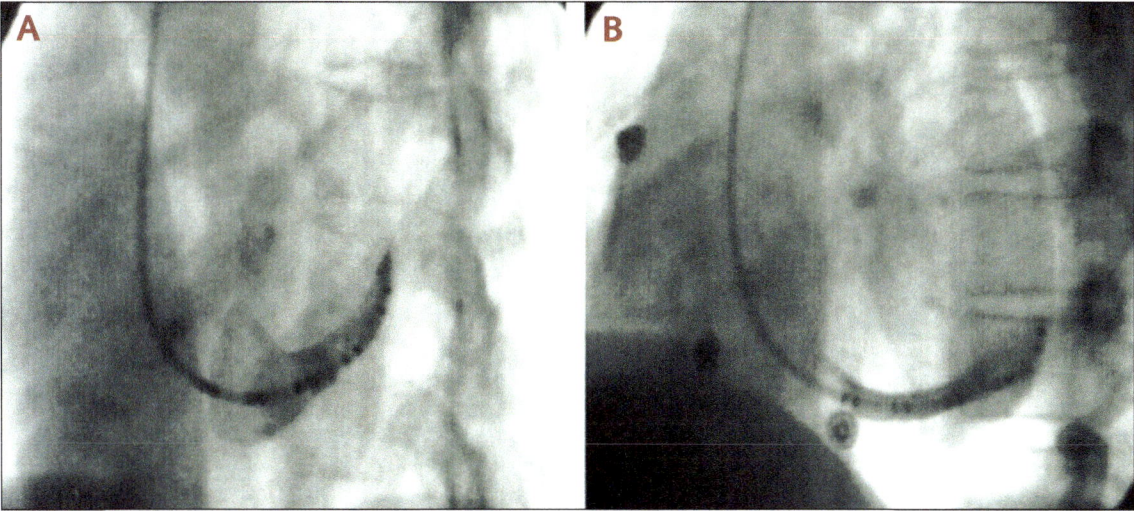

Figure 39.3 The variation in morphologies of coronary sinus (CS) ostia. Left anterior oblique projection of CS venography is demonstrated at the end systole. **Panel A:** Windsock morphology. **Panel B:** Tubular morphology. *Source:* Adapted with permission from Ong MG, et al.[48]

Electrophysiology of the Atrioventricular Node

The existence of dual-AV nodal physiology underlies the occurrence of AVNRT. The compact AV node consists of a loose transitional zone of cells blending and extending into the surrounding atrial myocardium.[49] These transitional cells are found in Koch's triangle and merge with the compact node. Previous studies have described at least two distinct groups of atrionodal connections to the compact AV node that may result from different cell types and anisotropic conduction.[50-53] It has been suggested that the posterior nodal extension, with node-like tissue that distributes toward the CS and tricuspid annulus (right posterior extenwsion), is involved in the tachycardia circuit of most patients with AVNRT (slow pathway input).[54] However, in some patients with AVNRT, the posterior extension distributing toward the mitral annulus (left posterior extension) also has been observed.[55] The fast pathway input is usually located anteriorly and in close proximity to the His bundle. Nevertheless, in rare cases, functionally fast pathway input may be located in the posteroseptal right atrium.[56,57]

The fast pathway conducts more rapidly, usually with a relatively longer refractory period, whereas the slow pathway conducts more slowly, usually with a relatively shorter refractory period. Previous studies have demonstrated the difference in the site of earliest atrial activation during retrograde conduction over the fast and slow pathways. They have also discovered concealed entrainment of the tachycardia (by atrial stimulation delivered outside the AV node to the posteroseptal right atrium and CS) and selective elimination of fast or slow pathway conduction (by ablation in the atrium remote from the compact AV node). These observations indicate that the fast and slow pathways represent conduction over different atrionodal connections rather than the previous manifestation of functionally longitudinal dissociation within the compact AV node. Thus, the electrogram characteristics inside Koch's triangle around the compact AV node display a relatively lower range of voltages exported and analyzed from the noncontact mapping system.[57] Koch's triangle also reveals a lower range of voltages than is found outside Koch's triangle during sinus rhythm and atrial pacing. This is possibly the result of transitional cell distribution, including multiple layers associated with a marked variability of fiber orientation, produced by longitudinal and circumferential fibers and anisotropic conduction.[32,58]

Dual-AV nodal physiology is normally evident in patients with AVNRT. It can be demonstrated by either 2 distinct ranges of PR interval during basic sinus rhythm or a jump (≥50 ms) in the H1-to-H2 interval at a critical range of A1-to-A2 coupling intervals (10 ms decrements). These abnormalities result in a discontinuity between the portion of the AV node conduction curve to the right of the jump in H1 to H2 (fast pathway conduction) and the portion of the AV node conduction curve to the left of the jump (slow pathway conduction) (Figure 39.4). However, dual-AV nodal physiology is not specific to patients with AVNRT; it has also been found in the healthy population. In addition, dual-AV nodal physiology cannot be demonstrated in some patients with AVNRT, which will be described in further detail below.

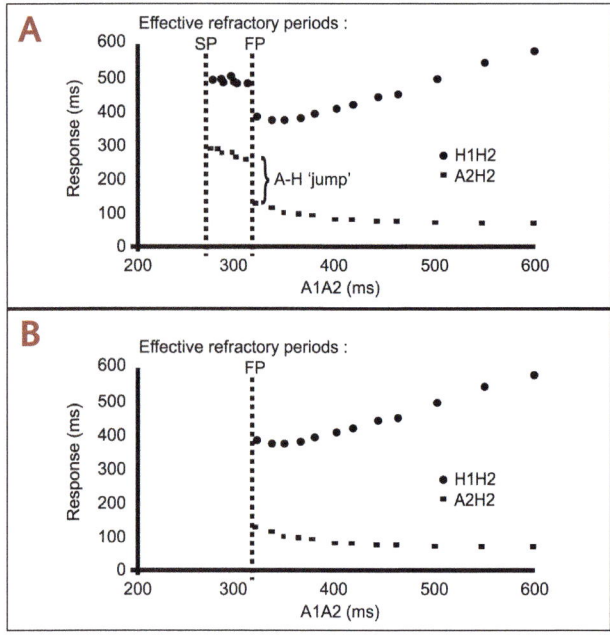

Figure 39.4 Antegrade conduction curves (**Panel A**) before ablation and (**Panel B**) after slow pathway ablation. The discontinuity in conduction curve was noted before ablation and disappeared after slow pathway ablation. FP = fast pathway; SP = slow pathway.

Diagnosis of AVNRT

AVNRT is diagnosed based on electrophysiological findings that include the following:

- No increase in the ventriculoatrial (VA) conduction interval during bundle branch block;

- Introduction of a single premature ventricular depolarization during the His refractory period that does not advance the atrial activation;

- No ventricular preexcitation during atrial pacing;

- Significant alternation of atrial activation with advancement of the time of retrograde His bundle activation; and

- Termination of tachycardia with VA block using ventricular extrastimulation.[50,59]

Traditionally, AVNRT has been categorized into typical or atypical subtypes. The classification of AVNRT is based on the anatomic site of earliest retrograde conduction as well as the ratio of atrio-Hisian/Hisio-atrial conduction time. Typical AVNRT (which accounts for 90% of patients with AVNRT) features anterograde conduction via a slow pathway and retrograde conduction via a fast pathway: so-called slow–fast AVNRT. Therefore, in typical AVNRT, the earliest retrograde atrial activation is usually identified in the anteroseptal region, in the vicinity of the His bundle recording (Figure 39.5).

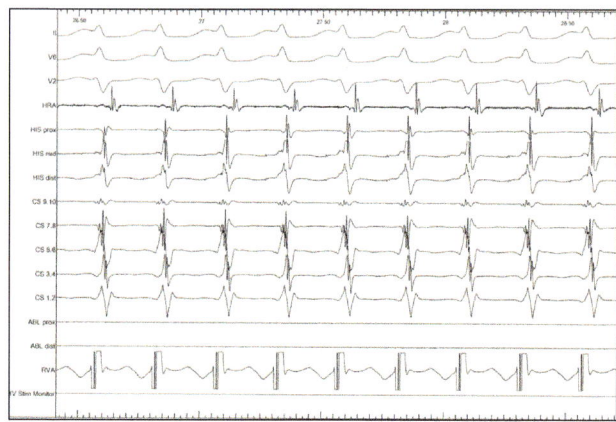

Figure 39.5 Intracardiac electrograms of typical AVNRT. Notice the concentric retrograde atrial activation and short ventriculoatrial interval during typical slow–fast AVNRT. The earliest atrial retrograde activation is noted in the distal His bundle electrogram.

In contrast, atypical AVNRT has anterograde conduction through a fast or slow pathway and retrograde conduction through a slow pathway (so-called fast–slow or slow–slow variants). Atypical AVNRT is also characterized by a longer Hisio-atrial interval during ventricular pacing than typical AVNRT and can be classified into two types: inferior and superior.[60] The inferior type, which accounts for more than 80% of patients with atypical AVNRT, exhibits earliest retrograde atrial activation at the inferoseptal right atrium or proximal CS, whereas the superior-type exhibits the earliest retrograde atrial activation at the right superior septum.[61] The retrograde slow pathway with a superoseptal exit has been described as exhibiting decremental conduction properties during ventricular pacing, and differs from the retrograde fast pathway, which usually exhibits little decremental properties.[62,63] In addition, the Wenckebach cycle length of the retrograde slow pathway that has a superoseptal atrial exit is significantly shorter than that of the retrograde slow pathway with an inferoseptal atrial exit. This difference in cycle length may reflect the heterogeneous electrophysiological properties of the anatomic substrates that are responsible for the retrograde slow pathway conduction with different atrial exits.[61]

Catheter Ablation for AVNRT

Catheter modification of the AV node has become the treatment of choice for drug-refractory AVNRT. The selective ablation of either retrograde fast pathway or slow pathway AVNRT has been studied. However, owing to the higher incidence of complete AV block after fast pathway ablation, ablation of the slow pathway has become the preferred technique. Several approaches have been taken for ablation of the antegrade slow pathway. These include an electrophysiological approach, an anatomic approach, and most commonly, a combination of both methods.

The Electrophysiological Approach

The electrophysiological approach uses electrogram patterns (commonly referred to as slow pathway potentials) as a guide for ablation. The slow pathway potentials have been variously described in the literature as the sharp potential[64] and the slow potential (Figure 39.6).[65] The slow potential can be recorded in the mid- or posterior septum, anterior to CS; in contrast, the sharp potential is recorded more posteriorly, around the CS ostium, and inferior to the ostium.

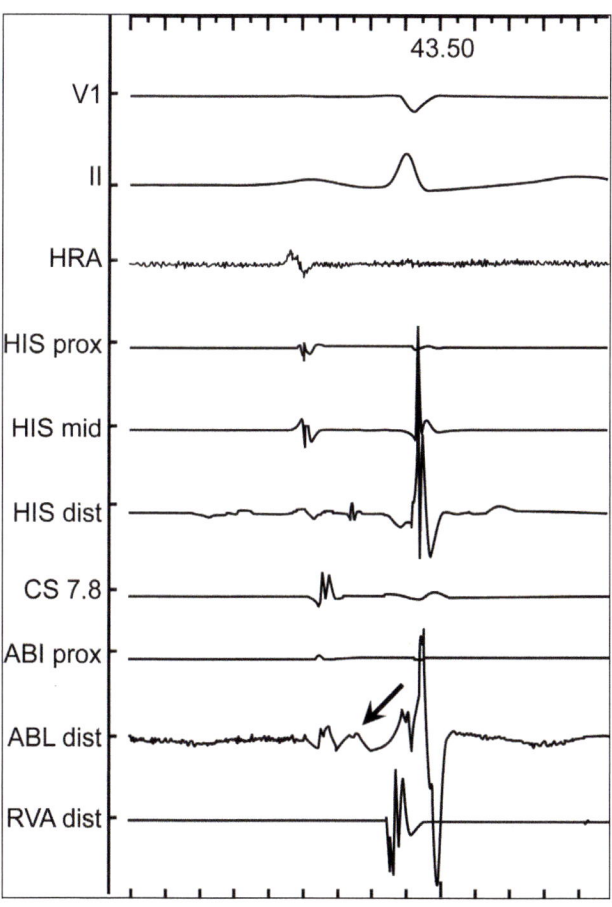

Figure 39.6 The slow pathway potentials. Note the slow potential (**arrow**) recorded from the ablation catheter placed at the posterior septum, anterior to the coronary sinus (CS) ostium.

It has been suggested that the slow potential represents the activation of posterior transitional cells and the posterior extension of the AV node, both of which correspond to the substrate of the slow AV nodal pathway. In contrast, the sharp potential seems to represent the activation of atrial fibers both above and below the CS ostium, which connect to the transitional cells approaching the posterior extension to the AV node.[64,66] It should be emphasized that the slow pathway potentials are *not* specific to individuals with AVNRT. Rather, the prevalence of slow pathway potentials recorded in the posteroseptal area did not differ between patients with or without AVNRT. Furthermore, the slow pathway potentials can be found outside Koch's triangle, along the tricuspid annulus, and may occur in regions of the right atrium.[67] Nevertheless, slow pathway potentials have been reportedly recorded at the successful ablation site in more than 90% of the patients.[64,65]

The Anatomic Approach

The other ablation method is the anatomic approach, in which the site of ablation is selected mainly on the basis of anatomic criteria.[68,69] In our laboratory, we suggest the sequential ablation sites, which start from the isthmus between the tricuspid annulus and the CS ostium (the usual site of slow pathway). They then proceed along the tricuspid edge of the CS ostium by moving the ablation catheter tip slightly in and out of the CS, the septum lower than CS ostium, moving higher up on the half of Koch's triangle along the septum, and applying one or two burns inside the first few centimeters of the CS and the left side of the septum (▶ Video 39.1). The presumed ablation site is considered optimal if the bipolar electrograms obtained from the distal electrodes show an AV ratio of 0.1–0.5 or a possible slow pathway potential.

Measures of Success

Previous studies have demonstrated similar high success rates and low incidence of AV block using both anatomic and electrophysiological approaches.[64,68] Notably, posterior displacement of the fast pathway has been observed in some patients. This effect was identified by early activation of the posteroseptal or midseptal region during retrograde fast pathway conduction in typical AVNRT. This variation is associated with a high risk of AV block during ablation in the posteroseptal region.[56]

Although patients with the atypical (fast–slow and slow–slow) forms of AVNRT have different electrophysiological characteristics from those with typical (slow–fast) AVNRT,[60] the ablation approach does not differ much. In patients with inferior type of atypical AVNRT, placing the radiofrequency catheter ablation at the inferoseptal right atrium or proximal CS (retrograde slow pathway) is well tolerated and effective in eliminating the retrograde slow pathway.[59] On the contrary, in those with superior-type AVNRT, conventional slow pathway ablation at the right inferior septum is usually ineffective. Otomo et al showed that ablation at the right midseptum, at a distance from the earliest retrograde atrial activation site, successfully eliminated tachycardia inducibility in 7 out of 9 (78%) patients with superior-type AVNRT. The success of ablation at the right midseptum (not at the superoseptum, where the earliest retrograde atrial activation was recorded) may have resulted from partial damage to the retrograde slow pathway.[61]

The presence of junctional rhythm has been considered to be a sensitive marker of successful slow pathway ablation. It is present in more than 90% of successful ablation sites. The junctional rhythm is more rapid at the anterior part of the node and less rapid at the posterior part. In rare cases, junctional rhythm is absent despite multiple radiofrequency applications delivered over a large area in Koch's triangle, and successful ablation can be achieved in the absence of a junctional rhythm. Our previous study showed that patients without junctional rhythm during successful slow pathway ablation had several characteristics: predominantly posterior locations of the ablation site, larger atrial-to-ventricular electrogram amplitude ratio, shorter duration of the atrial electrogram, and a lower incidence of a multicomponent or slow pathway potential than patients with junctional rhythm.[70]

As soon as junctional acceleration is observed during radiofrequency energy delivery, the ablation should be continued for a total of 45 to 60 seconds. Vigilant surveillance of the atrio-Hisian interval should continue during rapid atrial pacing.[71]

It is well established that, to manage the arrhythmia substrates, radiofrequency energy causes heat-induced tissue necrosis. Therefore, inadequate temperatures for heating tissue will lead to unsuccessful ablation. However, target temperatures greater than 50°C may not provide additional benefit, and the relatively low temperature required for successful slow pathway ablation may help to limit lesion size and the occurrence of complete AV block.[72,73] Therefore, careful power titration with automatic power adjustment is useful for achieving the predetermined target temperature and preventing such a complication. Subthreshold stimulation, delivered to the slow pathway region that terminates AVNRT, can safely and effectively guide slow pathway ablation.[74,75]

Complications of AVNRT Ablation

The success rate of slow pathway ablation is high; even so, transient or complete heart block requiring permanent pacing still occurs occasionally. The incidence rate is reportedly higher in patients with abnormal AV node anatomy node, especially if they also have posterior displacement of the fast pathway or compact AV node.[56,57] The occurrence of junctional rhythm with VA block during energy delivery usually predicts impending AV block after slow pathway ablation. Therefore, energy delivery should be terminated immediately as soon as VA block occurs. Nevertheless, previous study has suggested that, in patients with atypical AVNRT, junctional rhythm with VA block is not associated with a risk of impending AV block; instead, it may indicate the successful elimination of retrograde slow pathway conduction.[76]

In addition, ablation to avoid a short stimulation–His bundle interval (fast pathway area) by pace mapping Koch's triangle may reduce the risk of complete AV block.[77,78] However, this method is time consuming and depends on the pacing output and tissue contact of the ablation catheter. One recent study has shown that ablation at the target sites where the duration between the earliest atrial deflection on the His bundle electrogram and the beginning of the atrial signal on the distal ablation catheter is longer than 20 ms (reflecting electrical distance between ablation catheter and His bundle) can avoid permanently damaging AV conduction.[79]

Apart from ablation-induced permanent AV block, there have been reports of inappropriate sinus tachycardia[11,13] and postural orthostatic tachycardia syndrome (POTS)[80] as complications of successful radiofrequency catheter ablation of AVNRT. The mechanisms by which these complications occur are not well understood. However, it has been suggested that slow pathway ablation can damage the vagal fibers supplying the sinoatrial and AV nodal area, resulting in disruption of normal autonomic regulation.[11,13,80]

Cryoablation of AVNRT

Although the risk for AV block is very small during ablation procedures for AVNRT, it is considered a severe and devastating condition owing to the young age of the patients and the benign nature of the arrhythmia. Therefore, cryoenergy application was developed to avoid this complication. The main advantage of cryoablation is that, unlike radiofrequency energy ablation, it can create a lesion that is initially reversible and may prevent the complication of complete heart block. Although transient PR prolongation and 2:1 AV block were occasionally observed during cryoablation, complete recovery of AV nodal conduction resumed upon rewarming, possibly because the AV node was particularly resistant to cryothermal injury.[81,82] Also, because junctional rhythm occurs during radiofrequency ablation as a result of thermal injury to the slow pathway, during cryoablation, no junctional rhythm is observed.[83] Several studies have demonstrated that, in patients with AVNRT, cryoablation has a similarly high success rate but is associated with a significantly higher recurrence rate than ablation with radiofrequency energy. Thus, considering the very low incidence of permanent AV block using either energy form, the high recurrence rate after cryoablation may limit its use in AVNRT ablation.[84-86]

Endpoints of AVNRT Ablation

The well-accepted endpoint of AVNRT ablation is noninducibility of AVNRT and the abolition of dual-AV node physiology. However, modification of the slow pathway conduction properties with no more than one echo beat is considered an acceptable endpoint (Figure 39.7). In some patients in the electrophysiological laboratory, tachycardia may not be readily initiated using programmed stimulation alone in the baseline state, so administration of drugs (such as isoproterenol or atropine) to increase autonomic tone may be required.

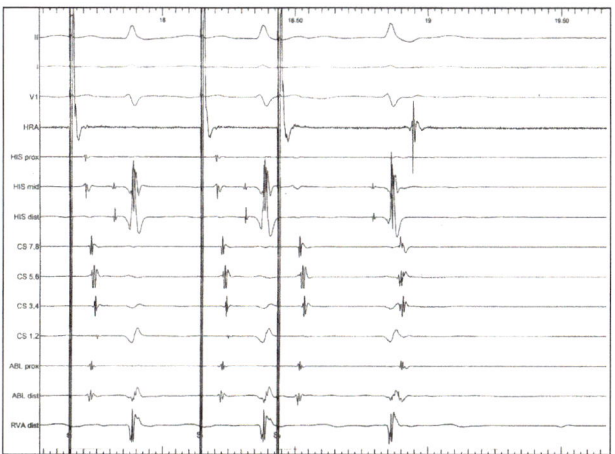

Figure 39.7 The presence of one slow–fast echo beat after modification of slow pathway. It is considered an acceptable ablation endpoint if no sustained tachycardia is inducible.

Previous studies have demonstrated that isoproterenol facilitates the initiation of AVNRT by shortening the refractory period of the retrograde fast pathway while prolonging antegrade slow pathway conduction.[87] Isoproterenol can be especially helpful for initiating tachycardia in patients without baseline VA conduction.[88] Nevertheless, in some patients, AVNRT cannot be reproducibly initiated despite administering isoproterenol with or without atropine. Frequently, this is because of mechanical trauma to the slow pathway during catheter manipulation around the CS ostium. In this case, the endpoint of noninducibility of AVNRT is difficult to establish. Hence, the elimination of dual-AV nodal physiology may be necessary to prevent recurrences.[89-91] In rare cases of scarcely inducible AVNRT and absent dual-AV nodal physiology, an alternative endpoint must be used. Alternative indications of successful ablation include (1) disappearance of a PR:RR ratio greater than 1 during atrial pacing at the maximum rate of 1:1 AV conduction; (2) modification of Wenckebach cycle length; and (3) shortening of the fast pathway's effective refractory period.[92]

Dual-AV nodal physiology may persist in some patients even after successful ablation of AVNRT. The electrophysiological characteristics after slow pathway modification with a preserved slow pathway include lengthening of the Wenckebach cycle length, eliminating the longest atrio-Hisian intervals,[93] decreasing the window of cycle length with 1:1 slow pathway conduction and an effective refractory period (ERP),[94] and decreasing the number of consecutive beats with conduction over the slow pathway before a final beat is blocked.[92] Previous study has demonstrated that persistent dual-AV nodal physiology (with or without echo beats) is not associated with higher recurrence rates of AVNRT than complete elimination of dual-AV nodal physiology, that is, if AVNRT remained noninducible with or without isoproterenol administration.[95]

Unusual Manifestations of AVNRT

AVNRT with Eccentric Retrograde Coronary Sinus Activation

AVNRT with eccentric retrograde CS activation consists of typical or atypical AVNRT whose earliest retrograde atrial activation is recorded within the CS distal to the ostium (Figure 39.8). In several previous reports, eccentric retrograde coronary activation has been demonstrated to occur in 6% to 8% of patients.[96,97] In this group, the tachycardia circuit may involve the left posterior nodal extension, in which case a left-sided ablative procedure is occasionally needed.[97-102] Nevertheless, a standard right atrial approach can successfully ablate AVNRT in most patients with eccentric retrograde coronary sinus activation.[96,103-105]

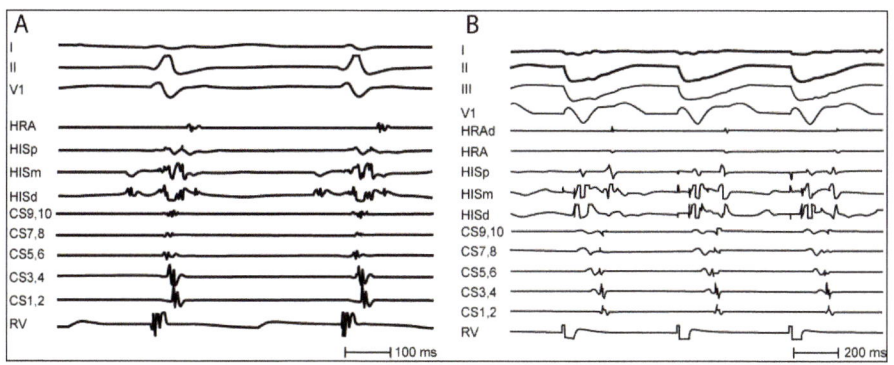

Figure 39.8 Intracardiac tracings of eccentric typical AVNRT. **Panel A:** The earliest atrial activation at coronary sinus (CS) 5,6 is noted during AVNRT. **Panel B:** right ventricular (RV) pacing before ablation shows earliest retrograde atrial activation at CS 5,6. *Source:* Adapted with permission from Ong MG, et al.[105]

A previous study from our group showed that, in all patients with eccentric retrograde atrial activation, the usual successful ablation site was located at the slow pathway on the right atrial septum. However, another study demonstrated that, in some patients, ablation targeting the earliest retrograde atrial activation inside the CS was necessary.[100,102] We found that, among patients with retrograde eccentric CS conduction, there were more females and cases of atypical AVNRT. In addition, more VA block occurred after ablation and tachycardia induction by right ventricular pacing/extrastimuli in eccentric rather than in concentric retrograde atrial activation. A shorter antegrade fast functional refractory period of the AV node was demonstrated in the atypical eccentric group as compared with the atypical concentric group. The mechanism for the retrograde left atrial exit has been unknown until now. It could be the result of nodal extensions, multiple atrionodal connections or anisotropic conduction (or both), nodal-type tissue around the mitral annulus, or the myocardial connections between left atrium and CS musculature.[56,96,101-106]

AVNRT with Multiple AV Nodal Pathways

Dual-AV nodal pathway physiology can be demonstrated in the vast majority of patients with inducible AVNRT. However, in some patients with AVNRT, multiple anterograde and retrograde AV nodal pathways with multiple discontinuities in the AV nodal function curve were observed.[50,59] The multiple anterograde AV nodal pathways were defined by AV nodal conduction curves with two or more discontinuities. We found that the incidence of triple anterograde pathways and quadruple anterograde pathways was 4.2% and 1%, respectively. Compared with patients with dual anterograde AV nodal pathways, those with multiple anterograde AV nodal pathways had a longer tachycardia cycle length, longer effective and functional refractory periods of the anterograde fast pathway, poorer retrograde VA conduction properties, and a higher incidence of multiple types of AVNRT.[50]

Regarding the multiple retrograde AV nodal pathways, we demonstrated that, among 550 consecutive patients with AVNRT, 11 (2%) had triple retrograde AV nodal pathways that consisted of fast, intermediate, and slow AV nodal pathways.[59] The retrograde fast pathway was defined when the earliest retrograde atrial activation was recorded at the His bundle area and revealed little or no decremental conduction during ventricular extrastimulus testing. The retrograde intermediate pathway was defined when the earliest retrograde atrial activation was recorded at the CS ostium (or simultaneously at the His bundle area and at the CS ostium) and revealed minimal degree of decremental conduction during ventricular extrastimulus testing. The retrograde slow pathway was defined as the retrograde conduction that occurred after a sudden increment of VA conduction time greater than 50 ms. In this pathway, the earliest retrograde atrial activation from the His bundle area shifted to the CS ostium in response to changes in cycle length or coupling interval and revealed decremental conduction.

Among the 11 patients with triple retrograde AV nodal pathways observed in our laboratory, only 1 patient had triple anterograde AV nodal pathways. Also, of 26 patients with multiple anterograde AV nodal pathways, only 1 had triple retrograde AV nodal pathways. It is still controversial whether multiple anterograde and retrograde AV nodal pathways originate from anatomically different pathways or from anisotropic conduction–induced functional pathways. Regarding these anatomically different pathways, the proximal AV node may include several pathways with varying lengths and electrophysiological properties when one considers its complex histology.[107,108] In contrast, the marked heterogeneity of the transitional cells and their connections produces a nonuniform structure. It is therefore conceivable that the nonuniform properties of the AV node can produce both anterograde and retrograde anisotropic conduction and longitudinal dissociation.[32]

We explored the possible anatomic site of the multiple anterograde and retrograde AV nodal pathways. We did so by using the stepwise upward method for mapping and ablation along the right atrial septum adjacent to the septal leaflet of the tricuspid valve, extending from the CS ostium to the recording site at the His bundle area. Among 21 patients with triple antegrade AV nodal pathways, 10 patients had 2 anterograde slow pathways simultaneously eliminated at a single ablation site; the other patients had either 2 anterograde slow pathways eliminated separately at different ablation sites or 1 residual slow pathway eliminated after ablation at a single or different ablation sites. Among 8 patients with retrograde dual-AV nodal pathways, 6 had anterograde and retrograde slow pathways simultaneously eliminated at a single ablation site; the other 2 patients had anterograde and retrograde slow pathways eliminated separately at different ablation sites. The requirement of performing ablation at different sites to eliminate different pathways can be explained by the presence of anatomically different anterograde or retrograde multiple pathways. In addition, we observed that the slow pathways with much longer functional refractory periods were located at a more inferior–posterior area in Koch's triangle. On the other hand, for the patients who had successful ablation of multiple anterograde or retrograde slow pathways at a single site, anisotropic conduction over the low septal area of the right atrium could explain the presence of multiple anterograde and retrograde AV nodal pathways.

AVNRT with Continuous AV Nodal Function Curves

Although dual-AV nodal physiology is recommended as a substrate for AVNRT, some patients with AVNRT may have continuous atrio-Hisian conduction curves. These curves are missing an atrio-Hisian jump after applying 2 extrastimuli and 2 driven cycle lengths during atrial pacing from the high right atrium and CS ostium.[109] Several possible mechanisms explain the continuous AV node function curve in AVNRT. First, the functional refractory period of the atrium limits the prematurity with which atrial premature depolarization encounters the effective refractory period of the AV node, which produces inability to dissociate the fast and slow AV nodal pathways. Second, the refractory periods of the fast and slow pathways may be similar, and therefore, faster atrial pacing rates, multiple atrial extrastimuli, or administration of drugs such as propranolol, verapamil, or digoxin may be required to dissociate them.[110-112] Third, the difference in conduction time between the fast and slow pathways may be too minimal.[54,113] In patients with a continuous atrio-Hisian conduction curve, a significant shortening of the maximal atrio-Hisian interval during atrial pacing after radiofrequency ablation suggests that AVNRT has been successfully eliminated.

AVNRT with Preexisting Prolonged PR Interval

In previously reported series, AVNRT was associated with preexisting prolonged PR interval in 2% to 3% of the patients referred for AVNRT ablation.[114-117] Both slow pathway ablation in patients with dual-pathway physiology, and retrograde fast pathway ablation in patients without dual-pathway physiology, were effective and well tolerated in patients with a prolonged PR interval.[118] However, slow pathway ablation was associated with a significant risk of a delayed higher-degree AV block in patients who had AVNRT and a prolonged PR interval at baseline.[117] In contrast, in patients with a first-degree AV block without demonstrable dual-pathway physiology, retrograde fast pathway ablation was associated with a higher intraprocedural risk of complete AV block but did not result in the development of higher-degree AV block during long-term follow-up.[119,120] Furthermore, after completely eliminating the slow pathway, the shortening of anterograde fast pathway ERP and shortest 1:1 conduction cycle length were greater in patients with a long–fast pathway ERP.[121] Therefore, in such cases, long-term follow-up is necessary in order to detect delayed higher-degree AV block.

References

1. Spodick DH. Normal sinus heart rate: sinus tachycardia and sinus bradycardia redefined. *Am Heart J.* 1992;124(4):1119-1121.
2. Boineau JP, Canavan TE, Schuessler RB, et al. Demonstration of a widely distributed atrial pacemaker complex in the human heart. *Circulation.* 1988;77(6):1221-1237.
3. Boineau JP, Schuessler RB, Hackel DB, et al. Widespread distribution and rate differentiation of the atrial pacemaker complex. *Am J Physiol.* 1980;239(3):H406-H415.
4. Boineau JP, Schuessler RB, Mooney CR, et al. Multicentric origin of the atrial depolarization wave: the pacemaker complex. Relation to dynamics of atrial conduction, P-wave changes and heart rate control. *Circulation.* 1978;58(6):1036-1048.
5. Sanchez-Quintana D, Cabrera JA, Farre J, et al. Sinus node revisited in the era of electroanatomical mapping and catheter ablation. *Heart.* 2005;91(2):189-194.
6. Petrescu CI, Niculescu V, Ionescu N, et al. Considerations on the sinus node microangioarchitecture. *Rom J Morphol Embryol.* 2006;47(1):59-61.
7. Krahn AD, Yee R, Klein GJ, Morillo C. Inappropriate sinus tachycardia: evaluation and therapy. *J Cardiovasc Electrophysiol.* 1995;6(12):1124-1128.
8. Cossu SF, Steinberg JS. Supraventricular tachyarrhythmias involving the sinus node: clinical and electrophysiologic characteristics. *Prog Cardiovasc Dis.* 1998;41(1):51-63.
9. Castellanos A, Moleiro F, Chakko S, et al. Heart rate variability in inappropriate sinus tachycardia. *Am J Cardiol.* 1998;82(4):531-534.
10. Bauernfeind RA, Amat YLF, Dhingra RC, et al. Chronic nonparoxysmal sinus tachycardia in otherwise healthy persons. *Ann Intern Med.* 1979;91(5):702-710.
11. Guo H, Wang P, Xing Y, et al. Delayed injury of autonomic nerve induced by radiofrequency catheter ablation. *J Electrocardiol.* 2007;40(4):355 e351-e354.
12. Pappone C, Stabile G, Oreto G, et al. Inappropriate sinus tachycardia after radiofrequency ablation of para-Hisian accessory pathways. *J Cardiovasc Electrophysiol.* 1997;8(12):1357-1365.
13. Skeberis V, Simonis F, Tsakonas K, et al. Inappropriate sinus tachycardia following radiofrequency ablation of AV nodal tachycardia: incidence and clinical significance. *Pacing Clin Electrophysiol.* 1994;17(5 Pt 1):924-927.
14. Shen WK. How to manage patients with inappropriate sinus tachycardia. *Heart Rhythm.* 2005;2(9):1015-1019.
15. Lee RJ, Kalman JM, Fitzpatrick AP, et al. Radiofrequency catheter modification of the sinus node for "inappropriate" sinus tachycardia. *Circulation.* 1995;92(10):2919-2928.
16. Kalman JM, Lee RJ, Fisher WG, et al. Radiofrequency catheter modification of sinus pacemaker function guided by intracardiac echocardiography. *Circulation.* 1995;92(10):3070-3081.
17. Jayaprakash S, Sparks PB, Vohra J. Inappropriate sinus tachycardia (IST): management by radiofrequency modification of sinus node. *Aust N Z J Med.* 1997;27(4):391-397.
18. Man KC, Knight B, Tse HF, et al. Radiofrequency catheter ablation of inappropriate sinus tachycardia guided by activation mapping. *J Am Coll Cardiol.* 2000;35(2):451-457.
19. Marrouche NF, Beheiry S, Tomassoni G, et al. Three-dimensional nonfluoroscopic mapping and ablation of inappropriate sinus tachycardia. Procedural strategies and long-term outcome. *J Am Coll Cardiol.* 2002;39(6):1046-1054.
20. Shen WK, Low PA, Jahangir A, et al. Is sinus node modification appropriate for inappropriate sinus tachycardia with features of postural orthostatic tachycardia syndrome? *Pacing Clin Electrophysiol.* 2001;24(2):217-230.

21. Boyett MR, Honjo H, Kodama I. The sinoatrial node, a heterogeneous pacemaker structure. *Cardiovasc Res.* 2000;47(4):658-687.
22. Dobrzynski H, Li J, Tellez J, et al. Computer three-dimensional reconstruction of the sinoatrial node. *Circulation.* 2005;111(7):846-854.
23. Lin D, Garcia F, Jacobson J, et al. Use of noncontact mapping and saline-cooled ablation catheter for sinus node modification in medically refractory inappropriate sinus tachycardia. *Pacing Clin Electrophysiol.* 2007;30(2):236-242.
24. Koplan BA, Parkash R, Couper G, Stevenson WG. Combined epicardial–endocardial approach to ablation of inappropriate sinus tachycardia. *J Cardiovasc Electrophysiol.* 2004;15(2):237-240.
25. Callans DJ, Ren JF, Schwartzman D, et al. Narrowing of the superior vena cava–right atrium junction during radiofrequency catheter ablation for inappropriate sinus tachycardia: analysis with intracardiac echocardiography. *J Am Coll Cardiol.* 1999;33(6):1667-1670.
26. Durante-Mangoni E, Del Vecchio D, Ruggiero G. Right diaphragm paralysis following cardiac radiofrequency catheter ablation for inappropriate sinus tachycardia. *Pacing Clin Electrophysiol.* 2003;26(3):783-784.
27. Vatasescu R, Shalganov T, Kardos A, et al. Right diaphragmatic paralysis following endocardial cryothermal ablation of inappropriate sinus tachycardia. *Europace.* 2006;8(10):904-906.
28. Rubenstein JC, Kim MH, Jacobson JT. A novel method for sinus node modification and phrenic nerve protection in resistant cases. *J Cardiovasc Electrophysiol.* 2009;20(6):689-691.
29. Gomes JA, Mehta D, Langan MN. Sinus node reentrant tachycardia. *Pacing Clin Electrophysiol.* 1995;18(5 Pt 1):1045-1057.
30. Weisfogel GM, Batsford WP, Paulay KL, et al. Sinus node re-entrant tachycardia in man. *Am Heart J.* 1975;90(3):295-304.
31. Spach MS, Dolber PC, Heidlage JF. Interaction of inhomogeneities of repolarization with anisotropic propagation in dog atria. A mechanism for both preventing and initiating reentry. *Circ Res.* 1989;65(6):1612-1631.
32. Spach MS, Josephson ME. Initiating reentry: the role of nonuniform anisotropy in small circuits. *J Cardiovasc Electrophysiol.* 1994;5(2):182-209.
33. Gomes JA, Hariman RJ, Kang PS, Chowdry IH. Sustained symptomatic sinus node reentrant tachycardia: incidence, clinical significance, electrophysiologic observations and the effects of antiarrhythmic agents. *J Am Coll Cardiol.* 1985;5(1):45-57.
34. Engelstein ED, Lippman N, Stein KM, Lerman BB. Mechanism-specific effects of adenosine on atrial tachycardia. *Circulation.* 1994;89(6):2645-2654.
35. Kay GN, Chong F, Epstein AE, et al. Radiofrequency ablation for treatment of primary atrial tachycardias. *J Am Coll Cardiol.* 1993;21(4):901-909.
36. Sperry RE, Ellenbogen KA, Wood MA, et al. Radiofrequency catheter ablation of sinus node reentrant tachycardia. *Pacing Clin Electrophysiol.* 1993;16(11):2202-2209.
37. Sanders WE Jr, Sorrentino RA, Greenfield RA, et al. Catheter ablation of sinoatrial node reentrant tachycardia. *J Am Coll Cardiol.* 1994;23(4):926-934.
38. Ivanov MY, Evdokimov VP, Vlasenco VV. Predictors of successful radiofrequency catheter ablation of sinoatrial tachycardia. *Pacing Clin Electrophysiol.* 1998;21(1 Pt 2):311-315.
39. Ho SY, Anderson RH. How constant anatomically is the tendon of Todaro as a marker for the triangle of Koch? *J Cardiovasc Electrophysiol.* 2000;11(1):83-89.
40. Lev M, Widran J, Erickson EE. A method for the histopathologic study of the atrioventricular node, bundle, and branches. *AMA Arch Pathol.* 1951;52(1):73-83.
41. Widran J, Lev M. The dissection of the atrioventricular node, bundle and bundle branches in the human heart. *Circulation.* 1951;4(6):863-867.
42. Langberg JJ, Leon A, Borganelli M, et al. A randomized, prospective comparison of anterior and posterior approaches to radiofrequency catheter ablation of atrioventricular nodal reentry tachycardia. *Circulation.* 1993;87(5):1551-1556.
43. Kay GN, Epstein AE, Dailey SM, Plumb VJ. Selective radiofrequency ablation of the slow pathway for the treatment of atrioventricular nodal reentrant tachycardia. Evidence for involvement of perinodal myocardium within the reentrant circuit. *Circulation.* 1992;85(5):1675-1688.
44. Hummel JD, Strickberger SA, Man KC, et al. A quantitative fluoroscopic comparison of the coronary sinus ostium in patients with and without AV nodal reentrant tachycardia. *J Cardiovasc Electrophysiol.* 1995;6(9):681-686.
45. Ueng KC, Chen SA, Chiang CE, et al. Dimension and related anatomical distance of Koch's triangle in patients with atrioventricular nodal reentrant tachycardia. *J Cardiovasc Electrophysiol.* 1996;7(11):1017-1023.
46. Doig JC, Saito J, Harris L, Downar E. Coronary sinus morphology in patients with atrioventricular junctional reentry tachycardia and other supraventricular tachyarrhythmias. *Circulation.* 1995;92(3):436-441.
47. Okumura Y, Watanabe I, Yamada T, et al. Comparison of coronary sinus morphology in patients with and without atrioventricular nodal reentrant tachycardia by intracardiac echocardiography. *J Cardiovasc Electrophysiol.* 2004;15(3):269-273.
48. Ong MG, Lee PC, Tai CT, et al. Coronary sinus morphology in different types of supraventricular tachycardias. *J Interv Card Electrophysiol.* 2006;15(1):21-26.
49. Anderson RH, Ho SY. The architecture of the sinus node, the atrioventricular conduction axis, and the internodal atrial myocardium. *J Cardiovasc Electrophysiol.* 1998;9(11):1233-1248.
50. Tai CT, Chen SA, Chiang CE, et al. Multiple anterograde atrioventricular node pathways in patients with atrioventricular node reentrant tachycardia. *J Am Coll Cardiol.* 1996;28(3):725-731.
51. McGuire MA, Bourke JP, Robotin MC, et al. High resolution mapping of Koch's triangle using sixty electrodes in humans with atrioventricular junctional (AV nodal) reentrant tachycardia. *Circulation.* 1993;88(5 Pt 1):2315-2328.
52. Hocini M, Loh P, Ho SY, et al. Anisotropic conduction in the triangle of Koch of mammalian hearts: electrophysiologic and anatomic correlations. *J Am Coll Cardiol.* 1998;31(3):629-636.
53. McGuire MA, de Bakker JM, Vermeulen JT, et al. Atrioventricular junctional tissue. Discrepancy between histological and electrophysiological characteristics. *Circulation.* 1996;94(3):571-577.
54. McGuire MA, Robotin M, Yip AS, et al. Electrophysiologic and histologic effects of dissection of the connections between the atrium and posterior part of the atrioventricular node. *J Am Coll Cardiol.* 1994;23(3):693-701.
55. Inoue S, Becker AE. Posterior extensions of the human compact atrioventricular node: a neglected anatomic feature of potential clinical significance. *Circulation.* 1998;97(2):188-193.
56. Engelstein ED, Stein KM, Markowitz SM, Lerman BB. Posterior fast atrioventricular node pathways: implications for radiofrequency catheter ablation of atrioventricular node reentrant tachycardia. *J Am Coll Cardiol.* 1996;27(5):1098-1105.
57. Lee PC, Tai CT, Lin YJ, et al. Noncontact three-dimensional mapping guides catheter ablation of difficult atrioventricular nodal reentrant tachycardia. *Int J Cardiol.* 2007;118(2):154-163.
58. Sanchez-Quintana D, Davies DW, Ho SY, et al. Architecture of the atrial musculature in and around the triangle of Koch:

its potential relevance to atrioventricular nodal reentry. *J Cardiovasc Electrophysiol*. 1997;8(12):1396-1407.
59. Tai CT, Chen SA, Chiang CE, et al. Electrophysiologic characteristics and radiofrequency catheter ablation in patients with multiple atrioventricular nodal reentry tachycardias. *Am J Cardiol*. 1996;77(1):52-58.
60. Lee PC, Hwang B, Tai CT, et al. The specific electrophysiologic characteristics in children with the atypical forms of atrioventricular nodal reentrant tachycardia. *Cardiology*. 2007;108(4):351-357.
61. Otomo K, Nagata Y, Taniguchi H, et al. Superior type of atypical AV nodal reentrant tachycardia: incidence, characteristics, and effect of slow pathway ablation. *Pacing Clin Electrophysiol*. 2008;31(8):998-1009.
62. Heidbuchel H, Jackman WM. Characterization of subforms of AV nodal reentrant tachycardia. *Europace*. 2004;6(4):316-329.
63. Otomo K, Suyama K, Okamura H, et al. Participation of a concealed atrio-Hisian tract in the reentrant circuit of the slow-fast type of atrioventricular nodal reentrant tachycardia. *Heart Rhythm*. 2007;4(6):703-710.
64. Jackman WM, Beckman KJ, McClelland JH, et al. Treatment of supraventricular tachycardia due to atrioventricular nodal reentry, by radiofrequency catheter ablation of slow-pathway conduction. *N Engl J Med*. 1992;327(5):313-318.
65. Haïssaguerre M, Gaita F, Fischer B, et al. Elimination of atrioventricular nodal reentrant tachycardia using discrete slow potentials to guide application of radiofrequency energy. *Circulation*. 1992;85(6):2162-2175.
66. McGuire MA, de Bakker JM, Vermeulen JT, et al. Origin and significance of double potentials near the atrioventricular node. Correlation of extracellular potentials, intracellular potentials, and histology. *Circulation*. 1994;89(5):2351-2360.
67. Niebauer MJ, Daoud E, Williamson B, et al. Atrial electrogram characteristics in patients with and without atrioventricular nodal reentrant tachycardia. *Circulation*. 1995;92(1):77-81.
68. Wathen M, Natale A, Wolfe K, et al. An anatomically guided approach to atrioventricular node slow pathway ablation. *Am J Cardiol*. 1992;70(9):886-889.
69. Jazayeri MR, Hempe SL, Sra JS, et al. Selective transcatheter ablation of the fast and slow pathways using radiofrequency energy in patients with atrioventricular nodal reentrant tachycardia. *Circulation*. 1992;85(4):1318-1328.
70. Hsieh MH, Chen SA, Tai CT, et al. Absence of junctional rhythm during successful slow-pathway ablation in patients with atrioventricular nodal reentrant tachycardia. *Circulation*. 1998;98(21):2296-2300.
71. Liberman L, Hordof AJ, Pass RH. Rapid atrial pacing: a useful technique during slow pathway ablation. *Pacing Clin Electrophysiol*. 2007;30(2):221-224.
72. Strickberger SA, Daoud EG, Weiss R, et al. A randomized comparison of fixed power and temperature monitoring during slow pathway ablation in patients with atrioventricular nodal reentrant tachycardia. *J Interv Card Electrophysiol*. 1997;1(4):299-303.
73. Strickberger SA, Zivin A, Daoud EG, et al. Temperature and impedance monitoring during slow pathway ablation in patients with AV nodal reentrant tachycardia. *J Cardiovasc Electrophysiol*. 1996;7(4):295-300.
74. Willems S, Rostock T, Shenasa M, et al. Sub-threshold stimulation in variants of atrioventricular nodal re-entrant tachycardia: electrophysiological effects and impact for guidance of slow pathway ablation. *Eur Heart J*. 2004;25(14):1249-1256.
75. Willems S, Weiss C, Hofmann T, et al. Subthreshold stimulation in the region of the slow pathway during atrioventricular node reentrant tachycardia: correlation with effect of radiofrequency catheter ablation. *J Am Coll Cardiol*. 1997;29(2):408-415.
76. Fujiki A, Sakamoto T, Sakabe M, et al. Junctional rhythm associated with ventriculoatrial block during slow pathway ablation in atypical atrioventricular nodal re-entrant tachycardia. *Europace*. 2008;10(8):982-987.
77. Delise P, Bonso A, Coro L, et al. Pace mapping of the triangle of Koch: a simple method to reduce the risk of atrioventricular block during radiofrequency ablation of atrioventricular node reentrant tachycardia. *Pacing Clin Electrophysiol*. 2001;24(12):1725-1731.
78. Delise P, Sitta N, Bonso A, et al. Pace mapping of Koch's triangle reduces risk of atrioventricular block during ablation of atrioventricular nodal reentrant tachycardia. *J Cardiovasc Electrophysiol*. 2005;16(1):30-35.
79. Stuhlinger MC, Etsadashvili K, Stuhlinger X, et al. Duration of the A(H)–A(Md) interval predicts occurrence of AV-block after radiofrequency ablation of the slow pathway. *J Interv Card Electrophysiol*. 2011;31(3):207-215.
80. Kanjwal K, Karabin B, Sheikh M, et al. New onset postural orthostatic tachycardia syndrome following ablation of AV node reentrant tachycardia. *J Interv Card Electrophysiol*. 2010;29(1):53-56.
81. Lemola K, Dubuc M, Khairy P. Transcatheter cryoablation part II: clinical utility. *Pacing Clin Electrophysiol*. 2008;31(2):235-244.
82. Skanes AC, Klein G, Krahn A, Yee R. Cryoablation: potentials and pitfalls. *J Cardiovasc Electrophysiol*. 2004;15(Suppl 10):S28-S34.
83. Skanes AC, Dubuc M, Klein GJ, et al. Cryothermal ablation of the slow pathway for the elimination of atrioventricular nodal reentrant tachycardia. *Circulation*. 2000;102(23):2856-2860.
84. Collins KK, Dubin AM, Chiesa NA, et al. Cryoablation versus radiofrequency ablation for treatment of pediatric atrioventricular nodal reentrant tachycardia: initial experience with 4-mm cryocatheter. *Heart Rhythm*. 2006;3(5):564-570.
85. Zrenner B, Dong J, Schreieck J, et al. Transvenous cryoablation versus radiofrequency ablation of the slow pathway for the treatment of atrioventricular nodal re-entrant tachycardia: a prospective randomized pilot study. *Eur Heart J*. 2004;25(24):2226-2231.
86. Deisenhofer I, Zrenner B, Yin YH, et al. Cryoablation versus radiofrequency energy for the ablation of atrioventricular nodal reentrant tachycardia (the CYRANO study): results from a large multicenter prospective randomized trial. *Circulation*. 2010;122(22):2239-2245.
87. Hatzinikolaou H, Rodriguez LM, Smeets JL, et al. Isoprenaline and inducibility of atrioventricular nodal re-entrant tachycardia. *Heart*. 1998;79(2):165-168.
88. Yu WC, Chen SA, Chiang CE, et al. Effects of isoproterenol in facilitating induction of slow-fast atrioventricular nodal reentrant tachycardia. *Am J Cardiol*. 1996;78(11):1299-1302.
89. Chen SA, Wu TJ, Chiang CE, et al. Recurrent tachycardia after selective ablation of slow pathway in patients with atrioventricular nodal reentrant tachycardia. *Am J Cardiol*. 1995;76(3):131-137.
90. Li HG, Klein GJ, Stites HW, et al. Elimination of slow pathway conduction: an accurate indicator of clinical success after radiofrequency atrioventricular node modification. *J Am Coll Cardiol*. 1993;22(7):1849-1853.
91. Kelly PA, Mann DE, Adler SW, et al. Predictors of successful radiofrequency ablation of extranodal slow pathways. *Pacing Clin Electrophysiol*. 1994;17(6):1143-1148.
92. Baker JH 2nd, Plumb VJ, Epstein AE, Kay GN. PR/RR interval ratio during rapid atrial pacing: a simple method for

confirming the presence of slow AV nodal pathway conduction. *J Cardiovasc Electrophysiol.* 1996;7(4):287-294.
93. Posan E, Gula LJ, Skanes AC, et al. Characteristics of slow pathway conduction after successful AVNRT ablation. *J Cardiovasc Electrophysiol.* 2006;17(8):847-851.
94. Kaltman JR, Rhodes LA, Wieand TS, et al. Slow pathway modification for atrioventricular nodal reentrant tachycardia. *Am J Cardiol.* 2004;94(10):1316-1319.
95. Khairy P, Novak PG, Guerra PG, et al. Cryothermal slow pathway modification for atrioventricular nodal reentrant tachycardia. *Europace.* 2007;9(10):909-914.
96. Chen J, Anselme F, Smith TW, et al. Standard right atrial ablation is effective for atrioventricular nodal reentry with earliest activation in the coronary sinus. *J Cardiovasc Electrophysiol.* 2004;15(1):2-7.
97. Hwang C, Martin DJ, Goodman JS, et al. Atypical atrioventricular node reciprocating tachycardia masquerading as tachycardia using a left-sided accessory pathway. *J Am Coll Cardiol.* 1997;30(1):218-225.
98. Gonzalez MD, Contreras LJ, Cardona F, et al. Demonstration of a left atrial input to the atrioventricular node in humans. *Circulation.* 2002;106(23):2930-2934.
99. Kilic A, Amasyali B, Kose S, et al. Atrioventricular nodal reentrant tachycardia ablated from left atrial septum: clinical and electrophysiological characteristics and long-term follow-up results as compared to conventional right-sided ablation. *Int Heart J.* 2005;46(6):1023-1031.
100. Otomo K, Okamura H, Noda T, et al. "Left-variant" atypical atrioventricular nodal reentrant tachycardia: electrophysiological characteristics and effect of slow pathway ablation within coronary sinus. *J Cardiovasc Electrophysiol.* 2006;17(11):1177-1183.
101. Nam GB, Rhee KS, Kim J, et al. Left atrionodal connections in typical and atypical atrioventricular nodal reentrant tachycardias: activation sequence in the coronary sinus and results of radiofrequency catheter ablation. *J Cardiovasc Electrophysiol.* 2006;17(2):171-177.
102. Otomo K, Nagata Y, Uno K, et al. Atypical atrioventricular nodal reentrant tachycardia with eccentric coronary sinus activation: electrophysiological characteristics and essential effects of left-sided ablation inside the coronary sinus. *Heart Rhythm.* 2007;4(4):421-432.
103. Jaïs P, Haïssaguerre M, Shah DC, et al. Successful radiofrequency ablation of a slow atrioventricular nodal pathway on the left posterior atrial septum. *Pacing Clin Electrophysiol.* 1999;22(3):525-527.
104. Sorbera C, Cohen M, Woolf P, Kalapatapu SR. Atrioventricular nodal reentry tachycardia: slow pathway ablation using the transseptal approach. *Pacing Clin Electrophysiol.* 2000;23(9):1343-1349.
105. Ong MG, Lee PC, Tai CT, et al. The electrophysiologic characteristics of atrioventricular nodal reentry tachycardia with eccentric retrograde activation. *Int J Cardiol.* 2007;120(1):115-122.
106. Chauvin M, Shah DC, Haïssaguerre M, et al. The anatomic basis of connections between the coronary sinus musculature and the left atrium in humans. *Circulation.* 2000;101(6):647-652.
107. Janse MJ, Anderson RH, McGuire MA, Ho SY. "AV nodal" reentry: Part I: "AV nodal" reentry revisited. *J Cardiovasc Electrophysiol.* 1993;4(5):561-572.
108. Sherf L, James TN, Woods WT. Function of the atrioventricular node considered on the basis of observed histology and fine structure. *J Am Coll Cardiol.* 1985;5(3):770-780.

109. Tai CT, Chen SA, Chiang CE, et al. Complex electrophysiological characteristics in atrioventricular nodal reentrant tachycardia with continuous atrioventricular node function curves. *Circulation.* 1997;95(11):2541-2547.
110. Wu D, Denes P, Dhingra R, et al. The effects of propranolol on induction of A-V nodal reentrant paroxysmal tachycardia. *Circulation.* 1974;50(4):665-677.
111. Spurrell RA, Krikler DM, Sowton E. Concealed bypasses of the atrioventricular mode in patients with paroxysmal supraventricular tachycardia revealed by intracardiac electrical stimulation and verapamil. *Am J Cardiol.* 1974;33(5):590-595.
112. Wellens HJ, Duren DR, Liem DL, Lie KI. Effect of digitalis in patients with paroxysmal atrioventricular nodal tachycardia. *Circulation.* 1975;52(5):779-788.
113. Wu D. A-V nodal re-entry. *Pacing Clin Electrophysiol.* 1983;6(5 Pt 2):1190-1200.
114. Sra JS, Jazayeri MR, Blanck Z, et al. Slow pathway ablation in patients with atrioventricular node reentrant tachycardia and a prolonged PR interval. *J Am Coll Cardiol.* 1994;24(4):1064-1068.
115. Reithmann C, Hoffmann E, Grunewald A, et al. Fast pathway ablation in patients with common atrioventricular nodal reentrant tachycardia and prolonged PR interval during sinus rhythm. *Eur Heart J.* 1998;19(6):929-935.
116. Verdino RJ, Burke MC, Kall JG, et al. Retrograde fast pathway ablation for atrioventricular nodal reentry associated with markedly prolonged PR intervals. *Am J Cardiol.* 1999;83(3):455-458, A9-A10.
117. Li YG, Gronefeld G, Bender B, et al. Risk of development of delayed atrioventricular block after slow pathway modification in patients with atrioventricular nodal reentrant tachycardia and a pre-existing prolonged PR interval. *Eur Heart J.* 2001;22(1):89-95.
118. Lee SH, Chen SA, Tai CT, et al. Atrioventricular node reentrant tachycardia in patients with a prolonged AH interval during sinus rhythm: clinical features, electrophysiologic characteristics and results of radiofrequency ablation. *J Interv Card Electrophysiol.* 1997;1(4):305-310.
119. Reithmann C, Remp T, Oversohl N, Steinbeck G. Ablation for atrioventricular nodal reentrant tachycardia with a prolonged PR interval during sinus rhythm: the risk of delayed higher-degree atrioventricular block. *J Cardiovasc Electrophysiol.* 2006;17(9):973-979.
120. Pasquie JL, Scalzi J, Macia JC, et al. Long-term safety and efficacy of slow pathway ablation in patients with atrioventricular nodal re-entrant tachycardia and pre-existing prolonged PR interval. *Europace.* 2006;8(2):129-133.
121. Lee SH, Chen SA, Tai CT, et al. Atrioventricular node reentrant tachycardia in patients with a long fast pathway effective refractory period: clinical features, electrophysiologic characteristics, and results of radiofrequency ablation. *Am Heart J.* 1997;134(3):387-394.
122. Lee PC, Chen SA, Hwang B. Atrioventricular node anatomy and physiology: implications for ablation of atrioventricular nodal reentrant tachycardia. *Curr Opin Cardiol.* 2009;24(2):105-112.

Video Legend

Video 39.1 The commonly successful slow pathway ablation site. The right anterior oblique view (**A**) and left anterior oblique view (**B**) show the position of the ablation catheter, which is placed at the posterobasal area of Koch's triangle.

CHAPTER 40

CATHETER ABLATION OF ACCESSORY AV PATHWAYS
(WOLFF–PARKINSON–WHITE SYNDROME AND VARIANTS)

Hiroshi Nakagawa, MD, PhD; Warren M. Jackman, MD

Introduction

Ventricular preexcitation and the various forms of AVRT result from antegrade or retrograde conduction over one or more accessory AV connections.[1-3] Antiarrhythmic drugs have been used to suppress conduction across APs to prevent AVRT or depress AP conduction during preexcited AF. However, antiarrhythmic drugs are either ineffective or poorly tolerated in many patients. As a result, surgical ablation (1970s), and later catheter ablation (1980s), of APs were developed as curative therapy for AVRT and rapid preexcited AF.[4-13] The high success rate (> 90%) and low incidence of complications (< 5%) in catheter ablation have led this modality to become first-line therapy for arrhythmias associated with APs.

A number of approaches have been developed for catheter ablation of APs.[8-16] In this chapter, we describe our current approach to mapping and ablation of various types of APs.[9,17-20]

Approach to Catheter Mapping (Localization) of APs

The presence of antegrade accessory AV pathway conduction is confirmed by progressive preexcitation during decremental atrial pacing.[1-3] We generally perform decremental pacing from two widely separate sites (RAA and posterolateral CS), since one atrial pacing site far from the AP may not demonstrate clear preexcitation. A change in the morphology of the preexcited QRS or the ventricular activation sequence on changing the atrial pacing site suggests the presence of two or more APs.

The presence of retrograde AP conduction is suggested by an eccentric retrograde atrial activation sequence, but the retrograde activation sequence for anteroseptal and posteroseptal APs is similar to the sequence during retrograde conduction over the fast and slow AV nodal pathways, respectively. The presence of more than one route from the ventricle to the atrium is often suggested by ventricular pacing at two widely separate sites close to the base. Confirmation of retrograde AP conduction can be obtained by para-Hisian ventricular pacing (with intermittent HB capture, Figure 40.1)[21,22] and by advancing atrial activation during AVRT using a late ventricular extrastimulus delivered close to the site of earliest atrial activation.[1,2]

Our approach to localize APs for ablation is based on the possibilities that: (1) an AP may have an oblique course (atrial and ventricular insertions are located at different sites along the AV groove)[19,20,23] and (2) multiple pathways may be present. As a result, we map the annular region during antegrade AP conduction (atrial pacing) as well as during retrograde AP conduction (ventricular pacing). We also perform differential atrial pacing (atrial pacing at two sites close to the annulus on

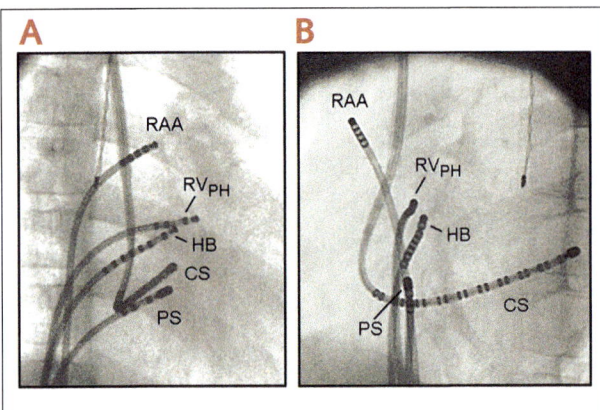
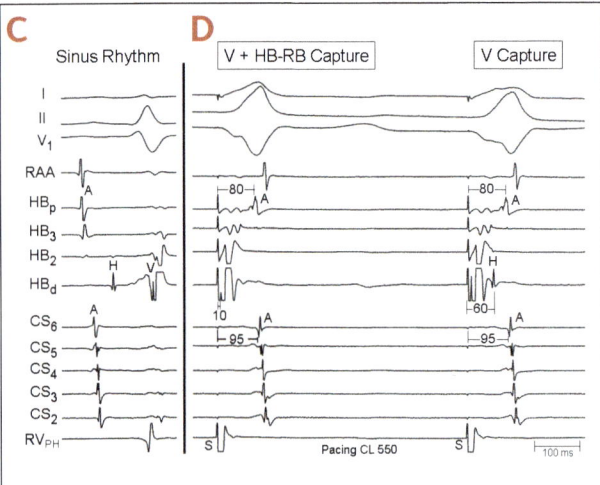
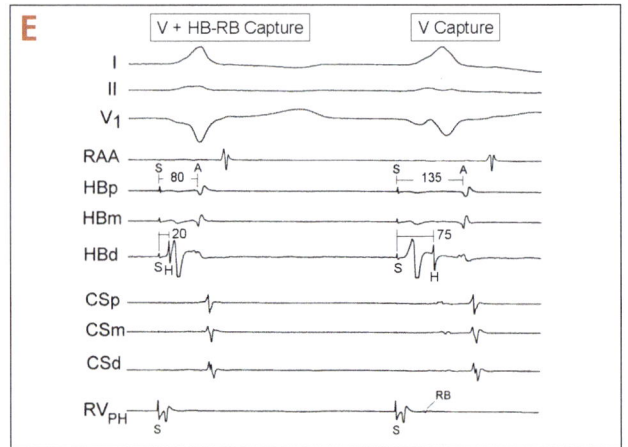

Figure 40.1 Para-Hisian pacing in a patient with a concealed anteroseptal AP before and after AP ablation. **Panels A and B**: Radiographs showing electrode catheter positions in the RAO (A) and LAO (B) projections. HB-deflectable octapolar electrode catheter (1 mm spacing) positioned to record HB potential from the distal pairs of electrodes. RV_{PH}-deflectable quadripolar electrode catheter (1 mm spacing) positioned for basal septal RV pacing with intermittent capture of proximal right bundle branch (HB-RB capture). Three other catheters are positioned at the RAA, CS, and posteroseptal tricuspid annulus (PS). **Panels C and D**: Before ablation, electrograms (EGMs) recorded during sinus rhythm (C) and para-Hisian pacing (D). The loss of HB-RB capture (right complex) resulted in delay in HB activation (S-H from 10 ms to 60 ms) and widening of QRS complex. However, the stimulus-atrial (S-A) intervals and retrograde atrial activation sequence are unchanged, indicating retrograde conduction over a single AP. **Panel E**: After ablation, the S-A interval was longer but retrograde atrial activation was early in the HB EGMs similar to before ablation. With HB-RB capture (left complex), the S-H interval was 20 ms. Without HB-RB capture (right complex, only ventricular capture), the S-H interval lengthened by 55 ms (20 ms to 75 ms). The S-A intervals also lengthened by 55 ms (80 ms to 135 ms) with no change in atrial activation sequence, indicating retrograde conduction over the AV node. *Source:* Modified with permission.[22]

opposite sides of the site of earliest antegrade ventricular activation, Figure 40.2) and differential ventricular pacing (ventricular pacing at two sites close to the annulus on opposite sides of the site of earliest retrograde atrial activation, Figure 40.3) to identify an oblique course of a single AP and presence of more than one AP (more than one antegrade ventricular or retrograde atrial activation sequence).[19,20]

With a single AP having an oblique course, differential ventricular pacing produces two different local V-A intervals (≥15 ms difference) measured at the site of earliest retrograde atrial activation. The ventricular pacing site that produces a ventricular wavefront propagating from the direction of the ventricular end of the AP (concurrent direction, Figure 40.2A) results in an artificially short local V-A interval at the site of earliest atrial activation (Figure 40.2A, C, E, and G). Because ventricular activation and AP activation are propagating simultaneously in the same direction, the ventricular potential overlaps and masks the AP activation potential and may even mask the atrial potential (Figure 40.2C, E, and G). Pacing from

the opposite side, reversing the direction of the ventricular wavefront (countercurrent direction), causes the ventricular wavefront to propagate away from the AP shortly after activating its ventricular end (Figure 40.2B). This increases the local V-A interval along the length of the AP, exposing the AP potential and the atrial activation sequence (Figure 40.2D, F, and H).[19,20]

With an oblique course, differential atrial pacing produces two different local A-V intervals (≥15 ms difference), measured at the site of earliest ventricular activation (Figure 40.3). Atrial pacing from the direction of the atrial insertion (concurrent atrial wavefront) shortens the local A-V interval at the site of earliest ventricular activation and produces overlapping atrial and AP potentials, masking the AP potential and occasionally even masking the site of earliest ventricular activation (Figures 40.3A and C).

Pacing from the opposite side, reversing the direction of the atrial wavefront (countercurrent direction), causes the atrial wavefront to propagate away from the AP shortly after activating its atrial end (Figure 40.3B). The

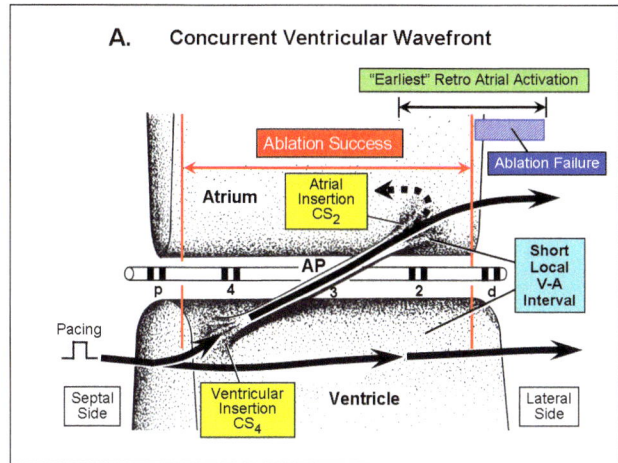
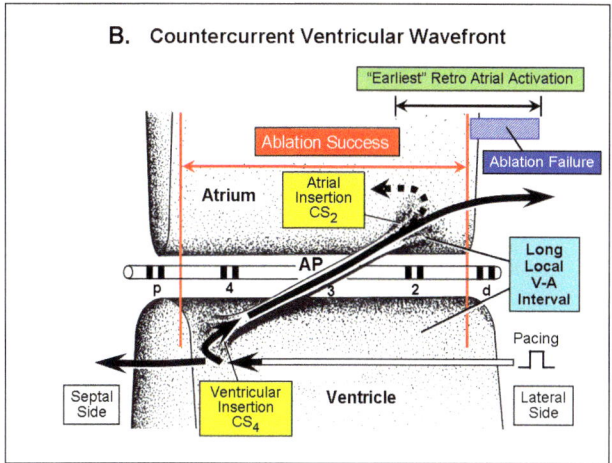
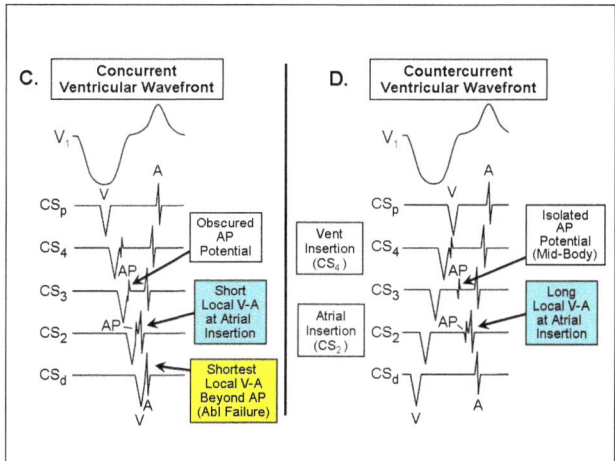
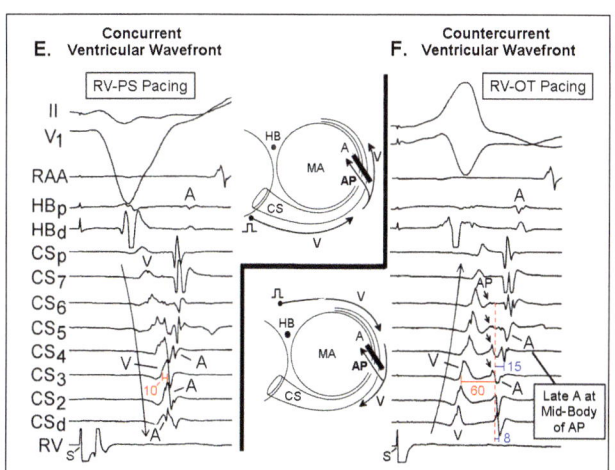
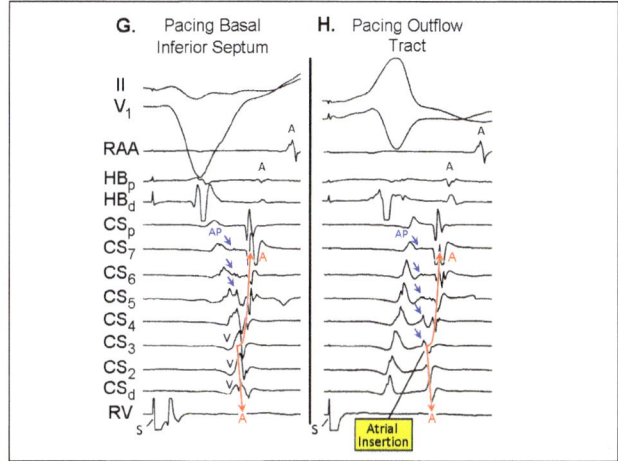

Figure 40.2 Effects of the oblique course in a left free-wall AP on the timing of ventricular (V), atrial (A), and accessory pathway (AP) potentials by reversing the direction of the ventricular wavefront. Modified with permission.[19]

A-V interval all along the AP is increased, exposing the AP potential and the ventricular activation sequence (Figure 40.3D).[19,20]

During antegrade or retrograde AP conduction, the ability to record an isolated AP potential (with an isoelectric interval between the atrial and AP potentials and between the AP and ventricular potentials) indicates an oblique course. The absence of an oblique course would produce fusion between the atrial, AP, and ventricular potentials unless the atrial or ventricular insertion of the AP are located far from the annulus, such as in Ebstein's anomaly.

Differential atrial and ventricular pacing was tested in 114 consecutive patients with a single AP (left free-wall AP in 65 patients, right free-wall AP in 22 patients, posteroseptal AP in 21 patients, and anteroseptal AP in 6 patients).[19] Reversing the direction of ventricular or atrial activation increased the local V-A or local A-V interval by ≥ 15 ms in 99 (87%) of the 114 patients, suggesting that the majority of APs have an oblique course. Separating

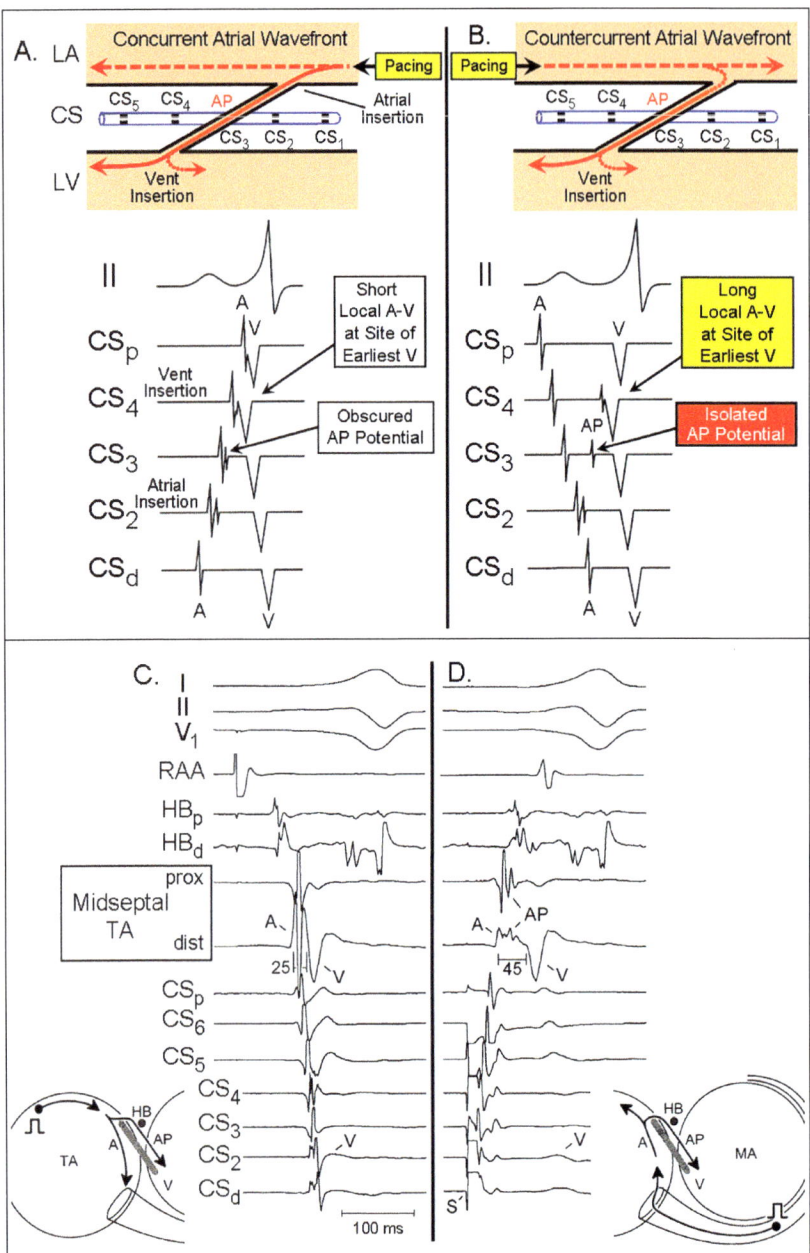

Figure 40.3 Effects of the oblique course in a left free-wall AP on the timing of atrial (A), ventricular (V), and accessory pathway (AP) potentials by reversing the direction of the atrial wavefront. *Source:* Modified with permission.[19]

the atrial and ventricular potentials by differential pacing exposed an AP potential in 102 of 114 (89%) patients. Ablation was attempted in 111 of the 114 patients, and an AP potential was recorded in 99 of these 111 patients. By targeting the AP potential in the 99 patients, AP conduction was eliminated with a median of only 1 RF application (range 1–11 applications). In contrast, a median of 4.5 RF applications (range 1–18 applications) were required in the 12 patients where an AP potential was not recorded, despite separating the atrial and ventricular potentials using differential pacing (Figure 40.4A).[19,20] These data strongly support the AP potential as the optimal target for ablation and suggest that the absence of an AP potential may indicate unusual anatomy.

In the same study, 60 of the 111 patients undergoing ablation had 1–3 prior failed ablation procedures. The number of RF applications required to eliminate AP conduction was not significantly greater for the 60 patients who had a prior failed ablation than for the 51 patients undergoing their first ablation procedure (median 1 RF application for both groups, Figure 40.4B).[19] AP conduction was eliminated by only 1 or 2 RF applications in 41 of the 60 patients with prior failed ablation. In these 41 patients, differential pacing showed an oblique course, exposing an AP potential for the ablation target. In most, there were low amplitude fractionated atrial potentials located 2 to 10 mm beyond the atrial insertion of the AP (blue hatched box in Figure 40.1), indicating the location of previous ablation sites. The consistent finding of fractionated EGMs at this site suggests that an oblique AP course may lead to placing unsuccessful RF applications beyond the atrial insertion of the AP when using two

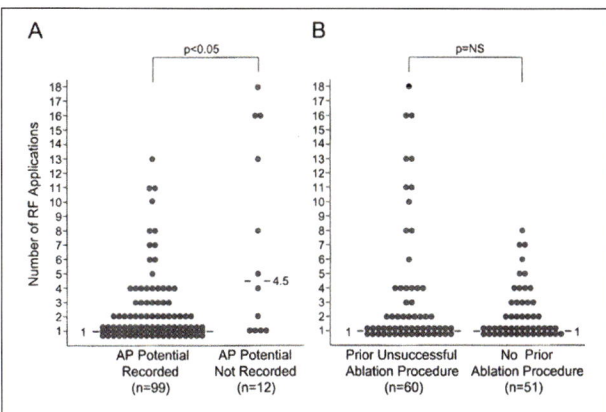

Figure 40.4 Comparison of number of RF applications required to eliminate AP conduction between 99 patients with AP potential recording and 12 patients without AP potential recording at the ablation site (**Panel A**) and between 60 patients with prior unsuccessful ablation procedure and 51 patients without unsuccessful ablation procedure (**Panel B**). Source: Modified with permission.[19]

common approaches for localizing APs (the site of earliest retrograde atrial activation and the shortest local V-A interval). During retrograde AP conduction, atrial activation propagates rapidly in the same direction as the AP, due to parallel atrial fiber orientation (Figure 40.2).[20] This rapid atrial propagation causes bipolar EGMs to identify "earliest" retrograde atrial activation over a wide range, extending beyond the atrial insertion of the AP (black arrow, "Earliest" Retro Atrial Activation in Figure 40.2A). RF applications in the distal half of this region (blue hatched area in Figure 40.2A) are likely to fail to eliminate AP conduction.[20]

Another common target for ablation, the shortest local V-A interval, is also misleading in the presence of an oblique course. This is due to the difference in conduction velocity between the atrial and ventricular wavefronts along the mitral and tricuspid annulus. With a concurrent ventricular wavefront, ventricular activation initially precedes the atrial activation near the atrial insertion of the AP (CS_2 EGM in Figure 40.2A and C). However, the velocity of the atrial wavefront parallel to the annulus is greater than the velocity of the ventricular wavefront. The local V-A interval shortens progressively beyond the atrial insertion of the AP, as the atrial wavefront catches the ventricular wavefront (CS_d EGM in Figure 40.2A, C, E, and G). The shorter (even negative) local V-A interval beyond the atrial insertion of the AP may explain the location of the fractionated atrial EGMs in the majority of patients with a prior failed ablation procedure.

For most APs along the mitral annulus (posteroseptal and left free-wall pathways), the direction from ventricular insertion to atrial insertion follows a counterclockwise orientation (as viewed in the LAO projection, Figure 40.5). For many of the APs along the tricuspid annulus (especially anteroseptal pathways), the direction from ventricular insertion to atrial insertion follows a clockwise orientation (as viewed in the LAO projection, Figure

40.5). Therefore, for many anteroseptal and right anterior paraseptal APs, the ventricular insertion is located toward the right free wall, allowing ablation away from the septum to reduce the risk of AV block.[19]

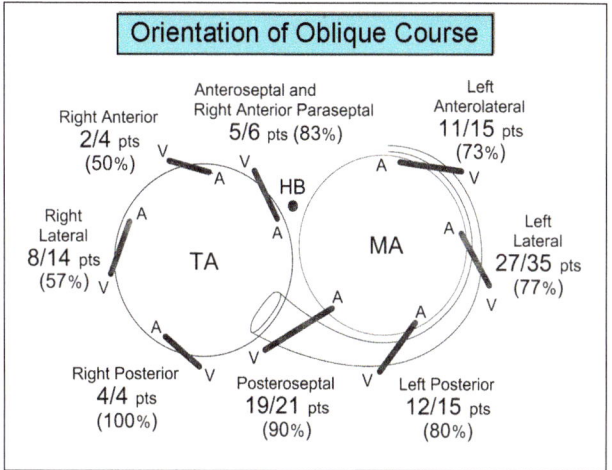

Figure 40.5 Orientation of oblique course of 114 APs in 8 anatomical regions. A = atrial end; HB = His bundle; MA = mitral annulus; TA = tricuspid annulus; V = ventricular end. Source: Modified with permission.[19]

To acquire optimal ventricular pacing sites close to the annulus for reversing the direction of the ventricular wavefront, we use a deflectable catheter with small, closely spaced bipolar electrodes. These pacing sites differ for APs in different locations (Figure 40.6). For left anterolateral and lateral pathways, a counterclockwise ventricular wavefront can be achieved by pacing from the inferobasal right ventricular septum (close to the tricuspid annulus, Figure 40.6A) or from the MCV (Figure 40.6C). A clockwise left ventricular wavefront can be achieved either by pacing at the inferior aspect of the distal RVOT (or proximal pulmonary artery, Figure 40.6B) or the anterior aspect of the great cardiac vein (or anterior interventricular vein, Figure 40.6D). For posteroseptal APs, the counterclockwise ventricular wavefront is obtained by pacing at the inferobasal right ventricular septum (Figure 40.6A). The clockwise ventricular wavefront is obtained by pacing from the posterior coronary vein or further lateral coronary vein (Figure 40.6D). For right free-wall APs, the counterclockwise ventricular wavefront is obtained by pacing at the inferobasal right ventricular septum (Figure 40.6E). The clockwise ventricular wavefront is obtained by pacing the basal right ventricular free wall anterior to the AP (Figure 40.6F).[19] For anteroseptal and right anterior paraseptal APs, the counterclockwise ventricular wavefront is obtained by pacing the basal anterior right ventricular septum (Figure 40.6G), similar to the site used for para-Hisian pacing.[20-22] The clockwise ventricular wavefront is obtained by pacing the basal anterolateral right ventricular free wall (Figure 40.6H).

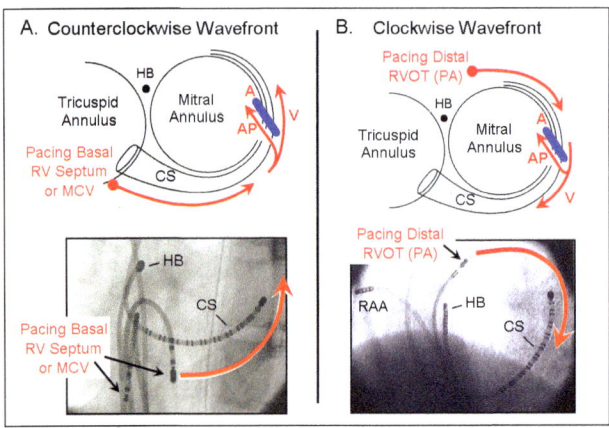
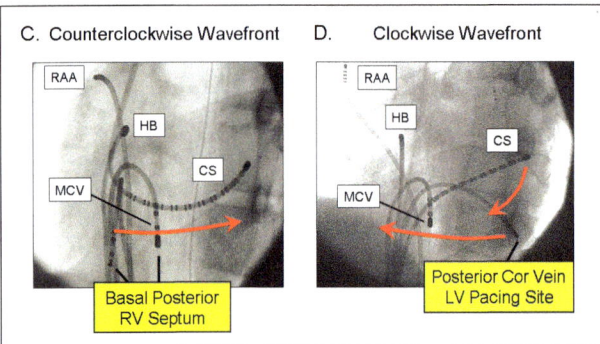
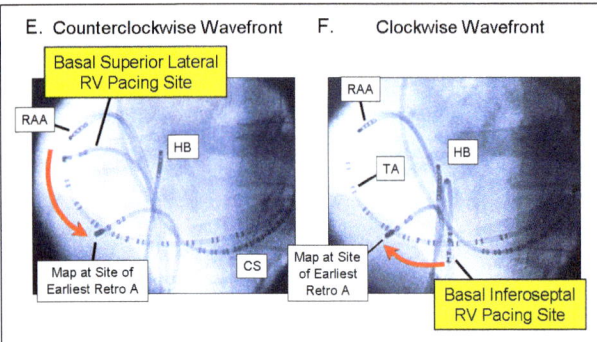
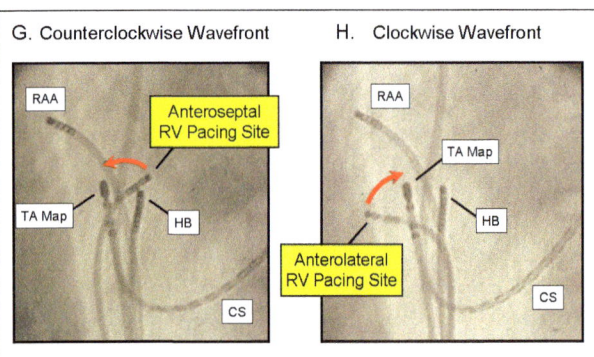

Figure 40.6 Radiographs in the LAO projection demonstrating two different ventricular pacing sites to produce clockwise and counterclockwise ventricular wavefronts along the mitral annulus for the left free-wall and posteroseptal APs (**Panels A–D**) and along the tricuspid annulus for the right free-wall APs (**Panels E, F**) and the right anteroseptal and right anterior APs (**Panels G, H**). CS = coronary sinus; HB = His bundle; MA = mitral annulus; MCV = middle cardiac vein; RAA = right atrial appendage; TA = tricuspid annulus. *Source:* Modified with permission.[19]

To summarize our approach in identifying the optimal site for ablation, we begin with a brief map during atrial pacing and during ventricular pacing to identify the approximate location of earliest antegrade ventricular activation and earliest retrograde atrial activation. We then perform differential atrial and ventricular pacing to identify a single pathway versus multiple pathways (change in activation sequence) and whether the AP(s) has or have an oblique course (significant increase in local A-V and V-A intervals). High-density mapping is performed using an ablation catheter during pacing at the atrial and ventricular sites, which increase the local A-V and local V-A intervals, to locate an isolated AP potential. The site recording an isolated AP potential is located in the middle region of the oblique course. The AP potential is validated by dissociation of the AP potential from the local atrial and ventricular potentials (Figures 40.7 and 40.8).[20] An antegrade AP potential is validated during atrial pacing using ventricular extrastimuli, gradually shortening the coupling intervals. Advancing the local ventricular potential without affecting the timing or morphology of the AP potential dissociates the AP potential from the local ventricular potential (Figure 40.7A). With an earlier ventricular extrastimulus, advancing the AP potential without affecting the timing or morphology of the atrial potential in the mapping EGM and any surrounding EGMs (such as the adjacent CS EGMs) dissociates the AP potential from the local atrial potential (Figure 40.7B). A retrograde AP potential is validated during ventricular pacing using atrial extrastimuli. Advancing the local atrial potential without affecting the timing or morphology of the AP potential dissociates the AP potential from the local atrial potential (Figures 40.8A and 40.8B). With an earlier atrial extrastimulus, advancing the AP potential without affecting the timing or morphology of the ventricular potential dissociates the AP potential from the local ventricular potential (Figure 40.8C).[17,18,20]

Approach to Catheter Ablation of Accessory Pathways

We generally prefer to perform mapping and ablation during ventricular or atrial pacing, rather than during AVRT. AVRT may not be sustained or well tolerated. In some patients, AVRT degenerates into AF. Most importantly, when ablation is performed during AVRT, the catheter is often dislodged when AVRT terminates after only a few seconds into the RF application, due to the enhanced contraction of the first post-tachycardia beat. AP conduction may not return immediately to guide subsequent RF applications, and the incomplete lesion may lead to ablation failure.

Final mapping is performed using an ablation catheter, recording both filtered bipolar EGMs (30–500 Hz) and two unfiltered unipolar EGMs (1–500 Hz) from the ablation tip electrode and the second electrode. After localizing

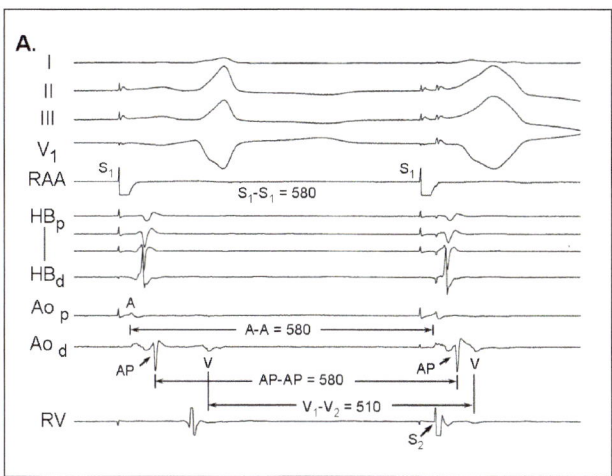
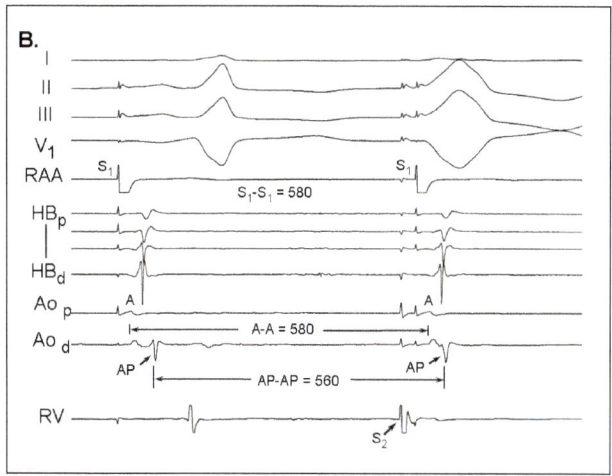

Figure 40.7 Validation of antegrade AP potential recorded in the non-coronary cusp (NCC) (Ao$_d$) using ventricular extrastimuli in a patient with an epicardial left anteroseptal AP. Mapping catheter in the NCC of the aortic valve (Ao$_d$) recorded a large, sharp AP potential (AP). **Panel A:** During RAA pacing at cycle length 580 ms (S$_1$–S$_1$ = 580), a late ventricular extrastimulus (S$_2$) advanced the local ventricular potential in the NCC EGMs by 70 ms (V$_1$–V$_2$ = 510 ms) without changing the timing or morphology of the AP potential, dissociating the AP potential from the local ventricular potential. **Panel B:** An earlier S$_2$ advanced the AP potential by 20 ms (AP–AP = 560 ms) without changing the timing of morphology of the atrial potential (A–A = 580 ms in RAA and Aod EGMs), dissociating the AP potential from the local atrial potential. *Source:* Modified with permission.[20]

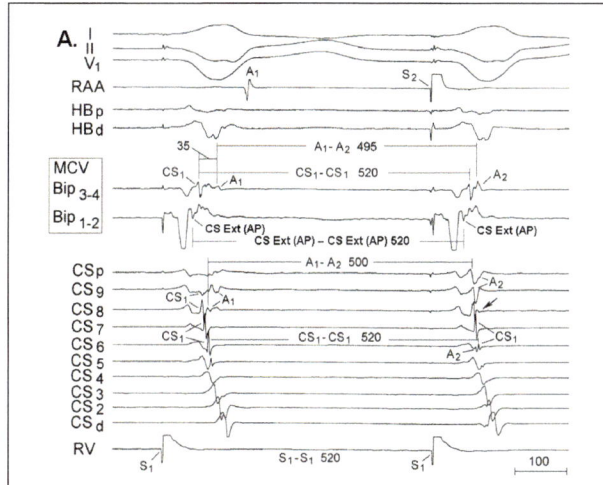
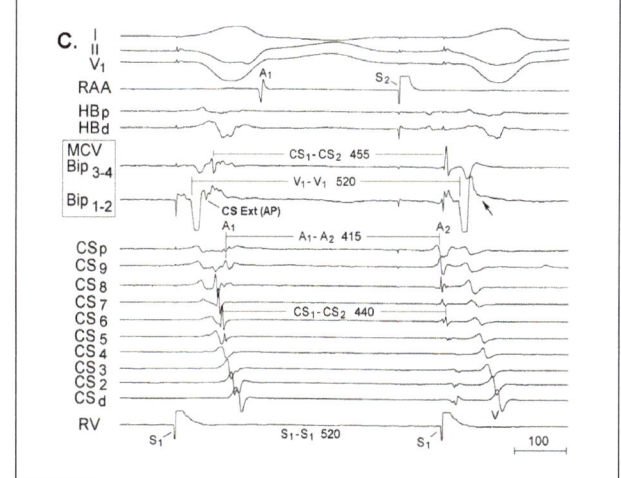
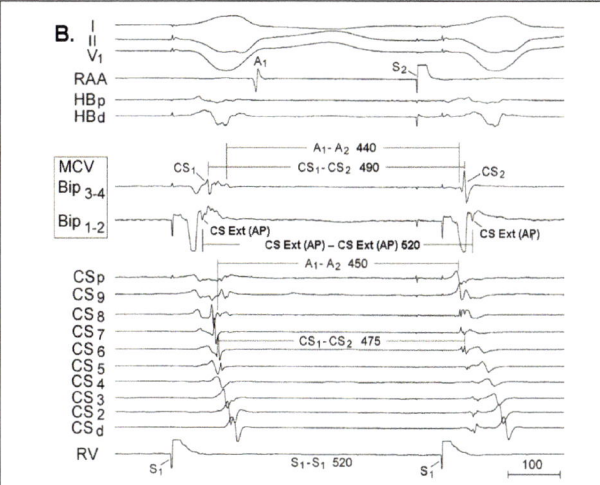

Figure 40.8 Validation of retrograde AP potential recorded in the MCV. **Panel A:** During right ventricular pacing at cycle length 520 ms (S$_1$–S$_1$ = 520), the earliest retrograde potential was recorded from the MCV, CS Ext (AP), in EGM MCV-Bip$_{1-2}$. This potential was followed by a CS myocardial potential at the MCV orifice (CS$_1$ in MCV-Bip$_{3-4}$). Leftward propagation of CS myocardial potentials (CS$_1$ in EGM CS$_9$ to CS$_7$) preceded the left atrial potential (A$_1$). A late atrial extrastimulus (S$_2$) advanced atrial activation by 25 ms in the MCV-Bip$_{3-4}$ EGM (A$_1$–A$_2$ = 495 ms) without changing the timing and morphology of CS$_1$ potentials, dissociating CS$_1$ from the local left atrial activation. **Panel B:** An earlier S$_2$ advanced both atrial activation (A$_1$–A$_2$ = 440 ms) and CS myocardial activation (CS$_1$–CS$_1$ = 490 ms) in MCV-Bip$_{3-4}$ without changing the timing or morphology of the CS Ext (AP) potential, dissociating CS Ext (AP) from the local left atrial activation and activation of CS myocardium. **Panel C:** A further earlier S$_2$ advanced CS Ext (AP), resulting in loss of the CS Ext (AP) potential (arrow) without changing the local ventricular potentials (V$_1$–V$_1$ 520 ms), dissociating CS Ext (AP) from local ventricular activation. *Source:* Modified with permission.[26]

the isolated AP potential, and confirming the AP origin using extrastimuli, the ablation catheter is positioned to record a large, sharp AP potential on the unipolar EGM from the ablation tip electrode (Figure 40.9).[20] Localization using just a bipolar EGM may be misleading, because a sharp AP potential may be recorded from the second (ring) electrode.

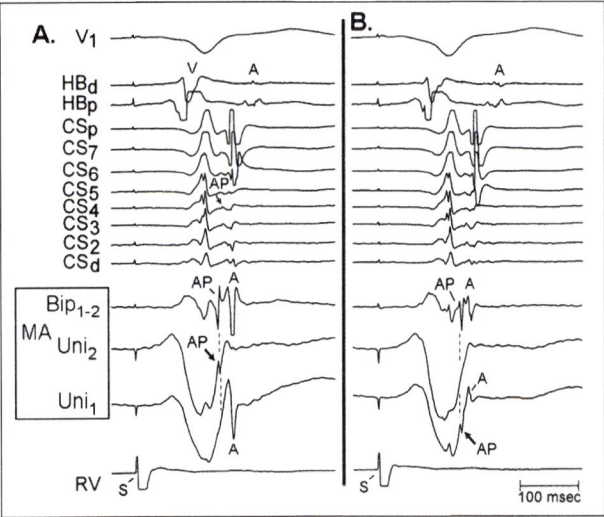

Figure 40.9 AP potential recorded from an ablation catheter positioned across the mitral annulus (MA) in a patient with a left posterolateral AP. **Panel A:** During RV pacing, a large, sharp AP potential was recorded in the bipolar (Bip$_{1-2}$) EGMs and unipolar EGMs from the second ring electrode (Uni$_2$) but not from the distal ablation electrode (Uni$_1$). **Panel B:** After the ablation catheter was positioned toward the ventricle, the AP potential was then generated from the distal ablation electrode (Uni$_1$). A single RF application at this site eliminated AP conduction. Source: Modified with permission.[20]

RF energy is delivered at 30–40 W for 60 seconds, but terminating the RF application immediately for a 5–10 ohm (Ω) increase in impedance above the lowest value. If AP conduction is not eliminated, we still continue the RF application for the full 60 seconds, because the AP potential, which was recorded before the RF application, may have represented activation of a branch of the AP. Earlier termination of the RF application, may lead to late recovery of conduction over that branch of the AP and long-term ablation failure.

In the event that an AP potential is not indentified during mapping, we target earliest antegrade ventricular activation (QS pattern on the unipolar EGM at the site of earliest activation) or earliest retrograde atrial activation.[11] These pathways are often atypical anatomically and may require more extensive ablation.

For 30 to 60 minutes following ablation, programmed atrial and ventricular stimulation is performed to confirm the absence of antegrade and retrograde AP conduction and elimination of the inducibility of AVRT. To confirm the absence of retrograde AP conduction, it is best to perform ventricular stimulation at a basal ventricular site (near the annulus) close to the location of the AP. For anteroseptal, right anterior, and posteroseptal APs, the para-Hisian site (basal anterior RV septum) is optimal. Para-Hisian pacing with intermittent HB capture differentiates between retrograde fast AV nodal pathway conduction and retrograde conduction over an anteroseptal or right anterior AP (Figure 40.1E), and differentiates between retrograde conduction over the slow AV nodal pathways and retrograde conduction over a posteroseptal AP (Figure 40.10).[20-22]

Accessory Pathways with Unusual or Unexpected Anatomy

APs are occasionally located at sites that are unexpected and not usually explored during the mapping procedure, or that require a unique approach for localization and ablation (Figure 40.11).[20,24,25] In general, the atrial and/or ventricular insertions of these pathways are located epicardially, relatively far from the mitral or tricuspid annulus.

Epicardial Posteroseptal APs (CS Myocardial–Ventricular Connections)

The true CS, between the CS ostium and the Vieussens valve, is a muscular chamber with extensive muscular (and therefore electrical) connections to the left atrium (Figure 40.12).[26-28] The CS myocardium occasionally extends a centimeter or more onto the MCV, posterior coronary vein, or other veins entering the true CS.[27] A myocardial (and electrical) connection rarely forms between the epicardial surface of the left ventricle and the myocardial extension along the veins (CS Myocardial–Ventricular Connection), forming an "epicardial posteroseptal AP" (Figure 40.12).[26] These connections also result from CS diverticula, which are muscular chambers attached to the epicardial surface of the left ventricle and connect to the true CS through a neck that also has myocardium along its surface.[26] This anatomy is a common finding in posteroseptal APs, and a frequent cause for ablation failure. We found this anatomy in 42 of 212 (20%) patients with a posteroseptal or left posterior AP and no prior attempt at ablation, but in 144 of 306 (47%) patients with one or more previous failed ablation procedures. The finding of a steep negative delta wave in ECG lead II in a patient with a posteroseptal AP (V_1–V_2 transition and negative delta wave in lead aVF) is specific, but only moderately sensitive (70%), for an epicardial location.[29]

During antegrade conduction (Figure 40.13A), earliest endocardial ventricular activation (downstroke of the unfiltered unipolar EGM) is usually recorded more than 25 ms after the onset of far-field activation and 1–3 cm apical to the mitral annulus. Endocardial activation is recorded nearly simultaneously on the right and left sides of the interventricular septum, when the AP is formed by a CS myocardial extension along the MCV. Earliest ventricular

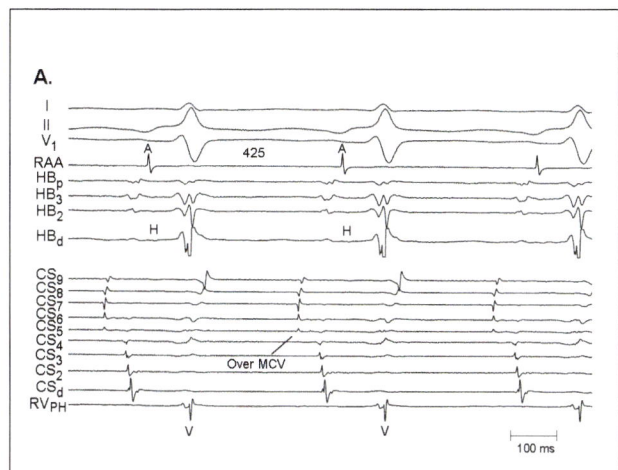
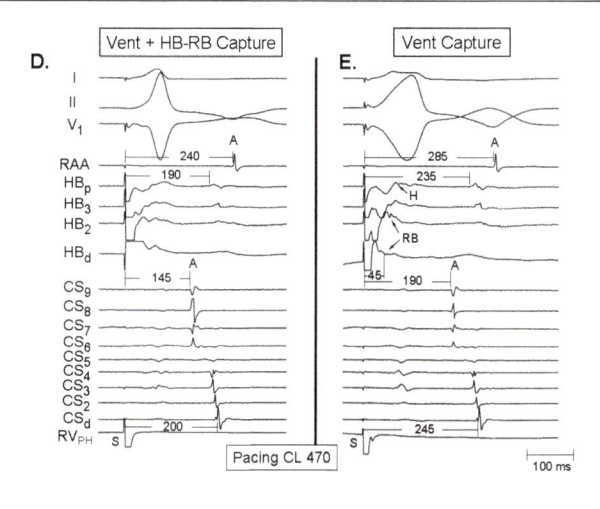
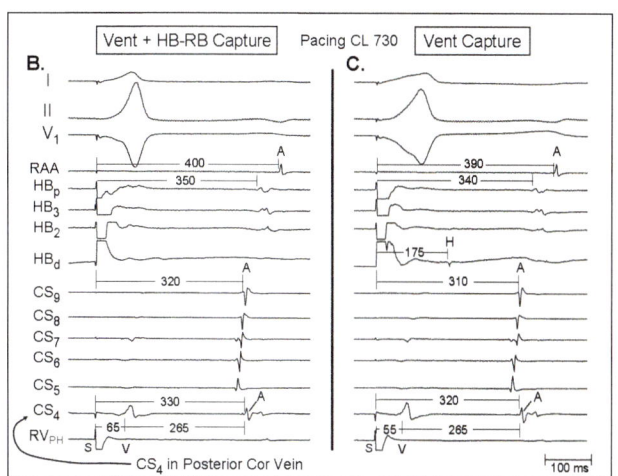

Figure 40.10 Para-Hisian pacing in a patient with permanent form of junctional reciprocating tachycardia (PJRT) resulting from an epicardial posteroseptal AP with long conduction time. **Panel A:** Orthodromic AVRT (PJRT) with cycle length (CL) 425 ms. **Panels B** and **C:** Before ablation, the loss of HB-RB capture resulted in a marked increase in S-H interval to 175 ms and 10 ms decrease in S-A intervals with identical atrial activation sequence, indicating retrograde conduction over a single AP with long conduction time. The 10 ms decrease in S-A interval resulted from a 10 ms decrease in S-V interval close to the site of the AP (65 ms to 55 ms). **Panels D** and **E:** Following ablation in the orifice of the middle cardiac vein (MCV), ventricular pacing continued to produce V-A conduction with the same atrial activation sequence as the tachycardia. However, the loss of HB-RB capture resulted in a 45 ms increase in S-A intervals, similar to the 45 ms increase in S-RB and S-H intervals, with no change in atrial activation sequence, indicating retrograde conduction over the slow AV nodal pathway with the same atrial activation sequence as the AP. *Source:* Modified with permission.[22]

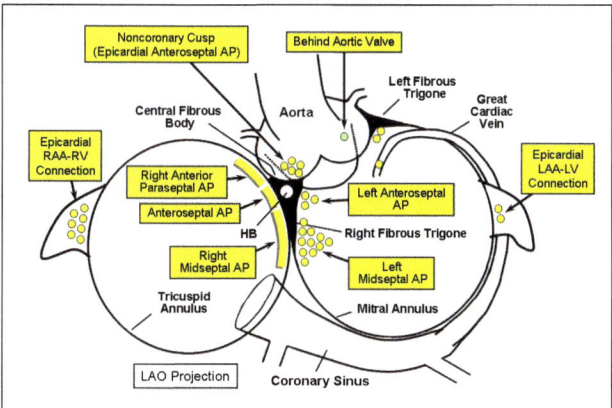

Figure 40.11 Schematic representation of unusual locations of APs. **Circles** represent the successful ablation sites for individual patients. *Source:* Modified with permission.[20]

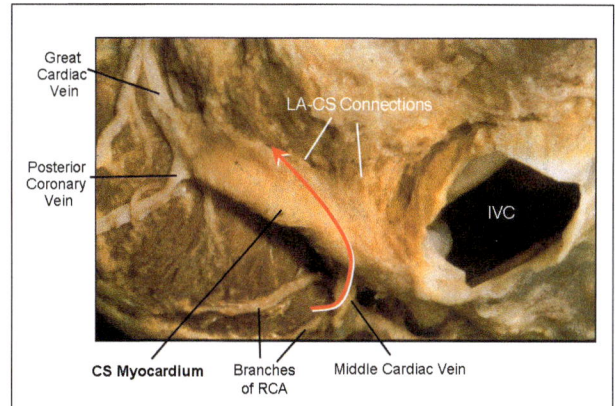

Figure 40.12 Photograph of a human heart showing CS, great cardiac vein, posterior coronary vein, CS myocardium, left atrial (LA)–CS connections, and the relationship between the MCV and distal branches of the RCA located very close to the coronary artery. *Source:* Modified with permission.[20]

activation (usually ≤15 ms after the onset of far-field activation) is recorded from the MCV, other coronary vein, or neck of a CS diverticulum, and is preceded by a distinct potential (similar to an AP potential) resulting from antegrade activation of the CS myocardial extension.[26]

During retrograde conduction over epicardial posteroseptal APs (Figure 40.13B), a characteristic pattern of three distinct potentials is recorded from the coronary venous system.[20,26] The first potential (#1 CS Extn in Figure 40.14), similar to an AP potential, is recorded from the MCV (or other coronary vein or CS diverticulum) and is generated by retrograde activation of the CS myocardial extension. The second potential (#2 CS Myo in Figure 40.14) is often smaller and is recorded along the floor of the proximal CS. This potential begins over the orifice of the MCV (or other vein or diverticulum) and propagates leftward due to the fiber orientation in the CS.[20,26] As another result of fiber orientation, the CS myocardium activates the left atrium at a location 2 to 4 cm leftward of the MCV (or other) orifice. The parallel orientation of the CS myocardium and the left atrium results in rapid left atrial activation in the leftward direction (Figure 40.13B). The third potential (#3 LA in Figure 40.14) is generated by the late left atrial activation recorded near the orifice of the MCV. Left atrial activation in the rightward (septal) direction is delayed due to slowing of conduction during the reversal in direction of activation (Figure 40.13B).

CS angiography (balloon occlusion technique) is useful to delineate the coronary venous anatomy associated with an epicardial posteroseptal AP. We initially inject contrast into the great cardiac vein with the balloon occluded to produce antegrade filling all the venous branches of the true CS. CS diverticula are also visualized due to their contraction, which fill the diverticula with blood from the CS (Video 40.1). We then inject contrast into the proximal CS (balloon occlusion) for retrograde visualization of the venous branches or diverticula related to AP conduction. CS angiography reveals totally normal venous anatomy in 70% of the patients with a CS myocardial–ventricular connection.[26] The proximal portion of the coronary vein (associated with AP conduction) exhibits vigorous contraction during atrial systole, due to activation of the CS myocardial extension. A CS diverticulum is found in only 20% of patients, and a distorted coronary vein (associated with the AP) is identified in the remaining 10% of patients.

In the majority of patients who had a failed ablation procedure, RF energy had been applied endocardially to the site of earliest retrograde atrial activation at the posterolateral mitral annulus.[30] Due to the extensive connections between the CS myocardium and the left atrium (Figure 40.12), ablation at the posterolateral mitral annulus resulted only in a shift in the site of earliest retrograde atrial activation toward the septum (rightward shift). At the end of the failed ablation procedure, many of these patients were incorrectly thought to have had two

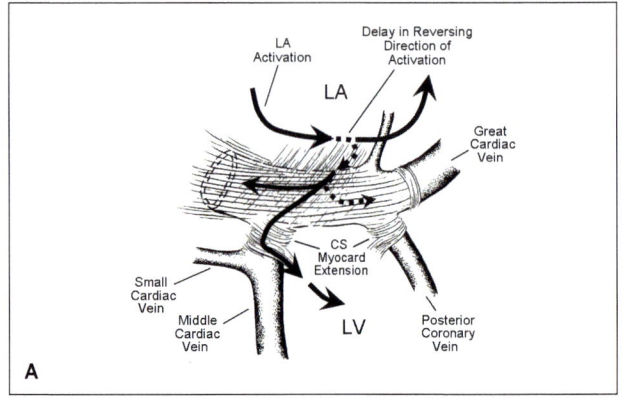

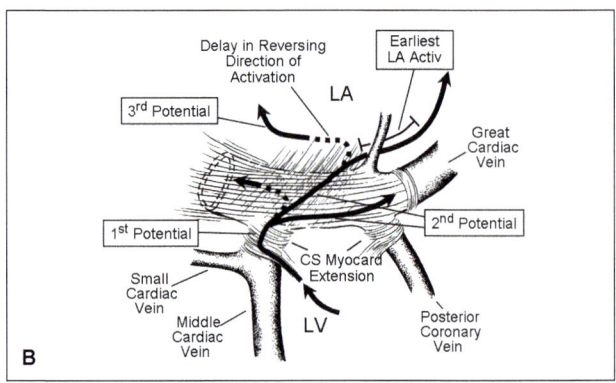

Figure 40.13 Schematic representation of antegrade (**Panel A**) and retrograde (**Panel B**) conduction over an epicardial posteroseptal AP resulting from the connection between an extension of CS myocardium along the MCV and epicardial LV. *Source:* Modified with permission.[20]

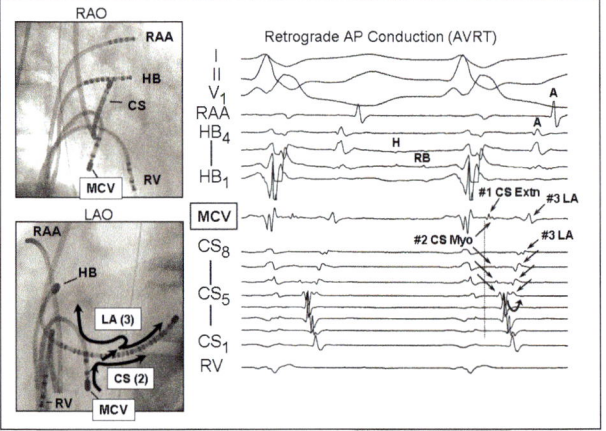

Figure 40.14 Recordings of a characteristic pattern of three distinct potentials in the MCV (MC) and CS during AVRT in a patient with an epicardial posteroseptal AP. See text. *Source:* Modified with permission.[20]

APs, a left posterolateral pathway (successfully ablated) and a posteroseptal pathway (failed ablation). Because of the extensive CS–LA connections, the optimal ablation site is within the MCV (or other coronary vein or neck of CS diverticulum) at the site recording the largest, sharpest potential generated by the CS myocardial extension on the unipolar ablation tip EGM. Before ablation, we perform coronary arteriography to determine the proximity of any significant coronary artery to the ideal ablation site within the MCV, other coronary vein, or neck of a CS diverticulum (Figure 40.15). RF ablation (RFA) is safe when coronary arteriography shows that the site recording the largest, sharpest CS myocardial extension potential is located at least 4–5 mm from the closest significant coronary artery.[31-33] Saline-irrigated RF electrodes are recommended to provide adequate electrode cooling, since cooling by blood flow is limited within the small vein. We begin the RF application at 10–15 W and increase power as required up to 25 W. It is important to terminate the RF application as quickly as possible when an impedance rise occurs, even a very small rise (3–5 Ω increase above the lowest value), to prevent adherence of the electrode to the vein. AP conduction is usually eliminated by 1 or 2 RF applications, with a low long-term recurrence, when ablation is performed at the site of a sharp unipolar CS extension potential.[20,26]

We found that an RF application in a coronary vein located within 2 mm of a coronary artery is associated with a high risk (> 50%) of arterial stenosis or occlusion (Figure 40.16).[31,34] When the optimal ablation site in the vein is located within 3–4 mm of a significant coronary artery, cryoablation is recommended.[34,35] In our early experience, we found an acute efficacy using cryoablation alone in 9 (75%) of 12 patients with long-term success in only 8 (67%) of 12 patients. Acute success has improved with larger cryoablation electrodes, but recurrence of AP conduction remains higher than with RFA.

Left Midseptal Accessory Pathways

It was thought initially that accessory pathways would not be located along the septal mitral annulus between the HB and the level of the CS ostium ("left midseptal region"), because the right fibrous trigone is devoid of atrial tissue (Figure 40.11). However, we have found the AP in the left midseptal region in 11 patients.[20,24] A clue that an AP is located at the midseptal mitral annulus is the simultaneous recording of "earliest" retrograde atrial activation in the HB and proximal CS EGMs (Figure 40.17), suggesting that activation originated at a site equidistant from the HB and proximal CS. A far-field AP potential, preceding atrial activation, is often recorded when a mapping catheter is positioned at the roof of the CS ostium and pushed upward (Figure 40.17C). Ablation should not be performed at the roof of the CS ostium with vertical pressure (close to the atrial side of the midseptal mitral annulus), because ablation at this site usually fails or only transiently eliminates AP conduction, and there is a significant risk of AV block. Mapping along the mitral annulus (posterior to the HB and anterior to the CS) reveals a large, sharp AP potential (Figure 40.17D), and ablation at this site eliminated AP conduction in all 11 patients without AV block.[20,24]

Epicardial Anteroseptal Accessory Pathways

An epicardial location for an anteroseptal AP should be suspected when endocardial recordings exhibit only far-field early antegrade ventricular activation and only far-field early retrograde atrial activation.[20,24,25] Far-field activation is identified by the unfiltered unipolar EGM, which shows an initial positive component. In patients with an epicardial anteroseptal AP, the unfiltered unipolar EGM recorded all along the tricuspid annulus shows local activation (rapid downstroke) beginning at least 20 ms after the onset of the far-field potential (Figure 40.18A–C) and may exhibit a tiny far-field AP potential (Figure 40.18C). Ablation at these sites usually fails, or only transiently eliminates AP conduction. Since the NCC of the aortic valve is located just opposite the anterior paraseptal tricuspid annulus (Figure 40.18D and E), the EGM recorded from the NCC may reveal a sharp AP potential, indicating a location close to the AP (Figure 40.18F; validation of this potential in Figure 40.7A and B). Ablation within the NCC at the site recording a sharp unipolar AP potential was successful in eliminating AP conduction in all 5 patients with this pattern of EGMs

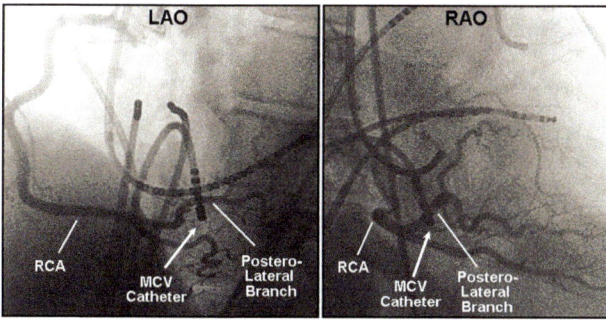

Figure 40.15 Right coronary arteriography with an ablation catheter positioned in the MCV. The ablation electrode (AP recording site) is located very close to (< 2 mm) the posterolateral branch of the right coronary artery. Cryoablation was performed from the MCV to avoid arterial injury, eliminating AP conduction. *Source:* Modified with permission.[20]

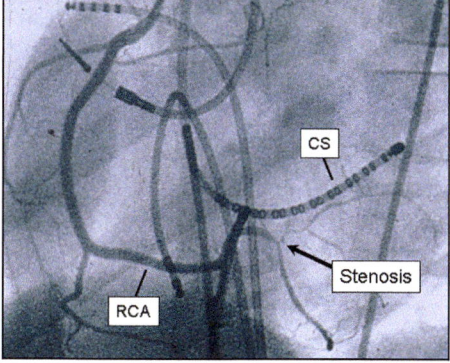

Figure 40.16 Significant narrowing of the distal right coronary artery in a 14-year-old male who underwent RFA at the floor of the CS ostium at another hospital. *Source:* Modified with permission.[20]

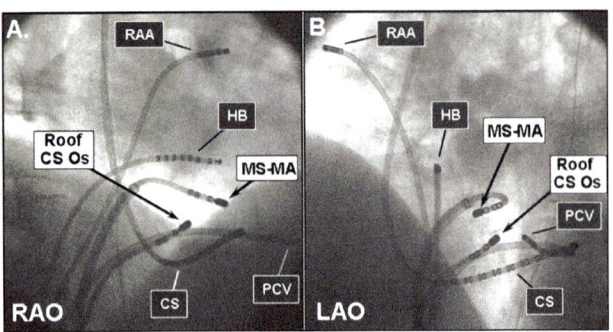
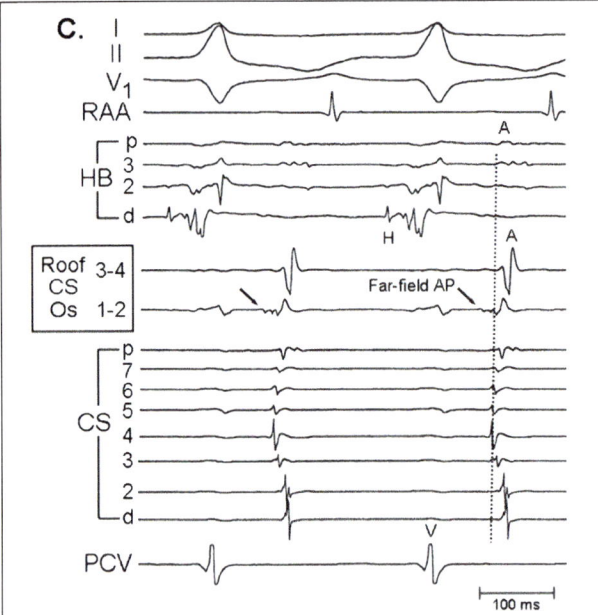
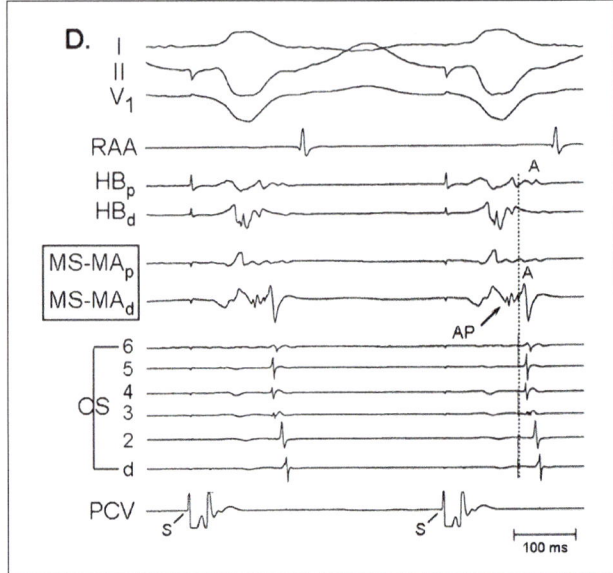

Figure 40.17 Ablation of a left midseptal AP. Catheter positions in the RAO (**Panel A**) and LAO (**Panel B**) projections. **Panel C:** During AVRT, the timing of retrograde atrial activation is similar in the HB region and the proximal CS (CSp) EGMs, suggesting that activation originated at a site equidistant from these two regions. Mapping at the roof of CS ostium (Roof CS Os1-2) identifies a small, low-frequency (far-field) AP potential. **Panel D:** EGMs from the ablation catheter positioned at the midseptal mitral annulus (MS-MA) show a sharp, large AP potential. A single RF application at this site eliminated AP conduction. PVC = posterior coronary vein; RAA = right atrial appendage. *Source:* Modified with permission.[20]

(Figure 40.18G). The risk of AV block for ablation in the NCC appears low, similar to the low risk of block with endocardial ablation more than 5 mm anterior to the HB ("right anterior paraseptal APs," Figure 40.11).[20,21,25,36,37]

The risk of AV block is generally considered to be high for ablation of APs at the site recording a sharp HB potential (anteroseptal AP, Figure 40.11) or posterior to the HB and anterior to the CS (midseptal AP). Some investigators have advocated for the use of cryoablation to reduce this risk.[35] However, cryoablation is associated with a higher recurrence of AP conduction[35] and the risk of AV block still remains. Because the AV node is located on the atrial side of the tricuspid annulus, we have found that positioning the ablation catheter on the ventricular side of the tricuspid annulus, such that the unipolar tip EGM records a sharp AP potential with little or no atrial potential, allows the use of RF current without AV block (or even a single junctional extrasystole) in patients with right anteroseptal and midseptal APs. The use of RF energy on the ventricular side of the annulus results in high acute success with a low recurrence of AP conduction.[9,20] RBBB generally occurs with ablation when a sharp RBB potential is recorded with the AP potential in the unipolar tip EGM. However, RBBB does not appear to be clinically significant in these patients,

and is preferable to the risk of AV block with ablation on the atrial side of the tricuspid annulus.

There are several tools that are helpful for ablation of APs in general and especially useful for anteroseptal and midseptal APs. The use of general anesthesia with a paralytic agent allows 1- or 2-minute periods of apnea to help stabilize the catheter position during mapping and ablation. Recently, high-frequency jet ventilation has been used to eliminate motion of the diaphragm during mapping and ablation. Another tool is para-Hisian pacing.[20-22] In patients with both retrograde AP conduction and retrograde AV node conduction, mapping can be performed during selective retrograde AP conduction by ventricular pacing at the para-Hisian site (anterior basal RV septum close to the HB) without HB capture (Figure 40.1D). After ablation, para-Hisian pacing with intermittent HB capture can be used to confirm that the retrograde conduction is occurring only over the AV node (absence of retrograde AP conduction, Figure 40.1E). Another tool for ablation of septal APs is to position the ablation catheter underneath the anterior leaflet (right subclavian venous approach) or the septal leaflet (femoral venous approach) of the tricuspid valve, and maneuvering the catheter tip to the annulus while remaining underneath the leaflet. This provides a stable catheter position on the ventricular side of the annulus during

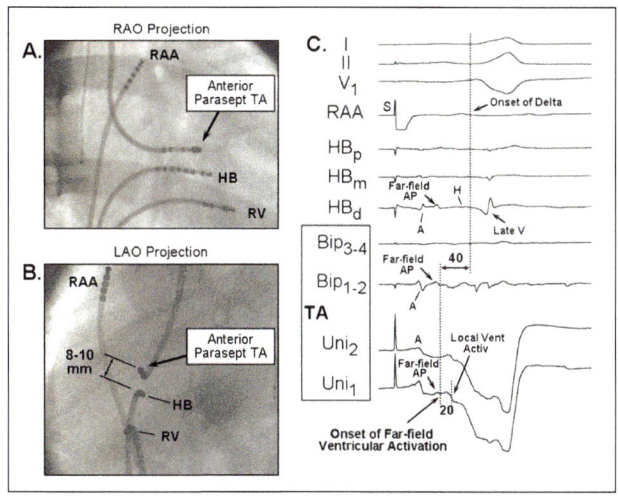
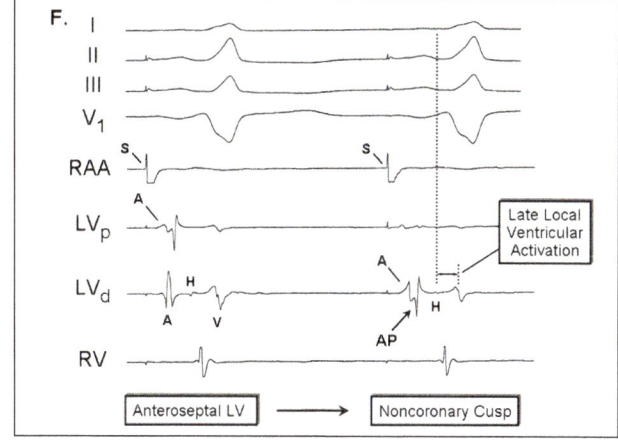
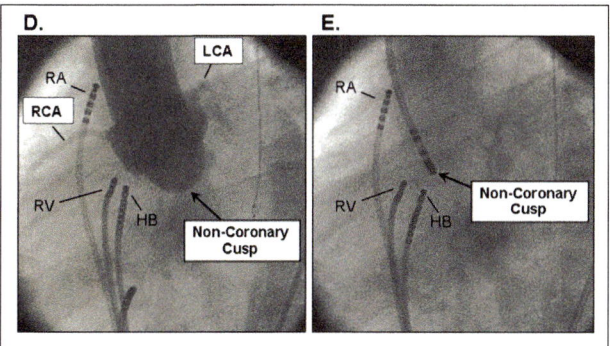
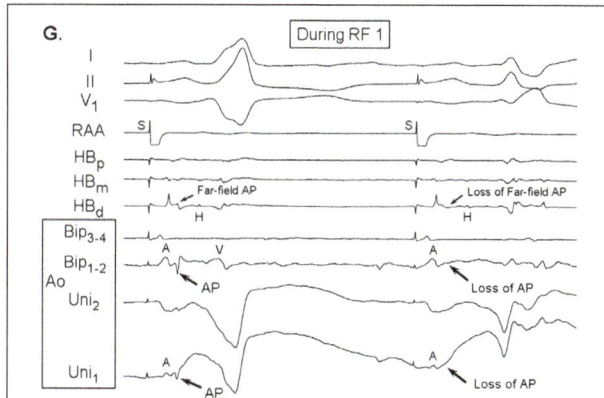

Figure 40.18 Ablation of an epicardial anteroseptal AP. **Panels A, B,** and **C:** Mapping at the anterior paraseptal tricuspid annulus (TA) during right atrial appendage (RAA) pacing, demonstrating far-field ventricular activation beginning 40 ms before the onset of delta wave but local ventricular activation beginning only 20 ms before the delta wave. This site is located 8 to 10 mm anterior to the HB region (HB). **Panels D** and **E:** Aortogram in the LAO projection, showing the mapping catheter is located at the septal side of the NCC. Note close proximity to the HB catheter at the anterior paraseptal tricuspid annulus region. **Panel F:** When the ablation catheter is pulled back from the anteroseptal LV to the NCC, a large, sharp AP potential is recorded. Note late local ventricular activation at this site—an indication that this AP has an oblique course. **Panel G:** A single RF application in the NCC at site recording a large, sharp AP potential from the tip unipolar EGM (Uni$_1$) eliminates AP conduction without affecting AV nodal conduction (no prolongation of A-H interval). *Source:* Modified with permission.[20]

ablation of anteroseptal and midseptal APs, respectively, with a low risk of AV block.[9,20,36-38]

Ablation of left anteroseptal APs may be associated with a higher risk of AV block. We used the retrograde transaortic approach for ablation of left anteroseptal APs in 3 patients. Even with apnea, there was significant movement of the catheter during each cardiac cycle. AV block (resolving after several months) occurred in 1 of the 3 patients.

Right and Left Appendage Connections

AP conduction can be produced by a connection between the right atrial appendage (RAA) or left atrial appendage (LAA) and the epicardial surface of the ventricle underlying the appendage (Figure 40.5A). These connections are located more than 1 cm apical to the tricuspid or mitral annulus.[20,39-41] Endocardial mapping along the annulus records late local activation (rapid downstroke of the unfiltered unipolar EGM), beginning at least 30–40 ms after the onset of the far-field potential. Retrograde atrial activation is recorded earlier close to the orifice of the appendage, but still long after the onset of far-field activation. Antegrade ventricular activation is recorded earlier at sites 1 to 3 cm apical of the annulus, but also long after the onset of far-field activation. Positioning the mapping catheter inside the atrial appendage locates earliest retrograde atrial activation and earliest antegrade ventricular activation, usually beginning within 10 ms of the onset of far-field retrograde atrial and antegrade ventricular activation, respectively. An AP potential is not recorded, because these pathways result from a direct epicardial connection between the atrial appendage and the ventricular myocardium. Ablation within the atrial appendage was successful in 6 of 7 patients with an RAA connection, but generally required isolation of a segment of the atrial appendage surrounding the attachment to the ventricle using a large number of RF applications (4 to 17, median 8).[20,39] It was helpful to use a saline-irrigated ablation electrode because of low blood flow around the electrode in the heavily trabeculated appendage. In 1 of the 7 patients, a steam pop produced perforation of the appendage requiring surgery, suggesting that RF power should be limited (15–25 W). Ablation was unsuccessful in both patients with an LAA connection. Surgical ablation was successful in these 2 patients and 1 patient with RAA connections.[29,39,40] A percutaneous epicardial approach may prove useful for catheter ablation of these connections,[42] although the width of the connection may limit complete ablation using this approach.

References

1. Gallagher JJ, Pritchett ELC, Sealy WC, et al. The preexcitation syndromes. *Prog Cardiovasc Dis.* 1987;20:285-327.
2. Gallagher JJ, Sealy WC, Kasell J, et al. Multiple accessory pathways in patients with the pre-excitation syndrome. *Circulation.* 1976;54:571-590.
3. Wellens HJ, Durrer D. Wolff-Parkinson-White syndrome and atrial fibrillation. *Am J Cardiol.* 1974:34:777-782.
4. Sealy WC, Hattler BG, Blumenschein SD, et al. Surgical treatment of Wolff-Parkinson-White syndrome. *Ann Thorac Surg.* 1969;8:1-11.
5. Iwa T, Magara T, Watanabe Y, et al. Interruption of multiple accessory conduction pathways in the Wolff-Parkinson-White syndrome. *Ann Thorac Surg.* 1980;30:313-325.
6. Guiraudon GM, Klein GJ, Gulamhusein S, et al. Surgical repair of Wolff-Parkinson-White syndrome: a new closed-heart technique. *Ann Thorac Surg.* 1984;37:67-71.
7. Cox JL, Gallaher JJ, Cain ME. Experience with 118 consecutive patients undergoing operation for the Wolff-Parkinson-White syndrome. *J Thorac Cardiovasc Surg.* 1985;90:490-501.
8. Borggrefe M, Budde T, Podzeck A, Breithardt G. High frequency alternating current ablation of an accessory pathway in humans. *J Am Coll Cardiol.* 1987;10:576-582.
9. Jackman WM, Wang X, Friday KJ, et al. Catheter ablation of accessory atrioventricular pathways (Wolff-Parkinson-White syndrome) by radiofrequency current. *N Engl J Med.* 1991;324:1605-1611.
10. Calkins H, Sousa J, Rosenheck S, et al. Diagnosis and cure of the Wolff-Parkinson-White syndrome or paroxysmal supraventricular tachycardias during a single electrophysiologic test. *N Engl J Med.* 1991;324:1612-1618.
11. Haïssaguerre M, Dartigues JF, Warin JF, Le Metayer P, Montserrat P, Salamon R. Electrogram patterns predictive of successful catheter ablation of accessory pathways: value of unipolar recording mode. *Circulation.*1991;84:188-202.
12. Kuck KH, Schluter M, Geiger M, Siebels J, Duckeck W. Radiofrequency current catheter ablation of accessory atrioventricular pathways. *Lancet.* 1991;337:1557-1561.
13. Lesh MD, Van Hare GF, Schamp DJ, et al. Curative percutaneous catheter ablation using radiofrequency energy for accessory pathway in all locations: results in 100 consecutive patients. *J Am Coll Cardiol.*1992;19:1303-1309.
14. Calkins H, Kim YN, Schmaltz S, et al. Electrogram criteria for identification of appropriate target sites for radiofrequency catheter ablation of accessory atrioventricular connections. *Circulation.* 1992;85:565-573.
15. Silka MJ, Kron J, Halperin BD, et al. Analysis of local electrogram characteristics correlated with successful radiofrequency catheter ablation of accessory atrioventricular pathways. *Pacing Clin Electrophysiol.* 1992;15:1000-1007.
16. Swartz JF, Tracy CM, Fletcher RD. Radiofrequency endocardial catheter ablation of accessory atrioventricular pathway atrial insertion sites. *Circulation.* 1993;87:487-499.
17. Jackman WM, Friday KJ, Scherlag BJ, et al. Direct endocardial recording from an accessory atrioventricular pathway: localization of the site of block, effect of antiarrhythmic drugs, and attempt at nonsurgical ablation. *Circulation.* 1983;68:906-916.
18. Jackman WM, Friday KJ, Yeung Lai Wah, et al. New catheter technique for recording left free-wall accessory AV pathway activation: identification of pathway fiber orientation. *Circulation.* 1988;78:598-611.
19. Otomo K, Gonzakez MD, Beckman KJ, et al. Reversing the direction of paced ventricular and atrial wavefronts reveals an oblique course in accessory AV pathways and improves localization for catheter ablation. *Circulation.* 2001;104:550-556.
20. Nakagawa H, Jackman WM. Catheter ablation of paroxysmal supraventricular tachycardia. *Circulation.* 2007;116:2465-2478.
21. Hirao K, Otomo K, Wang X, et al. Para-Hisian pacing: New method for differentiating between retrograde conduction over an accessory AV pathway and the AV node. *Circulation.* 1996;94:1027-1035.
22. Nakagawa H, Jackman WM. Para-Hisian pacing: Useful clinical technique to differentiate retrograde conduction between accessory atrioventricular pathways and atrioventricular nodal pathways. *Heart Rhythm.* 2005;2:667-672.
23. Becker AE, Anderson RH, Durrer D, Wellens HJ. The anatomical substrates of Wolff-Parkinson-White syndrome: a clinicopathologic correlation in seven patients. *Circulation.* 1978;57:870-879.
24. Arruda M, Wang X, McClelland JH, et al. Unusual locations for left-sided accessory pathways. *PACE.* 1994;17:42. (Abstract)
25. Po SS, Beckman KJ, Nakagawa H, et al. Epicardial anteroseptal and left anteroseptal accessory AV pathways. *PACE.* 2002;25:536. (Abstract)
26. Sun Y, Arruda MS, Otomo K, et al. Coronary sinus-ventricular accessory connections producing posteroseptal and left posterior accessory pathways: incidence and electrophysiological identification. *Circulation.* 2002;106:1362-1367.
27. von Ludihnghausen M, Schott C. Microanatomy of the human coronary sinus and its major tributary. In Meerbaum S, ed. *Myocardial Perfusion and Reperfusion, Coronary Venous Retroperfusion.* Darmstadt, Germany: Steinkopff Verlag; 1990:93-122.
28. Chauvin M, Shah DC, Haïssaguerre M, Marcellin L, Brechenmacher C. The anatomical basis of connections between the coronary sinus musculature and the left atrium in humans. *Circulation.* 200;101:647-652.
29. Arruda MS, McClelland JH, Wang X, et al. Development and validation of an ECG algorithm for identifying accessory pathway ablation site in Wolff-Parkinson-White syndrome. *J Cardiovasc Electrophysiology.* 1998:9:2-12.
30. Morady F, Strickberger A, Man KC, et al. Reasons for prolonged or failed attempts at radiofrequency catheter ablation of accessory pathways. *J Am Coll Cardiol.* 1996;27:683-689.
31. Sun Y, Po S, Arruda M, et al. Risk of coronary artery stenosis with venous ablation for epicardial accessory pathways. *PACE.* 2001;24:266. (Abstract)
32. Paul T, Kakavand B, Blaufox AD, Saul JP. Complete occlusion of the left circumflex coronary artery after radiofrequency catheter ablation in an infant. *J Cardiovasc Electrophysiol.* 2003;14:1004-1006.
33. Takahashi Y, Jaïs P, Hocini M, et al. Comparison of cryothermia and radiofrequency current in safety and efficacy of catheter ablation within the canine coronary sinus close to the left

circumferential coronary artery. *J Cardiovasc Electrophysiol.* 2005;16:1-9.
34. Aoyama H, Nakagawa H, Pitha JV, et al. Comparison of cryothermia and radiofrequency current in safety and efficacy of catheter ablation within the canine coronary sinus close to the left circumferential coronary artery. *J Cardiovasc Electrophysiol.* 2005;16:1-9.
35. Friedman PL, Dubuc M, Green MS, et al. Catheter cryoablation of supraventricular tachycardia: results of the multicenter prospective "frosty" trial. *Heart Rhythm.* 2004;1:129-138.
36. Kuck KH, Schluter M, Gursoy S. Preservation of atrioventricular nodal conduction during radiofrequency current catheter ablation of midseptal accessory pathways. *Circulation.* 1992;86:1743-1752.
37. Haïssaguerre M, Marcus F, Poquet F, Gencel L, Le Metayer P, Clementy J. Electrocardiographic characteristics and catheter ablation of parahisian accessory pathways. *Circulation.* 1994;90:1124-1128.
38. Tada H, Naito S, Nogami A, Taniguchi K. Successful catheter ablation of an anteroseptal accessory pathway from the noncoronary sinus of Valsalva. *J Cardiovasc Electrophysiol.* 2003;14:544-546.
39. Arruda M, McClelland J, Beckman K, et al. Atrial appendage-ventricular connections: a new variant of pre-excitation. *Circulation.* 1994;90:I-126. (Abstract)
40. Milstein S, Dunnigan A, Tang C, Pineda E. Right atrial appendage to right ventricle accessory atrioventricular connection: a case report. *Pacing Clin Electrophysiol.* 1997;20:1877-1880.
41. Goya M, Takahashi A, Nakagawa H, Iesaka Y. A case of catheter ablation of accessory atrioventricular connection between the right atrial appendage and right ventricle guided by a three-dimensional electroanatomical mapping system. *J Cardiovasc Electrophsyiol.* 1999:10;1112-1118.
42. Schweikert RA, Saliba WI, Tomassoni G, et al. Percutaneous pericardial instrumentation for endo-epicardial mapping of previously failed ablation. *Circulation.* 2003;108:1329-1335.

Video Legend

Video 40.1 CS angiography (balloon occlusion technique) in the RAO (**A**) and LAO (**B**) projections, demonstrating a CS diverticulum. Notice vigorous contraction of the diverticulum, indicating a muscular chamber.

CHAPTER 41

ATRIAL FLUTTER: RIGHT ATRIAL AND LEFT ATRIAL FLUTTER

Steven M. Markowitz, MD; Bruce B. Lerman, MD

Mapping Strategies for Atrial Flutter and Macroreentrant Atrial Tachycardias

Successful catheter ablation of atrial flutter (AFL) and macroreentrant atrial tachycardias requires accurate identification of the tachycardia circuit or its critical components. Mapping therefore constitutes the first step in an effective ablation strategy. The initial goal in mapping an atrial tachycardia (AT) is to distinguish macroreentry from a focal mechanism.

Before embarking on extensive mapping, observations about the tachycardia and pacing maneuvers provide useful information about mechanism. Characteristics of the flutter wave on the surface ECG do not necessarily distinguish focal from macroreentrant rhythms.[1] While the presence of isoelectric segments between P waves has been proposed as a characteristic of focal rhythms, it is not uncommon for macroreentrant rhythms to demonstrate isoelectric segments due to zones of slow conduction that are "electrically silent" on the surface ECG. Conversely, focal rhythms might not demonstrate isoelectric segments if the tachycardia is rapid or there are bystander zones of slow conduction. Variability in the AT cycle length exceeding 15% suggests a focal mechanism, but the absence of variability is consistent with either mechanism.[2] Termination of the tachycardia with adenosine (unrelated to premature beats or tachycardia acceleration) is also consistent with a focal mechanism due to triggered activity, whereas transient suppression with adenosine is characteristic of focal automaticity.[3] Reentrant ATs are insensitive to adenosine. These adenosine-insensitive reentrant circuits may comprise large pathways ("macroreentry") or may be localized to relatively small areas ("microreentry").[4]

Activation mapping is the traditional technique to define a macroreentrant AT. If mapping is complete, macroreentrant tachycardias should demonstrate electrical activation that spans the TCL with areas of adjacent "early" and "late" activation. Conventional multipolar or roving catheters may be sufficient to define a tachycardia circuit without the need for EAM. For example, right AFL dependent on the CTI is readily identified with a multipolar catheter around the tricuspid annulus, a catheter at the inferior septum or CS, and one at the His bundle. This configuration will reveal counterclockwise or clockwise activation around the tricuspid annulus that occupies the TCL (Figure 41.1). Slow conduction or prior block in the CTI could result in craniocaudal activation of the lateral RA during other tachycardias; therefore, confirmation through entrainment mapping is required to confirm participation of the CTI in the tachycardia circuit.

Conventional mapping techniques also identify common forms of left AFL.[2] In the case of perimitral reentry, mapping along the mitral annulus reveals that the superior and inferior aspects of the annulus are activated in opposite directions. For example, in counterclockwise mitral flutter, the superior annulus is activated in the lateral to septal direction, while the inferior annulus is activated in the septal to lateral direction. If mapping shows that the posterior and anterior walls of the LA are activated in opposite directions, a roof-dependent tachycardia is suggested. Complex fractionated and low-amplitude EGMs may be found in myopathic atria and represent areas of slow conduction. Complex EGMs may be found in critical zones of slow conduction that participate in a tachycardia circuit

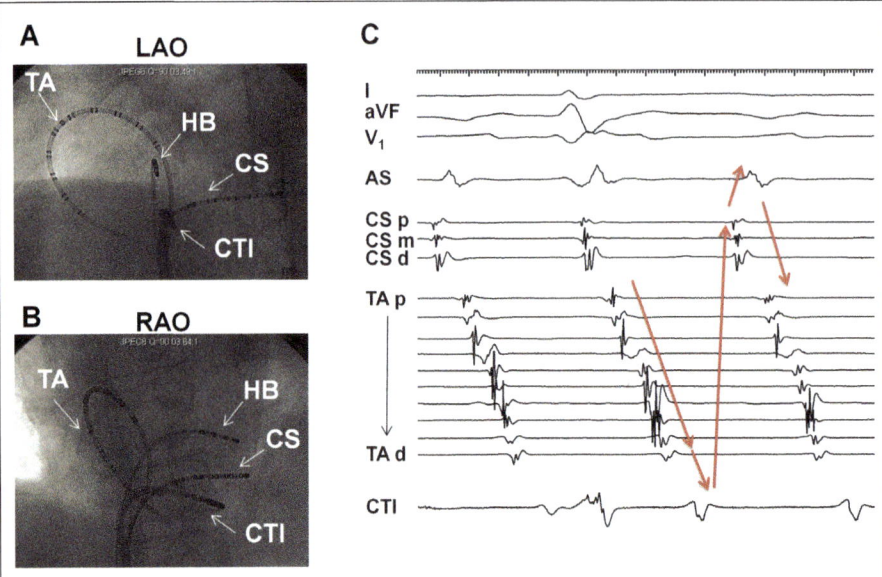

Figure 41.1 Intracardiac activation sequence of counterclockwise, isthmus-dependent right AFL. **Panels A** and **B:** Catheter positions in the LAO and RAO orientations show a duodecapolar catheter around the tricuspid annulus (TA), CS catheter, quadripolar catheter in the His bundle (HB) region, and catheter in the CTI. **Panel C:** The activation sequence is descending along the lateral RA wall (TA proximal to distal), followed by activation of the CTI, proximal CS, and anterior septum (AS).

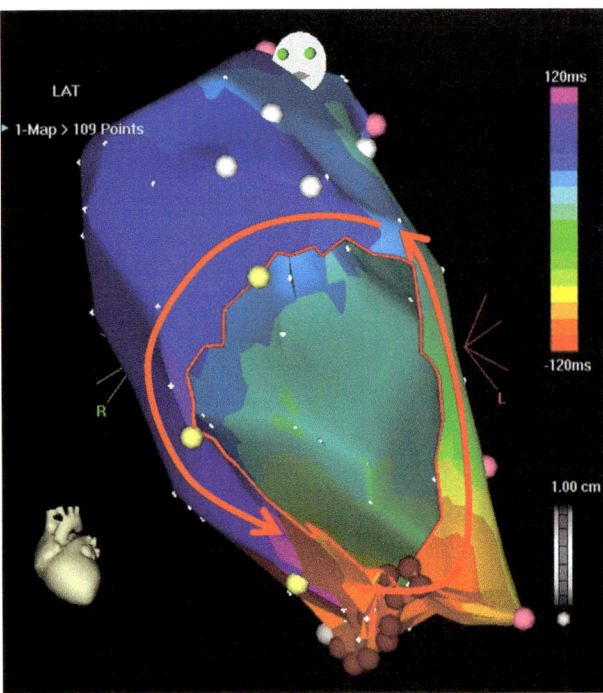

Figure 41.2 Electroanatomical map (EAM) of counterclockwise isthmus-dependent right AFL. The entire atrial cycle length of 240 ms is accounted for in the EAM. The isochrones indicate propagation of the impulse around the tricuspid annulus. There are adjacent zones of early and late activation. **Red tags** show ablation points in the CTI.

but also can exist in bystander zones, which can be verified through entrainment techniques.

EAM is an important adjunct to activation mapping of complex arrhythmias and facilitates identification of sites for ablation. Contact EAM registers multiple points in three-dimensional space and allows a graphical presentation of activation patterns or voltage. A characteristic of macroreentrant rhythms in EAMs is a zone of adjacent "early" and "late" activation (Figure 41.2). To avoid misleading EAMs, it is important to verify that sampled points span the TCL. Noncontact EAM uses a multielectrode array to compute virtual unipolar EGMs in the chamber of interest. The noncontact technology is particularly useful for nonsustained arrhythmias that are difficult to map with sequential contact mapping.

Entrainment mapping is a crucial technique to identify areas that participate in the tachycardia circuit, particularly when EAMs are misleading or inconclusive. Sites with concealed entrainment where the postpacing interval is less than 20 to 30 ms greater than the TCL are considered to participate in the tachycardia circuit (Figure 41.3). The ability to demonstrate entrainment with return cycle equal to the AT cycle length in two opposite segments of one chamber will identify a macroreentrant circuit. For example, fulfillment of entrainment criteria in the lateral and septal mitral annulus will identify perimitral reentry (Figure 41.4, ▶ Video 41.1). Likewise, fulfillment of entrainment criteria in the anterior and posterior LA will identify a roof-dependent left AT.

A basic principle in ablation of AFLs is to identify a critical isthmus and create conduction block by ablating between two nonconducting barriers. Examples of fixed barriers include the valve annuli, inferior or superior vena cavae, and areas of scar that could be due to underlying atrial myopathy, surgical incisions, or prior ablation lesions. Verification of conduction block in the critical isthmus is an important endpoint because termination of a tachycardia and noninducibility are less robust endpoints and generally are associated with higher recurrence rates if not accompanied by conduction block.[5,6]

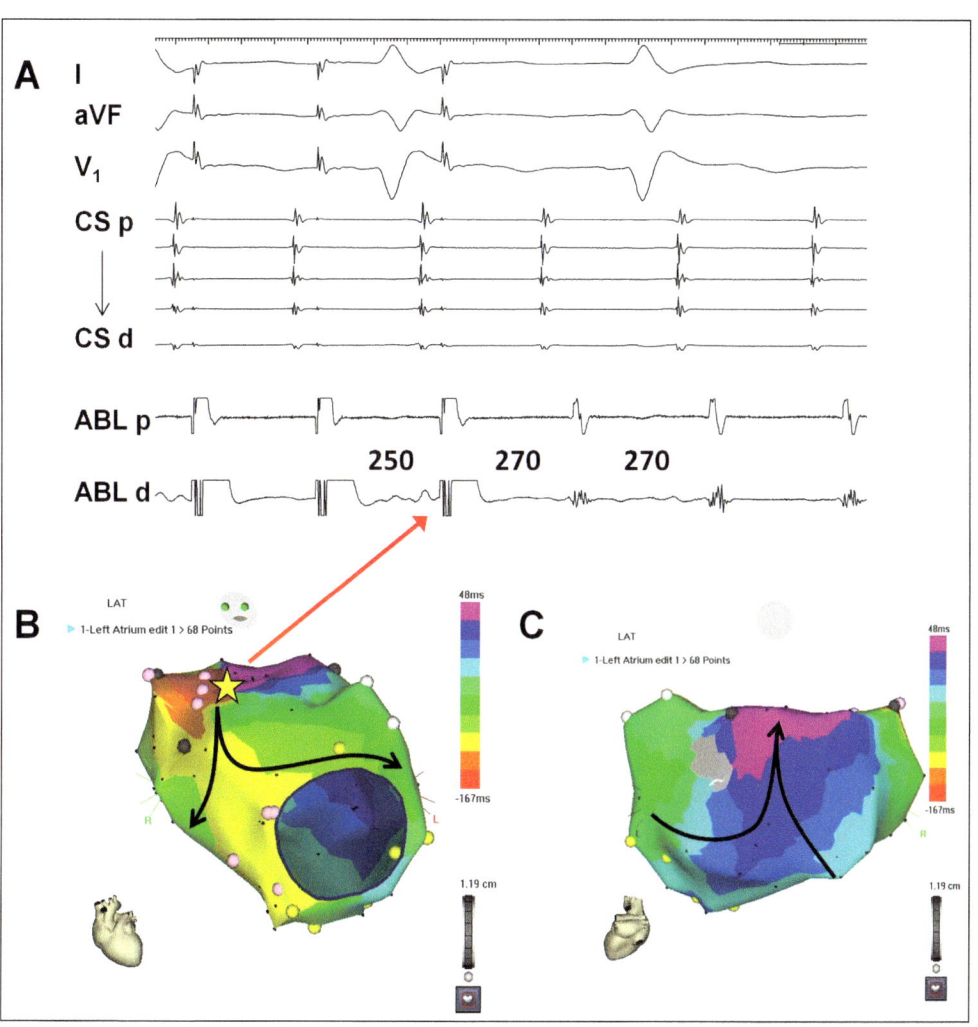

Figure 41.3 Roof-dependent left AFL. **Panel A:** Concealed entrainment is demonstrated during pacing from the roof, as indicated by the intracardiac activation sequence during pacing identical to that during tachycardia. In this location, the postpacing interval is identical to the TCL. **Panels B** and **C:** EAMs in the anteroposterior and posteroanterior orientations show a descending wavefront on the anterior wall and an ascending wavefront on the posterior wall.

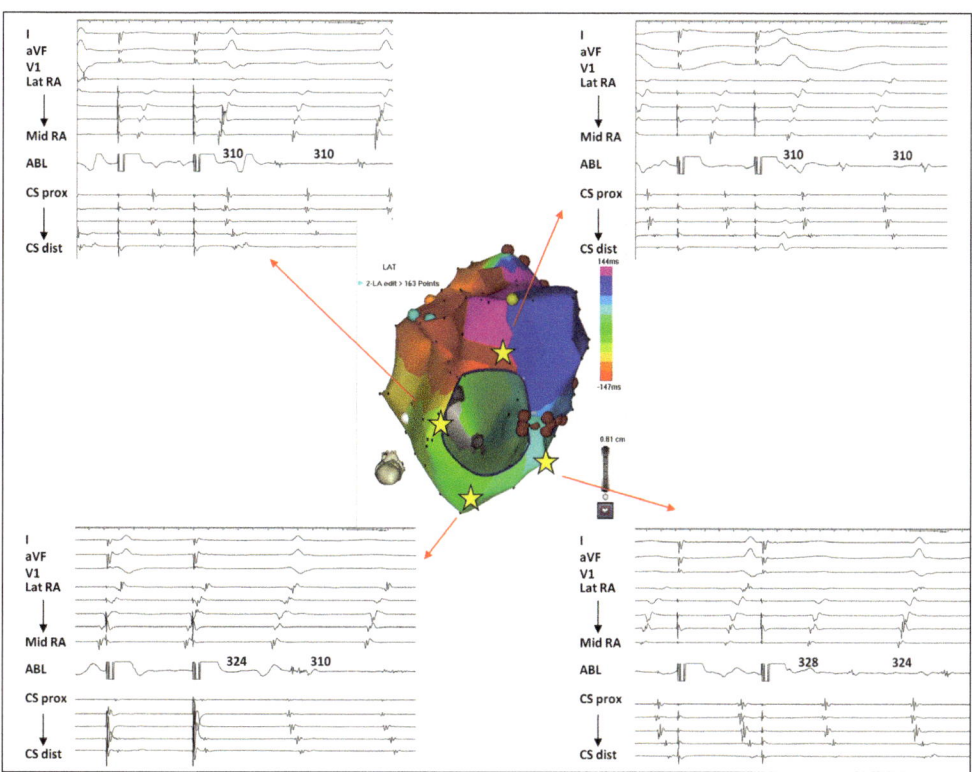

Figure 41.4 Perimitral reentry. Counterclockwise reentry around the mitral annulus is shown in an EAM of the LA. Activation mapping demonstrates lateral to septal activation of the superior annulus and septal to lateral activation of the inferior annulus. Entrainment mapping from lateral, anterior, septal, and inferior annular sites each show postpacing intervals consistent with participation in the tachycardia circuit.

Ablation Techniques for Atrial Flutters

Most catheter ablation for AFLs is accomplished with radiofrequency (RF) energy. Historically, 4 mm–tip electrodes were the technology initially available for RF. Large-electrode catheters (8 mm and 10 mm) are useful for creating linear lesions, particularly across the CTI.[7] Another advantage of a larger surface area electrode is cooling of the electrode due to surrounding blood flow; these electrodes will typically require higher power for effective lesion formation. Internally or externally irrigated electrodes have proved useful for mapping and ablating complex ATs. The smaller electrode sizes (3.5 to 4 mm) reduce far-field EGMs compared to larger-tip electrodes. Active irrigation permits the delivery of higher power without the limitation of excessively high tip-tissue interface temperatures.

Cryotherapy with large-tip electrodes have demonstrated efficacy for ablation of typical flutter in the CTI.[8-10] A cryoablation catheter with a 6.5 mm–tip electrode has been evaluated in several trials, and larger electrodes of 8 or 10 mm are also effective in CTI ablation. Cryotherapy offers the advantage of catheter stability due to formation of an "ice ball" at the catheter tip during active freezing. Another property of cryoablation is the absence of pain during therapeutic freezing.

Cavo-tricuspid Isthmus-dependent Flutters

The CTI-dependent flutters include counterclockwise and clockwise reentry around the tricuspid annulus, as well as lower loop reentry.[11,12] Counterclockwise CTI-dependent flutter gives rise to the characteristic "typical" flutter morphology on the surface ECG, with a "sawtooth" pattern in the inferior leads (superior flutter wave axis) and a positive P wave in lead V_1. Clockwise CTI-dependent flutter often causes an inferior flutter wave axis and negative P wave in lead V_1. Entrainment mapping of these two variants shows reentry around the tricuspid annulus, but variations have been reported in which peritricuspid tissue falls outside the critical parts of the tachycardia circuit. The wavefront may traverse either anterior or posterior to the SVC.[13] A zone of conduction block is present in the crista terminalis or posterior RA.[14,15] In the case of lower loop reentry, conduction occurs posterior to the IVC across the crista terminalis, but as with the "typical" variants described above, the CTI is a critical part of the tachycardia circuit.[12] Lower loop reentry may interconvert with typical AFL. The CTI may also serve as a common corridor for a figure-eight circuit involving simultaneous reentry around the tricuspid annulus and the IVC. Reentry confined to the CTI (intraisthmus reentry) can occur in patients with previous CTI ablation and is characterized by fractionated and prolonged potentials in the CTI.[16]

Ablation of these flutter variants is performed in the CTI, which is an accessible location and usually the shortest isthmus with fixed anatomical barriers. Various techniques have been employed to achieve complete ablation of the CTI. With RF energy, sequential focal ablations along the isthmus may be performed, whereas some operators prefer to drag the catheter from the tricuspid annulus to the IVC with continuous application of RF current. With 8 mm–tip catheters, up to 70 W is delivered, whereas 10 mm–tip catheters may require up to 100 W. With solid electrode catheters, target tip temperatures of 60° to 70° are typically employed. With open or closed irrigation catheters, power may be titrated up to 50 W (either manually or through a temperature-controlled mode), limited by a maximal tip temperature generally not exceeding 43°. It is customary to titrate power to achieve a fall in impedance of 5 to 10 ohm (Ω). In addition, reduction in EGM amplitude is used as an indicator of effective local ablation. Energy is usually applied at each point along the isthmus for at least 30 seconds. The central isthmus (6 o'clock position in the LAO projection) is the preferred location for ablation in the CTI because of its thinner wall and shorter length compared to the septal and lateral aspects.[17] An alternative technique is to target areas in the CTI with the largest voltage, which may establish CTI block with limited focal lesions.[18]

Anatomical variants could influence the choice of procedural techniques and the outcomes of CTI ablation. Imaging of the CTI with ICE,[19] magnetic resonance imaging,[20] CT,[21] EAM,[22] and RA angiography[23] have all been employed to reveal anatomical details, such as the length of the CTI, the presence of a prominent Eustachian ridge, or the presence of a deep sub-Eustachian recess. In some patients, a deep sub-Eustachian fossa forms a recess between the tricuspid annulus and the IVC. Successful ablation will require delivery of energy within this recess, which might be limited by high temperatures due to poor convective cooling of the electrode from low blood flow. Another challenge in some patients is the presence of thick muscle bundles in the CTI, which could limit the ability to obtain transmural lesions. Eschar formation on the endocardium can also limit energy delivery. In these cases, a new line parallel to the incomplete one might be necessary. Another technique in resistant cases is to orient the ablation catheter parallel to the isthmus (lateral to septal) instead of the usual perpendicular direction (caval to annular). For difficult cases or instances of recurrent conduction in the CTI, a gap in the line can be identified to (re)establish conduction block (Figure 41.5). The gap can be localized with contact or noncontact EAM.

Assessment of Conduction Block in the CTI

Regardless of technique, the endpoint of ablation is to achieve complete bidirectional conduction block in the CTI. Various methods have been described to verify bidirectional conduction block in the CTI.

1. *Activation mapping.* After bidirectional block is achieved, pacing from the septal aspect of the ablation line should reveal craniocaudal activation of the lateral RA wall. This can be easily assessed with a multipolar mapping catheter around the tricuspid annulus (Figure 41.6). For convenience, pacing is often performed from the posterior septum or proximal CS. Fusion of wavefronts in the lateral wall or early activation of the low lateral RA would indicate that conduction proceeds across the CTI. Likewise, pacing from the lateral aspect of the ablation line (or low lateral RA) will reveal craniocaudal activation of the septum. If a multipolar catheter is not positioned along the septum, the septal activation pattern can be inferred by the timing of activation in catheters at the His bundle and proximal CS. If the distal electrodes of a multipolar catheter are not positioned

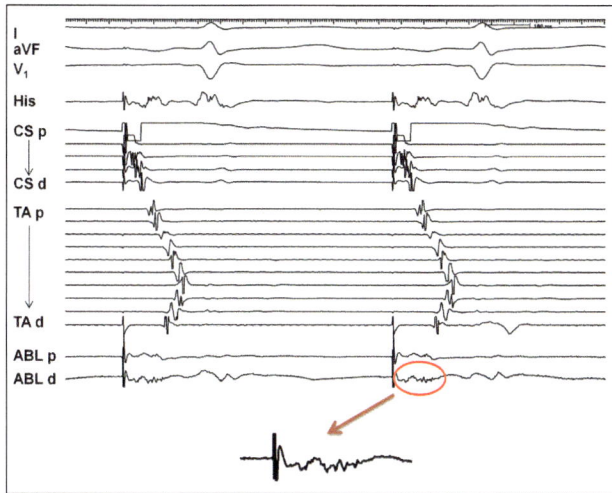

Figure 41.5 Gap in CTI identified as a complex, fractionated EGM.

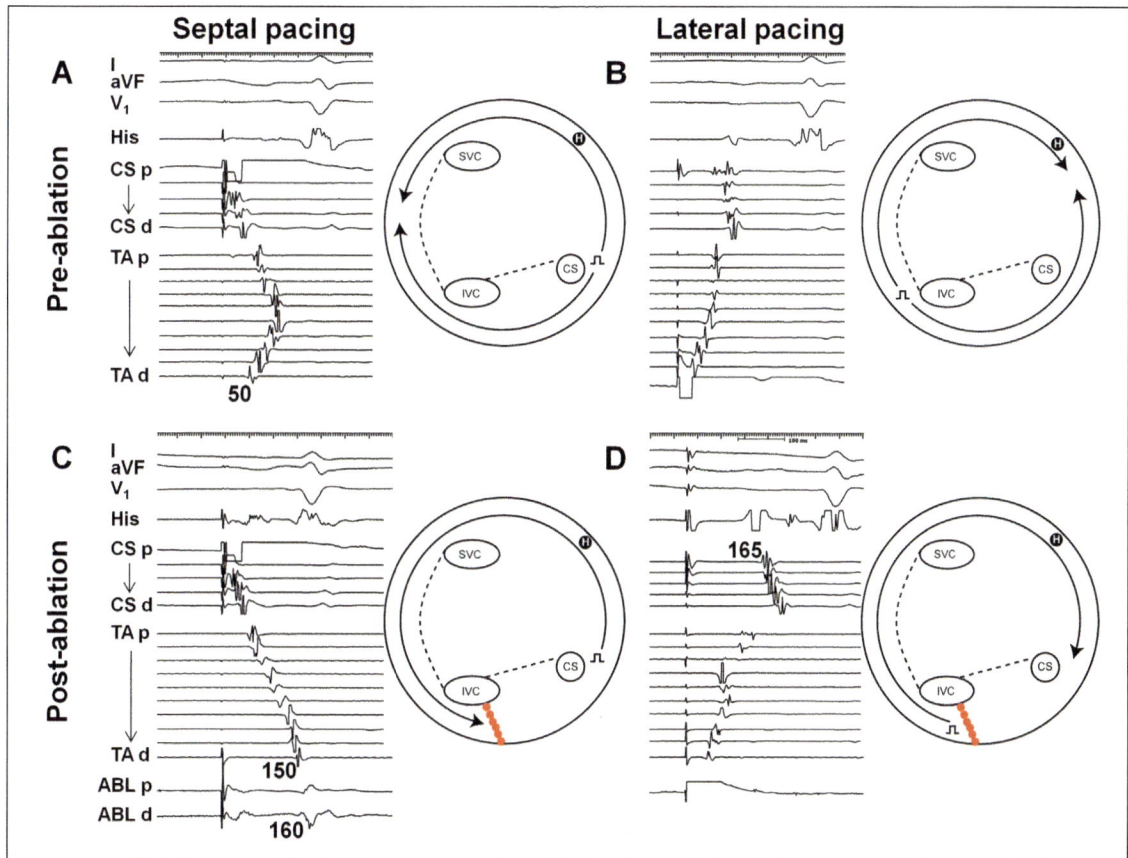

Figure 41.6 Evaluation of line of block in the CTI. **Panel A:** Before ablation, pacing from the proximal CS gives rise to fusion of wavefronts in the lateral RA (stimulation to low lateral RA 50 ms). **Panel B:** Pacing from the low lateral RA causes activation of the proximal CS before the atrial EGM on the His bundle catheter (**circle with H**). **Panel C:** After ablation, pacing from the proximal CS causes counterclockwise activation about the triscuspid annlus, with late activation of the low lateral RA (150 ms). Double potentials are recorded on the mapping catheter in the CTI, with the second component activated later than any EGM around the tricuspid annulus (160 ms). **Panel D:** During pacing lateral to the ablation line, activation of anterior septum (on the His bundle catheter) precedes activation of the proximal CS (165 ms).

adjacent to the ablation line, it is useful to position the roving ablation catheter just lateral (or septal) to the line to confirm late activation on the opposite side of the line. While the ablation catheter is moved from septal to lateral to the line, there should be a sudden change in activation from early to late during pacing from the inferior septum.

2. *Double potentials.* If conduction block is present, mapping along the ablation line during pacing from one side should reveal double potentials separated by isoelectric intervals (Figure 41.5C).[24] These double potentials should be found along the entire length of the line, whereas the presence of complex continuous EGMs indicate the presence of breakthrough conduction. Separation of double potentials of at least 90 ms is associated with conduction block, but the isoelectric interval may shorten in the presence of isoproterenol.

3. *Change in EGM polarity.* During pacing from one side of the ablation line, reversal of the bipolar EGM polarity just opposite to the line can be demonstrated when conduction block is achieved.[27] Unipolar recordings opposite the ablation line can also indicate conduction block.[28] A monophasic R wave in the unipolar EGM signifies conduction toward but not away from the electrode and can be observed in an electrode just adjacent and lateral to the line of block during pacing from the septal side, whereas a biphasic (RS, rS) pattern is consistent with conduction across the isthmus.

4. *Differential pacing.* This maneuver may be used to identify components of double potentials or complex EGMs on an ablation line and distinguish slow conduction from complete conduction block.[29] The technique is performed by pacing adjacent and farther away from the ablation line and comparing activation times to the EGMs on or near the line. If conduction block is present, those components activated on the opposite side of the line will occur later when pacing is close to the line, because the wavefront circulates around the tricuspid annulus. When pacing is performed farther away from the line, a shorter activation time results for those components across the line. In contrast, if conduction persists through the isthmus, then pacing close to the line results in shorter activation time to the opposite time.

Errors in Interpreting Conduction Block in the Cavotricuspid Isthmus

1. *Slow conduction.* Slow conduction through the CTI may allow a wavefront to propagate in the craniocaudal direction opposite to the pacing site, which might erroneously suggest conduction block in the CTI (Figure 41.7). Slow conduction can be distinguished from conduction block by careful interrogation of the ablation line to demonstrate double potentials along the length of the line. Activation opposite the pacing site should be recorded as close as possible to the ablation line and should occur later than any other site around the tricuspid annulus. As the isthmus is scanned from lateral to septal, abrupt changes in activation should be demonstrated as the catheter crosses the completed line. In the case of complex or

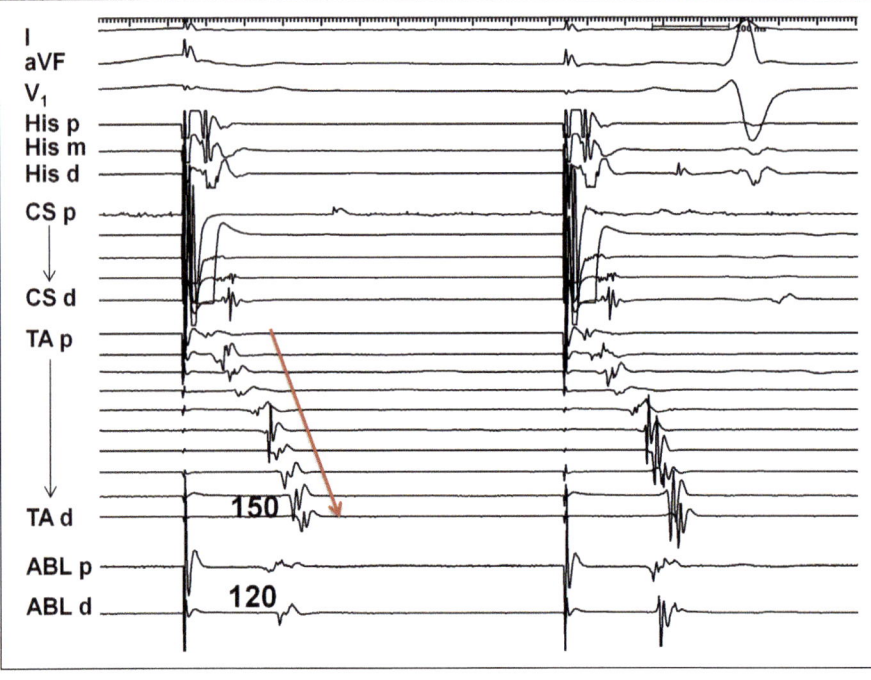

Figure 41.7 Slow conduction in the CTI after incomplete ablation produces a descending wavefront in the lateral wall during pacing from the proximal CS, which could be misinterpreted as conduction block in the isthmus. When the ablation catheter is positioned medial to the multipolar catheter, slow conduction through the isthmus becomes apparent since the ablation catheter is activated before the low lateral RA.

double EGMs, the techniques of differential pacing will identify if a component is activated via slow conduction or around the tricuspid annulus.

2. *Transcristal conduction.* If conduction occurs across the low crista terminalis, pacing from the septal aspect of the ablation line might result in early activation of the low lateral RA wall, which might be misinterpreted as conduction across the CTI. A multipolar mapping catheter positioned adjacent to or across the CTI might reveal earlier activation at the low lateral RA, but later activation just lateral to the CTI (Figure 41.8).

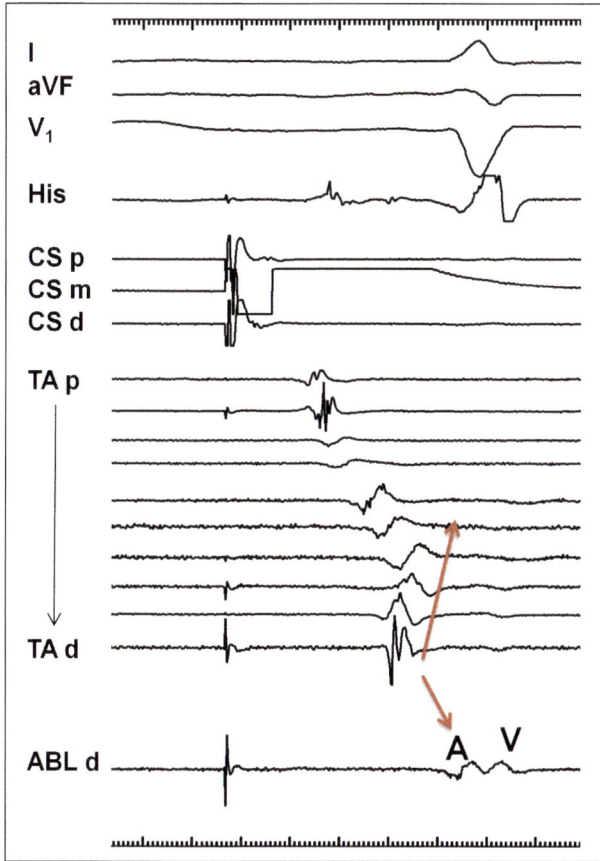

Figure 41.8 Transcristal conduction during CS pacing causes earlier activation of the low lateral RA (TA-d) compared to more proximal electrodes, which might erroneously suggest conduction through the CTI. When the ablation catheter is positioned just lateral to the ablation line, activation is even later than the low lateral RA.

This situation emphasizes the importance of recording as close as possible to the ablation line and the value of scanning the line for double potentials. More detailed mapping along the posterior RA behind the IVC might also demonstrate conduction across the crista terminalis. Altering the site of pacing will distinguish transcristal conduction from transisthmus conduction: If transcristal conduction is present, pacing posterior to the IVC will result in shorter conduction times to the lateral RA, whereas pacing just septal to the ablation line will result in the longer conduction times.[30] The converse holds if conduction proceeds through the CTI. It is also useful to position a multipolar catheter across the entire CTI (from lateral to septal) in order to identify the two distinct wavefronts.

3. *Malposition of the multipolar catheter.* If some poles of the multipolar catheter are posterior to the crista terminalis, there may be an ascending or complex activation pattern during septal pacing. This occurs because during low septal pacing the wavefront propagates in an ascending direction in the posteroseptal RA and in a descending direction in the anterolateral RA.

Outcomes of Ablation for CTI-dependent Atrial Flutter

Acute Success

Demonstration of bidirectional conduction block in the CTI has been shown to be a superior procedural endpoint compared to acute termination and noninducibility of AFL. In most studies, the acute success of RFA in the CTI exceeds 85%, and is generally more than 90%. A multicenter study of an 8 mm–tip catheter demonstrated an acute success rate of 88%, using an endpoint of bidirectional isthmus block.[31] In another multicenter trial with 8 and 10 mm–tip catheters, acute success was 93%.[32] A meta-analysis of 158 studies including over 10,000 patients yielded the following conclusions: Ablation with larger-tip (8 or 10 mm) or irrigated catheters generated an acute success rate of 93%.[6] There was only a trend toward higher acute success with larger-tip catheters over the smaller electrodes (4 and 6 mm). Cryoablation resulted in similar acute success rates as RFA.

Early resumption of conduction across the isthmus occurs in approximately 15% of patients, with most resumption of conduction occurring within 20 minutes of the ablation.[33,34] Isoproterenol can also identify latent conduction across the isthmus in approximately 16% of patients.[35]

Late Success and Recurrences

In several large cohort or multicenter studies, late recurrences of CTI-dependent AFL after RFA with large-tip or irrigated catheters occur at rates of 3% to 13%. A meta-analysis demonstrated that recurrent AFL occurs in 7% of patients who underwent ablation with larger-tip or irrigated catheters, and recurrences are more common with smaller-tip RF catheters.[6] Recurrent CTI-dependent AFL tends to occur within 6 months of the ablation procedure without substantial increases in recurrence rates during longer follow-up.

The meta-analysis also showed that cryoablation yields similar long-term success rates compared to RFA (11% recurrent AFL with cryoablation versus 7% with large tip/irrigated RF, a difference that was not statistically significant).[6] In one multicenter randomized study, RFA and cryoablation with an 8 mm–tip catheter had similar acute success in producing bidirectional isthmus block (approximately 90%), but persistence of bidirectional block 3 months after ablation was lower with cryoablation (65%) compared to RFA (85%), and there were more clinical recurrences of common AFL in the cryotherapy group.[36]

Catheter ablation for CTI-dependent AFL has been shown to be superior to antiarrhythmic drugs as first-line therapy. A trial of 104 patients with a single episode of CTI-dependent flutter randomized patients to catheter ablation or cardioversion and amiodarone.[37] This study demonstrated that CTI-dependent flutter recurred at a rate of 30% among patients treated with amiodarone versus 4% among those who underwent catheter ablation, with average follow-up of 13 months. The rate of AF was similar in the two treatment groups (18% for the amiodarone group and 25% for the ablation group). Another randomized study of 61 patients with at least two episodes of CTI-dependent AFL showed that patients who underwent catheter ablation as first-line therapy were more likely to remain in sinus rhythm and less likely to have rehospitalizations after an average of 21 months.[38]

Atrial Fibrillation

AF commonly occurs after ablation of right AFL, with an incidence of 10% to 50%, and the likelihood of AF increases over time following flutter ablation.[6,39] The most consistent predictor of recurrent AF after flutter ablation is a history of preexisting AF. Other predictors reported in various studies include depressed left ventricular function, hypertension, younger age, LA enlargement, and induction of AF at EP study. During long-term follow-up, AF occurs in approximately 50% of patients with preexisting AF, and most of these recurrences occur early after ablation. In contrast, AF will eventually occur in 20% to 25% of patients without evidence of this arrhythmia preablation, and the incidence increases gradually with longer follow-up. This phenomenon has been interpreted to mean that many patients with isolated AFL will develop progressive electrical disease that predisposes to AF. Among patients treated with class IC or III antiarrhythmic drugs for AF who undergo ablation of CTI-dependent AFL, the recurrence rate of AF is also substantial in the long term and approaches 50%.

Complications

The overall complication rate for AFL ablation averages 2.6% among various studies in the literature.[6,31] The most common complications are vascular access issues, complete heart block, and pericardial effusion. Cerebrovascular events, peripheral thromboembolism, and pulmonary embolism have also been reported. Thromboembolism can occur as a result of ablation-mediated conversion of AFL to sinus rhythm. This complication can be mitigated by careful attention to anticoagulation prior to the ablation or by excluding a thrombus with a TEE. Systemic anticoagulation is conventionally continued for at least one month after active conversion of AFL, and long-term anticoagulation is considered for patients at high risk for developing AF who have thromboembolism risk factors. Myocardial infarction can occur because of injury to the right coronary artery in the atrioventricular groove. Skin burns have rarely been reported with the use of high-power generators using larger-tip electrodes.

RA Free-wall Reentry

Reentry isolated to the RA free wall occurs most commonly in patients with prior lateral right atriotomies, although reentry in the lateral wall can occur in the absence of prior surgery.[40-44] This arrhythmia requires a line of block in the lateral wall, which is identified as a line of double potentials (Figure 41.9). Entrainment anterior and posterior to this line, as well as by the inferior and superior vena cavae, will confirm participation in the tachycardia circuit. A critical isthmus exists between the inferior end of the line and the IVC, and isthmuses can also be found between the line and the lateral tricuspid annulus, or between the line and the SVC. Each isthmus is a potential target for ablation, depending on the specific anatomical considerations of the case. Following ablation from the lateral wall to the IVC, confirmation of conduction block along the lateral wall can be confirmed by pacing from either side of the line, and descending wavefronts should be demonstrated on the opposite side of the line. Another variant of lateral wall reentry involves a gap within scar in the lateral RA, which can be treated by ablation within this localized gap (Figure 41.9).

Upper Loop Reentry

Upper loop reentry refers to reentry around the SVC and an adjacent line of block in the lateral RA wall. This tachycardia has been described with noncontact and contact EAM, which demonstrates conduction across a gap in the crista terminalis.[45] As with other forms of RA reentry, the upper reentrant loop may coexist with a second loop in the RA (such as a circuit around the tricuspid annulus) to produce a dual-loop tachycardia. Only small series of upper loop reentry have been reported in the literature, possibly because of the difficulty in defining this reentrant circuit or because this circuit can be less stable than CTI-dependent flutters. The strategy employed in

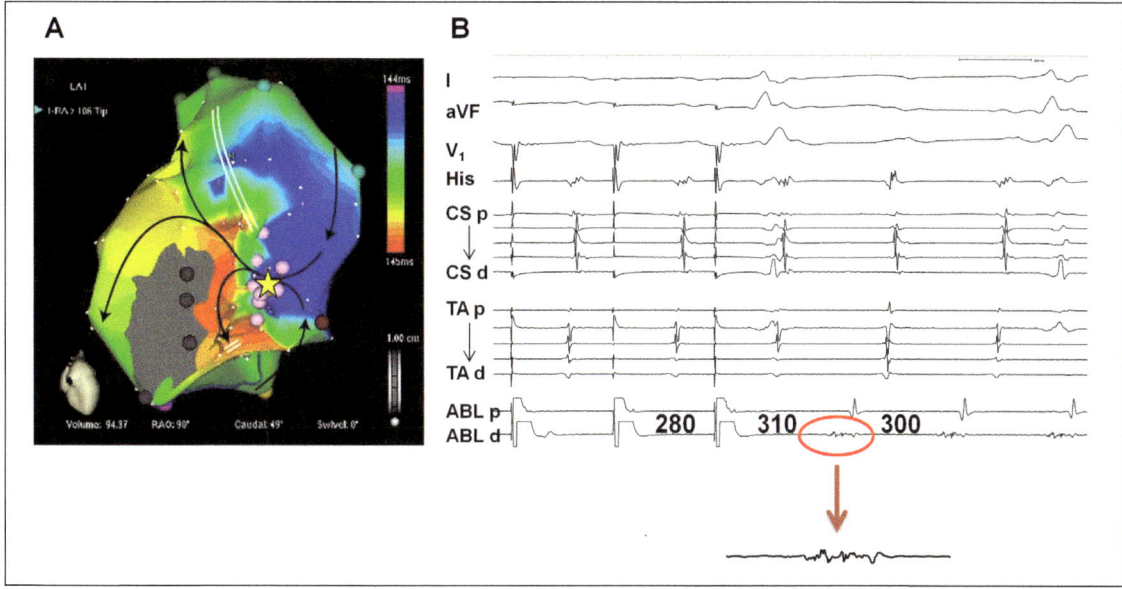

Figure 41.9 Reentry in the lateral RA. **Panel A:** EAM shows reentry involving a gap in the lateral wall of the RA (**star**). A line of block is present in the lateral wall (**double lines**) and an area of scar is identified in the low lateral RA (**gray zone**). **Panel B:** The EGM in the gap is highly fractionated, and entrainment is consistent with participation in the tachycardia circuit. A single ablation in the lateral wall gap terminates the tachycardia and prevents reinduction.

ablating these tachycardias is to target the gap in the crista terminalis or to ablate from the SVC to a conduction barrier in the high RA.

Right Atrial Septal Reentry

Reentry in the RA septum has been described in patients with repaired atrial septal defects[41] and following mitral valve surgery.[46] In reported cases, periseptal reentry often becomes evident during or after ablation of CTI-dependent reentry. Various ablation strategies have been used to eliminate reentry around a septal patch, including ablation from the septal patch to the SVC, IVC, or tricuspid annulus.

Dual Loop Right Atrial Tachycardias

Dual loop tachycardias may occur in the RA and consist of two circuits that share a common isthmus. One common variant is reentry around the tricuspid annulus and another around the IVC. This form of dual loop reentry is effectively treated by ablation in the CTI, which is the common isthmus for both loops. Another common form of dual loop tachycardia is reentry around the tricuspid annulus (as in typical AFL) and reentry around a line of block in the lateral RA.[47,48] This type of reentry can be encountered in patients with lateral atriotomies who appear to have ECGs suggestive of typical AFL. Ablation in the CTI will not terminate the tachycardia but will cause an abrupt (and sometimes subtle) change in the RA activation and/or flutter wave morphology, a clue that a second circuit is present. Entrainment can then confirm the presence of a second tachycardia circuit in the lateral wall and will show that the septal aspect of the annulus no longer participates in the arrhythmia. Although ablation could be performed in the common isthmus between the atriotomy in the lateral wall and the tricuspid annulus, this lesion set can be technically challenging because of poor catheter stability. Often, this form of dual loop reentry is treated by separate ablations in the CTI and between the atriotomy and the IVC.

Left Atrial Macroreentry

Most macroreentrant arrhythmias in the LA occur in patients with atrial myopathies, following atrial surgery, and after catheter ablation of AF or MAZE procedures for AF. Reentry occurs around anatomical obstacles or lines of block, such as the mitral annulus, pulmonary vein ostia, atriotomy scars, or RF lines, as well as patchy scars in the LA.[43,49-51] Circuits can be complex and consist of multiple loops. The most common variants of LA macroreentry are mitral annular flutter and roof-dependent AT.

In mitral annular flutter, reentry occurs clockwise or counterclockwise around the annulus (Figure 41.4). The goal for ablation is to create a linear lesion from the mitral annulus to another electrically silent area, such as an isolated pulmonary vein. Tissue between the lateral mitral annulus and the LIPV is known as the "mitral isthmus." Creation of transmural lesions in the mitral isthmus may be difficult from the endocardial surface, because the mitral isthmus can be relatively thick and the circumflex artery and its branches produce local cooling.[52,53] Ablation may therefore require multiple lesions on the endocardial surface.[54] Because endocardial ablation will often leave epicardial gaps, ablation within the CS is needed in up to 70% of patients. With a combined endocardial/epicardial approach, block in the mitral isthmus can be achieved in >90% of patients. Ablation in the CS is typically performed with power settings of 20 to 30 W and irrigation rates of 17 to 60 mL/min. A risk of ablation in the mitral isthmus, as with ablation in other locations in the LA, is cardiac tamponade, which can be avoided by limiting power to ≤42 W during endocardial ablation.

Line of block should be verified along the mitral isthmus, because conduction gaps in this line are proarrhythmic.[55] Conduction block can be demonstrated by pacing on either side of the ablation line using a CS catheter and one on the opposite side of the line in the LA. The LAA is a stable location for a catheter anterior to the ablation line. If conduction block is present, pacing anterior to the line will give rise to proximal-to-distal CS activation as the impulse propagates counterclockwise around the annulus (Figure 41.10). Similarly, pacing from the CS catheter just lateral to the line will cause delay to the anterior LA (and septal to lateral propagation along the superior mitral annulus), as the impulse propagates clockwise around the annulus. Double potentials along the line also support the presence of a line of block. The technique of "differential pacing" may be used to demonstrate conduction block. In this technique, pacing is performed from distal and proximal poles of a CS catheter, and conduction times to the anterior LA are compared. In the case of complete conduction block, pacing from the distal poles will result in a longer conduction time around the mitral annulus compared to proximal pacing.

One alternative approach to interrupting perimitral flutter is an "anterior" mitral line, which is created anterior to the LAA between the anterior/anterolateral mitral annulus and the ostium of the LSPV.[56] Another approach involves transsecting the anterior LA between the mitral annulus and a completed roof line between the superior PVs.[57] This latter approach may be technically difficult and achieves complete conduction block in fewer patients. In addition, this line can create significant conduction delays in activation of the LAA, which could adversely affect emptying of this structure.

In "roof-dependent" left AFL, the impulse propagates down the posterior wall and up the anterior wall, or the circuit is reversed. Ablation is accomplished as a linear lesion connecting the right and left superior pulmonary veins. As with mitral flutter, isolation of the pulmonary veins is needed to anchor the new ablation line. A linear lesion along the posterior wall would also interrupt this form of reentry. During ablation along the roof, caution is advised when the ablation catheter is oriented perpendicular to the roof, and the operator should be vigilant to temperature rises, high impedance,

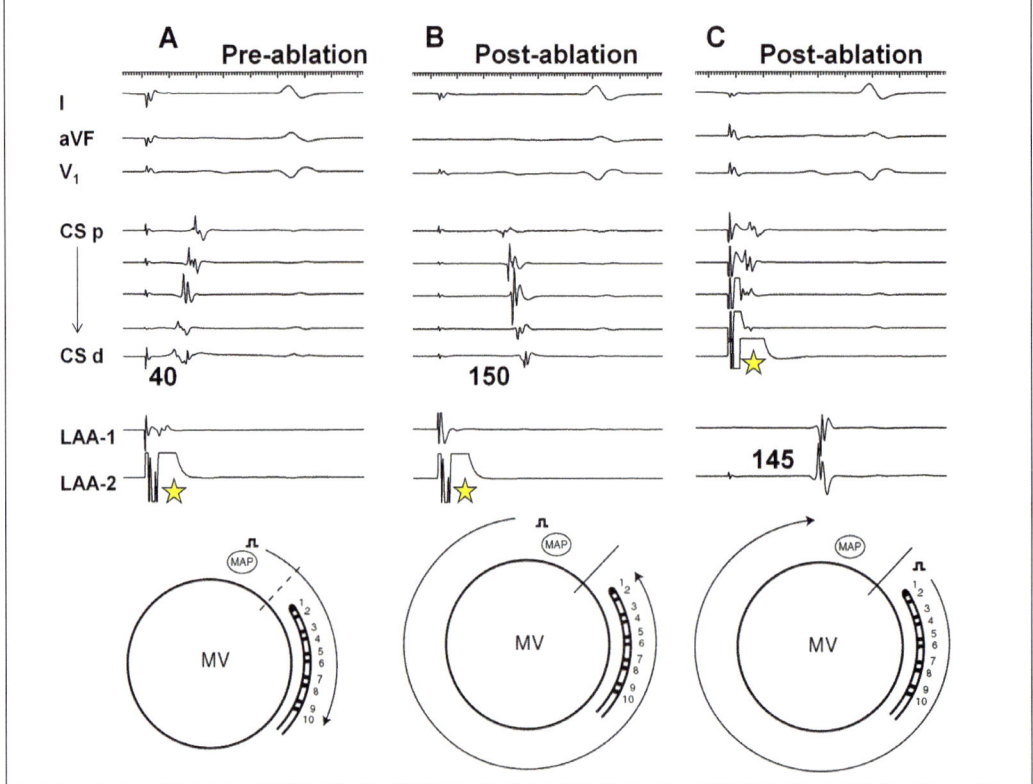

Figure 41.10 Line of block in the mitral isthmus. **Panel A:** At baseline, pacing from the LAA results in earlier activation in the distal CS. **Panel B:** After completion of the mitral line, pacing from the appendage causes counterclockwise activation of the mitral annulus, and the distal electrode on the CS catheter, which is just lateral to the line, is activated late. **Panel C:** Pacing from the distal CS causes late activation of the appendage, as the wavefront propagates clockwise around the mitral annulus.

and steam pops, which could lead to perforation. RFA along the posterior wall poses a risk of esophageal injury, which can manifest as ulceration, atrial-esophageal injury, and dysmotility. This risk is minimized by reducing power and duration of energy application in the vicinity of the esophagus (for example, to a maximum of 30 to 35 W with an irrigated electrode). Line of block along the roof is demonstrated by pacing adjacent to the line and recording an ascending wavefront on the opposite side. For example, pacing may be performed from the anterior LA (or the LAA), and the wavefront in the posterior wall should be ascending if conduction block is present. Double potentials should also be recorded along the line while pacing on one side of the line or during sinus rhythm (Figure 41.11).[58] Deployment of a roof line with complete line of block can be achieved with an acute success rate of > 95%.

the right pulmonary veins and the mitral annulus. This tachycardia can be treated with a linear lesion through the septum, between the septum primum and the right pulmonary veins, or between the septum primum and the mitral annulus.

Macroreentrant Atrial Tachycardias after Ablation of Atrial Fibrillation

The incidence and types of macroreentrant atrial tachycardias that occur after catheter or surgical ablation of AF depend on the lesion sets employed during the initial AF ablation procedure.[60] Atrial macroreentry is uncommon (< 5% of patients) after segmental PVI in the absence of extensive linear lesions or ablation of complex fractionated EGMs. After wide encircling antral ablation, atrial tachycardias occur more commonly, in up to 25% of patients. Gaps in the encircling PVI lesions are a common source of atrial tachycardias. Common macroreentrant rhythms after AF ablation are roof-dependent LA flutter and perimitral flutter. In fact, the addition of linear lesions in the LA roof or mitral isthmus during the initial AF ablation procedure may be proarrhythmic due to gaps in the ablation lines. One of the strongest predictors of developing perimitral flutter after AF ablation is the performance of mitral isthmus ablation during the AF procedure.[61] Activation and entrainment mapping are required to delineate the reentrant circuits and identify ablation targets, which typically are gaps in previously created lines. Commonly, the clinical atrial tachycardia is not present or inducible during the ablation procedure. In such cases, identifying gaps and reinforcing the previous ablation lines, including pulmonary vein re-isolation, is usually the best strategy.

Ablation of complex fractionated EGMs during AF ablation introduces additional complex substrate for both macroreentrant rhythms and small reentrant circuits (also known as "localized reentry"). Localized reentry can occur at previously ablated pulmonary vein ostia as well as at other previously treated sites in the body of the LA. The hallmark of localized reentry is a highly fractionated, long-duration EGM that occupies a large percentage of the TCL, and participation of this site in the tachycardia circuit can be confirmed with entrainment criteria.[4,62,63] Focal ablation at such sites is usually successful in interrupting localized reentrant rhythms.

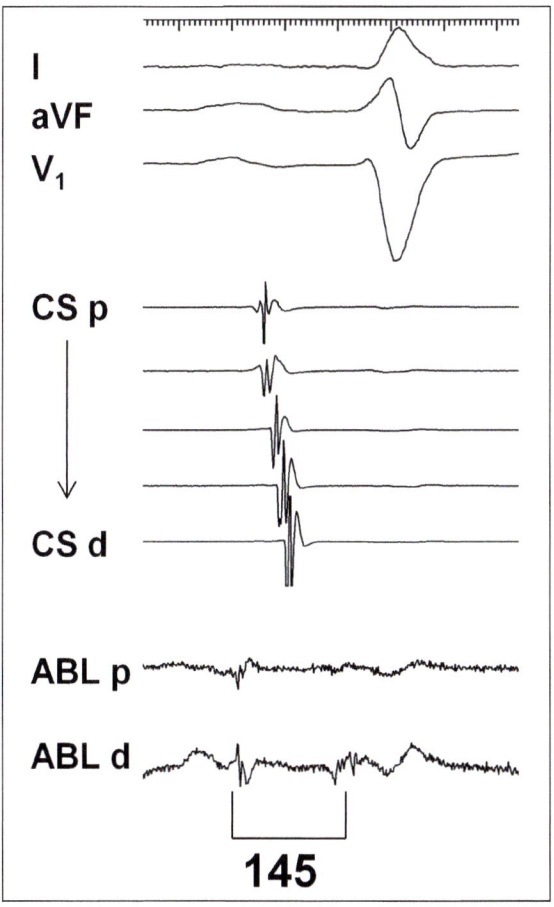

Figure 41.11 Line of block in the LA roof. Low-amplitude double potentials are present during sinus rhythm, separated by 145 ms.

Conclusions

Successful ablation of macroreentrant ATs requires identification of a critical isthmus through the techniques of activation and entrainment mapping. Linear lesions are usually required unless a focal gap can be identified through a region of scar or incomplete line of block.

Left Septal Flutter

Reentry confined to the LA septum has been reported in small series of patients without previous cardiac surgery, typically among patients with AF treated with antiarrhythmic drugs.[59] Boundaries of the reentrant circuit are

Conduction block in the ablation line can be verified through activation mapping, double potentials, and differential pacing. Confirmation of conduction block is an important endpoint that is associated with higher long-term success in ablation of macroreentrant circuits.

References

1. Shah D. ECG manifestations of left atrial flutter. *Curr Opin Cardiol*. 2009;24:35-41.
2. Jaïs P, Matsuo S, Knecht S, et al. A deductive mapping strategy for atrial tachycardia following atrial fibrillation ablation: importance of localized reentry. *J Cardiovasc Electrophysiol*. 2009;20:480-491.
3. Iwai S, Markowitz SM, Stein KM, et al. Response to adenosine differentiates focal from macroreentrant atrial tachycardia: validation using three-dimensional electroanatomic mapping. *Circulation*. 2002;106:2793-2799.
4. Markowitz SM, Nemirovksy D, Stein KM, et al. Adenosine-insensitive focal atrial tachycardia: evidence for de novo micro-re-entry in the human atrium. *J Am Coll Cardiol*. 2007;49:1324-1333.
5. Poty H, Saoudi N, Nair M, Anselme F, Letac B. Radiofrequency catheter ablation of atrial flutter. Further insights into the various types of isthmus block: application to ablation during sinus rhythm. *Circulation*. 1996;94:3204-3213.
6. Perez FJ, Schubert CM, Parvez B, Pathak V, Ellenbogen KA, Wood MA. Long-term outcomes after catheter ablation of cavo-tricuspid isthmus dependent atrial flutter: a meta-analysis. *Circ Arrhythm Electrophysiol*. 2009;2:393-401.
7. Feld GK. Radiofrequency ablation of atrial flutter using large-tip electrode catheters. *J Cardiovasc Electrophysiol*. 2004;15:S18-23.
8. Daubert JP, Hoyt RH, John R, et al. Performance of a new cardiac cryoablation system in the treatment of cavotricuspid valve isthmus-dependent atrial flutter. *Pacing Clin Electrophysiol*. 2005;28 Suppl 1:S142-145.
9. Feld GK, Daubert JP, Weiss R, Miles WM, Pelkey W. Acute and long-term efficacy and safety of catheter cryoablation of the cavotricuspid isthmus for treatment of type 1 atrial flutter. *Heart Rhythm*. 2008;5:1009-1014.
10. Moreira W, Timmermans C, Wellens HJ, et al. Long term outcome of cavotricuspid isthmus cryoablation for the treatment of common atrial flutter in 180 patients: a single center experience. *J Interv Card Electrophysiol*. 2008;21:235-240.
11. Kalman JM, Olgin JE, Saxon LA, Fisher WG, Lee RJ, Lesh MD. Activation and entrainment mapping defines the tricuspid annulus as the anterior barrier in typical atrial flutter. *Circulation*. 1996;94:398-406.
12. Yang Y, Cheng J, Bochoeyer A, et al. Atypical right atrial flutter patterns. *Circulation*. 2001;103:3092-3098.
13. Santucci PA, Varma N, Cytron J, et al. Electroanatomic mapping of postpacing intervals clarifies the complete active circuit and variants in atrial flutter. *Heart Rhythm*. 2009;6:1586-1595.
14. Olgin JE, Kalman JM, Fitzpatrick AP, Lesh MD. Role of right atrial endocardial structures as barriers to conduction during human type I atrial flutter. Activation and entrainment mapping guided by intracardiac echocardiography. *Circulation*. 1995;92:1839-1848.
15. Friedman PA, Luria D, Fenton AM, et al. Global right atrial mapping of human atrial flutter: the presence of posteromedial (sinus venosa region) functional block and double potentials: a study in biplane fluoroscopy and intracardiac echocardiography. *Circulation*. 2000;101: 1568-1577.
16. Yang Y, Varma N, Badhwar N, et al. Prospective observations in the clinical and electrophysiological characteristics of intra-isthmus reentry. *J Cardiovasc Electrophysiol*. 2010;21:1099-1106.
17. Cabrera JA, Sanchez-Quintana D, Farre J, Rubio JM, Ho SY. The inferior right atrial isthmus: further architectural insights for current and coming ablation technologies. *J Cardiovasc Electrophysiol*. 2005;16:402-408.
18. Gula LJ, Redfearn DP, Veenhuyzen GD, et al. Reduction in atrial flutter ablation time by targeting maximum voltage: results of a prospective randomized clinical trial. *J Cardiovasc Electrophysiol*. 2009;20: 1108-1112.
19. Morton JB, Sanders P, Davidson NC, Sparks PB, Vohra JK, Kalman JM. Phased-array intracardiac echocardiography for defining cavotricuspid isthmus anatomy during radiofrequency ablation of typical atrial flutter. *J Cardiovasc Electrophysiol*. 2003;14:591-597.
20. Kirchhof P, Ozgun M, Zellerhoff S, et al. Diastolic isthmus length and 'vertical' isthmus angulation identify patients with difficult catheter ablation of typical atrial flutter: a pre-procedural MRI study. *Europace*. 2009;11:42-47.
21. Saremi F, Pourzand L, Krishnan S, et al. Right atrial cavotricuspid isthmus: anatomic characterization with multi-detector row CT. *Radiology*. 2008;247:658-668.
22. Kottkamp H, Hugl B, Krauss B, et al. Electromagnetic versus fluoroscopic mapping of the inferior isthmus for ablation of typical atrial flutter: a prospective randomized study. *Circulation*. 2000;102:2082-2086.
23. Da Costa A, Romeyer-Bouchard C, Dauphinot V, et al. Cavotricuspid isthmus angiography predicts atrial flutter ablation efficacy in 281 patients randomized between 8 mm- and externally irrigated-tip catheter. *Eur Heart J*. 2006;27:1833-1840.
24. Shah DC, Takahashi A, Jaïs P, Hocini M, Clementy J, Haïssaguerre M. Local electrogram-based criteria of cavotricuspid isthmus block. *J Cardiovasc Electrophysiol*. 1999;10:662-669.
25. Tada H, Oral H, Sticherling C, et al. Double potentials along the ablation line as a guide to radiofrequency ablation of typical atrial flutter. *J Am Coll Cardiol*. 2001;38:750-755.
26. Tada H, Ozaydin M, Chugh A, et al. Effects of isoproterenol and amiodarone on the double potential interval after ablation of the cavotricuspid isthmus. *J Cardiovasc Electrophysiol*. 2003;14:935-939.
27. Tada H, Oral H, Sticherling C, et al. Electrogram polarity and cavotricuspid isthmus block during ablation of typical atrial flutter. *J Cardiovasc Electrophysiol*. 2001;12:393-399.
28. Villacastin J, Almendral J, Arenal A, et al. Usefulness of unipolar electrograms to detect isthmus block after radiofrequency ablation of typical atrial flutter. *Circulation*. 2000;102:3080-3085.
29. Shah D, Haïssaguerre M, Takahashi A, Jaïs P, Hocini M, Clementy J. Differential pacing for distinguishing block from persistent conduction through an ablation line. *Circulation*. 2000;102:1517-1522.
30. Anselme F, Cribier A, Saoudi N. Positional pacing to discriminate transverse crista terminalis conduction from incomplete clockwise isthmus block during typical atrial flutter ablation. *Circulation*. 2000;102:3013.
31. Calkins H, Canby R, Weiss R, et al. Results of catheter ablation of typical atrial flutter. *Am J Cardiol*. 2004;94:437-442.
32. Feld G, Wharton M, Plumb V, Daoud E, Friehling T, Epstein L. Radiofrequency catheter ablation of type 1 atrial flutter using large-tip 8 or 10 mm electrode catheters and a

high-output radiofrequency energy generator: results of a multicenter safety and efficacy study. *J Am Coll Cardiol.* 2004;43: 1466-1472.
33. Mittal S, Das MK, Stein KM, et al. Frequency of subacute resumption of isthmus conduction after ablation of atrial flutter. *Am J Cardiol.* 2001;87:1113-1116, A1119.
34. Bru P, Duplantier C, Bourrat M, Valy Y, Lorillard R. Resumption of right atrial isthmus conduction following atrial flutter radiofrequency ablation. *Pacing Clin Electrophysiol.* 2000;23:1908-1910.
35. Nabar A, Rodriguez LM, Timmermans C, Smeets JL, Wellens HJ. Isoproterenol to evaluate resumption of conduction after right atrial isthmus ablation in type I atrial flutter. *Circulation.* 1999;99:3286-3291.
36. Kuniss M, Vogtmann T, Ventura R, et al. Prospective randomized comparison of durability of bidirectional conduction block in the cavotricuspid isthmus in patients after ablation of common atrial flutter using cryothermy and radiofrequency energy: the CRYOTIP study. *Heart Rhythm.* 2009;6:1699-1705.
37. Da Costa A, Thevenin J, Roche F, et al. Results from the loire-ardeche-drome-isere-puy-de-dome (ladip) trial on atrial flutter, a multicentric prospective randomized study comparing amiodarone and radiofrequency ablation after the first episode of symptomatic atrial flutter. *Circulation.* 2006;114: 1676-1681.
38. Natale A, Newby KH, Pisano E, et al. Prospective randomized comparison of antiarrhythmic therapy versus first-line radiofrequency ablation in patients with atrial flutter. *J Am Coll Cardiol.* 2000;35:1898-1904.
39. Gilligan DM, Zakaib JS, Fuller I, et al. Long-term outcome of patients after successful radiofrequency ablation for typical atrial flutter. *Pacing Clin Electrophysiol.* 2003;26:53-58.
40. Akar JG, Kok LC, Haines DE, DiMarco JP, Mounsey JP. Coexistence of type I atrial flutter and intra-atrial re-entrant tachycardia in patients with surgically corrected congenital heart disease. *J Am Coll Cardiol.* 2001;38:377-384.
41. Delacretaz E, Ganz LI, Soejima K, et al. Multi atrial macrore-entry circuits in adults with repaired congenital heart disease: entrainment mapping combined with three-dimensional electro-anatomic mapping. *J Am Coll Cardiol.* 2001; 37:1665-1676.
42. Kall JG, Rubenstein DS, Kopp DE, et al. Atypical atrial flutter originating in the right atrial free wall. *Circulation.* 2000;101:270-279.
43. Markowitz SM, Brodman RF, Stein KM, et al. Lesional tachycardias related to mitral valve surgery. *J Am Coll Cardiol.* 2002;39:1973-1983.
44. Stevenson IH, Kistler PM, Spence SJ, et al. Scar-related right atrial macroreentrant tachycardia in patients without prior atrial surgery: electroanatomic characterization and ablation outcome. *Heart Rhythm.* 2005;2:594-601.
45. Tai CT, Huang JL, Lee PC, Ding YA, Chang MS, Chen SA. High-resolution mapping around the crista terminalis during typical atrial flutter: new insights into mechanisms. *J Cardiovasc Electrophysiol.* 2004;15:406-414.
46. Roberts-Thomson KC, Kalman JM. Right septal macroreentrant tachycardia late after mitral valve repair: importance of surgical access approach. *Heart Rhythm.* 2007;4:32-36.
47. Shah D, Jaïs P, Takahashi A, et al. Dual-loop intra-atrial reentry in humans. *Circulation.* 2000;101:631-639.
48. Seiler J, Schmid DK, Irtel TA, et al. Dual-loop circuits in postoperative atrial macro re-entrant tachycardias. *Heart.* 2007;93:325-330.
49. Jaïs P, Shah DC, Haïssaguerre M, et al. Mapping and ablation of left atrial flutters. *Circulation.* 2000;101:2928-2934.
50. Ouyang F, Ernst S, Vogtmann T, et al. Characterization of reentrant circuits in left atrial macroreentrant tachycardia: critical isthmus block can prevent atrial tachycardia recurrence. *Circulation.* 2002;105:1934-1942.
51. Fiala M, Chovancik J, Neuwirth R, et al. Atrial macroreentry tachycardia in patients without obvious structural heart disease or previous cardiac surgical or catheter intervention: characterization of arrhythmogenic substrates, reentry circuits, and results of catheter ablation. *J Cardiovasc Electrophysiol.* 2007;18:824-832.
52. Becker AE. Left atrial isthmus: anatomic aspects relevant for linear catheter ablation procedures in humans. *J Cardiovasc Electrophysiol.* 2004;15:809-812.
53. Wittkampf FH, van Oosterhout MF, Loh P, et al. Where to draw the mitral isthmus line in catheter ablation of atrial fibrillation: histological analysis. *Eur Heart J.* 2005;26:689-695.
54. Jaïs P, Hocini M, Hsu LF, et al. Technique and results of linear ablation at the mitral isthmus. *Circulation.* 2004;110: 2996-3002.
55. Matsuo S, Wright M, Knecht S, et al. Peri-mitral atrial flutter in patients with atrial fibrillation ablation. *Heart Rhythm.* 2010;7:2-8.
56. Tzeis S, Luik A, Jilek C, et al. The modified anterior line: an alternative linear lesion in perimitral flutter. *J Cardiovasc Electrophysiol.* 2010;21:665-670.
57. Sanders P, Jaïs P, Hocini M, et al. Electrophysiologic and clinical consequences of linear catheter ablation to transect the anterior left atrium in patients with atrial fibrillation. *Heart Rhythm.* 2004;1:176-184.
58. Hocini M, Jaïs P, Sanders P, et al. Techniques, evaluation, and consequences of linear block at the left atrial roof in paroxysmal atrial fibrillation: a prospective randomized study. *Circulation.* 2005;112:3688-3696.
59. Marrouche NF, Natale A, Wazni OM, et al. Left septal atrial flutter: electrophysiology, anatomy, and results of ablation. *Circulation.* 2004;109:2440-2447.
60. Gersenfeld EP, Marchlinski FE. Mapping and ablation of left atrial tachycardias occurring after atrial fibrillation ablation. *Heart Rhythm.* 2007;4:S65-72.
61. Matsuo S, Wright M, Knecht S, et al. Peri-mitral atrial flutter in patients with atrial fibrillation ablation. *Heart Rhythm.* 2010;7:2-8.
62. Gerstenfeld EP, Callans DJ, Sauer W, Jacobson J, Marchlinski FE. Reentrant and nonreentrant focal left atrial tachycardias occur after pulmonary vein isolation. *Heart Rhythm.* 2005;2:1195-1202.
63. Sanders P, Hocini M, Jaïs P, et al. Characterization of focal atrial tachycardia using high-density mapping. *J Am Coll Cardiol.* 2005;46:2088-2099.

Video Legend

Video 41.1 Demonstration of reentry around the mitral annulus in a 57-year-old man with muscular dystrophy and spontaneous atrial tachycardia. A propagation map of the LA obtained with the Ensite Velocity system is displayed in the LAO orientation. Counterclockwise reentry is demonstrated around the mitral annulus. Catheter ablation was performed in the "mitral isthmus" between the mitral annulus and the left inferior pulmonary vein. Additional ablation was performed in the CS (rightmost lesions in the image) to achieve block in the mitral isthmus.

CHAPTER 42A

Atrial Fibrillation: Linear Catheter Ablation

Carlo Pappone, MD, PhD; Vincenzo Santinelli, MD

Introduction

The mechanisms of initiation and perpetuation of AF are complex and depend on multiple factors, of which the most important are triggers and substrate,[1] as firstly reported in our long-term extensive experience.[2-16] Addressing AF substrate in addition to triggers is key to achieving maintenance of sinus rhythm with catheter ablation in many patients with AF. Potential substrate targets have been described and include ganglionated plexi and sites with complex fractionated EGMs and high dominant frequency. At present, it is not known whether the targeting of a specific substrate is superior to another, nor is it clear if these substrates may be related in any way. The preliminary encouraging results reported by the Bordeaux group in patients with paroxysmal AF by PVI alone[17] encouraged electrophysiologists to also include patients with persistent or long-lasting persistent AF and enlarged left atria, but poor results were reported in the long-term after PVI alone. What became clear was that catheter ablation of triggers alone (PVI) in the vast majority of patients with AF is insufficient to maintain long-term sinus rhythm.[18] In the atrium are several functional and anatomical areas of slow conduction (substrate) that permit transformation of ectopic activity into reentrant circuits, which maintain continuous fibrillatory activity. By creating a linear conduction block, linear catheter ablation should be able to interrupt potential areas available for AF propagation; thus, the linear lesion approach should be effective in most patients with AF. As a result, linear catheter ablation of AF has grown worldwide in recent years, resulting in a movement toward inclusion of many patients with structural heart disease and more persistent forms of AF.[19] A large number of different ablation approaches have been performed including circumferential pulmonary vein ablation (CPVA), , targeting of fractionated EGMs, compartmentalizing the atria with linear lesions, and various combinations and modifications of these lesion sets, but the optimal ablation strategy for patients with AF is still an issue of debate.[19] Initially, PVI was proposed by the Bordeaux group in patients with paroxysmal AF to eliminate AF triggers,[14] but this strategy alone was insufficient in the majority of patients with more persistent forms.[17] Simultaneously to the Bordeaux group, and in contrast to the initiating triggers theory, a different approach was first proposed by our group more than 10 years ago.[2,3] This approach was based on both triggers and substrate elimination by contiguous circumferential lesions around the PV ostia and added linear lesion lines guided by nonfluoroscopic mapping systems (CPVA). We first demonstrated that the benefit of added linear lesions is also extended to the modification of vagal tone by shortening the atrial refractory period.[5] Our lesion set was performed to partially reproduce the surgical maze procedure, in which elimination of all hypothetical biatrial functional reentrant circuits was able to prevent the perpetuation of AF with multiple biatrial incisions, PVI, and a critical mass reduction using amputation of both atrial appendages (atria compartmentalization). Unfortunately, the broad use of transcutaneous linear ablation of AF was initially limited by the difficulty inherent in creating transmural contiguous linear lesions under fluoroscopy alone. Indeed, clinical failure of percutaneously placed lesion lines may be the result of insufficient lesion extension and/or geometry, or ablation failure may be due to noncontiguous lesions without achievement of linear conduction block. In contrast to trigger elimination as proposed by the Bordeaux group,[17] deployment of linear ablation lines is very challenging without nonfluoroscopic mapping systems, and complete bidirectional block needs to be validated particularly in persistent AF where complex substrates are present. Contiguous transmural linear lesions require both stable temperature and energy delivery on the tip, which can be realized only by continuous catheter stability during each point-by-point RF application. If the catheter contact is continuously varying beat-by-beat, the lesion line necessarily becomes incomplete or the lesions will be nontransmural. Nonfluoroscopic systems, by allowing online monitoring of catheter and lesion positioning and tracking, are effective in creating transmural and contiguous lesions while reducing procedural and fluoroscopic times as well as RF energy application like closed-heart surgical procedure. Therefore, being very familiar with electroanatomically guided linear ablation in our laboratory, we have been able to deploy effective, contiguous lesions, ensuring continuity and transmurality, which translates into a long-term success rate that is equally high in patients with previously persistent and paroxysmal AF. From 1999 to 2010, we have performed more than 25,000 AF ablation procedures using linear catheter ablation strategy, and in the last 3 years, when linear catheter ablation in addition to PVI has been used by other electrophysiologists, a better outcome has been reported even in patients with persistent AF, approaching 90% success considering repeat procedures.[18] Therefore, in our experience electroanatomically guided linear ablation with activation mapping and differential pacing for lesion validation has substantially improved the outcome of patients with AF, including those with frequent recurrences or persistent AF. We have also developed newer technology, including remote magnetic ablation, to deploy contiguous sequential lesion lines more effectively and safely, thus avoiding unnecessary and potentially proarrhythmic lesions.[20-23] We believe that linear catheter ablation using fluoroscopy alone and without use of 3D electroanatomic systems is technically challenging and may frequently result in incomplete lesions, which facilitate the development of incessant atrial tachycardias.[19] To limit potentially excessive linear ablation in patients with long-lasting AF, it is necessary to determine how much substrate should be eliminated during the index procedure to minimize the proarrhythmic risk. Although linear ablation is technically challenging, this strategy is indeed necessary in almost all patients with AF. Therefore, incessant new ATs may represent the future challenge of all electrophysiologists "embarking linear ablation."[19] An extensive experience is required when using new 3D electroanatomic navigation, remote mapping and ablation systems, and new catheter ablation tools with energy sources alternative to RF energy. In addition, it will be necessary to accurately identify selective areas of slow conduction or vagal hyperactivity, actively participating in the AF generation to minimize the linear ablation amount. Important measures need to be taken to prevent potential complications using linear catheter ablation; in particular, the power should be limited inside the CS, isolating the LAA should be avoided, and single RF applications should be shortened (20 seconds), particularly on the posterior wall, to minimize potentially serious complications. Despite the large amount of RF energy required to cure AF, our 10-year experience with electroanatomically guided linear catheter ablation with activation mapping indicates that linear ablation is effective and well tolerated with an acceptable risk–benefit ratio. All targets can be accurately visualized and rapidly reached, which facilitates the placement of contiguous conduction block lines quickly and efficiently, greatly limiting postablation incessant AT development (6%). Even so, further studies are needed in a larger population of patients to identify which targets are unnecessary and which are essential to maintain a stable sinus rhythm. Despite the reported high success rates, we believe that in patients with persistent long-lasting AF and enlarged atria (> 50 mm), excessive linear ablation needs to be limited to avoid potentially serious complications and proarrhythmias. The need of multiple linear lesions to eliminate all potential targets perpetuating arrhythmia usually requires repeated, time-consuming procedures, which may increase complication rates.[18,19] Since persistent AF requires excessive additional linear ablation, arrhythmia progression should be limited by early catheter ablation when the arrhythmia is paroxysmal.[7] Unlike lone AF, progression from paroxysmal to persistent AF is relatively rapid in patients with comorbidities, particularly in heart failure patients.[7] Therefore, identification of patients at risk of arrhythmia progression may be useful for early catheter ablation.

Linear Catheter Ablation in CPVA

Step 1. CPVA

In our laboratory, a standard set of linear lesions is performed by irrigated tip catheters as the initial ablation step in patients with paroxysmal or persistent AF undergoing CPVA, while in patients with long-lasting persistent AF, we perform standard and additional linear lesions, which are guided by 3D AM systems (Figure 42A.1). Contiguous lesion lines are usually but not routinely validated, as reported in the modified CPVA approach. The standard set of lesions includes PV disconnection, mitral isthmus line, and posterior lines (Figures 42A.2 and 42A.3). Ablation is performed with a maximum power output of 30 W using an irrigation rate of 10 to 30 mL/min (0.9% saline) for the PVs, 35 W and an irrigation rate of 30 to 50 mL/min in the LA, and up to 30 W in the RA. RF

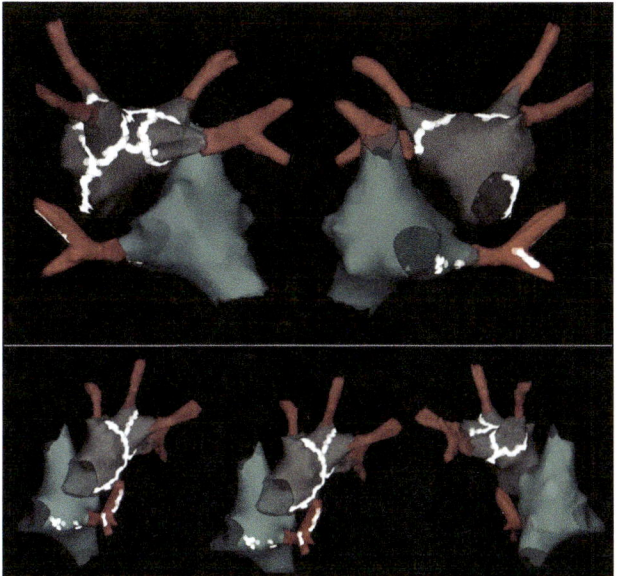

Figure 42A.1 Electroanatomic 3D (NavX) reconstruction of the LA in different projections showing the standard set of linear lesions, as performed in CPVA and additional lesions including CS disconnection. RFA lesions are shown as **white dots**.

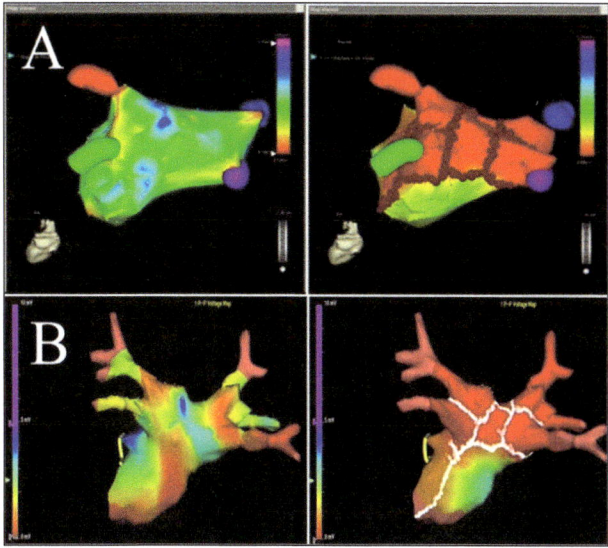

Figure 42A.2 Electroanatomic maps using the CARTO system (**Panel A**) or NavX (**Panel B**) before (**left**) and after CPVA (**right**). Ablated area is depicted in **red**.

current is applied within the CS with a maximum of 25 W and a manually adjusted irrigation rate to keep the tip temperature below 42°C. In cases of high impedance, the power setting is reduced up to 20 W. The duration for one RF application is set to 30 seconds.

PV Disconnection

Circumferential lines are aimed at PV-atrial junction outside the ostia, an area considered as the antrum. The lesions are performed to encircle the left and right PVs individually or as ipsilateral pairs in accordance with the venous anatomy and operator's preference to electrically disconnect all PVs. We have recently demonstrated that complete distal electrical isolation can be safely obtained by potential abatement (> 90% reduction of EGM amplitude) and EGM amplitude decrease of < 0.1 mV around and within the encircled areas (Figure 42A.4), as validated by Lasso catheter (Figure 42A.5).[24] Rapid PVI is achieved by good catheter stability and optimal wall contact that results in rapid elimination of atrial EGMs during each RF energy application, usually within 15 seconds, depending on the local effect. Residual signals require further RF applications before moving on to the next ablation site.

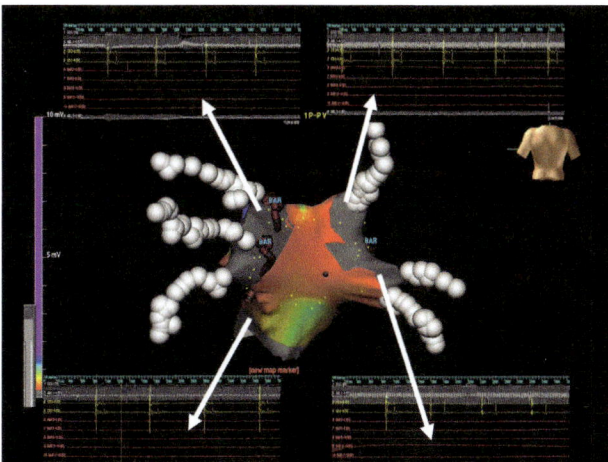

Figure 42A.3 Posterior view of an electroanatomic map of the LA acquired after CPVA showing that PVs are electrically isolated (**gray area**). Note that no PV potentials are recorded after ablation around PV ostia (**arrows**).

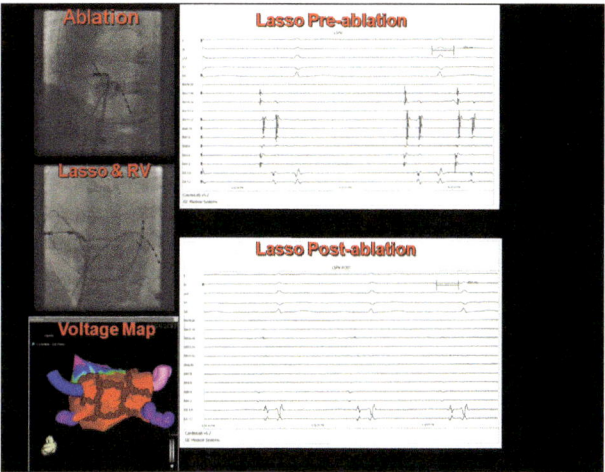

Figure 42A.4 Example of validation with the circular mapping catheter (Lasso) positioned at the ostium of PVs in a patient with paroxysmal AF. Note that no PV potentials are recorded on Lasso catheter after ablation during sinus rhythm.

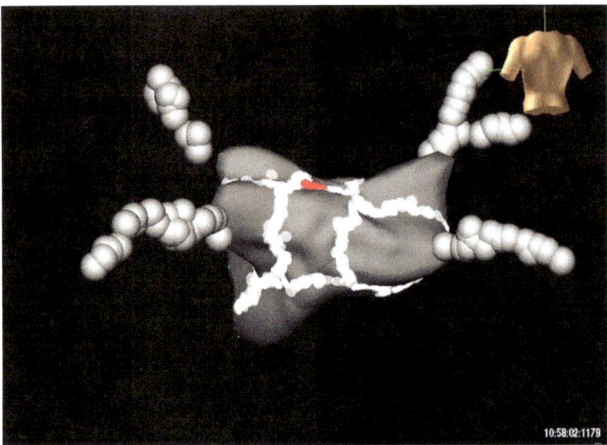

Figure 42A.5 The figure shows a 3D electroanatomic map with posterior lines connecting superior and inferior PVs.

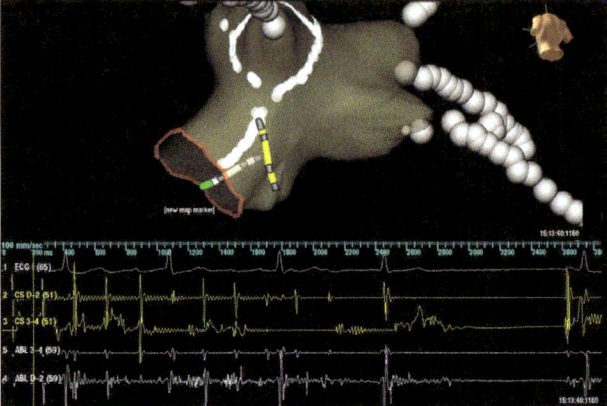

Figure 42A.7 RF applications on the mitral isthmus line gap terminates perimitral atrial MRT.

Posterior and Mitral Isthmus Lines

Ablation lines are performed point-by-point along the back and the roof of the LA between the two sets of PVs connecting the superior and inferior PVs and the mitral valve annulus (Figure 42A.6). The mitral isthmus line is deployed by creating a linear ablation line joining the lateral mitral annulus to the LIPV to further reduce the substrate as well as to prevent postablation left atrial MRTs[25] (Figure 42A.7). Completeness of the mitral isthmus line (bidirectional mitral isthmus conduction block) is an important EP endpoint. It is validated during CS pacing by endocardial and CS mapping, looking for widely spaced double potentials across the line of block and confirmed by differential pacing.[11] The minimum double-potential interval at the mitral isthmus during CS pacing after block is achieved is > 150 ms, depending on the atrial dimensions and the extent of scarring and lesion creation.[11] During the procedure, we attempt to eliminate all potential vagal reflexes, which enhances the efficacy of the procedure in the long-term outcome. If a reflex is elicited, RF energy is delivered until such reflexes are abolished, or for up to 30 seconds. The endpoint for ablation at these sites is defined as termination of the reflex. Failure to reproduce reflexes with repeat RF is considered confirmation of denervation.[5]

Step 2. Endocardial Coronary Sinus Ablation

Point-by-point linear ablation of the CS begins along its endocardial aspect and is usually completed from within the vessel. The ablation catheter is dragged along the endocardium of the inferior LA after looping the catheter in such a way as to position it parallel to the CS catheter. After achieving a 270- to 360-degree loop in the LA, ablation is started at the inferior LA along the posterior mitral annulus, near to the CS ostium up to the lateral LA (4 o'clock in the LAO projection). The endpoint is complete elimination of sharp potentials within the CS.

Step 3. Endocardial Septum Ablation

Linear ablation of the IAS starts from the anterior aspect of the lesion encircling the RSPV up to the anterior mitral annulus (Figure 42A.8). Ablation is sequentially point-by-point performed with the aim of transecting areas of complex fractionated EGMs, which are frequently found in this region. Like CS ablation, the endpoint is elimination of local EGMs or, alternatively, to prolong the cycle length by at least 20 ms, in this region; validation of complete conduction block across this lesion is not routinely performed. During ablation of the anterior septum, areas near to the His bundle are intentionally avoided.

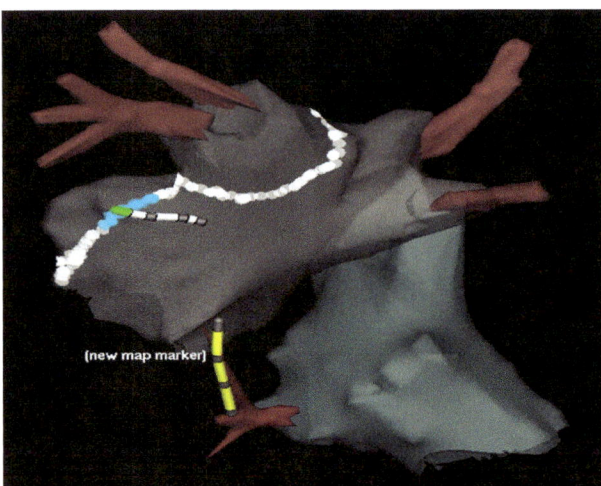

Figure 42A.6 Example of the mitral isthmus line represented by a linear lesion joining the lateral mitral annulus to the LIPV.

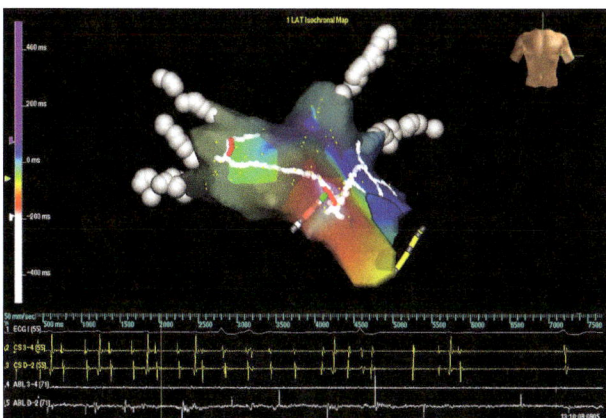

Figure 42A.8 Example of linear ablation of IAS resulting in termination of intermediate atrial tachycardia in a patient with persistent AF.

Step 4. Left Atrial Ablation

Ablation is typically performed beginning from the lesion encircling the LSPV, and the lesion is extended inferiorly and superiorly. The endpoint is complete elimination of local endocardial EGMs bordering the LAA posteriorly, inferiorly, and anteriorly to increase the CL of sharp potentials characteristically found within the LAA; complete isolation of the LAA is intentionally avoided.

Step 5. Epicardial Coronary Sinus Ablation

Ablation within the CS is performed if CS potentials persist and usually RF applications start distally (4 o'clock in LAO view) up to the ostium by targeting local sharp potentials (Figure 42A.9). Finally, further RF applications are deployed around the coronary ostium from the RA. CS disconnection is validated by the dissociation or abolition of sharp potentials in its first 3 cm.

Step 6. Right Atrium Ablation

Patients with persistent AF undergo ablation of the cavotricuspid isthmus. After ablation around the CS ostium, a linear lesion may be deployed between the inferior vena cava and the tricuspid annulus isthmus to create a bidiretional conduction block across the isthmus. Validation of bidirectional block is performed during sinus rhythm. Superior vena cava isolation is not routinely performed, but only when there is presence of an arrhythmogenic source.

Step 7. Atrial Linear Ablation

Point-by-point linear ablation is performed at sites showing continuous electrical activity, complex fractionated potentials, sites with a gradient of activation (significant EGM offset between the distal and proximal recording bipoles on the map electrode), or regions with a CL shorter than the mean LAA AF cycle length. Ablation at these sites is performed to achieve local prolongation of CL, with synchronous activation at distal and proximal bipoles indicating passive activation of this local area. At each site, 20 to 60 seconds of RF are delivered before moving.

AFCL During Linear Ablation

The effect of RF applications is continuously monitored by assessing potential changes of AF cycle length (AFCL) before and after each ablation step by averaging 10 consecutive cycles and at the time of AF termination. The AFCL is determined within the CS and the RAA and LAA. An individual site is considered to have a significant impact if its ablation results in termination of AF or prolongation of the AFCL (evaluated in the LAA except if specified otherwise) by 20 ms or more, when compared to the highest AFCL during the previous steps. Termination of AF is defined as a transition to SR or conversion to AT. Particularly in patients with frequent paroxysmal AF or persistent AF, LAA (Figure 42A.9), CS, and IAS (Figure 42A.8) are considered as key areas for linear lesions, suggesting that their inclusion in linear ablation strategies to prevent recurrent AF after CPVA or persistent AF may be useful to improve the clinical outcome in such a patient population.

Intermediate Atrial Tachycardias During Linear Ablation

AT not only represents linear ablation–induced proarrhythmia but also may be considered as a transition between AF and sinus rhythm in long-standing persistent AF successfully treated with linear catheter ablation. AT development depends on the percent of ablated area; its occurrence is more frequent in patients undergoing an extensive stepwise approach including PVI and additional

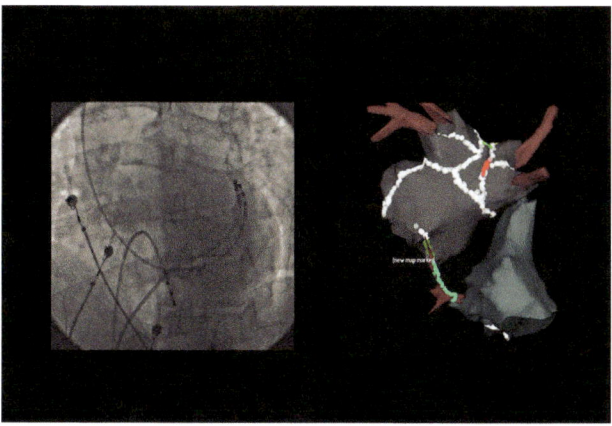

Figure 42A.9 After the standard set of lesions in a patient with long-lasting AF, additional epicardial CS ablation is shown. On the **left**, a fluoroscopic image in the LAO projection showing catheter position during ablation within CS. On the **right**, a 3D EAM is depicted.

linear ablation. When, during the procedure, AF converts to a regular atrial arrhythmia, conventional activation and entrainment mapping are performed to differentiate a focal from a macroreentrant mechanism. In our experience, during stepwise ablation, prolongation of AFCL occurs gradually, with the largest increments being in the IAS, CS region, and LAA region, which results in the conversion to SR with or without intermediate organized tachycardia. After conversion, multiple ATs may develop, but conventional mapping techniques usually show a limited number of critical structures from which they arise. Focal ATs are frequently located at the PVs, LAA, and CS regions originating at any part of their (circumferential or longitudinal) connection with the LA. Atrial MRTs are usually perimitral or roofline, and rarely, the CTI is involved.

In experienced centers, extensive linear catheter ablation can be performed with high success rates even in patients with enlarged atria and comorbidities using an approach mainly focused to organize left atrial activity, followed by appropriate mapping and ablation of intermediate atrial tachycardias. Despite preliminary encouraging results in persistent long-standing AF by a stepwise approach, the procedure is challenging and time-consuming, and many lines need to be validated. Therefore, we believe that early catheter ablation including PVI and less extensive linear ablation (as performed in CPVA), may be considered as a new indication in patients with frequent episodes of AF and those with comorbidities who are at risk to rapidly progress to persistent AF, which is associated with lower success rates and higher complication rates requiring repeat procedures.

The Future of Linear Catheter Ablation of AF

Electroanatomically guided linear ablation strategy of AF is safe and effective in patients with both paroxysmal and persistent AF. Therefore, it is not surprising that this strategy, which includes PVI and additional linear lesion lines, is increasingly performed in many EP laboratories even in patients with long-standing AF and comorbidities. However, lesions lines, particularly in challenging targets, such as the mitral isthmus line, need to be validated to prevent proarrhythmia development after the procedure. As a result, linear lesions need to be performed in highly specialized centers that are very familiar with 3D electroanatomic navigation and ablation systems to correctly place point-by-point contiguous sequential RF applications using irrigated-tip catheters, without creating gaps and incomplete lines. Currently, linear ablation by remote magnetic irrigated-tip catheters may be considered as an important technical advancement to increase efficacy while minimizing complications, but such strategy is costly and also requires high-experience centers.

References

1. Fuster V, Ryden LE, Cannom DS, et al. ACC/AHA/ESC 2006 guidelines for the management of patients with atrial fibrillation: a report of the American College of Cardiology/American Heart Association Task Force on Practice Guidelines and the European Society of Cardiology Committee for Practice Guidelines (Writing Committee to Revise the 2001 Guidelines for the Management of Patients with Atrial Fibrillation): developed in collaboration with the European Heart Rhythm Association and the Heart Rhythm Society. *Circulation*. 2006;114:e257-e354.
2. Pappone C, Rosanio S, Oreto G, et al. Circumferential radiofrequency ablation of pulmonary vein ostia: a new anatomic approach for curing atrial fibrillation. *Circulation*. 2000; 102:2619-2628.
3. Pappone C, Oreto G, Rosanio S, et al. Atrial electroanatomic remodeling after circumferential radiofrequency pulmonary vein ablation: efficacy of an anatomic approach in a large cohort of patients with atrial fibrillation. *Circulation*. 2001;104:2539-2544.
4. Pappone C, Santinelli V. Pulmonary vein isolation by circumferential radiofrequency lesions in atrial fibrillation. From substrate to clinical outcome. *Ann Ist Super Sanita*. 2001;37:401-407.
5. Pappone C, Santinelli V, Manguso F, et al. Pulmonary vein denervation enhances long-term benefit after circumferential ablation for paroxysmal atrial fibrillation. *Circulation*. 2004; 109:327-334.
6. Pappone C, Rosanio S, Augello G, et al. Mortality, morbidity, and quality of life after circumferential pulmonary vein ablation for atrial fibrillation: outcomes from a controlled nonrandomized long-term study. *J Am Coll Cardiol*. 2003; 42:185-197.
7. Pappone C, Radinovic A, Manguso F, et al. Atrial fibrillation progression and management. A 5-year prospective follow-up study. *Heart Rhythm*. 2008;5:1501-1507.
8. Pappone C, Santinelli V. How to perform encircling ablation of the left atrium. *Heart Rhythm*. 2006;3:1105-1109.
9. Pappone C, Santinelli V. Towards a unified strategy for atrial fibrillation ablation? *Eur Heart J*. 2005;26:1687-1688.
10. Pappone C, Santinelli V. Atrial fibrillation ablation: state of the art. *Am J Cardiol*. 2005;96:59L-64L.
11. Pappone C, Manguso F, Vicedomini G, et al. Prevention of iatrogenic atrial tachycardia after ablation of atrial fibrillation: a prospective randomized study comparing circumferential pulmonary vein ablation with a modified approach. *Circulation*. 2004;110:3036-3042.
12. Lang CC, Santinelli V, Augello G, et al. Transcatheter radiofrequency ablation of atrial fibrillation in patients with mitral valve prostheses and enlarged atria: safety, feasibility, and efficacy. *J Am Coll Cardiol*. 2005;45:868-872.
13. Pappone C, Augello G, Sala S, et al. A randomized trial of circumferential pulmonary vein ablation versus antiarrhythmic drug therapy in paroxysmal atrial fibrillation: the APAF study. *J Am Coll Cardiol*. 2006;48:2340-2347.
14. Pappone C, Augello G, Sala S, et al. A randomized trial of circumferential pulmonary vein ablation versus antiarrhythmic drug therapy in paroxysmal atrial fibrillation: the APAF study. *J Am Coll Cardiol*. 2006;48:2340-2347.
15. Wilber DJ, Pappone C, Neuzil P, et al. Comparison of antiarrhythmic drug therapy and radiofrequency catheter ablation in patients with paroxysmal atrial fibrillation: a randomized controlled trial. *JAMA*. 2010;303:333-340.

16. Oral H, Pappone C, Chugh A, et al. Circumferential pulmonary-vein ablation for chronic atrial fibrillation. *N Engl J Med.* 2006;354:934-941.
17. Haïssaguerre M, Jaïs P, Shah DC, et al. Spontaneous initiation of atrial fibrillation by ectopic beats originating in the pulmonary veins. *N Engl J Med.* 1998;339:659-666.
18. Haïssaguerre M, Sanders P, Hocini M, et al. Catheter ablation of long-lasting persistent atrial fibrillation: critical structures for termination. *J Cardiovasc Electrophysiol.* 2005;11:1125-1137.
19. Cappato R, Calkins H, Chen S, et al. Worldwide survey on the methods, efficacy and safety of catheter ablation for human atrial fibrillation. *Circulation.* 2005;111:1100-1105.
20. Pappone C, Vicedomini G, Manguso F, et al. Robotic magnetic navigation for atrial fibrillation ablation. *J Am Coll Cardiol.* 2006;47:1390-1400.
21. Pappone C, Santinelli V. Remote navigation and ablation of atrial fibrillation. *J Cardiovasc Electrophysiol.* 2007;Suppl 1:S18-S20.
22. Pappone C, Santinelli V. Safety and efficacy of remote magnetic ablation for atrial fibrillation *J Am Coll Cardiol.* 2008;51:1614-1615.
23. Pappone C, Vicedomini G, Frigoli E, et al. Irrigated-tip magnetic catheter ablation of AF. A long-term prospective study in 130 patients. *Heart Rhythm.* 2011;8:8-15.
24. Augello G, Vicedomini G, Saviano M, et al. Pulmonary vein isolation after circumferential pulmonary vein ablation: comparison between Lasso and three-dimensional electroanatomical assessment of complete electrical disconnection. *Heart Rhythm.* 2009;6:1706-1713.
25. Mesas CE, Pappone C, Lang CC, et al. Left atrial tachycardia after circumferential pulmonary vein ablation for atrial fibrillation. *J Am Coll Cardiol.* 2004;44:1071-1079.

CHAPTER 42B

Atrial Fibrillation: Focal and Map-guided Ablation

Mauricio S. Arruda, MD; Ashish A. Bhimani, MD

Overview of AF Ablation

AF ablation techniques have evolved to improve procedural efficacy and safety over the years since the procedure was first introduced in the late 1990s.[1,2] The finding of PV triggers provided an accessible target in trying to eliminate AF. There have been several ablation strategies designed to electrically isolate the PVs from the LA, which have shown success in reducing or eliminating AF. Additionally, over time, new techniques have been developed to enhance the success of catheter ablation, particularly for more advanced stages of AF. Catheter ablation has been recognized as a potentially curative therapeutic option for AF, and its role is supported by the current guideline statements.[3-6]

PV Triggers

Atrial ectopic activity arising from the musculature of the PVs is responsible for the initiation of most paroxysmal episodes of AF.[7-9] Haïssaguerre et al showed that ablation targeting the sites of spontaneous triggers could reduce AF, and in a landmark 1998 study, 94% of the triggers identified were from the PVs.[1] The structure of the PVs is quite variable, in number, orientation, size, and shape of their ostia.[10] Most PVs include an extension of atrial myocardial sleeves between 4 and 19 mm beyond the PV os.[11] The morphology of these sleeves includes different combinations of fiber orientation and thickness, with variable circumferential coverage and predominance toward the upper PVs (see Figure 42B.1A).[11,12] The myocardial sleeves show unique electrophysiological properties, including a predisposition to ectopic firing, which can initiate and potentially perpetuate AF.[13-16] These muscular sleeves also demonstrate rich neural innervations[17] (see Figure 42B.1B) as well as connections with sleeves of the ipsilateral PV,[18] both of which have important implications for ablation strategies. The morphology of the LA-PV connections, the PV structure, and the PV myocardial sleeves appears to be associated with AF, as patients with AF show a greater number of connections and greater PV ectopy.[19] Dilatation of the PV os occurs to a greater extent in patients with AF and may also impact PV ectopy.[20,21] Whether differences in PVs in patients with and without AF are a true cause or an effect is unknown. What is clear is that PV ectopy is a major contributor in the initiation of paroxysmal AF and for its recurrence following an ablation procedure. In addition, it may play at least some role in the maintenance of AF. Therefore, ablation targeting these PV triggers was a logical initial approach at controlling AF (see Figure 42B.1, C and D),[1,22] and it is still the cornerstone of today's ablation strategies.

EGM-guided AF Ablation Strategies—Targeting the PVs

Focal PV Trigger Ablation

PV triggers consist of ectopy or focal tachycardia that can initiate or possibly sustain AF. The key in identifying the PV triggers during sinus rhythm is recognizing PV ectopy and the reversal of conduction pattern from PV to LA rather than passive activation of LA to PV (see Figure 42B.1C). If PV ectopy is not seen spontaneously, provocative maneuvers can be performed.[2,23,24] Valsalva, carotid sinus massage, and deep breathing are useful physiologic maneuvers, while isoproterenol, adenosine, or atrial pacing may also elicit PV ectopy.

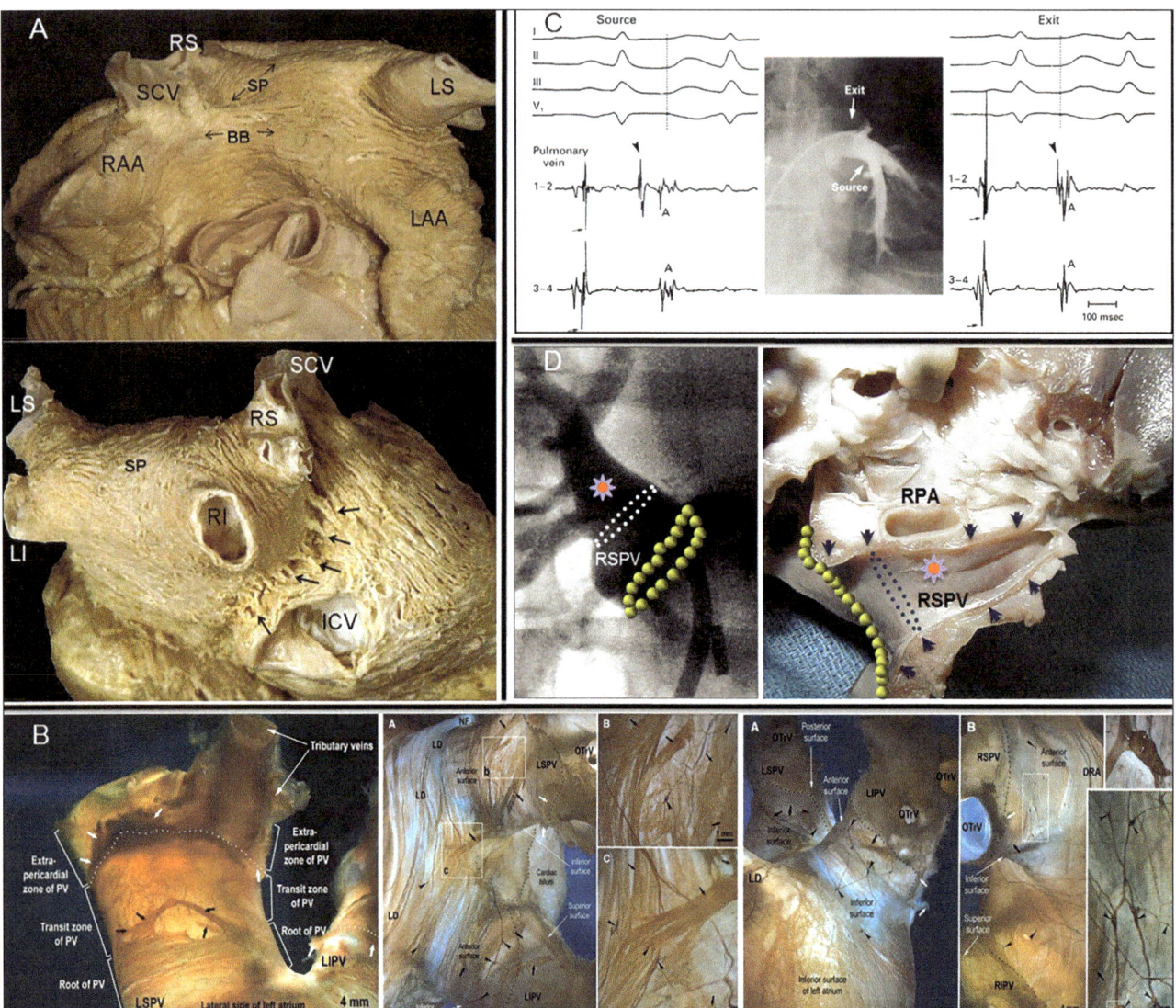

Figure 42B.1 Electroanatomic implications for ablation of AF. **Panel A:** A human heart dissected by Ho et al,[12] with myocardial fiber extensions surrounding the PVs and SVC, lateral ridge between left superior (LS) PV, and the LAA. *Source:* Ho SY et al.[12] **Panel B:** The extensive neural network of human PVs by Pauza et al,[17] with a high density of neuron fibers at the PV antra. *Source:* Vaitkevicius R et al.[17] **Panel C:** PV potentials (**arrows**) as ectopic electrical sources of AF described by Haïssaguerre et al.[1] *Source:* Haïssaguerre M et al.[1] Reprinted with permission from Massachusetts Medical Society. **Panel D:** Evolution of AF ablation over time from targeting focal PV trigger sites to electrical isolation at LA-PV junction. **Arrows** indicate myocardium along the RSPV; note proximity of right pulmonary artery (RPA).

During AF, a shorter cycle length within the PV than in the LA proper can identify spontaneous PV tachycardia. If the PV was activated passively from AF, the cycle length in the PV would be the same or longer than in the atrium.[25]

Ectopic PV activity may be localized by some typical ECG patterns;[26-28] however, endocardial activation mapping is typically performed to localize PV trigger sites. The mapping resolution required is highly dependent on the frequency of PV ectopic sites and is determined by the number and distribution of electrodes. Multielectrode circular or basket catheters can help identify sites of earliest ectopic activity. In Haïssaguerre's initial study, earliest PV activity preceded the ectopic P wave by 106 ± 24 ms.[1]

Pulmonary vein EGMs can typically be identified as a local high-frequency signal and are often separated from the far-field left atrial EGMs due to slow conduction between the LA and PV. However, this is not always straightforward, as the catheter in the PV or at the PV os may record a complex EGM. It is important to identify local EGMs representing PV activity and distinguish this from far-field phenomena including activity in adjacent PVs, the LA, the LAA, the SVC, or the vein of Marshall.[24] Pacing maneuvers can take advantage of the typical decremental conduction seen at the PV ostia, such that introducing premature stimuli from different locations may separate the PV potential from far-field potentials.[24] Pacing from different locations may move the relative positions of PV or non-PV potentials helping to distinguish the true PV potential[24,29] (see Figures 42B.5 and 42B.6). Note that distinguishing PV potentials can become confounded by PV ostial edema that begins after ablation has already taken place.[24]

Once the culprit PV and earliest activity are mapped, ablation is performed with the goal to eliminate the ectopic activity. The key next step in focal PV trigger ablation is to look for additional triggers as elimination of one trigger site will often unmask other triggers, in either the same PV, other PVs, or non-PV sites. The endpoint is for reduction and/or elimination of PV ectopy that initiates or sustains AF.[30] This ablation strategy showed that 60% of patients maintained sinus rhythm at one year.[31] However, several limitations led to the development of more evolved approaches. Successful ablation of induced PV triggers or tachycardias can only be achieved if the clinical ectopy is seen during the EP procedure. Secondary triggers not present during the ablation procedure may account for recurrence of AF.[32] Additionally, another major drawback of trigger ablation is the long-term complication of PV stenosis. Early studies of focal AF ablation showed that 31% of PVs exhibited increased PV flow by Doppler within 3 days of the ablation procedure.[33] The rate of severe symptomatic PV stenosis was lower at approximately 5%, but the complication can be devastating with limited treatment options.[34] To circumvent the limitations of ablation targeting the focal PV triggers, an ablation strategy was adopted to isolate the culprit PV, which would obviate the need for mapping the actual trigger or ablating within the PV. We had the opportunity to investigate the formation of acute and chronic RF lesions in experimental models designed to assess different approaches for circumferential PVI showing the risks of thermal injury within the PVs[35,56] (see Figure 42B.2). Although RF energy is the gold standard for AF ablation, alternative energy sources such as cryothermal energy,[36] laser, and high-frequency ultrasound have been used clinically, but are the beyond the scope of this chapter.

Segmental PV Isolation

Segmental PVI was developed with a goal of ablating to electrically isolate the myocardial sleeves along the PVs. The myocardial sleeves are variable in the extent of the circumference they cover, and achieving isolation only requires ablation in areas of myocardial extension. Circular catheters with 10-20 electrodes, available in fixed 15, 20, and 25 mm or variable diameters, can be used for circumferential PV ostial mapping.[37,38]

The circular catheter is placed into the PV os, and once in a stable position, a roving ablation catheter is moved to areas of earliest activation. These sites are ablated until

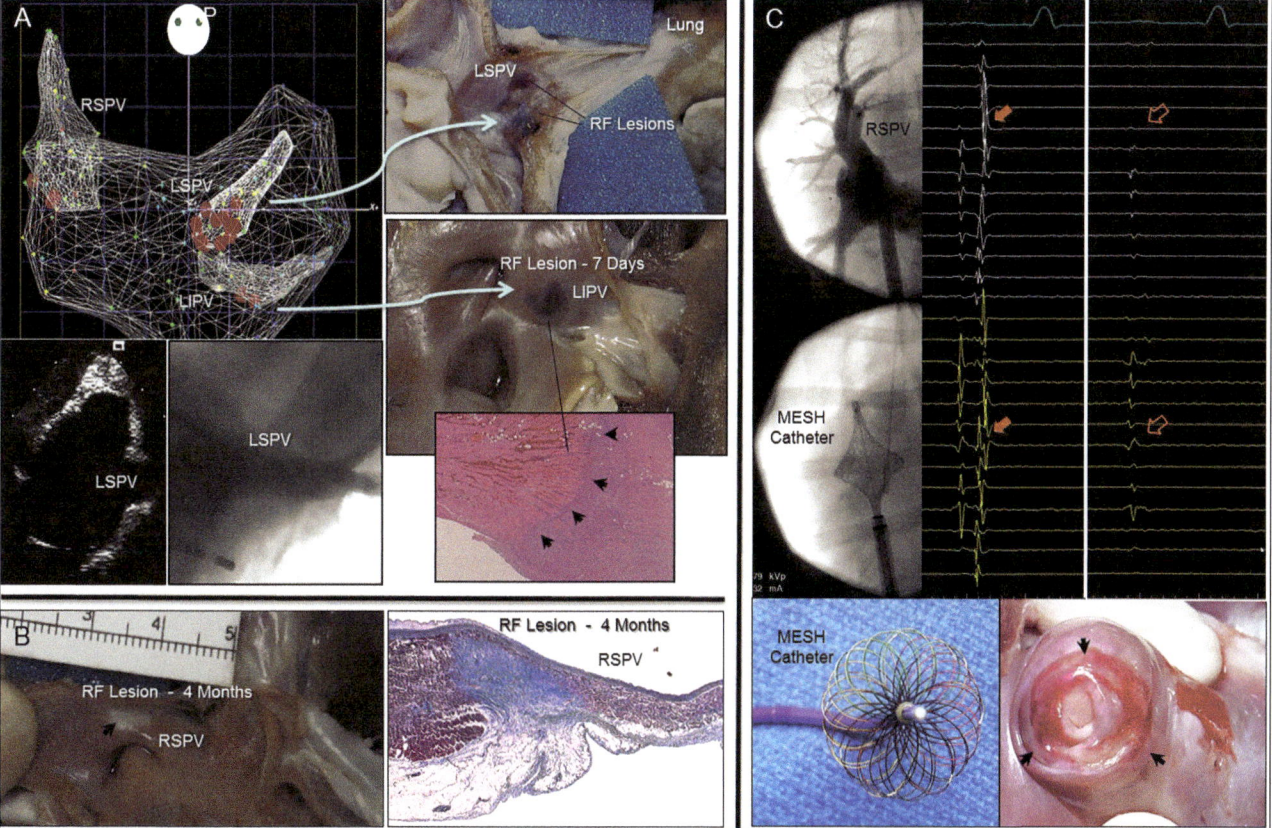

Figure 42B.2 Feasibility and safety of circumferential PVI in an experimental canine model. Note the gross and microscopic aspects of acute and chronic RF lesions in (**A**) and (**B**), respectively; these were created by conventional point-by-point RF ablation guided by EAM, ICE, and angiography. A circumferential mesh catheter designed for mapping and RF ablation was evaluated, and (**C**) shows the angiography of the RSPV, EGMs pre- and postablation, and the resulting gross circumferential RF lesion.

electrical isolation is achieved. Another method to identify effective ablation sites is the localization of polarity reversal, where PV potentials change polarity as they move out radially from the bipolar EGM corresponding to a muscular connection. These sites can be used as targets for segmental ablation with reassessment of the PV potentials after each ablation. It may lead to AF organization or cycle length slowing.[39]

The procedure endpoint is to achieve segmental isolation of the culprit[40] or, empirically, all four PVs. At times, there are electrical connections between two PVs,[18] and in this circumstance, it is necessary to isolate any connected PVs. Checking for electrical reconnection with adenosine infusion does add some value,[41] but testing for noninducibility of AF by rapid atrial pacing or isoproterenol administration appears to be less meaningful than successful PVI.[42]

The segmental ostial ablation approach has several limitations. The muscular connections are often identified within the PV so the risk of PV stenosis still exists. Additionally, some PV triggers exist just on the atrial side of the LA-PV junction and are not excluded by segmental ostial ablation, leading to AF recurrences.

Circumferential PV Antral Isolation

In order to address the limitations of segmental ostial ablation, full circumferential ablation was started as a promising approach; however, as ablation was done near or just within the PV os, there remained a significant risk for PV stenosis, particularly to the LSPV. The key step in improving outcomes was to perform ablation at the level of the PV antrum to include proximal triggers and develop a more reliable line of conduction block while avoiding PV stenosis.[43] This was subsequently extended to large circumferential exclusions of each pair of ipsilateral PVs en bloc in what is described as a wide-area circumferential ablation and has shown good initial outcomes.[44]

Antral ablation has been shown in numerous studies to be a superior strategy to segmental ostial ablation.[45-47] Arentz and colleagues compared a wide-area circumferential against a segmental ostial ablation and showed a significant improvement in AF-free survival in addition to shorter fluoroscopy times.[48] Of note, PV reconnection accounted for 86% of AF recurrences.[49]

Current techniques aiming at antral PV electrical isolation rely on reconstructions of the LA and PV for an anatomical ablation approach, multielectrode circular catheters to provide a direct EGM guidance strategy, or a combination of both strategies (see Figures 42B.3, 42B.5, and 42B.7).

3D Electroanatomic Mapping, ICE, and CT/MRI Image Integration

For any anatomic-guided ablation strategy, some type of imaging or structural mapping is required. 3D electroanatomic mapping can be performed with mapping systems that incorporate direct data from catheter locations in real space with electrical data recorded from the catheter tips or structural data from MRI or CT. Carto (Biosense Webster, Diamond Bar, CA) and NavX (St. Jude Medical, St. Paul, MN) are the two most commonly used systems (see Figures 42B.3, 42B.4, 42B.5, 42B.6, 42B.7, 42B.8, 42B.9, 42B.11, and 42B.12). A virtual geometry of the LA and PVs can be created by multisite recordings that can be displayed as activation or voltage maps and integrated to the patient's own cardiac CT, MR, or even rotational fluoroscopy imaging.[50] Ultimately, these maps can improve procedural efficacy and outcome.[51] Real-time assessment of catheter positions in relation to PV and LA structures may facilitate PVI as well as placement of linear ablation lesions (▶ Video 42B.1 and ▶ Video 42B.2). Even though imaging and 3D maps facilitate anatomical lesion sets, it is important to remember that they do not ensure complete PV electrical isolation.[52]

ICE is a real-time imaging modality that can greatly assist with fluoroscopy and 3D EAM to determine appropriate anatomical locations. PV angiography may be imprecise, whereas ICE guidance may allow better definition of the anatomy at the PV os and antrum, which is variable and not always distinct. Concurrent ICE imaging may guide ablation at the PV antrum rather than in the PV os.[53] ICE can assist throughout the PVI procedure, including safe transseptal puncture, precise visualization of the PV ostia, and maintenance of the ablation catheter in the antrum; this technique has been adopted with good safety and efficacy.[53] Marrouche and colleagues studied the use of ICE to guide the adjustment of power on an irrigated-tip RFA catheter during PVI and noted a reduced incidence of pulmonary stenosis in addition to greater efficacy using the ICE-guided approach.[54] Additionally, ICE has been used in its own mapping system to reconstruct LA and PV 3D geometry (CartoSound) identifying anatomical landmarks to guide AF ablation.[55] The use of ICE and CT/MRI to guide AF ablations is illustrated in some of our procedures (see Figures 42B.4A, 42B.5, 42B.7, and 42B.8 and ▶ Video 42B.3 and ▶ Video 42B.4).

EGM-guided PV Antral Isolation

While an anatomic-guided PV antral ablation set can be a useful first step, it is recommended to use an EGM-guided approach to demonstrate electrical isolation of all the PVs (see Figures 42B.3, 42B.4, 42B.5, 42B.6, 42B.10, 42B.11, and 42B.12). The EGMs originating from the PVs have some distinct properties allowing them to be recognized;[22] identifying these PV potentials was described earlier. The PV antrum is not strictly anatomically defined but is the area outside the os, usually 5 to 10 mm away, in which PV potentials can still be recorded. If ablation is performed in the setting of AF, organized PV potentials can be targeted at sites of

Chapter 42B: Atrial Fibrillation: Focal and Map-guided Ablation • 531

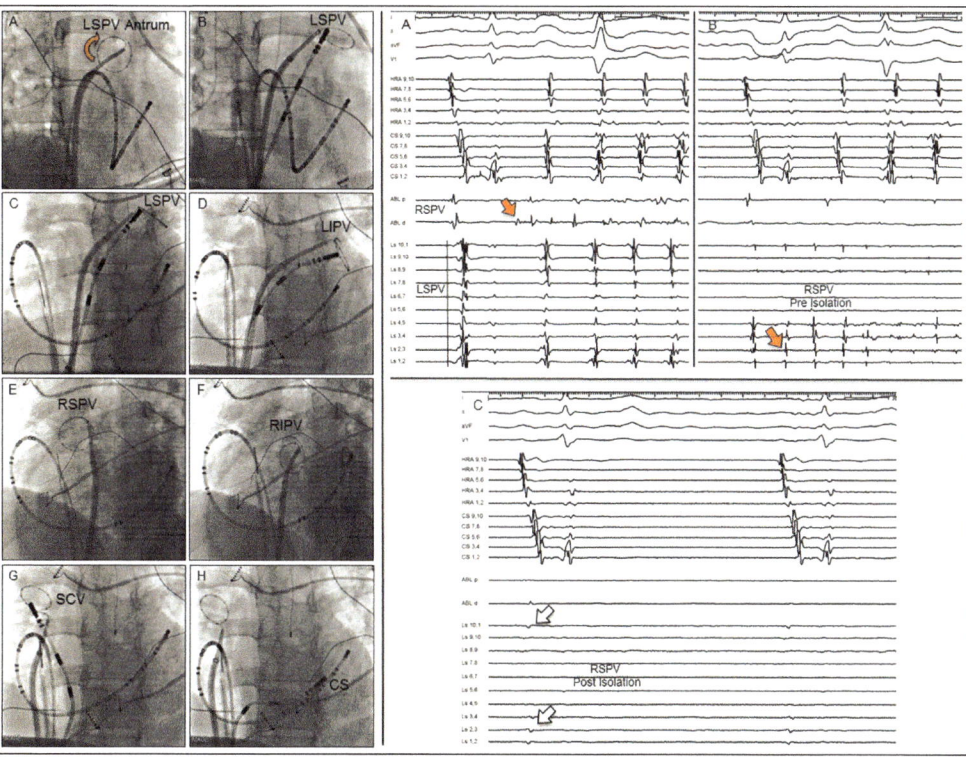

Figure 42B.3 Positioning of electrode catheters under fluoroscopy. **Left panels:** A catheter spans the RA free wall and CS. A circular catheter and an irrigated tip ablation catheter (RMT-Stereotaxis) are moving. Simultaneous clockwise rotation while advancing the circular catheter facilitates the posterior approach to the LSPV in (**A**). Note the ablation catheter targeting the circular catheter at PV ostia in (**B–D**) and the position of the circular catheter to right-sided PVs in (**E**) and (**F**). The ablation catheter is targeting the SVC in panel (**G**) and the CS in (**H**). **Right panels:** EGM-guided PV electrical isolation. Note that firing from the RSPV (**arrow**) preceded the LSPV in (**A**); the circular catheter (Ls) was positioned in the RSPV and recorded AF initiation in (**B**); note the electrical isolation of RSPV at the **hollow arrows** in (**C**).

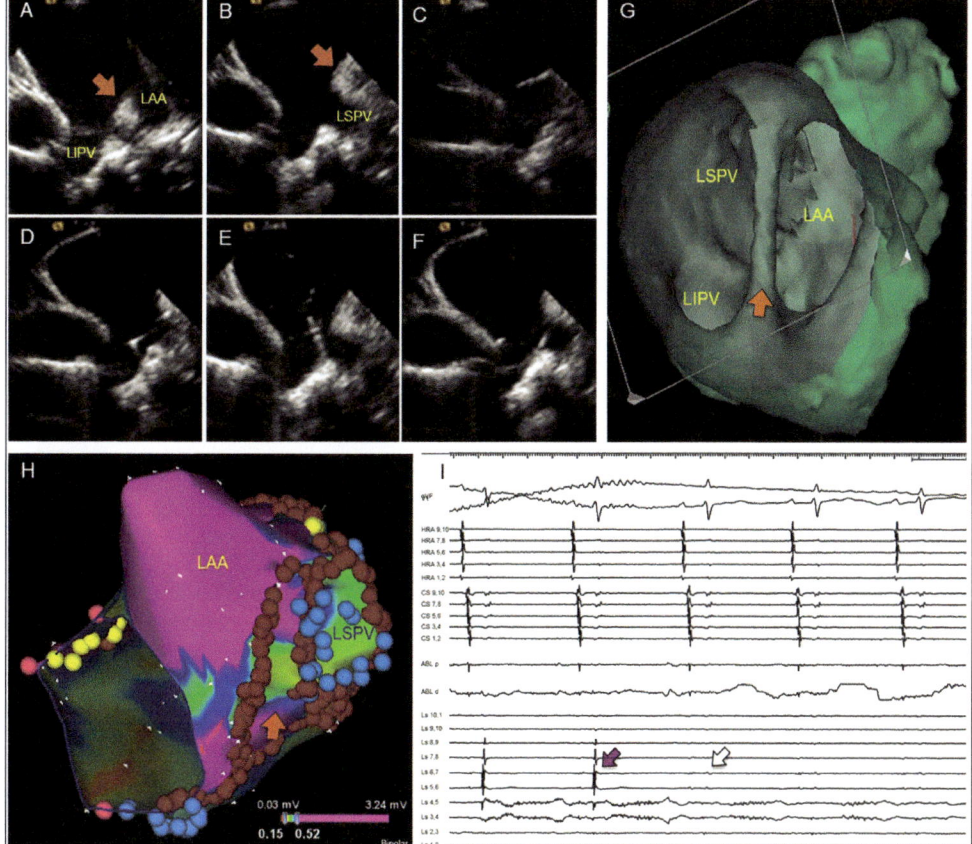

Figure 42B.4 ICE showing LA, LSPV, LIPV, and LAA (**A–F**). Note the prominent lateral ridge between LAA and LSPV (**arrows**), with the circular catheter at the common PV os (**C, E**), at the LSPV os (**D**), and at the LIPV os (**F**); note the ablation catheter at the carina (**E**). Cardiac CT showing an endoscopic view of left-sided PVs, LAA, and the ridge (**arrow**). A 3D voltage map of the LA showing an ablation lesion set (**H**). Note red tags indicating ablation along both sides of the ridge (**arrow**). Additional RF delivery (**blue tags**) was required to electrically isolate the LSPV, shown by the **arrows** in (**I**).

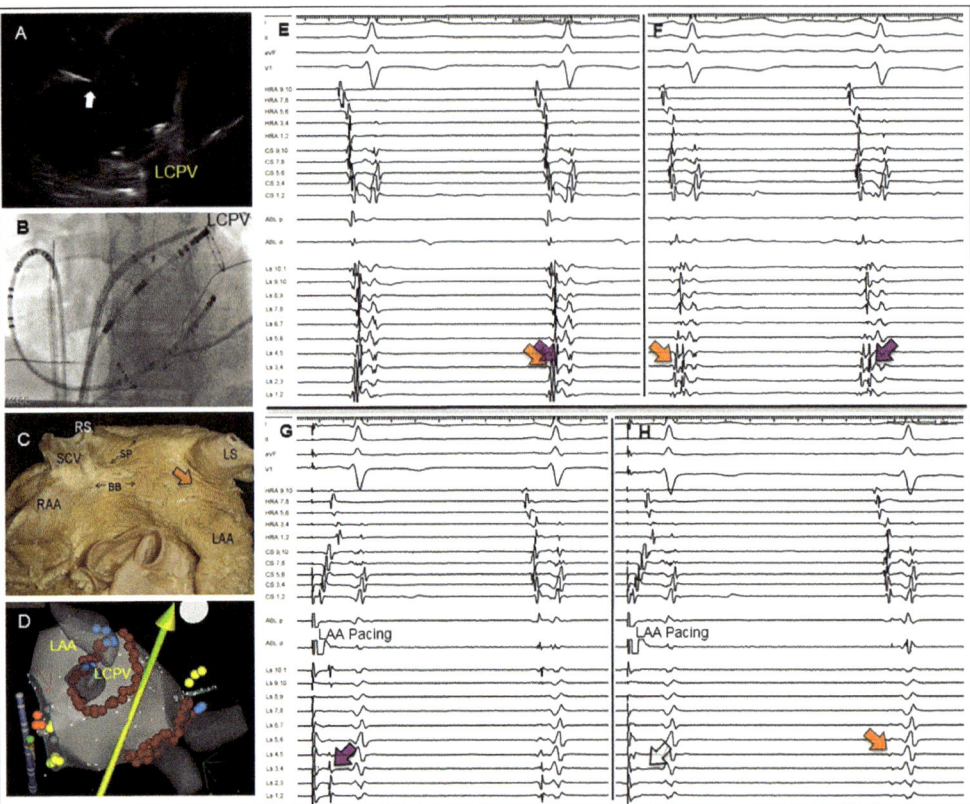

Figure 42B.5 Electrical isolation of a left common PV (LCPV). Note the circular catheter at the LCPV (**A, B**); also, tenting of the fossa ovalis on ICE prior to second transeptal puncture is shown at the arrow in (**A**). The epicardial aspect of a human heart[12] with an **arrow** indicating the lateral ridge is seen in (**C**). 3D anatomical map of LA shows the ablation lesion set in (**D**). Note PV potentials prior to ablation of LCPV, **arrows** in (**E**); their separation after initial ablation (**red tags** in D) shown in (**F**); residual PV potentials with additional ablation (**blue tags**) ruled in by pacing from the LAA in (**G**) and finally with electrical isolation of LCPV, **arrows** in (**H**).

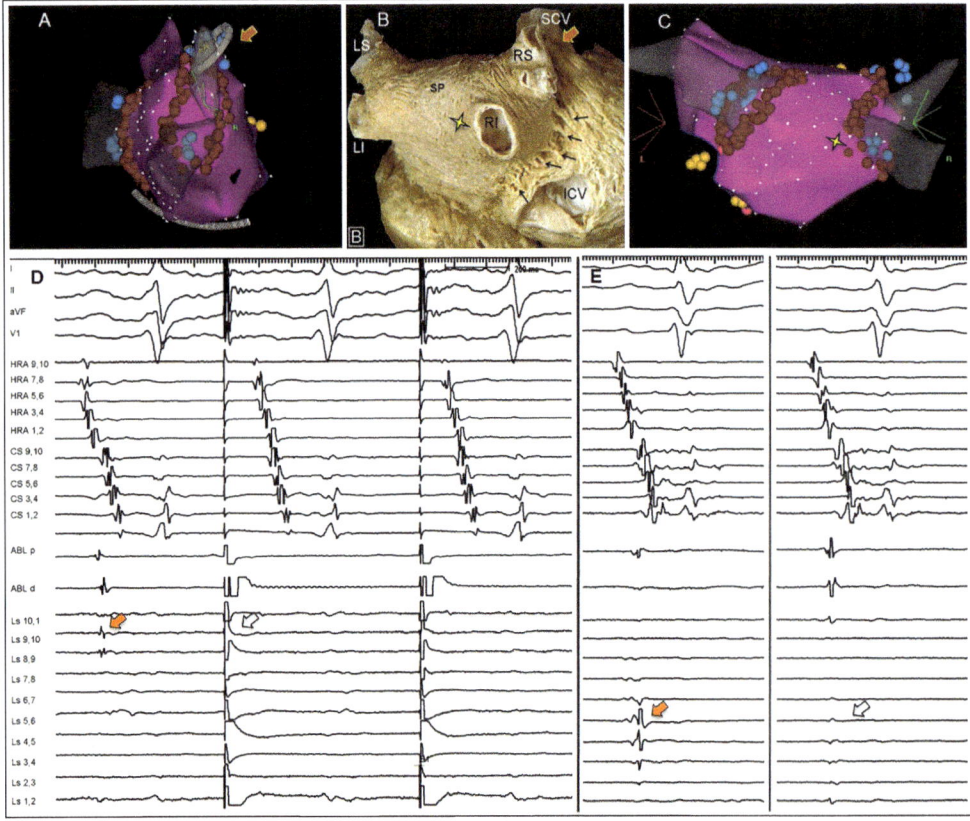

Figure 42B.6 Pacing maneuvers to differentiate far field from PV potentials. 3D voltage map of LA showing ablation lesion set (**A, C**). Note residual potential in the RSPV, **arrow** in (**D**); pacing from the SVC, **hollow arrow** in (**D**), and **arrows** in (**A, B**) confirmed SVC far-field potential. Also note the close proximity of the RSPV and SVC myocardium in (**B**).[12] On the other hand, the residual potentials in the RIPV, **arrow** in (**E**) located at a site, **star** in (**C, B**) were indeed PV potentials. Note PVI after additional ablation, **hollow arrow** in (**E**).

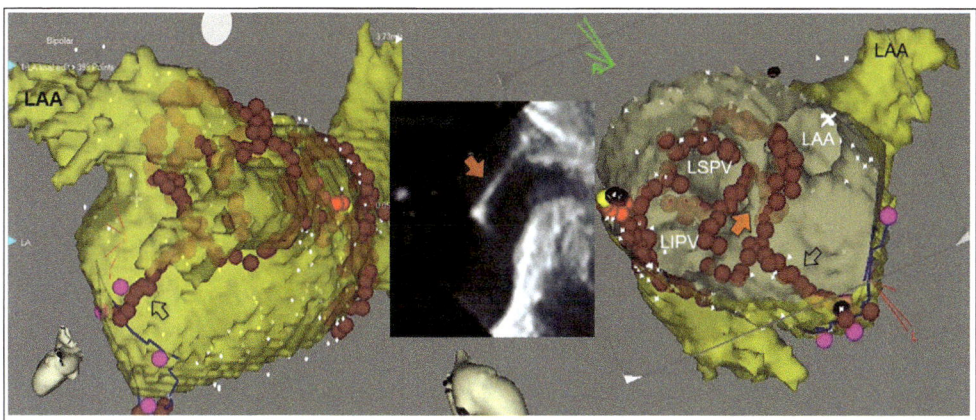

Figure 42B.7 Cardiac CT merge with 3D EAM to guide AF ablation lesion set. Note **red tags** indicating ablation along both sides of the ridge, **arrow** in the **right panel**, also indicated on ICE imaging, **center panel**. Mitral isthmus ablation line (**hollow arrows**).

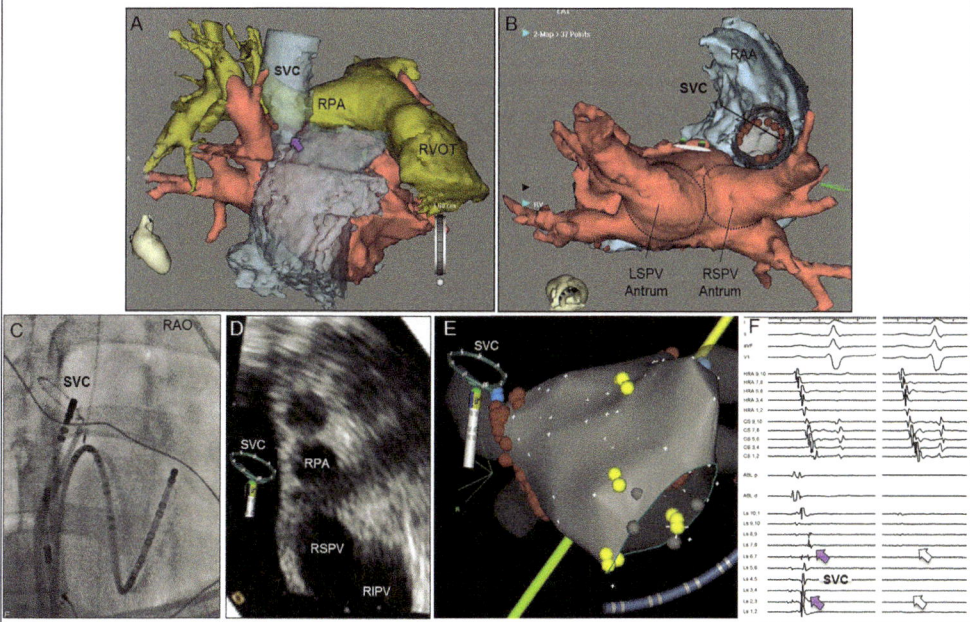

Figure 42B.8 Multiple imaging modalities can facilitate EGM-guided SVC isolation. Cardiac CT (**A, B**), fluoroscopy (**C**), ICE (**D**), and 3D EAM (**E**) indicating SVC isolation at the level of the inferior border of the right pulmonary artery (RPA), **arrows** and circular catheter position. Note SVC potentials, **arrows** in (**F**), and SVC isolation after ablation, **hollow arrows** in (**F**).

earliest activation. If PV activity is disorganized, then circumferential ablation can be done empirically and this will often cause changes in PV potentials (in cycle length or morphology) as active ablation is impacting the PV-LA connections directly.[29] Antral ablation is performed at each segment where PV potentials were recorded, which often ends up in a circumferential ablation lesion set. Subsequently, the circular catheter is placed just distal to the ablated area to ensure that no PV potentials are recorded in the antrum and then the PV itself to confirm entrance conduction block in sinus rhythm or with CS pacing.[53] An expandable electrode mesh catheter can facilitate mapping and ablating around the PVs (see Figure 42B.5).[56]

Remote Navigation

Remote navigation technologies have entered the field as an alternative means to precisely maneuver the ablation catheter during AF ablation procedures. Two systems are clinically available: the Stereotaxis Magnetic Navigation System (Niobe, St. Louis, MO) and the Sensei Robotic Catheter System (Hansen Medical, Mountain View, CA). The benefits from a clinical efficacy standpoint include better catheter maneuverability and more stable catheter positioning. Some argue that there is less effective contact without manual pressure, but initial clinical studies suggest equal efficacy to the conventional approach.[57] Also, there appears to be a reduction of fluoroscopy exposure to the patient by approximately one-third[57,58] in addition to a significant decrease in exposure to the operator. The development of an open-irrigated ablation catheter has improved magnetic-navigation AF ablation outcomes.[59,60] It may be safer than the conventional manual approach since virtually no significant pericardial effusion has been reported. We have utilized the Stereotaxis system successfully as illustrated in Figures 42B.3, 42B.4, 42B.5, and 42B.8. Ultimately, larger clinical trials are required to assess whether remote navigation can lead to superior outcomes.

AF Ablation Endpoint and Limitations

There should be an emphasis that the endpoint of PVI, regardless of which techniques above are utilized, should be complete electrical isolation of the PVs, as recommended by the HRS/EHRA/ECAS consensus statement on AF ablation.[6]

It is established that wider circumferential antral ablation leads to better outcomes; however, the ablation procedure can be more complex and time-consuming. The myocardial connections are thicker and more robust in the antrum as opposed to at the PV os, and the wider the circumferential ablation set, the greater the number of lesions required to achieve PV electrical isolation.[52] In addition, there may be a higher risk of recurrent iatrogenic reentrant tachyarrhythmias as a consequence of either an incomplete ablation lesion set or recovery of PV conduction.[52]

Adjunctive EGM-guided Ablation Strategies

Non-PV Triggers

Automatic triggers similar to those found in the PVs can be seen in non-PV sites. There is evidence that non-PV trigger sites may account for 14% of trigger sites in patients undergoing a repeat procedure for paroxysmal AF.[61] The SVC is often the culprit non-PV site followed by triggers in the crista terminalis, ligament of Marshall, CS, and rarely, a persistent left SVC (LSVC), the sinus node region, IVC, and LAA.[62] An LSVC is a distinct entity that, when present, can be a source of non-PV triggers. As most patients do not have an LSVC, they are significantly less common than SVC triggers. Due to the predominance of SVC triggers—12% in our initial experience—we evaluated the role of empiric SVC electrical isolation in a nonrandomized study of 407 patients; we found it to be safe and effective as an adjunct to PVI alone (see Figure 42B.8).[63] It is important to at least recognize while performing the ablation procedure that automatic AF triggers can exist outside the PVs.

Targeting Complex Fractionated Atrial Electrograms (CFAEs) in Atrial Fibrillation

CFAEs have been identified during surgical epicardial mapping as local sites in AF expressing slow conduction, functional conduction block and pivot points, and as potentially key locations for the maintenance of AF.[64] These complex electrical activities exhibit short cycle lengths and heterogeneous temporal and spatial patterns.[65] Despite extensive experimental and clinical investigation, CFAEs remain poorly understood, and the role of targeting atrial sites exhibiting CFAEs as an adjunctive approach for AF ablation is also uncertain. Nadamanee has performed mapping and ablation of CFAEs as a substrate modifying strategy without PVI.[66] To further modify the substrate that maintains long-standing AF, investigators have been evaluating the adjunctive role of CFAE ablation compared to conventional PVI. Oral et al randomized patients undergoing ablation for chronic AF to (1) linear LA lesions across CFAEs (nonencircling) or (2) large-area circumferential ablation (encircling), with both groups allowing linear mitral isthmus, posterior wall, or roof lesions; they found that outcomes in the two groups were similar.[67] Haïssaguerre et al have described a stepwise sequential ablation approach for patients with long-lasting persistent AF that includes PVI, linear ablation across the roof and along the isthmus between the mitral annulus and the LIPV, and ablation of the CFAE sites.[68]

We evaluated the adjunctive role of CFAE ablation to an EGM-guided PV antrum isolation (PVAI) in a prospective, randomized study including patients presenting for ablation of long-standing persistent AF.[69] In comparing the groups who underwent PVAI and adjunctive CFAE ablation to PVAI alone and their long-term results with an average follow-up of 16.3 months, the adjunct of extensive CFAE ablation at the LA, CS, and sometimes RA, in addition to PVAI, led to a significant increase in maintaining sinus rhythm from 40% to 61% ($P = 0.03$) after a single procedure and without antiarrhythmic drugs. The combination also showed a nonsignificant trend toward overall increased maintenance of sinus rhythm with any number of procedures and on antiarrhythmic drugs from 83% to 94% ($P = 0.17$), when compared to conventional PVAI alone. For the group receiving the hybrid approach, the first step was PVAI, which was performed in AF. Typically there were minimal changes in the level of fragmentation in the anterior LA, CS, and RA; in addition, AF rarely converted into sinus rhythm during PVAI. Following completion of empirical PVAI, we extensively targeted sites exhibiting CFAEs. A multielectrode circular catheter was used for mapping CFAEs in the LA and RA and a multielectrode linear catheter for mapping CFAEs in the CS and SVC-RA junction. We defined CFAEs as atrial sites exhibiting continuous electrical activity, fragmented electrical activity (complex EGMs with ≥2 deflections), or atrial EGMs with cycle length ≤120 ms. Targeting ablation at sites exhibiting CFAE as an adjunctive approach to PVI is illustrated in Figures 42B.9, 42B.10, 42B.11, and 42B.12.

Given the somewhat underwhelming results from CFAE-based ablations, Narayan and colleagues attempted to identify several different types of CFAEs that may correspond to different mechanisms.[70] Their recent study suggests that CFAEs with discrete monopolar action potentials, short cycle lengths, pansystolic activation, narrow spectral dominant frequency, and low-signal amplitude

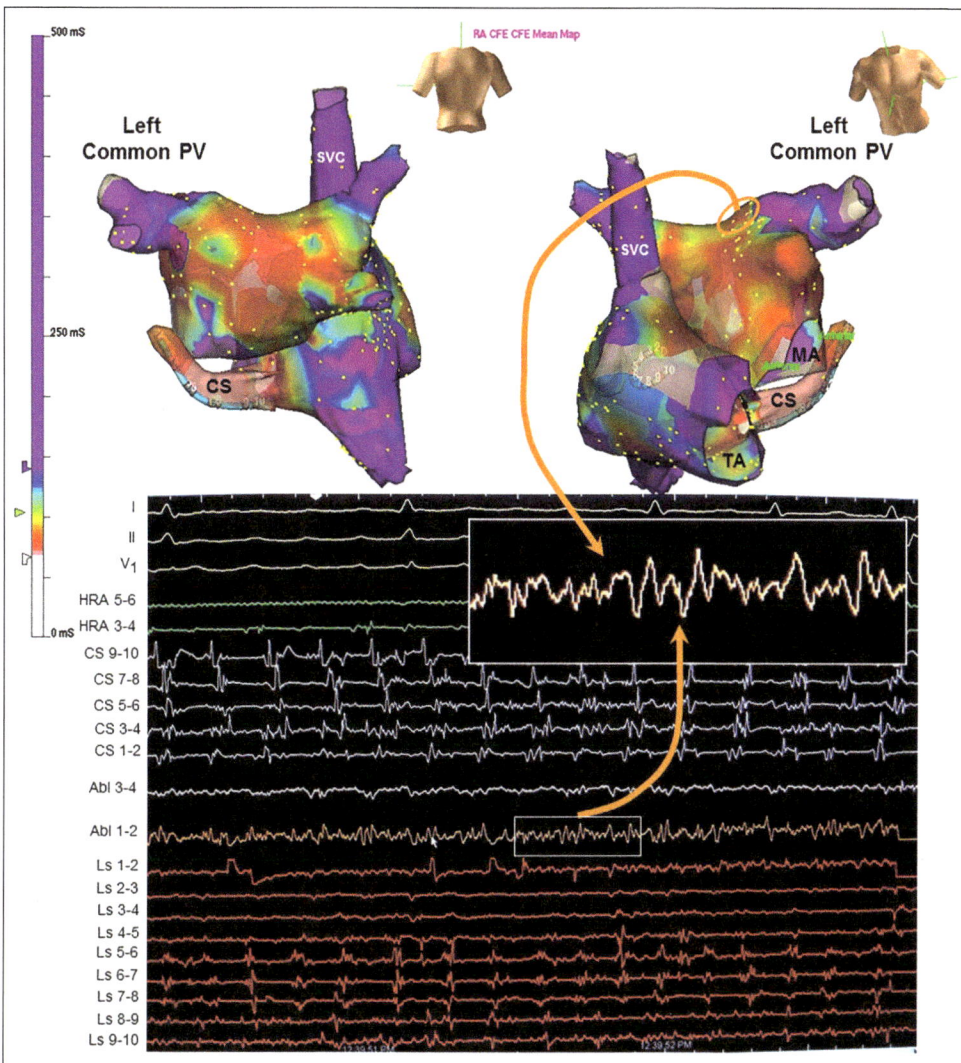

Figure 42B.9 3D EAM of the RA, LA, and CS exhibiting the degree of CFAE, from highest fractionation (**white sites**, such as the anteroseptal LA and CS) to no fractionation (**purple sites**). Note CFAEs at the antrum of the LCPV (**arrows**).

are consistent with rapid localized AF drivers, and targeting these so-called type 1 CFAEs for ablation may lead to greater success in reducing or eliminating AF.[70]

It has been suggested that targeting ganglionated plexi can be helpful in AF, and that CFAEs may be related to these sites. The typical endocardial stimulation sites used to identify the ganglionated plexi seem to have a spatial correlation to three major LA areas exhibiting CFAEs,[71,72] and preliminary data regarding ablation at sites of ganglionated plexi does show some early success.[73]

Targeting Sites with Dominant Frequency in Atrial Fibrillation

There is now significant evidence for the existence of local rotors, microreentrant circuits with regular activity, that are distributed in the atria, each with a different frequency, that contribute to the maintenance of AF.[74-77] The rotor foci can be measured in the frequency domain, and when these rotors are faster than surrounding activity, they are termed a site of dominant frequency. A key investigation by Sanders et al[78] revealed that dominant frequency sites were stable, spatially distributed with a higher propensity for PV location in paroxysmal AF, and that when standard ablation happened to be performed at these sites, AF was likely to be successfully terminated. Interestingly, a nonrandomized study showed that either circumferential PVI or CFAE-guided ablation both led to a significant reduction in dominant frequencies of similar magnitude.[79]

Shih-Ann Chen and colleagues explored the relationship of dominant frequency to CFAE sites in relation to AF ablation success, and they showed that fractionated activity was related spatially to sites of maximum dominant frequency, and patients with greater dominant frequency gradients within the LA had higher success rates of ablation.[80] Only one published study to date has prospectively evaluated the role of real-time dominant frequency identification and ablation targeted to these sites.[81] Atienza et al studied dominant frequency sites in 50 patients with paroxysmal or persistent AF. Maximum dominant frequency sites

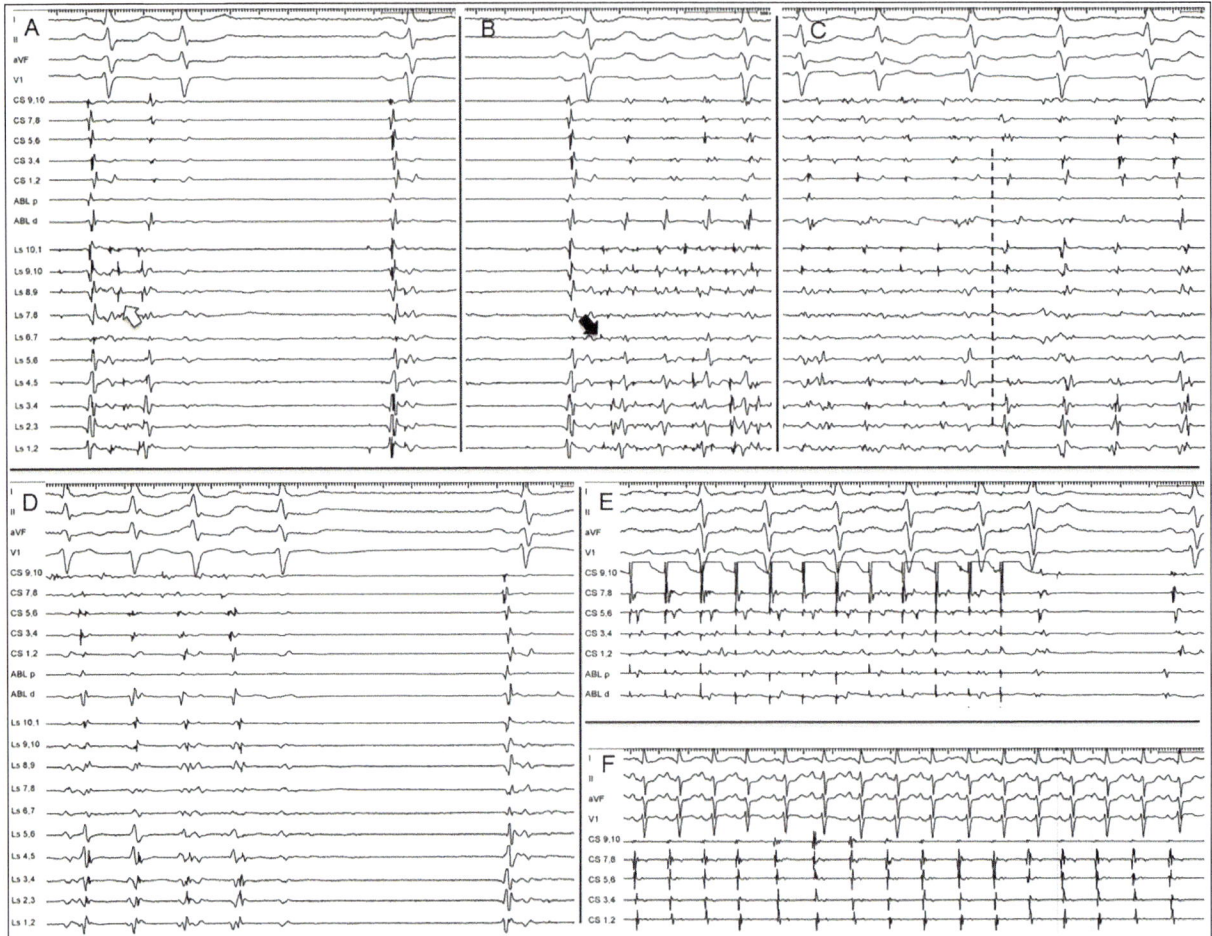

Figure 42B.10 AF ablation using a sequential EGM-guided strategy. Note short local coupling PAC on the LSPV (Ls) recordings and AF initiation (**arrows** in **A, B**); during PVI, AF organized into a residual tachyarrhythmia (**dotted line** in **C**), which terminated during ablation (**D**). After isolation of all PVs, rapid atrial pacing (**E**) and isoproterenol administration at 20 mcg/min (**F**) failed to induce AF or AFL.

were identified as those with a frequency signal 20% higher than surrounding atria, and using a real-time color-coded map, these areas were targeted for ablation. All patients subsequently received a standard PVI. RF ablation of maximum dominant frequency sites did result in a reduced dominant frequency and dominant frequency gradient, and the success rate of this feasibility study was freedom from AF in 88% of paroxysmal AF and in 56% of persistent AF patients at 9 months of follow-up. Additionally, patients with maximum dominant frequency sites that could not be ablated had a significantly higher AF recurrence rate (70% vs 12%).[81]

In summary, there is evidence that dominant frequency sites are related to the rotor mechanisms that may contribute to the underlying pathophysiology of AF, and it is clear that the pattern of dominant frequency sites is different with paroxysmal versus persistent AF. Patients with paroxysmal AF have a greater degree of dominant frequency gradients[78,79] and dominant frequency sites are more likely to be located in the PVs, whereas patients with persistent AF have a more homogenous distribution of frequencies and more non-PV locations of dominant frequency sites.[80,81] Dominant frequency sites seem to be correlated with areas of CFAE,[80] although the definite relationship and mechanisms are not entirely clear. In nonrandomized, mostly restrospective studies, ablation at dominant frequency sites does appear to correlate with ablation success. It is not clear that targeting dominant frequency sites, however, has any advantage over other accepted adjunctive techniques in addition to PVI. Further randomized study of a dominant frequency-targeted strategy may help clarify the role of using dominant frequency in AF ablation.

Ablation of AF Nests Guided by Real-time Spectral Mapping in Sinus Rhythm

Pachon et al have developed a system for real-time spectral mapping using fast Fourier transform in sinus rhythm. This mapping strategy identifies sites in which the unfiltered, bipolar atrial EGMs contain unusually high frequencies, namely fibrillar myocardium or the so-called

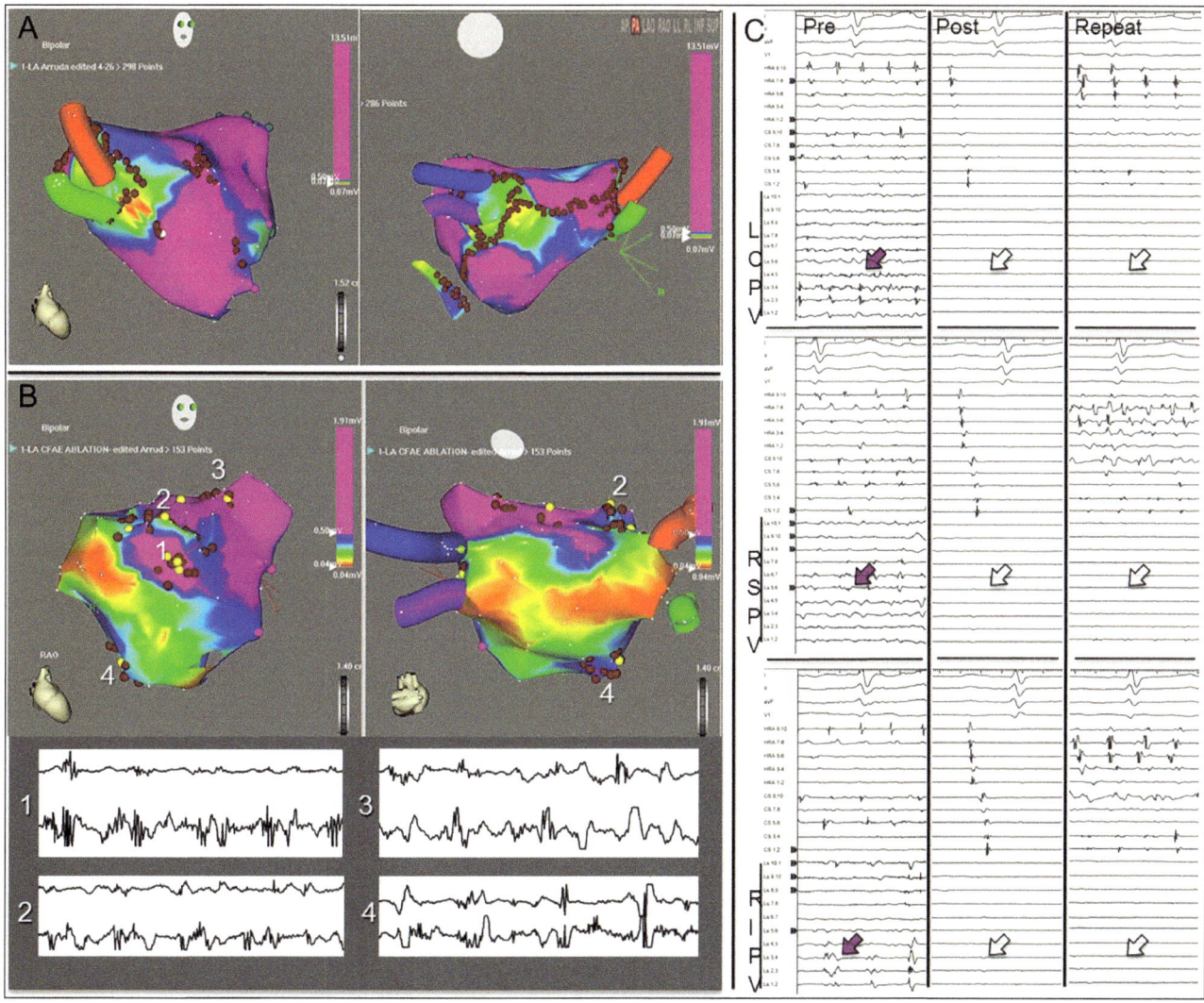

Figure 42B.11 EGM-guided ablation of long-standing persistent AF. 3D voltage map of LA prior to first ablation procedure, showing preexisting scar at PV antra and ablation lesion set (**A**) including PVI, LA roof and mitral isthmus lines, and along the atrial aspect of the CS. Note PV electrical activity (Pre) and its absence (Post) (**arrows** in **C panels**). AF recurred, and the 3D voltage map obtained during the second procedure is shown in **B**. Note the extensive scar, but importantly, the PVs remained isolated from the first procedure. Sites exhibiting CFAE were ablated (**1, 2, 3,** and **4** in **B**) on the map and EGMs, respectively. This patient has remained in sinus rhythm, off antiarrhythmic drugs, for more than 2 years.

AF nest. The investigators described a new AF ablation approach targeting solely the atrial sites exhibiting the AF nests, without intentional PVI. In their series, 94.1% of patients were maintained in sinus rhythm at 9.9 ± 5 months postprocedure. However, 41.1% remained on a previously ineffective antiarrhythmic drug.[82]

In an attempt to further modify the AF substrate and to improve long-term ablation success, we evaluated the adjunctive role of AF nest ablation to an EGM guided PVAI in a prospective randomized study in patients with long-standing persistent AF (see Figure 42B.13).[83] AF nest ablation had a favorable impact on the long-term outcome following a single procedure without antiarrhythmic drugs as it decreased overall recurrences in 10% as compared to PVAI. In a median follow-up of 11.5 months, only 11% of patients recurred with AF and 25% with an organized AT.

Summary

The cornerstone of AF ablation is PV electrical isolation. The evolving technologies applied to catheters, imaging, 3D EAM, and remote navigation systems have greatly contributed to current AF ablation strategies. Numerous adjunctive approaches including ablation of sites exhibiting CFAEs, ablation of sites with dominant frequencies in AF and high frequencies in sinus rhythm, ablation of non-PV triggers, and autonomic nervous system modulation, seem to have a favorable impact on procedural outcomes. Since AF ablation strategies are evolving, the procedure is often tailored to the individual patient and their burden of AF, as well as the operator's own preferences and experiences. Importantly, procedural safety and efficacy continue to improve and further investigations may optimize current strategies to achieve a safer and more effective ablation of AF.

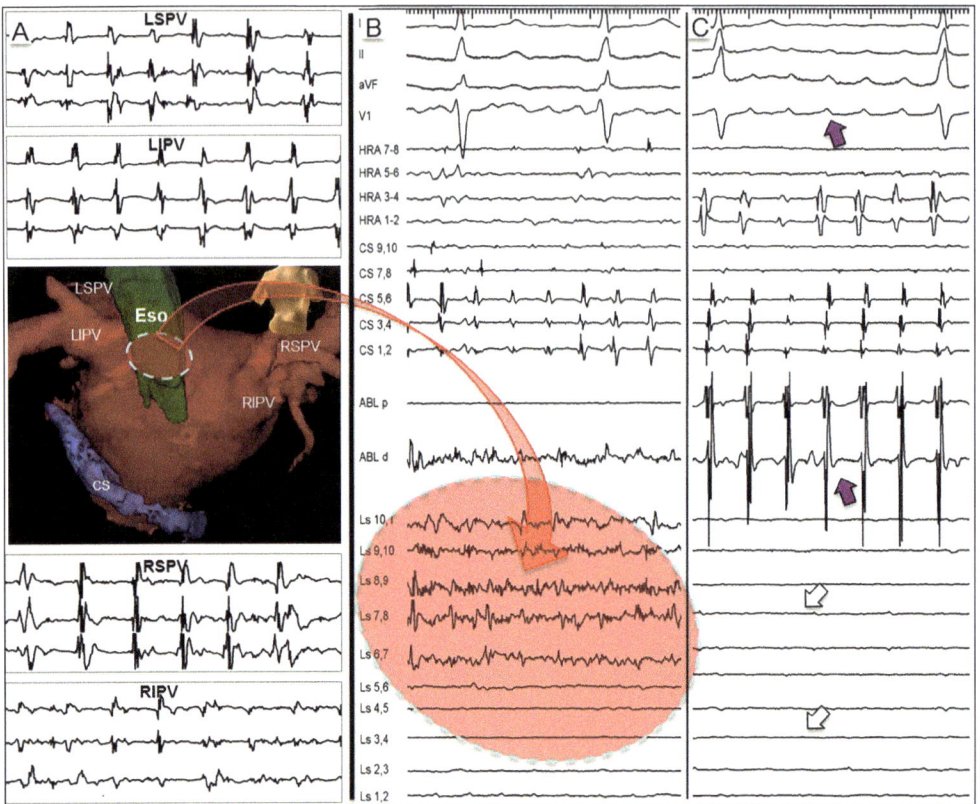

Figure 42B.12 The adjunct of CFAE ablation to reisolation of PVs in a repeat procedure. Segmented cardiac CT showing the LA, PVs, CS, and esophagus. The residual PV potentials (**A**) were easily eliminated. Note the extensive low-amplitude CFAE on the circular catheter at the posterior wall, in close proximity to the esophagus (**shaded area, B**). Low RF power was delivered at these CFAE sites, organizing AF into an atypical flutter (**C**). PVs were isolated, (**hollow arrow, C**). Recurrent atypical flutter was successfully treated with dofetilide.

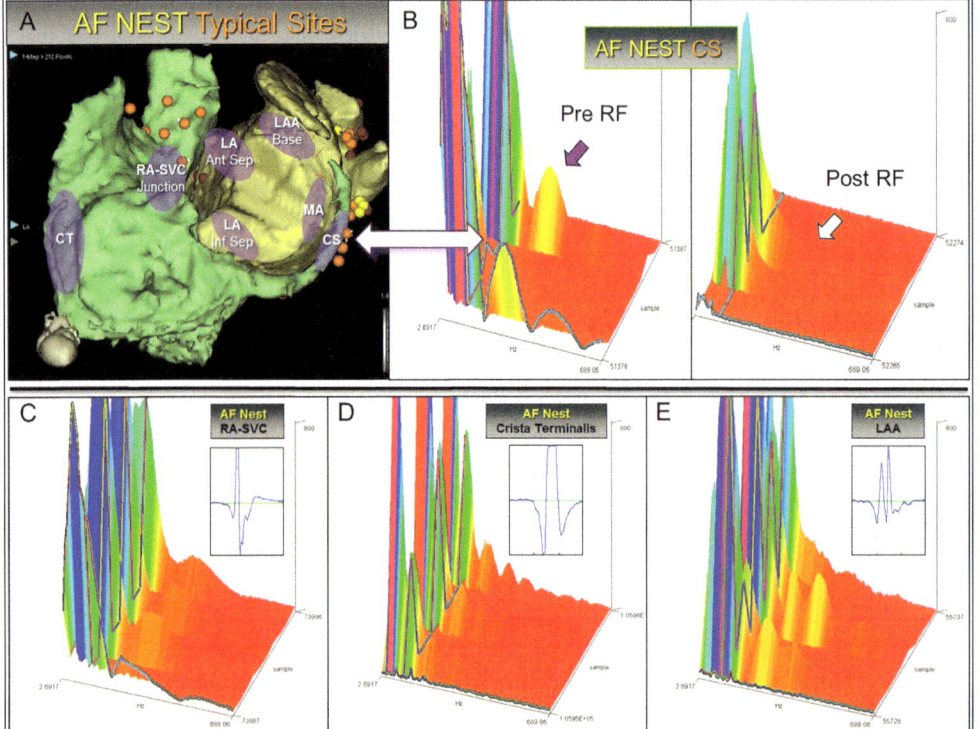

Figure 42B.13 Real-time spectral mapping in sinus rhythm as an adjunct to PVI: targeting sites exhibiting high frequencies, namely fibrillar myocardium or AF nest. Cardiac CT showing the anatomical distribution of AF nest outside the PV antra (**shaded areas, A**). Note AF nest in the CS preablation, with local spectral normalization postablation (**arrows, B**). **C, D,** and **E** illustrate the AF nests at the RA-SVC junction, crista terminalis, and base of the LAA, respectively.

References

1. Haïssaguerre M, Jaïs P, Shah DC, et al. Spontaneous initiation of atrial fibrillation by ectopic beats originating in the pulmonary veins. *N Engl J Med.* 1998;339(10):659-666.
2. Chen SA, Tai CT, Tsai CF, Hsieh MH, Ding YA, Chang MS. Radiofrequency catheter ablation of atrial fibrillation initiated by pulmonary vein ectopic beats. *J Cardiovasc Electrophysiol.* 2000;11(2):218-227.
3. Camm AJ, Kirchhof P, Lip GY, et al. Guidelines for the management of atrial fibrillation: the Task Force for the Management of Atrial Fibrillation of the European Society of Cardiology (ESC). *Eur Heart J.* 2010;31(19):2369-2429.
4. Fuster V, Ryden LE, Cannom DS, et al. 2011 ACCF/AHA/HRS focused updates incorporated into the ACC/AHA/ESC 2006 guidelines for the management of patients with atrial fibrillation: a report of the American College of Cardiology Foundation/American Heart Association Task Force on Practice Guidelines developed in partnership with the European Society of Cardiology and in collaboration with the European Heart Rhythm Association and the Heart Rhythm Society. *J Am Coll Cardiol.* 2011;57(11):e101-198.
5. Fuster V, Ryden LE, Cannom DS, et al. ACC/AHA/ESC 2006 guidelines for the management of patients with atrial fibrillation: full text: a report of the American College of Cardiology/American Heart Association Task Force on practice guidelines and the European Society of Cardiology Committee for Practice Guidelines (Writing Committee to Revise the 2001 guidelines for the management of patients with atrial fibrillation) developed in collaboration with the European Heart Rhythm Association and the Heart Rhythm Society. *Europace.* 2006;8(9):651-745.
6. Calkins H, Kuck KH, Cappato R, et al. HRS/EHRA/ECAS Expert consensus statement on catheter and surgical ablation of atrial fibrillation: recommendations for patient selection, procedural techniques, patient management and follow-up, definitions, endpoints, and research trial design. *Heart Rhythm.* 2012. doi:10.1016/j.hrthm.2011.12.016.
7. Chen S-A, Chen Y-J, Yeh H-I, Tai C-T, Chen Y-C, Lin C-I. Pathophysiology of the pulmonary vein as an atrial fibrillation initiator. *PACE.* Jul 2003;26(7 Pt 2):1576-1582.
8. de Bakker JMT, Ho SY, Hocini M. Basic and clinical electrophysiology of pulmonary vein ectopy. *Cardiovascular Research.* May 2002;54(2):287-294.
9. Nattel S. Basic electrophysiology of the pulmonary veins and their role in atrial fibrillation: precipitators, perpetuators, and perplexers. *J Cardiovasc Electrophysiol.* 2003;14(12):1372-1375.
10. Lin WS, Prakash VS, Tai CT, et al. Pulmonary vein morphology in patients with paroxysmal atrial fibrillation initiated by ectopic beats originating from the pulmonary veins: implications for catheter ablation. *Circulation.* 2000;101(11):1274-1281.
11. Hassink RJ, Aretz HT, Ruskin J, Keane D. Morphology of atrial myocardium in human pulmonary veins: a postmortem analysis in patients with and without atrial fibrillation. *J Am Coll Cardiol.* 2003;42(6):1108-1114.
12. Ho SY, Cabrera JA, Tran VH, Farre J, Anderson RH, Sanchez-Quintana D. Architecture of the pulmonary veins: relevance to radiofrequency ablation. *Heart.* 2001;86(3):265-270.
13. Chen SA, Hsieh MH, Tai CT, et al. Initiation of atrial fibrillation by ectopic beats originating from the pulmonary veins: electrophysiological characteristics, pharmacological responses, and effects of radiofrequency ablation. *Circulation.* 1999;100(18):1879-1886.
14. Jaïs P, Hocini M, Macle L, et al. Distinctive electrophysiological properties of pulmonary veins in patients with atrial fibrillation. *Circulation.* 2002;106(19):2479-2485.
15. Kumagai K, Ogawa M, Noguchi H, Yasuda T, Nakashima H, Saku K. Electrophysiologic properties of pulmonary veins assessed using a multielectrode basket catheter. *J Am Coll Cardiol.* 2004;43(12):2281-2289.
16. Fynn SP, Kalman JM. Pulmonary veins: anatomy, electrophysiology, tachycardia, and fibrillation. *PACE.* 2004;27(11):1547-1559.
17. Vaitkevicius R, Saburkina I, Rysevaite K, et al. Nerve supply of the human pulmonary veins: an anatomical study. *Heart Rhythm.* 2009;6(2):221-228.
18. Cabrera JA, Ho SY, Climent V, Fuertes B, Murillo M, Sanchez-Quintana D. Morphological evidence of muscular connections between contiguous pulmonary venous orifices: relevance of the interpulmonary isthmus for catheter ablation in atrial fibrillation. *Heart Rhythm.* 2009;6(8):1192-1198.
19. Nakagawa H, Aoyama H, Beckman KJ, et al. Relation between pulmonary vein firing and extent of left atrial-pulmonary vein connection in patients with atrial fibrillation. *Circulation.* 2004;109(12):1523-1529.
20. Pan N-H, Tsao H-M, Chang N-C, Chen Y-J, Chen S-A. Aging dilates atrium and pulmonary veins: implications for the genesis of atrial fibrillation. *Chest.* 2008;133(1):190-196.
21. Perez-Lugones A, Schvartzman PR, Schweikert R, et al. Three-dimensional reconstruction of pulmonary veins in patients with atrial fibrillation and controls: morphological characteristics of different veins. *PACE.* 2003;26(1 Pt 1):8-15.
22. Haïssaguerre M, Shah DC, Jaïs P, et al. Mapping-guided ablation of pulmonary veins to cure atrial fibrillation. *J Am Cardiol.* 2000;86(9A):9K-19K.
23. Ashar MS, Pennington J, Callans DJ, Marchlinski FE. Localization of arrhythmogenic triggers of atrial fibrillation. *J Cardiovasc Electrophysiol.* 2000;11(12):1300-1305.
24. Asirvatham SJ. Pulmonary vein-related maneuvers: part I. *Heart Rhythm.* 2007;4(4):538-544.
25. Takahashi Y, O'Neill MD, Jonsson A, et al. How to interpret and identify pulmonary vein recordings with the Lasso catheter. *Heart Rhythm.* 2006;3(6):748-750.
26. Teh AW, Kistler PM, Kalman JM. Using the 12-lead ECG to localize the origin of ventricular and atrial tachycardias: part 1. Focal atrial tachycardia. *J Cardiovasc Electrophysiol.* 2009;20(6):706-709; quiz 705.
27. Kistler PM, Roberts-Thomson KC, Haqqani HM, et al. P-wave morphology in focal atrial tachycardia: development of an algorithm to predict the anatomic site of origin. *J Am Coll Cardiol.* 2006;48(5):1010-1017.
28. Kistler PM, Sanders P, Fynn SP, et al. Electrophysiological and electrocardiographic characteristics of focal atrial tachycardia originating from the pulmonary veins: acute and long-term outcomes of radiofrequency ablation. *Circulation.* 2003;108(16):1968-1975.
29. Takahashi Y, O'Neill MD, Jonsson A, et al. How to interpret and identify pulmonary vein recordings with the Lasso catheter. *Heart Rhythm.* 2006;3(6):748-750.
30. Shah DC, Haïssaguerre M, Jaïs P, et al. Electrophysiologically guided ablation of the pulmonary veins for the curative treatment of atrial fibrillation. *Ann Med.* 2000;32(6):408-416.
31. Haïssaguerre M, Jaïs P, Shah DC, et al. Catheter ablation of chronic atrial fibrillation targeting the reinitiating triggers. *J Cardiovasc Electrophysiol.* 2000;11(1):2-10.
32. Marchlinski FE, Callans D, Dixit S, et al. Efficacy and safety of targeted focal ablation versus PV isolation assisted by magnetic electroanatomic mapping. *J Cardiovasc Electrophysiol.* 2003;14(4):358-365.

33. Yu WC, Hsu TL, Tai CT, et al. Acquired pulmonary vein stenosis after radiofrequency catheter ablation of paroxysmal atrial fibrillation. *J Cardiovasc Electrophysiol*. 2001;12(8):887-892.
34. Saad EB, Marrouche NF, Saad CP, et al. Pulmonary vein stenosis after catheter ablation of atrial fibrillation: emergence of a new clinical syndrome. [Summary for patients in *Ann Intern Med*. 2003;138(8):1; PMID: 12693916]. *Ann Inten Med*. 2003;138(8):634-638.
35. Arruda M, Wang Z, Patel A, et al. Circumferential radiofrequency catheter ablation of pulmonary vein ostea: feasible but potentially harmful. *PACE*. April 2000;23(4):1.
36. Moreira W, Manusama R, Timmermans C, et al. Long-term follow-up after cryothermic ostial pulmonary vein isolation in paroxysmal atrial fibrillation. *J Am Coll Cardiol*. 2008;51(8):850-855.
37. Yamane T, Date T, Kanzaki Y, et al. Segmental pulmonary vein antrum isolation using the "large-size" Lasso catheter in patients with atrial fibrillation. *Circulation*. 2007;71(5): 53-760.
38. Hsu L-F, Jaïs P, Hocini M, et al. High-density circumferential pulmonary vein mapping with a 20-pole expandable circular mapping catheter. *PACE*. 2005;28 Suppl 1:S94-98.
39. Haïssaguerre M, Sanders P, Hocini M, et al. Changes in atrial fibrillation cycle length and inducibility during catheter ablation and their relation to outcome. *Circulation*. 2004;109(24):3007-3013.
40. Pak H-N, Kim JS, Shin SY, et al. Is empirical four pulmonary vein isolation necessary for focally triggered paroxysmal atrial fibrillation? Comparison of selective pulmonary vein isolation versus empirical four pulmonary vein isolation. *J Cardiovasc Electrophysiol*. 2008;19(5):473-479.
41. Matsuo S, Yamane T, Date T, et al. Reduction of AF recurrence after pulmonary vein isolation by eliminating ATP-induced transient venous re-conduction. *J Cardiovasc Electrophysiol*. 2007;18(7):704-708.
42. Chang S-L, Tai C-T, Lin Y-J, et al. The efficacy of inducibility and circumferential ablation with pulmonary vein isolation in patients with paroxysmal atrial fibrillation. *J Cardiovasc Electrophysiol*. 2007;18(6):607-611.
43. Pappone C, Rosanio S, Oreto G, et al. Circumferential radiofrequency ablation of pulmonary vein ostia: A new anatomic approach for curing atrial fibrillation. *Circulation*. 2000;102(21):2619-2628.
44. Pappone C, Oreto G, Rosanio S, et al. Atrial electroanatomic remodeling after circumferential radiofrequency pulmonary vein ablation: efficacy of an anatomic approach in a large cohort of patients with atrial fibrillation. *Circulation*. 2001;104(21):2539-2544.
45. Fiala M, Chovancik J, Nevralov R, et al. Pulmonary vein isolation using segmental versus electroanatomical circumferential ablation for paroxysmal atrial fibrillation: over 3-year results of a prospective randomized study. *J Interv Card Electrophysiol*. 2008;22(1):13-21.
46. Liu X, Dong J, Mavrakis HE, et al. Achievement of pulmonary vein isolation in patients undergoing circumferential pulmonary vein ablation: a randomized comparison between two different isolation approaches. *J Cardiovasc Electrophysiol*. 2006;17(12):1263-1270.
47. Marrouche NF, Dresing T, Cole C, et al. Circular mapping and ablation of the pulmonary vein for treatment of atrial fibrillation: impact of different catheter technologies. *J Am Coll Cardiol*. 2002;40(3):464-474.
48. Arentz T, Weber R, Burkle G, et al. Small or large isolation areas around the pulmonary veins for the treatment of atrial fibrillation? Results from a prospective randomized study. *Circulation*. 2007;115(24):3057-3063.
49. Lo L-W, Tai C-T, Lin Y-J, et al. Mechanisms of recurrent atrial fibrillation: comparisons between segmental ostial versus circumferential pulmonary vein isolation. *J Cardiovasc Electrophysiol*. 2007;18(8):803-807.
50. Nolker G, Asbach S, Gutleben KJ, et al. Image-integration of intraprocedural rotational angiography-based 3D reconstructions of left atrium and pulmonary veins into electroanatomical mapping: accuracy of a novel modality in atrial fibrillation ablation. *J Cardiovasc Electrophysiol*. 2010;21(3):278-283.
51. Bertaglia E, Bella PD, Tondo C, et al. Image integration increases efficacy of paroxysmal atrial fibrillation catheter ablation: results from the CartoMerge Italian Registry. *Europace*. 2009;11(8):1004-1010.
52. Hocini M, Sanders P, Jaïs P, et al. Prevalence of pulmonary vein disconnection after anatomical ablation for atrial fibrillation: consequences of wide atrial encircling of the pulmonary veins. *Eur Heart J*. 2005;26(7):696-704.
53. Verma A, Marrouche NF, Natale A. Pulmonary vein antrum isolation: intracardiac echocardiography-guided technique. *J Cardiovasc Electrophysiol*. 2004;15(11):1335-1340.
54. Marrouche NF, Martin DO, Wazni O, et al. Phased-array intracardiac echocardiography monitoring during pulmonary vein isolation in patients with atrial fibrillation: impact on outcome and complications. *Circulation*. 2003;107(21):2710-2716.
55. Packer DL, Johnson SB, Kolasa MW, Bunch TJ, Henz BD, Okumura Y. New generation of electro-anatomic mapping: full intracardiac ultrasound image integration. *Europace*. 2008;10(suppl 3):iii35-iii41.
56. Arruda MS, He DS, Friedman P, et al. A novel mesh electrode catheter for mapping and radiofrequency delivery at the left atrium-pulmonary vein junction: a single-catheter approach to pulmonary vein antrum isolation. *J Cardiovasc Electrophysiol*. 2007;18(2):206-211.
57. Saliba W, Reddy VY, Wazni O, et al. Atrial fibrillation ablation using a robotic catheter remote control system: initial human experience and long-term follow-up results. *J Am Coll Cardiol*. 2008;51(25):2407-2411.
58. Schmidt B, Tilz RR, Neven K, et al. Remote robotic navigation and electroanatomical mapping for ablation of atrial fibrillation: considerations for navigation and impact on procedural outcome. *Circulation: Arrhythmia Electrophysiol*. 2009;2(2):120-128.
59. Chun KRJ, Wissner E, Koektuerk B, et al. Remote-controlled magnetic pulmonary vein isolation using a new irrigated-tip catheter in patients with atrial fibrillation. *Circulation: Arrhythmia Electrophysiol*. 2010;3(5):458-464.
60. Pappone C, Vicedomini G, Frigoli E, et al. Irrigated-tip magnetic catheter ablation of AF: a long-term prospective study in 130 patients. *Heart Rhythm*. 2011;8(1):8-15.
61. Gerstenfeld EP, Callans DJ, Dixit S, Zado E, Marchlinski FE. Incidence and location of focal atrial fibrillation triggers in patients undergoing repeat pulmonary vein isolation: implications for ablation strategies. *J Cardiovasc Electrophysiol*. 2003;14(7):685-690.
62. Arruda M, Natale A. The adjunctive role of nonpulmonary venous ablation in the cure of atrial fibrillation. *J Cardiovasc Electrophysiol*. 2006;17:S37-S43.
63. Arruda M, Mlcochova H, Prasad SK, et al. Electrical isolation of the superior vena cava: an adjunctive strategy to pulmonary vein antrum isolation improving the outcome of AF ablation. *J Cardiovasc Electrophysiol*. 2007;18(12):1261-1266.
64. Konings KT, Smeets JL, Penn OC, Wellens HJ, Allessie MA. Configuration of unipolar atrial electrograms during

electrically induced atrial fibrillation in humans. *Circulation.* 4 1997;95(5):1231-1241.
65. Jaïs P, Haïssaguerre M, Shah DC, Chouairi S, Clementy J. Regional disparities of endocardial atrial activation in paroxysmal atrial fibrillation. *PACE.* 1996;19(11 Pt 2):1998-2003.
66. Nademanee K, McKenzie J, Kosar E, et al. A new approach for catheter ablation of atrial fibrillation: mapping of the electrophysiologic substrate. *J Am Coll Cardiol.* 2004;43(11):2044-2053.
67. Oral H, Chugh A, Good E, et al. Randomized comparison of encircling and nonencircling left atrial ablation for chronic atrial fibrillation. *Heart Rhythm.* 2005;2(11):1165-1172.
68. Haïssaguerre M, Sanders P, Hocini M, et al. Catheter ablation of long-lasting persistent atrial fibrillation: critical structures for termination. *J Cardiovasc Electrophysiol.* 2005;16(11):1125-1137.
69. Elayi CS, Verma A, Di Biase L, et al. Ablation for longstanding permanent atrial fibrillation: results from a randomized study comparing three different strategies. *Heart Rhythm.* 2008;5(12):1658-1664.
70. Narayan SM, Wright M, Derval N, et al. Classifying fractionated electrograms in human atrial fibrillation using monophasic action potentials and activation mapping: evidence for localized drivers, rate acceleration, and nonlocal signal etiologies. *Heart Rhythm.* 2011;8(2):244-253.
71. Katritsis D, Giazitzoglou E, Sougiannis D, Voridis E, Po SS. Complex fractionated atrial electrograms at anatomic sites of ganglionated plexi in atrial fibrillation. *Europace.* 2009;11(3):308-315.
72. Lu Z, Scherlag BJ, Lin J, et al. Autonomic mechanism for complex fractionated atrial electrograms: evidence by fast Fourier transform analysis. *J Cardiovasc Electrophysiol.* 2008;19(8):835-842.
73. Po SS, Nakagawa H, Jackman WM. Localization of left atrial ganglionated plexi in patients with atrial fibrillation. *J Cardiovasc Electrophysiol.* 2009;20(10):1186-1189.
74. Kumagai K, Khrestian C, Waldo AL. Simultaneous multisite mapping studies during induced atrial fibrillation in the sterile pericarditis model: insights into the mechanism of its maintenance. *Circulation.* 1997;95(2):511-521.
75. Mansour M, Mandapati R, Berenfeld O, Chen J, Samie FH, Jalife J. Left-to-right gradient of atrial frequencies during acute atrial fibrillation in the isolated sheep heart. *Circulation.* 2001;103(21):2631-2636.
76. Berenfeld O, Mandapati R, Dixit S, et al. Spatially distributed dominant excitation frequencies reveal hidden organization in atrial fibrillation in the Langendorff-perfused sheep heart. *J Cardiovasc Electrophysiol.* 2000;11(8):869-879.
77. Sahadevan J, Ryu K, Peltz L, et al. Epicardial mapping of chronic atrial fibrillation in patients: preliminary observations. *Circulation.* 2004;110(21):3293-3299.
78. Sanders P, Berenfeld O, Hocini M, et al. Spectral analysis identifies sites of high-frequency activity maintaining atrial fibrillation in humans. *Circulation.* 2005;112(6):789-797.
79. Lemola K, Ting M, Gupta P, et al. Effects of two different catheter ablation techniques on spectral characteristics of atrial fibrillation. *J Am Coll Cardiol.* 2006;48(2):340-348.
80. Lin Y-J, Tsao H-M, Chang S-L, et al. Role of high dominant frequency sites in nonparoxysmal atrial fibrillation patients: Insights from high-density frequency and fractionation mapping. *Heart Rhythm.* 2010;7(9):1255-1262.
81. Atienza F, Almendral J, Jalife J, et al. Real-time dominant frequency mapping and ablation of dominant frequency sites in atrial fibrillation with left-to-right frequency gradients predicts long-term maintenance of sinus rhythm. *Heart Rhythm.* 2009;6(1):33-40.
82. Pachon MJ, Pachon ME, Pachon MJ, et al. A new treatment for atrial fibrillation based on spectral analysis to guide the catheter RF-ablation. *Europace.* 2004;6(6):590-601.
83. Arruda M, Natale A. Ablation of permanent AF: adjunctive strategies to pulmonary veins isolation: targeting AF NEST in sinus rhythm and CFAE in AF. *J Interv Card Electrophysiol.* 2008;23:51-57.

Video Legends

Video 42B.1 CARTO map showing the ablation catheter approaching the LSPV os to target specific PV potentials. The catheter manipulation is via Stereotaxis magnetic navigation. The LSPV has two distal branches, which are cut out in addition to the true os where the LASSO is sitting. The overall voltage of the LA is normal.

Video 42B.2 CARTO map showing the ablation catheter moving along the anteroinferior aspect of the LIPV os. During the rotation of the map, the marked ablation points can be seen surrounding the LSPV and part of the LIPV ostia. The CS catheter is visible in the posterior rim of the mitral valve annulus, and the LASSO catheter is sitting in the os of the LSPV. The LSPV also has two distal branches, which are cut out of the map.

Video 42B.3 Intracardiac echocardiography movie showing the LASSO positioned at the os of the LSPV os (the LIPV lies below). There are small bubbles from the ablation catheter, which is at the superior rim of the LSPV os.

Video 42B.4 Intracardiac echocardiography movie showing the LASSO positioned at the LSPV os (the LIPV lies below). There are small bubbles from the ablation catheter, which is at the carina between the LSPV and LIPV.

CHAPTER 42C

Laser and Cryothermal Balloon Ablation of Pulmonary Veins to Treat Atrial Fibrillation

Thorsten Lewalter, MD, PhD; Rangadham Nagarakanti, MD; Sanjeev Saksena, MBBS, MD

Introduction

The development of catheter ablation occurred over three decades ago. Inadvertently performed during a direct current cardioversion in 1979 by Vedel and Fontaine, it led to direct-current shock energy becoming the first evaluated energy source for percutaneous ablation.[1] Scheinman and Gonzalez first published its use in animal studies and later reported its use in clinical procedures using intracardiac shock delivery for AV nodal ablation.[2,3] Holt and Boyd reported on the barotrauma associated with this method and provided cinematographic evidence of a major shock wave being generated.[4] Modification of the direct-current waveform was undertaken by Fontaine in an attempt to avoid this potential risk.[5] However, the advent of radiofrequency energy use with contact catheter ablation methods proved to be more easily controlled without these adverse physical effects.[6] Early dose-response studies on radiofrequency ablation have been undertaken by Marcus and others.[6-8] Several groups performed detailed studies in normal and diseased ventricular myocardium in animals and later in human tissues.[8-10] Since that time, radiofrequency ablation has become the standard method in routine clinical care of these patients undergoing catheter ablation at any venue in the heart. Radiofrequency ablation requires contact between the delivery electrode(s) and the tissue surface in the chamber being ablated. This is not readily achieved at many cardiac chamber sites, and other options, such as irrigation of the tip or multiple electrode configurations, are being explored. The biophysics of radiofrequency ablation are now well understood and indicate that there is uneven energy delivery at the electrode tissue interface with potential for charring, tissue vaporization, and thromboembolism. This has been seen in clinical practice and has fostered the continued search for new energy sources for catheter ablation. Nowhere is this more important than in catheter ablation of atrial fibrillation (AF), where multiple experiences have identified a substantial complication profile for radiofrequency energy-based techniques.[11,12] In a prior chapter, we reviewed the basic science and experimental studies for new energy sources (Chapters 20 and 21). Here we will discuss the available experimental and clinical experience with two such technologies: laser and cryothermal ablation.

Laser Ablation

Laser ablation of tachyarrhythmias was first performed in humans in the mid-1980s as an intraoperative procedure with argon and Nd-YAG energy sources. In this clinical experience, both supraventricular and ventricular tachycardia ablation was performed.[13-16] Catheter ablation with laser energy raised special issues and challenges.[17] Several years would elapse before these were successfully being resolved and new device systems were developed. Pulsed laser ablation with tip- and side-firing prototype catheter systems were tested, and successful pilot experiences in supraventricular tachyarrhythmias were reported.[18] More recently, a laser balloon catheter system with endoscopic guidance has been in clinical trials for AF ablation.

Mechanisms of Laser Ablation

Laser energy produces thermal ablation that is associated with cellular damage and tissue destruction. Lesions differ with different laser energy sources, as discussed in Chapter 21. Argon laser ablation produced tissue coagulation necrosis, vaporization, and crater formation. Nd-YAG laser ablation lesions produced more coagulation and often maintained tissue architecture. Pulsed energy delivery often obviated the detrimental effects of tissue vaporization and permitted controlled ablation.[19,20] More recently, diode lasers have been used for ablation. This technology is discussed in more detail in Chapter 21.

Clinical Experience with Laser Ablation in Atrial Fibrillation

The recent development of a laser balloon catheter for atrial ablation has led to its application in patients with atrial fibrillation for pulmonary vein isolation procedures. The device and procedure are discussed in this section.

Laser Balloon Device

The Endoscopic Ablation System with Adaptive Contact (CardioFocus Inc, Marlborough, MA) consists of the following components: delivery sheath, balloon system, endoscope, lesion generator, and cooling console (Figure 42C.1A). The delivery sheath is a deflectable 12-Fr internal diameter sheath with a 180° deflection capability. The balloon system is a compliant balloon with adjustable diameters and a flexible tip. Contained within the balloon are multiple lumina within the central shaft for the endoscope, lesion generator, and cooling conduits. The balloon is constantly cooled with circulating D_2O.

The balloon is positioned at the pulmonary vein (PV) ostium and inflated to provide good contact. A 2-Fr endoscope is located at the proximal portion of the balloon and provides real-time visualization of the face of the balloon. Regions of the balloon in contact with blood appear red, and regions in contact with tissue are white. The lesion generator consists of an optical fiber within the central shaft that generates a 30° arc of light that is projected onto regions of the balloon with wall contact. This arc serves as an aiming beam for laser delivery and can be easily advanced/retracted and rotated along the balloon face with endoscopic visualization (Figure 42C.1B). Once an appropriate location is selected, laser energy (980 nm) is delivered through the same optical fiber to ablate the target tissue.

Ablation Procedure

The laser balloon PV ablation procedure requires standard transseptal access and the use of a circumferential mapping catheter to document electrical activity of the PVs. After documentation of the PV potentials in a given vein, the laser balloon system is placed at the PV ostium. Balloon position and pressure are adjusted to expose a circumferential ring of myocardium antral to the respective PV. Since the catheter shaft obstructs a portion of the total PV circumference, rotation of the balloon is required to complete ablation of the respective PV. Veins are ablated using laser applications with a duration of 20 seconds at an energy level between 7.5 (posterior areas of the vein) to a maximum of 12 W (anterior positions, carina between veins and carina to the left atrial appendage). Ablation points are applied in an overlapping manner, including 50% of each

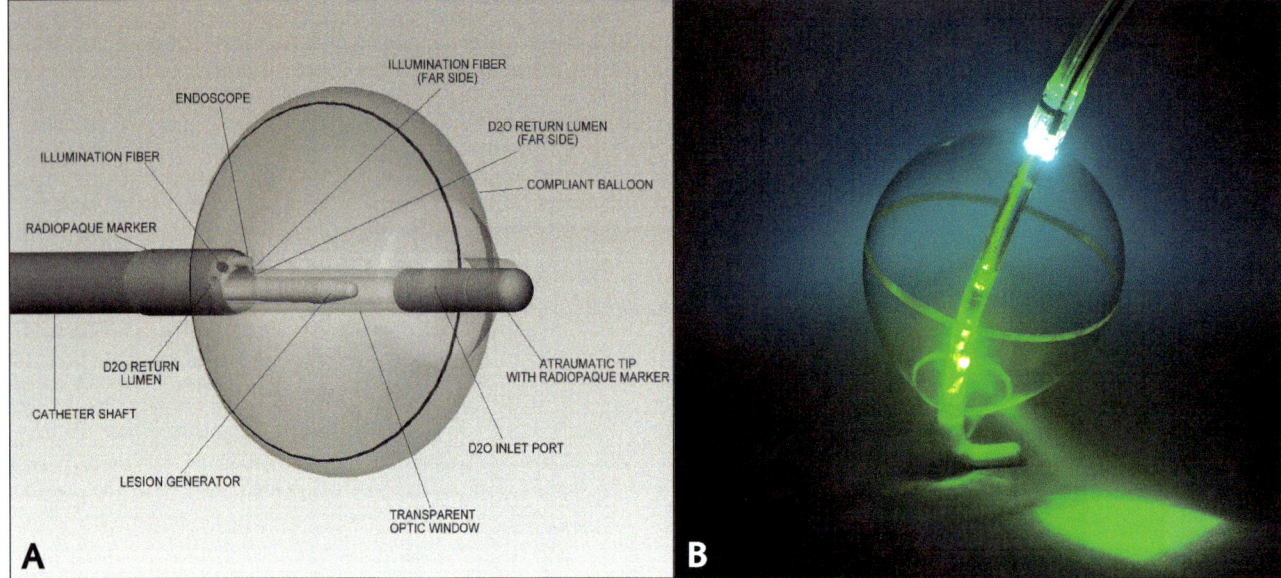

Figure 42C.1 The endoscopic ablation system consists of a nonsteerable, compliant balloon that is filled and flushed with D_2O (**Panel A**). The catheter shaft contains a 2-Fr fiberoptic endoscope connected to a 980-nm laser diode source delivering laser energy. In **Panel B**, the aiming beam is activated to highlight the desired ablation spot. *Source:* Courtesy of CardioFocus, Inc.

adjoining lesion in the ablation line. Temperature monitoring is continuously performed with an esophageal temperature probe. Laser deliveries are stopped when an esophageal temperature rise > 40°C is documented. During ablation along the right superior PV, phrenic nerve pacing is continuously performed (20 mA, 5 ms) via a diagnostic catheter placed in the superior caval vein.

After completion of the circumferential ablation line, LA to PV conduction is assessed using a multipolar mapping catheter. Gap mapping and gap ablation are performed if electrical PV isolation is not achieved after completion of the ablation line. Thirty minutes after initial complete electrical disconnection, recurrent PV potentials and gaps in the ablation line are identified. For gap mapping, a duodecapolar mapping catheter can be positioned distal to the inflated balloon to demonstrate real-time PV isolation during repeat laser energy application (Figures 42C.2, 42C.3, and 42C.4).

Comparison of Laser and Radiofrequency Ablation

Radiofrequency (RF) catheter ablation has a significant recurrence rate that is often related to the process of reconnection of acutely successful disconnected veins.[21,22] Laser balloon ablation is one of the latest technological approaches to increase the clinical success of PV disconnection.[23] This specific ablation technique is of great interest because it has shown a high persisting disconnection rate.[24] In contrast to these electrophysiological findings, the clinical recurrence rate after long-term follow-up was as high as 40%.[25-27] Possible explanations for these results of laser ablation may relate to (1) use of a different ablation and energy strategy while using the laser balloon among these patient groups, or (2) a possibility that late reconnection of pulmonary veins plays a role in laser-ablated patients.

Following these early experiences, Schmidt and co-workers could demonstrate that using a "high-dose"

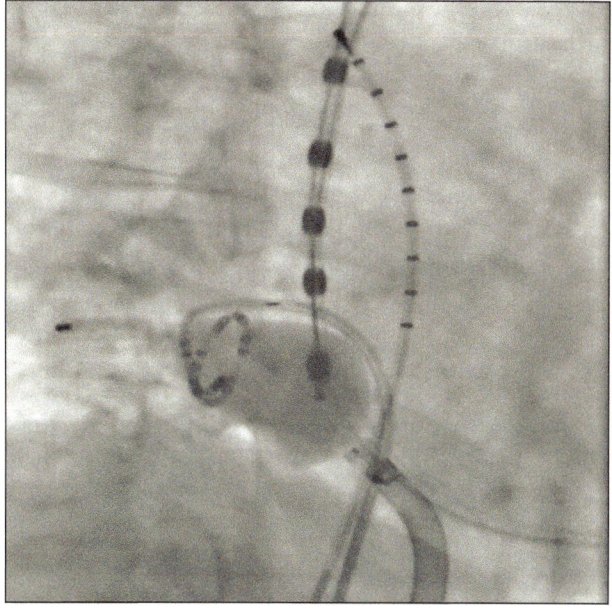

Figure 42C.2 X-ray in 30° right anterior oblique position depicting the laser balloon in the right inferior PV with a 20-polar diagnostic catheter riding on top of the balloon for gap mapping. In addition, a 10-polar catheter is used for phrenic nerve stimulation. A multipolar esophageal probe is used for temperature monitoring.

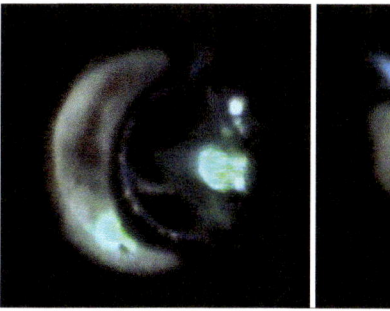
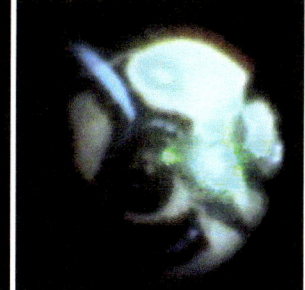

Figure 42C.3 The 20-polar mapping catheter riding on top of the laser balloon can be identified in the endoscopic view. Gap localization can be performed by direct visualization of the bipoles with gap signals.

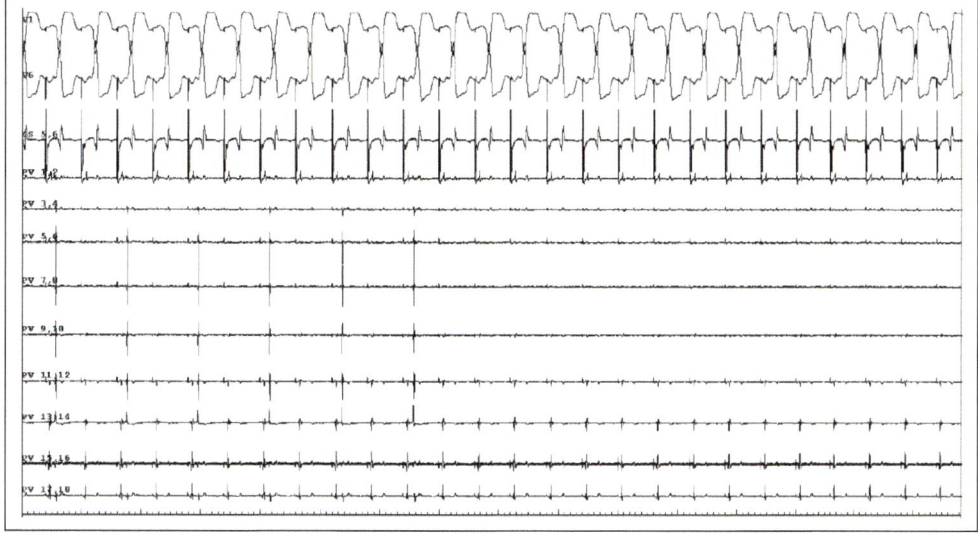

Figure 42C.4 This figure displays the surface ECG (V_1 and V_6) and the intracardiac bipolar recordings from the coronary sinus (CS 1/2) and from the right inferior PV (PV 1/2 to 17/18). Performing CS pacing on the left side, a 2:1 conduction from the left atrium (LA) to the PV is documented with a PV spike detection after every second LA capture. During laser application, complete online disconnection can be observed in the PV electrograms. (Paper speed 16 mm/sec.)

concept versus a moderate or conventional energy application level with the laser balloon significantly increased the single procedure success to as much as 80%, where success is defined as patients being AF-free one year after their laser ablation.[28] Table 42C.1 summarizes the available data on laser catheter balloon ablation from the literature. Note that studies confirm the viability of this approach in clinical application for PV isolation, and one-year follow-up data are competitive with currently available radiofrequency ablation methods.

Conclusion

The laser balloon concept is a new technical approach for PV disconnection. Aside from the fact that energy application is performed using laser light, a unique feature of this ablation concept is the use of intracardiac endoscopy. The early clinical studies indicate that a high rate of success for clinical single procedures can be achieved with the laser balloon ablation using high energy levels.

Cryothermal Ablation

Cryothermia has been used for intraoperative surgical ablation and mapping of tachyarrhythmias for over three decades. A variety of surgical probes was developed for ablation in atrial and ventricular tissues. Subsequently, there has been a sustained technologic effort to develop catheter-based cryothermal ablation devices. Early developments led to prototype passive-tip catheter ablation systems, and more recently, anatomically configured balloon ablation catheters. This section will review the technology and current application of cryothermal catheter technology for ablation of cardiac arrhythmias, including supraventricular tachycardias and AF.

Physics of Cryothermal Ablation

Cryothermal ablation has been achieved by the use of cryoprobes or cryocatheter devices. These devices usually utilize expanding nitrous oxide gas as the refrigerant that cools the cryoprobe or catheter electrode. Tissue contact with the cryoablation device surface results in rapid tissue cooling with ice crystals forming inside the cells, resulting in cellular injury and subcellular organelle damage and even rupture. Cellular changes up to −40°C may be reversible, and "ice-mapping" to demonstrate arrhythmogenic tissues has been used in intraoperative studies. Cooling to a range of −60°C to −80°C results in irreversible cellular death. At these temperatures, mitochondrial destruction occurs within 1 minute followed by cellular death.[29] Tissue inflammation and necrosis from microvascular circulatory changes have also been reported.

The cryoablation lesion formation progresses through three phases: the freeze/thaw phase, the inflammatory phase, and the fibrosis phase. Following the freeze or thaw, progressive mitochondrial damage and significant depletion of glycogen storage in the cells occur. This is followed by surrounding microvascular disruption causing the hemorrhagic-inflammatory phase, followed by replacement fibrosis. A key aspect of the cryolesion is the maintenance of cellular architecture and avoidance of tissue perforation. This has significant potential to improve safety of ablation lesions.

Cryoablation Catheter Systems

The first cryoablation catheters system (Freezor, CryoCath Technologies Inc, Montreal, Canada) was approved in 2003 (Figure 42C.5). It had a 7-Fr diameter catheter body with a 6 mm tip ablation/mapping electrode. It has, in addition, four mapping proximal electrodes with a 2-5-2 mm spacing. With this device, the ablation tip temperatures can reach as low as −80°C.

Preclinical Studies

Initial studies examined the effects of cryothermia on the atrioventricular nodal tissue for the treatment of atrioventricular reentrant tachycardia in a canine model.[30] As discussed previously, since the tissue changes were reversible up to a temperature of −40°C, this device offered the

Table 42C.1 Clinical trials of laser balloon catheter ablation

Study or Clinical Trial	N	Inclusion Criteria	Intervention	Length of Follow-up (average)	Results
Reddy et al, 2009	30	Paroxysmal AF patients	Visually guided/endoscopic Laser balloon ablation system	12 months	60% of patients free of AF at 12 months
Schmidt et al, 2010	30	Paroxysmal AF patients	Visually guided/endoscopic Laser balloon ablation system	168 days	80% of patients free of AF
Dukkipati et al, 2011	56	Paroxysmal AF patients	Visually guided/endoscopic Laser balloon ablation system	12 months	71.2% of patients free of AF at 12 months
Dukkipati et al, 2013	200	Paroxysmal AF patients	Visually guided/endoscopic Laser balloon ablation system	12 months	60.2% of patients free of AF at 12 months

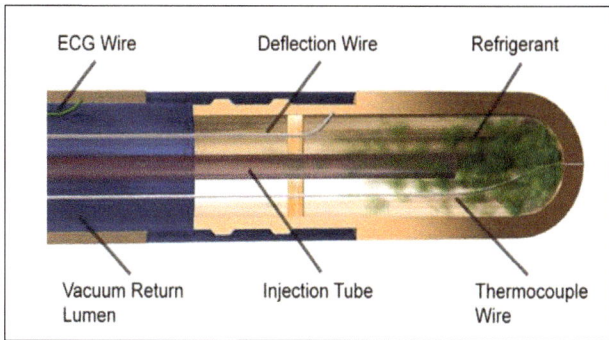

Figure 42C.5 The anatomy of the cyroablation catheter tip (Freezor, Medtronic CryoCath Technologies Inc, Montreal, Canada) with an ablation/mapping electrode.

unique possibility of catheter-based "ice mapping" to identify successful sites for irreversible ablation. Irreversible ablation was then achieved by cooling to –60°C and –70°C.

Compared to RF ablation, cryoablation is associated with lack of pain during energy delivery, more homogenous lesion formation, less destruction to surrounding vasculature, and preserved tissue integrity with a lower risk of thrombus formation.[31-33]

Clinical Applications

Cryoablation has been used in treatment of various supraventricular arrhythmias for the last three decades. Early intraoperative ablation was predominantly performed with point-to-point application of cryothermal energy. Cox et al first performed cryoablation of atrioventricular node reentrant tachycardia in eight patients.[34] Nine 3 mm cryolesions (at –60°C for 2 min) were placed around the triangle of Koch. No AVNRT was observed during the 5-year follow-up period. This experience expanded to other supraventricular tachycardias and ventricular tachycardia (discussed in other sections of this text).

More recent studies have examined catheter cryoablation techniques. A prospective, randomized clinical trial in patients with recurrent narrow QRS-complex tachycardia suggestive of AV nodal reentry tachycardia compared catheter-based cryoablation with RF catheter ablation. This study showed a procedural success rate of 91% in the RF group and 93% in the cryoablation group.[34] Another multicenter prospective clinical trial demonstrated that catheter-based cryoablation was a safe and effective alternative for RF ablation for treatment of AV nodal reentry tachycardia in 103 patients and AV reentrant tachycardia in 51 patients, and it permitted successful AV junction ablation for AF in 12 patients.[35] Acute procedural success was achieved in 83% of the overall group, and long-term success after 6 months was 91%. Because of lesion reversibility, it was very useful for mapping prior to ablation of septal accessory pathways in close proximity to the conduction system.[36] Cryomapping (cooling the catheter tip to –30°C) successfully identifies ablation targets and the electrophysiologic effects of cryomapping were reversible within minutes in 94% of the attempts. Cryothermal energy has also been used in the treatment of various other forms of tachycardias including atrial flutter, focal atrial tachycardia, and ventricular outflow tract tachycardia.[37,38]

Cryothermal Balloon Ablation for Atrial Fibrillation

Point-to-point RF ablation for PV isolation is associated with technical difficulties. The cryoballoon catheter was designed with the aim of facilitating more complete and uniform PV isolation. Currently, one balloon system (Arctic Front, Medtronic, Inc, Minneapolis, MN) is clinically available for PV isolation (Figure 42C.6). The Arctic Front system includes an over-the-wire balloon

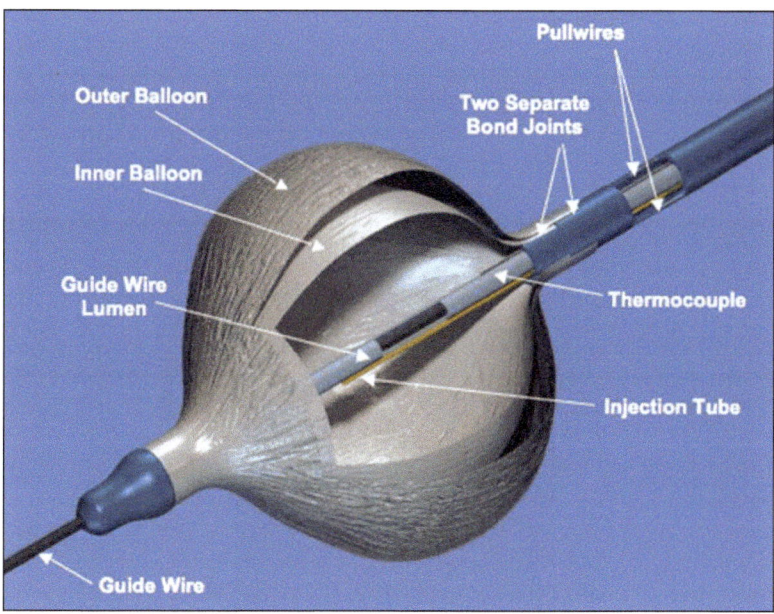

Figure 42C.6 The anatomy of the cryoballoon ablation catheter system. It consists of an over-the-wire catheter with deflection mechanism and a balloon tip, which is cooled using N_2O.
Source: Courtesy of Arctic Front, Medtronic, Inc, Minneapolis, MN.

catheter with deflection mechanism (Arctic Front cryoballoon) that is cooled using nitrous oxide (N_2O), a 14-Fr FlexCath steerable sheath, the Freezor MAX single-point cryoablation catheter used to provide additional ablations as needed, and the CryoConsole, which houses the coolant and electrical and mechanical components that run the system. During a cryoablation procedure, pressurized liquid N_2O is delivered from a tank. The liquid refrigerant travels in an ultra-fine tube through the coaxial umbilical and the shaft of the cryoablation catheter to the tip of the catheter. The liquid refrigerant vaporizes as it is sprayed into the tip. As it vaporizes, it absorbs heat from the surrounding tissue, thereby cooling and freezing the target tissue. The warmed refrigerant is vacuumed back to the CryoConsole through a large lumen within the shaft of the catheter and the coaxial umbilical.

Currently, two sizes of the cryoballoon catheter are available: 28 mm and 23 mm diameter. The balloon shaft size is 10.5-Fr. The shaft has a central lumen that can accommodate a wire for support and also used for contrast and saline injection.

Pulmonary Vein Isolation with Cryoballoon Technology

After transseptal puncture is performed under fluoroscopy and intracardiac echocardiogram (ICE) guidance, the cryoballoon catheter is introduced using over-the-wire technique into the left atrium using a 14-Fr FlexCath steerable sheath. The wire is then used to engage the vein first. The balloon is inflated outside the vein and advanced over the wire to occlude the vein (Figures 42C.7, 42C.8). Occlusion is confirmed by injecting the contrast. Intracardiac echocardiography with color Doppler flow mapping can also be used to confirm occlusion.

Once occlusion of the vein is confirmed, freezing is performed, usually for 5 to 6 minutes. A dip in the temperature curve is usually observed, indicating successful occlusion. PV isolation is usually achieved with one freeze in most patients.[39] Most operators apply one additional lesion after isolation. During the cryoablation of right-sided pulmonary veins, continuous phrenic nerve stimulation is performed via quadripolar catheter usually positioned in the superior vena cava (SVC) for continuous phrenic nerve stimulation.

After ablation, PV isolation is assessed using a circular mapping catheter. Instead of the wire, a small-caliber circular mapping catheter can be advanced in the central lumen of the balloon catheter shaft and can be used to confirm isolation.[40] Entrance block is demonstrated by left atrial pacing from the left atrial appendage (LAA) and the coronary sinus (CS), and exit block confirmed by pacing within the pulmonary veins. This is repeated by administration of IV adenosine in all the veins, and confirmation of block is documented. If complete isolation of the PVs cannot be achieved, a standard point-by-point

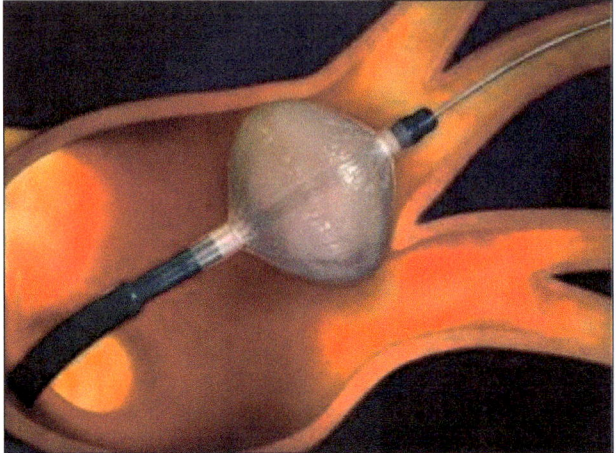

Figure 42C.7 Occlusion of the pulmonary vein with the inflated cryoballoon. *Source:* Courtesy of Medtronic, Inc, Minneapolis, MN.

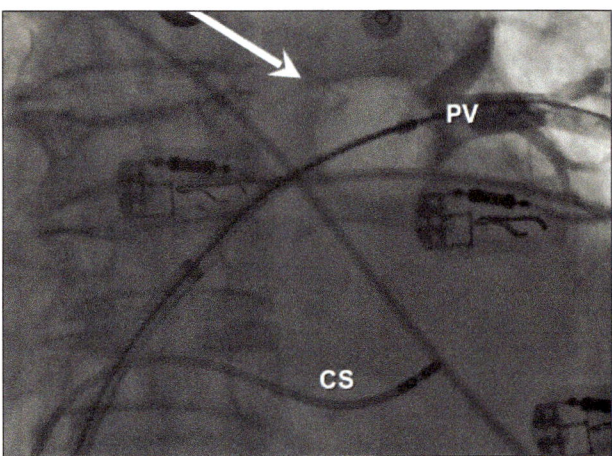

Figure 42C.8 Fluoroscopy and contrast venography demonstrating occlusion of the left superior PV with the inflated cryoballoon.

radiofrequency ablation catheter is used for complete isolation of the PVs.

Efficacy of Cryoballoon AF Ablation

There have been multiple published clinical reports of cryoballoon ablation of AF (Table 42C.2). In an early report, 57 consecutive paroxysmal AF patients underwent cryoballoon ablation with successful isolation of 84% of the targeted PVs.[40] In an other report, 21 paroxysmal symptomatic patients underwent cryoballoon ablation with successful isolation of 95% of targeted PVs.[41] Intermittent Holter monitoring demonstrated that 86% of these patients remained free of AF after 6 months.[41] In a larger series, 293 paroxysmal AF and 53 persistent AF patients underwent cryoballoon ablation.[42] 97% of the PVs were isolated and sinus rhythm was maintained in 74% and 42% of the patients with paroxysmal and persistent AF, respectively.[42] These trials demonstrated feasibility of cryoballoon PV isolation for AF ablation.

Table 42C.2 Clinical trials of cryoballoon catheter ablation

Study or Clinical Trial	N	Inclusion Criteria	Intervention	Length of Follow-up (average)	Results
Klein 2008	21	Highly symptomatic paroxysmal AF and at least one unsuccessful try of anti-arrhythmic therapy	Cryoablation (Arctic Front CryoCath)	6 months	86% of patients free of AF at 6 months
Neumann 2008	346	Symptomatic and drug refractory paroxysmal or persistent AF	Cryoablation (Arctic Front CryoCath)	12 months	Maintenance of sinus rhythm in 74% of patients with paroxysmal AF and 42% of those with persistent AF
STOP-AF 2010	245	At least 2 episodes of documented AF in previous 2 months or treatment failure with at least one anti-arrhythmic drug	Randomization (2:1) to Cryoablation (Arctic Front CryoCath) vs anti-arrhythmic drug therapy	12 months	69.9% of cryo patients were free of AF and did not require administration of a non-study drug or interventional procedure for treatment of AF
Kojodjojo 2010	177	Symptomatic medically refractory persistent or paroxysmal AF	28 mm cryoballoon ablation (Arctic Front) ($n = 124$) vs radiofrequency ablation ($n = 53$) (nonrandomized)	13 months	77% of PAF treated with cryo free of AF and 48% of persistent AF treated with cryo free of AF
Kühne 2010	50	Symptomatic paroxysmal AF	28 mm cryoballoon ablation (Arctic Front) ($n = 25$) or open irrigated radiofrequency ablation ($n = 25$)	12 months	88% of patients in cryoballoon group and 92% in RF group were free of AF
FREEZE-AF (ongoing)	Goal 244	At least two episodes of PAF in past 3 months; failure of at least one antiarrhythmic drub	Cryoablation (Arctic Front CryoCath) vs radiofrequency ablation		

The Sustained Treatment of Paroxysmal Atrial Fibrillation (STOP AF) trial was the most comprehensive study for the efficacy and safety of the cryoballoon catheter AF ablation.[43] Two hundred forty-five patients with drug-refractory paroxysmal atrial fibrillation were randomized in a 2:1 fashion to cryoballoon PV isolation or antiarrhythmic drug therapy. Isolation of PVs was achieved with only cryoballoon in 90.8%, with ≥3 PVs isolated in 98.2% of the patients. Repeat cryoablation procedure was performed in 19% of the patients within the 90-day blanking period. The success rate at 12-month follow-up was 69.9%.

Comparison with Conventional Radiofrequency Catheter Ablation

A case-controlled study compared 20 paroxysmal AF patients who underwent their first PV isolation using cryoballoon to 20 matched RF ablation patients. At 3 to 6 months follow-up, daily monitoring demonstrated success rate was 55% with cryoballoon only, compared to 45% in the RF-only group.[44] The efficacy of using the strategy of a larger cryoballoon for antral PV isolation was performed by Kojodjojo et al.[45] They used 28 mm cryoballoon ablation catheters to isolate PVs in 124 patients with paroxysmal and persistent AF and compared them to RF ablation. At one-year follow-up, freedom from AF was noted in 77% of paroxysmal and 48% of persistent AF patients after a single cryoballoon procedure. In the RF group, 72% of the patients with paroxysmal remained free of AF. The procedural and fluoroscopic times with cryo-ablation were shorter than RF ablation.[45] These results were reproduced in a recent study by Kühne at al.[46] Fifty-five paroxysmal AF patients were studied: 25 patients underwent PV isolation using a 28 mm cryoballoon and 25 patients underwent open-irrigation RF catheter ablation. The number of procedures was not different in the 2 groups (1.2 ± 0.4 in cryoablation vs 1.3 ± 0.6 in RF ablation). The success rate was 88% in the cryoballoon group and 92% in the RF group at one-year follow-up.

The Freeze AF trial is currently ongoing and compares cryoballoon catheter ablation with open-irrigation RF ablation in a randomized clinical study including 244 patients with paroxysmal AF.[46]

Limitations and Complications of Cryoballoon Ablation of AF

Phrenic Nerve Palsy (PNP)

The most common complication of cryoballoon ablation is phrenic nerve palsy. PNP was noted to occur during isolation of the right superior and less commonly the right inferior PV. In the STOP AF trial, PNP was reported in

29 out of 259 procedures (11.2%).[44] Only four patients had persistent PNP at 12 months. In a recent meta-analysis, the incidence is estimated at 6.38%,[48] PNP recovered in the majority of patients with time, and it lasted more than a year in only 0.37%.

Pulmonary Vein Stenosis

Pulmonary vein stenosis was noted in 3.1% of patients in the STOP AF study.[44] This is most likely due to ablation in the tubular portion of the pulmonary vein. Therefore, it is advisable and most operators have started to use a 28 mm balloon ablation catheter regardless of the size of the PV in order to reduce the risk of PV stenosis.

Atrioesophageal (AE) Fistula

There are recent isolated reports of incidence of AE fistulas with cryoballoon catheter ablation. Studies have shown that cold temperatures in the esophageal lumen predict esophageal lesions after PV isolation. A minimum esophageal temperature of 12°C predicted lesions with 100% sensitivity and 92% specificity. It is important to note that the balloon temperatures did not predict esophageal temperatures.

Bacterial Endocarditis

There was an isolated report of bacterial mitral valve endocarditis with embolic cerebral infarcts on post-cryoballoon AF ablation procedure day 5. The authors suggested that the unusually lengthy cryoapplication and the exchanges of multiple catheters may have played a role.

Conclusion

Cryotechnology is a viable technology used in management of variable cardiac arrhythmia disorders. Cryoballoon catheter isolation of pulmonary veins is a safe and effective technique for management of paroxysmal AF patients. It has limited success rate in persistent AF. Major procedural complications related to cryoballoon ablation include PNP and PV stenosis.

References

1. Vedel J, Frank R, Fontaine G, et al. Bloc auriculo-ventriculaire intra-Hisian definitive induit au cours d'une exploration endoventriculaire droite. *Arch Mal Coeur.* 1979;72:107.
2. Gonzalez R, Scheinman MM, Margaretten W, Rubenstein M. Closed chest electrode catheter technique for His bundle ablation in dogs: *Am J Physiol.* 1981;241(2):H283-H287.
3. Scheinman MM, Morady F, Hess DS, Gonzalez R. Catheter induced ablation of the atrioventricular junction to control refractory supraventricular arrhythmias. *JAMA.* 1982;248(7): 851-855.
4. Holt PM, Boyd EG. Physical and experimental aspects of ablation with direct current shocks. In Saksena S, Goldschlager N (eds). *Electrical Therapy for Cardiac Arrhythmias.* Philadelphia, PA: WB Saunders & Co.; 1989:619-633.
5. Fontaine G, Frank R, Gallais Y, et al. Fulguration and radiofrequency in ventricular tachycardia. *Arch Mal Coeur Vaiss.* 1994;87(11 Suppl):1589-1607.
6. Huang SK, Bharati S, Graham AR, Lev M, Marcus FI, Odell RC. Closed chest catheter desiccation of the atrioventricular junction using radiofrequency energy—a new method of catheter ablation. *J Am Coll Cardiol.* 1987;9(2):349-358.
7. Huang SK, Bharati S, Lev M, Marcus FI. Electrophysiologic and histologic observations of chronic atrioventricular block induced by closed-chest catheter desiccation with radiofrequency energy. *Pacing Clin Electrophysiol.* 1987;10(4 Pt 1): 805-816.
8. An H, Saksena S, Janssen M, Osypka P. Radiofrequency ablation of ventricular myocardium using active fixation and passive contact catheter delivery systems. *Am Heart J.* 1989;118:69-77.
9. Haines DE, Watson DD. Tissue heating during radiofrequency catheter ablation: a thermodynamic model and observations in isolated perfused and superfused canine right ventricular free wall. *Pacing Clin Electrophysiol.* 1989; 12(6):962-976.
10. Nath S, DiMarco JP, Mounsey JP, Lobban JH, Haines DE. Correlation of temperature and pathophysiological effect during radiofrequency catheter ablation of the AV junction. *Circulation.* 1995;92(5):1188-1192.
11. Baman TS, Jongnarangsin K, Chugh A, et al. Prevalence and predictors of complications of radiofrequency catheter ablation for atrial fibrillation. *J Cardiovasc Electrophysiol.* 2011;22(6): 626-631.
12. Cappato R, Calkins H, Chen SA, et al. Updated worldwide survey on the methods, efficacy, and safety of catheter ablation for human atrial fibrillation. *Circ Arrhythm Electrophysiol.* 2010;3(1):32-38.
13. Saksena S, Hussain SM, Gielchinsky I, Gadhoke A, Pantopoulos D. Intraoperative mapping-guided argon laser ablation of malignant ventricular tachycardia. *Am J Cardiol.* 1987;59:78-83.
14. Svenson RH, Gallagher JJ, Selle JG, et al. Neodymium-YAG laser photocoagulation: a successful new map-guided technique for the intraoperative ablation of ventricular tachycardia. *Circulation.* 1987;76(6):1319-1328.
15. Saksena S, Hussain SM, Gielchinsky I, Pantopoulos D. Intraoperative mapping-guided argon laser ablation of supraventricular tachycardia in Wolff-Parkinson-White syndrome. *Am J Cardiol.* 1987;60:196-199.
16. Saksena S, Gielchinsky I. Argon laser ablation or modification of the atrioventricular conduction system in refractory supraventricular tachycardia. *Am J Cardiol.* 1990;66:767-770.
17. Saksena S, Ciccone J, Chandran P, Pantopoulos D, Lee B, Rothbart ST. Laser ablation of normal and diseased human ventricle. *Am Heart J.* 1986;112:52-60.
18. Saksena S. Catheter ablation of tachycardias with laser energy: issues and answers. *Pacing Clin Electrophysiol.* 1989;12: 196-203.
19. Haines DE. Thermal ablation of perfused porcine left ventricle in vitro with the neodymium-YAG laser hot tip catheter system. *Pacing Clin Electrophysiol.* 1992;15(7):979-985.
20. Ciccone J, Saksena S, Pantopoulos D. Comparative efficacy of continuous and pulsed argon laser ablation of human diseased ventricle. *Pacing Clin Electrophysiol.* 1986;9:697-704.
21. Weber H, Sagerer-Gerhardt M. Open-irrigated laser catheter ablation: relationship between the level of energy, myocardial

thickness, and collateral damages in a dog model. *Europace.* 2014 Jan;16(1):142-148.
22. Calkins H, Brugada J, Packer DL, et al. HRS/EHRA/ECAS expert consensus statement on catheter and surgical ablation of atrial fibrillation: recommendations for personnel, policy, procedures and follow-up. A report of the Heart Rhythm Society (HRS) Task Force on Catheter and Surgical Ablation of Atrial Fibrillation. *Heart Rhythm.* 2007;4:816-861.
23. Ouyang F, Antz M, Ernst S, et al. Recovered pulmonary vein conduction as a dominant factor for recurrent atrial tachyarrhythmias after complete circular isolation of the pulmonary veins: lessons from double Lasso technique. *Circulation.* 2005;111:127-135.
24. Reddy VY, Neuzil P, Natale A, et al. Visually-guided balloon catheter ablation of atrial fibrillation: experimental feasibility and first-in-human multicenter clinical outcome. *Circulation.* 2009;120:12-20.
25. Dukkipati SR, Neuzil P, Reddy VY, et al. Visual balloon-guided point-by-point ablation: reliable, reproducible, and persistent pulmonary vein isolation. *Circ Arrhythm Electrophysiol.* 2010;3:266-273.
26. Schmidt B, Metzner A, Kuck KH, et al. Feasibility of circumferential pulmonary vein isolation using a novel endoscopic ablation system. *Circ Arrhythm Electrophysiol.* 2010;3: 481-488.
27. Metzner A, Schmidt B, Fuernkranz A, et al. One-year clinical outcome after pulmonary vein isolation using the novel endoscopic ablation system in patients with paroxysmal atrial fibrillation. *Heart Rhythm.* 2011;8:988-993.
28. Metzner A, et al. Acute and long-term clinical outcome after endoscopic pulmonary vein isolation: Results from the first prospective, multicenter study. *J Cardiovasc Electrophysiol.* 2013;24(1):7-13.
29. Bordignon S, et al. Energy titration strategies with the endoscopic ablation system: lessons from the high-dose vs. low-dose laser ablation study. *Europace.* 2013;15(5):685-689.
30. Whittaker DK. Mechanisms of tissue destruction following cryosurgery. *Ann R Coll Surg Engl.* 1984;66(5):313-318.
31. Holman W, et al. Cryosurgical ablation of atrioventricular nodal reentry: histologic localization of the proximal common pathway. *Circulation.* 1988;77:1356-1362.
32. Lustgarten DL, Keane D, Ruskin J. Cryothermal ablation: mechanism of tissue injury and current experience in the treatment of tachyarrhythmias. *Prog Cardiovasc Dis.* 1999; 41(6):481-498.
33. Khairy P, Chauvet P, Lehmann J, et al. Lower incidence of thrombus formation with cryoenergy versus radiofrequency catheter ablation. *Circulation.* 2003;107:2045-2050.
34. Cox J, Holman W, Cain M. Cryosurgical treatment of atrioventricular node reentrant tachycardia. *Circulation.* 1987; 76:1329-1336.
35. Kimman GP, Theuns DAMJ, Szili-Torok T, Scholten MF, Res JC, Jordaens LJ. CRAVT: a prospective, randomized study comparing transvenous cryothermal and radiofrequency ablation in atrioventricular nodal re-entrant tachycardia. *Eur Heart J.* 2004;25:2232-2237.
36. Friedman PL, Dubuc M, Green MS, et al. Catheter cryoablation of supraventricular tachycardia: results of the multicenter prospective "frosty" trial. *Heart Rhythm.* 2004; 1(2):129-138.
37. Gaita F, Montefusco A, Riccardi R, et al. Acute and long-term outcome of transvenous cryothermal catheter ablation of supraventricular arrhythmias involving the perinodal region. *J Cardiovasc Med.* 2006;7(11):785-792.
38. Manusama R, Timmermans C, Limon F, Philippens S, Crijns HJGM, Rodriguez LM. Catheter-based cryoablation permanently cures patients with common atrial flutter. *Circulation.* 2004;109(13):1636-1639.
39. Obel OA, d'Avila A, Neuzil P, Saad EB, Ruskin JN, Reddy VY. Ablation of left ventricular epicardial outflow tract tachycardia from the distal great cardiac vein. *J Am Coll Cardiol.* 2006;48(9):1813-1817.
40. Van Belle Y, Janse P, Rivero-Ayerza MJ, et al. Pulmonary vein isolation using an occluding cryoballoon for circumferential ablation: feasibility, complications, and short-term outcome. *Eur Heart J.* 2007;28(18):2231-2237.
41. Klein G, Oswald H, Gardiwal A, et al. Efficacy of pulmonary vein isolation by cryoballoon ablation in patients with paroxysmal atrial fibrillation. *Heart Rhythm.* 2008;5(6):802-806.
42. Neumann T, Vogt J, Schumacher B, et al. Circumferential pulmonary vein isolation with the cryoballoon technique results from a prospective 3-center study. *J Am Coll Cardiol.* 2008;52(4):273-278.
43. Packer D, Irwin JM, Champagne J, et al. Cryoballoon ablation of pulmonary veins for paroxysmal atrial fibrillation: first results of the North American Arctic Front STOP-AF pivotal trial. *J Am Coll Cardiol.* 2010;55:E3015-E3016.
44. Linhart M, Bellmann B, Mittmann-Braun E, et al. Comparison of cryoballoon and radiofrequency ablation of pulmonary veins in 40 patients with paroxysmal atrial fibrillation: a case-control study. *J Cardiovasc Electrophysiol.* 2009;20(12): 1343-1348.
45. Kojodjojo P, O'Neill MD, Lim PB, et al. Pulmonary venous isolation by antral ablation with a large cryoballoon for treatment of paroxysmal and persistent atrial fibrillation: medium-term outcomes and non-randomised comparison with pulmonary venous isolation by radiofrequency ablation. *Heart.* 2010;96(17):1379-1384.
46. Kühne M, Suter Y, Altmann D, et al. Cryoballoon versus radiofrequency catheter ablation of paroxysmal atrial fibrillation: biomarkers of myocardial injury, recurrence rates, and pulmonary vein reconnection patterns. *Heart Rhythm.* 2010;7(12):1770-1776.
47. Luik A, Merkel M, Hoeren D, Riexinger T, Kieser M, Schmitt C. Rationale and design of the FreezeAF trial: a randomized controlled non-inferiority trial comparing isolation of the pulmonary veins with the cryoballoon catheter versus radiofrequency isolation. *Am Heart J.* 2010;159 (4):555-560.
48. Andrade JG, Khairy P, Guerra PG, et al. Efficacy and safety of cryoballoon ablation for atrial fibrillation: a systematic review of published studies. *Heart Rhythm.* 2011;8(9):1444-1451.

CHAPTER 43

Ventricular Tachycardia in the Apparently Normal Heart: Optimizing Safety and Results with Ablative Therapy

Amit Noheria, MBBS, SM; Mohamed Nosair, MD; Traci L. Buescher, RN;
Christopher J. McLeod, MBChB, PhD; Samuel J. Asirvatham, MD

Background

RF ablative therapy for ventricular tachycardia (VT) has exponentially increased over the last two decades. While most procedures are done for patients with ischemic heart disease and as palliative therapy to treat frequent ICD shocks, an increasing number are also performed in patients with structurally normal-appearing hearts.[1-3] The clinical presentation of ventricular arrhythmias in structurally normal hearts varies from frequent PVCs to repetitive nonsustained VT to paroxysmal sustained monomorphic VT, and occasionally PVCs triggering polymorphic VT and ventricular fibrillation.[4,5]

The sites that are primarily responsible for PVCs and VT and therefore targets for ablation in structurally normal hearts are the RVOT and sometimes the LVOT and the infrahisian conduction system. The RVOT and LVOT are anatomically complex; an intimate knowledge of their regional anatomy and their relations to neighboring structures that may be damaged during ablation is essential to optimize safety and efficacy when targeting sites in this area. Though somewhat infrequent, the mitral annular region can also be a substrate for idiopathic PVCs and VT similar to the outflow tracts.[6,7] Abnormal triggered activity is thought to be the mechanism for the idiopathic outflow tract and mitral annular arrhythmias. Fascicular VT, typically arising from the region of the left posterior fascicle, is the second most common VT after the outflow tracts in patients without obvious structural heart disease.[1] The anatomy and actual pathological substrate for fascicular VT is less well understood than outflow tract arrhythmia, but familiarity with both the anatomy and physiology of this arrhythmia is important to avoid some frequent pitfalls that lead to incomplete success and/or complications. More recently, endocavitary VT involving the papillary muscle or moderator band have been described and share several clinical similarities with fascicular VT.[8-11]

In this chapter, we review the relevant regional, fluoroscopic, and echocardiographic anatomy, highlight salient ECG features, and offer detailed, comparative discussion of the approaches to mapping and ablation for these arrhythmias. The focus is on the basis for avoiding collateral damage and inexact methods for targeting the arrhythmogenic substrate based on correlative anatomic information. Interspersed in this chapter are brief tables emphasizing the key points to remember.

Idiopathic Outflow Tract Ventricular Tachycardia

The ventricular arrhythmias originating from the outflow tract region and presenting as frequent PVCs, nonsustained VTs, and/or paroxysmal sustained monomorphic VTs in otherwise structurally normal hearts have a similar adenosine-sensitive arrhythmogenic substrate. The mechanism for the idiopathic outflow tract arrhythmias is calcium-dependent triggered activity; these arrhythmias are catecholamine dependent and are usually provoked with exercise.[12] Idiopathic outflow tract VT is treatable by targeting the focal origin site in the outflow tract with RFA.

Anatomy of the Ventricular Outflow Tracts

Invasive electrophysiologists need to be thoroughly familiar with the complex anatomic and EP associations of the RVOT and LVOT and the supra-semilunar valve regions, as well as their relationships to the proximate anatomic structures that include the coronary arteries and the AV conduction system (Figure 43.1). The most important anatomical considerations to be attentive to during EP study and ablation for outflow tract VT are outlined here.[13]

Though complex, the RVOT and LVOT have a consistent relationship to each other in the normal heart (Figures 43.2 and 43.3). The right ventricular inflow is located anterior and to the right of the LV inflow. The course of the RVOT runs anterior to the LVOT. The distal part of the RVOT and pulmonic valve are slightly to the left compared to the distal LVOT and aortic valve. As the ascending aorta becomes the arch, it thus continues to be rightward of the pulmonary trunk. The aortic annulus, besides being to the right and posterior, is also caudal to the pulmonic annulus. Thus, the posterior part of the muscular infundibular RVOT is directly anterior to the aortic valve. The RVOT can be pictured as a cylindrical tube that wraps anteriorly around the LVOT, with the lowest and most rightward portion being contiguous with the tricuspid annulus on the IVS. This site overlies the bundle of His and the proximal RBB. Thus, the most rightward portion of the RVOT is commonly the bundle of His region. Notably, the RVOT is superior to, and does not take part in, forming the IVS. The myocardium of the proximal part of the posterior RVOT is in continuity with the LVOT and the adjacent anterior IVS. The more distal posterior RVOT myocardium lies directly anterior to the RCC and LCC of the aortic valve. Due to the leftward course of the RVOT going from the proximal to the distal part, the most leftward site in this region is the supravalvar myocardium above the anterior leaflet of the pulmonic valve.

The pulmonic valve and the supravalvar part of the pulmonary artery are a known site for origin of ventricular arrhythmias. The pulmonic valve is located anteriorly and

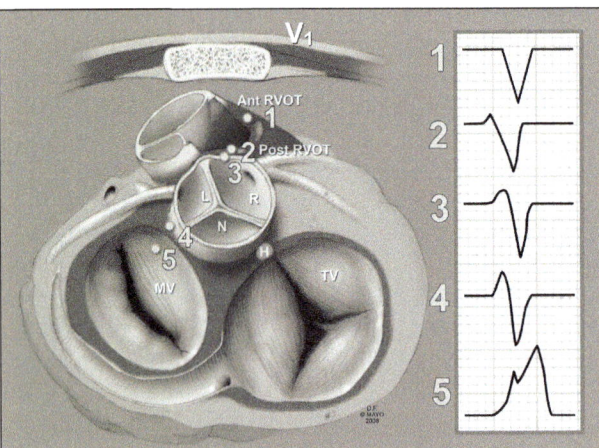

Figure 43.1 Illustration showing the important relationships of the semilunar valves with the coronary arteries and the conduction system. Also depicted are 5 anatomic sites of origin of outflow tract or supra-semilunar valve arrhythmia and the correlating manifest complex in lead V$_1$ of surface ECG. Because lead V$_1$ is an anterior and rightward lead, the amplitude of an initial R wave increases when the focus is relatively more posterior or leftward (see text for details). Ant RVOT = anterior RVOT; post RVOT = posterior RVOT; R = RCC; L = LCC; N = NCC; MV = mitral valve; TV = tricuspid valve; H = bundle of His. *Source:* Adapted from Tabatabaei N, Asirvatham SJ. Supravalvular arrhythmia: identifying and ablating the substrate. *Circ Arrhythm Electrophysiol.* 2009;2(3):316-326. By permission of Mayo Foundation for Medical Education and Research. All rights reserved.

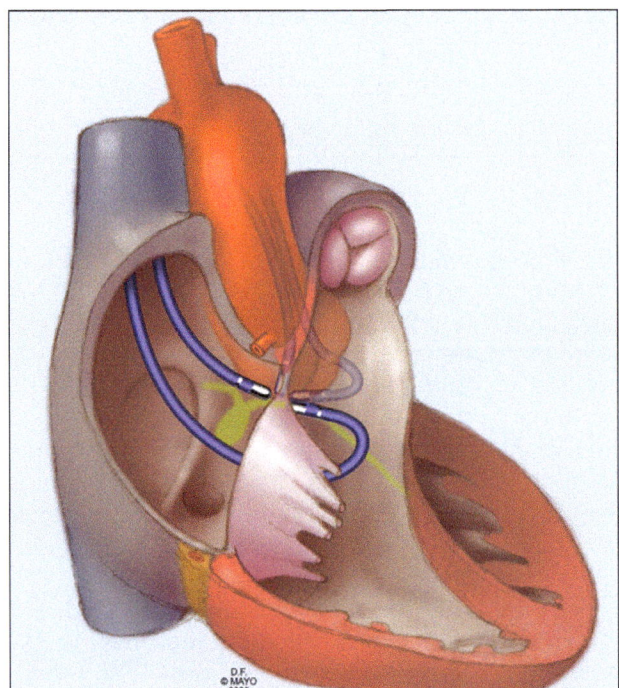

Figure 43.2 Illustration of the heart in the RAO projection with the anterior walls removed to depict the relationship between the right and the LVLVOTs and the semilunar valves (see text for details). The compact AV conduction system is depicted in **yellow**. Note the location of the bundle of His on the membranous septum at the confluence of the anterior and septal tricuspid leaflets and the right and noncoronary aortic cusps. Catheters are positioned at bundle of His region (1) antegrade at the commissure of tricuspid valve leaflets, (2) flexed retrograde under the septal leaflet of the tricuspid valve, or (3) placed supra- or (4) infra-aortic valve between the RCC and NCC. *Source:* Adapted from Suleiman M, Asirvatham SJ. Ablation above the semilunar valves: when, why, and how? Part II. *Heart Rhythm.* 2008;5(11):1625-1630. By permission of Mayo Foundation for Medical Education and Research. All rights reserved.

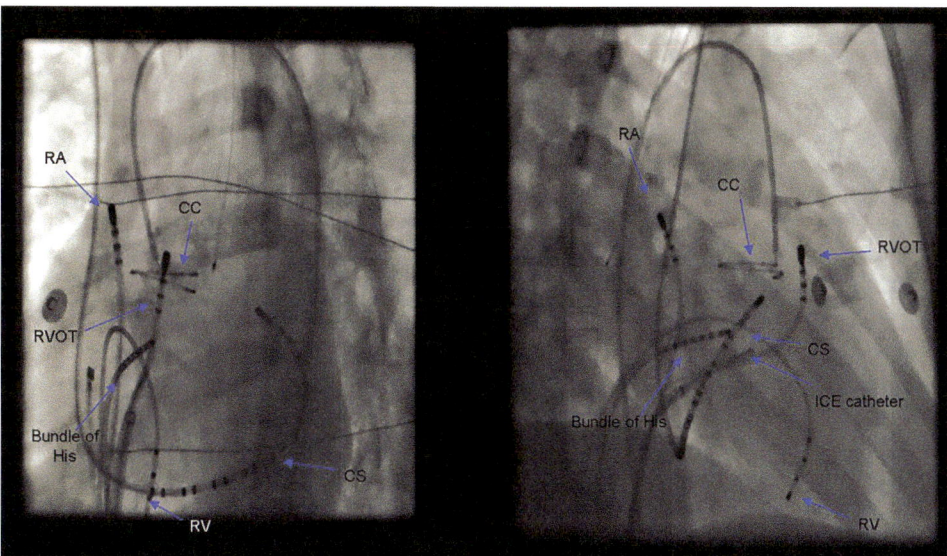

Figure 43.3 Orientation of intracardiac catheters as seen on fluoroscopy during a VT ablation procedure. A circumferential mapping catheter is placed in the aortic root and a quadripolar catheter in the RVOT. Note the immediate anterior proximity of the posterior wall of the RVOT to the LCC and RCC region. The CS catheter was introduced from the internal jugular vein. The left panel is the LAO view and the right panel is the RAO view. The various catheters are labeled. CS = coronary sinus; CC = circumferential catheter; RA = right atrium; RV = right ventricle; RVOT = right ventricular outflow tract.

to the left in relation to the LVOT and the aortic valve. As the pulmonic valve is in the anterior part of the heart and is superficially located just below the pericardium, there are no important structures in this location associated with the anterior cusp. The right cusp of the pulmonic valve can have a variable relationship with the distal portion of the RAA. The posterior pulmonic cusp has important anatomic relations that must be well recognized by the electrophysiologist performing ablation at this site. As the left main coronary artery courses leftward and anteriorly from its origin above the left aortic cusp to its bifurcation at the anterior epicardial surface, it passes just adjacent to the posterior cusp of the pulmonic valve (Figure 43.1).[14] The distal portion of the LAA is also proximate to the posterior pulmonic cusp.

The aortic valve occupies a central position at the base of the heart; all three aortic sinuses of Valsalva have important anatomic relationships, understanding of which is pertinent for the interventional electrophysiologist. The RCC lies posterior to the posterior infundibular portion of the RVOT. Inferiorly, the RCC is contiguous with the anterior part of the LVOT. There is physical continuity or proximity between the myocardium that extends above the RCC, the myocardium of the anterior LVOT, and that of the posterior RVOT. Posterior to the RCC is the NCC with the membranous IVS at the junction of the two cusps. This is the site of penetration of bundle of His into the ventricular myocardium (Figure 43.1). The NCC is situated posteriorly in the aortic annulus and is closely related to the anterior part of the IAS. The noncoronary sinus, as opposed to the right and left aortic sinuses, is usually devoid of myocardial extensions and has muscular connections with the ventricular myocardium only in rare cases.[13] Instead, the fibrous mitral–aortic continuity connects the posterior part of the LVOT with the LV inflow and the mitral annulus. The LCC has proximity to the left main coronary artery as it courses anteriorly from its ostium adjacent to the posterior pulmonic valve cusp. The depth of the LCC is close to the epicardial site of junction of the anterior interventricular and great cardiac veins. The commissure between the LCC and RCCs is immediately posterior to the distal RVOT and caudal to the posterior pulmonic annulus.[15-17]

Supravalvar Myocardial Extensions

It has been clearly established that myocardial sleeves frequently extend beyond the cardiac valves into the great vessels for variable distances.[14,18,19] These myocardial sleeves extend fairly symmetrically above each of the 3 pulmonic valve cusps and the length of these extensions into the pulmonary artery varies from a few mm up to more than 2 cm. Myocardial sleeves usually extend above the aortic valve, but their distribution above the 3 cusps is quite asymmetric. The myocardial extensions are much more common and are extend a longer distance above the RCC as compared to the LCC. It is rare for ventricular muscle to extend above the NCC, though the noncoronary aortic sinus at its junction with the right coronary aortic sinus can have some ventricular myocardium. Occasionally, ventricular muscle sleeves can extend into the valve cusps themselves.

> **Points to Remember #1**
> **Anatomy of the Outflow Tracts**
>
> - The distal RVOT and pulmonic valve lie anterior and to the left of the aortic valve and LVOT.
> - The septum of the outflow tract is posterior to the RVOT and anterior to the LVOT.
> - Supravalvar myocardial extensions may represent the arrhythmogenic substrate targeted above the semilunar valves.
> - Catheter ablation in one outflow tract may successfully target an arrhythmia originating from the other outflow tract; for example, ablation in the RCC may be the optimal site to ablate a posterior RVOT arrhythmia.

Electrocardiographic Features of Outflow Tract Arrhythmia

A 12-lead ECG of the target PVC or VT is typically available and should be sought for review prior to invasive mapping. It is imperative that the electrophysiologist attempts to localize the specific region that will need to be mapped in detail and targeted for ablation by carefully analyzing the ECG. The classic ECG appearance of VT originating from the RVOT is LBBB pattern and a strong inferior axis.[20,21] The ablationist, however, needs to critically assess this overall assumption to recognize exceptions and to glean the specific outflow tract site from the ECG, including origin from sites in the aortic valve cusps.

Specific ECG Lead Findings

Inferior Leads

LBBB-pattern inferior-axis VT may be seen from the anterior tricuspid annulus and anterior free wall of the right ventricle. Qualitatively, the height of the R waves in the inferior leads is significantly taller with RVOT origin versus anterior right ventricular origin. However, because of the variation in myocardial mass and cardiac position, any exact cut-off for the inferior R-wave amplitude to distinguish the two sites would be unreliable.

Leads aVR and aVL

Lead aVR tends to be negative with right ventricular origin, while lead aVL is often negative with left ventricular origin. However, since both these leads are superiorly directed, origin of the depolarization vector from the cranial location of the outflow tracts will manifest as negative polarity in both these leads. Thus, almost all outflow tract arrhythmias present with a unique simultaneous negative deflection (QS pattern) in leads aVR and aVL. This feature helps distinguish the two main causes of LBBB-pattern inferior-axis arrhythmia, and in the case of origin from the left side–RBBB-pattern inferior-axis, namely, outflow tract and anterior ventricular origins.

Lead I

In some of the earlier literature, the leftward sites of the RVOT were referred to as septal locations,[20] but as discussed earlier in this chapter, the septal outflow tract is the region between the RVOT and LVOT incorporating the posterior RVOT and the anterior LVOT. It is better to refer to the leftward portion of the RVOT simply as left-sided or peripulmonic valve region.[13,22-24] Thus, the outflow tract can be visualized as a quadrilateral with the superior and leftward portions residing on the left side of the body (Figure 43.2). Lead I is often helpful to ascertain the origin of the arrhythmia in the left or right portion of the RVOT. A QS pattern in lead I suggests origin on the left side of the body in the peripulmonic valve region, whereas a prominent R wave in lead I suggests origin in the free wall of the RVOT on the right side.

R Wave in Lead V1

With outflow tract VTs, lead V_1 may show the typical QS morphology (LBBB pattern) of RVOT origin to the rsR' (RBBB pattern) of LVOT origin. Various degrees of an initial R wave may be present in what is otherwise an LBBB morphology arrhythmia, and this yields critical clues to the exact site of origin (Figure 43.1). Lead V_1 is placed on the right side of the body on the anterior chest wall. Thus, RVOT arrhythmia originating in the free-wall portion anteriorly and on the right side will yield a typical LBBB pattern with absence of any significant R wave.[25] When the arrhythmia originates either on the left side of the body (peri/suprapulmonic valve region) or posteriorly (posterior RVOT and anterior LVOT/coronary cusps), then an R wave is present in lead V_1.[26] Thus, the differential diagnosis for an initial R wave in V_1 in what otherwise appears to be a outflow tract VT includes origin from:

- Peripulmonic valve region
- Posterior/septal RVOT
- RCC
- LCC
- Anterior/septal LVOT

Precordial R Transition

The precordial lead of transition from an rS complex to a dominant R wave may also be helpful in distinguishing LVOT from RVOT origin. Since the LVOT lies on the right side of the body and is posterior to the RVOT, a relatively taller R wave in the left-sided precordial leads (V_2, V_3, etc.) will be noted and result in an "early" transition in the precordial leads.[27]

Peri-His Bundle Origin

As mentioned above, generally, the vast majority of outflow tract sites show simultaneous QS complexes in aVR and aVL. An important exception is with peri-His bundle origin PVCs or VT. Because the bundle of His lies at the transition site between the outflow tracts and the right ventricular inflow (Figures 43.1 and 43.2), lead aVL is either isoelectric or slightly positive.

Correlating Surface ECG with the Anatomic Site of Outflow Tract Arrhythmia Origin

VTs arising from the RVOT classically have LBBB pattern with an inferior axis. Usually, infrapulmonic valve RVOT free-wall origin does not cause R waves in lead V_1. Arrhythmias arising from the region above the pulmonic valve located to the left and those from the posterior locations in the RVOT and the LVOT/coronary cusps will generate an initial R wave in lead V_1 (Figure 43.1).

Simultaneous analysis of leads I and V_1 may help narrow down the differential diagnosis of outflow tract VT with an R wave in V_1. Since peripulmonic valve and parts of the LCC lie on the left side of the body, a QS pattern in lead I will be observed for origin from these areas.[28] Additionally, lead III will be more positive than lead II. Some VTs originating in the LCC, however, have an rS pattern in lead I. Origin in the NCC, on the other hand, presents with a bifid R wave in lead I.[29] Origin either in the RCC or the posterior RVOT usually manifests with a low-amplitude and isoelectric QRS complex in lead I and a small initial R wave in lead V_1, and it is thus difficult to differentiate between these two sites by ECG.[29,30] As the site of origin becomes more posterior, the initial R wave in V_1 becomes larger. Origins in some parts of the LCC and the aorto-mitral continuity have larger R waves in V_1. Origin of tachycardia from the mitral annulus or posterior LVOT will have a tall R wave in V_1 (RBBB pattern). An "early" precordial R-wave transition in leads V_1 or V_2 can thus be used to distinguish an LVOT origin from RVOT. In cases with the precordial R transition in lead V_3, a ratio in lead V_2 of R-wave amplitude proportion (R/R+S) in VT vs sinus rhythm ≥ 0.6 distinguishes origin in LVOT from RVOT.[27]

Epicardial as opposed to endocardial arrhythmia has been shown to have a slurred initial component of the precordial QRS complex. Epicardial VT can thus be distinguished by a pseudodelta wave (onset of surface QRS to earliest rapid precordial deflection) ≥ 34 ms and intrinsicoid deflection time (onset of surface QRS to peak or R wave in lead V_2) ≥ 85 ms.[31] Furthermore, epicardial sites in the region of great cardiac vein–anterior interventricular vein junction as opposed to endocardial sites in the outflow tracts have a broader R wave in lead V_1 (> 75 ms) or a precordial maximal deflection index (time from QRS onset to earliest maximum deflection in any precordial lead as a proportion of QRS duration) > 0.55.[32,33]

There are several limitations in using surface ECG to determine the site of origin of outflow tract VTs; for example, anterior versus posterior site on the same cusp may change the size and shape of the R wave in V_1. Moreover, differences in body habitus, orientation of the heart, and variation in lead placement can significantly affect the V_1 R wave, and thus invasive EP mapping is useful to accurately localize the site of origin.[21]

Localization of Intracardiac Catheters in the Outflow Tracts

Electrophysiological catheters are placed based on physician preference in various locations within the heart such as the right atrium, the bundle of His, the ventricles (right and/or left as deemed necessary), and the CS. An

> **Points to Remember #2**
> **ECG Correlates of Outflow Tract Arrhythmia**
>
> - Classic RVOT arrhythmia has an LBBB pattern (QS in lead V_1) with an inferior axis.
> - An R wave in lead V_1 suggests outflow tract origin that is either leftward or posterior to the RVOT anterior/free wall.
>   - The pulmonic valve lies leftward in the body; peripulmonic valve origin has an initial small R wave in lead V_1.
>   - The posterior RVOT, the coronary cusps, and the anterior LVOT are located posteriorly, and arrhythmias from these sites also have an initial R wave in lead V_1.
>   - Origin from posterior LVOT or from the mitral annulus presents with tall R wave in lead V_1 (RBBB pattern).
> - Outflow tract arrhythmia with an R wave in V_1 but positive in lead I is more likely to be posterior in origin, whereas QS complex in lead I suggests leftward origins in the peripulmonic valve region and parts of LCC.
> - An "early" precordial R-wave transition suggests an LVOT rather than an RVOT origin.
> - Epicardial origin of outflow tract arrhythmia is characterized by a precordial pseudodelta wave, a longer time to intrinsicoid deflection (lead V_2), and a broad initial R wave in lead V_1.
> - Nearly all outflow tract VTs have QS complexes in both lead aVR and lead aVL. However, peri-His bundle ventricular arrhythmia has an isoelectric or positive R wave in lead aVL.

appropriately placed His bundle catheter demarcates the septal region (Figures 43.2, 43.3, 43.4, 43.5, 43.6, 43.7, 43.8, and 43.9). This helps to avoid inadvertent injury to the normal conduction system in addition to providing reference information on ablation catheter location. The CS catheter allows mapping of VTs originating around the mitral annular region (Figure 43.4) and the aorto-mitral continuity when advanced all the way into the superior mitral annulus region. The RAO and the LAO are the most commonly used fluoroscopic views (Figures 43.3, 43.4, 43.5, 43.6, 43.7, 43.8, and 43.9). These are nonobtrusive and necessary to assess the orientation and positioning of the intracardiac catheters.

For RVOT mapping, the catheter is usually inserted through the femoral vein (Figures 43.3 and 43.7). Once in the ventricle, application of a clockwise torque flexes the tip of the catheter to enter the RVOT. Mapping of the anterior region of the RVOT can be done by continued clockwise torque application. Mapping of the posterior RVOT can be more difficult because this requires counterclockwise torque that results in poor contact and can lead to prolapse back into the ventricle. Use of a guide sheath can help stabilize the catheter for mapping the posterior RVOT.[21] Catheter placement into the LVOT is typically done using a retrograde approach by cannulating the femoral artery (Figures 43.3, 43.4, 43.5, and 43.6). For mapping below the cusp, the catheter is advanced gently with the tip curved to avoid damage to the valve leaflets. The LVOT can also be approached transseptally using venous access and atrial septal puncture.

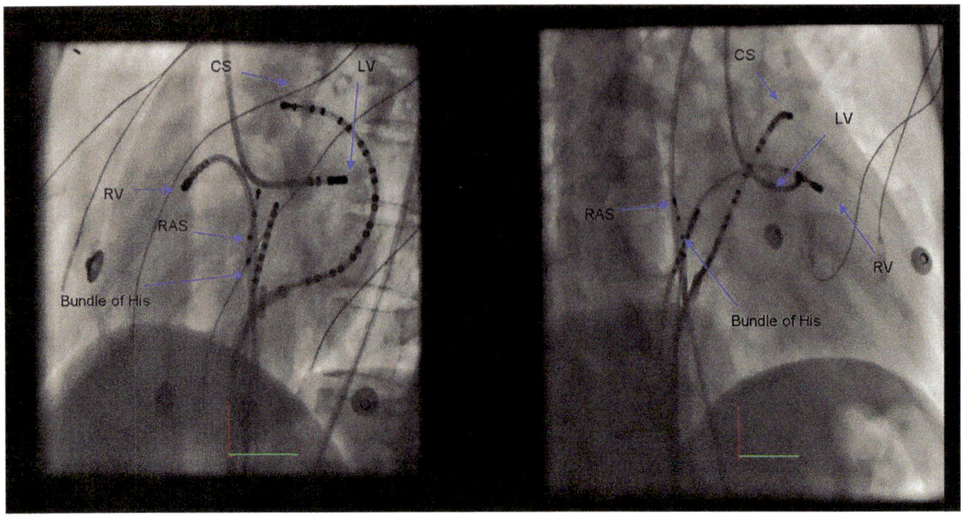

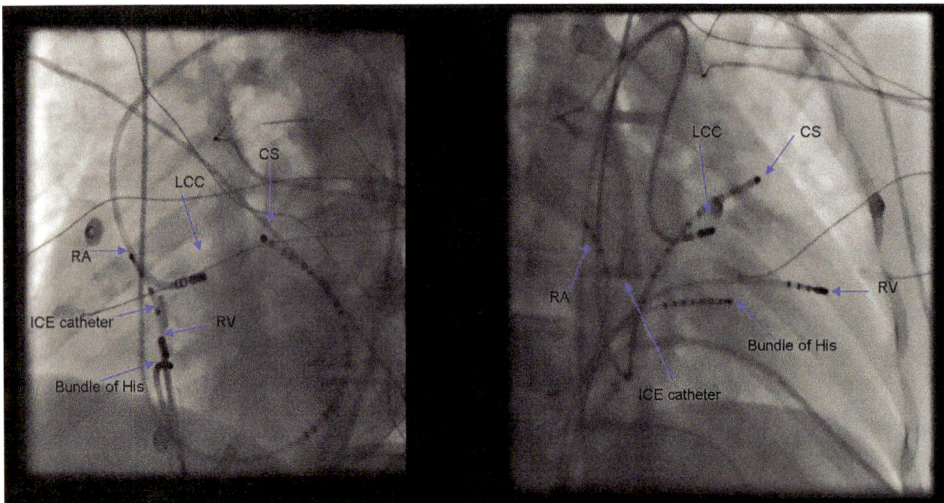

Figure 43.4 Orientation on fluoroscopy of the mapping/ablation catheter inserted via the retrograde aortic approach and advanced to the left ventricle. Earliest signals were recorded in the left ventricle near the mitral valve annulus at the 3 o'clock position. Successful ablation took place at this site. The CS catheter was introduced from the right femoral vein with distal poles advanced to the anterior interventricular vein. The left panel is LAO and the right panel is RAO. CS = coronary sinus; LV = left ventricle; RAS = right atrial septum; RV = right ventricle.

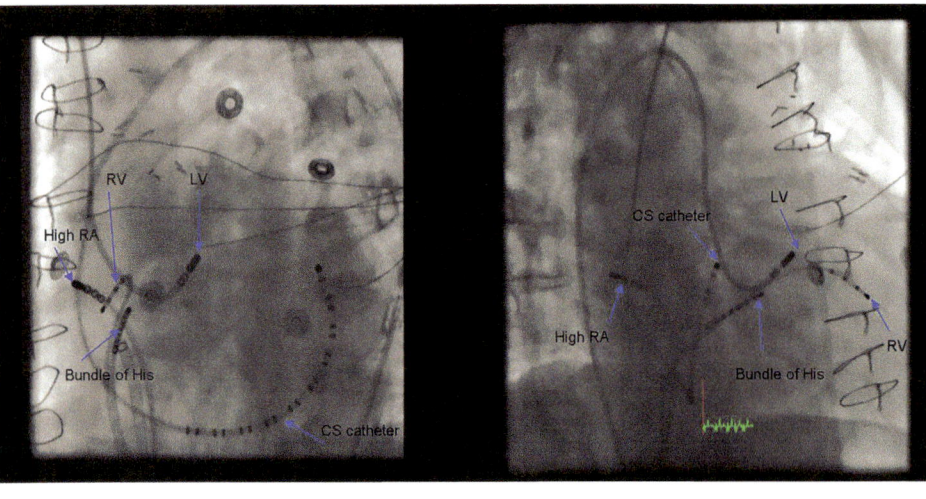

Figure 43.5 Orientation on fluoroscopy of mapping catheter inserted via the femoral artery and advanced to the LCC. The left panel is LAO and the right panel is RAO. CS = coronary sinus; LCC = left coronary cusp; RA = right atrium; RV = right ventricle.

Figure 43.6 Orientation on fluoroscopy of the mapping catheter introduced retrograde from the femoral artery into the aorta and located across the aortic valve at the anterolateral LVOT. The left panel is LAO and the right panel is RAO. CS = coronary sinus; LV = left ventricle; RA = right atrium; RV = right ventricle.

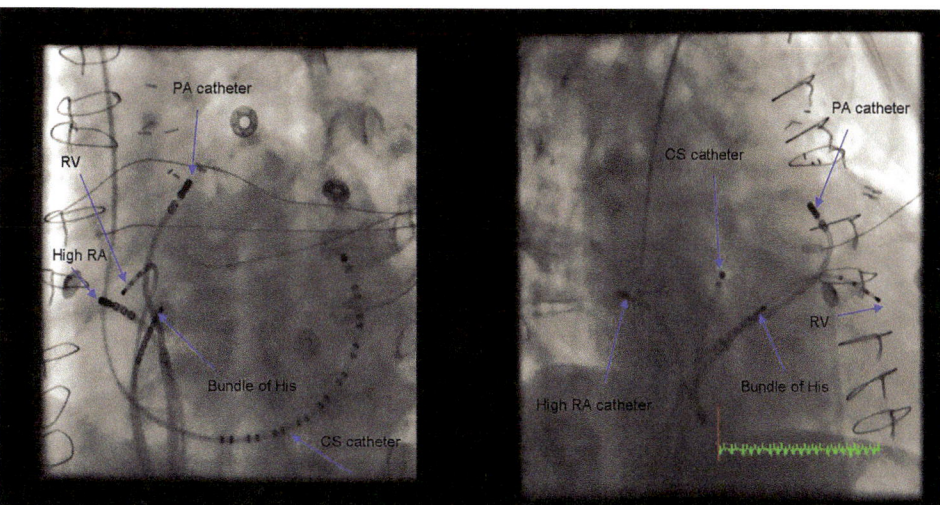

Figure 43.7 Orientation on fluoroscopy of the mapping/ablation catheter advanced to the pulmonary artery just beyond the pulmonic valve. At this site, early sharp near-field signals were recorded. In order to avoid arterial injury, ablation was performed just below the pulmonary valve. The left panel is LAO and the right panel is RAO. CS = coronary sinus; PA = pulmonary artery; RA = right atrium; RV = right ventricle.

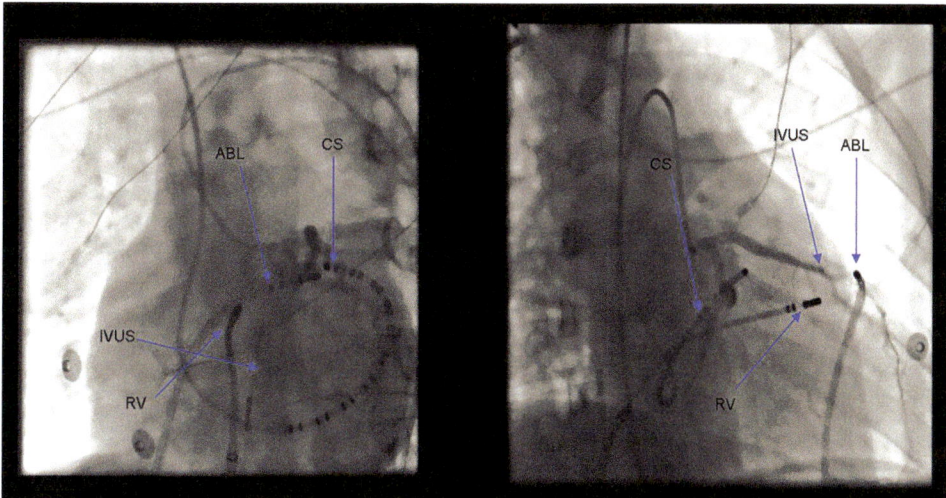

Figure 43.8 Orientation on fluoroscopy of the mapping/ablation catheter inserted into the pericardial space for epicardial mapping. Earliest signals were recorded near the mid portion of the left anterior descending coronary artery. Intravascular ultrasound and left coronary angiography was utilized to monitor the artery during energy application. The left panel is LAO and the right panel is RAO. ABL = ablation catheter; CS = coronary sinus; IVUS = intravascular ultrasound; RV = right ventricle.

The fluoroscopic views are correlated with the local EGMs to ascertain the location of the catheter. A methodical approach using fluoroscopic guidance is needed in order to systematically map the entire region of interest. The CS catheter in the RAO view marks the region of the AV groove, and in reference to this catheter, the ventricles are anterior and the atria posterior (Figures 43.3, 43.4, 43.5, 43.6, 43.7, 43.8, and 43.9). The bundle of His catheter in the LAO view helps to delineate the position of the IVS (Figures 43.3, 43.4, 43.5, 43.6, 43.7, 43.8, and 43.9). A catheter placed in the RVOT would assume a leftward position in the LAO view as it is advanced toward the pulmonic valve (Figures 43.3 and 43.7). In the RAO view, the catheter would be more superior on the anterior wall and move posteriorly when on the posterior wall. Recall that the position of the catheter in the posterior RVOT is just anterior to the right and also the LCCs. When mapping the RCC with the retrograde aortic approach, the catheter would appear to point rightward in the LAO view and anteriorly in the RAO view. As the catheter is moved toward the LCC, this will appear to point leftward in the LAO view (Figure 43.5). The catheter would move infero-posteriorly in the RAO view as is moved into the NCC.

The EGMs recorded in the RCC may originate in the RVOT but still appear large and near-field. An atrial EGM, if observed, may arise from the RAA. At the NCC, a large atrial EGM is typically recorded and a ventricular signal may or may not be present due to the

> **Points to Remember #3**
> **Localization of Catheter in the Aortic Valve Cusps**
>
> - A combination of EGM analysis and fluoroscopy can help define catheter location in the 3 aortic valve cusps.
>   - The RCC is anterior in the RAO view and rightward in the LAO view, and is typically associated with a large ventricular EGM and a small far-field atrial EGM.
>   - The LCC is mid/anterior in RAO and leftward in the LAO view, and can be associated with a large ventricular and a smaller atrial EGM.
>   - The NCC is posterior in RAO and mid position in LAO, and is associated with a large atrial EGM with a small or far-field ventricular EGM.

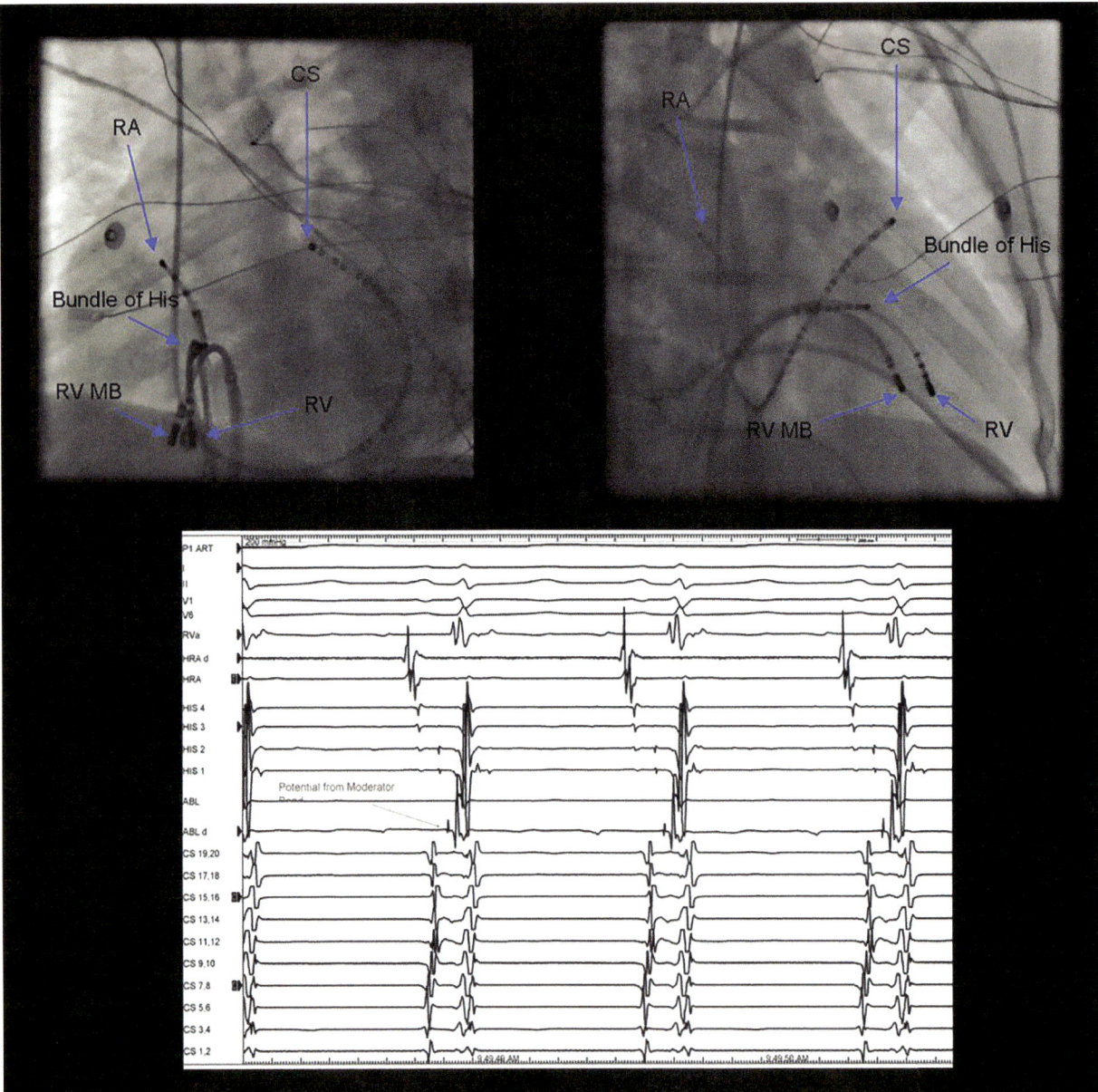

Figure 43.9 The top panels depict position of catheters on fluoroscopy with the mapping/ablation catheter on the moderator band in the right ventricle. The bottom panel shows the corresponding fascicular potential at the moderator band preceding the ventricular activation. The top left panel is LAO and the top right panel is RAO. CS = coronary sinus; RA = right atrium; RV = right ventricle; RV MB = right ventricular moderator band.

presence of the fibrous mitral-aortic continuity. A far-field and small ventricular EGM may represent distal LVOT activation. The EGM in the LCC is variable. As the retrograde arterial catheter is advanced into the proximal LVOT, it would move leftward in the LAO view and anteriorly in the RAO view (Figure 43.6).

Intracardiac Echocardiography

Fluoroscopy alone is sometimes inadequate for performing complex interventions. ICE is being used widely in procedures requiring precise visualization of intracardiac structures, especially for transseptal punctures to perform left atrial procedures.[28] To visualize the left ventricle and the mitral apparatus, the ICE catheter is advanced apically into the right ventricle and positioned against the IVS with clockwise rotation. The RVOT can be visualized in its long axis with a cross-sectional view of the pulmonic valve by withdrawing the ICE catheter to the base of the right ventricle and rotating the shaft to align the view with the RVOT. Alternatively, the ICE catheter tip can be positioned in the right atrium at the level of the outflow tracts to visualize the RVOT and the LVOT. The aortic valve and the aortic root in cross section with the coronary ostia can be visualized from this location.[34]

ICE permits accurate positioning of the ablation catheter on intracavitary structures such as the moderator band and the papillary muscles, and in the aortic cusps where care needs to be taken to not injure the coronary ostia during ablation. In addition to permitting accurate localization of ablation catheters, ICE can help titrate the amount and duration of energy delivered by monitoring the progression of the lesion as ablation is performed, and thus avoid unnecessary tissue injury. Details regarding ICE have been discussed elsewhere in a separate chapter.

> **Points to Remember #4**
> **Intracardiac Echocardiography**
> - The location of the mapping catheter in the outflow tracts and the semilunar valve cusps can be visualized with ICE.
> - ICE helps to assess distance to the coronary ostia and arteries and prevent coronary arterial injury during RFA.
> - The precise position of the ablation catheter in the semilunar valve annuli can be defined. The catheter tip should be deep in the cusp and deflected onto the myocardium rather than the valve leaflet to avoid valve perforation.

Principles of Mapping

Mapping strategies for VT have witnessed great advancements over the past two decades. This exponential growth comes from the increased understanding of mechanisms underlying VT as well as synergistic developments in mapping technology. Effective mapping techniques for both VT with structural heart disease and idiopathic VT have grown alongside and have enabled strategies for treating VT.

Isolated Trigger/Automatic Focus

VTs related to a macroreentry circuit related to myocardial scar are discussed in a separate chapter. Here we discuss idiopathic VTs assuming the underlying trigger to be an isolated focus. While presuming an arrhythmia to be arising from an isolated focus, however, it is difficult to exclude the presence of a microreentry circuit with certainty.

Mapping and ablation of an idiopathic automatic VT targets a fairly localized arrhythmogenic substrate that encompasses the trigger focus. Identifying the earliest site of activation with intracardiac EGMs preceding the ventricular activation on surface ECG is used to localize the trigger focus. Mapping at the site most proximate to the focus will give a completely negative deflection on the unipolar EGM as the activation wavefront moves away from this site of origin in all directions. This can be followed by pace mapping to confirm the site of the focus by pacing at the identified site of earliest activation. If the correct site is being paced, the EP characteristics of the depolarization wavefront, including the morphology on surface ECG, should exactly match the arrhythmia wavefront.

Earliest Activation Mapping

The commonly used principle of earliest activation mapping is based on recording the timing of the EGMs using the ablation catheter at different sites during the tachycardia, and comparing it to a preset reference signal in order to determine the earliest possible signal. Typically, the site of origin of the tachycardia is defined by the earliest bipolar recording at the distal tip of the mapping catheter, which usually precedes the surface QRS by 20–50 ms, and the unipolar signal at the site having a QS pattern (Figure 43.10).

A key limitation in using the earliest site of noticeable activation to localize the trigger/automatic focus is in cases where the arrhythmia originates at a distinct focus and

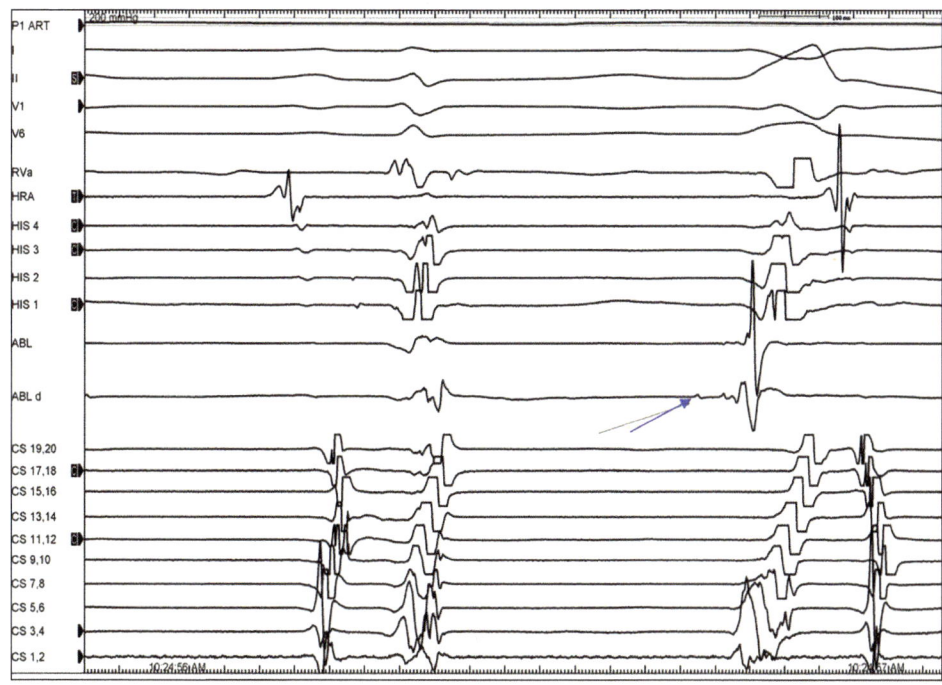

Figure 43.10 The **blue arrow** points to the early signal recorded on the ablation catheter positioned just below the LCC in the LVLVOT during the clinical PVC. The early potential occurred 65 ms preceding the QRS onset on surface ECG. This early signal is absent during the normal sinus beat. Ablation at this site was successful in the elimination of this PVC.

travels across insulated tissue to exit at a separate site. A common scenario is an origin within the conduction system, for example fascicular VT, from where it conducts down into the ventricular myocardium and exits at a separate site that can be mistaken as the earliest site of activation. Another example is VT with a focus above a semilunar valve where, due to the presence of tissue with variable conductivity (fibrous valve tissue and conducting muscular tissue), the activation wavefront makes an exit below the valve. In such a scenario, the exit below the valve may appear to be the earliest site, yet the arrhythmia would recur after the site is ablated, as the focus conducts to another exit site. Placing an electrode above the valve to observe any fragmented diastolic potentials during sinus rhythm or during arrhythmia can usually alert the electrophysiologist to the possibility of the focus being above the valve (see section on mapping above semilunar valves).

Myocardial tissue can continue from one outflow tract to the other; therefore, the defined earliest site of activation relative to neighboring myocardium can sometimes be misleading. For example, if the true origin of the arrhythmia is in the supravalvar aortic cusps with the activation wavefront exiting to both the infravalvar LVOT and the infundibular RVOT, an early site relative to all neighboring RVOT myocardium may be found in the posterior subpulmonic valve RVOT. A careful analysis of the EGM at this site should, however, identify far-field signals that give a clue of an earlier site at a related location.[13] Ablation only at the earliest RVOT site will only lead to a change in the exit site and the surface ECG morphology of the arrhythmia.

Detecting the earliest site of activation can be done using multiple techniques:

- *Point-to-point mapping.* This method relies on a single mapping electrode and is done by moving the catheter to multiple locations to map the PVC or VT of interest at each site and zoning in on the early area. The site of the earliest activation potential as compared to the surface ECG is usually the desired site of ablation, although there are exceptions as discussed above. Point-to-point mapping alone, however, is a very time-consuming process, so other techniques to reduce procedural time have been developed.
- *Multielectrode mapping.* This method uses the same principles as above, but uses multiple electrodes along the catheter tip to allow mapping at multiple points simultaneously. However, because it is difficult to establish good contact between all electrodes and the endocardial surface, multielectrode mapping requires careful interpretation and registration of points. Failure of an electrode to have contact with the surface could appear as absence of near-field signals.
- *Basket mapping.* This involves an inflatable basket-shaped catheter with multiple electrodes over its surface. The inflation allows the basket electrodes to make contact with the endocardial surface, thereby sampling many more sites with each mapped signal.
- *Electroanatomic mapping.* This involves the 3D localization of the catheter by triangulating decremental electromagnetic fields and integrating this information with the local EGMs. The activation sequence mapped using the techniques described above can then be displayed using 3D computer graphics. The principles of electroanatomic mapping and related techniques are reviewed elsewhere.[35,36]

Because of the overlapping nature of the outflow tracts, care must be taken to use only the signals originating from the specific outflow tract being mapped to yield accurate results. When mapping the peri-semilunar valve regions, both near-field and far-field signals may be noted, often separated by an isoelectric period. It is advisable to take only the near-field signals for the purposes of activation mapping. If the "first" signal is registered, and that is a far-field signal from activation on the side of the valve opposite to the mapping catheter, then the composite map will be unable to identify whether the true site of earliest activation is below or above the valve.

Pace Mapping

Pacing at the exit site of an arrhythmia should reproduce an exact or near exact match of the arrhythmia activation morphology on surface ECG.[37] Pace mapping is valuable in confirming the results of activation mapping that identify the earliest site of activation, and is commonly used for localizing the origin site of an arrhythmia. Pace mapping helps identify falsely picked signals from adjacent structures during activation mapping; pacing at these inaccurate sites leads to a pace map dissimilar from the arrhythmia. However, it is tricky to rely on pace mapping alone for successful ablation because of the likelihood that large areas could have acceptable pace map characteristics and the precision to localize the focal site is limited. This lack of precision is amplified by capture of distant sites at high pacing outputs.

As with activation mapping, pace mapping is also hampered by the limitations of a disparate exit site being misidentified as the true focus. For example, in case of an arrhythmia from the RCC region, a perfect pace map could be obtained at the breakthrough site in the posterior RVOT. However, after ablation at this RVOT site the ventricular arrhythmia may possibly continue with a different morphology due to exit of the focus to the left ventricle. Conversely, the possibility of exit to the other outflow tract should be considered when pacing from the aortic cusp yields a poor pace map despite an early near-field signal at the location. Ablation should target the earliest near-field signal despite a poor pace map at this site.[13]

> **Points to Remember #5**
> **Electrophysiologic Mapping of Outflow Tract Arrhythmia**
>
> - Earliest activation mapping is used to identify the focal site of outflow tract arrhythmia.
> - Breakthrough of an arrhythmia originating above the semilunar valves to a location below the valve or of a focus in one outflow tract to the other outflow tract can lead to misidentification of the exit site as the site of origin.
> - A match of pacing at the identified site with the arrhythmia morphology is used to confirm the focus of arrhythmia. Pace mapping is less accurate, however, above the semilunar valves and in the vicinity of conduction tissue.
> - Attention should be paid to the output being used for pace mapping and preferably the lowest output that captures only the local site should be used.

Mapping and Ablation at Some Unique Outflow Tract Locations

Most of the outflow tract tachycardias originate from the RVOT, and some others from the LVOT. Though these are usually mapped to endocardial sites, some have the earliest activation on the epicardial surface. As discussed before, the epicardial arrhythmia surface ECG morphology as opposed to endocardial outflow tract sites is characterized by a pseudodelta wave ≥ 34 ms, precordial maximum deflection index > 0.55, R wave in lead V_1 > 75 ms, and intrinsicoid deflection time in lead V_2 ≥ 85 ms.[31-33] Ablation in the left CS and occasionally the noncoronary sinus can target most of the epicardial outflow tract foci.[29] However, mapping and ablation in the epicardial coronary veins[32,38,39] or on the epicardial surface[33] with pericardial access is sometimes needed. Because of the intervening RVOT between the LVOT epicardial surface and the pericardial space, it might be difficult to approach the earliest site from the pericardial access. Nevertheless, most of the earliest epicardial sites are mapped in the distal great cardiac vein, great cardiac vein–anterior interventricular vein junction, or proximal anterior interventricular vein.

Mapping Above the Semilunar Valves: Importance of Near-field and Far-field Signals

As described previously, the 12-lead ECG might provide some clues as to the location of the focus in the peripulmonic valve region or the aortic cusps. However, the interpretation of EGMs obtained during mapping above the semilunar valves can be complex, and the presence of myocardium in the supravalvar region must be kept in mind. Near-field and far-field potentials are typically recorded when mapping for the arrhythmia focus above a semilunar valve. Typically, in sinus rhythm, there is an early far-field signal likely representing outflow tract activation that might be followed by an isoelectric period and a distinct sharp near-field potential representing local supravalvar myocardium activation. If, during the arrhythmia, the sharp near-field signal occurs first and is followed by the far-field signal, the operator can be certain that the supravalvar myocardium is the arrhythmogenic substrate for that arrhythmia. If any far-field signal precedes the near-field potential, even though the near-field potential might appear early, it is possible that the exact site of origin is not being mapped and the true site is possibly in a different cusp. Even though supravalvar myocardium might be present in the location being mapped and gets activated late during sinus rhythm, a far-field signal before the near-field activation during arrhythmia likely represents the responsible focus elsewhere.[16,17,21]

Mapping in the Epicardial Coronary Veins

Anatomically, the CS passes continue as the great cardiac vein in the anterior left AV sulcus in close proximity to the circumflex artery. The great cardiac vein turns anteriorly along the epicardial surface of the anterobasal LVOT, under the base of the LAA, and continues as the anterior interventricular vein adjacent to the left anterior descending artery. Several case reports have demonstrated successful mapping and ablation of idiopathic VT through the great cardiac vein after failure of ablation from various endocardial (LVOT, aortic valve cusps, LAA) and epicardial (pericardial access) locations.[38,39] In a large consecutive series of idiopathic VT ablations, the earliest ventricular activation during arrhythmia was mapped in the coronary veins in 14% of cases.[32] Ablation at the earliest site in the coronary veins resulted in long-term success in 67% of cases. Most ablation sites are in the distal great cardiac vein or proximal anterior interventricular vein where the activation precedes the earliest endocardial activation in the LCC. Occasionally mitral annular sites can be targeted in the proximal great cardiac vein or even the middle cardiac vein.[32,33] Even though it is favorable to ablate in the coronary veins in certain circumstances, caution is warranted due to potential for complications. Complications of ablating in the epicardial veins include vein stenosis, vein rupture, venous thrombosis, and of even more concern, coronary artery damage causing arterial stenosis. Cryoablation is likely safer than RFA when ablating in the branches of the CS. The maximum recommended power for RFA (if it is used) is 20 W.

> **Points to Remember #6**
> **Ablating Outflow Tract VT from Epicardial Veins**
>
> - The junction of the great cardiac and anterior interventricular veins represents a unique site for targeting epicardial outflow tract arrhythmia.
> - The arrhythmogenic substrate targeted in the great cardiac vein may be the mitral annular myocardium adjacent to these veins.
> - Due to their proximity with the coronary arteries, coronary angiography is routinely performed to assess safety of ablation in the coronary veins.
> - Saline flush through a sheath in the coronary vein or using internally or externally irrigated catheter may allow greater energy delivery in the coronary venous sites.
> - Epicardial ablation through pericardial access can be considered when achieving optimal energy delivery is not possible via the venous system.

Mapping in the Pericardial Space

While most VTs can be mapped and ablated via the endocardial approach, up to 30% of patients will need supplementary epicardial mapping and ablation. As discussed previously, the arrhythmia morphology on the 12-lead ECG can point toward an epicardial site of origin. If an endocardial approach has been attempted previously and failed, this can be a clue to start with an epicardial approach right away. If there is a contraindication to access the endocardial left ventricle, such as an endocavitary thrombus, the epicardial approach can still be used.

Epicardial access is generally obtained through the subxiphoid percutaneous puncture as described by Sosa et al.[40] Under fluoroscopy the needle is inserted about 2–3 cm below the xiphoid process. There are two possible approaches to enter the pericardial space. The needle can be directed superiorly at a shallow angle, which will aid in obtaining access to the anterior epicardial space over the anterior aspect of the ventricles. This approach is generally done using the RAO projection. Otherwise, the needle can be directed posteriorly aiming toward the left shoulder, accessing the pericardium over the inferior aspect of the ventricles. The LAO projection is particularly useful for this approach. A slight negative pressure might be felt as the needle enters the pericardial sac. Access to the pericardial space is confirmed with injection of contrast (< 1 cm^3) that shows sluggish layering in the sac, and tenting at the site of needle entry can be seen. Then the guidewire is inserted, over which the introducer sheath is advanced into the pericardial sac.

Epicardial mapping can be performed using fluoroscopy (Figure 43.8) with/without electroanatomic mapping systems. The pacing thresholds in general are higher in the pericardial space. Epicardial fat and catheter instability may contribute to these high thresholds. Pace mapping and entrainment mapping can still be performed in normal tissue with unipolar pacing, as thresholds may be around 10 mA using a pulse width of 2 ms.[41] It is not certain if bipolar pacing is less effective than unipolar pacing in the epicardial region. Areas with myocardial scar will have low-amplitude EGMs. However, it is also necessary to recognize that epicardial fat will produce similar low-amplitude regions and can be a potential barrier to pacing and ablation. With ablation in the pericardial space, the electrode temperature will increase substantially even with low-power RF applications due to the absence of cooling from blood flow. Higher temperatures (> 60°C) can usually be tolerated because thrombus formation and charring is a lesser concern, as there is no potential for arterial embolization. Internally irrigated cooled-tip catheters are preferred over externally irrigated catheters to avoid saline infusion in the pericardial space. Cryoablation is also feasible as the absence of blood flow favors formation of lesions, but this has not been adequately studied.

Epicardial mapping is a useful technique, but it is important to recognize that it will not lead to success in all endocardial ablation failures. Several complications can occur with the epicardial approach. Bleeding into the pericardial space, puncture into the ventricle, coronary artery injury, and phrenic nerve injury have all been reported, and caution must be sought to avoid these morbid complications. Epicardial access is particularly difficult in the presence of adhesions in a patient with previous cardiac surgery.

> **Points to Remember #7**
> **Epicardial Mapping for Outflow Tract Arrhythmia**
>
> - The myocardium of the ventricular outflow tract can be accessed epicardially through the coronary venous system or through pericardial access.
> - Pericardial access for mapping and ablation are rarely useful for LVOT arrhythmia because the LVOT is separated from the epicardial surface by the RVOT.
> - Catheter location in the transverse sinus of the pericardial space may allow mapping of the posterior supra-aortic valvar ascending aorta, including the NCC region.
> - Epicardial fat, higher pacing thresholds, ineffective energy delivery, and excessive heating can limit epicardial mapping and ablation.

Non-outflow Tract Idiopathic Ventricular Tachycardias

Idiopathic Fascicular Ventricular Tachycardia

Idiopathic LV tachycardia or fascicular VT is the second most common type of VT after outflow tract arrhythmias in patients with structurally normal hearts. Fascicular VT usually presents clinically as repetitive monomorphic tachycardia in young adults aged 15–40 years, and a majority (60%–70%) of cases are males. Rarely, fascicular triggers can induce (idiopathic) ventricular fibrillation. Most episodes of fascicular VT occur at rest, but VT can easily be induced by exercise and emotional stress. The most common form of fascicular VT originating from the posterior fascicular region of the left ventricle, thus presenting on ECG with RBBB morphology, and left axis deviation has been known for at least 4 decades.[42,43] This tachycardia can be entrained from either the atria or the ventricles and is known to be inducible with exercise, atrial premature complexes, and ventricular pacing. The mechanism that is thus postulated for this tachycardia is reentry involving the Purkinje fiber network. Belhassen et al demonstrated as early as 1981 that fascicular VT could be terminated with intravenous verapamil, a finding that has been subsequently replicated, confirmed, and recognized as an identifying feature for idiopathic fascicular VT.[44]

Electrocardiographic Features

Due to the propagation of the ventricular activation wavefront at least partially via the conduction system, the QRS duration of fascicular VT is relatively narrow and usually ranges from 110 to 150 ms. Moreover, the standard QRS morphology criteria used to differentiate VT from SVT are inapplicable for fascicular VT as they assume ventricular activation in VT to be independent of the conduction system. These features are the hallmark of fascicular VT and lend to the difficulty in differentiating it from SVT with aberrant conduction.

In current literature, the predominant classification of fascicular VT is based on the site of origin. The most common presentation arising from the posterior fascicle of the left ventricle manifests with an RBBB pattern and left axis deviation, and the earliest LV myocardial activation occurs in the apical inferoposterior IVS. The less common left anterior fascicular VT is characterized by RBBB pattern and right axis deviation with the earliest ventricular myocardial activation in the anterolateral left ventricle. A rare form from the left upper septum can manifest with a normal QRS morphology and duration or an RBBB pattern.

Electrophysiologic Activation Mapping: The Purkinje and Pre-Purkinje Potentials

Endocardial EP mapping during fascicular VT reveals a very short VH interval indicative of a pseudo-interval due to origin of the arrhythmia in the LV fascicles with anterograde conduction to the ventricles and retrograde activation of the bundle of His. There are 2 distinct potentials that can be seen before the ventricular activation on surface ECG: the presystolic Purkinje potential (PP) and the mid to late diastolic pre-Purkinje potential (pre-PP).[45,46] The relative time by which PP and pre-PP precede the onset of QRS complex usually varies between 5 to 30 ms and 30 to 70 ms, respectively. The PP is a brief, sharp, and high-frequency potential preceding the local ventricular myocardial activation and the surface QRS during tachycardia. The PP represents the activation of the posterior (or the anterior) fascicle and is also present before ventricular activation during sinus rhythm (Figure 43.9). The PP is activated bidirectionally proximal and distal from the earliest site during fascicular VT.[47] The pre-PP is usually a dull, lower-frequency potential preceding the PP during tachycardia. The pre-PP is recorded proximally to the earliest PP and is activated in the direction toward the earliest PP site.[47] During sinus rhythm, the pre-PP is captured orthodromically following the PP.

Anatomic Substrate for Fascicular Tachycardia

The primary postulated mechanism of fascicular VT is reentry involving the Purkinje fiber network. The pre-PP likely represents excitation of a specialized zone that has decremental properties and is sensitive to verapamil. The close relation between the fast Purkinje fibers and the verapamil-sensitive decremental fibers set the stage for a reentrant mechanism. Entrainment maneuvers have demonstrated this pre-Purkinje potential (pre-PP) to be an essential part of the reentry circuit, and ablation at the site of the pre-PP successfully terminates VT in all cases.[45] During endocardial electrophysiological mapping of the left posterior fascicular VT, the PP can be recorded from an area of 2 to 3 cm^2 in the posteroapical left IVS.[46,48] As a corollary, the PP for left anterior fascicular VT is mapped endocardially in the anterolateral wall of the left ventricle.[49] The pre-PP can be mapped in a smaller zone within the PP region.[45]

Ablation of Fascicular Tachycardia

Mapping of fascicular VT is usually done during tachycardia to localize the earliest ventricular activation site and the preceding PP and pre-PP potentials. There are 2 possible targets for ablation, the pre-PP or the earliest PP.[45,47] Application of 1 or 2 RF lesions at these sites leads to termination of the tachycardia, noninducibility with isoproterenol, and long-term success. Ablation at these sites carries the risk of AV block or LBBB. The earliest PP is located ~1 cm proximal from the earliest site of ventricular activation.[48] Ablation at only the early ventricular activation sites is either acutely unsuccessful or has late recurrence of the tachycardia, suggesting that targeting the early ventricular activation site in this form of VT is not sufficient.

Pace mapping in general is less useful in fascicular VT than for focal tachycardias. Pace mapping helps guide to the general site for ablation, but a pace map match is not essential for success. In one study, pacing from the successful site of ablation showed a match to the VT morphology in only 9.6 ± 2.1 of the 12 ECG leads.[50] This less than complete pace map is probably explained by the capture of a pathway within the Purkinje network that is not included in the reentry circuit and direct capture of the adjacent myocardium. However, in some cases when the VT is not easily inducible, pace mapping must be relied upon. Alternatively, using an electroanatomic map to tag the bundle of His, fascicles, and sinus breakout points in sinus rhythm, a linear lesion 1 cm proximal to the sinus breakout point and perpendicular to the direction of the left posterior fascicle can be applied empirically.[51] This approach causes modification of the Purkinje network and causes a rightward shift of the QRS axis in the limb leads without a complete left posterior fascicular block. Another approach targeting orthodromically activated pre-PP region during sinus rhythm has also been described.[52]

> **Points to Remember #8**
> **Fascicular Ventricular Tachycardia**
>
> - A reentrant circuit comprising a verapamil-sensitive slow conducting decremental zone and the fast fascicular fibers is the postulated mechanism of fascicular VT with no single true earliest site.
> - Earliest site of ventricular myocardial activation is rarely an appropriate target site for fascicular VT, because the true substrate can be several centimeters proximal given the insulated nature of the conduction system.
> - During 3D electroanatomic mapping, the Purkinje potential should be specifically annotated and analyzed for appropriateness of ablative therapy.
> - Near-field Purkinje potentials can be confirmed for relevance to fascicular VT with low-output pacing at that location. If near the true arrhythmia substrate, the stimulus to QRS onset interval is the same as the observed potential to QRS onset interval in VT, and the pace map matches the tachycardia QRS morphology.
> - Terminal fibers of the Purkinje network may be found in the papillary muscles, and mapping of these endocavitary structures may be required with the help of ICE.

Ventricular Tachycardia Due to Interfascicular Reentry

It is important to distinguish idiopathic fascicular VT from interfascicular reentrant VT, which is an entity mainly seen in patients with ischemic scar-related substrate. Interfascicular VT involves a reentrant circuit using retrograde conduction over one fascicle, anterograde conduction over the other fascicle, and slow conduction over scarred ventricular myocardium between the two fascicles. It typically has an RBBB morphology and left or right axis deviation during the tachycardia, but His bundle depolarization precedes the ventricular depolarization as opposed to His bundle activation shortly after surface QRS onset in fascicular VT.

Idiopathic Ventricular Tachycardia from Endocavitary Structures

LV papillary muscle VT is another important entity that is often confused with fascicular VT.[8,9,53] Ventricular arrhythmia from the papillary muscles is more common in older patients and patients with structural heart disease, and often presents with PVCs and pleomorphic ectopy rather than monomorphic VT.[11] Nonetheless, some patients with structurally normal hearts have been shown to have VT originating in the papillary muscles.[10] The close proximity of the LV papillary muscles to the fascicles leads to similar QRS morphologies on ECG in papillary muscle VT and fascicular VT. Posteromedial papillary origin has the appearance of left posterior fascicular VT, and anterolateral papillary muscle resembles left anterior fascicular VT. However, the QRS duration is longer for papillary muscle arrhythmia (150 ± 15 ms) compared to fascicular VT (127 ± 11 ms).[11] Moreover, instead of rsR' in lead V_1 and presence of Q waves in the limb leads with fascicular VT, papillary muscle arrhythmia usually presents as a monophasic R or qR complex in lead V_1 and may not have Q waves in the limb leads. In addition, mapping at the effective ablation site is not necessarily associated with a Purkinje potential, and when present the Purkinje potential might lag the earliest activation site.

In addition to LV papillary muscles, structures in the right ventricle including the moderator band and right ventricular papillary muscles can also give rise to VT.[8,9,54] ICE is useful for mapping and ablation at the endocavitary structures to enable appropriate catheter positioning.

Idiopathic Ventricular Tachycardia Originating from the Mitral Annulus

VT originating at the region of the mitral annulus represents approximately 5% of all idiopathic forms of VT.[7] The mechanism for the idiopathic mitral annular VTs is automatic triggered activity, and these are known to be sensitive to adenosine and verapamil. The "dead-end" remnants of the AV conduction system close to the aortomitral continuity and remnants of the AV ring in the posterior mitral annulus are hypothesized to be responsible for these arrhythmias.[7,55]

Specific ECG patterns can help recognize VT originating from the mitral annulus. In a case series of 19 patients with mitral annular VT, the site of origin was categorized as the anterolateral annulus (58%), posterior annulus (11%), and posteroseptal annulus (31%).[7] All mitral annular sites produce an RBBB pattern with an S wave (RS complex) in V_6. There was a very early precordial transition from negative to positive usually by lead V_1 and, in the case of posteroseptal mitral annular VT, by lead V_2. The QRS morphology from the different mitral annular locations parallels the delta wave of the preexcited QRS complexes from mitral annular accessory pathways.[6] The anterolateral mitral annular VT had positive polarity in the inferior leads and negative in leads I and aVL. The posteroseptal mitral annular VT was differentiated from the posterior annular VT by a larger Q wave in lead III compared to lead II, and a monophasic R in I (instead of Rs complex) with a negative component of the R wave in V_1 (instead of monophasic R). The ECG and/or activation mapping help in accurately localizing the origin of the arrhythmia around the mitral annulus. Pace mapping is then used to confirm the focal site of origin and determining the best site for RFA. In addition, the presence of low-amplitude presystolic potentials on local EGM during VT or PVCs helps confirm the correct site.[56]

Guiding Principles to Avoid Complications During Ablation

In addition to the potential adverse events generally associated with invasive electrophysiology and ablation, the ablationist needs to be cognizant of and avoid site-specific complications relevant to VT ablation in the structurally normal heart.[17,57]

Coronary Arterial Damage

The development of the ventricular outflow tracts and proximal coronary arterial vasculature is closely connected. This results in a complex overlapping pattern of the outflow tracts and the proximal coronary arteries (Figure 43.1). Ablation in proximity to coronary veins warrants coronary angiography and/or intravascular ultrasound to define the anatomy and ensure safety. Specific locations where a propensity for arterial damage and possible myocardial injury exist include:

- *Posterior peripulmonic valve RVOT.* The left main coronary artery is closely related to the posterior RVOT at or above the annulus of the pulmonic valve. This relationship occurs because of the nature of the spiral septum that separates the two outflow tracts and semilunar valves. The left main coronary artery arises above the LCC, and since the pulmonic valve lies cranial and leftward of the aortic valve, the posterior RVOT in this region is the immediate anterior neighbor of this artery.

- *Above the coronary cusps.* The coronary artery ostia arise ~15 mm above the depth of the coronary cusps. If the ablation catheter is well seated and deep in the coronary cusp, damage to the coronary artery ostium is unlikely. However, fluoroscopically, it can be difficult to determine whether a catheter has actually cannulated the artery and wedged in the vasculature rather than the assumed location in the depths of the respective coronary cusp. Gentle deflection of the catheter will usually help make the correct determination as the catheter tip should be freely mobile in the cusp but not in the artery. ICE with images usually viewed from the anterior tricuspid annulus location clearly identifies selective arterial cannulation.[58]

 Even if unrecognized prior to RF energy delivery, the operator must be cognizant of the possibility of arterial cannulation. A sudden increase in temperature, even at low power (typically less than 5 W), and an abrupt increase in the impedance strongly suggest ablation in the artery and should prompt the operator to turn off energy delivery immediately.

- *Epicardial veins.* An uncommon but well-recognized site for ablation of epicardial outflow tract tachycardia near the region of the LCC is the junction of the great cardiac and the anterior interventricular veins. The regional anatomy of these venous structures with the corresponding coronary arteries (proximal left circumflex, left anterior descending, and the diagonal branches) is highly variable and cannot be reliably predicted. As a result, left coronary angiography is essential prior to delivering energy in the vicinity of the great cardiac vein and anterior interventricular venous system.[59,60]

Damage to the Cardiac Conduction System

The AV conduction system may be damaged inadvertently during ablation of fascicular VT as well as outflow tract VT.

- *Fascicular ventricular tachycardia.* At times, the proximal His-Purkinje conduction system is incorrectly targeted for ablation when the actual culprit site of origin is in the distal Purkinje system, for example, the left posterior fascicle. This often can occur when right ventricular mapping is performed without LV mapping. For example, a left posterior fascicular tachycardia will show a relatively early retrograde His bundle EGM that may precede the surface QRS, giving the impression of the arrhythmogenic focus at the site of either the compact AV node or the His bundle. Ablation at this site would result in AV block. This misrepresentation can be readily clarified by mapping the LV conduction system.[48,49,61]

 Occasionally, even with mapping the LV conduction system, the true site of origin of the fascicular focus or localized reentry may be difficult to appreciate. For example, if the left posterior fascicular focus encounters anterograde conduction delay or block to the left ventricle, then retrograde conduction may exit via the right bundle or the left anterior fascicle and the earliest ventricular EGMs might be identified in the right or anterolateral left ventricle. Thus a left posterior fascicular arrhythmia presenting as LBBB tachycardia due to exit via the right bundle may result in incorrect ablation of the right bundle.

- *Ventricular outflow tract tachycardia.* The penetrating bundle of His has a consistent relationship with the outflow tracts. The commissure between the right and NCC lies directly adjacent and to the left of the commissure between the septal and anterior leaflets of the tricuspid valve. The meeting of these commissures marks the region of the membranous IVS and is the anatomic location of the bundle of His (Figures 43.1 and 43.2). Therefore, ablation in the RCC posteriorly or in the NCC at its junction with the right cusp may injure the bundle of His during ablation of supraaortic valvar tachycardia. Additionally, ablation at more posterior locations in the NCC may injure the fast pathway input to the compact AV node.

Damage to the Valvular Apparatus

When ablating above the semilunar valves, care with catheter positioning and titration of RF energy is required to prevent perforation or damage to the semilunar valve apparatus. To avoid coronary arterial injury during ablation in a coronary cusp, the operator advances the catheter to the depth of the cusp to maximize the distance from the coronary arterial ostium. If, however, pressure on the cusp is maintained during ablation, tissue heating may result in leaflet perforation. To avoid this complication, once in the depth of the cusp the catheter should be deflected to face the target outflow tract myocardium in the aortic wall prior to delivering RF energy.

Cardiac Perforation

While cardiac perforation may occur during catheter manipulation or energy delivery in a variety of arrhythmia ablation procedures, specific caution to avoid outflow tract perforation is needed. When ablating, for example, in the free wall of the RVOT, transient pulmonic regurgitation may effectively cool the catheter tip. Thus, the thermistor/thermocouple-based recordings underestimate the tissue temperature. Aggressive upward power titration due to perceived inadequate energy delivery in such a case may result in tissue vaporization and a "steam pop" causing perforation.[62,63]

Refractory Ventricular Arrhythmias

Occasionally, it might be challenging to terminate the induced VT during mapping and ablation, or the VT might not be hemodynamically tolerated. In some cases, energy delivery during ablation of fascicular VT may result in induction of VF.

Conclusion

While ventricular tachycardia is most commonly associated with ischemic heart disease or dilated cardiomyopathy, a substantial number of patients with structurally normal hearts present for ablation of VT. A thorough understanding of the regional anatomy of the outflow tract and fascicular conduction system is a prerequisite for safe and effective ablation in these regions. In this chapter, we have outlined an approach for the practicing electrophysiologist that begins with an appreciation of the background regional anatomy, continues with detailed inspection of the 12-lead ECG, and is followed by a plan with potential pitfalls to avoid for accurately mapping and localizing the focal site of the arrhythmia prior to safe energy delivery for ablation.

References

1. Latif S, Dixit S, Callans DJ. Ventricular arrhythmias in normal hearts. *Cardiology Clin.* 2008;26(3):367-380, vi.
2. Soejima K, Stevenson WG. Catheter ablation of ventricular tachycardia in patients with ischemic heart disease. *Curr Cardiol Rep.* 2003;5(5):364-368.
3. Tedrow U, Stevenson WG. Strategies for epicardial mapping and ablation of ventricular tachycardia. *J Cardiovasc Electrophysiol.* 2009;20(6):710-713.
4. Sheldon SH, Gard JJ, Asirvatham SJ. Premature ventricular contractions and non-sustained ventricular tachycardia: association with sudden cardiac death, risk stratification, and management strategies. *Indian Pacing Electrophysiol J.* 2010;10(8):357-371.
5. Takahashi Y, Sanders P, Ho SY, Haïssaguerre M. Pseudo-fascicular activity originating from the right ventricular outflow tract. *J Cardiovasc Electrophysiol.* 2004;15(11):1341.
6. Kumagai K, Yamauchi Y, Takahashi A, et al. Idiopathic left ventricular tachycardia originating from the mitral annulus. *J Cardiovasc Electrophysiol.* 2005;16(10):1029-1036.
7. Tada H, Ito S, Naito S, et al. Idiopathic ventricular arrhythmia arising from the mitral annulus: a distinct subgroup of idiopathic ventricular arrhythmias. *J Am Coll Cardiol.* 2005;45(6):877-886.
8. Abouezzeddine O, Suleiman M, Buescher T, et al. Relevance of endocavitary structures in ablation procedures for ventricular tachycardia. *J Cardiovasc Electrophysiol.* 2010;21(3): 245-254.
9. Madhavan M, Asirvatham SJ. The fourth dimension: endocavitary ventricular tachycardia. *Circ Arrhythm Electrophysiol.* 2010;3(4):302-304.
10. Yamada T, Doppalapudi H, McElderry HT, et al. Electrocardiographic and electrophysiological characteristics in idiopathic ventricular arrhythmias originating from the papillary muscles in the left ventricle: relevance for catheter ablation. *Circulation.* 2010;3(4):324-331.
11. Good E, Desjardins B, Jongnarangsin K, et al. Ventricular arrhythmias originating from a papillary muscle in patients without prior infarction: a comparison with fascicular arrhythmias. *Heart Rhythm.* 2008;5(11):1530-1537.
12. Kim RJ, Iwai S, Markowitz SM, Shah BK, Stein KM, Lerman BB. Clinical and electrophysiological spectrum of

idiopathic ventricular outflow tract arrhythmias. *J Am Coll Cardiol.* 2007;49(20):2035-2043.
13. Asirvatham SJ. Correlative anatomy for the invasive electrophysiologist: outflow tract and supravalvar arrhythmia. *J Cardiovasc Electrophysiol.* 2009;20(8):955-968.
14. Gami AS, Noheria A, Lachman N, et al. Anatomical correlates relevant to ablation above the semilunar valves for the cardiac electrophysiologist: a study of 603 hearts. *J Interventional Cardiac Electrophysiol.* 2011;30(1):5-15.
15. Habib A, Lachman N, Christensen KN, Asirvatham SJ. The anatomy of the coronary sinus venous system for the cardiac electrophysiologist. *Europace.* 2009;11 Suppl 5:v15-v21.
16. Suleiman M, Asirvatham SJ. Ablation above the semilunar valves: when, why, and how? Part II. *Heart Rhythm.* 2008;5(11):1625-1630.
17. Suleiman M, Asirvatham SJ. Ablation above the semilunar valves: when, why, and how? Part I. *Heart Rhythm.* 2008;5(10):1485-1492.
18. Hasdemir C, Aktas S, Govsa F, et al. Demonstration of ventricular myocardial extensions into the pulmonary artery and aorta beyond the ventriculo-arterial junction. *PACE.* 2007;30(4):534-539.
19. Talreja D, Gami AS, Edwards W, Friedman P, Packer D, Asirvatham SJ. The presence of ventricular muscular extensions into the pulmonary artery and aorta beyond the semilunar valves. *PACE.* 2001;24:734.
20. Jadonath RL, Schwartzman DS, Preminger MW, Gottlieb CD, Marchlinski FE. Utility of the 12-lead electrocardiogram in localizing the origin of right ventricular outflow tract tachycardia. *Am Heart J.* 1995;130(5):1107-1113.
21. Tabatabaei N, Asirvatham SJ. Supravalvular arrhythmia: identifying and ablating the substrate. *Circ Arrhythm Electrophysiol.* 2009;2(3):316-326.
22. Friedman PA, Asirvatham SJ, Grice S, et al. Noncontact mapping to guide ablation of right ventricular outflow tract tachycardia. *J Am Coll Cardiol.* 2002;39(11):1808-1812.
23. Sehar N, Mears J, Bisco S, Patel S, Lachman N, Asirvatham SJ. Anatomic guidance for ablation: atrial flutter, fibrillation, and outflow tract ventricular tachycardia. *Indian Pacing Electrophysiol J.* 2010;10(8):339-356.
24. Srivathsan KS, Bunch TJ, Asirvatham SJ, et al. Mechanisms and utility of discrete great arterial potentials in the ablation of outflow tract ventricular arrhythmias. *Circ Arrhythm Electrophysiol.* 2008;1(1):30-38.
25. Dixit S, Gerstenfeld EP, Callans DJ, Marchlinski FE. Electrocardiographic patterns of superior right ventricular outflow tract tachycardias: distinguishing septal and free-wall sites of origin. *J Cardiovasc Electrophysiol.* 2003;14(1):1-7.
26. Callans DJ, Menz V, Schwartzman D, Gottlieb CD, Marchlinski FE. Repetitive monomorphic tachycardia from the left ventricular outflow tract: electrocardiographic patterns consistent with a left ventricular site of origin. *J Am Coll Cardiol.* 1997;29(5):1023-1027.
27. Betensky BP, Park RE, Marchlinski FE, et al. The V(2) transition ratio: a new electrocardiographic criterion for distinguishing left from right ventricular outflow tract tachycardia origin. *J Am Coll Cardiol.* 2011;57(22):2255-2262.
28. Hynes BJ, Mart C, Artman S, Pu M, Naccarelli GV. Role of intracardiac ultrasound in interventional electrophysiology. *Curr Opin Cardiol.* 2004;19(1):52-57.
29. Kanagaratnam L, Tomassoni G, Schweikert R, et al. Ventricular tachycardias arising from the aortic sinus of valsalva: an under-recognized variant of left outflow tract ventricular tachycardia. *J Am Coll Cardiol.* 2001;37(5):1408-1414.
30. Ouyang F, Fotuhi P, Ho SY, et al. Repetitive monomorphic ventricular tachycardia originating from the aortic sinus cusp: electrocardiographic characterization for guiding catheter ablation. *J Am Coll Cardiol.* 2002;39(3):500-508.
31. Berruezo A, Mont L, Nava S, Chueca E, Bartholomay E, Brugada J. Electrocardiographic recognition of the epicardial origin of ventricular tachycardias. *Circulation.* 2004;109(15):1842-1847.
32. Baman TS, Ilg KJ, Gupta SK, et al. Mapping and ablation of epicardial idiopathic ventricular arrhythmias from within the coronary venous system. *Circulation.* 2010;3(3):274-279.
33. Daniels DV, Lu YY, Morton JB, et al. Idiopathic epicardial left ventricular tachycardia originating remote from the sinus of Valsalva: electrophysiological characteristics, catheter ablation, and identification from the 12-lead electrocardiogram. *Circulation.* 2006;113(13):1659-1666.
34. Morton JB, Kalman JM. Intracardiac echocardiographic anatomy for the interventional electrophysiologist. *J Interv Card Electrophysiol.* 2005;13 Suppl 1:11-16.
35. Asirvatham S, Narayan O. Advanced catheter mapping and navigation system. In: Huang S, Wood M, eds. *Catheter Ablation of Cardiac Arrhythmias.* Philadelphia, PA: Saunders/Elsevier; 2006:135-161.
36. Gurevitz OT, Glikson M, Asirvatham S, et al. Use of advanced mapping systems to guide ablation in complex cases: experience with noncontact mapping and electroanatomic mapping systems. *PACE.* 2005;28(4):316-323.
37. Dixit S, Callans DJ. Mapping for ventricular tachycardia. *Cardiac Electrophysiol Rev.* Nov 2002;6(4):436-441.
38. Stellbrink C, Diem B, Schauerte P, Ziegert K, Hanrath P. Transcoronary venous radiofrequency catheter ablation of ventricular tachycardia. *J Cardiovasc Electrophysiol.* 1997;8(8):916-921.
39. Obel OA, d'Avila A, Neuzil P, Saad EB, Ruskin JN, Reddy VY. Ablation of left ventricular epicardial outflow tract tachycardia from the distal great cardiac vein. *J Am Coll Cardiol.* 2006;48(9):1813-1817.
40. Sosa E, Scanavacca M, d'Avila A, Pilleggi F. A new technique to perform epicardial mapping in the electrophysiology laboratory. *J Cardiovasc Electrophysiol.* 1996;7(6):531-536.
41. Soejima K, Couper G, Cooper JM, Sapp JL, Epstein LM, Stevenson WG. Subxiphoid surgical approach for epicardial catheter-based mapping and ablation in patients with prior cardiac surgery or difficult pericardial access. *Circulation.* 2004;110(10):1197-1201.
42. Cohen HC, Gozo EG Jr, Pick A. Ventricular tachycardia with narrow QRS complexes (left posterior fascicular tachycardia). *Circulation.* 1972;45(5):1035-1043.
43. Zipes DP, Foster PR, Troup PJ, Pedersen DH. Atrial induction of ventricular tachycardia: reentry versus triggered automaticity. *Am J Cardiol.* 1979;44(1):1-8.
44. Belhassen B, Rotmensch HH, Laniado S. Response of recurrent sustained ventricular tachycardia to verapamil. *Br Heart J.* 1981;46(6):679-682.
45. Tsuchiya T, Okumura K, Honda T, et al. Significance of late diastolic potential preceding Purkinje potential in verapamil-sensitive idiopathic left ventricular tachycardia. *Circulation.* 1999;99(18):2408-2413.
46. Francis J, Venugopal K, Khadar SA, Sudhayakumar N, Gupta AK. Idiopathic fascicular ventricular tachycardia. *Indian Pacing Electrophysiol J.* 2004;4(3):98-103.
47. Aiba T, Suyama K, Aihara N, et al. The role of Purkinje and pre-Purkinje potentials in the reentrant circuit of verapamil-sensitive idiopathic LV tachycardia. *PACE.* 2001;24(3):333-344.

48. Nakagawa H, Beckman KJ, McClelland JH, et al. Radiofrequency catheter ablation of idiopathic left ventricular tachycardia guided by a Purkinje potential. *Circulation.* 1993;88(6):2607-2617.
49. Nogami A, Naito S, Tada H, et al. Verapamil-sensitive left anterior fascicular ventricular tachycardia: results of radiofrequency ablation in six patients. *J Cardiovasc Electrophysiol.* 1998;9(12):1269-1278.
50. Nogami A, Naito S, Tada H, et al. Demonstration of diastolic and presystolic Purkinje potentials as critical potentials in a macroreentry circuit of verapamil-sensitive idiopathic left ventricular tachycardia. *J Am Coll Cardiol.* 2000;36(3):811-823.
51. Chen M, Yang B, Zou J, et al. Non-contact mapping and linear ablation of the left posterior fascicle during sinus rhythm in the treatment of idiopathic left ventricular tachycardia. *Europace.* 2005;7(2):138-144.
52. Ouyang F, Cappato R, Ernst S, et al. Electroanatomic substrate of idiopathic left ventricular tachycardia: unidirectional block and macroreentry within the Purkinje network. *Circulation.* 2002;105(4):462-469.
53. Lin D, Ilkhanoff L, Gerstenfeld E, et al. Twelve-lead electrocardiographic characteristics of the aortic cusp region guided by intracardiac echocardiography and electroanatomic mapping. *Heart Rhythm.* 2008;5(5):663-669.
54. Crawford T, Mueller G, Good E, et al. Ventricular arrhythmias originating from papillary muscles in the right ventricle. *Heart Rhythm.* 2010;7(6):725-730.
55. Kurosawa H, Becker AE. Dead-end tract of the conduction axis. *Int J Cardiol.* 1985;7(1):13-20.
56. Badhwar N, Scheinman MM. Idiopathic ventricular tachycardia: diagnosis and management. *Curr Problems Cardiol.* 2007;32(1):7-43.
57. Sacher F, Tedrow UB, Field ME, et al. Ventricular tachycardia ablation: evolution of patients and procedures over 8 years. *Circ Arrhythm Electrophysiol.* 2008;1(3):153-161.
58. Asirvatham SJ, Bruce CJ, Friedman PA. Advances in imaging for cardiac electrophysiology. *Coronary Artery Dis.* 2003;14(1):3-13.
59. Asirvatham S. Anatomy of the coronary sinus. In: Yu CM, Auricchio HD, eds. *Cardiac Resynchronization Therapy.* Oxford: Blackwell/Futura; 2006:211-238.
60. Lachman N, Syed FF, Habib A, et al. Correlative anatomy for the electrophysiologist, Part II: cardiac ganglia, phrenic nerve, coronary venous system. *J Cardiovasc Electrophysiol.* 2011;22(1):104-110.
61. Haïssaguerre M, Shah DC, Jaïs P, et al. Role of Purkinje conducting system in triggering of idiopathic ventricular fibrillation. *Lancet.* 2002;359(9307):677-678.
62. Haines DE. The biophysics of radiofrequency catheter ablation in the heart: the importance of temperature monitoring. *PACE.* 1993;16(3 Pt 2):586-591.
63. Nath S, Haines DE. Biophysics and pathology of catheter energy delivery systems. *Progress Cardiovasc Dis.* 1995;37(4):185-204.

CHAPTER 44

Ventricular Tachycardia with Ischemic and Nonischemic Heart Disease

William W.B. Chik, MBBS, MD, PhD; Ioan Liuba, MD, PhD;
Pasquale Santangeli, MD, PhD; Francis E. Marchlinski, MD

Introduction

Catheter ablation has emerged as an important therapeutic option for patients with ventricular tachycardia (VT) to reduce or prevent shocks from implantable cardioverter-defibrillators (ICDs).[1,2] Although ICDs reduce sudden cardiac death and improve survival, they are not a cure and do not prevent recurrences of ventricular tachyarrhythmias and shocks associated with significant morbidity.[1,3] Considerable evolution of ablation techniques followed pioneering studies establishing the reentrant mechanism of postinfarction scar-related VT circuits.[4,5] The success of obliterating the underlying substrate harboring surviving channels of myocardial bundles within dense infarct scar and border zone by surgical resection of the endocardium and subendocardium led to initial attempts of radiofrequency (RF) ablation therapy postinfarction.[6] This chapter will review our present approach to catheter ablation of VT in ischemic and nonischemic heart disease, its implications on ablation procedural techniques, and endpoints.

Anatomic and Electrophysiologic Substrate

Ventricular Tachycardia in Ischemic Cardiomyopathy

Sustained VT in patients with coronary artery disease (CAD) is almost always associated with previous myocardial infarction (MI).[7] The time interval between infarction and the first episode of VT can range between days and more than 30 years. The anatomic substrate consists of bundles of surviving myocardial fibers embedded in fibrotic tissue. Fibrosis distorts the tissue architecture and reduces the intercellular coupling promoting heterogeneous slow conduction and unidirectional block, which increases the propensity to reentrant arrhythmias. In addition to fibrosis, the remodeling of the connexin and ion channel expression and distribution also contributes to the arrhythmogenicity.

Ventricular Tachycardia in Nonischemic Cardiomyopathy

Myocardial fibrosis also exists in patients with nonischemic cardiomyopathy (NICM). Necropsy studies in patients with idiopathic dilated cardiomyopathy (IDCM) showed grossly visible scars in 14% of patients, whereas histological examination revealed multiple patchy areas of replacement fibrosis in 35% and 57% of sectioned right and left ventricles, respectively.[8] Hypertrophied and atrophic myocytes, myofiber disarray, nuclear changes, and cytoskeletal disorganization were also observed.[9] Consistent with pathologic findings, gadolinium-enhanced cardiac magnetic resonance imaging (MRI) detects fibrosis in 40%–50% of patients with IDCM.[10,11] Similar findings have been reported in other NICMs. Myocyte loss with replacement by fibrofatty tissue, extending from epicardial or intramural layers then progressing to the endocardium, have been reported in arrhythmogenic right ventricular cardiomyopathy (ARVC).[12] The structural abnormalities are more pronounced in the right ventricle (RV), but the left ventricle (LV) was also involved in up to 76% of cases.[13-15] Patients with sarcoidosis and Chagas disease initially demonstrate inflammatory infiltrates and variable degrees of myocyte damage, later replaced by fibrous scars.[16] Interstitial and replacement fibrosis have also been reported in patients with hypertrophic cardiomyopathy (HCM).[17,18] As in the setting of CAD, the deposition of collagen tissue in patients with NICM increases the likelihood of reentrant VT. In a minority of cases, monomorphic VTs are due to bundle branch reentry.

It is important to stress that the distribution of fibrosis in patients with NICM is different than that reported for patients with CAD. Nonischemic scars are smaller and less well circumscribed than following MI (Figure 44.1). In addition, the scars in NICM are distributed predominantly intramurally or subepicardially,[19,20] typically located in the basal lateral areas of the LV and in the interventricular septum.[21,22] These features have important consequence for mapping and ablation strategy, as will be discussed.

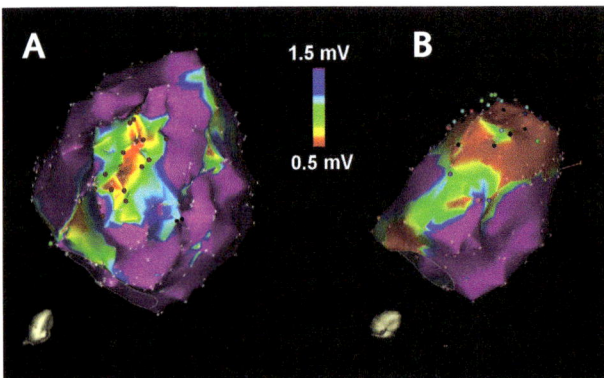

Figure 44.1 Inferior projections of the voltage map of the LV in a patient with idiopathic cardiomyopathy (**Panel A**) and a patient with prior MI (**Panel B**). Both patients had scars in the inferior wall. However, the scar in the patient with NICM was smaller and patchier.

Ablation Techniques and Endpoints

Patient Selection

According to the current guidelines,[23] catheter ablation is generally recommended in patients with recurrent monomorphic VTs, including VTs requiring frequent ICD shocks for termination of incessant VT. The need of complete withdrawal or reduction of antiarrhythmic medications due to undesirable side effects may necessitate ablation. Of note, most patients with NICM and VT qualify for ICD therapy based on either primary or secondary prevention criteria for sudden cardiac death. Therefore, as in the setting of CAD, ablation does not remove the need for an ICD, as the risk of recurrence after VT ablation due to the progression of the cardiomyopathic process exists.[24]

Preprocedural Assessment

As previously detailed in earlier chapters, thorough assessment of the existing arrhythmia substrate should be performed prior to ablation. The 12-lead ECG is scrutinized for evidence of advanced atrioventricular (block suggesting involvement of the interventricular septum in the disease process; a left bundle branch block indicates septal or a more generalized involvement of the LV).[25] The 12-lead ECG of all spontaneous VTs should be sought whenever possible in order to regionalize the origin of VT and to look for specific features suggesting a possible epicardial exit for the VT as will be detailed in the following paragraphs. When 12-lead ECG of the VT is not available, analysis of the VT morphology in stored device electrograms (EGMs) for patients with ICDs can help differentiate between "clinical" and "nonclinical" VTs (different VTs are often associated with different EGM morphologies) and the identification of exit sites for clinical VTs during pace mapping.[26]

Baseline transthoracic echocardiography (TEE) is performed to assess the LV size and function. In addition, concomitant valvular disease such as aortic stenosis (retrograde transaortic access) and other cardiomyopathic processes should be assessed. In patients with concomitant atrial fibrillation who have not been anticoagulated, intracardiac echocardiography (ICE) or contrast enhanced echocardiography can be helpful to exclude the presence of LV thrombus.

Cardiac MRI is routinely performed in our center, even in patients with implanted devices to assess the extent, distribution, and transmurality of myocardial fibrosis. Extensive intramural and/or epicardial fibrosis increase the likelihood of VT originating in regions remote from endocardium and consideration for epicardial mapping and ablation.

Coronary arterial anatomy and potential risk for ischemia should be assessed in most patients before ablation with functional noninvasive imaging and/or coronary angiography. Preventable procedure-related mortality is often due to inadequate assessments of underlying ischemic burden and excessive volume overload during prolonged ablation procedures.[27]

Anesthesia and Hemodynamic Support

General anesthesia is associated with hypotension and may inhibit VT inducibility.[28] Conscious sedation is therefore preferred at the beginning of the ablation procedure. However, if hemodynamically unstable VTs are anticipated with multiple cardioversions, general anesthesia may be necessary at the outset. The presence of advanced underlying structural heart disease in patients with inducible scar-related VT could severely compromise intraoperative cardiac output. The use of inotropes for hemodynamic support in this setting may be at the cost of increased myocardial oxygen consumption and reduction in cardiac perfusion to vital organs. Hemodynamic monitoring of filling pressure and early proactive hemodynamic support strategies are of critical importance, especially in the context of an additional large saline load imposed by the use of external irrigated-tip catheters. For patients with advanced cardiomyopathies and decompensated heart failure, early deployment of mechanical circulatory support devices including percutaneous insertion of intra-aortic balloon pump (IABP), left ventricular assist devices (LVAD) (ie, TandemHeart®, CardiacAssist, Inc., Pittsburgh, PA; and Impella®, ABIOMED, Danvers, MA) to facilitate adequate mapping of potentially hemodynamically unstable VT should be considered.

Approach to Ablation and Mapping of Ischemic Ventricular Tachycardia

The fundamental concept underpinning VT ablation is to perform detailed mapping to accurately define the VT circuit and the underlying arrhythmogenic substrate with the goal of optimizing RF ablation application. The primary focus of the mapping strategy is inherently dependent on the arrhythmia presentation: (1) activation and entrainment mapping for hemodynamically *stable* VT; (2) substrate mapping for hemodynamically *unstable* VT.

Activation and Entrainment Mapping

In patients with hemodynamically tolerated VT, activation and entrainment mapping are used with the goal of identifying the critical slowly conducting channels that maintain reentry circuits. Anistropic conduction in surviving channels of muscle bundles located within the scar creates the slow conduction responsible for reentrant VT.[4,29,30] Isthmus sites bound by more dense fibrosis or valve annuli can be characterized by activation mapping and entrainment maneuvers in hemodynamically stable VT.[5] In reentrant VT, mid-diastolic signals suggest recordings from critical components during continuous circuit activation that may be amenable to limited ablation for VT elimination.[31] In contrast for focal VT, earliest activation is generally 10–60 ms preceding the surface QRS complex.[32] Corridors of slow conduction within scar characteristic of a reentrant VT isthmus are marked by isolated high-frequency, low-amplitude electrograms recorded during mid-diastole. Occasionally, the signals are characterized by low-amplitude fragmented electrograms spanning all of diastole.[33,34]

Entrainment mapping by pacing at rates just shorter than the tachycardia cycle length (CL) confirms the presence of a reentrant circuit when a fixed relationship with the subsequent but not the preceding QRS complex is seen. Entrainment criteria consistent with a critical VT isthmus as opposed to bystander sites when pacing at sites of diastolic activation during VT include: (1) demonstration of fixed concealed QRS fusion during continuous pacing with QRS during pacing matching that of the VT; (2) stimulus to QRS interval (stim-QRS) within 30 ms of local electrogram to QRS (EGM-QRS) interval; and (3) return CL (postpacing interval, PPI) within 30 ms of the tachycardia CL[15,35] (Figure 44.2). In addition, ablation at sites demonstrating a stim-QRS interval < 70% of the VT CL is more likely to be successful in perturbing the tachycardia consistent with pacing within the isthmus (Table 44.1). In ischemic VT, RF energy delivery at sites satisfying the above entrainment criteria often terminates the tachycardia within 20–30 seconds of ablation.[36,37] Possible mechanisms for failure

Table 44.1 Targets for VT ablation

Entrainment mapping strategy: Ideal target sites are within the infarct zone (bipolar voltage < 0.5 mV) and during VT have components inscribed early in diastole (< 70% of the VT cycle length before the onset of the QRS).
Pacing "entrainment mapping" from these target sites results in the following:
• Concealed entrainment with pacing during VT
• PPI = VT cycle length ± 30 ms
• Stimulus-QRS interval during pacing = electrogram − QRS during VT ± 20 ms
Substrate mapping strategy: "Anchor points" for linear lesions are determined by pace mapping to match VT morphologies in the infarct border zone. Linear ablation is applied through these anchor points from the dense scar (< 0.5 mV) to normal tissue (> 1.5 mV) or to an anatomic barrier. Also target in sinus rhythm:
• Slow conduction areas as indexed by multicomponent fractionated signals
• Sites with stimulus-QRS interval > 40–70 ms during pace mapping
• Sites showing QRS morphology 12/12 match for VT with pace map
• Late potentials
• Channels of excitable abnormal substrate separated by unexcitable abnormal substrate
• Channels of higher voltage surrounded by lower voltage between or within dense scar
Mapping triggers for PMVT: Pace mapping at sites to match the surface ECG morphology of trigger beats. Sites typically display early Purkinje activation, both in sinus rhythm and during trigger PVCs.

to interrupt the tachycardia circuit may include: (1) inability to deliver effective lesions due to poor electrode tip–tissue contact or insufficient power and/or duration to achieve sufficient lesion depth (particularly if circuits are maintained by intramural or mid-myocardial scar within the interventricular septum); (2) broad isthmus requiring more extensive ablation; and (3) erroneous interpretation of the isthmus location due to incomplete/inaccurate mapping[38] (Table 44.2).

Substrate Mapping

Detailed activation and entrainment mapping cannot be used in VT associated with hemodynamic instability, unreliable inducibility, spontaneous termination of non-sustained runs, and nonuniform cycle lengths and/or morphologies during attempts at entrainment mapping. Multiple recent trials indicate that only one-third of patients have exclusively mappable VT circuits.[1] For postinfarction VT, 31% had unmappable VT and 38% had both mappable and unmappable VT.[1,39] Similarly, in patients with NICM, less than 50% of induced VT was hemodynamically stable and amenable to entrainment mapping. When entrainment mapping is not feasible, an alternative strategy to identify the sinus rhythm or pace mapping footprints of the VT circuit is necessary.

We first described the concept of substrate mapping in sinus rhythm to target the footprints of VT within the scar defined by voltage mapping in 2000.[33] The initial ablation strategy was modeled after the surgical subendocardial scar resection, which prevented VT recurrence in > 90% of patients.[40] Electroanatomic mapping utilized magnetic field-based or electrical impedance-based triangulation of a catheter's location in three-dimensional space to create color-coded voltage maps in sinus rhythm as the catheter roves and records electrical signals within a cardiac chamber. We initially demonstrated that in patients without structural heart disease, 95% of bipolar electrograms recorded during endocardial mapping in sinus rhythm have a voltage amplitude > 1.5 mV.[33] We therefore defined abnormal endocardium as contiguous electrograms with bipolar voltage < 1.5 mV. Dense scar was arbitrarily defined as regions with a bipolar voltage of < 0.5 mV, whereas the border zone between dense scar and healthy myocardium is identified as the area with a voltage between 0.5 mV and 1.5 mV[33] (Figure 44.1). Dense scar has also been identified on the basis of electrical unexcitability during high-output pacing.[41] Verma et al[42] and Hsia et al[30] showed that most isthmus regions of the VT circuit in patients with post-myocardial infarction VT are located in the dense scar (< 0.5 mV), whereas exit sites from the VT circuit are situated in the border zone as the VT circuit leaves the scar and engages normal myocardium. Once the myocardial scar has been accurately identified, ablation targets within the scar are chosen based upon identification of (1) channels, (2) sites of good pace maps associated with long stim-QRS times, and (3) locations of abnormal electrogram morphologies (fractionated electrograms or, more importantly, electrograms with late components inscribed to sinus QRS) (Table 44.1).

12-lead ECG Analysis of VT to Identify VT Exit

The QRS morphology during VT is determined by ventricular geometry and activation pattern. The exit site of a macroreentrant isthmus in reentrant VT can be deduced from the QRS complex. A left bundle branch block (LBBB) pattern suggests VT exiting from the interventricular septum or right ventricle. Right bundle branch block (RBBB) pattern indicates a left ventricular free-wall exit. A narrow QRS complex typically originates from a septal exit site. Positive precordial concordance is consistent with a basal origin, whereas negative concordance defines an apical origin. Frontal (superoinferior) axial

Table 44.2 Troubleshooting the difficult case

Problem	Causes	Solution
Unmappable VT Poor hemodynamic stability during VT Noninducible	Ventricular dysfunction Autonomically or ischemically mediated	Slow VT rate with drugs, support BP with atrial pacing, pressors, balloon pump, mechanical circulatory support devices Noncontact mapping, substrate mapping, optimize filling pressures Programmed stimulation on dopamine or isoproterenol, substrate mapping during sinus rhythm, linear ablation
Ineffective radiofrequency RF delivery	Small lesion size Poor catheter contact Low current delivery Wide isthmus Wrong site Misdiagnosis	Improve contact by changing catheter reach, change approach (transseptal from retrograde aortic) Longer duration irrigated radiofrequency RF ablation Linear lesion or lesion cluster to block wide isthmus Continue mapping to better define circuit Consider bundle branch or fascicular reentry
Diffuse area of early activation	Intramural or epicardial site of origin	Transcutaneous pericardial approach for epicardial mapping, map right ventricular septum

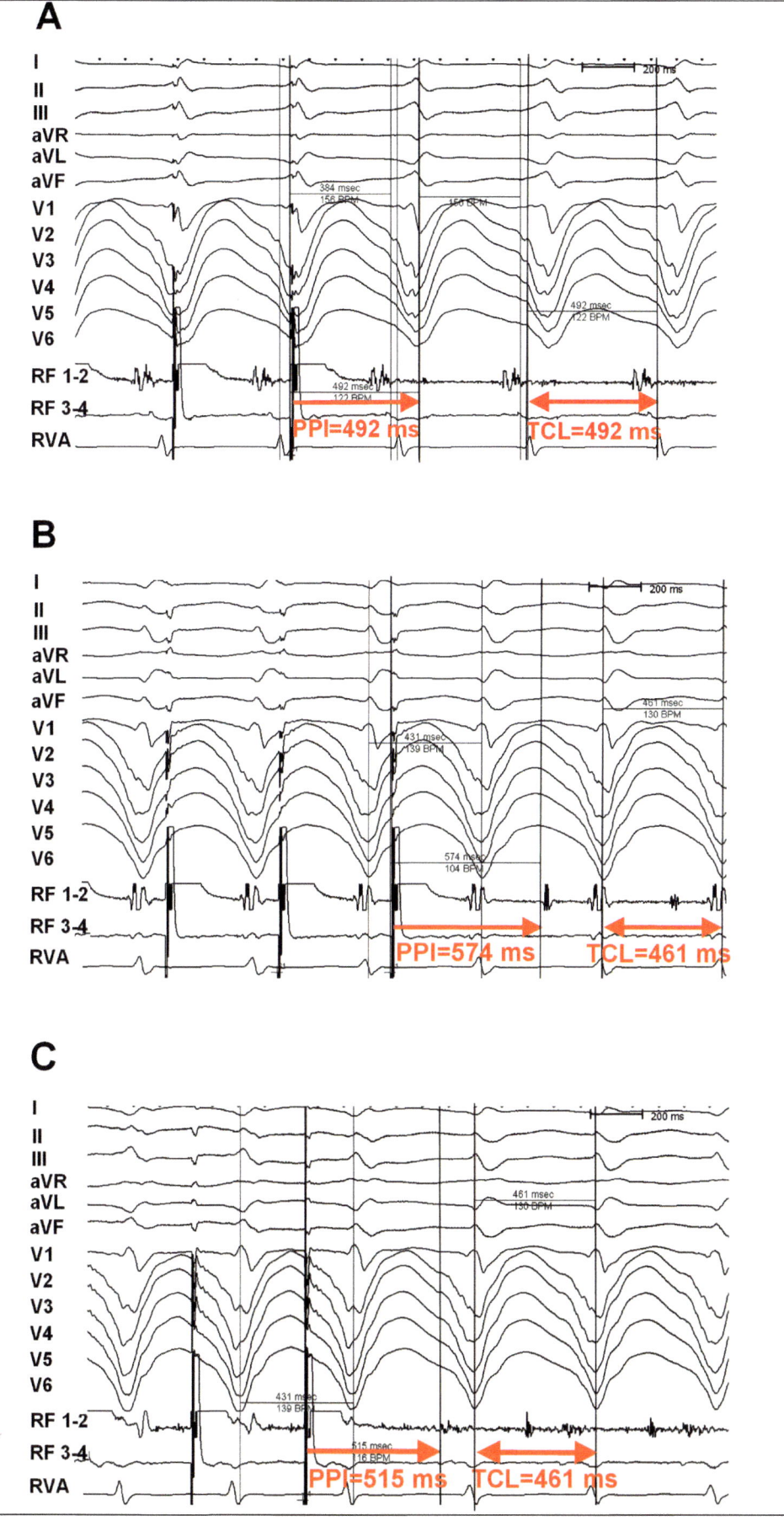

Figure 44.2 Panel **A:** Entrainment during postmyocardial infarction VT from the critical isthmus. The QRS morphology during pacing was identical to the one during tachycardia (concealed fusion). A long stimulus-QRS was consistent with pacing at the entrance of the isthmus. The local potential (**arrow**) was the last component of a long-duration, multicomponent EGM. The postpacing interval (PPI) was measured from the stimulus artifact to this local potential. The first component, which was larger in amplitude, was accelerated at the pacing rate during entrainment, suggesting a far-field recording. The PPI (492 ms) equaled the tachycardia cycle length (TCL). Collectively, these findings indicated that the pacing is done from a protected isthmus. **Panel B:** Concealed fusion during entrainment from a site demonstrating a double potential. The first potential was accelerated to the pacing CL, indicating far-field activity and that the sharp component represents local activity. The much longer PPI than TCL with the presence of concealed fusion suggested a bystander pathway. **Panel C:** Entrainment with manifest fusion (seen mostly in the precordial leads) with PPI that was longer than TCL, consistent with pacing from a site remote from the reentrant circuit.

plane examination provides useful clues for a superior exit in an inferiorly directed VT (positive QRS in inferior leads), while an inferior exit correlates with a superiorly directed VT (negative QRS inferiorly). The exit is frequently regionalized to scar border zone (0.5–1.5 mV).

Pace Mapping during Sinus Rhythm

Pace mapping in sinus rhythm attempts to replicate the 12-lead surface QRS morphology of the VT by delivering threshold pacing stimulus from various pacing sites. Sites of good 12-lead pace map morphology match in a scar-related reentrant circuit, with short stimulus to QRS interval identifying VT exit sites from scar.[43] A long stimulus-QRS time during pace mapping provide valuable additional clues to identify slowly conducting channels consistent with stimulation from a VT isthmus area.[44] In the setting of idiopathic VT with a homogenous myocardium without significant fibrosis, paced point source breakout in mapping can be particularly helpful in locating the focal generation of a wavefront during VT.

Pace mapping ECG is assessed with regard to both degree of concordance between paced QRS and clinical VT QRS and the stimulus-QRS interval (Figure 44.3). At sites in close proximity to the origin of VT, the paced QRS morphology is expected to mimic that of the VT. A long stimulus-QRS suggests proximity to regions of slow conduction and increases the likelihood that the pacing site is close to the reentrant circuit.[45] It should be noted, however, that the 1.5 mV bipolar voltage cutoff is a statistical definition of abnormal, with 95% of endocardial signals having that amplitude. The 1.5 mV cutoff has not been validated with pathological analysis or MRI imaging in patients with NICM.

Late Potential Mapping

Tagging of sites with abnormal fractionated EGM and EGM with split or late potentials is highly specific (albeit less sensitive) for unmasking VT circuits.[46,47] In patients with postinfarction VT, the majority of confirmed isthmuses are expected to demonstrate isolated late potentials in sinus rhythm.[48] However, late potentials are less frequently encountered in the setting of NICM compared with coronary artery disease.[49] This finding may be due to the fact that functional regions of conduction block have a more important role than areas of fixed scar in the mechanism of rapid NICM VT or VF compared to ischemic VT.

Localizing Conducting Channels

Identification of relatively higher voltage "channels" within a scar can be identified on electroanatomic mapping (EAM) by lowering the usual bipolar voltage cutoff for scar (< 1.5 mV) to pinpoint regions of preserved

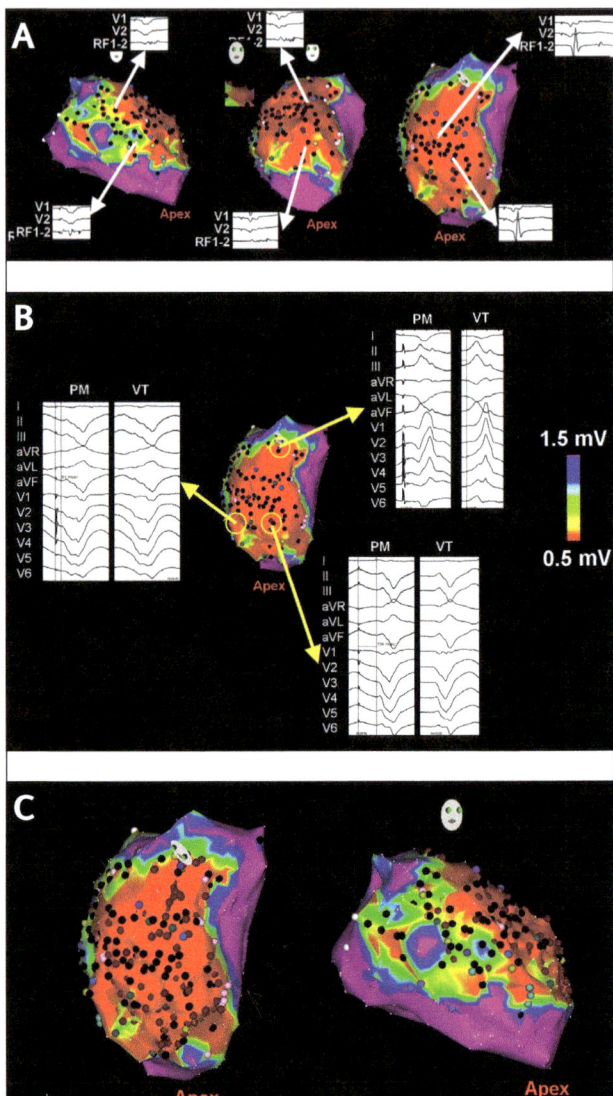

Figure 44.3 **Panel A:** RAO, AP, and superior projections of the left ventricle voltage maps in a patient with anteroseptal MI and apical aneurysm. A large area of scar involving the anterolateral wall and the interventricular septum was present. Clusters of fractionated EGMs and late potentials were noted. **Panel B:** Different VTs were induced and mapped to the apical, septal, and basal aspects of the scar. The paced QRS (PM) and QRS during VT were compared at the 3 locations. **Purple** corresponded to areas of normal voltage (> 1.5 mV) or healthy myocardium and **red** indicated dense scar (< 0.5 mV). The border zone was depicted in **rainbow colors**. **Panel C:** The final lesion set with ablations (**brown dots**) targeted the exit sites of the VT and abnormal EGMs.

voltage within the denser scar.[30,50] Not all channels are specific for the protected VT isthmus. Identification of voltage channels that also harbor isolated late potentials (ILPs) during sinus rhythm mapping may be more specific for clinical VT isthmus sites.[51] Targeting critical clinical VT isthmus associated with late potentials may be a more successful approach than extensive empiric ablation of all identified channels, especially in poorly tolerated or noninducible VTs. Putative intra-isthmus and exit sites by substrate mapping can be confirmed to be in the reentrant circuit by limited activation mapping and entrainment.

Radiofrequency Ablation Techniques for Ischemic Ventricular Tachycardia

After the characterization of the arrhythmogenic substrate, ablation is performed during VT, if VT is tolerated, or during sinus rhythm if VT is poorly tolerated. As discussed previously, ablation at isthmus sites identified by entrainment during VT typically terminates VT within 20–30 seconds, thereby confirming that the target site is a critical part of the reentrant circuit. Additional RF application is usually applied surrounding the initial successful target site. At our institution, ICE is routinely utilized to ensure adequate catheter tip–tissue contact during RF applications. If no termination of VT occurs despite 30 seconds or more of RF ablation, energy delivery is typically discontinued to minimize the likelihood of ablating noncritical areas of the surviving myocardium and worsening of LV impairment. Additional activation and entrainment mapping is typically performed to determine whether a broad isthmus is present that may require multiple or linear lesions.

For poorly tolerated VTs, linear RF lesions are placed transecting low-voltage regions and extending from the dense scar to healthy myocardium or connecting to anatomic boundaries. Linear lesions may be placed along the scar border to interrupt VT exit sites or cross through channels. In addition, clusters of lesions can be created at regions displaying fractionated electrograms and late potentials (Figure 44.3). This approach usually results in extensive ablation and substrate modification.

Open-irrigated RF electrode catheters enable greater power delivery, resulting in greater lesion size and deeper penetration in myocardial scar while reducing the incidence of coagulum and thrombus formation.[52] Internal irrigation catheters may be considered in patients with severely decompensated heart failure where intravascular volume expansion is poorly tolerated. The conventional 3.5 mm electrode tip is preferred to the large 8 mm tip as it preserves spatial resolution during mapping over small channels of surviving tissue within large regions of scar and reduces the gradient in temperature across the electrode tip surface, which could be a nidus for coagulum formation. For endocardial ablation, we generally use irrigated-tip ablation catheters with power between 30 W and 50 W and maximum temperature of 42–45°C. An impedance drop of ~10% or ~12–18 ohm during 60–120 seconds of energy application is targeted. In regions of mid-myocardial or intraseptal scars, longer lesions of 120–240 seconds were delivered. RF is ceased if a sudden drop in impedance occurs or if impedance rises by greater than 10, suggesting either thrombus and/or steam pops or catheter instability, to avoid complications.

Ablation Endpoints for Ischemic Ventricular Tachycardia

Termination of scar-related VT during RF energy delivery at effective target sites can be gratifying, but acute success of the procedure should ideally be assessed by endpoints that are widely accepted, clearly defined, and reliably reproducible, and possess predictive value for long-term outcomes. Noninducibility of VT by programmed electrical stimulation (PES) at end of procedure has been traditionally used to define acute success.[23] This can be subclassified into (1) noninducibility of all clinical VTs, (2) modification of induced VT CL ≥ clinical VT CL, and (3) noninducibility of all VTs.[23] When clinical VT (defined as induced VT with the same 12-lead ECG QRS morphology and CL as spontaneous VT) or presumed clinical VTs have been documented and can be induced at the onset of ablation, noninducibility on PES immediately postprocedure should represent the minimum endpoint of ablation procedures as this confers a lower risk (up to 37%) of recurrence compared with persistently inducible clinical VT (up to 80%).[53,54] In contrast, induction of faster "nonclinical" VT did not impact negatively on subsequent spontaneous recurrences.[55] Standardized PES protocol may be composed of up to 3 extrastimuli delivered from at least 2 ventricular sites (including LV) with the shortest coupling intervals of 180–200 ms or to refractoriness.[23] If VT induction initially required additional pacing sites or catecholamine infusion, these should be repeated following ablation. In the multicenter Cooled RF study, Calkins and colleagues affirmed that 89% of patients with ≥1 clinical VT still inducible postablation had a fourfold increased risk of failure.[56] Della Bella et al demonstrated in a single-center study that ablation of clinical VT (but not all inducible VT) significantly reduced the incidence of VT storm and cardiac mortality, notwithstanding a higher likelihood of recurrent sporadic VT.[54]

VT modification is defined as noninducibility of all clinical VT, but multiple other monomorphic VTs (MMVTs) remain inducible. For patients without 12-lead ECG documentation or VT morphologies inferred from limited telemetry and/or ICD stored EGMs, a strategy to abolish VTs with a slower CL than the clinical have led to a lower risk of recurrent VT.[57,58] This is further supported by 2 multicenter studies, THERMOCOOL® VT Ablation Trial[1] and Euro-VT-Study,[59] which showed that induction of only VT more rapid than the clinical VT did not predict a higher risk of VT recurrence. Noninducibility of any VT is known to be associated with a lower recurrence rate in single-center studies.[54,60] Conversely, induction of any VT confers a twofold increased risk of recurrence.[1] However, for unstable patients with incessant VT (VT storm), a reasonable clinical endpoint may be restoration of stable sinus rhythm and reduction of ICD shocks, irrespective of VT inducibility on PES. Furthermore, postablation PES should be avoided in hemodynamically unstable patients with substantial ischemic burden at risk to cardiopulmonary deterioration.[23] Frankel and colleagues[61] suggested that postablation PES may not be feasible or fail to predict VT recurrences due to a combination of factors including patient's hemodynamic instability following a prolonged procedure, alteration in autonomic tone, level of sedation/general anesthesia, subsequent changes/cessation of antiarrhythmic medications, and evolution (microcirculatory changes) or regression (healing and resolution of edema) of ablation lesion sets over time.[61] Hence, Frankel et al utilized noninvasive programmed stimulation (NIPS) performed (via the patients' existing ICD) in patients who did not have inducible clinical VT or spontaneous VT recurrence in the week following the ablation procedure. They found that inducibility of clinical VT at NIPS identified a group of patients at high risk of recurrence in whom further treatment may be warranted to avoid ICD shocks and reduce mortality. Furthermore, noninducibility of clinical VT at NIPS allows accurate prediction of likely VT-free survival at 12 months.[61]

Outcomes of Ischemic Ventricular Tachycardia Ablation

Multiple studies have demonstrated the benefit of catheter ablation in postinfarct recurrent drug-refractory VT patients.[1,36,53,56,62-64] The benefit of an earlier intervention with catheter ablation has also been evaluated in 3 recent randomized trials.[2,65,66] The Substrate Mapping and Ablation in Sinus Rhythm to Halt Ventricular Tachycardia (SMASH-VT) trial was a multicenter, randomized trial including patients undergoing ICD implantation for secondary prevention of sudden cardiac death.[2] A total of 128 patients were randomized to catheter ablation or optimal medical therapy; of note, antiarrhythmic drugs were not allowed in the control arm of this trial. At the end of 2-year follow-up, appropriate ICD intervention due to recurrent sustained VT occurred in 12% of patients in the ablation group and 33% of those in the control group (HR = 0.35, 95% CI 0.15 to 0.78, $P = 0.007$). The multicenter Catheter Ablation of Stable Ventricular Tachycardia before Defibrillator Implantation in Patients with Coronary Artery Disease (VTACH) trial was a randomized trial of catheter ablation versus standard medical therapy focused on patients with previous MI and reduced LV ejection fraction (ie, $\leq 50\%$) undergoing secondary-prevention ICD implant due to a documented episode of hemodynamically tolerated sustained VT.[65] After a mean follow-up of 22.5 ± 9 months, patients allocated to catheter ablation had significantly longer time to arrhythmia recurrence compared to those randomized to ICD only, and lower 2-year VT recurrence rates (53% vs 71%, HR = 0.61, 95% CI 0.37 to 0.99, $P = 0.045$). In a recent indirect comparison meta-analysis, Santangeli et al have quantitatively evaluated whether early intervention with catheter ablation might improve the arrhythmia-free survival compared to a "delayed" intervention after having failed antiarrhythmic drug therapy.[67] Remarkably, this pooled analysis failed to disclose a difference in long-term success rates between the 2 ablation strategies, with an odds ratio for VT-free survival (early vs delayed VT ablation) of 1.28 (95% CI 0.53 to 3.09, $P = 0.58$). In addition, the 2 strategies appeared substantially equivalent in terms of mortality benefit.[67] It is important to emphasize that all of the above studies adopted a limited substrate-based ablation approach aimed at targeting predominantly the clinical VT(s). Recent evidence supports a more extensive substrate-based approach, aimed at abolishing all the potential VT circuits within the scar, which might translate to a striking improvement in VT-free survival compared to classical limited substrate ablation.[68-70] In a prospective multicenter study, Di Biase et al assessed the value of an extensive endo-epicardial substrate modification, so-called "scar homogenization" strategy, versus a more limited substrate-based ablation in a series of 92 patients with postinfarct VT storm.[68] After a mean follow-up of 25 ± 10 months, the VT recurrence rate was 47% in patients who underwent limited substrate ablation versus 19% in patients who underwent endo-epicardial scar homogenization. Jaïs et al[69] reported a VT recurrence rate of 32% when abnormal high-frequency sharp signals indicative of abnormal local electrical activity (LAVA) were targeted for ablation, versus 75% without LAVA elimination at a median follow-up of 22 months. These recent studies support the concept that an extensive substrate-based ablation targeting not only the clinical VT(s) but also all the other potential arrhythmogenic areas within the scar is important to increase the long-term VT-free survival.

Ablation Endpoints for Nonischemic Cardiomyopathies

In a recent study on 45 patients with NICM and VT, Piers et al[71] showed that noninducibility of any VT after ablation (defined as complete procedural success) was associated with an 18% VT recurrence rate during a mean follow-up period of 25 months. In contrast, partial success (noninducibility of clinical VTs with persistent inducibility of nonclinical VTs) and failure (persistent inducibility of clinical VTs) was associated with 77% and 73% recurrence rates, respectively. These data suggest that partial procedural success is not superior to failure and that complete noninducibility should be pursued whenever possible. However, this endpoint is more difficult to achieve in patients with NICM. Other endpoints used in our institution are inability to capture at high-pacing output at sites targeted by ablation, change in the paced QRS morphology after ablation as compared to preablation, and elimination of late potentials within the scar.

Epicardial Mapping and Ablation

Approximately 30% of patients with VT in the setting of NICM require transcutaneous epicardial mapping and ablation.[24] This is consistent with MRI studies reporting that scars in patients with NICM are more often intramural and/or subepicardial.[19] In ischemic VT, epicardial circuits are more common in inferior infarcts.[72] The clues suggesting a need for epicardial mapping and ablation include (1) the absence of a sizable area of endocardial bipolar-voltage abnormality and the presence of large regions of endocardial unipolar abnormality, defined as confluent regions of unipolar voltage < 8.3 mV in LV and < 5.5 mV in RV (Figures 44.4 and 44.5);[73] (2) distinctive 12-lead ECG features during VT (presence of Q waves and QS complexes in lead I and inferior leads);[74-76] and (3) failed prior endocardial ablations. ICE may also identify the nonendocardial substrates as areas of increased echogenicity.[77]

Epicardial access is obtained using the technique described by Sosa et al.[78] This technique is discussed in detail in Chapter 45. In patients who had undergone endocardial ablation in the same procedure or on chronic warfarin, anticoagulation is commonly interrupted and reversed. After access to the pericardial space is confirmed, a short sheath is advanced with the dilator over the guidewire followed by insertion of the ablation catheter. During epicardial mapping, bipolar electrogram voltage of < 1 mV are considered abnormal consistent with the presence of scar. However, apart from low-voltage amplitude, true epicardial scars demonstrate a high incidence of fractionated electrograms and late potentials.[79] Ablation follows the same principles outlined above. Finally, caution should be exercised to avoid phrenic nerve and coronary artery injury during epicardial ablation. High-output pacing from the intended site of ablation to identify phrenic nerve and coronary angiograms to look for major coronary arteries located within 10 mm of the selected ablation site may be undertaken. When necessary, the phrenic nerve can be displaced away from the epicardium by inflating a balloon in the pericardial space or by introducing an air/saline mix until phrenic nerve capture is lost or until the blood pressure begins to drop because of cardiac compression.[80]

Immediate Postprocedural Care

Following catheter ablation, protamine is administered to reverse anticoagulation and the sheaths can be pulled out once the activated clotting time is less than 180 seconds. Anticoagulation with heparin is resumed 6 hours after the sheath removal and is continued for 24–48 hours. If the patient does not have indication for long-term anticoagulation, aspirin is administered for 6 weeks.

Once epicardial ablation has been performed, intrapericardial corticosteroids are infused (2 mg/kg triamcinolone or equivalent) to minimize the risk for pericardial adhesions. The pigtail drain is generally left in overnight and removed the following morning after significant effusions are excluded on transthoracic echocardiography. Echocardiography is repeated 3–4 hours later, and if no further pericardial bleeding has

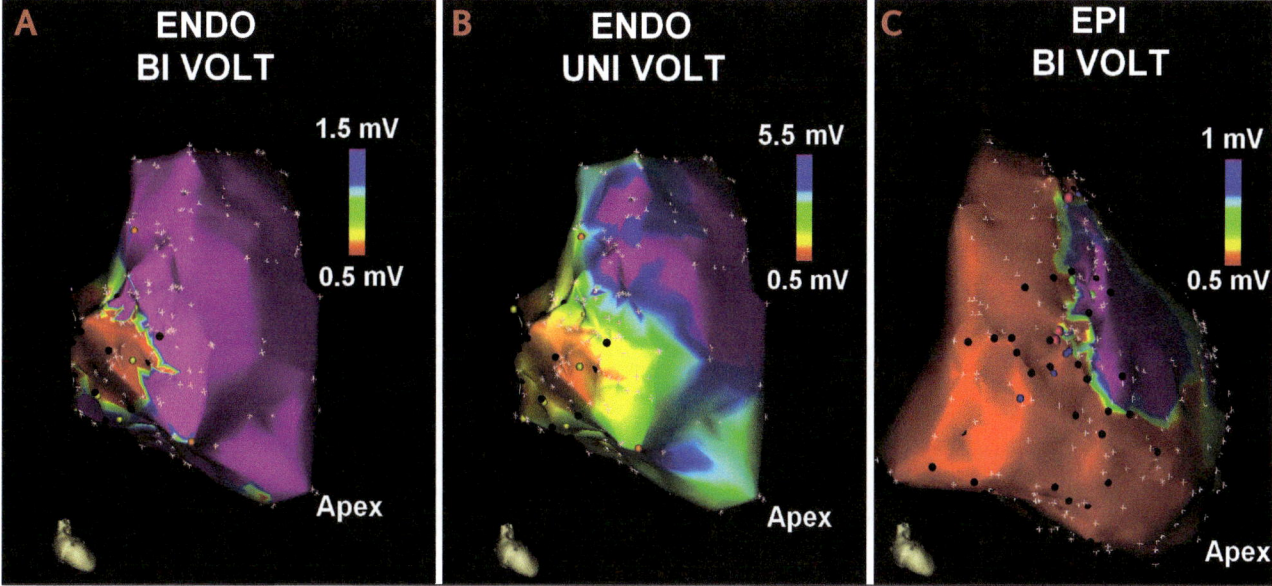

Figure 44.4 RAO projection of sinus rhythm voltage maps of the right ventricle from a patient with arrhythmogenic right ventricular cardiomyopathy. **Violet** represented areas of preserved bipolar voltage (>1.5 mV in **Panel A** and >1 mV in **Panel C**) and unipolar voltage (>5.5 mV in **Panel B**), respectively. **Red** represented dense electroanatomic scars (<0.5 mV in **Panels A** and **C** and <3.5 mV in **Panel B**). **Rainbow colors** depicted the border zone. **Panel A** showed a basal area of abnormal endocardium. Endocardial unipolar voltage map in **Panel B** suggested a much greater area of abnormal epicardium extending up to the pulmonic valve and anteriorly to the apical region. This was subsequently confirmed during epicardial voltage mapping (**Panel C**).

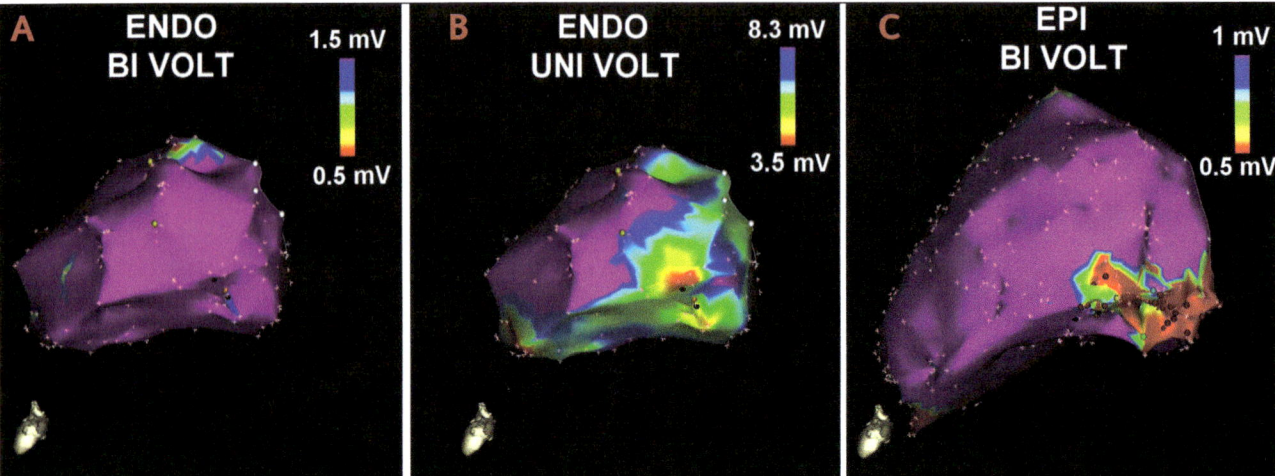

Figure 44.5 Left lateral projection of LV from a patient with idiopathic DCM and recurrent MMVT. **Panels A** and **B** showed endocardial bipolar and unipolar voltage maps in sinus rhythm, respectively. **Panel C** showed corresponding epicardial bipolar voltage map. **Purple-coded** regions indicated areas of preserved bipolar voltage (>1.5 mV in **Panel A** and >1 mV in **Panel C**) and unipolar voltage (>8.3 mV in **Panel B**), respectively. **Red-coded** areas represented dense scars (<0.5 mV). **Rainbow colors** highlighted the border zone. Endocardial bipolar voltage was normal in **Panel A**. Unipolar low-voltage areas in **Panel B** extended from the mitral valve to the apex and inferiorly. Epicardial bipolar voltage map in **Panel C** confirmed the existence of an area of abnormal voltage located at the basal and apex. Pace mapping suggested an exit at the epicardial basal scar, and ablations performed at this location were successful.

occurred, anticoagulation may be initiated in patients with extensive endocardial ablation with careful monitoring for late bleeding.

Procedural Complications

Procedural risk of VT ablation is inherently higher owing to the extent of ablation frequently required in the systemic circulation, significant underlying structural heart disease, and comorbidities. In experienced centers, major complications are reported in 3.6%–10% of patients.[71,81] Local vascular complications (large hematoma, arterial pseudoaneurysm, and AV fistula) occur in 2% of patients. Cardiac tamponade, strokes (due to ablation-related thrombus formation or mechanical plaque dislodgement), and complete heart block occur at a rate of ~1% each.[23,82] Coronary artery embolism and valvular injuries have been reported. Coronary arteries can be damaged during RF ablation, leading to arterial thrombosis or spasm. A distance of at least 5 mm between ablation catheter and epicardial artery on coronary angiography at the target site is recommended. Epicardial ablations are associated with risks of pericardial bleeding and inadvertent RV puncture.[83] Procedural-related mortality rate is estimated at 0%–3% and is predominantly related to exacerbation of heart failure and myocardial ischemia or recurrent VT.[81] Contributory factors to cardiogenic shock include ablations in viable myocardium, injury to valvular structures, fluid load from externally irrigated catheters, and repeated hemodynamically unstable VT.[82] The potential for complications highlight the importance of restricting ablation to areas of low-voltage or scar.

Catheter Ablation for Specific Nonischemic Cardiomyopathies

Dilated Cardiomyopathy

Dilated cardiomyopathy is a heterogeneous group of NICMs characterized by impaired systolic function and dilatation of one or both ventricles. An underlying etiology can be identified in approximately 50% of patients, whereas the remaining 50% are considered idiopathic. Idiopathic dilated cardiomyopathy (IDCM) is an important cause of heart failure, thromboembolism, arrhythmias, and sudden cardiac death. Sustained monomorphic VT occurs in only 5% of patients.[84] The predominant mechanism of VT is scar-related reentry. Less commonly, VT is due to bundle branch reentry or focal activity. As mentioned previously, scarring with variable degrees of atrophic myocytes, myofiber disarray, nuclear changes, and cytoskeletal disorganization are often present in these patients. The endocardial electrophysiologic substrate of MMVT in the setting of NICM is characterized by confluent areas of low-voltage EGMs distributed predominantly in the basal left ventricular region and in close proximity to the mitral and aortic annuli.[85] These regions usually involve less than 25% of the left ventricular surface. In patients with epicardial VTs, the epicardial electroanatomic scar is usually larger than endocardial.[79] Importantly, endocardial unipolar electrograms, due to their wider field of view, can detect the presence of an epicardial substrate. Data from our laboratory indicate that confluent regions of low unipolar voltage, that is, <8.3 mV for LV free wall and septum and <5.5 mV for the RV free wall, suggest epicardial scarring and the need for epicardial mapping even when the endocardial voltage is normal (Figure 44.4).[73,79]

Standard mapping and ablation techniques are used for ablation of VT in patients with IDCM. The acute success rate, when defined as noninducibility of any VT, ranges between 38% and 73%.[71,81,85]

Arrhythmogenic Right Ventricular Dysplasia

Arrhythmogenic right ventricular cardiomyopathy (ARVC) is a rare inherited myocardial disease characterized by replacement of the myocardium by fibrofatty tissue that predispose to ventricular arrhythmias and sudden cardiac death. VT occurs in up to 64% of patients.[14] It usually originates in the right ventricle and exhibits left bundle branch block morphology. Reentry is the predominant mechanism, as suggested by the fact that tachycardia can be initiated by programmed stimulation and be entrained.[86] Dysplastic regions in patients with ARVC are manifested as contiguous low-voltage, long-duration EGMs.[87] A good correlation has been reported between low-voltage areas delineated by EAM and histopathologic findings of myocyte loss and fibrofatty replacement.[87] As with other NICM, the endocardial low-voltage abnormalities are adjacent to the tricuspid and/or pulmonic valve, extending for a variable distance toward the apex, involving both the right ventricular free wall and occasionally extending to the interventricular septum.[88] Consistent with pathological findings suggesting predominant epicardial/mid-myocardial involvement in the disease process, we have noted that the epicardial scar burden is greater than the endocardial scar burden.[89,90] The epicardial scar typically has a predominantly perivalvular distribution that matched the endocardial scar (Figure 44.5).

The acute success rate of ablation ranges in different studies between 50% and 90%.[91] The variable outcomes reported in different studies can be attributed to differences in mapping techniques, procedural endpoints, and operator experience. Owing to the more extensive epicardial substrate, more aggressive ablation strategies targeting both the epicardium and the endocardium are often required. In a series of 13 consecutive ARVC patients who had previously undergone unsuccessful endocardial ablation, repeat ablation targeting epicardial circuits was associated with a long-term success rate of 77%.[89] Of note, the areas targeted by ablation in this study were situated opposite normal endocardium in 77% of patients, often separated by > 1 cm from the corresponding endocardial surface. This thickening, along with the presence of mid-myocardial scarring, may explain why endocardial-only ablation was not effective during the index ablation procedure. This concept is further supported by the results of a study by Bai et al,[92] in which 49 patients with ARVC were assigned to either endocardial-only or combined endocardial and epicardial ablation approach. After a follow-up of 3 years, 52% and 85% of patients, respectively, were free of VT recurrences and did not experience ICD therapy. Of note, 22% and 69% of patients, respectively, were off all antiarrhythmic medications. Collectively, these data indicate that combined endocardial and epicardial ablation is associated with better long-term results in terms of freedom from arrhythmia recurrence.

Chagas Disease

Chagas disease is a widespread tropical disease that affects millions of people in Latin America. The causative organism, *Trypanosoma cruzi*, is commonly transmitted to humans and animals by insect vectors. Chronic Chagasic cardiomyopathy is the most severe manifestation of Chagas disease and one of the most arrhythmogenic cardiomyopathies.[93] Sudden cardiac death, usually due to VT/VF, occurs in 51%–65% of patients.[15] Histologic examination demonstrates inflammatory infiltrates, variable degrees of cellular damage, and marked reparative fibrosis. The histologic changes most frequently occur at the apex, the basal inferolateral wall, in the posterior left ventricular wall, and in the conduction system.[15] EAM demonstrates low-voltage areas consistent with scars in all patients with VT, commonly with larger epicardial than endocardial scars. VT is most likely due to reentry as reproducibly induced with programmed stimulation and can be entrained.[94] Limited data exist on ablation in patients with Chagas cardiomyopathy. Initial attempts at endocardial ablation were associated with disappointing results. d'Avila[94] described a series of 24 consecutive patients who underwent endocardial ablation between 1991 and 1996. After an average of 26 months of follow-up, only 17% of patients remained VT free. The utility of epicardial mapping and ablation in patients with Chagasic cardiomyopathy was demonstrated by Sosa et al.[95] Fourteen of the 18 inducible VTs in 10 patients had an epicardial origin. Six patients underwent epicardial ablation and 4 patients underwent endocardial ablation. The earliest activation site during VT was more frequently situated on the epicardium. In addition, epicardial mid-diastolic and continuous electrical activity was noted in all patients. Patients who underwent epicardial ablation had no recurrences after a follow-up of 5–9 months. In contrast, 2 patients who underwent endocardial ablation had VT recurrences. These limited data suggest that the arrhythmogenic substrate in patients with Chagas cardiomyopathy and VT is often located on the epicardium and that epicardial mapping and ablation should be considered as the initial ablation strategy.

Sarcoidosis

Sarcoidosis is a multisystem inflammatory disease of unknown etiology characterized by nonnecrotizing granuloma formation, most commonly in the lungs, the thoracic lymph nodes, and the heart.[15] The predominant sites of myocardial involvement are the basal aspect of the ventricular septum, the left ventricular free wall and papillary muscles, the right ventricular free wall, and the atrial walls.[96] Patients with cardiac sarcoidosis are at increased risk of sudden cardiac death, which occurs secondary to bradyarrhythmias and reentrant VT.[97,98] EAM demonstrates confluent endocardial and/or epicardial regions of low-amplitude EGMs in both ventricles.[98,99] Isolated potentials can be recorded during sinus rhythm at effective ablation sites.[99,100] VTs in patients with cardiac sarcoidosis are often difficult to control by pharmacologic therapy only. In a study by Jefic et al[99] of 42 patients with cardiac sarcoidosis, 21 (50%) developed ventricular arrhythmias, 9 of whom (43%) did not respond to immunosuppressive and antiarrhythmic agents. Most patients are likely to require adjunctive catheter ablation in addition to ICD implantation (Figure 44.6). Mapping relies on substrate, activation, entrainment, and pace mapping. In the studies by Koplan et al[98] and Jefic et al,[99] the medium-term success rates for ablation were 25% and 56%, respectively.

Special Considerations for Patients with Septal Substrates: Alternative Ablation Techniques and Outcomes

Recent evidence has highlighted the presence of isolated intramural substrates in a substantial proportion of patients with nonischemic dilated cardiomyopathies.[22] Haqqani et al reported a prevalence of isolated septal substrates of 11.6% in a consecutive series of patients with nonischemic dilated cardiomyopathies referred for VT ablation at the University of Pennsylvania over an 11-year period.[22] These patients were typically characterized by both left and right bundle branch block VT morphologies, and catheter ablation was often performed from both sides of the septum. Patients with isolated septal substrates appear to have a significantly lower acute and long-term procedural success compared to those with nonseptal substrates, due to the inability to target deep intra-myocardial substrates with current RF ablation tools. In these cases, alternative approaches to conventional RF ablation can be of particular value. Such approaches include transcoronary (arterial or venous) chemical ablation with ethanol, coil embolization of septal coronary artery branches, bipolar RF ablation, long duration (> 3 minute) RF application, and RF ablation with needle-tip catheters.

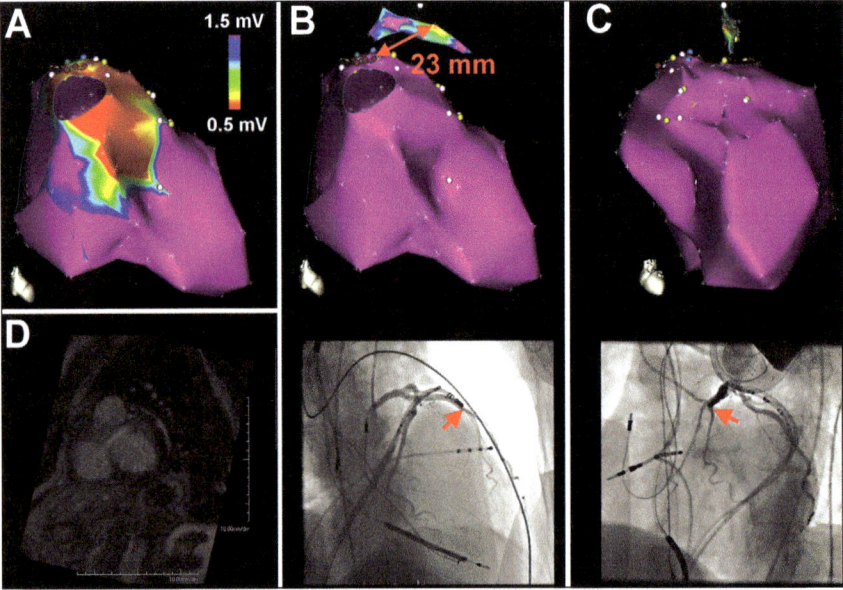

Figure 44.6 **Panel A** shows a modified RAO view of sinus rhythm bipolar voltage map from a patient with cardiac sarcoidosis who was diagnosed with complete heart block, necessitating initial pacemaker implantation and subsequent ICD upgrade due to recurrent MMVT. Scar was seen in close proximity to the aortic and mitral valve annuli in the basal interventricular septum. In the EP laboratory, VT was induced and activation mapping of the LV and the aortic cusps were performed with earliest activation mapped to the periaortic region below the junction of the LCC and RCC. Pace mapping was good. However, ablation (**brown dots**) failed to interrupt the tachycardia. Mapping was then extended to the adjacent coronary venous system and the earliest site was identified in the proximal aspect of the anterior interventricular vein (AIV), approximately 23 mm away from the earliest endocardial activation. However, coronary angiography revealed that the site of earliest epicardial activation was directly overlying a moderate-sized diagonal branch (**arrow**) of the left anterior descending artery, thereby precluding catheter ablation. **Panels B** (RAO) and **C** (LAO) illustrated the intimate relationships between the sites of earliest activation in the LV and AIV with the coronary arterial anatomy. This case illustrated two important clinical features in sarcoidosis: the presence of cardiac conduction abnormalities and VT, which in the setting of nonischemic cardiomyopathy should raise the suspicion of cardiac sarcoidosis. This may be related to the strong predilection for mid-myocardial scars in the basal aspect of interventricular septum with epicardial extensions in patients with sarcoidosis. **Panel D** highlighted a basal anteroseptal scar seen on cardiac MRI with late-gadolinium enhancement due to sarcoidosis.

Needle RF Ablation

Sapp et al modified a retractable needle-tipped catheter initially designed for intramyocardial drug delivery through the application of a connector pin to the proximal catheter end and by incorporating a thermocouple in the distal tip of the needle.[101] In a preclinical study, 3 swine underwent ablation in the left ventricle with both the novel needle catheter (power starting at 9–10 W and manually titrated up to maintain the tip temperature at or below 90°C) or a 4 mm nonirrigated catheter (power starting at 2–10 W and manually titrated up to maintain the tip temperature at or below 60°C). At pathological analysis, needle ablation lesions typically spared the endocardial surface, with minimal endocardial disruption and no evidence of thrombus. A small central area of pallor (3.3 ± 0.5 mm diameter) was highlighted. Serial sections through the central area of pallor demonstrated long and narrow lesions with a uniform diameter (4.4 ± 0.1 mm) and extended the whole length of the needle (ie, 10 mm). Standard RF ablations were typically wider (8.5 ± 0.2 mm) and shallower (5.7 ± 0.4 mm).[101] A clinical study evaluating the benefit of needle RF ablation for recurrent VT that has failed conventional RF ablation has also reported successful elimination of VT not responding to endocardial ablation alone.[102]

Bipolar RF Ablation

Sivagangabalan and colleagues first demonstrated the superior efficacy of bipolar ablation in creating transmural ablations involving the interventricular septum using a postinfarct ovine model.[103] Koruth et al compared bipolar with sequential unipolar ablation both in vitro in a preparation of porcine ventricular tissue in a saline bath and in vivo in a heterogeneous group of patients with either atypical septal atrial flutter ($n=3$), septal VT ($n=4$), or left ventricle free-wall VT ($n=2$). In the preclinical model, bipolar RF ablation results in a higher rate of transmural lesions (82% vs 33%, $P = 0.001$). In the clinical model, all patients with atypical septal atrial flutter were successfully terminated during the index procedure, although all had either atrial flutter or atrial fibrillation recurrences over follow-up. In the subgroup of patients with VT, 5/6 septal and 2/3 left free-wall VTs were successfully terminated with bipolar RF ablation. However, VT-free survival at 1 year was achieved in only 50% of cases in both groups.[104]

Ethanol Ablation

The first human demonstration of the feasibility of transcoronary arterial ethanol ablation of VT was provided by Brugada et al in a series of 3 patients with postinfarct VT.[105] A total of 1.5–6 mL of ethanol (96% concentration) was injected into the selected coronary artery supplying blood to the myocardial area responsible for VT, and coronary angiography was repeated after a waiting period of 10 minutes to assess for patency. Periprocedural complications were limited to transient episode atrioventricular block in 1 of the patients.[105] In a subsequent study, Brugada's group reported on a larger series of 12 patients with postinfarct VT. The coronary artery supplying blood to the site of origin of the VT was identified in 10/12 cases (83%). After a follow-up of 2–44 months, 70% of patients remained free from recurrent VT.[106]

Coronary Coil Embolization

The UCLA group has recently reported the feasibility of coronary coil embolization in 2 patients with septal VT refractory to conventional RF ablation.[107] Mapping within the coronary arterial system was carried out through selective cannulation of septal perforator branches of the left anterior descending coronary artery with dedicated recording wires. After confirmation of the septal site of origin of the VT, an over-the-wire balloon was inflated in a septal perforator branch and cold saline was injected, resulting in acute termination of the VT. The balloon catheter was exchanged for a microcatheter and occlusive coils were deployed in the septal perforator branch, resulting in noninducibility of VT.[107] Further studies on larger populations of patients are warranted to better evaluate the safety and long-term outcomes of this approach.

Key Ongoing Clinical Trials on Catheter Ablation of VT

The main focus of ongoing clinical trials on catheter ablation of VT is to determine whether an early intervention with ablation in patients at high risk of recurrent VT might improve long-term outcome. The ASPIRE trial will include 350 patients with postinfarct VT that have had at least 1 appropriate ICD shock despite antiarrhythmics. These patients are randomized to further antiarrhythmic drugs or catheter ablation. Freedom from recurrent VT, occurrence of VT storm, and hospitalization for VT are the primary endpoints in this trial. The PARTITA trial evaluates whether early ablation (after a first appropriate ICD shock) improves VT-free survival compared to a more delayed ablation strategy that waits for a high burden of recurrent VT. The trial will include 586 patients with either ischemic or nonischemic cardiomyopathy. The primary trial endpoints are freedom from appropriate ICD shock and survival free from heart failure hospitalization. The VANISH trial will evaluate whether catheter ablation is more effective than high-dose amiodarone in ischemic cardiomyopathy patients experiencing an appropriate ICD shock despite antiarrhythmic drug therapy. Patients will be randomized to either catheter ablation or high-dose amiodarone. If high-dose amiodarone fails, patients will be switched to mexiletine.

The primary endpoint is a composite of death and appropriate ICD therapy. The STRATUM VT trial will evaluate the optimal ablation strategy in patients with ischemic cardiomyopathy and VT. In particular, traditional VT mapping and ablation will be compared to substrate-based ablation and infarct border zone modification using a single-arm step-wise approach. The main endpoint is acute and mid-term (6 months) efficacy.

Conclusion

Catheter ablation in ischemic and nonischemic heart disease has an evolving but definitive place in the treatment paradigm for VT. Although typically used as the treatment of last resort for drug refractory arrhythmias, the success of the therapy would suggest that it should be considered much earlier in the patient's clinical course. Strategies for ablating mappable and unmappable VT have been defined. Ablation therapy has emerged as an important alternative option to antiarrhythmic medication. New catheter technologies allowing for creation of deeper ablation lesions that can interrupt intramural reentry circuits, image integration of tissue scar architecture, and optimizing ablation electrode–tissue contact may further improve both the acute and long-term success of VT ablation therapies.

References

1. Stevenson WG, Wilber DJ, Natale A, et al. Irrigated radiofrequency catheter ablation guided by electroanatomic mapping for recurrent ventricular tachycardia after myocardial infarction: the multicenter thermocool ventricular tachycardia ablation trial. *Circulation*. Dec 16 2008;118(25):2773-2782.
2. Reddy VY, Reynolds MR, Neuzil P, et al. Prophylactic catheter ablation for the prevention of defibrillator therapy. *N Engl J Med*. Dec 27 2007;357(26):2657-2665.
3. Moss AJ, Greenberg H, Case RB, et al. Long-term clinical course of patients after termination of ventricular tachyarrhythmia by an implanted defibrillator. *Circulation*. Dec 21 2004;110(25):3760-3765.
4. Josephson ME, Harken AH, Horowitz LN. Endocardial excision: a new surgical technique for the treatment of recurrent ventricular tachycardia. *Circulation*. Dec 1979;60(7):1430-1439.
5. Stevenson WG, Khan H, Sager P, et al. Identification of reentry circuit sites during catheter mapping and radiofrequency ablation of ventricular tachycardia late after myocardial infarction. *Circulation*. Oct 1993;88(4 Pt 1):1647-1670.
6. Fenoglio JJ Jr, Pham TD, Harken AH, Horowitz LN, Josephson ME, Wit AL. Recurrent sustained ventricular tachycardia: structure and ultrastructure of subendocardial regions in which tachycardia originates. *Circulation*. Sep 1983;68(3):518-533.
7. Josephson ME, Zimetbaum P, Huang D, Sauberman R, Monahan KM, Callans DS. Pathophysiologic substrate for sustained ventricular tachycardia in coronary artery disease. *Jpn Circ J*. Jun 1997;61(6):459-466.
8. Roberts WC, Siegel RJ, McManus BM. Idiopathic dilated cardiomyopathy: analysis of 152 necropsy patients. *Am J Cardiol*. Dec 1 1987;60(16):1340-1355.
9. Nakayama Y, Shimizu G, Hirota Y, et al. Functional and histopathologic correlation in patients with dilated cardiomyopathy: an integrated evaluation by multivariate analysis. *J Am Coll Cardiol*. Jul 1987;10(1):186-192.
10. Iles L, Pfluger H, Lefkovits L, et al. Myocardial fibrosis predicts appropriate device therapy in patients with implantable cardioverter-defibrillators for primary prevention of sudden cardiac death. *J Am Coll Cardiol*. Feb 15 2011;57(7):821-828.
11. McCrohon JA, Moon JC, Prasad SK, et al. Differentiation of heart failure related to dilated cardiomyopathy and coronary artery disease using gadolinium-enhanced cardiovascular magnetic resonance. *Circulation*. Jul 8 2003;108(1):54-59.
12. Kies P, Bootsma M, Bax J, Schalij MJ, van der Wall EE. Arrhythmogenic right ventricular dysplasia/cardiomyopathy: screening, diagnosis, and treatment. *Heart Rhythm*. Feb 2006;3(2):225-234.
13. Basso C, Corrado D, Marcus FI, Nava A, Thiene G. Arrhythmogenic right ventricular cardiomyopathy. *Lancet*. Apr 11 2009;373(9671):1289-1300.
14. Muir AR, Elliott PM. Arrhythmogenic right ventricular cardiomyopathy. In: Saksena S, Camm AJ, eds. *Electrophysiological Disorders of the Heart*. 2nd ed. Philadelphia, PA: Elsevier/Saunders; 2012:845-853.
15. Issa ZF, Miller JM, Zipes DP. Ventricular tachycardia in nonischemic dilated cardiomyopathy. *Clinical Arrhythmology and Electrophysiology: A Companion to Braunwald's Heart Disease*. 2nd ed. Philadelphia, PA: Elseiver/Saunders; 2012:594-600.
16. Teixeira AR, Nitz N, Guimaro MC, Gomes C, Santos-Buch CA. Chagas disease. *Postgraduate Medical Journal*. Dec 2006;82(974):788-798.
17. Moon JC, Reed E, Sheppard MN, et al. The histologic basis of late gadolinium enhancement cardiovascular magnetic resonance in hypertrophic cardiomyopathy. *J Am Coll Cardiol*. Jun 16 2004;43(12):2260-2264.
18. de Jong S, van Veen TA, van Rijen HV, de Bakker JM. Fibrosis and cardiac arrhythmias. *J Cardiovasc Pharmacol*. Jun 2011;57(6):630-638.
19. Bluemke DA. MRI of nonischemic cardiomyopathy. *AJR Am J Roentgenol*. Oct 2010;195(4):935-940.
20. Winterfield JR, Mahapatra S, Wilber DJ. Catheter ablation of ventricular arrhythmias: targets, tactics, and tools. *Curr Opin Cardiol*. May 2013;28(3):344-353.
21. Hsia HH, Marchlinski FE. Characterization of the electroanatomic substrate for monomorphic ventricular tachycardia in patients with nonischemic cardiomyopathy. *Pacing Clin Electrophysiol*. Jul 2002;25(7):1114-1127.
22. Haqqani HM, Tschabrunn CM, Tzou WS, et al. Isolated septal substrate for ventricular tachycardia in nonischemic dilated cardiomyopathy: incidence, characterization, and implications. *Heart Rhythm*. Aug 2011;8(8):1169-1176.
23. Aliot EM, Stevenson WG, Almendral-Garrote JM, et al. EHRA/HRS Expert Consensus on Catheter Ablation of Ventricular Arrhythmias: developed in a partnership with the European Heart Rhythm Association (EHRA), a Registered Branch of the European Society of Cardiology (ESC), and the Heart Rhythm Society (HRS); in collaboration with the American College of Cardiology (ACC) and the American Heart Association (AHA). *Heart Rhythm*. Jun 2009;6(6):886-933.
24. Bogun F, Morady F. Ablation of ventricular tachycardia in patients with nonischemic cardiomyopathy. *J Cardiovasc Electrophysiol*. Nov 2008;19(11):1227-1230.

25. Deyell MW, Callans D. How we ablate ventricular tachycardia in non-ischemic left ventricular cardiomyopathy. *Journal of Innovations in Cardiac Rhythm Management.* 2011;2:558-565.
26. Yoshida K, Liu TY, Scott C, et al. The value of defibrillator electrograms for recognition of clinical ventricular tachycardias and for pace mapping of post-infarction ventricular tachycardia. *J Am Coll Cardiol.* Sep 14 2010;56(12):969-979.
27. Garcia FC, Valles E, Dhruvakumar S, Marchlinski FE. Ablation of ventricular tachycardia. *Herzschrittmachertherapie & Elektrophysiologie.* Dec 2007;18(4):225-233.
28. Mandel JE, Hutchinson MD, Marchlinski FE. Remifentanil-midazolam sedation provides hemodynamic stability and comfort during epicardial ablation of ventricular tachycardia. *J Cardiovasc Electrophysiol.* Apr 2011;22(4):464-466.
29. Miller JM, Tyson GS, Hargrove WC 3rd, Vassallo JA, Rosenthal ME, Josephson ME. Effect of subendocardial resection on sinus rhythm endocardial electrogram abnormalities. *Circulation.* May 1 1995;91(9):2385-2391.
30. Hsia HH, Lin D, Sauer WH, Callans DJ, Marchlinski FE. Anatomic characterization of endocardial substrate for hemodynamically stable reentrant ventricular tachycardia: identification of endocardial conducting channels. *Heart Rhythm.* May 2006;3(5):503-512.
31. de Bakker JM, van Capelle FJ, Janse MJ, et al. Reentry as a cause of ventricular tachycardia in patients with chronic ischemic heart disease: electrophysiologic and anatomic correlation. *Circulation.* Mar 1988;77(3):589-606.
32. Joshi S, Wilber DJ. Ablation of idiopathic right ventricular outflow tract tachycardia: current perspectives. *J Cardiovasc Electrophysiol.* Sep 2005;16 Suppl 1:S52-58.
33. Marchlinski FE, Callans DJ, Gottlieb CD, Zado E. Linear ablation lesions for control of unmappable ventricular tachycardia in patients with ischemic and nonischemic cardiomyopathy. *Circulation.* Mar 21 2000;101(11):1288-1296.
34. Haqqani HM, Kalman JM, Roberts-Thomson KC, et al. Fundamental differences in electrophysiologic and electroanatomic substrate between ischemic cardiomyopathy patients with and without clinical ventricular tachycardia. *J Am Coll Cardiol.* Jul 7 2009;54(2):166-173.
35. Josephson ME. Electrophysiology of ventricular tachycardia: a historical perspective. *Pacing Clin Electrophysiol.* Oct 2003;26(10):2052-2067.
36. El-Shalakany A, Hadjis T, Papageorgiou P, Monahan K, Epstein L, Josephson ME. Entrainment/mapping criteria for the prediction of termination of ventricular tachycardia by single radiofrequency lesion in patients with coronary artery disease. *Circulation.* May 4 1999;99(17):2283-2289.
37. Stevenson WG, Friedman PL, Sager PT, et al. Exploring postinfarction reentrant ventricular tachycardia with entrainment mapping. *J Am Coll Cardiol.* May 1997;29(6):1180-1189.
38. Haqqani HM, Marchlinski FE. Electrophysiologic substrate underlying postinfarction ventricular tachycardia: characterization and role in catheter ablation. *Heart Rhythm.* Aug 2009;6(8 Suppl):S70-76.
39. Callans DJ, Zado E, Sarter BH, Schwartzman D, Gottlieb CD, Marchlinski FE. Efficacy of radiofrequency catheter ablation for ventricular tachycardia in healed myocardial infarction. *Am J Cardiol.* Aug 15 1998;82(4):429-432.
40. Miller JM, Marchlinski FE, Harken AH, Hargrove WC, Josephson ME. Subendocardial resection for sustained ventricular tachycardia in the early period after acute myocardial infarction. *Am J Cardiol.* Apr 1 1985;55(8):980-984.
41. Soejima K, Stevenson WG, Maisel WH, Sapp JL, Epstein LM. Electrically unexcitable scar mapping based on pacing threshold for identification of the reentry circuit isthmus: feasibility for guiding ventricular tachycardia ablation. *Circulation.* Sep 24 2002;106(13):1678-1683.
42. Verma A, Marrouche NF, Schweikert RA, et al. Relationship between successful ablation sites and the scar border zone defined by substrate mapping for ventricular tachycardia post-myocardial infarction. *J Cardiovasc Electrophysiol.* May 2005;16(5):465-471.
43. Josephson ME, Waxman HL, Cain ME, Gardner MJ, Buxton AE. Ventricular activation during ventricular endocardial pacing. II. Role of pace-mapping to localize origin of ventricular tachycardia. *Am J Cardiol.* Jul 1982;50(1):11-22.
44. Brunckhorst CB, Delacretaz E, Soejima K, Maisel WH, Friedman PL, Stevenson WG. Identification of the ventricular tachycardia isthmus after infarction by pace mapping. *Circulation.* Aug 10 2004;110(6):652-659.
45. Stevenson WG, Sager PT, Natterson PD, Saxon LA, Middlekauff HR, Wiener I. Relation of pace mapping QRS configuration and conduction delay to ventricular tachycardia reentry circuits in human infarct scars. *J Am Coll Cardiol.* Aug 1995;26(2):481-488.
46. Cassidy DM, Vassallo JA, Buxton AE, Doherty JU, Marchlinski FE, Josephson ME. The value of catheter mapping during sinus rhythm to localize site of origin of ventricular tachycardia. *Circulation.* Jun 1984;69(6):1103-1110.
47. Dukkipati SR, d'Avila A, Soejima K, et al. Long-term outcomes of combined epicardial and endocardial ablation of monomorphic ventricular tachycardia related to hypertrophic cardiomyopathy. *Circ Arrhythm Electrophysiol.* Apr 1 2011;4(2):185-194.
48. Bogun F, Good E, Reich S, et al. Isolated potentials during sinus rhythm and pace-mapping within scars as guides for ablation of post-infarction ventricular tachycardia. *J Am Coll Cardiol.* May 16 2006;47(10):2013-2019.
49. Nakahara S, Tung R, Ramirez RJ, et al. Characterization of the arrhythmogenic substrate in ischemic and nonischemic cardiomyopathy implications for catheter ablation of hemodynamically unstable ventricular tachycardia. *J Am Coll Cardiol.* May 25 2010;55(21):2355-2365.
50. Arenal A, del Castillo S, Gonzalez-Torrecilla E, et al. Tachycardia-related channel in the scar tissue in patients with sustained monomorphic ventricular tachycardias: influence of the voltage scar definition. *Circulation.* Oct 26 2004;110(17):2568-2574.
51. Mountantonakis SE, Park RE, Frankel DS, et al. Relationship between voltage map "channels" and the location of critical isthmus sites in patients with post-infarction cardiomyopathy and ventricular tachycardia. *J Am Coll Cardiol.* May 21 2013;61(20):2088-2095.
52. Yokoyama K, Nakagawa H, Wittkampf FH, Pitha JV, Lazzara R, Jackman WM. Comparison of electrode cooling between internal and open irrigation in radiofrequency ablation lesion depth and incidence of thrombus and steam pop. *Circulation.* Jan 3 2006;113(1):11-19.
53. Borger van der Burg AE, de Groot NM, van Erven L, Bootsma M, van der Wall EE, Schalij MJ. Long-term follow-up after radiofrequency catheter ablation of ventricular tachycardia: a successful approach? *J Cardiovasc Electrophysiol.* May 2002;13(5):417-423.
54. Della Bella P, Riva S, Fassini G, et al. Incidence and significance of pleomorphism in patients with postmyocardial infarction ventricular tachycardia. Acute and long-term outcome of radiofrequency catheter ablation. *Eur Heart J.* Jul 2004;25(13):1127-1138.
55. Gonska BD, Cao K, Schaumann A, Dorszewski A, von zur Muhlen F, Kreuzer H. Catheter ablation of ventricular

tachycardia in 136 patients with coronary artery disease: results and long-term follow-up. *J Am Coll Cardiol.* Nov 15 1994;24(6):1506-1514.
56. Calkins H, Epstein A, Packer D, et al. Catheter ablation of ventricular tachycardia in patients with structural heart disease using cooled radiofrequency energy: results of a prospective multicenter study. Cooled RF Multi Center Investigators Group. *J Am Coll Cardiol.* Jun 2000;35(7):1905-1914.
57. Soejima K, Suzuki M, Maisel WH, et al. Catheter ablation in patients with multiple and unstable ventricular tachycardias after myocardial infarction: short ablation lines guided by reentry circuit isthmuses and sinus rhythm mapping. *Circulation.* Aug 7 2001;104(6):664-669.
58. Ventura R, Klemm HU, Rostock T, et al. Stable and unstable ventricular tachycardias in patients with previous myocardial infarction: a clinically oriented strategy for catheter ablation. *Cardiology.* 2008;109(1):52-61.
59. Tanner H, Hindricks G, Volkmer M, et al. Catheter ablation of recurrent scar-related ventricular tachycardia using electro-anatomical mapping and irrigated ablation technology: results of the prospective multicenter Euro-VT-study. *J Cardiovasc Electrophysiol.* Jan 2010;21(1):47-53.
60. Carbucicchio C, Santamaria M, Trevisi N, et al. Catheter ablation for the treatment of electrical storm in patients with implantable cardioverter-defibrillators: short- and long-term outcomes in a prospective single-center study. *Circulation.* Jan 29 2008;117(4):462-469.
61. Frankel DS, Mountantonakis SE, Zado ES, et al. Noninvasive programmed ventricular stimulation early after ventricular tachycardia ablation to predict risk of late recurrence. *J Am Coll Cardiol.* Apr 24 2012;59(17):1529-1535.
62. Della Bella P, De Ponti R, Uriarte JA, et al. Catheter ablation and antiarrhythmic drugs for haemodynamically tolerated post-infarction ventricular tachycardia; long-term outcome in relation to acute electrophysiological findings. *Eur Heart J.* Mar 2002;23(5):414-424.
63. Morady F, Harvey M, Kalbfleisch SJ, el-Atassi R, Calkins H, Langberg JJ. Radiofrequency catheter ablation of ventricular tachycardia in patients with coronary artery disease. *Circulation.* Feb 1993;87(2):363-372.
64. Stevenson WG, Friedman PL, Kocovic D, Sager PT, Saxon LA, Pavri B. Radiofrequency catheter ablation of ventricular tachycardia after myocardial infarction. *Circulation.* Jul 28 1998;98(4):308-314.
65. Kuck KH, Schaumann A, Eckardt L, et al. Catheter ablation of stable ventricular tachycardia before defibrillator implantation in patients with coronary heart disease (VTACH): a multicentre randomised controlled trial. *Lancet.* Jan 2 2010;375(9708):31-40.
66. Schreieck J, Schneider MAE, Röhling M, et al. Preventive ablation of post infarction ventricular tachycardias: results of a prospective randomized study. *Heart Rhythm.* 2004;1(Suppl):S35-S37.
67. Santangeli P, Di Biase L, Al-Ahmad A, et al. Primary ablation for ventricular tachycardia: when and how? *Card Electrophysiol Clin.* 2011;3(4):675-688.
68. Di Biase L, Santangeli P, Burkhardt DJ, et al. Endo-epicardial homogenization of the scar versus limited substrate ablation for the treatment of electrical storms in patients with ischemic cardiomyopathy. *J Am Coll Cardiol.* Jul 10 2012;60(2):132-141.
69. Jaïs P, Maury P, Khairy P, et al. Elimination of local abnormal ventricular activities: a new end point for substrate modification in patients with scar-related ventricular tachycardia. *Circulation.* May 8 2012;125(18):2184-2196.
70. Vergara P, Trevisi N, Ricco A, et al. Late potentials abolition as an additional technique for reduction of arrhythmia recurrence in scar related ventricular tachycardia ablation. *J Cardiovasc Electrophysiol.* Jun 2012;23(6):621-627.
71. Piers SR, van Huls van Taxis CF, Tao Q, et al. Epicardial substrate mapping for ventricular tachycardia ablation in patients with non-ischaemic cardiomyopathy: a new algorithm to differentiate between scar and viable myocardium developed by simultaneous integration of computed tomography and contrast-enhanced magnetic resonance imaging. *Eur Heart J.* Feb 2012;34(8):586-596.
72. Sosa E, Scanavacca M, d'Avila A, Oliveira F, Ramires JA. Nonsurgical transthoracic epicardial catheter ablation to treat recurrent ventricular tachycardia occurring late after myocardial infarction. *J Am Coll Cardiol.* May 2000;35(6):1442-1449.
73. Hutchinson MD, Gerstenfeld EP, Desjardins B, et al. Endocardial unipolar voltage mapping to detect epicardial ventricular tachycardia substrate in patients with nonischemic left ventricular cardiomyopathy. *Circ Arrhythm Electrophysiol.* Feb 2011;4(1):49-55.
74. Bazan V, Bala R, Garcia FC, et al. Twelve-lead ECG features to identify ventricular tachycardia arising from the epicardial right ventricle. *Heart Rhythm.* Oct 2006;3(10):1132-1139.
75. Bazan V, Gerstenfeld EP, Garcia FC, et al. Site-specific twelve-lead ECG features to identify an epicardial origin for left ventricular tachycardia in the absence of myocardial infarction. *Heart Rhythm.* Nov 2007;4(11):1403-1410.
76. Valles E, Bazan V, Marchlinski FE. ECG criteria to identify epicardial ventricular tachycardia in nonischemic cardiomyopathy. *Circ Arrhythm Electrophysiol.* Feb 2012;3(1):63-71.
77. Bala R, Ren JF, Hutchinson MD, et al. Assessing epicardial substrate using intracardiac echocardiography during VT ablation. *Circ Arrhythm Electrophysiol.* Oct 2011;4(5):667-673.
78. Sosa E, Scanavacca M, d'Avila A, Pilleggi F. A new technique to perform epicardial mapping in the electrophysiology laboratory. *J Cardiovasc Electrophysiol.* Jun 1996;7(6):531-536.
79. Cano O, Hutchinson M, Lin D, et al. Electroanatomic substrate and ablation outcome for suspected epicardial ventricular tachycardia in left ventricular nonischemic cardiomyopathy. *J Am Coll Cardiol.* Aug 25 2009;54(9):799-808.
80. Di Biase L, Burkhardt JD, Pelargonio G, et al. Prevention of phrenic nerve injury during epicardial ablation: comparison of methods for separating the phrenic nerve from the epicardial surface. *Heart Rhythm.* Jul 2009;6(7):957-961.
81. Tokuda M, Tedrow UB, Kojodjojo P, et al. Catheter ablation of ventricular tachycardia in nonischemic heart disease. *Circulation.* Oct 1 2012;5(5):992-1000.
82. Natale A, Raviele A, Al-Ahmad A, et al. Venice Chart International Consensus document on ventricular tachycardia/ventricular fibrillation ablation. *J Cardiovasc Electrophysiol.* Mar 2010;21(3):339-379.
83. d'Avila A. Epicardial catheter ablation of ventricular tachycardia. *Heart Rhythm.* Jun 2008;5(6 Suppl):S73-75.
84. Stevenson WG, Soejima K. Catheter ablation for ventricular tachycardia. *Circulation.* May 29 2007;115(21):2750-2760.
85. Hsia HH, Callans DJ, Marchlinski FE. Characterization of endocardial electrophysiological substrate in patients with nonischemic cardiomyopathy and monomorphic ventricular tachycardia. *Circulation.* Aug 12 2003;108(6):704-710.
86. Jacquemet V, Henriquez CS. Loading effect of fibroblast-myocyte coupling on resting potential, impulse propagation, and repolarization: insights from a microstructure model. *Am J Physiol Heart Circ Physiol.* May 2008;294(5):H2040-2052.
87. Marra MP, Leoni L, Bauce B, et al. Imaging study of ventricular scar in arrhythmogenic right ventricular cardiomyopathy: comparison of 3D standard electroanatomical voltage

mapping and contrast-enhanced cardiac magnetic resonance. *Circ Arrhythm Electrophysiol.* Feb 2012;5(1):91-100.
88. Marchlinski FE, Zado E, Dixit S, et al. Electroanatomic substrate and outcome of catheter ablative therapy for ventricular tachycardia in setting of right ventricular cardiomyopathy. *Circulation.* Oct 19 2004;110(16):2293-2298.
89. Garcia FC, Bazan V, Zado ES, Ren JF, Marchlinski FE. Epicardial substrate and outcome with epicardial ablation of ventricular tachycardia in arrhythmogenic right ventricular cardiomyopathy/dysplasia. *Circulation.* Aug 4 2009;120(5):366-375.
90. Haqqani HM, Tschabrunn CM, Betensky BP, et al. Layered activation of epicardial scar in arrhythmogenic right ventricular dysplasia: possible substrate for confined epicardial circuits. *Circ Arrhythm Electrophysiol.* Aug 1 2012;5(4):796-803.
91. Arbelo E, Josephson ME. Ablation of ventricular arrhythmias in arrhythmogenic right ventricular dysplasia. *J Cardiovasc Electrophysiol.* Apr 2010;21(4):473-486.
92. Bai R, Di Biase L, Shivkumar K, et al. Ablation of ventricular arrhythmias in arrhythmogenic right ventricular dysplasia/cardiomyopathy: arrhythmia-free survival after endo-epicardial substrate based mapping and ablation. *Circ Arrhythm Electrophysiol.* Aug 1 2011;4(4):478-485.
93. Biolo A, Ribeiro AL, Clausell N. Chagas cardiomyopathy—where do we stand after a hundred years? *Prog Cardiovasc Dis.* Jan-Feb 2010;52(4):300-316.
94. d'Avila A, Splinter R, Svenson RH, et al. New perspectives on catheter-based ablation of ventricular tachycardia complicating Chagas' disease: experimental evidence of the efficacy of near infrared lasers for catheter ablation of Chagas' VT. *J Interv Card Electrophysiol.* Aug 2002;7(1):23-38.
95. Sosa E, Scanavacca M, d'Avila A, et al. Endocardial and epicardial ablation guided by nonsurgical transthoracic epicardial mapping to treat recurrent ventricular tachycardia. *J Cardiovasc Electrophysiol.* Mar 1998;9(3):229-239.
96. Doughan AR, Williams BR. Cardiac sarcoidosis. *Heart.* Feb 2006;92(2):282-288.
97. Jacobson JT, Lin D, Verdino R, Cooper J, Marchlinski FE. Ablation of ventricular tachycardia associated with nonischemic structural heart disease. In: Wilber DJ, Packer D, Stevenson WG, eds. *Catheter Ablation of Cardiac Arrhythmias: Basic Concepts and Clinical Applications.* 3rd ed. Malden, MA: Blackwell; 2008:342-363.
98. Koplan BA, Soejima K, Baughman K, Epstein LM, Stevenson WG. Refractory ventricular tachycardia secondary to cardiac sarcoid: electrophysiologic characteristics, mapping, and ablation. *Heart Rhythm.* Aug 2006;3(8):924-929.
99. Jefic D, Joel B, Good E, et al. Role of radiofrequency catheter ablation of ventricular tachycardia in cardiac sarcoidosis: report from a multicenter registry. *Heart Rhythm.* Feb 2009;6(2):189-195.
100. Issa ZF, Miller JM, Zipes DP. Ventricular tachycardias in nonischemic dilated cardiomyopathy. *Clinical Arrhythmology and Electrophysiology: A Companion to Braunwald's Heart Disease.* 2nd ed. Philadelphia, PA: Elseiver/Saunders; 2009:478-486.
101. Sapp JL, Cooper JM, Soejima K, et al. Deep myocardial ablation lesions can be created with a retractable needle-tipped catheter. *Pacing Clin Electrophysiol.* May 2004;27(5):594-599.
102. Sapp JL, Beeckler C, Pike R, et al. Initial human feasibility of infusion needle catheter ablation for refractory ventricular tachycardia. *Circulation.* Nov 19, 2013;128(21):2289-2295.
103. Sivagangabalan G, Barry MA, Huang K, et al. Bipolar ablation of the interventricular septum is more efficient at creating a transmural line than sequential unipolar ablation. *Pacing Clin Electrophysiol.* Jan 2010;33(1):16-26.
104. Koruth JS, Dukkipati S, Miller MA, Neuzil P, d'Avila A, Reddy VY. Bipolar irrigated radiofrequency ablation: a therapeutic option for refractory intramural atrial and ventricular tachycardia circuits. *Heart Rhythm.* Dec 2012;9(12):1932-1941.
105. Brugada P, de Swart H, Smeets JL, Wellens HJ. Transcoronary chemical ablation of ventricular tachycardia. *Circulation.* Mar 1989;79(3):475-482.
106. Nellens P, Gursoy S, Andries E, Brugada P. Transcoronary chemical ablation of arrhythmias. *Pacing Clin Electrophysiol.* Sep 1992;15(9):1368-1373.
107. Tholakanahalli VN, Bertog S, Roukoz H, Shivkumar K. Catheter ablation of ventricular tachycardia using intracoronary wire mapping and coil embolization: description of a new technique. *Heart Rhythm.* Feb 2013;10(2):292-296.

CHAPTER 45

Epicardial Ablation

Wendy S. Tzou, MD; Francis E. Marchlinski, MD

Introduction

Contemporary management of ventricular tachycardia (VT) has increasingly incorporated catheter ablation (Figure 45.1). This strategy has largely been used for patients with drug-refractory VT in the setting of chronic ischemic heart disease, but has also included those with nonischemic structural heart disease, as well as with idiopathic VT and structurally normal hearts. In the majority of patients with structural heart disease, the etiology of VT is reentry via scarred myocardium, with critical circuit elements localized to the subendocardium.[1,2] Endocardial ablation is usually successful in eliminating or mitigating VT episodes, particularly with now widely used cooled- or irrigated-tip ablation catheters. The irrigated tip allows for more radiofrequency energy to be applied to the myocardial surface without overheating, allowing the radiofrequency energy to penetrate enough to target VTs that are deeper than subendocardial tissue. However, in as many as 32% of cases, essential circuit components are localized to the epicardium or subepicardium and require epicardial mapping and ablation.[2-4] With development of a percutaneous method for accessing the pericardial space,[5] epicardial mapping and ablation can typically be performed in the electrophysiology laboratory.

In this chapter, we detail an approach for identifying appropriate indications and techniques for performing epicardial mapping and ablation.

Clues to Identifying Epicardial Origin of VT

Type of Structural Heart Disease

In our and others'[6] clinical experience, most patients who require epicardial ablation to eliminate VT have will have nonischemic right or left ventricular cardiomyopathy (Figure 45.2). Patients with arrhythmogenic right ventricular cardiomyopathy/dysplasia (ARVC/D) uniformly have more epicardial than endocardial scar and VT substrate, and epicardial mapping and ablation will be required in the majority of patients despite the observed thinning of the right ventricle.[7-9] Many patients with nonischemic left ventricular cardiomyopathy from an idiopathic process, Chagas disease, and/or prior myocarditis will frequently have epicardial involvement with the VT substrate. Importantly there is more variability in the distribution of fibrosis, and some patients will have scar confined to the endocardium and/or mid-myocardium. Almost uniformly, the areas of fibrosis are predominantly basal and can variably involve anterior, inferior, septal, or

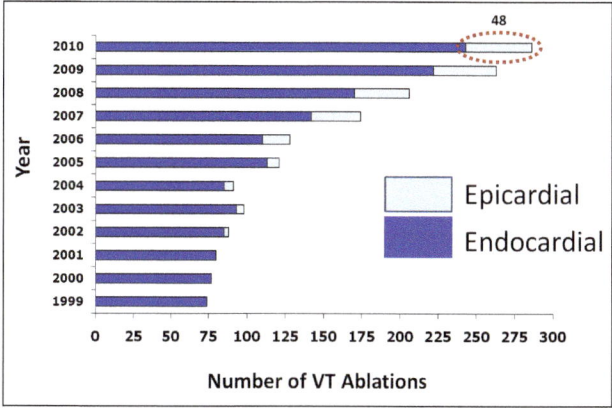

Figure 45.1 Bar graph depicting the progressive increase in number of endocardial and epicardial ablations for ventricular tachycardia (N = 1,686 ablation procedures from 1999 to 2010). Currently at least one in six VT ablation procedures access the epicardium to eliminate VT.

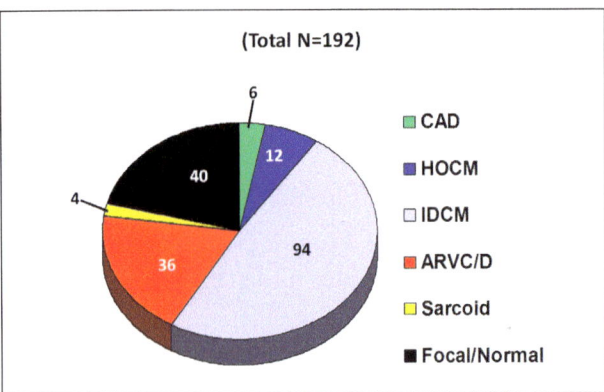

Figure 45.2 Number of epicardial ablations for VT by underlying disease substrate, performed at the Hospital of the University of Pennsylvania, 1999–2010 (N = 192). Most VT ablations were performed for nonischemic right or left ventricular cardiomyopathy (**highlighted**). Epicardial ablation was uncommonly required in patients with coronary artery disease. ARVC/D = arrhythmogenic right ventricular cardiomyopathy/dysplasia; HOCM = hypertrophic obstructive cardiomyopathy; IDCM = idiopathic dilated cardiomyopathy.

lateral left ventricle; however, the basolateral left ventricle remains the most common area of involvement.[7,10-12] Although most VTs due to prior infarction can be successfully targeted from the endocardium, as many as 15%–30% of such cases may also be successfully or more easily targeted with epicardial ablation, suggesting a larger macroreentrant VT circuit with both endocardial and epicardial components even in this setting.[2-4,6,13]

Surface ECG Clues

A 12-lead ECG tracing of VT can provide valuable insight into whether an epicardial approach should be utilized in an ablation procedure, particularly in the setting of nonischemic cardiomyopathy or idiopathic VT (Table 45.1). Criteria suggestive of an epicardial origin include those that identify a delay in the initial QRS activation during VT, indicating that onset of activation is further from the endocardial Purkinje network. A pseudodelta wave (PdW, time from QRS onset to earliest fast deflection in any precordial lead) ≥ 34 ms; intrinsicoid deflection time (IDT, time from QRS onset to peak R wave in V_2) ≥ 85 ms; and shortest RS (time of QRS onset to nadir of first S wave in any precordial lead) ≥ 121 ms all suggest an epicardial VT origin.[14] These criteria have been demonstrated to be generally useful in identifying epicardial left ventricular VT, although the sensitivity and specificity are variable and sometimes much poorer than expected depending on VT site of origin, particularly when from the apex or basal inferior or lateral left ventricle.[11,15] Site-specific criteria have been generated for left ventricular epicardial VT origin in the absence of ischemic cardiomyopathy and include (1) Q wave in lead I for both basal and apical superior VTs, and (2) Q wave in the inferior leads for basal and apical inferior VTs (Table 45.1).[15] A four-step algorithm for identifying epicardial VT in the setting of nonischemic cardiomyopathy with basal lateral left ventricular involvement was recently developed, prospectively evaluating previously proposed ECG criteria.[11] Using this algorithm, the absence of inferior Q waves, a precordial pseudodelta of ≥ 75 ms, a maximum deflection index (MDI, calculated by dividing QRS-onset-to-maximum-precordial-deflection time by total QRS duration) of ≥ 0.59, and presence of Q wave in lead I identified basal lateral epicardial VT origin with 93% sensitivity and 86% specificity.[11]

Table 45.1 Clues suggesting epicardial origin of VT based on underlying disease

Structural heart disease	NICM > ARVC/D ~ Idiopathic > Ischemic CM
Surface ECG findings	
ARVC	Inferior origin: Q waves in II, III, and aVF
	Anterior-basal origin: Q waves in V_2 and I [Bazan, 2006]
NICM	PdW ≥ 34 ms
	IDT ≥ 85 ms
	Shortest RS ≥ 121 ms [14 – Berruezzo et al]
	Absent inferior Q waves + PdW ≥ 75 ms + MDI > 0.59 + Q in lead I [11 – Vallès et al]
	Superior origin: Q wave in I
	Inferior origin: Q waves in II, III, and aVF [15, 16 – Bazan et al]
Idiopathic LV VT	MDI ≥ 0.55 [17 – Daniels et al]
Cardiac imaging	MRI: Epicardial delayed enhancement
	Contrast-enhanced CT: Perfusion defect
	ICE: increased epicardial echogenicity
Endocardial mapping/ablation	Absence of early or mid-diastolic potentials;
	Absence of isthmus sites;
	Endocardial ablation → delayed or lack of VT termination
	Abnormal unipolar > bipolar voltage distribution

ARVC/D = arrhythmogenic right ventricular cardiomyopathy/dysplasia; CT = computed tomography; ICE = intracardiac echocardiography; IDT = intrinsicoid deflection time; LV = left ventricle; MDI = maximum deflection index; MR = magnetic resonance imaging; NICM = nonischemic cardiomyopathy; PdW = pseudodelta wave. See text for details.

Similar criteria have been developed for right ventricular epicardial VTs. Q waves in II, III, and aVF suggest inferior right ventricular involvement; a Q wave in V_2 and Q wave in lead I predict anterior-basal epicardial right ventricular origin.[16] Notably, the non-site-specific criteria for left ventricular epicardial VT[14] are not helpful for differentiating epicardial VT from the right ventricle.[16] All such findings should be tempered by the fact that presence of diffuse or extensive scar or concomitant antiarrhythmic drug use can confound interpretation. As anticipated,

ECG criteria have not been helpful in identifying epicardial VT origin in the setting of prior infarction.

In the setting of idiopathic outflow tract VT, a maximum deflection index (MDI) ≥ 0.55, calculated by dividing QRS onset to maximum precordial deflection time by total QRS duration,[17] is suggestive of an epicardial site of origin. Finally, for tachycardias originating adjacent to the septum, a dramatic pattern break in V_2 may suggest epicardial origin, with either a large S wave if from the superior septum or large R wave if from the inferior septum (Figure 45.3).

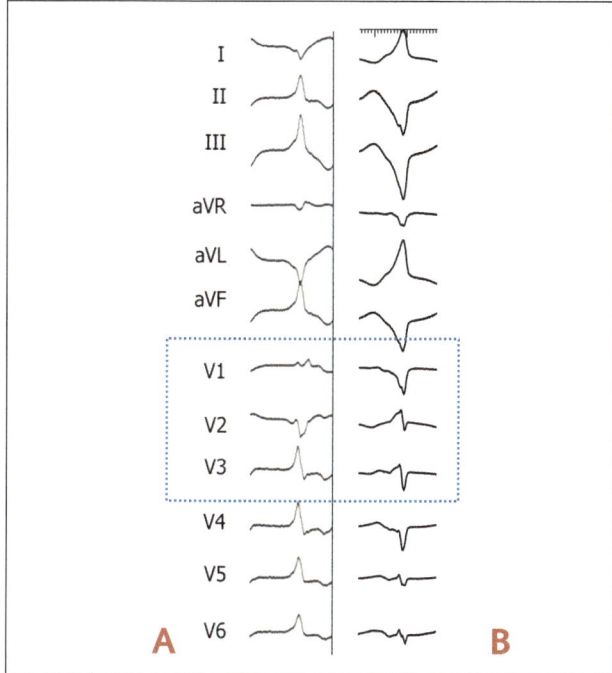

Figure 45.3 Morphologies of VT taken from patients with sites of origin from (**A**) the basal superior septum and (**B**) the basal inferior septum. Note the "pattern break" (**dashed box**) for each patient in leads V_1–V_3, with disparate V_2 R- and S-wave magnitudes compared to those seen in leads V_1 and V_3.

Imaging Clues in the Setting of Structural Heart Disease

Cardiac magnetic resonance imaging (MRI), although more costly and generally less accessible than traditional noninvasive imaging tools (ie, echocardiography and nuclear scintigraphy), is more sensitive in identifying nontransmural and epicardial versus midmyocardial or endocardial scar in both the left and right ventricles.[18-21] Presence of an ICD or pacemaker has long been viewed as a contraindication for performing an MRI, but experiences at several centers, including our own, have shown that it can be done safely.[22,23] Recent developments have also made contrast-enhanced computed tomography (CT), with or without positron emission tomography, potentially helpful in identifying scar and potential VT substrate.[24,25] In the absence of contraindications, most patients presenting for VT ablation at our facility, particularly those with nonischemic substrate, undergo cardiac MRI imaging to identify the presence and extent of nonendocardial abnormalities.

Intracardiac echocardiography (ICE), which can be performed at the time of mapping and ablation, is an additional resource that can quickly help to identify presence of epicardial VT substrate. Specifically, areas of increased epicardial echogenicity seen on ICE have been shown to correlate with areas of low-voltage and abnormal electrograms on epicardial mapping, even when endocardial bipolar mapping is unrevealing.[26]

Clues from Endocardial Mapping and Ablation

Once endocardial mapping and ablation have commenced in the EP laboratory, several clues may indicate the need for additional epicardial work (Table 45.1). During endocardial VT mapping in the setting of structural heart disease, if (1) there is an absence of early or mid-diastolic potentials with detailed activation mapping; (2) there is an absence of isthmus sites identified with entrainment mapping; and/or (3) endocardial ablation from regions with the best entrainment and/or activation times results in delayed termination or fails to terminate VT, adjunctive epicardial mapping with possible ablation is likely necessary. Additionally, if the endocardial bipolar voltage map in sinus rhythm reveals a paucity of areas with low voltage or abnormal electrograms, epicardial mapping to identify more extensive substrate may be indicated. In the case of basal left ventricular VT, and/or in the setting of true idiopathic or left ventricular outflow tract VT, a multipolar catheter in the distal coronary sinus, extending to the great cardiac vein/anterior interventricular vein junction, can be helpful. Earlier recorded activation during VT than that recorded from the LV endocardium, or identification of better pace map matches for VT from this region, each may indicate that epicardial access is needed. Although basal LV epicardial VT can sometimes be targeted via the coronary venous system, proximity of the coronary arteries often prohibits safe ablation.

Another useful tool for identifying potential epicardial substrate during endocardial procedures is the presence of abnormal unipolar endocardial voltage. The wider field of view of the unipolar electrogram allows for identification of abnormal substrate deeper than the normal endocardium. In the left ventricle, endocardial unipolar voltage < 8.3 mV was found to correlate well with abnormal overlying epicardial bipolar voltage among patients with nonischemic cardiomyopathy[27] (Figure 45.4). Similarly, for the right ventricle, endocardial unipolar voltage < 5.5 mV predicted regions of abnormal overlying right ventricular epicardium among patients with ARVC or cardiomyopathy in the absence of coronary artery disease (Figure 45.5).[28]

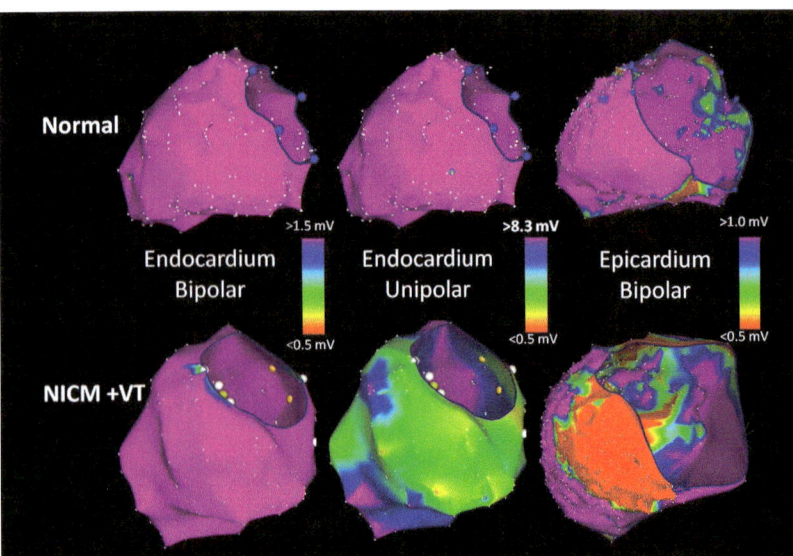

Figure 45.4 Electroanatomic left ventricular maps in posterior-lateral projection are compared from a patient with idiopathic VT and structurally normal heart ("Normal," **top row**) and a patient with nonischemic cardiomyopathy and VT ("NICM +VT," **bottom row**). The endocardial bi- and unipolar and epicardial bipolar voltage maps are all normal for the Normal patient. The endocardial bipolar voltage map from the NICM +VT patient also is normal (**bottom left panel**). However, in contrast, the NICM +VT endocardial unipolar voltage map, using an abnormal cut-off of < 8.3 mV, suggests extensive periannular abnormality in the mid-myocardium and/or epicardium (**bottom middle panel**). These findings are corroborated by a corresponding area of bipolar voltage abnormality on the epicardium of the same patient (**bottom right panel**). Source: Figure adapted with permission from Hutchinson et al. Circ Arrhythm Electrophysiol. 2011;4:49-55.

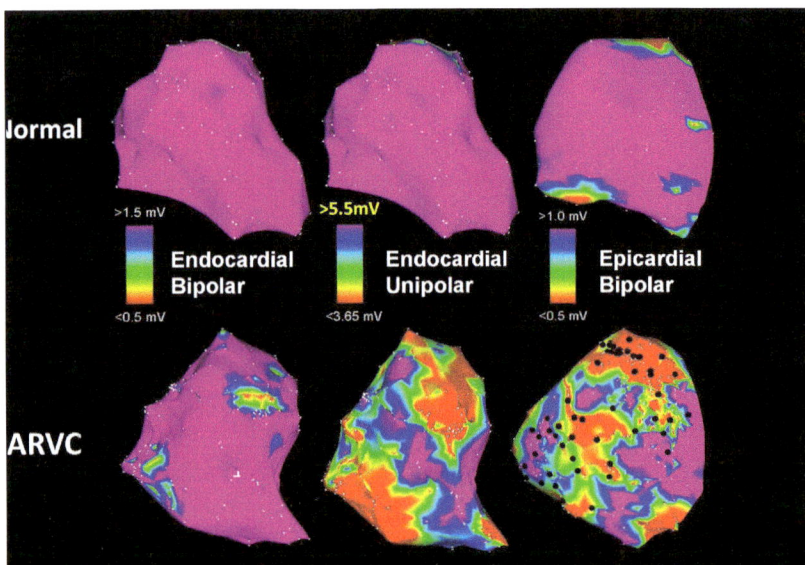

Figure 45.5 Right-lateral projections of right ventricular electroanatomic voltage maps are displayed from a normal patient ("Normal," **top row**) and a patient with arrhythmogenic right ventricular cardiomyopathy ("ARVC," **bottom row**). The endocardial bipolar and unipolar and epicardial bipolar voltage maps from the Normal patient are unremarkable. The endocardial bipolar voltage map from the ARVC patient reveals only small areas of patchy abnormalities along the basal anterior and inferior free wall (**bottom left panel**). However, the endocardial unipolar map (**bottom middle panel**) suggests extensive mid-myocardial and/or epicardial abnormality (cut-off for abnormal < 5.5 mV) that is corroborated on the subsequent epicardial bipolar voltage map (**bottom right panel**). Source: Adapted from Polin et al. Heart Rhythm. 2011;8:76-83, with permission pending from Elsevier.

Obtaining Epicardial Access

Using the technique developed by Sosa and colleagues, subxiphoid, percutaneous access to the pericardial space can be performed with reasonably low risk and without surgical assistance.[5,6] Patients are placed under conscious sedation or general anesthesia, depending on clinical circumstances. If left ventricular endocardial ablation has been performed beforehand, or if patients are on chronic warfarin, anticoagulation is fully reversed. With a 17–18-gauge Tuohy needle inserted just below the rib margin and to the left of the xiphoid process, advancing posteriorly and aiming for the left shoulder or region of the apex will generally allow access to the inferior right ventricle, typically the middle or apical third, where major coronary vessels can be avoided (Figure 45.6A).[29] Alternatively, advancing with a relatively shallow angle and aiming for the right ventricular apex can also be performed, which will allow one to enter the pericardial space over the anterior right ventricle. The former approach may lead to greater risk of liver and diaphragmatic vessel laceration; however, these can usually be avoided by carefully advancing the needle using fluoroscopic guidance and, if necessary, applying gentle traction to move more inferiorly located structures out of the way of the advancing needle.[30] The anterior approach may pose greater risk of right ventricular or distal coronary artery laceration. In general, we prefer the inferior approach. However, depending on the anticipated focus of mapping and ablation, the strategy may differ. For instance, in a patient in whom the area of focus is the inferior right ventricle, an anterior puncture may provide greater maneuverability in the site of interest. In patients with prior cardiac surgery or with prior myocarditis, however, adhesions tend to form anteriorly; thus, a more inferior approach may be more successful.[3]

The pericardial space, in most patients, is a potential space with < 50 mL of pericardial fluid, which can make access challenging. Injecting small amounts of contrast dye once nearing the heart border can help identify when the needle has contacted the parietal pericardium and is visualized as tenting. Additionally, the transmission of the beating heart frequently can be palpable through the shaft of the needle when the heart border has been encountered, and occasionally, ventricular ectopic beats may occur as the needle makes contact with myocardium.

Indications that the needle has passed through the outer pericardial layer include (1) a "popping" sensation transmitted through the needle and (2) distribution of contrast diffusely around the cardiac silhouette with additional, small injection (≤ 1 mL). In the left anterior oblique projection, one then advances a long, soft- or J-tipped guidewire through the needle lumen (Figure 45.6B). It is critical to observe the wire tracking along borders of both right and left ventricles to confirm that access to the pericardial space and not the right ventricle has been obtained. Carrying out this portion of the procedure only in the right anterior oblique or anterior-posterior projection can be misleading, as a wire in the RVOT can appear very similar to a wire tracking along the lateral left ventricle border. If the right ventricle has been entered, the pericardium may still be safely accessed by removing the wire, slightly retracting the needle, and then readvancing the wire. In most circumstances, as long as right ventricle cannulation occurs only with needle and/or wire, laceration of the right ventricular free wall has not occurred, and anticoagulation has been fully reversed, significant bleeding can be avoided.[6] Once pericardial access has been confirmed, a long sheath (7.5 Fr or greater) can be advanced with the dilator over the guidewire.

Difficulty in access may arise when adhesions are present, either from prior cardiac surgery, epicardial patches, myocarditis, or pericarditis, including from prior epicardial ablation.[6,13] Often, with blunt dissection using the guidewire, or a fully deflected catheter, with or without additional support from a stiff, steerable sheath (eg, a short Agilis, St. Jude Medical, St. Paul, MN), adhesions from prior inflammation can be dissected.[13] Pericarditis from epicardial ablation can often be mitigated in advance by infusing intrapericardial corticosteroids at the end of the case.[6,31] In our and others' experience, it has been far more challenging to successfully and safely penetrate adhesions associated with prior surgery.[3] Frequently, dense adhesions are noted anteriorly over the site of valve replacement surgery, but the rest of the epicardium is usually accessible. Patients with prior coronary surgery are especially challenging since disruption of coronary grafts would be life-threatening. Some success has been reported with access obtained via a hybrid approach, using surgical subxiphoid pericardial window or lateral or anterior thoracotomy prior to epicardial mapping and ablation.[6,32] Consistently the most difficult regions to expose are the anterolateral walls and apex, access to which will usually be inadequate using any subxiphoid approach, whether percutaneous or surgical.[32] If access to these regions is necessary, the most success has been reported using anterior thoracotomy, although even then multiple thoracotomies are sometimes required to achieve adequate exposure.[32] Finally, although percutaneous epicardial access has been successfully performed in patients who have undergone prior coronary artery bypass surgery,[13,32] a hybrid or open-chest approach with direct visualization and protection of grafts prior to further instrumentation is recommended.

Epicardial Ablation

After epicardial access has been secured with a sheath, any ablation catheter can then be advanced and maneuvered with usually little difficulty about the ventricles. Pericardial reflections, marking the junctions of the visceral and parietal layers of the serous pericardium, are encountered at the very base of the heart, around the roots of the great vessels, and thus may limit maneuverability somewhat.[30] However, they usually do not significantly hinder ventricular mapping or ablation. Access to the basal anterior-lateral left and

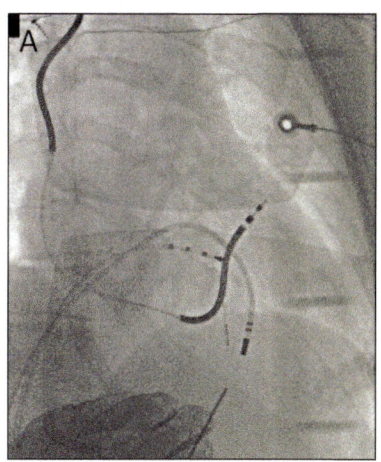
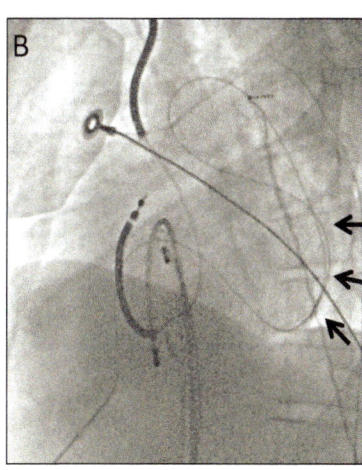

Figure 45.6 Fluoroscopic images acquired in the process of successful pericardial access for epicardial mapping and ablation. Initial approach to the heart border in the right anterior oblique view (**A**) is aimed at the tip of the mapping catheter, which has been placed at the distal inferior right ventricle. Once one documents that access to the pericardial space has been achieved, in the left anterior oblique view (**B**), a guidewire advanced via the needle into the space (**black arrows**) should be observed to cross the plane of the right ventricle and track along borders of both ventricles. See text for details.

right ventricles may be limited by overhanging atrial appendages, which can be recognized by the appearance of atrial electrograms on bipolar recordings. Either irrigated- or nonirrigated-tip radiofrequency or cryoablation catheters may be used. Larger lesions, particularly over areas with epicardial fat, tend to be achievable with either cooled-tip radiofrequency or cryoablation systems, however.[33-37] If an open-irrigated radiofrequency system is used, it is advisable to aspirate periodically from the sideport of the sheath to prevent hemodynamically significant fluid accumulation within the pericardial space. Because there are few concerns for thrombus formation in the nonvascular space, the irrigation flow rate can be decreased to 1–2 mL/min during mapping, and then increased to 10–17 mL/min during ablation.

Mapping strategies as previously described for the endocardium can then be employed, with the following caveats. In contrast to the endocardium, where normal voltage is defined as ≥ 1.5 mV, normal epicardial voltage is defined as < 1 mV, corresponding to ≥ 95% of normal epicardial left ventricular signals recorded at a distance of at least 1 cm from the defined large vessel coronary vasculature.[7,38] Dense scar is still defined by areas with voltage < 0.5 mV.[7] Associated abnormal characteristics other than low voltage include increased width (> 80 ms duration); split electrograms (≥ 2 distinct components separated by > 20 ms isoelectric segment[s]); or late potentials (distinct onset after the QRS).[7] The presence and typical distributions of epicardial fat should be considered in interpreting data. Low voltage in the absence of associated abnormal electrograms, particularly if in the predicted distribution of a major coronary artery or valve annulus, should lead one to suspect location within fat rather than abnormal epicardial tissue.[7,13,39]

Care should be made to avoid damage to the coronary arteries or phrenic nerve. Our approach is to perform coronary angiography prior to any epicardial VT ablation, including ablation from the coronary sinus, as the left circumflex artery often closely follows the venous course. Typically, the ablation catheter is positioned at the site of interest on the epicardium during the angiogram, so that direct visualization and distance estimations can be made. Generally, ablation within 12 mm of any proximal or large coronary artery is avoided, although ablation as close as 5 mm may be performed depending on clinical circumstances.[29,40] Complications including both acute and late occlusion, as well as transient occlusion due to vasospasm, have been reported but can generally be avoided.[37,41]

The same is also generally true for the phrenic nerve, which usually courses along the lateral left ventricle (Figure 45.7A). Its position can be delineated with bipolar pacing at 20 mA, 2 ms pulse-width, and areas of diaphragmatic stimulation are marked using the electroanatomic mapping system (Figure 45.7B).[42] However, because this structure is not adherent to the epicardial surface, it can be lifted away to avoid damage caused by ablation that would otherwise be too close in proximity. This can be accomplished by using either a large, peripheral angioplasty or vascular balloon catheter (Figure 45.7C) or by insufflation of a combination of air and saline.[42,43] When a balloon is used, additional pericardial access is needed, either via another percutaneous puncture or using retained guidewires through the previously placed sheath. A steerable sheath, such as an Agilis (St. Jude Medical), will allow greater ease in positioning the balloon catheter in the desired location. Success has been reported using balloon sizes of 18–25 × 40–60 mm.[42,43] Alternatively, injecting a mixture of air and saline, each alternating in 20 mL

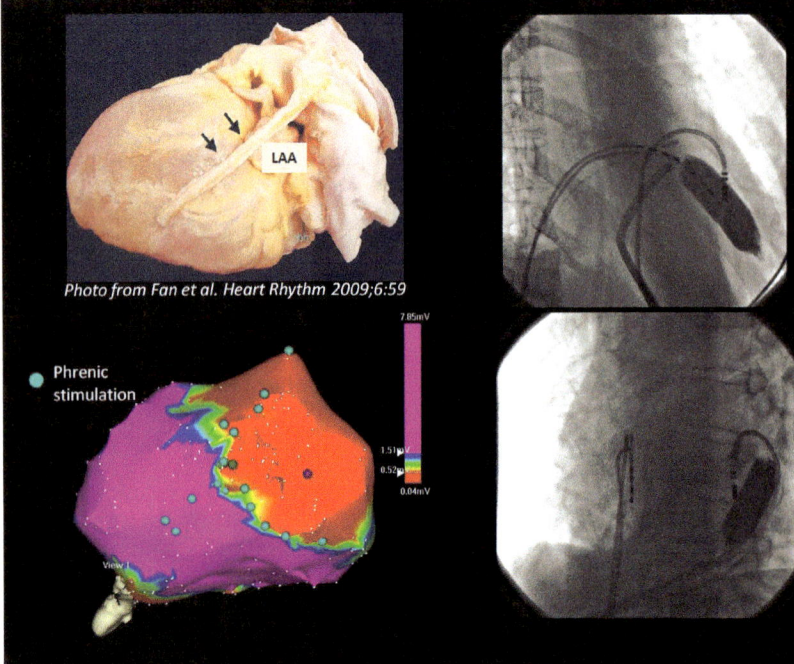

Figure 45.7 Anatomic specimen of the heart in left lateral view (**A**) illustrates the course of the phrenic nerve (**black arrows**) along the top of the left atrial appendage (LAA) and along the lateral left ventricle (LV). Photo courtesy of Dr. Yen Ho and adapted from Fan et al. *Heart Rhythm.* 2009;6:59-64, with permission pending from Elsevier. Electroanatomic LV map in left lateral projection (**B**) is annotated where phrenic nerve stimulation has occurred with high-output pacing (**teal dots**) and through the region of interest for ablation, in this patient with nonischemic cardiomyopathy and ventricular tachycardia. Shown on fluoroscopy in right anterior oblique (**C, top**) and left anterior oblique (**C, bottom**) views, a peripheral angioplasty balloon has been introduced via additional access and sheath to the pericardial space and inflated to lift the phrenic nerve away from the lateral LV, such that ablation in that region can safely be performed. See text for additional details.

volumes, to total volumes of approximately 248 ± 32 mL air and 278 ± 27 mL saline, has been reported to be successful in separating the phrenic nerve from the lateral left ventricular wall without significant hemodynamic compromise.[43] We have found it difficult to titrate such air/saline combinations to maintain adequate separation of the phrenic nerve away from the epicardium over a series of required burns when performing epicardial substrate ablation. Lack of phrenic nerve capture with high-output pacing should be confirmed with either method before each ablation lesion.

Using radiofrequency ablation, typical settings for nonirrigated ablation are power limited to 50 W for 60 to 120 seconds with a maximum temperature of 50°C to 80°C, targeting an impedance drop of 10 to 15 ohms. For irrigated ablation power of 20–50 W, maximum temperature of 42°C to 45°C is commonly employed.[4,37,42] Although it has not been as well utilized in humans as radiofrequency ablation has, animal studies suggest that at least equivalent lesion size can be achieved with epicardial cryoablation as irrigated-tip radiofrequency ablation via 4-minute freeze cycles to temperatures of <−75°C, particularly when freezing energy is delivered through a larger surface area.[36,44] Some animal data suggest that cryoablation can be performed safely closer to coronary arteries than can standard radiofrequency ablation, but further studies are needed to confirm this.[36]

Because of the anatomic constraints described above, targets for epicardial substrate-based ablation differ slightly from those for endocardial ablation. The usual endocardial strategy of applying linear ablation sets that transect arrythmogenic areas within scar and border zone and anchor to either healthy tissue borders or to valve annulus[38] is usually limited by proximity of the coronary arteries. Abnormal substrate should be carefully characterized, with areas of abnormal electrograms marked on the electroanatomic map. Pace mapping can be performed simultaneously in and around the abnormal substrate to define approximate VT exit site(s) or sites with a long stimulus to QRS interval that suggest participation as a critical component of the VT circuit.[45] In general, the combination of LPs in sinus rhythm, a long-stimulus QRS during pace mapping, and a good pace map QRS match suggest the likelihood of proximity to a VT circuit.[7] Substrate-based ablation can then be performed guided by these sites, extended in clusters to incorporate surrounding late potentials within a 3 cm distance. When possible, additional ablation incorporating these cluster sets is performed to linearly transect the substrate or extend as a line to an anatomic boundary, but no closer than 1 cm to a coronary vessel or site demonstrating phrenic nerve capture with 10–20 mA pacing output (Figure 45.8).

Endpoints for epicardial ablation are similar to those for endocardial ablation, with acute success judged by lack of inducibility with programmed stimulation up to triple extrastimuli. Occasionally, additional ablation on the endocardium must ensue after epicardial ablation; this is often true for deeper, mid-myocardial circuits. Anticoagulation is resumed for the duration of left heart intravascular instrumentation, with a sheath maintained in the pericardium, to allow for (1) drainage should pericardial bleeding occur, and (2) additional epicardial mapping and ablation as needed.

Using this approach, we have observed a 71% success rate in eliminating recurrent, sustained VT an average of 1–2 years following epicardial VT ablation for left ventricular NICM. We have demonstrated a nearly 90% intermediate-term success for ablation of VT in the setting of ARVC.[7,9] Multicenter studies that have included

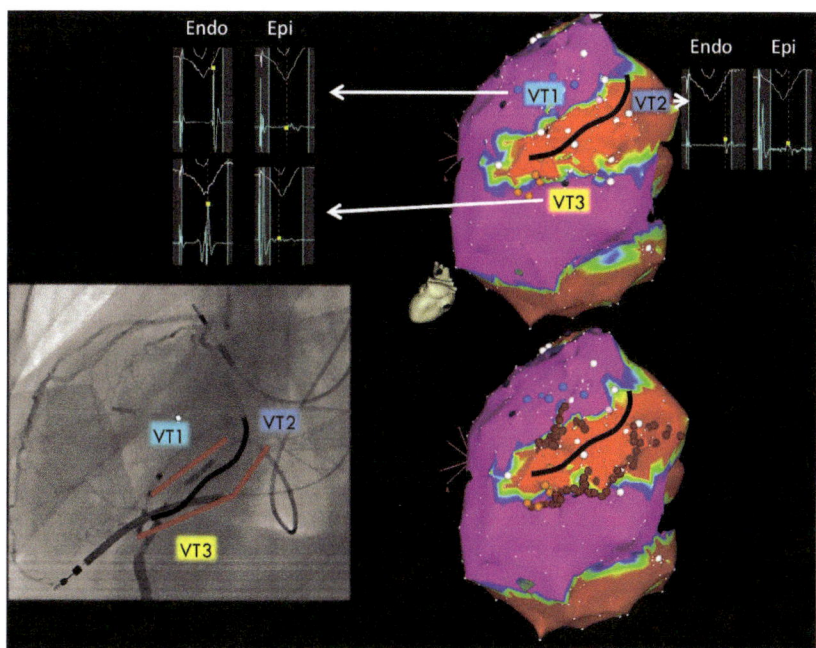

Figure 45.8 Coronary angiogram in a patient with nonischemic cardiomyopathy and ventricular tachycardia (VT) is shown in left lateral view in **panel A**. Transposed on the fluoroscopic image and electroanatomic epicardial map (**B**) are the exits for three different VTs (VT1, VT2, and VT3), determined by entrainment mapping, and their relative position to the obtuse marginal coronary artery (highlighted with **black line** in A and B). Also shown are endocardial (Endo) and epicardial (Epi) electrograms at the sites of each VT. **Red lines** in A indicate the proposed ablation strategy, based on the area of abnormal epicardial voltage and electrograms (**B**). **Panel C** shows the final epicardial map after ablation, again in relation to the obtuse marginal coronary artery position.

patients with a greater variety of substrates (these as well as ischemic and hypertrophic cardiomyopathy) report similar results.[6,46]

Once mapping and ablation are completed, we typically infuse intrapericardial steroids (2 mg/kg triamcinolone or equivalent) to dwell for a period of 10 minutes, to help prevent pericarditis and secondary development of adhesions should a repeat epicardial attempt be required.[31]

Other Potential Complications

Hemopericardium

The most common complication related to epicardial access is bleeding, with major intrapericardial bleeding (> 80 mL) reported in 4.5% of cases; more than half of those are due to right ventricle puncture with initial access.[6] However, epicardial vessel perforation and disruption of tissue from dissection of preexistent pericardial adhesions also can lead to acute hemopericardium.[47] In the unique situation of distal coronary artery perforation, balloon occlusion just proximal to the site of bleeding has been reported to obtain successful hemostasis and may be considered when appropriate to prevent open surgical repair.[47,48] Hemopericardium occurring after epicardial access and during mapping and ablation may be due to (1) rebleeding due to catheter or sheath disruption of thrombus over the site of earlier injury; (2) myocardial bleeding or perforation (eg, during epicardial right ventricular free-wall ablation) due to steam pop; (3) ruptured hemorrhagic epicardial bleb following ablation; (4) new injury with mapping or sheath manipulation; and/or (5) delayed bleeding with re-initiation of heparin due to earlier micro-injury.

Most of these cases can be managed conservatively, with complete reversal of anticoagulation and/or platelet or blood factor transfusions as needed. Additionally, taking care to not manipulate a sheath, particularly if stiff, in the pericardial space without a guidewire, catheter, or dilator through it may help to minimize potential trauma. Continuous surveillance with ICE and repeated drainage of pericardial fluid as needed are important in ascertaining whether operative repair is needed. If, after 30 minutes, frankly bloody fluid is continuously aspirated from the pericardial space (> 500 mL total), or if ICE shows continued effusion despite aggressive aspiration, surgical intervention is likely necessary. Evidence for double right ventricle puncture—where the pericardial space was accessed after entering and then exiting the right ventricular cavity—may not be apparent until after removal of the sheath and catheter, which potentially block the bleeding. Pericardial bleeding in this situation is typically brisk and necessitates surgical repair.[47]

Hemopericardium occurring late after the procedure may also occur, and usually as a consequence of associated pericarditis. These effusions are typically small and amenable to treatment with nonsteroidal anti-inflammatory agents, except in the setting of anticoagulation, where the effusions may be substantial and lead to hemodynamic compromise. Administration of intrapericardial steroids at the end of a case may help to prevent such occurrences.[47] Additionally, we routinely perform serial echocardiography after the procedure, especially if anticoagulation is initiated.

Damage to Adjacent Structures

In the process of obtaining epicardial access, other acute bleeding complications may result from diaphragmatic vessel perforation, which, although rare, can lead to major intra-abdominal bleeding.[3] Liver laceration and hematoma may also occur, as the left lobe of the liver typically crosses the midline and may lie in the trajectory of an advancing needle. In the event that the needle is aimed too far laterally, the pleural space may be inadvertently accessed; pneumothorax can occur in this setting, although rarely.

Lung injury has also been reported in the setting of ablation, given its close proximity, particularly along the lateral surfaces of the heart. Taking care to ensure catheter tip contact and orientation against the epicardial surface and away from the lungs can minimize this effect.[37]

Summary

Epicardial mapping and ablation are frequently necessary for the ablative treatment of VT. This is particularly true among patients with ARVC and nonischemic cardiomyopathy. Access to the epicardium can be achieved percutaneously with relative ease and generally without surgical assistance. Additionally, mapping and ablation are performed using the same general concepts as for the endocardium, with a few modifications. Important caveats include being mindful of preventing injury to coronary arteries and the phrenic nerve, as well as other potentially serious bleeding complications. When performed in experienced hands, outcomes with epicardial ablation in the appropriate patient populations have been promising.

References

1. Miller JM, Tyson GS, Hargrove WC, Vassallo JA, Rosenthal ME, Josephson ME. Effect of subendocardial resection on sinus rhythm endocardial electrogram abnormalities. *Circulation*. 1995;91:2385-2391.
2. Kaltenbrunner W, Cardinal R, Dubuc M, et al. Epicardial and endocardial mapping of ventricular tachycardia in patients with myocardial infarction. Is the origin of the tachycardia always subendocardially localized? *Circulation*. 1991;84:1058-1071.

3. Sosa E, Scanavacca M. Epicardial mapping and ablation techniques to control ventricular tachycardia. *J Cardiovasc Electrophysiol.* 2005;16:449-452.
4. Tedrow U, Stevenson WG. Strategies for epicardial mapping and ablation of ventricular tachycardia. *J Cardiovasc Electrophysiol.* 2009;20:710-713.
5. Sosa E, Scanavacca M, d'Avila A, Pilleggi F. A new technique to perform epicardial mapping in the electrophysiology laboratory. *J Cardiovasc Electrophysiol.* 1996;7:531-536.
6. Sacher F, Roberts-Thomson K, Maury P, et al. Epicardial ventricular tachycardia ablation: a multicenter safety study. *J Am Coll Cardiol.* 2010;21:2366-2372.
7. Cano O, Hutchinson M, Lin D, et al. Electroanatomic substrate and ablation outcome for suspected epicardial ventricular tachycardia in left ventricular nonischemic cardiomyopathy. *J Am Coll Cardiol.* 2009;54(9):799-808.
8. Soejima K, Stevenson WG, Sapp JL, Selwyn AP, Couper G, Epstein LM. Endocardial and epicardial radiofrequency ablation of ventricular tachycardia associated with dilated cardiomyopathy. *J Am Coll Cardiol.* 2004;43:1834-1842.
9. Garcia F, Bazan V, Zado ES, Ren JF, Marchlinski FE. Epicardial substrate and outcome with epicardial ablation of ventricular tachycardia in arrhythmogenic right ventricular cardiomyopathy/dysplasia. *Circulation.* 2009;120:366-375.
10. Hsia HH, Callans DJ, Marchlinski FE. Characterization of endocardial electrophysiological substrate in patients with nonischemic cardiomyopathy and monomorphic ventricular tachycardia. *Circulation.* 2003;108:704-710.
11. Vallès E, Bazan V, Marchlinski FE. ECG criteria to identify epicardial ventricular tachycardia in nonischemic cardiomyopathy. *Circ Arrhythm Electrophysiol.* 2010;3:63-71.
12. Haqqani HM, Tschabrunn CM, Tzou WS, et al. Isolated septal substrate for ventricular tachycardia in nonischemic dilated cardiomyopathy: incidence, characterization, and implications. *Heart Rhythm.* 2011 Aug;8(8):1169-1176.
13. Sosa E, Scanavacca M, d'Avila A, Ramires JAF. Nonsurgical transthoracic epicardial approach in patients with ventricular tachycardia and previous cardiac surgery. *J Interv Card Electrophysiol.* 2004;10:281-288.
14. Berruezo A, Mont L, Nava S, Chueca E, Bartholomay E, Brugada J. Electrocardiographic recognition of the epicardial origin of ventricular tachycardias. *Circulation.* 2004;109:1842-1847.
15. Bazan V, Gerstenfeld EP, Garcia F, et al. Site-specific twelve-lead ECG features to identify an epicardial origin for left ventricular tachycardia in the absence of myocardial infarction. *Heart Rhythm.* 2007;4:1403-1410.
16. Bazan V, Bala R, Garcia F, et al. Twelve-lead ECG features to identify ventricular tachycardia arising from the epicardial right ventricle. *Heart Rhythm.* 2006;3:1132-1139.
17. Daniels DV, Lu YY, Morton JB, et al. Idiopathic epicardial left ventricular tachycardia originating remote from the sinus of Valsalva: electrocardiographic characteristics, catheter ablation, and identification from the 12-lead electrocardiogram. *Circulation.* 2006;113:1659-1666.
18. Jerosch-Herold M, Kwong RY. Optimal imaging strategies to assess coronary blood flow and risk for patients with coronary artery disease. *Curr Opin Cardiol.* 2008;23:599-606.
19. Ashikaga H, Sasano T, Dong J, et al. Magnetic resonance based anatomical analysis of scar-realted ventricular tachycardia: implications for catheter ablation. *Circ Res.* 2007;101:939-947.
20. Bogun FM, Desjardins B, Good E, et al. Delayed-enhanced magnetic resonance imaging in nonischemic cardiomyopathy: utility for identifying the ventricular arrhythmia substrate. *J Am Coll Cardiol.* 2009;53:1138-1145.
21. Yokokawa M, Tada H, Koyama K, et al. The characteristics and distribution of the scar tissue predict ventricular tachycardia in patients with advanced heart failure. *PACE.* 2009;32:314-322.
22. Nazarian S, Roguin A, Zviman MM, et al. Clinical utility and safety of a protocol for noncardiac and cardiac magnetic resonance imaging of patients with permanent pacemakers and implantable-cardioverter defibrillators at 1.5 Tesla. *Circulation.* 2006;114:1277-1284.
23. Naehle CP, Strach K, Thomas D, et al. Magnetic resonance imaging at 1.5-T in patients with implantable cardioverter-defibrillators. *J Am Coll Cardiol.* 2009;54:549-555.
24. Tian J, Jeudy J, Smith MF, et al. Three-dimensional contrast-enhanced multidetector CT for anatomic, dynamic, and perfusion characterization of abnormal myocardium to guide ventricular tachycardia ablations. *Circ Arrhythm Electrophysiol.* 2010;3:496-504.
25. Tian J, Smith MF, Chinnadurai P, et al. Clinical application of PET/CT fusion imaging for three-dimensional myocardial scar and left ventricular anatomy during ventricular tachycardia ablation. *J Cardiovasc Electrophysiol.* 2009;20:597-604.
26. Bala R, Cano O, Hutchinson MD, et al. Unique epicardial substrate in nonischemic cardiomyopathy: echo signature, electrogram correlates and outcome with substrate based ablation. *Circulation.* 2008;118:S826.
27. Hutchinson MD, Gerstenfeld EP, Desjardins B, et al. Endocardial unipolar voltage mapping to detect epicardial ventricular tachycardia substrate in patients with nonischemic left ventricular cardiomyopathy. *Circ Arrhythm Electrophysiol.* 2011 Feb;4(1):49-55.
28. Polin GM, Haqqani H, Tzou W, et al. Endocardial unipolar voltage mapping to identify epicardial substrate in arrhythmogenic right ventricular cardiomyopathy/dysplasia. *Heart Rhythm.* 2011 Jan;8(1):76-83.
29. Sosa E, Scanavacca M, d'Avila A, Oliveria F, Ramires JAF. Nonsurgical transthoracic epicardial catheter ablation to treat recurrent ventricular tachycardia occurring late after myocardial infarction. *J Am Coll Cardiol.* 2000;35:1442-1449.
30. Lachman N, Syed FF, Habib A, et al. Correlative anatomy for the electrophysiologist, Part I: the pericardial space, oblique sinus, transverse sinus. *J Cardiovasc Electrophysiol.* 2010;21:1421-1426.
31. d'Avila A, Neuzil P, Thiagalingam A, et al. Experimental efficacy of pericardial instillation of anti-inflammatory agents during percutaneous epicardial catheter ablation to prevent postproceure pericarditis. *J Cardiovasc Electrophysiol.* 2007;18:1178-1183.
32. Michowitz Y, Mathuria N, Tung R, et al. Hybrid procedures for epicardial catheter ablation of ventricular tachycardia: value of surgical access. *Heart Rhythm.* 2010 Nov;7(11):1635-1643.
33. Haines DE, Verow AF. Observations on electrode-tissue interface temperature and effect on electrical impedance during radiofrequency ablation of ventricular myocardium. *Circulation.* 1990;82:1034-1038.
34. Thiagalingam A, Pouliopoulos J, Barry MA, et al. Cooled needle catheter ablation creates deeper and wider lesions than irrigated tip catheter ablation. *J Cardiovasc Electrophysiol.* 2005;16:508-515.
35. Nakagawa H, Yamanashi WS, Pitha JV, et al. Comparison of in vivo tissue temperature profile and lesion geometry for radiofrequency ablation with a saline-irrigated electrode versus temperature control in a canine thigh muscle preparation. *Circulation.* 1995;91:2264-2273.
36. d'Avila A, Aryana A, Thiagalingam A, et al. Focal and linear endocardial and epicardial catheter-based cryoablation of

normal and infarcted ventricular tissue. *PACE*. 2008;31: 1322-1331.
37. d'Avila A, Houghtaling C, Gutierrez P, et al. Catheter ablation of ventricular epicardial tissue: a comparison of standard and cooled-tip radiofrequency energy. *Circulation*. 2004; 109:2363-2369.
38. Marchlinski FE, Callans DJ, Gottlieb CD, Zado ES. Linear ablation lesions for control of unmappable ventricular tachycardia in patients with ischemia and nonischemic cardiomyopathy. *Circulation*. 2000;101:1288-1296.
39. Dixit S, Narula N, Callans DJ, Marchlinski FE. Electroanatomic mapping of human heart: epicardial fat can mimic scar. *J Cardiovasc Electrophysiol*. 2003;14:1128.
40. Aliot EM, Stevenson WG, Almendral-Garrote JM, et al. EHRA/HRS expert consensus on catheter ablation of ventricular arrhythmias. *Heart Rhythm*. 2009;6:886-933.
41. Roberts-Thomson KC, Seller J, Steven D, et al. Percutaneous access of the epicardial space for mapping ventricular and supraventricular arrhythmias in patients with and without prior cardiac surgery. *J Cardiovasc Electrophysiol*. 2010; 21:406-411.
42. Fan R, Cano O, Ho SY, et al. Characterization of the phrenic nerve course within the epicardial substrate of patients with nonischemic cardiomyopathy and ventricular tachycardia. *Heart Rhythm*. 2009;6:59-64.
43. Di Biase L, Burkhardt JD, Pelargonio G, et al. Prevention of phrenic nerve injury during epicardial ablation: comparison of methods for separating the phrenic nerve from the epicardial surface. *Heart Rhythm*. 2009;6:957-961.
44. Hashimoto K, Watanabe I, Okumura Y, et al. Comparison of endocardial and epicardial lesion size following large-tip and extra-large-tip transcatheter cryoablation. *Circ J*. 2009; 73:1619-1626.
45. Stevenson WG, Sager PT, Natterson PD, Saxon LA, Middlekauf HR, Wiener I. Relation of pace mapping QRS configuration and conduction delay to ventricular tachycardia reentry circuits in human infarct scars. *J Am Coll Cardiol*. 1995;26:481-488.
46. Dukkipati SR, d'Avila A, Soejima K, et al. Long-term outcomes of combined epicardial and endocardial ablation of monomorphic ventricular tachycardia related to hypertrophic cardiomyopathy. *Circ Arrhythm Electrophysiol*. 2011;4:185-194.
47. Koruth JS, d'Avila A. Management of hemopericardium related to percutaneous epicardial access, mapping and ablation. *Heart Rhythm*. 2011;8:1652-1657.
48. Hsieh CHC, Ross DL. Case of coronary perforation with epicardial access for ablation of ventricular tachycardia. *Heart Rhythm*. 2011;8:318-321.

CHAPTER 46

Ventricular Fibrillation

Ashok J. Shah, MD; Daniel Scherr, MD; Xingpeng Liu, MD;
Nicolas Derval, MD; Michel Haïssaguerre, MD

Introduction

Ventricular fibrillation (VF) underlies the majority of potentially preventable sudden cardiac deaths all over the world. Due to strikingly lethal characteristics and momentary presence, VF has been mapped and studied, by and large, in animal hearts or models.[1-13] Moreover, VF is likely to be mechanistically varied in comparison to the sustained monomorphic reentrant ventricular arrhythmias. Reentry involving the substrate and the Purkinje-myocardium junction and the migratory propagation of vortices are the likely mechanisms describing the role of ventricular myocardium in the maintenance of arrhythmia.[7-9] The recently described role of triggers initiating these arrhythmias in structurally normal and diseased hearts is conceptually important.[13-16] This chapter discusses ablation of primary VF (excluding VF occurring due to degeneration of VT) in normal and diseased hearts involving triggers like distal Purkinje network in idiopathic VF and LQTS and substrate like RVOT myocardium in Brugada syndrome.

Mapping of Purkinje Triggers Initiating VF and Postablation Monitoring

Mapping of arrhythmogenic triggers in Purkinje arborization and/or contiguous myocardium has been extensively discussed in Chapter 32 in different subsets of patients with normal and diseased hearts presenting with complex ventricular arrhythmias, eg, idiopathic PMVT/VF; VF in LQTS, Brugada, and early repolarization syndromes; VF associated with ischemic and amyloid heart diseases; and VF associated with nonischemic dilated cardiomyopathies. The discussion includes a description of a special multipolar mapping catheter (PentaRay®, Biosense Webster, Diamond Bar, CA), procedural techniques, description of study population and outcomes of mapping in each of the above-mentioned subsets. The readers are referred to Chapter 32 for pertinent details.

Postablation, the patients remain in the hospital for a variable period depending on their clinical situation associated with VF. All of them stay at least 3 days postprocedure on continuous telemetry. On follow-up at our center, 12-lead ECG, stress test, and 24-hour ambulatory telemonitoring are performed at 1, 3, 6, and 12 months postprocedure and every 6 months to 1 year thereafter. If the patients are referred from a distance, they will be followed up by the referring physician. Finally, all patients who agree have an implantable cardioverter-defibrillator (ICD) at discharge. Besides the clinical history of recurrent symptoms, we rely on ICD logs for recurrence of VF (sustained/nonsustained) episodes (syncope/presyncope, etc.).

RF Catheter Ablation of VF Triggers: Insights from Clinical Studies

Ablation of Triggers of Idiopathic PMVT/VF

Procedural Technique

Knecht et al[17] diagnosed and ablated the site of origin of ventricular ectopy (Figure 46.1) initiating polymorphic VT and VF in 38 patients with idiopathic VF (Chapter 32). Ablation of monomorphic ectopy was performed at the earliest site (Purkinje network in 33 patients, and myocardium in 5 patients) observed during mapping by the use of RF energy with a target temperature of 50°C and a maximum power of 50 W using 4 mm tip nonirrigated ablation catheter (Celsius® THERMOCOOL catheter, Biosense Webster). In cases wherein the desired power could not been delivered, an externally irrigated 3.5 mm tip catheter (THERMOCOOL, Biosense Webster) was used. For this purpose, manual titration of the saline perfusate ranging from 10 to 60 mL/min was performed to achieve the required power. In all cases, ablation was extended approximately 1 cm² around the targeted site involving the distal Purkinje network and/or myocardium. It might have been even larger when varying morphologies of clinical ectopies—isolated or in repetitive form—were documented.

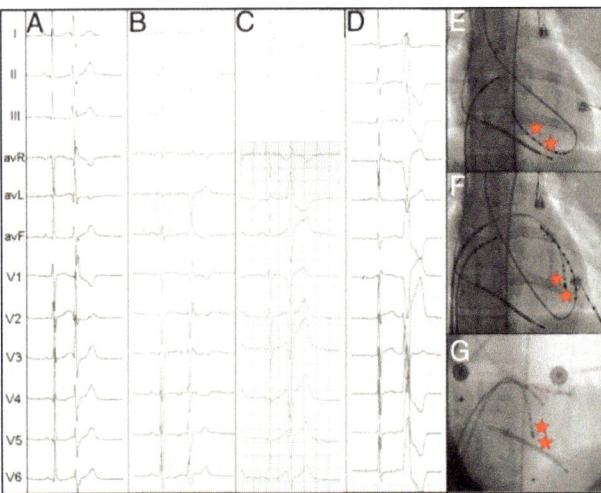

Figure 46.1 Triggered VF 12-lead ECGs (**left**) and their corresponding location in the anteroposterior fluoroscopic view (**right, red asterisks**). The origin of ventricular premature beat (VPB) triggering ventricular fibrillation (VF) was the left Purkinje either at the posterior (**A**) or the anterior (**B**) insertion, the right Purkinje (**C**), and the RVOT (**D**). Related fluoroscopic views with a decapolar catheter inserted in the left ventricle (**E, F**), an ablation catheter inserted in the right ventricle (**G**), and a quadripolar catheter inserted at the His position (**E, F,** and **G**).

Ventricular premature beat originating in the left Purkinje system (**A** and **B** and related anteroposterior fluoroscopic view) produce more variable 12-lead ECG patterns, reflecting the more complex and extended Purkinje arborization on the left. VPBs originating in the right Purkinje system (**C** and related anteroposterior fluoroscopic view) typically have an LBBB pattern with left superior axis. Ventricular premature beat originating from the RVOT (**D**) have the classical aspect with an LBBB pattern and an inferior axis. *Source: J Am Coll Cardiol.* 2009;54(6):522-528. Figure reproduced with permission from Elsevier (March 16, 2011).

Procedural Endpoints

The procedural endpoint was abolition of all clinical ventricular ectopies and unstable ventricular arrhythmias.

Procedural Outcomes and Safety

The median durations of RF energy delivery, fluoroscopy, and total procedural time were 14 minutes, 28 minutes, and 135 minutes, respectively. Typically, 5 to 7 RF energy applications were made at and around (~1 cm) the region of interest to minimize the risk of recurrence. Thirty patients (81%) had clinical ectopy at the time of the procedure, whereas 8 patients (19%) did not. Of 5 patients with myocardial-origin ectopies, 4 patients were successfully ablated in the RVOT. A mean of 1.7 ± 2.0 ectopic morphologies were targeted per patient. Ectopies were abolished successfully in all patients. Ablation at successful sites often resulted in transient polymorphic VT and/or VF in most patients but required shock in 5 patients (Video 46.1). After ablation, 1 patient developed transient LBBB. Six patients developed intraventricular conduction defects not meeting the established criteria for BBB. None of the patients developed any other complication.

Follow-up Results

All patients were followed for a median duration of a little over 5 years. The efficacy of the ablation procedure was judged on the basis of clinical history of syncope/presyncope, follow-up ECGs, Holter monitoring, and interrogation of defibrillator. The latter was available in 37 of 38 patients to retrieve arrhythmia logs. Thirty-one patients did not have recurrence off antiarrhythmic drugs. Repeat ablation procedure was required after median 2 years in 5 of 7 patients whose ICD logs showed frequent VF recurrence refractory to antiarrhythmic medication. Four of these 5 patients had new morphology ectopy, whereas 1 patient had the same clinical morphology of the ectopy triggering VF as previously ablated. These patients had no subsequent recurrence of VF or documented ectopies over a follow-up period of median 28 months. One of the 2 patients with VF recurrence who were not reablated responded to previously ineffective quinidine therapy. Arrhythmia resolved spontaneously in the other. Electrical storm recurred in 3 of 12 patients who presented with storm before undergoing ablation. Ectopic beats recurred in 3 patients, 1 of whom underwent successful reablation for symptoms. In the other 2 patients, ectopies continued to persist without initiating arrhythmia while on verapamil and quinidine therapy, respectively.

Ablation of Triggers of PMVT/VF Associated with Long QT Syndrome and Ablation of Triggers and Substrate in Brugada Syndrome

Procedural Technique and Endpoints

Ablation has been reported in 7 patients experiencing polymorphic VT and VF associated with LQTS and Brugada syndrome.[15] Similar procedural technique and endpoints as described previously for idiopathic VF were adopted for mapping and ablation.

Procedural Outcomes and Safety

The procedural and fluoroscopy durations were 169 ± 57 minutes and 42 ± 21 minutes, respectively (▶ Video 46.2).

Long QT Syndrome: Ventricular ectopy initiating the arrhythmia originated in Purkinje arborization in 3 of 4 patients (distal arborization in 2 and posterior fascicle in 1). In the remaining patient, the ventricular ectopy originated from RVOT myocardium and was successfully ablated by 6 minutes of RF application. Successful ablation of Purkinje ectopies was preceded by a flurry of ectopies and polymorphic VT before elimination of ectopic activity. Different morphologies were progressively eliminated by ablation at multiple sites using 12 to 24 minutes of RF energy application. Postablation, Purkinje potential was not observed preceding the local EGM. There was no evidence of block within the HPS or ventricular conduction delay on surface ECG.

Brugada Syndrome: Ventricular ectopy initiating the arrhythmia originated in right ventricular distal Purkinje arborization in 1 of 3 patients and was eliminated after 10 minutes of RF energy application. In the other 2 patients, RVOT myocardial triggers responsible for originating the arrhythmia were successfully ablated by 7 to 10 minutes of RF energy application. VF, which was induced previously from the RVA, could not be induced with 2 extrastimuli in any of the 3 patients, indicating a change in the arrhythmogenic RVOT myocardial substrate. No conduction disturbances were observed.

Follow-up Results

Long QT Syndrome. During follow-up of mean 4 years, 2 patients have remained free from recurrent VF leading to syncope or sudden cardiac death off antiarrhythmic drugs. One patient died unexpectedly during sleep after 5 years (unpublished data) and another continues to experience recurrent ectopies on β-blocker therapy without VF, syncope, or sudden cardiac death. Although ventricular ectopies recurred in all, the daily ectopic burden was substantially reduced in 6 patients.

Brugada Syndrome. During follow-up of mean 4 years, all patients have remained free from recurrent VF leading to syncope or sudden cardiac death off antiarrhythmic drugs (unpublished data). In 1 patient, the ECG pattern of Brugada syndrome was abolished immediately after ablation of the substrate in the anteroseptal and lateral RVOT.[18] The ECG has shown no reappearance of Brugada pattern after an almost 7-year follow-up period, suggesting a potential role of ablation in curing the primary electrical disorder (Figure 46.2).

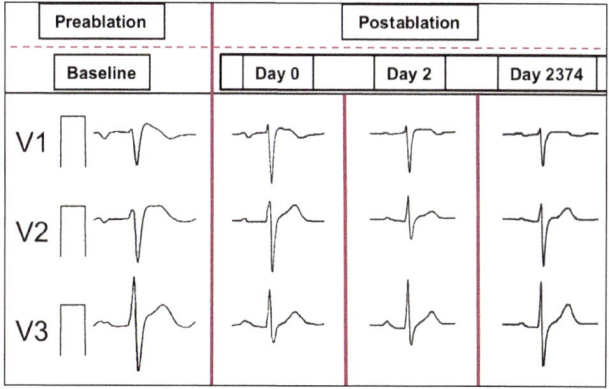

Figure 46.2 Abolition of Brugada syndrome ECG by regional ablation.

Ablation of Triggers of PMVT/VF Associated with Early Repolarization Syndrome

Procedural Technique and Endpoints

Ablation has been reported in 8 patients experiencing recurrent, drug-refractory VF associated with early repolarization syndrome without any structural cardiac abnormality.[19] Similar procedural technique and endpoints as described previously for idiopathic VF were adopted for mapping and ablation. A total of 26 ectopic patterns were mapped either to the ventricular myocardium (16 patterns) or to Purkinje tissue (10 patterns). In 6 subjects with early repolarization recorded only in inferior leads, all ectopic beats originated from the inferior ventricular wall. In 2 subjects with widespread early repolarization, as recorded by both inferior and lateral leads, ectopic beats originated from multiple regions.

Procedural Outcomes

Catheter ablation eliminated all ectopic beats in 5 subjects but failed to control them in 3 subjects. Multiple morphologies of ectopic beats and widespread presence of triggering foci in a small number of patients with early repolarization syndrome treated with catheter ablation may make catheter ablation therapy less appealing.

Ablation of Triggers of PMVT/VF in Ischemic Heart Disease

Several centers have reported their experience in ablation of triggers of VF arising in the setting of acute and chronic myocardial infarction.[16,20,21] We prefer to discuss ablation therapy targeting triggers of polymorphic ventricular arrhythmias and VF arising acutely (< 1 week), delayed (> 1 week), and remotely (> 6 months) after myocardial infarction.

Part A. Arrhythmia Onset < 1 Week after Acute Myocardial Infarction

Procedural Technique and Endpoints

Bansch et al[16] mapped and ablated refractory VF storm within 1 week of acute myocardial infarction in 4 patients. Left ventricular mapping has been described in detail in Chapter 32. Ablation of ectopy originating the storm was performed with a nonirrigated 7-Fr, 4 mm tip electrode via a retrograde transaortic approach with or without anterograde transseptal approach. Purkinje-origin ectopies were targeted in 3 of 4 patients using power limited to 50 W and temperature limited to 55°C during each application lasting 120 seconds maximum. The procedural endpoint was abolition of electrical storm and all clinical ventricular ectopies initiating the storm.

Procedural Outcomes and Safety

In 3 of 4 patients with intraprocedural clinical ectopy, successful ablation of the focal source in the distal Purkinje network suppressed the ectopies after 6–21 RF applications in the inferomedial (2 patients) and anteromedial (1 patient) left ventricle. In the remaining patient, a well-matched site of pace mapping was ablated with 30 RF applications in both anteromedial and inferomedial left ventricle. No complications including conduction abnormalities were noted.

Follow-up Results

All patients were monitored intensively on β-blockers (+ amiodarone in 1 patient for concomitant atrial fibrillation) during hospitalization. Except for 1 patient, all of them underwent implantation of a defibrillator before discharge from the hospital. At mean follow-up of 15 ± 13 months, all patients have remained free from ventricular tachyarrhythmia based on the clinical history and ICD logs.

Part B. Arrhythmia Onset > 1 Week after Acute Myocardial Infarction

Procedural Technique and Endpoints

In an unpublished work by Szumowski et al (personal communication), mapping and ablation of Purkinje-origin ectopy (Figure 46.3) initiating polymorphic VT and/or VF storm after a mean period of 10 days post acute coronary syndrome were performed in 14 patients (Chapter 32). Ablation was performed using 8 mm tip RFA catheter with a target temperature of 55°C to 65°C and a maximum power of 70 W. If sufficient power could not be applied, a 4 mm irrigated-tip catheter with saline perfusion at 15 to 30 mL/min was used with maximum power of 35 W and temperature of 48°C.

The procedural endpoints were to abolish Purkinje-origin ectopy or terminate the arrhythmia. Applications consolidating the abolition of culprit foci were aimed to minimize recurrence. All patients were followed in the hospital for 3 to 5 days postablation.

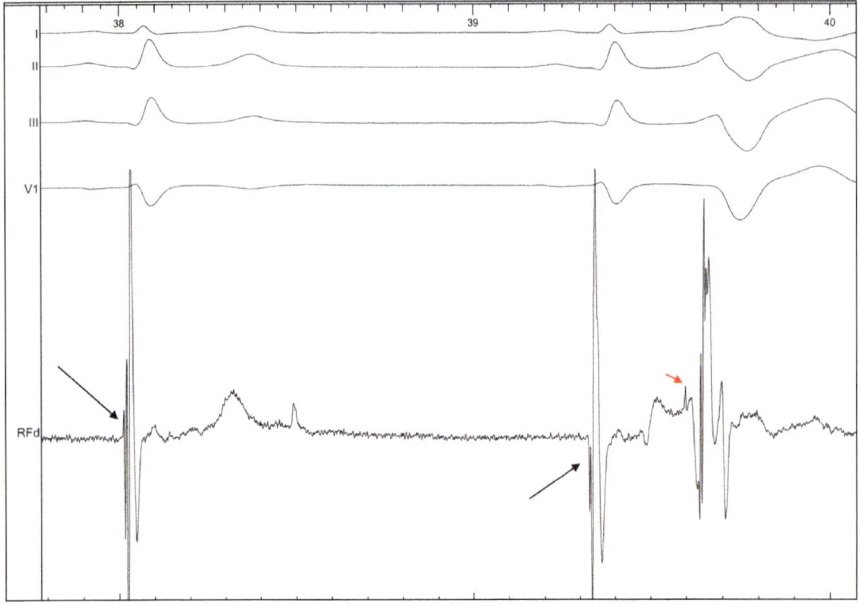

Figure 46.3 Purkinje-triggered ectopy. Distal Purkinje potential is marked by **black arrows** in sinus rhythm. During an ectopic beat, Purkinje potential distinctly stands out preceding the local ventricular EGM.

Procedural Outcomes and Safety

Successful abolition of the culprit foci and clinical arrhythmia was achieved in 13 of 14 patients after mean 26 ± 10 minutes of RF application in the peripheral Purkinje network. Ablation was unsuccessful in the remaining patient, who expired one day after the procedure. In 2 patients, ventricular MRT was inducible at the end of the ablation of clinical arrhythmia, necessitating further appropriate ablation. Defibrillators were implanted in 12 of 13 successfully ablated survivors. No other complications, including conduction disturbances, were observed.

Follow-up Results

Follow-up data on arrhythmia recurrence included clinical history, Holter, and ICD logs. Aggressive (≥ 3 times) Holter monitoring was performed in a patient without ICD. After a mean follow-up of 30 ± 24 months, 1 patient developed monomorphic VT and underwent a successful second procedure. None of the patients developed recurrent polymorphic VT/VF/electrical storm. Three patients died due to heart failure.

Part C. Arrhythmia Onset > 6 Months after Acute Myocardial Infarction

Procedural Technique and Endpoints

Marrouche et al[20] reported mapping and ablation of refractory electrical storm occurring > 6 months after acute coronary event without any identifiable precipitant in 8 patients (Chapter 32). RFA was performed with a cooled-tip ablation catheter (NaviStar, Biosense Webster) with maximum power of 60 W and temperature of 55°C. The RF current was applied for a maximum of 120 seconds at a time. For patients with inducible PVCs, the earliest activation site of the PVC was targeted. For those patients without inducible PVCs, ablation was performed along the scar border zone in locations where the Purkinje-like potentials were identified.

Ablation was considered acutely successful if no ventricular ectopy could be documented 30 minutes after the last lesion. If they recurred, more RF lesions were applied in the target region. Abolition of Purkinje-like potentials was the endpoint in patients without intraprocedural ectopies.

Procedural Outcomes and Safety

Intraprocedural ectopy was observed and successfully ablated in 5 of 8 patients with preceding Purkinje-like potential in scar border zone. Fast monomorphic VT was subsequently induced with programmed ventricular stimulation and successfully ablated again in the scar border zone in 2 of these 5 patients. In the remaining 3 patients without intraprocedural ectopy, ablation targeted areas with Purkinje-like potential observed during sinus rhythm along the scar border zone. Programmed stimulation led to the development of unstable monomorphic VT postablation in 1 patient. VF storm acutely subsided after ablation in the scar border zone in all patients (anteroseptal, 5 patients; posteroseptal, 2 patients; lateral, 1 patient) without any complications.

Follow-up Results

Seven patients had an implantable defibrillator. At a mean follow-up time of 10 ± 6 months, 1 patient (the one with an LVAD) experienced a single episode of VF and died later of septic shock. Another patient developed a slow, hemodynamically stable monomorphic VT, which resulted in shock therapy. Later, it was successfully ablated. Nonsustained episodes of monomorphic VT occurred in 3 patients without any device intervention. No deaths reportedly occurred due to arrhythmia or heart failure.

Ablation of Triggers of PMVT/VF in Amyloid Heart Disease

Procedural Technique and Endpoints

Mlcochova et al[22] described successful mapping and ablation of ventricular ectopy triggering polymorphic VT/fibrillation and electrical storm in 2 patients with amyloid heart disease (Chapter 32). Ablation was performed using irrigated 4 mm tip ThermoCool Shower Catheter (Biosense Webster) at the site of earliest activation in the ventricle during ectopy. Postablation arrhythmia induction was attempted.

Procedural Outcomes and Safety

Patient 1: After 25 applications of RF energy at the myocardial focus of origin of ectopy, complete elimination was achieved without inducibility of sustained ventricular arrhythmia and substantial improvement in the patient's hemodynamic status. A defibrillator was implanted before discharge from the hospital.

Patient 2: Ablation was performed in the proximal Purkinje network (posterior fascicle) with elimination of clinical ectopy within 2 seconds of RF delivery and no intraprocedural inducibility. There were no recurrences of ventricular ectopy and polymorphic VT or VF postablation. However, the in-hospital course was complicated by sepsis and multiorgan failure due to an underlying medical disorder. Three weeks later, she died in the hospital from prolonged asystole.

Follow-up Results

No ventricular arrhythmias have been recorded 8 months postablation in patient 1.

Ablation of Triggers of PMVT/VF in Nonischemic Dilated Cardiomyopathy

Procedural Technique and Endpoints

Sinha et al[23] reported ablation of triggers of refractory VF in 5 patients with nonischemic dilated cardiomyopathy (Chapter 32). RFA was performed with a cooled-tip ablation catheter (NaviStar ThermoCool, Biosense Webster), with maximum power of 40 W and temperature of 50°C. Maximum application duration was 60 seconds at a time. For patients with ectopies, the earliest activation site was targeted. In patients without inducible PVCs, RF ablation was performed along the scar border zone, where Purkinje-like potentials were identified. No ablation was undertaken in 1 patient without scar and ectopies/arrhythmia.

If there were no ectopies within 30 minutes of the last RF lesion, ablation was considered successful. If ectopies recurred during that time, more RF lesions were applied in the target region. In patients without intraprocedural ectopy, the endpoint was abolition of all detectable Purkinje-like potentials.

Procedural Outcomes and Safety

Four of 5 patients underwent ablation. Since all the patients who underwent ablation had scar on the posterior mitral annular region, the number of RF lesions (mean 11 ± 8) in the posterolateral and posteroseptal left ventricle varied depending on the scar size.

In the patient who underwent mapping and ablation of the triggering extrasystole, ablation was successfully performed at the earliest site with Purkinje-like potential in the scar border zone. There were no ectopies or inducible ventricular arrhythmias 30 minutes after ablation. In 3 patients without any ectopy, Purkinje-like potentials in 7 different regions in the scar border zone were successfully ablated.

No complications including conduction disturbances following ablation were noted, although the lesion was applied in clear vicinity of the left bundle as evident by intracardiac recording in 2 patients.

Follow-up Results

Patients were followed up at 3, 6, and 12 months after RFA, and defibrillators were interrogated to detect stored ventricular arrhythmias at each follow-up visit. Recurrence of arrhythmias was defined by delivery of ICD therapy due to ventricular dysrhythmia. During a mean follow-up of 12 ± 5 months, the patient who did not have posterior mitral scar, and consequently did not receive any treatment with ablation, had 4 episodes of VF that resulted in shocks. Among the 4 patients with ablation of Purkinje-like potential, 1 experienced a single nonsustained episode of VF without ICD intervention. No deaths were reported.

RF Catheter Ablation of VF Triggers: Excerpts from Clinical Case Reports

Purkinje and myocardial triggers have been implicated in sporadic individual case reports, besides a series of patients, on initiation of VF by focal sources followed by successful ablation of the foci to cure the arrhythmia. In 1997, Ashida et al[24] showed that the isolated ventricular extrasystoles that initiated idiopathic polymorphic VT were exactly replicated by pace mapping at the septal site of the RVOT. RFA at this site abolished the arrhythmia and episodes of syncope off antiarrhythmic agents. Since extrasystoles persisted, the authors believed ablation to have altered the local substrate so as to render it incapable of sustaining the arrhythmia. The authors were the first to report focal ablation therapy as a cure for unmappable arrhythmias. Several years later, Kusano et al[25] and Takatsuki et al[26] separately demonstrated successful ablation of focal RVOT ectopy initiating recurrent idiopathic VF resulting in cure. Both activation and pace mapping were helpful in localization of the trigger source. Later, Saliba et al[27] demonstrated the role of a focal trigger in the initiation of idiopathic VF in a patient with late systolic potential in sinus rhythm, which resembled Purkinje potential and preceded the ectopy. In 2004, Pasquié et al[28] reported fever as a trigger for idiopathic VF storm initiated by the ectopy in the anterior right ventricular distal Purkinje network, ablation of which successfully abolished the refractory arrhythmia. In the same year, when Li et al[29] reported successful ablation of Purkinje-origin ectopy initiating VF post aortic valve repair in a teenage girl, Betts et al[30] used a noncontact mapping system to localize and ablate focal triggers in a patient with idiopathic VF. Nogami et al[31] nicely demonstrated reentry within the Purkinje tree as an essential mechanism for maintenance of idiopathic VF. The authors successfully abolished the arrhythmia by breaking the reentrant circuit without necessarily ablating the earliest Purkinje potential. Several reports involving trigger ablation of VF arising from different regions of the right and left ventricles of the structurally normal and diseased hearts followed.[32-41] The tissue that generated Purkinje potentials preceding the ectopy initiating VF were histopathologically studied by Nogami et al.[42] The authors demonstrated Purkinje cells in the tissue where successful RF energy application abolished ischemic VF. A report involving myocardial trigger from the right ventricular septum 1 cm away from the septal infarct zone without preceding Purkinje potential elucidated the importance of right ventricular triggers in ischemic VF.[43] Nakagawa et al[44] successfully ablated the focal triggers from the RVOT in Brugada syndrome patients experiencing VF storm initiated by monomorphic extrasystole. Trigger ablation cured VF in patients with varied structural heart diseases like bacterial endocarditis of the aortic valve, status post replacement, and chronic human herpes virus-6 myocarditis.[45] Recently, in a patient with nonischemic dilated cardiomyopathy, Kirubakaran et al[46] demonstrated noncontact mapping of the ectopy initiating VF from the left ventricular outflow tract followed by successful focal ablation of the trigger.

RF Catheter Ablation of VF Triggers: Insights from Animal Studies

Although clinical studies had demonstrated the curative potential of endocardial RFA in patients with Brugada syndrome experiencing recurrent polymorphic VT/VF, Morita et al[47] studied the efficacy of ablation in curing arrhythmia in a canine model of pinacidil- and pilsicainide-induced Brugada syndrome with spontaneous ventricular arrhythmias. The RF energy was applied at the site of earliest activation of the ectopy, initiating the arrhythmia both epicardially and endocardially. The authors optically mapped the electrical activity on the epicardium and transmurally and found that the extrasystoles originating in the electrically heterogeneous epicardial layer of Brugada syndrome were responsible for the associated ventricular arrhythmias. Multiple foci existed in each tissue. Only RF lesions applied to the epicardium successfully eliminated the ectopy initiating the arrhythmia, and eventually the arrhythmia, without altering the underlying electrical heterogeneity. Endocardial lesions failed to eliminate the ectopy or the arrhythmia.

Procedural Limitations

In order to map and then ablate VF using the methods that have been described, it is essential that there is accurate documentation of the triggering ectopic beat, with a 12-lead ECG. Due to the unpredictable nature of triggering beats, the optimal time for ablation is often at the time of an electrical storm when the ectopies tend to be frequent. Indeed, the procedural outcome can be influenced by the situation when there are no clinical ectopies at the time of ablation. When performing the EP study, care needs to be taken when manipulating the intracardiac catheters not to inadvertently "bump" the right or left bundle, as this conceals ipsilateral Purkinje activation during sinus rhythm. Mechanical ablation of the triggering beats might be another possibility with manipulation of the catheter.

Conclusions

Purkinje arborization and myocardial triggers play a crucial role in focal arrhythmogenesis of VF in structurally normal and diseased hearts. The focal sources initiating refractory, incessant, or recurrent VF can be successfully and safely eliminated by RF energy with good acute and medium-term outcomes.

References

1. Moe GK, Harris AS, Wiggers CJ. Analysis of the initiation of fibrillation by electrographic studies. *Am J Physiol*. 1941;134:473.
2. Waldo AL, Kaiser GA. Study of ventricular arrhythmias associated with acute myocardial infarction in the canine heart. *Circulation*. 1973;47:1222-1228.
3. Hoffman BF. Genesis of cardiac arrhythmias. *Prog Cardiovasc Dis*. 1966;8:219-229.
4. Friedman PL, Stewart JR, Fenoglio JJ Jr, Wit AL. Survival of subendocardial Purkinje fibers after extensive myocardial infarction in dogs. *Circ Res*. 1973;33:597-611.
5. Friedman PL, Stewart JR, Wit AL. Spontaneous and induced cardiac arrhythmias in subendocardial Purkinje fibers surviving extensive myocardial infarction in dogs. *Circ Res*. 1973;33:612-626.
6. Myerburg RJ, Stewart JW, Hoffman BF. Electrophysiological properties of the canine peripheral conducting system. *Circ Res*. 1970;26:361-372.
7. Berenfeld O, Jalife J. Purkinje-muscle reentry as a mechanism of polymorphic ventricular arrhythmias in a 3-dimensional model of the ventricles. *Circ Res*. 1998;82:1063-1077.
8. Janse MJ. Focus, reentry, or "focal" reentry? *Am J Physiol Heart Circ Physiol*. 2007;292:2561-2562.
9. Overholt ED, Joyner RW, Veenstra RD, Rawling D, Wiedmann R. Unidirectional block between Purkinje and ventricular layers of papillary muscles. *Am J Physiol*. 1984;247:H584-H595.
10. Tabereaux PB, Walcott GP, Rogers JM, et al. Activation patterns of Purkinje fibers during long-duration ventricular fibrillation in an isolated canine heart model. *Circulation*. 2007;116:1113-1119.
11. Damiano RJ Jr, Smith PK, Tripp HF Jr, et al. The effect of chemical ablation of the endocardium on ventricular fibrillation threshold. *Circulation*. 1986;74:645-652.
12. Dosdall DJ, Tabereaux PB, Kim JJ, et al. Chemical ablation of the Purkinje system causes early termination and activation rate slowing of long-duration ventricular fibrillation in dogs. *Am J Physiol Heart Circ Physiol*. 2008;295:H883-H889.
13. Haïssaguerre M, Shah DC, Jaïs P, et al. Role of Purkinje conducting system in triggering idiopathic sudden cardiac death. *Lancet*. 2002;359:677-678.
14. Haïssaguerre M, Shoda M, Jaïs P, et al. Mapping and ablation of idiopathic ventricular fibrillation. *Circulation*. 2002;106:962-967.
15. Haïssaguerre M, Extramiana F, Hocini M, et al. Mapping and ablation of ventricular fibrillation associated with long-QT and Brugada syndromes. *Circulation*. 2003;108:925-928.
16. Bansch D, Oyang F, Antz M, et al. Successful catheter ablation of electrical storm after myocardial infarction. *Circulation*. 2003;108:3011-3016.
17. Knecht S, Sacher F, Wright M, et al. Long-term follow-up of idiopathic ventricular fibrillation ablation: a multicenter study. *J Am Coll Cardiol*. 2009;54:522-528.
18. Shah AJ, Hocini M, Lamaison D, Sacher F, Derval N, Haïssaguerre M. Regional substrate ablation abolishes Brugada syndrome. *J Cardiovasc Electrophysiol*. 2011;22:1290-1291.

19. Haïssaguerre M, Derval N, Sacher F, et al. Sudden cardiac arrest associated with early repolarization. *N Engl J Med.* 2008;358:2016-2023.
20. Marrouche NF, Verma A, Wazni O, et al. Mode of initiation and ablation of ventricular fibrillation storms in patients with ischemic cardiomyopathy. *J Am Coll Cardiol.* 2004;43:1715-1720.
21. Peichl P, Cihák R, Kozeluhová M, Wichterle D, Vancura V, Kautzner J. Catheter ablation of arrhythmic storm triggered by monomorphic ectopic beats in patients with coronary artery disease. *J Interv Card Electrophysiol.* 2010;27:51-59.
22. Mlcochova H, Saliba WI, Burkhardt DJ, et al. Catheter ablation of ventricular fibrillation storm in patients with infiltrative amyloidosis of the heart. *J Cardiovasc Electrophysiol.* 2006;17:426-430.
23. Sinha AM, Schmidt M, Marschang H, et al. Role of left ventricular scar and Purkinje-like potentials during mapping and ablation of ventricular fibrillation in dilated cardiomyopathy. *Pacing Clin Electrophysiol.* 2009;32:286-290.
24. Ashida K, Kaji Y, Sasaki Y. Abolition of torsade de pointes after radiofrequency catheter ablation at right ventricular outflow tract. *Int J Cardiol.* 1997;59:171-175.
25. Kusano KF, Yamamoto M, Emori T, Morita H, Ohe T. Successful catheter ablation in a patient with polymorphic ventricular tachycardia. *J Cardiovasc Electrophysiol.* 2000;11:682-685.
26. Takatsuki S, Mitamura H, Ogawa S. Catheter ablation of a monofocal premature ventricular complex triggering idiopathic ventricular fibrillation. *Heart.* 2001;86:E3.
27. Saliba W, Abul Karim A, Tchou P, Natale A. Ventricular fibrillation: ablation of a trigger? *J Cardiovasc Electrophysiol.* 2002;13:1296-1299.
28. Pasquié JL, Sanders P, Hocini M, et al. Fever as a precipitant of idiopathic ventricular fibrillation in patients with normal hearts. *J Cardiovasc Electrophysiol.* 2004;15:1271-1276.
29. Li YG, Gronefeld G, Israel C, Hohnloser SH. Catheter ablation of frequently recurring ventricular fibrillation in a patient after aortic valve repair. *J Cardiovasc Electrophysiol.* 2004;15:90-93.
30. Betts TR, Yue A, Roberts PR, Morgan JM. Radiofrequency ablation of idiopathic ventricular fibrillation guided by noncontact mapping. *J Cardiovasc Electrophysiol.* 2004;15:957-959.
31. Nogami A, Sugiyasu A, Kubota S, Kato K. Mapping and ablation of idiopathic ventricular fibrillation from the Purkinje system. *Heart Rhythm.* 2005;2:646-649.
32. Darmon JP, Bettouche S, Deswardt P, et al. Radiofrequency ablation of ventricular fibrillation and multiple right and left atrial tachycardia in a patient with Brugada syndrome. *J Interv Card Electrophysiol.* 2004;11:205-209.
33. Yu CC, Tsai CT, Lai LP, Lin JL. Successful radiofrequency catheter ablation of idiopathic ventricular fibrillation presented as recurrent syncope and diagnosed by an implanted loop recorder. *Int J Cardiol.* 2006;110:112-113.
34. Enjoji Y, Mizobuchi M, Shibata K, et al. Catheter ablation for an incessant form of antiarrhythmic drug-resistant ventricular fibrillation after acute coronary syndrome. *Pacing Clin Electrophysiol.* 2006;29:102-105.
35. Kohsaka S, Razavi M, Massumi A. Idiopathic ventricular fibrillation successfully terminated by radiofrequency ablation of the distal Purkinje fibers. *Pacing Clin Electrophysiol.* 2007;30:701-704.
36. Okada T, Yamada T, Murakami Y, Yoshida N, Ninomiya Y, Toyama J. Mapping and ablation of trigger premature ventricular contractions in a case of electrical storm associated with ischemic cardiomyopathy. *Pacing Clin Electrophysiol.* 2007;30:440-443.
37. Srivathsan K, Gami AS, Ackerman MJ, Asirvatham SJ. Treatment of ventricular fibrillation in a patient with prior diagnosis of long QT syndrome: importance of precise electrophysiologic diagnosis to successfully ablate the trigger. *Heart Rhythm.* 2007;4:1090-1093.
38. Uemura T, Yamabe H, Tanaka Y, et al. Catheter ablation of a polymorphic ventricular tachycardia inducing monofocal premature ventricular complex. *Intern Med.* 2008;47:1799-1802.
39. Naik N, Juneja R, Sharma G, Yadav R, Anandraja S. Malignant idiopathic ventricular fibrillation "cured" by radiofrequency ablation. *J Interv Card Electrophysiol.* 2008;23:143-148.
40. Kataoka M, Takatsuki S, Tanimoto K, et al. A case of vagally mediated idiopathic ventricular fibrillation. *Nat Clin Pract Cardiovasc Med.* 2008;5:111-115.
41. Suh WM, Fowler SJ, Yeh T, Krishnan SC. Successful catheter ablation of focal ventricular fibrillation originating from the right ventricle. *J Interv Card Electrophysiol.* 2009;26:139-142.
42. Nogami A, Kubota S, Adachi M, Igawa O. Electrophysiologic and histopathologic findings of the ablation sites for ventricular fibrillation in a patient with ischemic cardiomyopathy. *J Interv Card Electrophysiol.* 2009;24:133-137.
43. Takahashi Y, Takahashi A, Isobe M. Ventricular fibrillation initiated by premature beats from the ventricular myocardium not associated with the Purkinje system after myocardial infarction. *Heart Rhythm.* 2008;5:1458-1460.
44. Nakagawa E, Takagi M, Tatsumi H, Yoshiyama M. Successful radiofrequency catheter ablation for electrical storm of ventricular fibrillation in a patient with Brugada syndrome. *Circ J.* 2008;72:1025-1029.
45. Bode K, Hindricks G, Piorkowski C, et al. Ablation of polymorphic ventricular tachycardias in patients with structural heart disease. *Pacing Clin Electrophysiol.* 2008;31:1585-1591.
46. Kirubakaran S, Gill J, Rinaldi CA. Successful catheter ablation of focal ventricular fibrillation in a patient with nonischemic dilated cardiomyopathy. *Pacing Clin Electrophysiol.* 2011;34:e38-e42.
47. Morita H, Zipes DP, Morita ST, Lopshire JC, Wu J. Epicardial ablation eliminates ventricular arrhythmias in an experimental model of Brugada syndrome. *Heart Rhythm.* 2009;6:665-671.

Video Legends

Video 46.1 The onset of RFA at the earliest Purkinje source of the ectopy-initiating VF triggers short-lasting bursts of polymorphic VT/VF. They gradually become infrequent and eventually disappear during RF application with the elimination of the ectopic beats.

Video 46.2 The Purkinje potential just precedes the QRS complex (< 15 ms) and appears fused with the early part of the local ventricular EGM in sinus rhythm. During clinical ectopy, the sharp Purkinje potential clearly precedes both the QRS complex and the local ventricular EGM, confirming that the Purkinje network is the trigger/source of the ectopic beat.

CHAPTER 47

COMPLICATIONS OF CATHETER ABLATION AND THEIR MANAGEMENT

Riccardo Cappato, MD; Luigi De Ambroggi, MD

Introduction

Catheter ablation has been proven to be an effective cure for the treatment of patients with supraventricular and ventricular tachyarrhythmias. Safety of the treatment varies in relation to several factors, including type of arrhythmia, site of ablation, methodology used, experience of the center, and patient characteristics (underlying heart disease, comorbidities, age).

Incidence and Type of Complications

AV Junctional Ablation

The incidence of complications reported by the Multicenter European Radiofrequency Survey (MERFS)[1] in 900 patients undergoing AV junctional catheter ablation was 3.2%. Among this group, severe complications occurred in 17 patients (1.8%). One patient died suddenly 7 days after the procedure, most likely from a malignant ventricular arrhythmia. Three other patients developed torsades de pointes after successful interruption of AV junction despite effective ventricular pacing. The authors were unable to state whether arrhythmic events after RFA were due to a direct proarrhythmic effect of the energy applied or solely due to the induction of complete AV block by the ablative procedure. Since the occurrence of torsades de pointes often appears to be bradycardia-dependent, the authors recommended pacing the ventricle at a sufficiently high rate after successful ablation of AV junction.

An increased incidence of sudden death has been observed in other retrospective or prospective studies.[2-4] In particular, Geelen et al[4] reported a 6% incidence of VF or sudden death within 1 month after catheter ablation of AV junction when pacing rates were lower than 70 bpm, compared with no incidents of sudden death when pacing rates were set at 90 bpm for 1 to 3 months after the procedure.

In the 1998 NASPE Prospective Catheter Ablation Registry,[5] major complications (death due to pacemaker malfunction in 1 patient, hematomas, significant tricuspid regurgitation) occurred in 5 of 646 patients (0.8%) undergoing AV junctional catheter ablation.

AV Nodal Reentry Tachycardia Ablation

In 815 patients, the MERFS reported a high incidence (8%) of procedure-related complications.[1] Nevertheless, no deaths were reported, and the majority of complications reported (41 of 65) were due to unwanted induction of complete AV block. Of note, a 6.2% incidence of complete AV block was reported when catheter ablation of fast pathway was attempted, whereas the incidence of complete AV block was only 2.1% in patients in whom catheter ablation of slow pathways was attempted. The incidence was highest (16%) when catheter ablation of both pathways was attempted in a single session after failure of initial site.

A much lower complication rate (2.2%) than in MERFS was reported by the NASPE registry[5] in 1,197 patients who underwent initial slow pathway catheter ablation (fast pathway ablation was required in 17 (1.5%) patients). Complete AV block was induced in 0.74% of patients and second-degree AV block in 0.16%; other significant complications included hematoma or significant bleeding, deep vein thrombosis, pneumothorax, and pulmonary embolus.

A similar rate of complication (3%) was recently reported in a systematic review and meta-analysis of the safety and efficacy of radiofrequency catheter ablation of AV node-dependent SVT in adult patients.[6]

Accessory Pathway Ablation

The incidence of complications reported by MERFS in 2,222 patients was 4.4%.[1] Severe complications occurred in 2.3%, the most common being due to complete AV block, mainly observed in patients with a right anteroseptal AP, and cardiac tamponade. Considering the relatively high incidence of cardiac tamponade (0.72%) and clinical significant pericardial effusion (54%) observed in this group, the authors suggested that there is a specific risk of this type of complication during catheter ablation of the AP. Three procedure-related deaths (0.13%) were also reported.

The NASPE registry reported on AP catheter ablation in 654 patients: major complications included cardiac tamponade (7 patients), acute coronary occlusion with myocardial infarction (1 patient), complete AV block (1 patient), femoral artery pseudoaneurysm (1 patient), pericarditis (2 patients), and pneumothorax (1 patient).

A similar rate of adverse events (2.8%) was found in a recent meta-analysis.[6]

Atrial Flutter Ablation

In the MERFS report, the number of patients who underwent catheter ablation of AFL was relatively low.[1] Three of 141 patients (2.1%) had severe complications; perforation and cardiac tamponade occurred in 1 patient. Thus, although the experience was limited, catheter ablation of AFL did not appear to carry an increased risk with respect to other types of ablative procedures more commonly performed.

The NASPE registry reported on 477 patients undergoing ablation of the tricuspid valve annulus-inferior vena caval isthmus for AFL.[5] The flutter was described as typical counterclockwise in 62.4% and typical clockwise flutter in 37.6%. Significant complications included cardiac tamponade (1 patient), complete AV block (2 patients), AV Wenckebach conduction (1 patient), new significant tricuspid regurgitation (1 patient), hemopneumothorax (1 patient), and bleeding/hematoma (3 patients).

Adverse events rate was low also in a meta-analysis evaluating catheter ablation in 1,323 patients.[6] The most common complications were AV block (0.4%) and pericardial effusion (0.3%); no procedure-related deaths were reported.

Atrial Tachycardia Ablation

In the NASPE registry, 216 patients undergoing atrial tachycardia were reported.[5] The tachycardia focus was localized to the RA in 149 patients, the LA in 43, and the septum in 44 (10 patients had more than one focus). Significant complications (3%) included cardiac tamponade (2 patients), pacemaker lead damage (1 patient), transient complete AV block (1 patient), right atrial to aortic fistula (1 patient), and aspiration pneumonia (1 patient).

Atrial Fibrillation Ablation

Catheter ablation of atrial fibrillation (AF) is a quite complex interventional EP procedure. Ablation risks may vary with the experience of the operator and support team. However, it could be expected that a higher risk of procedure-related complications associate with AF ablation than with ablation of most other cardiac arrhythmias. Several factors may precipitate major or even fatal complications. These include transseptal puncture, prolonged catheter manipulation in the LA and large doses of cumulative RF energy delivered in the LA in the context of high level of systemic anticoagulation. In a recent survey, transseptal catheterization was shown to be a cause of death in 0.2% of procedures.[7]

Major adverse events have been reported in up to 6% of patients undergoing AF ablation.[8-15] In a recently published worldwide survey on catheter ablation for AF,[16] data were analyzed from 85 centers that reported to have performed 20,825 procedures on 16,309 patients with AF between 2003 and 2006. A major complication occurred in 741 patients (4.5%). A detailed list of the different complications reported with their relative incidence is outlined in Table 47.1. There were 25 procedure-related deaths, 37 strokes, 115 transient ischemic attacks, and 213 episodes of tamponade. Altogether, 216 PVs presented significant

Table 47.1 Major complications reported in 16,309 patients

Type of Complication	Number of Pts	Rate (%)
Death	25	0.15
Tamponade	213	1.31
Pneumothorax	15	0.09
Hemothorax	4	0.02
Sepsis, abscesses, or endocarditis	2	0.01
Permanent diaphragmatic paralysis	28	0.17
Total femoral pseudoaneurysm	152	0.93
Total artero-venous fistulae	88	0.54
Valve damage	11	0.07
Atrium-esophageal fistulae	6	0.04
Stroke	37	0.23
Transient ischemic attack	115	0.71
Pulmonary vein stenoses requiring intervention	48	0.29
TOTAL	744	4.56

Source: Adapted from table 7, *Circ Arrhythm Electrophysiol.* 2010;3:32-38.[16]

(> 50%) stenosis (assessed by means of pre- and postablation PV angiography in 71.3% and MRI in 28.7% of centers), which resulted in the need for a corrective intervention in 48 patients.

Tamponade was the most frequent adverse event, but its rate was comparable to values commonly observed during catheter ablation of other arrhythmogenic substrates.[1,3,5] Death and stroke did not differ with respect to a previous survey[11] that reported data observed between 1995 and 2002, while transient ischemic attacks and PV stenoses were reduced by at least twofold and threefold, respectively. Atrial–esophageal fistulas were not reported in the previous survey and presented with a 0.04% rate in the second survey.

Data relevant to the incidence and cause of intra- and postprocedural deaths occurring in patients undergoing catheter ablation of AF between 1995 and 2006 were collected from 162 of 546 identified centers worldwide[17] (Tables 47.2 and 47.3). In this study, the incidence of death associated with catheter ablation of AF was 1 per 1,000 patients. Cardiac tamponade was the most frequent fatal complication leading to intraoperative irreversible pump failure secondary to myocardial hypoperfusion, postoperative early cardiac arrest, or sudden pericardial bleeding occurring 50 days after the procedure (1 patient). Development of atrial–esophageal fistula was the second most frequent cause of death. This complication has been reported to occur between 10 and 23 days after the ablation procedure, and to be fatal in the majority.[14,18-20] Causes of death in patients with atrial–esophageal fistulas include cerebral air embolism, massive gastrointestinal bleeding, and septic shock.[21] While atrial–esophageal fistula is a rare event, mucosal lesions of the esophagus have been frequently described using endoscopy after PVI,[22] and also morphological changes of the periesophageal connective tissue and the posterior wall of the LA were observed by endosonography in 27% of 30 patients following PVI.[23]

Ischemic brain or myocardial damage was the third most frequent cause of death in our survey.[17] Modes of death associated with this complication included intraprocedural acute myocardial infarction as well as intra- or postprocedural stroke. Other causes of death included extra-pericardial bleeding mostly due to subclavian or PV

Table 47.2 Causes and proportions of death in 32,569 patients from 162 centers

Cause of Death	Intraoperative Number	Postoperative Number	Total Number	Proportion %
Early death (within 30 days from procedure)				
• Tamponade with subsequent cardiac arrest	5	2	7	21.8
• Atrial–esophageal fistula	0	5	5	15.6
• Peripheral embolism				
– Stroke	2	1	3	9.4
– Myocardial infarction	1	0	1	3.1
• Massive pneumonia	0	2	2	6.3
• Extra-pericardial pulmonary vein perforation	1	0	1	3.1
• Irreversible torsades de pointes	1	0	1	3.1
• Septicemia (3 weeks after procedure)	0	1	1	3.1
• Sudden respiratory arrest	1	0	1	3.1
• Acute pulmonary vein occlusion of both lateral veins	0	1	1	3.1
• Hemothorax	0	1	1	3.1
• Anaphylaxis	1	0	1	3.1
Late death (after 30 days from procedure)				
• Complications from prior perioperative events				
– Stroke			2	6.3
– Tracheal compression from subclavian hematoma			1	3.1
– Acute respiratory distress syndrome			1	3.1
– Esophageal perforation from intraoperative TEE probe			1	3.1
• Acutely precipitating events				
– Tamponade with subsequent cardiac arrest in prior stroke			1	3.1
– Intracranial bleeding under oral anticoagulation therapy in prior stroke			1	3.1

Source: With permission from Elsevier.[17]

Table 47.3 Fatality rates according to type of complication

Complication	Death / Overall Events Number	Rate %
• Tamponade	7/331	2.3
• Atrio-esophageal fistula	5/7	71.4
• Massive pneumonia	2/2	100.0
• Peripheral embolism		
– Stroke	3/59	5.1
– Myocardial infarction	1/3	33.3
• Torsades de pointes	1/1	100.0
• Septicemia (3 weeks after procedure)	1/3	33.3
• Sudden respiratory arrest	1/1	100.0
• Acute pulmonary vein occlusion of both lateral veins	1/6	16.7
• Internal bleeding (includes hemothorax, subclavian hematoma, and extrapericardial pulmonary vein perforation)	3/21	14.3
• Anaphylaxis	1/6	16.7
• Acute respiratory distress syndrome	1/1	100.0
• Esophageal perforation from intraoperative TEE probe	1/1	100.0
• Intracranial bleeding under oral anticoagulation therapy in prior stroke	1/4	25.0

Source: With permission from Elsevier.[17]

perforation and massive pneumonia refractory to antibiotic therapy. Conditions such as torsades de pointes, sudden respiratory arrest, and acute respiratory distress syndrome appear to be unspecific causes of death; it is likely that they represented the final event of unrecognized causes ultimately leading to fatal outcome. Some of the complications leading to death in this series, such as bleeding from the subclavian access site, are clearly unrelated to catheter ablation of AF and could be observed for EP procedures requiring the same access; however, it is possible that the anticoagulation strategies utilized for the purpose of this specific procedure may have influenced the outcome.

The larger prevalence of causes of death such as tamponade, peripheral embolism, and internal bleeding reflects a higher frequency in these complications, but their probability of causing death once they have developed is small compared to that of less common complications such as atrial-esophageal fistula, septicemia, and acute respiratory distress syndrome.

Center experience did not appear to influence the incidence of death. Carto-guided left atrial ablation and Lasso-guided PVI were not associated with different risks of death. A 2.5-fold increase in death rate observed in patients undergoing irrigated- or cooled-tip ablation versus 4 mm tip ablation raises some concern with regard to the potential harm of the first type of catheter, although this difference did not reach statistical significance. Careful prospective monitoring is advised to exclude a greater degree of harm with use of more powerful ablation catheters.

Atrial Tachyarrhythmias after AF Ablation

New-onset atrial tachyarrhythmias are commonly observed (5% to 25%) in patients who have undergone AF ablation.[12,13] The variability in the frequency of occurrence and the mechanism of the tachycardia appear to be dependent on the type of ablation procedure used. Centers utilizing wide-area circumferential PV ablation combined with additional linear lesions in the LA report a higher prevalence of macroreentrant atypical flutters and an overall incidence of organized left atrial tachycardias that is three times that observed with PVI procedures alone.[13,24-26] Centers that utilize PVI alone have reported a low incidence of recurrent regular atrial tachycardias, and these arrhythmias have been predominantly focal left atrial tachycardias originating from reconnected PVs.[25,26]

Up to 50% of these tachycardias appear to resolve spontaneously during the "healing phase" postablation.[24] If the tachyarrhythmias persist after a 2- to 3-month blanking period and are recurrent and symptomatic, repeat ablation procedures are appropriate. Depending on the underlying mechanism, the ablation strategy may require isolation of the reconnected PV segment (for focal tachycardias of PV origin) or may involve targeting the zone of slow conduction or a well-defined anatomic isthmus for macroreentrant flutter.[25]

Ventricular Tachycardia Ablation

The MERFS reported on 320 patients from 23 institutions who underwent catheter ablation for VT.[1] The rate of complications was 7.6% (24 patients) and was significantly higher when compared to catheter ablation of the AV node and of APs reported in the same survey. One patient with remote anterior myocardial infarction had perforation with cardiac tamponade, underwent cardiac surgery, and died 2 hours after surgery due to pump failure. Of note, among the complications, the prevalence of thromboembolic events reported was remarkably high (2.8%). Tentative explanations offered by the authors were: (1) ablation of VT was often a long-lasting procedure and (2) some thromboembolic complications might have been related to a preexisting ventricular thrombus not detected by echocardiography.

The NASPE registry reported on 201 patients with VT due to various underlying substrates (coronary heart disease, NICM, idiopathic VT) who underwent attempted catheter ablation.[5] Significant complications (cardiac tamponade, respiratory failure, sepsis, worsening congestive heart failure, pericarditis) occurred in 3.8%. No deaths related to the procedure were reported.

Calkins et al[27] reported a procedure-related mortality of 2.7% in 146 patients with mappable VT and ablation performed with an irrigated catheter. The rate of major complications was 8%, including 4 strokes (2.7%) and 4 cardiac tamponade (2.7%).

More recently, the Multicenter Thermocool Ventricular Tachycardia Ablation Trial[28] enrolled 231 patients with recurrent VT in the setting of ICM. Procedure mortality was 3% with 6 of 7 deaths related to uncontrollable VT and 1 due to tamponade with myocardial infarction. Nonfatal complications occurred in 7% of patients, including heart failure and vascular complications; there were no strokes.

In the SMASH-VT multicenter study,[29] no procedure-related mortality was reported among the group of 64 patients undergoing VT ablation after ICD implantation.

The higher incidence of thromboembolic events in VT patients compared with patients with supraventricular arrhythmias might be related to the site of ablation, longer procedure time, multiple RF current applications, presence of severe atherosclerotic aortic lesions, and the possible existence of mural thrombus not detected by TTE.[30] Thus, TTE and TEE should be used for routine screening of mural thombi in the cardiac chambers, particularly in patients with ICM and LV dysfunction. For patients with severe atherosclerotic aortic disease, catheter access via transseptal approach should be considered to avoid embolic complications. To make large transmural lesions without unfavourable heating injury and thromboembolic complications, a cooled RFA catheter is preferable.

Epicardial Ablation

A percutaneous epicardial mapping approach allows to ablate in the EP laboratory many VTs originating from the subepicardium, in which the endocardial ablation is unsuccessful.[30,31] VT epicardial ablation[32] has additional risks compared with endocardial approach. In approximately 30% of cases, pericardial bleeding of some extent is recognized[33] and is mostly due to unintentional RV puncture or lesion of pericardial vessels. Mild bleeding usually resolves with repeated aspirations of the pericardial space and rarely required surgical intervention. To prevent the laceration, the sheath should never be left without a catheter inside. Puncture of a subdiaphragmatic vessel causing intra-abdominal bleeding has been reported and can require surgery.[33,34] Hepatic laceration and bleeding are also potential risks.

RF injury to coronary artery can cause acute thrombosis.[35] Severe coronary artery spasm was also reported during epicardial mapping.[36] The long-term consequences of ablation near the coronary arteries are unknown.

The left phrenic nerve is susceptible to injury along its course adjacent to the lateral LV wall. To prevent the phrenic nerve damage, moving the nerve away from the myocardium by injection of air into the pericardial space or placement of a balloon catheter between the ablation site and the nerve has been reported.[37,38]

After the procedure, symptoms of pericarditis can be observed in about one-third of patients.[34] Symptoms usually disappear within a few days with anti-inflammatory medications. In a swine model of ablation-related pericarditis, intrapericardial instillation of corticosteroids has been shown to reduce inflammation.[39] This practice has been adopted by several laboratories prior to removing the epicardial sheaths, but the results are still controversial.

Management of Main Complications

Cardiac Tamponade

Clinical manifestations of cardiac tamponade may appear either as a gradual decrease of blood pressure associated with tachycardia, dyspnea, paradoxical pulse, or jugular venous distension, or as an abrupt, dramatic fall of blood pressure and shock. In the first case, fluid administration may return the blood pressure to normal (at least for some time). However, careful vigilance is required from the operators, who should have easy access to echocardiographic imaging and experience in gaining pericardial access for prompt drainage. A continuous monitoring of systemic arterial pressure should be performed during and following some procedures as AF ablation. The development of hypotension in any patient should be assumed to indicate tamponade until proven otherwise by immediate echocardiography. An early sign of cardiac tamponade is a reduction of the excursion of the cardiac silhouette on fluoroscopy with a simultaneous fall in blood pressure. The majority of episodes of cardiac tamponade can be managed successfully by immediate percutaneous drainage and reversal of anticoagulation with protamine.

Atrial–esophageal Fistula

The development of an atrial–esophageal fistula is one of the most serious complications of AF ablation.[12,13,16] Atrial–esophageal fistula typically presents late after the ablation procedure (2 to 4 weeks), and early diagnosis is difficult. Patients often present to their primary care physicians or general cardiologists with a constellation of vague symptoms, including dysphagia, odynophagia, recurrent neurological ischemia likely due to air emboli, persistent fever, chills, bacteremia, fungemia, and melena. Presentations that are more dramatic are septic shock or death. If suspected, the best diagnostic modalities are CT or MR imaging of the esophagus. Although a barium swallow may detect a fistula, its sensitivity is low. If a fistula is suspected, is it important to avoid endoscopy because insufflation of the esophagus has been demonstrated to lead to massive air emboli through the fistula, leading to stroke and myocardial infarction. Though mortality of this complication is very high, survival following rapid surgical correction has been reported.[40] It appears that survival may depend on rapid diagnosis and prompt surgical intervention. There has been 1 case report of a favorable outcome after placement of an esophageal stent.[41]

Because of the severe consequences of an atrial–esophageal fistula, it is quite important to avoid this complication. Currently, a number of different approaches are being employed with this aim. The most common practice[12] decreases power delivery, limiting energy to 25 to 35 W, decreases tissue contact pressure, and moves the ablation catheter every 10 to 20 seconds when close to the esophagus. However, owing to the rarity of this complication, it remains unproven whether these practices lower or eliminate the risk of esophageal injury.

Phrenic Nerve Injury

Phrenic nerve injury is an important, even though rare, complication of ablation procedures, specifically when performed for atrial fibrillation. In fact, the right phrenic nerve has a close anatomic relationship to the RSPV and the SVC as it runs along the posterior and posterolateral wall of the RA.[42] This proximity makes the nerve potentially vulnerable to thermal injury during endocardial RF delivery within or in close proximity to those structures.[43,44]

Permanent nerve damage may be preceded by transient loss of function, allowing for early recognition and prevention by close monitoring in most patients.

Phrenic nerve damage can be asymptomatic or can cause dyspnea, hiccups, atelectasis, pleural effusion, cough, and thoracic pain.[12] When suspected, the diagnosis can be confirmed by fluoroscopy showing unilateral diaphragmatic paralysis. Strategies to prevent phrenic nerve damage include high-output pacing to establish whether the phrenic nerve can be captured from the proposed ablation site before ablation; phrenic nerve mapping by pacing along the SVC to identify the location of the phrenic nerve; ensuring proximal/antral ablation when ablating around the RSPV; and fluoroscopic monitoring of diaphragmatic excursion during ablation, with/without phrenic nerve pacing from the SVC and above the ablation site during energy delivery. Energy delivery should be interrupted immediately when diaphragmatic movement stops. In most reports, phrenic nerve function recovered between 1 day and more than 12 months. However, there have been some cases of permanent phrenic nerve injury. There is no active treatment known to aid phrenic nerve healing.

PV Stenosis

PV stenosis is a well-recognized complication of AF ablation resulting from thermal injury to PV musculature.[45-47] To reduce the risk of PV stenosis when ablation is performed near the PV ostium, the anatomy should be clearly defined. To localize the PV ostium and to avoid ablation inside the vein, angiography of the PVs, ICE, 3D mapping systems with integration of CT or MRI scan anatomic information, and impedance measurements using the ablation catheter has been used.[47-49] Whatever monitoring/imaging technique is used, the decisive factor in avoiding PV stenosis seems to be a precise knowledge of the anatomy of the LA, coupled with the ability to further define the anatomy and identify the location of lesion deployment. Avoidance of lesion placement within the venous structure is critical.[50]

At selected sites, titration of energy delivery may avoid excessive tissue disruption and subsequent narrowing. The use of alternative energy delivery tools, such as balloon technology or energy sources for ablation like cryoenergy, ultrasound, or microwave, will need additional evaluation to determine if they may help to further reduce or even eliminate the risk of PV stenosis.

Symptoms are more likely associated with severe stenoses (> 70%), but even severe PV stenosis or total occlusion may be asymptomatic, particularly if only a single vein is involved. The clinical manifestation of PV stenosis may be quite insidious. The most frequent symptoms include cough, dyspnea, hemoptysis, or recurrent and drug-resistant pneumonia.[47,50,51] Symptoms may develop both early and/or late after the procedure with most patients presenting within 2 to 6 months.[49] To diagnose PV stenosis, transesophageal Doppler-echocardiography, lung scan, CTm, or MRI may be used.[47,50,52,53]

Significant PV stenosis in symptomatic patients should be treated by angioplasty and/or stenting.[54] Angioplasty is associated with a high restenosis rate of 45%, a problem not completely resolved by stenting.[54] Surgical interventions may be considered for clinically important PV occlusion where angioplasty and stenting have failed. In asymptomatic patients with two or more stenosed pulmonary veins, invasive therapy might be considered to prevent pulmonary hypertension during exercise.[55] Whether patients with one PV stenosis and no or minimal clinical symptoms should be treated is questionable.

Coronary Arteries Injury

Thermal injury to the coronary arteries has been described during ablation of VT, mainly with the epicardial approach,[34-36] and of AF.[56]

To prevent coronary injury, prior to an epicardial ablation procedure, direct visualization of the relation between the ablation site and adjacent coronary arteries should be obtained by coronary angiography. Based on available experimental and clinical data, a distance of more than 5 mm between the ablation catheter and an epicardial artery is generally accepted.[30,31] In patients who developed an acute coronary occlusion after ablation, coronary angioplasty with stenting was reported to be the treatment of choice.[35]

Takahashi et al[56] described a case of acute occlusion of the left circumflex coronary artery following RF energy delivery in CS to complete the linear lesion between the posterolateral mitral annulus and the LIPV for the treatment of AF. A more posterior mitral isthmus line may avoid this complication, but may increase the risk of injury to the esophagus. Haïssaguerre's group has suggested the reduction of energy power if RF applications are needed inside the CS to complete the line of block.[57]

Thromboembolism

Thromboembolism is one of the most serious complications of ablation procedures and is a potential cause of cerebral, coronary, or peripheral vascular compromise. Therefore, careful attention to anticoagulation of patients before, during, and after ablation procedures, in particular for AF ablation, is critical to avoid the occurrence of thromboembolic events. In addition to performing an optimal anticoagulation, there is a consensus[12] that patients with persistent AF who are in AF at the time of ablation should undergo TEE to search for an atrial thrombus, regardless of whether they have been anticoagulated with warfarin prior to ablation. This reflects the risk that catheter manipulation throughout the LA during an AF procedure could dislodge an *in situ* thrombus that would result in a thromboembolic complication.

To avoid thromboembolic events, in accordance with the most recent guidelines,[12,13] intense anticoagulation is performed during the procedure with a loading dose of unfractionated heparin followed by a standard infusion (10 U/kg/hr) to maintain the activated clotting time around 300 seconds. After the procedure, heparin or subcutaneous low-molecular-weight heparin (eg, enoxaparin) is administered until a therapeutic range of INR is achieved using warfarin, which is recommended to be continued for at least 3 months or long term in patients at risk (CHADS2 score ≥2). In some laboratories, oral anticoagulation is not discontinued before ablation, and the procedure is conducted under therapeutic INR values. In these cases, IV heparin is still administered to prevent clot formation during sheath and catheter manipulation.[58]

Thromboembolic events typically occur within 24 hours of the ablation procedure with the high-risk period extending for the first 2 weeks following ablation.[59] Although silent cerebral thromboembolism has been reported following AF ablation,[60,61] its incidence is not exactly known.

A number of potential explanations for the development of thromboembolic complications have been proposed. These include the development of thrombi on stationary sheaths or ablation catheters positioned within the LA, char formation at the tip of the ablation catheter and at the site of ablation, and disruption of a thrombus located in the atrium prior to the ablation procedure. Treatment of a thromboembolic event will vary according to the location of the embolus. Peripheral arterial embolization may be amenable to surgical thrombectomy, whereas cerebral embolization has traditionally been managed conservatively and the consequences accepted. However, there is growing interest in aggressive early management of such events, with either thrombolytic drugs or percutaneous interventional techniques.

Air Embolism

Air emboli may enter the arterial system during sheath/catheter exchanges, aspiration, irrigation, or continuous infusion of sheaths.[62,63] A common presentation of air embolism during AF ablation is acute inferior ischemia and/or heart block. This reflects preferential downstream migration of air emboli into the RCA. Supportive care usually results in complete resolution of symptoms and signs of inferior ischemia within minutes. Air emboli may also travel to cerebral circulation and may lead to neurologic manifestations. Prompt MRI or CT scans obtained before the intravascular air is rapidly absorbed may show multiple serpiginous hypodensities representing air in the cerebral vasculature, with or without acute infarction.

Air emboli are best prevented by proper attention to technique.[13] Caution should be exercised when exchanging the sheaths and catheters. The sheaths should routinely be flushed intermittently and also after each catheter withdrawal. If sheaths are continuously irrigated throughout the procedure, air bubbles should be avoided, and automatic pumps capable of detecting air in the tubing should be used. It should be noted that some sheaths, particularly those with a larger diameter, may not have tight hemostatic valves. As the catheter is withdrawn, air may be aspirated into the sheath. This risk may easily be prevented by simultaneously aspirating blood from the sideport of the sheath during catheter withdrawal.

According to the recommendations of HRS/EHRA/ECAS,[12] treatment should be initiated immediately in the laboratory if cerebral air embolism is suspected. The most important initial step is to maximize cerebral perfusion by the administration of fluids and supplemental oxygen, which increases the rate of nitrogen absorption from air bubbles. It may be beneficial to briefly suspend the patient in a head-down position.[64] Treatment with hyperbaric oxygen may reverse the condition and minimize endothelial thromboinflammatory injury if it is started within a few hours. Heparin appears to limit injury in animal models of cerebral arterial air embolism.

Mitral Valve Damage

Catheter entrapment in the mitral valve apparatus is an uncommon complication associated with ablation procedures that require deployment of catheters in the LA, as for AF ablation.[16,65,66] In a recent worldwide survey on 16,309 patients undergoing catheter ablation for AF,[16] mitral valve damage was reported in 11 (0.07%) subjects, of whom 7 required surgery.

Entrapment may result from inadvertent positioning of the circular electrode catheter into the ventricle with counterclockwise rotation of the catheter, resulting in entrapment of the circular catheter in the mitral valve apparatus. When suspected, it is important to confirm the diagnosis with echocardiography. Although successful freeing of the catheter has been reported with gentle catheter manipulation and advancing the sheath into the ventricle, great caution must be used, as it is possible to tear the mitral valve apparatus. It is recommended that if gentle attempts to free the catheter fail, elective surgical removal of the catheter should be performed.[12]

Vascular Complications

Access vascular complications are common and include groin hematoma, retroperitoneal bleed, development of a femoral arterial pseudoaneurysm, or a femoral A-V fistula. The incidence of vascular complications varies in different reports and is higher after ablation procedures requiring more intense anticoagulation protocols.[12,14,16,67,68] In our worldwide survey on ablation procedures, incidence of femoral pseudoaneurysm and A-V fistulae were found to be 0.93% and 0.54%, respectively.[16]

The high incidence of vascular access complications is likely related to the number and size of venous catheters used and to the fact that in most EP laboratories patients are fully anticoagulated during and following the ablation procedure, with interruption of anticoagulation for less than 4 to 6 hours to allow for sheath removal. Although vascular complications rarely cause long-term disability or death, they are important because they prolong hospitalization, cause inconvenience and discomfort to the patient, and may require transfusions. The risk of vascular complications can be minimized by technical proficiency with vascular access, avoidance of very large sheaths, and care with anticoagulation. Large hematomas usually can be managed conservatively. Echo-guided manual compression and percutaneous or surgical closure are all effective treatments of femoral arteriovenous fistulae or pseudoaneurysms.

Conclusions

The increasing number of patients receiving catheter ablation of AF prompts for parallel development of appropriate standard of safety. The increasing experience developed during the last 10 years of practice has not resulted in a significant reduction of the complication rate. Awareness about the risk of procedure-related complications may contribute to limit their occurrence and consequences. Patients and referring physicians should be informed about the risk of complication at time of decision.

References

1. Hindricks G, on behalf of the Multicentre European Radiofrequency Survey (MERFS) investigators of the Working Group on Arrhythmias of the European Society of Cardiology. *Eur Heart J.* 1993;14:1644-1653.
2. Morady F, Calkins H, Langberg JJ, et al. A prospective randomized comparison of direct current and radiofrequency ablation of the atrioventricular junction. *J Am Coll Cardiol.* 1993;21:102-109.
3. Calkins H, Yonh P, Miller JM, et al, for the Atakr Multicenter Investigators Group. Catheter ablation of accessory pathways, atrioventricular nodal reentrant tachycardia, and the atrioventricular junction. Final results of a prospective, multicenter clinical trial. *Circulation.* 1999;99:262-270.
4. Geelen P, Brugada J, Andries E, Brugada P. Ventricular fibrillation and sudden death after radiofrequency catheter ablation of the atrioventricular junction. *Pacing Clin Electrophysiol.* 1997;20:343-348.
5. Scheinman MM, Huang S. The 1998 NASPE Prospective Catheter Ablation Registry. *Pacing Clin Electrophysiol.* 2000;23:1020-1028.
6. Spector P, Reynolds MR, Calkins H, et al. Meta-analysis of ablation of atrial flutter and supraventricular tachycardia. *Am J Cardiol.* 2009;104:671-677.
7. De Ponti R, Cappato R, Curnis A, et al. Trans-septal catheterization in the electrophysiology laboratory. Data from a multicenter survey spanning 12 years. *J Am Coll Cardiol.* 2006;47:1037-1042.
8. Stabile G, Bertaglia E, Senatore G, et al. Catheter ablation treatment in patients with drug-refractory atrial fibrillation: a prospective, multi-center, randomized, controlled study (Catheter Ablation for the Cure of Atrial Fibrillation Study). *Eur Heart J.* 2006;27:216-221.
9. Wazni OM, Marrouche NF, Martin DO, et al. A. Radiofrequency ablation vs antiarrhythmic drugs as first-line treatment of symptomatic atrial fibrillation: a randomized trial. *JAMA.* 2005;293:2634-2640.
10. Pappone C, Augello G, Sala S, et al. A randomized trial of circumferential pulmonary vein ablation versus antiarrhythmic drug therapy in paroxysmal atrial fibrillation: the APAF study. *J Am Coll Cardiol.* 2006;48:2340-2347.
11. Cappato R, Calkins H, Chen SA, et al. Worldwide survey on the methods, efficacy and safety of catheter ablation for human atrial fibrillation. *Circulation.* 2005;111:1100-1105.
12. Calkins H, Brugada J, Packer DL, et al. HRS/EHRA/ECAS Expert Consensus statement on catheter and surgical ablation of atrial fibrillation: recommendations for personnel, policy, procedures and follow up. *Heart Rhythm.* 2007;4:816-861.
13. Natale A, Raviele A, Arenz T, et al. Venice chart: international consensus document on atrial fibrillation ablation. *J Cardiovasc Electrophysiol.* 2007;18:560-580.
14. Dagres N, Hindricks G, Kottkamp H, et al. Complications of atrial fibrillation ablation in a high-volume center in 1,000

procedures: still cause for concern? *J Cardiovasc Electrophysiol.* 2009;20:1014-1019.
15. Wilber DJ, Pappone C, Neuzil P, et al, for the ThermoCool AF Trial Investigators. Comparison of antiarrhythmic drug therapy and radiofrequency catheter ablation in patients with paroxysmal atrial fibrillation. A randomized controlled trial. *JAMA.* 2010;303:333-340.
16. Cappato R, Calkins H, Chen SA, et al. Updated worldwide survey on the methods, efficacy, and safety of catheter ablation for human atrial fibrillation. *Circ Arrhythm Electrophysiol.* 2010;3:32-38.
17. Cappato R, Calkins H, Chen SA, et al. A. Prevalence and causes of fatal outcome in catheter ablation of atrial fibrillation. *J Am Coll Cardiol.* 2009;53:1798-1803.
18. Cummings JE, Schweickert RA, Saliba WI, et al. Atrial-esophageal fistulas after radiofrequency ablation. *Annals Int Med.* 2006;144:572-574.
19. Pappone C, Oral H, Santinelli V, et al. Atrio-esophageal fistula as a complication of percutanoeus transcatheter ablation of atrial fibrillation. *Circulation.* 2004;109:2724-2726.
20. Scanavacca MI, d'Avila A, Parga J, Sosa E. Left atrial-esophageal fistula following radiofrequency catheter ablation of atrial fibrillation. *J Cardiovasc Electrophysiol.* 2004;15:960-962.
21. Doll N, Borger MA, Fabricius A, et al. Esophageal perforation during left atrial radiofrequency ablation: is the risk too high? *J Thorac Cardiovasc Surg.* 2003;125:836-842.
22. Schmidt M, Nolker G, Marschang H, et al. Incidence of oesophageal wall injury post-pulmonary vein antrum isolation for treatment of patients with atrial fibrillation. *Europace.* 2008;10:205-209.
23. Zellerhoff S, Ullerich H, Lenze F, et al. Damage to the esophagus after atrial fibrillation ablation. Just the tip of the iceberg? High prevalence of mediastinal changes diagnosed by endosonography. *Circ Arrhythm Electrophysiol.* 2010;3:155-159.
24. Chugh A, Oral H, Lemola K, et al. Prevalence, mechanisms, and clinical significance of macroreentrant atrial tachycardia during and following left atrial ablation for atrial fibrillation. *Heart Rhythm.* 2005;2:464-471.
25. Gerstenfeld EP, Callans DJ, Dixit S, et al. Mechanisms of organized left atrial tachycardias occurring after pulmonary vein isolation. *Circulation.* 2004;110:1351-1357.
26. Ouyang F, Antz M, Ernst S, et al. Recovered pulmonary vein conduction as a dominant factor for recurrent atrial tachyarrhythmias after complete circular isolation of the pulmonary veins: lessons from double Lasso technique. *Circulation.* 2005;111:127-135.
27. Calkins H, Epstein A, Packer D, et al. for the Coled RF Multi Center Investigators Group. Catheter ablation of ventricular tachycardia in patients with structural heart disease using cooled radiofrequency energy: results of a prospective multicenter study. *J Am Coll Cardiol.* 2000;35:1905-1914.
28. Stevenson WG, Wilber DJ, Natale A, et al, for the Multicenter ThermoCool VT Ablation Trial Investigators. Irrigated radiofrequency catheter ablation guided by electroanatomic mapping for recurrent ventricular tachycardia after myocardial infarction. *Circulation.* 2008;118:2773-2782.
29. Reddy VY, Reynolds MR, Neuzil P, et al. Prophylactic catheter ablation for prevention of defibrillator therapy. *N Engl J Med.* 2007;357:2657-2665.
30. Natale A, Raviele A, Al-Ahmad A, et al, for the Venice Chart members. Venice chart international consensus document on ventricular tachycardia/ventricular fibrillation ablation. *J Cardiovasc Electrophysiol.* 2010;21:339-379.
31. Aliot EM, Stevenson WG, Almendral-Garrote JM, et al. EHRA/HRS expert consensus on catheter ablation of ventricular arrhythmias. *Europace.* 2009;11:771-817.
32. Sosa E, Scanavacca M, d'Avila A, Oliveira F, Ramires JA. Nonsurgical transthoracic epicardial catheter ablation to treat recurrent ventricular tachycardia occurring late after myocardial infarction. *J Am Coll Cardiol.* 2000;35:1442-1449.
33. d'Avila A. Epicardial catheter ablation of ventricular tachycardia. *Heart Rhythm.* 2008;5:S73-S75.
34. Sosa E, Scanavacca M. Epicardial mapping and ablation techniques to control ventricular tachycardia. *J Cardiovasc Electrophysiol.* 2005;16:449-452.
35. Rober-Thomson KC, Steven D, Seiler J, et al. Coronary artery injury due to catheter ablation in adults, presentations and outcomes. *Circulation.* 2009;120:1465-1473.
36. d'Avila A, Gutierrez P, Scanavacca M, et al. Effects of radiofrequency pulses delivered in the vicinity of the coronary arteries: implications for nonsurgical transthoracic epicardial catheter ablation to treat ventricular tachycardia. *Pacing Clin Electrophysiol.* 2002;25:1488-1495.
37. Buch E, Vaseghi M, Cesario DA, Shivkumar K. A novel method for preventing phrenic nerve injury during catheter ablation. *Heart Rhythm.* 2007;4:95-98.
38. Matsuo S, Jaïs P, Knecht S, et al. Images in cardiovascular medicine. Novel technique to prevent left phrenic nerve injury during epicardial catheter ablation. *Circulation.* 2008;117:e471.
39. d'Avila A, Neuzil P, Thiagalingam A, et al. Experimental efficacy of pericardial instillation of anti-inflammatory agents during percutaneous epicardial catheter ablation to prevent postprocedure pericarditis. *J Cardiovasc Electrophysiol.* 2007;18:1178-1183.
40. Pappone C, Oral H, Santinelli V, et al. Atrio-esophageal fistula as a complication of percutaneous transcatheter ablation of atrial fibrillation. *Circulation.* 2004;109:2724-2726.
41. Bunch TJ, Nelson J, Foley T, et al. Temporary esophageal stenting allows healing of esophageal perforations following atrial fibrillation ablation procedures. *J Cardiovasc Electrophysiol.* 2006;17:435-439.
42. Sanchez-Quintana D, Cabrera JA, Climent V, Farré J, Weiglein A, Ho SY. How close are the phrenic nerves to cardiac structures? Implications for cardiac interventionalists. *J Cardiovasc Electrophysiol.* 2005;16:309-313.
43. Bunch TJ, Bruce GK, Mahapatra S, et al. Mechanisms of phrenic nerve injury during radiofrequency ablation at the pulmonary vein orifice. *J Cardiovasc Electrophysiol.* 2005;16:1318-1325.
44. Lee BK, Choi KJ, Kim J, Rhee KS, Nam GB, Kim YH. Right phrenic nerve injury following electrical disconnection of the right superior pulmonary vein. *Pacing Clin Electrophysiol.* 2004;27:1444-1446.
45. Robbins IM, Colvin EV, Doyle TP, et al. Pulmonary vein stenosis after catheter ablation of atrial fibrillation. *Circulation.* 1998;98:1769-1775.
46. Taylor GW, Kay GN, Zheng X, Bishop S, Ideker RE. Pathological effects of extensive radiofrequency energy application in the pulmonary veins in dogs. *Circulation.* 2000;101:1736-1742.
47. Saad EB, Rossillo A, Saad CP, et al. Pulmonary vein stenosis after radiofrequency ablation of atrial fibrillation. Functional characterization, evolution, and influence of the ablation strategy. *Circulation.* 2003;108:3102-3107.
48. Kistler, PM, Early MJ, Harris S, et al. Validation of three-dimensional cardiac image integration: use of integrated CT image into electroanatomical mapping system to perform catheter ablation of atrial fibrillation. *J Cardiovasc Electrophysiol.* 2006;17:341-348.

49. Lang CC, Gugliotta F, Santinelli V, et al. Endocardial impedance mapping during circumferential pulmonary vein ablation of atrial fibrillation differentiates between atrial and venous tissue. *Heart Rhythm*. 2006;3:171-178.
50. Packer DL, Keelan P, Munger TM, et al. Clinical presentation, investigation, and management of pulmonary vein stenosis complicating ablation for atrial fibrillation. *Circulation*. 2005;111:546-554.
51. Ernst S, Ouyang F, Goya M, et al. Total pulmonary vein occlusion as a consequence of catheter ablation for atrial fibrillation mimicking primary lung disease. *J Cardiovasc Electrophysiol*. 2003;14:366-370.
52. Jander N, Minners J, Arentz T, et al. Transesophageal echocardiography in comparison with magnetic resonance imaging in the diagnosis of pulmonary vein stenosis after radiofrequency ablation therapy. *J Am Soc Echocardiogr*. 2005;18:654-659.
53. Dill T, Neumann T, Ekinci O, et al. Pulmonary vein diameter reduction after radiofrequency catheter ablation for paroxysmal atrial fibrillation evaluated by contrast-enhanced three-dimensional magnetic resonance imaging. *Circulation*. 2003;107:845-850.
54. Quereshi AM, Prieto LR, Latson LA, et al. Transcatheter angioplasty for acquired pulmonary vein stenosis after radiofrequency ablation. *Circulation*. 2003;108:1336-1342.
55. Arentz T, Weber R, Jander N, et al. Pulmonary hemodynamics at rest and during exercise in patients with significant pulmonary vein stenosis after radiofrequency catheter ablation for drug resistant atrial fibrillation. *Eur Heart J*. 2005;26:1410-1414.
56. Takahashi Y, Jaïs P, Hocini M, et al. Acute occlusion of the left circumflex coronary artery during mitral isthmus linear ablation. *J Cardiovasc Electrophysiol*. 2005;16:1104-1107.
57. Jaïs P, Hocini M, Hsu LF, et al. Technique and results of linear ablation at the mitral isthmus. *Circulation*. 2004;110:2996-3002.
58. Di Biase L, Burkhardt JD, Mohanty P, et al. Periprocedural stroke and management of major bleeding complications in patients undergoing catheter ablation of atrial fibrillation: the impact of periprocedural therapeutic international normalized ratio. *Circulation*. 2010;121(23):2550-2556.
59. Oral H, Chugh A, Ozaydin M, et al. Risk of thromboembolic events after percutaneous left atrial radiofrequency ablation of atrial fibrillation. *Circulation*. 2006;114:759-765.
60. Lickfett L, Hackenbroch M, Lewalter T, et al. Cerebral diffusion-weighted magnetic resonance imaging: a tool to monitor the thrombogenicity of left atrial catheter ablation. *J Cardiovasc Electrophysiol*. 2006;17:1-7.
61. Gaita F, Caponi D, Pianelli M, et al. Radiofrequency catheter ablation of atrial fibrillation: a cause of silent thromboembolism? Magnetic resonance imaging assessment of cerebral thromboembolism in patients undergoing ablation of atrial fibrillation. *Circulation*. 2010;122:1667-1673.
62. Lesh MD, Coggins DL, Ports TA. Coronary air embolism complicating transseptal radiofrequency ablation of left free-wall accessory pathways. *Pacing Clin Electrophysiol*. 1992;15:1105-1108.
63. Hinkle DA, Raizen DM, McGarvey ML, Liu GT. Cerebral air embolism complicating cardiac ablation procedures. *Neurology*. 2001;56:792-794.
64. Krivonyak GS, Warren SG. Cerebral arterial air embolism treated by a vertical head-down maneuver. *Catheter Cardiovasc Interv*. 2000;49:185-187.
65. Wu RC, Brinker JA, Yuh DD, Berger RD, Calkins HG. Circular mapping catheter entrapment in the mitral valve apparatus: a previously unrecognized complication of focal atrial fibrillation ablation. *J Cardiovasc Electrophysiol*. 2002;13:819-821.
66. Kesek M, Englund A, Jensen SM, Jensen-Urstad M. Entrapment of circular mapping catheter in the mitral valve. *Heart Rhythm*. 2007;4:17-19.
67. Cheema A, Dong J, Dalal D, et al. Long-term safety and efficacy of circumferential ablation with pulmonary vein isolation. *J Cardiovasc Electrophysiol*. 2006;17:1080-1085.
68. Prudente LA, Moorman JR, Lake D, et al. Femoral vascular complications following catheter ablation of atrial fibrillation. *J Interv Card Electrophysiol*. 2009;26:59-64.

SECTION 2C

INTERVENTIONAL ELECTROPHYSIOLOGY PROCEDURES

Surgical Ablation

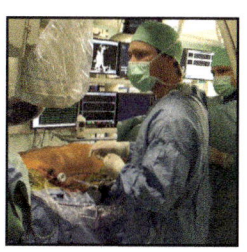 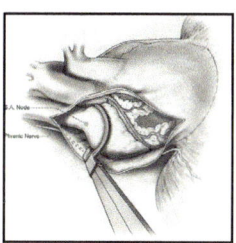 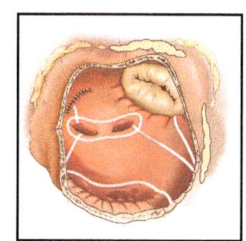 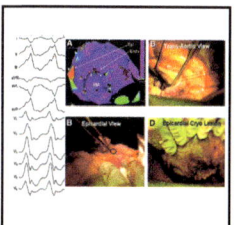

CHAPTER 48

Ventricular Tachycardia with Hybrid Endocardial and Epicardial Approaches

Nimesh D. Desai, MD, PhD; Michael A. Acker, MD

Historical Context

Open surgical techniques for treatment of cardiac arrhythmias date back to 1969, with open ablation of Wolff-Parkinson-White syndrome as described by Sealy.[1] During the 1970s, there was a significant interest in surgical ablation of ventricular arrhythmias and techniques developed primarily for treatment of postinfarct scar-related VTs.[2-8] In the predefibrillator and percutaneous coronary intervention (PCI) eras, such patients typically underwent coronary bypass grafting and resection of scar or ventricular aneurysms, which served as arrhythmogenic foci. Early approaches involved fairly broad resection of infarcted myocardium and border zones such that myocardial function was deleteriously impacted by these procedures and carried a high mortality.[9,10]

Part of the evolution of these procedures was the development of surgical endocardial and epicardial mapping systems in order to identify VT foci for a more targeted ablation.[11-13] Techniques were eventually developed for isolated endocardial scar excision, which proved to be effective without compromising myocardial function. The less aggressive myocardial resection operations mandated careful endocardial mapping to ensure the focus of arrhythmia was truly excised. Over time, cryotherapy was also successfully used to achieve the same results without extensive myocardial excision and further decreased perioperative mortality and morbidity.[14-16]

Techniques for ventricular aneurysm resection also evolved over time. The more recent use of ventricular aneurysmectomy with circular endoventricular patch reconstruction as described by Dor has been shown to provide excellent protection from recurrent ventricular arrhythmias while excising the ventricular aneurysm.[17] Cryoablation of the residual endocardial scar during the Dor procedure is an important adjunct among patients with ventricular arrhythmia.

Current Rationale for Surgical Access

With the introduction of implantable devices, such as implantable cardioverter-defibrillators (ICDs), and the tremendous success of percutaneous catheter-based endocardial approaches to ventricular arrhythmias, open surgery has been reserved as a last-resort operation in patients with multiple failed endocardial lesions and life-threatening ventricular arrhythmias.[18-23] Increasingly, such patients have also been treated with percutaneous catheter-based epicardial ablation.

First described by Sosa and colleagues, this emerging technique has evolved from experimental stages to a well-developed and frequently successful procedure over a relatively short period of time.[24] Continued innovation in the development of steerable catheters and improved mapping and visualization techniques may allow this technique to expand, and a larger proportion of patients may be successfully ablated via the percutaneous epicardial approach.

There are, however, cases where epicardial access is not feasible via a subxiphoid percutaneous catheter-based technique due to loss of the pericardial potential space from adhesions, either from pericarditis or, more likely, from previous open heart surgery. Catheter-based epicardial ablation also may not be feasible in situations where the ventricular tachycardia (VT) substrate is in close proximity to the native coronary arteries, previous bypass grafts, or phrenic nerve. In these cases, surgical access to the epicardium may play an important role. Complex, often nonischemic, anatomic substrates may require ablation in intracardiac or epicardial locations that are difficult to access with a catheter, such as those in close proximity to valvular structures.[25] In the largest multicenter study examining epicardial VT ablation, Sacher and colleagues reported that among 136 patients with planned percutaneous pericardial access, 20 required surgical access to the epicardium.[26]

Epicardial VT ablation on the beating heart may be achieved by 3 possible approaches, including an open subxiphoid approach, a left thoracotomy approach, or a thoracoscopic approach. Additionally, for complex endocardial and epicardial surgical ablation, a full sternotomy with cardiopulmonary bypass and cardioplegic arrest with preoperative mapping and/or endocardial ablation remains a last-resort option. Subxiphoid and left anterior thoracotomy approaches are used most commonly in hybrid procedures (Figure 48.1).[27]

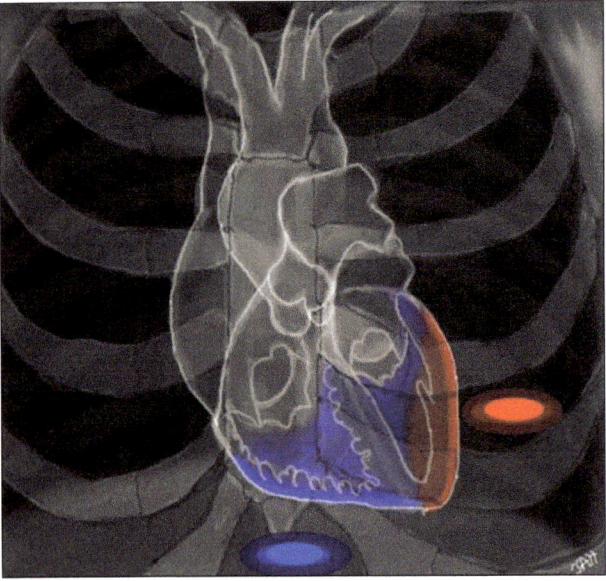

Figure 48.1 Schematic demonstration of the potential exposed area with each approach (**red:** anterior thoracotomy; **blue:** subxiphoid). *Source:* Reprinted from Michowitz Y, et al,[27] with permission.

Surgical Approaches

Subxiphoid Approach

In the subxiphoid, a pericardial window is typically accomplished using general anesthesia with the patient in the supine position. In a patient who cannot tolerate general anesthesia, a combination of local anesthesia and mild sedation is theoretically feasible, although it may not be well tolerated for prolonged procedures. Typically, pericardial access can be achieved with a 4- to 5-cm incision starting from the lower edge of the sternum at the most caudal part of the xiphoid. Frequently, either dividing or preferably excising the xiphoid completely can improve exposure to the pericardial space. The upper portion of the linea alba is divided in the midline, and the preperitoneal space is entered. Care is taken to avoid opening the peritoneum; if it is inadvertently opened, it should be closed with absorbable sutures prior to proceeding. In a patient under general anesthesia, placement of a retractor, such as a Favaloro retractor used for internal mammary artery harvest, can facilitate exposure by providing anterior and superior retraction of the chest wall. Blunt dissection is carried down to the pericardium, and typically a plane between the pericardium and the posterior aspect of the sternum is developed with blunt dissection. The pericardium is then opened anteriorly. The pericardial incision is extended anteriorly as far as is visible, inferiorly to the diaphragm and then in both directions laterally as far as can be safely reached. Once the potential space is opened, a sheath may be inserted to provide mapping and ablation catheter access. Typically, these functions are performed using fluoroscopic guidance as direct visualization is limited (Figure 48.2).[28]

As there may be severe adhesions in patients with previous cardiotomy, care is taken at this point to perform sharp dissection either with scissors or low-energy electrocautery to free the adhered epicardial surface from the pericardium. It is critical to enter the correct plane between the diaphragmatic surface of the heart and pericardium. Once the pericardial space has started to open, it may be possible to further extend the working area using blunt dissection with finger. Extreme care must be taken in the presence of a coronary artery bypass graft to the posterior descending artery, which is invariably adherent to the pericardium. Performing blunt dissection maneuvers should be avoided in this case, and careful scissor dissection is preferable. In general, only the inferior wall and potentially the basal portion of the inferolateral wall are accessible to the subxiphoid approach. Should it be required, extending the incision superiorly into a partial or full sternotomy may provide partial access to the anterior wall.

Left Anterior Thoracotomy Approach

The left thoracotomy approach to the pericardium is made via several different potential incisions and anesthetic strategies. Limited anterior thoracotomy is preferable, as it minimizes postoperative pain. It is performed with the patient in the supine position with an inflatable bump on the left side. This particular approach to the heart has become increasingly popular in cardiac surgery for performance of transapical aortic valve replacement and surgical anesthetic techniques have become highly standardized. Typically, a 5- to 8-cm incision is used in the fourth or

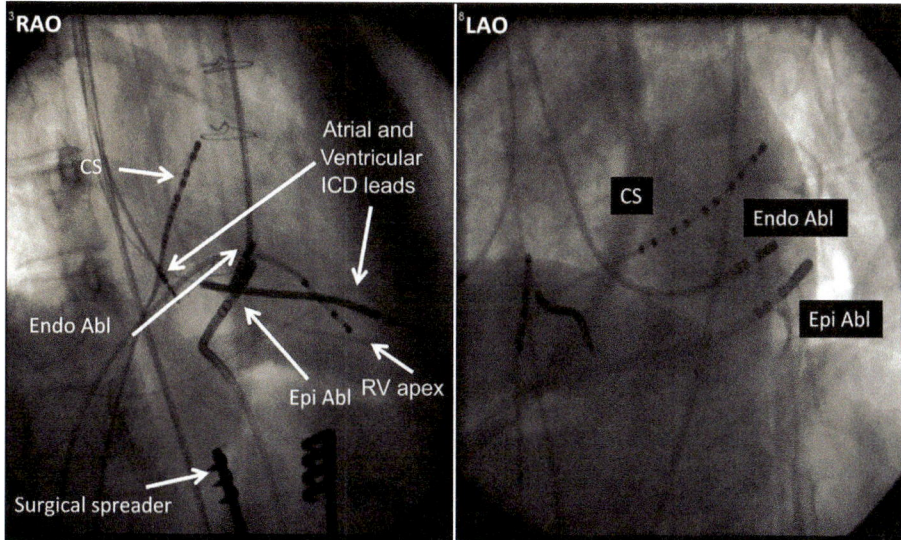

Figure 48.2 Fluoroscopic view during VT ablation with surgical subxiphoid access. **Left Panel:** Right anterior oblique (RAO) view with an ablation catheter on the site of interest on the endocardial side (Endo Abl) via a retrograde aortic approach. Another catheter (Epi Abl) is placed on the epicardial side of the same spot and has been introduced via surgical approach. Note the surgical spreader (**bottom**). **Right Panel:** Left anterior oblique (LAO) view of the same site. CS = coronary sinus catheter; ICD = implantable cardioverter-defibrillator; RV apex = catheter placed at the apex of the right ventricle; VT = ventricular tachycardia. Source: Reprinted from Soejima K, et al,[28] with permission.

fifth interspaces. In stable patients who can tolerate single-lung ventilation, use of a double-lumen endotracheal tube with deflation of the left lung is preferable but not necessary. In cases where this is not feasible, it may be possible to perform the surgery with standard intubation and dual-lung ventilation. The anterior thoracotomy approach will typically give access to the apex, anterior wall, and the more anterior portions of the lateral wall. Preoperative electrophysiologic mapping correlated to a preoperative chest CT scan can assist in the determination of the precise location of the incision and identification of the correct rib interspace to enter the chest.

In cases where multiple segments of the heart, in particular the lateral and inferolateral walls, need to be accessed, a larger left thoracotomy performed with the patient in the left lateral decubitus position with double-lumen endotracheal tube and single-lung ventilation is preferred. This approach may not be well tolerated in severe cardiomyopathy patients with compromised reserve. The primary advantage of a full lateral thoracotomy is that it provides access to the entire left side of the heart. With all left-sided approaches, care must be taken to avoid injury to the phrenic nerve. With a limited anterolateral thoracotomy, the pericardial space is always entered anterior to the phrenic nerve. With the full lateral thoracotomy, the pericardial space can be entered anterior or posterior to the phrenic nerve. With left-sided approaches, it is extremely important to be knowledgeable about the patient's coronary anatomy as well as the location of the bypass grafts. There is typically a significant amount of adhesion along the course of an internal mammary artery graft, and its location should be identified with a preoperative contrast-enhanced, cardiac-gated CT angiogram. Care must be taken to completely avoid the graft, as injury would usually necessitate going on cardiopulmonary bypass and repairing or revising the graft.

Thoracoscopic Approach

An evolving area of interest is in the performance of epicardial ablation using only port access from the left chest. This procedure can be performed either in the supine position with a bump under the left side or a full thoracotomy with the patient in the lateral decubitus position. Use of single-lung ventilation is mandatory, and this technique may not be suitable for a marginal patient. However, it is less invasive and does not carry the pain and morbidity of a major thoracotomy incision.

When accessing the heart using thoracoscopic instrumentation, particularly in the redo setting where there may be significant adhesions and scar tissue, extreme care must be taken to enter the pericardium in a safe manner. In the opinion of many in the field, previous thoracic surgery is a contraindication to a thoracoscopic approach. Although clinical experience with this approach is limited, animal studies support feasibility (Figure 48.3).[29] However, great care should be taken in redo patients.

Sternotomy Approach

In cases where endocardial surgical access is required, operations are performed via full sternotomy approach with cardiopulmonary bypass with cold cardioplegic arrest of the heart. Access to the ventricular myocardium for surgical endocardial ablation in this situation is typically through the aortic valve. An unusual variant is the development of mid-myocardial scar in which there is significant thickening of basal aspect of the interventricular septum, which requires combined endocardial and epicardial ablation.[25]

Energy Sources

Several different energy sources have been proposed to perform cardiac ablation. Each technology has its own

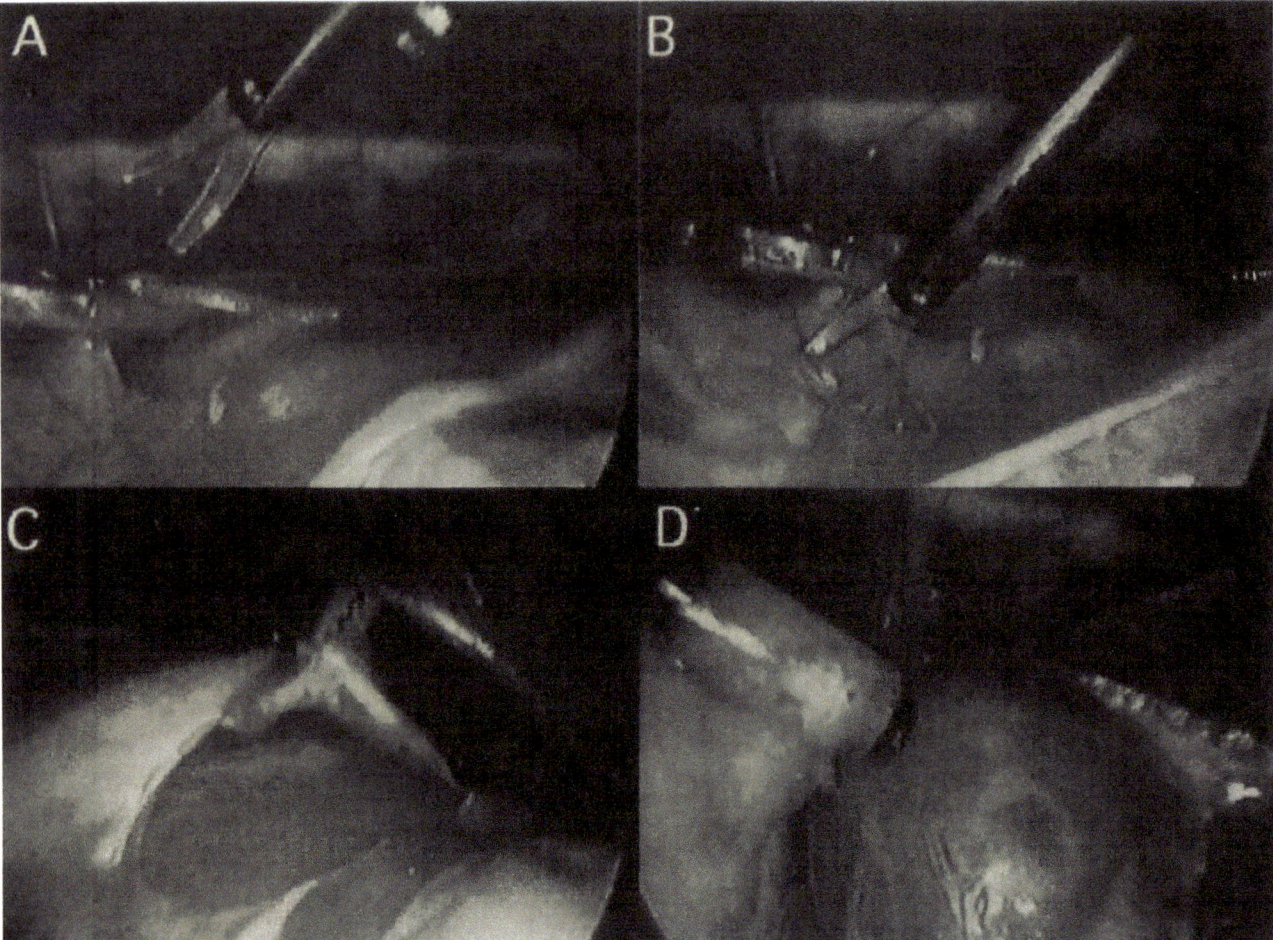

Figure 48.3 Thoracoscopic entry in to the pericardium with a longitudinal incision into the pericardium (**Panels A and B**). Application of ablation probe to the myocardium (**Panels C and D**). *Source:* Reprinted from Watanabe G, et al,[29] with permission.

unique benefits and limitations. The main goals of myocardial tissue ablation are to achieve a transmural lesion leading to a complete electrical disconnection and to maintain cardiac anatomy such that the fibrous skeletal structure of the heart remains intact and a stable scar forms without perforation or aneurysmal formation. This allows creation of a scar that is not arrhythmogenic and provides a controlled ablation without significant collateral tissue damage. Energy sources used on the beating heart also require the ability to overcome the heat-sink effect of flowing endocardial blood, which dissipates thermal energy. An ideal energy source would also be able to perform ablation either near or even on top of the epicardial coronary arteries without causing thrombosis or endothelial damage to the artery. While no one specific technology can currently achieve all of these goals, there are several energy sources available. It is important to note that while transmurality may be very difficult to achieve on a beating heart via the epicardial approach, most patients have had ablation at the corresponding location with the endocardial approach, and epicardial ablation must be able to extend to the endocardial lesion to achieve full transmurality.

Cryoablation

Surgical cryoablation has traditionally been a commonly used approach to surgical VT ablation. Cryoablation procedures have traditionally been performed on the empty heart with cardiopulmonary bypass and, when needed, cardioplegic arrest.[30] Cryoablation causes the necrosis of cardiac tissue by freezing. Based on the Joule–Thomson effect, as the gas is compressed through the probe, there is dramatic drop in pressure resulting in a rapid expansion of the gas with a concomitant decrease in temperature.[31] In the freezing phase, ice crystals form intracellularly at temperatures below –5°C, resulting in swelling and bursting of cell membranes, mitochondria, and organelles. Additionally, ice formation in the fluid surrounding the cells causes intracellular dehydration. These events eventually lead to cell death and active inflammation. There is also an induction of apoptosis, which results in additional necrosis.[32] This is followed by immune-modulated formation of stable scar.

Cryoablation maintains the structural integrity of the tissues being ablated including maintenance of the collagenous structure of the tissue.[33] Despite cell death, the resulting fibrous scar maintains strength and does not dilate or rupture. Other than the area being ablated, it does not have a significant effect on the contractile function of the surrounding tissues.[34] It also creates a homogenous scar that is not arrhythmogenic and shows low myocardial potentials with normal electrical activity in the surrounding tissues.[34]

There are two widely used energy sources for cryoablation: liquid nitrogen and argon. Liquid nitrogen can achieve a maximum low temperature of −100°C, while the more recently available argon can achieve a temperature of −192°C.[34,35] Lesions are usually performed with 60- to 180-second freeze times. Due to the heat sink effect from flowing blood in a warm beating heart, cryosurgery has generally been less successful on the full, warm, beating heart.[36,37]

Cryotherapy can be achieved on the heart from the sternotomy, subxiphoid, thoracotomy, and thoracoscopic approaches. Historically, cryothermy probes were large, rigid probes placed during open sternotomy procedures. Current-generation cryothermal probes are available in a variety of shapes and sizes and are also available in the form of flexible, malleable linear probes (Figure 48.4).[36] Additionally, catheters designed for percutaneous intracardiac approaches may also be used.

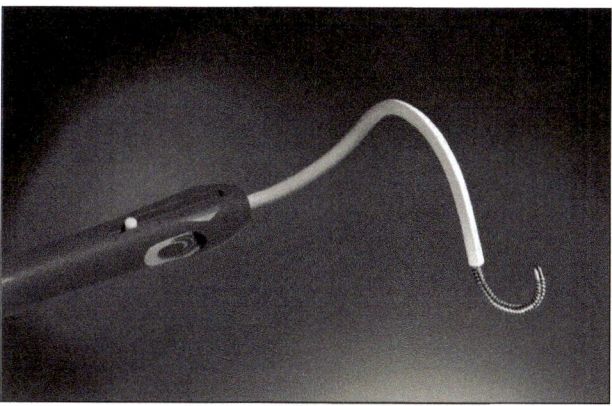

Figure 48.4 SurgiFrost CryoSurgical® probe. Hand-held probe with 60-mm flexible freezing segment and 170-mm malleable shaft. Ablation zone can be adjusted by insulation sleeve. *Source:* Reprinted from Doll, et al,[36] with permission.

Radiofrequency Ablation

Radiofrequency ablation is performed by applying high-frequency (> 500 kHz) electromagnetic energy to cardiac tissue to achieve thermal injury.

Thermal injury typically occurs when the myocardial cells are heated above 50°C.[38] The radiofrequency energy is provided from a generator and can be applied to the heart using standard ablation catheters or various pen-like or linear probe devices. Ablation can be achieved through median sternotomy, subxiphoid, thoracotomy, and thoracoscopic approaches. There are specific probes designed for thoracoscopic use that have articulating ablation heads and smaller profiles. Some probes, in addition to ablation, can also perform epicardial mapping, pacing, and sensing.

Surgical devices for cardiac tissue ablation may be generally categorized into unipolar, unipolar irrigated, bipolar, and bipolar irrigated. Unipolar approaches typically achieve myocardial ablation when the tissue temperature reaches above 50°C. They frequently require 30 to 90 seconds to achieve a lesion 4–5 mm deep.[39] On a beating heart, these probes have difficulty penetrating myocardial tissue due to the endocardial heat sink. One of the drawbacks of nonirrigated unipolar energy ablation is the formation of surface char that contacts the interface with the electrode tip, which has an insulating effect and causes a rapid rise in impedance.[40] Irrigation with saline allows for achievement of optimal ablation temperature and will typically increased depth by 1 to 2 mm.[41] Temperature controls are also present on most devices to ensure appropriate heating. Achieving a full transmural lesion in tissue greater than 4 mm, which would be required for most ventricular muscle ablation, is not reliable with current unipolar technologies.[42] This is in part due to an endocardial heat sink effect limiting its thermal injury. Unipolar approaches to surgical atrial fibrillation ablation have been associated with esophageal perforation due to the close proximity of posterior left atrial tissue to the esophagus.[43,44]

Bipolar ablation techniques are standard for surgical ablation of the pulmonary veins and employ clamp-like devices, which would not be suitable for ventricular ablation. A more recent innovation is the development of pen-like and linear bipolar ablation probes (Figure 48.5).[45] These bipolar ablation probes are capable of creating a lesion up to 20 mm in length and employ two discrete, linear radiofrequency electrodes placed in parallel on the ablation head. Radiofrequency energy is delivered between the two linear probes, causing a maximum focus of energy deeper in the myocardium between the two probes. These technologies have recently been shown in animal studies to reliably produce transmural lesions in myocardial tissue up to 6 mm.[42] Ablation time is typically 15 to 60 seconds.

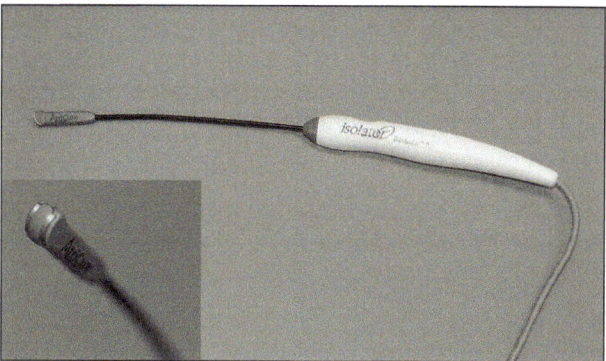

Figure 48.5 AtriCure Isolator Bipolar Pen®. Hand-held probe with two parallel electrodes (**Inset**). *Source:* Reprinted from Sakamoto, et al,[45] with permission.

High-intensity Focused Ultrasound

High-intensity focused ultrasound (HIFU) is a fairly new technology used for arrhythmia ablation. HIFU is specifically designed for epicardial ablation of nonblood-contacting cardiac tissue on a full, warm, beating heart. This technology uses ultrasound energy at 3.8 to 6.4 MHz with a power output of 15 to 130 W, can be focused at various depths, and can achieve uniform ablation from the endocardial surface to the epicardial surface.[46] The acoustic energy results in oscillation and collision of molecules, generating mechanical heat with limited thermal injury to the contact surface between the probe and the myocardium. The ability to focus the ultrasonic energy at varying depths allows the creation of uniform lesions. The technology was originally devised for AF ablation, for which there is an encircling probe to ablate around the pulmonary veins.[47] A handheld ablation wand is also available that could be used through the minimal access, full sternotomy, or thoracoscopic approaches (Figure 48.6).[47] Ablation time with the wand is typically 80 seconds. The device is irrigated with room temperature normal saline, which enhances acoustic coupling. HIFU has been shown in beating-heart animal models to ablate myocardium over 14 mm thick.[48] It is also highly effective at ablating through adipose tissue. As ultrasonic energy is 30 times more rapidly absorbed by tissue than blood, this technology may also allow for ablation of cardiac tissue that is in close proximity to epicardial coronary arteries.[48] In a study by Koruth and colleagues, a HIFU probe was placed directly over the LAD in an in-vivo beating heart porcine model (Figure 48.7).[48] At eight weeks of follow-up, histologic studies showed myocardial ablation depths of over 15 mm and up to 22.7 mm. With intentional direct ablation of the coronary artery itself, 21% showed no significant tissue injury, and tissue injury severe enough to cause thrombus formation and myocardial necrosis occurred in only one of 33 specimens. The ability to ablate through myocardial fat and to ablate near or even on epicardial coronary arteries without damage is unique to this technology. At present there is no data on the use of this technology for ventricular tachyarrhythmias ablation in humans, but it may represent a potential new form of ablation. This technology is not currently commercially available and further development for clinical application is still in the developmental stage.

Results of Hybrid VT Ablation

Due to the infrequent and complex nature of these cases, there are no large, multicenter studies to date to determine efficacy of hybrid catheter/surgical VT ablation. The results of hybrid procedures for VT ablation are dependent to some extent on the indication for hybrid procedure and the complexity of the lesions being ablated.

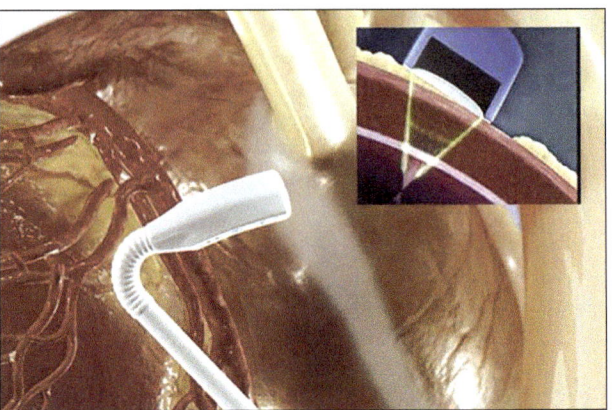

Figure 48.6 St. Jude Epicor High Intensity Focused Ultrasound Probe®. Ultrasonic energy is focused to varying tissue depths for full-thickness ablation (Inset). *Source:* Reprinted from Villamizar, et al,[47] with permission.

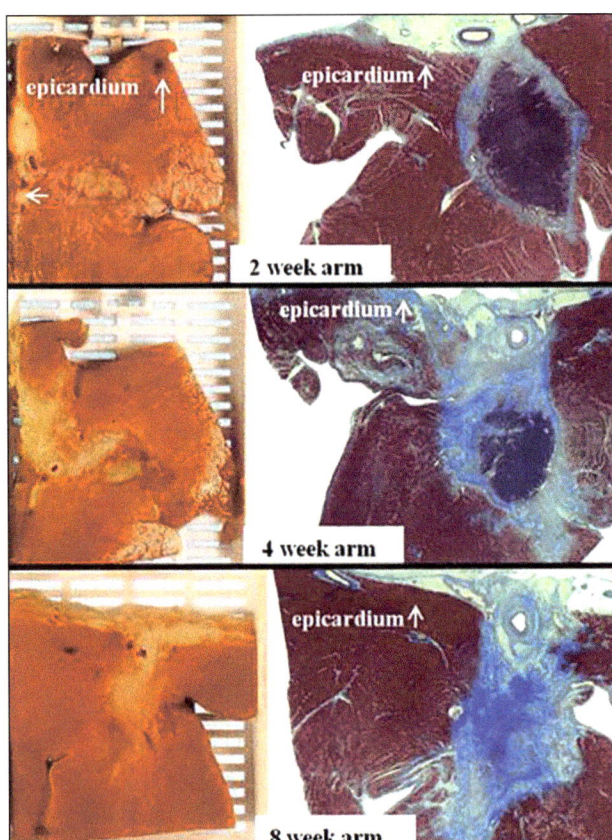

Figure 48.7 Gross Histology at 2, 4, and 8 weeks post-HIFU epicardial ablation directly on the LAD. *Source:* Reprinted from Koruth, et al,[48] with permission.

In general, the patients are divided into two groups: (1) those who do not have suitable percutaneous epicardial access due to presence of epicardial adhesions, or close proximity of ablation target to coronary arteries or phrenic nerve, and (2) those with complex, typically nonischemic pathology, which require multimodal ablation including surgical endocardial and epicardial approaches.

Inadequate Epicardial Access

The first report of a planned hybrid intervention with surgical access to the pericardial space via subxiphoid incision was described by Soejima and colleagues in Boston.[28] They performed this procedure in six patients who either had failure of previous percutaneous epicardial access (three patients, of which two had previous cardiac surgery) or in patients with previous cardiac surgery in which percutaneous epicardial access was not attempted. Two of the patients had previous epicardial defibrillation patches placed. Among these patients, four had nonischemic cardiomyopathy and two had ischemic cardiomyopathy with previous CABG. Using the subxiphoid approach, the pericardium was entered and blunt dissection was performed to create a potential pericardial space allowing for insertion of a sheath and standard catheter mapping ablation systems were employed. They did not use any form of direct visualization but rather used fluoroscopy and performed the procedure similar to standard percutaneous epicardial access approaches. All procedures were performed in an electrophysiology lab. The inferoposterior aspect of the left ventricle was mapped in all patients, and in four of six patients the anterior lateral LV was also accessible. Procedural success was achieved in 4 of 6 patients, and there were no major complications.

In the largest hybrid series to date, Michowitz and colleagues performed hybrid ablation on 14 patients in the electrophysiology lab.[49] Of these, 11 were performed via a subxiphoid approach and three were performed by a limited anterior thoracotomy. There were 10 patients with an ischemic substrate and four patients with nonischemic substrate. Cardiac surgery had been performed in 12 of 14 patients. In the two patients who did not have previous cardiac surgery, one had failed access, and one the area of ablation was in close proximity to the coronary arteries and phrenic nerve. All patients had failed two or more antiarrhythmic drugs, and 13 of 14 patients had previous endocardial ablation. In cases with subxiphoid access, catheters similar to percutaneous epicardial approaches were employed with electroanatomic mapping for guidance. In the left anterior thoracotomy cases, ablation was performed under direct visualization with electro-anatomic mapping guidance. Ablations were performed on the beating heart without cardiopulmonary bypass. Overall, eight of 14 patients achieved acute procedural success. One patient had a recurrence 120 days after the procedure for an overall success rate of 50%.

Complex Anatomic Substrate

Among patients with nonischemic, scar-related VT, there exists a small subset of patients who cannot be successfully ablated using catheter-based endocardial or epicardial approaches. Nonischemic, scar-related VT is particularly challenging from the catheter-based perspective as the VT focus may be in close proximity to the left-sided valvular structures, deep within the myocardium or on the epicardial surface in an inaccessible location or in close proximity to the coronary arteries. In such cases, after failed endocardial and percutaneous epicardial catheter-based ablation, open surgery may be required. This is typically performed via a full sternotomy on an arrested heart and may require open ablation inside cardiac chambers in addition to epicardial ablation.

The largest series to date of nonischemic VT patients was published by Anter et al from the Hospital of the University of Pennsylvania.[50] They examined 527 patients who underwent VT ablation, of which 8 had a nonischemic significant ventricular arrhythmia refractory to medications and endocardial and/or epicardial radiofrequency ablation. Among the eight patients, six had dilated cardiomyopathy and two patients had hypertrophic cardiomyopathy. Patients underwent the hybrid procedure due to extreme complexity of the anatomic substrate of the VT focus. None of the patients had previous heart surgery. Patients typically had 3 to 16 defibrillator shocks in the three months preceding surgery and were on 1 to 3 antiarrhythmic drugs. These patients had undergone on average, 1.5 endocardial ablation procedures and one epicardial ablation procedure. Among the six patients in the series who underwent epicardial mapping, the abnormal substrate was typically opposite to the site of the endocardial ablation lesions with the intervening myocardial thickness ranging from 15 to 32 mm. In four patients who underwent cardiac MRI, mid-myocardial scar was identified in the septum in three cases and on the inferior wall in one case. A variety of approaches to surgical ablation were employed. In all cases, cryothermy was used as the energy source, and lesions were performed at least 0.5 cm away from major epicardial coronary vessels. On average, 5 cryothermy applications were performed per patient, with a mean cryoablation time of 18 ± 6 minutes. All procedures were performed on cardiopulmonary bypass, with six of eight patients requiring cardioplegic arrest. The surgical procedures were performed in the operating room and were guided with the preoperative electrophysiologic mapping studies. Intraoperative late, three patients had epicardial ablation only, and five patients had both endocardial and epicardial cryoablation (Figures 48.8 and 48.9). Six of eight patients survived to discharge, indicative of the extremely high-risk nature of this patient population. Two mortalities were related to heart failure and sepsis.

The authors identified four key elements to success in this extremely challenging patient population, including a detailed characterization of the underlying arrhythmia mechanism using mapping, sophisticated cardiac imaging, surgical access via sternotomy, and cardiopulmonary bypass with cold blood cardioplegia. The authors also noted the importance of using previous radiofrequency lesions on the endocardial surface for guiding open intracardiac surgical ablation. This appears to be less useful for the epicardial approach where the previous lesions are not visible.

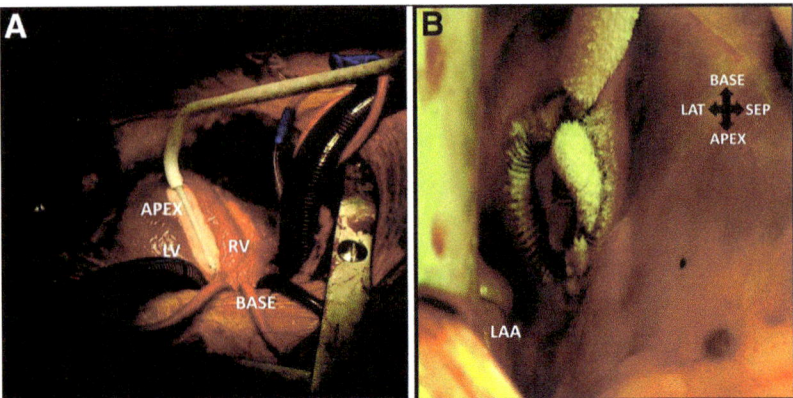

Figure 48.8 Two approaches to epicardial cryoablation. **Panel A:** The cryoprobe was aligned in its entire length along the anterior interventricular septum, ensuring a safe distance from the left anterior descending coronary artery. **Panel B:** The cryoprobe was coiled to create a circular lesion at the anterolateral left ventricular (LV) base between the branches of the circumflex artery. Sep indicates septum; Lat, lateral wall; RV, right ventricle, and LAA, left anterior ascending. *Source:* Reprinted from Anter E, et al,[50] with permission.

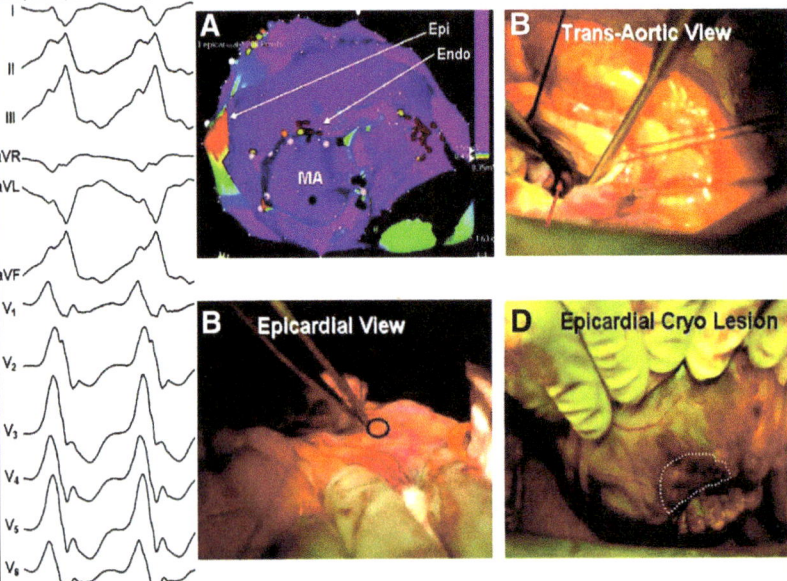

Figure 48.9 Ventricular tachycardia morphology (right bundle, right inferior) and cardiac images in a patient with hypertrophic cardiomyopathy. Endocardial (Endo) and epicardial (Epi) electroanatomic mapping revealed normal voltage and thick basal left ventricle (distance between Epi and Endo surface >3 cm (**Panel A**). At surgical ablation, prior radiofrequency lesions were visualized epicardially (**Panel B, black circle**) and endocardially, through the transaortic approach (**Panel C, red arrow**). Epi and Endo cryothermy applications were made over prior radiofrequency lesions, resulting in large, confluent basal epicardial lesions (**Panel D, dotted area**). MA indicates mitral annulus. *Source:* Reprinted from Anter E, et al,[50] with permission.

Future Directions

In summary, the vast majority of VT can be approached via a percutaneous endocardial ablation. Increasingly, percutaneous epicardial approaches into the pericardial space have also proliferated, allowing a fairly minimally invasive approach to treat more complex arrhythmia substrates. In the small subset of patients in whom epicardial access is not feasible due to adhesions or proximity to cardiac structures, or in patients with very complex lesions not fully curable with traditional catheter-based techniques, surgical approaches guided by a sophisticated electrophysiologic map in conjunction with prior catheter-based intervention can successfully eliminate life-threatening arrhythmias. Today, most of these hybrid-type procedures are performed either through a median sternotomy with cardiopulmonary bypass on an arrested heart in the case of complex, nonischemic VT, or via a subxiphoid or limited anterior thoracotomy approach for cases with inadequate percutaneous epicardial access. Emerging technologies, such as thoracoscopic approaches and the development of energy sources that can safely ablate in close proximity to coronary arteries, will further increase the number of patients who can benefit from hybrid therapies while minimizing invasiveness and morbidity. However, the gold standard for arrhythmia ablation during surgery still remains mapping guided endocardial ablation with or without left ventricular aneurysemctomy.[51–53] Map-guided endocardial ablation with or without left ventricular aneurysmectomy via sternotomy with cardiopulmonary bypass also remains an important option in complex arrhythmia ablation.[51–53]

References

1. Sealy WC, Hattler BG Jr, Blumenschein SD, Cobb FR. Surgical treatment of Wolff-Parkinson-White syndrome. *Ann Thorac Surg.* 1969;8(1):1-11.
2. Mickleborough LL, Mizuno S, Downar E, Gray GC. Late results of operation for ventricular tachycardia. *Ann Thorac Surg.* 1992;54:832-839.
3. Kron IL, Lerman B, DiMarco JP. Surgical management of sustained ventricular arrhythmias presenting within eight weeks of acute myocardial infarction. *Ann Thorac Surg.* 1986;42(1):13-16.

4. Shumway SJ, Johnson EM, Svendsen CA, et al. Surgical management of ventricular tachycardia. *Ann Thorac Surg.* 1997;63:1589-1591.
5. Cox JL. Anatomic-electrophysiologic basis for the surgical treatment of refractory ischemic ventricular tachycardia. *Ann Surg.* 1983;198:119-129.
6. Cabrol A, Guiraudon G, Laughlin L, et al. Resection of left ventricular aneurysms and fibrous plaques. *J Cardiovasc Surg (Torino).* 1974;15(1):72-73.
7. Bourke JP, Campbell RW, McComb JM, et al. Surgery for postinfarction ventricular tachycardia in the pre-implantable cardioverter defibrillator era: Early and long term outcomes in 100 consecutive patients. *Heart.* 1999;82:156-162.
8. Hammon JW Jr. Excisional surgery for patients with ventricular tachyarrhythmias. *J Card Surg.* 1987;2(3):361-368.
9. Lee R, Mitchell JD, Garan H, et al. Operation for recurrent ventricular tachycardia. Predictors of short- and long-term efficacy. *J Thorac Cardiovasc Surg.* 1994;107:732-742.
10. Gallagher JJ, Selle JG, Svenson RH, et al. Surgical treatment of arrhythmias. *Am J Cardiol.* 1988;61:27A-44A.
11. Haines DE, Lerman BB, Kron IL, DiMarco JP. Surgical ablation of ventricular tachycardia with sequential map-guided subendocardial resection: electrophysiologic assessment and long-term follow-up. *Circulation.* 1988;77(1):131-141.
12. Pagé PL, Cardinal R, Shenasa M, et al. Surgical treatment of ventricular tachycardia. Regional cryoablation guided by computerized epicardial and endocardial mapping. *Circulation.* 1989;80(3 Pt 1):I124-I134.
13. Manolis AS, Rastegar H, Payne D, et al. Surgical therapy for drug-refractory ventricular tachycardia: Results with mapping-guided subendocardial resection. *J Am Coll Cardiol.* 1989;14:199-208.
14. Camm J, Ward DE, Cory-Pearce R, et al. The successful cryosurgical treatment of paroxysmal ventricular tachycardia. *Chest.* 1979;75:621-624.
15. Frapier JM, Hubaut JJ, Pasquié JL, Chaptal PA. Large encircling cryoablation without mapping for ventricular tachycardia after anterior myocardial infarction: Long-term outcome. *J Thorac Cardiovasc Surg.* 1998;116:578-583.
16. Guiraudon GM, Thakur RK, Klein GJ, et al. Encircling endocardial cryoablation for ventricular tachycardia after myocardial infarction: Experience with 33 patients. *Am Heart J.* 1994;128:982-989.
17. Dor V, Montiglio F, Sabatier M, et al. Left ventricular shape changes induced by aneurysmectomy with endoventricular circular patch plasty reconstruction. *Eur Heart J.* 1994;15(8):1063-1069.
18. Josephson ME. Catheter ablation of arrhythmias. *Ann Intern Med.* 1984;101(2):234-237.
19. Fisher JD, Brodman R, Waspe LE, Matos JA, Kim SG. Catheter ablation of tachycardias. *Arch Mal Coeur Vaiss.* 1985;78 Spec No:43-47.
20. Scheinman M. Interventional electrophysiology: catheter ablation for patients with cardiac arrhythmias. *Cardiol Clin.* 1986;4(3):543-550.
21. Josephson ME, Miller JM, Marchlinski FE, Buxton AE. Nonpharmacologic therapy of ventricular tachycardia. *Clin Cardiol.* 1988;11(3 Suppl 2):II17-21.
22. Lim HS, Singleton CB, Alasady M, McGavigan AD. Catheter ablation for ventricular tachycardia. *Intern Med J.* 2010;40(10):673-681.
23. Kessler EJ, Knight BP. Catheter ablation for ventricular tachycardia: indications and techniques. *Expert Rev Cardiovasc Ther.* 2007;5(5):977-988.
24. Sosa E, Scanavacca M, d'Avila A, Pilleggi F. A new technique to perform epicardial mapping in the electrophysiology laboratory. *J Cardiovasc Electrophysiol.* 1996;7(6):531-536.
25. Hsia HH, Callans DJ, Marchlinski FE. Characterization of endocardial electrophysiological substrate in patients with nonischemic cardiomyopathy and monomorphic ventricular tachycardia. *Circulation.* 2003;108(6):704-710.
26. Sacher F, Roberts-Thomson K, Maury P, et al. Epicardial ventricular tachycardia ablation a multicenter safety study. *J Am Coll Cardiol.* 2010;55(21):2366-2372.
27. Michowitz Y, Mathuria N, Tung R, et al. Hybrid procedures for epicardial catheter ablation of ventricular tachycardia: value of surgical access. *Heart Rhythm.* 2010;7(11):1635-1643.
28. Soejima K, Couper G, Cooper JM, Sapp JL, Epstein LM, Stevenson WG. Subxiphoid surgical approach for epicardial catheter-based mapping and ablation in patients with prior cardiac surgery or difficult pericardial access. *Circulation.* 2004;110(10):1197-1201.
29. Watanabe G, Misaki T, Nakajima K, Ueda T, Yamashita A. Thoracoscopic radiofrequency ablation of the myocardium. *Pacing Clin Electrophysiol.* 1998;21(3):553-558.
30. Garratt C, Camm AJ. The role of cryosurgery in the management of cardiac arrhythmias. *Clin Cardiol.* 1991 Feb;14(2):153-159.
31. Budman H, Shitzer A, Del Giudice S. Investigation of temperature fields around embedded cryoprobes. *J Biomech Eng.* 1986 Feb;108(1):42-48.
32. Lustgarten DL, Keane D, Ruskin J. Cryothermal ablation: mechanism of tissue injury and current experience in the treatment of tachyarrhythmias. *Prog Cardiovasc Dis.* 1999;41(6):481-498.
33. Iida S, Misaki T, Iwa T. The histological effects of cryocoagulation on the myocardium and coronary arteries. *Jpn J Surg.* 1989;19:319-325.
34. Klein GJ, Harrison L, Ideker RF, et al. Reaction of the myocardium to cryosurgery: Electrophysiology and arrhythmogenic potential. *Circulation.* 1979;59:364-372.
35. Doll N, Kiaii BB, Fabricius AM, et al. Intraoperative left atrial ablation (for atrial fibrillation) using a new argon cryocatheter: early clinical experience. *Ann Thorac Surg.* 2003;76(5):1711-1715.
36. Doll N, Meyer R, Walther T, Mohr FW. A new cryoprobe for intraoperative ablation of atrial fibrillation. *Ann Thorac Surg.* 2004;77(4):1460-1462.
37. Gallegos RP, Rivard AL, Rajab TK, et al. Transmural atrial fibrosis after epicardial and endocardial argon-powered CryoMaze ablation. *J Card Surg.* 2011;26(2):240-243.
38. Lall SC, Damiano RJ Jr. Surgical ablation devices for atrial fibrillation. *J Interv Card Electrophysiol.* 2007;20(3):73-82.
39. Williams MR, Garrido M, Oz MC, Argenziano M. Alternative energy sources for surgical atrial ablation. *J Card Surg.* 2004;19(3):201-206.
40. Nakagawa H, Yamanashi WS, Pitha JV, et al. Comparison of in vivo tissue temperature profile and lesion geometry for radiofrequency ablation with a saline-irrigated electrode versus temperature control in a canine thigh muscle preparation. *Circulation.* 1995;91(8):2264-2273.
41. Petersen HH, Chen X, Pietersen A, Svendsen JH, Haunsø S. Tissue temperatures and lesion size during irrigated tip catheter radiofrequency ablation: an in vitro comparison of temperature-controlled irrigated tip ablation, power-controlled irrigated tip ablation, and standard temperature-controlled ablation. *Pacing Clin Electrophysiol.* 2000;23(1):8-17.
42. Schuessler RB, Lee AM, Melby SJ, et al. Animal studies of epicardial atrial ablation. *Heart Rhythm.* 2009;6(12 Suppl):S41-45.

43. Dagres N, Kottkamp H, Piorkowski C, et al. Rapid detection and successful treatment of esophageal perforation after radiofrequency ablation of atrial fibrillation: lessons from five cases. *J Cardiovasc Electrophysiol.* 2006;17(11):1213-1215.
44. Kottkamp H, Piorkowski C, Tanner H, et al. Topographic variability of the esophageal left atrial relation influencing ablation lines in patients with atrial fibrillation. *J Cardiovasc Electrophysiol.* 2005;16(2):146-150.
45. Sakamoto S, Voeller RK, Melby SJ, et al. Surgical ablation for atrial fibrillation: the efficacy of a novel bipolar pen device in the cardioplegically arrested and beating heart. *J Thorac Cardiovasc Surg.* 2008;136(5):1295-1301.
46. Ninet J, Roques X, Seitelberger R, et al. Surgical ablation of atrial fibrillation with off-pump, epicardial, high-intensity focused ultrasound: results of a multicenter trial. *J Thorac Cardiovasc Surg.* 2005;130(3):803-809.
47. Villamizar NR, Crow JH, Piacentino V 3rd, et al. Reproducibility of left atrial ablation with high-intensity focused ultrasound energy in a calf model. *J Thorac Cardiovasc Surg.* 2010;140(6):1381-1387.
48. Koruth JS, Dukkipati S, Carrillo RG, et al. Safety and efficacy of high-intensity focused ultrasound atop coronary arteries during epicardial catheter ablation. *J Cardiovasc Electrophysiol.* 2011;22(11):1274-1280.
49. Michowitz Y, Mathuria N, Tung R, et al. Hybrid procedures for epicardial catheter ablation of ventricular tachycardia: value of surgical access. *Heart Rhythm.* 2010;7(11):1635-1643.
50. Anter E, Hutchinson MD, Deo R, et al. Surgical ablation of refractory ventricular tachycardia in patients with nonischemic cardiomyopathy. *Circ Arrhythm Electrophysiol.* 2011;4(4):494-500.
51. Dor V, Sabatier M, Montiglio F, Rossi P, Toso A, Di Donato M. Results of nonguided subtotal endocardiectomy associated with left ventricular reconstruction in patients with ischemic ventricular arrhythmias. *J Thorac Cardiovasc Surg.* 1994;107(5): 1301-1307
52. Baravelli M, Cattaneo P, Rossi A, et al. Low-risk profile for malignant ventricular arrhythmias and sudden cardiac death after surgical ventricular reconstruction. *Pacing Clin Electrophysiol.* 2010;33(9):1054-1062.
53. Saksena S, Hussain SM, Wasty N, Gielchinsky I, Parsonnet V. Long-term efficacy of subendocardial resection in refractory ventricular tachycardia: relationship to site of arrhythmia origin. *Ann Thorac Surg.* 1986;42(6):685-689.

CHAPTER 49A

Surgical Ablation for Atrial Fibrillation: The Cox-Maze IV Procedure

Timo Weimar, MD; Ralph J. Damiano, Jr., MD

Introduction

The significant limitations of pharmacological therapy of atrial fibrillation (AF) have led to the development and proliferation of interventional approaches for the treatment of AF over the last two decades.[1-4] The most promising and successful options have included catheter ablation and surgery.

One of the most effective interventional techniques in the management of symptomatic drug-refractory AF has been the Cox-Maze procedure (CMP), introduced by Dr. James L. Cox in 1987.[4-6] His surgical approach was based on the theoretical and experimental studies of Moe and Allessie, suggesting multiple nonstationary macroreentrant circuits as the cause for sustained AF.[7] The final version of his cut-and-sew technique, termed the CMP-III, intended to block these macroreentrant circuits by creating a biatrial lesion set.[4] This procedure has proved to be highly efficacious with a 97% freedom from symptomatic AF and became the gold standard in the surgical therapy of AF for more than a decade.[8] Moreover, the incidence of stroke, the most feared complication of AF, has been strikingly low following this procedure.[8,9]

Development of the Cox-Maze IV Procedure

The Maze procedure was clinically introduced after extensive animal investigation at Washington University in St. Louis.[4-6] Unlike other historical attempts to address AF, such as the left atrial isolation procedure, His bundle ablation, the corridor procedure, or the atrial transection procedure, the Cox-Maze procedure successfully restored both AV synchrony and sinus rhythm, thus potentially reducing the risk of thromboembolism and stroke.[9-12] The operation consisted of creating surgical incisions in both the right and left atria. These incisions were placed in a pattern that allowed the propagation of the sinoatrial node impulse throughout both atria (Figure 49A.1). This resulted in an electrical activation of most of the atrial myocardium and preservation of atrial transport function in most patients.

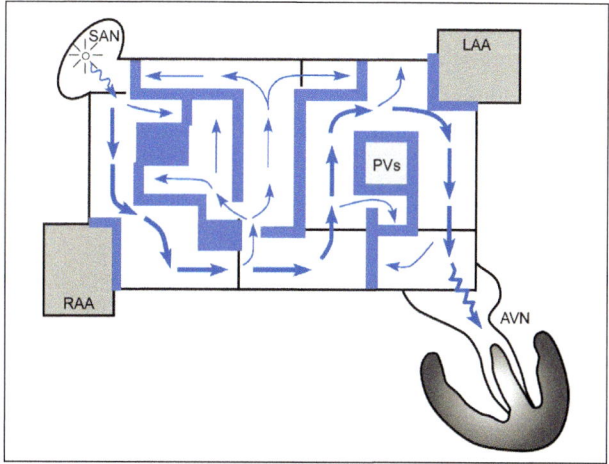

Figure 49A.1 Propagation of the sinus impulse throughout both atria in the original Cox-Maze procedure. *Source:* Cox JL, Schuessler RB, D'Agostino HJ, Jr., et al.[4] Used with permission from Elsevier.

The original version, the Maze I procedure, was modified due to problems with late chronotropic incompetence and a high incidence of pacemaker implantations. The Maze II procedure was technically difficult to perform, and was soon replaced by the final iteration known as the Cox-Maze III procedure (Figure 49A.2).[13]

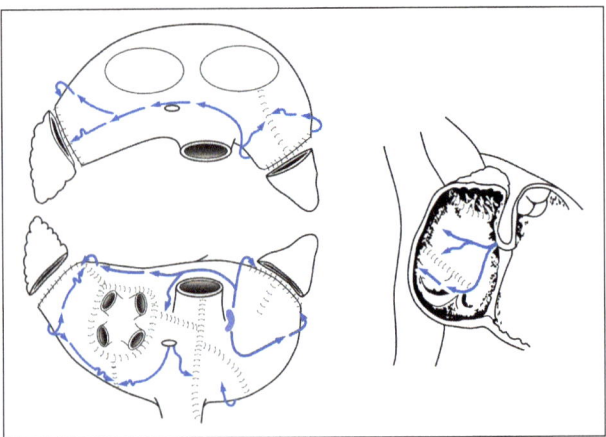

Figure 49A.2 The original cut-and-sew Cox-Maze procedure III. Source: Cox JL, Schuessler RB, D'Agostino HJ, Jr., et al.[4] Used with permission from Elsevier.

The Cox-Maze III procedure, often referred to as the "cut-and-sew Maze," became the gold standard for the surgical treatment of AF with excellent long-term success rates and a low postoperative risk of stroke.[8,14-16] In our series at Washington University, 97% of 198 consecutive patients who underwent the procedure with a mean follow-up of 5.4 years were free from symptomatic AF. There was no difference in the cure rates between patients undergoing a stand-alone Cox-Maze procedure and those undergoing concomitant procedures.[8] There was also no difference in success rates between paroxysmal or persistent AF.[8]

Although the Cox-Maze III procedure was effective in eliminating AF, it was technically difficult and lengthy, and few cardiac surgeons still perform this operation today. At most centers, the surgical incisions have been replaced with linear lines of ablation using a variety of energy sources. These ablation-assisted procedures have greatly expanded the field of AF surgery in the past decade.[17] With present ablation technology, surgery can be performed with low mortality and limited access incisions while preserving the high success rates of the traditional procedure.[18]

In our laboratory, bipolar radiofrequency (RF) energy has been found to be able to create reliable transmural lines of ablation in seconds while minimizing the risk of collateral damage to surrounding tissue.[19-21] Since the energy is applied within the jaws of a clamp, it is inherently safer than unipolar sources.[22] It has been used successfully to replace most of the surgical incisions of the Cox-Maze III procedure. In 2002, our group introduced an ablation-assisted procedure, termed the Cox-Maze IV, which closely resembled the original lesion set of the Cox-Maze III and has now been performed in more than 360 patients.[23] The shortcoming of bipolar RF energy is that it requires clamping of the tissue to perform an effective ablation. This is difficult near the valve annuli; because of this limitation, a unipolar source, usually cryoablation, was used in these areas.

Ablation Technologies

The two preferred alternative energy sources used at our institution to perform the biatrial lesion set of the CMP-IV are bipolar RF and cryoablation. They have both been extensively studied in our laboratory and have been found to effectively and safely create transmural lesions.[19-21]

Bipolar RF Energy

RF energy uses alternating current in the range of 100 to 1,000 kHz. This frequency is high enough to prevent rapid myocardial depolarization and the induction of ventricular fibrillation, yet low enough to prevent tissue vaporization and perforation. Resistive RF energy can be delivered by either unipolar or bipolar electrodes. The lesion size created by thermal injury depends on electrode-tissue contact area, the interface temperature, and the current and voltage (power), as well as the duration of delivery. The depth of the lesion can be limited by char formation, epicardial fat, myocardial and endocavity blood flow, and tissue thickness.

Bipolar clamps, which are used to perform a CMP-IV, have been found to be the most reliable devices for creating transmural lesions in our laboratory. Bipolar ablation has been shown to be capable of creating transmural lesions on the beating heart both in animals and humans with short ablation times between 5 and 20 seconds.[19,20,24] Another advantage of bipolar RF energy is its safety profile. A number of clinical complications of unipolar RF devices have been reported. These include coronary artery injuries, cerebrovascular accidents, and esophageal perforation leading to atrioesophageal fistula.[22,25-28] Bipolar RF technology has eliminated most of this collateral damage, and there have been no injuries described with these devices despite extensive clinical use.

Cryoablation

Cryoablation has been used for ablation of arrhythmias for more than 3 decades and has an excellent safety profile.[29-31] It is unique in that it destroys myocardial tissue by freezing rather than heating. Ice formation is the source of tissue injury and the mode of ablation in modern devices. The onset of ice formation at the cryoprobe provides cryoadhesion to maintain and ensure tissue contact and creates an area at which heat is extracted from the tissue. As heat is removed by various cryogens, such as nitrous oxide, argon, or liquid oxygen, extracellular fluid freezes at −20°C, creating a hyperosmotic environment that causes cell shrinkage and ultimately cell death.[32] Rapid freezing to −40°C induces expansion of intracellular ice formation that disrupts organelles and cell membranes even before osmotic imbalance occurs.[33] A fast rate of cooling will increase cell death, while slowly thawing the tissue is also effective in prolonging the mechanisms of cell destruction.[32]

As opposed to other unipolar energy sources that resulted in severe complications, such as esophageal perforation, when applied endocardially, cryoenergy has an excellent safety profile.[22,29] Moreover, it is the only available energy source that does not disrupt tissue collagen, thus preserving normal tissue architecture and allowing a safe ablation close to valvular tissue or the fibrous skeleton of the heart with a low arrhythmogenic potential.[34-36] Cryoablation has a well-defined efficacy and safety profile and is generally safe except around the coronary arteries.[37,38]

The potential disadvantage of cryoablation, however, is the relatively long time required to create lesions (1 to 3 minutes). There is also difficulty in creating lesions on the beating heart due to the "heat sink" of the circulating blood volume.[39] Furthermore, if blood is frozen during epicardial ablation on the beating heart, it coagulates, creating a potential thromboembolic risk.

Surgical Technique

A variety of surgical procedures are currently performed to ablate AF. They can be grouped into three broad categories: pulmonary vein isolation, left atrial lesion sets, and the Cox-Maze procedure. The following section will summarize the performance of the ablation-assisted CMP-IV.

The CMP-IV can be performed either through a median sternotomy or a less invasive right minithoracotomy.[18,24,40] After initiating normothermic cardiopulmonary bypass, the right and left pulmonary veins (PVs) are bluntly dissected. If the patient is in AF, amiodarone is administered, and the patient is electrically cardioverted after a left atrial thrombus is ruled out by intraoperative transesophageal echocardiography. Pacing thresholds are obtained from each pulmonary vein. Using a bipolar RF ablation device, the PVs are isolated by ablating a cuff of surrounding atrial tissue. Proof of electrical isolation is confirmed by demonstrating exit and/or entrance block from each PV.

The right atrial lesion set is performed on the beating heart (Figure 49A.3). A single incision is usually made in the right atrial free wall, but recently a three purse-string approach has been adopted to eliminate this incision in patients undergoing a minithoracotomy approach. All ablations are performed with the bipolar RF clamp except for two endocardial ablation lines to the tricuspid annulus. These are performed with a linear cryoprobe that is cooled to −60°C for 2 to 3 minutes.

The left-sided lesion set is performed via a standard left atriotomy under cardioplegic arrest (Figure 49A.4). Our group has shown that isolating the entire posterior left atrium with connecting ablation lines between the upper and lower pulmonary veins, termed the box lesion set, which resembles more closely the original CMP-III lesion set, resulted in a significantly higher drug-free freedom from AF at 6 and 12 months.[40] Cryoablation is used to connect the lesion to the mitral annulus and complete the left atrial isthmus line. It is important to remember that the coronary sinus needs to be ablated in line with the endocardial ablation in order to create a complete left atrial isthmus line. This is usually done with either the bipolar RF clamp or a linear cryoprobe placed epicardially over the coronary sinus. The left atrial appendage is amputated, and a final ablation is performed using the bipolar clamp through the amputated left atria appendage into one of the left pulmonary veins.

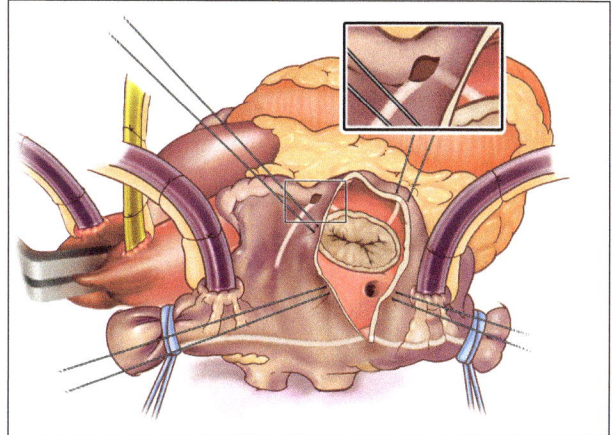

Figure 49A.3 Right atrial lesion set of the Cox-Maze procedure IV. *Source:* Damiano, RJ, Jr., Schwartz FH, Bailey MS, et al.[23] Reprinted with permission from Elsevier.

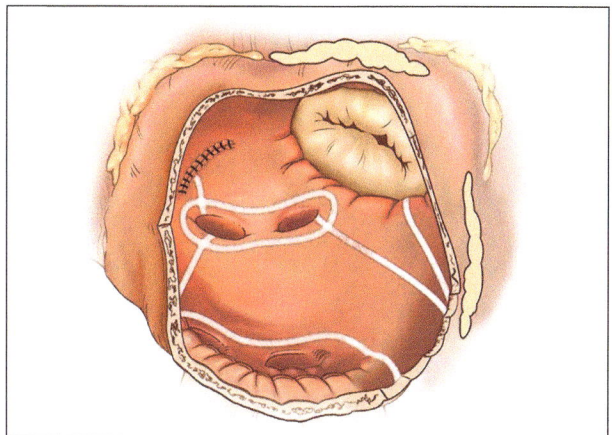

Figure 49A.4 Left atrial lesion set of the Cox-Maze procedure IV. *Source:* Damiano, RJ, Jr., Schwartz FH, Bailey MS, et al.[23] Reprinted with permission from Elsevier.

In patients undergoing a right minithoracotomy, cryoablation is more extensively applied to complete the posterior left atrial isolation, and the left atrial appendage is oversewn from the inside.[18]

Clinical Outcome

A propensity analysis performed by our group has shown that there was no significant difference in the freedom from AF at 3, 6, or 12 months between the Cox-Maze-III and -IV groups.[41] However, the CMP-IV has significantly shortened operative time and lowered complication rates.[17,41] A Kaplan-Meier estimate of freedom from symptomatic AF for our entire CMP series was 85% at 10 years (Figure 49A.5). In 100 patients undergoing a stand-alone CMP-IV for lone AF (31% paroxysmal and 69% persistent or longstanding persistent AF), we reported a freedom from AF of 90% and freedom from AF off antiarrhythmic medication of 84% at 2 years with no intraoperative mortality and no postoperative strokes (Figure 49A.6).[42]

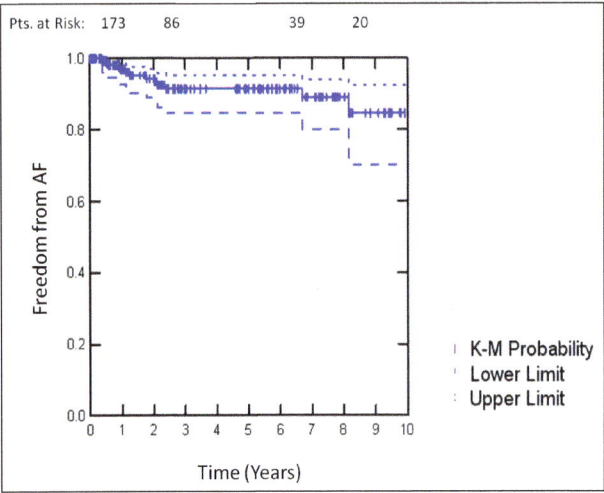

Figure 49A.5 Kaplan-Meier (K-M) Analysis of freedom from atrial fibrillation (AF) for the Cox-Maze procedure (III+IV). Pts = patients.

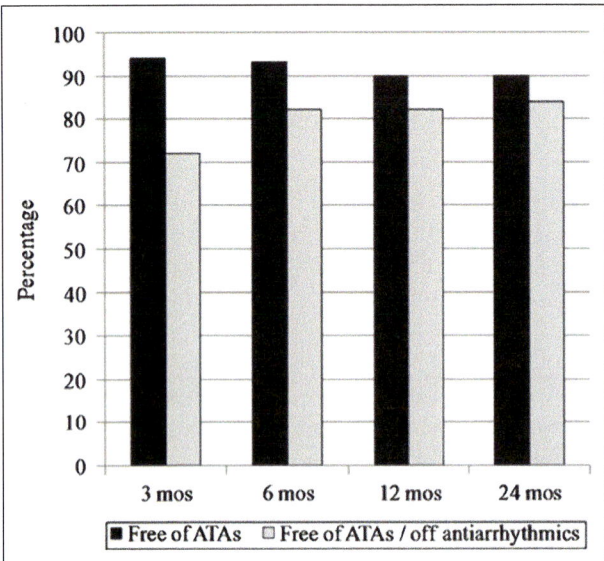

Figure 49A.6 Freedom from atrial tachyarrhythmias (ATAs) and freedom from ATAs off antiarrhythmic drugs following a stand-alone Cox-Maze IV procedure.

Moreover, 84% of patients were free from anticoagulation therapy with warfarin. In this series, we found that isolating the entire posterior left atrium, as has been our practice since 2005, resulted in a 1-year freedom from AF of 96%, with 86% also being off antiarrhythmic drugs. In the entire CMP-IV series including concomitant cardiac procedures, the freedom from AF was 89% and the freedom from AF off antiarrhythmic drugs was 78% at one year.[23] The majority of these patients had prolonged monitoring, and failure was considered any episode of AF, atrial flutter, or atrial tachycardia longer than 30 seconds. There was no difference in success rates for patients with paroxysmal compared to persistent or longstanding, persistent AF.[23,42]

The CMP-IV should be considered for symptomatic patients with AF who either have failed previous interventions or who are poor candidates for catheter ablation. In 40 patients who had failed a mean of 2.6 ± 1.3 (range: 1–6) previous catheter ablations for AF or atrial flutter, freedom from AF was 92% and freedom from AF off antiarrhythmics was 84% at 12 months following a stand-alone CMP-IV, respectively.

Indications for the Cox-Maze IV Procedure

The indications for surgical ablation that have been defined in the recent consensus statement presently include:[43]

1. All symptomatic patients with documented atrial fibrillation undergoing other cardiac surgical procedures.

2. Selected asymptomatic patients with atrial fibrillation undergoing cardiac surgery in which the ablation can be performed with minimal risk in experienced centers.

3. Stand-alone surgery should be considered for symptomatic patients with atrial fibrillation who either prefer a surgical approach, have failed one or more attempts of catheter ablation, or are not candidates for catheter ablation.

There is still controversy regarding the referral of patients for surgery with medically refractory, symptomatic atrial fibrillation in lieu of less invasive catheter ablation. In our opinion, there are relative indications for surgery that were not included in the consensus statement:

1. Patients with AF who develop a contraindication to long-term anticoagulation and have a high risk for stroke (CHADS score ≥ 2) are excellent candidates for surgery. The Cox-Maze procedure is able not only to eliminate AF in most of these patients, but also amputates the left atrial appendage, which is known to be one of the main sources of atrial thrombus formation. The stroke rate following the procedure off anticoagulation has been remarkably low, even in patients with high CHADS scores.

2. Patients with longstanding AF who have suffered a cerebrovascular accident despite adequate

anti-coagulation. These patients are at high risk for repeat neurological events.[44] In our experience with over 200 patients with a stand-alone CMP, there was only 1 late stroke, with more than 80% of patients off anticoagulation at last follow-up. This is remarkable in that almost 20% of patients had experienced a cerebrovascular accident before surgery. Comment: It is not a statement comparing results, rather pointing out that such a low stroke rate (sentence before) is remarkable in a patient group that had already experienced cerebrovascular accidents in the past.

3. Patients with a clot in the left atrial appendage are not candidates for catheter ablation and should be considered for surgical ablation.

Preoperative Management

Besides a documentation of the patient's heart rhythm prior to surgery, a preoperative transthoracic and an intraoperative transesophageal echocardiogram should be performed to determine left atrial diameter and to evaluate for the presence of a left atrial thrombus. Left atrial size is a significant predictor of failure in our series and others and is important to define prior to ablation surgery.[23,45] It is our policy in patients with a left atrial size ≥ 7 cm to perform a left atrial reduction procedure. A cardiac catheterization is performed both to provide information about the presence of coronary artery disease and to define the anatomical location of the circumflex coronary artery. The latter information is critical to safely perform the left atrial isthmus lesion and the ablation of the coronary sinus. In patients who have failed catheter ablation, a chest CT is indicated to assess for pulmonary vein stenosis.

Postoperative Management

Following surgery, patients are started on antiarrhythmic drugs when they resume normal sinus rhythm. Amiodarone is our drug of choice if postoperative atrial tachyarrhythmias (ATAs) occur. In our series, over 40% of patients experience ATAs, including AF, atrial flutter, or atrial tachycardia, during the first month.[46] Antiarrhythmics are discontinued at 2 months if the patient is in normal sinus rhythm as documented by ECG or prolonged monitoring.

Anticoagulation with warfarin should be started postoperatively with a targeted INR of 2.0–2.5. Anticoagulation is discontinued at 3 months if prolonged monitoring shows no ATAs and echocardiography shows no atrial stasis or thrombus.

Postoperative sinus node dysfunction occurs in approximately 5% of patients, many of whom have had a history of sick sinus syndrome. In patients developing postoperative bradycardia or slow junctional rhythms, antiarrhythmic medication should be discontinued and pacemaker implantation should be considered after 5–7 days.

In our institution, patients are followed with prolonged electrocardiographic monitoring at 3, 6, and 12 months and annually thereafter. Success rates should be defined as freedom from ATAs and antiarrhythmic medication documented by prolonged monitoring of at least 24 hours. A recurrence of any ATAs > 30 seconds is considered a failure, according to the recent consensus statement.[43]

Conclusion

The biatrial lesion set of the CMP has been simplified and shortened by alternative energy sources. This procedure provides a benchmark for the excellent long-term success rate of a stand-alone surgical ablation technique and allows for comparison to the variety of new procedures that are presently performed for surgical ablation of AF, including left atrial lesion sets and pulmonary vein isolation.

The CMP-IV has excellent long-term results and a low risk of stroke even with improved follow-up and stricter definitions of failure. With its low operative risk, the CMP-IV should be considered as an option in lone AF patients who fail catheter ablation and remain symptomatic or in patients with medically refractory symptomatic AF who are poor candidates for catheter ablation.

References

1. Marcus GM, Sung RJ. Antiarrhythmic agents in facilitating electrical cardioversion of atrial fibrillation and promoting maintenance of sinus rhythm. *Cardiology*. 2001;95:1-8.
2. Wann LS, Curtis AB, January CT, et al. 2011 ACCF/AHA/HRS focused update on the management of patients with atrial fibrillation (updating the 2006 guideline): A report of the American College of Cardiology Foundation/American Heart Association Task Force on Practice Guidelines. *Circulation*. 2011;123:104-123.
3. Oral H, Knight BP, Tada H, et al. Pulmonary vein isolation for paroxysmal and persistent atrial fibrillation. *Circulation*. 2002;105:1077-1081.
4. Cox JL, Schuessler RB, D'Agostino HJ, Jr., et al. The surgical treatment of atrial fibrillation. III. Development of a definitive surgical procedure. *J Thorac Cardiovasc Surg*. 1991;101:569-583.
5. Cox JL, Schuessler RB, Boineau JP. The surgical treatment of atrial fibrillation. I. Summary of the current concepts of the mechanisms of atrial flutter and atrial fibrillation. *J Thorac Cardiovasc Surg*. 1991;101:402-405.
6. Cox JL, Canavan TE, Schuessler RB, et al. The surgical treatment of atrial fibrillation. II. Intraoperative electrophysiologic mapping and description of the electrophysiologic basis of atrial flutter and atrial fibrillation. *J Thorac Cardiovasc Surg*. 1991;101:406-426.
7. Moe GK, Rheinboldt WC, Abildskov JA. A computer model of atrial fibrillation. *Am Heart J*. 1964;67:200-220.

8. Prasad SM, Maniar HS, Camillo CJ, et al. The Cox Maze III procedure for atrial fibrillation: Long-term efficacy in patients undergoing lone versus concomitant procedures. *J Thorac Cardiovasc Surg.* 2003;126:1822-1828.
9. Cox JL, Ad N, Palazzo T. Impact of the Maze procedure on the stroke rate in patients with atrial fibrillation. *J Thorac Cardiovasc Surg.* 1999;118:833-840.
10. Williams JM, Ungerleider RM, Lofland GK, Cox JL. Left atrial isolation: New technique for the treatment of supraventricular arrhythmias. *J Thorac Cardiovasc Surg.* 1980;80:373-380.
11. Guiraudon GM, Campbell, CS, et al. Combined sinoatrial node atrioventricular node isolation: A surgical alternative to His bundle ablation in patients with atrial fibrillation. *Circulation.* 1985;72:220.
12. Scheinman MM, Morady F, Hess DS, Gonzalez R. Catheter-induced ablation of the atrioventricular junction to control refractory supraventricular arrhythmias. *JAMA.* 1982;248:851-855.
13. Cox JL, Boineau JP, Schuessler RB, et al. Modification of the maze procedure for atrial flutter and atrial fibrillation. I. Rationale and surgical results. *J Thorac Cardiovasc Surg.* 1995;110:473-484.
14. McCarthy PM, Gillinov AM, Castle L, 3rd, et al. The Cox-Maze procedure: The Cleveland Clinic experience. *Semin Thorac Cardiovasc Surg.* 2000;12:25-29.
15. Raanani E, Albage A, David TE, et al. The efficacy of the Cox/Maze procedure combined with mitral valve surgery: A matched control study. *Eur J Cardiothorac Surg.* 2001;19:438-442.
16. Schaff HV, Dearani JA, Daly RC, et al. Cox-Maze procedure for atrial fibrillation: Mayo Clinic experience. *Semin Thorac Cardiovasc Surg.* 2000;12:30-37.
17. Melby SJ, Zierer A, Bailey MS, et al. A new era in the surgical treatment of atrial fibrillation: The impact of ablation technology and lesion set on procedural efficacy. *Ann Surg.* 2006;244:583-592.
18. Lee AM, Clark K, Bailey MS, et al. A minimally invasive Cox-Maze procedure: Operative technique and results. *Innovations (Phila).* 2010;5:281-286.
19. Prasad SM, Maniar HS, Schuessler RB, Damiano RJ, Jr. Chronic transmural atrial ablation by using bipolar radiofrequency energy on the beating heart. *J Thorac Cardiovasc Surg.* 2002;124:708-713.
20. Prasad SM, Maniar HS, Diodato MD, et al. Physiological consequences of bipolar radiofrequency energy on the atria and pulmonary veins: A chronic animal study. *Ann Thorac Surg.* 2003;76:836-841; discussion 841-832.
21. Gaynor SL, Ishii Y, Diodato MD, Prasad SM, et al. Successful performance of Cox-Maze procedure on beating heart using bipolar radiofrequency ablation: A feasibility study in animals. *Ann Thorac Surg.* 2004;78:1671-1677.
22. Doll N, Borger MA, Fabricius A, et al. Esophageal perforation during left atrial radiofrequency ablation: Is the risk too high? *J Thorac Cardiovasc Surg.* 2003;125:836-842.
23. Damiano RJ, Jr., Schwartz FH, Bailey MS, et al. The Cox-Maze IV procedure: Predictors of late recurrence. *J Thorac Cardiovasc Surg.* 2011;141:113-121.
24. Gaynor SL, Diodato MD, Prasad SM, et al. A prospective, single-center clinical trial of a modified Cox Maze procedure with bipolar radiofrequency ablation. *J Thorac Cardiovasc Surg.* 2004;128:535-542.
25. Kottkamp H, Hindricks G, Autschbach R, et al. Specific linear left atrial lesions in atrial fibrillation: Intraoperative radiofrequency ablation using minimally invasive surgical techniques. *J Am Coll Cardiol.* 2002;40:475-480.
26. Gillinov AM, Pettersson G, Rice TW. Esophageal injury during radiofrequency ablation for atrial fibrillation. *J Thorac Cardiovasc Surg.* 2001;122:1239-1240.
27. Laczkovics A, Khargi K, Deneke T. Esophageal perforation during left atrial radiofrequency ablation. *J Thorac Cardiovasc Surg.* 2003;126:2119-2120; author reply 2120.
28. Damiano RG, Pagé P, Leung TK, et al. Surgical radiofrequency ablation induces coronary endothelial dysfunction in porcine coronary arteries. *Eur J Cardiothorac Surg.* 2003;23:277-282.
29. Mack CA, Milla F, Ko W, et al. Surgical treatment of atrial fibrillation using argon-based cryoablation during concomitant cardiac procedures. *Circulation.* 2005;112:I1-6.
30. Holman WL, Ikeshita M, Douglas JM, Jr., et al. Cardiac cryosurgery: Effects of myocardial temperature on cryolesion size. *Surgery.* 1983;93:268-272.
31. Lall SC, Damiano RJ, Jr. Surgical ablation devices for atrial fibrillation. *J Interv Card Electrophysiol.* 2007;20:73-82.
32. Mazur P. Cryobiology: The freezing of biological systems. *Science.* 1970;168:939-949.
33. Gage AA, Baust J. Mechanisms of tissue injury in cryosurgery. *Cryobiology.* 1998;37:171-186.
34. Holman WL, Ikeshita M, Douglas JM, Jr., et al. Ventricular cryosurgery: Short-term effects on intramural electrophysiology. *Ann Thorac Surg.* 1983;35:386-393.
35. Wetstein L, Mark R, Kaplan A, et al. Nonarrhythmogenicity of therapeutic cryothermic lesions of the myocardium. *J Surg Res.* 1985;39:543-554.
36. Lustgarten DL, Keane D, Ruskin J. Cryothermal ablation: Mechanism of tissue injury and current experience in the treatment of tachyarrhythmias. *Prog Cardiovasc Dis.* 1999;41:481-498.
37. Gage AM, Montes M, Gage AA. Freezing the canine thoracic aorta in situ. *J Surg Res.* 1979;27:331-340.
38. Holman WL, Ikeshita M, Ungerleider RM, et al. Cryosurgery for cardiac arrhythmias: Acute and chronic effects on coronary arteries. *Am J Cardiol.* 1983;51:149-155.
39. Aupperle H, Doll N, Walther T, et al. Ablation of atrial fibrillation and esophageal injury: Effects of energy source and ablation technique. *J Thorac Cardiovasc Surg.* 2005;130:1549-1554.
40. Voeller RK, Bailey MS, Zierer A, et al. Isolating the entire posterior left atrium improves surgical outcomes after the Cox Maze procedure. *J Thorac Cardiovasc Surg.* 2008;135:870-877.
41. Lall SC, Melby SJ, Voeller RK, et al. The effect of ablation technology on surgical outcomes after the Cox-Maze procedure: A propensity analysis. *J Thorac Cardiovasc Surg.* 2007;133:389-396.
42. Weimar T, Bailey MS, Watanabe Y, et al. The Cox-Maze IV procedure for lone atrial fibrillation: A single center experience in 100 consecutive patients. *J Interv Card Electrophysiol.* 2011.
43. Calkins H, Brugada J, Packer DL, et al. HRS/EHRA/ECAS Expert Consensus Statement on catheter and surgical ablation of atrial fibrillation: Recommendations for personnel, policy, procedures and follow-up. A report of the Heart Rhythm Society (HRS) task force on catheter and surgical ablation of atrial fibrillation. *Heart Rhythm.* 2007;4:816-861.
44. Hart RG, Halperin JL. Atrial fibrillation and thromboembolism: A decade of progress in stroke prevention. *Ann Intern Med.* 1999;131:688-695.
45. Gillinov AM, Sirak J, Blackstone EH, et al. The Cox Maze procedure in mitral valve disease: Predictors of recurrent atrial fibrillation. *J Thorac Cardiovasc Surg.* 2005;130:1653-1660.
46. Ishii Y, Gleva MJ, Gamache MC, et al. Atrial tachyarrhythmias after the maze procedure: Incidence and prognosis. *Circulation.* 2004;110:II164-168.

CHAPTER 49B

Surgical Ablation for Atrial Fibrillation: The Cryosurgical Cox-Maze Procedure Using Argon-based Cryoprobes

Niv Ad, MD

Introduction

The Cox-Maze procedure remains the gold standard for the nonmedical treatment of atrial fibrillation.[1] Its perceived complexity led to a major shift of the surgical approach, in which all surgical incisions were replaced with ablation lines applied to the atrial tissue using different energy sources.[2,3] As a result, we are witnessing a significant increase in the number of surgical ablation procedures performed and multiple modifications to the original procedure using different surgical ablation techniques.

A little over 10 years ago, James L. Cox, MD, was the first to perform a full Cox-Maze III using cryoblation techniques by utilizing the older generation nitrous oxide-based platform.[4] A newer generation argon-based system was introduced since and is now being widely used. The argon-based cryoprobe is a device built on the principle of the Joule-Thomson effect and is capable of producing significantly colder probe temperatures compared to the nitrous oxide-based systems.

Cryosurgical ablation is defined as the use of freezing temperature to obtain a specific response in tissue. The severity of the tissue response and destruction is directly related to the intensity of the freezing energy.[5] While minor freezing injury causes inflammation, the tissues have the potential to recover, whereas severe freezing kill cells and results in significant destruction of tissue. Studies have shown that cell death following cryoablation is induced by direct cell necrosis and vascular stasis that develops only during the thawing period.

Many types of cryogenic agents, devices, and freezing techniques have been used to treat a variety of pathologies.

The understanding of the mechanism of the injury helped to develop the devices. In 1961, Cooper and Lee developed a device that was capable of cooling liquid nitrogen that could be applied on tissue.[6] In recent years, a number of devices using the Joule-Thomson (J-L) effect were developed utilizing argon (–186°C) and nitrous oxide (–89.5°C). These new devices facilitated soft tissue ablation and, more recently, the treatment of atrial fibrillation.[7,8]

In the past 5 years, we have established a very active surgical ablation program utilizing different energy sources. During this time frame, 600 surgical ablation procedures were performed as stand-alone procedures or concomitantly with other surgical procedures. In our most recent experience (18 months), we have performed almost all our surgical ablations using argon-based cryoprobes.

In this chapter, our surgical approach and results will be discussed, focusing on first-time cryosurgical Cox-Maze III procedure in patients having surgery for stand alone atrial fibrillation or concomitant with another procedure.

The CryoCox-Maze III Lesion Set

In all cases the Cox-Maze III lesion set was applied.[15–17]

Right Atrial Lesions

Lesions are applied to the right atrium following the initiation of cardiopulmonary bypass, but on a beating heart (Figure 49B.1). If the concomitant procedure requires right atriotomy (tricuspid valve surgery or closure of an atrial septal defect), then an incision along the lateral aspect of the right atrial free wall would be applied. Following the atriotomy, lesions across the right-sided AV groove will be applied to incorporate the tricuspid annular commissural areas between the septal and the anterior leaflets and between the anterior and the posterior leaflets (lesions 1 and 2).

To complete the right-sided lesions, cryoablations are applied cephalad into the superior vena cava (lesion 3) and caudally into the inferior vena cava (lesion 4) and across the crista terminalis and the interatrial septum (lesion 5). If a right atrial incision is not required, the right-sided lesions are applied as described in a prior publication, utilizing multiple purse strings.[18]

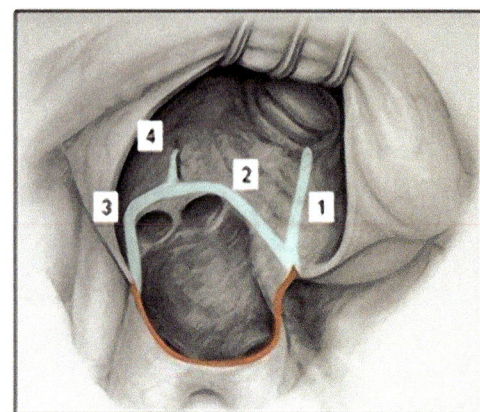

A

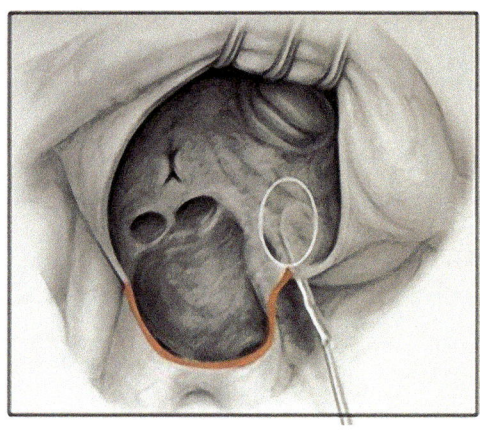

B

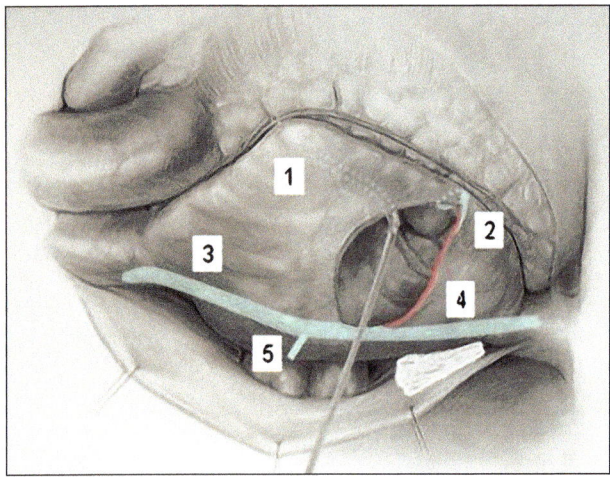

Figure 49B.1   CryoCox-Maze III: right atrial cryolesions.

Figure 49B.2   CryoCox-Maze III: left atrial cryolesions. All cryolesions are applied for 120 seconds on both the left and the right atria. The left atrial appendage was managed in all cases.

Left Atrial Lesions

The left atrial lesions (Figure 49B.2) are applied following the application of a cross clamp and myocardial arrest, or when a minimally invasive approach is used with fibrillatory arrest and systemic cooling to 32°C. A vertical left atriotomy is then applied over the right pulmonary veins. A lesion across the left atrial isthmus toward the mitral valve annulus at the P2 area across the mitral valve isthmus (lesion 1). A box lesion is then completed by encircling all 4 pulmonary veins using multiple cryoenergy applications (lesions 2 and 3). The left-sided lesions are then completed by connecting the box to the base of the left atrial appendage (lesion 4). An epicardial lesion over the coronary sinus to overlap the endocardial mitral isthmus is performed last (Figure 49B.2B).

Management of the Left Atrial Appendage

The left atrial appendage is managed either by amputation or exclusion using either an epicardial or endocardial approach. Transesophageal echocardiography is used in all cases to confirm the adequacy of left atrial appendage control in the operating room.

Patients

All our surgical ablation patients are followed prospectively using a unique data platform. This chapter presents data related specifically to first-time surgery in patients having the CryoCox-Maze III procedure performed using an argon-based cryosystem.[9,10]

At follow-up, rhythm was verified using ECGs and 24-hour Holter monitor for all patients. Health-related quality of life (HRQL) (SF-12)[11] and symptom and severity (AF Symptom Frequency and Severity Checklist)[12] was collected prior to surgery and then at 6 months. In addition, HRQL was collected at 12 and 24 months postoperatively.

The prospective follow-up was done in conjunction with patients' respective cardiologists in an effort to have patients followed by the same protocol. Our protocol recommends that patients stop their respective class I/III antiarrhythmics at 3 months post surgery when noted to be in sinus rhythm. Long-term monitoring is then recommended at 6 months post surgery, or sooner if symptomatic. At the completion of the long-term monitoring, if the patient is noted to be in sinus rhythm without other indications for warfarin, we recommend the discontinuation of warfarin and initiation of daily aspirin.[10]

Health-related quality of life was evaluated at baseline and follow-up using the Short-Form 12, which has long been considered a reliable and validated instrument for use across many disease populations and is easy to administer, being particularly adept for use in self-report situations.[11] The family of Short Form instruments has been used and validated in the cardiac surgery population. The instrument measures eight concepts and two summary measures: physical component summary (PCS) and mental component summary (MCS). Scores range from 0 to 100 and the summary scores are standardized to a mean of 50 and a standard deviation of 10.[11] A higher score means better HRQL and can be compared against age group norms. Our program is currently structured so that all patients who undergo the surgical ablation procedures are asked to participate in our HRQL program where they complete a survey preoperatively and then at 3, 6, and 12 months postoperatively, and yearly thereafter.

In addition, to capture patients' perceptions of their atrial fibrillation symptoms and the corresponding severity of these symptoms, we administer the Atrial Fibrillation Symptom Checklist: Frequency and Severity (V.3). This survey consists of 16 symptom items. The maximum frequency score is 64 and the maximum severity score is 48. Higher scores indicate more symptoms and a higher degree of severity when experiencing the symptom.[12]

The STS definitions were used for the major adverse cardiac events (MACE), which included in-hospital mortality, stroke, reoperation for bleeding, prolonged ventilation, renal failure with and without dialysis, and readmission within 30 days.[13] Rhythm status for patients who underwent the Cox-Maze III/IV procedure was verified by ECG and 24-hour Holter monitor. The Heart Rhythm Society defines failure as documented atrial arrhythmias >30 seconds, and this definition was used to determine the return to sinus rhythm rate at 6 and 12 months.[14] The Social Security Death Index was searched for any follow-up deaths.

Data Analysis

Chi square and paired *t*-tests were used to determine differences between HRQL scores at baseline, 6 months, and 12 months as well as to determine any differences between baseline and 6-month symptom and severity scores. Kaplan-Meier survival analysis was conducted to determine survival over time. All statistical analysis and data management was completed in SAS/STAT® software, version 9.1.3 of the SAS System for Windows (Cary, NC).

Results

Concomitant CryoCox-Maze III procedure in a first-time surgical intervention was performed for 149 patients by multiple surgeons (Figure 49B.3, Table 49B.1). In 25 patients (17%) the procedure performed through a right mini-thoracotomy (6-cm incision). Different types of concomitant procedures were performed as described in Table 49B.2. There were 3 operative deaths (within 30 days), both unrelated to the cryosurgical procedure. There were 2 permanent strokes, of which one was completely resolved and one TIA, documented within 30 days. Table 49B.3 includes details regarding other morbidities and outcome that were captured perioperatively.

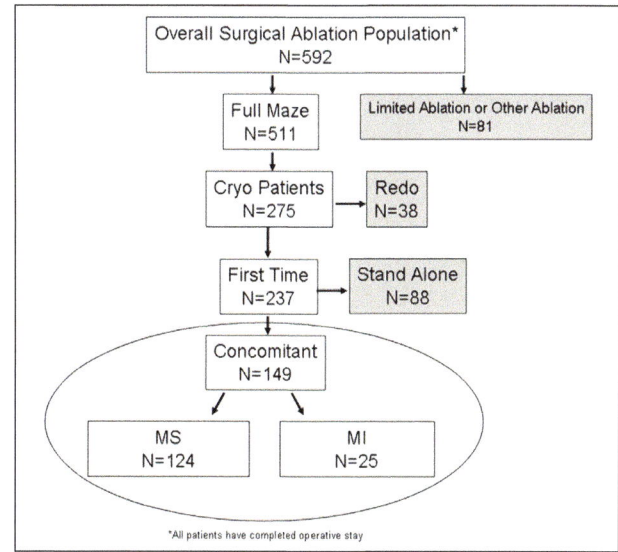

Figure 49B.3 Study population slide.

Table 49B.1 Patient characteristics (*N* = 149)

	No Redo N (%) Mean (SD) *N* = 149
Age >75 years	26 (17%)
Long-standing Persistent/Permanent Afib	64 (43%)
Months Duration	69.9 (79.3)
Persistent Afib	70 (47%)
Months Duration	6.4 (12.1)
Paroxysmal	12 (8.1%)
Months Duration	23.5 (38.9)
History of Other Atrial Arrhythmia	3 (3%)
Thromboembolic Event	22 (15%)
Pacemaker Preop	14 (9%)
LA Size > 5.5 cm²	28 (19%)
EF < 35%	13 (9%)
Euro Score (Additive)	5.7 (2.6)
CHADS Score	1.7 (1.2)
Hemorrhagic Score*	1.9 (1.3)

*Hemorrhagic Score Calculation= [1.6*age > 60 (0,1)] + [1.3* female (0,1)] + [2.2* history of malignancy (0,1)] (Higher score indicates an increased risk for bleeding/maximum score would be 5.1)

Table 49B.2 Concomitant procedures with the Cryothermia Cox-Maze procedure

Concomitant Procedure	N (%)
CABG only	17 (11%)
Valve only	88 (59%)
Valve + CABG	32 (21%)
Other*	12 (9%)
Total	149

CABG = coronary bypass grafting surgery; *ASD (atrial septal defect) repair = percardiectomy, ascending aorta aneurysm repair.

Table 49B.3 Selected perioperative morbidities

Selected Perioperative Morbidities	N = 149
Days of Hospital Stay (op to DC)	9.0 (7.5)
Length of Stay > 10 days	35 (23%)
Infection-Sternum Deep	0
Infection-Sternum Superficial	0
Permanent Stroke	2 (1.5%)
Transient Stroke	1 (<1%)
Operative Death*	3 (2%)
Prolonged Ventilator	17 (11%)
Readmit to ICU	6 (4%)
Readmit to Hosp < 30 days	21 (14%)
Renal Failure	8 (5%)
Reoperation for Bleeding	4 (3%)
Reoperation for Valve Dysfunction	1 (<1%)
Rewire Sternum	2 (1%)

During follow-up, the return to sinus rhythm was found to be acceptable and comparable to previous reports. The return to sinus rhythm at 12 months post withdrawal of class I or class III antiarrhythmic drugs was found to be 83%. As described in Figure 49B.4, the success rate is being maintained through 24 months following the procedure, although the number of patients at follow-up is somewhat small. At one year, we have data regarding 57 patients, with 53 patients not due.

During follow-up of 12 months, 6 patients died, none of which had a documented cause of death related to the Cox-Maze procedure. There were 7 major bleeding events related to anticoagulation, which required blood transfusions. No embolic strokes were documented; however, one bleeding stroke secondary to head trauma was documented. At 24 months, none of the patients in stable sinus rhythm were on warfarin.

Of interest, we noticed significant differences in periprocedural outcomes and the long-term success rate among the different surgeons. The findings suggest that the results may be directly related to the experience of the surgeon in applying the Cox-Maze lesion set. Six different surgeons performed the procedures; 5 surgeons each performed fewer than 20 concomitant CryoCox-Maze III procedures, and the success rate captured at 12 months is below 70%. One surgeon performed over 90 first-time CryoCox-Maze III procedures with a success rate approaching 95% at 12 months off antiarrhythmic medications.

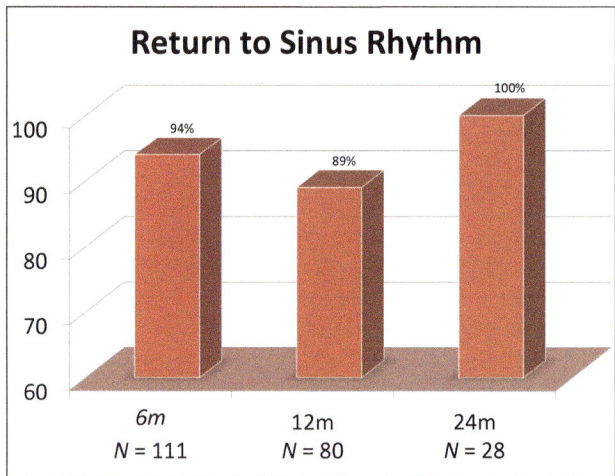

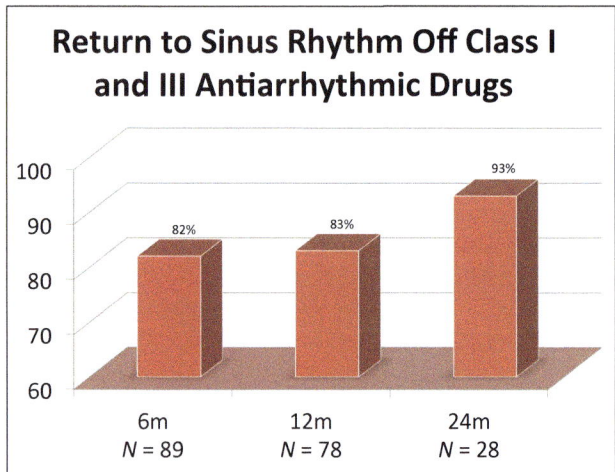

Figure 49B.4 Return to sinus rhythm on and off antiarrhythmic medications at 6, 12, and 24 months.

Health-related Quality of Life

All domains (physical functioning, mental, and general health) of health-related quality of life had improved by 12 months; however, only the improvement in the physical functioning domain was significant ($P \leq 0.001$). The physical functioning component improved by 16% at 12 months, surpassing their age-group norms (47.24 vs 44.66).

Patients' perceptions of the frequency and severity of their symptoms had also significantly improved by 6

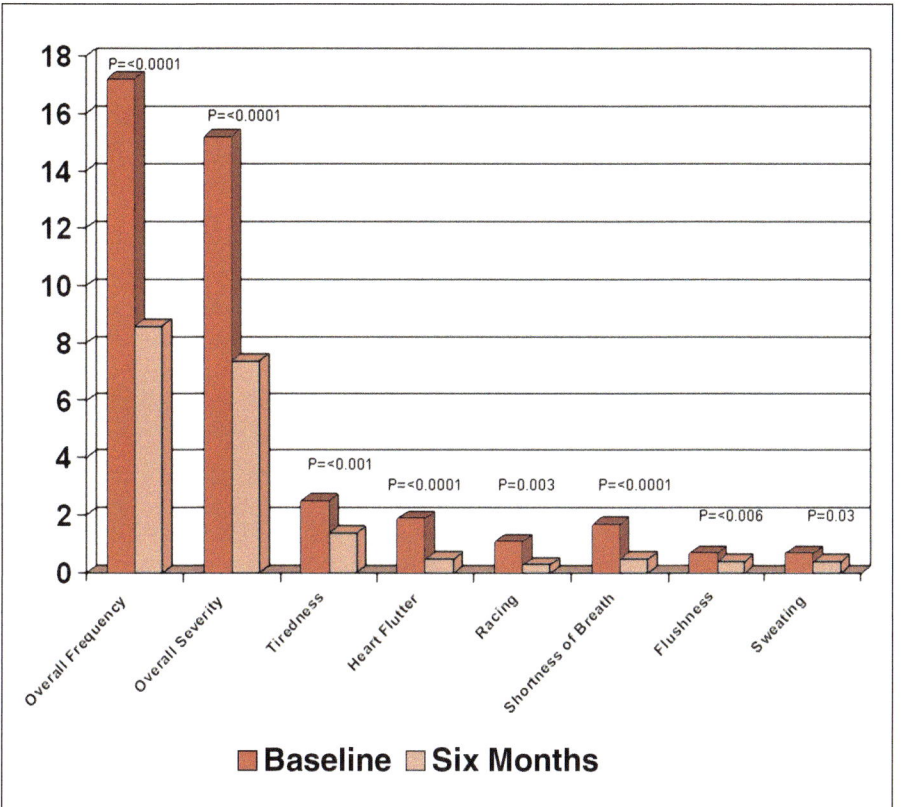

Figure 49B.5 Atrial fibrillation symptom frequency and severity checklist from baseline to 6 months.

months ($P \leq 0.0001$). Their perceptions of the frequency and severity of their symptoms had decreased by 51%. The symptoms that were noted to show the most improvement were as follows: feelings of tiredness, heart fluttering, heart racing, and having trouble catching their breath ($P \leq 0.0001$; $P \leq 0.0001$; $P = 0.0003$; $P \leq 0.0001$; Figure 49B.5).

Discussion

This chapter is focused on the cryosurgical Maze III procedure (CryoCox-Maze III) in a concomitant set up. As mentioned, the semiflexible argon-based cryoprobes allow the application of all Maze III lesion set using a median sternotomy or a right mini-thoracotomy approach. The results of the CryoCox-Maze III procedure are essentially the same as the cut-and-sew Maze procedure, especially when the procedure is being performed by an experienced operator. The 12-month results following a first-time CryoCox-Maze III procedure when performed concomitantly with other cardiac surgical procedure (valve, coronary bypass surgery, repair of a congenital anomaly, or a combination) suggest that the procedure is safe and effective.

When the original cut-and-sew Maze procedure was modified, different energy sources were introduced, with the most common one being radiofrequency. The use of cryothermal energy to treat cardiac arrhythmias surgically was very common early on, with reports dating back to the 1970s.[19] The appropriate use of the current generation of cryothermia requires the heart-lung machine and myocardial arrest in most cases. Interestingly, despite the fact that unipolar or unidirectional energy sources, such as cryothermal or radiofrequency, share the same limitation of the inability to create a reliable transmural lesion when applied epicardially on a full beating heart, this method of utilizing radiofrequency is very popular among surgeons.[20] Recent reports do raise some concerns related to the reliability of bipolar radiofrequency energy, especially in patients with a thick left atrial wall and in those in whom conduction block was not assessed during the procedure.[21] Recent publications related to limited left atrial ablation suggest that the limited lesion set to the left atrium is very ineffective in patients with a larger atrial size and nonparoxysmal atrial fibrillation. Thus, surgeons should be very hesitant in using the current available devices on a beating heart and should wait for the next generation of devices that would be more efficient and effectively applied on a full beating heart.

Cryoablation was found very safe and as effective as the cut-and-sew techniques, especially when performed with cardiopulmonary bypass support and on an arrested heart.[22] In this series, we performed all cases while the patients were supported by cardiopulmonary bypass and all left-sided lesions following myocardial arrest were achieved. The perioperative outcome suggest that the addition of the CryoCox-Maze III procedure did not result in increased periprocedural complications and were consistent with our previous reports.

The cryoablation process is the easiest to understand of all the ablation technologies that exist today. Cryoablation is based on the concept of heat being transferred from the tissue by thermal conduction only. Current devices use the rapid expansion of either nitrous oxide gas (N_2O) or argon gas (ie, the Joule-Thomson effect) to achieve probe temperatures of about −75°C for N_2O and about −186°C for argon, which are at or near the boiling points of these gases. Heat is being transferred from the tissue into the contacting probe to form an ice ball that expands with time. Myocytes within the frozen tissue that reach temperatures below about −20°C are lethally damaged. In the absence of a heat sink, such as with an endocardial lesion applied during mitral valve surgery, it requires about 2 minutes to achieve lethal temperatures through the full thickness of the atrial wall.[5-8] Neither cryoablation system appears capable of achieving lethal endocardial temperatures when the ablation probes are applied to the epicardium of a beating heart, because the blood pool within the atrium provides a heat source that maintains endocardial tissues above freezing.[23]

In our institute, we have developed a unique registry (the implementation paper) to capture important data related to surgical ablation and patient care. In the current report, we have shown that when the full Cox-Maze lesion set is applied with cryoablation, the success rate resembles the original reports with a follow-up that is totally in line with the Heart Rhythm Society guidelines.[14]

Follow-up and accurate reporting of data using, at minimum, ECG and Holter monitoring is challenging; in this series, data could not be retrieved for 8% of our patients at 12 months despite repeated efforts. The issue of longer monitoring is also challenging due to combined factors of patients' compliance and insurance coverage (in the United States). We offer 1 week of monitoring to all our patients, but not all of them enroll for a variety of reasons. The primary reason is that patients do not wish to wear a monitor at the requested time. We have reported our results using this methodology in the past, and currently, we have about 189 patients who were monitored at 6 months with a success rate around 91% while off antiarrhythmic medications.[24]

Our reports of success resemble the results from the cut-and-sew Cox-Maze procedure, which reports success rates of over 90%; however, these reports do not take into account the use of antiarrhythmic drugs, despite the fact that the HRS guidelines are very specific and current reports should describe the results on and off antiarrhythmic drugs. In this series, the 12-month results show that 83% of the patients maintained sinus rhythm off antiarrhythmic drugs. Interestingly, if we review the results by the level of experience of the surgeons, the results appear to improve as the experience level increases. This fact is important and brings into discussion an important variable such as surgeon training and knowledge.

All patients, as well as the subgroup of patients presented here, are evaluated for quality of life together using the Short Form 12 (SF-12) as well as a specifically designed tool to assess the frequency and severity of atrial fibrillation-related symptoms. Based on the SF-12 surveys, we found that in general quality of life is improved; however, only the physical scores increased by a statistically significant amount. When using the more specific atrial fibrillation assessment tool to measure the frequency and the severity of the symptoms, a significant improvement was captured when compared to baseline scores. This highlights the somewhat limited capacity of a generic quality of life tool such as the SF-12 or -36 when applied to atrial fibrillation. Cardiac surgeons and electrophysiologists should consider using more specific assessment tools when measuring quality of life post surgery or catheter ablation for atrial fibrillation. It is also important to note that all patients in this group have had a concomitant procedure and some improvement in the quality of life and their symptoms may be unrelated only to the ablation of their atrial fibrillation.

References

1. Prasad SM, Maniar HS, Camillo CJ, et al. The Cox Maze III procedure for atrial fibrillation: long-term efficacy in patients undergoing lone versus concomitant procedures. *J Thorac Cardiovasc Surg.* 2003;126(6):1822-1828.
2. Viola N, Williams MR, Oz MC, Ad N. The technology in use for the surgical ablation of atrial fibrillation. *Semin Thorac Cardiovasc Surg.* 2002;14(3):198-205.
3. Aupperle H, Doll N, Walther T, et al. Histological findings induced by different energy sources in experimental atrial ablation in sheep. *Interact Cardiovasc Thorac Surg.* 2005;4(5):450-455.
4. Cox JL, Ad N. New surgical and catheter-based modifications of the Maze procedure. *Semin Thorac Cardiovasc Surg.* 2000;12(1):68-73.
5. Gage AA, Baust JM, Baust JG. Experimental cryosurgery investigations in vivo. *Cryobiology.* 2009;59:229-243.
6. Cooper IS, Lee AS. Cryostatic coagulation: A system for producing a limited controlled region of cooling or freezing of biological tissue. *J Nerv Ment Dis.* 1961;133:259-263.
7. Cox JL, Ad N. The importance of cryoablation of the coronary sinus during the maze procedure. *Semin in Thorac and Cardiovasc Surg.* 2000;12:20-24.
8. Doll N, Fabricius AM, Meyer R, et al. Surgical treatment of atrial fibrillation with argon-based cryotechnology. *Future Cardiol.* 2005;1(3):381-391.
9. Hunt S, Henry L, Ad N. Using multiple databases to produce comprehensive follow-up in an effort to enhance evaluation of outcome measurements: Cox-Maze III/IV procedure (Maze) exemplar. *J Healthc Qual.* 2011;33(3):50-63.
10. Ad N, Henry L, Hunt S. The implementation of a comprehensive clinical protocol improves long-term success after surgical treatment of atrial fibrillation. *J Thorac Cardiovasc Surg.* 2010;139(5):1146-1152.
11. Ware J, Kosinski M, Turner-Bowker D, Gandek B. *How to Score Version 2 of the SF-12 Health Survey.* Lincoln, RI: Quality Metric Inc., 2002.

12. Jenkins LS. *Test-Specifications for the Bubien and Kay (Revised Jenkins) Symptom Checklist: Frequency and Severity.* Baltimore: University of Maryland Press, 1993.
13. Society of Thoracic Surgeons National Adult Cardiac Surgery Database. 2007. Further information may be obtained at http://www.sts.org/doc/8242.
14. A report of the Heart Rhythm Society (HRS) Task Force on Catheter Ablation of Atrial Fibrillation developed in partnership with European Heart Rhythm Association (EHRA) and the European Cardiac Arrhythmia (ECAS); in collaboration with the American College of Cardiology (ACC), American Heart Association (AHA), and the Society of Thoracic Surgeons (STS). HRS/EHRA/ECAS Expert consensus statement on catheter and Cox-Maze III/IV procedure of atrial fibrillation: Recommendations for personnel, policy, procedures and follow-up. *Europace.* 2007;9(6):330-379.
15. Cox JL, Scussler RB, D'Agostino HJ Jr, et al. The surgical treatment of atrial fibrillation: III Development of a definite surgical procedure. *J Thorac Cardiovasc Surg.* 1991;101:569-583.
16. Cox JL. The surgical treatment of atrial fibrillation: IV. Surgical technique. *J Thorac Cardiovasc Surg.* 1991;101:584-592.
17. Cox JL, Boineau JP, Schuessler RB, et al. Modifications of the Maze procedure for atrial flutter and atrial fibrillation. I. Rationale and surgical results. *J Thorac Cardiovasc Surg.* 1995;110:473-483.
18. Ad N. The multi-purse string Maze procedure: a new surgical technique to perform the full Maze procedure without atriotomies. *J Thorac Cardiovasc Surg.* 2007;134(3):717-722.
19. Gallagher JJ, Sealy WC, Anderson RW, et al. Cryosurgical ablation of accessory atrioventricular connections: a method for correction of the pre-excitation syndrome. *Circulation.* 1977;55(3):471-479.
20. Miyagi Y, Ishii Y, Nitta T, et al. Electrophysiological and histological assessment of transmurality after epicardial ablation using unipolar radiofrequency energy. *J Card Surg.* 2009;24(1):34-40.
21. Benussi S, Galanti A, Zerbi V, et al. Electrophysiologic efficacy or irrigated bipolar radiofrequency in the clinical setting. *J Thorac Cardiovasc Surg.* 2010;139:1131-1136.
22. Moten SC, Rodriguez E, Cook RC, et al. New ablation techniques for atrial fibrillation and the minimally invasive cryo-Maze procedure in patients with lone atrial fibrillation. *Heart Lung Circ.* 2007;16 Suppl 3:S88-S93.
23. Aupperle H, Doll N, Walther T, et al. Histological findings induced by different energy sources in experimental atrial ablation in sheep. *Interact Cardiovasc Surg.* 2005;4:450-455.
24. Ad N, Henry L, Hunt S, et al. The Cox Maze III procedure success rate: Comparison by electrocardiogram, 24-hour Holter monitoring and long-term monitoring. *Ann Thorac Surg.* 2009;88(1):101-105.

CHAPTER 49C

Surgical Ablation for Atrial Fibrillation: Left Antral Pulmonary Vein Isolation, Ganglionic Plexi Ablation, and Excision of the Left Atrial Appendage

Randall K. Wolf, MD; Sandra Burgess, BS, BA

Introduction

Approximately 14 years ago, the treatment strategies for atrial fibrillation (AF) began to change. Some electrophysiologists initiated catheter ablation for lone (structurally normal heart) AF.[1] Reported success with the Haïssaguerre technique led some cardiac surgeons to begin concomitant surgical left atrial isolation for treatment of AF as an adjunct to open heart surgery for valve or coronary artery bypass graft procedures.

More recently, a divergence of recommended treatments has evolved for patients with lone AF. For patients who tolerate the symptoms or have few symptoms, rate and/or rhythm control is widely prescribed. For patients with symptomatic lone AF, catheter-based ablation has been recommended.

Since 1999, my colleagues and I have diligently pursued a minimally invasive surgical, beating-heart, left atrial isolation technique that is offered to patients with lone AF. We began clinical cases in 2003. In 2005, we reported our initial experience with video-assisted bilateral pulmonary vein isolation and left atrial appendage exclusion for the minimally invasive treatment of AF (Wolf technique).[2] Pulmonary vein (PV) isolation was achieved bilaterally using a dry radiofrequency device (AtriCure Inc., West Chester, OH). The left atrial appendage was removed with a surgical stapler (Ethicon Endo-Surgery, Blue Ash, OH).

At average 3-month follow-up in 23 patients, 21 were free of AF by objective endpoints (ECG and 7-day continuous Holter monitoring). The short-term cure rate was 91%.

In 2004, we then began two projects simultaneously: First, we undertook to demonstrate this minimally invasive surgical technique to other thoracic surgeons, and second, we investigated options for new instruments that could improve the technique.

Over the last eight years, we have added pacing for block, testing entrance and exit block, ganglionic plexi testing and isolation,[3] and use of a bipolar pen for isolation.

After demonstrating the technique to surgeons in the United States, Europe, South America, and Asia, more single-center reports were published using the Wolf technique, with similar encouraging short-term results.[4-6] With over 12,000 minimally invasive left antral pulmonary vein isolation procedures performed to date, the Wolf technique to treat AF has become more widely practiced.

Recently, the Atrial Fibrillation Catheter Ablation Versus Surgical Ablation Treatment (FAST) Trial—the first randomized, controlled study comparing surgical ablation with the Wolf technique (minimally invasive surgical bilateral left atrial antral isolation and excision of the left atrial appendage) to catheter ablation—was reported with 1-year follow-up.[7] Even though 67% of patients had a previous catheter ablation, the surgical results were far superior to catheter ablation with respect to absence of AF at one year (65.6% for surgery vs 36.5%

for catheter ablation). In addition, all surgical patients had removal of the left atrial appendage (LAA), which obviates the need for continued anticoagulation.[8]

At present, patients with lone AF can initially choose between a catheter-based or a minimally invasive surgical approach. Minimally invasive surgery to treat lone AF also can benefit patients who have a contraindication to warfarin, heparin, or antiarrhythmic medications or a history of cerebral events. There are several energy sources that have been used in open-type MAZE procedures that are now being used as energy sources for minimally invasive approaches. These include dry bipolar radiofrequency (RF), wet bipolar RF, monopolar RF, cryotherapy, and high-intensity focused ultrasound (HIFU). It should be clearly understood that energy sources that seem to perform adequately during on-pump procedures with the heart empty may not provide transmural lesions in the beating heart. However, dry bipolar RF results in complete transmural lesions and no histological damage to surrounding tissues on the beating heart.[9] (Figure 49C.1). These findings are explained by the fact that circulating blood in the beating heart acts as an infinite heat sink, making transmural lesions problematic. Using a bipolar clamp and dry RF, there is no heat sink as the blood is excluded from the treated area. In addition, using a dry bipolar clamp there is minimal lateral thermal spread, so the energy application is limited to the treated area.

Each surgeon should ponder the following questions in choosing a minimally invasive surgical AF procedure:

- What energy source is utilized?
- What surgical technique is employed?
- Is the left atrial appendage addressed?
- Is intraoperative EP testing performed?

Energy Source Considerations

A key question for surgeons regarding energy sources is: Does the energy source reliably create transmural lesions without skip lesions on the beating heart? This is important as we compare results: If some procedures do not create transmural lesions, results will be difficult to interpret. This is particularly true with all types of pens. In the FAST trial, additional lines, which were created with a bipolar pen, actually decreased the efficacy of the surgical procedure. As predicted, epicardial pen use does not provide a reliable transmural lesion that a bipolar clamp provides. A pen provides energy to only the epicardial surface without isolating the heat sink of circulating blood on the endocardial surface, while the bipolar clamp provides circumferential transmural lesions, both epicardial and endocardial, without a blood interface.[10]

Considerations About Surgical Technique

The definition of minimally invasive AF surgery varies widely. Examples include:

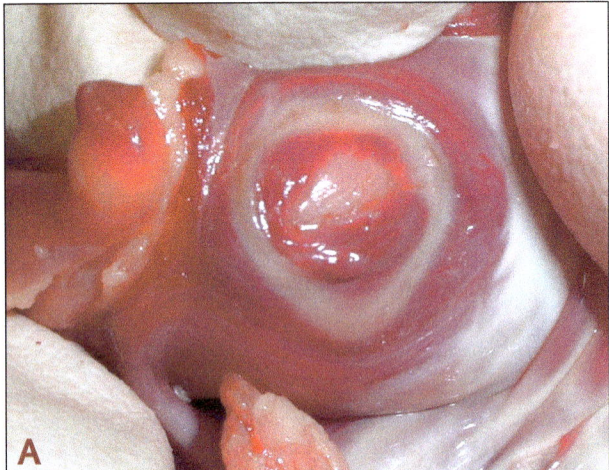

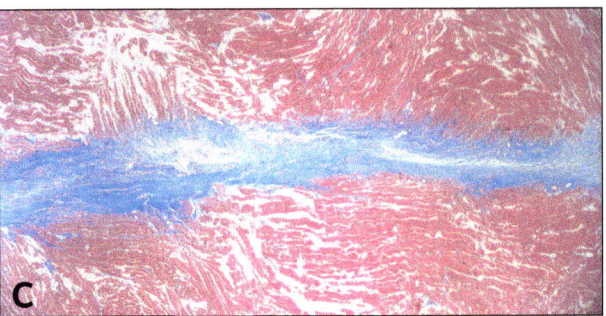

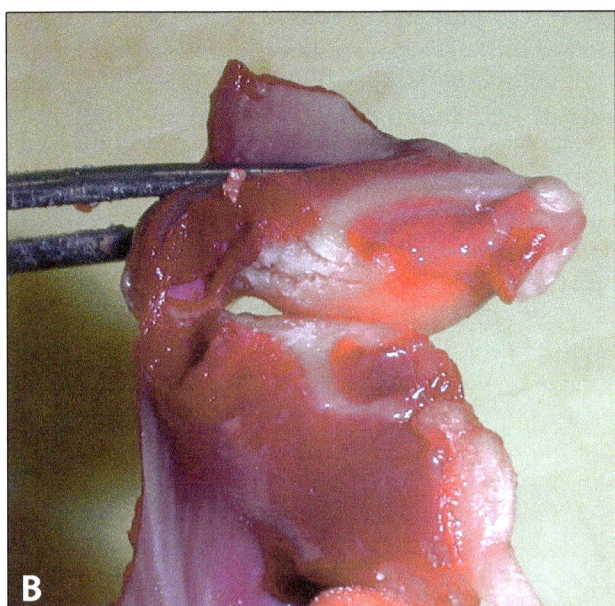

Figure 49C.1 Encircling PV isolation created epicardially utilizing dry bipolar RF on the beating heart. (**Panel A**) Endocardial lesion is shown to be transmural in the acute porcine model. (**Panel B**) Gross dissection revealing transmural lesion. (**Panel C**) Trichrome stain documenting transmurality with no skip lesions.

- On-pump, opened left atrium (LA) with cross-clamp and cardioplegia through a small right thoracotomy with application of cryothermia.[11,12]
- Unilateral totally thoracoscopic PV isolation utilizing microwave. This technology was finally removed from the market, as results were poor.
- Partial or full sternotomy off-pump utilizing HIFU.[13]
- Bilateral video-assisted thoracoscopic surgery (VATS) utilizing bipolar RF clamps.[2, 4-6, 14]

It must be kept in mind that patients who choose a minimally invasive AF surgical approach generally are otherwise in good health. There is no room for error and the mortality must be zero. Our current bilateral VATS Wolf technique is designed to allow cardiac surgeons to achieve minimally invasive surgical AF cures safely, without mastering all thoracoscopic skills. The bilateral working ports are deliberately positioned directly over the pulmonary veins and on the left side over the LAA to allow direct (3D) visualization of these important structures. This increases the safety margin, especially early in the surgeon's experience. As individual experience increases, totally thoracoscopic procedures can evolve, although we have not seen any difference in discomfort after the procedure or difference in length of stay with the totally endoscopic technique. Discomfort comes from the port sites and manipulation between the ribs, not from the working port with a soft tissue retractor. The risks without a working port increase, with no additional benefit. In the FAST trial, there were an increased number of procedural complications, which can be attributed to increased risks when not using working ports. For example, the FAST trial's authors reported complications, including bleeding, necessitating sternotomy, as well as one instance of cardiac tamponade in a group of 61 patients.[7] We have not encountered these complications in more than 1,000 cases due to our use of working ports.

Addressing the Left Atrial Appendage (LAA)

The various "minimally invasive" techniques used currently also differ in LAA treatment. We have been a strong proponent of LAA exclusion or excision.

Some patients are referred because of inability to tolerate anticoagulants in the background of transient ischemic attacks (TIAs) or stroke. The main reason for surgical referral in this subgroup of patients is to exclude the LAA as a source of repeated cerebral embolic events. With these minimally invasive surgical AF techniques, it seems prudent to reduce the stroke rate by excluding or removing the LAA. In the FAST trial, there were two cerebral vascular events in the catheter ablation group in the postoperative 12-month period. These problems are absent in the postop Wolf technique patients, as the LAA has been removed.

Intraoperative Electrophysiologic Testing (EP)

We believe intraoperative EP testing is of paramount importance. Ganglionic plexi (GP) isolation also addresses one of the plausible mechanisms of AF. We were the first to test for GP activity about the LA and isolate these GPs during our minimally invasive AF procedure, with the assistance of Dr. Ben Scherlag, and using his techniques.[15-17] A map has been developed to record the epicardial position of these GPs in each patient. The GPs are isolated both with the bipolar clamp and with a bipolar pen. We also test after isolation of the GPs (Figure 49C.2).

The second part of the intraoperative EP testing is designed to objectively document PV block after PV isolation. In addition to adding objectivity to the procedure, by learning these EP techniques, the surgeon will speak the same language as the electrophysiologist. We recommend the electrophysiologist be involved with the testing if possible. In Wolf technique cases referred after failed catheter ablation for AF, the nonisolated PVs are identified at the time of testing during the minimally invasive surgical AF procedure. In addition to providing a map for the surgical ablation procedure, this provides helpful feedback to the electrophysiologist and helps ensure consistency when reporting results.

Patient Selection and Preoperative Testing

The ideal patient for minimally invasive surgical treatment is listed in Table 49C.1.

Table 49C.1 Candidates for the Wolf technique

Documented AF
Failed catheter ablation
LA less than 6 cm
History of TIA or stroke
Inability to take anticoagulants
Patient desire to be rid of anticoagulants or antiarrhythmics
No significant valvular disease
No significant obstructive coronary artery disease

AF must be objectively documented preoperatively. If it has not been, 7-day continuous Holter monitoring is recommended. We have found other arrhythmias in patients labeled with AF, including recurrent nonsustained ventricular tachycardia. These patients must be referred for proper work-up and certainly would not benefit from a surgical AF procedure. Any history of

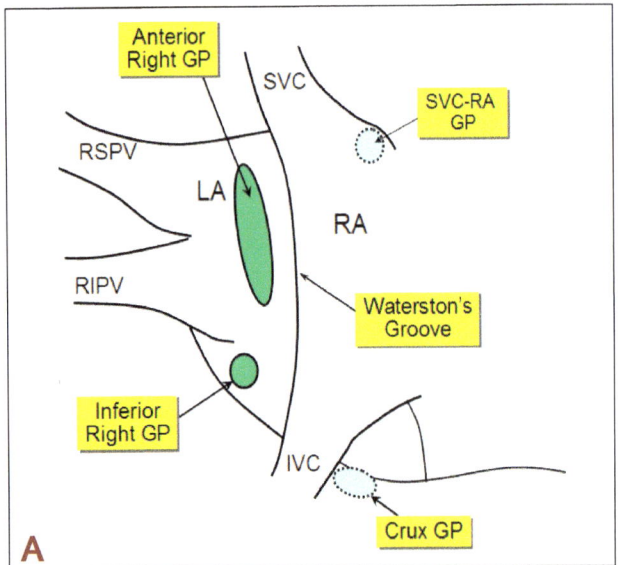
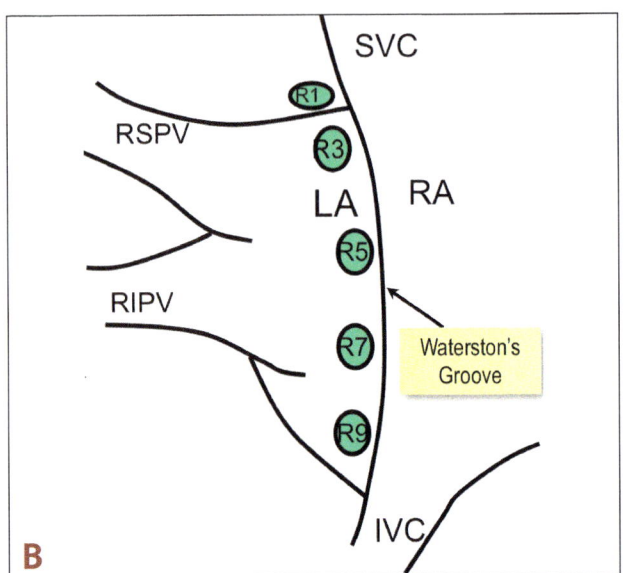
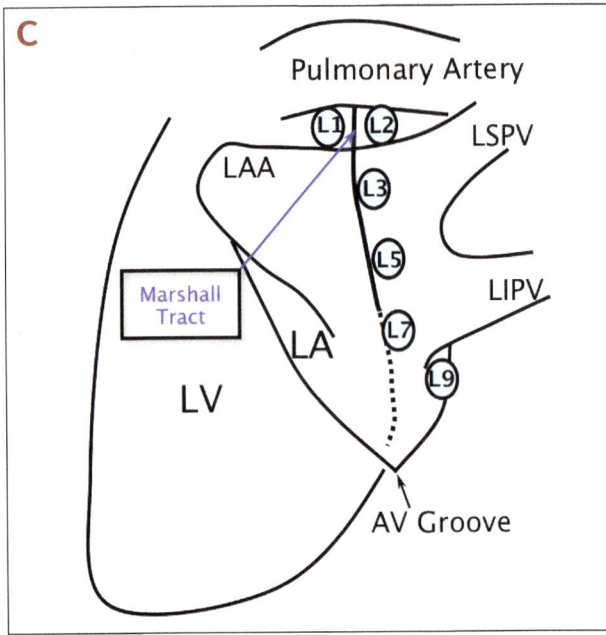
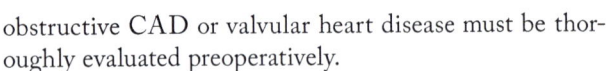

Figure 49C.2 Representative map of ganglionated plexi activity about the left atrium. **Panel A:** Schematic of right-side surgical view and GP areas. **Panel B:** Schematic of right-side surgical view with GP test sites. **Panel C:** Schematic of left-side surgical view with GP test sites.

obstructive CAD or valvular heart disease must be thoroughly evaluated preoperatively.

Our routine preoperative work-up is described in Table 49C.2.

Table 49C.2 Preoperative work-up

Imaging Test	Purpose
ECG	Document rhythm
Echocardiogram	Measure size of LA, confirm valve function
64-slice CT	Visualize anatomy of PVs, LAA; identify possible thrombus, PV stenosis, coronary anatomy pathology
7-day Holter monitoring, if needed	Document AF burden

All patients undergo 64-slice CT one to two days prior to the minimally invasive surgical procedure to rule out significant coronary artery disease, pulmonary vein stenosis (in patients with a history of catheter ablation), thrombus in the LAA, and to evaluate the PV anatomy. We have reported on the value of preop 64-slice CT scanning.[18] A 60-second delayed image of the LAA on 64-slice CT reliably rules out LAA thrombus. We no longer rely on intraoperative transesophageal echocardiography, as the preoperative CT gives additional information and is noninvasive and helps tremendously in planning the procedure by documenting posterior PV branches and anomalous coronary anatomy. A 64-slice CT scan with delayed imaging is more sensitive and specific than transesophageal echocardiography for ruling out LAA thrombus.

Surgical Approach

Although catheter-based techniques are the least invasive approach to the heart, it can be argued that epicardial discrete surgical isolation of the antrum (as opposed to current extensive endocardial ablative techniques) is much less invasive on the heart itself. This difference in approach helps to account for the low proarrhythmia rate following minimally invasive antrum exclusion surgically with a clamp versus catheter ablation, as left atrial flutter is unusual after the Wolf technique. Another advantage of this minimally invasive surgical approach is that it reliably treats the autonomic nerves, which are epicardial.[3,5,15-17]

Preparation

A double lumen endotracheal tube is used for selective lung ventilation, and a central line is placed. External defibrillator pads are placed in the appropriate vector. Sequential compression stockings are placed on the lower extremities. A warmer is used to control body temperature during the procedure.

Right Side

Place the patient in the left lateral decubitus position, at 45°–60°, with the right arm on an arm holder (Allen Medical Systems, Acton, MA). Document the external anatomy. Place the first port in the sixth or seventh intercostal space (ICS) in the mid-axillary line. From the scope view, identify the fourth ICS. Make a 4–6 cm working port in the fourth ICS with cautery on 30–40 watts and carry it anteriorly (Figure 49C.3). The incision should comfortably fit the surgeon's three fingers. Divide the serratus anterior in the direction of the muscle fibers. Use caution posteriorly to retract the fat pad containing the axillary nerve, artery, and vein with a finger when carrying the incision over the axillary contents. A medium soft-tissue retractor is inserted through the working port. Using soft tissue retraction (STR) with this setup, the surgeon can directly visualize the pericardium. Turn the cautery down to 20–30 watts. Open the pericardium a few centimeters anterior and parallel to the right phrenic nerve (a plastic sucker may be used to insulate the heart from the cautery). Be certain to visualize the phrenic nerve during pericardial opening and throughout the procedure. This way, the surgeon can avoid contact, traction, compression, or electrocautery injury to the phrenic nerve. Pericardial stay sutures (2–3) are placed in the lateral cut pericardial edge and are anchored as posteriorly as possible using suture snares through separate stab sites. The superior pericardial stay suture is placed adjacent to the superior vena cava (SVC) and right pulmonary artery (RPA). This improves direct visualization and access. An inferior pericardial stay suture is placed adjacent to the inferior aspect of the inferior pulmonary vein (IPV). If necessary, an additional stay suture may be placed adjacent to the bifurcation of the right pulmonary veins. It is extremely important at this stage to verify adequate visualization directly through the incision and endoscope. Ensure that all of the relevant anatomical structures can be clearly visualized (SVC, right superior pulmonary vein [RSPV], right inferior pulmonary vein [RIPV], IVC, RPA).

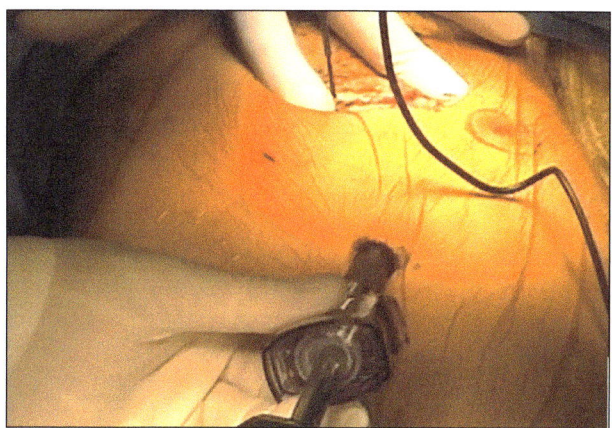

Figure 49C.3 Right-side surgical view with head at the top and feet at the bottom. Working port incision is lateral to right breast and port site is in the 7th intercostal space.

Initial Dissection

Bluntly develop a space just inferior to the RIPV and lateral to the IVC into the oblique sinus. Verify that a Wolf suction instrument (Scanlan International, St. Paul, MN) freely falls into the oblique sinus through this opening. Use the scope to check the access angle for the dissector device. A sponge stick can be used to gently retract the heart medially as needed for access and visualization. Roll the SVC medially with the suction or with an endoscopic knittner, but do not grasp the SVC.

The Wolf Lumitip™ Dissector Manufactured by AtriCure

Create a second working port (10 mm) either medially or laterally to the scope port for dissector use, allowing the dissector to be lined up for direct in-line access with the appropriate port site. The dissector is shown in Figure 49C.4. In this procedure, no hands are placed in the chest. The dissector acts as the surgeon's index finger around the back of the heart. Do not use a trocar with the dissector. The GlidePath Transfer Guide™ is attached to the dissector by inserting the dissector tip into the GlidePath hood. Then the dissector/GlidePath is introduced with no articulation through the port site into the pericardial space.

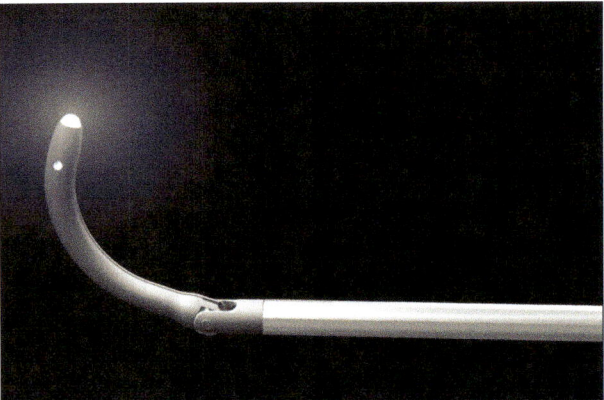

Figure 49C.4 Wolf Lumitip™ Dissector with GlidePath Transfer Guide (AtriCure Inc.).

Dissector Placement

Bluntly retract the SVC medially with a sponge stick or endoscopic knittner to help gain exposure and visualization of the superior aspect of the RPA. Feed the dissector tip into the oblique sinus just lateral to the IVC (Figure 49C.5). Advance the distal end of the dissector tip posteriorly and sweep it medially into position behind the right pulmonary veins. Articulate the lighted dissector to pass between the RSPV and RPA using the lighted tip as a guide.

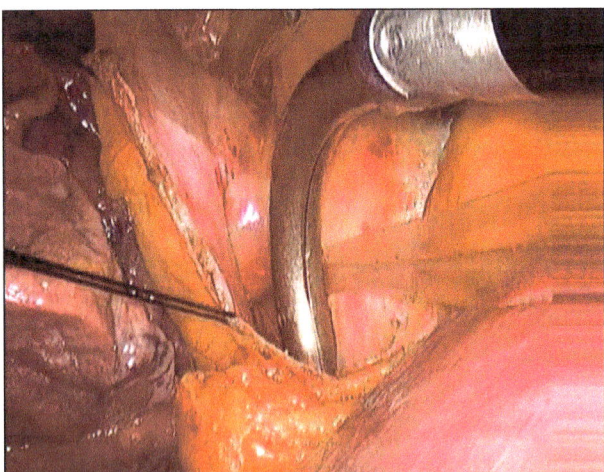

Figure 49C.5 Right-side intraoperative photograph of lighted dissector being placed in the oblique sinus.

Grasp the GlidePath and remove the lighted dissector. (Figure 49C.6). Traction on the GlidePath will advance the Isolator® lower jaw until its posterior tip is visible superior to the RSPV. Make sure to apply adequate tension to the red rubber catheter to help lead the lower jaw into place.

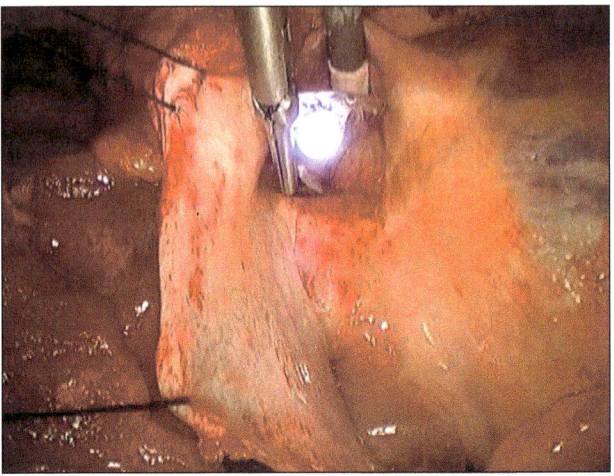

Figure 49C.6 Right-side intraoperative photograph with lighted dissector around the back of the heart with lighted dissector tip between right pulmonary artery and right superior pulmonary vein.

Antral Ablation

Right Side

Transmural and contiguous lesions are created to electrically isolate the antrum from the remainder of the heart. After completing the ablation, place the AtriCure pen on the previously recorded locations of the RSPV, RIPV, and the bifurcation of RPVs. Map and record the epicardial ECG. If the ECG recording shows quiescence in all locations on the PVs, then PV antral isolation is complete.

On the right side during clamp applications, perform additional three burns after herniating the Waterson's groove fat pad into the clamp. This provides for more medial isolation of the left antrum and usually treats all the GPs except level 9 on the right.

Place a bipolar pacing lead inside the pericardium on the right side. Before the minimally invasive surgical procedure some patients have been continuously out of rhythm for more than a year. These patients are often on medications that poison the conduction system to slow the ventricular response to AF. When patients in such a state are cardioverted they often have slow conduction. Temporary pacing for 1–5 days allows time for the conduction system to recover while medications are held.

GP Ablation Right Side

The GPs are isolated both with the bipolar clamp applied medial to Waterston's groove fat pad and with a bipolar pen directly over any remaining positive GPs. We also test after isolation of the GPs.

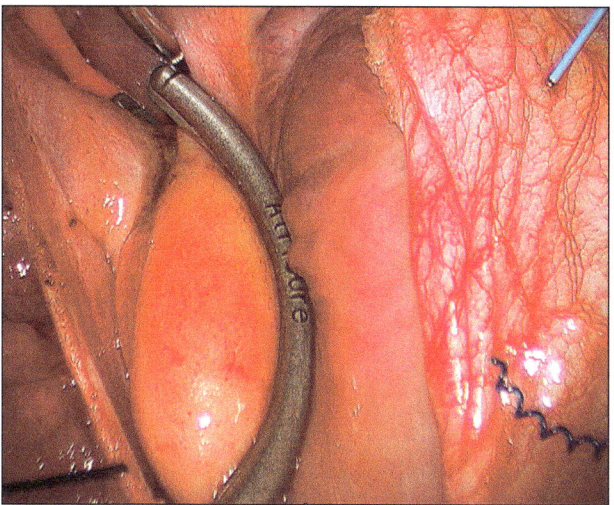

Figure 49C.7 Right-side intraoperative photograph with Isolator™ clamp (AtriCure Inc.) in position for second set of abalations medial to Waterston's groove. This application encompasses GPs 1, 3, 5, and 7 on the right. The Wolf suction device (Scanlan International, St. Paul, MN) is seen superiorly ensuring all antral tissue is inside the black line on the clamp. A bipolar pacing lead (Medtronic Inc.) is seen medially. The pacing lead is held in place simply by pressure between the epicardium and the pericardium.

Left Side

The same patient position is utilized and the access ports and exposure are identical to the right side (Figure 49C.8). The dissection and ablation are performed similar to the right side, except on the left side the ligament of Marshall must be divided. The position of the ligament of Marshall is seen in Figure 49C.9. Passing and placement of the Isolator clamp is similar to the right side. The left-sided isolator clamp is seen in position in Figure 49C.10.

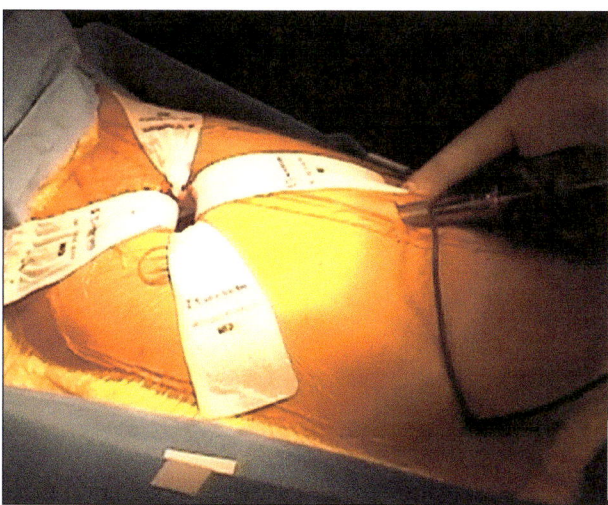

Figure 49C.8 Intraoperative photograph with the patient left side up with head to the left. The working port (6 cm long) with soft tissue retractor is in the fourth intercostal space lateral to the left breast. The camera port is just anterior to the left scapular border in the seventh intercostal space.

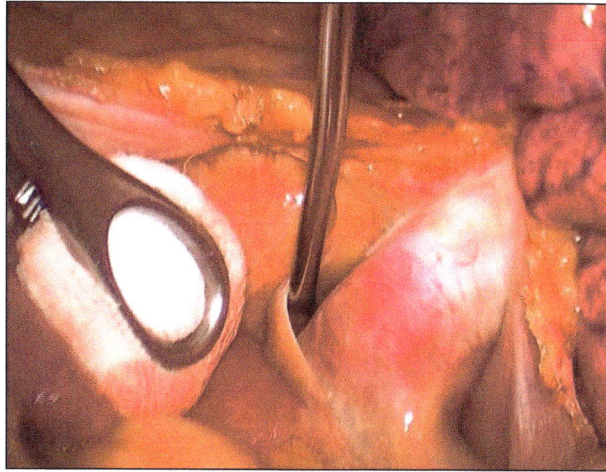

Figure 49C.9 Left-side intraoperative photograph with head to the top. Visualized is the Wolf suction device (Scanlan International, St. Paul, MN) between the ligament of Marshall and the RPV. Sponge stick is retracting the LAA medially.

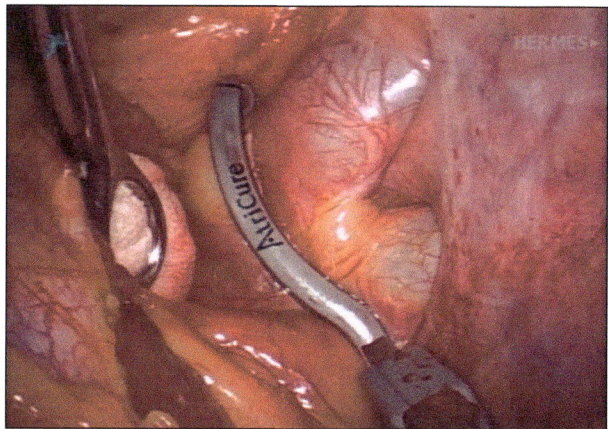

Figure 49C.10 Left-sided thoracoscopic view with head of patient to the top. Classic pulmonary venous branching is depicted. The left-sided isolator clamp is placed well medially on the left atrial antrum. A sponge stick retracts the LAA.

Exclusion of the Left Atrial Appendage (LAA)

After the left PVs have been isolated, the LAA is excluded. The Echelon Flex™ Endopath Stapler (Ethicon Endo-Surgery) is used with a thick tissue load (green, staple height 4.8 mm). The stapler should be introduced through the most posteriorly located inferior port site. The stapler is fired across the base of the LAA to excise the LAA (Figure 49C.11). The entire LAA can be seen removed in Figures 49C.12 and 49.13. We remove the LAA in all cases as it is of paramount importance in dramatically decreasing the risk of AF-related stroke. In addition, the active focus of AF is observed in the LAA in 15%–20% of patients. The pericardium should be closed on the left side to avoid herniation of the heart.

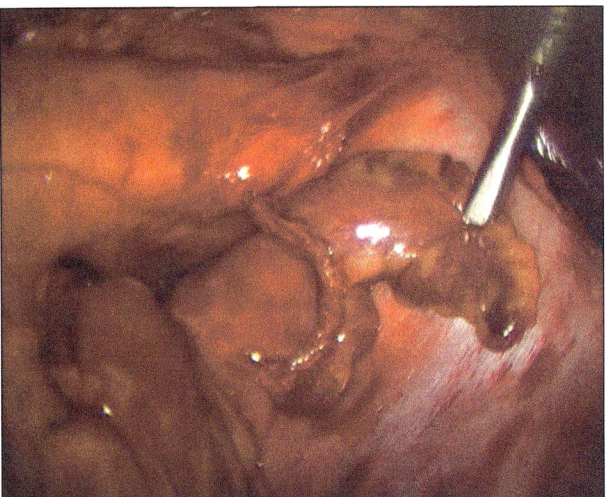

Figure 49C.12 Left-side intraoperative photograph with a grasper removing the entire LAA.

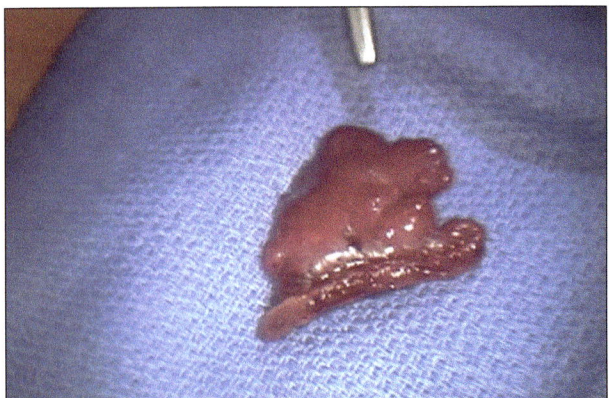

Figure 49C.13 Left-side intraoperative photograph with excised LAA.

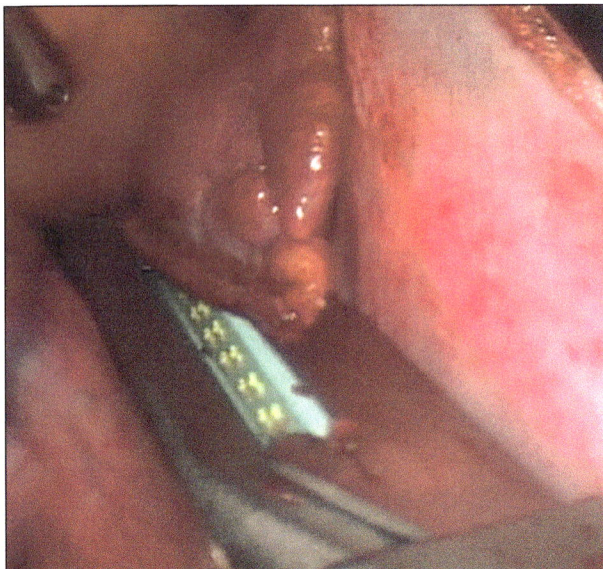

Figure 49C.11 Left-side intraoperative photograph with stapler stapling and excising the LAA at the base (Ethicon Endo-Surgery Inc.).

The completed left side is seen in Figure 49C.14. The working port incision measures 6 cm. One of the inferior ports is utilized for chest tube placement.

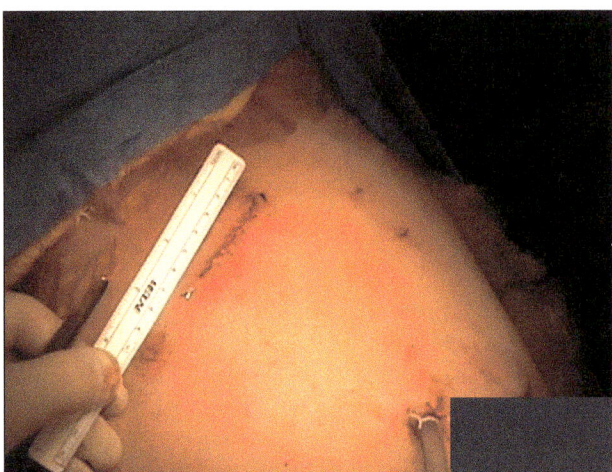

Figure 49C.14 Left-side intraoperative photograph at the conclusion of the procedure. The working port measures 6 cm. One of the inferior ports is utilized for chest tube placement.

Postoperative Considerations

Temporary pacing postoperatively is quite helpful. It is utilized for bradycardia, junctional rhythm, and for diagnostics. In more than 1,000 cases, we have placed only three pacemakers, all in patients who were recommended to have a pacemaker before the procedure. The relatively high need for permanent pacemakers in other series can be explained by surgeons not using a temporary wire (most slow heart rhythms postop resolve after a few days) and by the use of additional lines made with a pen. Pen lines across the roof can result in destruction of the Bachmann's bundle or damage to the artery of the sinus node. The artery to the sinus node traverses the roof of the LA in 30% of cases.

Various strategies exist for weaning off antiarrhythmics and anticoagulants. Home ECG monitoring should be considered to assess AF postoperatively after antiarrhythmics are weaned. Check-ups are performed at 8 to 14 days, 3, 6, and 12 months postoperatively, and annually. This follow-up routine ensures proper weaning of medications, timely cardioversions if needed, and better assessment of absence of AF at 1 year and subsequent years.

Conclusions

Recently we reviewed 157 patients who are now 1 to 8 years out from the Wolf technique. The patients' ages ranged from 15 to 87 years old. The AF-free rate for paroxysmal AF was 92%; for persistent AF, 85%; and for longstanding persistent AF, 75%. The follow-up included

7-day continuous Holter monitoring. There were no deaths (personal review). This follow-up exceeded the minimum follow-up screening recommendations as listed in the HRS/EHRA/ECAS Catheter and Surgical Ablation consensus statement.[19]

The Wolf technique is much more than just PV isolation. It is a truly minimally invasive approach and includes bilateral antrum isolation as per Pappone[20] and a partial cardiac denervation as per Jackman and Scherlag.[15-17] In cases referred after failed catheter ablation for AF, the nonisolated PVs are identified at the time of testing during the minimally invasive surgical AF procedure. In addition to providing a map for the surgical ablation procedure, this provides helpful feedback to the electrophysiologist and helps ensure consistency when reporting results.

The LAA is removed with this technique. The removal of the appendage serves two purposes. First, it obviates the need for continued anticoagulation, and second, it removes the source of triggers in up to 15% of patients. Average postoperative hospital stay is 2 days. After the procedure, we discontinue anticoagulants, even if the patient is in AF. If the patient is still in AF at 1 month, antiarrhythmics are prescribed and cardioversion is performed. Cardioversion is routinely performed postoperatively without anticoagulation.

In over 1,000 cases, there have been no strokes or TIAs. If the patient has failed 2 postop cardioversions and antiarrhythmic therapy and is at least 6 months' postprocedure, we recommend EP mapping and ablation. The Wolf technique has been utilized in over 12,000 patients, and other investigators are finding similar high success rates compared to catheter ablation.[4-6] In contrast to catheter ablation techniques, this minimally invasive surgical technique is accomplished without prolonged operating time; there is no fluoroscopy, there are few complications, proarrhythmia is uncommon, and success is superior to catheter ablation for AF.

Haïssaguerre recently reported the success of one catheter ablation at 5 years in a study population not representative of patients with AF at large, as it consisted predominantly of younger, healthier, nonobese patients with relatively smaller atria and paroxysmal or recent progression to persistent AF.[21] Nevertheless, the 5-year AF-free rate was only 29%.

Currently patients with paroxysmal, persistent, and long-standing persistent AF are evaluated for treatment. If the LA is less than 6 cm and/or the length of time in continuous AF is less than 5 years, we consider the minimally invasive surgical approach.

There is interest in a hybrid procedure, consisting of a catheter-based approach performed simultaneously with a Wolf technique or other minimally invasive surgical variation. The hypothesis is that combining a minimally invasive surgical technique and catheter ablation will lead to a better cure rate. However, this type of hybrid procedure also has many disadvantages, including a much longer procedure time, greater expense, and the potential complications of both minimally invasive surgery and catheter-based ablation. Potential complications include esophageal fistula, emergency sternotomy, and neurological injury.[22-24]

Rather than a hybrid procedure, the Wolf technique alone can deliver good results in 75% or more of all patients. In the interest of reducing costs and expanding access to care, we feel it is better to initially perform the minimally invasive surgical option.[25] For patients with AF postop at least 6 months, we then recommend catheter ablation. This model has worked well for us.

Previous CABG is not a contraindication to the Wolf technique, provided there is no graft in the vicinity of the LAA. A patent circumflex graft is a contraindication to the minimally invasive surgical procedure. Some patients benefit from simply LAA excision. LAA excision alone has been presented prospectively by Ohtsuka and was found to be safe and effective.[26] These are patients that are not good candidates for the Wolf technique, but cannot take anticoagulants. Patients who have been continuously out of rhythm for even 7 years are able to maintain sinus rhythm after the minimally invasive surgical procedure if the LA is less than 5.5 cm preoperatively. The treatment to cure AF continues to evolve rapidly, and patients are benefiting from the tremendous amount of focus on this common problem.

References

1. Haïssaguerre M, Jaïs P, Shah DC, et al. Spontaneous initiation of atrial fibrillation by ectopic beats originating in the pulmonary veins. *N Engl J Med.* 1998;339(10):659-666.
2. Wolf RK, Schneeberger EW, Osterday R, et al. Video-assisted bilateral pulmonary vein isolation and left atrial appendage exclusion for atrial fibrillation. *J Thorac Cardiovasc Surg.* 2005;130(3):797-802.
3. Mehall JR, Kohut RM Jr, Schneeberger EW, et al. Intraoperative epicardial electrophysiologic mapping and isolation of autonomic ganglionic plexi. *Ann Thorac Surg.* 2007;83(2):538-541.
4. Wudel JH, Chaudhuri P, Hiller JJ. Video-assisted epicardial ablation and left atrial appendage exclusion for atrial fibrillation: extended follow-up. *Ann Thorac Surg.* 2008;85:34-38.
5. Edgerton JR, Jackman WM, Mack MJ. Minimally invasive pulmonary vein isolation and partial autonomic denervation for surgical treatment of atrial fibrillation. *J Interv Card Electrophysiol.* 2007;20:89-93.
6. McClelland JH, Duke D, Reddy R. Preliminary results of a limited thoracotomy: new approach to treat atrial fibrillation. *J Cardiovasc Electrophysiol.* 2007;18:1289-1295.
7. Boersma LV, Castella M, van Boven W, et al. Atrial Fibrillation Catheter Ablation Versus Surgical Ablation Treatment (FAST): A 2-center randomized clinical trial. *Circulation.* 2012;125(1):23-30.
8. Holmes DR, Schwartz RS. Left atrial appendage occlusion eliminates the need for warfarin. *Circulation.* 2009;120:1919-1926.
9. Aupperle H, Doll N, Walther T, et al. Histological findings induced by different energy sources in experimental atrial

ablation in sheep. *Interact Cardiovasc Thorac Surg.* 2005;4(5):450-455.
10. Author's personal observation in the acute porcine model.
11. Ad N, Henry L, Friehling T, Wish M, Holmes SD. Minimally invasive stand-alone Cox-Maze procedure for patients with nonparoxysmal atrial fibrillation. *Ann Thorac Surg.* 2013 Sep;96(3):792-798; discussion 798-799.
12. Rodriguez E, Cook RC, Chu MWA, Chitwood WR. Minimally invasive biatrial CryoMaze operation for atrial fibrillation. *Op Tech Thorac Cardiovasc Surg.* 2009;14(3):208-223.
13. Klinkenberg TJ, Ahmed S, Ten Hagen A, et al. Feasibility and outcome of epicardial pulmonary vein isolation for lone atrial fibrillation using minimal invasive surgery and high intensity focused ultrasound. *Europace.* 2009 Dec;11(12):1624-631.
14. Wang JG, Li Y, Shi JH, Han J, Cui YQ, Luo TG, Meng X. Treatment of long-lasting persistent atrial fibrillation using minimally invasive surgery combined with irbesartan. *Ann Thorac Surg.* 2011 Apr;91(4):1183-1189.
15. Patterson E, Po SS, Scherlag BJ, Lazzara R. Triggered firing in pulmonary veins initiated by in vitro autonomic nerve stimulation. *Heart Rhythm.* 2005;2:634-631.
16. Scherlag BJ, Yamanashi W, Patel U, et al. Autonomically induced conversion of pulmonary vein focal firing into atrial fibrillation. *J Am Coll Cardiol.* 2005;45:1878-1886.
17. Schauerte P, Scherlag BJ, Patterson E, et al. Focal atrial fibrillation experimental evidence for a pathophysiologic role of the autonomic nervous system. *J Cardiovasc Electrophysiol.* 2001;12:592-599.
18. Meyer C, Hall J, Mehall J, et al. Impact of preoperative 64-slice CT scanning on mini-Maze atrial fibrillation surgery. *Innovations.* 2007;2:169-175.
19. Calkins H, Kuck KH, Cappato R, et al. 2012 HRS/EHRA/ECAS Expert Consensus Statement on Catheter and Surgical Ablation of Atrial Fibrillation: recommendations for patient selection, procedural techniques, patient management and follow-up, definitions, endpoints, and research trial design. *Europace.* 2012;14(4):528-606.
20. Augello G, Vicedomini G, Saviano M, et al. Pulmonary vein isolation after circumferential pulmonary vein ablation: comparison between Lasso and three-dimensional electroanatomical assessment of complete electrical disconnection. *Heart Rhythm.* 2009 Dec;6(12):1706-1713.
21. Weerasooriya R, Khairy P, Litalien J, et al. Catheter ablation for atrial fibrillation: are results maintained at 5 years of follow-up? *J Am Coll Cardiol.* 2011;57:160-166.
22. Cappato R, Calkins H, Chen SA, et al. Prevalence and causes of fatal outcome in catheter ablation of atrial fibrillation. *J Am Coll Cardiol.* 2009;53(19):1798-1803.
23. Sacher F, Monahan KH, Thomas SP, et al. Phrenic nerve injury after atrial fibrillation catheter ablation: characterization and outcome in a multi-center study. *J Am Coll Cardiol.* 2006;47(12):2498-2503.
24. Bai R, Patel D, Di Biase L, et al. Phrenic nerve injury after catheter ablation: should we worry about this complication? *J Cardiovasc Electrophysiol.* Sep 2006; 17(9):944-948.
25. Boersma LV, Castella M, van Boven M, et al. Atrial Fibrillation Catheter Ablation Versus Surgical Ablation Treatment (FAST): A 2-Center Randomized Clinical Trial *Circulation.* 2012;125(1):23-30.
26. Ohtsuka T, Ninomiya M, Nonaka T, Hisagi M, Ota T, Mizutani T. Thoracoscopic stand-alone left atrial appendectomy for thromboembolism prevention in nonvalvular atrial fibrillation. *J Am Coll Cardiol.* 2013 Jul 9;62(2):103-107.

CHAPTER 49D

Surgical Ablation for Atrial Fibrillation: Extended Left Atrial Lesion Set

James R. Edgerton, MD; Karen L. Roper, PhD; Stuart J. Head, MD, PhD

Introduction

Recent advances in our understanding of the mechanisms of atrial fibrillation (AF), along with the development of new enabling technology, have made less-invasive interventional treatments possible. We review the progress that has been made in the development of modern minimally invasive approaches for AF treatment, with particular focus on the "Dallas lesion set." A description of the lesion set and review of our data shows the promise of this approach. Finally, we discuss future possibilities including the potential for improved outcomes using hybrid procedures.

The Cox-Maze Procedure

Generally regarded as the "gold standard" surgical treatment of AF, the Cox-Maze approach was initiated by James Cox in the late 1980s. It involved creating a "maze" of incisions through the left atrium to disrupt the reentrant circuits responsible for AF. The technique prevented reoccurrence of AF in up to 98% of patients.[1] Yet despite advancements in the technique over the ensuing years, the Cox-Maze III procedure remains technically difficult to perform. Because the incision set requires on-bypass open heart surgery, the associated morbidity of this time-consuming surgery makes the procedure too complex to be applied to all patients with AF.

In the landmark article by Haïssaguerre,[2,3] paroxysmal AF was shown to be triggered by single ectopic beats originating from within the pulmonary veins (PVs) and to a lesser extent in the right atrium. Once induced, AF persists until the circuits terminate (either spontaneously or via drugs or other interventions). If AF termination occurs spontaneously, followed by a return to normal sinus rhythm, it is termed "intermittent" AF. It can be initiated repetitively, but requires a "trigger" each time new episodes are induced. Such discovery focused attention on pulmonary vein isolation (PVI), thus opening the door for alternative minimally invasive procedures. As scientific knowledge about the special electrical properties of the PVs evolved, so did the availability of new enabling technology to create transmural, electrically isolating scars on the atria. At present, energy sources used for intraoperative ablation include cryotherapy, radiofrequency, and ultrasound. There is little difference in the results so long as the ablation creates transmural lesions and complete conduction block.[4]

Further development of catheter-based technology allowed for transvascular endocardial ablation. Catheter treatment strategies that offer a minimal access treatment of AF using electrical isolation and/or ablation of the PVs have since been brought to rapid focus. The goal of such ablation is to electrically isolate triggers and to prevent propagation of the initiating wavefront, reentry around anatomic obstacles, and/or reduction of the critical mass of tissue required for multiple wavelet reentry.[1-3]

Initial studies of catheter ablation focused largely on the left atrium, because initiation and perpetuation of AF are partly dependent on anatomic and functional obstacles that exist there. By one estimate, 90% of intermittent or "paroxysmal" AF can be cured by a properly performed isolation of the PVs.[5] In further study of left atrial ablation, however, Haïssaguerre found that while the ablation technique organized local electrical activity and led to stable sinus rhythm during the procedure, sustained AF remained inducible in most patients. The lesions failed to produce evidence of a significant linear conduction block/delay in all but 4 of 45 patients.[6]

Subsequent research confirmed that ablation of these triggering foci, while beneficial in the treatment of AF, entails significant recurrence rates. The contribution of the posterior left atrium is increasingly recognized as a source of non-PV triggering foci and as a substrate for maintaining AF. The posterior wall of the left atrium adjacent to the PV antrum has a shorter mean cycle length and greater number of discharges than other portions of the atrium.[7] Accordingly, electrophysiologists began to perform wide antral encircling ablation, which increased success.[8] In one study, circumferential PVI alone restored sinus rhythm in just 43.2% of patients with long-standing persistent AF.[9] In short, it has become increasingly evident that persistent (continuing for 7 days without termination) or long-standing persistent AF (eg, "continuous"; defined as persistent AF for a year or longer) may not be successfully treated by PVI alone, since the mechanisms for initiation and maintenance of AF lie in the changed left atrial substrate beyond the PVs. From a pathophysiological perspective, this is explained by structural and electrical remodeling of the atrial myocardium, which can then initiate and sustain AF independent of the PVs in patients with persistent AF. In these patients, the augmented number and location of drivers for fibrillation necessitates additional linear ablation strategies, and sometimes multiple procedures with a commensurate shift toward posterior wall and left atrial appendage isolation. Indeed, the Cox-Maze III emphasized the importance of right- and left-sided isthmus lesions, particularly of the left-sided isthmus, which includes ablation over the coronary sinus.

Today, it is widely accepted that additional substrate modification is required to effectively address persistent AF using catheter ablation. These additional lesions in the left atrium involve the left atriotomy from the PV encircling incision down to the mitral valve annulus posteriorly and ablation of coronary sinus conduction at the same point. Cox[5] added that since this additional lesion is now becoming easier to perform, there is little reason not to add it in patients with intermittent AF as well.

Because of the challenges presented in reliably encircling the PV antra and of creating multiple linear ablations with a catheter, the feasibility of minimally invasive surgical epicardial PVI and exclusion of the left atrial appendage was initially described by Wolf in 2005.[10] These procedures were performed off-pump using bilateral video-assisted thoracoscopic vein isolation with a bipolar radiofrequency device.

Pulmonary Vein Isolation Inadequate for Persistent and Long-standing Persistent AF

A number of our own findings support the contention that PVI alone is inadequate for persistent and long-standing persistent AF due to the substrate changes induced by electrical remodeling. Video-assisted bilateral PV antral isolation with confirmation of block and partial autonomic denervation was performed in 74 patients with follow-up at 6 months. A successful return to normal sinus rhythm for patients classified as persistent and long-standing persistent AF remained at 81.5% by ECG and dropped to only 56.5% by longer-term monitoring.[11] In a larger study involving 5 surgical centers, 114 patients underwent the identical bilateral PV antral electrical isolation as in the prior study, with targeted autonomic denervation of the left atrium with selective left atrial appendectomy. Once again, the patients with persistent AF had a low success rate at 6-month follow-up, especially with longer-term monitoring. Normal sinus rhythm was found in only 18/32 (56.3%) of persistent cases, and only 11/22 (50%) of the long-standing patients.[12]

Others have reported that long-term success of PVI is poor when compared directly to other lesion sets.[13,14] Such findings make clear that PV antral isolation and partial autonomic denervation are not adequate treatment in patients with persistent and long-standing persistent AF, with the associated changes in the left atrial substrate that occur in these conditions.[15] Because of electrical remodeling, the left atrium produces a shortened refractory period and a shortened fibrillatory interval;[16] atrial fibrosis may also be present.[17] It is apparent that elimination of the PV triggers alone is inadequate treatment for persistent and long-standing persistent AF. A more extensive lesion set is necessary—one that extends beyond PVI to include targets along the left atrium substrate, and that can be performed epicardially on the beating heart.

Justification of the Lesion Set

The largest challenge to replicating the Cox-Maze III lesion set on the full beating heart is making the connection to the mitral annulus. The other connecting lesions can be done through the transverse sinus. When connection lines to the mitral annulus are added, however, the success rates are shown to be comparable with the cut-and-sew maze: Jeanmart and colleagues reported an AF-free rate of 69.7% with an endocardial box lesion plus a connecting line to the mitral annulus.[18] However, incorporation of the mitral valve isthmus can be challenging.

In traditional techniques, the connection to the mitral valve is ablated across the left atrial isthmus. However, there are 3 inhibitors to doing this on the full beating heart. First, the traditional connection is to the posterior annulus, but visualization behind the full, beating heart's left atrium is very limited. Secondly, when working epicardial to endocardial, there is the risk of collateral damage to the circumflex coronary artery overlying the mitral valve. Third, the coronary sinus, which is used as the epicardial landmark for the mitral annulus, is unreliable, and may leave a gap.[19] This leads to a significant risk of incomplete ablation or introducing atrial flutter, because of reentry or electrical bridging by tissue.[20-22]

The Dallas Lesion Set

To address these problems, the Dallas Lesion Set[23] was developed. The set replicates the left atrial lesions of the Cox-Maze III. The problem of connecting to the mitral valve is addressed by connecting to the anterior annulus at the left fibrous trigone. The mitral valve touches the aortic valve at the left fibrous trigone, which lies at the junction of the left and the noncoronary cusps of the aortic root. Thus an epicardial landmark is available,[24] and visualization is excellent (Figure 49D.1).

This lesion set interrupts conduction around the mitral annulus and is expected to interrupt circuits causing left atrial tachycardias in other ablation procedures.[25] The other left atrial connecting lesions are done in the transverse sinus. A linear lesion is made from the right superior PV to the left superior PV, and a line is made from the left superior PV to the base of the amputated left atrial appendage. This completes all the left atrial lines of the Cox-Maze III.

Description of Surgical Technique

The procedure is elsewhere described in detail.[26-28] Briefly, the patient is positioned supine on the operating table. He is intubated with a double lumen endotracheal tube to allow selective ventilation. The right side is approached first. A 5-mm port is placed in the third intercostal space at the mid-axillary line, and CO_2 is insufflated to expand the space by compressing the lung and depressing the diaphragm. Next, two 11-mm ports are placed, one at about the second intercostal space at the mid-clavicular line and one at about the sixth intercostals space at the mid-axillary line. Working through these, the pericardium is opened. Next, the PV antrum is electrically isolated using a bipolar radiofrequency clamp. Antral isolation is confirmed by mapping the PVs for entrance block using a pacing and sensing pen. The pen is also used to deliver high-frequency stimulation to locate active ganglionated plexi.[27] If ablation is insufficient or active ganglionated plexi are recognized, the pen is used to deliver radiofrequency energy to fully ablate the area.

The superior vena cava (SVC) is fully mobilized to allow access to the transverse sinus behind the SVC. The fat pad that lies behind the SVC is dissected to expose the muscular dome of the left atrium in the transverse sinus. A linear radiofrequency device is introduced in the most caudal port. The device is advanced to the dome and utilized to place a linear burn from the right superior PV across the

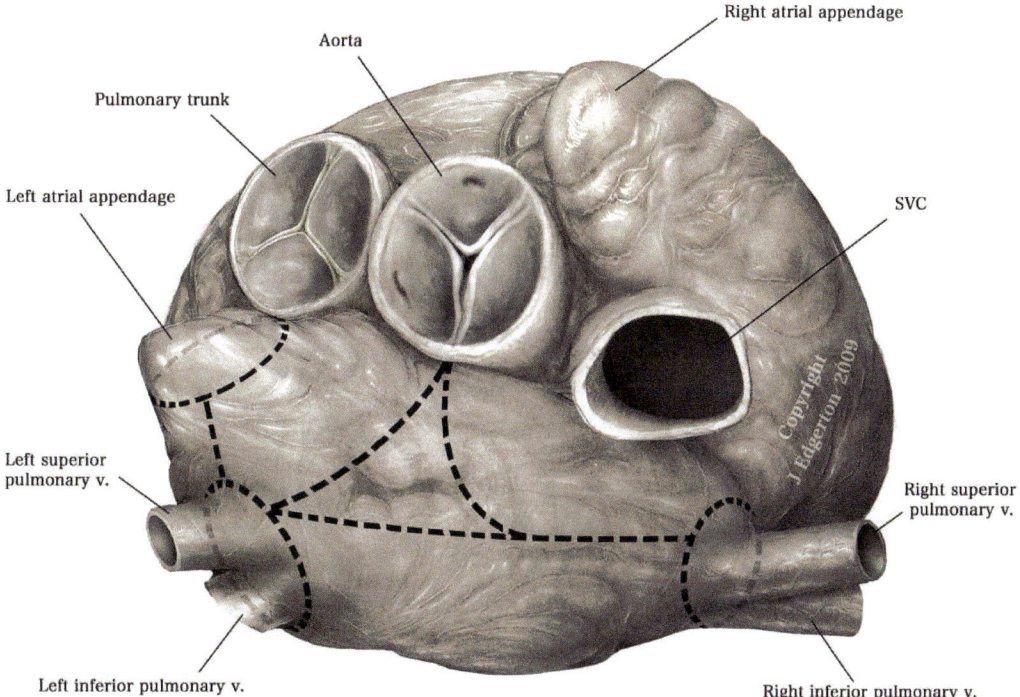

Figure 49D.1   The Dallas Lesion Set. SVC = superior vena cava; v = vein.

dome to the left superior PV, as high as possible on the dome. The device is redirected to the landmark junction of the left coronary cusp of the aorta, and the noncoronary cusp at the left fibrous trigone. Accurate positioning can be checked by transesophageal echocardiography, where the left fibrous trigone of the aortic annulus touching the mitral annulus can be visualized in themed-esophageal, long-access, 140° view. Ablation of a linear line from the fibrous trigone to the previously applied line across the dome is performed. When the lesion is insufficient, the sensing/ablating pen can again be used to perform additional ablation. After applying this lesion, the procedure through the right thoracoscopic approach is completed. The pericardium is closed, and a long catheter continuously infusing pain medication is tunneled beneath the pleura. All equipment is extracted, a soft silastic chest tube is placed, and the incisions are closed.

The access on the left side is similar to that on the right side, only more posterior. The left pericardium is opened posterior to the phrenic nerve. Caution should be taken to avoid nerve damage to the phrenic nerve, and the recurrent laryngeal nerve on the left, which courses beneath the aorta. A suture is placed in the pericardium to protect the phrenic nerve and to open the pericardium so the atrial appendage can be exposed.

Similar to the lesions applied on the right side, the sensing pen is introduced to obtain a baseline electrogram. Furthermore, the ligament of Marshall is divided, the PVs are encircled with a bipolar radiofrequency clamp, and three ablations are performed, each time on a slightly different location high on the antrum. When the lesions are sufficient, the sensing pen should not be able to detect any transmitted electrical activity in the PVs, thus confirming entrance block. Any other active ganglionated plexi can be ablated through radiofrequency energy through the sensing/ablating device.

Further lesions are performed with the linear ablation device. To achieve visualization of the transverse sinus, the atrial appendage and the pulmonary artery are retracted. The linear device is placed upon the dome of the left atrium, and a line is placed on the dome as far posterior as possible, connecting the right superior PV and the left superior PV. Completing the ablations, the linear device is redirected to the left, where a line is placed between the trigone and the right superior PV. An inverted triangle of viability is now formed on the atrial dome, in which no conducted atrial activity will be recorded with the sensing pen if the lesions are continuous and transmural. Pacing in this triangle when the patient is in sinus rhythm is a test to ensure exit block is present.

Finally, a stapler device is introduced to remove the atrial appendage. To ensure correct placement and guiding of the device, the transesophageal echocardiogram is used. The amputated appendage is thereafter withdrawn through the stapler. A pain medication infusion catheter is placed subpleural, a soft chest tube is introduced, and the pericardium (and subsequently the wounds) are closed.

Our Results

The Dallas Lesion Set is being adopted by increasing numbers of dedicated surgeons worldwide, but has been performed by only a small group of dedicated surgeons. Early results have been published on 30 of our patients with a mean age of 58 years.[26] The group included 10 patients with persistent AF and 20 with long-standing persistent AF. Data related to ECG, long-term monitoring, and the use of antiarrhythmic drugs was collected 6 months postoperative, and follow-up was 100%. Procedure-related complications did not occur during follow-up, nor were there any deaths. Efficacy measured at 6 months was available for all patients and showed a success rate indicated by the number of patients in sinus rhythm, of 90% in persistent AF patients, and 75% in long-standing persistent AF patients. The use of antiarrhythmic drugs was unnecessary in 78% of persistent AF and 47% of long-standing persistent AF cases.

Further results of a multicenter registry including 124 patients showed less optimal safety assessment, but outcomes remained satisfactory. Operative mortality was only 0.8%, and procedure-related complications were at a minimum of 10% (renal failure, pericarditis, pneumothorax, pleural effusion, reoperation for bleeding). Again, a high success rate was measured. After 6 months, normal sinus rhythm was achieved in 71%–94%, depending on previous catheter ablation and measurement by ECG or long-term monitoring. One-year success rate obtained by long-term monitoring demonstrated a success rate of 63% in a group that had previously undergone catheter ablation ($n = 21$). Data by ECG even showed a success of 86% in patients who had not been ablated before. It can be concluded from these reported results that the Dallas Lesion Set is a safe procedure, and has a significant success rate in patients with paroxysmal, persistent, or long-standing persistent AF. Since our study, research has shown a significant increase in adverse events following catheter ablation of the PV alone, as compared to surgical ablation of the PV, ganglionated plexi, and left atrial appendage

The Future: Hybrid Endocardial/Epicardial Approach

Our quest has been to increase the success rate of the surgical ablation, especially in patients who present with persistent AF and long-standing persistent AF. The Dallas lesion set is safe and effective and provides an improved, minimally invasive surgical approach for these challenging patients. Further frontiers are likely to use hybrid approaches, combining the strengths of epicardial and endocardial ablation. One is more likely to be transmural when burning inside out and outside in simultaneously. The potential for improved outcomes through hybrid ablation also derives from combining expertise levels. Surgeons are very good at making linear lesions and electrophysiologists at mapping for completeness and "spot welding" gaps in lines. The demonstration of the efficacy of this approach awaits the completion of trials currently underway.

References

1. Damiano RJ, Gaynor SL, Bailey M, et al. The long-term outcome of patients with coronary disease and atrial fibrillation undergoing the Cox Maze procedure. *J Thorac Cardiovasc Surg*. 2003;126.
2. Haïssaguerre M, Jaïs P, Shah DC, et al. Spontaneous initiation of atrial fibrillation by ectopic beats originating in the pulmonary veins. *N Engl J Med*. 1998;339:659-666.
3. Jaïs P, Haïssaguerre M, Shah DC, et al. A focal source of atrial fibrillation treated by discrete radiofrequency ablation. *Circulation*. 1997;95:572-576.
4. Hazel SJ, Paterson HS, Edwards JR, Maddern GJ. Surgical treatment of atrial fibrillation via energy ablation. *Circulation*. 2005;111(8):e103-e106.
5. Cox JL. Surgical treatment of atrial fibrillation: a review. *Europace*. 2004;5:20-29.
6. Haïssaguerre M, Jaïs P, Shah DC, Pradeau V, et al. Right and left atrial radiofrequency catheter therapy of parosysmal atrial fibrillation. *J Cardiovasc Electrophysiol*. 1996;7:1132-1144.
7. Wu TJ, Doshi RN, Huang HL, et al. Simultaneous biatrial computerized mapping during permanent atrial fibrillation in patients with organic heart disease. *J Cardiovasc Electrophysiol*. 2002;13:571-577.
8. Pappone C, Rosanio S, Oreto G, et al. Circumferential radiofrequency ablation of pulmonary vein ostia: a new anatomic approach for curing atrial fibrillation. *Circulation*. 2000;102:2619-2628.
9. Tilz RR, Chun KR, Schmidt B, et al. Catheter ablation of long-standing persistent atrial fibrillation: a lesson from circumferential pulmonary vein isolation. *J Cardiovasc Electrophysiol*. 2010;21(10):1085-1093.
10. Wolf RK, Schneeberger EW, Osterday R, et al. Video assisted bilateral pulmonary vein isolation and left atrial appendage exclusion for atrial fibrillation. *J Thorac Cardiovasc Surg*. 2005;130:797-802.
11. Edgerton JR, Edgerton ZJ, Weaver T, et al. Minimally invasive pulmonary vein isolation and partial autonomic denervation for surgical treatment of atrial fibrillation. *Ann Thorac Surg*. 2008;86:35-39.
12. Edgerton JR, McClelland, JH, Duke D, et al. Minimally invasive surgical ablation of atrial fibrillation: Six-month results. *J Thorac Cardiovasc Surg*. 2009;138:109-114.
13. Gillinov AM, Bhavani S, Blackstone EH, et al. Surgery for permanent atrial fibrillation: impact of patient factors and lesion set. *Ann Thorac Surg*. 2006;82:502-513.
14. Wisser W, Seebacher G, Fleck T, et al. Permanent chronic atrial fibrillation: is pulmonary vein isolation alone enough? *Ann Thorac Surg*. 2007;84:1151-1157.
15. Gillinov AM, Bhavani S, Blackstone EH, et al. Surgery for permanent atrial fibrillation: impact of patient factors and lesion set. *Ann Thorac Surg*. 2006;82:502-514.
16. Wijffels MC, Kirchhof CJ, Dorland R, et al. Electrical remodeling due to atrial fibrillation in chronically instrumented conscious goats: roles of neurohumoral changes, ischemia, atrial stretch, and high rate of electrical activation. *Circulation*. 1997;96:3710-3720.
17. Nattel S, Shiroshita-Takeshita A, Cardin S, Pelletier P. Mechanisms of atrial remodeling and clinical relevance. *Curr Opin Cardiol*. 2005;20:21-25.
18. Jeanmart H, Casselman F, Beelen R, et al. Modified maze during endoscopic mitral valve surgery: The OLV Clinic Experience. *Ann Thorac Surg*. 2006;82:1765-1769.
19. Shinbane JS, Lesh MD, Stevenson WG, et al. Anatomic and electrophysiologic relation between the coronary sinus and mitral annulus: implications for ablation of left-sided accessory pathways. *Am Heart J*. 1998;135:93-98.
20. Antz M, Otomo K, Arruda M, Scherlag BJ, Pitha J, Tondo C, Lazzara R, Jackman WM. Electrical conduction between the right atrium and the left atrium via the musculature of the coronary sinus. *Circulation*. 1998;98:1790-1795.
21. Cox JL. Atrial fibrillation II: rationale for surgical treatment. *J Thorac Cardiovasc Surg*. 2003; 126:1693-1699.
22. Jaïs P, Hocini M, Hsu L-F, et al. Technique and results of linear ablation at the mitral isthmus. *Circulation*. 2004;110:2996-3002.
23. Edgerton JR. Total thoracoscopic ablation of atrial fibrillation using the Dallas Lesion Set, partial autonomic denervation, and left atrial appendectomy. *Operative Techniques in Thoracic and Cardiovascular Surgery*. 2009;14:224-242.
24. Edgerton JR, Jackman WM, Mack MJ. A new epicardial lesion set for minimal access left atrial maze: the Dallas lesion set. *Ann Thorac Surg*. 2009;88:1655-1657.
25. Lockwood D, Nakagawa H, Peyton MD, et al. Linear left atrial lesions in minimally invasive surgical ablation of persistent atrial fibrillation: Techniques for assessing conduction block across surgical lesions. *Heart Rhythm*. 2009;6:S50-S63.
26. Edgerton JR, Jackman WR, Mahoney C, Mack MJ. Totally thoracoscopic surgical ablation of persistent AF and long-standing persistent atrial fibrillation using the "Dallas" lesion set. *Heart Rhythm*. 2009;6:S64-S70.
27. Vincenzi FF, West TC. Release of autonomic mediators in cardiac tissue by direct subthreshold electrical stimulation. *J Pharmacol Exp Ther*. 1963;141:185-194.
28. Boersma LV, Castella M, van Boven W, et al. Atrial Fibrillation Catheter Ablation Versus Surgical Ablation Treatment (FAST): A 2-Center Randomized Clinical Trial. *Circulation*. 2012;125(1):23-30.

CHAPTER 49E

Surgical Ablation for Atrial Fibrillation: Ganglionic Ablation

Rishi Arora, MD; Richard Lee, MD, MBA

Introduction

Both the extrinsic and intrinsic cardiac autonomic nervous system (ANS) innervate mammalian hearts. The extrinsic ANS is the input from the brain and spinal cord. The intrinsic ANS is composed of a complex neural network, characterized by numerous clusters of autonomic ganglia and interconnecting neurons/nerves.[1-3] Ganglionated plexi (GPs) embedded in the epicardial fat pads act as "integration centers" to modulate the autonomic interactions between the extrinsic and intrinsic ANS.[1,4,5] The anatomical location of the GPs alone raises suspicion for a role in initiation and maintenance of atrial fibrillation (AF). However, a growing body of both basic science and clinical research supports the idea that the GPs play a critical role in AF. Therefore, GPs represent a potential target for treatment and cure of AF.

This chapter reviews the basic science and clinical work investigating the role of the GPs in causing and treating AF. Subgroups of AF patients with vagal dominance and initiation of AF events during bradycardia have been well documented by Coumel and others. They are discussed elsewhere in this text and are not the subject of the current topic.

Basic Science Investigation

Complexity and Heterogeneity of the Mechanisms Underlying AF

The pathophysiology of AF is complex and multifactorial. Various mechanisms that involve remodeling at the molecular, ion-channel, gap-junction, and structural levels are thought to play roles in the creation of AF substrate.[6-10] Alterations in expression of ion channels such as I_{CaL}, I_{to}, I_{Na}, and I_{K1} have been demonstrated in experimental and/or clinical models of AF. The aforementioned changes in ion-channel expression, as well as changes in gap-junction expression,[11-13] have been shown to contribute to changes in refractoriness and conduction, that in turn contribute to AF substrate.

In addition to the contribution of ion-channel and gap-junction alterations to altered atrial refractoriness and conduction, primary structural abnormalities are also thought to play an important role in the creation of electrophysiologic substrate for AF. An important structural abnormality that has been studied extensively for its role in creating electrophysiologic abnormalities in the atrium is fibrosis.[6,14-19] The pathophysiology of fibrosis is complex and thought to be at least partially related to the inflammation and oxidative stress that are observed in the setting of AF. Several signaling pathways, including the angiotensin II and transforming growth factor-β (TGF-β) pathways,[14] have been invoked for their possible contribution to fibrotic substrate in the atria. Chronic atrial stretch has also been shown to activate pathways that may result in the creation of fibrosis. Importantly, structural abnormalities, such as stretch and fibrosis, may in turn lead to secondary alterations in the ion-channel and gap-junction expression in the atria,[20] thereby further perpetuating conditions that may be necessary for the genesis and maintenance of AF.

In addition to the above-mentioned factors, neurohumoral factors have also been invoked for their possible contribution to the creation of electrophysiologic substrate for AF.[21,22] Studies using the pacing-induced heart failure of AF—a model that results in marked fibrosis in the atria—suggest that reversal of structural, as well as ion-channel, alterations in this model does not entirely eliminate the propensity for AF. The persistent AF substrate noted in this model suggests that additional mechanisms, such as alterations in neurohumoral signaling, may be at play. An important neurohumoral factor that has been studied fairly extensively for its involvement in AF is the autonomic nervous system.

Potential Role of the Autonomic Nervous System in the Creation of Substrate for AF—Insights from Cellular, Ex-vivo, and In-vivo Data

Earlier studies suggested that exercise-induced AF may be sympathetically driven; in contrast, the parasympathetic nervous system may be contributing to AF in young patients with no structural heart disease.[23] Sympathetic activation of the heart is thought to be pro-arrhythmic by increasing both calcium (Ca^{2+}) entry and the spontaneous release of Ca^{2+} from the sarcoplasmic reticulum.[24,25] Animal studies show that vagal stimulation contributes to the genesis of AF by nonuniform shortening of atrial effective refractory periods, thereby setting up substrate for reentry. Vagal stimulation can also lead to the emergence of focal triggers in the atrium.[26] More recently, as explained below, both the parasympathetic and the sympathetic nervous system have been shown to play a role in AF. Below we discuss how the sympathetic and parasympathetic nervous systems contribute to the creation of AF substrate.

Both reentry and triggered activity have been proposed as arrhythmogenic mechanisms in the pulmonary veins (PV). Electrophysiological studies on isolated PV cardiomyocytes show that these cells possess a unique ion-channel profile.[27,28] PV myocytes appear to have the ability to sustain automatic as well as triggered activity, especially in the presence of b-adrenergic stimulation.[27] Since b-adrenergic/Gs signaling enhances If and ICa-L, the presence of these currents in PV myocytes suggests their possible involvement in atrial arrhythmogenesis. The PVs are also very sensitive to vagal stimulation.[29] Given that muscarinic (M2)–Gi signaling attenuates If and activates IK-ACh, the presence of IK-ACh in PV myocytes[30] further suggests roles for these currents in the genesis of atrial arrhythmias. Indeed, the presence of constitutively active IK-ACh (IKH) in PV myocytes in the setting of AF indicates a role for IK-ACh in shortening atrial refractoriness even in the absence of vagal stimulation.[30]

Recent studies also indicate that abnormal calcium (Ca^{2+}) regulation may underlie PV arrhythmogenic activity. Both b-adrenergic as well as cholinergic stimulation appear to create conditions for enhanced calcium release in the PVs, with resulting substrate for triggered activity. For example, Honjo et al[31] have demonstrated enhanced isoproterenol-mediated ectopic activity within myocardial sleeves of the PVs in the presence of ryanodine; this ectopic activity is attenuated by the inhibition of sodium–calcium exchanger (NCX). More recent studies suggest that a rise in Cai precedes the upstroke in Vm at the site of focal PV discharge.[32] Thus, spontaneous Cai release in the PV muscle sleeves may induce triggered activity—especially given PV myocytes have a less-negative resting membrane potential than LA myocytes. In related studies, Patterson et al propose that the elevated Cai drives INCX (inward) in the absence of significant outward (repolarizing) membrane currents, initiating an early after-depolarization (EAD) and triggered arrhythmia.[33]

The intact PVs (and the surrounding posterior left atrium [PLA]) also demonstrate a unique electrophysiological profile. Using high-resolution optical mapping, we have recently described marked heterogeneity of conduction and repolarization in normal canine PVs, with demonstration of substrate for functional reentry.[34] In these experiments, microreentry within the PVs could be sustained only in the presence of isoproterenol or acetylcholine, indicating that although substrate for reentry exists within normal PVs, it is not sufficient to allow the emergence of sustained focal "drivers" in the baseline state. Other conditions, including sympathomimetic or cholinergic stimulation, therefore appear to be necessary to promote development of sustained focal activity in the PVs.

In vivo animal data also suggest that these PV foci appear to be at least partially modulated by the autonomic nervous system, with sympathetic stimulation (eg, with isoproterenol) being frequently utilized to "bring out" these triggers in clinical studies. Clinical studies have demonstrated a change in sympathetic–parasympathetic balance, measured by heart-rate variability, after ablation of PV triggers.[35] Several investigators have also noted significant Bezold-Jarisch-like reflexes during radiofrequency ablation of the PV tissues.[36] More recently, Pappone et al have suggested that altering vagal input to the left atrium and the PVs, as measured by the elimination of vagal reflexes on PV stimulation, may improve efficacy of ablation procedures for AF.[37]

The greater ability of vagal maneuvers or cholinergic drugs to cause AF in normal dogs, as compared to sympathetic stimulation alone,[38] and the heightened vagal responses observed during PV stimulation/ablation suggest that vagal innervation may indeed be a key player in the genesis of focal AF (at least in normal hearts). Sharifov et al showed that although acetylcholine alone could induce AF in all the dogs that were studied, acetylcholine-induced AF was facilitated by isoproterenol, which decreased the concentration of acetylcholine required for AF induction and maintenance.[38] The physiology studies conducted by Patterson et al[39-41] further suggest that adrenergic influences may be playing an important modulatory role in creating adequate substrate for AF, helping provide a necessary "catalyst" for the emergence of focal drivers in the presence of an increased vagal tone. In their proposed model, Patterson et al[40] suggest that Ca^{2+} transient triggering can generate rapid discharges under conditions in which atrial repolarization is abbreviated by the activation of IKAch (eg, by vagal stimulation) and the Ca^{2+} transient is augmented by b-adrenergic stimulation. The synergism between the two limbs of the autonomic nervous system in the creation of AF substrate is supported by our recent data, where we have shown that parasympathetic and sympathetic nerves are colocalized in the atrium[42] and that vagal responsiveness is altered in the setting of β-blockade.[29]

Recent studies suggest that the autonomic nervous system may also be playing a role in the genesis of AF in diseased hearts. Jayachandran et al demonstrated a heterogeneous increase in sympathetic innervation in the atria in dogs subjected to rapid atrial pacing for prolonged periods of time.[43] Ogawa et al[44] have recently shown increased sympathetic and vagal nerve discharge prior to the onset of atrial arrhythmias in dogs with pacing-induced congestive heart failure. There is also evidence of sympathetic hyperinnervation in patients with AF.[45] Studies from our own laboratory indicate increased sympathetic as well as parasympathetic nerve growth in the atria of dogs with pacing-induced congestive heart failure.[46] This nerve growth is accompanied by an increase in downstream signaling molecules involved in both the sympathetic and parasympathetic signaling cascade

Peculiar Autonomic Innervation of the Pulmonary Veins and Posterior Left Atrium

Elegant studies by Armour and Randall several years ago demonstrated the presence of an intricate pattern of autonomic innervation in the heart.[47-49] Armour et al[3] showed that autonomic nerves were concentrated in GPs around great vessels such as the PVs, with the atria being innervated by at least 5 major atrial fat pads, most of which were located on the posterior surface of the atria. More recently, Hou et al[4,50] suggested the presence of an intricate, interconnecting neural network in the left atrium that may contribute to substrate for focal AF. A recent human study described heterogeneity of nerve distribution in the region of the pulmonary veins and surrounding left atrium.[51] Regional heterogeneity of nerve distribution could contribute to heterogeneity in conduction velocity and refractoriness, which in turn may create substrate for AF.

We compared the distribution and physiology of sympathetic and parasympathetic nerves among the PVs and the rest of the left atrium.[52] The PLA was the most richly innervated with nerve bundles containing parasympathetic and sympathetic fibers (see Figure 49E.1); nerve bundles were located in fibrofatty tissue as well as in surrounding myocardium. Parasympathetic predominated over sympathetic fibers within bundles.

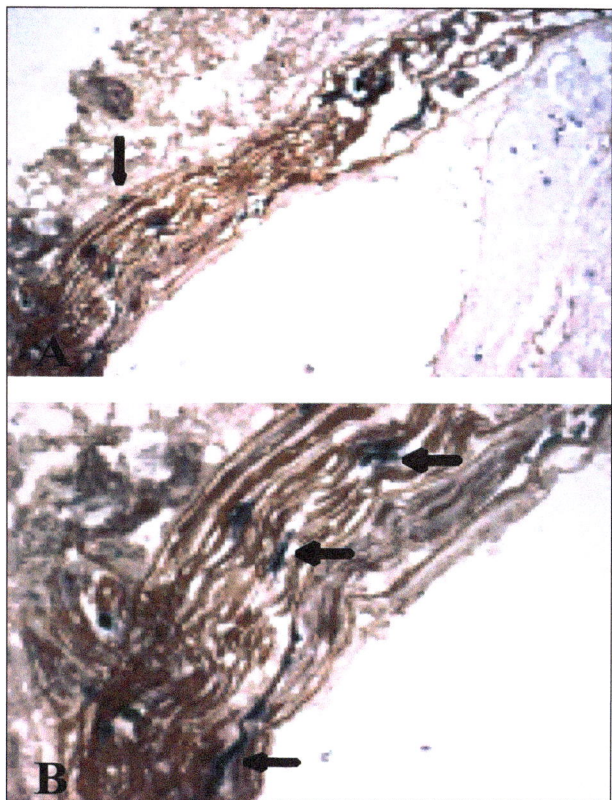

Figure 49E.1 A single nerve trunk/bundle in the left atrium. **Panels A and B** are at 10× and 40×, respectively, and are double stained for parasympathetic nerves (**stained brown**) and sympathetic nerves (**stained blue; arrows**). *Source:* Arora R, Ulphani JS, Villuendas R, et al.[42]

M2-receptor distribution was also most pronounced in the posterior left atrium. Following application of tropicamide—a muscarinic receptor blocker—to the PLA, vagal-induced shortening of the effective refractory period (ERP) was significantly attenuated not just in the PLA but also remotely from the site of application in the PVs and the left atrial appendage. In a related study, we discovered a particularly high concentration of parasympathetic fibers in the ligament of Marshall.[53] The ligament of Marshall could be traced back to a major branch of the left cervical vagus nerve. Ablation of the ligament of Marshall led to an attenuation of vagal-induced ERP shortening in the left-sided PVs and the PLA.

Related data from our laboratory shows differences in autonomic responsiveness between the PVs, the PLA, and the rest of the left atrium.[29] In response to vagal stimulation, we demonstrated a greater decrease in refractory periods in the PVs and PLA as compared to the rest of the left atrium. This heterogeneity of vagal responses was found to correlate with differences in the pattern of distribution of IKAch in each of the regions studied. We also discovered that with vagal stimulation and/or β-blockade, there was evidence of regional conduction delay in the PVs with a significant change in activation direction. Similar activation changes were not seen in the PLA and left atrial appendage.

Clinical Evidence

The clinical evidence of the role that the autonomic ganglia (AG) play in atrial fibrillation lags behind the basic science evidence. However, the data continue to grow in support of an integral role.

Catheter Ablation

One of the earliest reports was limited to an abstract evaluating 26 consecutive patients in persistent/chronic AF refractory to 2 or more antiarrhythmic drugs.[54] GP sites were identified by a 20% increase in R-R interval and ablated. The PVs were not electrically isolated. At a median of 6-month follow-up, 84% of patients remained in sinus rhythm. Since that time, the standard definition of a positive response has shifted to AV block, asystole, or an increase in R-R interval of at least 50%. However, Verma et al demonstrated that pulmonary vein isolation effectively eliminates preprocedurally identified AG in both first time a repeat ablation patients.[55] The suggestion is that an anatomical approach eliminates the AG and any role that they may play in AF.

As enthusiasm for GPs has grown, some authors have recommended identifying and ablating GPs prior to anatomical PV isolation.[56] In a series of 83 patients, a success rate of 86% was reported with a mean follow-up of 86% using this approach. In a series of 297 patients, Pappone et al found that complete vagal denervation, along with the percentage of left atrial isolation, were the only predictors of AF recurrence at 12 months.[37]

At the same time that support has grown for the GP ablation, an appreciation for complex fractionated atrial electrograms (CFAEs) in AF has grown, and CFAEs have become independent targets for treatment.[57,58] However, there is some data suggesting that the CFAEs are linked to the GPs.

In a series of 32 patients, Katritsis et al mapped CFAEs at sites where GPs are commonly located.[59] In nearly 70% of patients, CFAEs were identified at the GP sites. In the remaining 11 patients, only 1 had a CFAE on the atrial wall, suggestion that a correlation exists between the two entities. The authors recommended initiation of CFAE ablation at the GP sites.[59]

Although the majority of reports support GP ablation in AF, there is some disagreement. In a small study of 18 patients with vagal-mediated AF, 17 of 18 patients still had inducible AF after successful GP ablation.[60] Furthermore, in a reproduction of the Platt study,[54] Lemery found only a 50% success after ablation of the GPs alone.[61,62] In addition, Pokusalov et al reported only a 38.2% success rate at two years in patient who underwent GP ablation alone.[63]

Although there is still a great deal of uncertainty of the role of the GP in catheter ablation, more evidence suggests that there will continue to be a role in the future. The long-term durability of GP ablation, as well as the role of GP ablation as stand-alone therapy, remain areas for future investigation.

Surgical Ablation

Since the GPs are epicardial structures, it makes some sense that they should be targets in the surgical treatment of the disease. However, historically, AF surgery has been strictly based on an anatomic approach. The classic cut-and-sew Maze procedure has long been the gold standard for the treatment of AF, successfully restoring sinus rhythm at rates above 90%.[64] The original technique actually created the lines of block by cutting the atrial tissue and sewing it back together, which anatomically obliterates any potential reentrant circuit. However, in the original procedure, virtually every GP is destroyed as a byproduct. Probably for this reason, the GPs have been virtually ignored in the open procedure.

In the current era, the vast majority of Maze procedures are performed with the new ablation technologies, such as bipolar radiofrequency ablation or cryothermia.[65-67] These technologies allow the scars of the Maze to be created without dividing the tissue, yet usually leaves the areas of the GPs structurally intact. In general, although the outcomes remain excellent with this approach, most reports suggest slightly less favorable outcomes than previous reports.[68-71] Limited data suggest that the GPs may play a role. One report by Isomura suggests an improvement in the rate of sinus rhythm restoration from 75% to 88% when identification and ablation of the GPs are added to the Maze lesion set when using alternate energy sources.[72] In addition, in patients undergoing the Maze with bipolar radiofrequency ablation, Onorati et al reported an increase in success from 52% to 83% in patients that received an additional dissection and excision of the GPs.[73] However, most reports suggest success above 80% without intervening on the GPs.[64,74] Although there may be some residual autonomic effects, innervation is clearly disrupted after the Maze.[75] However, the denervation may not be sustained, and reinnervation may occur over time.[76] More investigation needs to be done.

Most of the work on GPs in the surgical literature has been produced during minimally invasive pulmonary vein isolation via small bilateral thoracotomies. In this procedure, in addition to a pulmonary vein ablation, GPs are routinely tested and ablated when positive.[77-80]

There have been two GP maps described with minimally invasive surgery.[77,81] The one we favor is an anatomical one that tests medially and laterally above the PVs, at the veins, and below (Figure 49E.2).

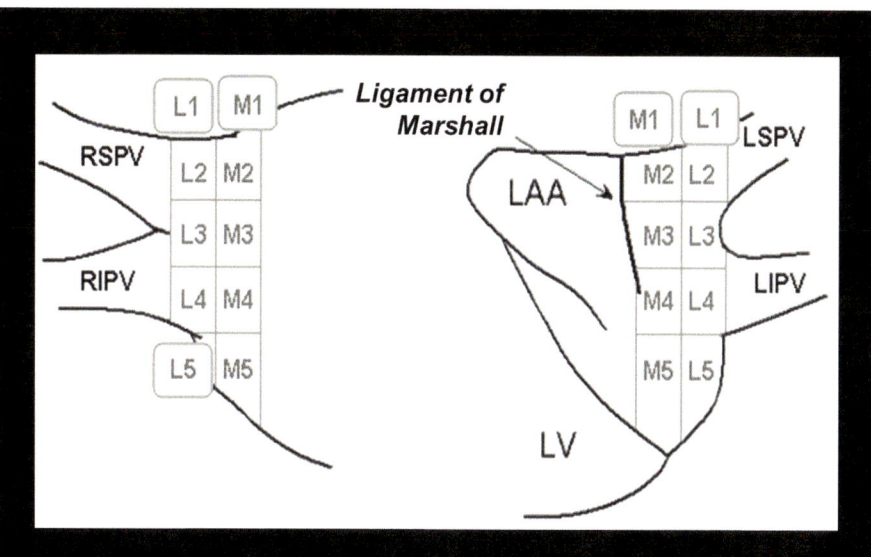
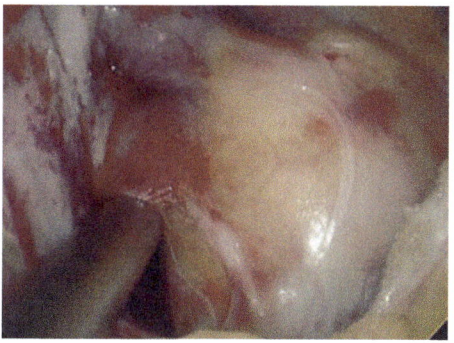
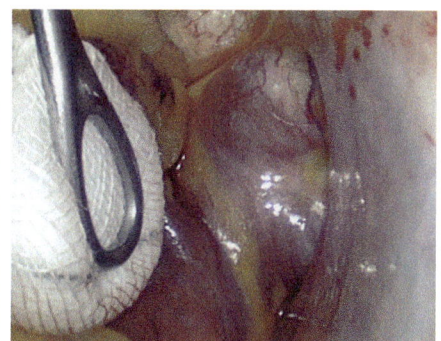

Figure 49E.2 The illustration demonstrates the 10 functional areas tested for active GPs (5 medial, 5 lateral) in each set of pulmonary veins. The pictures demonstrate the in-vivo view of the right (**left picture**) and left (**right picture**) pulmonary veins and location of the GPs.

In a series of 41 patients, active GPs, defined as sites with an increase in R-R interval of greater than 50% (Figure 49E.3), were found in all patients undergoing minimally invasive surgery for AF. Active sites were found bilaterally in 24 and unilaterally in 17, with a mean of 5 GPs on the right and 2.7 on the left. More than 50% had active sites on the right along the atrioventricular groove and the ligament of Marshall.[81]

Circumferential "island" creation around the PVs are effective at elimination of the GPs, and in one series was effective in elimination of 79% of GP activity.[82] This has led most minimally invasive AF surgeons to add GP ablation as a routine part of their procedure.[77-80]

In a recent report, Katrisis and coworkers undertook a randomized clinical trial of catheter ablation in 242 patients with paroxysmal and persistent AF using a circumferential pulmonary vein isolation (PVI) technique and compared it to left atrial ganglionic plexus ablation (LGP) alone or the two techniques in combination.[83] In this report, rhythm control was achieved in 56%, 48%, and 74% patients in the PVI, LGP, and PVI + LGP groups, respectively ($P = 0.004$). PVI + LGP ablation strategy compared with PVI alone yielded a hazard ratio of 0.53 (95% confidence interval: 0.31 to 0.91; $P = 0.022$) for recurrence of AF or atrial tachycardia. In a surgical ablation series, Zheng et al studied 139 patients with

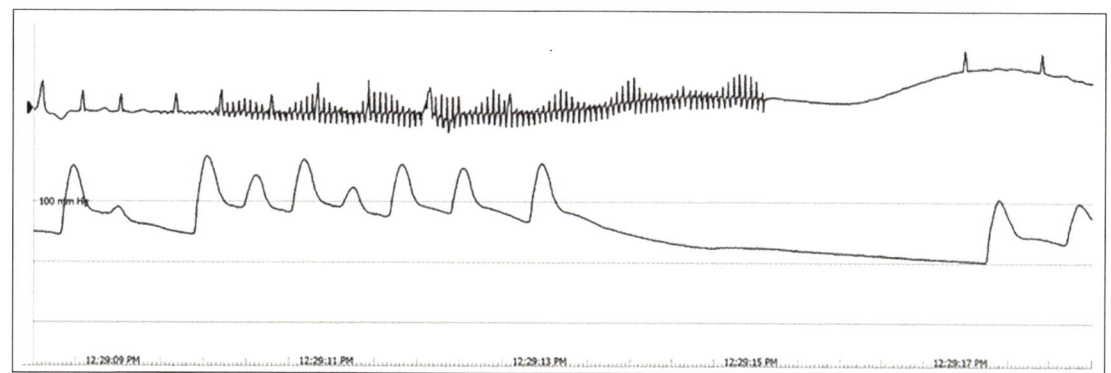

Figure 49E.3 This demonstrates a positive ganglionic plexus. Direct pacing of the area resulted in a period of asystole.

paroxysmal and persistent AF, with PVI and GP ablation. The success rate of minimally invasive surgical PVI with GP ablation was 51.8% for paroxysmal AF, 28.2% for persistent AF, and 28.6% for long-standing, persistent AF after initial procedure. Patients with AF duration of less than 24 months, left atrial diameter < 40 mm, and no early recurrences of AF had more favorable outcomes.[84]

Both types of approaches to GP ablation suggest an inherent efficacy and a potential additive value to the standard PVI approach. However, concern exists regarding the occurrence of parasympathetic reinnervation of the ganglia that could result in attrition of efficacy. Canine studies show parasympathetic reinnervation of the atrium occurring in relatively short periods of a few weeks after GP ablation.[85] This results in restoration of the electrophysiologic effects seen with thoracic nerve stimulation. However, the intra-atrial effects of such reinnervation are still unclear. Experimental studies indicate that vagus nerve stimulation in canines involves biatrial atrial neural pathways in its effects.[86] Sympathetic reinnervation has been widely demonstrated after myocardial infarction or even after cardiac transplant. Such recovery could potentially limit the initial benefit or result in attrition of long-term benefit of this procedure as a stand-alone intervention or as an added-on procedure to established techniques such as the Cox-Maze procedure.

Conclusion

The autonomic nervous system clearly plays a role in the initiation and maintenance of AF. We have great insight into the extent and mechanism of the influence of the GPs, but the complete picture remains unclear. Further investigation, both in basic science and clinical research, should provide a clearer view. Inevitably, modulation of the GPs will play a role in a more effective treatment of AF in the future.

References

1. Lin J, Scherlag BJ, Niu G, et al. Autonomic elements within the ligament of Marshall and inferior left ganglionated plexus mediate functions of the atrial neural network. *J Cardiovasc Electrophysiol*. 2009;20:318-324.
2. Ardell J. Structure and function of mammalian intrinsic cardiac neurons. In: Armour J, Ardell J, eds. *Neurocardiology*, 2nd ed. New York: Oxford University Press; 1994:95-114.
3. Armour JA, Murphy DA, Yuan BX, Macdonald S, Hopkins DA. Gross and microscopic anatomy of the human intrinsic cardiac nervous system. *Anat Rec*. 1997;247:289-298.
4. Hou Y, Scherlag BJ, Lin J, et al. Interactive atrial neural network: Determining the connections between ganglionated plexi. *Heart Rhythm*. 2007;4:56-63.
5. Lin J, Scherlag BJ, Lu Z, et al. Inducibility of atrial and ventricular arrhythmias along the ligament of Marshall: role of autonomic factors. *J Cardiovasc Electrophysiol*. 2008;19:955-962.
6. Burstein B, Nattel S. Atrial fibrosis: mechanisms and clinical relevance in atrial fibrillation. *J Am Coll Cardiol*. 2008;51:802-809.
7. Burstein B, Nattel S. Atrial structural remodeling as an antiarrhythmic target. *J Cardiovasc Pharm*. 2008;52(1):4-10.
8. Nattel S. Defining "culprit mechanisms" in arrhythmogenic cardiac remodeling. *Circulation*. 2004;94:1403-1405.
9. Nattel S, Shiroshita-Takeshita A, Brundel BJ, Rivard L. Mechanisms of atrial fibrillation: lessons from animal models. *Prog Cardiovasc Dis*. 2005;48:9-28.
10. Nattel S, Shiroshita-Takeshita A, Cardin S, Pelletier P. Mechanisms of atrial remodeling and clinical relevance. *Curr Opin Cardiol*. 2005;20:21-25.
11. Gollob MH. Cardiac connexins as candidate genes for idiopathic atrial fibrillation. *Curr Opin Cardiol*. 2006;21:155-158.
12. Gollob MH, Jones DL, Krahn AD, et al. Somatic mutations in the connexin 40 gene (GJA5) in atrial fibrillation. *N Engl J Med*. 2006;354:2677-2688.
13. Guerra JM, Everett TH 4th, Lee KW, Wilson E, Olgin JE. Effects of the gap junction modifier rotigaptide (ZP123) on atrial conduction and vulnerability to atrial fibrillation. *Circulation*. 2006;114:110-118.
14. Cardin S, Li D, Thorin-Trescases N, Leung TK, Thorin E, Nattel S. Evolution of the atrial fibrillation substrate in experimental congestive heart failure: angiotensin-dependent and -independent pathways. *Cardiovasc Res*. 2003;60:315-325.
15. Shinagawa K, Li D, Leung TK, Nattel S. Consequences of atrial tachycardia-induced remodeling depend on the preexisting atrial substrate. *Circulation*. 2002;105:251-257.
16. Shi Y, Li D, Tardif JC, Nattel S. Enalapril effects on atrial remodeling and atrial fibrillation in experimental congestive heart failure. *Cardiovasc Res*. 2002;54:456-461.
17. Li D, Shinagawa K, Pang L, et al. Effects of angiotensin-converting enzyme inhibition on the development of the atrial fibrillation substrate in dogs with ventricular tachypacing-induced congestive heart failure. *Circulation*. 2001;104:2608-2614.
18. Li D, Melnyk P, Feng J, et al. Effects of experimental heart failure on atrial cellular and ionic electrophysiology. *Circulation*. 2000;101:2631-2638.
19. Li D, Fareh S, Leung TK, Nattel S. Promotion of atrial fibrillation by heart failure in dogs: atrial remodeling of a different sort. *Circulation*. 1999;100:87-95.
20. Cha TJ, Ehrlich JR, Zhang L, Nattel S. Atrial ionic remodeling induced by atrial tachycardia in the presence of congestive heart failure. *Circulation*. 2004;110:1520-1526.
21. Olshansky B. Interrelationships between the autonomic nervous system and atrial fibrillation. *Prog Cardiovasc Dis*. 2005;48:57-78.
22. Parthenakis FI, Patrianakos AP, Skalidis EI, et al. Atrial fibrillation is associated with increased neurohumoral activation and reduced exercise tolerance in patients with non-ischemic dilated cardiomyopathy. *Int J Cardiol*. 2007;118:206-214.
23. Chen PS, Tan AY. Autonomic nerve activity and atrial fibrillation. *Heart Rhythm*. 2007;4:S61-S64.
24. Bers DM. Cardiac excitation-contraction coupling. *Nature*. 2002;415:198-205.
25. Ter Keurs HE, Boyden PA. Calcium and arrhythmogenesis. *Physiol Rev*. 2007;87:457-506.
26. Nemirovsky D, Hutter R, Gomes JA. The electrical substrate of vagal atrial fibrillation as assessed by the signal-averaged electrocardiogram of the P wave. *Pacing Clin Electrophysiol*. 2008;31:308-313.
27. Chen YJ, Chen SA, Chen YC, et al. Effects of rapid atrial pacing on the arrhythmogenic activity of single

cardiomyocytes from pulmonary veins: implication in initiation of atrial fibrillation. *Circulation.* 2001;104:2849-2854.
28. Melnyk P, Ehrlich JR, Pourrier M, Villeneuve L, Cha TJ, Nattel S. Comparison of ion channel distribution and expression in cardiomyocytes of canine pulmonary veins versus left atrium. *Cardiovasc Research.* 2005;65:104-116.
29. Arora R, Ng J, Ulphani J, et al. Unique autonomic profile of the pulmonary veins and posterior left atrium. *J Am Coll Cardiol.* 2007;49:1340-1348.
30. Ehrlich JR, Cha TJ, Zhang L, et al. Characterization of a hyperpolarization-activated time-dependent potassium current in canine cardiomyocytes from pulmonary vein myocardial sleeves and left atrium. *J Physiol.* 2004;557:583-597.
31. Honjo H, Boyett MR, Niwa R, et al. Pacing-induced spontaneous activity in myocardial sleeves of pulmonary veins after treatment with ryanodine. *Circulation.* 2003;107:1937-1943.
32. Chou CC, Nihei M, Zhou S, et al. Intracellular calcium dynamics and anisotropic reentry in isolated canine pulmonary veins and left atrium. *Circulation.* 2005;111:2889-2897.
33. Patterson E, Po SS, Scherlag BJ, Lazzara R. Triggered firing in pulmonary veins initiated by in vitro autonomic nerve stimulation. *Heart Rhythm.* 2005;2:624-631.
34. Arora R, Verheule S, Scott L, et al. Arrhythmogenic substrate of the pulmonary veins assessed by high-resolution optical mapping. *Circulation.* 2003;107:1816-1821.
35. Hsieh MH, Chiou CW, Wen ZC, et al. Alterations of heart rate variability after radiofrequency catheter ablation of focal atrial fibrillation originating from pulmonary veins. *Circulation.* 1999;100:2237-2243.
36. Tsai CF, Chen SA, Tai CT, et al. Bezold-Jarisch-like reflex during radiofrequency ablation of the pulmonary vein tissues in patients with paroxysmal focal atrial fibrillation. *J Cardiovasc Electrophysiol.* 1999;10:27-35.
37. Pappone C, Santinelli V, Manguso F, et al. Pulmonary vein denervation enhances long-term benefit after circumferential ablation for paroxysmal atrial fibrillation. *Circulation.* 2004;109:327-334.
38. Sharifov OF, Fedorov VV, Beloshapko GG, Glukhov AV, Yushmanova AV, Rosenshtraukh LV. Roles of adrenergic and cholinergic stimulation in spontaneous atrial fibrillation in dogs. *J Am Coll Cardiol.* 2004;43:483-490.
39. Patterson E, Lazzara R, Szabo B, et al. Sodium-calcium exchange initiated by the Ca^{2+} transient: an arrhythmia trigger within pulmonary veins. *J Am Coll Cardiol.* 2006;47:1196-1206.
40. Patterson E, Po SS, Scherlag BJ, Lazzara R. Triggered firing in pulmonary veins initiated by in vitro autonomic nerve stimulation. *Heart Rhythm.* 2005;2:624-631.
41. Patterson E, Yu X, Huang S, Garrett M, Kem DC. Suppression of autonomic-mediated triggered firing in pulmonary vein preparations, 24 hours postcoronary artery ligation in dogs. *J Cardiovasc Electrophysiol.* 2006;17:763-770.
42. Arora R, Ulphani JS, Villuendas R, et al. Neural substrate for atrial fibrillation: implications for targeted parasympathetic blockade in the posterior left atrium. *Am J Physiol Heart Circ Physiol.* 2008;294:H134-H144.
43. Jayachandran JV, Sih HJ, Winkle W, Zipes DP, Hutchins GD, Olgin JE. Atrial fibrillation produced by prolonged rapid atrial pacing is associated with heterogeneous changes in atrial sympathetic innervation. *Circulation.* 2000;101:1185-1191.
44. Ogawa M, Zhou S, Tan AY, et al. Left stellate ganglion and vagal nerve activity and cardiac arrhythmias in ambulatory dogs with pacing-induced congestive heart failure. *J Am Coll Cardiol.* 2007;50:335-343.
45. Hamabe A, Chang CM, Zhou S, et al. Induction of atrial fibrillation and nerveسprouting by prolonged left atrial pacing in dogs. *Pacing Clin Electrophysiol.* 2003;26:2247-2252.
46. Belin RJ, Mottl S, Goldstein J, et al. Molecular Basis for sympathetic remodeling in the left atrium in the ventricular tachypacing canine model of congestive heart failure [abstract]. *Circulation.* 2007;116:II-251.
47. Armour JA, Randall WC. Functional anatomy of canine cardiac nerves. *Acta Anat.* 1975;91:510-528.
48. Randall WC, Armour JA, Geis WP, Lippincott DB. Regional cardiac distribution of the sympathetic nerves. *Fed Proc.* 1972;31:1199-1208.
49. Armour JA, Hageman GR, Randall WC. Arrhythmias induced by local cardiac nerve stimulation. *Am J Physiol.* 1972;223:1068-1075.
50. Hou Y, Scherlag BJ, Lin J, et al. Ganglionated plexi modulate extrinsic cardiac autonomic nerve input: effects on sinus rate, atrioventricular conduction, refractoriness, and inducibility of atrial fibrillation. *J Am Coll Cardiol.* 2007;50:61-68.
51. Chevalier P, Tabib A, Meyronnet D, et al. Quantitative study of nerves of the human left atrium. *Heart Rhythm.* 2005;2:518-522.
52. Arora R, Ulphani JS, Villuendas R, et al. Neural substrate for atrial fibrillation: implications for targeted parasympathetic blockade in the posterior left atrium. *Am J Physiol Heart Circ Physiol.* 2008;294:H134-H144.
53. Ulphani JS, Arora R, Cain JH, et al. The ligament of Marshall as a parasympathetic conduit. *Am J Physiol Heart Circ Physiol.* 2007;293:H1629-H1635.
54. Platt M, Mandapati R, Scherlag B, et al. Limiting the number and extent of radiofrequency applications to terminate atrial fibrillation and subsequently prevent its inducibility [abstract]. *Heart Rhythm.* 2004;1:IS-II.
55. Verma A, Saliba WI, Lakkireddy D, et al. Vagal responses induced by endocardial left atrial autonomic ganglion stimulation before and after pulmonary vein antrum isolation for atrial fibrillation. *Heart Rhythm.* 2007;4:1177-1182.
56. Po SS, Nakagawa H, Jackman WM. Localization of left atrial ganglionated plexi in patients with atrial fibrillation. *J Cardiovasc Electrophysiol.* 2009;20:1186-1189.
57. Nademanee K, McKenzie J, Kosar E, et al. A new approach for catheter ablation of atrial fibrillation: mapping of the electrophysiologic substrate. *J Am Coll Cardiol.* 2004;43:2044-2053.
58. Nademanee K, Lockwood E, Oketani N, Gidney B. Catheter ablation of atrial fibrillation guided by complex fractionated atrial electrogram mapping of atrial fibrillation substrate. *J Cardiol.* 2010;55:1-12.
59. Katritsis D, Giazitzoglou E, Sougiannis D, Voridis E, Po SS. Complex fractionated atrial electrograms at anatomic sites of ganglionated plexi in atrial fibrillation. *Europace.* 2009;11:308-315.
60. Danik S, Neuzil P, d'Avila A, et al. Evaluation of catheter ablation of periatrial ganglionic plexi in patients with atrial fibrillation. *Am J Cardiol.* 2008;102:578-583.
61. Pokushalov E. The role of autonomic denervation during catheter ablation of atrial fibrillation. *Curr Opin Cardiol.* 2008;23:55-59.
62. Lemery R, Birnie D, Tang AS, Green M, Gollob M. Feasibility study of endocardial mapping of ganglionated plexuses during catheter ablation of atrial fibrillation. *Heart Rhythm.* 2006;3:387-396.
63. Pokushalov E, Romanov A, Artyomenko S, et al. Ganglionated plexi ablation for longstanding persistent atrial fibrillation. *Europace.* 2010;12:342-346.

64. McCarthy PM, Kruse J, Shalli S, et al. Where does atrial fibrillation surgery fail? Implications for increasing effectiveness of ablation. *J Thorac Cardiovasc Surg.* 2010;139:860-867.
65. Gammie JS, Laschinger JC, Brown JM, et al. A multi-institutional experience with the CryoMaze procedure. *Ann Thorac Surg.* 2005;80:876-880; discussion 80.
66. Gillinov AM, McCarthy PM, Blackstone EH, et al. Bipolar radiofrequency to ablate atrial fibrillation in patients undergoing mitral valve surgery. *Heart Surg Forum.* 2004;7:E147-E152.
67. Gaynor SL, Diodato MD, Prasad SM, et al. A prospective, single-center clinical trial of a modified Cox Maze procedure with bipolar radiofrequency ablation. *J Thorac Cardiovasc Surg.* 2004;128:535-542.
68. Srivastava V, Kumar S, Javali S, et al. Efficacy of three different ablative procedures to treat atrial fibrillation in patients with valvular heart disease: a randomised trial. *Heart Lung Circ.* 2008;17:232-240.
69. Jessurun ER, van Hemel NM, Defauw JJ, et al. A randomized study of combining maze surgery for atrial fibrillation with mitral valve surgery. *J Cardiovasc Surg (Torino).* 2003;44:9-18.
70. Khargi K, Deneke T, Haardt H, et al. Saline-irrigated, cooled-tip radiofrequency ablation is an effective technique to perform the maze procedure. *Ann Thorac Surg.* 2001;72:S1090-1095.
71. de Lima GG, Kalil RA, Leiria TL, et al. Randomized study of surgery for patients with permanent atrial fibrillation as a result of mitral valve disease. *Ann Thorac Surg.* 2004;77:2089-2094; discussion 2094-2095.
72. Isomura T, Hoshino J, Fukada Y, et al. Surgical treatment for atrial fibrillation using ablation devices and ablation of autonomic ganglion plexi. *Kyobu Geka.* 2010;63:303-307.
73. Onorati F, Curcio A, Santarpino G, et al. Routine ganglionic plexi ablation during Maze procedure improves hospital and early follow-up results of mitral surgery. *J Thorac Cardiovasc Surg.* 2008;136:408-418.
74. Prasad SM, Maniar HS, Camillo CJ, et al. The Cox Maze III procedure for atrial fibrillation: long-term efficacy in patients undergoing lone versus concomitant procedures. *J Thorac Cardiovasc Surg.* 2003;126:1822-1828.
75. Lall SC, Melby SJ, Voeller RK, et al. The effect of ablation technology on surgical outcomes after the Cox-Maze procedure: a propensity analysis. *J Thorac Cardiovasc Surg.* 2007;133:389-396.
76. Mabuchi M, Imamura M, Kubo N, et al. Sympathetic denervation and reinnervation after the maze procedure. *J Nucl Med.* 2005;46:1089-1094.
77. Beyer E, Lee R, Lam BK. Point: Minimally invasive bipolar radiofrequency ablation of lone atrial fibrillation: early multicenter results. *J Thorac Cardiovasc Surg.* 2009;137:521-526.
78. Edgerton JR, Brinkman WT, Weaver T, et al. Pulmonary vein isolation and autonomic denervation for the management of paroxysmal atrial fibrillation by a minimally invasive surgical approach. *J Thorac Cardiovasc Surg.* 2010;140:823-828.
79. Han FT, Kasirajan V, Kowalski M, et al. Results of a minimally invasive surgical pulmonary vein isolation and ganglionic plexi ablation for atrial fibrillation: single-center experience with 12-month follow-up. *Circ Arrhythm Electrophysiol.* 2009;2:370-377.
80. Sirak J, Jones D, Sun B, Sai-Sudhakar C, Crestanello J, Firstenberg M. Toward a definitive, totally thoracoscopic procedure for atrial fibrillation. *Ann Thorac Surg.* 2008;86:1960-1964.
81. Mehall JR, Kohut RM Jr, Schneeberger EW, Taketani T, Merrill WH, Wolf RK. Intraoperative epicardial electrophysiologic mapping and isolation of autonomic ganglionic plexi. *Ann Thorac Surg.* 2007;83:538-541.
82. McClelland JH, Duke D, Reddy R. Preliminary results of a limited thoracotomy: new approach to treat atrial fibrillation. *J Cardiovasc Electrophysiol.* 2007;18:1289-1295.
83. Katrisis D, Pokushalov E, Romanov A, et al. Autonomic denervation added to pulmonary vein isolation for paroxysmal atrial fibrillationa randomized clinical trial. *J Am Coll Cardiol.* 2013;62(24):2318-2325.
84. Zheng S, Li Y, Han J, Zhang H, Zeng W, et al. Long-term results of a minimally invasive surgical pulmonary vein isolation and ganglionic plexi ablation for atrial fibrillation. *PLoS ONE.* 2013;9(1):10.1371.
85. Sakamoto SC, Schuessler R, Anson ML, Aziz A, Lall SC, Damiano RJ Jr. Vagal denervation and reinnervation after ablation of ganglioniated plexi. *J Thorac Cardiovasc Surg.* 2010;139:444-452.
86. Moss E, Cardinal R, Yin Y, Page P. Bilateral atrial ganglionic plexus involvement in atrial responses to left-sided plexus stimulation in canines. *Cardiovasc Res.* 2013;99(1):194-202.

CHAPTER 49F

Surgical Ablation for Atrial Fibrillation: Hybrid Atrial Fibrillation Procedures

Mark La Meir, MD, PhD; Laurent Pison, MD, PhD

Introduction

A cardiac hybrid procedure combines the treatment options available in the catheterization room with those available in the operating room. The purpose of this collaboration is to improve patient outcome by providing knowledge and technical skills of both the cardiologist and the cardiac surgeon. One of the areas in which hybrid approaches are currently being developed is in treatment of atrial fibrillation (AF). The key requirement for a successful hybrid AF program is structural communication. In the majority of AF centers, a heart team comprised of electrophysiologists (EPs) and cardiac surgeons does not exist. The electrophysiologist is the rhythm expert who has an important patient population to treat and has sophisticated mapping systems to improve the quality of endocardial ablations. Cardiac surgeons don't have sufficient numbers of lone AF patients to treat and don't have access to intraoperative mapping. This makes surgery for lone AF rare and rather elementary. But, the surgeon has one major advantage in that surgical techniques are not as limited as EP techniques by the vascular access, and therefore the surgeon potentially has a better choice of ablation tools.

If we understand and accept these differences, how can we design a procedure that will give an optimal patient outcome—an outcome that not only should be measured by the success rate of the procedure, but also by its complication rate?

The idea of performing a combined procedure has been published.[1-3] Furthermore, the utility of an epicardial touch-up to complete electrical isolation of an atrial lesion or to ablate vagal nerve endings has been described.[4,5] In a small study, a percutaneous epicardial catheter ablation (PECA) was successfully performed in 4 repeat-ablation procedures of persistent AF and 1 of permanent AF.[6] Based on their experience, the authors concluded that the ideal PECA candidates are patients who need repeat-ablation procedures with a high risk for pulmonary vein stenosis as well as patients with a history of a failed endocardial ablation (because the epicardial tissue at the junction between the left atrial appendage (LAA) and the left-sided pulmonary veins are covered with a myocardial layer, unlike the pulmonary veins). Other potential candidates for PECA are patients requiring a difficult transseptal puncture during a repeat procedure or patients with a suspicious left atrial mass. A hybrid PECA could avoid thromboembolism by limiting the endocardial manipulations.[7]

Understanding the current limitations of a catheter-based ablation, what to think about the utility of combining a minimally invasive epicardial procedure with an endocardial procedure in a patient with AF? In other words, what are the advantages and disadvantages of a single percutaneous procedure and a single surgical procedure alone? What could be the advantages and disadvantages of a dual endocardial and epicardial procedure (DEEP)?

The answer, as often in medicine, depends on objective data and subjective feelings, upon the experience of the individual and the center, and the will to change and innovate.

Current Treatment of Lone AF: Transmurality and Lesion Set

Historically, the MAZE-III procedure, introduced by Cox, has been the surgical treatment of choice for medically refractory atrial fibrillation.[8] This procedure was developed as a salvage procedure because AF mapping data at that time was ambiguous and difficult to analyze. Based on the principles of critical mass and the anatomy of the heart, its purpose was to eliminate all potential reentrant circuits that could rotate around the thoracic veins and valve annuli, by subdividing large areas of contiguous tissue and leaving a pathway for the sinus node to activate both atria and the atrioventricular node.[9] It soon was called the gold standard and provided the essential foundation for the development of catheter techniques in the treatment of AF.[10] Technically challenging, the "cut and sew" Maze was not routinely performed by the majority of surgeons and, because of the invasiveness, rarely accepted by the EPs.

The knowledge that AF is often initiated from ectopic beats at foci in the pulmonary veins (PVs), radically changed the treatment options for patients with AF.[11,12] The use of catheter-based radiofrequency (RF) ablations to isolate the PVs became widespread. Some groups even suggested that pulmonary vein isolation (PVI) by catheter-based RF ablation can be considered as a first-line treatment of AF in patients without heart disease.[13,14] As the nonsurgical techniques were rapidly evolving, surgeons adapted and started to treat AF with fewer lesions on the atria than the traditional Cox-Maze procedure. The electrophysiologists' growing knowledge and experience made it possible to reduce the invasiveness of the surgical procedure by replacing the incisions with epicardial and endocardial catheter ablation lines. Realizing the necessity for continuous transmural lesions but wanting to reduce the burden of a cardiopulmonary bypass, Dr. Cox initiated a study to surgically recreate the atrial incisions of the MAZE-III without the use of cardiopulmonary bypass. This tunneling technique would allow for the immediate assessment of electrophysiologic and mechanical function for any type of procedure using the "maze principle."[15] Because it was still too complex, it was never translated into clinical practice, and catheter ablation (percutaneous and surgical) became the standard of treatment. The potential of catheter-based surgical ablation was confirmed by the work of Damiano. He replaced the "cut-and-sew" lesions through lesions created with ablation tools. The Cox-Maze IV procedure tremendously facilitated the surgery of AF.[16]

Transmurality

Catheter-based treatment of AF changed the concept of long-lasting transmural lesions, since replacing the "cut-and-sew" lesions with lesions created by an energy source no longer guaranteed the quality of the lesions. The importance of long-lasting continuous transmural lesions has been demonstrated with the Maze procedure. In patients experiencing atrial arrhythmias after surgical "cut-and-sew" Maze, approximately one-third have AF secondary to pulmonary vein reconduction. Moreover, incisional atrial flutter seems to be a common finding in this group of patients. Catheter-based mapping and ablation of these arrhythmias is feasible and effective.[17] The concept that atrial lesions must be transmural and continuous to successfully cure AF was elegantly demonstrated in a study that determined the effect of residual gaps on conduction properties of atrial tissue.[18] Canine right atria were divided with a bipolar radiofrequency ablation clamp, leaving a gap that was progressively narrowed. Conduction velocities at varying pacing rates and AF frequencies were measured before and after ablations. Conduction velocities were slowed through residual gaps, but propagation of wavefronts during pacing and AF occurred through the majority of residual gaps, down to sizes as small as 1.1 mm. Therefore, leaving viable tissue in ablation lines for the treatment of AF could account for failures. These findings have been confirmed in electrophysiologists' and surgeons' clinical practice. Recovery of conduction in previously ablated muscle fascicles is a common finding in patients with recurrent AF after segmental ostial ablation.[19] Recovered PV conduction is a dominant factor for recurrent atrial tachyarrhythmias after complete circular isolation of the PVs.[20] Acute and chronic PV reconnection after AF ablation is related to anatomical sites.[21]

Bipolar surgical clamps also have demonstrated failures in isolating PVs. Recurrent atrial arrhythmias after minimally invasive surgical PV isolation occur in up to 40% of patients during a minimal follow-up of 12 months. PV reconnection accounts for most recurrences. One study demonstrated that on average 25.6% of PVs reconnected, with a conduction delay between the left atrium and the PV.[22] One of the challenges with which we are confronted when assessing conduction block across surgical ablation lines is the mistake most surgeons make by checking for entrance and exit block immediately after ablation, without rechecking after a 30-minute delay. This concept of temporary block has been described by Benussi et al.[23] We demonstrated that the reason for failure of long-lasting block after initial proven exit and entrance block of the PVs could be related to a mechanical clamping-induced ischemia.[24]

These findings clearly demonstrate that PV isolation, the basis of most AF ablation strategies, is not guaranteed chronically and is often the reason for relapse.[25,26]

Lesion Set

Given the difficulty to predict whether the ablation points or lines will be chronically transmural, it makes sense to avoid the full lesion set of the Cox-Maze procedure as a standard lesion set for the patient with lone AF. Incomplete lines can cause iatrogenic proarrhythmia, therefore, every linear lesion should be accurately checked. Given this difficulty there is a clear tendency to minimize the ablation to mostly PV isolation alone, even in patients with nonparoxysmal atrial fibrillation. Although success rates are acceptable, some groups propose a more patient-tailored approach for persistent and long-lasting persistent AF.[27] In general, paroxysmal atrial fibrillation is amenable to catheter ablation with limited atrial tissue destruction causing electrical isolation of the PVs. Persistent and long-lasting forms of AF probably necessitate more extensive atrial tissue ablation in order to restore SR. Success rates for catheter ablation without concomitant antiarrhythmic therapy can be as high as 85%–89% at 1 year for paroxysmal AF, and 66%–80% for persistent AF.[28-31] But, a second and even a third procedure is frequent in patients with persistent and long-lasting persistent AF. A major issue with more extensive AF ablation is the increase of incidence of atrial tachycardias (ATs). Extensive substrate modification generates focal areas of slow conduction and low voltage capable of sustaining localized reentry.[32,33] Ascertaining bidirectional block after linear ablation and minimizing the volume of tissue ablation can help reduce the incidence of ATs.

Recent Surgical Literature

The surgical literature on the thoracoscopic treatment of lone AF with follow-up longer than 1 year is limited, certainly if we take publications presenting the results in accordance with the Heart Rhythm Society Guidelines.[34] Often, the minimally invasive approach to lone AF has been the video-assisted bilateral mini-thoracotomy or thoracoscopic PV island creation and LAA removal or exclusion, usually with ganglionic plexus evaluation and destruction. The percentage of success reported with this technique ranged from 42% to 91%, with a follow-up ranging from 6 to 40 months.[35] Edgerton et al reported a prospective, nonrandomized study of consecutive patients with symptomatic PAF undergoing a video-assisted, minimally invasive surgical ablation procedure.[36] The procedure consisted of bilateral, epicardial PVI with bipolar radiofrequency, partial autonomic denervation, and in 88% excision of the LAA. There were no major complications. At 1-year follow-up, freedom from atrial fibrillation/flutter/tachycardia was 80.8%.

Yilmaz et al studied 30 patients operated with a similar technique, but with a mixture of AF.[37] Freedom from AF was obtained in 77% of the patients during a mean follow-up of 11.6 months. Two patients underwent a conversion to sternotomy during the thoracoscopic procedure because of bleeding.

Castellá et al operated on 34 patients after unsuccessful catheter ablations.[38] A bilateral thoracoscopic PVI with a bipolar-radiofrequency clamping device was performed. Two patients were converted to thoracotomy because of bleeding. After 1-year follow-up, sinus rhythm was maintained in 82% of patients treated for PAF without use of antiarrhythmic drugs (AAD), in 60% of patients with persistent AF, and in 20% of patients with long-standing persistent AF. Left atrial size greater than 45 mm and AF type were preoperative factors that significantly influenced outcome in the univariate logistic regression analysis.

In another study published by Bagge et al, 43 patients with symptomatic AF were referred for thoracoscopic epicardial PV isolation and ganglionated plexi ablation using RF energy.[39] Overall, 25 of 33 patients (76%) followed up for 12 months had no AF episodes on 24-hour Holter recordings. The corresponding figures were 79% for patients with PAF, 100% for persistent AF, and 57% for permanent AF. The most common complication was bleeding events (9%) during pulmonary vein dissection.

The FAST Trial—the first randomized trial (two-center) designed to compare the efficacy and safety of radiofrequency catheter ablation (CA) versus minimally invasive surgical ablation (SA) in specific subgroups of patients with symptomatic AF refractory to at least 1 AAD—was published in 2012.[40] The inclusion criteria were left atrial (LA) diameter of 40–44 mm in association with hypertension, LA diameter ≥ 45 mm, or a prior unsuccessful CA procedure. Exclusion criteria included long-standing persistent AF, LA diameter > 65 mm, and left ventricular ejection fraction < 45%. One hundred twenty-four patients (mean age 56 years, mean LA diameter 43 mm) with AF (paroxysmal in 67%) were randomly assigned to CA ($n = 63$) or SA ($n = 61$). A prior unsuccessful CA procedure had been performed in 67% of patients. In the CA group, an LA ablation line was made at the roof in 48% of patients, at the mitral isthmus in 27%, and in the right atrium in 23%. In the SA group, additional lines were created in 31% of patients. Sinus rhythm at 12 months was achieved significantly more often in the SA group (65.6%) than in the CA group (36.5%). The complication rate was significantly higher in the SA group (34.4%) than in the CA group (15.9%). The rate of procedural serious adverse events (SAEs) was significantly higher in the SA group (23%) than in the CA group (3.2%). During the 12 months of follow-up, the rates of SAEs were similar in the SA and CA groups (11.5% versus 12.6%, respectively). These findings highlighted the greater efficacy, but greater risk of a minimally invasive surgical ablation compared to catheter ablation.

How Can Complications Related to Catheter and Surgical Ablation Be Reduced?

Eliminating AF with an ablation procedure has several hypothetical advantages. These include improvement in quality of life, decreased stroke risk, decreased heart failure risk, and improved survival. Since this hypothesis has not been systematically evaluated as part of large, randomized clinical trials, it is as yet unproven. Adverse events in catheter ablation will affect its clinical utility. Cappato et al reported the rate of complications in a worldwide survey on 16,309 patients undergoing catheter ablation.[41] A major complication occurred in 741 patients (4.5%). There were 25 procedure-related deaths (0.15%), 37 strokes (0.23%), 115 transient ischemic attacks (0.71%), and 213 episodes of tamponade (1.31%).

Reducing the number of complications and simultaneously improving the success rate is certainly the ultimate goal of any AF procedure. The European Society of Cardiology guidelines recommend to take several important considerations before considering an ablation procedure in symptomatic patients: success rate (which will be related on the stage of the disease), operator's experience, complication rate, potential treatment alternatives, and the patient's preference.[42]

Based upon the experience of the FAST Trial and the worldwide survey, what are the complications to avoid, and how can a dual endocardial-epicardial procedure help?

Thromboembolism

The risk of thromboembolism, most importantly transient ischemic attack and stroke, could be lowered if we are able to replace a number of endocardial ablations by transmural lesions on the epicardial surface of the left atrium. Epicardial ablation of the right and left antrum of the PVs with a bipolar clamp, with exclusion of the ligament of Marshall and, if necessary, a roof and inferior line, can be reliably done with a minimum risk for embolic events. Our group investigated the occurrence of cerebral microembolic signals (MES) as a surrogate marker for the risk of neurological impairment marker by using transcranial doppler (TCD) monitoring to detect MES in the middle cerebral arteries, which represent 40% of the cerebral blood flow.[43] Two different PVI methods, a percutaneous endocardial RF ablation and a thoracoscopic epicardial ablation using RF energy, were compared. An average of 5 (± 6) MES were detected during epicardial PVI procedure versus 3,908 (± 2,816) MES during percutaneous endocardial PVI procedure. During the ablation application period, respectively, 1 (± 1) and 2,566 (± 2,296) cerebral MES were detected. We also studied the incidence of MES as a risk factor for neurological complications during 3 percutaneous endocardial ablation procedure strategies: segmental PVI using a conventional RF ablation catheter (CRF), segmental PVI using an irrigated-tip RF catheter (IRF), and circumferential PVI with a cryoballoon catheter (CB).[44] The total number of cerebral MES differed significantly among the 3 PVI groups; 3,908 cerebral MES were measured with use of the CRF catheter, 1,404 cerebral MES with use of the IRF catheter, and 935 cerebral MES with use of the CB catheter. These studies clearly demonstrated that the thromboembolic load in endocardial procedures can be significantly reduced by limiting the number of endocardial ablations regardless of the catheter and energy source used.

Pulmonary Vein Stenosis

Pulmonary vein stenosis is a well-known complication and depending on the ablation site with regards to the PV ostium. Pulmonary vein stenosis has been described in up to 10% for focal PV ablation and less than 5% for segmental PV isolation. In patients with symptomatic and severe PV stenosis, balloon dilatation and stent implantation has been performed. The incidence of PV restenosis is acceptable with drug eluting stents.[45] There is no available literature on PV stenosis after epicardial surgical PV ablation, suggesting that this is a safe procedure with regard to the risk of PV stenosis.

Atrioesophageal Fistula Formation

This was first described in open-heart surgery with endocardial RF ablation of the posterior wall of the left atrium.[46] Due to the anatomical relationship between the esophagus and the posterior left atrium, similar complications can occur with any endocardial catheter ablation. Although specific imaging can reduce the risk, the frequency is 0.05% to < 1%.[47] The dreadful consequences of an oesophageal perforation are mostly lethal. The only reliable and safe way to avoid oesophageal injury during ablation is to have an anatomical real-time view of the esophagus and to ablate from the epicardium toward the endocardium. During thoracoscopy the esophagus can always be visualized at the level of the posterior left atrium through the bulging of the transesophageal echo probe. Knowing the exact position of the esophagus and having the possibility to direct the ablation energy from the epicardium toward the endocardium is a guarantee to protect the esophagus. It is therefore possible to safely create an inferior line, a line which could increase the success rate of the procedure.[48,49]

Tamponade

Cardiac tamponade is the most common potentially lethal complication associated with AF ablation. It can occur in up to 6% of procedures and is related to extensive intracardiac catheter manipulation and ablation, as well as to the need for systemic anticoagulation. A misdirected transseptal puncture, overheating during energy delivery, and direct mechanical trauma (the LAA) can lead to cardiac perforation. During the hybrid procedure the pericardium is opened thereby avoiding the risk for tamponade (but not the risk for bleeding).

Phrenic Nerve Injury

The anatomical relationship between the right phrenic nerve, the anterior part of the right superior pulmonary vein (RSPV), and the superior caval vein is well known, as is the proximity of the left phrenic nerve to the LAA.[50] A multicenter study reported that phrenic nerve injury rarely occurred (0.48%) after AF catheter ablation.[51] Phrenic nerve injury can be avoided by pacing before energy delivery in these areas. If phrenic nerve capture is documented, energy delivery should be limited, thereby potentially diminishing the transmurality and completeness of the lesion at these sites. Phrenic nerve injury has also been described in the minimal invasive surgical approach for the treatment of AF.[52] This is related to the opening of the pericardium too close to the phrenic nerve, to the use of cautery in the vicinity of the phrenic nerve, or to the manipulation. Since the phrenic nerve is always visualized during surgery, this complication could be avoided by increasing the surgeon's vigilance. A hybrid procedure could avoid phrenic nerve injury by retracting the pericardium at the level of the RSPV and so protect the phrenic nerve during endocardial application of energy.

Postprocedural Arrhythmias

Atrial tachycardias of new onset may be observed in 5% to 25% of patients who have undergone catheter ablation or surgical ablation of AF. A hybrid procedure could improve the transmurality and continuity of the ablation lines by performing ablations from the epicardial surface, confirming strong endpoints measured from the endocardium and if necessary complete a lesion with an endocardial touch-up. An epicardial ablation checked by an endocardial approach will certainly give the strongest indicator for a transmural continuous lesion.

Virtual Imaging

The knowledge of anatomy to the electrophysiologist is crucial in AF procedures.[53] Direct visualization of the heart with thoracoscopy can certainly increase this knowledge. The real-time anatomy of the PVs, the posterior left atrium, the LAA, the coronary sinus (CS), the esophagus, the phrenic nerves, and sometimes the positioning of the endocardial catheters could improve the quality of the lesion and avoid complications. LAA potentials masquerading PV potentials can be elegantly demonstrated by removing the LAA from the left superior PV.[54,55]

Radiation Exposure During Catheter Ablation

The increasing availability of mapping systems significantly reduces fluoroscopy time and the need for biplane fluoroscopy. The use of remote navigation systems also significantly reduces radiation exposure of the patients and the EPs who perform these procedures. An epicardial ablation with direct videoscopic visualization reduces the total number of endocardial applications, thereby further reducing fluoroscopy time.

Surgical Bleeding

A thoracoscopic procedure necessitates dissection of pericardial reflections around both caval veins and PVs. This dissection can be challenging and injury to major vessels or heart is possible. An endocardial access can reduce this risk, since an endocardial touch-up is always possible. Therefore, if the surgical ablation is incomplete because of a risk for bleeding due to the anatomy or to the amount of epicardial fat, the surgeon does not feel forced to push the surgical risk of his procedure.

Left Atrial Appendage

Exclusion or excision of the LAA could reduce the stroke rate in patients treated for AF.[55] Expensive endocardial exclusion devices are available. The endocardial positioning of the device leaves foreign material in the heart. This could explain the remaining stroke risk for patients with an implanted device.[56] An epicardial surgical excision or exclusion of the LAA avoids intracardiac foreign material, is less expensive, and will eliminate the LAA as a potential inducer of AF.

Hybrid AF

The experience with a hybrid dual endocardial–epicardial approach for the treatment of AF was started in 2007 in 3 patients with a history of persistent AF. In all patients a monolateral right thoracoscopic approach was performed, and microwave was used as the energy source to create an epicardial box lesion (Flex10, Maquet, Getinge, Sweden). An important conduction delay between the posterior wall of the left atrium and the left atrium could be measured after the epicardial microwave lesion, but no exit or entrance block. In order to make this incomplete epicardial surgical ablation line continuous and transmural, a complementary endocardial isolation of one or more pulmonary veins and/or the roof and inferior line was necessary. It was therefore decided to perform a transvenuous endocardial mapping during the same procedure, and touch up the mapped gaps with an irrigated radiofrequency 3.5 mm-tip catheter (THERMOCOOL, Biosense Webster, Diamond Bar, CA). Even after multiple epi and endocardial ablations we were unable to create a long-lasting exit block from the box. The energy source for the surgical ablation was changed to monopolar radiofrequency (Cobra AdhereXL™ surgical system, AtriCure, West Chester, OH). Nineteen consecutive patients (mean 60.8 ± 8.6 years, 84.2% male) underwent a right unilateral minimally invasive hybrid procedure. Ten patients (52.6.6%) had long-standing persistent AF while 4

(21.1%) had persistent and 5 (26.3%) paroxysmal AF.[57] In 17 patients, one or more PVs (mostly the left superior PV) were not isolated, and an endocardial touch-up was needed. It was possible to complete all the procedures as planned without any conversion to cardiopulmonary bypass. No patient died during the follow-up. At 1 year, 7/19 (36.8%) patients were in sinus rhythm with no episode of AF and off antiarrhythmic drugs. Among patients with long-standing persistent AF, 20% (2/10) were in sinus rhythm and off AAD, 50% (2/4) in persistent and 60% (3/5) in paroxysmal AF. Based on this experience, we concluded that 1-year results combining a percutaneous endocardial radiofrequency procedure with a right thoracoscopic epicardial monopolar radiofrequency box lesion were not satisfactory, particularly in patients with LSP and persistent AF. The concept of combining a percutaneous endocardial approach with a thoracoscopic epicardial approach was safe and technically feasible, but creation of an electrically isolated box lesion from the epicardium with monopolar energy could not be assured. This probably explains the relatively low success rate at long-term follow-up.

To prevent recurrences of AF, it is necessary for a device to be able to produce a transmural continuous lesion, since even small 1-mm gaps in lesions will increase the likelihood of AF.[18] An epicardial ablation on the beating heart is challenging because the atrial wall muscle thickness is variable and can be covered with an epicardial layer of fat. Moreover, the circulating intracavitary blood acts as a potential heat sink. Schuessler et al tested the effect of epicardial ablation on the beating heart in domestic pigs using 9 different unidirectional devices.[58] With these devices, all the energy is applied by a single transducer on a single heart surface. The authors concluded that the percentage of transmural lesions varied for a minimum of 5% up to 100% for the different devices tested, and that none of the devices tested demonstrated the ability to penetrate the atrial wall at its thickest dimensions. The most consistent devices for creating transmural epicardial lesions have been bipolar radiofrequency clamps.[59,60] Clamping of the pulmonary veins between the two jaws excludes the effect of circulating blood on delivery of power thereby eliminating the heat-sink cooling effect to the tissue. Therefore, these clamps can be used from the epicardium on the beating or nonbeating heart to isolate PVs.

In order to use this technology, we redesigned the single-step hybrid procedure to a bilateral thoracoscopic approach. Our initial experience in 26 patients has been reported.[61] We performed a stepwise ablation as described in ▶ Video 49F.1. All procedures were performed in the cathlab (Figure 49F.1).

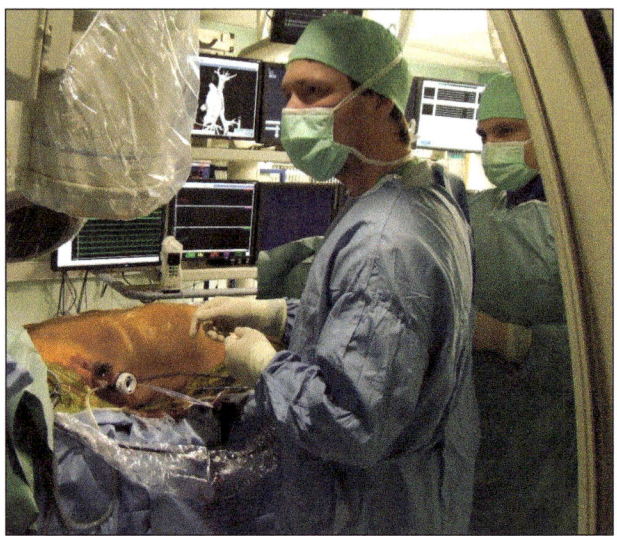

Figure 49F.1 Hybrid AF procedure performed in the cathlab. Cardiac surgeon and electrophysiologist are side-by-side during an AF ablation.

In all patients, bipolar ablation of all the PVs was performed. It is important to position the bipolar clamp in order to isolate the carina region of the PVs (Figure 49F.2) since many PV triggers commonly originate from this region.[62] Furthermore, the ligament of Marshall should be ablated while clamping the antral portion of the left PVs (Figure 49F.3). Figure 49F.4 shows a Carto 3 (Biosense Webster) mapping of the posterior left atrium after ablation. In 22 patients, a bipolar unidirectional radiofrequency pen was used to make a roof and inferior line, to create a box lesion (Figure 49F.5). Only in 16 (77%) were we able to demonstrate entrance and exit block in the box from the endocardial side. After endocardial toucsh-up in 5 patients, we were able to complete the isolation of the box. In 3 patients, there was a clear gap at the junction of the right superior PV with the roof of the left atrium. In 1 patient, an incomplete lesion occurred due to a gap in the lateral portion of the roof line, and in another patient an incomplete lesion occurred due to a gap in the middle of the inferior line. In 3 patients, a left isthmus line was made epicardially using a bipolar unidirectional radiofrequency pen, starting from the ablation line around the left inferior PV and going toward the CS. This line was then completed by an endocardial touch-up from the CS toward the mitral annulus. The combined left isthmus line could easily be verified on fluoroscopy by showing the ablated CS with a surgical forceps. In all patients, a bidirectional block could be measured. Three patients needed a right isthmus line. In 7 patients, the LAA was stapled. There were no major complications.

The complete DEEP lesion set is comparable to the Cox-Maze IV (Figure 49F.6). All lines were created epicardially except both isthmus lines, which were made endocardially.

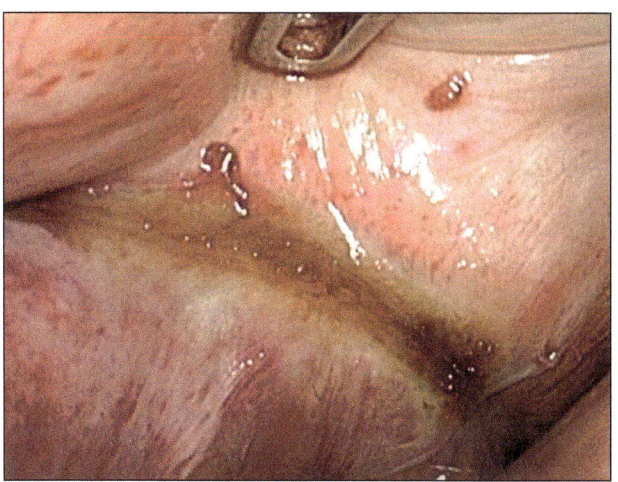

Figure 49F.2 Right thoracoscopic view: visualization of the ablation lesion created with a bipolar clamp at the antrum of RPV, just proximal of the carina.

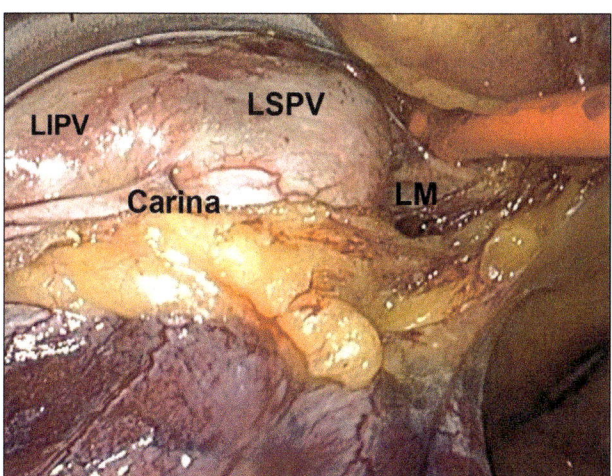

Figure 49F.3 Left thoracoscopic view: clamping of the LPV and the LM with a bipolar clamp.

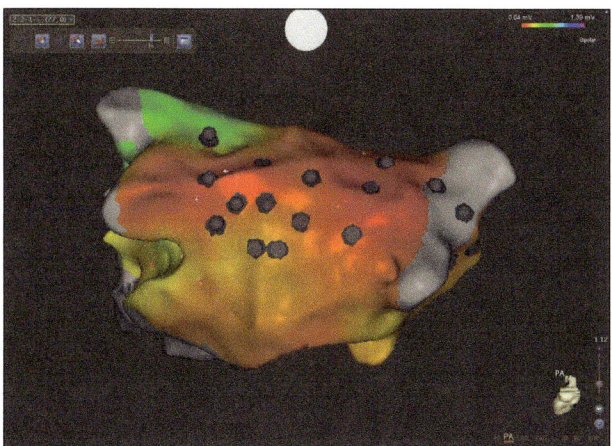

Figure 49F.4 CARTO 3 voltage map of the posterior left atrium after the thoracoscopic epicardial box lesion.

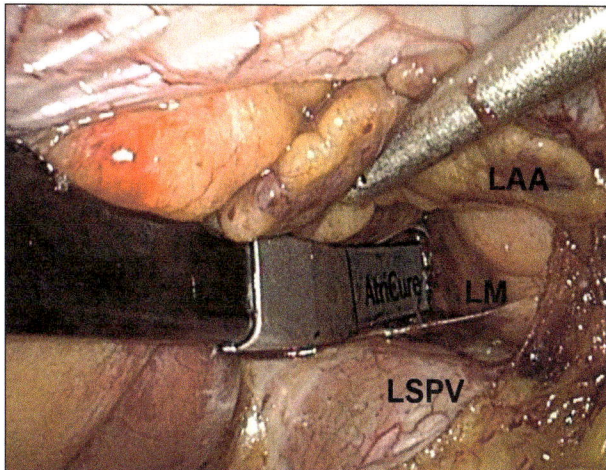

Figure 49F.5 Left thoracoscopic view: roofline, connecting the LSPV with the RSPV using a bipolar unidirectional ablation device.

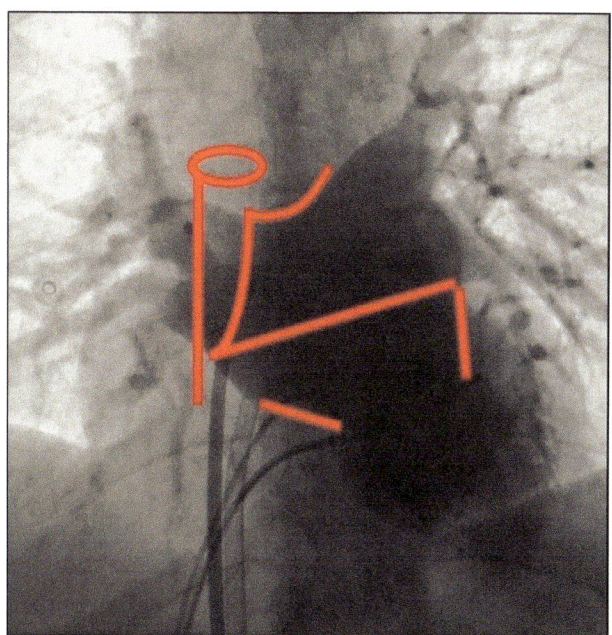

Figure 49F.6 Left atrial angiography with illustration of the combined epicardial and endocardial lesion set. The final ablated area is comparable to a Cox-Maze IV.

In 23% of patients, the epicardial lines created with linear ablation devices were not transmural and necessitated an endocardial touch-up ablation, confirming the importance of endocardial mapping, and the advantage to ablate on both sides of the atrial wall during catheter treatment of AF. The single-procedure success rate (sinus rhythm without AAD and/or repeat procedure) was 79% at 1 year for paroxysmal and 90% for persistent AF patients. The overall single-procedure success rate was 83% at 1 year. In our experience, the possibility to perform an endocardial touch-up in a setting of epicardial lesions, and the very low complication rate, seems to be one of the major advantages of this single-step dual epicardial–endocardial approach.

The single-step hybrid procedure can also have an advantage in patients where a repeat catheter ablation procedure is needed. Many patients that are candidates for an epicardial treatment of AF will have had a previous endocardial procedure. The possibility to map the patient endocardially first, including knowledge of which veins have been isolated and which have not, can have important consequences for the treatment strategy. If all pulmonary veins have been electrically isolated, the epicardial procedure should be focused on linear lesions to compartmentalize the posterior left atrium and (mostly) exclusion of the LAA. Therefore, the thoracoscopic procedure can be limited to the left side. If the pulmonary veins have been isolated on the left side, the thoracoscopic procedure could be limited to the right side, if exclusion of the LAA is not needed.

Complex fractionated electrograms (CFAE) probably are important in AF.[63,64] In a group of patients with long-standing persistent AF, we mapped the CFAE prior and after epicardial isolation of the PVs and posterior left atrium (Figure 49F.7). Interestingly, all CFAE were gone except the CFAE at the base of the LAA and at the lateral septum. These CFAE were endocardially targeted with a cooled irrigated RF catheter (Figure 49F.8).

There can be concerns about the single-step hybrid procedure. Depending on the lesion set, this procedure can become time-consuming. Furthermore, this hybrid treatment might represent a "logistical nightmare" since it requires a multidisciplinary team approach.[65] Finally, we must understand the importance of timing between the surgical and electrophysiological procedures. In a simultaneous epicardial–endocardial procedure, we may be confronted with false-negative results because of transient bidirectional block, as well as with false-positive results because of early inducible arrhythmias, which could require further maturation of the lesions.

A sequential hybrid procedure during the same hospital stay has been proposed by Mahapatra et al.[66] Fifteen patients with persistent or long-standing persistent AF who failed at least one catheter ablation and one AAD were treated. This group was matched categorically to 30

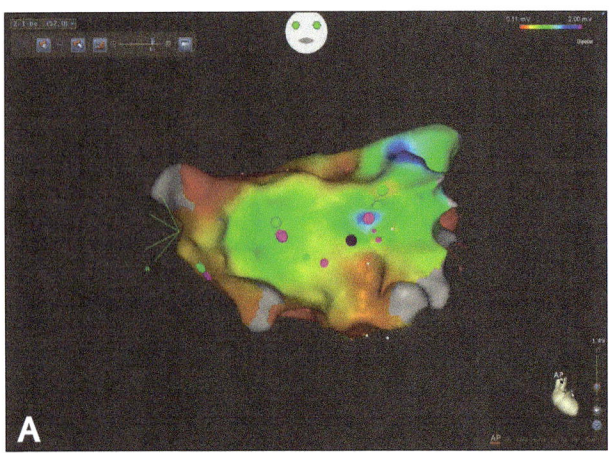 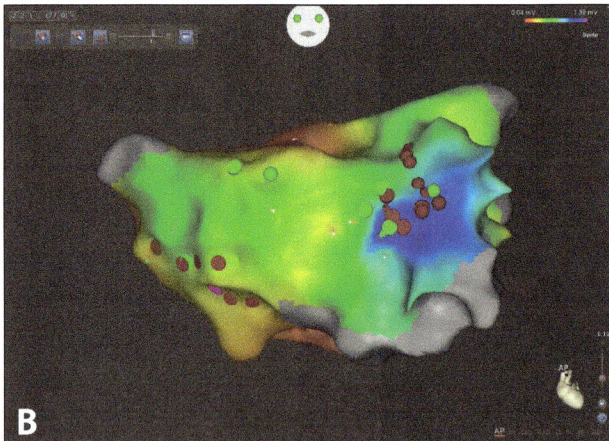

Figure 49F.7 **Panel A:** Carto 3 image of anterior CFAE before epicardial ablation of the posterior wall of the left atrium. **Panel B:** Carto 3 of anterior CFAE after epicardial box lesion. Endocardial ablation points (**red dots**).

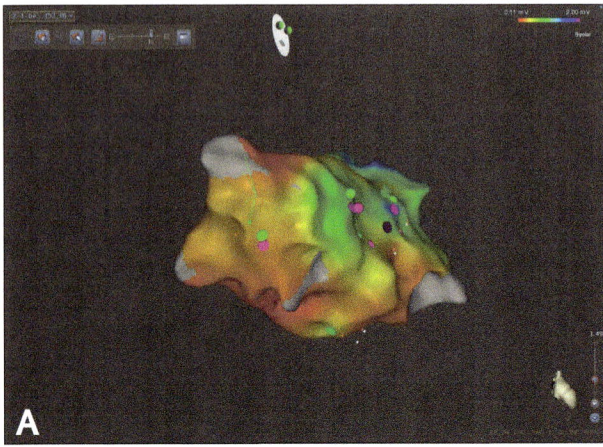 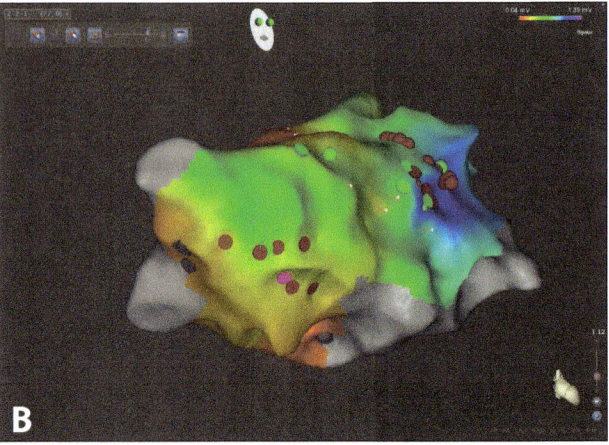

Figure 49F.8 **Panel A:** Carto 3 of septal CFAE before epicardial ablation of the posterior wall of the left atrium. **Panel B:** Carto 3 of septal CFAE after epicardial box lesion. Endocardial ablation points (**red dots**).

patients who had previously failed at least one catheter ablation and underwent a repeat catheter ablation. Five patients had 7 inducible atrial flutters that were mapped during the sequential catheter procedure and ablated. After a mean follow-up of 20.7 ± 4.5 months, 86.7% of patients of the sequential hybrid group were free of any atrial arrhythmia and off all AAD, compared to 53.3% of the catheter-alone patients.

The literature related to the hybrid treatment (staged or as a single-step procedure) of lone AF with follow-up longer than 1 year is limited. Furthermore, it has not yet been established whether the hybrid approach will produce more favorable outcomes regardless of the type of AF. There are currently only 9 papers with > 10 patients and a follow-up of at least 12 months.[57,61,66-72] Freedom from AF off AAD at latest follow-up ranged from 85.7% to 92% in papers employing bipolar RF and from 36.8% to 88.9% in those utilizing monopolar RF. With specific reference to AAD-free success rate by the type of AF, it ranged from 60% to 91.6% in paroxysmal AF, from 50% to 77.7% in persistent AF and from 20% to 100% in long-standing persistent AF.

These results are comparable to the success rates of the Cox-Maze IV procedure and success rates after repeat catheter ablations.

Conclusion

There is a role for both surgical and catheter ablation in the optimal treatment of atrial fibrillation. The challenge with AF surgery is the development of an off-pump thoracoscopic ablation procedure that can create transmural lesions in a reliable and safe manner. Therefore, intraoperative electrophysiological assessment of the triggers and substrates of AF in a step-by-step approach, with verification of conduction block over the ablation lines (and maybe inducibility) are needed to guarantee a high success rate. The challenge with percutaneous catheter ablation, in patients with persistent or long-standing persistent AF, is the low success rate inherent to the technique and the approach.

The combination of an EP procedure and a surgical procedure as two complementary ablation techniques, performed in conjunction, could improve long-term success rates, reduce complication rates, morbidity, and mortality related to atrial fibrillation.

A hybrid endocardial–epicardial approach for the treatment of AF combines the efficacy of surgical ablation with the knowledge of endocardial mapping and, if necessary, short and focused endocardial ablations. The hybrid approach has the potential to increase success rates and lower complication rates, but is still actively evolving and for the time being relatively untested in a controlled environment.

References

1. Nitta T. Surgery for atrial fibrillation: a worldwide review. *Semin Thorac Cardiovasc Surg.* 2007;19(1):3-8.
2. Byrne JG, Leacche M, Vaughan DE, Zhao DX. Hybrid cardiovascular procedures. *JACC Cardiovasc Interv.* 2008;1(5):459-468.
3. Bisleri G, Curnis A, Bottio T, Mascioli G, Muneretto C. The need of a hybrid approach for the treatment of atrial fibrillation. *Heart Surg Forum.* 2005;8(5):E326-E330.
4. Reddy VY, Neuzil P, D'Avila A, Ruskin JN. Isolating the posterior left atrium and pulmonary veins with a "box" lesion set: use of epicardial ablation to complete electrical isolation. *J Cardiovasc Electrophysiol.* 2008;19(3):326-329.
5. Scanavacca M, Pisani CF, Hachul D, et al. Patients with paroxysmal atrial fibrillation selective atrial vagal denervation guided by evoked vagal reflex to treat. *Circulation.* 2006;114:876-885.
6. Pak HN, Hwang C, Lim HE, Kim JS, Kim YH. Hybrid epicardial and endocardial ablation of persistent or permanent atrial fibrillation: a new approach for difficult cases. *J Cardiovasc Electrophysiol.* 2007;18(9):917-923.
7. Jong-Il C, Hui-Nam P, Young-Hoon K. Hybrid epicardial and endocardial catheter ablation in a patient with atrial fibrillation and suspicious left atrial thrombus *Circ J.* 2009;73:384-387.
8. Cox JL, Schuessler RB, D'Agostino HJ Jr, et al. The surgical treatment of atrial fibrillation. III. Development of a definitive surgical procedure. *J Thorac Cardiovasc Surg.* 1991;101(4):569-583.
9. Schuessler RB, Damiano RJ Jr. Mechanisms of human atrial fibrillation: Lessons learned from 20 years of atrial fibrillation surgery. *J Interv Card Electrophysiol.* 2007;20(3):59-64.
10. Cox JL. Cardiac surgery for arrhythmias. *J Cardiovasc Electrophysiol.* 2004;15(2):250-262.
11. Haïssaguerre M, Jaïs P, Shah DC, et al. Spontaneous initiation of atrial fibrillation by ectopic beats originating in the pulmonary veins. *N Engl J Med.* 1998;339:659-666.
12. Chen SA, Hsieh MH, Tai CT, et al. Initiation of atrial fibrillation by ectopic beats originating from the pulmonary veins: electrophysiological characteristics, pharmacological responses, and effects of radiofrequency ablation. *Circulation.* 1999;100:1879-1886.
13. Wazni OM, Marrouche NF, Martin DO, et al. Radiofrequency ablation vs antiarrhythmic drugs as first-line treatment of symptomatic atrial fibrillation: a randomized trial. *JAMA.* 2005;293:2634-2640.
14. Verma A, Natale A, Padanilam BJ, et al. Why atrial fibrillation ablation should be considered first-line therapy for some patients. *Circulation.* 2005;112:1214-1222.
15. Lee R, Nitta T, Schuessler RB, Johnson DC, Boineau JP, Cox JL. The closed heart MAZE: a nonbypass surgical technique. *Ann Thorac Surg.* 1999;67(6):1696-1702.
16. Damiano RJ Jr, Bailey M. The Cox-Maze IV procedure for lone atrial fibrillation. *MMCTS.* 2007 July 23; doi:10.1510/mmcts.2007.002758.
17. Wazni OM, Saliba W, Fahmy T, et al. Atrial arrhythmias after surgical maze: findings during catheter ablation. *J Am Coll Cardiol.* 2006;3;48(7):1405-1409.
18. Melby SJ, Lee AM, Zierer A, et al. Atrial fibrillation propagates through gaps in ablation lines: implications for ablative treatment of atrial fibrillation. *Heart Rhythm.* 2008;5(9):1296-1301.

19. Lemola K, Hall B, Cheung P, et al. Mechanisms of recurrent atrial fibrillation after pulmonary vein isolation by segmental ostial ablation. *Heart Rhythm.* 2004;1:197-202.
20. Ouyang F, Antz M, Ernst S, et al. Recovered pulmonary vein conduction as a dominant factor for recurrent atrial tachyarrhythmias after complete circular isolation of the pulmonary veins: lessons from double lasso technique. *Circulation.* 2005;111:127-135.
21. Rajappan K, Kistler PM, Earley MJ, et al. Acute and chronic pulmonary vein reconnection after atrial fibrillation ablation: a prospective characterization of anatomical sites. *Pacing Clin Electrophysiol.* 2008;31:1598-1605.
22. Kron J, Kasirajan V, Wood M, Kowalski M, Han F, Ellenbogen K. Management of recurrent atrial arrhythmias after minimally invasive surgical pulmonary vein isolation and ganglionic plexi ablation for atrial fibrillation. *Heart Rhythm.* 2010;7:445-451.
23. Benussi S, Galanti A, Zerbi V, Privitera Y, Iafelice I, Alfieri O. Electrophysiologic efficacy of irrigated bipolar radiofrequency in the clinical setting. *J Thorac Cardiovasc Surg.* 2010;139:1131-1136.
24. Pison L, La Meir M, van Opstal J, Crijns HJ. Transient clamp-induced mechanical block of pulmonary vein potentials. *J Thorac Cardiovasc Surg.* 2011;141(2):e15-e16.
25. Nademanee K, Gidney BA. Pulmonary vein isolation without reconnection: a decade of trying. *J Cardiovasc Electrophysiol.* 2010;21(7):738-740.
26. Chun KRJ, Bansch D, Ernst S, et al. Pulmonary vein conduction is the major finding in patients with atrial tachyarrhythmias after intraoperative maze ablation. *J Cardiovasc Electrophysiol.* 2007;18:1-6.
27. O'Neill MD, Jaïs P, Takahashi Y, et al. The stepwise ablation approach for chronic atrial fibrillation–evidence for a cumulative effect. *J Interv Card Electrophysiol.* 2006;16:153-167.
28. Jaïs P, Cauchemez B, Macle L, et al. Catheter ablation versus antiarrhythmic drugs for atrial fibrillation: The A4 study. *Circulation.* 2008;118:2498-2505.
29. Wazni OM, Marrouche NF, Martin DO, et al. A. Radiofrequency ablation vs antiarrhythmic drugs as first-line treatment of symptomatic atrial fibrillation: A randomized trial. *JAMA.* 2005;293:2634-2640.
30. Pappone C, Augello G, Sala S, et al. A randomized trial of circumferential pulmonary vein ablation versus antiarrhythmic drug therapy in paroxysmal atrial fibrillation: The APAF Study. *J Am Coll Cardiol.* 2006;48:2340-2347.
31. Stabile G, Bertaglia E, Senatore G, et al. Catheter ablation treatment in patients with drug-refractory atrial fibrillation: A prospective, multi-centre, randomized, controlled study (Catheter Ablation For The Cure Of Atrial Fibrillation Study). *Eur Heart J.* 2006;27:216-221.
32. Shah AJ, Jadidi A, Liu X, et al. Atrial tachycardias arising from ablation of atrial fibrillation: a proarrhythmic bump or an antiarrhythmic turn? *Cardio Res Pract.* 2010;2010-950763, doi:10.4061/2010/950763.
33. Magnano AR, Argenziano M, Dizon JM, et al. Mechanisms of atrial tachyarrhythmias following surgical atrial fibrillation ablation. *J Cardiovasc Electrophysiol.* 2006;17(4):366-373.
34. Calkins H, Brugada J, Packer DL, et al. HRS/EHRA/ECAS expert consensus statement on catheter and surgical ablation of atrial fibrillation: recommendations for personnel, policy, procedures and follow-up. *Heart Rhythm.* 2007;4(6):816-861.
35. Gelsomino S, La Meir M, Lucà F, et al. Treatment of lone atrial fibrillation: a look at the past, a view of the present and a glance at the future. *Eur J Cardiothorac Surg.* 2012;41(6):1284-1294.
36. Edgerton JR, Brinkman WT, Weaver T, et al. Pulmonary vein isolation and autonomic denervation for the management of paroxysmal atrial fibrillation by a minimally invasive surgical approach. *J. Thorac Cardiovasc Surg.* 2010;140(4):823-828.
37. Yilmaz A, Van Putte BP, Van Boven WJ. Completely thoracoscopic bilateral pulmonary vein isolation and left atrial appendage exclusion for atrial fibrillation. *J Thorac Cardiovasc Surg.* 2008;136:521-522.
38. Castellá M, Pereda D, Mestres CA, Gómez F, Quintana E, Mulet J. Thoracoscopic pulmonary vein isolation in patients with atrial fibrillation and failed percutaneous ablation. *J Thorac Cardiovasc Surg.* 2010;140(3):633-638.
39. Bagge L, Blomström P, Nilsson L, Einarsson GM, Jidéus L, Blomström-Lundqvist C. Epicardial off-pump pulmonary vein isolation and vagal denervation improve long-term outcome and quality of life in patients with atrial fibrillation. *J Thorac Cardiovasc Surg.* 2009;137(5):1265-1271.
40. Boersma LV, Castella M, van Boven W, et al. Atrial Fibrillation Catheter Ablation versus Surgical Ablation Treatment (FAST): A 2-center randomized clinical trial. *Circulation.* 2012;125:23-30.
41. Cappato R, Calkins H, Chen SA, et al. Updated worldwide survey on the methods, efficacy, and safety of catheter ablation for human atrial fibrillation. *Circ Arrhythm Electrophysiol.* 2010;3:32-38.
42. Camm AJ, Kirchhof P, Lip GYH, et al. European Heart Rhythm Association, European Association for Cardio-Thoracic Surgery, Guidelines for the management of atrial fibrillation. *Eur Heart J.* 2010;31:2369-2429.
43. Sauren LD, La Meir M, de Roy L, et al. Increased number of cerebral emboli during percutaneous endocardial pulmonary vein isolation versus a thoracoscopic epicardial approach. *Eur J Cardiothorac Surg.* 2009;36(5):833-837.
44. Sauren LD, Van Belle Y, De Roy L, et al. Transcranial measurement of cerebral microembolic signals during endocardial pulmonary vein isolation: comparison of three different ablation techniques. *J Cardiovasc Electrophysiol.* 2009;20(10): 1102-1107.
45. De Potter TJ, Schmidt B, Chun KR, et al. Drug-eluting stents for the treatment of pulmonary vein stenosis after atrial fibrillation ablation. *Europace.* 2011;13(1):57-61.
46. Gillinov AM, Pettersson G, Rice TW. Esophageal injury during radiofrequency ablation for atrial fibrillation. *J Thorac Cardiovasc Surg.* 2001;122:1239-1240.
47. Pappone C, Oral H, Santinelli V, et al. Atrio-esophageal fistula as a complication of percutaneous transcatheter. *Circulation.* 2004;109;2724-2726.
48. Damiano RJ Jr, Voeller RK. Biatrial lesion sets. *J Interv Card Electrophysiol.* 2007;20:95-99.
49. Gillinov AM, Bhavani S, Blackstone EH, et al. Surgery for permanent atrial fibrillation: impact of patient factors and lesion set. *Ann Thorac Surg.* 2006;82(2):502-513; discussion 513-514.
50. Sánchez-Quintana D, Cabrera JA, Climent V, Farré J, Weiglein A, Ho SY. How close are the phrenic nerves to cardiac structures? Implications for cardiac interventionalists. *J Cardiovasc Electrophysiol.* 2005;16:309-313.
51. Sacher F, Monahan KH, Thomas SP, et al. Phrenic nerve injury after atrial fibrillation catheter ablation: Characterization and outcome in a multicenter study. *J Am Coll Cardiol.* 2006;47:2498-2503.
52. Han FT, Kasirajan V, Kowalski M, et al. Results of a minimally invasive surgical pulmonary vein isolation and ganglionic plexi ablation for atrial fibrillation: single center experience

53. Marchlinski FE, Leong-Sit P. Learning before burning: the importance of anatomy to the electrophysiologist. *Heart Rhythm*. 2009;6:1199-1201.
54. Shah D, Haïssaguerre M, Jaïs P, et al. Left atrial appendage activity masquerading as pulmonary vein potentials. *Circulation*. 2002;105:2821-2825.
55. Pison L, La Meir M, Maessen J, Crijns H. Seeing is believing: unmasking left atrial appendage activity recorded in the left superior pulmonary vein without stimulation. *J Cardiovasc Electrophysiol*. 2010;21:1417-1418.
56. Holmes DR, Reddy VY, Turi ZG, et al. Percutaneous closure of the left atrial appendage versus warfarin therapy for prevention of stroke in patients with atrial fibrillation: a randomised non-inferiority trial. *Lancet*. 2009;374:534-542.
57. La Meir M, Gelsomino S, Lorusso R, et al. The hybrid approach for the surgical treatment of lone atrial fibrillation: One-year results employing a monopolar radiofrequency source. *J Cardiothorac Surg*. 2012;7:71.
58. Schuessler RB, Lee AM, Melby SJ, et al. Animal studies of epicardial atrial ablation. *Heart Rhythm*. 2009;6(12, S1):S41-S45.
59. Melby SJ, Gaynor SL, Lubahn JG, et al. Efficacy and safety of right and left atrial ablations on the beating heart with irrigated bipolar radiofrequency energy: a long-term animal study. *J Thorac Cardiovasc Surg*. 2006;132(4):853-860.
60. Prasad SM, Maniar HS, Schuessler RB, Damiano RJ Jr. Chronic transmural atrial ablation by using bipolar radiofrequency energy on the beating heart. *J Thorac Cardiovasc Surg*. 2002;124(4):708-713.
61. Pison L, La Meir M, van Opstal J, Blaauw Y, Maessen JG, Crijns HJ. Hybrid thoracoscopic surgical and transvenous catheter ablation of atrial fibrillation. *J Am Coll Cardiol*. 2012;60:54-61.
62. Valles E, Fan R, Roux JF, et al. Localization of atrial fibrillation triggers in patients undergoing pulmonary vein isolation: importance of the carina region. *J Am Coll Cardiol*. 2008;52(17):1413-1420.
63. Nademanee K, Lockwood E, Oketani N, Gidney B. Catheter ablation of atrial fibrillation guided by complex fractionated atrial electrogram mapping of atrial fibrillation substrate. *J Cardiol*. 2010;55(1):1-12.
64. Elayi CS, Verma A, Di Biase L, et al. Ablation for long-standing permanent atrial fibrillation: results from a randomized study comparing three different strategies. *Heart Rhythm*. 2008;5(12):1658-1664.
65. Edgerton ZJ, Edgerton JR. A review of current surgical treatment of patients with atrial fibrillation. *Proc (Bayl Univ Med Cent)*. 2012;25:218-223.
66. Mahapatra S, LaPar DJ, Kamath S, Payne J, Bilchick KC, Mangrum JM et al. Initial experience of sequential surgical epicardial-catheter endocardial ablation for persistent and long-standing persistent atrial fibrillation with long-term follow-up. *Ann Thorac Surg*. 2011;91:1890-1898.
67. Krul SP, Driessen AH, van Boven WJ, et al. Thoracoscopic video-assisted pulmonary vein antrum isolation, ganglionated plexus ablation, and periprocedural confirmation of ablation lesions: first results of a hybrid surgical-electrophysiological approach for atrial fibrillation. *Circ Arrhythm Electrophysiol*. 2011;4:262-270.
68. La Meir M, Gelsomino S, Lucà F, et al. Minimally invasive surgical treatment of lone atrial fibrillation: Early results of hybrid versus standard minimally invasive approach employing radiofrequency sources. *Int J Cardiol*. 2013;167(4):1469-1475. doi:10.1016/j.ijcard.2012.04.044.
69. Zembala M, Filipiak K, Kowalski O, et al. Minimally invasive hybrid ablation procedure for the treatment of persistent atrial fibrillation: one year results. *Kardiol Pol*. 2012;70:819-828.
70. Muneretto C, Bisleri G, Bontempi L, Curnis A. Durable staged hybrid ablation with thoracoscopic and percutaneous approach for treatment of long-standing atrial fibrillation: a 30-month assessment with continuous monitoring. *J Thorac Cardiovasc Surg*. 2012;144:1460-1465.
71. Gehi AK, Mounsey JP, Pursell I, et al. Hybrid epicardial-endocardial ablation using a pericardioscopic technique for the treatment of atrial fibrillation. *Heart Rhythm*. 2013;10:22-28.
72. Bisleri G, Rosati F, Bontempi L, Curnis A, Muneretto C. Hybrid approach for the treatment of long-standing persistent atrial fibrillation: electrophysiological findings and clinical results. *Eur J Cardiothorac Surg*. doi:10.1093/ejcts/ezt115.

Video Legend

Video 49F.1 Stepwise approach hybrid AF.

CHAPTER 50

Surgical Ablation of Inappropriate Sinus Tachycardia

Timo Weimar, MD; Ralph J. Damiano, Jr., MD

Introduction

Inappropriate sinus tachycardia (IST) is an uncommon nonparoxysmal tachyarrhythmia that was first decribed in 1979 and has recently been acknowledged as a unique medical condition.[1,2] It is characterized by normal P-wave morphology in a structurally normal heart that suggests an endocardial activation pattern similar to normal sinus rhythm. The resting heart rate is usually elevated ≥ 100 bpm, and there is an exaggerated rate response to mild physical activity or emotional stress, without nocturnal normalization, that is generally out of proportion to physiological needs.[1-5] A population study from Europe suggested a prevalence of more than 1% meeting the diagnostic criteria of IST.[4]

Diagnosis of Inappropriate Sinus Tachycardia

Patients are primarily young women between 15 and 50 years of age. The clinical presentation of IST is highly variable. Associated symptoms include dyspnea; atypical precordial pain; cephalalgia; fatigue; occasional syncope and presyncope; palpitations; and incapacitating, incessant tachycardia. Although usually one or more of these symptoms bring the patient to medical attention, reproducibility and correlation of symptoms and heart rate can be challenging.

The P-wave morphology recorded on surface electrocardiogram (ECG) does not change during episodes of tachycardia. On 24-hour Holter monitor, the mean heart rate exceeds 100 bpm, daytime resting heart rate exceeds 95 bpm, or sinus rate from supine to upright position increases more than 25 to 30 bpm in a persistent manner.[6] When performing a Bruce protocol treadmill stress test, IST patients' heart rates usually exceed 130 bpm within Stage I of the test. Although these electrocardiographic and heart rate features provide some quantifiable parameters for IST, the diagnosis is not straightforward. Overall, IST is diagnosed by excluding more common reasons for sinus tachycardia such as heart failure or structural abnormalities, anemia, hyperthyroidism, orthostatic hypotension, diabetes mellitus, pheochromocytoma, hypovolemia, infections, anxiety disorders, and drug abuse.[4,7]

Pathomechanisms

The underlying mechanisms of IST are incompletely understood. The proposed potential pathology include enhanced automaticity of the sinus node, altered autonomic activity by increased sympathetic tone, hypersensitivity of sympathetic receptor or blunted parasympathetic tone,[6] and impairment of baroreflex sensitivity.[1,7-9] Furthermore, immunologic disorders involving antibodies generated against β-adrenergic receptors are discussed as possible mechanisms.[10] The extent to which each of these proposed mechanisms contributes to the manifestation of IST is unknown.

Management Strategies

Treatment options for IST have been suggested both by a consensus statement from a joint council of the American

College of Cardiology, American Heart Association, and the European Society for Cardiology for the management of patients with supraventricular arrhythmias in 2003 and more recently by Shen in 2005.[2,7]

Rate control with β-blockers is recommended and most commonly used as first-line therapy.[11] Alternatively, calcium-channel blockers may be used.[12] Unfortunately, these drugs are often insufficient to alleviate patients' symptoms. Ivabradine is a novel antiarrhythmic drug that selectively blocks the I_f-current and inhibits diastolic depolarization. It is highly specific for pacemaker cells in the sinus node and does not affect blood pressure, cardiac contractility, conduction, or ventricular repolarization. Recent reports on a small number of patients suggest a beneficial effect of ivabradine on IST with a significant decrease in tachycardia-associated symptoms.[13,14] However, the drug has so far been approved only for stable angina pectoris.[15]

Different percutaneous catheter ablation techniques and mechanical or chemical occlusion of the sinus node artery can provide a therapeutic alternative for patients refractory to medical management of IST. Radiofrequency catheter modulation of the sinoatrial (SA) node has had less compromising side effects than AV nodal ablation, but success rates have been low. Lee and colleagues reported 14 of 16 patients being free of IST after SA modulation.[16] However, 44% of those patients still complained about cardiac symptoms. Marrouche et al identified earliest sites of activation by three-dimensional nonfluoroscopic mapping and successfully ablated 79% of 39 patients with IST.[17] But again, 44% of those patients remained symptomatic. This confirms findings of Shen and colleagues, who recognized a persistence of cardiac symptoms despite decreased heart rates in IST patients receiving sinus node modification.[18] A reason for failure of the SA node ablation might be the fact that surviving epicardial structures of the SA node have been found at autopsy after recurrent IST.[19] Moreover, Man and Beaver observed a cranial to caudal migration of the activation site with each subsequent ablation performed endocardially or epicardially, respectively, reflecting another challenge when treating this disorder.[20,21] The existence of unique exit pathways for conduction from the SA node to the atrial myocardium may explain why ablation of the earliest area of activation might not properly correlate with the area of functional SA node that is ablated in these patients.[22,23] The vicinity of the targeted sites to the phrenic nerve, which occasionally results in nerve injury, is an additional challenge.[17,20,24] Shen et al recommend a multidisciplinary approach in the treatment of IST, including evaluation by an autonomic neurologist.[7] It is appropriate that a thorough work-up of the individual patient and trials of the above-mentioned medical strategies should be completed before considering invasive therapy like catheter ablation or surgical therapy.

Surgical Ablation of Inappropriate Sinus Tachycardia

Surgical treatment of IST has the advantage of completely isolating the SA node from the right atrium without the risk of collateral damage to the phrenic nerve. The first attempts to surgically treat IST by SA node excision in the 1990s were not successful, because most patients developed new foci of atrial or junctional tachycardia. A modification of the procedure by excising a portion of the right atrial wall at the SVC inflow that was identified as earliest site of activation by epicardial mapping terminated the IST, but a pacemaker implantation was necessary to control prolonged atrial pauses.[25] All of these procedures involved a median sternotomy and cardiopulmonary bypass.

At our institution, 13 patients underwent a surgical ablation for IST between 1987 and 2010 (Table 50.1). This represents the largest surgical series reported for the treatment of IST and reflects the fact that surgery is rarely used as a treatment option for this tachycardia. However, the introduction of alternative energy sources capable of creating transmural lines of ablation on the beating heart has allowed for the development of minimally invasive approaches, including a right minithoracotomy or video-assisted thoracoscopy, without the need for cardiopulmonary bypass.

Surgical Technique

Our early cases ($n = 7$) between 1987 and 2002 were performed through a median sternotomy using cardiopulmonary bypass with bicaval cannulation. An intraoperative mapping system was used to identify the area of earliest activation in the right atrium, and a circumferential incision was performed to isolate this area along with the region of the anatomical SA node from the remaining atrium.

In our recent series ($n = 6$) the incisions were partly or completely replaced by lines of ablation using cryoenergy or bipolar radiofrequency. A minimally invasive approach via a right minithoracotomy was used to isolate the sinus node along with the entire proximal right atrium with a bipolar radiofrequency clamp (Figure 50.1). In our laboratory, bipolar radiofrequency energy was found to be able to create reliable transmural lines of ablation on the beating heart in seconds while minimizing the risk of collateral damage to the surrounding tissue.[26-28] Cryoablation has been used for ablation of arrhythmias for over 3 decades and also has an excellent safety profile.[29-31] However, it is not as reliable in creating transmural lesions on the beating heart.[32]

Intraoperative administration of isoproterenol was used to induce sinus tachycardia with rates of 120 to 180 bpm. Circumferential ablations around the right atrium

Table 50.1 Patient characteristics

Patient (No.)	Age (years)	Gender	Duration of IST (years)	Medical Treatment	No. of Previous Catheter Ablations	Other EP Procedures
1	36	F	3	BB + AA	4	None
2	33	F	7	BB	1	None
3	30	F	12	BB	2	AVJ-ablation/pacemaker
4	42	F	10	BB	2	None
5	29	F	6	BB + AA	2	AVJ-ablation/pacemaker
6	25	F	1	BB	4	AVNRT-ablation
7	42	F	16	BB	3	AVNRT-ablation/pacemaker
8	25	F	1	BB	1	None
9	34	F	6	BB	1	AVNRT-ablation
10	52	M	2	BB + AA	2	None
11	42	F	2	BB + AA	0	None
12	26	M	6	BB + AA	4	AVNRT-ablation/pacemaker
13	20	F	2	BB + AA	3	AVN-ablation/pacemaker
Mean ± SD	35.5 ± 9.0		5.8 ± 4.6		2.2 ± 1.3	

AA = antiarrhythmic medication; AVJ = AV junction; AVN = atrioventricular nodal; AVNRT = atrioventricular nodal reentrant tachycardia; BB = β-blocker; EP = electrophysiological; IST = inappropriate sinus tachycardia; SD = standard deviation.

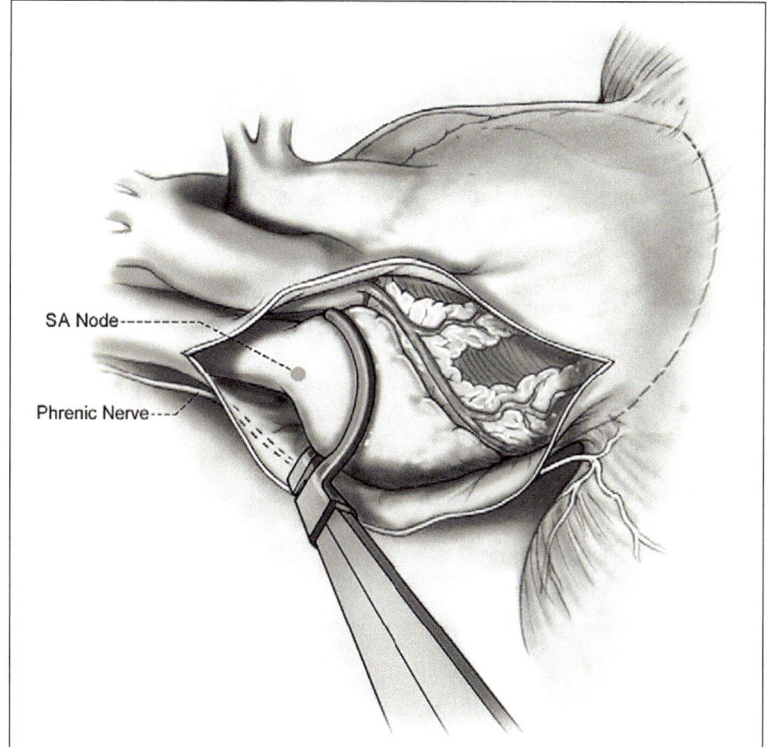

Figure 50.1 Bipolar radiofrequency clamp isolating the sinoatrial (SA) node complex while preserving the phrenic nerve. *Source:* Reprinted with permission from Beaver et al,[21] with permission from Elsevier.

were performed until an inversion of the P-wave morphology was seen in the inferior leads and blunting of the response to isoproterenol was achieved (Figure 50.2). The change in morphology of the P wave after SA node isolation indicates that atrial activation is driven by more caudally located pacemaker regions. A mean of 8.3 ± 1.5 ablations were necessary to completely isolate the SA node along with a generous cuff of surrounding right atrial tissue in this series. Bipolar pacing was used to confirm electrical isolation of the SA node and surrounding areas from the remaining right atrium in each case. In 2 patients, epicardial mapping was performed following ablation, which demonstrated a subsidiary pacemaker located in the lower right atrium producing a normal

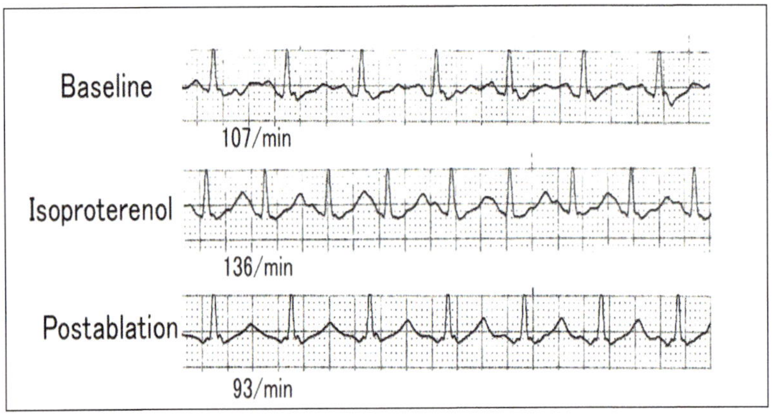

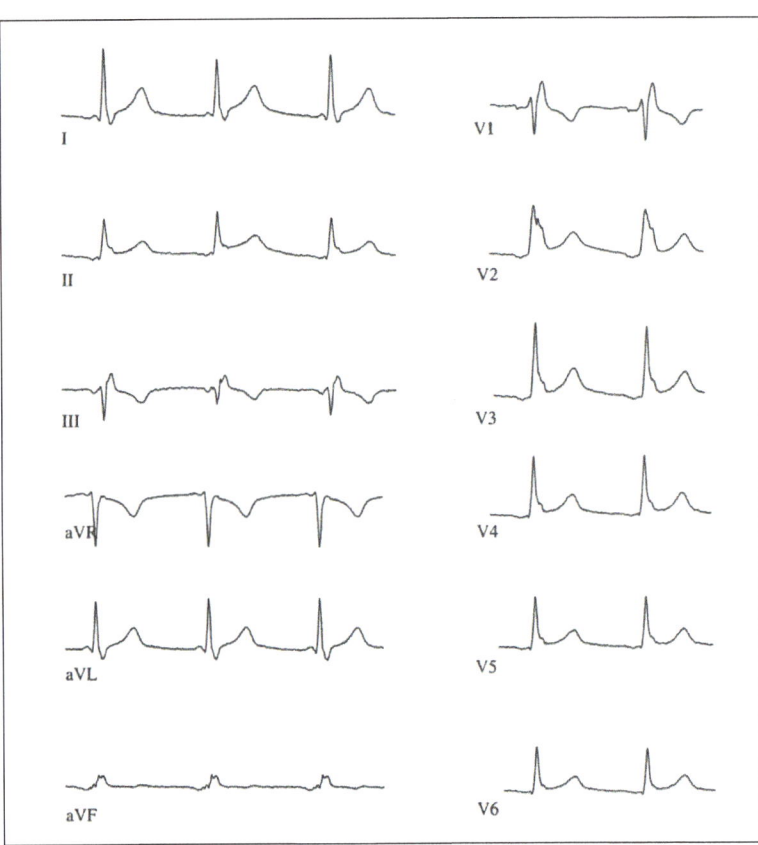

Figure 50.2 Inferior lead (II) of the intraoperative electrocardiogram of patient #10. The baseline EGM demonstrated an upright P wave with an increase in heart rate during administration of isoproterenol. After ablation there was no rate acceleration after isoproterenol administration and negative P-wave morphology.

Figure 50.3 Twelve-lead ECG showing stable postoperative atrial escape rhythm with negative P-wave morphology in inferior leads.

heart rate. However, mapping is not a necessary component of these cases except in situations where an ectopic pacemaker is suspected.

Clinical Outcome

Sinus tachycardia was eliminated in all patients in the immediate postoperative course as noted by ECG (Table 50.2). Nine patients had an atrial escape rhythm as shown in Figure 50.3. Two patients (15%) had a junctional rhythm and required postoperative pacemaker implantation. There were no operative deaths or major complications.

All 13 patients were available for follow up. After a mean follow-up time of 5.6 ± 5.7 years, 3 patients (23%) developed atrial tachyarrhythmias (atrial flutter, ectopic atrial tachycardia arising from the coronary sinus, and atrial fibrillation, respectively). Overall, 62% of patients were free of cardiac symptoms and 39% of patients were free from cardiac symptoms without the need for additional medical therapy. None of the patients receiving a minimally invasive approach in our more recent series have reported any tachycardia during the long-term follow-up period, and our success rate has been 100%.

Summary

Surgical isolation of the SA node for medically refractory IST can result in successful long-term prevention of

Table 50.2 Results of surgical ablation

Patient (No.)	Surgical Procedure	Postoperative Rhythm	Late Findings	Follow-up (Years)
1	SAN Isolation	AVJR / Pacemaker	Atrial Flutter	17
2	SAN Isolation	Atrial Escape Rhythm	Asymptomatic	14
3	SAN Isolation	Pacemaker	AF / Pacemaker	10
4	SAN Isolation (Cryoablation)	Atrial Escape Rhythm	Palpitations	10
5	SAN Isolation	Pacemaker	Palpitations	9
6	SAN Isolation (Cryoablation)	AVJR / Pacemaker	Asymptomatic	5
7	SAN Isolation (Cryoablation)	Atrial Escape Rhythm	Pacemaker	2
8	SAN Isolation (Bipolar RF)	Atrial Escape Rhythm	Asymptomatic	2
9	SAN Isolation (Bipolar RF)	Atrial Escape Rhythm	Asymptomatic	2
10	SAN Isolation (Bipolar RF)	Atrial Escape Rhythm	Asymptomatic	0.1
11	SAN Isolation (Bipolar RF)	Atrial Escape Rhythm	Asymptomatic	1.3
12	SAN Isolation (Bipolar RF+Cryo)	Atrial Escape Rhythm	Asymptomatic	0.1
13	SAN Isolation (Bipolar RF+Cryo)	Atrial Escape Rhythm	Asymptomatic	0.4
Mean ± SD				5.6 ± 5.7

AVJR = AV junction rhythm; RF = radiofrequency; SAN = sinoatrial node.

recurrent IST. However, approximately one-third of patients experience cardiac symptoms even without tachycardia recurrence or require pacemaker implantation.

The minimally invasive approach coupled with modern ablation technologies can reduce and simplify the surgical treatment of IST, avoid sternotomy, and allow completion of the procedure without cardiopulmonary bypass. This may make surgery a more attractive option for patients with IST refractory to medical management. Patients should be considered for surgical ablation of their IST if they have failed medical therapy and have recurrent symptomatic IST following catheter ablation, if they are poor candidates for catheter ablation.

References

1. Bauernfeind RA, Amat YLF, Dhingra RC, Kehoe R, Wyndham C, Rosen KM. Chronic nonparoxysmal sinus tachycardia in otherwise healthy persons. *Ann Intern Med.* 1979;91:702-710.
2. Blomstrom-Lundqvist C, Scheinman MM, Aliot EM, et al. ACC/AHA/ESC Guidelines for the Management of Patients with Supraventricular Arrhythmias—Executive Summary. A report of the American College of Cardiology/American Heart Association Task Force on Practice Guidelines and the European Society of Cardiology Committee for Practice Guidelines (Writing Committee to Develop Guidelines for the Management of Patients with Supraventricular Arrhythmias) developed in collaboration with NASPE-Heart Rhythm Society. *J Am Coll Cardiol.* 2003;42:1493-1531.
3. Cossu SF, Steinberg JS. Supraventricular tachyarrhythmias involving the sinus node: Clinical and EP characteristics. *Prog Cardiovasc Dis.* 1998;41:51-63.
4. Still AM, Raatikainen P, Ylitalo A, et al. Prevalence, characteristics and natural course of inappropriate sinus tachycardia. *Europace.* 2005;7:104-112.
5. Krahn AD, Yee R, Klein GJ, Morillo C. Inappropriate sinus tachycardia: Evaluation and therapy. *J Cardiovasc Electrophysiol.* 1995;6:1124-1128.
6. Castellanos A, Moleiro F, Chakko S, et al. Heart rate variability in inappropriate sinus tachycardia. *Am J Cardiol.* 1998;82:531-534
7. Shen WK. How to manage patients with inappropriate sinus tachycardia. *Heart Rhythm.* 2005;2:1015-1019.
8. Morillo CA, Klein GJ, Thakur RK, Li H, Zardini M, Yee R. Mechanism of 'inappropriate' sinus tachycardia. Role of sympathovagal balance. *Circulation.* 1994;90:873-877.
9. Leon H, Guzman JC, Kuusela T, Dillenburg R, Kamath M, Morillo CA. Impaired baroreflex gain in patients with inappropriate sinus tachycardia. *J Cardiovasc Electrophysiol.* 2005;16:64-68.
10. Chiale PA, Garro HA, Schmidberg J, et al. Inappropriate sinus tachycardia may be related to an immunologic disorder involving cardiac beta andrenergic receptors. *Heart Rhythm.* 2006;3:1182-1186.
11. Schulze V, Steiner S, Hennersdorf M, Strauer BE. Ivabradine as an alternative therapeutic trial in the therapy of inappropriate sinus tachycardia: A case report. *Cardiology.* 2008;110: 206-208.
12. Foster MC, Levine PA. Use of verapamil to control an inappropriate chronic sinus tachycardia. *Chest.* 1984;85:697-699.
13. Khan S, Hamid S, Rinaldi C. Treatment of inappropriate sinus tachycardia with ivabradine in a patient with postural orthostatic tachycardia syndrome and a dual chamber pacemaker. *Pacing Clin Electrophysiol.* 2009;32:131-133.
14. Zellerhoff S, Hinterseer M, Felix Krull B, et al. Ivabradine in patients with inappropriate sinus tachycardia. *Naunyn Schmiedebergs Arch Pharmacol.* 2010;382:483-486.
15. Borer JS, Fox K, Jaillon P, Lerebours G. Antianginal and antiischemic effects of ivabradine, an i(f) inhibitor, in stable

angina: A randomized, double-blind, multicentered, placebo-controlled trial. *Circulation*. 2003;107:817-823.
16. Lee RJ, Kalman JM, Fitzpatrick AP, et al. Radiofrequency catheter modification of the sinus node for "inappropriate" sinus tachycardia. *Circulation*. 1995;92:2919-2928.
17. Marrouche NF, Beheiry S, Tomassoni G, et al. Three-dimensional nonfluoroscopic mapping and ablation of inappropriate sinus tachycardia. Procedural strategies and long-term outcome. *J Am Coll Cardiol*. 2002;39:1046-1054.
18. Shen WK, Low PA, Jahangir A, et al. Is sinus node modification appropriate for inappropriate sinus tachycardia with features of postural orthostatic tachycardia syndrome? *Pacing Clin Electrophysiol*. 2001;24:217-230.
19. Sanchez-Quintana D, Cabrera JA, Farre J, Climent V, Anderson RH, Ho SY. Sinus node revisited in the era of electroanatomical mapping and catheter ablation. *Heart*. 2005;91:189-194.
20. Man KC, Knight B, Tse HF, Pelosi F, Michaud GF, Flemming M, Strickberger SA, Morady F. Radiofrequency catheter ablation of inappropriate sinus tachycardia guided by activation mapping. *J Am Coll Cardiol*. 2000;35:451-457.
21. Beaver TM, Miles WM, Conti JB, et al. Minimally invasive ablation of a migrating focus of inappropriate sinus tachycardia. *J Thorac Cardiovasc Surg*. 2010;139:506-507.
22. Fedorov VV, Schuessler RB, Hemphill M, et al. Structural and functional evidence for discrete exit pathways that connect the canine sinoatrial node and atria. *Circ Res*. 2009;104:915-923.
23. Stiles MK, Brooks AG, Roberts-Thomson KC, et al. High-density mapping of the sinus node in humans: Role of preferential pathways and the effect of remodeling. *J Cardiovasc Electrophysiol*. 2010;21:532-539.
24. Vatasescu R, Shalganov T, Kardos A, et al. Right diaphragmatic paralysis following endocardial cryothermal ablation of inappropriate sinus tachycardia. *Europace*. 2006;8:904-906.
25. Esmailzadeh B, Bernat R, Winkler K, Meybehm M, Pfeiffer D, Kirchhoff PG. Surgical excision of the sinus node in a patient with inappropriate sinus tachycardia. *J Thorac Cardiovasc Surg*. 1997;114:861-864.
26. Prasad SM, Maniar HS, Schuessler RB, Damiano RJ, Jr. Chronic transmural atrial ablation by using bipolar radiofrequency energy on the beating heart. *J Thorac Cardiovasc Surg*. 2002;124:708-713.
27. Prasad SM, Maniar HS, Diodato MD, Schuessler RB, Damiano RJ, Jr. Physiological consequences of bipolar radiofrequency energy on the atria and pulmonary veins: A chronic animal study. *Ann Thorac Surg*. 2003;76:836-841; discussion 841-832.
28. Gaynor SL, Ishii Y, Diodato MD, et al. Successful performance of Cox-Maze procedure on beating heart using bipolar RFA: A feasibility study in animals. *Ann Thorac Surg*. 2004;78:1671-1677.
29. Mack CA, Milla F, Ko W, et al. Surgical treatment of atrial fibrillation using argon-based cryoablation during concomitant cardiac procedures. *Circulation*. 2005;112:I1-6.
30. Holman WL, Ikeshita M, Douglas JM, Jr., Smith PK, Cox JL. Cardiac cryosurgery: Effects of myocardial temperature on cryolesion size. *Surgery*. 1983;93:268-272
31. Lall SC, Damiano RJ, Jr. Surgical ablation devices for atrial fibrillation. *J Interv Card Electrophysiol*. 2007;20:73-82.
32. Doll N, Kornherr P, Aupperle H, et al. Epicardial treatment of atrial fibrillation using cryoablation in an acute off-pump sheep model. *Thorac Cardiovasc Surg*. 2003;51:267-273.

CHAPTER 51

COMPLICATIONS OF SURGICAL ABLATION

Peyman Benharash, MD; Richard J. Shemin, MD

Overview of Techniques for Surgical Ablation

As the electroanatomic details of atrial fibrillation (AF) have been elucidated, a variety of surgical techniques have been developed to create anatomic lesion sets that create exit block from foci of AF generation and prevent the reentry of waves in both atria. The details of the lesions and the technical aspects of their creation are discussed elsewhere in this book. Briefly, the first generation of such modern techniques involves precise surgical incisions in the atria and scar formation to prevent macroreentrant circuits and create pulmonary vein isolation. The current lesion pattern is known as the Cox-Maze III. Naturally, these operations require great technical expertise and precision as the atria are both cut in multiple places and recreated with suture lines. The operative time and complexity of the operation as well as the proximity of many vital structures, such as the coronary arteries, valves, and the conduction system, have limited the widespread use of the cut-and-sew Maze operation. A variety of energy delivery techniques have been developed to deliver a collimated source of energy that is theoretically able to create a "perfect burn" on the atrium, creating electrically isolating lesions. Such lesions can be created with the application of cold or heat to cause tissue injury.

The "perfect burn" created by these alternate energy sources must be transmural; that is, permanently create electrically nonconducting tissue throughout the thickness of the atrium in a contiguous fashion. Secondly, the burn line must have sharp demarcations and must not create tissue damage beyond the application zone. The lesion sets of the Cox-Maze III procedure performed with energy sources is called the Cox-Maze IV operation.

It is important to understand how tissue can become electrically isolating with the use of any energy source. As discussed elsewhere, heating the tissue to the 50°C isotherm has been shown to render the tissue permanently electrically inactive. Application of cryogenic probes similarly causes irreversible cell death and electrical isolation. All energy sources are imperfect with regard to how their energy spreads. Therefore, at high enough powers it creates a transmural lesion, which will affect adjacent tissues and can cause injury, known as "collateral damage." Additionally, the circumferential transmission of all energy sources does not allow them to be fully directional. This problem has been somewhat addressed with the development of bipolar systems and directional focused antennae. However, the inability to completely control direction and spread of the energy sources has created a set of unique complications that will be discussed below.

Additionally, the variable apposition of the source and tissue creates another variable in the efficacy of the alternate energy sources. Application of energy in between clamps has certainly limited the energy spread and has improved tissue contact for better transmission of energy.

Complications of Surgical Approaches

Surgical ablation with or without the use of alternate energy sources has proven to be an effective treatment for AF. However, a number of significant complications can occur that are potentially life threatening. A discussion of the general complications of the surgical ablation will be followed by specifics of each technical category.

General Complications of Surgical Ablation

Efficacy

Failure of the Cox-Maze III or IV procedures to render the patient in sinus rhythm is an important but often overlooked complication. The high efficacy of the Cox-Maze operation has been demonstrated by numerous groups.[1-3] Clearly, the cure rate is very different in populations with paroxysmal AF when compared to the permanent type. Failure to achieve sinus rhythm can be divided into early and late phases.

Immediately after the operation, tissue injury, pericardial irritation, and exposure to the cardiopulmonary bypass circuit causes an intense local and systemic inflammatory response. Such inflammation may be responsible for early failure of the Cox-Maze operation.[4] Development of tachyarrhythmias in the postoperative period presents a challenging problem to the clinician. Although most of these arrhythmias are AF, atrial flutter and other supraventricular tachycardic rhythms have been seen.[5] The inflammation usually subsides within the first 2 to 3 months, and sinus rhythm is restored.

After the so-called "blanking period" (3 months), during which the inflammatory response subsides, variable cure rates are reported in the literature. While a long-term success rate of >89% has been reported by most of the large series,[3] it is important to note that the cure rate can be as low as 60% in patients with risk factors that include large left atrial size, duration of AF, permanent AF, and age.[6]

In a large series from University of Michigan, Romano and others have reported excellent cure rates in patients with large atria when a reduction atrioplasty is done in addition to the Cox-Maze procedure.[7]

The measurement of cure rate is problematic in a condition such as AF, which can be transient yet recurrent. Sampling the patients at a particular time point with tools such as ECG, phone calls, and surveys overestimates the cure rate, while a Kaplan-Mayer curve will underestimate this population. A Heart Rhythm Society task force on catheter and surgical ablation of AF has set forth a comprehensive set of guidelines and definitions in following patients who have had AF ablation.[8] Major points include at least a 12-month follow-up, absence of any atrial arrhythmia without the use of antiarrhythmic drugs, measurement of the quality of life, and recording of all major complications.

Heart Block and Conduction Disturbances

The use of cut-and-sew or alternate energy sources for the Cox-Maze operation can injure the sinoatrial or atrioventricular nodes or the conduction pathways between. Although this problem is usually temporary, about 5% of patients require a permanent pacemaker. This injury must be considered collateral damage and usually results from the spread of heat or cold energy to the right atrium and its junction with the superior vena cava. This complication is best avoided by deliberate placement of lesions away from the conduction tissue in a biatrial lesion set, keeping in mind the penumbral zone that is at risk around each lesion.

Most often, a properly performed procedure can still present with nodal dysfunction, especially in patients who have had prolonged periods of AF. This may be attributed to down-regulation of the sinus node in presence of long-term AF signals and pre-existing sinus node disease in some patients.

Thromboembolism

The transmural injury created by the lesions of the Cox-Maze procedure causes damage to the normally smooth and antithrombotic endocardium. Exposed myocardium, suture material, burnt tissue, and scar all attract platelets and cause fibrin deposition, leading to potential formation of clot. Additionally, it has been shown that surgery, exposure to cardiopulmonary bypass, and intravascular/intracardiac manipulation can cause derangements in the coagulation cascade and create a prothrombotic effect.[9] Moreover, atrial transport function does not return to normal immediately, and a period of relative stasis will exist inside the heart postoperatively. This is likely also the case with catheter ablation, although its true incidence is likely underreported. The frequent recurrence of atrial fibrillation during the "blanking period" also contributes to the thromboembolic risk after the Cox-Maze procedure.

Early anticoagulation with warfarin and/or aspirin is recommended in the postoperative period. Although individual preferences dictate anticoagulation protocols, we start warfarin on the same day of surgery as long as bleeding is not suspected. If the patient develops AF postoperatively, we tend to use heparin as a bridge until achieving an INR > 2.0.

The low incidence of perioperative and late thromboembolism is in part due to the exclusion of the left atrial appendage (LAA) as part of the Cox-Maze procedure.

Bleeding and Perforation

The Cox-Maze technique being a surgical procedure carries a finite risk of bleeding and perforation of vascular structures in the mediastinum. The cut-and-sew Maze procedure requires extensive suture lines in the back of the left atrium and relatively inaccessible areas once separated from bypass. Meticulous hemostasis is paramount in these operations and troublesome bleeding can cause significant harm to the patient and success of the operation.

Particular attention must be paid to the LAA regardless of the surgical approach. Removal or exclusion of the LAA reduces the risk of postoperative thromboembolism and is an important part of the Cox-Maze procedure. The friable appendage can tear during manipulation or can bleed in an immediate or delayed fashion in the postoperative period. Close attention to this issue during and following the operation is important in order to optimize patient outcomes.

Introduction of clamps and catheters inside and along the atrium can lead to inadvertent injury to the pulmonary veins, pulmonary artery, and the atrium itself. This is of particular significance in minimally invasive cases, and insertion of these catheters under videoscopic guidance is advised.

Pulmonary Vein Stenosis

With Haïssaguerre's landmark report[10] on the location of triggers in the pulmonary veins as the major focus for initiation of AF, much attention has been paid to creating a complete burn and isolating the pulmonary vein orifices from the left atrium. This is perhaps the most important part of any Cox-Maze procedure for paroxysmal AF. Ensuring adequate cell death around the pulmonary vein cuffs, however, is accompanied by a small chance of scarring and subsequent pulmonary vein stenosis. Although this complication has been observed with catheter ablation and early generation radiofrequency devices, modern series do not report this problem. Prevention is best accomplished by ensuring that the energy is applied to the antrum and not directly to the pulmonary veins when isolating the veins in pairs. The "box" lesion encompassing all four pulmonary veins prevents this injury.

Investigation of this problem would require CT/MRI or echocardiographic imaging of the pulmonary veins as they converge into the left atrium. Atypical segmental pulmonary edema, dyspnea, and hemoptysis may serve as clues to the diagnosis of pulmonary vein stenosis. Stenting of such strictures has not been successful and therefore augmentation of the pulmonary veins with a patch is generally preferred.

Coronary Artery and Sinus Injury

The lesions of the Cox-Maze procedure often come close to the coronary arteries. While injuries to the circumflex artery can occur and are recognized during the traditional cut-and-sew Maze operation, damage to the coronary arteries by the various energy sources can present in a delayed fashion. Direct injury to the circumflex artery during amputation of the LAA can lead to hemorrhage, thrombosis, or fistula formation to the left atrium.[11,12] Intraoperative detection of a new posterior wall motion abnormality should raise the suspicion for injury to the circumflex coronary artery. Cold and heat injury create intimal damage, clot formation, and delayed intimal hyperplasia, which can present as late at 1 year following the procedure. Angina following the Cox-Maze procedure should prompt investigation of the coronary arteries.

The coronary sinus is also at risk during the Cox-Maze procedure, as it runs in the left atrioventricular groove adjacent to the circumflex artery. While intraoperative injury can be recognized immediately, no reports of late coronary sinus strictures are found, likely due to the asymptomatic nature of this process. Although cryotherapy was thought to be safe with regards to coronary artery injury, many large series now report rare instances of such complication.[12-14] During epicardial application of cryothermy, it is important to have the retrograde cardioplegia catheter in the coronary sinus near the os to prevent inadvertent transmission to the coronary artery.

Esophageal Injury

The esophagus travels in the posterior mediastinum and runs behind the left atrium as it travels under the left main stem bronchus. A layer of pericardium separates the left atrial wall from the esophagus, making it prone to collateral damage. Although esophageal injury has not been found with the cut-and-sew Cox-Maze procedure, there are many reports of esophageal injury with alternate energy sources. A thin-walled organ, the esophagus is at risk of thermal or cold injury in particular due to the low flow state of bypass and presence of a transesophageal probe within the lumen. Unfortunately, such injury does not present itself immediately unless a direct mechanical disruption has occurred. In the postoperative period, the injured mucosa sloughs off and a transmural injury is created, leading to delayed rupture or fistulization into the left atrium.[15] This rare but often fatal complication is most often seen in unipolar, endocardial radiofrequency catheter-based procedures, but has been reported with endocardial application of thermal/cryo energy of surgical procedures.

Development of an atrioesophageal fistula can present with gastrointestinal hemorrhage, hemoptysis, or sequelae of intracardiac air such as stroke, air embolization, or cardiac arrest. A high index of suspicion must exist for prompt diagnosis of this problem, usually with a CT scan. If the patient survives the initial event, repair is undertaken, which includes the use of cardiopulmonary bypass and repair of the left atrium followed by buttressing of the esophageal perforation with a muscle flap after adequate debridement and wide drainage. Although literature reports only demonstrate esophageal injury with application of unipolar radiofrequency,[15] our group has encountered this problem with endocardial application of a cryoballoon during an electrophysiological catheter procedure.

Since the esophagus is in close proximity to the back of the left atrium, we recommend making the connecting lesions in the floor or roof of the left atrium to avoid close contact. There exist balloon devices that inflate in this region and create insulation during minimally invasive cases.[16]

Phrenic Nerve Injury

The phrenic nerve traverses the outside of the pericardium in its posterolateral aspect as it reaches the diaphragm. Without insulation, and given its long path length, it is prone to damage during the Cox-Maze procedure. This is particularly the case while ablating the pulmonary veins as they emerge through the pericardium. Phrenic nerve palsy can be temporary or permanent depending on the extent of injury. However, roughly 1% of patients undergoing the Cox-Maze operation develop this complication.

Again, shielding of the pericardium and application of the energy source at the confluence of pulmonary veins and the atrium is thought to reduce this complication. Close attention to the entire course of the cryoprobe is critical in avoiding inadvertent freezing of the pericardium near the phrenic nerve.

Fluid Retention

The neurohormonal mechanisms responsible for fluid homeostasis are altered after the Cox-Maze procedure. The systemic injury from surgery as well as removal of the atrial appendages are thought to be responsible for the marked fluid retention observed after the Cox-Maze procedure.[17,18] Furthermore, preservation of the right atrial appendage (RAA) has been shown to alleviate this problem.[19] In the current iteration of the Cox-Maze procedure, the RAA is preserved, while the LAA is removed to reduce the chance of thromboembolism.[20,21]

Additionally, activation of the renin-angiotensin-aldosterone system as well as high levels of antidiuretic hormone after surgery contributes to the fluid retention. It is important to initiate diuresis in these patients early, using furosemide. In our experience, addition of spironolactone is of great benefit, as it directly counteracts the effects of aldosterone and mitigates potassium wasting, which can predispose the patient to arrhythmias.

Considerations Related to Minimally Invasive Approaches

The surgeon must adapt his/her skills while performing surgical approaches with minimal access. Lack of optimal visualization can lead to certain complications that are specific to minimal access cases. Thoracoscopic ports are inserted in the intercostal spaces to create tracks in the chest wall for introduction of various instruments and cannulae. Due to the proximity of intercostal vessels and tunneling through the muscles of the chest wall, these sites can bleed after withdrawal of the ports and relief of the local tamponade. It is especially important to videoscopically examine each port site after removal of the ports to ensure perfect hemostasis.

In minimally invasive cases, split lung ventilation is used to optimize visualization and allow access to the heart and the great vessels. A recently recognized problem that occurs after the expansion of both lungs involves the development of a transient homogenous radiographic infiltrate in the deflated lung and is termed "down-lung syndrome." Although the exact pathogenesis of this problem remains elusive, it is thought to originate from ischemia-reperfusion injury and lack of positive intra-alveolar pressure. In most patients, this problem is self-limited and is of little clinical significance. Occasionally, the patient can develop severe hypoxemia and require temporary mechanical support.

In our experience, withdrawal of the transesophageal echocardiogram probe proximally along with deflation the endotracheal tube cuff while on bypass, or use of a bronchial blocker in place of a dual-lumen endotracheal tube, has nearly completely eliminated this problem. We believe the salutary effects of such maneuvers to emanate from increased bronchial artery flow and elimination of reperfusion injury.

Final Remarks

Surgical ablation of atrial arrhythmias has revolutionized the field of electrophysiology and has undoubtedly improved patients' quality of life by reducing the risk of thromboembolism and offering freedom from anticoagulation.

However, complications that occur with such relatively new techniques are unique and require familiarity for prompt diagnosis and treatment. In the above sections, the most commonly encountered surgical complications are presented. Since some of these problems are life threatening, the clinician must carry a high index of suspicion in order to institute immediate life-saving treatment. It is our opinion that meticulous surgical technique and knowledge of the pitfalls associated with the Cox-Maze procedures is mandatory and the best tool in our armamentarium in achieving excellent results.

References

1. Melby SJ, Zierer A, Bailey MS, et al. A new era in surgical treatment of atrial fibrillation: the impact of technology and lesion set on procedural efficacy. *Ann Thorac Surg.* 2006;244(4):588-592.
2. Damiano RJ, Voeller RK. Surgical and minimally invasive ablation for atrial fibrillation. *Curr Treat Options Cardiovasc Med.* 2006;8(5):371-376.
3. Gaynor SL, Diodato MD, Prasad SM, et al. A prospective, single-center clinical trial of a modified Cox-Maze procedure with bipolar radiofrequency ablation. *J Thorac Cardiovasc Surg.* 2004;128(4):535-542.
4. Ishii Y, Schuessler RB, Gaynor SL, et al. Inflammation of atrium after cardiac surgery is associated with inhomogeneity of atrial conduction and atrial fibrillation. *Circulation.* 2005;111(22):2881-2888.
5. Ishii Y, Gleva MJ, Gamache MC, et al. Atrial tachyarrhythmias after the Maze procedure: incidence and prognosis. *Circulation.* 2004;110(11 Suppl 1):II164-II168.

6. Gillinov AM, Sirak J, Blackstone EH, et al. The Cox Maze procedure in mitral valve disease: predictors of recurrent atrial fibrillation. *J Thorac Cardiovasc Surg.* 2005;130(6):1653-1660.
7. Romano MA, Bach DS, Pagani FD, Prager RL, Deeb GM, Bolling SF. Atrial reduction plasty Cox Maze procedure: extended indications for atrial fibrillation surgery. *Ann Thorac Surg.* 2004;77(4):1282-1287; discussion 1287.
8. Calkins H, Brugada J, Packer DL, et al. HRS/EHRA/ECAS expert consensus statement on catheter and surgical ablation of atrial fibrillation: recommendations for personnel, policy, procedures and follow-up. *Europace.* 2007;9(6):335-379.
9. Ad N, Pirovic EA, Kim YD, et al. Observations on the perioperative management of patients undergoing the Maze procedure. *Semin Thorac Cardiovasc Surg.* 2000;12(1):63-67.
10. Parolari A, Mussoni L, Frigerio M, et al. Increased prothrombotic state lasting as long as one month after on-pump and off-pump coronary surgery. *J Thorac Cardiovasc Surg.* 2005;130(2):303-308.
11. Haïssaguerre M, Jaïs P, Shah DC, et al. Spontaneous initiation of atrial fibrillation by ectopic beats originating in the pulmonary veins. *N Engl J Med.* 1998;339(10):659-666.
12. Nguyen-Do P, Bannon P, Leung DY. Coronary artery to the left atrial fistula after resection of atrial appendages. *Ann Thorac Surg.* 2004;78(2):e26-e27.
13. Roberts-Thomson KC, Steven D, Seiler J, et al. Coronary artery injury due to catheter ablation in adults: presentations and outcomes. *Circulation.* 2009;120(15):1465-1473.
14. Aoyama H, Nakagawa H, Pitha JV, et al. Comparison of cryothermia and radiofrequency current in safety and efficacy of catheter ablation within the canine coronary sinus close to the left circumflex coronary artery. *J Cardiovasc Electrophysiol.* 2005;16(11):1218-1226.
15. Gaita F, Riccardi R, Gallotti R. Surgical approaches to atrial fibrillation. *Card Electrophysiol Rev.* 2002;6(4):401-405.
16. Contreras-Valdes FM, Heist EK, Danik SB, et al. Severity of esophageal injury predicts time to healing after radiofrequency catheter ablation for atrial fibrillation. *Heart Rhythm.* 2011;8(12):1862-1868.
17. Kottkamp H, Hindricks G, Autschbach R, et al. Specific linear left atrial lesions in atrial fibrillation: intraoperative radiofrequency ablation using minimally invasive surgical techniques. *J Am Coll Cardiol.* 2002;40(3):475-480.
18. Omari BO, Nelson RJ, Robertson JM. Effect of right atrial appendectomy on the release of atrial natriuretic hormone. *J Thorac Cardiovasc Surg.* 1991;102(2):272-279.
19. Yoshihara F, Nishikimi T, Sasako Y, et al. Plasma atrial natriuretic peptide concentration inversely correlates with left atrial collagen volume fraction in patients with atrial fibrillation: plasma ANP as a possible biochemical marker to predict the outcome of the maze procedure. *J Am Coll Cardiol.* 2002;39(2):288-294.
20. Yoshihara F, Nishikimi T, Sasako Y, et al. Preservation of the right atrial appendage improves reduced plasma atrial natriuretic peptide levels after the maze procedure. *J Thorac Cardiovasc Surg.* 2000;119(4 Pt 1):790-794.
21. Mokadam NA, McCarthy PM, Gillinov AM, et al. A prospective multicenter trial of bipolar radiofrequency ablation for atrial fibrillation: early results. *Ann Thorac Surg.* 2004;78(5):1665-1670.

SECTION 2D

INTERVENTIONAL ELECTROPHYSIOLOGY PROCEDURES

Device Implantation: Intraoperative, Surgical, and Device Management

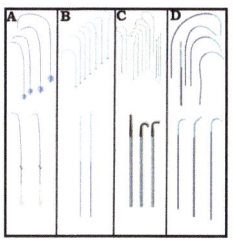
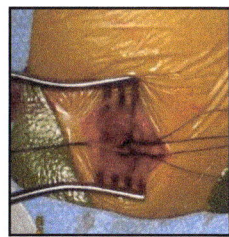
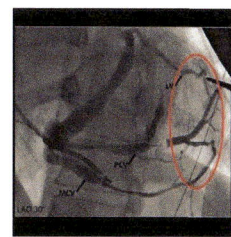
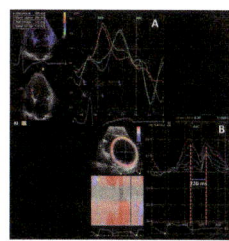

CHAPTER 52

Implantation Techniques for Permanent Pacemakers and Single- and Dual-Chamber Implantable Cardioverter-defibrillator Devices

Mark L. Blitzer, MD; Mark H. Schoenfeld, MD

Introduction

The purpose of this chapter is to provide the practicing clinician or student of the field with an overview of implantation techniques for pacemakers and defibrillators. A wide variety of strategies are used around the world, although certain fundamental principles should be acknowledged.[1] In specific cases, there may not be a single best approach. Therefore, the greater the array of techniques available in a physician's arsenal, the more likely it is that the physician can consistently provide implantation in a safe, effective, and timely manner.

Preoperative Planning

Attention to detail prior to the procedure is critical. A thorough review of the patient's history—including prior coronary artery disease, congestive heart failure, valvular heart disease, and dysrhythmias—is important. This prerequisite is no different than when consulting on patients prior to noncardiac surgery. Factors that will affect choice of anesthesia during the case, such as obesity or history of obstructive sleep apnea (OSA), are important to ascertain. All infectious issues should be resolved prior to surgery.

Antiplatelet and anticoagulation status must be analyzed. There are risks to continuing anticlotting medications, including development of a significant pocket hematoma or hemopericardium. However, these risks need to be balanced against the increased thromboembolic risks (stroke, deep venous thrombosis, or pulmonary embolus), if these medications are discontinued. These risks have been nicely quantified in a recent report.[2] For an elective procedure in a patient who is on aspirin for primary prevention, the drug is ordinarily discontinued for 5 to 7 days preoperatively. If the patient has established cardiovascular disease, the aspirin is continued. Clopidogrel is rarely discontinued since studies suggesting its importance after deployment of a drug-eluting stent have become more compelling.

Practice patterns vary markedly in terms of how to manage patients on warfarin.[3] For patients with persistent atrial fibrillation (AF) and a low CHADS-2 score, the drug is usually discontinued for 3 or 4 days preprocedure provided the baseline international normalized ratio (INR) is not excessive. Warfarin is reinitiated on the day of surgery. Managing patients at higher risk of adverse event with drug discontinuation, such as those with prior thromboembolic events or who have a mechanical valve in the mitral position, is more complicated. Many implanters would traditionally admit the patient and start intravenous heparin or administer low-molecular-weight heparin on an outpatient basis. This technique, particularly when the heparin is reintroduced postoperatively, has the highest risk of bleeding.[4] In response to this issue, many have investigated the possibility of maintaining warfarin without interruption periprocedurally. An increasingly large database supports the safety of this practice.[5,6] As ever, meticulous attention to pocket hemostasis and operator experience are important.

An antiseptic skin wash, eg, Phisohex® (Sanofi-Aventis, Bridgewater, NJ) or Hibiclens® (Molnlycke Health Care Inc., Norcross, GA), administered either at home or in-house successfully diminishes skin bacteria counts.[7] While it remains controversial whether this translates into reduced surgical site infections,[8,9] it is currently accepted as prudent practice. Recent data strongly support "decontaminating" the subgroup of patients who are staphylococcal carriers with mupirocin ointment to the nares twice daily for 5 days preoperatively along with chlorhexidine soap.[10]

A set of laboratory studies including complete blood count, chemistry panel, and prothrombin/partial thromboplastin are routinely obtained within 2 weeks of surgery. Patients with morning operating room times are kept fasting after midnight. Afternoon cases may be given clear liquid breakfasts. Most medications are continued on the morning of surgery with a small sip of water. For a type 2 diabetic patient, oral hypoglycemics—ie, sulfonylureas—and short-acting insulin are withheld on the morning of surgery. Of the oral agents that do not result in hypoglycemia, metformin and alpha-glucosidase inhibitors should be avoided on the morning of surgery, but thiazolidinediones may be continued. Metformin may only be resumed once normal renal function is confirmed postoperatively. The doses of longer-acting insulins are usually halved on the morning of surgery.

Room Set-up

Implantation of a permanent pacemaker (PPM) or implantable cardiac-defibrillator (ICD) can be safely performed in the catheterization lab, in a dedicated procedure room, or in the operating room. All venues require equal attention to meticulous sterile technique, quick access to supplies, and emergency plans for rare complications such as pneumothorax or cardiac tamponade. In addition to the operating physician, a circulating nurse and an x-ray technician must be present. An assistant such as a trainee or "scrub" tech facilitates the procedure. A field clinical engineer from the implanting company is often present, although this remains controversial and his or her role should be strictly and narrowly defined according to previously published guidelines.[11,12] Continuous telemetry, oximetry, and blood pressure readings either via an automated cuff or arterial line is mandatory. Vital signs should be easily visible to the implanting physician as well as nursing/anesthesia staff. It is important that communication among the team members should be maintained throughout.

External pacing/defibrillating pads should be placed for all ICD implants and a subset of PPM implants with recent symptomatic bradycardia or a left bundle branch block pattern. In the latter instance, passing a pacing lead into the right ventricle may mechanically traumatize the right bundle branch, resulting in complete heart block. Fixed fluoroscopic units provide more precise imaging and greater ability to perform cine "runs," but portable c-arms are usually adequate.

Sedation can be performed either by a dedicated nurse, usually with midazolam and fentanyl, or by an anesthesiologist. An anesthesiologist has more options available such as total intravenous anesthesia with drugs such as diprivan, laryngeal mask anesthesia, and, in rare instances, general endotracheal anesthesia. Anesthesiologists are also more adept with maintaining oral and nasal airways. The latter techniques are rarely needed for uncomplicated pacemaker implants but are more commonly used for ICD implants. This is particularly helpful during defibrillation threshold testing and can be crucial during lengthier procedures such as biventricular implants particularly in those patients with a history of OSA, an anatomically challenging airway, or a body habitus conducive to airway obstruction. Noninvasive blood pressure monitoring is adequate for most pacemakers and defibrillator implants. Arterial lines are occasionally used if a prolonged case or hemodynamic instability is anticipated.

Meticulous site preparation is, of course, mandatory. The use of hair clippers rather than shaving is preferred as it minimizes microabrasions that may allow ingress of bacteria.[13] Recent data suggest an advantage to preoperative skin preparation (prep) utilizing a combination cleanser including an alcohol-based component along with chlorhexidine, rather than the more commonly used povidine-iodine–based scrub and prep.[14] The prep should be allowed to dry fully to minimize risk of flammability in this oxygen-enriched environment. Prophylactic antibiotics are effective in reducing infection rates and should be given preoperatively such that adequate serum levels are present at the time of incision.[15] An antibiotic with activity against staphylococcal species such as cefazolin is appropriate. With penicillin-allergic patients or those colonized with methicillin-resistant *Staphylococcus aureus* (MRSA), vancomycin can be used as an alternative. Four sterile towels are placed in a parallelogram surrounding the incision site, an antimicrobially impregnated incise drape (eg, Ioban® [3M, St. Paul, MN]) is deployed, and a "thyroid" sterile drape is placed on top (above the towels).

Pacemakers can be implanted with equal ease from either left or right pectoral regions. Using the right side avoids the 0.5% risk of encountering a left-sided superior vena cava (SVC) that does not communicate with the right SVC. On the other hand, implanting the device on the right imposes postoperative movement restrictions on what is, for most patients, their dominant side. In general, devices should be placed contralateral to AV fistulas, mastectomies, and indwelling central lines. Knowledge of a patient's workplace and recreational interests may be important so that one can avoid placing an implant ipsilateral to where a rifle butt may be held by a hunter or a stringed instrument may be held by a musician. ICDs can also be placed on either side, but defibrillation thresholds tend to be lower from the left side,[16] and, in the case of biventricular implants, the coronary sinus is often easier to engage from the left. Therefore, the left side is preferable unless a specific contraindication is present.

The Incision

An incision of 3 to 4 cm for a PPM and 4 to 5 cm for an ICD is usually adequate to allow the device to be placed into the pocket while minimizing cosmetic concerns. A slightly longer incision is used in those patients with greater thickness of adipose tissue. A variety of incision locations may be used. An incision slightly medial and oblique to the delto-pectoral groove allows easy access to the cephalic vein as well as the ability to perform direct central venous punctures. The incision begins 2 fingerbreadths below the clavicle. If a cephalic vein approach is not going to be used, a more medial incision may be used. Approximately 20 cc of a local anesthetic is used prior to the incision. Some implanters prefer a mixture of 1% lidocaine with 0.5% marcaine. Marcaine is longer acting and may therefore be helpful in minimizing immediate postop discomfort. The local anesthetic is devoid of epinephrine.

The Pulse Generator Pocket

An additional 10 cc of local anesthetic is delivered from within the incision prior to developing the pocket. The pocket is created with Bovie electrocautery or blunt dissection using Metzenbaum scissors or "finger" dissection. The pocket can be formed either before or after the leads are placed. The pocket is created inferomedial to the incision so that the bulk of the device does not interfere with normal movement of the shoulder. The plane should be placed deep within the subcutaneous fat while trying to preserve the fascial covering over the pectoral muscle, which minimizes risk of pocket hematomas—an increasing issue with the current trend toward more aggressive use of antiplatelet medications. A pocket placed too superficially increases the risk of erosion and chronic pocket discomfort.

In rare instances, the use of hemostatic agents is necessary to prevent oozing from the pectoral muscle. Thrombin gels such as Floseal® (Baxter Health Care Corp., Deerfield, IL) or hemostatic meshes may be used and familiarity with at least one technique is prudent. In rare instances, alternative pocket locations are preferred. In patients with minimal subcutaneous tissue or in patients who have previously suffered a device erosion, a submuscular pocket may be used. In women with cosmetic concerns and sufficient breast tissue, a submammary implant may be employed. The leads are still placed through traditional means but then tunneled to the submammary pocket. The assistance of a plastic surgeon is usually preferred and the woman should be cautioned as to the interference the device in this location may cause with routine mammography. With any of these choices, the pocket should be copiously irrigated with an antibiotic containing solution before placing the device.

Venous Access

Venous access can be obtained either through a cephalic vein cutdown or puncture of the axillary or subclavian veins. The cephalic vein approach avoids any risk of pneumothorax and is likely less traumatic to the lead. The cephalic vein approach is successful in roughly 80% to 90% of attempts. For a cephalic vein cutdown, Metzenbaum scissors and Debakey forceps are used to dissect into the fat pad within the delto-pectoral groove. The cephalic vein is then isolated with 2-0 silk ties, proximally and

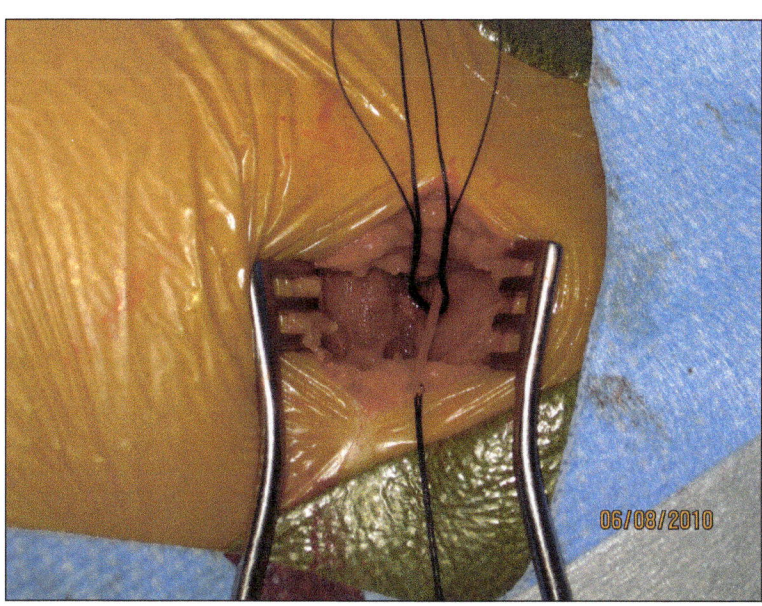

Figure 52.1 The cephalic vein is isolated with sutures proximally and distally. The deltoid muscle is noted lateral to the cephalic vein and the pectoral muscle is medial to it.

distally. The distal suture is tied off (Figure 52.1). This will minimize bleeding if the cephalic vein avulses during sheath and lead manipulation. The proximal suture is looped around the vein a second time. This is gently tightened after the leads have been placed, preventing back bleeding from the venotomy.

An opening is then made in the cephalic vein using either a #11 blade or Iris scissors, spanning approximately one-third of the circumference of the vein. The vein is tethered open with a vein pick (provided with the lead) or with curved Iris forceps. The lead is passed directly through the venotomy and into the heart. If the vein is large enough or sufficiently distensible, two leads may be passed directly through the cephalic. At times, venous valves, sub-branches, and tortuosity can make this difficult. If direct lead passage is unsuccessful, a J-tipped wire is advance through the venotomy into the right heart. The wire accompanying the introducer sheath is usually sufficient. Rarely, a hydrophilic wire is more successful due to superior handling characteristics and greater lubricity. Advancing the wire into the inferior vena cava (IVC) guarantees that it is appropriately in the venous system and not inadvertently in the arterial system.

A peel-away sheath is then placed over the wire, allowing introduction of the lead. When placing two leads, the sheath should be sized appropriately to allow retention of a wire for the second lead. Alternatively, a 5- or 6-Fr sheath can be passed over the first wire, a second wire placed, and the sheath removed. With two wires, the sheath size can be minimized, as one no longer needs to retain a wire. This results in less trauma to the vein and surrounding tissue. A sheath with a hemostatic valve is preferred as it minimizes the risk of air emboli, reduces the amount of back bleeding, and can be left in during placement of a second lead to minimize friction between the two leads.

If there is difficulty advancing the sheath, a series of increasing-sized dilators may be used to "size-up" the vein. At times, the cephalic vein invaginates around the sheath, and it is necessary to incise the vein on top of a dilator with a #11 blade to allow its smooth passage. The sheath should be gently curved to allow directional steering and more effective torquing. It should be advanced under fluoroscopic guidance or, at a minimum, using periodic to/fro movement to the wire to assure the sheath remains coaxial to the wire.

If the cephalic vein approach is unsuccessful or if it is the implanter's preference, a central vein may entered by direct needle puncture. Subclavian vein puncture particularly medially may be associated with subclavian crush syndrome resulting in premature lead failure due to repetitive scissoring on the lead within the subclavius muscle and costo-clavicular ligament. Puncture of the axillary vein (the section of vein before it crosses the first rib and enters the thoracic cavity) avoids this possibility and may minimize the risk of pneumothorax, given the extra-thoracic nature of the puncture.[17]

In anatomically challenging circumstances, additional techniques can be helpful to assist in successful venipuncture. One technique is to perform a venogram via an 18- or 20-gauge IV in the ipsilateral arm with 10 to 20 cc of dye followed by 20 cc of flush.[18] Repetitive "squeezing" of the ipsilateral upper arm often improves the density of opacification (Figure 52.2). It is worthwhile to routinely place an ipsilateral forearm intravenous catheter before beginning the procedure. In other situations, the puncture can be guided by a wire placed via the cephalic vein approach[19] or with the use of a sterile ultrasound probe.

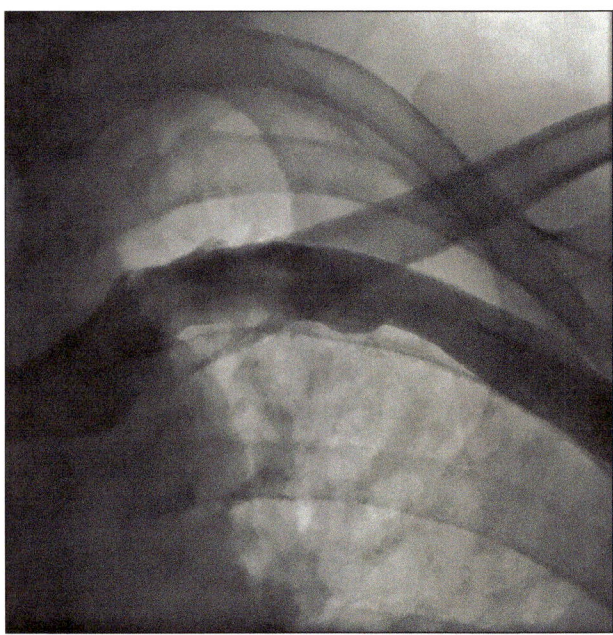

Figure 52.2 Left-sided venogram performed with 20 cc of dye injected through a left forearm intravenous catheter. The venogram demonstrates patency in the venous system and provides an anatomical roadmap for an axillary vein puncture.

For an axillary vein puncture, the patient is first placed in Trendelenburg position (or if the table does not allow this, a wedge is placed under the patient's feet). This promotes venous distention. The axillary vein is entered via a steep puncture at 45° aiming at the first rib just below where it crosses the clavicle. If the first pass is unsuccessful, the needle is withdrawn, the deflection angle subtly adjusted, and the needle readvanced. In this way, the surgeon can "walk" his way along the first rib. One can periodically observe the needle advancement in a caudally angulated view to better judge the depth of the needle tip relative to the first rib (Figure 52.3). If the puncture goes smoothly, a separate second puncture is performed for the second lead. If the first puncture is complicated, a wire can be retained during placement of the first lead. This can result in friction between the two leads but minimizes the risk of pneumothorax. Many surgeons routinely use a micro-puncture needle to gain venous access, which may

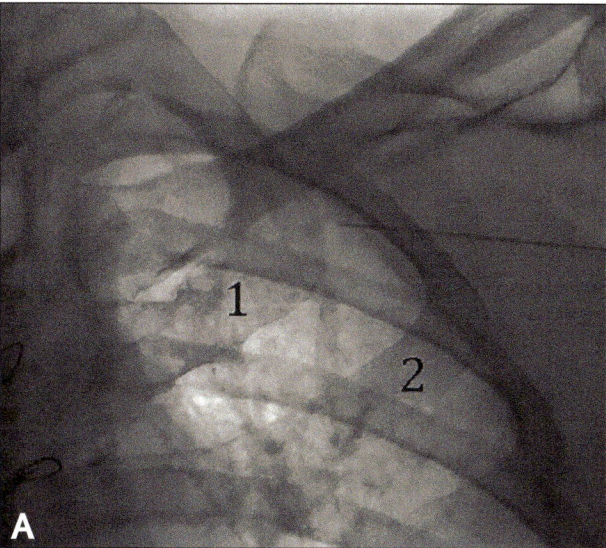 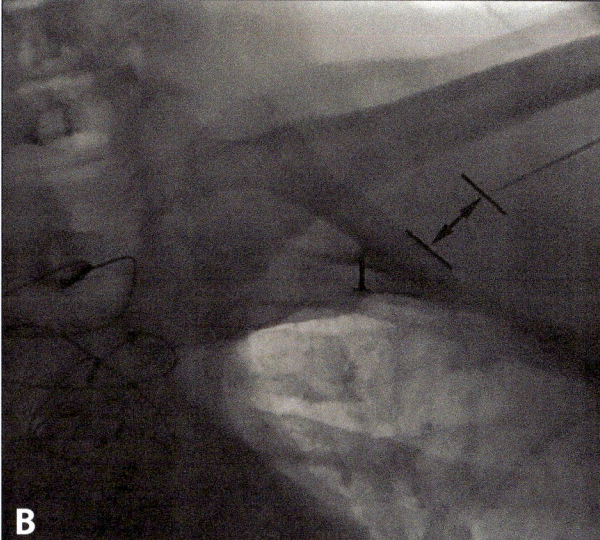

Figure 52.3 Approach to needle puncture of the axillary vein. **Panel A:** The needle is directed steeply downward toward the first rib, just beneath where it intersects the clavicle. **Panel B:** The depth of the needle tip is difficult to judge in an AP view. This caudal angulation demonstrates the needle tip is still a long distance from the first rib and will need to be advanced further to encounter the axillary vein. 1 = first rib, 2 = second rib.

decrease the risk of pneumothorax if the lung parenchyma is inadvertently entered.

At times, an implanter will need to add a new lead at a later date. This may occur due to lead failure or the need to upgrade a simpler system to a dual lead or a biventricular system. In a subset of these cases, the subclavian system will be occluded as demonstrated by venography. Several approaches are available to the implanter. These include placement of a wholly new system contralaterally, placement of the new lead(s) contralaterally and "tunneling" them across to the initial pocket, and extracting a preexisting lead to allow ipsalateral venous access. A new technique was recently described whereby the subclavian vein is punctured via a supraclavicular approach medial to the site of obstruction. The lead is sutured in place then tunneled over the clavicle and into the original pocket.[20]

In rare instances, such as congenital heart disease, recurrent endovascular infections, or SVC occlusion, endovascular leads cannot be placed. In these cases, modified techniques may be employed. One method utilizes a posterior subcutaneous array with an epicardial rate sensing lead and a standard generator.[21] A second method under development utilizes a novel subcutaneous array placed in a left parasternal location with a proprietary generator placed lateral to the point of maximal impulse.[22] This entirely subcutaneous ICD system may ultimately prove to have wider applicability in patients who do not require cardiac pacing.

Right Ventricular Lead Placement

With the sheath advanced fully into the subclavian vein, the ventricular lead is advanced into the right atrium. The straight stylet is removed and formed into a curve using fingers or a clamp. With the curved stylet advanced to the lead tip, the lead is gently advanced through the tricuspid valve, into the right ventricular outflow tract (RVOT) and past the pulmonary valve. In this way, the surgeon is certain the lead is traversing the right ventricle and not inadvertently in the coronary sinus or across an atrial or ventricular septal defect. The presence of premature ventricular contractions (PVCs) during advancement is also a good sign that the lead is not within the coronary sinus.

Alternatively, the lead tip can be directed to the lateral wall of the right atrium. With the lead tip against the lateral wall, the lead body is advanced to create a "loop" and then prolapsed through the tricuspid valve. Once in the RVOT, the curved stylet is replaced with a straight stylet. The lead is gently withdrawn awaiting a sudden drop where it falls down toward the right ventricular apex. The lead is then gently advanced (Figure 52.4). One should avoid pushing the straight stylet all the way to the tip of the lead when advancing toward the right ventricular apex. This will decrease the stiffness and "spear-like" characteristics of the lead and minimize the risk of perforation.

Leads routinely are packaged with a family of stylets with different properties. One often uses the "stiff" stylet to form into a curve and advance into the RVOT and the "soft" stylet to advance toward the apex. Great care must be exercised with manipulation of any stylet to avoid getting any blood on it lest it occlude the lumen of the lead and thereby prevent the passage of other stylets that might be required. Performing the right ventricular lead placement in a right anterior oblique (RAO) projection often allows a better sense of how close to the apex the lead is sited. A left anterior oblique (LAO) view can help rule out that the right ventricular lead has inadvertently entered the coronary sinus.

698 • *Section 2D: Device Implantation: Intraoperative, Surgical, and Device Management*

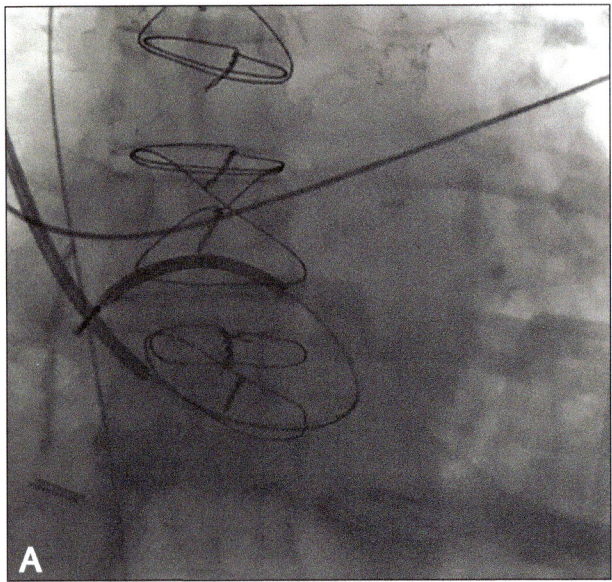
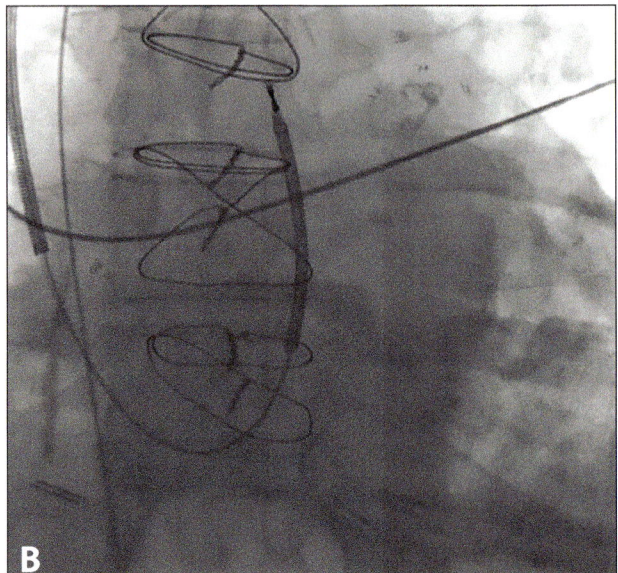
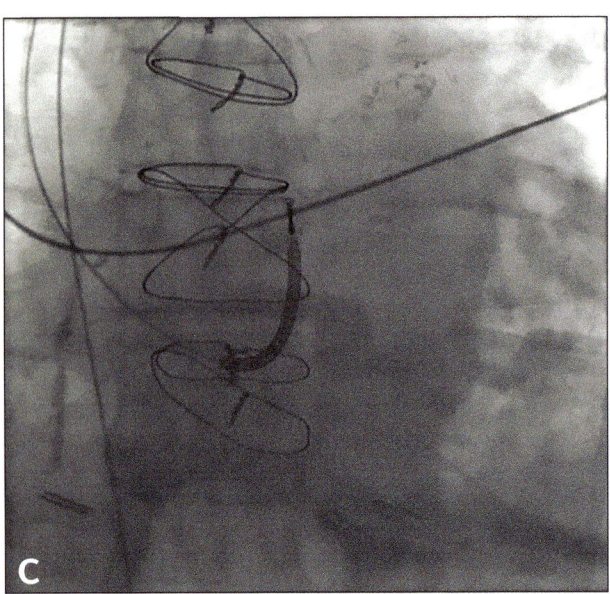
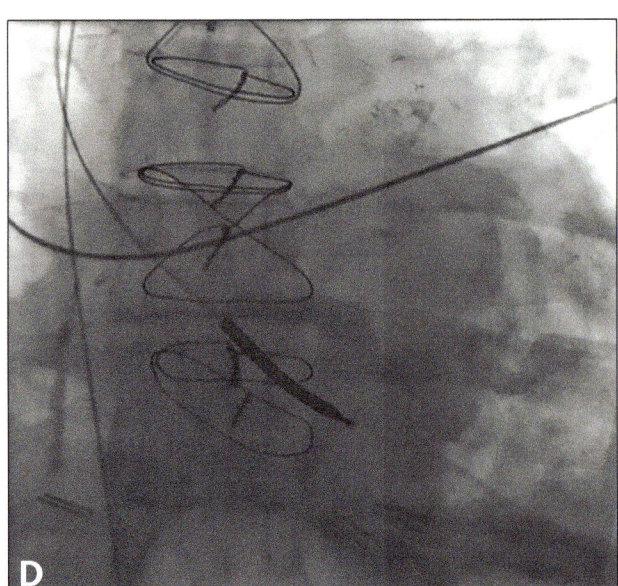
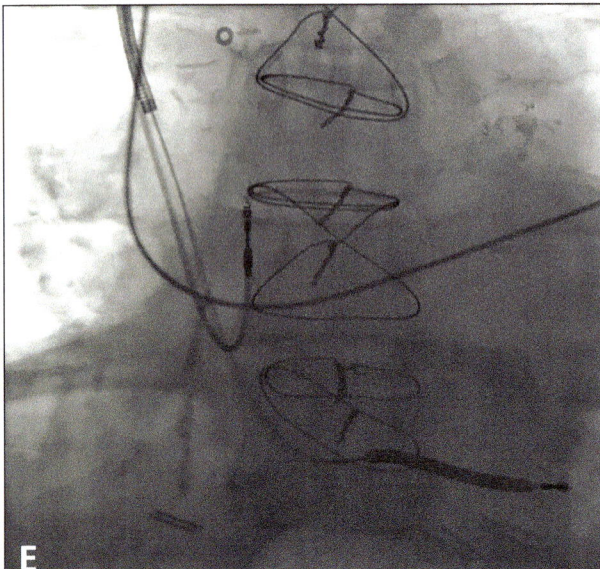

Figure 52.4 Positioning the right ventricular lead in the apex. **Panel A:** Either withdrawing the straight stylet several centimeters or using a gently curved stylet, one advances the right ventricular lead tip to the right atrium lateral wall and creates a loop heading toward the tricuspid valve. **Panel B:** Further advancement frees the tip of the lead, which crosses the valve and straightens in the RVOT. **Panel C:** Using a straight stylet, the lead is gently withdrawn. **Panel D:** With further withdrawal, the lead falls toward the apex. **Panel E:** The lead is gently advanced to its final position, seen here with the atrial lead also in place.

Typically, the morphology of RV apical pacing is that of left bundle branch block pattern with a superiorly directed axis. In a minority of patients, RV pacing results in a right bundle branch block pattern. Precordial transition of the QRS complex by lead V_3 indicates "safe" right ventricular lead placement, as opposed to septal or free wall perforation or inadvertent placement in the left ventricle or a coronary venous branch.[23]

Occasionally, there is a problem with a recently introduced lead (eg, a need to switch from a passive fixation to an active fixation lead) with loss of previously established venous access. In this situation, a #11 blade or Iris scissor may be used to slit the insulation of the lead to be sacrificed, and a guidewire is wedged through the breach and under the lead insulation. The lead and guidewire are then advanced as a unit so that the guidewire enters the vascular space. The guidewire is then fixed, and the lead advanced several additional centimeters so as to disengage it from the guidewire. The lead is removed, and an introducer can be advanced over the guidewire, providing access for a new lead.

Controversy remains as to the ideal location for the right ventricular lead. Traditionally, it was placed in the right ventricular apex. There now exists ample evidence that right ventricular apical pacing is hemodynamically disadvantageous, engendering a markedly dysnchronous contraction pattern and resulting in increased rates of congestive heart failure, particularly in those with left ventricular dysfunction.[24-26] A variety of small studies have suggested that the right ventricular septum or the RVOT might provide a better location.[27] The data to date are not conclusive, although interest in alternate sites is ongoing and several large studies are underway in an attempt to address these questions. Reasonable data exists that RVOT placement, particularly along the septal aspect, results in a narrower paced QRS complex. A LAO projection is necessary to prove the lead is along the septum, not the free wall. If the lead tip is located along the free wall, there is a higher risk of perforation, broader paced QRS, and increased incidence of intercostal muscle stimulation. Using a stylet with a secondary posteriorly directed curve 3 cm from its tip often helps position the lead along the septal surface.[28] Theoretically, direct Hisian pacing would be the most effective ventricular pacing site.[29] Unfortunately, technical constraints presently limit its use to very unique circumstances only.

Both passive fixation and active leads are reasonable choices. The chronic dislodgement rates between the two are not significantly different, despite an intuitive assumption that active fixation leads are more stable. An active fixation lead is necessary when placing the right ventricular lead in a position other than the apex. There is concern about a higher incidence of complications with use of an active fixation lead; for example, perforation or pericarditis. However, flexibility in placement sites is enhanced. An active fixation lead may also be a better choice in patients with significant tricuspid regurgitation or in patients where an AV nodal ablation procedure will be immediately performed following the pacemaker implant. In favor of passive fixation leads is their tendency to superior pacing and sensing thresholds. For pacemaker implants, a 52-cm atrial lead and a 58-cm ventricular lead are most commonly utilized for moderate or large sized patients. Shorter leads, such as a 46-cm atrial lead and a 52-cm ventricular lead, are often chosen for smaller patients to minimize excess lead coiled in the pocket.

Atrial Lead Placement

Typically, the atrial lead is placed in the right atrial appendage. An active fixation atrial lead is most commonly used. After advancing the lead into the right atrial body, the straight stylet is replaced with a preformed J-shaped stylet. This stylet pulls the lead tip up. With lead pullback and gentle torque, the lead tip easily enters the appendage where the helical coil can then be deployed. Some then gently torque the lead body/stylet unit an additional one-quarter or one-half clockwise turn to further entrench the lead tip. Prior to deployment, gently withdrawing the lead by 1 or 2 cm, and thus changing the J shape to more of an L shape, should demonstrate that the lead tip is "stuck." If the lead tip moves superiorally, it should be readvanced toward the IVC and withdrawn again at a slightly different angle until a more stable location is achieved. An appendage location is confirmed by the characteristic to-and-fro movement of the lead tip. One should try to minimize the number of times the helical screw is deployed. This will minimize the risk of damaging the screw mechanism and entrapping tissue in the coils, which may adversely affect the fixation mechanism.

Alternatively, a passive fixation atrial lead may be used. Most commonly, these leads have an intrinsic J-shape to them. The straight stylet straightens the lead for advancement into the low right atrium. The stylet is then partially withdrawn. This allows the lead to assume its J-shape. With gentle retraction, the lead falls into the appendage. The active fixation lead is favored in those patients who have undergone previous bypass surgery in whom the appendage is often truncated. Occasionally, the appendage is not accessible or pacing parameters are unacceptable. In these instances, lateral wall locations may be used. This often requires "custom-made" curves for the stylet. The surgeon can also consider septal or dual-site atrial pacing, which may minimize the risk of atrial arrhythmias.[30] If the patient is sufficiently awake, the slack on the leads should be assessed with respiratory excursion.

Lead Measurements

After an anatomically appropriate position is obtained, the lead parameters are analyzed. An injury current is desirable indicating appropriate pressure on the lead tip-myocardial interface with a passive fixation lead and appropriate "bite" when utilizing an active fixation lead (Figure 52.5). Absence of an injury current should prompt repositioning of the lead.[31] The lead should be tested at high output (eg, 10 V) to rule out extracardiac stimulation (ie, phrenic nerve or direct stimulation of the diaphragm or intercostal muscles). The impedance values should be within the range of acceptable values for that particular lead. Traditionally, desirable P waves were greater than 2.0 mV. With the greater sensitivity settings of modern pacemakers, smaller numbers are often acceptable. R waves should be greater than 5 mV. Smaller R waves are usually still acceptable in terms of appropriate ventricular fibrillation (VF) sensing in ICDs, but the risk of T wave oversensing is enhanced.

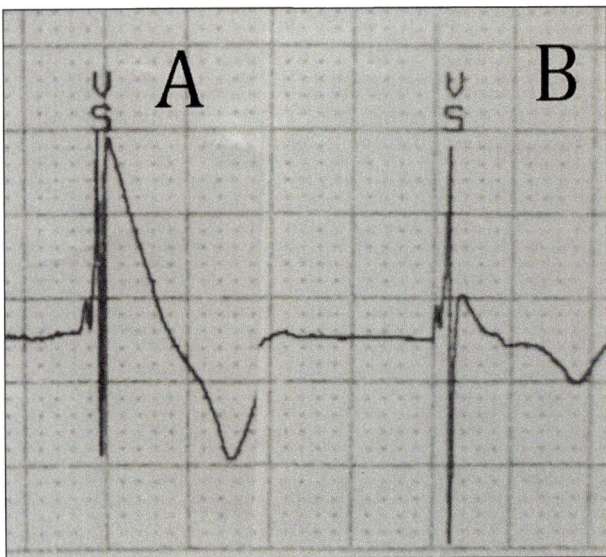

Figure 52.5 **Panel A:** Prominent injury current in an active fixation ventricular lead immediately after deployment of the screw mechanism. **Panel B:** Diminution in the injury current 10 minutes later accompanied by an improvement in the pacing threshold.

The capture threshold defined as the smallest voltage to successfully capture myocardium should be at or below 1.0 V. One should recognize that the pacing threshold often diminishes appreciably over the first few minutes, particularly if a significant injury current is present. A detailed understanding of the particular pacing requirements of the patient allows deviation from these ideal values. For example, there is less need for concern in a patient with a higher ventricular pacing threshold if atrioventricular conduction is robust and the need for ventricular pacing will be minimal.

Implanters often need to place atrial leads in patients with paroxysmal atrial fibrillation. If the patient is in AF at the time of the procedure, several techniques can be used. Some advocate electrically cardioverting the patient to sinus rhythm so that pacing and sensing thresholds may be accurately obtained. Once this portion of the procedure is complete, the patient may be purposefully returned to AF with rapid-burst atrial pacing if therapeutic anticoagulation had not been consistently maintained over the preceding 3 to 4 weeks. Alternatively, a site may be used that has reasonably sized fibrillatory waves that are over 1 mV. Several reports support this technique demonstrating favorable pacing and sensing thresholds in these patients when tested in sinus rhythm at a later date.[32,33]

Lead Tie-down and Pulse Generator Placement

After the leads are successfully placed, the leads need to be stabilized in position. Sutures should not be placed directly over unprotected leads as the suture will often damage the outer insulation. Instead, leads routinely come with suture sleeves. After lead placement, the suture sleeves are advanced to the venotomy in the cephalic vein (for cutdowns) or to the point where the lead enters the pectoral muscle (for axillary/subclavian punctures). Next, two or three silk sutures are placed around the suture sleeve and tightened. Either 0 silk or 2-0 silk may be used. This prevents lead migration. Some operators suture around the sleeve and underlying muscle with a single pass. Others create a preformed knot, thread it around the pin, advance the knot directly over the suture sleeve, and tie it. Then, a second "looser" knot is created to attach the suture sleeve to the muscle. With the latter method, damage to the muscle is minimized. With either technique, the surgeon should "tug" on the leads to assure lack of movement of the lead within the sleeve. Repeat fluoroscopy should be undertaken once anchoring has been performed to make sure that lead tip position and redundancy remain stable at baseline and with deep inspiration.

The leads are then placed into the header block of the pulse generator and set screws tightened with the included torque wrench. With certain manufacturers' devices, the wrench should engage the set screw before the lead is placed to allow air to escape so the lead is not "forced" out. Certain header blocks require 2 screws to be tightened for bipolar leads but most require just a single screw per lead. Once tightened, one should tug on the leads to assure stability within the header block. The generator is then placed within the pocket. Excess lead should be placed under the generator so that future generator replacements will not be compromised by inadvertent slicing of the lead(s).

Defibrillation Threshold Testing

With ICDs, after appropriate lead placement and connection to the device, defibrillation threshold testing (DFTs) is performed. There is controversy as to the necessity of routinely performing DFTs.[34-36] Those in favor argue that despite advances in ICD technology, high-DFT patients still account for up to 6.2% of implants. Knowledge of which patients fall within this subgroup allows remedial measures to be performed at the time of implant. Further, DFT trials assess the sensing accuracy and integrity of connections within the device. Intraoperative testing at lesser degrees of sensitivity allow more confident reprogramming of the device as an outpatient to less sensitive values if oversensing of T wave or myopotentials occurs.

Opponents of DFT testing cite the cost and the risk involved. Among the risks is the chance of stroke, particularly in those AF patients who are converted to sinus rhythm during testing. Other risks include death from cardiogenic shock/pulseless electrical activity and the potential for precipitating a need for prolonged resuscitation.[37] There is recent data that delivered shocks may have a long-term detrimental effect on mortality.[38] Others argue that it is the abnormal myocardial substrate that leads to ventricular arrhythmias and death, and not the shocks themselves that are the cause of the increased mortality.[39]

Many implanters routinely reinitiate AF if a shock converts a patient with persistent AF back to sinus rhythm. This can be done either with burst atrial pacing if an atrial lead is present or with a low output synchronized shock if no atrial lead exists. An R-wave synchronized shock often times to atrial repolarization and thus strikes the atrial vulnerable period in a manner similar to how a T-wave shock will induce VF.

To perform a DFT, typically the depth of anesthesia is augmented. VF is then purposefully induced with a low-energy shock delivered during the electrically vulnerable T wave. Other fibrillation inducers such as a 9 V direct current pulse between the RV coil and the device or a rapidly alternating (20 Hz) high output (15 V at 1.1 ms) current through the shocking coils may be used instead. The device is tested with "worst-case scenario" conditions. The sensing is set to a less than normal sensitivity value, and a shock energy is used that is well beneath the maximum output of the particular device. In the present era, with the routine use of an active "can," biphasic waveforms, and dual coil leads, elevated DFTs are rarely an issue. Characteristics that might suggest an enhanced risk for high DFTs include use of amiodarone, dilated cardio-myopathy, hypertrophic cardiomyopathy, lower ejection fraction, markedly enlarged left ventricular end-diastolic dimension, New York Heart Association Class III/IV congestive heart failure, and broad QRS complex.[40-42]

Traditionally, a rigorous step-down to failure approach was used, at times reconfirming success a second time at the lowest successful energy. Others prefer a simplified approach judging an acceptable DFT as two consecutive successful defibrillations at 10 J below the maximum output of the device or even a single successful shock at 15 to 20 J below the maximum output. Care should be taken that the induced arrhythmia is truly VF. If monomorphic ventricular tachycardia is inadvertently induced, neither the accuracy of the sensing nor the DFT is an adequate surrogate for measurements made during VF.

A stepwise approach should be taken in the rare case of elevated DFT (Table 52.1).[43] First, one should ascertain that no complication during the procedure may be affecting the DFT such as pneumothorax or pericardial effusion. Next, a retest can be performed, reversing the polarity of the shocking vector. Most studies have demonstrated that a shocking polarity using the right ventricular coil as the anode for phase 1 is superior.[44] This is a practice that most, but not all, manufacturers have adopted as the norm. In individual patients, however, polarity reversal, at times, can be helpful. If this is unsuccessful, the surgeon can retest removing the SVC coil from the shocking vector, particularly if the high voltage impedance is low (< 40 Ohms). If persistently unsuccessful, the surgeon should consider repositioning of the lead either deeper toward the apex if shallowly placed or to the RVOT if an adequate apical position was already established. Certain device manufacturers allow a "tuned" defibrillation waveform using a fixed pulse width rather than relying on a fixed tilt.[45,46] Often a shorter pulse width may prevent the reinduction of VF by removing residual charge at the "virtual electrode." Changing to a high output generator, if one is not already being used, is an additional option.

Table 52.1 Approach to the high DFT patient

Reprogramming Options
• Reverse polarity
• Remove SVC coil electronically
• Modify the waveform (change the tilt or use a fixed pulse width)
Lead Interventions
• Reposition a shallowly placed lead to the right ventricular apex
• Reposition an apical lead to the RVOT
• Mechanically remove the SVC coil (if unable to program it "off")
• Add a subcutaneous array or other coil (azygous, innominate, etc)
Device Interventions
• Change to a high output device
• Change to a device with programmable waveforms
Drug Interventions
• Stop drugs that elevate DFTs (amiodarone or mexiletine)
• Initiate a drug that lowers DFT (sotalol or dofetilide)

If all of the above modifications are unsuccessful, then placement of an additional electrode will usually be required. The goal is usually to provide a more posterior site for energy delivery that will better encompass the left ventricular mass. There may be ancillary changes to adding another electrode beyond the change in vector, including a change in shock impedance, which affects pulse width. Placement of an additional electrode is most commonly accomplished by placing a subcutaneous array posterolaterally around the left hemithorax. Studies have demonstrated an average of 9 J improvement in DFTs with this approach.[47] The array most commonly replaces the proximal coil in the shocking vector but other configurations are possible as well. In rare instances, for example in patients with right-sided implants, an additional lead can be placed in the azygous vein,[48] coronary sinus branch, or left subclavian vein.

One should be exceedingly careful not to over-test. Repeated DFT inductions can prove catastrophic to the unstable patient. It is often more prudent to stop testing and plan additional interventions on a future day after a period of recovery. Stopping amiodarone or beginning a drug known to lower DFTs like sotalol or dofetilide[49] is often quite effective as well.

An alternative to DFT testing that can minimize or even eliminate VF induction is upper limit of vulnerability (ULV) testing. The ULV is the least amount of shock energy delivered during the vulnerable period of the cardiac cycle that does not induce VF. The ULV is thought to correlate well with DFT_{90}, which represents the amount of energy that will successfully defibrillate the heart 90% of time.[50] The "vulnerable period" is estimated as the peak of the latest peaking monophasic T wave on the surface ECG. If VF is not induced at this coupling interval, the T wave is scanned with the same energy at –20 ms, +20 ms, and +40 ms from the T wave peak. Surrogate measurement taken from intracardiac electrograms and simplified scans are being investigated.

Closure

After the procedure is completed as described, a final brief fluoroscopic survey is obtained over the thorax. Multiple parameters are assessed. These include appropriate lead tip position, correct slack in the right atrium and right ventricular leads, absence of pneumothorax, pin tips beyond the cathodal connector within the header block (Figure 52.6), and absence of sponges within the pacemaker pocket. Closure of the wound then may be performed. Many surgeons use three continuous suture layers. The first layer consists of vertical sutures as a deep layer closing the pocket. An absorbable suture such as 2-0 vicryl is used with an SH- or CT-shaped needle. The second layer uses 3-0 vicryl to place horizontally oriented sutures within the dermis. For the third layer, 4-0 monocryl is used because of its characteristics as a monofilament-based suture material, which results in minimal tissue reaction and provides a particularly pleasing cosmetic result. The layer is begun with a deep knot. The needle tip is then reversed within the needle driver and backhanded so that it comes out within the wound just at the tip of the incision. A running subcuticular layer is then placed. Instead of placing a knot at the end of this layer, the bite begins within the wound but then exits through the skin about 1 cm beyond the incision. A final bite is performed reentering the last exit site and coming through the skin 1 cm further away. This layer remains simply by friction. Avoiding this final superficial knot minimizes the separation of the wound edges by the knot and minimizes risk of stitch abscess. New approaches involving alternative wound closure techniques[51] or placement of the generator in an antibacterial envelope are being studied in an attempt to minimize the chance of device-related infections.[52]

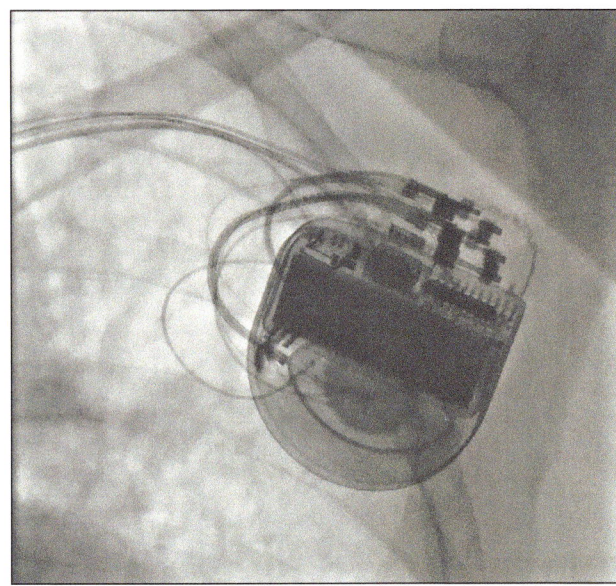

Figure 52.6 The pin tips of each of the five leads in this biventricular device are clearly visible beyond the cathodal connector block.

Steri-strips cut in thirds are applied, followed by a folded 4 × 4 and then a transparent medical dressing such as Tegaderm® (3M, St. Paul, MN). A pressure dressing may be applied overnight to minimize the possibility of a pocket hematoma particularly in patients on warfarin or clopidogrel.

Other closure techniques can be used instead such as a superficial skin closure using staples or biologic glue like Derma-Bond (Ethicon, Somerville, NJ). Derma-Bond has the advantage of providing a waterproof closure and avoids the need for Steri-strips and a final dressing.

Postoperative Care

The patient is sent to the recovery room to have a portable chest x-ray and ECG performed and to awaken from anesthesia. Patients are routinely kept overnight on bed rest and with an ipsilateral arm sling. The patient is discharged home the following day after a posteroanterior/lateral chest x-ray is obtained, the wound is inspected, and the device is interrogated to assure stability in lead parameters. The bio-occlusive dressing and 4 × 4 gauze is kept in place for 5 days and then removed by the patient. The wound is kept dry until then. The patient is asked to refrain from lifting the ipsilateral arm above shoulder height for 2 to 4 weeks and to avoid lifting more than 10 lb during that time.

Instructions regarding MRIs, other radiographic imaging, driving, recreational activities, cell phones, theft detectors, power tools, household appliances, and metal detectors are given both verbally as well as in writing on an instruction sheet. If applicable, return to work timing is discussed and a first follow-up visit is arranged in 2 to 4 weeks. Many implanters routinely give a prophylactic antibiotic course for 5 to 7 days post implant, but scientific data supporting this practice are limited. If antiplatelet or anticoagulant medications had been discontinued, the timing of resuming these medications is reviewed.

References

1. Hayes DL, Naccarelli GV, Furman S, et al. NASPE training requirements for cardiac implantable electronic devices: selection, implantation and follow-up. *Pacing Clin Electrophysiol*. 2003;26:1556-1562.
2. Tompkins C, Cheng A, Dalal D, et al. Dual antiplatelet therapy and heparin "bridging" significantly increase the risk of bleeding complications after pacemaker or implantable cardioverter-defibrillator device implantation. *J Am Coll Cardiol*. 2010;55:2376-2382.
3. van Hemel NM. Anticoagulation management during cardiac device surgery: many tastes tolerated? *Heart Rhythm*. 2009;6(9):1280-1281.
4. Michaud GF, Pelosi F Jr, Noble MD, et al. A randomized trial comparing heparin initiation 6h or 24h after pacemaker or defibrillator implantation. *J Am Coll Cardiol*. 2000;35: 1915-1918.
5. Ahmed IA, Gertner E, Nelson WB, et al. Continuing warfarin therapy is superior to interrupting warfarin with or without bridging anticoagulation therapy in patients undergoing pacemaker and defibrillator implantation. *Heart Rhythm*. 2010;7:745-749.
6. Giudici MC, Barold SS, Paul DL, Bontu P. Pacemaker and implantable cardioverter defibrillator implantation without the reversal of warfarin therapy. *Pacing Clin Electrophysiol*. 2004;27:358-60.
7. Edmiston CE, Krepel CJ, Seabrook GR, et al. Preoperative shower revisited: can high topical antiseptic levels be achieved on the skin surface before surgical admission? *J Am Coll Surg*. 2008;207(2):233-239.
8. Rao N, Cannella B, Crossett LS, et al. A preoperative decolonization protocol for *Staphylococcus aureus* prevents orthopedic infections. *Clin Orthop Relat Res*. 2008;466(6):1343-1348.
9. Webster J, Osborne S. Meta-analysis of preoperative antiseptic bathing in the prevention of surgical site infection. *Br J Surg*. 2006;93(11):1335-1341.
10. Bode LG, Kluytmans JA, Wertheim HF, et al. Preventing surgical-site infections in nasal carriers of *Staphylococcus aureus*. *N Engl J Med*. 2010;362:9-17.
11. Hayes JJ, Juknavorian R, Maloney JD. The role(s) of the industry employed allied professional. *Pacing Clin Electrophysiol*. 2001;24(3):398-399.
12. Lindsay BD, Estes NA, Maloney JD, et al. Heart rhythm society policy statement update: recommendations on the role of industry employed allied professionals (IEAPS). *Heart Rhythm*. 2008;5(11):e8-10.
13. Kjonniksen I, Andersen BM, Sondenaa VG, et al. Preoperative hair removal—a systematic literature review. *AORN J*. 2002;75:928-940.
14. Darouiche RO, Wall MJ, Itani KM, et al. Chlorhexidine-alcohol versus povidone-iodine for surgical-site antisepsis. *N Engl J Med*. 2010;362:18-26.
15. DaCosta A, Kirkorian G, Cucherat M, et al. Antibiotic prophylaxis for permanent pacemaker implantation: a meta-analysis. *Circulation*. 1998;97:1796-1801.
16. Friedman PA, Rasmussen MJ, Grice S, et al. Defibrillation thresholds are increased by right-sided implantation of totally transvenous implantable cardioverter defibrillators. *Pacing Clin Electrophysiol*. 1999;22(8):1186-1192.
17. Ramza BM, Rosenthal L, Hui R, et al. Safety and effectiveness of placement of pacemaker and defibrillator leads in the axillary vein guided by contrast venography. *Am J Cardiol*. 1997;80:892-896.
18. Calkins H, Ramza BM, Brinker J, et al. Prospective randomized comparison of the safety and effectiveness of placement of endocardial pacemaker and defibrillator leads using the extrathoracic subclavian vein guided by contrast venography versus the cephalic approach. *Pacing Clin Electrophysiol*. 2001;24:456-464.
19. Lau EW. Navigation by parallax in three-dimensional space during fluoroscopy: application in guide-wire directed axillary/subclavian vein puncture. *Pacing Clin Electrophysiol*. 2007;30:1054-1-66.
20. Antonelli D, Freedberg NA, Turgeman Y. Supraclavicular vein approach to overcoming ipsilateral chronic subclavian vein obstruction during pacemaker-ICD lead revision or upgrading. *Europace*. 2010;12(11):1596-1599.
21. Kowalski M, Nicolato P, Kalahasty G, et al. An alternative technique of implanting a nontransvenous implantable cardioverter-defibrillator system in adults with no or limited venous access to the heart. *Heart Rhythm*. 2010;7(11): 1572-1577.
22. Bardy GH, Smith WM, Hood MA, et al. An entirely subcutaneous implantable cardioverter-defibrillator. *N Engl J Med*. 2010;363:36-44.
23. Coman JA, Trohman RG. Incidence and electrocardiographic localization of safe right bundle branch block configurations during ventricular pacing. *Am J Cardiol*. 1995;76(11):781-784.
24. Wilkoff BL, Cook JR, Epstein AE, et al. Dual-chamber pacing or ventricular back-up pacing in patients with an implantable defibrillator: the dual chamber and VVI implantable defibrillator (DAVID) trial. *JAMA*. 2002;288:311531-311523.
25. Sweeney MO, Hellkamp AS, Ellenbogen KA, et al. Adverse effect of ventricular pacing on heart failure and atrial fibrillation among patients with normal baseline QRS duration in a clinical trial of pacemaker therapy for sinus node dysfunction. *Circulation*. 2003;107:2932-2937.
26. Tse HF, Yu C, Wong KK, et al. Functional abnormalities in patients with permanent right ventricular pacing: the effect of sites of electrical stimulation. *J Am Coll Cardiol*. 2002;40: 1451-1458.
27. Schoenfeld MH. Alternative site pacing to promote cardiac synchrony: has conventional pacing become unconventional. *J Am Coll Cardiol*. 2006;47:1946-1948.
28. Hillock RJ, Stevenson IH, Mond HG. The right ventricular outflow tract: a comparative study of septal, anterior wall, and free wall pacing. *Pacing Clin Electrophysiol*. 2007;30:942-947.
29. Occhetta E, Bortnik M, Magnani A, et al. Prevention of ventricular desynchronization by permanent para-Hisian pacing after atrioventricular node ablation in chronic atrial

fibrillation: a crossover, blinded, randomized study versus apical right ventricular pacing. *J Am Coll Cardiol.* 2006;47(10):1938-1945.
30. Saksena S, Prakash A, Ziegler P, et al. Improved suppression of recurrent atrial fibrillation with dual-site right atrial pacing and antiarrhythmic drug therapy. *J Am Coll Cardiol.* 2002;40(6):1140-1150.
31. Saxonhouse SJ, Conti JB, Curtis AB. Current of injury predicts adequate active lead fixation in permanent pacemaker/defibrillation leads. *J Am Coll Cardiol.* 2005;45(3):412-417.
32. Wiegand UK, Bode F, Bonnemeier H, et al. Atrial lead placement during atrial fibrillation. Is restitution of sinus rhythm required for proper lead function? Feasibility and 12 month functional analysis. *Pacing Clin Electrophysiol.* 2000;23:1144-1149.
33. Kindermann M, Frohlig G, Berg M, et al. Atrial lead implantation during atrial flutter or fibrillation. *Pacing Clin Electrophysiol.* 1998;21:1531-1538.
34. Kolb C, Tzeis S, Zrenner B. Defibrillation threshold testing: tradition or necessity? *Pacing Clin Electrophysiol.* 2009;32(5):570-572.
35. Blatt JA, Poole JE, Johnson GW, et al. No benefit from defibrillation threshold testing in the SCD-HeFT trial. *J Am Coll Cardiol.* 2008;52(7):551-556.
36. Russo AM, Sauer W, Gerstenfeld EP, et al. Defibrillation threshold testing: is it really necessary at the time of implantable cardioverter-defibrillator insertion? *Heart Rhythm.* 2005;2:456-461.
37. Birnie D, Tung S, Simpson C, et al. Complications associated with defibrillation threshold testing: the Canadian experience. *Heart Rhythm.* 2008;5(3):387-390.
38. Sweeney MO, Sherfesee L, DeGroot PJ, et al. Differences in effects of electrical therapy type for ventricular arrhythmias on mortality in implantable cardioverter-defibrillator patients. *Heart Rhythm.* 2010;7:353-760.
39. Bhavnani SP, Kluger J, Coleman, et al. The prognostic impact of shocks for clinical and induced arrhythmias on morbidity and mortality among patients with implantable cardioverter-defibrillators. *Heart Rhythm.* 2010;7:755-760.
40. Mainigi SK, Cooper JM, Russo AM, et al. Elevated defibrillation thresholds in patients undergoing biventricular defibrillator implantation: incidence and predictors. *Heart Rhythm.* 2006;3(9):1010-1016.
41. Lubinski A, Lewicka-Novak E, Zienciuk A, et al. Clinical predictors of defibrillation thresholds in patients with implantable cardioverter-defibrillators. *Kardiol Pol.* 2005;62(4):317-328.
42. Shukla HH, Flaker GC, Jayam V, et al. High defibrillation thresholds in transvenous biphasic implantable defibrillators: clinical predictors and prognostic implications. *Pacing Clin Electrophysiol.* 2003;26:44-48.
43. Mainigi SK, Callans DJ. How to manage the patient with a high defibrillation threshold. *Heart Rhythm.* 2006;3(4):492-495.
44. Kroll MW, Efimov IR, Tchou PJ. Present understanding of shock polarity for internal defibrillation: the obvious and non-obvious clinical implications. *Pacing Clin Electrophysiol.* 2006;29:885-891.
45. Denman RA, Umesan C, Martin PT, et al. Benefits of millisecond waveform durations for patients with high defibrillation thresholds. *Heart Rhythm.* 2006;3:536-541.
46. Natarajan S, Henthorn R, Burroughs J, et al. "Tuned" defibrillation waveforms outperform 50/50% tilt waveforms: a randomized multi-center study. *Pacing Clin Electrophysiol.* 2007;30(Suppl 1):S139-S142.
47. Osswald BR, De Simone R, Most S, et al. High defibrillation threshold in patients with implantable defibrillator: how effective is the subcutaneous finger lead? *Eur J Cardiothorac Surg.* 2009;35(3):489-492.
48. Cooper JA, Latacha MP, Soto GE, et al. The azygous defibrillator lead for elevated defibrillation thresholds: implant technique, lead stability, and patient series. *Pacing Clin Electrophysiol.* 2008;31(11):1405-1410.
49. Simon RD, Sturdivant JL, Leman RB, et al. The effect of dofetilide on ventricular defibrillation thresholds. *Pacing Clin Electrophysiol.* 2009;32(1):24-28.
50. Swerdlow C, Ahern T. Upper limit of vulnerability is a good estimator of shock strength associated with a 90% probability of successful defibrillation in humans with implantable cardioverter-defibrillators. *J Am Coll Cardiol.* 1996;27(5):1112-1118.
51. Grubb BP, Welch M, Karabin B, et al. Initial experience with a technique for wound closure after cardiac device implantation designed to reduce infection and minimize tissue scar formation. *Am J Ther.* 2012;19(2):88-91.
52. Bloom HL, Constantin L, De Lurgio DB, et al. Implantation success and infection in cardiovascular implantable electronic device procedures utilizing an antibacterial envelope. *Pacing Clin Electrophysiol.* 2011;34(2):133-142.

CHAPTER 53

Surgical Considerations in Device Implantation

Raj R. Kaushik, MD; Sanjeev Saksena, MBBS, MD

Introduction

Advances in device and lead technology have resulted in an evolution in the process of device system implantation over the last two decades. Epicardial lead systems, which were the norm a few decades ago, are now reserved for the patients who are not candidates for the transvenous systems, eg, patients with mechanical tricuspid prosthesis or infants and children who have size mismatch with lead caliber due to rapid growth and development. In such patients, implantation may be performed using sternotomies, anterolateral thoracotomies, or with minimally invasive thoracoscopic techniques, with or without robotic assistance. These instances are rare today, and lead and device implantation are almost exclusively performed by the transvenous approach.

This evolution of the device implant procedure has resulted in two key changes: first, physicians with training in cardiology and electrophysiology, but not necessarily surgery, are qualified to perform these procedures, and second, venues other than conventional surgical suites are now suitable for performance of these procedures. In order to have the requisite expertise, it is necessary for such operators to be facile with many surgical techniques and adequate availability of trained surgical personnel. (The details of the surgical aspects of the implant procedure are discussed in Chapter 52.)

The current permanent pacemaker (PM) or implantable cardioverter-defibrillator (ICD) device implant procedure in an adult or adolescent patient involves transvenous insertion of leads and creation of a subcutaneous or submuscular pocket for generator placement, usually in a pectoral location. The procedure requires use of appropriate surgical techniques and careful adherence to the surgical principles of planning and preparation to ensure success and minimize complications. Finally, the recent introduction of subcutaneous electrode systems in the subcutaneous implantable cardioverter-defibrillator (S-ICD) devices, originally developed as a transitional phase from epicardial to wholly intravascular leads, has required a revisiting of the surgical principles of extrathoracic surgery in the chest. In the instance of an abdominal implant, some other specific considerations apply, such as the tunneling of leads from a pectoral or femoral site.

Planning

Practice guidelines for patient selection for device implantation have been published and are discussed in Section 3.[1,2] These will help implanters determine whether the patient is suited for this therapy, as well as the choice of device and the appropriate lead system that needs to be implanted in the individual patient. The experience of the implanter and the frequency with which the implanter performs the procedures is related to the potential for complications. A minimum volume of device implants is needed to achieve and maintain competency. In current guidelines, this comprises at least 75 implantations as the primary operator. Exposure during clinical training to a cardiac surgical service or ongoing clinical exposure with an experienced implanter would be a definite asset to any implanter.

The venue for implantation has changed over the last two decades from the traditional operating suite to the catheterization or electrophysiology laboratory. Despite a much better fluoroscopy system in the catheterization laboratory, overhead lighting and systems for maintenance of sterility may need augmentation to facilitate optimal conditions. A hybrid suite would be ideal, as this provides all the requirements of both the catheterization laboratory room and the operating suite. Trained surgical support personnel are invaluable additions to the device implant team. Uncomplicated generator replacements can be discharged after a few hours of routine observation. In some healthcare systems, even primary implants of devices that have 1 or 2 leads are performed as 1-day procedures. We recommend keeping patients who undergo complex device procedures overnight to observe for appropriate device function and lead stability.

Patient Evaluation

All planned device recipients should be carefully evaluated for preexisting medical and surgical issues. Patients with a history of prior upper extremity thrombophlebitis may need to have a preoperative evaluation of the venous system for patency. A history of indwelling catheter placement should prompt such an examination as well. Any history of vascular anomalies or difficulty in obtaining access in the past may require a venous evaluation. Patients with a prior mastectomy should be prepared for the procedure on the contralateral side. Anatomical variations of the chest wall should be duly noted.

Patients maintained on oral anticoagulant therapy and/or antiplatelet therapy require special consideration, and their periprocedural management is a subject of active discussion and evolution.[3-8] Ideally, these agents should be discontinued for a sufficient period of time to allow for reducing risk of bleeding. In the instance of warfarin, this can be monitored by the international normalized ratio (INR) level. Dabigatran is often discontinued for 36 to 48 hours prior to the procedure, as are other agents such as apixaban and rivaroxaban. However, in many instances these medications may not be discontinued without significant risk of adverse events, eg, patients with mechanical valves who are on warfarin or patients on clopidogrel and aspirin due to recent drug-eluting stent placement. In such instances, surgical implantation of the device may need to be performed on continued therapy.

Traditionally, patients on oral anticoagulants were admitted to the hospital after discontinuation of the medications for the procedure and treated with IV heparin. In the case of warfarin, this occurred when the INR decreased to < 1.75 in our laboratory. Heparin is discontinued 3 or more hours prior to the procedure. After the procedure is performed, warfarin therapy is restarted.

More recently, we have chosen to continue the warfarin, maintain INR around 2.0, then performed the implant.[9,10] Meticulous attention to the surgical technique will minimize bleeding issues. Dabigatran and other factor Xa inhibitors should be discontinued for 36 to 48 hours and short-term bridging anticoagulation considered if essential.[11] Finally, perioperative antibiotic therapy is recommended for a minimum of 24 hours after the procedure and can be continued for longer periods up to 5 days in high-risk patients, eg, diabetics, immunosuppressed patients, or those with frequent cutaneous infections or concomitant steroid therapy.

Surgical Considerations for the Implant Procedure

Transvenous lead placement using the cephalic vein or axillary-subclavian vein route is currently the preferred route for introduction of the lead systems for purposes of demand pacing, cardiac resynchronization therapy, and primary or secondary defibrillator insertion indications. Occasionally, the external jugular or the internal jugular veins may be used due to extenuating circumstances. Herein, an intimate knowledge of the anatomy of these veins is imperative to any implanting physician. Pulse-generator implants are almost invariably pectoral implants as the first choice, as this is most acceptable from mechanical device-system stress, generator replacement considerations, and cosmetic and kinetic considerations for the patient.

Anatomic Considerations

The location and configuration of the thoracic vessels and their anatomic relationship to adjacent thoracic structures is relatively constant (Figure 53.1). Minor variations may occur due to chest wall deformities or healing of prior fractures involving the bony elements, such as the ribs or the clavicle. Major variations may be due to congenital anomalies, eg, persistent left-sided superior vena cava.

The anatomic landmarks for the upper-extremity veins and their course is of significant surgical importance. The cephalic vein courses up the lateral aspect of the arm; at the shoulder, the cephalic vein travels lateral to the biceps and between the pectoralis major and the deltoid, where it adjoins the deltoid branch of the thoracoacromial vein. Traveling posterior to the clavicular head of the pectoralis major in the infraclavicular fossa, it pierces the clavipectoral fascia and goes over the axillary artery to join the axillary vein just below the clavicular level. The axillary vein is a continuation of the basilic vein in the arm, and it starts at the lower border of the teres major, traveling to the outer border of the first rib, where it becomes the subclavian vein. Usually lying posterior to the pectoralis major, pectoralis minor, and the clavipectoral fascia, the subclavian vein lies medial or anteromedial to the artery and adjacent to the medial cord of the brachial plexus. The subclavian vein extends from the lateral border of the first rib to the medial border of the scaleneus anticus, where it joins the internal jugular vein to form the brachiocephalic vein. Through its course, the vein lies anteroinferior to the artery and is separated from it by the scalenus anticus and the phrenic nerve. Posteroinferior to the vein are the first rib and the pleura, and anterior to the vein are the clavicle and the subclavius. At the confluence of the internal jugular and the left subclavian veins, the thoracic duct drains into the vein.

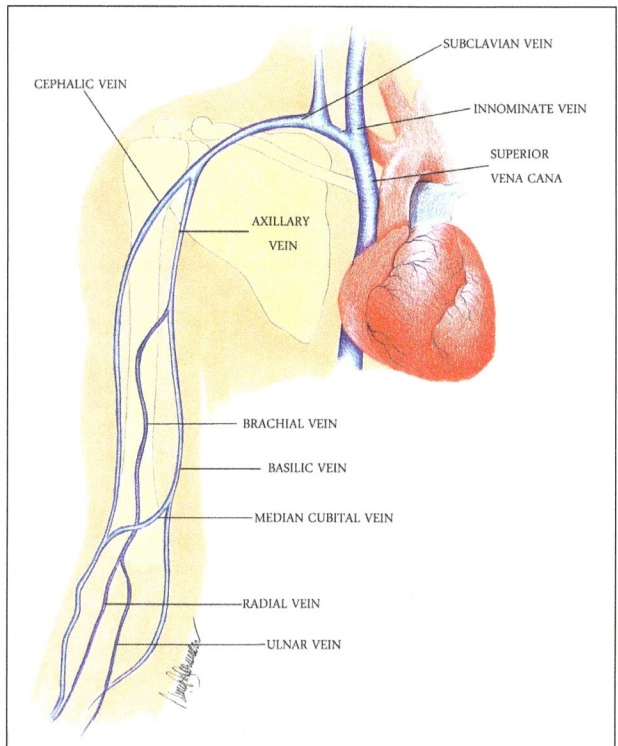

Figure 53.1 Veins of the upper extremity and shoulder region showing the location of individual veins schematically. *Source:* Reproduced from Rosen et al, *Crit Ultrasound J*, 2012;4:4.

Imaging Venous Anatomy

In any instance of concern with respect to the integrity or anatomic variability in the vasculature, an angiographic study should be performed before the procedure is commenced either preoperatively or prior to incision at surgery. Preoperative venograms may be necessary in patients with prior venous obstruction, anomalies, or recent thrombophlebitis.

Preparation of the Surgical Site

The infraclavicular region(s) are cleaned with antiseptic and isolated with sterile drapes. Conventional scrubbing with antiseptic is still performed for high-risk patients or those with poor local hygiene. Otherwise, chlorhexidine alone or chloraprep (2% chlorhexidine gluconate and 70% isopropyl alcohol) is used to cleanse the area. This affords adequate protection for the procedure. We prefer to prepare both sides, in the event of unexpected inability to gain adequate access on one side.

Vascular Access

Most people prefer to attempt the nondominant side for arm motion first unless there are extenuating circumstances, eg, mastectomy or left-sided superior vena cava. Details of the percutaneous vascular access technique are described below. In brief, cephalic vein isolation is achieved after local anesthesia is administered to the pectoral infraclavicular region and deltopectoral groove. After pectoral skin incision (straight or curved), the deltopectoral groove is dissected and the cephalic vein isolated with two temporary vascular ties to control antegrade and retrograde blood flow. Vascular access is achieved by anterior incision involving 25% to 50% of the vein diameter. In some instances, venous entry can be obtained with a needle puncture and guidewire insertion and sheath-dilator assembly.

Axillary or subclavian vein puncture is performed percutaneously, and a guidewire inserted followed by sheath-dilator assembly placement (Figure 53.2). We favor cephalic vein placement whenever possible to improve lead outcomes, reduce risk of perioperative complications of pneumothorax and local bleeding, and limit the possibility of subclavian crush injury to or fracture of the implanted lead.

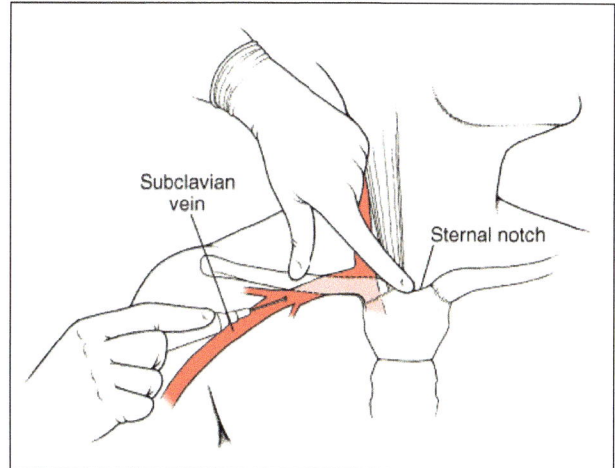

Figure 53.2 Technique of subclavian puncture. *Source:* From the *Merck Manual of Diagnosis and Therapy*, edited by Robert Porter. Copyright 2013. by Merck Sharp & Dohme Corp., a subsidiary of Merck & Co, Inc, Whitehouse Station, NJ. Available at http://www.merckmanuals.com/professional/critical_care_medicine/approach_to_the_critically_ill_patient/vascular_access.html. Accessed August 2014. Used with permission.

Use of multiple transvenous leads is now increasingly common. To insert more than one lead in the cephalic vein, it is necessary to pass the first lead into the thorax prior to attempting second and third lead placement. Frequently, leads can impinge on each other, with surface contact impeding free movement of each lead individually or placement of individual leads in target atrial or ventricular regions. In general, we prefer to fix the first lead in the target region with a stay suture placed on the suture sleeve prior to manipulation of a second lead. This process is repeated for a third lead. Many operators prefer to use separate cephalic and subclavian access or wholly subclavian insertion for 3-lead systems (Figure 53.3). We have successfully used cephalic access alone in such systems when the vein is large enough and prefer to use leads coated with surface lubricant when multiple leads are passed. In such leads, particular care may be needed to place extra stay sutures on the suture sleeve to prevent migration.

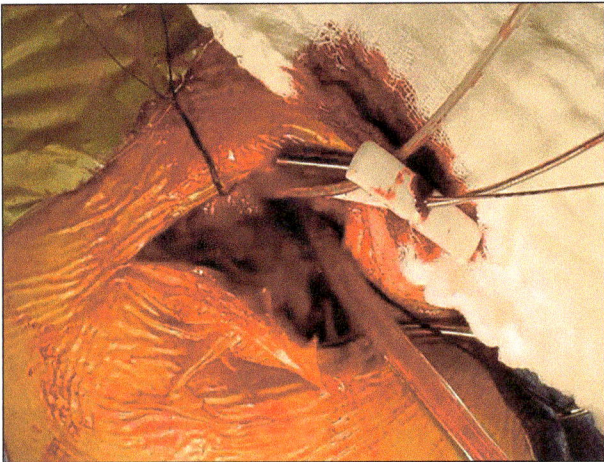

Figure 53.3 Multiple lead access being achieved by separate subclavian vein punctures for lead placement and a retained guidewire technique for placement of a third lead.

Retained-wire techniques are often used for multiple lead insertions. In such instances, a larger sheath upsized by 1- to 2-Fr sizes is used with the initial lead insertion, which is performed with a retained guidewire. While this approach is convenient for the operator, it does create a larger entry point into the vein than the lead caliber and produces adjacent and continuous entry points that form a large overall venous puncture site. Such a site is often associated with greater local bleeding after sheath removal and may require pursestring sutures around the venous entry site to control bleeding. This technique is not recommended in patients with severe heart failure and high venous pressures due to the risk of substantial and serious back-bleeding.

Other Access Techniques

The femoral vein can be used when the upper extremity veins cannot be utilized or lack sufficient capacity to accept the leads involved in the device system. This approach should be planned preoperatively, and the area appropriately prepared as described above. The femoral vein is accessed in the inguinal triangle, preferably below the inguinal ligament where it lies just medial to the midpoint between the anterior iliac spine and the pubic tubercle. Its position is just medial to the palpable femoral artery, which is usually used to localize the position, and percutaneous Seldinger puncture technique can access this vein. Sheath-dilator assemblies are used for individual leads, and a retained-wire technique is strongly discouraged due to risks of local bleeding and hematoma formation that can be difficult to control, particularly in obese patients and those on anticoagulant therapy. Iliac vein access has also been utilized.[12]

The jugular veins can also be accessed in the neck, if so required. External and internal jugular vein access can be obtained by percutaneous puncture as described elsewhere. External jugular vein insertion can also be achieved by a small shallow incision in the supraclavicular triangle with careful dissection in and around the vein and placement of stay sutures above and below the planned site of venous entry to control bleeding (Figure 53.4, A and B).

A needle puncture and guidewire insertion approach is preferable to venous wall incision even with the vein exposed. In both jugular vein insertion approaches, the lead must traverse the clavicle to reach the infraclavicular region where the device pocket is located. The risk of lead abrasion due to clavicular motion is significant, and care to avoid direct contact is necessary. Passing the lead below the clavicle is preferable, and protection of insulation by use of a suture sleeve may be considered.

Epicardial lead-system implantation was the original technique used by Senning for pacemaker implant, and now, with modifications to reduce its invasiveness, it can still be an option in patients with significant venous issues. Approaches to the epicardium using subcostal, subxiphoid, and anterolateral thoracotomies with minimally invasive approaches are well described.[13,14] Another established surgical approach utilizes video-assisted thoracoscopic visualization of the epicardium.[15,16]

Surgical Considerations and Technique(s) for Pectoral Device Implant

An incision is made in the infraclavicular fossa at the middle and outer third at an angle to the deltopectoral groove, almost parallel to the plane of the clavicle. This incision is deepened to the fascia and the deltopectoral groove is identified. Sharp dissection is preferable to blunt dissection. The knife and scissors cause less tissue damage than digital dissection; however, careless use may cause damage to the insulation of the lead, if a previous lead is present. The use of a well-grounded electrocautery is perfectly acceptable to facilitate dissection and achieve hemostasis. One should be careful to use it in short bursts to avoid heat damage to any leads. One should also keep the cautery away from the metallic lead connector pins to avoid endocardial injury.

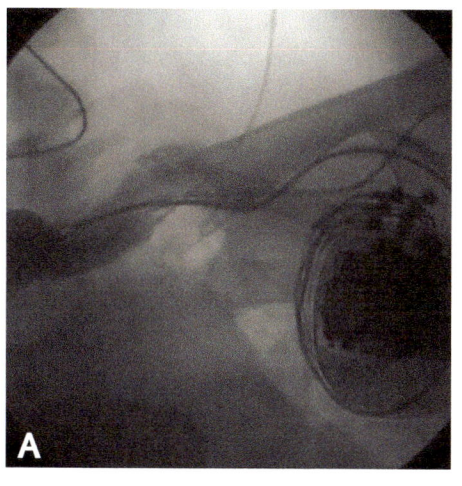
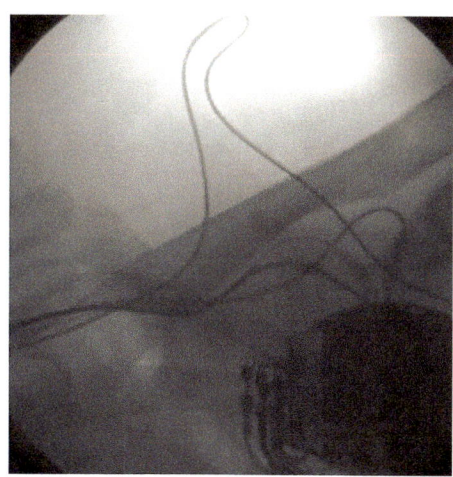
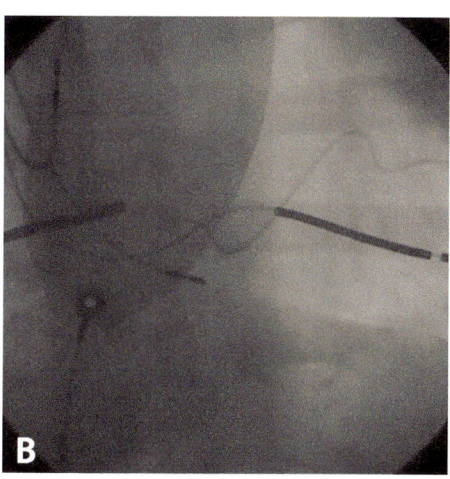
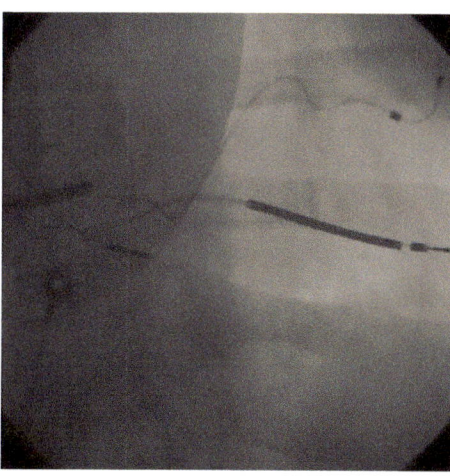

Figure 53.4 **Panel A:** Obstruction of left subclavian vein by a previously placed biventricular pacemaker-defibrillator system with 3 leads. The device's existing leads are inserted via the left subclavian vein, which is occluded laterally from the point of entry. The medial aspect of vein is collateralized and filled retrogradely from the jugular veins (**left panel**). The addition of an atrial lead for dual site right atrial pacing is accomplished using the external jugular vein for access (**right panel** and ▶ Video 53.1). **Panel B:** The 2 atrial leads are seen at the high right atrial appendage and coronary sinus ostium (**left panel**) and the right ventricular pacing and defibrillation lead with the lateral left ventricular pacing lead (**right panel**).

Access

Cephalic Vein

In our opinion, isolating the cephalic vein in the deltopectoral groove provides the best access for lead placement and should be attempted in all patients.[17] The vein is usually large enough to accommodate multiple leads and obviates multiple potential complications, namely, pneumothorax, hemothorax, arterial injury, and subclavian crush lead injury. It also preserves the axillary-subclavian axis for future revisions.

This vein can be exposed in the deltopectoral groove adjacent to the deltoid branch of the thoracoacromial artery. The vein can be isolated and cannulated directly with the leads, or a wire can be threaded, using fluoroscopic guidance, into the subclavian vein.

Axillary and Subclavian Veins

Familiarity with the course of these veins and the anatomical landmarks allows the operator to access the vein anywhere along its course by using the right technique. Accessing the axillary vein potentially avoids the risk of pneumothorax and subclavian crush (see Figures 53.1 and 53.2).

While accessing the vein with a needle (Figure 53.3), the operator must be careful to stay tangential to the first rib and at an acute angle with the vein. This will minimize the risk of violating the pleura. Linear movement without any lateral movement will avoid lacerating the vascular structures. If initially unsuccessful, repeat attempts may be made, reassessing the landmarks and repositioning the needle after full withdrawal. Lateral movement for repositioning should be avoided at all costs. Inadvertent arterial puncture can be handled with local pressure for a few minutes, and the procedure can be continued. If the subclavian vein is accessed too medially, one runs the risk of compression injury to the lead at the costoclavicular junction, either due to the subclavius or the costoclavicular ligament (the so-called subclavian crush syndrome).[18,19]

In this scenario, the pacing or defibrillation lead is trapped between the clavicle and the first rib in narrowest part, ie, the apex of triangle formed by these structures (Figure 53.5).

If unsuccessful after multiple attempts, dye injected into an ipsilateral peripheral vein may be helpful. We have also found an intraoperative Doppler probe placed on the surgical field invaluable in identifying the vein.[20]

After the vein has been accessed, guidewires are introduced, keeping the needle extremely steady, and fluoroscopic

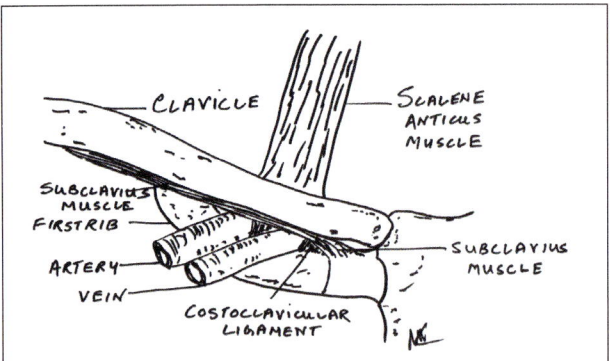

Figure 53.5 Anatomical site of subclavian crush injury.

confirmation of the position is obtained. For multiple leads, we prefer multiple wires being placed at this time, using the same or adjoining access point(s). The wires are followed by the introducer sheaths, through which the leads are placed in their appropriate positions using fluoroscopic guidance.

The appropriate positioning of the leads for their various purposes are discussed elsewhere in this book. Fluoroscopically guided lead placement in the heart is the rule, though occasional implants with ultrasound guidance have been described in special situations (eg, pregnant women).[21,22]

After positioning the leads appropriately, the sleeves are sutured to the underlying fascia. We advocate 3 nonabsorbable sutures tied down firmly but not too tightly, as this might damage the leads.

Device Pocket Creation

We delay the creation of the device pocket until after adequate access of the vein has been achieved. Using sharp dissection, we create a pocket on the pectoral fascia. We could accurately call this a suprafascial pocket, although it is subcutaneous. We find this plane the least vascular and easy to create, leaving an excellent cutaneous flap without any chance of buttonholing or devitalization. Hemostasis of the few bleeders encountered can be achieved using the electrocautery. The pocket should be slightly larger than the size of the generator to prevent tension on the flap thus created. Too large a pocket may allow space for accumulation of fluid and create a nidus for infection. This is particularly true in patients who are on anticoagulant and/or antiplatelet therapy. Excess mobility of the generator in the pocket may also lead to migration or the Twiddler's syndrome.

An esthetic choice for device pocket creation may be a submammary or an axillary pocket.[23-27] The dissection technique considerations should be adhered to, dissecting up to the fascia, and paying close attention to hemostasis (Figure 53.6).

Where the pocket is larger than the device, constant manipulation of the device can result in significant rotation and torsion damage to the leads, often producing functional disturbances.[28-30] This can be prevented by appropriately sizing the device pocket and, of course, offering patient education and counseling to prevent pocket manipulation.

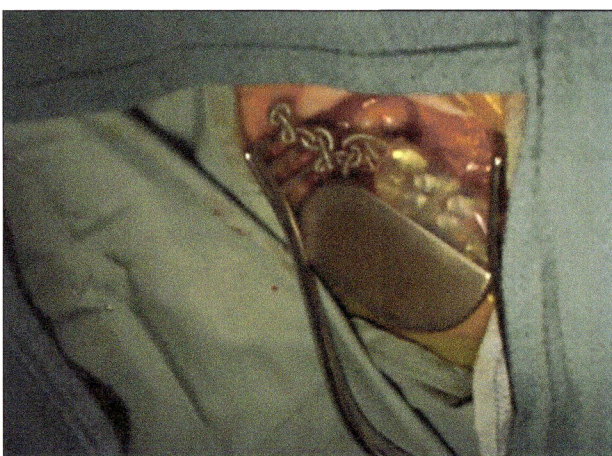

Figure 53.6 "Twiddling" of a pacemaker in the fairly large pocket with severe twisting of pacing leads requiring lead revision.

Lead Tunneling

In the event of infraclavicular lead insertion and pocket creation, tunneling of the lead or leads is obviated by the entry point of the leads being in close proximity to the device pocket. However, in the event of disparate sites, the lead(s) would have to be tunneled to the site of the generator pocket. Lead manufacturers have tunneling systems that are effective for single leads and short distances. Multiple leads and bifurcated or trifurcated leads pose a challenge, particularly under local infiltration analgesia and the awake patient. We have been successful in using a small thoracostomy tube to carry up to 3 leads without damaging them, tunneled subcutaneously from the lead insertion site to the pocket. This does require extensive infiltration with local analgesics and a short duration of deeper sedation. Care must be taken not to buttonhole the skin during the process. Occasionally, we have had to make bridging incisions to cover the distance.

Infection Control

Apart from prophylactic antibiotics, rigorous attention to sterility during the procedure is essential to minimize the risk of infection. The use of a povidone-iodine–impregnated plastic barrier over the incision site is the first step in reducing local infection. Some authors have advocated the use of local irrigation of the pocket with nonsystemic antibiotics. We follow a protocol of thorough irrigation with a pulsatile irrigator, first after all dissection has been completed and again after confirming adequate hemostasis, prior to placement of the generator in the pocket. We also advocate a change of gloves or double-gloving before the generator is brought onto the field.

Perioperative Surgical Complications

Perioperative complications of pacemaker implantation have been extensively studied and are not uncommon.[31]

Intraoperative Bleeding

Persistent bleeding may be encountered during the implant procedure, particularly in patients on concomitant oral anticoagulants and/or antiplatelet agents. Meticulous attention to the smallest bleeder is essential in these patients to prevent postoperative hematomas. Inadvertent arterial punctures can be dealt with by digital pressure for a few minutes. Respiratory or cardiovascular instability may indicate a more severe vascular injury such as a hemothorax. This may have to be ascertained and dealt with by introducing a thoracostomy tube and/or exploration. Meticulous attention to the details of vein access will avoid this disastrous complication.

Intrapericardial Bleeding

Persistent tachycardia with or without hemodynamic instability may be the first clinical signs indicative of intrapericardial bleeding. Ongoing progressive hemodynamic instability would necessitate a diagnostic echocardiogram to confirm pericardial bleeding as the cause. This may be due to immediate intra- or postoperative lead perforations. Another diagnostic indicator may be increasing thresholds and impedance of the implanted lead. In true cardiac perforation, fluoroscopy may reveal a distant migration of the lead. Surgical intervention would depend on the severity of the hemodynamic compromise. Slow bleeds may be dealt with by initiating needle pericardiocentesis, followed by catheter drainage. The preferred route would be a subxiphoid needle insertion, directed toward the left shoulder, under echocardiographic guidance and/or ECG monitoring. Hemodynamic collapse may require a thoracotomy to evacuate the blood, relieve tamponade, and repair the damage. The possibility of perforation may be minimized and even obviated by placement of the active fixation lead in the interventricular septum.

Postoperative Hematomas

These may be slow or rapidly progressive. Slow progress is usually indicative of venous or capillary bleeds. Fast-growing hematomas are indicative of arterial bleeds. Ultrasound imaging may provide insight into the extent of a hematoma in case of doubt. If the hematoma is of any significance, we advocate surgical exploration of the pocket to correct the cause, culture the contents, and thoroughly irrigate the pocket. We do not advocate aspiration for fear of introducing infection.

Pneumothorax

Creation of an intraoperative or postoperative pneumothorax is an infrequent but well-known complication of subclavian vein cannulation and the result of violating the pleura and puncturing the lung. Aspiration of air during the attempted vein puncture may have been noticeable in some instances but may occur even after an apparently uncomplicated procedure. Patients with emphysema, bullae, or small thoracic bone structure are particularly vulnerable. Use of micropuncture needles and preoperative or intraoperative venography to outline the course of the vein is helpful in reducing its incidence.

The clinical presentation of a pneumothorax may vary from absence of any symptoms, to mild chest pain or dyspnea, to difficulty in inspiration, to acute respiratory collapse. It should be remembered that the pneumothorax can manifest hours after the procedure. Persistent tachycardia with decreased oxygen saturation should raise suspicion of such an event. A chest radiograph is the definitive diagnostic study. We routinely advocate a chest x-ray at least 6 hours postprocedure. Tube thoracostomy is indicated if the pneumothorax is significant in size or impairing respiratory function. A symptomatic pneumothorax should be treated with a tube thoracostomy in the anterior axillary line away from the pocket site. A pneumothorax of less than 20% with no clinical effect may be observed with follow up. Spontaneous resorption may be observed in these patients. Follow-up radiographs to document this regression and/or lack of progress in size should be obtained before discharging the patient. This complication can be minimized by following all the tenets of implantation technique.

Lead Dislodgement

Displacement of the implanted lead system can occur during the procedure and also in the postoperative period. While lead displacement is more often seen in the immediate perioperative observation period, it can be seen up to 30 days after device system implantation. Later dislodgement is uncommon and may have a specific trigger.

Minimization of this complication is best achieved by careful selection of lead(s) and implant procedures to document lead stability. We prefer active-fixation leads in unfavorable anatomic situations, such as severe atrial or ventricular enlargement or tricuspid regurgitation. Larger-diameter leads may also provide more stability in such situations. Use of intraoperative maneuvers such as inspiration or coughing to document lead stability are encouraged.

Often this complication can result due to errors during the implant procedure, such as incomplete lead-tip stability, inadequate tip fixation during the implant, severe anatomic abnormalities such as atrial or ventricular dilatation, or physiologic disturbances such as tricuspid incompetence that limit lead-tip stability or placement site. Excessive movement by the patient, especially upper-extremity motion in the intra- or immediate postoperative period, predisposes to this complication. Shoulder and arm immobilizers can be employed for short periods of time, but this should not exceed a few days to avoid risk of shoulder mobility issues. Other preventive measures include avoidance of lifting heavy objects or other activities with excessive extremity motion, such as driving or reaching up above the head, until the lead system is fully healed in place.

In general, the right ventricular apex and right atrial appendage are preferred due to better lead stability, but currently few recent data exist to suggest that other lead placement sites are more vulnerable. Left ventricular epicardial lead placement via the coronary veins with the early generation leads had higher displacement rates, reaching up to 8% in some series, but newer lead-fixation designs have reduced this problem to much lower levels. Lead displacement requiring lead and/or system revision has prevalence rates that approximate 1% or less in the right ventricular apex, right atrium, and right ventricular outflow tract. Passive-fixation leads are more at risk, and active-fixation leads may be more desirable in such anatomic situations or as part of complex, multilead systems.

Displacement can manifest as a change in fluoroscopic position, excessive lead system/tip motion during the normal cardiac cycle, and change in electrical parameters during lead testing or fluoroscopic dislodgement. It should be addressed and remedied as soon as identified. This may involve re-exploration of a previously sutured pulse-generator pocket or postoperative detection on a chest radiograph or device testing. Lead dislodgement should be corrected immediately unless clinical circumstances dictate otherwise.

Late Complications

Device End of Life or Malfunction

Longer life expectancies in the patient cohort has led to a greater need for upgrades and replacements. Lead malfunction or disruption has similarly led to a need for replacements. Specific problems with certain lead systems, eg, Medtronic's Fidelis or St. Jude Medical's Riata, will need appropriate preparation for their management (Figure 53.7).

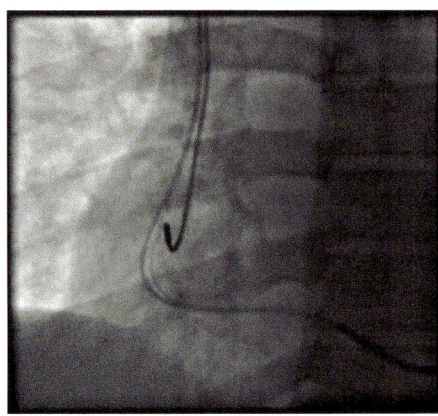

Figure 53.7 Exteriorization of conductors in a Riata lead (St. Jude Medical). The exteriorized element occupies most of the right atrial course of the lead.

Device System Infections

Clinical Presentation and Diagnosis

Infections of the device systems are late complications and can be devastating. They can occur from a few days after surgery to years after implantation. Causes of the infection can be local contamination of the pocket or systemic seeding of the foreign body. Clinical presentations range from minimal erythema at the pocket site, to unexplained fever, recurrent bacteremia, or systemic septic shock. A minimal erythematous reaction at the site of the pocket may be normal tissue reaction immediately after the procedure, but should be monitored closely. Persistent erythema with induration, if associated with systemic signs of fever should warn the clinician of a possible infection. Confirmation of the diagnosis would require hematological and bacteriological confirmation.

Late infection may be insidious or acutely fulminant. Systemic seeding may be the cause, causing an inflammatory sign at the pocket or a systemic manifestation. Hematological and bacteriological evidence of an infection without local signs may not be diagnostic of lead system infections, but should certainly be warning signs of this possibility. Further investigation would be warranted.

Diagnosis would depend on the clinician's ability to isolate the process with the system components. Pocket infections are locally self-evident with signs of erythema, induration, and possibly drainage from the site. Lead and device extrusion may also be evident. Occasionally, obvious signs or symptoms are lacking, and investigative procedures are necessary to document infection in the system.

Routine hematological evidence with leukocytosis would indicate the presence of an infection. Local signs at the device pocket site confirm the localization of an infection at this site. It is important to know that pocket infection is always accompanied by evidence of bacterial infection along the lead body, and thus, hematogenous dissemination.

In the absence of local signs, or to confirm lead infections, further investigation may be required. Transesophageal echocardiography may show evidence of vegetations along the lead course. Differentiation between thrombus formation along the leads—a normal occurrence in up to one-third of patients—and vegetations requires an experienced echocardiographer to identify important differences in appearance and location, as well as other confirmatory studies. Positive blood cultures establish systemic infection and favor vegetations. Gallium imaging, indium-labeled leukocyte imaging, and more rapid radio-imaging procedures are now available and may help in the localization of the site of active infection. In the presence of localizing signs, the diagnosis of device system infections may be straightforward. However, in their absence, the diagnosis can be challenging and may be a process of exclusion.

Treatment

Mild, superficial skin infections (eg, cellulitis at the incision site) with no significant systemic sequelae, negative blood cultures, and negative or inconclusive imaging studies can be treated with appropriate antibiotic therapy. Resolution of the clinical and/or inflammatory signs and the absence of any bacteremia indicate a cure of the infection. These patients still require constant monitoring for any resurgence of the infection.

Although some infections of device systems may respond to conservative therapy, the only definitive treatment necessitates extraction of the complete system. This may require the use of extraction devices, with their potential hazards, and sometimes even open thoracotomies and direct extraction using cardiopulmonary bypass. This subject is discussed in detail in Chapter 60. Some principles of device and lead explantation are discussed below.

Device and Lead Explantation

Device explantation for infection and/or system upgrades are common occurrences during the lifetime of patients with implanted cardiac rhythm management devices. Though relatively straightforward, careful attention to detail is imperative to maintain lead integrity and minimize the risk of infections. Dissection in these patients should be done extremely cautiously. Multiple leads pose the threat of lead damage during the process of dissection. We choose to use the electrocautery, at a very low setting, or a plasma blade, sparingly, to minimize the risk of thermal injury. Careful sharp dissection is performed to release these leads from the device, and if need be from each other. We also routinely irrigate the pocket with saline, using a pulsatile irrigator to reduce the risk of infections.

Explantation may also be performed for infected systems. In these instances, management of the pocket may be an issue. In the presence of significant tissue damage with infection, the tenets of open drainage and healing with secondary intention may be appropriate. However, this takes time, and wherever possible, we do completely excise all unhealthy tissue, thoroughly irrigate with a pulsatile irrigator, confirm hemostasis, and close primarily. We are always prepared to reopen the incision and let it heal by secondary intention, if required.

Lead extractions, though most often performed for infected systems, may also be performed to reduce the intravascular load, procure access, or reduce interference.[32] Leads implanted less than year prior to explantation may be extracted with simple traction. We advocate using a locking stylet on all these cases to prevent uncoiling the lead and insulation separation. If either of these occurs, extraction with a lead extractor may become more challenging.

Lead Repair

In extremely high-risk patients, where lead extraction or lead introduction may be fraught with problems, lead repair may be a viable alternative.[33] Insulation breaches that are accessible may be sealed with silicone adhesive. Damaged leads that are close to the connector can be spliced with a new connector after division of the lead.

Bridging Defibrillation Support Methods

ICD recipients are at risk of sudden death after explantation of these devices. If another device cannot be placed due to technical issues or an infection, preparation for bridging with a wearable defibrillator or a subcutaneous defibrillator should be considered. Adequate instructions as to its use and appropriate education should be part of the preoperative education.

Lead Extraction

Indwelling leads develop a thrombofibrotic reaction around them. This reaction adheres them to any surface they make contact with. The density of this adherence determines the difficulty in their extraction. The longer these leads are in place, the denser the adherence. Extraction devices, mechanical or energy-driven, cut the tissue around the lead to release it and facilitate extraction. Due to their ability to cause separation of tissue, their potential to damage the vascular components is significant, and the guidelines for their use should be closely followed.

Evaluating the lead position within the vascular structure facilitates the positioning of the bevel of the extractor and preparation for potential areas of problems. We evaluate all candidates for extraction with a CT angiogram, venous phase, or a conventional venogram. The course of the lead within the vasculature is closely analyzed. The points of particular interest are the innominate/subclavian-superior vena cava-atrial axis and the intracardiac course. In the operating suite, every patient is monitored with hemodynamic monitoring and continuous transesophageal echocardiography.

Planning lead extraction should incorporate site, personnel, patient, and device system evaluations.

Procedure Site

The traditional operating room is well equipped with the essential personnel and apparatus for dealing with any of the potential complications that may arise. However, the fluoroscopy system may be suboptimal. The cardiac catheterization suite, on the contrary, usually has excellent fluoroscopy, but is not usually ideal for emergent surgical intervention. A hybrid location, incorporating the best features of both sites, would be the most conducive for this procedure.

Personnel

Adequate training and allocation of responsibilities for all the personnel along with maintenance of their competence is essential, not only for the extraction, but also the ability to expeditiously deal with any potential complication. Surgical backup should be immediately available. Communication with all essential personnel is of the utmost importance.

Patient

An intimate knowledge of the patient's clinical status and comorbidities should be documented. A chest x-ray, CT scan, and a venogram may all be useful in assessing the potential for problems. The type, condition, and number of leads; their proximity and adherence to the surrounding structures; and vein patency are all information provided by these tests that may be helpful, particularly when additional or new lead implantations are planned.

Device

Dependency on pacing and the need for temporary pacing should be assessed on all the patients. A temporary pacing wire can be introduced via the jugular or the femoral route prior to the extraction, if needed. A permanent lead attached to the skin using the explanted generator or an alternate one can be used if longer term pacing is required.

Monitoring

Arterial pressure monitoring and continuous echocardiography using a transesophageal probe is used to monitor hemodynamic changes during the extraction. Slight fluctuations in blood pressure may indicate excessive traction on the lead that can be correlated with the echocardiogram. Persistent hemodynamic compromise during the procedure can be indicative of a more serious issue. Fluoroscopy combined with the transesophageal echocardiogram is invaluable in early identification of potential disasters. Expeditious intervention can improve results dramatically. A large bore venous access for fast fluid resuscitation is placed in the femoral vein prior to commencing lead extraction.

Fluoroscopy

Continuous fluoroscopy during any manipulation of the extracting tool(s) is essential. Laser lead-extraction systems are now widely used for these procedures, and a few principles of use are outlined here (more detail is available in Chapter 60).

Traction on the lead should be maintained to straighten the lead and maintain the parallel orientation of the extraction sheath to the lead. Sudden changes in resistance or hemodynamic instability should be evaluated for the possibility of the vascular wall being pulled into the tool with potential perforation. This can also be seen with invagination of the right ventricular wall at the lead tip. The tip of the bevel of an extraction laser sheath should be kept away from the adherent vessel wall at its attachment point(s). The extraction sheath should never be advanced up to or beyond the tip of the lead. In general, the sheath tip should be left about 5 mm short of the tip of the lead. Traction is usually sufficient to remove the remaining lead from the adherent tissues at its tip. At all times, evaluating hemodynamic stability and being prepared to take corrective action in the event of vascular damage cannot be stressed enough. Lead division and embolization can be addressed with a snare using the transfemoral venous route and is discussed elsewhere.

Lead Extraction Complications

Management of Complications

The literature is replete with complications of lead extraction.[34] Expeditious recognition and intervention are imperative to reduce procedure-related mortality, as some of the complications can be lethal (Table 53.1). A standard paradigm that can be followed if there is evidence of any hemodynamic compromise is outlined in Table 53.2. Institution of immediate hemodynamic support with fluids and/or inotropes and simultaneous assessment and evaluation of the type and severity of the injury are crucial. The proposed surgical intervention will depend on the type and site of injury. Sternotomy, a lateral thoracotomy, or a subxiphoid approach may be necessary to repair the damage. Patient survival is closely related to the promptness of intervention.

Table 53.1 Lead extraction complications

Major
- Death
- Vascular injury requiring surgical repair using thoracotomy or sternotomy with or without the use of cardiopulmonary bypass
- Cardiac injury requiring surgical repair using sternotomy with or without cardiopulmonary bypass
- Pulmonary embolism requiring surgical intervention
- Stroke

Minor
- Pericardial effusion not requiring surgery
- Hemothorax not requiring surgery
- Pocket hematomas
- Localized vascular injury at entry site
- Dislodged, migrated lead fragment with no sequelae

Table 53.2 Procedures for addressing lead-extraction complications

Management
- Clinical presentation: Cardiovascular compromise
- Identify the problem
- Fluoroscopy:
  - Reduction in heart size
  - New or increasing pleural effusion
- Echocardiography:
  - New or increasing pericardial effusion
- Intervention:
  - Immediate fluid resuscitation
  - Blood transfusion as needed
  - Inotropes as needed
  - Surgical intervention
- Tamponade: Pericardiocentesis or surgical drainage of effusion
  - Sternotomy for ongoing bleeding with suspected cardiac injury
- New or expanding right pleural effusion:
  - Sternotomy for suspected RA/SVC/RV injury and for CPB
  - High right thoracotomy for suspected brachiocephalic or high SVC injury

Surgical Wisdom

Experience is the best teacher. Awareness of specific issues regarding the patient and the lead system is important. Contrary to the popular truism, all patients and all leads are *not* created equal. Understanding individual differences in lead behavior can be crucial in modifying technique. While there has been a long series of leads that have shown a propensity for subnormal performance, of particular interest in recent years have been the Medtronic Sprint Fidelis lead and the St. Jude Medical Riata lead, which have shown higher than usual failure rates.[35-38] Recognition of the characteristic behavior and structural components of these leads will greatly facilitate their removal (see Figure 53.7).

Recent studies have defined this challenging condition better and reported conductor externalization ranging from 9% for 8-Fr leads and up to 32% for 7-Fr Riata leads.[36,37] In a recent report of 577 patients with the Riata 467 (84%) and Riata ST 89 (16%) leads, 53% were extracted for infection and 36% for lead malfunction. Extraction was successful in 99.1% of cases. Thirty-five percent were found to have externalized cables, and patients with these leads required laser sheath extraction more frequently.[38] These circumstances are discussed in Chapter 60.

Conclusions

Device implantations and extractions have greatly increased over the last two decades. Expanding indications for implantation and longer patient survival have contributed to almost half a million devices being implanted per year. A deeper understanding of the technical challenges and patient vagaries has allowed us to prevent potential problems and improve our experience. Technological lead and device improvements will further optimize our experience with this group of potentially sick patient population.

References

1. Tracy CM, Epstein AE, Darbar D, et al. 2012 ACCF/AHA/HRS focused update of the 2008 guidelines for device-based therapy of cardiac rhythm abnormalities. A report of the American College of Cardiology Foundation/American Heart Association Task Force on Practice Guidelines. *J Am Coll Cardiol.* 2012;60(14):1297-1313.
2. Epstein AE, DiMarco JP, Ellenbogen KA, et al. ACC/AHA/HRS 2008 guidelines for device based therapy of cardiac rhythm abnormalities: Executive summary. *Circulation.* 2008;117:2820-2840.
3. Cheng A, Nazarian S, Brinker JA, Tompkins C, Spragg DD, Leng CT, et al. Continuation of warfarin during pacemaker or implantable cardioverter–defibrillator implantation: A randomized clinical trial. *Heart Rhythm.* 2011;8:536-540.
4. Jamula E, Douketis JD, Schulman S. Perioperative anticoagulation in patients having implantation of a cardiac pacemaker or defibrillator: a systematic review and practical management guide. *J Thromb Haemost.* 2008;6:1615-1621.
5. Daubert JC, Mabo P. Continue or withhold oral anticoagulation in high-risk patients undergoing pacemaker or ICD implantation. *Eur Heart J.* 2009;30(15):1828a-1828c. DOI: http://dx.doi.org/10.1093/eurheartj/ehn491
6. Love CJ. Perioperative management of anticoagulation in patients undergoing cardiac rhythm device procedures: a bridge to nowhere? *Pacing Clin Electrophysiol.* 2010;33:383-384.

7. Tompkins C, Henrikson CA. Optimal strategies for the management of antiplatelet and anticoagulation medications prior to cardiac device implantation. *Cardiol J.* 2011;18:103-109.
8. Korantzopoulos P, Letsas KP, Liu T, Fragakis N, Efremidis M, Goudevenos JA. Anticoagulation and antiplatelet therapy in implantation of electrophysiological devices. *Europace.* 2011;13(12):1669-1680.
9. Goldstein DJ, Losquadro W, Sputnitz HM. Outpatient pacemaker procedures in orally anticoagulated patients. *Pacing Clin Electrophysiol.* 1998;21:1730-1734.
10. Gludici MC, Barold SS, Paul DL. Pacemaker and implantable cardioverter defibrillator implantation without reversal of warfarin therapy. *Pacing Clin Electrophysiol.* 2004;27:338.
11. Healey JS, Eikelboom J, Douketis J, Wallentin L, Oldgren J, Yang S, et al. Periprocedural bleeding and thromboembolic events with dabigatran compared with warfarin: results from the Randomized Evaluation of Long-term Anticoagulation Therapy (RE-LY) randomized trial. *Circulation.* 2012;126(3):343-348.
12. Ellestad MH, French J. Iliac vein approach to permanent pacemaker implantation. *Pacing Clin Electrophysiol.* 1989;12:1030-1033.
13. Lawrie GM, Kaushik R, Pacifico A. Right mini-thoracotomy as an adjunct to left sub-costal AICD implantation. *Ann Thorac Surg.* 1989;209 6:716-727.
14. Krasna MJ, Buser GA, Flowers JL, et al. Thoracoscopic versus laporoscopic placement of defibrillator patches. *Surg Laporosc Endosc.* 1996;5:91.
15. Frumin H, Goodman GR, Pleatman M: ICD implantation via thoracoscopy without the need for sternotomy or thoracotomy. *Pacing Clin Electrophysiol.* 1993;16(2):257-260.
16. Jutley RS, Waller DA, Loke I, Skehan D, Ng A, Stafford P, et al. Video-assisted thoracoscopic implantation of the left ventricular pacing lead for cardiac resynchronization therapy. *Pacing Clin Electrophysiol.* 2008;31:812-818.
17. Furman S. Venous cutdown for pacemaker implantation. *Ann Thorac Surg.* 1980;41:438.
18. Magney JE, Flynn DM, Parsons JA, et al. Anatomic mechanisms explaining damage to pacemaker leads, defibrillator leads and failure of central venous catheters adjacent to the sternoclavicular joint. *Pacing Clin Electrophysiol.* 1993;16:445-457.
19. Roelke M, O'Nunain SS, Osswald S, et al. Subclavian crush syndrome complicating transvenous cardioverter defibrillator systems. *Pacing Clin Electrophysiol.* 1995;18(5 Pt 1):973-979.
20. Gayle DD, Bailery CJ, Haistey WK, et al. A novel ultrasound-guided approach to the puncture of the extrathoracic subclavian vein for surgical lead placement. *Pacing Clin Electrophysiol.* 1996;19:700.
21. Güdal M, Kervancioğlu C, Oral D, Gürel T, Erol C, Sonel A. Permanent pacemaker implantation in a pregnant woman with the guidance of ECG and two-dimensional echocardiography. *Pacing Clin Electrophysiol.* 1987;10(3 Pt 1):543-545.
22. Pedrinazzi C; Gazzaniga P, Durin O, Tovena D, Inama G. Implantation of a permanent pacemaker in a pregnant woman under the guidance of electrophysiologic signals and transthoracic echocardiography. *J Cardiovasc Med (Hagerstown).* 2008;9(11):1169-1172.
23. Kolettis TM, Saxena A, Krol RB, Saksena S. Submammary implantation of a cardioverter-defibrillator with a nonthoracotomy lead system. *Am Heart J.* 1993;126:1222-1223.
24. Giudici MC, Meierbachtol CJ, Paul DL, Krupa RK, Vazquez LD, Serge Barold S. Submammary device implantation in women: A step-by-step approach. *J Cardiovasc Electrophysiol.* 2013;24:476-479.
25. Roelke M, Jackson G, Harthorne JW. Submammary pacemaker implantation: a unique tunneling technique. *Pacing Clin Electrophysiol.* 1994;17(11 Pt 1):1793-1796.
26. Al-Bataineh M, Sajadi S, Fontaine JM, Kutalek S. Axillary subpectoral approach for pacemaker or defibrillator implantation in patients with ipsilateral prepectoral infection and limited venous access. *J Interv Card Electrophysiol.* 2010;27(2):137-142.
27. Rosenthal E. A cosmetic approach for pectoral pacemaker implantation in young girls. *Pacing Clin Electrophysiol.* 2000;23(9):1397-1400.
28. Bayliss CE, Beanlands DS, Baird RJ. The pacemaker-Twiddler's syndrome: a new complication of implantable transvenous pacemakers. *Can Med Assoc J.* 1968;99:371-373.
29. Kumar A, McKay CR, Rahimtoola SH. Pacemaker Twiddler's syndrome: an important cause of diaphragmatic pacing. *Am J Cardiol.* 1985;56:797-799.
30. Mehta D, Lipsius M, Suri RS, Krol RB, Saksena S. Twiddler's syndrome with the implantable cardioverter-defibrillator. *Am Heart J.* 1992;123(4 Pt 1):1079-1082.
31. Parsonnet V, Bernstein AD, Lindsay B. Pacemaker implantation complication rates: an analysis of some contributing factors. *J Am Coll Cardiol.* 1989;13:917-921.
32. Wilkoff BL, Love CJ, Byrd CL, Bongiorni MG, Carrillo RG, Crossley GH 3rd, et al. Transvenous lead extraction: Heart Rhythm Society expert consensus on facilities, training, indications, and patient management. *Heart Rhythm.* 2009;6(7):1085-1104.
33. Mahapatra S, Homoud MK, Wang PJ, Estes NA 3rd. Durability of repaired sensing leads equivalent to that of new leads in implantable cardioverter defibrillator patients with sensing abnormalities. *Pacing Clin Electrophysiol.* 2003;26(12):2225-2229.
34. Wilkoff BL, Byrd CL, Love CJ, Hayes DL, Sellers TD, Schaerf R, et al. Pacemaker lead extraction with the laser sheath: results of the pacing lead extraction with the excimer sheath (PLEXES) trial. *J Am Coll Cardiol.* 1999;33:1671–1676.
35. Hauser RG, Maisel WH, Friedman PA, Kallinen LM, Mugglin AS, Kumar K, et al. Longevity of sprint fidelis implantable cardioverter-defibrillator leads and risk factors for failure—implications for patient management. *Circulation.* 2011;123:358-363.
36. Lorvidhaya P, Mendoza I, Sehli S, Atalay MK, Kim MH. Prospective evaluation of cinefluoroscopy and chest radiography for Riata lead defects: implications for future lead screening. *J Interv Card Electrophysiol.* 2013;38(2):131-135.
37. Hayes D, Freedman R, Curtis AB, Niebauer M, Neal Kay G, Dinerman J, Beau S. Prevalence of externalized conductors in Riata and Riata ST silicone leads: results from the prospective, multicenter Riata Lead Evaluation Study. *Heart Rhythm.* 2013;10(12):1778-1782.
38. Maytin M, Wilkoff BL, Brunner M, Cronin E, Love CJ, Grazia, et al. Multicenter experience with extraction of the Riata/Riata ST ICD lead. *Heart Rhythm.* 2014;11(9):1613-1618.

Video Legend

Video 53.1 Fluoroscopy showing a 4-lead implantable defibrillator system for multisite pacing in the right atrium and biventricular pacing and defibrillation back up in a 40-year-old patient with refractory congestive heart failure class 3, dilated cardiomyopathy, and refractory persistent atrial fibrillation after pulmonary vein ablation and antiarrhythmic drug therapy.

CHAPTER 54

Ventricular and Atrial Resynchronization Devices: Technology and Implantation Methods

Robert K. Altman, MD; Jagmeet P. Singh, MD, DPhil

Introduction

The incidence and prevalence of congestive heart failure (CHF) continues to rise to what has been referred to as epidemic proportions. Approximately 5.7 million people in the United States have heart failure, and it accounts for about 300,000 deaths each year, according to the National Heart Lung and Blood Institute of the National Institutes of Health.[1,2] Treatment of heart failure has improved dramatically over the preceding decades as a result of the introduction of neurohormonal directed pharmacotherapies, which have had an impact on the quality and length of life of patients with CHF. The introduction of ICD therapy, and the use of these devices for the primary prevention of sudden cardiac death in those at risk, has also altered the prognosis of the disease; ICDs are now recommended for treatment of CHF in various stages of the disease.[3] Despite these advances, the mortality from heart failure and the economic impact to society continues to be significant. The latter is driven in large part by frequent and expensive hospitalizations.[4] Cardiac resynchronization therapy (CRT) with biventricular pacing has been shown to improve quality of life, decrease heart failure hospitalizations, and improve mortality in an expanding subset of patients with CHF by improving the mechanical function of the heart, reducing arrhythmia, and promoting electrical and mechanical remodeling. Furthermore, CRT has been shown to improve left ventricular (LV) size and function, improve hemodynamics, and reduce mitral regurgitation in patients with systolic heart failure.[5-9]

In this chapter, we will review the rationale for CRT including the concepts of electrical and mechanical dyssynchrony, the current indications for CRT, as well as future directions for research. We will review the theory and technical aspects of LV lead implantation as well as the prevention, identification, and management of complications of CRT device implantation. The follow-up and optimization of these devices is discussed in another chapter. In addition, strategies for achieving interatrial synchronization will be discussed.

Cardiac Resynchronization Therapy and Electromechanical Dyssynchrony in Congestive Heart Failure

Current Indications and Future Directions for Cardiac Resynchronization Therapy

It was in 1996 that the first report regarding the addition of a LV lead was shown to improve hemodynamics in a patient with heart failure.[10] Subsequently, a number of small studies following this finding showed improved hemodynamics and LV function in patients with severe systolic heart failure with LV pacing.[11,12] Over the last decade a large number of patients in well-designed randomized trials have been shown to benefit from CRT in terms of functional status, quality of life, reduction in hospitalization, and mortality.[13-19] As a result, CRT is currently recommended by the American College of

Cardiology, the American Heart Association, and the Heart Rhythm Society for patients who have New York Heart Association (NYHA) class III or IV heart failure symptoms on optimal medical therapy, left ventricular ejection fraction (LVEF) less than or equal to 35%, and a QRS duration greater than or equal to 0.12 seconds.

With the recent results of the MADIT-CRT trial, the class I recommendations may soon expand to include less symptomatic patients. In fact, an FDA advisory panel recently voted unanimously to expand the indications for CRT to patients with Class II heart failure, or Class I in patients with ischemic cardiomyopathy with an LVEF of less than 30%, a QRS duration of > 130 ms, and a left bundle branch block.[13] Despite the growing indications, as many as 30% of patients who fit the current criteria for CRT devices are nonresponders in one or more outcome measures such as LV systolic function and reverse remodeling.[13-15,18,19] Identification of predictors of response to CRT, both in those patient populations who meet the current guidelines and those for whom the current guidelines do not apply, is a focus of ongoing research.

Dyssynchrony

Dyssynchrony refers to the loss of mechanical or electrical coordination between or within the various cardiac chambers (Figure 54.1). Atrioventricular (AV) dyssynchrony, interventricular dyssynchrony, and intraventricular (ie, dyssynchronous electromechanical activation of the left ventricle) dyssynchrony are all important targets of CRT. Using 3D mapping, Auricchio et al have defined the presence of intramural dyssynchrony, ie, the delay in normal conduction from endocardium to epicardium, which accounts for the surface appearance of a left bundle branch block in 24 patients with systolic heart failure.[20] Inter- and intra-atrial (AA) dyssynchrony has also been described in patients with cardiomyopathy and arrhythmia and may improve with CRT or atrial pacing strategies.

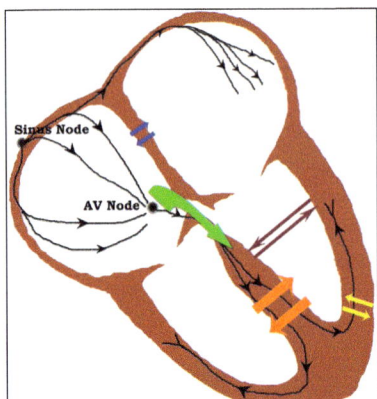

Figure 54.1 Electromechanical dyssynchrony: Atrioventricular dyssynchrony (**green arrow**), interventricular dyssynchrony (**orange arrows**), and intraventricular dyssynchrony (**purple arrows**) are direct targets of cardiac resynchronization therapy. Interatrial dyssynchrony (**blue arrows**) and intramural dyssynchrony (**yellow arrows**) have also been described in CHF.

AA Dyssynchrony

A delay between the activation of the right and left atrium (interatrial dyssynchrony) as well as dispersion of depolarization within each atrium (intra-atrial) is common and in some forms has been hypothesized to contribute to the development of atrial arrhythmias.[21] Thus pacing strategies to reduce dyssynchrony within the atrium have been developed. These include pacing from Bachmann's bundle, CS ostial pacing, as well as biatrial pacing from sites within the right atrium and the left atrium (via the coronary sinus). Where single site atrial pacing strategies in general have been shown ineffective in the prevention of atrial fibrillation,[22] there are some data, including small randomized trials, to suggest that compared to standard atrial pacing from the right atrial appendage, alternative pacing sites or biatrial pacing may reduce the incidence and recurrence of atrial fibrillation, especially in those undergoing pacemaker placement for sick sinus syndrome.[23,24] Furthermore, these techniques may improve hemodynamics and AV timing compared with single-site atrial pacing.[25-28] Other studies have not confirmed this benefit.[29] Techniques for implantation of these leads are discussed below.

AV Dyssynchrony

The delay between the activation of the atrial contraction, ventricular filling, and the initiation of ventricular contraction can have a profound effect on filling pressures and cardiac output, especially in patients with ventricular dysfunction, and may cause or worsen mitral regurgitation.[30,31] These changes may be of particular importance in obtaining maximum benefit for patients with CRT devices both to ensure adequate ventricular filling as well as to ensure a high percentage of biventricular pacing. There are a number of techniques including echocardiographic methods that are used for optimizing the AV delay and these are discussed elsewhere in this text.

Ventricular Dyssynchrony

In large-scale trials of patients with systolic heart failure, the prevalence of an intraventricular conduction delay (IVCD) was 33% to 50%; IVCD has also been shown to be an important predictor of outcome.[32,33] In many trials, QRS length also seems to be a predictor of response to CRT and, as mentioned above, is now an integral part of the guidelines for the implantation of CRT devices.[34,35] However, QRS duration alone is a more important marker for interventricular dyssynchrony than for intraventricular dyssynchrony, and 30% of patients with a prolonged QRS duration have no evidence of mechanical intraventricular dyssynchrony.[36] This might in part explain the approximately 30% incidence of nonresponders in large CRT trials that used prolonged QRS duration as an inclusion criteria.

Both interventricular and intraventricular dyssynchrony are targets of CRT. However, it is intraventricular dyssynchrony that best predicts a positive response to CRT. Bax et al summarized 24 trials using echocardiographic parameters to predict response to CRT. Only 2 had some value for interventricular dyssynchrony, yet all 24 had some predictive value for intraventricular dyssynchrony.[37]

Assessment of LV Dyssynchrony

Echocardiography is the most widespread technique used to assess mechanical dyssynchrony. Early attempts focused on M-mode echocardiography across the parasternal short axis to assess the difference in time to maximal systolic wall thickening between the anterior and posterior walls. Tissue Doppler imaging (TDI) is a technique in which the Doppler filter is set such that low frequency, high amplitude signals are detected. In this manner, the direction and velocity of contracting or relaxing myocardium can be obtained within various segments. The difference in time to peak velocities of various segments can be assessed and in many single center studies has been shown to be a good predictor of response to CRT. However, with TDI, passive myocardial motion cannot be distinguished between active contraction as is the case when assessing a patient with ischemic cardiomyopathy who might have segments of scar. In this case, contracting segments of myocardium may pull on adjacent segments causing translational motion of the scarred segment in the absence of myocardial contraction. This is an important limitation to this technique.

Speckle tracking is another echocardiographic technique that takes advantage of interference in ultrasound beams, which creates speckles in the two-dimensional echo images. Software tracks changes in the distance between individual speckles throughout the cardiac cycle. In this manner strain can be directly measured. Strain is the change in length divided by original length, which can only be calculated indirectly via TDI (by integrating the change in velocity of various segments). Strain can be measured longitudinally, circumferentially, and radially. Radial strain analysis has, in small studies, been the best predictor of response to CRT (Figure 54.2).[38]

Despite very promising results in small-scale trials, when tested prospectively in two multicenter trials, echocardiographic methods have not convincingly predicted response to CRT.[34,39] The PROSPECT and RethinQ trials were multicenter trials designed to assess the utility of dyssynchrony parameters in predicting response to CRT and, in the case of RethinQ, in patients with a narrow QRS. The PROSPECT trial was a nonrandomized prospective observational trial, which enrolled 426 patients undergoing device placement according to current selection criteria. Prior to implant subjects underwent dyssynchrony assessment using various methods to assess intra- and interventricular dyssynchrony including M-mode and TDI. At 6 months, endpoints including a clinical composite score (all-cause mortality, heart failure hospitalization, NYHA class, and patient global assessment) and 15% reduction in LV end-systolic volume were assessed. Despite site training in acquisition methods and a blinded core lab analysis, there was no single echocardiographic predictor of response

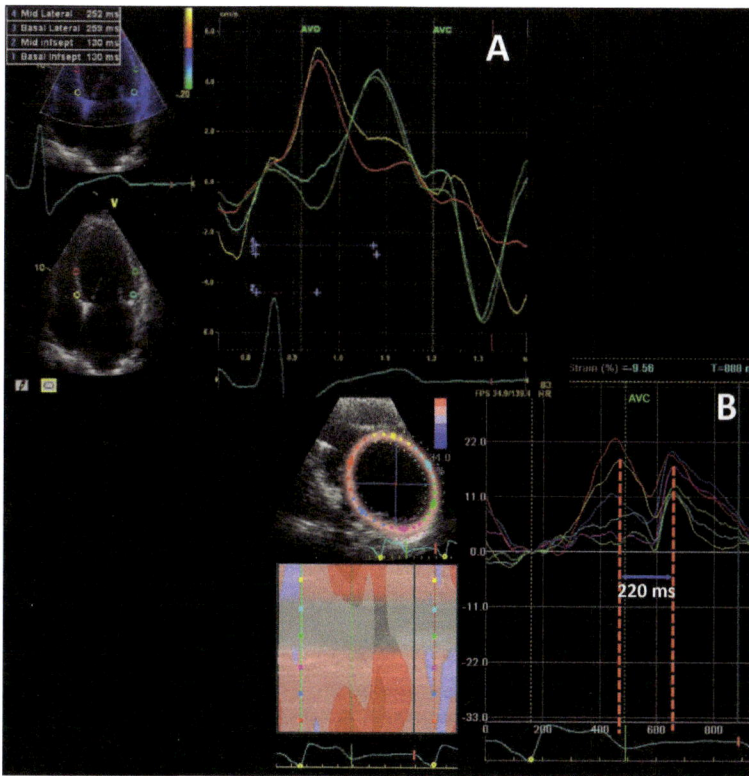

Figure 54.2 **Panel A:** Tissue Doppler imaging of longitudinal velocities in the 4-chamber view in a patient with LV intraventricular dyssynchrony. The velocities of the various segments are color-coded. There is a 129-ms delay between the time to peak velocity of the basal septal (**yellow**) versus the basal lateral (**blue**) segments.

Panel B: 2D radial strain images and segmental strain curves obtained by speckle tracking in the parasternal short axis view at the level of the papillary muscles in a patient with LV intraventricular dyssynchrony. There is a 220-ms difference in the time to peak strain between the anterior septum (**yellow**) and the posterior wall (**purple**).

to CRT. The RethinQ trial was a randomized multicenter trial designed to assess the utility of dyssynchrony parameters in predicting the response to CRT in patients with a narrow QRS. Two hundred and fifty subjects with NYHA class III or IV heart failure, EF less than or equal to 35%, and a QRS duration of less than 130 ms were randomized to CRT or no CRT. Dyssynchrony was assessed by M-mode and TDI parameters. At 6 months, the two groups showed no difference in the end point of increase in peak oxygen consumption of at least 1.0 mL/kg/min. While these two studies showed no dyssynchrony parameter to be predictive of CRT, this comes in contrast to myriad smaller studies that seemed to show some promise. This in part may be due to variability in study designs and in the methods used to obtain the data in these trials, as well as variability and poor standardization among readers. There are currently trials underway to address these issues; however, the role of echocardiography to predict response to CRT, especially in patients with a narrow QRS, remains uncertain.[33,39,40]

Other techniques, such as cardiac MRI and CT, offer the possibility of integrating measurements of dyssynchrony with the presence of scar and coronary venous anatomy for LV lead placement. Small-scale studies have shown promising results.[40-42] There remain no large-scale multicenter trials assessing these techniques.

Technical Aspects of Device Implantation

Alternative Atrial Pacing Strategies

Pacing from Bachmann's Bundle

Bachmann's bundle originates in the crest of the crista terminalis and has fibers that extend across the superior atrial septum as a band of atrial muscle that serves, during normal sinus rhythm, as the preferential path for electrical activation of the left atrium. Implantation at this site, via the right atrium, uses standard implantation techniques with active fix leads. There are some necessary modifications when attempting to fix the lead at this site. In general, a preformed J-stylet does not offer adequate reach and thus some straightening of the stylet is needed. The plane of the septum can be identified by placing the RV lead first after which, in the LAO position, when foreshortened, the lead will be parallel to the axis of the image. Once on the septum, the lead can be pulled back to hook against the roof of the atrium. In the RAO position, the lead should be confirmed to be anterior and then fixated. Pacing from this site will reveal a shortened and peaked P wave.[44]

Biatrial Pacing

Techniques for biatrial pacing involve placing a right atrial lead in the standard position of the right atrial appendage and a second lead either near the CS ostium (using an active fixation mechanism) or in the coronary sinus or an atrial coronary sinus branch that allows for left atrial capture. Techniques for locating and cannulating the CS ostium are described below. Once in place, the leads are connected to a Y-adapter with one lead acting as the anode and one as the cathode. In this manner, programming the device for bipolar atrial pacing achieves biatrial unipolar pacing, whereas programming the device to bipolar pacing would result from pacing from the cathode.[26,27]

Biventricular Devices and Leads

CRT devices have the capability of atrial pacing via a right atrial lead and biventricular pacing via the combination of a right and left ventricular lead. Most devices implanted are placed with implantable automatic cardioversion defibrillation (ICD) capabilities, as randomized trials have shown a trend toward decreased mortality in patients who received CRT-D versus CRT-P alone.[16] Furthermore, there is significant overlap of the clinical indications for CRT and for primary prevention of sudden cardiac death with ICD, and in the United States the majority of CRT implants are CRT-D devices.

Access and placement of the atrial and right ventricular/defibrillator leads utilize the same techniques for permanent pacemaker and ICD implantation discussed elsewhere in this text. However, it is worth noting that left-sided access is preferred both with respect to defibrillation thresholds as well as from a technical perspective as cannulation of the coronary sinus from this angulation is technically less challenging. However, right-sided devices can be implanted. Puncture at the axillary vein is preferred over the cephalic approach given its greater diameter and ability to accommodate a coronary sinus sheath to guide placement of the LV lead. Alternatively, the atrial and ventricular leads may be placed via the cephalic while the axillary or subclavian is then used to accommodate the coronary sinus sheath and the LV lead.

Generally, the RV lead is placed first in order to provide backup ventricular pacing if necessary. This is especially important in this population of patients with cardiomyopathy often with left bundle branch block who may have catheter-induced AV nodal block during the procedure. The right atrial lead is placed next prior to turning attention to the left ventricular lead. However, any lead order can be used depending on operator preference. Transvenous placement of the LV lead is the most commonly used approach and is successful in 80% to 90% of cases.

Left Ventricular Lead Location

The location of the LV coronary venous lead is an important determinant of response to CRT and is also important in minimizing complications. In the majority of patients with cardiomyopathy and left bundle branch block, it is the posterior free wall that is electrically and mechanically activated latest and thus should benefit from earlier activation via LV lead stimulation. In a substudy of the PATH-CHF-II trial, 30 patients underwent biventricular pacing both at a free wall stimulation site and at an anterior wall stimulation site. Acute changes in hemodynamics as measured by dP/dT and aortic pulse pressure changes. Among these patients, improved hemodynamic performance was observed for all patients at the LV free wall stimulation site. In the majority of patients, hemodynamics improved with the anterior site as well; however, in 37% of patients, the opposite response was observed for anterior wall placement.[45] These observations appear to extend to clinical outcomes as well. In a study of 233 consecutive patients who underwent LV lead implantation followed for 6 months, those with lateral and posterolateral lead locations had significant improvements in EF and functional capacity compared to those with anterior lead locations whose EF did not improve significantly.[46] However, while placement of the LV lead in the lateral wall seems to generate improved response to CRT, in many patients this does not tell the whole story. Even in patients with left bundle branch block and cardiomyopathy, from patient to patient there is a heterogeneous pattern of LV activation as demonstrated by TDI and noncontact LV mapping.[47,48]

In a recent subanalysis of the MADIT-CRT trial, the location of the LV lead was determined using coronary sinus venograms and chest x-rays in 799 patients and then classified along the short and long axis of the heart. The benefit of CRT was similar in patients with leads in the anterior, lateral, and posterior positions, whereas those with an apical location had an increased risk of heart failure and death compared to those with a midventricular or basal position.[49] The relationship of lead location in relation to LV scar and viability has also yet to be completely understood.[50,51] In the future, optimizing for nonresponders in CRT will at least in part likely rely on optimizing LV lead location to individual patient characteristics.

Coronary Venous Anatomy

The coronary sinus and its branches provide the epicardial venous access for LV lead implantation and thus is the major determinant of LV lead location. Conventional descriptions of venous anatomy focus on the anatomic path of the major coronary veins as they join the coronary sinus. While important, this description presents several problems for the implanter of an LV lead. First, there is a large amount of variability in the presence, size, angle of takeoff, and the course of first and second order tributaries off of the coronary sinus.[52] Second, conventional description of the venous anatomy does not focus on a vein's location in relation to the underlying myocardium, which is important in successful CRT. Thus, a complementary descriptive system that uses a segmental approach to describe the location of veins and tributaries is useful to aid in the identification of a suitable vein for LV lead placement. In this segmental approach, the vertical (longitudinal) axis of the heart is divided into three equal segments: basal, mid, and apical. The horizontal (short) axis is divided into anterior, lateral, and posterior segments making a 3 × 3 grid. Using these two descriptive approaches (segmental and conventional) in a complementary fashion, one can describe the location of a particular coronary venous branch both in terms of its relationship to other veins as well as with regard to its location and course over the myocardium. This information gives the implanter the necessary data to access the vein as well as whether it is in a suitable location for CRT (Figure 54.3).

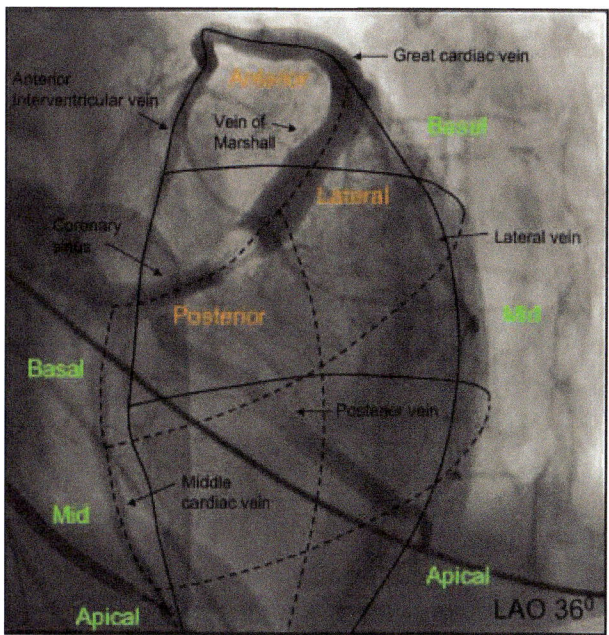

Figure 54.3 Balloon occlusive coronary venous angiogram in the left anterior oblique projection demonstrating the segmental approach to venous anatomy description. The vertical (longitudinal) axis of the heart is divided into three equal segments: basal, mid, and apical. The horizontal (short) axis is divided into anterior, lateral, and posterior segments, making a 3 × 3 grid. *Source:* Blendea D, Mansour M, Shah RV, et al. Usefulness of high-speed rotational coronary venous angiography during cardiac resynchronization therapy. *Am J Cardiol.* 2007;100(10):1561-1565. With permission from Elsevier.

The CS ostium opens into the posterior right atrium near the septum. The ostium is quite variable in its diameter from patient to patient, and factors such as the presence or absence of coronary artery disease can affect this.[52] At the ostium lies the Thebesian valve, which is present in some form in about 85% of patients. The morphology is variable. It can be a small crescentic valve at the inferior aspect of the ostium or may essentially cover the ostium completely as a membrane with fenestrations, and in turn can represent a technical barrier to cannulation (Figure 54.4).[53] In addition to a spectrum of normal anatomy, the CS ostium undergoes changes in patients who have a dilated cardiomyopathy with right atrial enlargement in which the CS ostium is angled more inferiorly and the sinus itself runs in a more vertical plane.

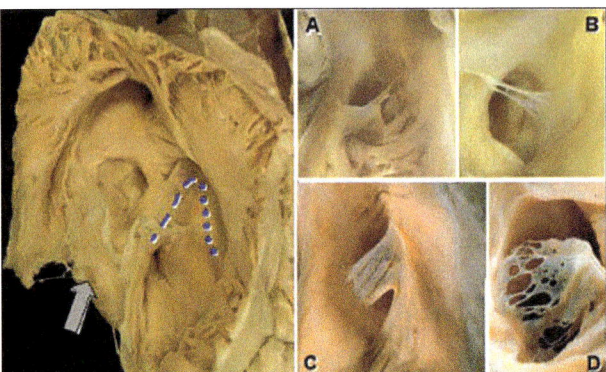

Figure 54.4 Thebesian valve and its variants. The main panel shows the Thebesian valve bordered inferiorly and posteriorly by the eustachian ridge. The orifice of the inferior caval vein (**arrow**) in this heart is guarded by a Chiari network that extends over the orifice of the coronary sinus. The small panels show examples of variations in morphology of the Thebesian valve: (**A**) crescent with fenestrations, (**B**) fine strand, (**C**) broad fibrous band, and (**D**) fenestrated valve almost covering the os. *Source:* Used with permission, Ho SY, Sánchez-Quintana D, Becker AE. A review of the coronary venous system: a road less travelled. *Heart Rhythm.* 2004;1(1):Figure 2, page 108. With permission from Elsevier.

The coronary sinus is approximately 4 to 7 cm long, runs in the AV groove, and is contiguous with the great cardiac vein, which completes the AV venous ring along the mitral annulus. The vein of Marshall or its remnant marks this transition from coronary sinus to great cardiac vein; in the absence of this vessel, Vieussen's valve marks this transition. This valve is present in 80% to 90% of hearts and in some cases may represent a barrier to access beyond the coronary sinus. The wall of the sinus is lined by a layer of atrial myocardium, or myocardial sleeve, which usually does not extend to the coronary sinus tributaries but may extend a few millimeters into the great cardiac vein.

Using the segmental classification, the area of LV epicardium is bordered posteriorly by middle cardiac vein, which runs posteriorly along the ventricular septum. The middle cardiac vein most often originates as a branch of the coronary sinus, but occasionally can have a separate ostium from the right atrium and extends to the apex. The anterior border is marked by the anterior interventricular vein, which runs along the anterior interventricular sulcus from the apex to the base and runs into the great cardiac vein. The basal border is comprised of the coronary sinus and the great cardiac vein as they run in the AV groove. These borders are fairly constant features, being present in more than 90% of hearts.[54]

The posterior cardiac vein arises usually distal to the middle cardiac vein, or the two may share a common ostium. Tributaries of this vein course from apex to base along the lateral wall of the LV. Near the apex of the heart, the small branches form tributaries with the small branches of the anterior interventricular venous system. Thus the lateral wall of the LV can sometimes be accessed via the branches of the posterior vein or via the branches of the anterior interventricular vein, which is important if access to the lateral veins is technically difficult. There are variable numbers of lateral cardiac veins with the posterolateral vein usually the largest; these represent the most frequent target for implantation of the LV lead. The posterolateral vein joins the main portion of the AV venous ring at the junction of the coronary sinus and the great cardiac vein (at the site of Vieussen's valve and the vein of Marshall). Using the segmental description, lateral veins can be described as anterior, lateral, or posterior. Segments coursing over the lateral wall give tributaries that course anteriorly and posteriorly, while segments that originate more anteriorly or posteriorly have tributaries that course medially or laterally.

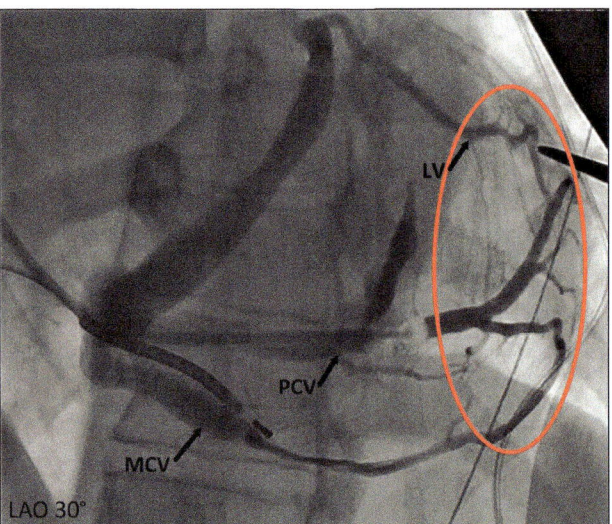

Figure 54.5 Coronary venous angiogram performed with balloon occlusion in the posterior cardiac vein. In this patient the middle cardiac vein (MCV), the posterior cardiac vein (PCV), and a lateral vein all anastamose over a segment of the mid- and apical-lateral wall (**circled in red**).

Summary

Using a combination of conventional venous anatomic descriptions and the segmental approach, a strategy for lead placement can be developed at the time of implantation that incorporates both the approach for the LV lead and its ultimate location. For instance, the lateral wall might be most directly reached in the main body or first order tributary of a lateral vein; however, technical considerations such as angle of takeoff or tortuosity make this approach difficult, and the same segmental area could be reached by advancing the lead to a distal tributary of a lateral branch of the anterior interventricular vein or the middle cardiac vein.

Left Ventricular Lead Implantation

Coronary Sinus Access

The first step in LV lead placement is location and cannulation of the CS ostium. Most operators take advantage of specially designed coronary sinus sheaths in order to access the ostium from the superior approach. There are a wide range of designs; however, most of these systems incorporate a long sheath with varying degrees of a J-shaped curve that when advanced into the right ventricle and pulled back with the dilator removed, assumes a configuration in which the tip of the catheter points posteriorly and superiorly. Given the generally inferior pointing CS ostium in the dilated right atrium and more vertical axis of the myopathic heart, this design may allow for direct cannulation of the coronary sinus. Fluoroscopic landmarks such as RCA calcification and radiographic lucency of fat running along the AV groove can assist in locating the ostium. Despite the wide range of shapes of these guides, frequently it is impossible to directly cannulate the ostium with the CS guide alone.

In these cases, a 0.035-inch guidewire advanced through the sheath tracking along the right atrial floor to point upwards or advanced into the right ventricle and pulled back can be used to enter the ostium after which the guide can be advanced over the wire. A deflectable or standard electrode catheter placed within the guide can be used for cannulation as well. Inner catheters have various shapes, which may be useful depending on the specific ranging from extending reach to angled upward or downward angulation. Conventional diagnostic catheters such as a multipurpose or LIMA catheter can be used effectively as well (Figure 54.6).

If the ostium is unable to be localized using these techniques, a contrast injection of the right atrium can sometimes demonstrate negative contrast in the area of the CS ostium. In more difficult cases, intracardiac ultrasound can be used to localize the CS ostium. Cannulation of the coronary sinus, once achieved, is suggested by the absence of PVCs, a characteristic rocking motion of the catheter, the path of the catheter crossing the spine in the LAO view, or more definitively by a contrast injection. Once cannulated, the sheath should be advanced to the mid body of the coronary sinus over a wire or electrode catheter. The sheath should never be advanced without a J-wire or electrode catheter in order to avoid coronary sinus dissection (see following). When resistance is encountered, the sheath should not be forced forward, as this will often result in either a coronary sinus dissection or the dislodgement of the guide from the coronary sinus as a redundant loop begins to form against the floor of the right atrium. Gentle clockwise or counterclockwise torque is sometimes required to align the guide with the trajectory of the sinus in order to advance it; more than one radiographic view (LAO and RAO) may be necessary. If resistance continues to be encountered, a contrast puff may elucidate a mechanical problem such as a curve at the junction of the great cardiac vein or a valve.

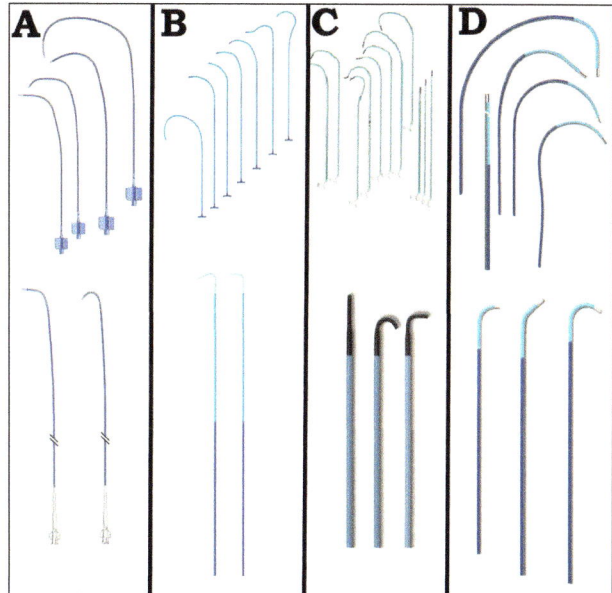

Figure 54.6 A sample of commercially available coronary sinus guiding catheters and subselection catheters. **Panel A:** Coronary sinus guide catheters and RAPIDO 6-Fr CS-IC 90 and CS-IC 50C subselection catheters. *Source:* Reproduced with permission of Boston Scientific Corporation. **Panel B:** ScoutPro 7-Fr Introducer System coronary sinus guide catheters and ScoutPro IC subselection catheters. *Source:* Reproduced with permission of Biotronik SE & Co. AG. **Panel C:** Attain Command coronary sinus guide catheters and Attain subselection catheters. *Source:* Reproduced with permission of Medtronic, Inc. **Panel D:** CPS Direct SL coronary sinus guide catheters and Aim SL subselection catheters. *Source:* Reproduced with permission of St. Jude Medical.

Coronary Venous Angiography

Defining the anatomy in this way provides a roadmap for lead placement and elucidates many technical challenges such as small venous diameters, sharp branch takeoff angles, valves, and tortuousities. Furthermore, it allows for the selection of an appropriately sized lead and, if necessary, a secondary catheter to further facilitate lead placement. Assessment of anatomy preprocedurally can be accomplished using cardiac computed tomography, magnetic resonance imaging, or real-time 3D echocardiography. These methods may give additional information relating venous anatomy to myocardial segmental function and scar. However, despite these possibilities, retrograde balloon occlusive angiography remains the standard method used intraprocedurally and will remain necessary to help guide lead placement.

Injections of contrast in the coronary venous system from the coronary sinus are against the direction of blood flow. Therefore, to avoid immediate washout of contrast, a balloon catheter is used to simultaneously occlude the sinus and inject contrast. Care must be taken to correctly size the balloon as underinflation leads to poorly visualized distal branches and overinflation can lead to dissection of the vessel. Furthermore, catheter stability is important in order to avoid to-and-fro motion, which can cause vessel dissection (see ▶ Video 54.1). In certain cases, advancing the balloon distally can secure more complete occlusion in patients with a dilated coronary sinus at the expense of excluding some branches from the venogram. Prior to performing the balloon occlusive angiography, a pre-angio "puff" should be performed with balloon down in order to be certain that there is no side branch occlusion when the balloon is inflated (see Video 54.1). Occasionally, venograms at various levels within the coronary sinus may need to be performed to be certain that all branches are visualized. Subselective angiograms may also be useful to better visualize more distal anatomy (Figure 54.5). Just as in coronary arteriography, it may be necessary to visualize the venous system in multiple angulations to define the path of potential target vessels. Usually, standard LAO and RAO orthogonal views with cranial and caudal angulations as necessary are required to minimize foreshortening and vessel overlap. However, it is worth noting that the optimal angulation to identify target vessels varies widely from patient to patient and multiple views or rotational angiography (see below) may be necessary (Figure 54.7). Longer cine images allow for delineation of initially unvisualized veins via collateral flow. Careful attention must be paid during injection to holding the balloon catheter in position, as backward motion of the inflated balloon results in suboptimal filling of the venous tree, may cause trauma to the vessel, and may result in the dislodgement of the guide catheter from the coronary sinus (see ▶ Video 54.2).

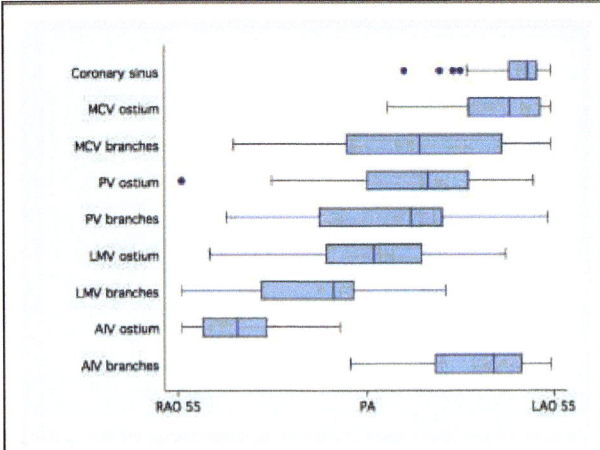

Figure 54.7 Horizontal box plot depicting the distribution among patients of the best angiographic views for the different segments of the coronary venous system. AIV = anterior interventricular vein; LAO = left anterior oblique; LMV = left marginal vein; MCV = middle cardiac vein; PA = posteroanterior; PV = posterior vein; RAO = right anterior oblique. *Source:* Used with permission from Blendea D, Mansour M, Shah RV, et al. Usefulness of high-speed rotational coronary venous angiography during cardiac resynchronization therapy. *Am J Cardiol.* 2007;100(10): Figure 4, page 1562. With permission from Elsevier.

Alternative methods for performing intraprocedural venography have been described. High-speed rotational coronary venous angiography (RCVA) acquires images over a 110-degree arc: from LAO 55 degrees to RAO 55 degrees in 4 seconds, at a rate of 30 frames per second (see ▶ Video 54.3). In a study of 49 patients comparing static angiography to RCVA, RCVA better classified the angle of takeoff of target branches, allowed for more frequent selection of the target branch after the first injections, and better defined second order tributaries with diameters suitable for lead implantation (see Video 54.3).[55] Whichever method is used, the goal is to obtain a roadmap to be used throughout the rest of the procedure for lead implantation.

Lead Placement and Tackling Tortuous Vessels and Stenoses

Once a suitable target vein is selected, an appropriate LV lead should be selected. Over-the-wire leads are now standard and allow for navigation of the venous system with guidewires followed by advancement of the lead to the target vein. For the most part, commercially available LV leads rely on passive fixation in the target vessel. There is a tradeoff between small-lead diameter allowing for increased maneuverability and inability to achieve fixation within a larger vein. This obstacle has been, in part, addressed by the use of preformed shapes that the lead assumes when the wire is withdrawn to improve stability. Leads that incorporate active fixation mechanisms are also currently available for cases in which suitable stability cannot be achieved in the desired location; however, lead removal, should this be necessary, might prove difficult with these leads (Figure 54.8).

Once the target vein and lead are selected, the over the wire lead is loaded onto a 0.014-inch interventional wire. Acute or complex angled takeoffs of target veins or tortuosity in the mid segments of the vessel are frequently encountered in the posterior and lateral veins and can make navigating the wire through the vein difficult. It is helpful to advance the CS guide as close to the takeoff as possible to provide support for the wire and to guide the wire tip. The lead itself can be torqued to guide the tip of the wire into the target vessel. The wire should then be advanced as far down the target vein as possible to provide adequate purchase for advancing the lead. A working knowledge of the properties of various interventional wires is useful and an implanter should become familiar with a variety of wires with different properties. Different wire constructions provide varying degrees of flexibility, tracking, steerability, lubricity, and support, which may be required for a given clinical situation. These properties often come at the expense of one another. For instance, a wire with a tapered core that provides increased tracking may allow for easy navigation into an acutely angled takeoff; however, this comes at the expense of support, which may result in prolapse of the wire once the tip enters the vessel. A stiff wire advanced as far as possible into the target vein can sometimes straighten the takeoff or

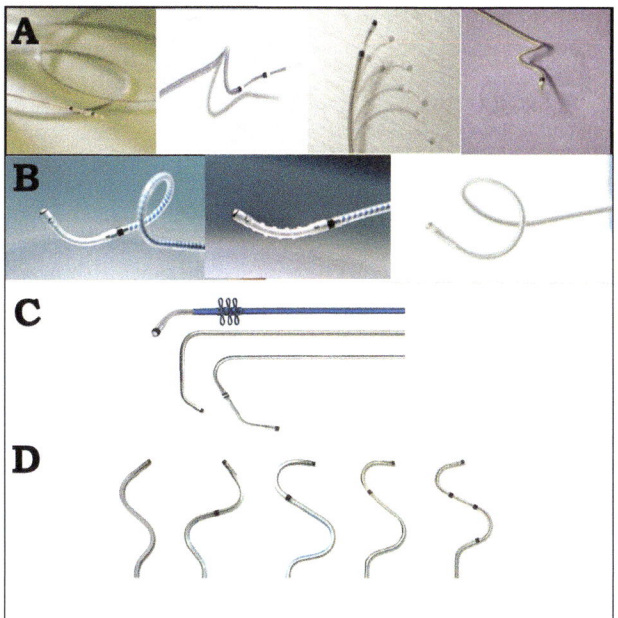

Figure 54.8 A sample of commercially available LV leads with various passive and active fixation mechanisms. **Panel A:** Easytrak and ACUITY LV leads. *Source:* Reproduced with permission of Boston Scientific Corporation. **Panel B:** Corox OTW LV leads. *Source:* Reproduced with permission of Biotronik SE & Co. AG. **Panel C:** Attain left heart LV leads. *Source:* Reproduced with permission of Medtronic, Inc. **Panel D:** Quicksite and Quickflex LV leads. *Source:* Reproduced with permission of St. Jude Medical.

tortuous segment sufficiently to allow for advancement of the lead over this wire.

The telescoping catheter technique can be used to provide enough support for lead placement in a difficult takeoff or to straighten a tortuous segment if the guidewire alone is not enough. In this technique, an appropriately shaped catheter is advanced through the CS guide to cannulate the segmental vein. The subselection catheter should be chosen based on the shape of the angled takeoff (Figure 54.6). If the technique is used to straighten a tortuous mid-segment of a vessel, a straight catheter may be useful. It may be necessary to use a larger diameter wire to advance the subselection catheter such as a standard 0.035-inch guidewire. Once the tip of the catheter enters the segmental vein, this wire can be advanced. Systems designed for this telescoping catheter technique are commercially available incorporating a peel-away sheath with a prefitted cutting system for the inner catheter to aid in removal once the LV lead is in place; some even have a deflectable tipped inner catheter (Figure 54.6).

Advancing the lead over the wire when resistance is encountered should be avoided, as this may result in trauma to the vessel or loss of coronary sinus access as the more proximal portion of the lead forms a redundant loop in the right atrium. In cases in which a wire can be placed, but the catheter not advanced due to tortuosity, the buddy wire technique can be used. In this technique, a stiff wire is placed as far as possible in the target vessel to straighten the segment. A second wire is then placed and the lead advanced over this second wire while the first wire remains in place to straighten the vessel. The first wire is then removed once the lead is advanced (Figure 54.9). This technique may also be used to maintain access to the coronary sinus when the target vessel is close to the ostium. This is often the case if the posterior cardiac vein is the target (which can sometimes share a common ostium with the middle cardiac vein, see Figure 54.9). In this case, the first wire is inserted far into the coronary sinus and great cardiac vein. The guide is then pulled back proximally until it is close to the ostium while being supported by the first wire so as not to lose coronary sinus access. A second wire is then placed into the target vessel and the lead advanced.

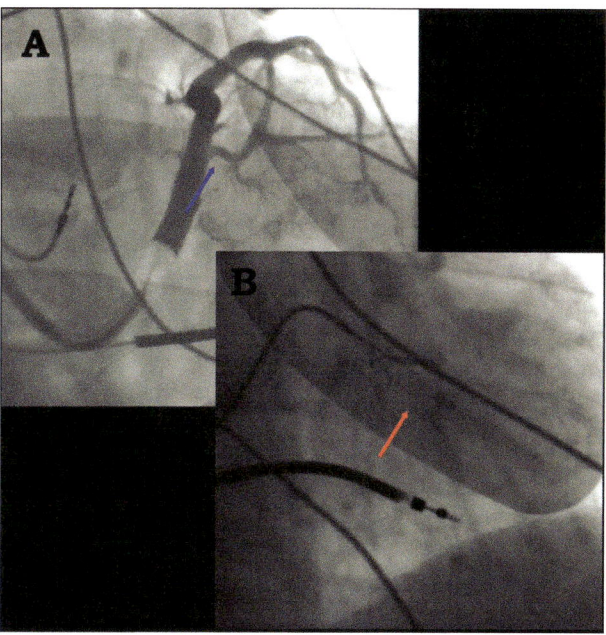

Figure 54.9 The buddy wire technique. **Panel A** shows an balloon occlusive retrograde venogram revealing a tortuous takeoff of a target lateral vein (**blue arrow**) into which it would be difficult to advance a lead. **Panel B** shows the vein with a balanced middle-weight wire used as a "buddy wire" to straighten the segment, which allowed passage of another guidewire (**red arrow**) over which a lead could be advanced.

Some operators have begun using interventional techniques to overcome obstacles in LV lead placement. Venous strictures and stenosis may be present from prior surgery posing a barrier to lead implantation. Balloon angioplasty in experienced hands can be employed to overcome this. Angioplasty has also been used to dilate small collateral veins to increase diameter enough to allow advancement of a lead to a desired location through collateral networks (ie, via the anterior interventricular vein). Stents have been used to straighten tortuous segments and have also been used as a lead fixation method in a larger caliber vein. Table 54.1 outlines some technical challenges to CS lead placement along with the strategies, outlined previously, that can be used to overcome them.

Table 54.1 Challenges and strategies for CS lead placement

Challenges	Strategy
Inadequate visualization of the coronary venous tree	• Subselective venous angiography
	• Rotational angiography
Difficult angle of takeoff in a target branch	• Advance CS guide close to the angle of takeoff
	• Subselection sheaths
Tortuous CS or venous branch	• Use of a straight subselection catheter
	• Use of a stiff wire to straighten the vessel
	• Buddy wire technique
Target vessel takeoff is close to the CS ostium	• Use of the buddy wire technique to maintain access to the coronary sinus as the CS guide is withdrawn
Venous strictures or stenosis	• Balloon venous angioplasty
Phrenic nerve stimulation	• Reposition in a different tributary
	• Explore various pacing configurations

CS = coronary sinus

Complications of LV Lead Placement

CRT device implantation using transvenous LV lead implantation has a high success rate and a complication rate that is generally comparable to that of other devices in similar sets of patients. In major trials of CRT, implant success was achieved between 87% to 95% of the time. In a systematic review of randomized clinical trials, the 30-day mortality for transvenous CRT systems was 0.7%, the rate of pneumothorax was 0.9%. There was coronary vein dissection, perforation, or tamponade in 2% of patients, with tamponade occurring in 0.4%. Bleeding or hematoma at the site occurred in 2.4% of patients.[56,57] The recognition and management of complications related to venous access and right atrial and right ventricular lead complications are discussed elsewhere in this text.

Phrenic Nerve Stimulation

The phrenic nerve runs along the lateral epicardial surface in most patients. Stimulation of the phrenic nerve by the LV lead can be recognized during the procedure with diaphragmatic contraction; however, it may not be recognized until the patient sits upright after the procedure is complete. If the stimulation is noticed during the procedure, the most reliable way to address this is with repositioning of the LV lead within the target vein. A secondary venogram may be useful to identify tertiary branches that may support the LV lead and were not seen during the primary venogram that will orient the lead in a different direction. Repositioning within the same branch may require a larger or smaller caliber lead to achieve fixation.

If the lead cannot be repositioned due to technical considerations, or if the phrenic nerve stimulation is recognized post procedurally, changes in device programming can sometimes overcome this issue. When there is a significant difference in phrenic nerve stimulation threshold and LV capture, the device can be programmed to avoid stimulation. This can sometimes be achieved by using a wider pulse width allowing for lower voltage stimulation of the LV. When multielectrode leads are used, electronic repositioning of the pacing vector or pacing site can sometimes overcome phrenic nerve stimulation as well. The advent of quadripolar leads greatly increased the versatility of electronic repositioning and reduced the need for adjusting lead location.

High Left Ventricular Pacing Thresholds

When stimulations thresholds are unacceptably high or LV capture cannot be achieved at all in the target vein, repositioning the lead in the manner described previously can sometimes overcome the problem. Often an alternative target vein selection is necessary. In this situation, further imaging to localize scar (which is the most common cause of high LV thresholds) may be useful. However, if there is no target vessel in the desirable area of myocardium, an alternative method of LV lead implantation may be necessary (see following).

Left Ventricular Lead Dislodgment

Causes of lead dislodgement include target vein-lead size mismatch, proximal position of the LV lead, or excessive slack in the LV lead. Dislodgement often occurs intraprocedurally even without these factors upon removal of the CS guide from the CS ostium. As the guide exits the ostium, it may fall to the right atrium floor, thereby pulling the lead out of position. Guidewire support should be maintained as the lead is pulled out of the ostium. Fluoroscopy should be used continuously as the guide is pulled back, and the operator must simultaneously watch the exiting guide and the distal LV lead tip during this process.

If the dislodgement occurs postprocedurally, it may sometimes be detected by a change in QRS morphology on a surface ECG, but is more often detected on routine device interrogation. Reattempt at LV lead positioning either in a small target vessel or with a larger diameter lead can solve this issue. However, in circumstances in which lead stability cannot be achieved in this manner, active fixation leads can be used, though as mentioned previously, lead removable, should this prove necessary, might be difficult. Also, a coronary stent in experienced hands can be used to fixate a lead to the vessel wall; however, this would make lead removal virtually impossible and may result in lead fracture. This should be reserved for refractory cases or patients on a transplant list. If stable lead positioning cannot be achieved, alternative methods for LV lead implantation should be considered.

Dissection and Perforation of the Coronary Sinus or Target Vessel

Dissection of the coronary sinus may occur during catheter cannulation or advancement, guidewire manipulation, or during retrograde balloon angiography and is detectable by the presence of contrast staining within the sinus (Figure 54.10). While dissection occurs commonly, it only rarely has serious consequences due to containment by the pericardium and the low pressure of the venous system. If the flap occludes the CS ostium or the true lumen cannot be determined, the procedure should be aborted and reattempted in 2 to 3 months, after which the majority of these dissections will have healed. However, if the true lumen can be found by probing gently with a floppy-tipped, 0.035-inch guidewire, then the sinus can be reengaged with a guide. In these circumstances venography can be performed though the guide, but retrograde balloon angiography should be avoided due to the risk of extending the dissection. Target vein dissection may occur due to guidewire or lead manipulation and may cause distal thrombosis, making it impossible to place the lead in the desired target vein. However, dissection itself should not necessarily cause the procedure to be aborted.

Venous perforation may also occur and is a more serious complication than dissection. It can be identified by contrast extravasation or by the free extravascular movement of the guidewire. Venous pressure is low and external compression by the resultant pericardial hematoma frequently tamponades the bleed making it self-limited. However, despite the slow nature of the bleed, cardiac tamponade may result, requiring pericardial drainage and sometimes surgical repair of the perforation.

Alternatives to Transvenous Left Ventricular Lead Placement

In large trials, successful transvenous lead implantation has been achieved in 87% to 95% of attempts. However, in real-world clinical circumstances, these numbers may be considerably lower. This is usually due to the limitations noted previously (difficult anatomy, target vein location, lead stability, LV thresholds, complications, or operator experience). In these cases, given the potential benefit of CRT, alternative methods of LV lead placement should be sought. Most commonly this involves the placement of a surgical epicardial lead either via a limited thoracotomy or video-assisted procedure. Just as in transvenous placement, in epicardial placement, lead location is an important determinant of outcome and should be carefully planned preprocedurally.

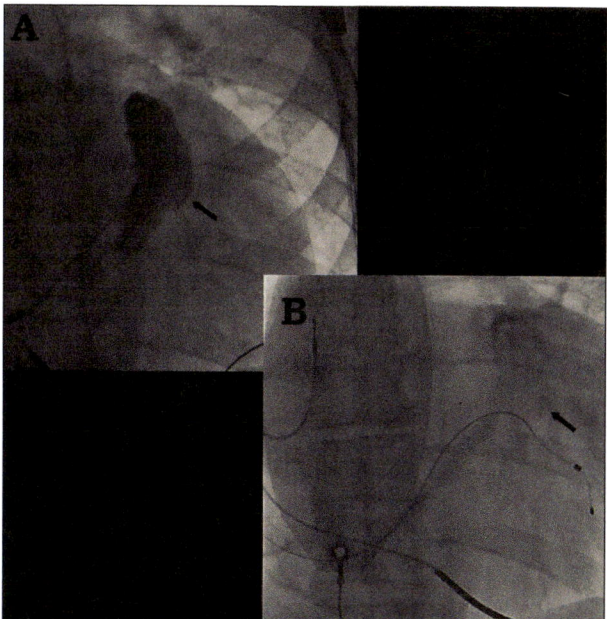

Figure 54.10 **Panel A:** A balloon occlusive retrograde venous angiogram revealing a coronary sinus dissection. Note the contrast staining of the coronary sinus (**arrow**). **Panel B:** The final position of a lead placed via the true lumen after the dissection. Note the persistent faint contrast staining (**arrow**).

Transseptal endocardial placement via the left atrium and through the mitral valve has been described.[58-60] Given the potential for thromboembolism, warfarin anticoagulation is used, and small studies show comparable outcomes to venous lead placement. However, this technique has not gained widespread use.

Summary

Cardiac resynchronization therapy improves quality of life, decreases heart failure hospitalizations, and improves mortality in an expanding subset of patients with CHF and left ventricular dysfunction by improving the mechanical function of the heart, reducing arrhythmia, and promoting electrical and mechanical remodeling. Factors that influence response to therapy include appropriate patient selection and successful placement and location of an LV lead. Transvenous placement of the LV lead can be achieved safely with few complications in the majority of patients who qualify for CRT. The procedure requires knowledge of the coronary venous anatomy and a unique subset of skills to cannulate the coronary sinus from the superior approach, navigate the venous system, and overcome anatomical barriers such as tortuosity.

In the remaining patients for whom LV lead placement cannot be achieved transvenously, surgical options exist and should be pursued. Retrospective studies comparing the outcome of those patients who underwent surgical epicardial LV lead placement to those who underwent coronary sinus lead placement have revealed that while surgical lead placement carries a higher up-front risk of complication, including renal failure, long-term survival was similar as was the rate of response to CRT. Thus, pursuing epicardial LV lead placement is a reasonable strategy in those for whom a coronary sinus lead cannot be placed.[61,62] Some authors have advocated for routine placement of biventricular devices in "hybrid suites" in which, after an attempt at coronary sinus lead placement fails, the epicardial lead can be placed during the same procedure, obviating the need for a staged procedure in which the pocket needs to be re-opened and the patient exposed to further risk of anesthesia and infection.[63]

Successful operators have an algorithm for lead implantation but also a willingness to be flexible in individualizing a strategy to each patient. This requires familiarity by the operator with an array of lead designs, guidewires, catheters, and techniques described above that might be useful in an individual clinical scenario.

References

1. McCullough PA, Philbin EF, Spertus JA, Kaatz S, Sandberg KR, Weaver WD. Confirmation of a heart failure epidemic: findings from the Resource Utilization Among Congestive Heart Failure (REACH) study. *J Am Coll Cardiol*. 2002;39(1):60-69.
2. Roger VL, Weston SA, Redfield MM, et al. Trends in heart failure incidence and survival in a community-based population. *JAMA*. 2004;292(3):344-350.
3. Hunt SA, Abraham WT, Chin MH, et al. ACC/AHA 2005 Guideline Update for the Diagnosis and Management of Chronic Heart Failure in the Adult: A Report of the American College of Cardiology/American Heart Association Task Force on Practice Guidelines (Writing Committee to Update the 2001 Guidelines for the Evaluation and Management of Heart Failure): Developed in Collaboration With the American College of Chest Physicians and the International Society for Heart and Lung Transplantation: Endorsed by the Heart Rhythm Society. *Circulation*. 2005;112(12):e154-235.
4. Connell JBO. The economic burden of heart failure. *Clinical Cardiology*. 2000;23(S3):III6-III10.
5. Leclercq C, Kass DA. Retiming the failing heart: principles and current clinical status of cardiac resynchronization. *J Am Coll Cardiol*. 2002;39(2):194-201.
6. Solis J, McCarty D, Levine RA, et al. Mechanism of decrease in mitral regurgitation after cardiac resynchronization therapy: optimization of the force-balance relationship. *Circ Cardiovasc Imaging*. 2009;2(6):444-450.
7. St John Sutton MG, Plappert T, Abraham WT, et al. Effect of cardiac resynchronization therapy on left ventricular size and function in chronic heart failure. *Circulation*. 2003;107(15):1985-1990.
8. Thijssen J, Borleffs CJ, Delgado V, et al. Implantable cardioverter-defibrillator patients who are upgraded and respond to cardiac resynchronization therapy have less ventricular arrhythmias compared with nonresponders. *J Am Coll Cardiol*. 2011;58(22):2282-2289.
9. Goldenberg I, Hall WJ, Beck CA, et al. Reduction of the risk of recurring heart failure events with cardiac resynchronization therapy: MADIT-CRT (Multicenter Automatic Defibrillator Implantation Trial With Cardiac Resynchronization Therapy). *J Am Coll Cardiol*. 2011;58(7):729-737.
10. Cazeau S, Ritter P, Bakdach S, et al. Four chamber pacing in dilated cardiomyopathy. *Pacing Clin Electrophysiol*. 1994;17(11):1974-1979.
11. Cazeau S, Ritter P, Lazarus A, et al. Multisite pacing for end-stage heart failure: early experience. *Pacing Clin Electrophysiol*. 1996;19(11):1748-1757.
12. Kass DA, Chen C-H, Curry C, et al. Improved Left ventricular mechanics from acute VDD pacing in patients with dilated cardiomyopathy and ventricular conduction delay. *Circulation*. 1999;99(12):1567-1573.
13. Moss AJ, Hall WJ, Cannom DS, et al. Cardiac-resynchronization therapy for the prevention of heart-failure events. *N Engl J Med*. 2009;361(14):1329-1338.
14. Abraham WT, Fisher WG, Smith AL, et al. Cardiac resynchronization in chronic heart failure. *N Engl J Med*. 2002;346(24):1845-1853.
15. Young JB, Abraham WT, Smith AL, et al. Combined cardiac resynchronization and implantable cardioversion defibrillation in advanced chronic heart failure: The MIRACLE ICD Trial. *JAMA*. 2003;289(20):2685-2694.
16. Bristow MR, Saxon LA, Boehmer J, et al. Cardiac-resynchronization therapy with or without an implantable defibrillator in advanced chronic heart failure. *N Engl J Med*. 2004;350(21):2140-2150.
17. Lozano I, Bocchiardo M, Achtelik M, et al. Impact of biventricular pacing on mortality in a randomized crossover study of patients with heart failure and ventricular arrhythmias. *Pacing Clin Electrophysiol*. 2000;23(11 Part 2):1711-1712.
18. Cleland JGF, Daubert J-C, Erdmann E, et al. The effect of cardiac resynchronization on morbidity and mortality in heart failure. *N Engl J Med*. 2005;352(15):1539-1549.
19. Cazeau S, Leclercq C, Lavergne T, et al. Effects of multisite biventricular pacing in patients with heart failure and intraventricular conduction delay. *N Engl J Med*. 2001;344(12):873-880.
20. Auricchio A, Fantoni C, Regoli F, et al. Characterization of left ventricular activation in patients with heart failure and left bundle-branch block. *Circulation*. 2004;109(9):1133-1139.
21. Papageorgiou P, Monahan K, Boyle NG, et al. Site-dependent intra-atrial conduction delay. Relationship to initiation of atrial fibrillation. *Circulation*. 1996;94(3):384-389.
22. Healey JS, Connolly SJ, Gold MR, et al. Subclinical atrial fibrillation and the risk of stroke. *N Engl J Med*. 2012;366(2):120-129.
23. Bailin SJ, Adler S, Giudici M. Prevention of chronic atrial fibrillation by pacing in the region of Bachmann's bundle: results of a multicenter randomized trial. *J Cardiovasc Electrophysiol*. 2001;12(8):912-917.
24. Saksena S, Prakash A, Ziegler P, et al. Improved suppression of recurrent atrial fibrillation with dual-site right atrial pacing and antiarrhythmic drug therapy. *J Am Coll Cardiol*. 2002;40(6):1140-1150; discussion 1151-1142.
25. Burri H, Bennani I, Domenichini G, et al. Biatrial pacing improves atrial haemodynamics and atrioventricular timing compared with pacing from the right atrial appendage. *Europace*. 2011;13(9):1262-1267.
26. Matsumoto K, Ishikawa T, Sumita S, et al. Beneficial effects of biatrial pacing on cardiac function in patients with bradycardia-tachycardia syndrome. *Circ J*. 2005;69(7):831-836.
27. Saksena S, Prakash A, Hill M, et al. Prevention of recurrent atrial fibrillation with chronic dual-site right atrial pacing. *J Am Coll Cardiol*. 1996;28(3):687-694.
28. Prakash A, Saksena S, Ziegler PD, et al. Dual site right atrial pacing can improve the impact of standard dual chamber pacing on atrial and ventricular mechanical function in patients with symptomatic atrial fibrillation: further observations from the

dual site atrial pacing for prevention of atrial fibrillation trial. *J Interv Card Electrophysiol.* 2005;12(3):177-187.
29. Hermida JS, Kubala M, Lescure FX, et al. Atrial septal pacing to prevent atrial fibrillation in patients with sinus node dysfunction: results of a randomized controlled study. *Am Heart J.* 2004;148(2):312-317.
30. Brecker SJD, Xiao HB, Sparrow J, Gibson DG. Effects of dual-chamber pacing with short atrioventricular delay in dilated cardiomyopathy. *The Lancet.* 1992;340(8831):1308-1312.
31. Nishimura RA, Hayes DL, Holmes DR, Tajik J. Mechanism of hemodynamic improvement by dual-chamber pacing for severe left ventricular dysfunction: An acute Doppler and catheterization hemodynamic study. *J Am Coll Cardiol.* 1995;25(2):281-288.
32. Wang NC, Maggioni AP, Konstam MA, et al. Clinical implications of QRS duration in patients hospitalized with worsening heart failure and reduced left ventricular ejection fraction. *JAMA.* 2008;299(22):2656-2666.
33. Moss AJ, Zareba W, Hall WJ, et al. Prophylactic implantation of a defibrillator in patients with myocardial infarction and reduced ejection fraction. *N Engl J Med.* 2002;346(12):877-883.
34. Chung ES, Leon AR, Tavazzi L, et al. Results of the Predictors of Response to CRT (PROSPECT) Trial. *Circulation.* 2008;117(20):2608-2616.
35. Unverferth DV, Magorien RD, Moeschberger ML, Baker PB, Fetters JK, Leier CV. Factors influencing the one-year mortality of dilated cardiomyopathy. *Am J Cardiol.* 1984;54(1):147-152.
36. Gabe BB, Martin JS, Sander GM, et al. Relationship between QRS duration and left ventricular dyssynchrony in patients with end-stage heart failure. *J Cardiovasc Electrophysiol.* 2004;15(5):544-549.
37. Bax JJ, Abraham T, Barold SS, et al. Cardiac resynchronization therapy: part 1—issues before device implantation. *J Am Coll Cardiol.* 2005;46(12):2153-2167.
38. Delgado V, Ypenburg C, van Bommel RJ, et al. Assessment of left ventricular dyssynchrony by speckle tracking strain imaging: comparison between longitudinal, circumferential, and radial strain in cardiac resynchronization therapy. *J Am Coll Cardiol.* 2008;51(20):1944-1952.
39. Beshai JF, Grimm RA, Nagueh SF, et al. Cardiac-resynchronization therapy in heart failure with narrow QRS complexes. *N Engl J Med.* 2007;357(24):2461-2471.
40. Van de Veire NR, Delgado V, Schuijf JD, van der Wall EE, Schalij MJ, Bax JJ. The role of non-invasive imaging in patient selection. *Europace.* 2009;11(suppl 5):v32-v39.
41. Taylor AJ, Elsik M, Broughton A, et al. Combined dyssynchrony and scar imaging with cardiac magnetic resonance imaging predicts clinical response and long-term prognosis following cardiac resynchronization therapy. *Europace.* 2010;12:708-713.
42. Ypenburg C, Westenberg JJ, Bleeker GB, et al. Noninvasive imaging in cardiac resynchronization therapy—part 1: selection of patients. *Pacing Clin Electrophysiol.* 2008;31(11):1475-1499.
43. Sakamoto S, Nitta T, Ishii Y, Miyagi Y, Ohmori H, Shimizu K. Interatrial electrical connections: the precise location and preferential conduction. *J Cardiovasc Electrophysiol.* 2005;16(10):1077-1086.
44. Bailin SJ. Atrial lead implantation in the Bachmann bundle. *Heart Rhythm.* 2005;2(7):784-786.
45. Butter C, Auricchio A, Stellbrink C, et al. Effect of resynchronization therapy stimulation site on the systolic function of heart failure patients. *Circulation.* 2001;104(25):3026-3029.
46. Antonio R, Atul V, Eduardo B S, et al. Impact of coronary sinus lead position on biventricular pacing. *J Cardiovasc Electrophysiol.* 2004;15(10):1120-1125.
47. Maurizio G, Massimo M, Paola G, et al. Is the left ventricular lateral wall the best lead implantation site for cardiac resynchronization therapy? *Pacing Clin Electrophysiol.* 2003;26(1p2):162-168.
48. Fung JWH, Yu CM, Yip G, et al. Variable left ventricular activation pattern in patients with heart failure and left bundle branch block. *Heart.* 2004;90(1):17-19.
49. Singh JP, Klein HU, Huang DT, et al. Left ventricular lead position and clinical outcome in the multicenter automatic defibrillator implantation trial-cardiac resynchronization therapy (MADIT-CRT) trial. *Circulation.* 2011;123(11):1159-1166.
50. Birnie D, deKemp RA, Ruddy TD, et al. Effect of lateral wall scar on reverse remodeling with cardiac resynchronization therapy. *Heart Rhythm.* 2009;6(12):1721-1726.
51. Riedlbauchova L, Brunken R, Jaber WA, et al. The impact of myocardial viability on the clinical outcome of cardiac resynchronization therapy. *J Cardiovasc Electrophysiol.* 2009;20(1):50-57.
52. Blendea D, Shah RV, Auricchio A, et al. Variability of coronary venous anatomy in patients undergoing cardiac resynchronization therapy: A high-speed rotational venography study. *Heart Rhythm.* 2007;4(9):1155-1162.
53. Ho SY, Sánchez-Quintana D, Becker AE. A review of the coronary venous system: a road less travelled. *Heart Rhythm.* 2004;1(1):107-112.
54. Singh JP, Houser S, Heist EK, Ruskin JN. The coronary venous anatomy: a segmental approach to aid cardiac resynchronization therapy. *J Am Coll Cardiol.* 2005;46(1):68-74.
55. Blendea D, Mansour M, Shah RV, et al. Usefulness of high-speed rotational coronary venous angiography during cardiac resynchronization therapy. *Am J Cardiol.* 2007;100(10):1561-1565.
56. NASPE Abstracts. *Pacing Clin Electrophysiol.* 2003;26(4p2):929-1126.
57. van Rees JB, de Bie MK, Thijssen J, Borleffs CJ, Schalij MJ, van Erven L. Implantation-related complications of implantable cardioverter-defibrillators and cardiac resynchronization therapy devices: a systematic review of randomized clinical trials. *J Am Coll Cardiol.* 2011;58(10):995-1000.
58. Leclercq F, Hager F-X, Macia J-C, Mariottini C-J, Pasquié J-L, Grolleau R. Left ventricular lead insertion using a modified transseptal catheterization technique: a totally endocardial approach for permanent biventricular pacing in end-stage heart failure. *Pacing Clin Electrophysiol.* 1999;22(11):1570-1575.
59. Jaïs P, Douard H, Shah Dc, Barold S, Barat J-L, Clémenty J. Endocardial biventricular pacing. *Pacing Clin Electrophysiol.* 1998;21(11):2128-2131.
60. Garrigue S, Jaïs P, Espil G, et al. Comparison of chronic biventricular pacing between epicardial and endocardial left ventricular stimulation using Doppler tissue imaging in patients with heart failure. *Am J Cardiol.* 2001;88(8):858-862.
61. Ailawadi G, Lapar DJ, Swenson BR, et al. Surgically placed left ventricular leads provide similar outcomes to percutaneous leads in patients with failed coronary sinus lead placement. *Heart Rhythm.* 2010;7(5):619-625.
62. Miller AL, Kramer DB, Lewis EF, Koplan B, Epstein LM, Tedrow U. Event-free survival following CRT with surgically implanted LV leads versus standard transvenous approach. *Pacing Clin Electrophysiol.* 2011;34(4):490-500.
63. Quigley RL. A hybrid approach to cardiac resynchronization therapy. *Ann Thorac Cardiovasc Surg.* 2011;17(3):273-276.

Video Legends

Video 54.1 In this video of a balloon occlusive coronary venous angiogram, the balloon partially obstructs the ostium of a lateral vein. This can sometimes be avoided by performing a pre-angio "puff" prior to balloon inflation.

Video 54.2 This cine loop of a balloon occlusive retrograde venous angiogram shows an unsteady balloon catheter. Such to-and-fro motion can cause vessel damage and dissection. *Source:* Courtesy of Dr. Jagmeet P. Singh, MD, DPhil.

Video 54.3 High-speed rotational coronary venous angiogram over a 110-degree arc from LAO 55 degrees to RAO 55 degrees at a rate of 30 frames per second.

CHAPTER 55

Organizing Best Practices in the Device Clinic

Melanie Turco Gura, MSN RN

Evidence-based Medicine and Best Practices

Clinicians deal daily with questions regarding the ordering and interpretation of diagnostic testing; the prognosis of the patient's disease; and the effectiveness, consequences, and costs of a specific intervention or therapy. For the clinician to validate the conducted systematic review and improve and evaluate the quality of care delivered, evidence-based medicine (EBM) should be applied.[1-2]

EBM is a relatively new paradigm for the healthcare system and describes the process of basing clinical decisions on the latest scientific evidence in the medical literature to provide the "best" possible care to patients.[3-5] *Best practice* is the term used to describe a program whose success is based on evidence. There is no universally accepted definition of a *best practice*. However, a best practice is one that, upon evaluation, demonstrates success, has had an impact, and can be replicated.[6] A commitment to using the best practices in any field is a commitment to using all the knowledge and technology at one's disposal to ensure success. In device clinics, best practice can be achieved through the application of EBM, clinical practices guidelines, and the standards of professional practice.

The Heart Rhythm Society (HRS) and the American College of Cardiology's (ACC) evidenced-based clinical practice guidelines and consensus statements act as a template for optimal care for patients with cardiovascular disease and arrhythmias.[1] They translate the best evidence into practice and, where evidence for specific strategies is weaker, apply clinical wisdom.[7] Applying the guidelines shown in Table 55.1 will allow the clinician to optimally treat patients with cardiovascular implantable electronic devices (CIEDs), resulting in a measurable impact on the patient's health and clinical outcomes. According to the HRS, in the device clinic, applying guidelines and "the provision of safe optimal care [are] contingent on the coordinated efforts of multiple disciplines, the acquisition of a defined specialized knowledge base and the application of knowledge and skills in rendering patient care and technical support services."[8] The HRS developed its Standards of Professional Practice for the Allied Professional in Pacing and Electrophysiology to articulate the scientific foundation, clinical skills, and technical knowledge requisite to providing and facilitating safe, quality patient care.[8]

The Device Clinic

Evolution

Since the introduction of implantable cardiovascular devices in 1958,[9] device technology has evolved significantly to produce complex devices that treat not only bradyarrhythmias, but also tachyarrhythmias and heart failure.[10-11] Cardiac pacemakers, implantable cardioverter-defibrillators (ICDs), cardiac resynchronization therapy (CRT) devices, implantable cardiovascular monitors (ICMs), and implantable loop recorders (ILRs) are currently referred to as cardiovascular implantable electronic devices (CIEDs).[11-13]

Table 55.1 Clinical practice guidelines and expert consensus documents for cardiology best practices

Title	Date Published	Web Address and Reference
HRS/EHRA/APHRS/SOLAECE Expert Consensus Statement on ICD Programming and Testing *Scope:* The consensus statement will focus on optimal programming for primary and secondary prevention ICDs, inappropriate shock avoidance programming (detection times, SVT discrimination, ATP), and use of defibrillation testing	(Currently in development–scheduled for publication 2015)	
HRS Expert Consensus Statement on Remote Monitoring *Scope:* The consensus statement will focus on providing a review of different modalities, indications, utility, implementation and remote monitoring of Cardiovascular Implantable Electronic Devices	(Currently in development–scheduled for publication 2015)	
HRS/ACC/AHA Expert Consensus Statement on the Use of Implantable Cardioverter-Defibrillator Therapy in Patients Who Are Not Included or Not Well Represented in Clinical Trials	May 9, 2014	http://dx.doi.org/10.1016/j.hrthm.2014.03.041
ACCF/HRS/AHA/ASE/HFSA/SCAI/SCCT/SCMR 2013 Appropriate Use. Criteria for Implantable Cardioverter-Defibrillators and Cardiac Resynchronization Therapy	April 2013	http://www.heartrhythmjournal.com/webfiles/images/journals/hrthm/Else_HRTHM_5178.pdf
A Report of the American College of Cardiology Foundation Appropriate Use Criteria Task Force, Heart Rhythm Society, American Heart Association, American Society of Echocardiography, Heart Failure Society of America, Society for Cardiovascular Angiography and Interventions, Society of Cardiovascular Computed Tomography, and Society for Cardiovascular Magnetic Resonance	April 2013	Russo AM, Stainback RF, *Heart Rhythm.* 2013;10(4):1-47.
2012 ACCF/AHA/HRS Focused Update Incorporated Into the AACF/AHA/HRS 2008 Guidelines for Device-Based Therapy of Cardiac Rhythm Abnormalities. Developed in Collaboration With the American Association for Thoracic Surgery, Heart Failure Society of America, and Society of Thoracic Surgeons	January 22, 2013	http://content.onlinejacc.org/article.aspx?articleid=1486116 Tracy CM, Epstein AE, Darbar D, DiMarco JP, et al. *JACC.* 2013;61(3)e6-75.
HRS/ACCF Expert Consensus Statement on Pacemaker Device and Mode Selection. Developed in partnership between the Heart Rhythm Society (HRS) and the American College of Cardiology Foundation (ACCF) and in collaboration with the Society of Thoracic Surgeons	September 2012	http://www.heartrhythmjournal.com/webfiles/images/journals/hrthm/hrt00812001344.pdf Gillis AM, Russo AM, Ellenbogen, KA et al. *Heart Rhythm.* 2012;9(8):1344-1365.
EHRA/HRS Expert Consensus Statement on Cardiac Resynchronization Therapy in Heart Failure: Implant and Follow-up Recommendations and Management	September 2012	http://dx.doi.org/10.1016/j.hrthm.2012.07.025
The Heart Rhythm Society (HRS)/American Society of Anesthesiologists (ASA) Expert Consensus Statement on the Perioperative Management of Patients with Implantable Defibrillators, Pacemakers, and Arrhythmia Monitors: Facilities and Patient Management. Developed as a joint project with the American Society of Anesthesiologists, and in collaboration with the American Heart Association (AHA) and the Society of Thoracic Surgeons (STS)	July 2011	http://www.hrsonline.org/content/download/1432/20125/file/2011-HRS_ASA Perioperative Management.pdf Crossley GH, Poole JE, Rozner MA, et al. *Heart Rhythm.* 2011;8(7):1114-1154.
The HRS Expert Consensus Statement on the Management of Cardiovascular Implantable Electronic Devices (CIEDs) in patients nearing end of life or requesting withdrawal of therapy. Developed in collaboration and endorsed by the American College of Cardiology (ACC), the American Geriatrics Society (AGS), the American Academy of Hospice and Palliative Medicine (AAHPM), the American Heart Association (AHA), the European Heart Rhythm Association (EHRA), and the Hospice and Palliative Nurses Association (HPNA)	May 14, 2010	http://www.hrsonline.org/content/download/1392/19393/file/2010-HRS Management of CIEDs in patients nearing end of life.pdf Lampert R, Hayes DL, Annas GJ, et al. *Heart Rhythm.* 2010;7(7):1008-1026.
Recommendations from the Heart Rhythm Society Task Force on Lead Performance Policies and Guidelines. Developed in collaboration with the American College of Cardiology (ACC) and the American Heart Association (AHA)	May 13, 2009	http://www.hrsonline.org/Practice-Guidance/Clinical-Guidelines-Documents/2009-Recommendations-on-Lead-Performance-Policies-and-Guidelines#axzz2MEK4s7K5 Maisel WH, Hauser RG, Hammill SC, et al. *Heart Rhythm.* 2009;6(6):869-884.

Title	Date Published	Web Address and Reference
ACC/AHA/HRS 2008 Guidelines for Device-Based Therapy of Cardiac Rhythm Abnormalities	May 15, 2008	http://www.hrsonline.org/content/download/9216/403794/file/2008-ACC-AHA-HRS Device Based Therapy_guidelines_full.pdf
		Epstein AE, DiMarco JP, Ellenbogen KA, et al. *Heart Rhythm.* 2008;5(6):e1-e62.
HRS/EHRA Expert Consensus on the Monitoring of Cardiovascular Implantable Electronic Devices (CIEDs): Description of Techniques, Indications, Personnel, Frequency and Ethical Consideration	May 14, 2008	http://www.hrsonline.org/content/download/1389/19336/file/2008-HRS-EHRA Monitoring of CIEDs.pdf
		Wilkoff BL, Auricchio A, Brugada J, et al. *Heart Rhythm.* 2008;5(6):907-926.
ACCF Training Statement: Task Force 6: Training in Specialized Electrophysiology, Cardiac Pacing, and Arrhythmia Management endorsed by the Heart Rhythm Society	January 2008	http://content.onlinejacc.org/cgi/content/full/51/3/374
		Naccarelli GV, Conti JB, DiMarco JP, Tracy CM; Heart Rhythm Society. *J Am Coll Cardiol.* 2008;51(3):374-380.[12]
HRS Policy Statement Update: Recommendations on the Role of Industry-Employed Allied Professionals (IEAPs)	November 2008	http://www.hrsonline.org/content/download/1428/20049/file/2008-HRS Role-of-IEAP.pdf
		Lindsay BD, Estes NAM III, Maloney JD, Reynolds DW. *Heart Rhythm.* 2008;5(11):e8-e10.
Recommendations from the Heart Rhythm Society Task Force on Device Performance Policies and Guidelines	September 2006	http://www.hrsonline.org/content/download/1393/19412/file/Recommendations of the Heart Rhythm Society Task Force on.pdf
		Carlson MD, Wilkoff BL, Maisel WH, et al. *Heart Rhythm.* 2006;1250-1273.
2003 NASPE (HRS) Standards of Professional Practice for the Allied Professional in Pacing and Electrophysiology	January 2003	http://www.hrsonline.org/content/download/1409/19701/file/2003-NASPE Allied Professional Statement.pdf
		Gura MT, Bubien RS, Belco KM, et al. *Pacing Clin Electrophysiol.* 2003;26(1 Pt 1):127-131.
ACC Expert Consensus Document on Ethical Coding and Billing Practices for Cardiovascular Medicine Specialists	March 1999	http://content.onlinejacc.org/cgi/content/full/33/4/1076
		Blankenshop JC, Bateman TM, Haines DE, et al. *J Am Coll Cardiol.* 1999;33(4):1076-1086.

ACCF = American College of Cardiology Foundation; NASPE = North American Society of Pacing and Electrophysiology.

As the indications for CIED implantation have broadened[14-18] and spurred increased utilization of device diagnostic data,[11] a paradigm shift has occurred—moving from simply testing the device to overall patient and device management. With the addition of remote monitoring access, the clinician also has the potential to improve patients' outcomes by reducing the time between onset and detection of clinical pathology and the appropriate therapeutic intervention.[19-22] The management of these patients and their devices has become a distinct and multifaceted medical service,[11] whereby device evaluation has evolved into enhanced patient monitoring and sophisticated disease management (Figure 55.1).

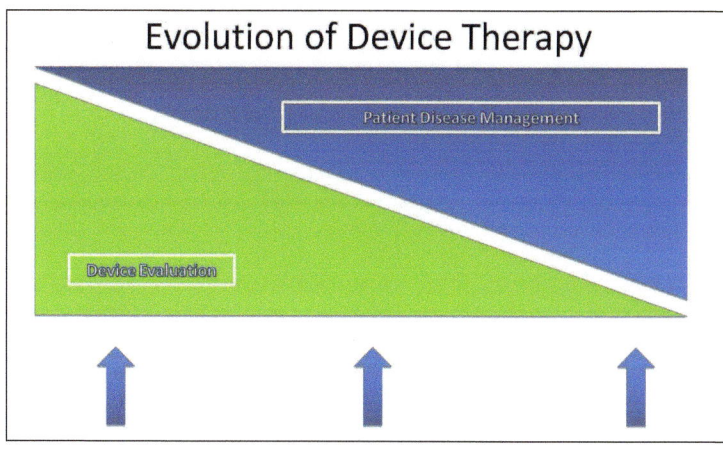

Figure 55.1 Evolution of device therapy from device testing to disease management. Source: Courtesy of Mike Hess, Medtronic Inc.

Purpose and Goals

The purpose of the device clinic is multifaceted. It aims to provide excellence in patient care by evaluating CIEDs and optimizing them for performance and patient safety, recognizing and correcting any CIED anomalies, monitoring cardiac arrhythmias and physiological parameters. The clinic also communicates these data to relevant healthcare providers (eg, helping them to plan for elective CIED replacement), maintains patient records, manages databases, and educates patients, their families, and cardiac-device clinician specialists.[10-11,23-25]

According to the 2008 HRS and European Heart Rhythm Association (EHRA) expert consensus statement on the monitoring of CIEDs,[11] the major goals of device clinics can be divided into four major groups: (1) patient related, (2) device related, (3) disease related, and (4) communication related.

Patient-related Goals

Patient-related goals include optimizing the patient's quality of life, optimizing device function to meet the patient's clinical requirements, identifying patients at risk, and initiating appropriate follow-up. Follow-up can involve field safety corrective actions, safety alerts, triaging of non-CIED–related health problems, and making the appropriate referrals.[11]

Device-related Goals

Device-related goals include documenting appropriate CIED function, identifying and correcting abnormal CIED behavior, maximizing pulse-generator longevity while maintaining patient safety, and recognizing appropriate end of battery life. It also involves organizing CIED replacement in a nonemergent manner and identifying leads at risk for failure.[11]

Disease-related Goals

Disease-related goals include documenting the characteristics and frequency of arrhythmias over time, correlating arrhythmias with patient symptoms, and determining the appropriateness of CIED response to these arrhythmias. Other goals include documenting, when available, hemodynamic status, transthoracic impedance, patient activity, and other physiological parameters over time as part of chronic disease monitoring of heart failure as well as monitoring the patient's response to therapy.[11]

Communication-related Goals

Communication-related goals include maintaining a patient database, timely communication to the patient and relevant healthcare providers of CIED and disease-related information, and providing technical expertise and education to the patient, the community, and colleagues.[11]

Facility Logistics Space

Regardless of whether the device clinic is based in an office or hospital, a dedicated space or area is essential.[25-27] Patients have a fundamental right to considerate care that safeguards them from harm while respecting their personal dignity.[28] Since the patient has the right to privacy and confidentiality, he or she should be examined in a private room. Sufficient space is required for assessing the patient, evaluating the device, and performing essential equipment storage. There should be adequate space to informally walk or exercise the patient to evaluate rate-adaptive pacing response and a designated 6-minute hall walk area for patients with CRT devices.[25] Necessary equipment includes the following:

- A patient examination table or chair (Figure 55.2);
- Programmers from different manufacturers for every device being followed;
- Magnets;
- Electrocardiographic (ECG) monitoring equipment (eg, the Paceart® System [Medtronic, Minneapolis, MN], an ECG machine, and a rhythm-strip recorder);
- A transtelephonic receiving location (more than one station may be necessary based on the volume of patients enrolled in the device clinic);
- Remote monitoring access stations to review and analyze transmissions;
- Chart/record storage (either computerized or on paper);
- CPR equipment, including an external defibrillator; and

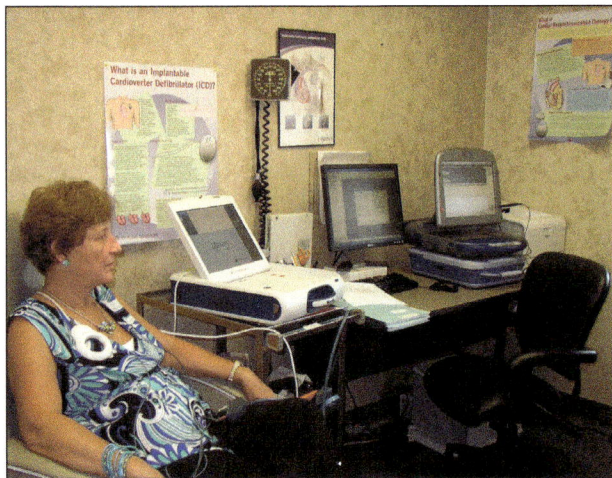

Figure 55.2 Patient evaluation room with nurse workstation and reclining chair. Workstation includes programmers and desktop computer for access to the Paceart System (Medtronic), the patient's electronic medical record, the Internet, and a printer.

- A patient/family education area (for teaching; viewing flip charts, heart and device models, and videos/DVDs; and storing patient literature).

Resources should be available to the device specialists, including manuals both in hard copy and accessible on the Internet. Contact information for technical support for each device manufacturer should be readily available.[25-27]

Personnel

The literature is replete with studies[29-33] substantiating that a nurse-managed, physician-directed clinic markedly improves patient outcomes. In the subspecialty of cardiac rhythm management, clinically employed allied professionals (including registered nurses, midlevel providers, technologists, and technicians) with specialized knowledge in CIED programming and follow-up can improve patient outcomes. They do so by implementing detailed protocols based on practice guidelines while complying with state, province, and country statutes. As directed by these regulations, they render patient care and technical support services in collaboration with and/or under the direct or indirect supervision of the physician.[9,11]

The basic device clinic staff should include a physician, nurse manager, cardiac device specialists (who are usually register nurses), technicians, and secretarial support. A well-defined organizational chart with a clear chain of command should be available.[10] The lines of clinical responsibility must be clearly defined in the job description (Figure 55.3). However, all individuals involved in the device clinic, including patients, device manufacturers, and the referring physician, have specific responsibilities.[11]

The HRS/EHRA 2008 Expert Consensus Statement on monitoring guidelines[11] recommends that some type of "care agreement" be implemented at the onset of the patient interaction. This agreement can be either written (Figure 55.4) or informal but should clearly identify the specific responsibilities of each party, including the patient. It is essential that patients and their family members realize that quality care for patients with CIEDs is a joint endeavor and that they must play an active role in their own care.

Roles and Responsibilities

Patient

Patient education commences during the preimplantation phase. Patients should understand their indications for device therapy and be familiar with the function of the device and any restrictions that apply during the perioperative period. It is imperative that they also comprehend the importance of device follow-up, including follow-up methods and schedules. It is then the responsibility of the patient and his or her family to thoroughly understand this information. If not, they should be encouraged to ask questions. They need to clearly recognize the importance of adhering to the follow-up schedule.[11]

The patient should carry the identification card at all times to facilitate care if the need arises. A temporary card should be received at implantation and a permanent card received from the manufacturer via mail shortly after the procedure. The patient's responsibility also includes notifying the device clinic if his or her contact information changes. It is crucial that contact information remain accurate to maintain appropriate and seamless follow-up and in the event of an advisory. Any change in the patient's medical condition, as shown in Table 55.2, should be communicated to the device clinic.[11]

Table 55.2 Responsibilities of patients with CIEDs

Clinical Information
• Symptom recurrence that existed prior to CIED implantation
• Cardiac and antiarrhythmic medication change
• Encounter with a different device clinic, especially if programming changes were made there
• Trauma near or at the pulse-generator site
• Requiring therapeutic radiation near or at the pulse-generator site
• Terminal illness
• Considerable change in mental status
• Planned invasive medical procedure or diagnosis of new clinical condition
• Exposure to a "shock" from an electrical source

Source: Adapted with permission from Wilkoff BL, Auricchio A, Brugada J, et al. *Heart Rhythm.* 2008;5(6):907-926.[11]

Implanting Physician/Follow-up Physician

In the device clinic, the physician who gives and signs off on any orders is responsible for all aspects of the patient–device evaluation encounter. The HRS strongly recommends that physicians in training who incorporate CIED implantation and follow-up into their clinical practice meet the training requirements described in the COCATS 3 (Core Cardiology Training Symposium, Bethesda, MD, June 1994) Task Force 6 document[13] and pass the American Board of Internal Medicine (ABIM) examination of Clinical Cardiac Electrophysiology (CCEP). However, the physician already in practice who decides to implant CIEDs should undergo appropriate training in a program accredited by the Accreditation Council for Graduate Medical Education (ACGME). Physicians who intend to implant ICD and CRT devices should have extensive experience with pacemaker implantation. The HRS also recommends that physicians meet the same training level 3 requirements specified in COCATS 3 Task Force 6 curriculum. Furthermore, as indicated in the curriculum, the HRS recommends that

Job Description Sample #1

Job Title: *Director of the Device Clinic*

Department: Device Clinic

General Summary of Duties: Manages, monitors, and coordinates the Pacemaker and Arrhythmia Services operations to ensure compliance with governmental regulations and to meet the standards of care established by the HRS, AHA, and ACC. Oversees the education, manages clinical practice, and conducts quality review of the clinical device clinic staff for all campuses of [*HOSPITAL/PRACTICE*] patient service and testing sites. Provides professional nursing care and facilitates the provision of technology-based interventions and therapies to in-office and hospital patients following [*HOSPITAL/PRACTICE*] established standards and practices.

Supervision Received: Reports to the Executive Committee

Supervision Exercised: Directs the Device Clinic Clinical/Secretarial Staff

Responsibilities:

- Promotes quality patient care
- Reviews and communicates standards of care for the allied professional in pacing and electrophysiology
- Facilitates collaboration between clinical and medical staff
- Promotes evidenced-based practice and research
- Monitors adherence to standards of practice and quality of care
- Monitors device advisories and compliance to recommendations and standards of care
- Promotes positive staff and community relations
- Provides clinical guidance to clinical staff
- Facilitates new staff clinical orientation
- Facilitates clinical professional education and educational in-services
- Facilitates learning experiences for clinical staff and students
- Coordinates nursing clinical professional efficiency and quality goals
- Ensures adherence to [*HOSPITAL/PRACTICE*] billing guidelines and practices
- Monitors clinical staff interventions to assure appropriateness of intervention

Knowledge, Skills, and Ability: The Director of the Device Clinic of [HOSPITAL/PRACTICE] must be proactive, compliant, and able to communicate clinical professional roles clearly and accurately to staff. Must possess the ability to work and lead people under all circumstances; must possess the ability to access and retrieve information from the computer; and needs to have expert knowledge of pacing and electrophysiology and the procedures, technology, and equipment involved in patient care.

Minimum Qualifications: RN licensure in the state of Ohio, MSN, OBN CTP, Advanced Practice Nurse Certificate of Authority in cardiology or adult medicine, demonstrated leadership, clinical competence, and teaching and communication skills. Must be a Certified Cardiac Device Specialist (CCDS from IBHRE).

Experience: Five [5] years' experience in pacing and electrophysiology, including device follow-up, and previous management experience.

Job Description Sample #2

Job Title: *Cardiac Rhythm Management Device Specialist*

Department: Device Clinic

General Summary of Duties: Provides professional nursing care for office/hospital patients following [*HOSPITAL/PRACTICE*] established standards and practices, consistent with [*HOSPITAL/PRACTICE*] mission values. Evaluates and manages patients with cardiac rhythm disorders and selected cardiovascular diseases. The RN must be able to demonstrate the professional nursing skills to evaluate patients with arrhythmias and the technical skills to evaluate patients with cardiac rhythm management devices.

Supervision Received: Director, Device Clinic

Supervision Exercised: None

Responsibilities:

- Promotes quality patient care by adhering to HRS and NASPE standards of care for the Allied Professional in Pacing and Electrophysiology
- Triages phone calls and gives verbal and written orders according to standing orders or established protocols
- Performs interrogation, evaluation, and reprogramming of all manufacturers' models of cardiac rhythm management devices
- Reviews remote, transtelephonic, and in-office evaluations and completes documentation according to [*HOSPITAL/PRACTICE*] protocols
- Provides patient and family education with appropriate documentation in EMR or Paceart
- Adheres to [*HOSPITAL/PRACTICE*] billing guidelines and practices
- Promotes positive staff and interoffice relations

Knowledge, Skills, and Ability: Acquires, maintains, and integrates knowledge of scientific principles and derived technology-based interventions and therapies in cardiac pacing, defibrillation, and electrophysiology to provide and facilitate the provision of safe, optimal patient care. Must demonstrate the technical knowledge and clinical skills to assist in the care of patients with heart rhythm disorders.

Minimum Qualifications: RN licensure in the state of Ohio. Certification by IBHRE as a Certified Cardiac Device Specialist (CCDS) preferred.

Experience: Five [5] years' experience as an RN and two [2] years in pacing and electrophysiology, including device follow-up.

Source: Adapted from Pacemaker and Arrhythmia Services. Courtesy of Melanie T. Gura, MSN, CNS, CCDS.

Figure 55.3 Job descriptions of device clinic staff.

Job Description Sample #3

Job Title: *Cardiac Device Technologist*

Department: Device Clinic

General Summary of Duties: Provides quality patient care for office/hospital patients following [HOSPITAL/PRACTICE] established standards and practices, consistent with NEOCS mission values. Assists in the evaluation of patients with cardiac implanted electronic devices.

Supervision Received: Director, Device Clinic

Supervision Exercised: None

Responsibilities:

- Promotes quality patient care by adhering to standards set by the Pacemaker and Arrhythmia Service
- Performs transtelephonic and remote transmissions and completes documentation according to department protocols
- Triages phone calls from device patients to the device RN
- Maintains patient device records
- Schedules patient appointments
- Performs ECGs as necessary
- Maintains stock inventory
- Promotes positive staff and interoffice relations

Knowledge, Skills, and Ability: Demonstrated technical knowledge to assist in the care of patients with cardiac implantable electronic devices. Basic computer skills.

Minimum Qualifications: Graduate of an accredited school of medical assisting, or certified cardiovascular technician with three [3] years' experience.

Source: Adapted from Pacemaker and Arrhythmia Services. Courtesy of Melanie T. Gura, MSN, CNS, CCDS.

Job Description Sample #4

Job Title: *Secretary*

Department: Device Clinic

General Summary of Duties: Provides clerical and administrative support to [*HOSPITAL/PRACTICE*] device clinic. Responsible for specific projects as well as helping coordinate and implement office procedures. Most work involves communication and word processing skills; medical background preferred.

Supervision Received: Director, Device Clinic

Supervision Exercised: None

Responsibilities:

- Uses a variety of software packages to produce correspondence and documents and maintain presentations, spreadsheets, and databases
- Devises and maintains device records
- Schedules patient appointments
- Triages patient phone calls
- Arranges meetings, books rooms, takes minutes, and keeps notes
- Acts as liaison with members of staff in other departments or external contacts
- Organizes and stores paperwork, documents, and computer-based information
- Promotes positive staff and interoffice relations

Knowledge, Skills, and Ability: Demonstrates organizational and project management skills. Displays the ability to manage pressure and conflicting demands and to prioritize tasks.

Minimum Qualifications: High school graduate with basic office skills and advanced computer skills. Good oral and written communication abilities.

Source: Adapted from Pacemaker and Arrhythmia Services. Courtesy of Melanie T. Gura, MSN, CNS, CCDS.

Figure 55.3 (continued) Job descriptions of device clinic staff.

CARDIOVASCULAR IMPLANTABLE DEVICES
Patient's Responsibilities and Rights

Importance of Pacemaker or ICD Monitoring/Follow-up

Consistent follow-up evaluations of your pacemaker or implantable cardioverter-defibrillator (ICD) are imperative for your safety and to assure normal function of your implanted device.

Regular follow-up is the best approach to discover real or impending complications with your implanted device and changes in your medical condition.

It is important for you to actively participate in your medical care with your healthcare team.

Your responsibilities as a patient with an implanted device include the following:

- Knowing the name of the manufacturer of your implanted device and the reason you had the device implanted.
- Understanding when and how to follow-up with your healthcare team.
- Notifying the device clinic with updated contact information, such as a change of address or telephone number.
- Notifying the device clinic when you cannot make your scheduled appointment, whether it is an in-person evaluation or an evaluation by phone.
- Notifying your doctor and/or device clinic if you experience:
  - A shock from your ICD
  - An external shock from an outside electrical source
  - Pain and/or any trauma on or near your device
  - Therapeutic radiation

Our responsibility as the healthcare team include the following:

- Creating and maintaining a follow-up schedule with you.
- Evaluating you and your device in person yearly or more frequently if clinical or device-related events occur.
- Notifying you in person or by phone of normal and abnormal evaluations and the physician's recommended plan of care.
- Notifying you of a manufactures' advisory via a certified letter.

DEVICE CLINIC • 555.555.5555

Your signature below acknowledges that you have reviewed and discussed this information with us and you agree to actively participate in the follow-up care of your implanted device.

NAME (Please print clearly)

SIGNATURE

DATE

WITNESS

Figure 55.4 Sample patient contract. *Source:* Adapted from Pacemaker and Arrhythmia Services. Courtesy of Melanie T. Gura.

each physician complete an examination of certification. The examination offered by the International Board of Heart Rhythm Examiners (IBHRE, previously known as NASPExAM®) is an appropriate alternative for the practicing physician who does not qualify for the CCEP examination offered by the ABIM.[13]

Clinically Employed Allied Professionals

Clinically employed allied professionals (CEAPs) are a diverse group of clinicians who come from multiple disciplines. The CEAP must demonstrate the requisite skills, knowledge, and abilities to perform specific tasks for evaluating patients with CIEDs. Although the HRS Standards of Professional Practice for the Allied Professional in Pacing and Electrophysiology address these clinicians' scope of activities,[9] the CEAP should also strive to become a Certified Cardiac Device Specialist (CCDS) credentialed by the IBHRE.[33] This specialty certification formally recognizes individuals who demonstrate that they have met predefined, standardized criteria for proficiency and knowledge in this area of expertise.[31] The credential of CCDS represents a standard of excellence for cardiac arrhythmia professionals.[34]

The CEAP may be responsible for the operation and administration of the device clinic, but as previously stated, the physician is ultimately responsible for all aspects of the patient encounter.[11,35] The CEAP is responsible for scheduling and maintaining appropriately timed follow-up of the patient and the device, as indicated by the patient's status, type of device, and type of follow-up. In general, CEAPs are responsible for maintaining patient records that include previous medical history, device indications, and the implantation record, which includes the device and lead model and serial numbers, implantation values, and access to prior evaluations, transmissions, remote downloads, and face-to-face evaluations.[11] With the advent of remote monitoring, a systematic process for incorporating and analyzing remote monitoring events is imperative. A plan should also be in place to address patient issues when the device clinic is closed after hours, on weekends, and during holidays.[11] In the event of a manufacture's advisory or field safety alert, the CEAP will facilitate the implementation of the corrective action, as directed by the physician.

Patient education commences during the preimplantation phase and is the ongoing responsibility of the CEAP. During encounters with patients, the CEAP should be able to answer questions the patients may have about device function, electrical myopotential interference, intimacy, and a variety of other areas of concern.

Industry Employed Allied Professionals

The industry employed allied professional (IEAP) applies to persons who are directly employed or contracted manufacturer representatives, field clinical engineers, and "technical specialists."[11,36-37] Traditionally, IEAPs have played a significant role in providing technical support to physicians and CEAPs during all phases of the patient–device evaluation continuum. Although their technical expertise is valuable to physicians and CEAPs, the physician maintains responsibility for evaluating the effectiveness of the device's programming, identifying any device malfunctions, and prescribing a plan of care and recommended intervention or action.[11,37]

In 2001, the HRS published a policy statement to provide guidance to IEAPs when rendering technical support.[36] The main beliefs of this document were incorporated into the 2008 HRS/EHRA Consensus Statement[11] and the HRS Policy Statement Update: Recommendations on the Role of Industry Employed Allied Professionals.[37] Since IEAPs are not licensed practitioners, any activity they perform must be carried out per order and under the supervision of a qualified physician. As defined in the policy statement, the role of the IEAP includes the following:[36]

1. The IEAP in the clinical environment is to provide technical support on the implant, use, and operation of their proprietary equipment specific to their company only.

2. The IEAP may participate in the implant procedure if trained in sterile techniques, but as a rule should not enter the sterile field.

3. The IEAP should perform technical support tasks in the office or clinic setting only under direct supervision of the physician. Direct supervision is defined as the physician being present physically in the office suite and available immediately if needed throughout the evaluation.

4. If the IEAP is requested by the physician to evaluate a device in the hospital setting, the physician who made the request needs to be available immediately by phone if he or she cannot provide direct supervision.

5. The IEAP may provide technical assistance to the CEAP under the supervision of the physician. However, the IEAP should not be viewed as replacing the physician. The required level of service or supervision set forth in relevant regulations applies to the physician and the scope of practice of the CEAP.

6. The IEAP provides expertise, may assist in training, and answers questions on their company-specific systems and equipment; however, they should not be viewed or used as unpaid employees of physicians in their practice, routinely retrieve patient information, or enroll patients in remote monitoring systems.

7. The IEAP should not provide clinical assistance in the clinical environment when alone, unsupervised

by an appropriately trained or experience physician. IEAPs should not provide technical assistance in a patient's home in the absence of a responsible physician.

8. The IEAP should not provide technical assistance for a competitive manufacturer's device unless during intraoperative device change.

9. Physicians ultimately have the final responsibility for both clinical oversight of the IEAP and appropriate billing in accordance with all local, state, and federal regulations and laws.

10. IEAPs must abide by specific hospital polices that pertain to their presence and clinical activity in a hospital setting.

11. If the guidelines conflict with state, provincial, or federal law or regulation, such law or regulation takes precedence and control, bearing in mind that the physician has overall responsibility for the patient being treated and for the CIED's function and programming.

Paradigm for Follow-up

The individual patient, the physician, and the CEAP together determine the follow-up paradigm.[11] Issues that will impact the paradigm consist of the patient's preference, the device clinic's resources, the cost-effectiveness of the type of follow-up, and the geographic location of the patient in relation to the device clinic. Many patients are unable to do remote monitoring and will need in-clinic evaluations instead. Barriers to remote monitoring include patient preference, technical difficulties with telephone lines, and patient's feelings of being overwhelmed by this technology. The CIED prescription for follow-up also must be individualized to the patient's clinical status.[11,23,25-27,38]

Table 55.3 describes in detail the types of CIED follow-up evaluations. Types of follow-up include in-person monitoring (either by a CEAP or physician), complete CIED evaluation, interrogation evaluation, periprocedural CIED evaluation/reevaluation, remote monitoring, patient-initiated remote transmission, CIED-initiated remote transmission, and transtelephonic monitoring (TTM) without interrogation.[11]

Frequency of Follow-up

The frequency of device follow-up will be individualized to the patient and determined by patient-related, device-related, and disease-related factors. Patient-related factors include cardiovascular symptoms, the stability of the

Table 55.3 Types of CIED follow-up

In-person monitoring	In-person CIED evaluation performed by a trained physician or CEAP in a designated device clinic, physician's office, or medical facility.
CIED complete evaluation	Consists of device interrogation, review of diagnostic data, programming parameters, and temporary programming for evaluating system function.
CIED interrogation evaluation	Performed either face-to-face or remotely. Data are reviewed without any programming changes or additional testing.
CIED periprocedural evaluation and reevaluation	Interrogation and review of CIED-specific data and function, with or without temporary reprogramming of a parameter prior to and/or following a procedure, test, or surgery.
Remote monitoring	CIED-capable devices transmit a device interrogation signal from the patient's home, using either wanded or wireless communication capabilities, to a remote data-collection site.
Patient-initiated remote transmission	CIED interrogation with data transmission initiated by the patient. It can be a scheduled follow-up transmission or an unscheduled transmission resulting from the patient's symptoms or reports of shock therapy.
CIED-initiated remote transmission	Automatic CIED interrogation with data transmission. Transmission triggers are either scheduled date and time or alerts sufficiently significant for HV shock therapy, AF burden, abnormal lead impedance, and device ERI.
Transtelephonic monitoring (TTM)	Limited to PMs, transmissions include initial rhythm strip, magnet mode rhythm strip, and rhythm strip postmagnet removal.

AF = atrial fibrillation; CEAP = clinically employed allied professional; CIED = cardiac implantable electronic device; ERI = elective replacement indicators; HV = high voltage; PM = pacemaker. *Source:* Wilkoff BL, Auricchio A, Brugada J, et al.[11]

rhythm, adjustment or change in medications (especially antiarrhythmic drugs or heart failure therapy), unstable or elevated stimulation thresholds, frequent ICD therapies, planned medical or surgical intervention, the patient's inability to accurately describe symptoms, and other medical or social issues. Device-related factors include the reliability of the CIED system, the age and complexity of the device, which arrhythmia or heart failure diagnostics are needed for optimal disease management, medications that influence stimulation or defibrillation thresholds, programmed parameters that influence battery longevity, stimulation thresholds, frequency of pacing, and frequency of high-voltage therapy.[11] Disease-related factors include, but are not limited to, the frequency and severity of the patient's symptoms and changes in cardiovascular therapy. The minimum recommended follow-up times are summarized in Table 55.4.

Table 55.4 Minimum frequency of CIED in-person or remote evaluations

Pacemaker/ICD/CRT	
In person	Within 72 hours of implantation of CIED
In person	2–12 weeks postimplantation of CIED
In person or remote	Every 3–12 months for pacemakers and CRT-Ps
In person	Annually until battery depletion
In person or remote	Every 1–3 months at signs of battery depletion
Implantable loop recorder	
In person or remote	Every 1–6 months depending on indication and symptoms
Implantable hemodynamic monitor	
In person or remote	Every 1–6 months depending on indication
In person or remote	More frequent assessment as clinically needed

CRT-P = cardiac resynchronization therapy pacemaker. *Source:* Adapted with permission from Wilkoff BL, Auricchio A, Brugada J, et al, their Table 3.[11]

Predischarge Evaluation

The patient should have a complete face-to-face device evaluation following implantation but before hospital discharge. The predischarge evaluation should document normal CIED function, record initial telemetry values, ensure the absence of operative complications (such as lead dislodgement, perforation of the lead, pneumothorax, and hemothorax), determine patient-specific programming features, educate the patient on restrictions and limitations, and emotionally support the patient and family.[11,23] A CIED identification card should be given to the patient as well as written discharge instructions (Figure 55.5), which include a return visit to the device clinic for wound evaluation and patient assessment.

Postdischarge Evaluation

Patients may be asked to return to the office or device clinic at 6 to 10 days after implantation for a wound evaluation and/or removal of surgical staples, if they were used to close the pocket. A second face-to-face evaluation should be conducted within 4 to 12 weeks postimplantation. Elements of this evaluation include a patient history, a focused physical examination, a complete device evaluation, and device optimization, such as adjusting voltage outputs or rate-modulation parameters. If a patient has a CRT, it also may be optimized at this time. (Refer to Chapter 56 herein for an in-depth description of device optimization, and to Chapter 57 for an in-depth description of CRT optimization.) In-person or remote follow-up should be done every 3 to 12 months subsequently, depending on patient-specific factors and type of CIED.[11] The postdischarge evaluation is the ideal setting for discussing the implementation of remote monitoring.

Device Evaluation Content

The content of the device evaluation will depend on the patient's clinical issues, the type of CIED implanted, and various technical factors. A systematic approach should be developed and consistently utilized by the CEAP who is assessing the patient and the device. After taking the patient's history and doing a focused physical examination of the pocket site, a free-running ECG rhythm strip and magnet strip for pacemakers should be evaluated and documented. Then, the CIED should be interrogated and a printout obtained of all programmed parameters and diagnostic data for review. This step becomes important if modifications have been made owing to a device encounter during a hospitalization or in another physician's office, or in case the diagnostics have been inadvertently cleared. Interrogating the device, either in person or remotely, will reveal several types of data: the battery voltage, battery impedance, lead impedance, a magnet rate for pacemakers (depending on manufacturer), the charge time for ICDs, the percentage paced and sensed, arrhythmias detected by the device, alerts, hemodynamic measurements, and capture thresholds (if available). In-person stimulation thresholds should be performed every 6 to 12 months, depending on the CIED type and the patient's clinical factors.[11,23-27] Table 55.5 lists the required content for CIED in-person or remote monitoring according to the HRS/EHRA Expert Consensus statement on the monitoring of CIEDs.[11]

DISCHARGE INSTRUCTIONS
ICD IMPLANTATION

When can I take a shower?

You may shower on _____.

How do I care for my incision?

Keep the area clean and dry. Do not scrub the incision. Steri-strips™ (3M Nexcare) (small tape strips) may be covering the wound or you may have staples. The device nurse will remove them at your 1-week office visit. You may wash with soap and water and let the water run gently over your incision. Gently towel-dry the incision. Do not use creams, ointment, or lotions on your incision.

When should I call the device clinic?

You should call the device clinic at 555-555-5555 if you have questions.

Call us if you have any of the following:

- Any sign of infection (eg, fever, increased redness, or swelling at incision site; drainage from incision; increased pain or tenderness at site of defibrillator or pacemaker)
- Shortness of breath
- Dizziness
- Fainting spells
- Swelling in the ankles
- Chest pains
- Prolonged hiccoughing
- Therapy received from the device
- Loss of consciousness before receiving therapy from the device
- Numbness or tingling of the arm closest to your device

What activities can I do?

- Do not lift heavy objects (those that weigh more than 10 pounds) until 6 weeks after your procedure.
- You may move your arms normally, but do not raise your arms above shoulder level until you are seen in the device clinic.
- No excessive stretching.
- Do not drive a motor vehicle until advised by your physician.
- You may resume sexual activity in approximately 3 weeks.
- Avoid activity that involves rough contact with your pulse generator.
- No golfing, swimming, tennis, or bowling for 8 weeks.
- Your physician will tell you when you can go back to work.

What is an ID Card?

You will receive a temporary ID card that has the name of the device manufacturer, the type of device and leads, the date of implantation, and the name of the physician who implanted the device. In about 4 to 6 weeks, you should receive a permanent ID card in the mail directly from the company. It is very important that you carry this ID card with you at all times in case you need medical therapy.

What electric equipment will interfere with my device?

- Cells phones should be used on the side opposite your device. They should not be placed directly against your chest or carried in your pocket on the same side as your device.
- Microwave ovens, heating pads, and electric blankets can be used and will not interfere with your device function. However, do not place a heating pad directly over your device.
- Avoid strong electric or magnetic fields, such as industrial equipment, high-intensity radio waves, and arc resistance welders.
- When passing through the entrance of a store that is equipped with antitheft devices, be sure to walk quickly through them, and do not linger between the panels.
- You CANNOT have an MRI.

When do I follow up?

Your device needs to be checked on _____
at the device clinic, located at _____.
Phone: _____.

A device evaluation will be scheduled about 6 to 8 weeks after your incision evaluation. It is critical to comply with your scheduled visit because adjustments will be made that can prolong the battery life of your device and promote optimal device function. You'll need follow-up evaluations approximately every 3 months. Depending on your device and your home phone line, you may be able to monitor your device with a special telephone transmitter or remote monitor. If you can use the transmitter/monitor, you may need to be seen in the device clinic only once a year.

What should I do if I receive device therapy?

- Stay calm, sit, or lie down if you are alone.
- If someone is touching you when your device discharges, they will not be harmed but may experience a tingling sensation similar to a bee sting.
- If you do not feel well within 5 to 10 minutes after a shock, or you receive 2 discharges, call 911.
- If you feel fine, you do not need to seek medical attention immediately but should call the device clinic during business hours.
- A defibrillation shock may feel like a kick in the chest but lasts for only a few seconds.
- Pacing therapy is usually painless, and you should not feel the impulses.

DEVICE CLINIC • 555.555.5555

Figure 55.5 Discharge instructions for ICD patients. *Source:* Adapted from Pacemaker and Arrhythmia Services. Courtesy of Melanie T. Gura.

Table 55.5 Content for in-person or remote monitoring of CIEDs

Pacemaker or ICD Required Parameters: In-person or Remote Monitoring: 3–6 Months (suggested)
• Battery voltage and battery impedance
• Magnet rate for pacemakers
• Charge time for ICDs
• Update current rhythm diagnosis and pacemaker dependency
Pacemaker/CRT-P In-person Follow-up: 6–12 Months (suggested)
• Battery voltage and impedance
• Magnet rate
• Pacing and sensing threshold(s) for atrium, right and left ventricles (all leads)
• Pacing lead impedance(s) for all leads
• Arrhythmias detected by device (eg, mode switching, high ventricular or atrial rate episodes)
• Percentage of pacing/sensing in each chamber
• Review of programmed parameters
• Review of any "safety" or automatic alerts
• Review of hemodynamic measurements or recordings of any other programmed parameters (eg, activity level, HRV, etc.) when available
ICD/CRT-D In-person Follow-up: 3–6 Months (suggested)
• Battery voltage and impedance
• Capacitor charge time
• Pacing and sensing threshold(s) for atrium, right and left ventricles (all leads)
• Pacing lead impedance(s) for all leads
• Shocking impedances for defibrillation leads
• Arrhythmias detected by device
• Percentage of pacing/sensing in each chamber
• Therapies required for termination of SVT/VT/VF
• Review of main programmed parameters
• Review of any device-triggered alerts
• Review of hemodynamic measurements when available
Implantable Loop Recorder: In-person or Remote Monitoring: 1–6 Months (suggested)
• Integrity of sensing
• Arrhythmias (symptomatic) recorded
• Arrhythmias (asymptomatic) stored
Implantable Hemodynamic Monitor: In-person or Remote Monitoring: 1 Week–3 Months (suggested)
• Battery function
• Integrity of lead
• Hemodynamic measurements of variable(s) being monitored
• Arrhythmias detected

HRV = heart rate variability; SVT = supraventricular tachycardia; VT = ventricular tachycardia; VF = ventricular fibrillation. *Source:* Adapted with permission from Wilkoff BL, Auricchio A, Brugada J, et al, their Table 4.[11]

Follow-up Data Management

The communication of device information and data presents a complex medical undertaking owing to the increased number of patients with CIEDs, the amount of data these devices generate, multiple encounters with patients over time, and geographical factors.[39] Maintaining follow-up data is the responsibility of the implanting and follow-up physician or institution.[11] Cost-effective and efficient tools that can access, filter, manage, and utilize patient data are important to these clinicians.[39] It is hoped that the use of all this health information technology will lead to safer and higher-quality care.[40]

When managing CIED-generated information, the best type of follow-up uses longitudinal stored and measured CIED data.[11] Currently, no one system can fulfill the complex needs of patient care in general; however, the most commonly used commercial system is the Paceart® database management system (Medtronic), which standardizes patient and device information.[25-27] The formatted report it generates is consistent with those of all device manufacturers (Figure 55.6). Ideally, this database should be integrated with the patient's electronic medical record (EMR) in order to give all clinicians access to the data. If this is not technically feasible, then acquired and transmitted data obtained from remote access monitoring can be stored in this system and electronically exported, stored as a virtual document, or scanned and placed in the EMR. Optimally, the longitudinal database can be utilized for scheduling patient visits (either face-to-face, remote, or TTM evaluations), tracking missed appointments, billing, generating productivity reports, and tracking implantable leads and devices. Access to patient data is critical in the event of an advisory or safety alert.[19,41]

Advisories, Safety Alerts, and Field Corrections

All manufacturers' devices are subject to unexpected failures. A device malfunction occurs when an implanted device fails to meet the performance specifications or otherwise function as intended.[41] Devices and leads may malfunction owing to physical or mechanical factors and software or firmware failures or anomalies. In a meta-analysis of both pacemaker and ICD registries spanning 1966 to 2005, Maisel[42] demonstrated that, despite continual efforts to improve CIEDs, pacemaker malfunction rates decreased since 1980 while ICD malfunction rates increased fourfold from 1998 to 2002 before substantially declining in the latter two years of the study.

Although no standardized, worldwide tracking measures have been devised, in the United States it is mandated[43-45] that manufacturers register and track their devices. Hospitals and outpatient treatment facilities are also required to report to the FDA whenever a device is

Table 55.6 FDA classification of device "recalls"

Advisory Class	Risk Level	Description	Examples
Class I	Highest risk	Comprises situations in which there is a reasonable probability that the use of, or exposure to, a volatile product will cause serious adverse health consequences or death	Lead failure, sudden output failure
Class II	Medium risk	Comprises situations in which the use of, or exposure to, a volatile product may cause temporary or medically reversible adverse health consequences or in which the probability of serious adverse health consequences is remote	Reduced battery longevity
Class III	Low risk	Comprises situations in which the use of, or exposure to, a volatile product is not likely to cause adverse health consequences	Mislabeling
Safety Alert or Safety Advisory	Less significant than class III	Any communication to inform CEAPs and physicians of a risk of substantial harm from a medical device in commercial use	

Source: Shein MJ, Brinker JA. Pacing the FDA and Regulatory Environment. In: Ellenbogen KA, Kay GN, Wilkoff BL, eds.[42]

thought to have caused or contributed to the death of a patient. If the device is thought to have caused patient injury, reports must be made to the manufacturer, who is then required to submit a report to the FDA.[44-46]

Device and lead recalls are usually initiated by the manufacturer and categorized by the FDA into three classes, depending on the risk of harm to the patient.[45-46] Table 55.6 describes how the FDA classifies recalls. In 2006, the HRS Task Force on Device Performance[37] recommended eliminating the term *recall* and substituting the terms *advisory* or *safety alert*. Note, however, that a safety alert or communication may indicate an equally life-threatening situation as a class I recall.[47] Device manufacturers are obligated to report to competent authorities all incidents or near incidents. Safety alerts and so-called field safety corrective actions are issued by the manufacturer directly to implantable device purchasers or users, usually after consulting with the FDA.[11]

Device clinics play a critical role in following up patients affected by a device alert or advisory.[20] In the event of an advisory, both the implanting and follow-up physician and the device clinic should receive an official notification letter from the manufacturer. Usually, the manufacturer's representative makes an in-person follow-up visit to discuss the technical aspects of the advisory, the manufacturer's recommendations to remedy the problem, and any steps to take to ensure the safety and care of the patients affected. If not, engineers in the manufacturer's technical support division should be consulted to discuss these issues. However, the final decision regarding patient management will rest with the implanting or follow-up physician.[48-49]

The manufacturer will have a list of at-risk patients, but it may be incomplete and reflect only the patients implanted by the physicians from that clinic. Ultimately, the device clinic staff is responsible for providing safe patient care. They will have a difficult time defending their actions during litigation if they did not correctly identify and appropriately handle an advisory that resulted in harm to a patient enrolled in their clinic for follow-up.[48] The device clinic can make use of a computerize database, which allows a search to be conducted to identify all patients with the affected device. This information can then be compared with the manufacturer's list. If the device clinic does not have a computerized database, the staff should conduct a chart-by-chart search. All affected patients should receive a letter from the device clinic concerning the recall and the manufacturers' and physicians' recommendations. Figure 55.7 shows sample letters sent to patients with a pacemaker or an ICD lead under advisory, respectively.

Patient Education

Patient education is the ongoing responsibility of the CEAP[11] and will be affected by the patient's health literacy (HL). HL has been described as the ability to obtain, process, and understand the basic information needed to make appropriate health decisions. Evidence has revealed that approximately 13% of the US population is competent in HL[50] and that the greatest problem exists among those with the greatest need: the elderly, minorities, and people in poor health.[51] HL reaches far beyond the patient's ability to read or complete academic education.[52] Rather, HL declines with age regardless of education[53] and has a significant impact on health outcomes. Patients often feel helpless in the healthcare system and vulnerable when asking questions to clarify information they receive.

Appropriate and timely assessment of the patient's HL capability and needs is an important first step in patient education. The CEAP needs to be aware of where patients are receiving their information and supply accurate information at the level appropriate for the patient (and guide them to the most reliable sources). Patient education is more than giving facts. Instead, it consists of sharing information, discussing concerns, addressing implications, and working with patients to determine how they intend to use the information in their plan of care.[52]

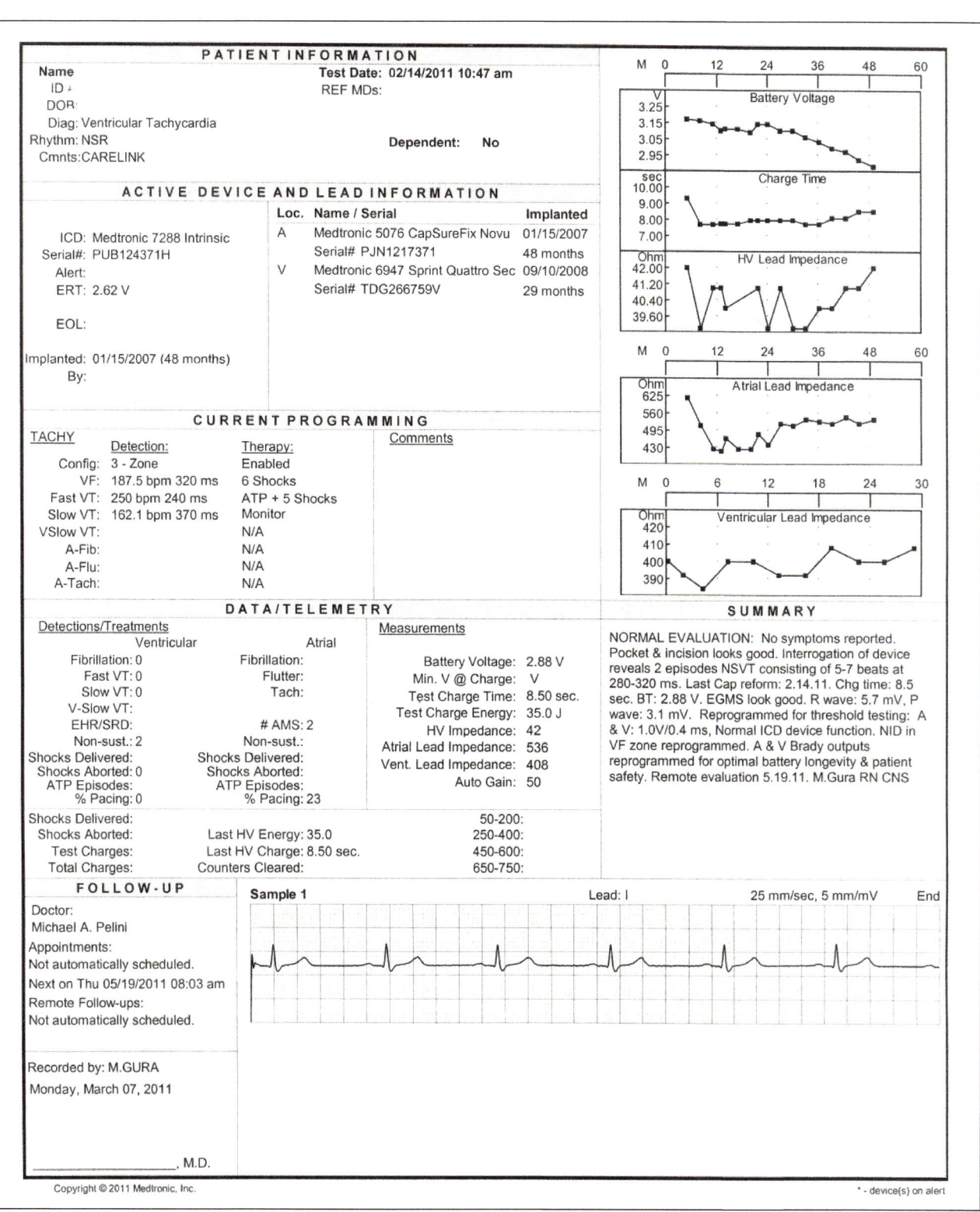

Figure 55.6 Paceart report.

Panel A:

Date:

Dear:

DEVICE MANUFACTURER'S NAME has recently notified our device clinic about important information regarding your pacemaker. You may have heard on television or in the newspaper about the possibility for a problem to occur.

Pacemakers, which are very dependable, complex devices, are manufactured to high reliability standards. However, these devices, like anything that is made, can sometimes be less than flawless.

Your pacemaker model has been identified as affected by a problem that could cause your pacemaker to work improperly. The problem identified by the manufacturer occurs rarely. We have reviewed the advisory and the manufacturer's recommendations very carefully, and we recommend the following:

- *List your recommendations.*

It is important that you continue to keep your regularly scheduled device evaluations.

Please call us at the device clinic at 555.555.5555 if you have any questions.

Sincerely,

PHYSICIAN NAME

A

Panel B:

Date

Dear:

DEVICE MANUFACTURER'S NAME has recently notified our device clinic about important information regarding your implantable cardioverter-defibrillator (ICD). You may have heard on television or in the newspaper about the possibility for a problem to occur.

Implantable cardioverter-defibrillators (ICD), which are very dependable, complex devices, are manufactured to high reliability standards. However, these devices, like anything that is made, can sometimes be less than flawless.

Your ICD model has been identified as affected by a problem that could cause your device to work improperly. The problem identified by the manufacturer occurs rarely. We have reviewed the advisory and the manufacturer's recommendation very carefully, and we recommend the following:

- *List your recommendations.*

If you feel a shock or hear a beeping sound from your ICD, please call us at the office, 555.555.5555, and we'll be happy to see you that same day during business hours. It is important that you continue to keep your regularly scheduled device evaluations.

Please call us at the device clinic at 555.555.5555 if you have any questions.

Sincerely,

PHYSICIAN NAME

B

Figure 55.7 Sample advisory notification letters for patients with pacemaker (**Panel A**) and ICD lead (**Panel B**) on advisory. *Source:* Adapted from Pacemaker & Arrhythmia Services. Courtesy of Melanie T. Gura.

Educational materials should be written at the simplest level possible, usually at about the sixth-grade level or below. Pictographs should be used to illustrate essential points, and information should be translated into the patient's language if possible. During the education encounter, the CEAP should review the information out loud with the patient, ask the patient to repeat the information, and ask questions to ensure comprehension. Patients should be encouraged to ask questions such as, What is my main problem? Why do I have this device? What should I do if I receive a shock?[54] By promoting HL, the CEAP can improve patient safety and quality of care. The patient information section of the HRS's website[55] has a plethora of patient literature that can be easily downloaded and printed. Device manufactures also offer educational literature, videos, DVDs, newsletters, and educational websites for patients. Figure 55.8 illustrates detailed instructions for patients on the implementation of remote monitoring.

Ethical Considerations

As the population of patients with CIEDs continues to grow, these devices are enhancing many patients' quality of life.[54] However, there comes a time when, despite the best and most advanced medical efforts, quality of life begins to diminish and patients no longer experience the benefits of medical intervention. It is then that the device clinic staff may receive a request from a patient to withdraw ICD or pacemaker therapy. There is also a standard medical, bioethical, and legal agreement stating that even a patient who is not terminally ill has the right to decline or have withdrawn any treatment, as long as the patient is cognitively competent and aware of the consequences.[11,57-58]

The HRS 2010 Expert Consensus Statement on the Management of CIEDs in patients nearing end of life or requesting withdrawal of therapy[58] addresses the appropriate ethical, legal, and religious principles involved and the logistics of deactivating the CIED. The basic assumptions of this document include the following:

1. The patient must have decision-making capacity and, if not, their "legally defined surrogate decision-maker" has the same right.

2. Advance directives should be encouraged.

3. CIED deactivation is neither physician-assisted suicide nor euthanasia.

4. The clinician and IEAP cannot be compelled to carry out the task when it conflicts with their personal views and values. However, the patient cannot be abandoned, and a colleague who is willing to perform the procedure should be involved.

Discussion of device deactivation should be ongoing, commencing prior to implantation and continuing over the course of the patient's illness. This should be considered part of the ongoing patient education process. However, if it is not, a thorough discussion should be

---

REMOTE MONITORING FOR DEVICES
Patient Instructions

Remote monitoring follow-up permits your healthcare team to evaluate your device from the comfort of your home. By enrolling in remote monitoring and following these guidelines, the device clinic can communicate with your device and gather important clinical and technical information. This allows us to monitor the function of your device and coordinate your medical care and treatment in a timely manner.

What you need:

1. A standard analog telephone line.
2. Your transmitter will arrive at your home in approximately 2 weeks from enrollment. Please notify us if have not received your transmitter by the day you are scheduled to transmit.

What to do:

1. Please review the written and audiovisual instructions that we have given to you and the instructions sent with the transmitter.
2. Do NOT send a transmission until the day you have been scheduled to send your first transmission.
3. On the day you are scheduled for your initial set up, please connect the monitor and perform the transmission according to the manufacturer's instructions before 10:00 a.m.
4. If you need assistance for the initial set up, please call your device manufacturer's technical support line.

   Boston Scientific. 866-484-3268
   Medtronic. 800-551-5544
   St. Jude Medical. 877-696-3754

5. We will call you in the afternoon of the same day or the following day to discuss the results of the transmission and to schedule your next follow-up appointment.

What you need to know about billing:

1. There is no charge for the remote transmitter.
2. Scheduled transmissions are reimbursed by Medicare or your insurance.
3. If you have questions about your billing statement, please contact _____.

Missed Follow-up Remotes

1. If you miss sending your remote transmission, we will call you to reschedule.
2. If we are unable to reach you by telephone, we will send a letter in the mail for you to call us to reschedule.
3. If we do not hear back from you, you will receive a certified letter from us.

DEVICE CLINIC • 555.555.5555

Figure 55.8 Patient instructions for implementation of remote monitoring. *Source:* Adapted from Pacemaker and Arrhythmia Services. Courtesy of Melanie T. Gura.

conducted preceding deactivation with the patient (if able) and his or her family or an official designee (eg, someone with power of attorney for health care). The physician must convey the details of the patient's medical status and the predicted outcome of decisions that involve the patient's CIED.[11] Documentation of the encounter should include several elements: the perception of the caregiver; a description of the patient's cognitive and psychological state and decision-making competence; communications with the family; that the consequences of deactivation (including relevant alternatives) have been discussed; and a written, signed, and witnessed consent by the patient or legal representative.[11,58]

The device clinic or center should have a clearly defined policy and procedure for withdrawing therapies. Deactivating an ICD and withdrawing pacemaker therapy require an order from the responsible physician (preferably written prior to deactivation) and should include the specific therapies to be deactivated or reprogrammed. If the hospital has electrophysiological (EP) expertise, the responsible physician (if not an EP expert) should arrange for a cardiac electrophysiologist or a CEAP with expertise in CIED programming to deactivate the device. If the facility (such as a nursing facility or hospice) has no EP expertise, then the responsible physician should consult the patient's CIED follow-up physician as to which therapies should be deactivated. However, if withdrawal of pacemaker therapy may be followed by the rapid death of the patient, "such deactivation may not always be appropriate."[58] Out of respect for religious beliefs and individual values, a clinician has the right not to participate in device deactivation; however, in such a case, the patient should not be abandoned, and arrangements should be made for another clinician to deactivate the device.[58]

Continuous magnet application or device reprogramming can be used to deactivate antitachycardia therapy, while deactivation of pacemaker therapies may require decreasing the lower rate limit, programming the output to subthreshold levels, or using specific pacing modes, such as OOO, ODO, and OSO.[11,58] After withdrawal from therapy, patients should also be offered the full range of individualized palliative care to treat symptoms associated with the progression of their underlying illness and new symptoms that may arise.

Reimbursement

Procedures and services that physicians perform are reported using the American Medical Association (AMA) Current Procedural Terminology (CPT®) coding system. The goal of the CPT system is to provide uniform language for accurately describing physicians' services.[59-61] Coding should be performed by trained personnel who are supervised and checked by experts and audited internally for accuracy. The HRS, the ACC, the AMA, and the device companies have numerous resources for coding.[57] These include printed billing and coding guide booklets, customer support lines, e-mail communications, physician websites, webcasts, and periodical course offerings with the most up-to-date information.

The CPT coding guidelines for CIED evaluations were completely revised for 2009 and parallel the current standard of care for follow-up practices. Evolving technology necessitated a modernization of relevant codes previously used to report CIED monitoring. The codes are now categorized by interrogation evaluations and programming evaluations. They are further distinguished as in-person or remote interrogations, as well as TTM. Remote and TTM monitoring now has a 90-day global billing concept, and ILRs and ICMs carry a 30-day global period. This means that the global period will start on the first submission of the code and will restart on Day 91 or 31.

Periprocedural programming codes for pacemakers and ICDs describe services that are rendered immediately before or after surgery, or alternatively, during a procedure or test. For example, an ICD may need to be deactivated before surgery and then reactivated following surgery. In this scenario, the periprocedural codes would be submitted twice—once for programming before surgery and once for reprogramming after surgery.[60]

It is also worth noting that once a patient is enrolled in remote monitoring, in-person interrogations are no longer billable during the 90-day global period. However, programming evaluations are billable within the remote global period. The rationale is that patients who are monitored remotely will eventually require a programming evaluation when they are seen in person. It should be noted that a complete device evaluation (including stimulation threshold testing) is considered "iterative" reprogramming without any change in the final parameters. When a patient is enrolled in TTM follow-up, TTM evaluations can be billed only on Day 91, even if performed on a monthly basis. However, an in-person interrogation can be separately billed during the TTM global period. The rationale is that TTM evaluations are more limited and an in-person interrogation is more extensive.[60] Table 55.7 gives the CPT codes and a description of the corresponding services.

One must be familiar with the requirements and levels of physician supervision that different CIED evaluations require. Physician supervision comprises three levels: personal, direct, and general supervision. Personal supervision indicates that the physician is in the room with the patient, even though someone else may be performing the procedure. An example requiring personal physician supervision is CPT code 93724, which uses noninvasive programmed stimulation (NIPS) through an antitachycardia pacemaker system. Direct supervision, which is necessary for CIED in-office evaluations, implies that the physician is in the office suite or on the same floor as the patient (if two different office spaces are utilized). General supervision refers to access to the physician by phone.[59]

Device evaluation CPT codes consist of two components: one professional and one technical. Global billing includes billing for both components and requires the physician to be the owner of the device clinic and to be the employer of the CEAP who is conducting the evaluation. For example, in the physician's office–based device clinic, a patient with a single-chamber ICD is evaluated in person. Iterative adjustments are made to the ICD to test the device's function and to select the optimal permanent programmed values, with physician analysis, review, and reporting performed, and the physician employing the CEAP. CPT code 93282 should be reported, as it is considered a global billing code for both components. However, if an IEAP evaluates the patient in the physician's office, only the professional component may be submitted because the IEAP is not an employee of the physician. A modifier-26 would be attached to the CPT code, indicating that the charge submitted is only for the professional component. So the correct coding would be 93282-26. A modifier-26 is used to denote the professional services of a physician and is usually reserved for the physician who interprets the procedure. The professional component refers to the physician's time, skill, and judgment in interpreting the results of the test.

If the device clinic is facility based, the physician would bill for the professional component with a modifier-26, while the facility would bill for the technical component. The technical component (TC) includes reimbursement for the facility use, equipment, and the technician and is identified by adding a modifier TC to the procedure code.[61]

Table 55.7 CPT codes and descriptions

CPT Code	CPT Code Description
Implantable Cardioverter-defibrillators	
93289	**Interrogation** device evaluation **(in-person)** with analysis, review, and report by a physician or other qualified healthcare professional, includes connection, recording, and disconnection per patient encounter; single-, dual-, or multiple-lead **ICD**, including analysis of heart rhythm–derived data elements.
	Use 93290 for monitoring physiologic cardiovascular data elements derived from an ICD.
93282	**Programming** device evaluation **(in-person)** with iterative adjustments of the implantable device to test the function of the device and select optimal permanent programmed values with analysis, review, and report by a physician or other qualified healthcare professional; **single**-lead **ICD** system.
	This code is not used for periprocedural reprogramming; refer to periprocedural section.
92383	**Programming** device evaluation **(in-person)** with iterative adjustments of the implantable device to test the function of the device and select optimal permanent programmed values with analysis, review, and report by a physician or other qualified healthcare professional; **dual**-lead **ICD** system.
	This code is not used for periprocedural reprogramming; refer to periprocedural section.
93284	**Programming** device evaluation **(in-person)** with iterative adjustments of the implantable device to test the function of the device and select optimal permanent programmed values with analysis, review, and report by a physician or other qualified healthcare professional; **multiple**-lead **ICD** system.
	This code is not used for periprocedural reprogramming; refer to periprocedural section.
93295	**Interrogation** device evaluation(s) **(remote)**, up to 90 days; single-, dual-, or multiple-lead ICD system with interim analysis, review(s), and report(s) by a physician or other quailed healthcare professional (report only once per 90 days).
	Use 93297 for **remote** monitoring of physiologic cardiovascular data elements derived from an **ICD**.
93296	**Interrogation** device evaluation(s) **(remote)**, up to 90 days; single-, dual-, or multiple-lead **PM** system or **ICD** remote data acquisition(s), receipt of transmission, and **technician** review, technical support, and distribution of results (report only once per 90 days).

(continued on next page)

Table 55.7 CPT codes and descriptions *(continued)*

CPT Code	CPT Code Description
Implantable Pacemaker	
93288	**Interrogation** device evaluation **(in-person)** with analysis, review, and report by a physician or other qualified healthcare professional; includes connection, recording, and disconnection per patient encounter; single-, dual-, or multiple-lead **PM** system.
93279	**Programming** device evaluation **(in-person)** with iterative adjustment of the implanted device to test the function of the device and select optimal permanent programmed values with analysis, review, and report by a physician or other qualified healthcare professional; **single**-lead PM system.
93280	**Programming** device evaluation **(in-person)** with iterative adjustment of the implanted device to test the function of the device and select optimal permanent programmed values with analysis, review, and report by a physician or other qualified healthcare professional; **dual**-lead PM system.
93281	**Programming** device evaluation **(in-person)** with iterative adjustment of the implanted device to test the function of the device and select optimal permanent programmed values with analysis, review, and report by a physician or other qualified healthcare professional; **multiple**-lead PM system.
93296	**Interrogation** device evaluation(s) **(remote)**, up to 90 days; single-, dual-, or multiple-lead **PM** system or **ICD** remote data acquisition(s); receipt of transmission and **technician** review, technical support, and distribution of results (report only once per 90 days).
93294	**Interrogation** device evaluation(s) **(remote)**, up to 90 days; single-, dual-, or multiple-lead **PM** system with interim analysis, review(s), and reports(s) by a physician or other qualified healthcare professional (report only once per 90 days).
93293	**Transtelephonic** rhythm-strip **pacemaker** evaluation(s); single-, dual-, or multiple-lead **PM** system; includes recording with and without magnet application with analysis, review(s), and reports(s) by a physician or other qualified healthcare professional, up to 90 days (report only once per 90 days).
Periprocedural	
93286	**Periprocedural** device evaluation **(in-person)** and programming of device system parameters before or after a surgery, procedure, or test with analysis, review, and report by a physician or other qualified healthcare professional; single-, dual-, or multiple-lead **PM** system.
93287	**Periprocedural** device evaluation **(in-person)** and programming of device system parameters before or after a surgery, procedure, or test with analysis, review, and report by a physician or other qualified healthcare professional, single-, dual-, or multiple-lead **ICD** system.
Implantable Loop Recorder	
93285	**Programming** device evaluation **(in-person)** with iterative adjustment of the implanted device to test the function of the device and select optimal permanent programmed values with analysis, review, and report by a physician or other qualified healthcare professional; **ILR** system.
93291	**Interrogation** device evaluation **(in-person)** with analysis, review, and report by a physician or other qualified healthcare professional; includes connection, recording, and disconnection per patient encounter; **ILR** system, including heart rhythm–derived data analysis.
93298	**Interrogation** device evaluation **(remote)** up to 30 days; **ILR** system, including analysis of recorded heart rhythm data, analysis, review(s), and report(s) by a physician or other qualified healthcare professional (report only once per 30 days).
93299	**Interrogation** device evaluation **(remote)** up to 30 days; **ILR** or **ICM** system, remote data acquisition(s), receipt of transmission, and **technician** review, technical support, and distribution of results (report only once per 30 days).
Implantable Cardiovascular Monitor	
93290	**Interrogation** device evaluation **(in-person)** with analysis, review, and report by a physician or other qualified healthcare professional; includes connection, recording, and disconnection per patient encounter; **ICM** system, including analysis of 1 or more recorded physiologic cardiovascular data elements from all internal and external sensors.
93297	**Interrogation** device evaluation **(remote)** up to 30 days; **ICM** system, including analysis of 1 or more recorded physiologic cardiovascular data elements from all internal and external sensors; analysis, review(s), and reports(s) by a physician or other qualified healthcare professional (report only once per 30 days).
93299	**Interrogation** device evaluation **(remote)** up to 30 days; **ILR** or **ICM** system, remote data acquisition(s), receipt of transmission, and **technician** review, technical support, and distribution of results (report only once per 30 days).

CPT = current procedural terminology; ICM = implantable cardiovascular monitor; ILR = implantable loop recorder; PM = pacemaker. *Sources:* The Heart Rhythm Society. *Coding Guide: 2013.* coding@HRSonline.org. Accessed April 7, 2013. *CPT 2013 Professional Edition.* American Medical Association; 2013.

Summary

The management of CIED patients has become a distinct and multifaceted medical service. Achieving best practice in the device clinic will depend on several operational undertakings. For example, practice guidelines and evidence-based medicine should be used as a template for providing optimal patient care. Also, appropriate follow-up of the CIED patient is necessary not only to provide appropriate disease management but also to maintain system integrity. Eventually, device monitoring will permit us to predict disease progression before it actually manifests in the patient.

References

1. Mayer D. *Essential Evidence-Based Medicine.* 2nd ed. Cambridge: Cambridge University Press; 2010.
2. Fineout-Overholt E, Hofstetter S. Teaching EBP: getting to the gold: how to search the best evidence. *Worldviews Evid Based Nurs.* 2005;2(4):207-211.
3. Kenney CK. *The Best Practice: How the New Quality Movement Is Transforming Medicine.* Philadelphia, PA: Public Affairs (Perseus); 2008.
4. Sackett DI, Tosenbert EM, Gray JA, et al. Evidence-based medicine: what is it and what it isn't. *BMJ.* 1996;312:71-72.
5. Slawson DC, Shaughnessy AF, Bennett JH. Becoming a medical information master: feeling good about not knowing everything. *J Fam Pract.* 1994; 38(5):505-513.
6. Perleth M, Jakuboski E, Busse R. What is "best practice" in health care? State of the art perspectives in improving the effectiveness and efficiency of the European healthcare system. *Health Policy.* 2001;56(2):235-250.
7. Malcolm J, Arnold O, Howlett JG, et al. Canadian Cardiovascular Society Consensus Conference guidelines on heart failure—2008 update: best practice for transition of care for heart failure patients, and the recognition, investigation and treatment of cardiomyopathies. *Can J Cardiol.* 2008;24(1)21-40.
8. Gura MT, Bubien RS, Belco KM, et al. North American Society of Pacing and Electrophysiology: standards of professional practice for the allied professional in pacing and electrophysiology. *Pacing Clin Electrophysiol.* 2003;26(1): 127-131.
9. Curtis A. A brief history of cardiac pacing. In: Curtis AB, ed. *Fundamentals of Cardiac Pacing.* Boston: Jones and Bartlett Publishers; 2010:1-11.
10. Jones S, Gammage M, Linker N, et al. Clinical guidance by consensus for the follow-up of implantable cardiac devices for cardiac rhythm management. *Heart Rhythm UK.* 2008;1-9.
11. Wilkoff BL, Auricchio A, Brugada J, et al. HRS/EHRA Expert Consensus on the Monitoring of Cardiovascular Implantable Electronic Devices (CIEDs): description of techniques, indications, personnel, frequency and ethical considerations. *Heart Rhythm.* 2008;5(6):907-926.
12. Hayes DL, Naccarelli GV, Furman S, et al. North American Society of Pacing and Electrophysiology. NASPE training requirements for cardiac implantable electronic devices: selection, implantation, and follow up. *Pacing Clin Electrophysiol.* 2003;26(7 Pt 1):1556-1562.
13. Naccarelli GV, Conti JB, DiMarco JP, Tracy CM; Heart Rhythm Society. Task Force 6: training in specialized electrophysiology, cardiac pacing, and arrhythmia management endorsed by the Heart Rhythm Society. *Heart Rhythm.* 2008;5(2):332-337.
14. Epstein AE, DiMarco JP, Ellenbogen KA, et al. ACC/AHA/HRS 2008 guidelines for device-based therapy of cardiac rhythm abnormalities. *JACC.* 2008;51(21):e1-e62.
15. Tracy, CM, Epstein AE, Darbar D., et al. 2012 ACCF/AHA/HRS focused Update Incorporated into the ACCF/AHA/HRS 2008 Guidelines for Device-Based Therapy of Cardiac Rhythm Abnormalities. A report of the American College of Cardiology Foundation/American Heart Association Task Force on Practice Guidelines and the Heart Rhythm Society. Developed in Collaboration with the American Association of Thoracic Surgery, Heart Failure Society of America and Society of Thoracic Surgeons. *JACC.* 2013;61(3)e6-75.
16. Gillis AM, Russo AM, Ellenbogen, KA, et al. HRS/ACCF Expert Consensus Statement on Pacemaker Device and Mode Selection. Developed in partnership between the Heart Rhythm Society (HRS) and the American College of Cardiology Foundation (ACCF) and in collaboration with the Society of Thoracic Surgeons. *Heart Rhythm.* 2012;9(8): 1344-1365.
17. Russo AM, Stainback RF. ACCF/HRS/AHA/ASE/HFSA/SCAI/SCCT/SCMR 2013 Appropriate use. Criteria for implantable cardioverter-defibrillators and cardiac Resynchronization Therapy. a report of the American College of Cardiology Foundation Appropriate Use Criteria Task Force, Heart Rhythm Society, American Heart Association, American Society of Echocardiography, Heart Failure Society of America, Society for Cardiovascular Angiography and Interventions, Society of Cardiovascular Computed Tomography, and Society for Cardiovascular Magnetic Resonance. *Heart Rhythm.* 2013;10(4):1-47.
18. Kusumoto FM, Calkins H, Boehmer, Buxton AE, et al. 2013 HRS/ACC/AHA Expert Consensus Statement on the Use of Implantable Cardioverter-Defibrillator Therapy in Patients Who Are Not Included or Not Well Represented in Clinical Trials. *Heart Rhythm,* 2014;11(7):1270-1300.
19. Maisel WH, Hauser RG, Hammill SC, et al. Recommendations from the Heart Rhythm Society Task Force on Lead Performance Policies and Guidelines: developed in collaboration with the American College of Cardiology (ACC) and the American Heart Association (AHA). *Heart Rhythm.* 2009; 6(6):869-884.
20. Crossley GH, Boyle A, Vitense H, et al. The CONNECT (Clinical Evaluations of Remote Notification to Reduce Time to Clinical Decision) trial: the value of wireless remote monitoring with automatic clinician alerts. *J Am Coll Cardiol.* 2011;57(10):1181-1189.
21. Movsowitz C, Mittal S. Remote patient management using implantable devices. *J Interv Card Electrophysiol.* 2011;31(1): 81-90.
22. Folino AF, Chiusso F, Zanotto G, et al. Management of alert messages in the remote monitoring of implantable cardioverter defibrillators and pacemakers: an Italian single-region study. *Europace.* 2011;13(3):1281-1291.
23. Lopera G, Curtis A. Follow-up. In: Curtis AB, ed. *Fundamentals of Cardiac Pacing.* Boston: Jones and Bartlett Publishers; 2010:149-170.
24. Love CL. Pacemaker troubleshooting and follow-up. In: Ellenbogen KA, Kay GN, Lau CP, Wilkoff BL, eds. *Clinical Cardiac Pacing, Defibrillation, and Resynchronization Therapy.* 3rd ed. Philadelphia: Saunders Elsevier; 2007.

25. Hayes DL, Tabatabacei N, Glikson M, Friedman PA. Follow-up. In: Hayes DL, Friedman PA. *Cardiac Pacing, Defibrillation and Resynchronization: A Clinical Approach.* 2nd ed. Hoboken, NJ: Wiley-Blackwell; 2008;572-616.
26. Schoenfeld MH. Pacemaker insertion, revision, extraction and follow-up. In: Saksena S, Camm AJ, eds. *Electrophysiological Disorders of the Heart.* Elsevier; 2005:767-808.
27. Schoenfeld MH, Blitzer ML. Follow-up assessments of the pacemaker patient. In: Ellenbogen KA, Wood MA, eds. *Cardiac Pacing and ICDs.* 5th ed. Oxford, UK: Blackwell Publishing; 2008:498-545.
28. Gura MT. Medical jurisprudence. In: Schuring L, Gura MT, Taibi B, eds. *Educational Guidelines: Pacing and Electrophysiology.* 2nd ed. Armonk, NY: Futura Publishing Co.; 1997:165-102.
29. DeBusk RF. Miller NH, Superko R, et al. A case-managed system for coronary risk factor modification after acute myocardial infarction. *Ann Intern Med.* 1994;120(9):721-729.
30. Patrice C, Beard M, Mashburn M. Nurse-managed clinics provide access and improved health care. *Nurse Pract.* 1993;18(5)15-57.
31. Grady KL, Dracup K, Kennedy G, et al. Team management of patients with heart failure. *Circulation.* 2000;102(19):2443-2456.
32. Bramlet DA, King H, Young L, et al. Management of hypercholesterolemia: practice patterns for primary care providers and cardiologists. *Am J Cardiol.* 1997;80(8B):39H-44H.
33. Davidson M. Effect of nurse-directed diabetes care in a minority population. *Diabetes Care.* 2003;26(8):2281-2287.
34. Chiu C. Certification of international allied professionals in cardiac pacing and electrophysiology: opportunities? *Can J Cardiol.* 2010;26(1):e24-e26.
35. Moulton L. New HRS/EHRA expert consensus on monitoring of cardiovascular implantable electronic devices: what this means for the allied professional. *EP Lab Digest.* 2008;8:28. http://www.eplabdigest.com/articles/New-HRSEHRA-Expert-Consensus-Monitoring-Cardiovascular-Implantable-Electronic-Devices. Accessed February 26, 2013.
36. Hayes JJ, Juknavorian R, Maloney JD. NASPE policy statement: the role(s) of the industry employed allied professional. *Pacing Clin Electrophysiol.* 2001;24(3):398-399.
37. Lindsay BD, Estes NAM, Maloney JD, Reynolds DW. Heart Rhythm Society policy statement update: recommendations on the role of industry employed allied professionals (IEAPs). *Heart Rhythm.* 2008;5(11):e8-e10.
38. Daubert JC, Saxon L, Adamson PB, Auricchio A, et al. 2012 EHRA/HRS expert consensus statement on cardiac resynchronization therapy in heart failure: implant and follow-up recommendations and management. *Heart Rhythm.* 2012;9(9):1524-1576.
39. Lewis K, Kumar S, Wilding E. Data management enhances device patient care. September 1, 2006. Medicaldevice-network.com. http://www.medicaldevice-network.com/features/feature737. Accessed February 26, 2013.
40. Chaudhry B, Wang J, Wu S, et al. Systematic review: impact of health information technology on quality, efficiency, and costs of medical care. *Ann Intern Med.* 2006;144 (10):742-752.
41. Carlson MD, Wilkoff BL, Maisel WH, et al. Recommendations from the Heart Rhythm Society Task Force on Device Performance Policies and Guidelines Endorsed by the American College of Cardiology Foundation (ACCF) and the American Heart Association (AHA) and the International Coalition of Pacing and Electrophysiology Organizations (COPE). *Heart Rhythm.* 2006;3(10):1250-1273.
42. Maisel WH. Pacemaker and ICD generator reliability: a meta-analysis of device registries. *JAMA.* 2006;295(16):1929-1934.
43. Furman S. Safe Medical Devices Act of 1990. *Pacing Clin Electrophysiol.* 1991;14:387-388.
44. Samuel FE Jr. Update: legislation. Safe Medical Devices Act of 1990. *Health Aff (Millwood).* 1991 Spring;10(1):192-195.
45. FDA Modernization Act of 1997. *JAMA.* 1998;297:381.
46. Medical Device Amendments of the Food, Drug, and Cosmetic Act. 21 CFR §860.7(e)(1)(1992).
47. Shein MJ, Brinker JA. Pacing the FDA and regulatory environment. In: Ellenbogen KA, Kay GN, Wilkoff BL, eds. *Clinical Cardiac Pacing.* Philadelphia: W.B. Saunders; 1995:809-820.
48. Sweesy MW, Forney RC, Erickson SL, Hull RW. *Arrhythmia Technologies: A Clinical Guide for Self-Assessment and Device Follow-up.* USA: Arrhythmia Technology Institute; 1998.
49. Levine PA. Guidelines to the routine evaluation, programming and follow-up of the patient with an implanted dual-chamber rate-modulated pacing system. Sylmar, CA: St. Jude Medical; 2003.
50. Shah LC, West P, Bremmeyr K, Savoy-Moore RT. Health literacy instrument in family medicine: the "newest vital sign" ease of use and correlates. *J Am Board Fam Med.* 2010;23:195-203.
51. Kirsch IS, Jungeblut A, Jenkins L, Kolstad A. Adult literacy in America: a first look at the findings of the National Adult Literacy Survey. 3rd ed. NCES 1993-275. Washington, DC: U.S. Department of Education National Center for Education Statistics; April 2002.
52. Dickerson PS. Health literacy: who knows what? *Ohio Nurse.* 2010; 393:1.
53. Baker DW, Gazmararian JA, Sudano J, Patterson M. The association between age and health literary among elderly persons. *J Gerontol B Psychol Sci Soc Sci.* 2000;55(6):S368-S374.
54. Fleming JM. A life-threatening communication gap. *Health Literacy.* March 1, 2007. http://www.rdhmag.com/articles/print/volume-27/issue-3/feature/health-literacy.html. Accessed February 26, 2013.
55. Heart Rhythm Society. Patient resources. http://www.hrsonline.org/Patient-Resources. Accessed February 26, 2013.
56. Goldberg Z, Lampert R. Implantable cardioverter-defibrillators: expanding indications and technologies. *JAMA.* 2006;295(7):809-818.
57. Kobza R, Erne P. End-of-life in ICD patients with malignant tumors. *Pacing Clin Electrophysiol.* 2007;30:845-849.
58. Lampert R, Hayes DL, Annas GJ, et al. HRS Expert Consensus Statement on the Management of Cardiovascular Implantable Electronic Devices (CIEDs) in patients nearing end of life or requesting withdrawal of therapy. *Heart Rhythm.* 2010;7(7):1008-1026.
59. Blankenship JC. Bateman TM, Haines DE, et al. ACC expert consensus document on ethic coding and billing practices for cardiovascular medicine specialist. American College of Cardiology. *J Am Coll Cardiol.* 1999;33(4):1076-1086.
60. The Heart Rhythm Society. *Coding Guide: 2013.* coding@HRSonline.org. Accessed June 26, 2013.
61. American Medical Association. *CPT 2013 Professional Edition.* American Medical Association; 2012.

CHAPTER 56

Postoperative Management and Follow-up of Cardiac Rhythm Management Devices

Bharat K. Kantharia, MD; Arti N. Shah, MD

Cardiac Rhythm Management

Cardiac rhythm management (CRM) devices, which include permanent pacemakers (PPMs) and implantable cardioverter-defibrillators (ICDs) are now being implanted in an increasing number of patients, in part due to an expansion of indications for CRM therapy. The incorporation of a left ventricular (LV) pacing lead, in addition to a right ventricular (RV) lead to both PPMs and ICDs, allows these devices to be used for cardiac resynchronization therapy (CRT-P, and CRT-D, respectively). CRT has now been demonstrated to improve heart failure symptoms, reduce hospitalizations for heart failure, and improve mortality in drug-refractory heart failure subpopulations.[1,2] Generally, placement of CRM devices is considered to be a very safe procedure. However, the safety of these procedures is still highly dependent on the operator as well as several patient factors. Favorable outcomes are highly dependent on meticulous attention to preoperative, procedural, and postprocedure care. The focus of this chapter will be on the postoperative management of patients undergoing CRM device insertion.

Postprocedure Care

Complications related to device insertion have been decreasing with improved training and experience of implanting physicians, better patient selection, and advances in CRM device technology. Postoperative complications can be classified as "acute" (within 24 hours), "subacute" (1–7 days), and "late," indicating that they occur later than 7 days (Table 56.1). By definition, complications requiring surgical intervention are classified as major complications. Bleeding requiring transfusion, strokes, and several other procedure-related complications also are considered major in the absence of surgical intervention. At any time after device implantation, infections that require surgical intervention are considered major complications. Infections at any time after device implantations, which require surgical intervention, are considered major complications.

Most CRM device implantation procedures are now performed in the cardiac catheterization or electrophysiology laboratory. These procedures are generally performed using local anesthesia and conscious sedation typically using agents such as midazolam and fentanyl. Supplemental anesthetic agents such as propofol, considered to be a general anesthetic, are commonly used selectively, such as at the time of defibrillation testing or during more extensive lead tunneling procedures. Less commonly, CRM implantation procedures are performed in the operating room or with the use of general anesthesia for the entire case. Like other routine surgery, the postoperative management of most of the patients undergoing CRM device implantation is comprised of multiple standard steps developed to optimize outcomes. Thus, postoperative complications are best discussed as part of postoperative routine and specific management steps.

Table 56.1 Common postoperative complications of CRM devices

Acute (within 24 hours)
- Bleeding and pocket hematoma
- Pneumothorax and hemothorax
- Perforation, pericardial effusion, and cardiac tamponade
- Lead dislodgement
- Device malfunction: failure to sense, failure to pace, inappropriate shocks, etc.

Subacute (1–7 days)
- Bleeding and pocket hematoma
- Pneumothorax and hemothorax
- Perforation, pericardial effusion, and cardiac tamponade
- Lead dislodgement
- Lead insulation failure and/or coil fracture
- Device malfunction: failure to sense, failure to pace, inappropriate shocks, etc.
- Vascular thrombosis: upper extremity swelling
- Infection

Chronic (more than 7 days)
- Lead insulation failure and/or coil fracture
- Device malfunction: failure to sense, failure to pace, inappropriate shocks, etc.
- Vascular thrombosis: upper extremity swelling
- Infection: pocket and skin infection, sepsis, and endocarditis
- Twiddler's syndrome

Routine Postoperative Evaluation

Following CRM device implantation, patients are generally observed in the recovery or the postoperative telemetry units with careful assessment of their vital signs, level of consciousness, pain, and cardiac rhythm. Analgesics such as acetaminophen with or without codeine are prescribed to minimize postoperative pain. Occasionally oxycodone or other narcotics are needed for more severe pain. Discomfort after CRM device implantation is variable and dependent on multiple factors such as age, comorbidities, procedure length, type of anesthesia, and individual patient pain tolerance. Those patients who undergo uneventful device generator replacements may be fed, ambulated, and discharged within a few hours of the procedure. By contrast, patients who undergo a new device and lead implantation or require a new lead or lead revision at the time of device replacement should be kept on bed rest for several hours. Generally these patients are kept overnight for pain control and assessment of their clinical status. Clinically appropriate monitoring allows early detection and treatment of any potential postprocedure complications.

On the day following implantation of a new ICD system or lead, it would be considered the current standard of care to clinically assess the patient, inspect the incision, obtain a 12-lead ECG, and obtain chest radiographs in the anteroposterior and lateral views. In addition, a comprehensive assessment of sensing, capture, and lead impedances should be performed. With these steps, several acute complications may be identified promptly and addressed. Pacing and sensing issues can be identified. Inadvertent placement of a ventricular lead through a patent foramen ovale into the left ventricle can be suspected by an abnormal ECG showing a right bundle branch block (RBBB) paced configuration rather than the standard left bundle branch block (LBBB) patterns found with RV pacing. Chest radiographs in the anteroposterior and lateral views (Figure 56.1) and a transthoracic echocardiogram (Figure 56.2) can identify this error in lead placement. Early postoperative recognition of the problem can prompt the removal and repositioning of the lead in the right ventricular apex in a timely manner, prior to chronic fixation of the lead in the left ventricle. Right ventricular lead perforation with left ventricular stimulation can also produce a RBBB pattern, and lead withdrawal and relocation may be necessary. Comprehensive assessment of CRM devices prior to hospital discharge can identify sensing issues as well. For example, in a patient with hypertrophic cardiomyopathy receiving an ICD for primary prevention of sudden death, device evaluation prior to discharge revealed T-wave oversensing (Figure 56.3), which could not be eliminated with reprogramming. A new rate-sensing lead had to be inserted to eliminate the risk of inappropriate ICD shocks.

Discharge Instructions

Patients are instructed to minimize ipsilateral arm movement for 6 to 8 hours immediately after the procedure and are commonly given a sling for short-term use. While a single dose of antibiotics is considered to be the standard of care immediately prior to the procedure, antibiotics are not given in the postoperative period based on current recommendations.[18] At our center, most patients are discharged home after being counseled regarding the need for daily dressing changes and for keeping the incision dry for 1 week following the procedure. Patients are instructed on recognition of early signs of complications, such as fever, local redness or pain, and swelling suggesting a pocket hematoma; they are given specific instructions to contact the medical team in such instances or if there are any other concerns. In general, driving should be avoided until recovery from the procedure is complete to avoid lead dislodgement or incision dehiscence.

Chapter 56: Postoperative Management and Follow-up of Cardiac Rhythm Management Devices

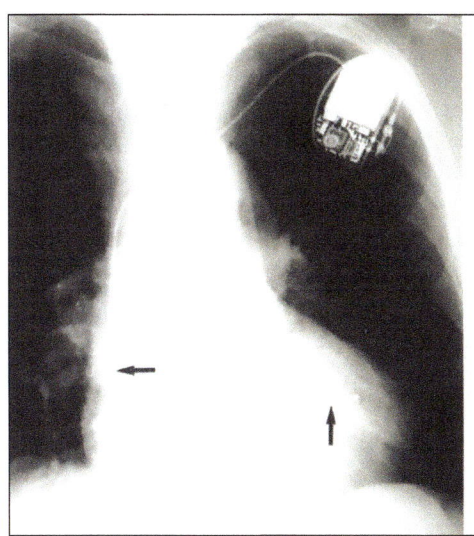
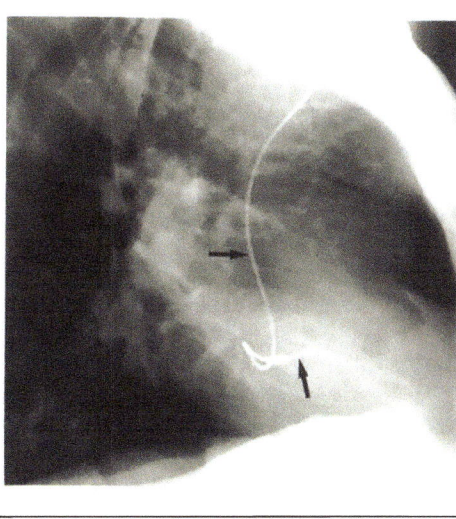

Figure 56.1 Following implantation of a single chamber pacemaker, postoperative chest radiographs (anteroposterior view on the left, and lateral view on the right) show the course of the lead (**black arrows**) through patent foramen ovale into the left ventricle.

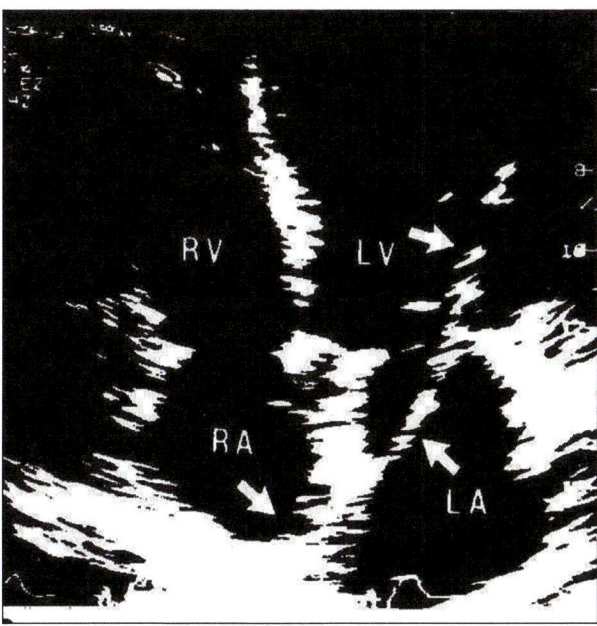

Figure 56.2 Apical 4-chamber view of transthoracic echocardiogram shows the course of the ventricular lead through patent foramen ovale from the right atrium (RA) into the left atrium (LA) and to the left ventricle (LV).

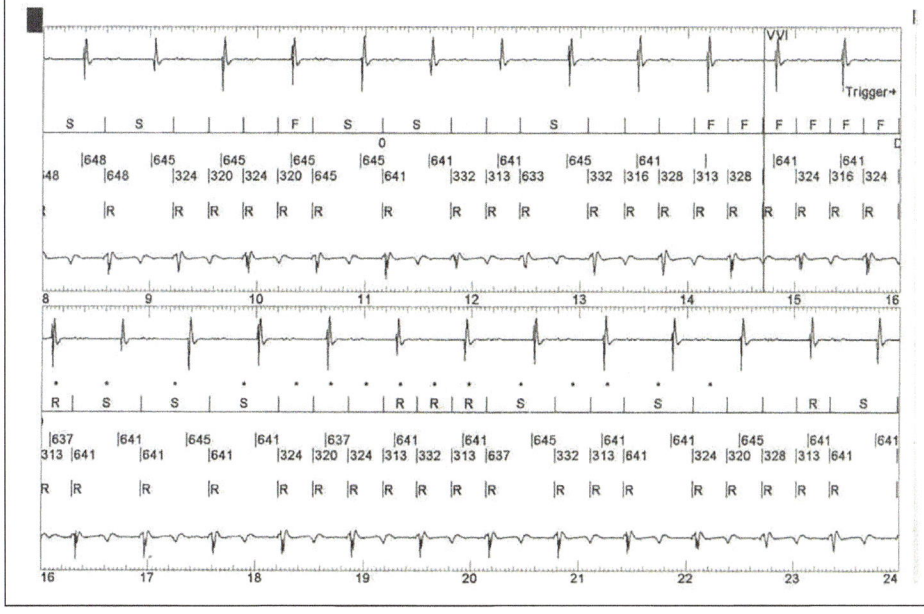

Figure 56.3 Interrogation of a dual-chamber ICD shows T-wave oversensing. The top, middle, and bottom panels are the atrial, marker, and ventricular channels, respectively. The device detected occurrence of multiple short, coupled R waves corresponding to T waves as fast (F) ventricular fibrillation rhythm (**right-hand corner of the top strip**); however, therapy was delivered, as failure to oversense T waves intermittently (**left-hand corner of the bottom strip**) resets the detection algorithm.

Driving Instructions

For those patients who receive ICD or CRT-D devices, instructions related to driving should be addressed prior to discharge. Patients should be counseled that impairment of consciousness potentially related to a spontaneous arrhythmic event is possible despite ICD insertion. Driving recommendations vary depending on whether the device is placed for primary or secondary prevention of sudden cardiac death and whether the patient has a standard or commercial license. Based on a scientific statement from the American Heart Association and the Heart Rhythm Society published in 2007,[3] "no driving" is recommended for those with a standard license for at least 1 week after implantation for patients receiving a primary prevention device to allow for recovery from implantation procedure. For patients receiving a device for secondary prevention with a standard license, driving is restricted for 6 months. In addition, driving is restricted for a period of 6 months also for any patient with a primary or secondary prevention device who receives appropriate shock therapy. In the absence of symptoms potentially related to cardiac arrhythmias, such as chest pain, dyspnea, palpitations, marked lightheadedness, frank loss of consciousness, and shocks from the ICD, these patients may continue to drive private automobiles. Those patients who receive ICDs for secondary prevention of sudden cardiac death are recommended not to drive for a minimum event-free period of 6 months. A similar recommendation is also made to those patients who are implanted with ICDs for primary prevention but subsequently get appropriately treated for VT and VF. Furthermore, patients who receive appropriate shocks for VT and VF are prohibited from driving school buses as well as public and commercial automobiles.

Management of Postoperative ICD Shocks

Patients and their family members are instructed to seek emergency medical attention in case of even a single shock from the ICDs in the postoperative follow-up period. This is due to the fact that in the acute and subacute postoperative follow-up period, an inappropriate shock may result from lead dislodgement or atrial fibrillation with rapid ventricular response, or appropriately from episodes of VT and VF.[4] All such situations require immediate attention and appropriate intervention. Before their discharge from the hospital, the patients are given their CRM identification cards as well as follow-up instructions.

Management of Postoperative Complications and In-hospital Care

In the following section, some specific issues and complications that may arise in the immediate postoperative period and their management are discussed.

Bleeding and Pocket Hematoma

Although it is difficult to ascertain the true incidence of postoperative pocket hematomas in general clinical practice, it is estimated to be approximately 2.0% to 5.0%.[5,6] In a systematic review of implantation-related complications of ICDs and CRTs reported in randomized clinical trials, van Rees et al noted the incidence of pocket hematomas in 2.2% of nonthoracotomy ICD recipients and 2.4% in the CRT device recipients.[5] The true incidence of pocket hematomas is likely to be higher, as most randomized trials reported only those hematomas requiring evacuation and drainage. In a study by Wiegand et al,[6] high-dose heparin, combined aspirin and thienopyridine treatment after coronary stenting, and low operator experience were found to be independent predictors for development of postoperative hematoma. In patients with atrial fibrillation, postoperative high-dose heparin substantially increases the hematoma rate without reducing the rate of embolic events within the first month after implantation of a CRM device.[6] Likewise, in patients with a mechanical aortic valve requiring anticoagulation, a minimalist strategy of simply withholding oral anticoagulation provides similar results of quality-adjusted life expectancy (QALE) as an aggressive strategy of administering perioperative subcutaneous low-molecular-weight heparin or intravenous heparin.[7] Although the latter aggressive approach provides greater QALE for patients with mechanical mitral valves who are at higher risk of stroke, the benefit is small. Elimination of postoperative use of low-molecular-weight heparin substantially reduces hematoma rates.[8]

Continuation of oral anticoagulation until the procedure does not necessarily increase complications such as hemoatomas. In a randomized, prospective trial of strategies for performing ICD implantation procedures on maintenance oral anticoagulant therapy continued on the day of the procedure versus stopping oral anticoagulants and transitioning with intravenous heparin, the incidence of postoperative hematomas was similar, indicating that continuation of oral anticoagulation within acceptable international normalized ratios (INRs) of around 2.0 can be safe at experienced centers.[9] Meticulous attention to hemostasis is required at the time of the procedure to obtain such outcomes. There are also commercially available topical products consisting of thrombin or fibrin sealant that may be used intraoperatively to reduce the risk of pocket hematomas when a lack of hemostasis occurs with conventional measures.[10]

Once pocket hematomas develop, they should be treated conservatively with local compressive bandage dressings. If the hematoma expands significantly or causes stretch and tension over the skin, thereby compromising skin capillary perfusion and leading to potential wound dehiscence and necrosis, or if the hematoma results in significant pain, then exploration and evacuation of the pocket becomes necessary. At the time of reopening and exploration of the pocket, besides removal of the entire collection of clots, the wound is thoroughly cleaned and inspected for any active bleeding, which may need cauterization or ligation. If the patient is treated with long-term anticoagulation, the interior of the wound may be treated with topical thrombin before closing it. Surgical intervention in the postoperative period is associated with a much higher risk (up to 15-fold) for pocket and device infection.[11] Pocket drainage with percutaneous aspiration is contraindicated due to the considerable risk of infection being introduced into the pocket from the skin.

Infection

Prevention

Postoperative infection is a major and feared complication of device insertion. It is more likely in prolonged, complex procedures. Preventative measures play an important role in avoiding this problem. With increasing operator experience and improved device technology to abbreviate the operative time, stricter sterilization and aseptic precautions taken at the time of implantation proc edure, and proper prophylactic antibiotic measures taken preoperatively, the infection rate related to CRM device implantation has decreased considerably. In clinical studies, specific precautions can reduce this complication. Preoperative antibiotic therapy administered within 1 hour of the procedure is recommended by current standards of care. Other clinical studies support the use of antiseptic impregnated skin barriers and double gloving during implant procedures. Other investigational approaches being considered are the use of antibiotic-impregnated device pouches for device placement within the pocket.

Management

Although it is difficult to estimate the true incidence of infection of CRM devices postoperatively, it is considered to be fairly low at less than 5%.[11-16] Among the clinical variables, presence of diabetes mellitus, heart failure, and renal insufficiency have been recognized as risk factors for postoperative infection of CRM devices.[17] The occurrence of infection correlates positively with fever within 24 hours before the implantation procedure, use of temporary pacing before the implantation procedure, and early reinterventions. Infection incidence negatively correlates with implantation of a new system and antibiotic prophylaxis.[11] Most CRM device-related infections in the acute and subacute setting occur from *Staphylococcus aureus* or *S. epidermis*, and rarely from other organisms such as *Enterococcus*, *Propionobacter*, *Pseudomonas*, and *Proteus* species. In most cases, periprocedure erythema and inflammation around the incision indicative of superficial infection can be treated safely with systemic and topical antibiotics. In the acute or subacute postoperative setting, when a deep device pocket is involved and there are no signs of improvement over time

despite a trial of antibiotic therapy, total removal of the entire system is necessary.[15,16] In one series, up to 5% of CRM devices needed to be removed within a short postoperative period.[12] Most CRM device-related infections with or without signs of generalized sepsis become apparent after 3 months of device implantation. In the event of device erosion through skin (Figure 56.4), total removal of the CRM device with attached leads is recommended. Total removal of the CRM system is also recommended in the event of device-related endocarditis. Vegetation on the leads and valves from CRM device-related endocarditis are better visualized by transesophageal echocardiography (▶ Video 56.1).

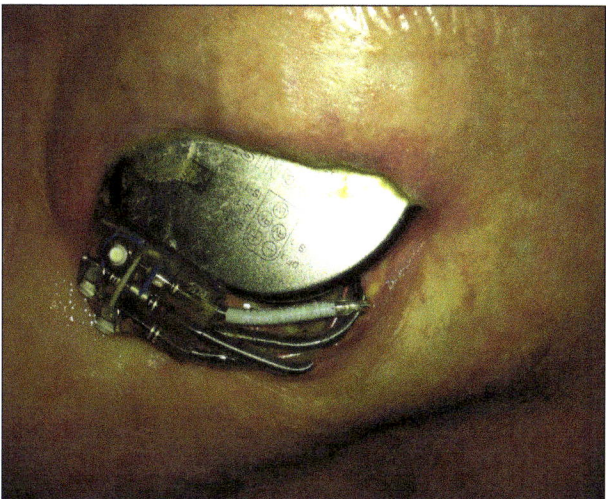

Figure 56.4 Frank erosion of infected ICD and the attached leads through the skin is visible.

Lead Dislodgement and Perforation

Dislodgement

Acute lead dislodgement usually occurs within 24 to 48 hours after implantation of CRM devices. The reported incidence of acute lead dislodgement varies from 1.8% to 4%.[11,12] While any type of leads may dislodge, the risks are higher with coronary sinus (CS) leads and passive fixation leads. The dislodgement rate also depends on the operator's experience and the implantation techniques. Specifically, appropriate positioning in stable regions, proper active fixation helix deployment, and securing leads with anchoring sleeves are important in reducing the risk of dislodgement. The routine practice of applying an arm immobilizer to minimize traction on the lead may minimize acute lead dislodgement. Failures to sense or pace, inappropriate lead impedance on device interrogation, or frequent ectopy are some of the signs that may indicate lead dislodgement. One such example is shown in ▶ Video 56.2. Dislodgement of a CS lead into the pulmonary artery in a patient in whom insertion of the CS lead was technically challenging was identified on postoperative day #3 due to loss of LV capture and frequent ventricular ectopic beats (Video 56.2). While gross displacement can be easily seen by chest radiography, microdislodgement of a lead may not be appreciated radiographically, even with use of multiple views. Lead dislodgement can impair accurate sensing. For example, inappropriate mode switching due to sensing of far-field R waves lead to detection of atrial lead dislodgement from its original site to the tricuspid annulus (Figure 56.5). This required lead repositioning. Immediate repositioning of the dislodged lead or its removal and replacement by a new lead if the active fixation mechanism is deemed to have failed is strongly recommended in such situations. Dislodgement of a right ventricular ICD lead may cause significant problems with appropriate sensing and therapy of VT and VF.

Perforation

The incidence of early postoperative lead perforation is very rare. In a large Mayo Clinic series comprising 4,280 patients who underwent PPM implantation, the incidence of detection of pericardial effusion related to lead perforation was 1.2%.[18] By multivariate analysis, the use of a temporary pacemaker, helical screw leads, and use of steroids were identified as the predictors of lead perforation.[18] Most immediate postoperative lead perforations are the perforations that occur during the time of surgery but are not recognized. In this situation, progressive accumulation of blood in the pericardial space may result in pain, and ultimately cardiac tamponade, necessitating emergent drainage of pericardial effusion either percutaneously (Video 56.3, Video 56.4, and Video 56.5) or surgically. In addition, the perforated lead requires repositioning. Abnormal pacing and sensing parameters, usually with marked difference in the unipolar and bipolar sensing, and inappropriate lead impedance on device interrogation occurs with lead perforation. In one series utilizing CT scans, up to 15% of cases of late lead perforation that were asymptomatic and posed no major performance issues were identified.[19] Although such late lead perforation may be truly "late," it may represent unrecognized asymptomatic acute perforation as well.

Pneumothorax and Hemothorax

Inadvertent injury to the lung resulting in pneumothorax can be prevented by accessing the extrathoracic venous system, for example via the cephalic vein by a surgical cutdown, or the axillary vein under fluoroscopic, venography, and ultrasound guidance.[20-22] However, for de novo CRM device implantation or at the time of device upgrades where the subclavian vein may be the only access point available for insertion of additional leads, the subclavian venous access may result in pneumothorax. Data derived from many large ICD and CRT trials in which the patients received nonthoracotomy devices indicate that the incidence of pneumothorax related to CRM device implantation in recent years has fallen relatively low. In one report, a pneumothorax was observed in 14 of 1,497 ICD implantations (0.9%) and in 30 of 3,300 CRT implantations (0.9%).[5] An upright chest x-ray must be routinely performed immediately upon completion of the procedure for all patients in whom subclavian vein was used primarily for venous access and if multiple attempts were made to access axillary vein. Use of micropuncture needles can be valuable in minimizing this risk.

Irrespective of the venous access point, all patients should undergo chest x-ray examination on the day after the procedure. Most small pneumothoraces that do not result in respiratory or hemodynamic compromise may be observed closely without any intervention, and they resolve spontaneously over a period of time. If there is no evidence of further increase in the size and severity of pneumothorax with follow-up chest x-rays over 24 to 48 hours, and if the patient has no symptoms or signs of respiratory distress, it is safe to discharge the patient home. These patients are followed up in an outpatient

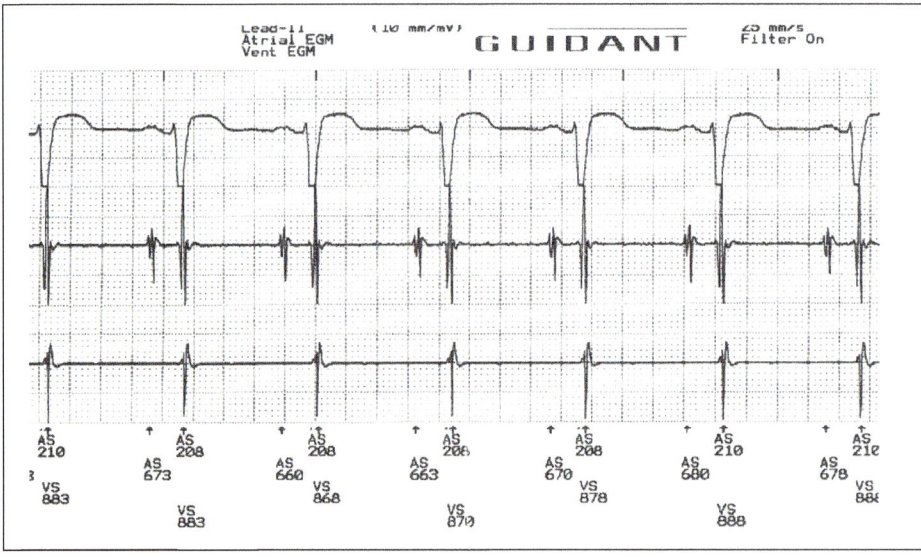

Figure 56.5 Interrogation of a dual-chamber ICD shows sensing of far-field R waves by the atrial lead. The top, middle, and bottom panels are the surface lead II, atrial, and ventricular channels. On the atrial channel, two atrially sensed events (AS) are seen in succession; the second one occurs in time with the ventricular sensed event (VS) and corresponds with the QRS complexes on the surface ECG. This occurred due to dislodgement of the atrial lead from its position in the right atrial appendage location to lower in the right atrium in the proximity of the tricuspid valve.

office in 7 to 10 days for further clinical and radiological evaluation of pneumothorax. On the other hand, medium to large pneumothoraces, and those resulting in pain, respiratory distress, and hemodynamic compromise, need to be treated surgically with insertion of chest drain.

Hemothorax is a relatively rare complication to occur in the postoperative follow-up period as it results from major vascular injury during surgery. These can be related to use of large-caliber sheaths and leads or to attempts to insert leads in stenosed and partially occluded subclavian veins. They can also occur as complications of lead extraction procedures and use of extraction devices. Most hemothoraces require surgical drainage, as prolonged observation for complete resorption is generally unsuccessful for moderate size or larger collections, which organize and can cause loculated collections and/or fibrosis in the pleural cavity.

Diaphragmatic Stimulation

Diaphragmatic stimulation can occur either if a ventricular lead penetrates through the ventricular wall and the paced stimuli causes direct diaphragmatic stimulation or if the pacing lead is positioned close to a phrenic nerve in the lateral right atrium or lateral left ventricular epicardium. In the former instance, interrogation of the device can show myopotentials detected on the ventricular electrogram channel. Appearance of new diaphragmatic stimulation in the acute postoperative setting indicates lead perforation or dislodgement; the ventricular or atrial lead must be promptly repositioned. In cases of CRT device implantations, diaphragmatic stimulation indicates left phrenic nerve capture by paced stimuli energy delivered through the coronary sinus lead. This may occur if the CS lead gets displaced from its original implant site, but it may also occur due to proximity of the left phrenic nerve occurring with particular body positions that could not be tested at the time of implantation. Administration of any muscle-relaxing agents at the time of CRT device implantation must be avoided so that phrenic nerve capture resulting in diaphragmatic contractions may be easily identified during lead threshold testing. In case of the phrenic nerve capture by the CS lead and unstable or unavailable alternative locations, new multipolar lead technology may be helpful. This offers options of different pacing site configurations that may help in resolving the issue rather than repositioning the lead.

Outpatient Device Follow-up

A comprehensive plan for follow-up after CRM device implant should be based on the Heart Rhythm Society and the European Heart Rhythm Association expert consensus document on monitoring of cardiovascular implantable electronic devices.[23] At minimum, patients with CRM devices should be seen at 1 week, 1 month, and 3 months initially after their implantations, and on a regular schedule thereafter (Table 56.2). Single-chamber pacemaker patients are seen annually, and dual-chamber pacemaker patients are seen every 6 months for the first 5 years. Frequency of these visits increases thereafter as battery longevity dictates and can approach monthly follow-ups near the end of the life of the device battery, especially in pacemaker-dependent patients. ICD patients are evaluated every 3 to 4 months, but alternate evaluations can be achieved with remote monitoring.

Clinic Visits: At each outpatient follow-up visit, the patients should receive a history and physical examination. Any specific issues related to CRM devices, for example, ICD shocks, anxiety, fear, depression, change in the health status, and so forth, must also be dealt with as necessary. The protocol of CRM device follow-up must not be rigid. There should be a regular and open communication link between the patients and the physicians and other healthcare providers. There should be provisions for the patients to be seen even at their unscheduled office visits and to make necessary changes in the device programming or performing any medical intervention as necessary. This practice is strongly encouraged in an event the patient receives ICD shocks, as appropriate reprogramming may be necessary. An example of a patient receiving an appropriate shock for a regular monomorphic VT event is shown in Figure 56.6. The patient was subsequently hospitalized on a regular telemetry unit. The device was reprogrammed to two zones, for VT and VF with overdrive antitachycardia pacing (ATP) programmed as initial therapies for the VT zone. Subsequent episodes of VT were successfully treated by the ATP therapies. Good teamwork between the physicians, specialist device nurses, other healthcare providers, and the industry support personnel is mandatory.

On the first outpatient visit (day 7–10 postimplantation), specific attention is paid to wound care. The Steri-strips, and when applicable the sutures, are removed. The pocket is also assessed for any evidence of hematoma and infection. Typically, the device is not interrogated unless necessary on the first visit within 7 to 10 days. The patient and the family are further counseled for standard CRM device care and follow-up. At this stage, the concept of an ICD support group is introduced to the patient and the family, all of whom are encouraged to participate in the ICD support group activities. On the next scheduled visit, the devices is interrogated and necessary programming adjustments are made (eg, adjusting parameters for rate-responsive pacing). In a nonpacemaker-dependent patient, reprogramming the device parameters including adjusting the timing of AV delays and reducing pacing outputs to provide adequate safety margin to conserve battery longevity is carried out. At the 3-month follow-up visit, further programming changes are made (eg, introducing an autocapture feature and/or reducing pacing current output in the pacemaker-dependent patient to provide adequate safety margin and yet minimizing battery drainage).

Table 56.2 Postoperative care of cardiac rhythm management (CRM) devices

OPERATIVE DAY #0: Clinical observation on a telemetry unit

- Sterile dressing over the incision
- Pressure dressing if ongoing treatment with anticoagulants
- Arm immobilizer/arm sling
- Portable chest x-ray to assess position of the leads and device generator, integrity of the device system, procedure-related complications such as pneumothorax
- 12-lead ECG to assess pacing characteristics

POSTOPERATIVE DAY #1: Predischarge clinical assessment; symptoms/signs of well-being, infection, bleeding, hematoma, dressing removal, assessment of the incision and device pocket area, etc.

- Analgesia; for example acetaminophen, with or without narcotics such as codeine, at 6–8 hourly intervals if necessary
- Arm immobilizer/arm sling and instructions to avoid arm movement above the shoulder level
- Chest x-ray (anteroposterior and lateral views)
- 12-lead ECG
- Device interrogation and adjustments in any parameters if necessary; for example "mode switch" for atrial arrhythmias
- Predischarge noninvasive program stimulation electrophysiology study and/or defibrillation threshold testing in patients with defibrillators implanted for secondary prevention of VT and VF to further adjust and add detection zones and therapies; for example, antitachycardia pacing for VT, in patients implanted with ICDs for secondary prevention of sudden cardiac death
- Predischarge counseling of patients (and family members) about CRM postoperative "Dos and Don'ts," especially strenuous activities (allow light movement at the shoulder area but do not lift heavy objects), bathing (allow shower but do not scrub directly on the incision area), indulgence in sexual activities, and, especially for patients with defibrillators about shocks, driving, etc.

POSTOPERATIVE DAYS #7–10: Outpatient clinic (office) visit

- Clinical assessment; symptoms/signs of well-being, infection, bleeding, hematoma, etc.
- Assessment of the incision, suture removal if necessary
- Device interrogation if clinically indicated; for example, lead dislodgement suspected
- Encourage moderate level of shoulder movement
- Counseling of patients (and family members) with defibrillators about shocks, driving, etc., and encourage participation in ICD support group activities

POSTOPERATIVE WEEKS #4–6: Outpatient clinic (office) visit

- Clinical assessment; symptoms/signs of well-being, infection etc.
- Assessment of the incision and device pocket area
- Device interrogation and adjustments in any parameters if necessary; for example, turning the pacing output when appropriate to conserve battery life, addition of monitor zones for ventricular tachycardia, antitachycardia pacing therapy, etc.
- Counseling of patients (and family members) with defibrillators about shocks, driving, etc., and encourage participation in ICD support group activities
- Set up remote monitoring of the CRM device if possible

POSTOPERATIVE MONTHS #3–4: Outpatient clinic (office) visit

- Clinical assessment; symptoms/signs of well-being, infection, etc.
- Assessment of the incision and device pocket area
- Device interrogation and adjustments in any parameters if necessary; for example, turning the pacing output when appropriate to conserve battery life, addition of monitor zones for ventricular tachycardia, antitachycardia pacing therapy, etc.
- Consideration of DFT testing in patients in whom amiodarone was just started around the time of implantation and considered to have full amiodarone loading and subsequent maintenance long-term amiodarone therapy
- Counseling of patients (and family members) with defibrillators about shocks, driving, etc., and encourage participation in ICD support group activities
- Set up remote monitoring of the CRM device if possible

POSTOPERATIVE MONTHS #6–7: Outpatient clinic (office) visit

- Clinical assessment; symptoms/signs of well-being, infection, etc.
- Assessment of the incision and device pocket area
- Device interrogation and adjustments in any parameters if necessary; for example, turning the pacing output when appropriate to conserve battery life, addition of monitor zones for ventricular tachycardia, antitachycardia pacing therapy, etc.
- Consideration of DFT testing, if not already done, in patients with long-term amiodarone therapy
- Counseling of patients (and family members) with defibrillators about shocks, driving, etc., and encourage participation in ICD support group activities
- Set up remote monitoring of the CRM device if possible

POSTOPERATIVE MONTH 12: Outpatient clinic (office) visit

- Clinical assessment; symptoms/signs of well-being, infection, etc.
- Assessment of the incision and device pocket area
- Device interrogation and adjustments in any parameters if necessary; for example, turning the pacing output when appropriate to conserve battery life, addition of monitor zones for ventricular tachycardia, antitachycardia pacing therapy, etc.
- Consideration of DFT testing, if not already done at previous follow-ups, in patients with long-term amiodarone therapy
- Counseling of patients (and family members) with defibrillators about shocks, driving, etc., and encourage participation in ICD support group activities
- Set up remote monitoring of the CRM device if possible
- Transthoracic echocardiogram in patients with CRT devices to assess cardiac function and guide programming of cardiac resynchronization pacing parameters when appropriate

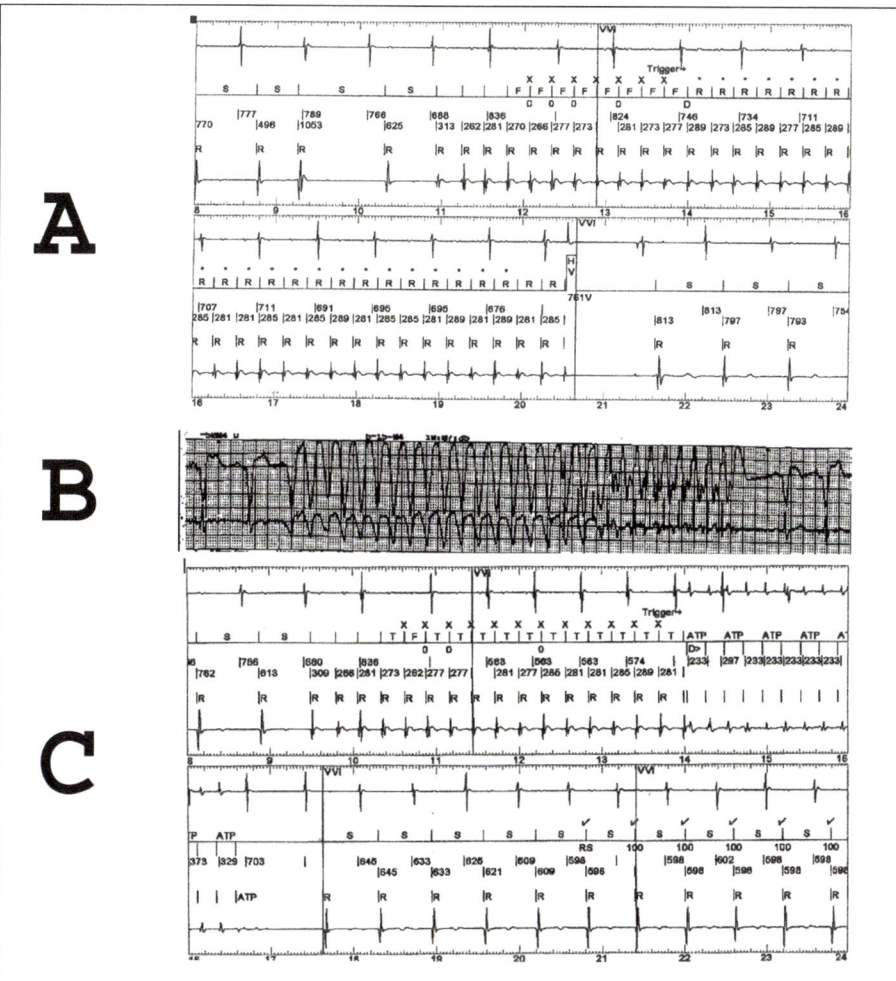

Figure 56.6 Interrogation of a dual-chamber ICD shows appropriate shock from a regular monomorphic ventricular tachycardia (VT) that was subsequently treated with overdrive antitachyardia pacing (ATP) therapies after reprogramming of the device. For the ICD interrogation strips (**A** and **B**), the top, middle, and bottom panels are the atrial, marker, and ventricular channels. A regular rapid VT with ventriculoatrial dissociation is clearly seen in **Panel A**. However, since the device was programmed for only one zone, this rhythm was determined to be ventricular fibrillation and appropriately treated with high-voltage shock to successfully restore sinus rhythm. The same arrhythmia after reprogramming the device to two zones (VT and VF) now falls into the VT zone and terminated to sinus rhythm with programmed ATP therapy. The whole episode as captured on regular telemetry in the hospital is shown in **Panel B**.

Empiric ICD Device Programming: Shock therapy delivery has been shown to be associated with worse cardiovascular outcomes, including mortality, in the MADIT-2 and SCD-HeFT studies.[25] Fully two-thirds of these shocks are not delivered appropriately. In patients with ICDs implanted for primary prevention, further fine-tuning of ICD programming is made to avoid inappropriate shocks (eg, programming the sudden onset criterion, and/or turn the morphology discriminators "ON" to avoid inappropriate shocks). To further limit inappropriate shocks, the Primary Prevention Parameters Evaluation (PREPARE) study's programming strategies can be considered.[26] In the PREPARE study, the devices were programmed as follows: (1) VT/VF rates ≥ 182 bpm; (2) VT/VF maintained for at least 30 of 40 beats; (3) ATP as first therapy for fast VTs with rates of 182 to 250 bpm; (4) SVT discriminators for rhythms ≥ 200 bpm; and (5) high-output first shock. Such key programming strategies were intended to detect only fast and sustained tachycardias and allow quick treatment for rapid ventricular tachyarrhythmias. Programming devices in this manner resulted in the morbidity index (the combined incidence of device-delivered shocks, arrhythmic syncope, and untreated sustained symptomatic VT/VF) to be significantly lower at 0.26 events/patient-year versus 0.69 events/patient-year in the control setting.[25] More recently, the MADIT-RIT study showed marked benefits of programming a single-shock-only zone above 200 bpm with a 2.5-second delay or a rhythm detection algorithm with a 60-second delay at heart rates of 170 to 199 bpm, a 12-second delay at a rate of 200 to 249 bpm, and a 2.5-second delay at ≥ 250 bpm.[27]

There are device manufacturers' specific discriminatory algorithms available for both single- and dual-chamber ICDs.[28] In the simplest terms, for the most part sudden onset of arrhythmia defines VT, and irregularity rather than stability in beat-to-beat cycle length defines atrial fibrillation in single-chamber devices. When the wavelets during tachycardia are uniform and match with the ones acquired during sinus rhythm, the arrhythmia is classified as supraventricular in origin; in contrast, when the wavelets are different and discordant, the device classifies the rhythm as ventricular in origin. For dual-chamber devices, the algorithms take atrial (A) and ventricular (V) rates in account to discriminate arrhythmias. For the most part, V > A defines VT, A > V defines atrial arrhythmias, and A = V would suggest SVT or VT and would need additional criteria to further define the arrhythmia.

Many times, despite such programming, patients continue to receive inappropriate therapies in the form of ATPs and shocks. To err on the side of caution, ICDs deliver programmed therapies for VT and VF even for SVTs when the ventricular rate is very rapid. This is highlighted in Figures 56.7 and 56.8. In this young patient with dilated nonischemic cardiomyopathy, a single-chamber ICD (Medtronic, Minneapolis, MN) was implanted for secondary prevention of VT and VF following successful resuscitation from cardiac arrest due to VT that degenerated to VF. She presented with multiple ICD shocks. The device interrogation showed both appropriate therapies (ATP for VT, Figure 56.7) and inappropriate therapies (shocks) for SVT with rapid ventricular rate (Figure 56.8). It is noteworthy that while the wavelet template match—a discriminatory criterion to diagnose the episode to be either from SVT or VT—was useful to correctly identify a somewhat slower and wider complex VT (Figure 56.7), the wavelet templates were not applied in spite of a high percentage of match to baseline sinus rhythm template for the episode of SVT because the rate was too fast, resulting in the patient receiving defibrillator shocks (Figure 56.8). Additional therapeutic options should be considered for patients who continue to receive ICD shocks, whether the shocks are appropriate or inappropriate, as both types of shocks are associated with marked increased in the subsequent risk of death, particularly death from progressive heart failure. An example of inappropriate shocks due to atrial flutter is shown in Figure 56.9. In this patient, a curative radiofrequency ablation of atrial flutter was performed, after which he never experienced inappropriate shocks from atrial flutter.

Outpatient Device Data Management: At each follow-up visit, systematic interrogation of the CRM device is performed, and the data is recorded and maintained, preferably electronically, in the patient's chart. Data on battery voltage, replacement indicators, pacing and high voltage lead impedances, pacing and sensing threshold, the percentage of pacing in different chambers, activity logs, the number of mode switches, and arrhythmia burden are collected. The modern devices also provide data on autonomic function, heart rate variability, and fluid status to reflect underlying heart failure status. In cases of ICDs, particular attention is paid to the event logs. All stored electrograms of appropriate and inappropriate shocks and overdrive antitachycardia pacing therapies are downloaded and scrutinized to take further actions such as medication changes, hospitalization for further treatment, and ablation of specific arrhythmias.

Remote Device Monitoring: Recently, most major device manufacturers have introduced their unique version of "remote monitoring" technology that allows home transmitters to interrogate devices and download and transmit collected and stored data using the Internet to a protected network.[28-31] Remote monitoring has not only rapidly shifted the paradigm in device follow-up, but also it allows early intervention in management of patients with CRM devices.[32] For many years, remote follow-up was limited only to pacemakers and was only available via transtelephonic monitoring (TTM), which could provide information, albeit limited, on battery status, pacing, and sensing.[1] With the advent of wireless devices and widespread Internet access, TTM is not preferred and is being phased out of clinical practice.

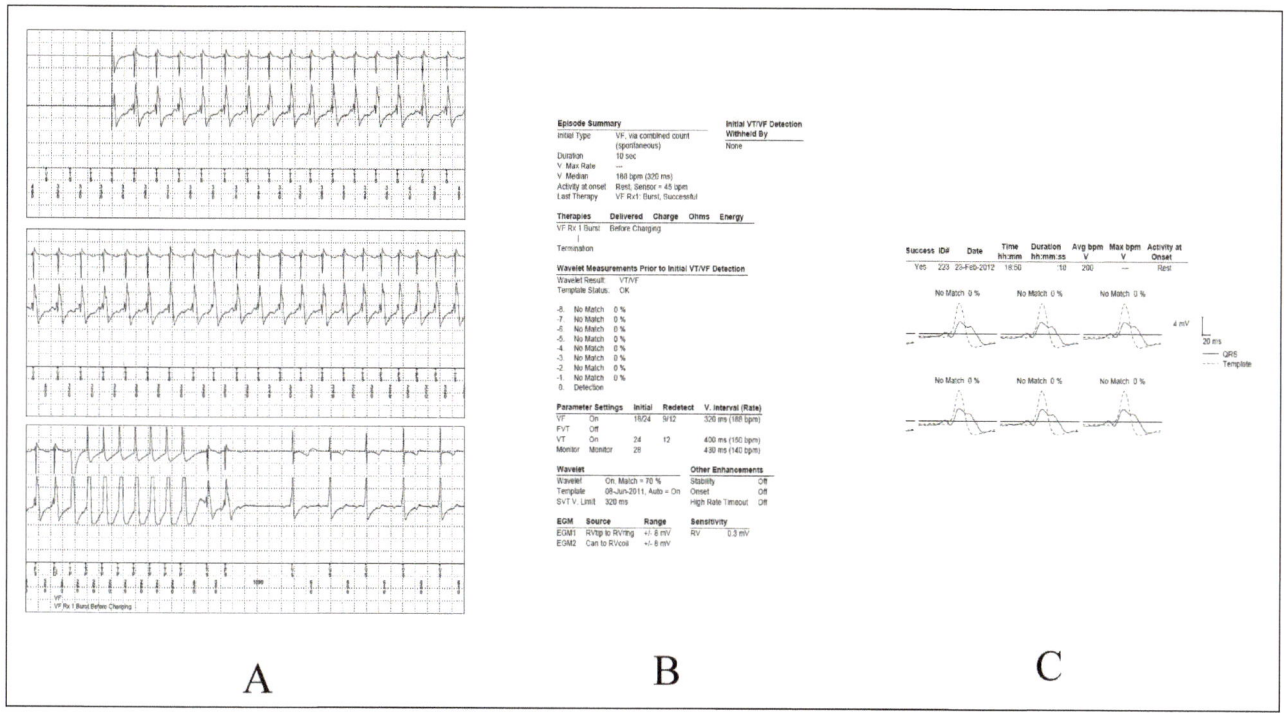

Figure 56.7 Interrogation of a single-chamber ICD shows episode detail with intracardiac electrograms (**A**), the episode summary (**B**), and wavelet template details (**C**). The device sensing algorithm correctly diagnosed the episode as ventricular tachyarrhythmia, and the programmed therapy, antitachycardia pacing (ATP) during device charging, was delivered. This terminated the tachycardia. Note total mismatch (0% match) of wavelets between the ones during arrhythmia and those acquired during sinus rhythm at baseline (**C**).

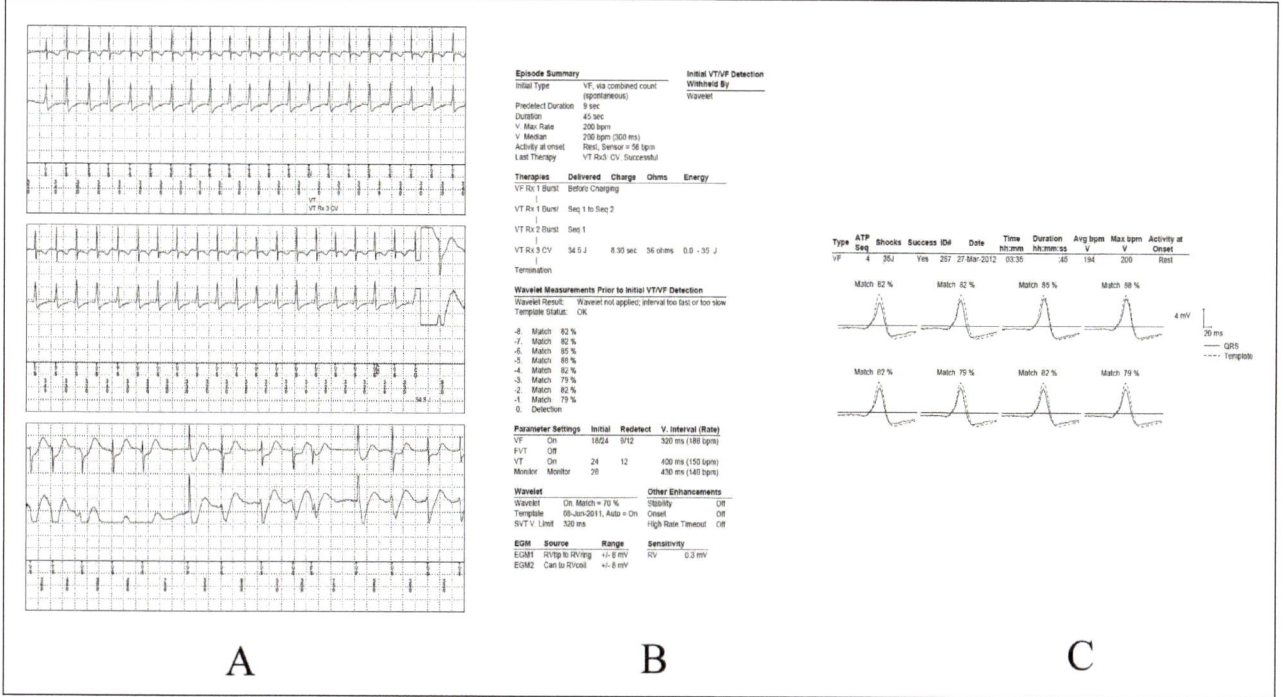

Figure 56.8 Interrogation of a single-chamber ICD shows episode detail with intracardiac electrograms (**A – left panel**), the episode summary (**B – middle panel**), and wavelet template details (**C – right panel**). The device sensing algorithm incorrectly diagnosed the episode as ventricular tachyarrhythmia, and the programmed therapy, antitachycardia pacing (ATP) and shocks, was delivered. This latter thereapy did terminate the tachycardia. Note high level of match (79%–88% match) of wavelets between the ones during arrhythmia and those acquired during sinus rhythm at baseline (**C**). However, the wavelet discriminators were not applied as the arrhythmia rate was too rapid, falling into VF zone (**B**).

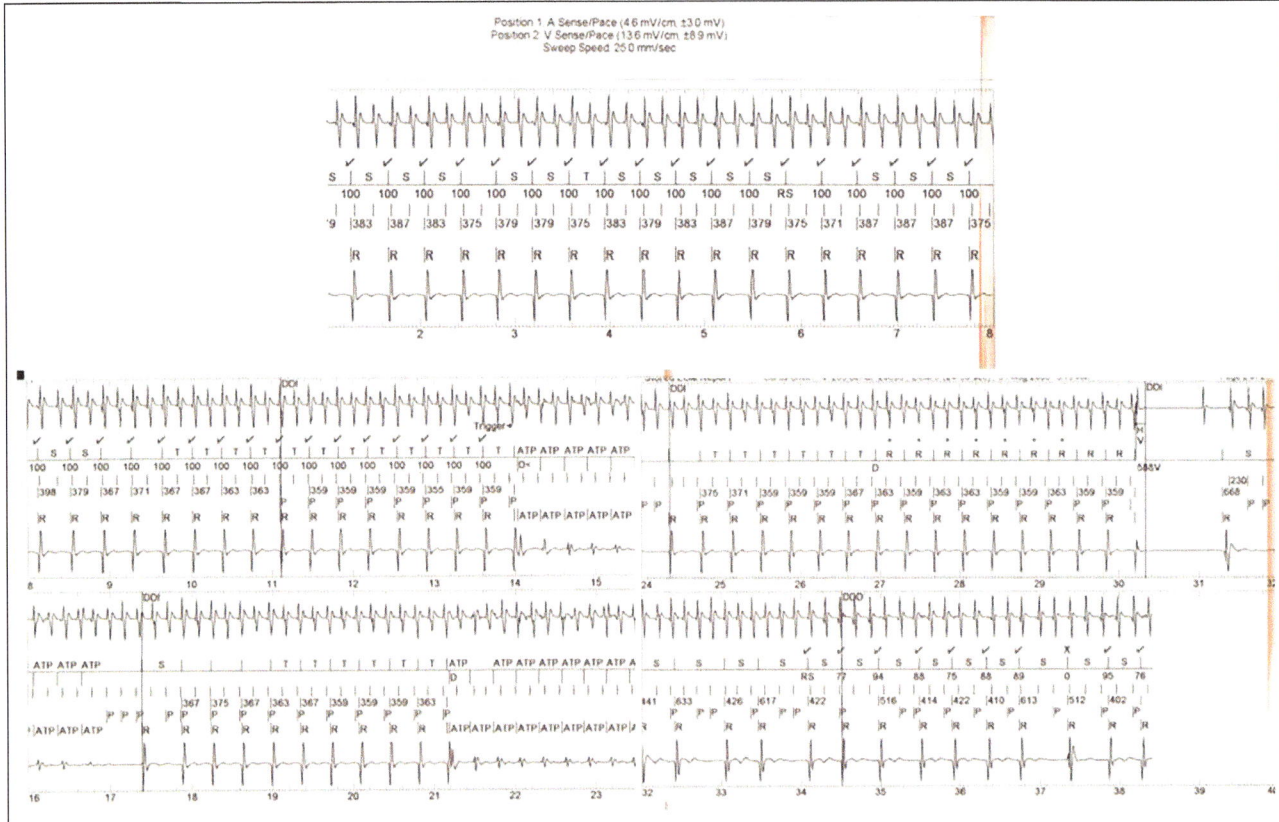

Figure 56.9 Interrogation of a dual-chamber ICD shows inappropriate shock for atrial flutter. For the ICD interrogation strips, the top, middle, and bottom panels are the atrial, marker, and ventricular channels. Atrial flutter with rapid ventricular response leads to determination of the ventricular rhythm by the device as ventricular tachycardia, and the device delivers overdrive antitachycardia pacing (ATP) therapies, which fail to terminate the tachycardia. As a result subsequently, a high voltage shock is delivered.

Conclusions

Due to ongoing progress and advancements made in device technology, it is easier to implant and follow-up CRM devices. The postoperative management and follow-up of patients with CRM devices, irrespective of whether inpatients or outpatients in office settings, remains complex. The physicians and healthcare providers should consider the challenges in the management of these patients with complex cardiac arrhythmias and their substrates as a continuum of overall care that begins much before the implantation of CRM devices. It is only with the understanding of the disease processes, the effects of various concomitant morbidities, the role of drugs and other nonpharmacological therapies, and detailed knowledge of the CRM devices' functionalities that the physicians and healthcare providers are able to deliver the best possible care to these patients.

References

1. Epstein AE, DiMarco JP, Ellenbogen KA, Estes NA 3rd, Freedman RA, et al. American College of Cardiology/American Heart Association Task Force on Practice Guidelines (Writing Committee to Revise the ACC/AHA/NASPE 2002 Guideline Update for Implantation of Cardiac Pacemakers and Antiarrhythmia Devices); American Association for Thoracic Surgery; Society of Thoracic Surgeons. *J Am Coll Cardiol*. 2008;51(21):e1-62. *Circulation*. 2008;117:e350–408.
2. Mond HG, Proclemer A. The 11th World Survey of Cardiac Pacing and Implantable Cardioverter-Defibrillators: Calendar Year 2009–A World Society of Arrhythmia's Project. *Pacing Clin Electrophysiol*. 2011;1-15.
3. Epstein AE, Baessler CA, Curtis AB, Estes NA 3rd, Gersh BJ, Grubb B, Mitchell LB; American Heart Association; Heart Rhythm Society. Addendum to "Personal and Public Safety Issues Related to Arrhythmias That May Affect Consciousness: Implications for Regulation and Physician Recommendations. A medical/scientific statement from the American Heart Association and the North American Society of Pacing and

Electrophysiology." Public safety issues in patients with implantable defibrillators. A Scientific statement from the American Heart Association and the Heart Rhythm Society. *Heart Rhythm.* 2007;4:386-393.

4. Kantharia BK, Patel JA, Nagra BS and Ledley GS. Electrical storm of monomorphic ventricular tachycardia after a cardiac resynchronization therapy defibrillator upgrade. *Europace.* 2006;8:625-628.

5. van Rees JB, de Bie MK, Thijssen J, Borleffs CJ, Schalij MJ, van Erven L. Implantation-related complications of implantable cardioverter-defibrillators and cardiac resynchronization therapy devices: a systematic review of randomized clinical trials. *J Am Coll Cardiol.* 2011;58:995-1000.

6. Wiegand UKH, LeJeune D, Boguschewski F, Bonnemeier H, Eberhardt F, Schunkert H, Bode F. Influence of patient morbidity, operation strategy, and perioperative antiplatelet/anticoagulation therapy. *Chest.* 2004;126:1177-1186.

7. Dunn AS, Wisnivesky J, Ho W, Moore C, McGinn T, Sacks HS. Perioperative management of patients on oral anticoagulants: a decision analysis. *Med Decis Making.* 2005;25(4):387-397.

8. Robinson M, Healey JS, Eikelboom J, Schulman S, Morillo CA, Nair GM, Baranchuk A, Ribas S, Evans G, Connolly SJ, Turpie AG. Postoperative low-molecular-weight heparin bridging is associated with an increase in wound hematoma following surgery for pacemakers and implantable defibrillators. *Pacing Clin Electrophysiol.* 2009;32(3):378-382.

9. Tolosana JM, Berne P, Mont L, Heras M, Berruezo A, Monteagudo J, Tamborero D, Benito B, Brugada J. Preparation for pacemaker or implantable cardiac defibrillator implants in patients with high risk of thrombo-embolic events: oral anticoagulation or bridging with intravenous heparin? A prospective randomized trial. *Eur Heart J.* 2009;30(15):1880-1884.

10. Milic DJ, Perisic ZD, Zivic SS, Stanojkovic ZA, Stojkovic AM, Karanovic ND, Krstic NH, Salinger SS. Prevention of pocket related complications with fibrin sealant in patients undergoing pacemaker implantation who are receiving anticoagulant treatment. *Europace.* 2005;7(4):374-379.

11. Klug D, Balde M, Pavin D, Hidden-Lucet F, Clementy J, Sadoul N, Rey JL, Lande G, Lazarus A, Victor J, Barnay C, Grandbastien B, Kacet S; PEOPLE Study Group. Risk factors related to infections of implanted pacemakers and cardioverter-defibrillators: results of a large prospective study. *Circulation.* 2007;116(12):1349-1355.

12. Grimm W, Flores BF, Marchlinski FE. Complications of implantable cardioverter defibrillator therapy: follow-up of 241 patients. *Pacing Clin Electrophysiol.* 1993;16(1 Pt 2):218-222.

13. Sohail MR, Uslan DZ, Khan AH, Friedman PA, Hayes DL, Wilson WR, Steckelberg JM, Stoner S, Baddour LM. Management and outcome of permanent pacemaker and implantable cardioverter-defibrillator infections. *J Am Coll Cardiol.* 2007;49;1851-1859.

14. Pavia S, Wilkoff B. The management of surgical complications of pacemaker and implantable cardioverter-defibrillators. *Curr Opin Cardiol.* 2000;16:66-71.

15. Wilkoff B. How to treat and identify device infections. *Heart Rhythm.* 2007;4:1467-1470.

16. Baddour LM, Epstein AE, Erickson CC, Knight BP, Levison ME, Lockhart PB, Masoudi FA, Okum EJ, Wilson WR, Beerman LB, Bolger AF, Estes NA 3rd, Gewitz M, Newburger JW, Schron EB, Taubert KA; American Heart Association Rheumatic Fever, Endocarditis, and Kawasaki Disease Committee; Council on Cardiovascular Disease in Young; Council on Cardiovascular Surgery and Anesthesia; Council on Cardiovascular Nursing; Council on Clinical Cardiology; Interdisciplinary Council on Quality of Care; American Heart Association. Update on cardiovascular implantable electronic device infections and their management: a scientific statement from the American Heart Association. *Circulation.* 2010;121:458-477.

17. Bloom H, Heeke B, Leon A, Mera F, Delurgio D, Beshai J, Langberg J. Renal insufficiency and the risk of infection from pacemaker or defibrillator surgery. *Pacing Clin Electrophysiol.* 2006;29:142-145.

18. Mahapatra S, Bybee KA, Bunch TJ, Espinosa RE, Sinak LJ, McGoon MD, Hayes DL. Incidence and predictors of cardiac perforation after permanent pacemaker placement. *Heart Rhythm.* 2005;2(9):907-911.

19. Hirschl DA, Jain VR, Spindola-Franco H, Gross JN, Haramati LB. Prevalence and characterization of asymptomatic pacemaker and ICD lead perforation on CT. *Pacing Clin Electrophysiol.* 2007;30(1):28-32.

20. Belott P. How to access the axillary vein. *Heart Rhythm.* 2006;3(3):366-369.

21. Burri H, Sunthorn H, Dorsaz PA, Shah D. Prospective study of axillary vein puncture with or without contrast venography for pacemaker and defibrillator lead implantation. *Pacing Clin Electrophysiol.* 2005;28 Suppl 1:S280-S283.

22. Fyke FE 3rd. Doppler guided extrathoracic introducer insertion. *Pacing Clin Electrophysiol.* 1995;18(5 Pt 1):1017-1021.

23. Gillis AM, Philippon F, Cassidy MR, Singh N, Dorian P, Love BA, Kerr CR; Canadian Working Group on Cardiac Pacing. Guidelines for implantable cardioverter defibrillator follow-up in Canada: a consensus statement of the Canadian Working Group on Cardiac Pacing. *Can J Cardiol.* 2003;19(1):21-37.

24. Wilkoff BL, Auricchio A, Brugada J, Cowie M, Ellenbogen KA, Gillis AM, Hayes DL, Howlett JG, Kautzner J, Love CJ, Morgan JM, Priori SG, Reynolds DW, Schoenfeld MH, Vardas PE; Heart Rhythm Society; European Heart Rhythm Association; American College of Cardiology; American Heart Association; European Society of Cardiology; Heart Failure Association of ESC; Heart Failure Society of America. HRS/EHRA expert consensus on the monitoring of cardiovascular implantable electronic devices (CIEDs): description of techniques, indications, personnel, frequency and ethical considerations. *Heart Rhythm.* 2008(6):907-925.

25. Poole JE, Johnson GW, Hellkamp AS, Anderson J, Callans DJ, Raitt MH, Reddy RK, Marchlinski FE, Yee R, Guarnieri T, Talajic M, Wilber DJ, Fishbein DP, Packer DL, Mark DB, Lee KL, Bardy GH. Prognostic importance of defibrillator shocks in patients with heart failure. *N Engl J Med.* 2008;359(10):1009-1017.

26. Wilkoff BL, Williamson BD, Stern RS, Moore SL, Lu F, Lee SW, Birgersdotter-Green UM, Wathen MS, Van Gelder IC, Heubner BM, Brown ML, Holloman KK; PREPARE Study Investigators. Strategic programming of detection and therapy parameters in implantable cardioverter-defibrillators reduces shocks in primary prevention patients: results from the PREPARE (Primary Prevention Parameters Evaluation) study. *J Am Coll Cardiol.* 2008;52:541-550.

27. Moss AJ, Schuger C, Beck CA, et al. Reduction in inappropriate therapy and mortality through ICD programming. *N Engl J Med.* 2012;367:2275-2283.

28. Tzeis S, Andrikopoulos G, Kolb C, Vardas PE. Tools and strategies for the reduction of inappropriate implantable cardioverter defibrillator shocks. *Europace.* 2008;10:1256–1265.

29. Burri H, Senouf D. Remote monitoring and follow-up of pacemakers and implantable cardioverter defibrillators. *Europace.* 2009;11:701-709.

30. Saxon LA, Hayes DL, Gilliam FR, Heidenreich PA, Day J, Seth M, Meyer TE, Jones PW, Boehmer JP. Long-term outcome after ICD and CRT implantation and influence of

remote device follow-up: the ALTITUDE survival study. *Circulation*. 2010;122:2359-2367.
31. Crossley GH, Boyle A, Vitense H, Chang Y, Mead RH; CONNECT Investigators. The CONNECT (Clinical Evaluation of Remote Notification to Reduce Time to Clinical Decision) trial: the value of wireless remote monitoring with automatic clinician alerts. *J Am Coll Cardiol*. 2011;57(10): 1181-1189.
32. Varma N, Epstein AE, Irimpen A, Schweikert R, Love C; TRUST Investigators. Efficacy and safety of automatic remote monitoring for implantable cardioverter-defibrillator follow-up: the Lumos-T Safely Reduces Routine Office Device Follow-up (TRUST) trial. *Circulation*. 2010;122(4):325-332.

Video Legends

Video 56.1 Large (> 2 cm) vegetations attached to the tricuspid valve and device leads are seen by transesophageal echocardiography.

Video 56.2 Cinefluoroscopy 3 days after implantation of a CRT-D system shows dislodgement of the coronary sinus-left ventricular lead, which takes the course into the right ventricle to main right pulmonary artery trunk.

Videos 56.3–56.5 Percutaneous pericardiocentesis was performed in a thin, elderly female who developed pericardial effusion and cardiac tamponade after implantation of a dual-chamber pacemaker. Pericardial access was obtained from subxiphoid approach. A guidewire was inserted up to the level of pericardial reflection under fluroscopy (clip 1), injection of dye into the pericardium confirmed pericardial effusion (clip 2), and after removal of blood from the pericardial space, the pericardial drain was left in situ (clip 3).

CHAPTER 57

Optimization of Cardiac Resynchronization Therapy: Techniques and Patient Selection

Kevin P. Jackson, MD; Brett D. Atwater, MD; James P. Daubert, MD

Introduction

Multiple randomized, controlled trials have shown that cardiac resynchronization therapy (CRT) provides hemodynamic and clinical benefits for patients with heart failure (HF). CRT has been associated with a 30% to 50% reduction in all-cause mortality or HF hospitalization among thousands of select patients enrolled in clinical trials.[1,2] Cost-effectiveness analyses have also demonstrated the attractiveness of CRT for eligible patients.[3] However, the benefit of CRT is not universal among patients with HF; up to 30% of patients implanted with current generation CRT devices fail to demonstrate clinical benefit, and up to 50% of patients fail to demonstrate echocardiographic response.[4]

Extensive work has identified several potential reasons for suboptimal CRT response (Figure 57.1). Broadly, these may be grouped into issues pertaining to patient selection, device implantation technique, and postoperative programming and patient management. The most common causes of CRT nonresponse are suboptimal atrioventricular interval timing; presence of a competing arrhythmia, including atrial fibrillation (AF), atrial flutter (AFL), or premature ventricular contractions (PVCs); anemia; and suboptimal left ventricular (LV) lead position. A multidisciplinary approach to the identification

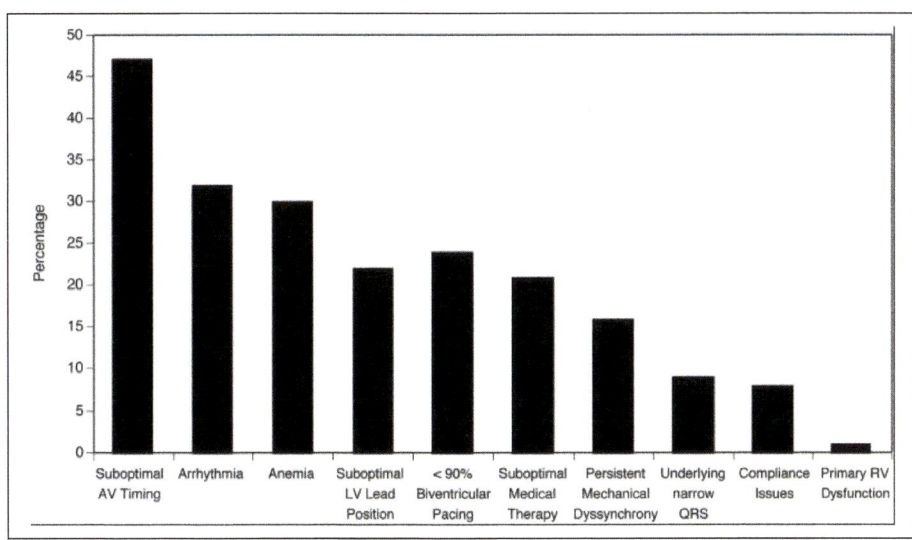

Figure 57.1 Potential reasons for suboptimal CRT response. AV = atrioventricular; LV = left ventricular; RV = right ventricular. *Source:* Mullens W, Grimm RA, Verga T, et al.[5]

and correction of these underlying conditions has been shown to improve the frequency of CRT response.[5] This chapter will review the current state of the art for optimal patient selection, device implantation techniques, and postimplant management of CRT patients. Optimization of these three phases of care can lead to improvements in response to CRT and patient outcomes (Table 57.1).

Table 57.1 Comprehensive approach to CRT optimization

Preoperative	• Patient selection
	• Dyssynchrony echocardiogram to identify latest activated LV segment
	• Cardiac MRI to identify transmural scar
Intraoperative	• Lead placement on latest mechanically activated LV segment
	• Lead placement on latest electrically activated LV segment (QLV)
	• Acute hemodynamic evaluation (dP/dt max)
Postoperative	• Titration of evidence-based medications
	• Management of arrhythmias (AF, PVC) resulting in suboptimal BiV pacing percentage
	• Echocardiographic-based optimization of device timing

Optimizing Patient Selection

Cardiac resynchronization therapy is meant to restore ventricular synchrony, and therefore it stands to reason that methods that identify and localize regions of significant dyssynchrony could improve our ability to select patients who will benefit from CRT. A variety of methods have been developed to identify and quantify ventricular dyssynchrony.

Presence of Electrical Dyssynchrony

Ventricular conduction delay is common among patients with HF and results in decreased stroke volume, worsening mitral regurgitation, and increased ventricular wall stress.[6] Conduction delay is frequently manifest on surface electrocardiogram (ECG) as prolongation of the QRS interval with left bundle branch block (LBBB), right bundle branch block (RBBB), or nonspecific intraventricular conduction delay (IVCD) patterns. Prolongation of the QRS interval independently predicts HF hospitalization and death among patients with systolic HF.[7]

The objective of CRT is to approximate normal ventricular conduction to deliver near simultaneous mechanical contraction of the RV, interventricular septum (IVS), and LV free wall. Delivery of properly timed CRT improves a variety of cardiac hemodynamics, including cardiac output, systolic pressure, mitral regurgitation, and left atrial pressure.[8]

The gold standard for identifying patients with dyssynchrony is the presence of QRS prolongation on surface ECG. The major clinical trials of CRT enrolled subjects with a minimum QRS duration of 120 to 150 ms, but the mean QRS in each study was substantially higher (Table 57.2).[1,9-12] Post-hoc analyses of the REVERSE and MADIT-CRT studies demonstrated that the clinical response to CRT was directly correlated to the baseline QRS duration.[13] A meta-analysis including over 5,800 subjects enrolled in 5 clinical trials showed that patients with a QRS duration ≥150 ms derived a significant reduction in clinical adverse events (risk ratio = 0.6, $P < 0.001$), while those with a QRS duration < 150 ms derived no such reduction (risk ratio = 0.95, $P = 0.49$).[14] Although the ECG (QRS prolongation and LBBB morphology) is the mainstay for identification of low-ejection fraction (EF) patients for CRT, it clearly has limitations, since not all implanted patients respond clinically or by echocardiography. Moreover, although non-LBBB patients generally have not responded to CRT,[15] this does not mean that all non-LBBB patients would be nonresponders. Identification of unique areas of late conduction or abnormal conduction due to scar or other factors may improve the response to CRT.

ECG-based methods have been developed to analyze detailed information about LV myocardial scar location, baseline, and biventricular paced electrical vectors, and the activation times of the RV and LV.[16,17] Baseline ECG characteristics associated with echocardiographic reverse remodeling after CRT included a low LV scar burden, as measured by the Selvester score, and prolonged LV activation time. After CRT implantation, ECG characteristics associated with response to CRT included biventricular-paced morphology with increasing R-wave amplitude in V_1 to V_2, and an axis shift from the left-axis deviation to right-axis deviation. The predicted probability of reverse remodeling ranged from < 20% for patients with adverse predictors to 99% for patients with positive predictors.

The majority of patients enrolled in clinical trials of CRT had a baseline LBBB ECG pattern. Retrospective subgroup analyses of these studies show that patients with non-LBBB patterns derived less clinical and echocardiographic benefit than patients with LBBB.[18] The largest report of the use of CRT in patients with non-LBBB was a retrospective subgroup analysis of the MADIT-CRT trial in which 13% of subjects had RBBB, and 17% had nonspecific IVCD.[19] While patients with LBBB had significantly reduced risk of death, HF event, or ventricular tachycardia, patients with non-LBBB had no significant reduction in any of these endpoints, although the study was not powered to detect differences in this subgroup. It is unclear whether clinical outcomes of CRT in patients with RBBB and IVCD are worse due to decreased efficacy of CRT or because of the higher rate of comorbid adverse predictors and disease severity. In a severely diseased conduction system, delay may be present in both the

Table 57.2 Inclusion/exclusion criteria and key baseline subject characteristics of major CRT trials

	Cardiac Rhythm	NYHA Class	QRS cutoff (msec)	Mean ± SD QRS (msec)	LVEF (%)	Mean ± SD LVEF (%)
MUSTIC (n = 67)	SR	III	≥150	176 ± 19	≤35	23 ± 7
PATH-CHF (n = 36)	SR	III, IV	≥120	175 ± 32	≤35	21 ± 7
MIRACLE (n = 453)	SR	III, IV	≥130	166 ± 20	≤35	22 ± 6
MIRACLE-ICD (n = 369)	SR	III, IV	≥130	164 ± 22	≤35	24 ± 1
CONTAK (n = 490)	SR	II-IV	≥120	158 ± 26	≤35	21 ± 7
COMPANION (n = 1520)	SR	III, IV	≥120	160	≤35	22
MADIT-CRT (n = 1820)	SR	I, II	≥130	159	≤30	24 ± 5
RAFT (n = 1798)	SR	II, III	≥120	158 ± 24	≤30	23 ± 6
REVERSE (n = 610)	SR	I, II	≥120	154 ± 24	≤40	27 ± 7

CRT = cardiac resynchronization therapy; LVEF = left ventricular ejection fraction; NYHA = New York Heart Association; SD = standard deviation; SR = sinus rhythm.

right and left bundle branches, with the manifest electrocardiographic pattern determined by the bundle with the slowest conduction. Extensive LV conduction delay is frequently present in patients with RBBB and left-axis deviation referred for CRT.[20] Prospective trials of CRT in patients with RBBB and IVCD may help determine if CRT offers clinical and echocardiographic advantages over ICD therapy alone.

Previous studies have shown that chronic RV apical pacing can cause LV dilation, reduced LVEF, and an increased chance of HF hospitalization and death in patients with baseline HF.[21] Thus, patients with underlying HF and depressed LVEF who are expected to receive >40% ventricular pacing may benefit from biventricular rather than RV-only pacing. The BLOCK-HF study evaluated patients with AV block destined to receive ventricular pacing who had an LVEF of 50% or less and randomized them to receive CRT or conventional dual-chamber RV pacing.[22] Results from this study showed that patients receiving CRT had a 22% reduction in death or hospitalization for HF compared to RV-paced patients. Therefore, patients with systolic HF and existing RV-only pacemakers or those undergoing device implantation with an expected requirement of ventricular pacing from their device appear to be good candidates for CRT.

Presence of Mechanical Dyssynchrony

Electrical dyssynchrony, manifested by prolongation of the QRS interval, and mechanical dyssynchrony may not always coexist. Bleeker and colleagues reported that up to 30% of HF patients with QRS duration <120 ms have significant mechanical dyssynchrony by echocardiographic TDI, and 20% to 30% of HF patients with QRS duration >120 ms may not have mechanical dyssynchrony.[23] Taken together, these data led to the belief that an imaging-based assessment of mechanical dyssynchrony may provide additional useful information when selecting patients for CRT.

Early single-center studies evaluating echocardiography for identification and quantitation of ventricular dyssynchrony used TDI techniques to assess septal and lateral LV wall motion.[24] A delay in activation from the septal to lateral wall of >65 ms or standard deviation of time to peak systolic velocity of 12 segments >33 ms predicted clinical improvement or echocardiographic response to CRT. Further, these small studies suggested that these cut-off values predicted CRT response better than electrocardiographic QRS duration. Newer methods using myocardial deformation analysis based on echocardiographic pixel "speckle" tracking can provide dyssynchrony information as well as identify areas of transmural scar, potentially allowing the implanting physician to target the LV lead to viable myocardium.[25]

The Predictors of Response to CRT (PROSPECT) study enrolled 498 patients from 53 international centers with LVEF ≤35%, QRS duration ≥130 ms, and NYHA class III or IV HF and evaluated 12 echocardiographic parameters as possible predictors of a positive response to CRT (Table 57.3).[26] Clinical outcomes were improved in 69% of patients, and LV end-systolic volume decreased by more than 15% in 56% of patients. However, no single echocardiographic dyssynchrony parameter predicted clinical or echocardiographic response to CRT. The core echocardiographic lab found high variability in the measurement of each echocardiographic parameter, and therefore it is unclear whether the negative results of this trial were due to technical or physiologic factors.

The Echocardiography Guided Cardiac Resynchronization Therapy (EchoCRT) study was designed to definitively evaluate the utility echocardiography to select patients for CRT.[27] Mechanical dyssynchrony was measured using both tissue Doppler imaging and radial strain analysis by speckle tracking as assessed by two-dimensional (2D) echocardiogram. Patients with mechanical dyssynchrony by echocardiogram, but minimal to no evidence of electrical dyssynchrony by ECG (QRS duration <130 ms), were randomized to CRT or standard

Table 57.3 Echocardiographic dyssynchrony measures in clinical trials of CRT in narrow QRS patients

Study	Echocardiographic Predictor	Echocardiography Type	Dyssynchrony Measure Description	Met Prespecified Criteria for Prediction of CRT Response?
PROSPECT	SPWMD	M-Mode	Septal-posterior wall motion delay	No
	IVMD	Pulsed Doppler	Interventricular mechanical delay	No
	LVFT/RR	Pulsed Doppler	LV filling time	No
	LPEI	Pulsed Doppler	LV preejection interval	No
	LLWC	M-Mode and Pulsed Doppler	Intraventricular dyssynchrony left lateral wall contraction	No
	TS-(lateral-septal)	Tissue Doppler Imaging	Delay between time to peak systolic velocity in ejection phase at basal septal and basal lateral segments	No
	TS-SD	Tissue Doppler Imaging	Standard deviation of time from QRS to peak systolic velocity in ejection phase for 12 LV segments (6 basal and 6 middle)	No
	PVD	Tissue Doppler Imaging	Peak velocity difference of maximum and minimum of time to peak velocity	No
	DLC	Tissue Doppler Imaging + SRI	Delayed longitudinal contraction	No
	Ts-peak displacement	Tissue Doppler Imaging	Maximum difference of time to peak systolic displacement for 4 segments	No
	Ts-peak (basal)	Tissue Doppler Imaging	Maximum difference of time to peak systolic velocity for 6 segments at basal level	No
	Ts-onset (basal)	Tissue Doppler Imaging	Maximum difference of time to onset of systolic velocity for 6 segments at LV base	No
ECHO-CRT	Ts-(lateral-septal)	Tissue Doppler Imaging	Opposing wall delay of 80 msec or more in apical four chamber or long axis views	No
	Radial strain	Speckle Tracking	Delay in anteroseptal to posterior wall of 130 msec or more	No

DLC = delayed longitudinal contraction; IVMD = interventricular mechanical delay; LLWC = left lateral wall contract; LPEI = left ventricular pre-ejection interval; LVFT/RR = left ventricular filling time/refill rate; PVD = peak velocity difference; SPWMD = septal-posterior wall motion delay; TS-SD = tissue synchrony standard deviation.

implantable cardioverter-defibrillator (ICD) therapy. The primary outcome was the composite of death from any cause or first hospitalization for worsening heart failure. The trial was stopped early due to excessive mortality in the CRT arm (11.1% vs 6.4%; hazard ratio, 1.81; $P = 0.02$). Largely based on the outcome of the EchoCRT trial, there currently is no role for echocardiographic evaluation of mechanical dyssynchrony as a selection tool for CRT in patients with systolic heart failure and "narrow" QRS duration.

Magnetic Resonance Imaging (MRI) for Scar Identification

Contrast-enhanced MRI offers excellent spatial resolution and is able to assess scar tissue noninvasively while offering the ability to assess mechanical dyssynchrony in three dimensions.[28] In a small study of 40 patients with NYHA class III or IV HF, LVEF ≤35%, QRS duration ≥120 ms, LBBB, and chronic coronary artery disease, patients with transmural posterolateral scar tissue showed a low response rate compared to patients without posterolateral scar (14%

vs 81%; $P < 0.05$).[29] Patients with severe baseline dyssynchrony on echocardiographic TDI (>65 ms delay between septal and lateral walls) in the absence of posterolateral scar on MRI had a response rate of 95% compared to 11% among patients with posterolateral scar and/or absent LV dyssynchrony on TDI. In a larger series of 559 consecutive patients who received CRT for existing clinical indications, patients with the LV lead placed in an area of scar ($n = 43$) based on cardiac MRI or who did not have a pre-procedure MRI ($n = 350$) had significantly higher risk of cardiovascular death or hospitalization, higher clinical composite score, and more advanced NYHA class than patients who had the LV lead placed in an area without scar on preprocedure MRI ($n = 166$).[30]

A small, single-center study examined the utility of MRI-guided LV lead placement in patients with LVEF ≤35%, NYHA Class III or IV HF, but without evidence of electrical dyssynchrony (QRS ≤120 ms).[31] A total of 60 patients were randomly assigned to optimal medical therapy or CRT-D implantation. At 6-month follow-up, the 6-minute walk distance increased significantly in the CRT group (146.3 meters to 249.0 meters), but not in the medical therapy group (120 meters to 90 meters) ($P < 0.0001$). Significant improvements were also found in the clinical composite score, NYHA class, and quality of life score in the patients randomly assigned to receive CRT but not in patients assigned to medical therapy. No randomized trial data is available on the use of cardiac MRI in patients without evidence of electrical dyssynchrony, however.

Clinical Characteristics of CRT "Super-responders" and Nonresponders

While no consistent definition exists of CRT super-response, in general, super-responders obtain >15% improvement in EF or >20% reduction in LV end-systolic volume. Following this definition, between 15% and 25% of CRT recipients receive super-response, and these patients enjoy dramatic improvements in HF symptoms and HF hospitalizations. In the MADIT-CRT trial, which enrolled patients with mildly symptomatic HF, QRS > 130 ms, and LVEF ≤30%, the cumulative probability of HF or all-cause death at 2 years was 4% in super-responders, 11% in responders, and 26% in hypo-responders ($P < 0.001$).[32] Characteristics of patients enrolled in MADIT-CRT who obtained CRT super-response included female sex (odds ratio [OR]: 1.96; $P = 0.001$), no prior myocardial infarction (OR: 1.80; $P = 0.005$), QRS duration ≥150 ms (OR: 1.79; $P = 0.007$), LBBB (OR: 2.05; $P = 0.006$), body mass index <30 kg/m^2 (OR: 1.51; $P = 0.035$), and smaller baseline LA volume index (OR: 1.47; $P < 0.001$).

Much effort has been spent identifying patient characteristics that reduce the likelihood of CRT response. In addition to male sex, ischemic cause of underlying cardiomyopathy, and lack of true LBBB on baseline ECG, AF and a high baseline PVC burden have been associated with reduced likelihood of response and warrant special consideration prior to CRT implantation. Of the 7,379 patients enrolled in randomized trials of CRT, only 272 (3.6%) had permanent AF, and therefore the data on the use of CRT in this population is limited. The presence of AF potentially reduces the benefit of CRT due to the competition of rapid, natively conducted beats with CRT pacing. Among patients with standard CRT implantation criteria and a history of atrial arrhythmia, the percentage biventricular pacing is a strong predictor of HF hospitalization and all-cause mortality (Figure 57.2).[33] Patients in this study with >92% biventricular pacing had a 66% reduction in HF hospitalization or all-cause mortality compared to patients with <92% biventricular pacing ($P < 0.001$). Slowing intrinsic conduction to allow adequate CRT pacing may require high-doses or multiple AV nodal agents. In addition, device counters are not able to reliably distinguish between pure CRT-paced beats and fully or partially fused beats.[34]

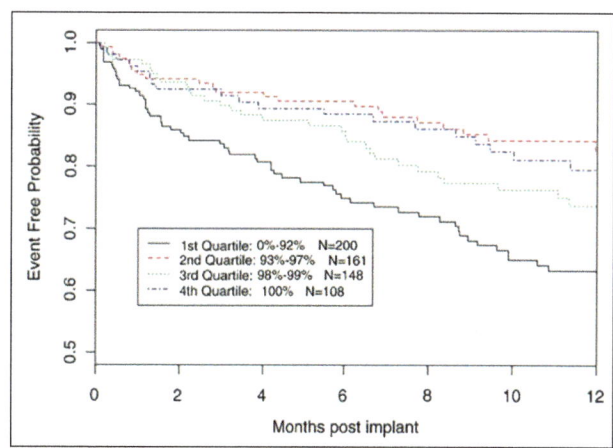

Figure 57.2 Survival free from heart failure hospitalization and all-cause mortality in patients with a history of atrial arrhythmia. Q2 to Q4 vs Q1, HR: 0.44, $P < 0.00001$; Q2 vs Q1, HR: 0.34, $P < 0.001$ *Source:* Koplan BA, et al.[33]

In patients with AF who otherwise meet criteria for CRT implantation, adequate rate control, and therefore maximal CRT pacing percentage, is best achieved with AV node ablation. Gasparini and colleagues showed that overall mortality was equivalent at 3 years in patients with CRT and AF who underwent AV node ablation versus patients with CRT in sinus rhythm.[35] Similarly, a meta-analysis of 3 studies comparing patients with permanent AF and CRT who underwent AV node ablation, mortality was decreased 58% in comparison to patients who did not undergo AV node ablation.[36]

Similar to AF, frequent PVCs are suspected to reduce the effectiveness of CRT by reducing the percentage of biventricular-paced beats and by causing fusion of some additional percentage of paced beats. In the MADIT-CRT trial, 15% of enrolled subjects had >5,000 PVCs on preimplant 24-hour Holter monitoring. Among patients with nonischemic cardiomyopathy, the RV outflow tract was the most common origin for PVCs. Although a high burden of PVCs is relatively common in CRT recipients, little work has been done investigating the role of PVC burden in predicting response to CRT therapy. One prospective, multicenter, nonrandomized observational study has assessed the effect of PVC ablation in CRT nonresponders.[37] Subjects were enrolled if they had < 5% improvement in the LVEF and/or LV end-systolic volume of < 10% with no associated improvement in clinical status 1 year after CRT implantation and had > 10,000 PVCs/day on Holter monitoring. Follow-up echocardiography 6 months after ablation revealed CRT response with improvements in mean LVEF (26.2 to 32.7%, $P < 0.001$), LV end-systolic volume (178 mL to 145 mL, $P < 0.001$), and median NYHA class (III to II, $P < 0.001$). Approximately one-third of patients had no improvement in LVEF after PVC ablation. These patients had a lower burden of PVCs and a higher percentage of biventricular pacing before ablation than patients who responded.

Summary of Current Guidelines for CRT Patient Selection

In 2012, the ACC/AHA/HRS organizations provided an update to their joint guidelines for device-based therapies of cardiac rhythm abnormalities.[38] This update incorporated new data for the use of CRT in patients with NYHA class II HF derived from the RAFT and MADIT-CRT studies. In addition, recommendations regarding the presence of LBBB and the degree of QRS prolongation have been included, reflecting the weight of evidence supporting CRT implantation in these populations. A summary of the Guideline recommendations is presented in Table 57.4.

Optimizing Device Implantation

Targeting the Left Ventricular Lead

While the use of echocardiographic dyssynchrony analysis to select patients for CRT implantation has not been supported by multicenter research trials, evidence suggests that preprocedure dyssynchrony evaluation can be used to effectively target the LV lead and improve the response rate to CRT. In the Targeted Left Ventricular Lead Placement to Guide Cardiac Resynchronization Therapy (TARGET) study, 220 patients were randomized to either standard LV lead placement or targeted placement based on the latest wall of activation on echocardiographic speckle-tracking analysis. More patients with an LV lead placed on or near the wall with latest activation had LV reverse remodeling after CRT than those with unguided LV lead placement (70% vs 55%, $P = 0.031$).[39] Similarly, the Speckle Tracking Assisted Resynchronization Therapy for Electrode Region (STARTER) found reduced HF hospitalization in patients with guided LV lead placement versus those without (11% vs 22%, $P = 0.031$).[40]

Development of Biventricular Pacing

In 1994, Cazeau and colleagues published the first case report of dedicated biventricular pacing for the treatment of congestive heart failure.[41] Using an epicardial lead placed on the LV free-wall via thoracotomy and endocardial leads placed in the RA, the LA via the coronary sinus (CS), and the RV, they demonstrated a decrease in pulmonary capillary wedge pressure and an increase in cardiac output with 4-chamber pacing. After 6 weeks of biventricular pacing, the patient had a profound diuresis and reported symptomatic improvement to NYHA functional class II. In 1998, Daubert and colleagues published a series of the first fully transvenous-placed biventricular pacing systems with LV leads inserted via the CS.[42]

Early implanters discovered quickly that a major limitation of effective biventricular pacing was the ability to insert, locate, and stabilize the LV lead in an appropriate branch of the CS. Despite improvements in implant technique and tools, failure rates for placement of LV leads at initial implant still range between 7.5% and 10% in major clinical trials.[2,43] Most of these implant failures are due to difficulty accessing the CS ostium or advancing the pacing lead into an adequate, stable position.

Anatomy of the Coronary Venous System

The coronary sinus runs in the posterior coronary groove between the LA and LV and the ostium opens into posteroseptal region of the RA near the tricuspid valve. The ostium itself is 5 to 15 mm in diameter and is partially covered by a Thebesian valve in approximately 60% of patients. In a small subset of patients, the ostium is completely enclosed by the valve with only small fenestrations allowing venous drainage, thereby presenting a major impediment to CS access. In addition, RA dilation may lead to an abnormally high insertion of the CS ostium, making access with a fixed-shape catheter or wire difficult.

Gross anatomic studies have shown a median of 6 LV veins draining into the CS, although not all may be suitable for placement of a LV pacing lead. The nearest branch to the CS ostium is the middle cardiac vein (MCV), which may be covered by a small valve or originate with a separate ostium. The MCV runs in the interventricular groove toward the ventricular apex and is usually not a suitable target for LV lead placement. Three distinct veins drain the lateral wall of the LV. The posterolateral branch, the most prominent and consistent of these veins, usually enters the CS within 1 centimeter of the ostium. The lateral marginal vein and lateral branches off the anterior interventricular vein (AIV) are variably present (Figure 57.3). In patients with prior myocardial infarction, first-order branches to the lateral wall off the CS are often diminutive or absent. For CRT implantation, where mid-lateral LV wall lead placement is generally preferred, this region was accessible from at least 2 CS tributaries (posterolateral and AIV) in greater than 85%

of patients. In approximately 20% of patients, the mid-lateral LV wall was also accessible from branches off of the middle cardiac vein.

Imaging of the cardiac venous system prior to LV lead placement is a critical aspect of the implant procedure. In most cases, this is accomplished after CS access via occlusive

Table 57.4 Guideline changes for CRT in the 2012 ACCF/AHA/HRS focused update

Class I	
1. CRT is indicated for patients who have LVEF less than or equal to 35%, sinus rhythm, LBBB with a QRS duration greater than or equal to 150 msec, and NYHA class II, III, or ambulatory IV symptoms on GDMT. *(Level of Evidence: A for NYHA class III/IV; Level of Evidence: B for NYHA class II)*	Modified recommendation (specifying CRT in patients with LBBB of ≥150 msec; expanded to include those with NYHA class II symptoms).
Class IIa	
1. CRT can be useful for patients who have LVEF less than or equal to 35%, sinus rhythm, LBBB with a QRS duration 120 to 149 msec, and NYHA class II, III, or ambulatory IV symptoms on GDMT.[16-18,20-22] *(Level of Evidence: B)*	New recommendation
2. CRT can be useful for patients who have LVEF less than or equal to 35%, sinus rhythm, a non-LBBB pattern with a QRS duration greater than or equal to 150 msec, and NYHA class III/ambulatory class IV symptoms on GDMT.[16-18,21] *(Level of Evidence: A)*	New recommendation
3. CRT can be useful in patients with atrial fibrillation and LVEF less than or equal to 35% on GDMT if a) the patient requires ventricular pacing or otherwise meets CRT criteria and b) AV nodal ablation or pharmacologic rate control will allow near 100% ventricular pacing with CRT.[23-26,48] *(Level of Evidence: B)*	Modified recommendation (wording changed to indicate benefit based on ejection fraction rather than NYHA class; level of evidence changed from C to B)
4. CRT can be useful for patients on GDMT who have LVEF less than or equal to 35% and are undergoing new or replacement device placement with anticipated requirement for significant (>40%) ventricular pacing.[25,27-29] *(Level of Evidence: C)*	Modified recommendation (wording changed to indicate benefit based on ejection fraction and need for pacing rather than NYHA class); class changed from IIb to IIa)
Class IIb	
1. CRT may be considered for patients who have LVEF less than or equal to 30%, ischemic etiology of heart failure, sinus rhythm, LBBB with a QRS duration of greater than or equal to 150 msec, and NYHA class I symptoms on GDMT.[20,21] *(Level of Evidence: C)*	New recommendation
2. CRT may be considered for patients who have LVEF less than or equal to 35%, sinus rhythm, a non-LBBB pattern with QRS duration 120 to 149 msec, and NYHA class III/ambulatory class IV on GDMT.[21,30] *(Level of Evidence: B)*	New recommendation
3. CRT may be considered for patients who have LVEF less than or equal to 35%, sinus rhythm, a non-LBBB pattern with a QRS duration greater than or equal to 150 msec, and NYHA class II symptoms on GDMT.[20,21] *(Level of Evidence: B)*	New recommendation
Class III: No Benefit	
1. CRT is not recommended for patients with NYHA class I or II symptoms and non-LBBB pattern with QRS duration less than 150 msec.[20,21,30] *(Level of Evidence: B)*	New recommendation
2. CRT is not indicated for patients whose comorbidities and/or frailty limit survival with good functional capacity to less than 1 year.[19] *(Level of Evidence: C)*	Modified recommendation (wording changed to include cardiac as well as noncardiac comorbidities)

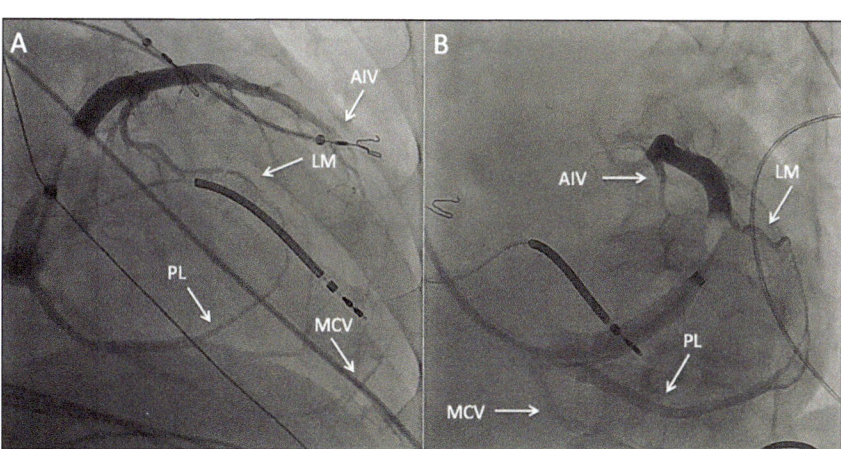

Figure 57.3 Branches of the coronary sinus for left ventricular lead placement. **Panel A:** Right anterior oblique (RAO) fluoroscopic projection showing the anterior interventricular vein (AIV), lateral marginal (LM), posterolateral (PL), and middle cardic vein (MCV). **Panel B:** Left anterior oblique (LAO) projection. *Source:* Courtesy of Dr. Kevin P. Jackson.

venography with a balloon-tipped catheter. Rotational venography may provide a more complete assessment of the CS branches and their takeoff, which can be difficult to appreciate in one- or two-view venograms. Multislice computed tomography (MSCT) has been used preprocedure to assess the cardiac vasculature prior to the implant procedure and correlates well with occlusive venograms.[44] In addition, MSCT may reveal a high takeoff of the CS ostium and aid in catheter selection for successful CS access.

Left Ventricular Lead Implantation

The first LV pacing leads were placed on the epicardial surface via a subxiphoid or thoracoscopic approach. Although operative morbidity was low, access to the lateral or posterolateral walls of the LV is difficult when there is only limited exposure. The development of endovascular LV pacing leads ushered in a new era for CRT; however, successful implantation was hampered by having to use stylet-driven pacing leads. The development of preshaped sheaths that follow the curvature of the lateral wall and floor of the RA allows easier access to the CS. In addition, device companies have improved LV lead design and shapes with smaller tip sizes and isodiametric lead bodies to aid in tracking the lead through small, tortuous side branches. Despite these advances, however, failure of LV lead placement in recent large clinical trials remains near 10%. Most of these implant failures are due to difficulty accessing the CS ostium or inability to advance the pacing lead into an adequate, stable position. In addition, LV lead dislodgement may occur both acutely or in the first few months after implantation. In the REVERSE trial, which reported complications out to 12 months, the rate of late LV lead dislodgement (between 1 and 12 months postimplant) was 3.4%.[45]

During the procedure, the implanting physician may be presented with limited options for LV lead placement. In 70% of patients, at least three suitable CS side branches are available; however, in patients with ischemic cardiomyopathy and extensive transmural scar, options may be more limited. In addition, women tend to have a smaller diameter in both the main CS and side branches, independent of LV end-diastolic diameter. Even when a posterior or lateral CS branch is present, anatomic characteristics such as a steep takeoff angle, small vessel diameter and extensive tortuosity may make lead implantation difficult or impossible.

Many implanting physicians use an "over-the-wire" technique for LV lead placement. This technique involves probing for the CS ostium with a soft-tipped wire through a preformed sheath, followed by advancement of the pacing lead into the target branch over an angioplasty wire. However, tortuous anatomy may make advancement of the sheath or LV lead using only a wire for support difficult or impossible. New catheter-based techniques using contrast injection to localize the CS ostium and telescoping delivery systems that allow direct advancement of the sheath into the target branch may allow more efficient, targeted LV lead placement.[46] These systems utilize inner directional catheters and guide sheaths to allow direct lead delivery into the target branch (Figure 57.4). Observational data have shown that CRT implant procedures using contrast injection through telescoping-catheter delivery systems result in fewer failed LV leads (1.9% vs

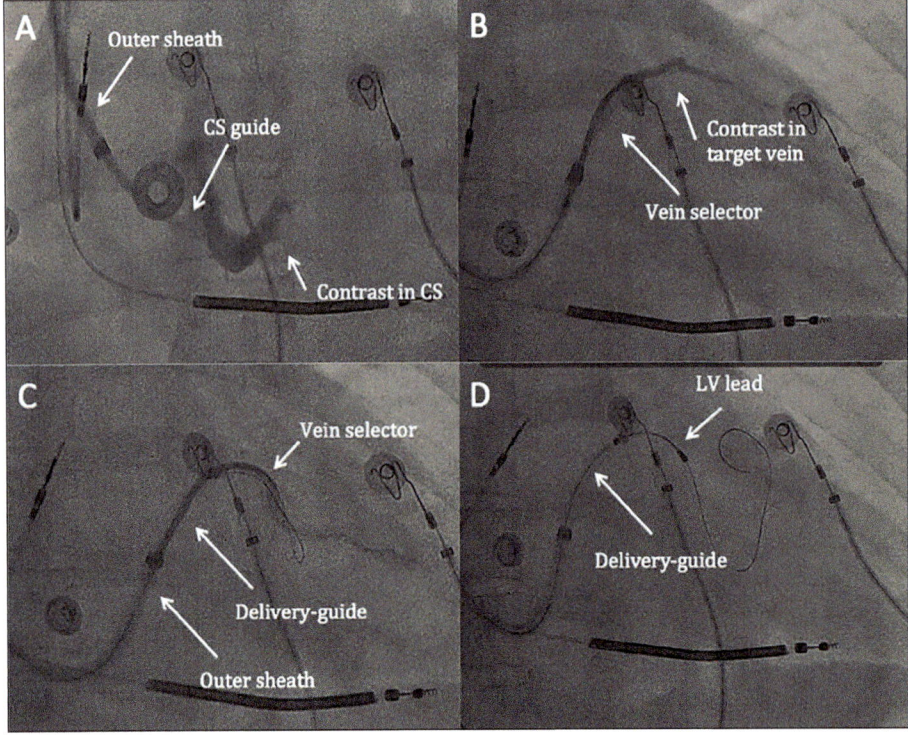

Figure 57.4 Steps in left ventricular lead implantation using telescoping catheters and contrast injection. **Panel A:** The CS is identified with contrast puffed through CS guide attached to a contrast injection system. The outer sheath is then advanced over the CS guide. **Panel B:** Once the outer sheath is in place in the mid-CS, the CS guide is removed. The vein selector is attached to the contrast injection system and inserted into the delivery guide. Both vein selector and deliver guide are advanced through the outer sheath. The target vein is identified with contrast injection through the vein selector. **Panel C:** The delivery guide is advanced over the vein selector into the target branch. **Panel D:** The LV lead is advanced over a wire through delivery guide into final position. *Source:* Courtesy of Dr. Kevin P. Jackson.

8.1%, $P = 0.02$), improved targeted lead placement and reduced fluoroscopic times compared to standard over-the-wire techniques.[47]

Acute Hemodynamic Response to CRT

Placement of an open-lumen catheter or pressure wire into the LV chamber during CRT implantation allows real-time assessment of hemodynamics with biventricular pacing, including measurement of stroke work and the maximum rate of left ventricular pressure (dP/dt_{max}). In small studies, positioning the LV lead in CS branches demonstrating maximal acute improvement in LV hemodynamics from baseline has translated to improved long-term clinical response rates.[48] Randomized, controlled trials of this technique are lacking, however.

Noninvasive measures of hemodynamic changes during CRT implantation are possible using standard echocardiography; however, technical considerations including procedure sterility and maintaining adequate imaging windows during prolonged implant procedures limit this technique. Newer imaging modalities, such as intracardiac echocardiography (ICE), may overcome these limitations.[49]

Measurement of Left Ventricular Electrical Activation

During the early era of CRT implantation, measurement of the electrical delay at the final implant location of the LV lead was common practice. With data that posterolateral or lateral LV sites were generally preferable, however, a strictly anatomic implant strategy became commonplace. Recently, there is renewed interest in measurement and placement of LV leads in sites of delayed electrical activation. Comprehensive mapping of electrical activation in patients with LBBB shows significant heterogeneity in the location of the line of functional block.[50] By measuring the electrical activation from the onset of ventricular activation on the surface ECG to the local activation on the LV lead, the implanting physician can optimize the lead location based on the site of latest electrical delay (QLV). Placement of the LV lead on sites of significant electrical delay, measured either as an absolute value (QLV > 95 ms) or as a percentage of the QRS duration (> 50%), results in improvements in both acute hemodynamic response and long-term clinical outcomes.[51,52]

Advancements in Left Ventricular Lead Technology

Optimizing the CRT implant procedure relies on multiple factors including proper patient selection, targeted lead placement, arrhythmia management and postimplant device optimization. Placing the lead in the target branch requires the proper tools, technique, and pacing leads capable of tracking tortuous anatomy and remaining stably positioned once deployed.

Recent advancements in CRT lead technology have improved stability and lead tracking into difficult target vessels. Early LV leads were straight and unipolar, and dislodgement rates were high. Current leads with angled or coiled distal tips allow "passive fixation" into the target vessel with lower rates of lead dislodgement. An "active fixation" lead utilizing an expandable mesh on the lead coating, which anchors the lead into the vessel, may further reduce lead dislodgment, although there are concerns in the event of subsequent need for removal.[53] Another recent advance has been the development of quadripolar LV pacing leads, allowing multiple pacing vectors configurations to overcome inadvertent phrenic nerve stimulation. Further advances in lead fixation and multi-electrode pacing are in development.

Left Ventricular Endocardial Pacing

Despite the tremendous progress made in the development of improved implantation instruments and methods, including balloon venoplasty and snare techniques, CRT implantation is unsuccessful in 5% to 10% of attempted cases. In these cases, the LV lead is usually implanted onto the LV epicardium through a thoracotomy. This approach has a higher morbidity and mortality than percutaneous implantation techniques, particularly in patients with prior cardiac surgery.[54,55] More recently, endocardial LV lead implantation through a transseptal approach has been described.[56-58] The use of this approach has been limited because of technical difficulty, the increased risk of thromboembolism associated with a lead inside the LV cavity, and concern about the interaction of a lead and the mitral valve. Better instruments for performing transseptal puncture from a left subclavian venous access are under development, but are not currently available. To reduce the risk of thromboembolism, operators are encouraged to use thin, polyurethane leads and continue lifelong anticoagulation with warfarin in patients undergoing LV endocardial LV lead placement.[59]

Although the LV endocardial lead has limitations, the technique has several advantages including (1) access to the entire left ventricle, allowing more precise targeting of lead position to areas with delayed activation; (2) better approximation of the physiologic transmural activation and repolarization sequence from endocardium to epicardium; and (3) faster LV impulse propagation. Acute hemodynamic studies in animals and humans have demonstrated improvements, dP/dT_{max}, stroke work, pulse pressure, and LV end-diastolic pressure with LV endocardial pacing compared to standard LV epicardial pacing.[60,61]

Large-scale clinical outcomes studies comparing LV endocardial lead placement to standard epicardial LV lead placement by the coronary sinus have not yet been performed.

Postimplant Optimization

Assessing Response to CRT

The definition of response to CRT has varied across clinical trials and in clinical practice. This has led to a broad range of reported response rates. In one of the early randomized, controlled trials of CRT, 34% of patients felt moderately or markedly improved in the control arm as compared with 60% in the CRT arm.[1] Improvements in the three coprimary endpoints of NYHA functional class, 6-minute hall walk, and HF QOL were all superior in the CRT arm, but improvement also occurred in these subjective measures in the "placebo" arm. For more objective secondary endpoints, such as maximal oxygen consumption (peak VO_2) or reduction in LV end-systolic dimension by echocardiography, the mean improvement in the control arm was negligible. In the MADIT-CRT trial, the non-CRT control group had a mean reduction in LV echocardiographic end-systolic volume (18 mL), though it was far less than the CRT arm (57 mL) at 1 year as compared to the baseline echocardiogram.[2] Nevertheless, the placebo effect of CRT must be accounted for when considering the response rate attributable to biventricular pacing. When considering the response rates from the large, randomized trials of CRT, the percentage nonresponse varies from about 20% to 30% for subjective measures, as opposed to 35% to 50% for echocardiographic measures (Figure 57.5).

A number of factors can contribute to the lack of improvement after CRT, whether defined as persistent, advanced heart failure symptoms or lack of ventricular remodeling. These include improperly programmed AV intervals, arrhythmias (especially PVCs or atrial fibrillation), poor lead position, an insufficient percentage of biventricular pacing, inadequate medical therapy, and lack of underlying wide QRS as contributors.[5] In evaluating a patient with poor response to CRT, analysis of each of these factors and corrective action where possible may improve outcomes.

Loss of Biventricular Pacing

Studies have shown that biventricular pacing should be delivered nearly 100% of the time in order to achieve an optimal response. In a large, observational database of over 80,000 patients, 40% of patients had < 98% biventricular pacing and 11% had < 90% pacing.[62] Atrial arrhythmias caused the most CRT loss overall, but in patients with < 90% biventricular pacing, too long of an AV interval (resulting in ventricular sensing) became the dominant cause (Table 57.5).

Table 57.5 Causes of loss of biventricular pacing

Cardiac arrhythmia:
Atrial fibrillation
Ventricular ectopic beats
Sinus tachycardia (causing upper rate behavior)
Excessively long AV interval programming
Fusion or pseudofusion of native conduction
Excessive interatrial conduction delay
Latency and delayed LV conduction

In order to accurately assess adequate LV capture, 12-lead electrocardiography is essential (Figure 57.6). A baseline ECG for future comparison should be established intraoperatively or at device follow-up when capture is confirmed by device interrogation. Analysis of the frontal plane axis as well as the R-wave pattern across the precordial leads can help identify proper LV pacing. In one algorithm proposed by Ammann and colleagues, the presence of either an R/S ratio ≥ 1 in V_1 or an R/S ratio ≤ 1 in lead I confirms the presence of LV capture with sensitivity and specificity of nearly 95%.[63] This algorithm works best when the LV lead is in a lateral position, however, as pacing from an inferior or posterior LV lead location results in absence of an R/S ratio ≤ 1 in lead I in a significant proportion of patients (24%–36%). In addition, if the RV lead is placed in the outflow tract, biventricular capture may demonstrate a mostly negative QRS complex in V_1 with a right-inferior, frontal-plane axis.

Atrial fibrillation is a common cause of failure to deliver effective biventricular pacing and of nonresponse to CRT. Several device-based algorithms have been developed to mitigate the loss of biventricular pacing, including ones that deliver biventricular pacing upon sensing an intrinsic activation, increase the lower pacing rate temporarily when sensed beats occur during AF, or seek to minimize the variation in R-R intervals.[64] It is important to realize, however, that counts of biventricular pacing through the device may overestimate fully paced complexes due to unrecognized fusion beats during AF. In a study of 19 patients with CRT and permanent AF in which device counters showed > 90% LV pacing, analysis of continuous Holter monitor tracings revealed complete biventricular capture in only 76%.[34] Therefore, in patients with AF where response is poor after CRT implant, device counters reporting an adequate biventricular pacing percentage may be unreliable, and AV node ablation should be considered.

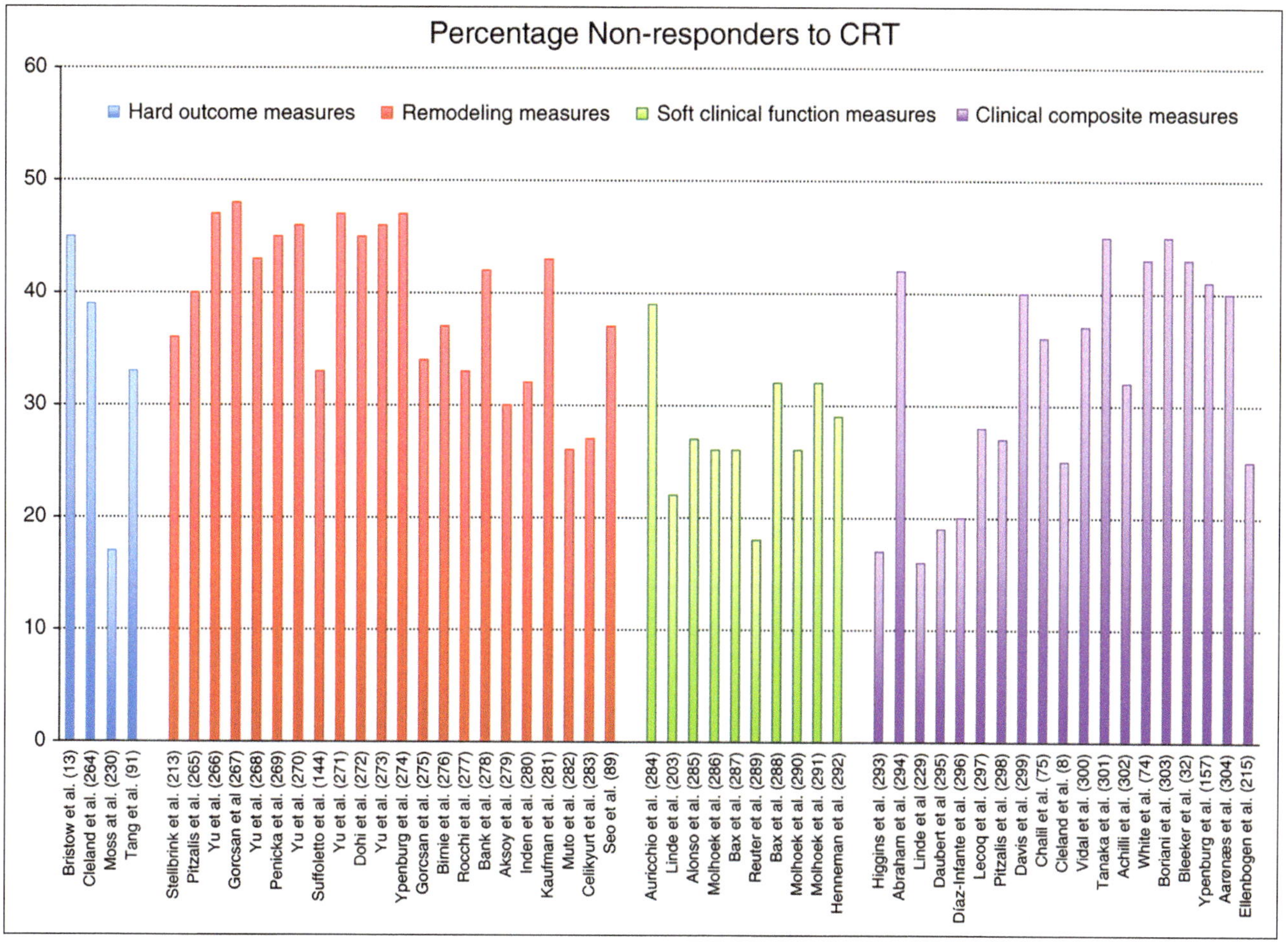

Chapter 57: Optimization of Cardiac Resynchronization Therapy: Techniques and Patient Selection • **777**

Figure 57.5 Percentage of patients with nonresponse to cardiac resynchronization therapy in major randomized, controlled trials. *Source:* Daubert JC, Saxon L, Adamson PB, et al. *Heart Rhythm.* 2012;9(9):1266, Figure 8.

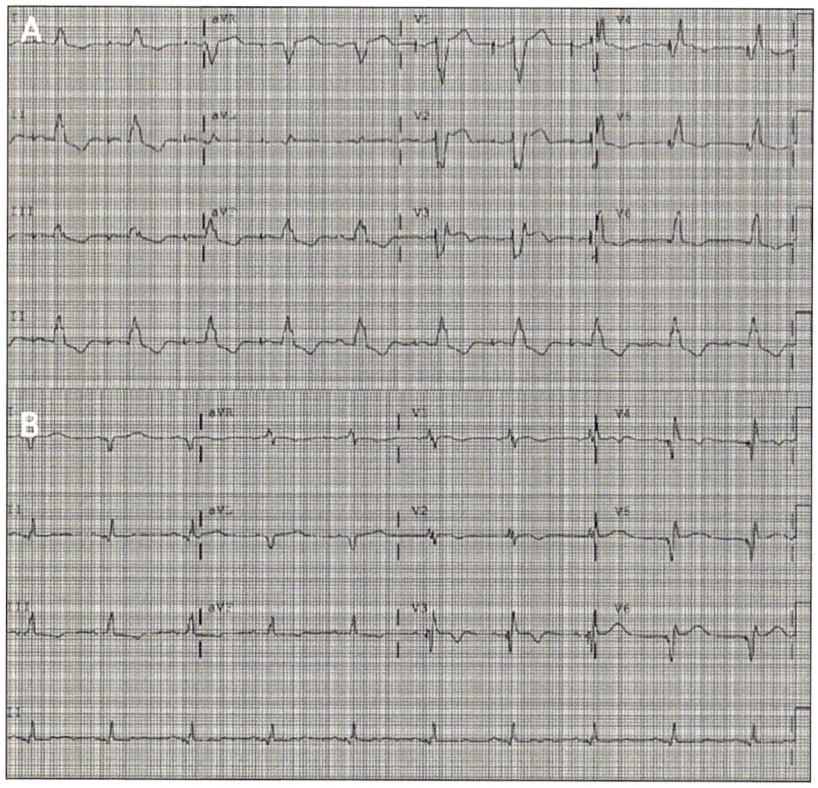

Figure 57.6 An example of analysis of the 12-lead ECG to determine adequate left ventricular pacing. **Panel A:** Baseline LBBB-like configuration in a patient with underlying AV block necessitating continuous RV pacing. **Panel B:** Post-CRT implant QRS morphology is dramatically different. Note the negativity in lead I and the R-wave in lead V1, reflecting activation away from the lateral wall of the left ventricle and from posterior to anterior. *Source:* Courtesy of Dr. James P. Daubert.

AV Interval Optimization

To ensure proper AV interval programming, a number of different methodologies have been proposed. The most established methodology uses echocardiographic examination of the mitral inflow pattern to evaluate the left-sided atrial and ventricular systolic and diastolic events from a mechanical perspective. In CRT, the AV interval must be short enough that pacing is uniformly delivered, yet not so short that left atrial contraction is preempted. One of the most common methodologies for selecting the optimal AV interval is the iterative method, which relies upon visual analysis of the passive (E-wave) and active (A-wave) components of the mitral valve inflow tracing. The first step is to determine the longest AV interval still providing ventricular capture; this will result in fusion of E and A waves, since the E wave is delayed. Next, the AV interval is shortened until the longest AV interval producing truncation of the A wave is found. The optimal AV delay is determined to be optimal when the E and A waves are distinct (no fusion) and there is no evidence of A wave truncation (Figure 57.7).

An alternative echocardiographic approach to AV interval optimization looks at left ventricular ejection rather than filling, comparing the aortic velocity time integral (VTI) with different programmed AV intervals. Measurement of cardiac output by aortic VTI can also be used to complement or verify iterative evaluation of the mitral inflows. Optimization of the AV interval by the aortic VTI method was compared in a small, randomized study (n = 40) to an empiric AV interval of 120 ms. Interestingly, the mean "optimal" AV delay was 119 ms, but the range of optimal delays was 60 to 200 ms. By clinical criteria (NYHA functional class and QOL score), the optimized group fared better, and there were trends toward more improvement in echocardiographic remodeling.[65] However, routine use of echocardiography to optimize AV delays is costly and time consuming and therefore not routinely employed in clinical practice.

Device-based algorithms to find and program optimal AV delays eliminate the need for echocardiography and have other potential advantages, including automation of the process to allow more frequent adjustments. The SmartDelay Determined AV Optimization (SMART-AV) trial compared outcomes in over 1,000 patients randomized to 3 different optimization methodologies: a device-based electrogram approach, an echo-based mitral inflow iterative approach, and a fixed AV delay of 120 ms.[66] The device-based electrogram approach had been validated against LV dp/dt and was found to outperform echocardiogram-based optimization techniques. However, in SMART-AV, no significant differences were found in the primary endpoint (LV end-systolic volume 6 months after implant) or other echocardiographic or clinical secondary outcomes. Similarly, the FREEDOM trial compared the device-based AV optimization performed every 3 months with a control group receiving CRT with a fixed AV interval (or one-time, echocardiographic-based optimization at investigator discretion) in 1,647 patients.[67] There was no significant difference between these groups for the primary endpoint of improvement in heart failure clinical composite score or secondary endpoints of heart failure class or 6-minute walk test.

An important and often overlooked aspect of AV interval optimization relates to whether the atrium is tracked or paced. Right atrial pacing may induce significant interatrial conduction delay depending on the location of the RA lead. Pacing from the RA free wall or appendage can augment the delay between the activation time at the RA lead and LA mechanical events. Atrial pacing during CRT has been found to be significantly less effective than atrial tracking using a VDD mode, a mode used in several early CRT trials.[68]

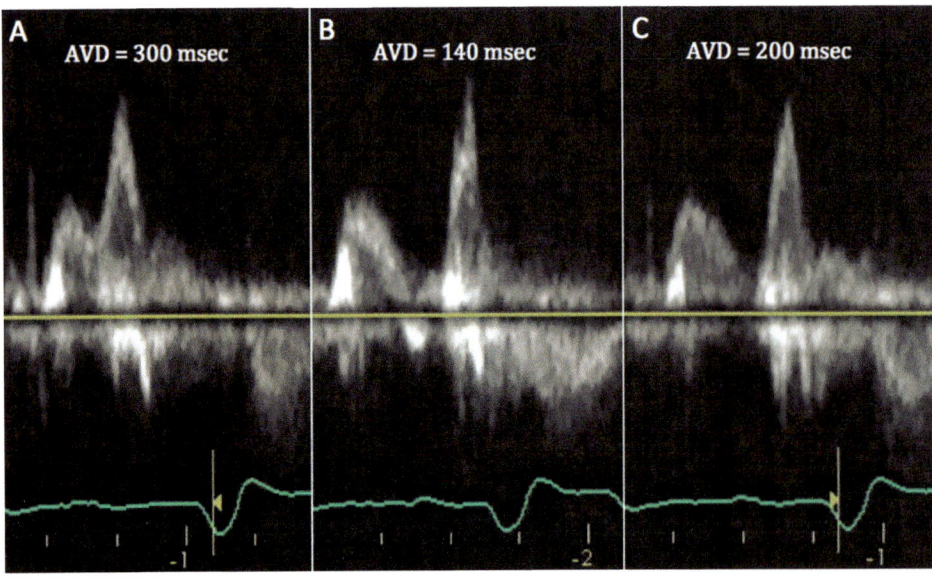

Figure 57.7 Echocardiographic evaluation of the mitral valve inflows to determine proper AV timing. **Panel A:** Long programmed AV interval results in fusion of the E and A waves. **Panel B:** Shortening of the AV interval results in truncation of the A wave. **Panel C:** Proper AV interval programming results in distinct E and A wave. AVD = trioventricular delay. *Source:* Courtesy of Dr. Kevin P. Jackson.

The American Society of Echocardiography recommends routine echocardiographic assessment after CRT; however, based on currently available evidence, routine optimization of the AV interval for all recipients of CRT devices is not justified.[69] Whether patients who are deemed to be nonresponders to CRT should undergo echocardiogram-based or device-based optimization is still a matter of debate. Preliminary data from the RESPONSE-HF trial (presented at the Heart Rhythm Society 2010 meeting) suggests that adjustment of the RV-to-LV timing (V–V interval) in patients who have received CRT and failed to improve NYHA class or have been hospitalized for congestive heart failure exacerbation do show clinical improvement after adjustment of the V–V interval. However, as discussed above, randomized, controlled trials of routine optimization in all patients has not shown clinical benefit to date.

References

1. Abraham WT, Fisher WG, Smith AL, et al. Cardiac resynchronization in chronic heart failure. *N Engl J Med*. 2002;346(24):1845-1853.
2. Moss AJ, Hall WJ, Cannom DS, et al. Cardiac-resynchronization therapy for the prevention of heart-failure events. *N Engl J Med*. 2009;361(14):1329-1338.
3. Linde C, Mealing S, Hawkins N, et al. Cost-effectiveness of cardiac resynchronization therapy in patients with asymptomatic to mild heart failure: insights from the European cohort of the REVERSE (Resynchronization Reverses remodeling in Systolic Left Ventricular Dysfunction). *Eur Heart J*. 2011;32(13):1631-1639.
4. Ghio S, Freemantle N, Scelsi L, et al. Long-term left ventricular reverse remodelling with cardiac resynchronization therapy: results from the CARE-HF trial. *Eur J Heart Fail*. 2009;11(5):480-488.
5. Mullens W, Grimm RA, Verga T, et al. Insights from a cardiac resynchronization optimization clinic as part of a heart failure disease management program. *J Am Coll Cardiol*. 2009;53(9):765-773.
6. Strickberger SA, Conti J, Daoud EG, et al. Patient selection for cardiac resynchronization therapy: from the Council on Clinical Cardiology Subcommittee on Electrocardiography and Arrhythmias and the Quality of Care and Outcomes Research Interdisciplinary Working Group, in collaboration with the Heart Rhythm Society. *Circulation*. 2005;111(16):2146-2150.
7. Baldasseroni S, Opasich C, Gorini M, et al. Left bundle-branch block is associated with increased 1-year sudden and total mortality rate in 5517 outpatients with congestive heart failure: a report from the Italian network on congestive heart failure. *Am Heart J*. 2002;143(3):398-405.
8. Nelson GS, Curry CW, Wyman BT, et al. Predictors of systolic augmentation from left ventricular preexcitation in patients with dilated cardiomyopathy and intraventricular conduction delay. *Circulation*, 2000;101(23):2703-2709.
9. Cazeau S, Leclercq C, Lavergne T, et al. Effects of multisite biventricular pacing in patients with heart failure and intraventricular conduction delay. *N Engl J Med*. 2001;344(12):873-880.
10. Young JB, Abraham WT, Smith AL, et al. Combined cardiac resynchronization and implantable cardioversion defibrillation in advanced chronic heart failure: the MIRACLE ICD Trial. *JAMA*. 2003;289(20): 2685-2694.
11. Higgins SL, Hummel JD, Niazi IK, et al. Cardiac resynchronization therapy for the treatment of heart failure in patients with intraventricular conduction delay and malignant ventricular tachyarrhythmias. *J Am Coll Cardiol*. 2003;42(8):1454-1459.
12. Bristow MR, Saxon LA, Boehmer J, et al. Cardiac-resynchronization therapy with or without an implantable defibrillator in advanced chronic heart failure. *N Engl J Med*. 2004; 350(21):2140-2150.
13. Gold MR, Thébault C, Linde C, et al. Effect of QRS duration and morphology on cardiac resynchronization therapy outcomes in mild heart failure: results from the Resynchronization Reverses Remodeling in Systolic Left Ventricular Dysfunction (REVERSE) study. *Circulation*. 2012;126(7):822-829.
14. Sipahi I, Carrigan TP, Rowland DY, Stambler BS, Fang JC. Impact of QRS duration on clinical event reduction with cardiac resynchronization therapy: Meta-analysis of randomized controlled trials. *Arch Intern Med*. 2011;171(16):1454-1462.
15. Goldenberg I, Kutyifa V, Klein HU, et al. Survival with cardiac-resynchronization therapy in mild heart failure. *N Engl J Med*. 2014;370(18):1694-1701.
16. Sweeney MO, van Bommel RJ, Schalij MJ, Borleffs CJ, Hellkamp AS, Bax JJ. Analysis of ventricular activation using surface electrocardiography to predict left ventricular reverse volumetric remodeling during cardiac resynchronization therapy. *Circulation*. 2010;121(5):626-634.
17. Ruschitzka F1, Abraham WT, Singh JP, et al. Cardiac-resynchronization therapy in heart failure with a narrow QRS complex. *N Engl J Med*. 2013;369(15):1395-1405.
18. Egoavil CA, Ho RT, Greenspon AJ, Pavri BB. Cardiac resynchronization therapy in patients with right bundle branch block: analysis of pooled data from the MIRACLE and Contak CD trials. *Heart Rhythm*. 2005;2(6):611-615.
19. Zareba W, Klein H, Cygankiewicz I, et al. Effectiveness of cardiac resynchronization therapy by QRS morphology in the Multicenter Automatic Defibrillator Implantation Trial–Cardiac Resynchronization Therapy (MADIT-CRT)/ Clinical Perspective. *Circulation*. 2011;123(10):1061-1072.
20. Fantoni C, Kawabata M, Massaro R, et al. Right and left ventricular activation sequence in patients with heart failure and right bundle branch block: a detailed analysis using three-dimensional non-fluoroscopic electroanatomic mapping system. *J Cardiovasc Electrophysiol*. 2005;16(2):112-119; discussion 120-121.
21. Wilkoff BL, Cook JR, Epstein AE, et al. Dual-chamber pacing or ventricular backup pacing in patients with an implantable defibrillator: The Dual Chamber and VVI Implantable Defibrillator (DAVID) trial. *JAMA*. 2002;288(24):3115-3123.
22. Curtis AB, Worley SJ, Adamson PB, Chung ES, Niazi I, Sherfesee L, Shinn T, Sutton MS; Biventricular versus Right Ventricular Pacing in Heart Failure Patients with Atrioventricular Block (BLOCK HF) Trial Investigators. Biventricular pacing for atrioventricular block and systolic dysfunction. *N Engl J Med*. 2013;368(17):1585-1593.
23. Bleeker GB, Schalij MJ, Molhoek SG, et al. Relationship between QRS duration and left ventricular dyssynchrony in patients with end-stage heart failure. *J Cardiovasc Electrophysiol*. 2004;15(5):544-549.
24. Yu CM, Fung JW, Zhang Q, et al. Tissue Doppler imaging is superior to strain rate imaging and postsystolic shortening on the prediction of reverse remodeling in both ischemic and nonischemic heart failure after cardiac resynchronization therapy. *Circulation*. 2004;110(1):66-73.
25. Becker M, Hoffmann R, Kühl HP, et al. Analysis of myocardial deformation based on ultrasonic pixel tracking to

determine transmurality in chronic myocardial infarction. *Eur Heart J.* 2006;27(21):2560-2566.
26. Chung ES, Leon AR, Tavazzi L, et al. Results of the Predictors of Response to CRT (PROSPECT) Trial. *Circulation.* 2008;117(20):2608-2616.
27. Ruschitzka F, Abraham WT, Singh JP, et al. Cardiac-resynchronization therapy in heart failure with a narrow QRS complex. *N Engl J Med.* 2013;369(15):1395-1405.
28. Kim RJ, Fieno DS, Parrish TB, et al. Relationship of MRI delayed contrast enhancement to irreversible injury, infarct age, and contractile function. *Circulation.* 1999;100(19):1992-2002.
29. Bleeker GB, Kaandorp TA, Lamb HJ, et al. Effect of postero-lateral scar tissue on clinical and echocardiographic improvement after cardiac resynchronization therapy. *Circulation.* 2006;113(7):969-976.
30. Leyva F, Foley PW, Chalil S, et al. Cardiac resynchronization therapy guided by late gadolinium-enhancement cardiovascular magnetic resonance. *J Cardiovasc Magn Reson.* 2011;13:29.
31. Foley PW, Patel K, Irwin N, et al. Cardiac resynchronisation therapy in patients with heart failure and a normal QRS duration: the RESPOND study. *Heart.* 2011;97(13):1041-1047.
32. Hsu JC, Solomon SD, Bourgoun M, et al. Predictors of super-response to cardiac resynchronization therapy and associated improvement in clinical outcome: the MADIT-CRT (Multicenter Automatic Defibrillator Implantation Trial with Cardiac Resynchronization Therapy) study. *J Am Coll Cardiol.* 2012;59(25):2366-2373.
33. Koplan BA, Kaplan AJ, Weiner S, Jones PW, Seth M, Christman SA. Heart failure decompensation and all-cause mortality in relation to percent biventricular pacing in patients with heart failure: Is a goal of 100% biventricular pacing necessary? *J Am Coll Cardiol.* 2009;53(4):355-360.
34. Kamath GS, Cotiga D, Koneru JN, et al. The utility of 12-lead Holter monitoring in patients with permanent atrial fibrillation for the identification of nonresponders after cardiac resynchronization therapy. *J Am Coll Cardiol.* 2009;53:1050-1055.
35. Gasparini M, Auricchio A, Metra M, et al. Long-term survival in patients undergoing cardiac resynchronization therapy: the importance of performing atrio-ventricular junction ablation in patients with permanent atrial fibrillation. *Eur Heart J.* 2008;29(13):1644-1652.
36. Ganesan AN, Brooks AG, Roberts-Thomson KC, Lau DH, Kalman JM, Sanders P. Role of AV nodal ablation in cardiac resynchronization in patients with coexistent atrial fibrillation and heart failure: a systematic review. *J Am Coll Cardiol.* 2012;59(8):719-726.
37. Lakkireddy D, Di Biase L, Ryschon K, et al. Radiofrequency ablation of premature ventricular ectopy improves the efficacy of cardiac resynchronization therapy in nonresponders. *J Am Coll Cardiol.* 2012;60(16):1531-1539.
38. Tracy CM, Epstein AE, Darbar D, et al. 2012 ACCF/AHA/HRS focused update of the 2008 guidelines for device-based therapy of cardiac rhythm abnormalities. *Circulation.* 2012;126(14):1784-1800.
39. Khan FZ, Virdee MS, Palmer CR, et al. Targeted left ventricular lead placement to guide cardiac resynchronization therapy: the TARGET study: a randomized, controlled trial. *J Am Coll Cardiol.* 2012;59(17):1509-1518.
40. Saba S, Marek J, Schwartzman D, et al. Echocardiography-guided left ventricular lead placement for cardiac resynchronization therapy: results of the Speckle Tracking Assisted Resynchronization Therapy for Electrode Region trial. *Circ Heart Fail.* 2013; 6(3):427-434.
41. Cazeau S, Ritter P, Bakdach S, et al. Four chamber pacing in dilated cardiomyopathy. *Pacing Clin Electrophysiol.* 1994;17(11 Pt 2):1974-1979.
42. Daubert JC, Ritter P, Le Breton H, et al. Permanent left ventricular pacing with transvenous leads inserted into the coronary veins. *Pacing Clin Electrophysiol.* 1998;21(1 Pt 2):239-245.
43. Tang AS, Wells GA, Talajic M, et al. Cardiac-resynchronization therapy for mild-to-moderate heart failure. *N Engl J Med.* 2010;363(25):2385-2395.
44. Van de Veire NR, Schuijf JD, Bleeker GB, Schalij MJ, Bax JJ. Magnetic resonance imaging and computed tomography in assessing cardiac veins and scar tissue. *Europace.* 2008;10 Suppl 3:iii110-iii113.
45. Daubert C, Gold MR, Abraham WT, et al. Prevention of disease progression by cardiac resynchronization therapy in patients with asymptomatic or mildly symptomatic left ventricular dysfunction: insights from the European cohort of the REVERSE (Resynchronization Reverses Remodeling in Systolic Left Ventricular Dysfunction) trial. *J Am Coll Cardiol.* 2009;54(20):1837-1846.
46. Worley SJ. CRT delivery systems based on guide support for LV lead placement. *Heart Rhythm.* 2009;6(9):1383-1387.
47. Jackson KP, Hegland DD, Frazier-Mills C, et al. Impact of using a telescoping-support catheter system for left ventricular lead placement on implant success and procedure time of cardiac resynchronization therapy. *Pacing Clin Electrophysiol.* 2013;36(5):553-558.
48. Duckett SG, Ginks M, Shetty AK, et al. Invasive acute hemodynamic response to guide left ventricular lead implantation predicts chronic remodeling in patients undergoing cardiac resynchronization therapy. *J Am Coll Cardiol.* 2011;58(11):1128-1136.
49. Saksena S, Simon AM, Mathew P, Nagarakanti R. Intracardiac echocardiography-guided cardiac resynchronization therapy: technique and clinical application. *Pacing Clin Electrophysiol.* 2009;32(8):1030-1039.
50. Auricchio A, Fantoni C, Regoli F, et al. Characterization of left ventricular activation in patients with heart failure and left bundle-branch block. *Circulation.* 2004;109(9):1133-1139.
51. Gold MR, Yu Y, Singh JP, et al. The effect of left ventricular electrical delay on AV optimization for cardiac resynchronization therapy. *Heart Rhythm.* 2013;10(7):988-993.
52. Singh JP, Fan D, Heist EK, et al. Left ventricular lead electrical delay predicts response to cardiac resynchronization therapy. *Heart Rhythm.* 2006;3(11):1285-1292.
53. Cronin EM, Ingelmo CP, Rickard J, et al. Active fixation mechanism complicates coronary sinus lead extraction and limits subsequent reimplantation targets. *J Interv Card Electrophysiol.* 2013;36(1):81-86.
54. Mair H, Jansens JL, Lattouf OM, Reichart B, Dabritz S. Epicardial lead implantation techniques for biventricular pacing via left lateral mini-thoracotomy, video-assisted thoracoscopy, and robotic approach. *Heart Surg Forum.* 2003;6(5):412-417.
55. Gabor S, Prenner G, Wasler A, Schweiger M, Tscheliessnigg KH, Smolle-Jüttner FM. A simplified technique for implantation of left ventricular epicardial leads for biventricular re-synchronization using video-assisted thoracoscopy (VATS). *Eur J Cardiothorac Surg.* 2005;28(6):797-800.
56. Jaïs P, Douard H, Shah DC, Barold S, Barat JL, Clémenty J. Endocardial biventricular pacing. *Pacing Clin Electrophysiol.* 1998;21(11 Pt 1):2128-2131.
57. Jaïs P, Takahashi A, Garrigue S, et al. Mid-term follow-up of endocardial biventricular pacing. *Pacing Clin Electrophysiol.* 2000;23(11 Pt 2):1744-1747.

58. Leclercq F, Hager FX, Macia JC, et al. Left ventricular lead insertion using a modified transseptal catheterization technique: A totally endocardial approach for permanent biventricular pacing in end-stage heart failure. *Pacing Clin Electrophysiol.* 1999;22(11):1570-1575.
59. Purevjav E, Varela J, Morgado M, et al. Nebulette mutations are associated with dilated cardiomyopathy and endocardial fibroelastosis. *J Am Coll Cardiol.* 2010;56(18):1493-1502.
60. van Deursen C, van Geldorp IE, Rademakers LM, et al. Left ventricular endocardial pacing improves resynchronization therapy in canine left bundle-branch hearts. *Circ Arrhythm Electrophysiol.* 2009;2(5):580-587.
61. Derval N, Steendijk P, Gula LJ, et al. Optimizing hemodynamics in heart failure patients by systematic screening of left ventricular pacing sites: the lateral left ventricular wall and the coronary sinus are rarely the best sites. *J Am Coll Cardiol.* 2010;55(6):566-575.
62. Cheng A, Gold MR, Waggoner AD, et al. Potential mechanisms underlying the effect of gender on response to cardiac resynchronization therapy: insights from the SMART-AV multicenter trial. *Heart Rhythm.* 2012;9(5):736-741.
63. Ammann P, Sticherling C, Kalusche D, et al. An electrocardiogram-based algorithm to detect loss of left ventricular capture during cardiac resynchronization therapy. *Ann Intern Med.* 2005;142(12 Pt 1):968-973.
64. Aktas MK, Jeevanantham V, Sherazi S, et al. Effect of biventricular pacing during a ventricular sensed event. *Am J Cardiol.* 2009;103(12):1741-1745.
65. Kerlan JE, Sawhney NS, Waggoner AD, et al. Prospective comparison of echocardiographic atrioventricular delay optimization methods for cardiac resynchronization therapy. *Heart Rhythm.* 2006;3(2):148-154.
66. Ellenbogen KA, Gold MR, Meyer TE, et al. Primary results from the SmartDelay determined AV optimization: a comparison to other AV delay methods used in cardiac resynchronization therapy (SMART-AV) trial: a randomized trial comparing empirical, echocardiography-guided, and algorithmic atrioventricular delay programming in cardiac resynchronization therapy. *Circulation.* 2010;122(25):2660-2668.
67. Abraham WT, Gras D, Yu CM, Guzzo L, Gupta MS; FREEDOM Steering Committee. Rationale and design of a randomized clinical trial to assess the safety and efficacy of frequent optimization of cardiac resynchronization therapy: the Frequent Optimization Study Using the QuickOpt Method (FREEDOM) trial. *Am Heart J.* 2010;159(6):944-948.
68. Bernheim A, Ammann P, Sticherling C, et al. Right atrial pacing impairs cardiac function during resynchronization therapy: acute effects of DDD pacing compared to VDD pacing. *J Am Coll Cardiol.* 2005;45(9):1482-1487.
69. Gorcsan J 3rd, Abraham T, Agler DA, et al. Echocardiography for cardiac resynchronization therapy: recommendations for performance and reporting—a report from the American Society of Echocardiography Dyssynchrony Writing Group endorsed by the Heart Rhythm Society. *J Am Soc Echocardiogr.* 2008;21(3):191-213.

CHAPTER 58

Radiologic Aspects of Cardiovascular Implantable Electronic Devices

John C. Evans, MD; Karin Chia, MBBS, MD, PhD; Mintu P. Turakhia, MD;
Henry H. Hsia, MD; Paul Zei, MD; Marco V. Perez, MD;
Paul J. Wang, MD; Amin Al-Ahmad, MD

Introduction

Radiography is an integral tool in the evaluation of patients with cardiovascular implantable electronic devices (CIEDs).[1,2] Radiography is used for device identification, evaluation of the location of leads, identification of procedural complications, and procedural planning in patients with existing systems that need upgrade. In addition, radiography can also be used in some instances to identify device system abnormalities.

The most common type of radiographic imaging used for device patients is the chest x-ray (CXR). In addition to plain film radiography, more advanced modalities of imaging can be critical for procedural planning. Tomographic images can provide insight into of the cardiac venous anatomy for cardiac resynchronization therapy, as well as an evaluation of patency of venous access in select cases.[3,4] This chapter will focus on the application of various radiographic modalities for evaluation of patients with implantable cardiac devices.

The Chest X-ray

A systematic approach is required to examine the chest radiograph for preprocedural planning, postoperative follow-up, and troubleshooting for device evaluations. The entire radiograph should be evaluated with a thorough inspection of all anatomic structures, including bony landmarks, cardiac silhouette, great vessels, trachea, and lung parenchyma, as well as the diaphragmatic position. The device should likewise be inspected in a systematic fashion. We recommend evaluation proceeding from the device generator to the header and then following the length of each lead.

Postimplantation Chest Radiograph

All patients should receive a posteroanterior (PA) and lateral chest radiograph or x-ray (CXR) within 24 hours of device placement. Because a single PA view may only provide a 2-dimensional (2D) localization, lateral imaging is also generally recommended. Two views are essential for determining the lead position in the heart, as certain appearances can be indistinguishable in the PA view (Figure 58.1). Radiographs performed in this initial early postoperative period can be done without ipsilateral arm elevation to avoid the risk of lead dislodgement. Although the bony and soft tissue structures of the arm may obstruct the evaluation of the lung parenchyma, it does not sufficiently alter the evaluation of the leads.

784 • Section 2D: Device Implantation: Intraoperative, Surgical, and Device Management

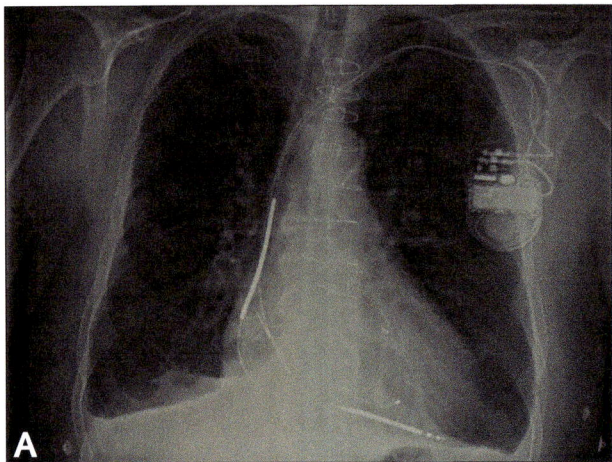

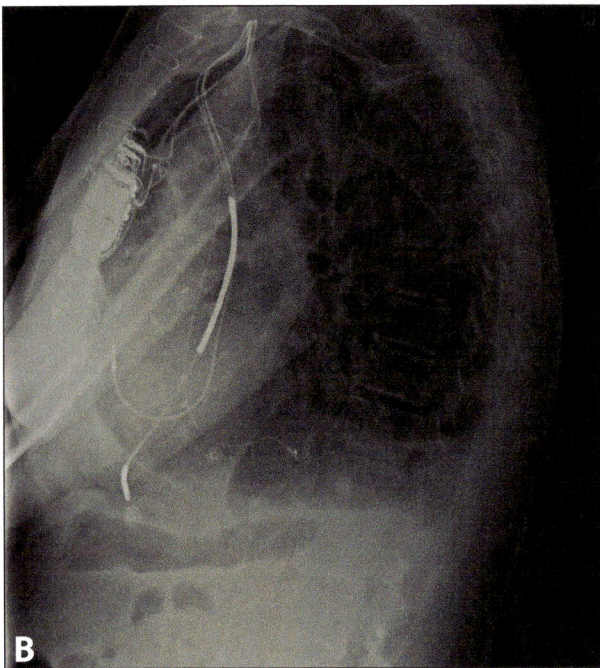

Figure 58.1 PA (**Panel A**) and lateral (**Panel B**) CXR of a biventricular ICD. Notice the similar course of the coronary sinus (CS) and RV leads in the AP view, and that the lateral view nicely demonstrates that the CS lead is posterior to the heart, whereas the RV lead is anterior.

Complications

As well as serving as a comparison for future evaluations, the initial postimplantation x-ray is imperative to evaluate for complications. A CXR is performed to evaluate for pneumothorax immediately after the procedure whenever venous access is obtained by venopuncture (Figure 58.2A). In addition, rarely a right-sided pneumothorax can be seen when there is perforation of an active fixation lead through the RA and overlying pleura (Figure 58.2B).[5,6] Perforations, although often symptomatic, can also be discovered with the postoperative CXR (Figure 58.3). Other complications that can be apparent on CXR are pleural and pericardial effusion.[7]

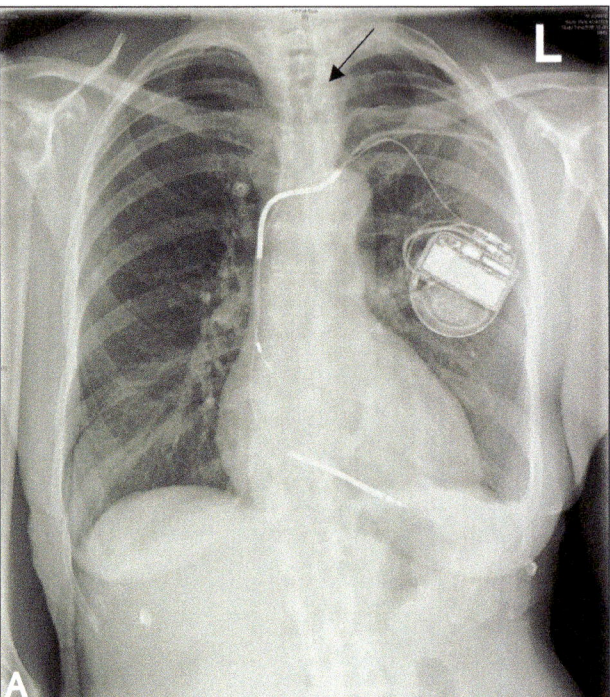

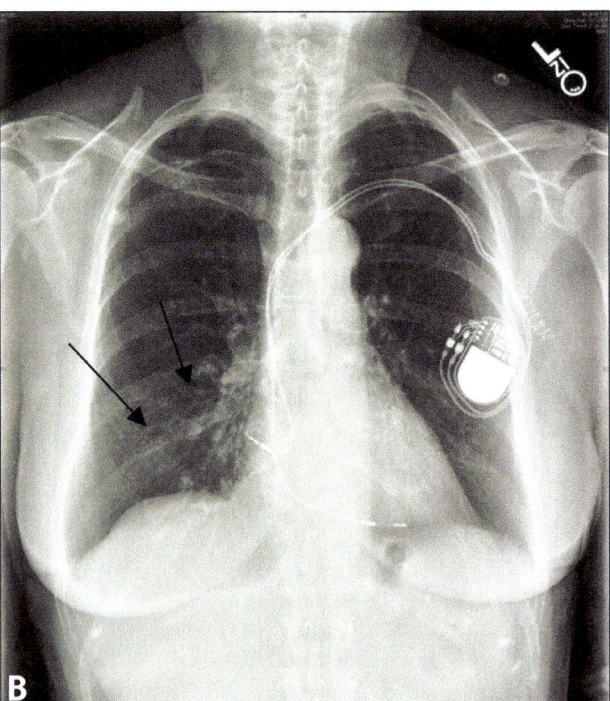

Figure 58.2 Pneumothoraces with arrows at lung margin. **Panel A:** Left-sided pneumothorax likely caused by the left-sided venipuncture. **Panel B:** Right-sided pneumothorax with a left-sided device. The likely culprit is the RA lead that can be seen abutting the right lung and pleura.

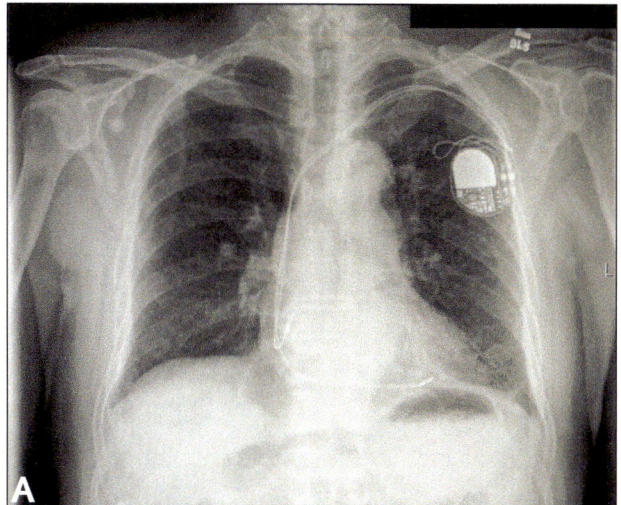

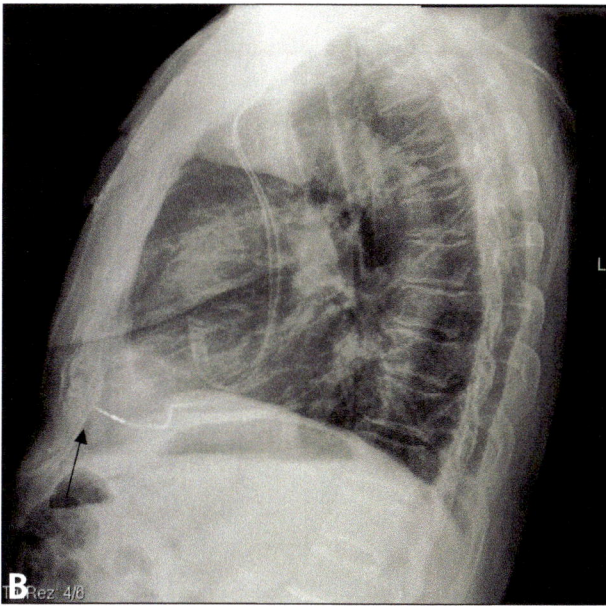

Figure 58.3 Perforation of the right ventricular lead on chest radiography. This provides another example of the importance of orthogonal views. In the PA view, the perforation is not evident (**Panel A**). In the lateral view, the RV lead tip is outside the cardiac silhouette (**Panel B**).

Postimplant Lead Assessment

When performing a chest radiograph for device evaluation, optimal viewing is not the same as for evaluation of the native anatomic structures. To maximize the clinical information that can be gathered from the CXR, it is important to have an image that delineates the implanted structures well. With digital images, the contrast can be adjusted to focus on the leads and generator. Inversion of the x-ray such that it is seen as a "negative" making radio-opaque material black on a white background is helpful when examining the course of the leads in the chest (Figure 58.4). When digital images are not available, increased penetration of x-rays may make the implanted materials more easily distinguishable from the soft tissue.

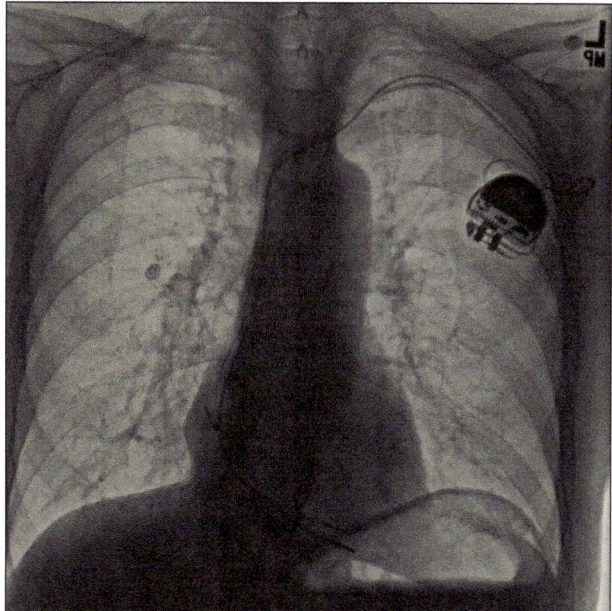

Figure 58.4 This inverted image provides excellent contrast with the overlying tissue to be able to follow the entire course of the leads.

The most important aspects of lead assessment in the postimplant period are evaluation of slack and distal electrode positions. Even in the setting of the new implant, it is important to follow the leads back to the pocket to ensure the appropriate lead is connected to the corresponding header, as well as recognizing abandoned leads when they are present.

As noted before, whenever inspecting the leads, the entire length should be evaluated. Immediately postimplant, lead fracture is extremely unlikely, but the lead should be evaluated for any sharp bend that may predispose to future fracture. The length of the lead should also be evaluated for an appropriate amount of slack. There should be modest amount of slack, but not so much that the lead interferes with other structures (such as the tricuspid valve, which could result in significant tricuspid regurgitation). The angle of the "J" can be evaluated in the evaluation of slack in a lead placed in the RAA. Optimally, the angle formed by the portion of the lead entering the RA from the SVC just prior to the curvature of the J and the portion extending from the distal tip of the lead should be an acute angle to ensure that there is not too much tension on the lead predisposing to dislodgement (Figure 58.5). The ventricular lead will optimally have three to four regions of alternating convexity in the heart (Figure 58.6). There is typically convexity as it enters the SVC–RA junction, changing within the body of the RA, and then curve again over the tricuspid valve. Often there will be a fourth curvature within the ventricle as well. If there is too little slack in any lead, dislodgement may be more likely (Figure 58.7). Additionally, excess slack should be left in pediatric patients to accommodate growth and avoid dislodgement in the future. The lead redundancy needs to be balanced

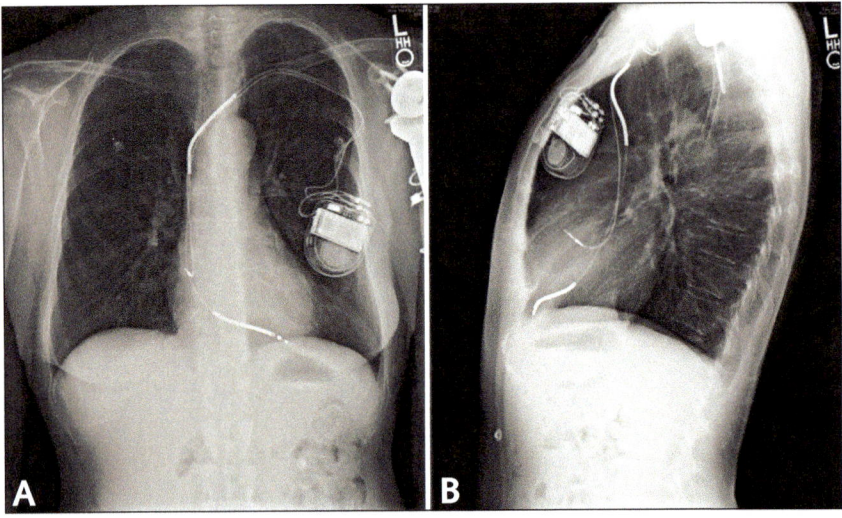

Figure 58.5 Atrial leads should have at least the bend demonstrated. Notice that the angle of the lead tip and the body of the lead going up into the IVC is approximately approaching 90 degrees, but still an acute angle. Any less slack would be unacceptable.

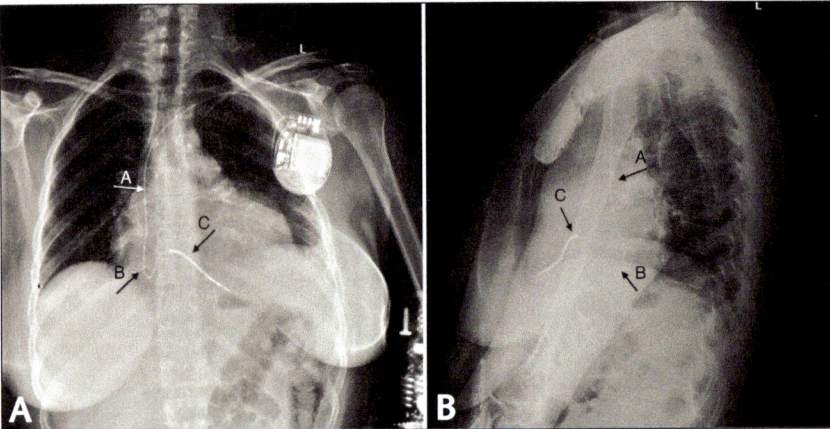

Figure 58.6 This patient's lead has redundancy that demonstrates the curvatures that should be seen in a ventricular lead. Convexities of the lead are labeled as it enters the SVC–RA junction (**Arrow A**), changing within the body of the RA (**Arrow B**), and over the tricuspid valve (**Arrow C**). Adequate slack for the RV lead has been classically described as a "lady's slipper" in the AP view, with a "heel" along the RA, the "arch" representing slack along the tricuspid valve, and the "toe" in the right ventricle.

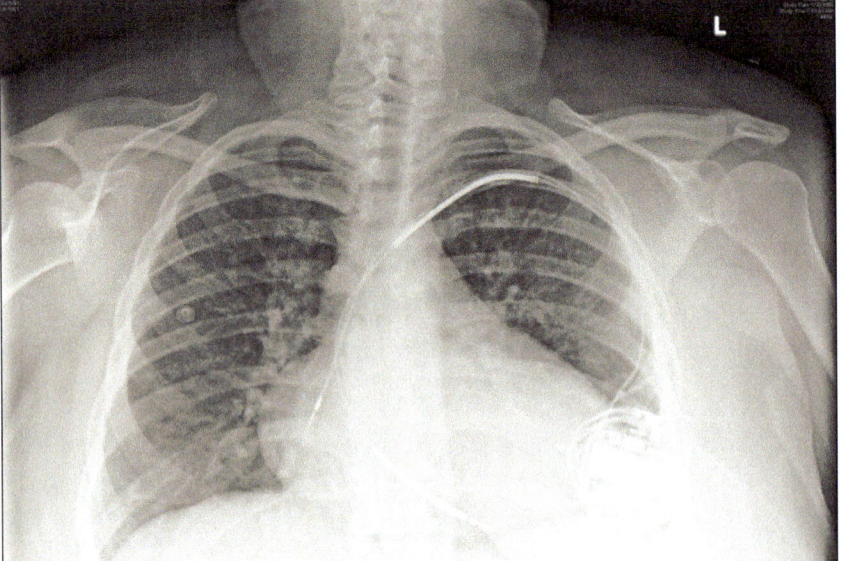

Figure 58.7 Unacceptable traction on the leads in a patient with large body habitus and breast shadows. Remarkably, there was considerable redundancy of the lead on fluoroscopy when the patient returned to a supine position in the electrophysiology laboratory. When patients like this first sit upright, there can be shifting of the tissues, pulling the device can downward and removing redundant slack from the leads.

against the propensity for prolapse.[8] It is worth mentioning that during the implant, it is often useful to use different imaging projections such as the RAO, LAO, and AP views in order to ensure proper lead placement in complementary views. In addition, a "final fluoro" of the leads from the tip to the device and would be useful as well.

The distal tip location of all leads can be approximated by using the PA and lateral CXR. The tip of an atrial lead in the RAA, the most common placement, will be directed anteromedially (Figure 58.8). Other common placements include septal and lateral RA placement. The tip in these positions may be oriented more posteriorly, and there may be less J on the lead depending on how low in the atrium it is attached (Figure 58.9). Because it was once thought to reduce atrial fibrillation,[9] some patients will have atrial pacing from the LA with a lead tip in the body of the CS. When this LA lead is present, the lead is often split after the header to provide both RA and LA pacing (Figure 58.10). Dislodged RA leads are often easily identified with a loss of the J-shaped redundancy and the leads are often prolapsed into the RV (Figure 58.7, Figure 58.11). Another clue to dislodgement on the CXR, even if not prolapsed into the ventricle, is that the lead may be in a position other than that intended.

RV lead-tip position is also readily recognized. The three most common locations for RV lead placement are apical, septal, and in the RV outflow tract (RVOT) (Figure 58.12). In the most traditional location, the apex, the tip of the lead, will be directed downward in the PA view with its tip between spine and apex. Often the tip will be directed anteriorly in the lateral view, but the body of the lead should not lie in a predominantly posterior position. When the lead is primarily lying in the posterior portions of the cardiac silhouette, one must consider that the lead has crossed an intracardiac shunt to reside in the left ventricle (Figure 58.13). LV lead placements must be

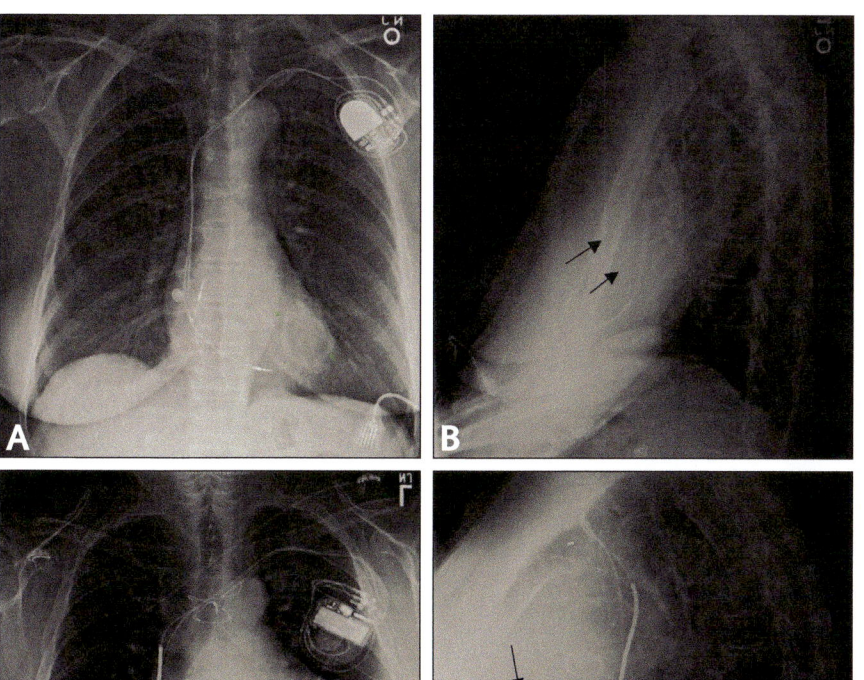

Figure 58.8 This x-ray demonstrates the location of atrial lead in the RAA. Notice that the lead is directed medially in the AP view (**Panel A**) and anteriorly in the lateral view (**Panel B**).

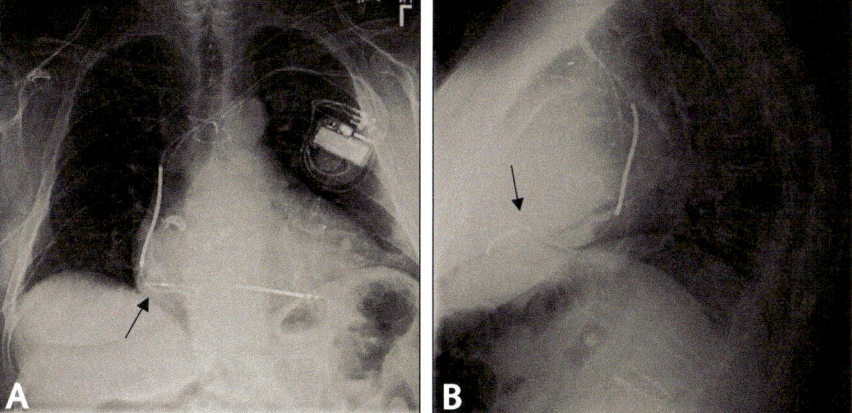

Figure 58.9 Notice that the atrial lead is not in the appendage. Here it is in the low lateral RA (**arrows**).

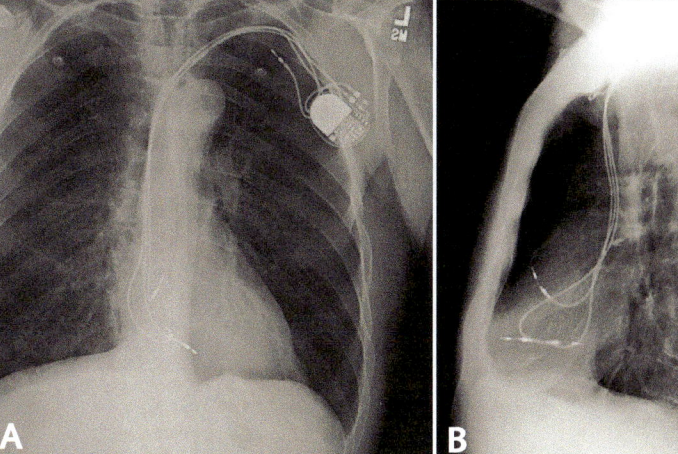

Figure 58.10 This x-ray demonstrates three leads: the RA lead with the J in the RAA, the RV lead with its tip in the mid ventricle, and a lead at the os of the CS that could be used to pace the LA. At the pocket, this LA lead is not connected to the device, but could be attached to the RA lead via y-connector.

788 • Section 2D: Device Implantation: Intraoperative, Surgical, and Device Management

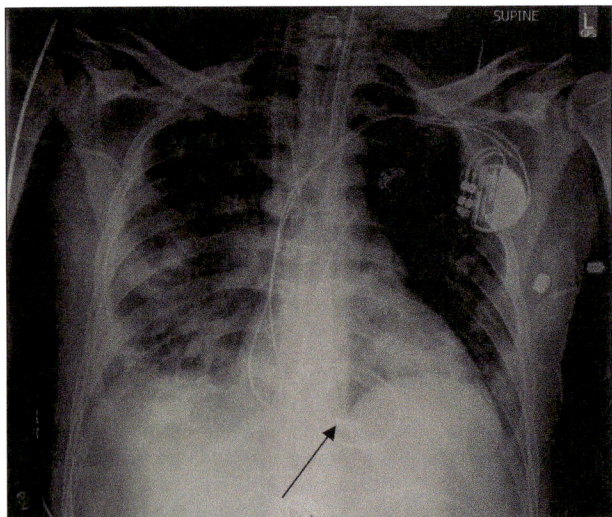

Figure 58.11 Notice that the atrial lead has fallen from the RAA and is into the right ventricle.

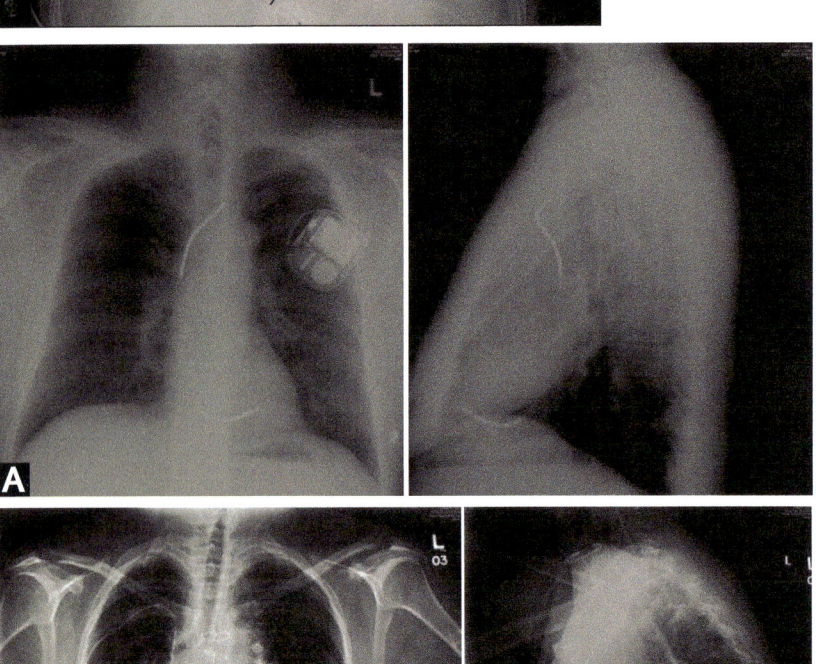

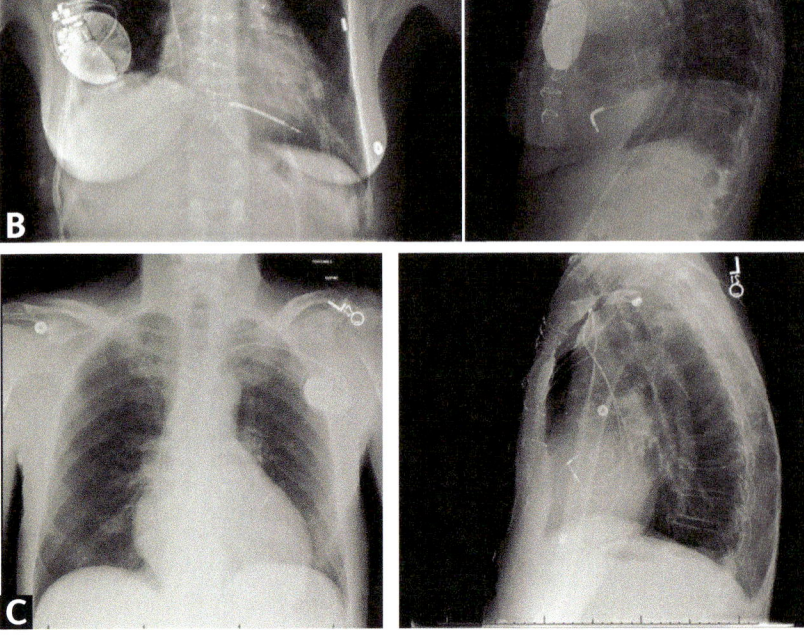

Figure 58.12 Contrasting an apical position of the RV lead (**Panel A**) with septal positioning (**Panel B**) and RVOT (**Panel C**). The septal position does extend to apically in this case and the tip is usually directed posteromedially. At the apex, the tip of the lead is downward in PA view with its tip between spine and apex and anteriorly in the lateral view. The RVOT placement leaves the lead superiorly on the CXR and directed posteriorly in the lateral view.

identified because of their implications on thromboembolic complications and long-term anticoagulation. RVOT lead placement is identified with a lead directed upward in the PA view, and the upward portion of the body of the lead typically lies in an anterior position with the tip directed posteriorly. Septal positions are recognized in that they do not extend to the apex. Septal tip positioning is usually directed posteromedially, but can vary based on the orientation of the heart within the chest. Dislodged leads in the ventricle are not as readily identified as those in the atrium, but the biggest clue is often that the lead tip is located in a position other than where it was initially placed (Figure 58.14). Thus, it is possible for leads to dislodge but to not be readily identifiable on the CXR.

The left ventricle is a posterior structure. Ideally, CS leads for cardiac resynchronization therapy should have a posterior course, but their appearance will vary depending on the branch selected for lead placement (Figure 58.15).

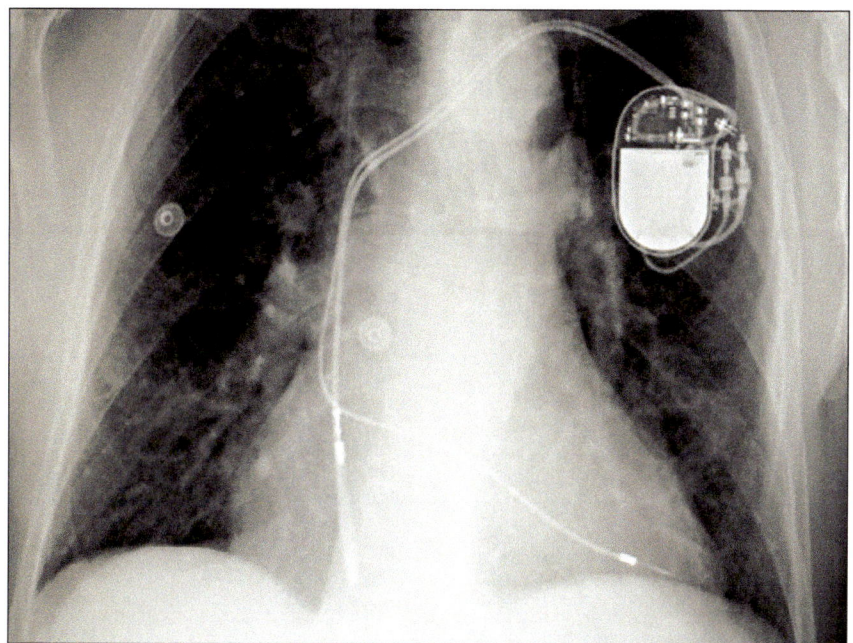

Figure 58.13 In this CXR, the ventricular lead crosses the midline more superiorly than typically seen because it is crossing at the level of a patent foramen ovale and entering the left ventricle.

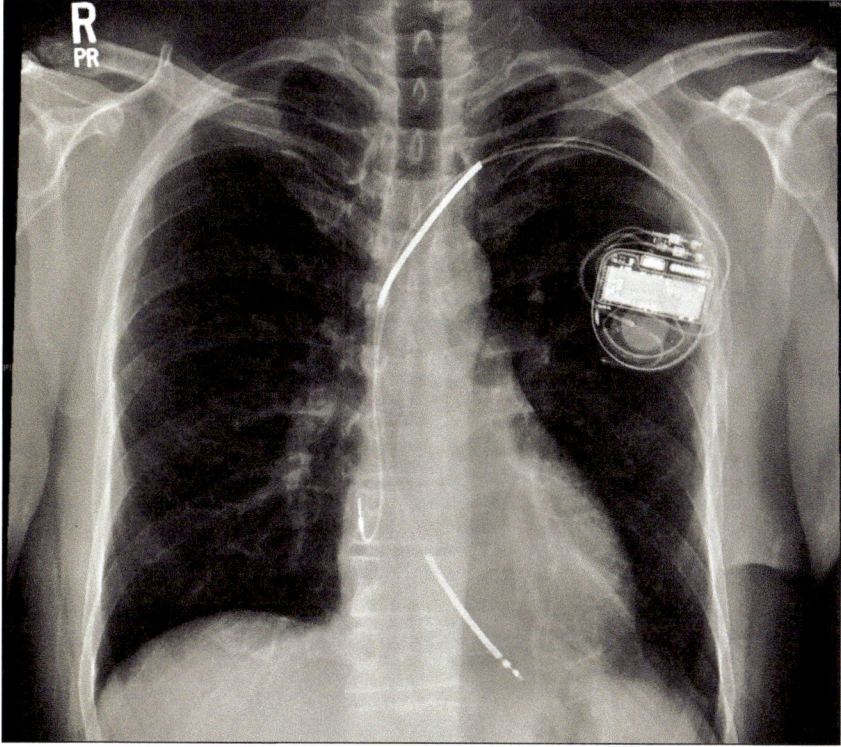

Figure 58.14 Dislodged RV ICD lead. Most of the lead, including the distal coil, remains in the right ventricle, but the lead was originally in a very apical position. The lack of lead redundancy raises suspicion that this lead has pulled back.

The most common selection is a lateral branch off the CS. In these cases, the lead follows the body of the CS and leaves the AV groove before reaching the anterior interventricular vein (AIV) (Figure 58.15C). When placed in a branch of the middle cardiac vein, the lead will run inferiorly along the border of the heart, but when appropriately placed in a lateral branch of this vein, the tip should head posteriorlaterally away from the apex of the heart (Figure 58.15B). Some patients will have the leads placed in lateral branches off of the AIV as well. Such leads will course around the CS and then superiorly to the anterior interventricular vein, and then deviate either posteriorly or laterally away from the apex via one of the AIV's lateral branches (Figure 58.15A).

Anatomic variants of the CS are beyond the scope of this chapter and often require epicardial lead placement.

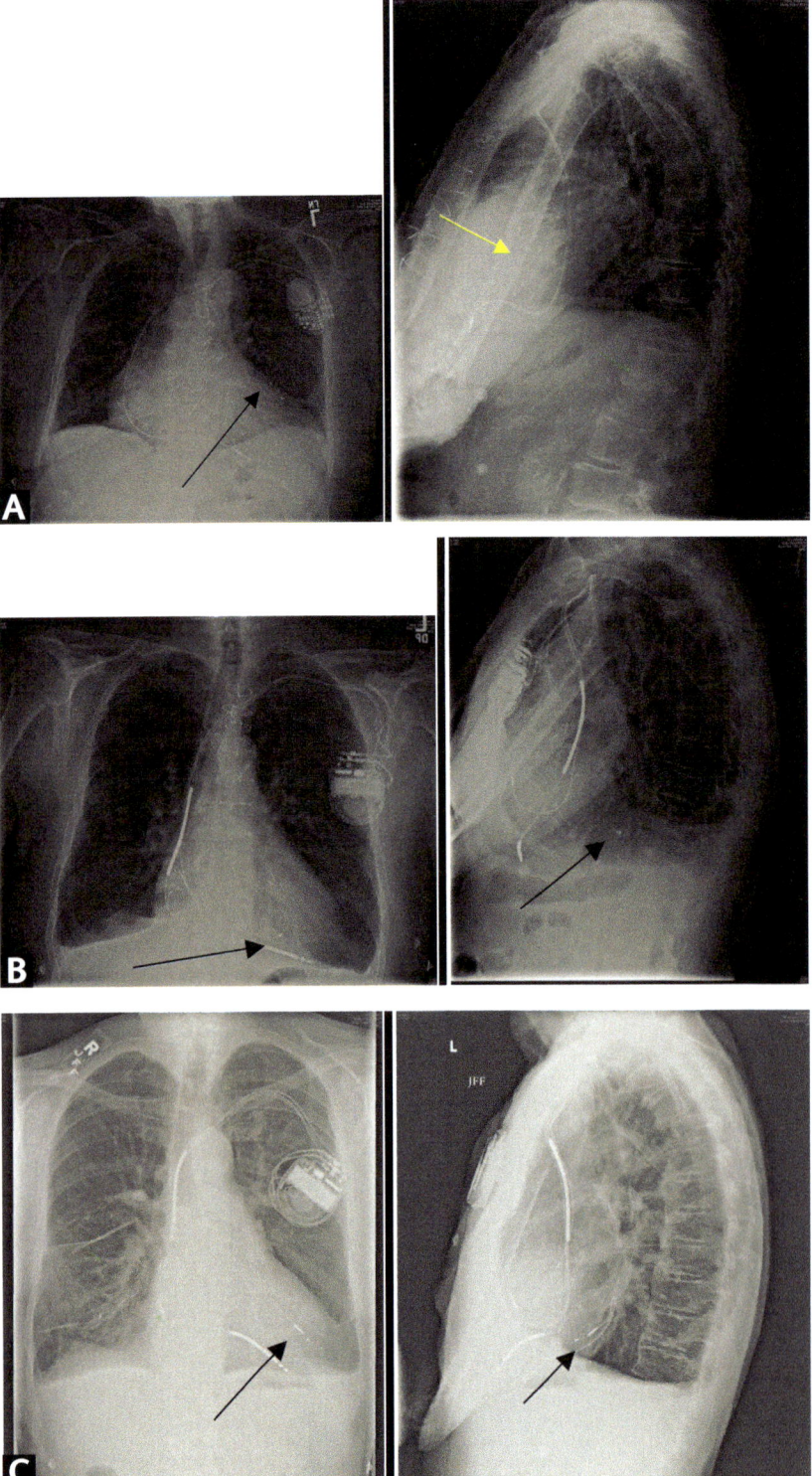

Figure 58.15 Three patients with CS leads placed in different locations. In **Panel A**, the LV lead goes superiorly to the anterior interventricular vein and out a lateral branch. In **Panel B**, the lead goes to a lateral branch of the middle cardiac vein. In **Panel C**, the lateral vein leaves the CS posteriorly.

One other common variant of the anatomy is the persistent superior vena cava (SVC) in which the left-sided brachiocephalic vessels drain directly into the body of the CS.[10] Apart from the large CS, the anatomy of the heart is normal and thus the distal tip will have a similar position as described above, but the course of the leads will be directed into the CS and into the RA at the CS os rather than from the SVC (Figure 58.16).

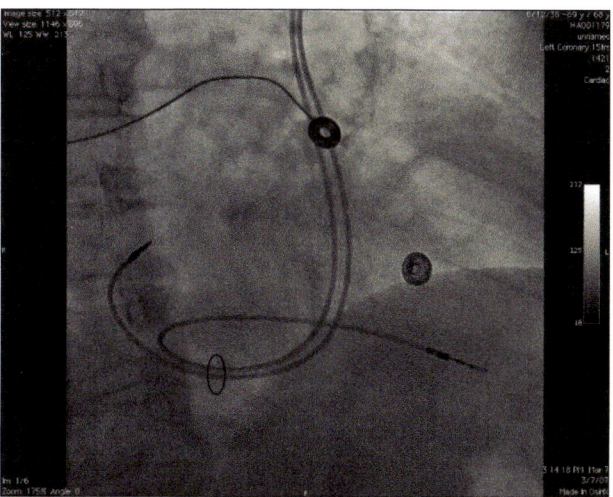

Figure 58.16 Flouroscopic image of leads entering the lateral CS via a persistent left superior vena cava. The leads separate at the CS os (**oval**) in the RA to head to the RAA and right ventricle.

Device Recognition

The posterior-anterior (PA) CXR film can be used to identify both the type of device and manufacturer when a patient presents for evaluation with little knowledge of their device. As noted previously, the x-ray should be evaluated systematically regardless of the clinical context. The manufacturer of the device can readily be identified from inspection of the header on x-ray, which will help in identifying the programmer to use for device interrogation. The type of device can readily be recognized by the position and appearance of leads, but it is important to note that abandoned leads may be left in place, so it is necessary to see how many leads are connected at the header. An evaluation for the type of device should start at the header to identify the number of leads connected to the generator. ICD leads with an IS-1 connector will have individual connectors for the pace-sense portion and the connectors for the high-energy defibrillation coils, thus a dual coil lead will often have three connections at the header. New IS-4 connectors have the pace sense and coil connectors integrated into one connector (Figure 58.17). An attempt should be made to follow the leads from the header to the lead tips, but this is often difficult with the generator overlying loops of lead. After leaving the header,

there may be numerous leads or coils attached in a single port. Adapters are typically used to integrate leads for pacing or defibrillation, as in the example of simultaneous right and LA pacing. Adapters are also used to connect subcutaneous arrays or other additional coils to devices in patients with elevated defibrillation thresholds (DFT). Again, these adapters and additional materials typically are coiled in the pocket and are even more difficult to identify (Figure 58.18).

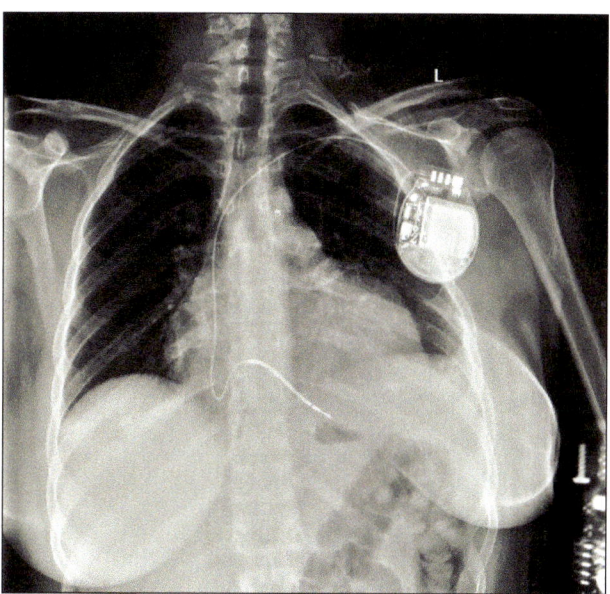

Figure 58.17 IS-4 lead with a single connection of lead at the header.

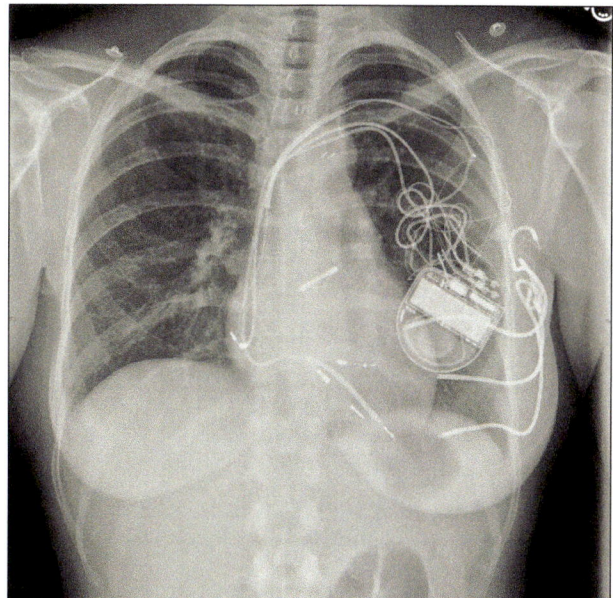

Figure 58.18 Patient with numerous wires in the pocket. There is a capped RV pace-sense lead, an ICD lead with a capped pace-sense lead, a functioning RV pace sense lead, an atrial lead, and a subcutaneous array. The subcutaneous array is connected via y-connector to the SVC coil of the ICD lead.

792 • Section 2D: Device Implantation: Intraoperative, Surgical, and Device Management

Devices are manufactured with a radio-opaque marker to identify the manufacturer (see Table 58.1). This marker can usually be identified with the PA view of the device, but if the can is situated out of the frontal plane, an oblique film may be needed to see the identification. Magnification of the header can aid in identifying this marker. Once the manufacturer is identified, all other device information can be obtained from the manufacturer-specific programmer. Newer MRI conditional devices can also be identified, as they will have specific x-ray markers on the leads as well as the device (Figure 58.19).

Table 58.1 Radiographic identification of manufacturers' pacemaker and defibrillator pulse generators

Manufacturer	Description of Radiographic Features	Example
Biotronik	All devices have Biotronic logo as well as a 2-letter code identifying the device. ICD and CRT devices also include the year of manufacture. *Source:* Courtesy of Biotronik.	PPM / ICD
Boston Scientific	Devices have the letters BSC or BOS followed by a 3-digit number indicating the model of the device. *Source:* Courtesy of Boston Scientific.	
Sorin	The x-ray ID is a series of 3 letters: For ICDs: S = Sorin, D = Defibrillator For pacemakers: S = Sorin, P = Pacemaker The last letter denotes the model. *Source:* Courtesy of Sorin.	ICD / PPM
Medtronic	Medtronic logo followed by a 3-letter code signifying the family of devices. *Source:* Courtesy of Medtronic.	

| St. Jude Medical | SJM logo and an alphanumeric identification or a pacesetter logo. *Source:* Courtesy of St. Jude Medical. | 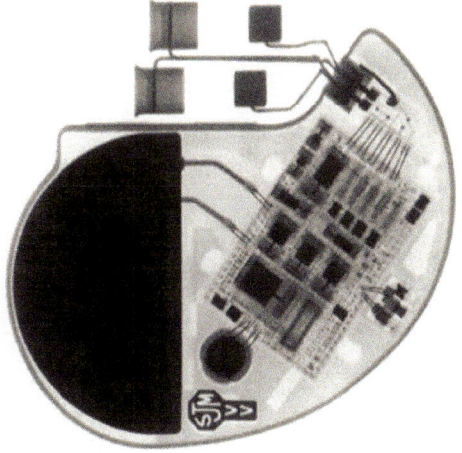
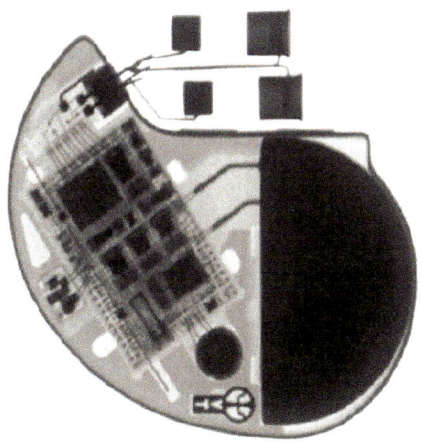 |

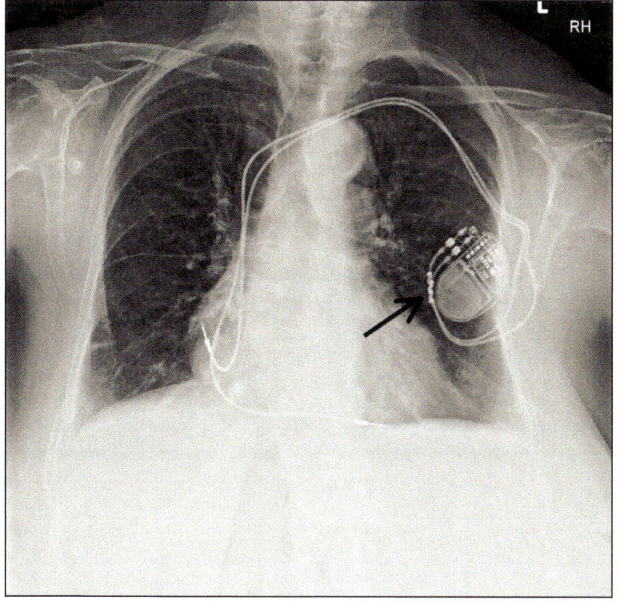

Figure 58.19 MRI conditional device with the clear x-ray markers on the leads (**arrow**).

Leads, Coils, and Patches

Several characteristics of the leads can be identified on x-ray including the polarity and means of fixation. Polarity is readily identified by the appearance of the tip electrode. Bipolar electrodes will have an electrode pair at the tip, whereas the unipolar leads will just have a single electrode at the tip (Figure 58.20). In addition, there will be a corresponding number of connector pins at the generator. VDD leads can be identified by their sensing bipole within the RA, which is located several centimeters proximal to the pacing tip (Figure 58.21). These VDD leads will typically be bifurcated with two connections at the header of the device. Active fixation leads have a screw-in mechanism, so these leads are readily recognized from the radio-opaque screw at the tip. In contrast, passive fixation leads are typically identified by their lack of such a mechanism (Figure 58.22).

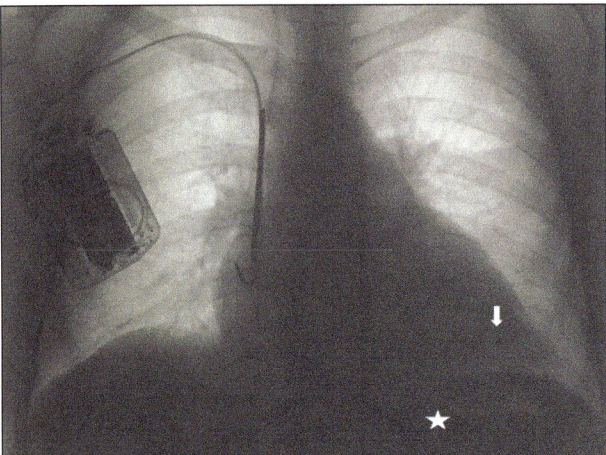

Figure 58.20 Patient with biventricular device; the left ventricular lead (**arrow**) is a unipolar lead, while the RV lead is bipolar.

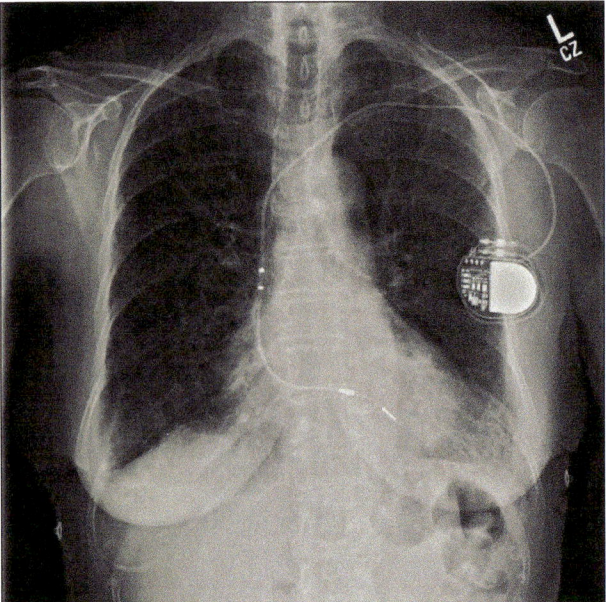

Figure 58.21 VDD lead. Notice the bipole on the body of the lead for atrial sensing. The lead also splits for insertions for the atrial lead pin and ventricular lead pin.

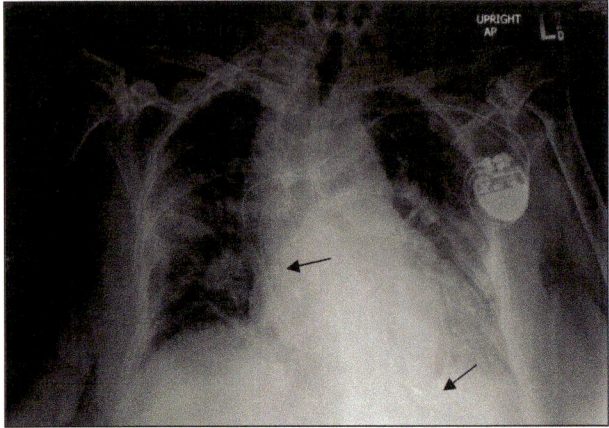

Figure 58.22 Active fixation lead with the screw readily visible in the atrium. There is no such screw in the passive fixation ventricular lead.

The other materials connected to the header must be identified as well. Epicardial pacing leads can be identified on the surface of the heart and tunneled back to the generator and thus will not follow the same course as the endovascular leads. There are differing mechanisms for the fixation of epicardial leads including screws and sutures (Figure 58.23).

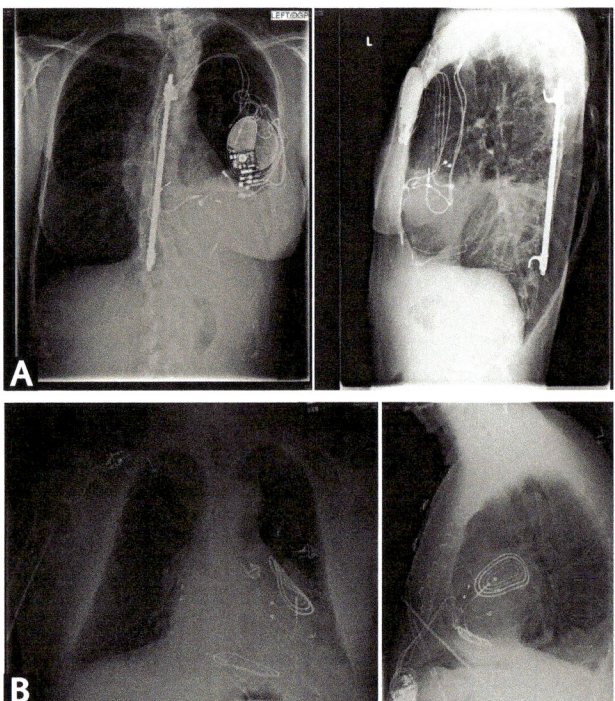

Figure 58.23 **Panel A:** Epicardial biventricular ICD with abandoned endocardial dual chamber pacemaker. The bipolar atrial lead is sewn onto the atrium and there are screw-in leads for the RV and LV. Also notice the epicardial defibrillator patches placed anteriorly and inferiorly. **Panel B:** Another epicardial BiV ICD system with both types of pacing leads and patches with concentric rings.

Epicardial defibrillator patches also can be seen on CXRs (Figure 58.23). Although they were once commonly used for high-energy delivery in defibrillators, their use has been largely supplanted by high-energy coils placed endovascularly in the right ventricle. In addition, more coils can be added to address high defibrillation thresholds. In addition to subcutaneous locations (Figure 58.18), additional coils may be placed in the azygos vein,[11-13] CS,[14] or epicardially (Figure 58.24).

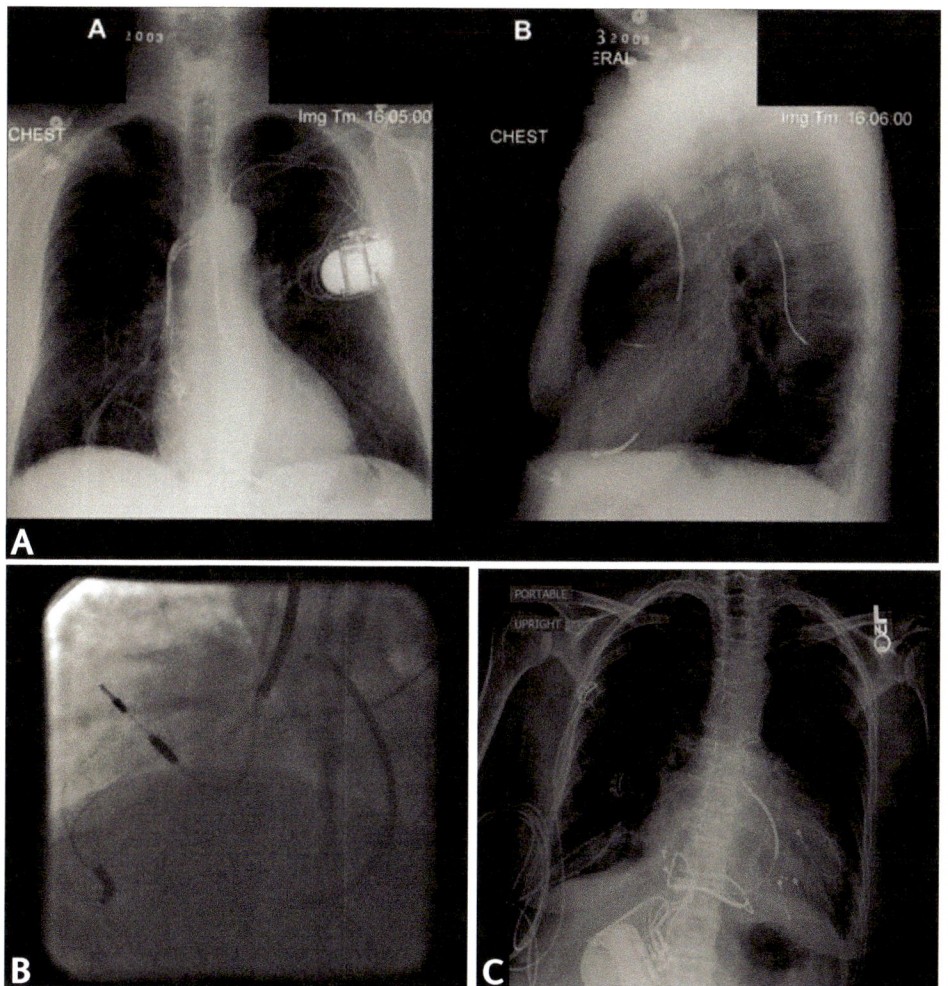

Figure 58.24 Defibrillator coils placed in the azygos vein (**Panel A**), CS (**Panel B**), and pericardial space (**Panel C**). *Sources:* Panel A: Dilling-Boer D, et al.[7] Used with permission. Panel B: Zerbe F et al.[10] Used with permission.

Troubleshooting

The CXR is also a critical tool in the evaluation of malfunctioning devices. Although not all problems will be apparent on the plain film, many issues including header connections and lead abnormalities may be apparent.

One potential issue, although avoidable at implantation, is problems with the lead connection at the header. Loose connections at the header can result in either failure to deliver pacing output or failure to capture the myocardium. It is important to make certain that the connector pin can be seen completely in the connector block (Figure 58.25). Another problem that has been reported is air in the header connector leading to over-sensing. Clinically, this over-sensing of electrical noise occurs within several days of implant and can lead to failure to pace or inappropriate therapy in high-energy devices. "Burping" the residual air within the header at the time of implantation before the insertion of lead pins is important because it can eliminate the air trapping. The air will typically dissipate and not necessitate reoperation, so it is important to recognize that the pins are appropriately placed in the header.

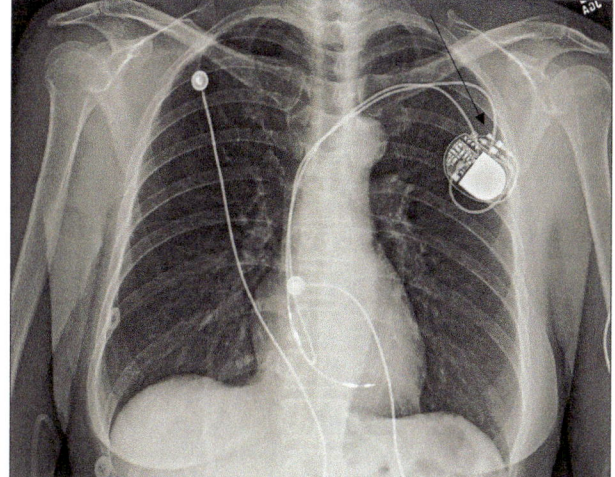

Figure 58.25 Device with lead pins not properly screwed into the header. The pin does not extend to the back of the header.

Lead issues can present with numerous clinical scenarios including failure to capture or sensing abnormalities. Before they are clinically evident, lead problems may be identified by changing lead impedance or numerous short sensing interval episodes. In the evaluation of either scenario, the entire length of the lead should be inspected for lead integrity. Areas of lead discontinuity likely represent lead fracture (Figure 58.26). Typically, the compression on the lead on the suture sleeve tie downs may be apparent on CXR, but it usually is not problematic (Figure 58.27). Although lead insulation is not radioopaque and cannot be seen on the x-ray, sudden kinks in the course of leads may identify the site problems with the integrity of the insulation as well as predisposing to lead fracture (Figure 58.28).

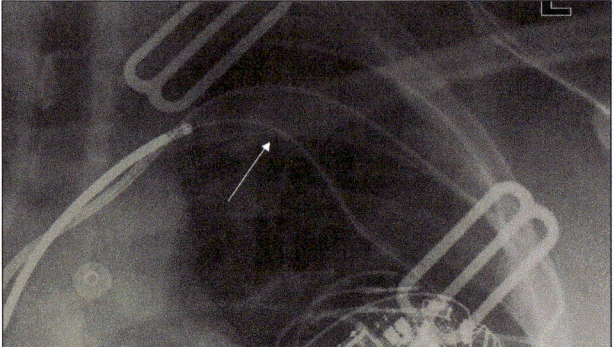

Figure 58.28 Crush injury to a lead at its insertion under the clavicle. The lead has been revised with the addition of a lead placed more laterally in the axillary vein.

Dislodgement of leads may also be apparent on the CXR. Although addressed previously, it is important to remember that assessing the positioning of the distal tip is critical in troubleshooting of devices. If possible, the tip location should be compared to the tip location in the CXR taken postoperatively.

Specific leads may require additional follow-up. The Teletronics atrial lead 330-801 has been recalled for potential fracture of the lead with protrusion of the retention wire from the lead. This lead should be followed radiographically annually, and high-resolution fluoroscopy is indicated because the protrusion may be foreshortened or too fine to see on plain film radiography (Figure 58.29).[15] Another lead that has recently been the subject of a recall is the Riata lead; in this lead externalization of the conductor cables can occur along the length of the lead. This can be seen using either an x-ray or a fluoroscopic examination (Figure 58.30).

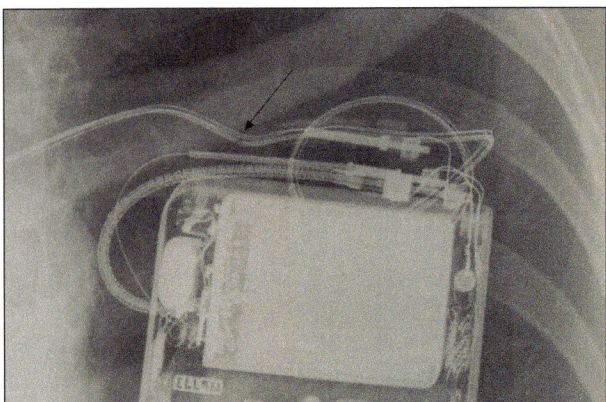

Figure 58.26 Lead fracture is easily recognized with discontinuity of the lead.

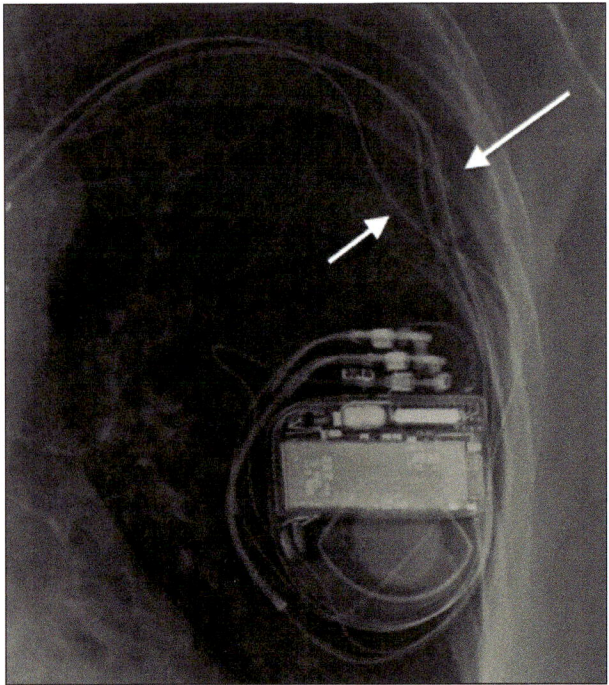

Figure 58.27 Impression of suture sleeve tie-down on the lead.

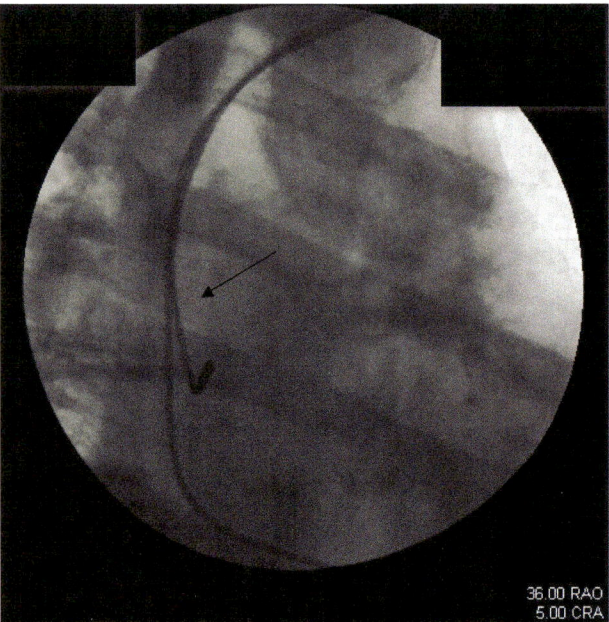

Figure 58.29 High-resolution fluoroscopy demonstrating the protruding retention wire from a Teletronics lead.

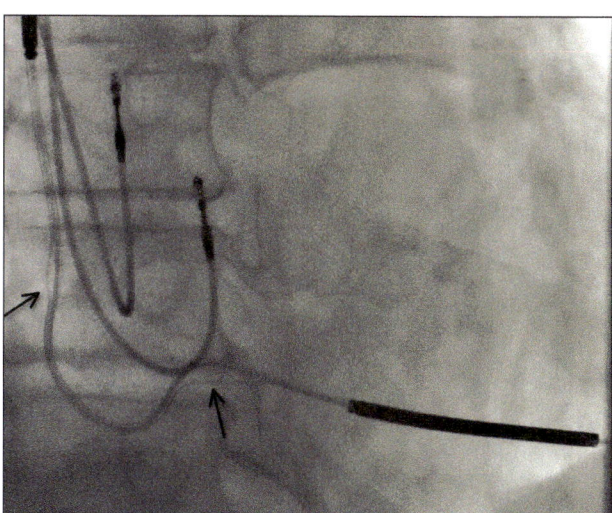

Figure 58.30 Riata lead with externalization of the inner cable (**arrows**).

Preprocedural Assessment

The final clinical scenario to be addressed is the evaluation of the device in preparation for repeat procedures. This is important for a simple generator change as well as pocket or lead revisions and device upgrades as preoperative awareness of positioning and access can greatly aid in planning a procedure. Most often, vendors will have information on the device and leads in place, but it is important to note that in patients who have had multiple procedures, some information may not be available.

When incising a pocket, it is important to know how the device is situated. The plain film can be used to identify the orientation of the device including the direction of the header and the direction the leads exit from the header. This information can be particularly important for generator changes performed without the aid of fluoroscopy, especially when devices are unexpectedly positioned with the header inferiorly (Figure 58.23A). The other important information that can be obtained from evaluating the x-ray is the relative positioning of the lead with respect to the generator making sure no coils of lead are susceptible to inadvertent damage from dissection into the pocket. The lateral x-ray can sometimes identify coils of lead that may be superficial to the generator as well.

It is very important to identify the number and type of all leads, even those that have been capped and abandoned (Figure 58.31). This information is critical in the planning of future venous access and the extraction of endovascular hardware. It is also important to recognize retained leads that have been cut short because their removal may require a femoral approach or an open surgical approach (Figure 58.32). Portions of leads can also be retained after extraction. The CXR will also readily reveal fragments of leads that remain in the body (Figure 58.33).

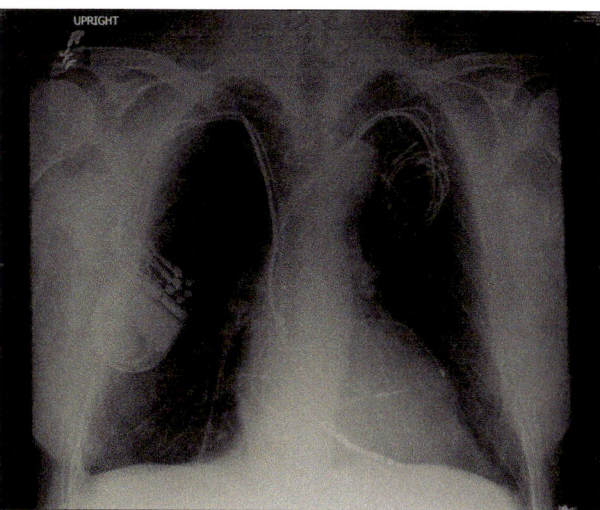

Figure 58.31 This patient was referred for extraction due to device infection and persistent bacteremia. He has a biventricular system with 3 active leads on the right as well as 4 capped leads on the left.

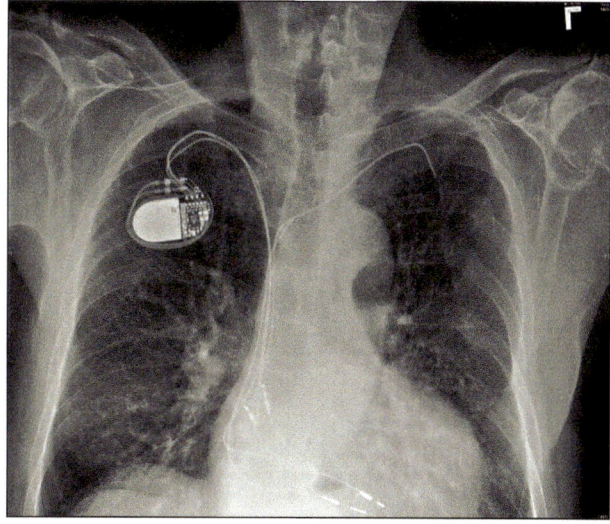

Figure 58.32 Retained cut leads on the left with a device reimplanted on the right chest. This patient was referred for complete extraction for persistent infection.

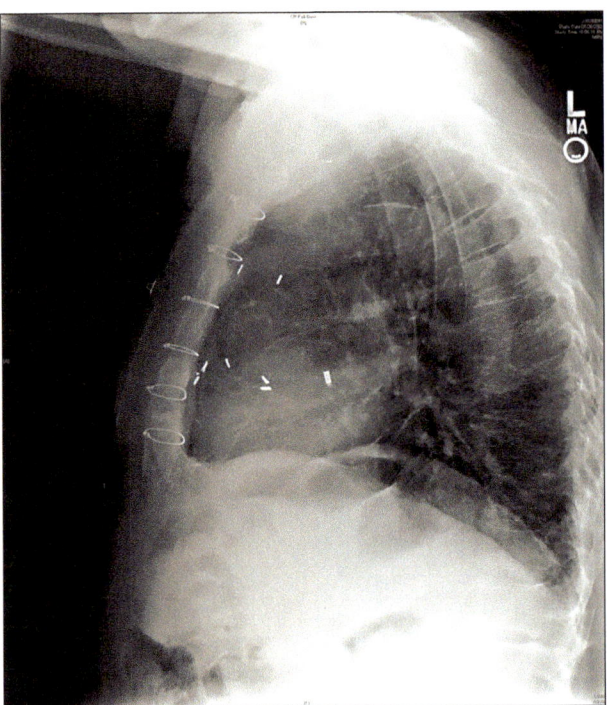

Figure 58.33 Retained lead tip after extraction of lead.

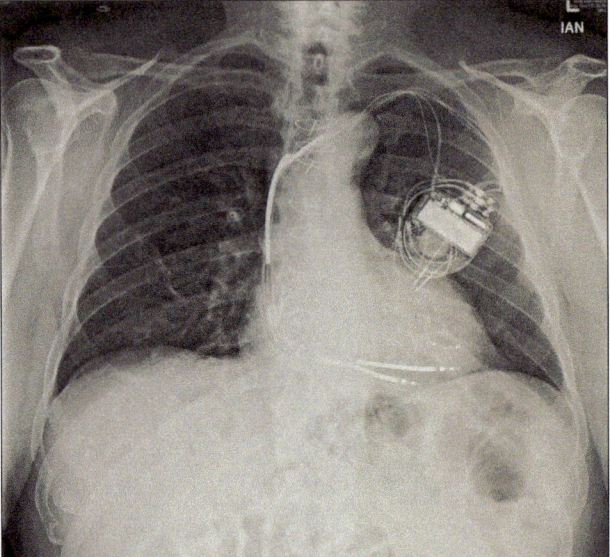

Figure 58.34 Comparison of access. Laterally, there is a capped, fractured RV ICD lead and a RA lead. The ICD lead was revised and access was obtained more medially in the axillary on the first rib. The patient later presented for upgrade to biventricular device and the LV lead was inserted via a subclavian approach as he was partially occluded distally.

Identification of prior venous access site can also be very helpful in planning future venous access. The most common sites of access include: subclavian or medial axillary, lateral axillary, and cephalic veins. The biggest clue to the identification of the access site is from the direction of the leads, especially if the suture sleeve can be identified. Subclavian access may have a bend in the contour of the lead as it passes under the clavicle, and the suture sleeve, if identified, is often near the midclavicular line parallel and inferior to the clavicle. The medial axillary approach over the first rib should have a similar suture sleeve location, but the bend at the clavicle should be absent, as the lead is already intravascular and free to move at that location (Figure 58.34). The lateral axillary and cephalic approaches will have suture sleeves and venous entry points that are more laterally located. The lateral axillary approach may be deeper on the lateral x-ray if done from a completely extrathoracic approach, but this is often difficult to visualize with overlying device and bones, such as the humerus. The cephalic will likely be directed more superiorly in its initial course (Figure 58.35). Although quite uncommon, internal jugular access can also be identified because the leads are tunneled across the clavicle.

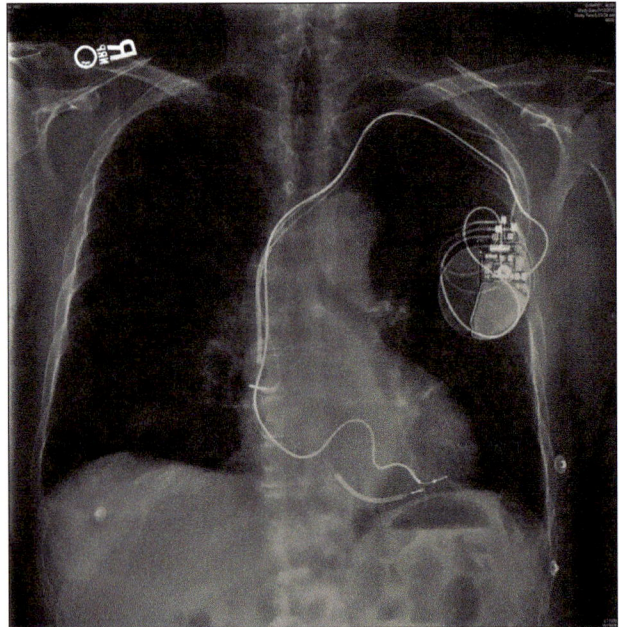

Figure 58.35 Biventricular device with RV ICD lead in the cephalic vein and LV and RA leads entering the lateral axillary vein.

Other Imaging Modalities

As discussed earlier in the chapter, chest radiography is the primary radiographic tool used to evaluate device implant and function, but there are roles for many other imaging modalities as well.[16] Echocardiography is important for the evaluation of complications such as effusions due to lead perforation and vegetations on leads due to infection. Three-dimensional (3D) imaging can be very important in demonstrating the anatomy of the heart itself and the vasculature, as well as surrounding structures.

Although MRI conditional devices are now approved,[17,18] the limitation of the magnetic resonance over the heart has made computed tomography (CT) the mainstay of 3D imaging. CT can help define both the vascular and cardiac anatomy in patients with cardiac devices or with an indication for a device. From a preprocedural standpoint, fluoroscopic venography is usually the preferred method to determine if vessels are patent, but if there is a preexisting CT scan, it can be used to determine vessel patency. In patients with previous surgery or congenital disease, the CT can verify that the os of the CS opens into the RA (see Figure 58.39).

CT scan can provide 3D information that will aid in the localization of leads. This localization is especially important in the case of congenital heart disease where the 2D information is insufficient. In some congenital conditions, such as dextrocardia (Figure 58.36), the plain films can be sufficient because the anatomy is as expected except for left right reversal.

In many congenital conditions, such as those with single ventricle or other conditions with significant mixing of venous and systemic blood, endocardial devices will be contraindicated due to the risk of thromboembolic complications and infection. Plain radiographs can be sufficient to evaluate epicardial hardware in these situations. Transposition of the great vessels, whether congenitally or surgically corrected, is a condition with separate pulmonary and systemic circulations and shunts, and many of these patients will have endocardial devices. L-TGA may often go unrecognized on plain film, and CT can better define the anatomy (Figure 58.38). In D-transposition with an arterial switch, the anatomy will be very similar to "normal hearts," but with an atrial switch procedure, such as the Sennig or Mustard, CT can be helpful in assessing

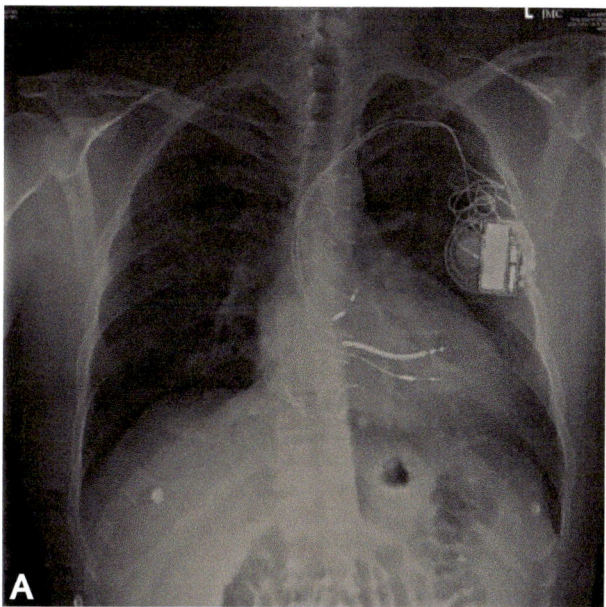

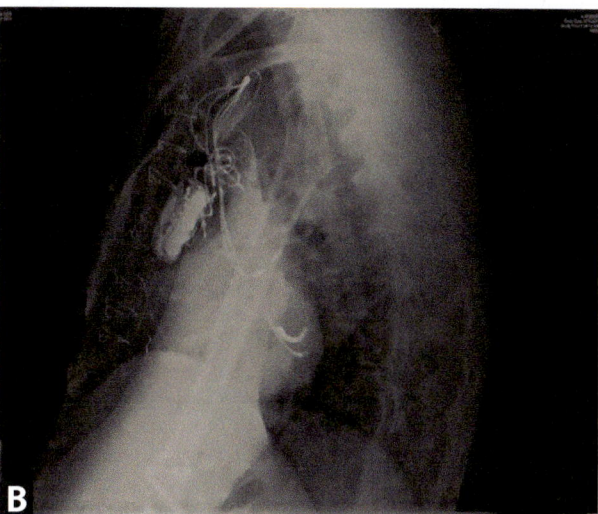

Figure 58.37 Chest radiograph, PA view (**Panel A**) and lateral view (**Panel B**), of a patient with a Mustard procedure for d-TGA. The ventricular leads (both a defibrillator lead and a pace-sense lead) are in the posteriorly situated left/ systemic ventricle.

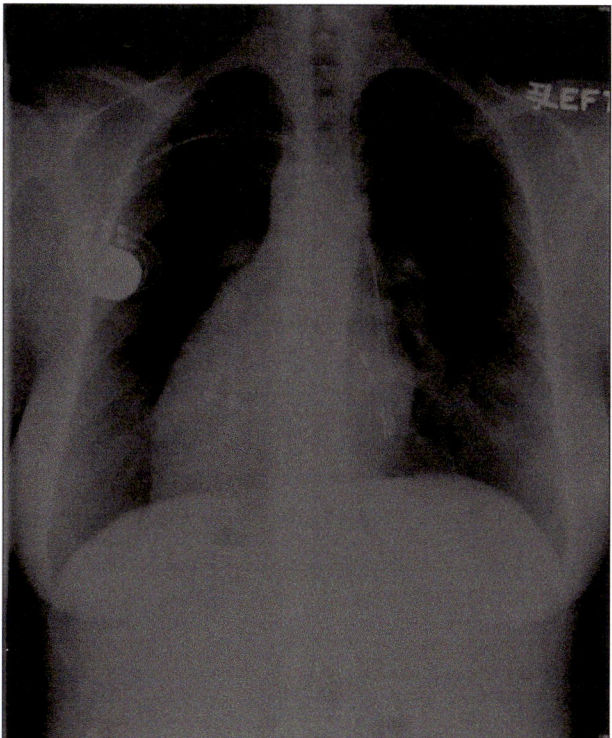

Figure 58.36 Mirror image dextrocardia with situs inversus. The gastric bubble is seen below the heart on the right side.

lead positions (Figure 58.37). Finally, CS anatomy can be variable in congenital heart disease, so any preexisting CT can be reviewed to detect whether the CS will be readily accessible (Figure 58.38).

There are times when the anatomy is unclear in structurally normal hearts as well. The CT can be necessary to identify courses of leads when the CXR appearance is atypical (Figure 58.39). A CT is recommended if there is an atypical course to any lead, as some very serious complications, such as inadvertent lead placement in the left heart, can only be definitively determined with 3D imaging.

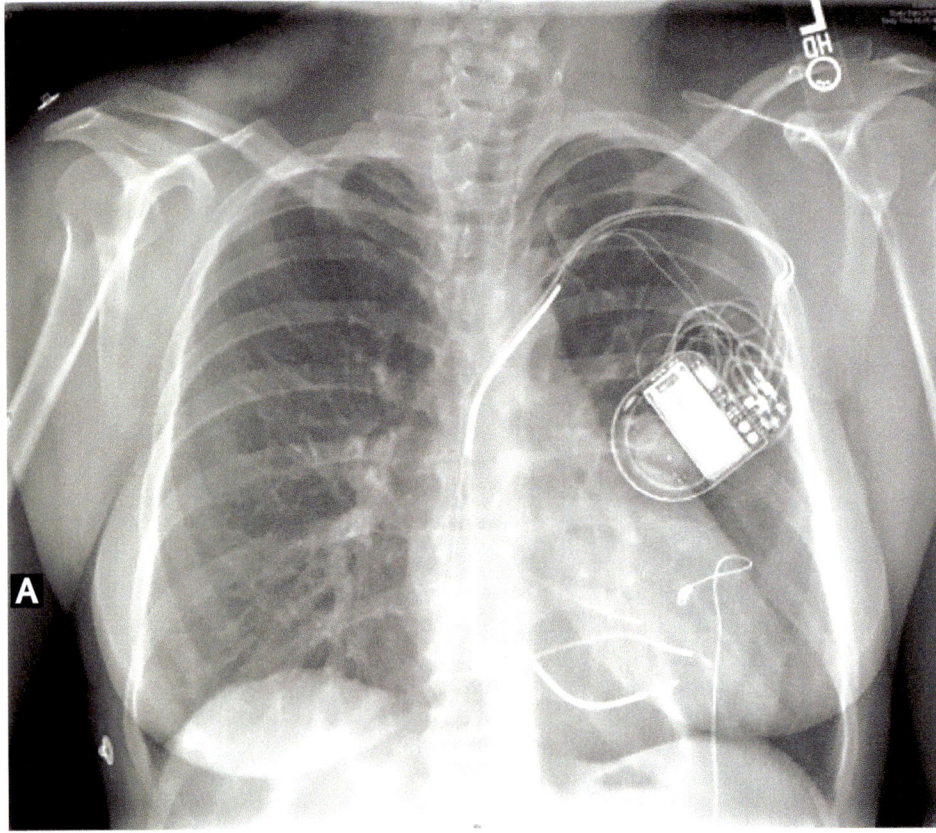
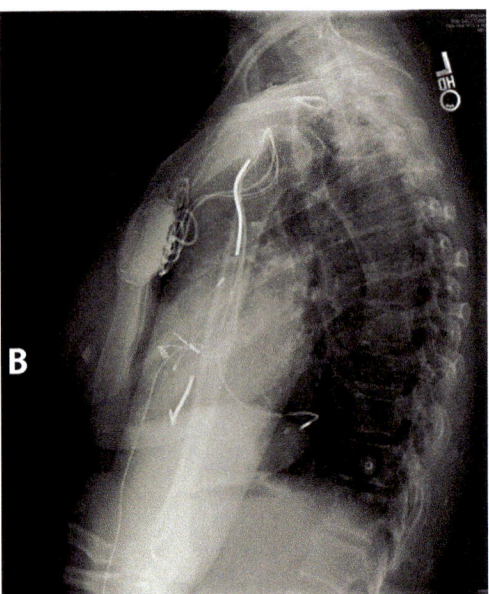
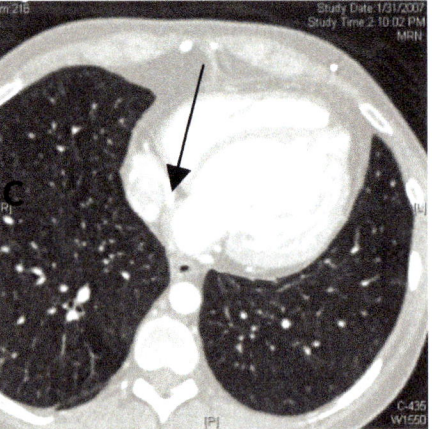

Figure 58.38 Chest radiograph (**Panels A & B**) and CT (**Panel C**) from a patient with L-transposition. The radiograph demonstrates a biventricular with the defibrillator lead in the anterior left/pulmonic ventricle. It is difficult to recognize the L-TGA from the radiograph. The CT demonstrates the highly trabeculated right/systemic ventricle is situated posteriorly. Of note, the os of the CS (**arrow**) can be seen as it enters the RA, which is helpful to know in preoperative planning.

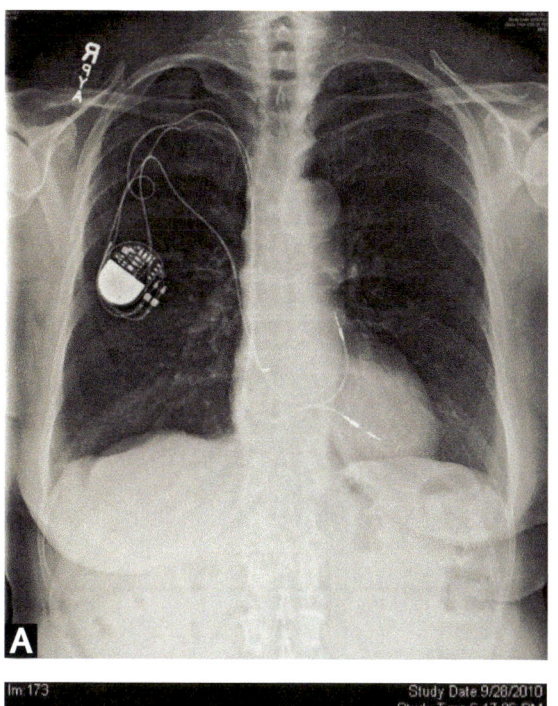
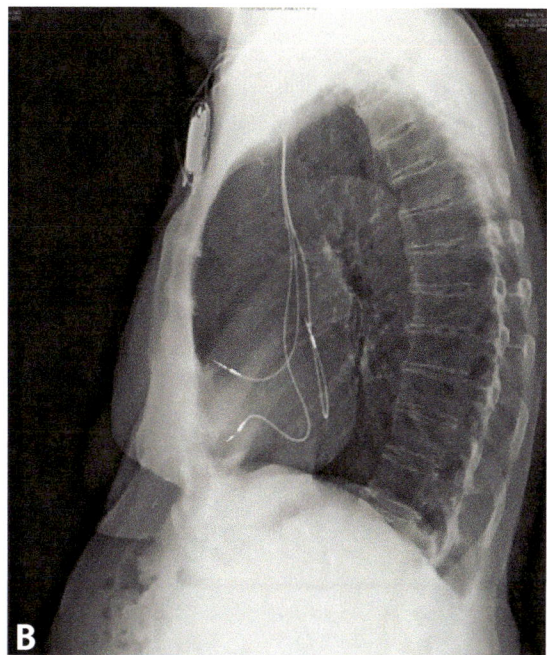
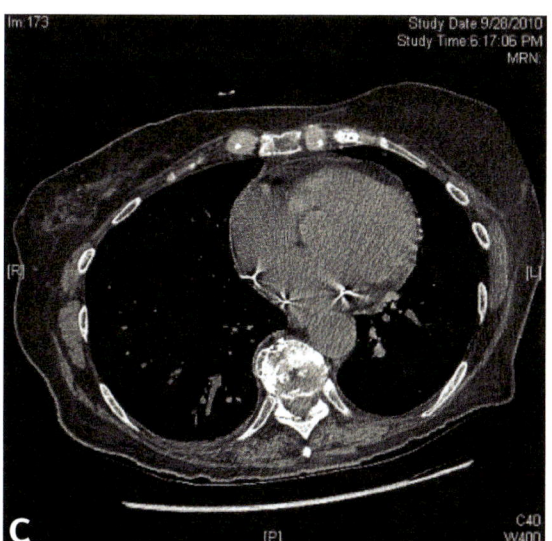
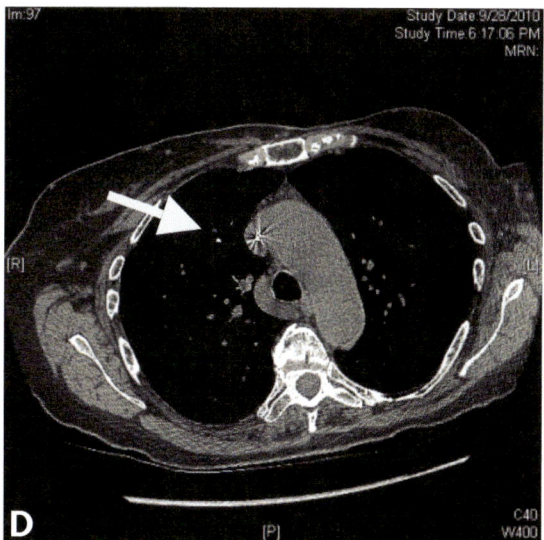
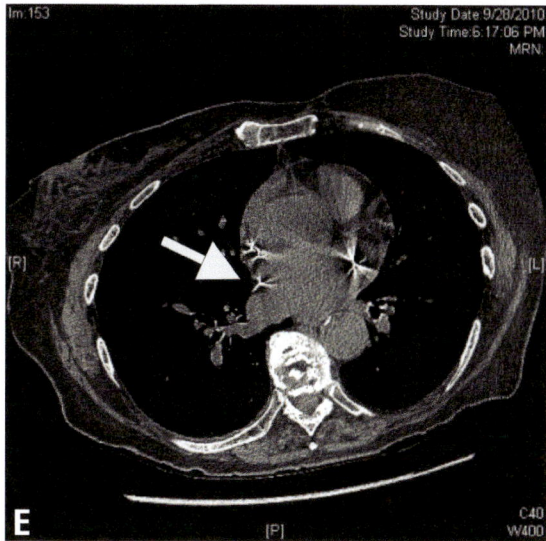

Figure 58.39 The chest radiograph (**Panels A & B**) demonstrates a lead with a very unusual course not following the major vasculature with its distal tip in the left chest. The CT demonstrates this lead coursing through the lung parenchyma (**Panel C**), into the right superior pulmonary vein (**Panel D**), and terminating in the LA (**Panel E**).

Conclusion

Radiography is an essential tool with device implantation. The plain film is instrumental in preprocedural planning in patients that currently have devices, and in postprocedural assessment of the patients with new implants. Along with device interrogation, the plain film is also very helpful in troubleshooting device malfunction. Occasionally, the 2D information provided by the chest radiograph is insufficient, and other modalities such as echocardiography and CT will aid in assessing the patient, their device, and potential complications.

References

1. Steiner RM, Tegtmeyer CJ. The radiology of cardiac pacemakers. *Cardiovasc Clin.* 1983;14(2):63-95.
2. Burney K, Burchard F, Papouchado M, Wilde P. Cardiac pacing systems and implantable cardiac defibrillators (ICDs): a radiological perspective of equipment, anatomy and complications. *Clin Radiol.* 2004;59(8):699-708.
3. Joshi SB, Blum AR, Mansour M, Abbara S. CT applications in electrophysiology. *Cardiol Clin.* 2009;27(4):619-631.
4. Hemminger EJ, Girsky MJ, Budoff MJ. Applications of computed tomography in clinical cardiac electrophysiology. *J Cardiovasc Comput Tomogr.* 2007;1(3):131-142.
5. Ho WJ, Kuo CT, Lin KH. Right pneumothorax resulting from an endocardial screw-in atrial lead. *Chest.* 1999;116(4):1133-1134.
6. Van Herendael, H, Willems, R. Contralateral pneumothorax after endocardial dual-chamber pacemaker implantation resulting from atrial lead perforation. *Acta Cardiol.* 2009;64(2):271-273.
7. Dilling-Boer D, Ector H, Willems R, Heidbuchel H. Pericardial effusion and right-sided pneumothorax resulting from an atrial active-fixation lead. *Europace.* 2003;5(4):419-423.
8. Berul CI, Villafane J, Atkins DL, et al. Pacemaker lead prolapse through the pulmonary valve in children. *Pacing Clin Electrophysiol.* 2007;30(10):1183-1189.
9. Mirza I, Holt P, James S. Permanent left atrial pacing: a 2-year follow-up of coronary sinus leads. *Pacing Clin Electrophysiol.* 2004;27(3):314-317.
10. Zerbe F, Bornakowski J, Sarnowski W. Pacemaker electrode implantation in patients with persistent left superior vena cava. *Br Heart J.* 1992;67:65-66.
11. Cesario D, Bhargava M, Valderrábano M, Fonarow GC, Wilkoff B, Shivkumar K. Azygos vein lead implantation: a novel adjunctive technique for implantable cardioverter defibrillator placement. *J Cardiovasc Electrophysiol.* 2004;15(7):780-783.
12. Cooper JA, Smith TW. How to implant a defibrillation coil in the azygos vein. *Heart Rhythm.* 2009;6(11):1677-1680
13. Cooper JA, Latacha MP, Soto GE, et al. The azygos defibrillator lead for elevated defibrillation thresholds: implant technique, lead stability, and patient series. *Pacing Clin Electrophysiol.* 2008;31(11):1405-1410.
14. Faheem O, Padala A, Kluger J, Zweibel S, Clyne CA. Coronary sinus shocking lead as salvage in patients with advanced CHF and high defibrillation thresholds. *Pacing Clin Electrophysiol.* 2010;33(8):967-972.
15. Woo G, Burkart T, Miles W, Saxonhouse S, Conti J. Detection of a retention wire fracture in an asymptomatic patient 18 years after implantation. *Pacing Clin Electrophysiol.* 2010;33(2): 246-247.
16. Sierra M, Machado C. Magnetic resonance imaging in patients with implantable cardiac devices. *Rev Cardiovasc Med.* 2008;9(4):232-238.
17. Roguin A, Schwitter J, Vahlhaus C, Lombardi M, Brugada J, Vardas P, Auricchio A, Priori S, Sommer T. Magnetic resonance imaging in individuals with cardiovascular implantable electronic devices. *Europace.* 2008;10(3):336-346.
18. Pulver AF, Puchalski MD, Bradley DJ, et al. Safety and imaging quality of MRI in pediatric and adult congenital heart disease patients with pacemakers. *Pacing Clin Electrophysiol.* 2009;32(4):450-456.

CHAPTER 59

Device-based Monitoring for Arrhythmias

Paul D. Ziegler, MS; Douglas A. Hettrick, PhD;
Rangadham Nagarakanti, MD; Sanjeev Saksena, MBBS, MD

Introduction

When implantable devices for the treatment of cardiac arrhythmias were first introduced more than 50 years ago, their function was limited to the delivery of the intended therapy. Over the subsequent decades, implantable devices have become much more sophisticated, both in their ability to deliver appropriate and novel therapies as well as their capability to provide a wealth of monitoring and diagnostic information aimed at helping clinicians manage patients with arrhythmias.

While the initial diagnostic features focused primarily on monitoring the performance and function of the device itself, modern cardiac rhythm devices have advanced diagnostic features that permit a detailed view of the arrhythmia and its characteristics. Today's implantable devices are also capable of monitoring more than just device function and the presence of arrhythmias. The addition of novel sensors has permitted devices to monitor new physiologic variables such as acceleration (as a surrogate of patient activity) and intrathoracic impedance (as a surrogate of fluid accumulation). Future devices are likely to integrate these various diagnostic measures into a unified score, which assesses a patient's risk for different cardiac conditions.

The availability of these features now allows implantable cardiac monitoring devices to provide important diagnostic information, record data that is of value integrated into patient medical records, and allows evaluation of the clinical status and disease progression in specific cardiac disorders. This chapter will discuss the current state of device-based monitoring for cardiac arrhythmias such as atrial tachycardia/atrial fibrillation (AT/AF), syncope, and heart failure (HF) as well as their clinical applications.

Atrial Arrhythmias

Atrial arrhythmias comprise a significant component of the global cardiovascular disease burden, and their incidence is increasing rapidly due to the aging of the population. Recent projections indicate that the prevalence of AF could exceed 12 million people in the United States by 2050.[1] They occur concomitantly with bradycardias, supraventricular tachycardias, and ventricular tachyarrhythmias and are frequently observed in these populations when an implantable device is prescribed for therapeutic purposes.

Atrial tachyarrhythmias may cause symptoms of tiredness, palpitations, and dizziness and consequently contribute to reduced quality of life. However AT/AF episodes can also be completely asymptomatic in many patients,[2,3] and the percentage of patients with only asymptomatic episodes has been shown to increase after patients undergo an AF ablation procedure.[4] A study of pacemaker patients showed that 38% of patients with episodes lasting longer than 48 hours were completely asymptomatic.[5] Whether AT/AF is symptomatic or asymptomatic, it also increases the risk of stroke in the presence of clinical risk factors; it is estimated that approximately 15% of strokes occur in patients with AT/AF.[6] Furthermore, AT/AF leads to more hospital admissions than any other arrhythmia[7] and increases

803

mortality.[8] Management of this arrhythmia with drugs, catheter or surgical ablation, and implantable devices requires an accurate assessment of the arrhythmia burden both at baseline and after treatment.

Regardless of the chosen AF treatment strategy, implantable device diagnostics can provide valuable information to help evaluate treatment efficacy and guide clinical decisions. Other important clinical considerations for monitoring patients with AT/AF include:

- The physician needs to evaluate whether the patient's symptoms are caused by AT/AF. When confirmed, symptoms may be related to rapid or irregular ventricular response to AT/AF, loss of atrial contribution to cardiac output, or rapid atrial rates. In all instances, rhythm monitoring is valuable in assessing symptoms. If the patient's symptoms are not the result of AT/AF, other potential causes for these complaints can be explored.

- If a rhythm-control strategy is selected, the objective is to reduce the total duration (burden) of AT/AF that a patient has over a given period of time.

- In contrast, a rate-control strategy requires maintenance of physiologically appropriate ventricular rates during the AT/AF episodes, which is associated with improvement of these symptoms.[9]

- Measurement of symptomatic or asymptomatic AT/AF episodes can be used to assess the need to initiate or discontinue anticoagulation therapy.

Comprehensive monitoring allows physicians to quantify and objectively assess the efficacy of their rhythm and rate control therapies. Optimization of treatment strategies based on AT/AF diagnostics may lead to improved patient outcomes.

Overview of Monitoring Methods

Monitoring of atrial arrhythmias can be challenging, particularly for patients with paroxysmal atrial fibrillation, because the abnormal rhythm occurs in an unpredictable and sporadic manner. A variety of techniques are available for monitoring these patients including symptom-based recording, external monitoring systems, and implantable monitoring devices. Each method has its own set of advantages and disadvantages, as discussed below.

Symptoms

Symptom-based monitoring of AT/AF is relatively inexpensive and clinically relevant, since the treatment goal is often to reduce symptoms. However, identification of patients with AT/AF based on symptoms is complicated by the fact that patients are frequently unaware that they are having the arrhythmia. Numerous studies have shown that the correlation between symptoms and rhythm status is poor. That is, the vast majority of AT/AF episodes are asymptomatic, and most symptoms attributed to AT/AF are not actually associated with the arrhythmia.[2,3,10,11] Consequently, even if patients employ external recorders to document their rhythm status at the time of symptoms, most atrial arrhythmias will fail to be detected due to the absence of symptoms.

External Devices

Whether AT/AF is symptomatic or asymptomatic, current anticoagulation guidelines[12] are the same, since the stroke risk has been shown to be similar for both types of arrhythmia.[13] External recorders were developed to both help identify asymptomatic AF and assist with the correlation between symptoms and rhythm status. Advantages of these external systems are that the procedure is noninvasive and the cost is moderate. However, the bulky size of these devices can interfere with showering and daily activities, while the adhesive electrodes can irritate the skin. Patient compliance with these systems can be quite low as a result,[10,14] and they are difficult to use over extended periods. Consequently, external monitoring is typically performed intermittently and for short durations (1–21 days), which increases the opportunity for missing paroxysmal episodes of asymptomatic AT/AF.

Implantable Therapeutic Devices

Devices such as pacemakers, implantable cardioverter-defibrillators (ICDs), and cardiac resynchronization therapy (CRT) devices are capable of monitoring atrial arrhythmias continuously over the lifetime of the device with both a high sensitivity and specificity for AT/AF detection.[15,16] Although these devices require an invasive implant procedure, patient compliance is generally not an issue, and the devices rarely interfere with normal daily activities. Patients can communicate with many modern implantable devices via an external activator to record the occurrence of symptoms within the memory of the device. This symptom information can then be retrieved later by the clinician when the device is interrogated via telemetry. However, the use of the monitoring capabilities afforded by these sophisticated devices is limited to those AF patients with a comorbid condition requiring device therapy.

Implantable Devices for Monitoring Only

Recently, small subcutaneous devices have been developed that also have AF detection capabilities with both high sensitivity and specificity.[17,18] These devices allow the benefits of continuous monitoring to be extended to a broader population of AF patients than just those with traditional device indications. These devices are currently about the size of a USB memory stick and do not have intracardiac leads. Because the bipolar recording electrodes are generally located on the surface of the device itself, reliable detection of P waves can be challenging from the subcutaneous space. Consequently, detection of AF is accomplished by analyzing the irregularity and unpredictability of R-R intervals. As with other implantable devices, patients are able to indicate the presence of symptoms by activating an external, hand-held device. The expected longevity of these devices is typically around 3 years.

Comparison of Monitoring Methods

The ability to detect patients who have asymptomatic AT/AF depends on two factors: the degree of monitoring rigor employed and the amount of AT/AF that the patient has to find. A single ECG snapshot would be sufficient to identify a patient who has permanent AT/AF, whereas all but the most rigorous monitoring methods will fail to identify a patient with very brief and sporadic episodes. Several studies have quantified the ability to identify patients with paroxysmal AT/AF via symptoms, intermittent external monitoring, and continuous monitoring with implantable devices.[19,20] Symptom-based and intermittent external monitoring methods were shown to have significantly lower sensitivity (range 31%–71%) and negative predictive value (range 21%–39%) for identification of patients with AT/AF (Figure 59.1) and underestimated AT/AF burden compared to continuous monitoring. The reported efficacy of clinical procedures such as pulmonary vein ablation for the treatment of AT/AF can vary greatly depending on how the arrhythmia is monitored. One study reported a success rate of 70% on the basis of symptoms alone, but only 50% when intermittent external monitoring was also considered.[10] These results were achieved despite the fact that 47% of the patients did not complete the external monitoring protocol and compliance with the monitoring schedule was only 42%. Such results highlight the clinical need for continuous monitoring that does not rely upon patient symptoms or patient compliance.

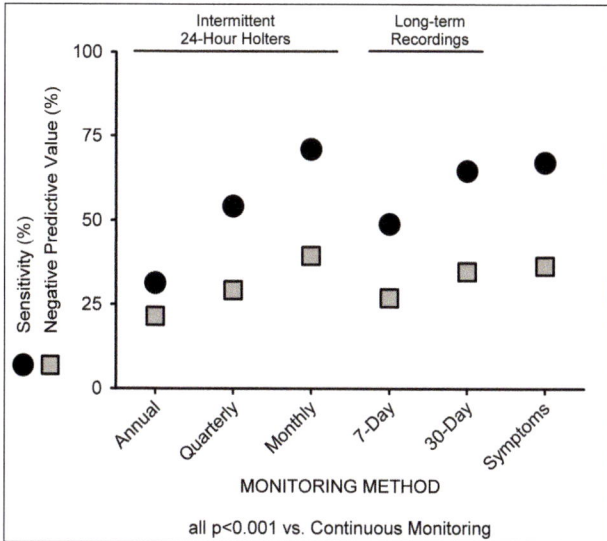

Figure 59.1 Sensitivity and negative predictive value of various intermittent AT/AF monitoring strategies. *Source:* Ziegler PD, Koehler JL, Mehra R.[19] Used with permission from Elsevier.

Device-based Arrhythmia Diagnostics

While implantable devices are capable of continuously monitoring cardiac rhythms over the life of the device, there are two important reasons why this information must be condensed and summarized. First, memory limitations within the device would not permit continuous storage of electrogram and other data for each cardiac cycle. A patient experiences approximately 100,000 heartbeats per day, and 6 months may elapse between follow-up visits, at which time the data can be extracted from the device via telemetry. This means the device might monitor more than 18 million heartbeats between office visits. Secondly, this amount of data would be far too much for clinicians to process and interpret for each patient. The challenge for device manufacturers is to convert this vast amount of *detection information* into *diagnostic information* that is manageable by both the device and the clinician.

To accomplish this, the device stores atrial arrhythmia information in a hierarchical fashion. Extremely detailed information is only stored for a small subset of the episodes, while very general information is tabulated across all episodes. For example, one of the most memory-intensive pieces of information is the electrogram (EGM) waveform. This data can be crucial for the clinician to verify that the device is detecting correctly and aids in troubleshooting when it is not. Because this information requires extensive amounts of memory as well as additional power consumption, only small portions of electrograms from a select number of episodes are stored by the device. On the other end of the spectrum, a continuous running tally of the duration of all AT/AF episodes is important so the physician can assess the AT/AF burden experienced by the patient. Between these two extremes are a variety of other parameters that may be tabulated per episode, per day, or per follow-up period. The goal is to strike a balance between providing enough information to be clinically useful in managing the patient without providing so much data as to overwhelm the clinician. Specific examples of device diagnostics used for monitoring rhythm control, rate control, and anticoagulation management of patients with AT/AF will be presented in the remainder of this section.

Rhythm Control

The prevalence of AT/AF among patients with implantable devices is quite high; it is therefore important that these devices have diagnostic information to convey the particular arrhythmia characteristics of each individual patient. A large study of more than 140,000 patients with ICD and CRT devices showed that 40% had device-detected AT/AF over a follow-up period of 1.6 ± 1.0 years.[21] While the overall prevalence of AT/AF was similar between device types, there was more paroxysmal AT/AF among ICD patients but more persistent and permanent AT/AF among CRT patients. A separate analysis of more than 50,000 CRT-D patients showed that 32% had at least one day with greater than 6 hours of AT/AF over a follow-up of 2.1 ± 1.6 years.[22] Among these device patients with AT/AF, 34% were characterized as paroxysmal, 47% were classified as persistent, while the remaining 19% had permanent AT/AF. A striking finding of this analysis was that the impact of AT/AF on mortality was similar between patients with paroxysmal, persistent, and permanent AT/AF in the presence of systolic heart failure. This finding demonstrates that even paroxysmal AT/AF (defined as at least one day with >6 hours of AT/AF) is associated with decreased survival. Interestingly, the authors also found that patients with very short paroxysms of AT/AF (never more than 6 hours on a single day) had a similar survival to patients with no recorded AT/AF (Figure 59.2). Consequently, knowledge of the patient's rhythm status may be useful to inform clinical decisions regarding rhythm control strategies and could potentially impact patient outcomes.

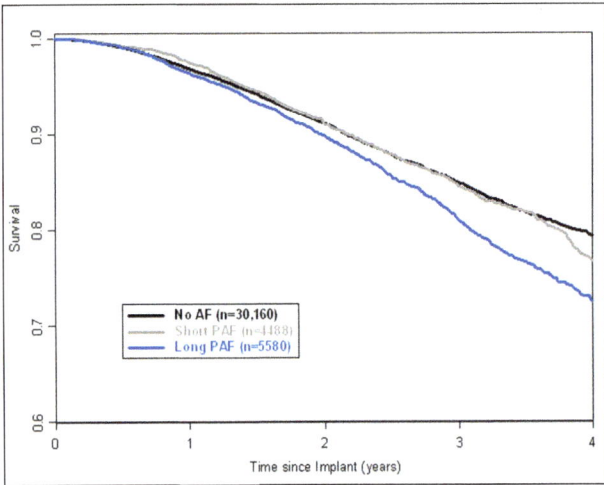

Figure 59.2 Survival curves for patients with short paroxysmal AT/AF (no day with more than 6 hours of AT/AF) and long paroxysmal AT/AF (at least one day with more than 6 hours of AT/AF) compared to patients with no AT/AF.

Validation of Rhythm Control

Regardless of the particular rhythm control treatment, accurate monitoring of the rhythm is vitally important. Some of the diagnostic information that can be used to evaluate the efficacy of rhythm control is shown in Figure 59.3. Validation of the actual cardiac rhythm status is important to establish the true reliability of a rhythm control strategy. For example, observations from hybrid therapy trials involving implantable pacemakers have validated that sinus rhythm or atrial pacing is maintained during long-term follow-up in over 80% of patients with paroxysmal AF and 75% of patients with persistent AF.[23,24]

Recent analyses from the AFFIRM trial now suggest that the degree of quantitative restoration of sinus rhythm may be more predictive of cardiovascular outcomes than simple reversion to sinus rhythm on a given day of follow-up.[25] Correlation of symptoms with the rhythm is another important aspect of this validation technique. In the Natural History of AF Study, Strickberger and colleagues noted that only 8% of patients could accurately report symptoms that correctly correlated with normal sinus rhythm or AF.[2]

One of the key rhythm control quantitative diagnostics is the measurement of the AT/AF burden (ie, the percentage of time spent in an atrial arrhythmia). This parameter can be monitored continuously for up to 14 months before data is overwritten on a first in, first out basis. Additional insight into the status of rhythm control is provided by histograms of the longest AT/AF episode duration and episode start times (Figure 59.4). Electrogram validation to support the accuracy of such measurements is critical. Far-field R waves or underdetection of AF electrograms is often noted and can give spurious values. There is also an innate variability in serial measurements of AT/AF burden that needs to be determined before interpreting data.[26] Absolute measurements in an individual need to considered in this context.

Progression of the AF Disease State

Important insights into the progression of the AF disease state and arrhythmia progression can be obtained from such measures. Our prior studies have shown that AT/AF burden does not inevitably increase in all patients with AF. In fact, subpopulations that show increase or plateau behavior with respect to quantitation of AT/AF burden can be identified on long-term monitoring.[27] Increasing burden is seen when there is a comorbidity of documented cardiovascular disease. In contrast, atrial premature beat density seems unrelated to this comorbidity. Transition to persistent AF is not necessarily preceded by high burden but may actually be preceded by virtually no AF events, strongly supporting the idea that an increasingly vulnerable substrate is the primary abnormality that can be engaged by even low-density ectopy or brief arrhythmia.[28] Monitoring noted that the initial episodes of persistent AF are actually self-terminating after approximately 15 to 18 days, but rapid reinitiation occurs with rapidly decreasing likelihood of self-termination.[29] This suggests acceleration of the arrhythmia complexity, probably related to rapid remodeling of the substrate.

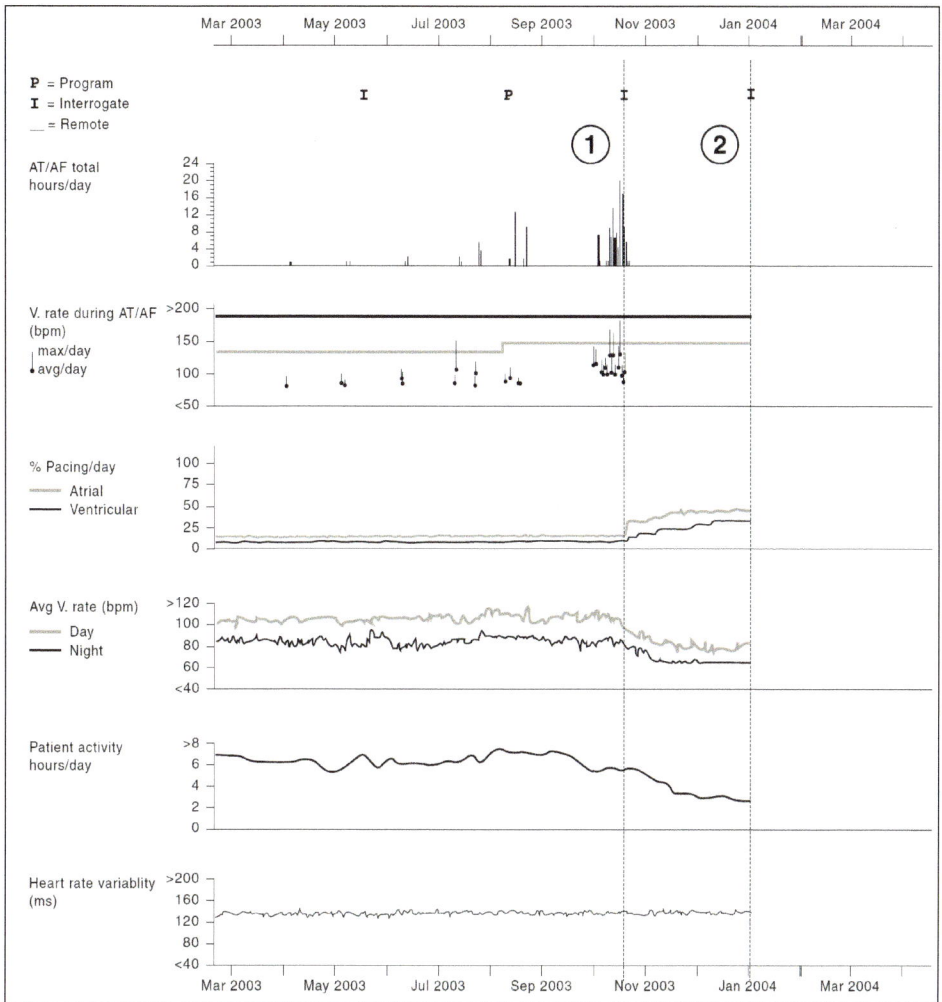

Figure 59.3 Example of trending diagnostic information from an implantable cardiac device. Daily values are tabulated over the most recent 14-month period. *Source:* Reproduced with permission of Medtronic, Inc.

AT/AF Durations	Episodes	AT/AF Start Times	Episodes
>72 hr	0	09:00-12:00	0
48 hr to 72 hr	0	12:00-15:00	0
24 hr to 48 hr	0	15:00-18:00	1
12 hr to 24 hr	0	18:00-21:00	0
4 hr to 12 hr	0	21:00-00:00	1
1 hr to 4 hr	3	00:00-03:00	0
10 min to 1 hr	0	03:00-06:00	0
1 min to 10 min	2	06:00-09:00	3
<1 min	0		

Figure 59.4 Histogram diagnostic data for the duration and start times of AT/AF episodes are available in many implantable devices.

AF Ablation

There are several difficulties in assessing the success of AF ablation procedures. First, what is the definition of success? Is it freedom from symptomatic episodes or freedom from both symptomatic and asymptomatic episodes? If asymptomatic episodes are considered, what level of rigor should be employed for rhythm monitoring? It has been shown that different monitoring modalities produce very different results in terms of the apparent percentage of patients free from AT/AF recurrence.[19,20,30,31] The only way to know the full truth and to make accurate comparisons is to monitor the patient continuously, particularly since studies have shown that the percentage of patients with only asymptomatic episodes increases significantly following AF ablation procedures.[4]

Few ablation studies have utilized continuous arrhythmia monitoring because until recently, continuous monitoring was only available in the subgroup of ablation patients who had clinical indications for pacemakers, ICDs, and CRT devices. One such study monitored 14 pacemaker patients both before and after a pulmonary vein isolation procedure (Figure 59.5).[30] This important study showed that patients may remain in sinus rhythm for many months following an ablation procedure but can later experience unpredictable recurrences that would be challenging to detect with intermittent monitoring methods. With the advent of subcutaneous monitoring devices, more data is beginning to emerge regarding the true state of rhythm control following ablative procedures in a broader population of AF patients.

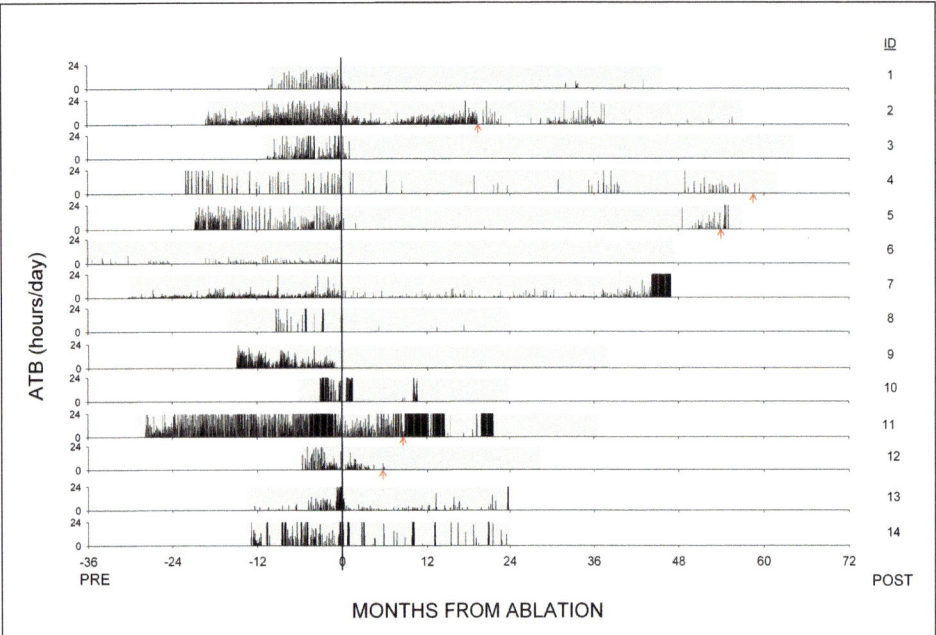

Figure 59.5 Data from 14 patients with implantable pacemakers who underwent pulmonary vein isolation for atrial fibrillation. Preablation data is to the left of time 0 and post-ablation data is to the right of time 0. Shading represents the extent of follow-up for each individual patient. *Source:* Martinek M, Aichinger J, Nesser HJ, et al.[30] Used with permission.

Antiarrhythmic Drugs

The effect of antiarrhythmic drug therapy can also be assessed with implantable devices. Several trials have recently looked at the efficacy of an investigational pharmacologic compound in patients with permanent pacemakers capable of continuous AT/AF monitoring.[32,33] These studies showed a dose-dependent decrease in AT/AF burden with budiodarone relative to a baseline treatment period with placebo (Figure 59.6). Use of device-recorded AT/AF burden as an endpoint may allow for quicker development of new pharmacologic therapies since it permits a more quantitative assessment of antiarrhythmic effect, as opposed to endpoints such as time to first symptomatic recurrence. Device diagnostics such as the episode start time histogram (Figure 59.4) may also provide an indication regarding the adequacy of antiarrhythmic medication dosage and frequency of administration.

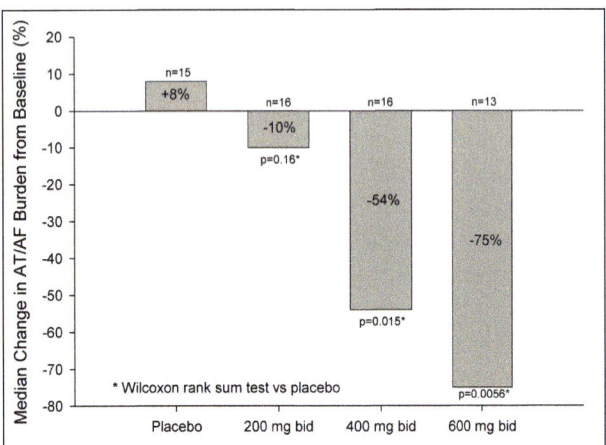

Figure 59.6 AT/AF burden data from drug trial investigating the dose response relative to placebo.

Rate Control

A rate-control treatment strategy involves maintaining the ventricular rate during AT/AF within acceptable ranges while at rest and during exercise. Typically, the AF guidelines recommend a ventricular rate during AF below 80 beats per minute (bpm) while at rest and below 115 bpm during moderate exercise.[12] Several large randomized trials, including the AFFIRM study,[9] have shown no difference in survival between the treatment strategies of rhythm control or rate control for patients with atrial fibrillation. Consequently, rate control remains a viable treatment strategy for many AF patients.

Despite the perception that it may be easier to control a patient's rate than their rhythm, the incidence of poor rate control among AF patients with ICD and CRT devices has been shown to be high. In a retrospective analysis of 56,299 device patients with paroxysmal (n = 35,345) or persistent (n = 20,954) AT/AF, the percentage with average ventricular rates during AT/AF above 80 bpm were 74% and 34%, respectively (Figure 59.7).[34] While poor rate control was relatively common among these device patients, it is likely that inadequate rate control is even more prevalent among patients without implantable devices for several reasons. First, the implantable devices in this study were capable of continuously monitoring the ventricular rate during AT/AF and provided diagnostic information summarizing the data. Therefore, physicians are more likely to be aware when the ventricular rate during AT/AF is not optimally controlled compared to patients in whom this data is not available. Secondly, AF patients with implantable devices have some treatment options for rate control that are not available to nondevice patients such as AV node ablation and more aggressive pharmacologic therapies since these devices can also provide pacing support for drug-induced bradycardia. The maintenance of adequate rate control is of particular importance for AF patients with implantable devices for several reasons, as discussed below.

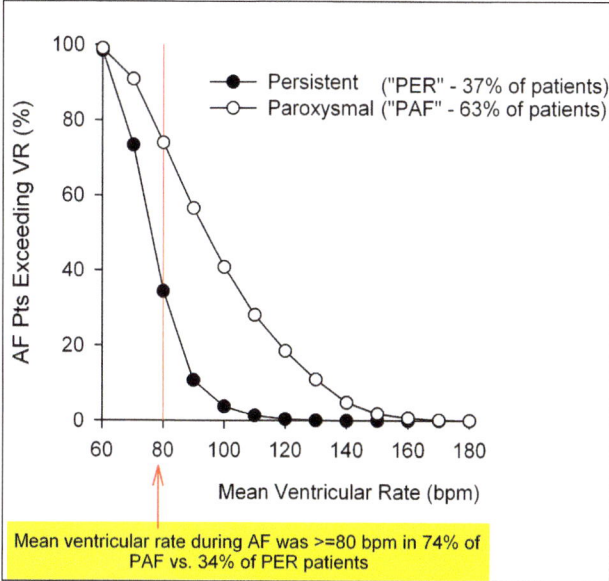

Figure 59.7 The percentage of patients exceeding various mean ventricular rate indicates that patients with paroxysmal AT/AF have worse rate control during AT/AF compared to persistent AT/AF patients.

Limiting Symptoms and Heart Failure Exacerbation

Ventricular rates that are rapid and irregular can cause symptoms of palpitations, dyspnea, or angina. This lack of rate control may lead to heart failure in many patients with AF. The RACE II study[35] recently reported no difference in the composite endpoint of cardiovascular death, heart failure hospitalization, stroke, systemic embolism, bleeding, and life-threatening arrhythmias between patients with permanent AF who were randomized to a lenient versus strict rate-control strategy. On the surface, these results may suggest that more strict control of ventricular rate is not warranted. However, several limitations with this study may have masked the true benefit of more rigorous rate control. Most notably, the patient population studied in this trial appeared to be able to tolerate high resting heart rates quite well as evidenced by a high average resting heart rate at baseline (96 bpm), yet only a small percentage of patients (< 10%) had prior heart failure hospitalizations. Also, all enrolled patients were required to be capable of exercising (ie, physically active) in order to be eligible for randomization to the strict rate control arm. Furthermore, heart failure was not a significant comorbidity in the studied population, with 65% of patients in NYHA Class I and less than 5% of patients classified above NYHA Class II. In contrast, patients in whom ventricular rate control may be most critical are those who cannot tolerate high ventricular rates and have a significant degree of heart failure. Another limitation was that one-third of patients in the strict rate control arm did not meet their rate control targets, thereby making it difficult to truly assess the potential benefits of strict rate control and consequently this issue remains largely unanswered.

Several device diagnostics can aide in the management of patients who are symptomatic during periods of poor rate control. Many devices provide a comprehensive summary of the average and maximum ventricular rate during AT/AF for each day over the past 14 months (Figure 59.8). This provides a means for the physician to determine if symptoms correlate with high ventricular rates. Devices are also capable of tracking the heart rates during day and night separately, which can be helpful in monitoring patients with heart failure, as their heart rates at night tend to be elevated during periods of decompensation.

Reducing Inappropriate Shocks

One of the leading causes of inappropriate device shocks in ICD patients is poor rate control during AT/AF.[36] Although relatively infrequent, implantable devices may misinterpret the rapid and irregular ventricular conduction during AT/AF as being a life-threatening ventricular arrhythmia. Because it is often too late to prevent an inappropriate shock by learning about the existence of rapidly conducted AT/AF at the next regularly scheduled office visit, many modern implantable devices have the ability to wirelessly transmit a notification to the clinic when the ventricular rate during AT/AF exceeds a programmable threshold (Figure 59.9). By learning about the existence of poor rate control almost in real time, the physician has a greater chance of being able to intervene in a timely manner, thus potentially preventing an unnecessary and painful electric shock.

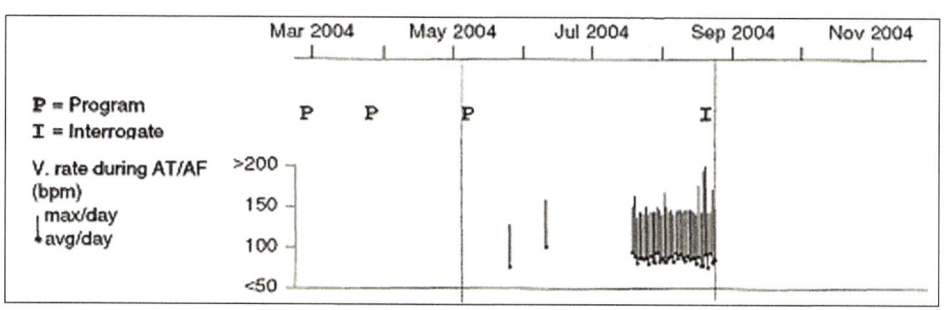

Figure 59.8 Device diagnostics can report the mean and maximum ventricular rates during AT/AF for each day that a patient experiences AT/AF over the past 14 months.

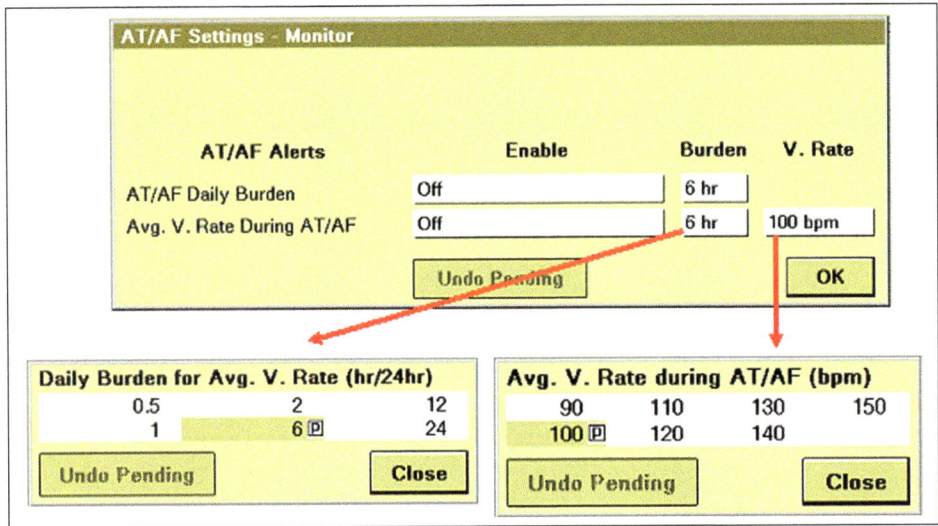

Figure 59.9 Implantable devices can be programmed to automatically notify physicians when certain conditions are met. The parameters for high ventricular rate notification are shown here (any day with at least 6 hours of AT/AF and an average ventricular rate during AT/AF of at least 100 bpm).

Maintaining Biventricular Pacing

Biventricular pacing with CRT devices is used to synchronize contractions of the left and right ventricle, thereby mitigating the effects of heart failure. However, rapid intrinsic ventricular rates during AT/AF can inhibit the delivery of CRT therapy.[37] Consequently, adequate control of the ventricular rate is needed to permit CRT devices to provide maximal therapy. In addition to the diagnostics described previously for ventricular rate during AT/AF, devices can also report the percentage of atrial and ventricular pacing each day (Figure 59.10). Monitoring this diagnostic can provide another clue as to the adequacy of ventricular rate control.

The importance of maintaining a very high percentage of biventricular pacing was highlighted in a retrospective analysis of 10,830 CRT-D patients with permanent and persistent AT/AF.[38] The authors divided patients into quartiles based on their percentage of biventricular pacing and found that decreased biventricular pacing was significantly associated with increased mortality, even after controlling for age and gender (Figure 59.11). Furthermore, reduced biventricular pacing was correlated with poorer rate control (Figure 59.12), emphasizing the need to adequately control ventricular rate in this patient population. It is important to note that a reduction in biventricular pacing of only a few percent is enough to significantly increase the risk of mortality.

Anticoagulation

Continuous monitoring of rhythm status is critically important for managing an appropriate anticoagulation regimen for AF patients. Device diagnostics can be helpful in aiding in both the decision to initiate anticoagulation as well as the decision to discontinue its use, when appropriate.

Initiation of Anticoagulation

Current guidelines recommend the use of anticoagulation therapy for patients with stroke risk factors and AT/AF, regardless of the AT/AF burden or the presence/absence of symptoms.[12] Therefore, identification of patients with even relatively brief episodes of AT/AF may be important. Prior studies have shown that continuous monitoring with implantable devices is particularly well suited for this purpose.[19,20]

One patient population in whom evidence of AT/AF frequently prompts the initiation of oral anticoagulants is those who have suffered a prior stroke since, by definition, these patients automatically have a $CHADS_2$ score of at least 2. Several studies with short-term external monitoring have shown that more intensive cardiac monitoring following a cryptogenic stroke results in increased detection of patients with AF.[39-41] A study utilizing long-term, continuous arrhythmia monitoring to detect previously undiagnosed AT/AF in cardiac device patients with a prior history of thromboembolic events revealed that AT/AF was present in 28% of the cohort.[42] The study found that the majority of these patients with newly detected atrial

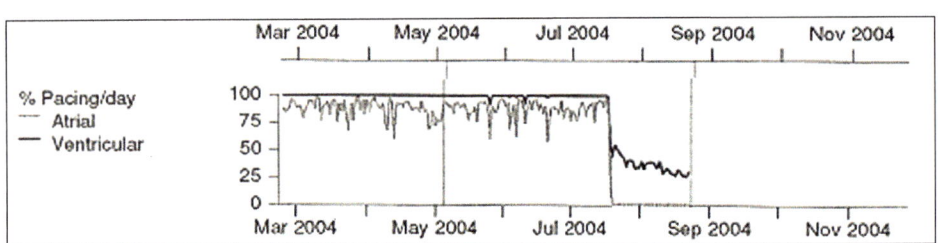

Figure 59.10 Device diagnostics can report the percentage of atrial and ventricular pacing delivered for each day over the past 14 months.

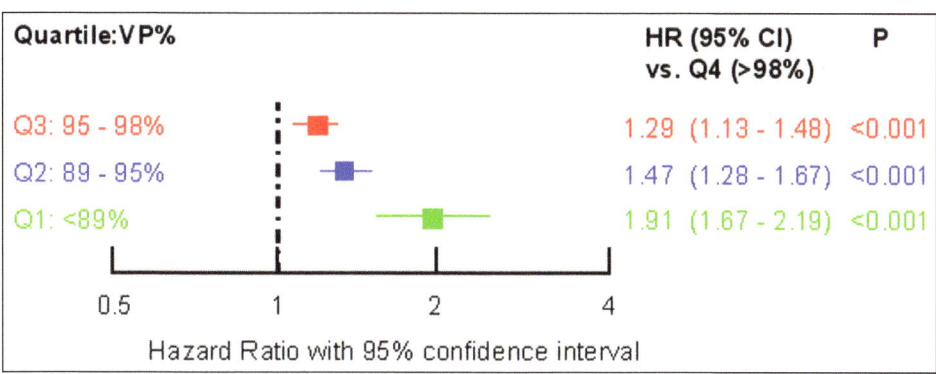

Figure 59.11 The risk of mortality increased with successive quartiles of decreased biventricular pacing in CRT-D patients after adjusting for patient age and gender.

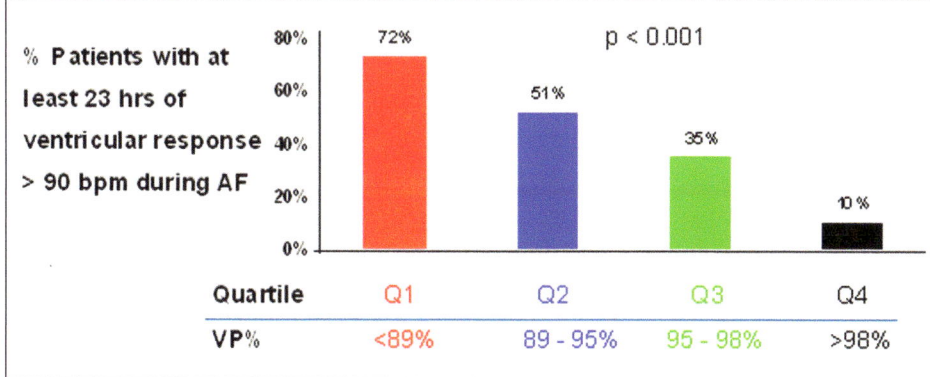

Figure 59.12 Poor ventricular rate control (as measured by the percentage of patients with at least one day with a ventricular rate during AT/AF above 90 bpm) is associated with progressively decreased biventricular pacing percentages.

arrhythmias experienced at least one day with greater than 6 hours of AT/AF. However, the arrhythmia episodes occurred infrequently with 73% of patients experiencing AT/AF episodes on less than 10% of the follow-up days. In fact, only 11% of patients experienced AT/AF episodes on the majority of follow-up days, and therefore, detection of AT/AF would be unlikely with standard intermittent monitoring techniques. A prospective study is being conducted in cryptogenic stroke patients without a cardiac rhythm device indication who have received a subcutaneous monitor capable of detecting AF.[43]

Figure 59.13 shows the atrial arrhythmia burden data from a patient who had frequent AT/AF episodes both before and after the occurrence of a thromboembolic event. However, the patient remained in sinus rhythm for 12 consecutive days immediately following the event until the resumption of the next AT/AF episode. Short-term monitoring for 24 hours, 48 hours, or even 7 days at the time of the stroke would have failed to detect AT/AF in this patient. The importance of timely identification of AT/AF in patients with prior stroke was highlighted in a study by Kamel et al, which showed that stroke patients with newly diagnosed AF have a much higher risk of recurrent stroke than patients with either no AF or previously known AF.[44]

While the exact relationship between AT/AF burden and stroke risk is not fully understood, data from implantable devices can be used to gain a better understanding. Several studies have examined the impact of quantitative measures of AT/AF on stroke risk in device patients. A sub-study of the MOde Selection Trial (MOST) reported that the composite endpoint of nonfatal stroke and death was significantly higher in patients having at least

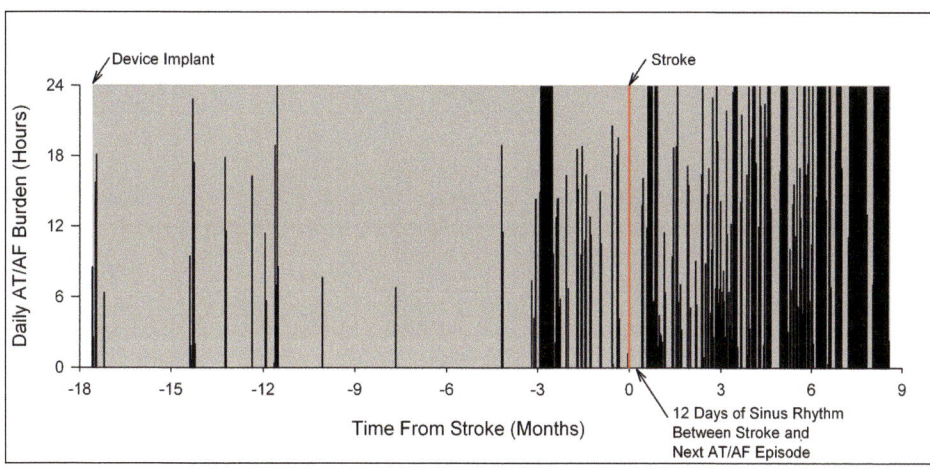

Figure 59.13 Despite having significant AT/AF both before and after an ischemic stroke, this patient was in sinus rhythm for 12 consecutive days immediately following the stroke. Short-term cardiac monitoring may have failed to detect AT/AF in this patient.

5-minute episodes of high-rate atrial arrhythmias.[45] A study by Capucci et al showed that atrial arrhythmias lasting longer than 24 hours increased the risk of thromboembolic events by a factor of three compared to those with shorter or no episodes.[46] The TRENDS study reported that an arrhythmia burden of at least 5.5 hours on any of 30 prior days conferred twice the risk of thromboembolic events compared to no AT/AF burden.[47] Taken together, these studies suggest that quantitative AT/AF burden detected by implantable devices is a risk factor for thromboembolism, and that the burden threshold for increased risk may be relatively low.

Figure 59.14 shows the arrhythmia burden data from a patient with no history of AT/AF but three risk factors for stroke. The device recorded no atrial arrhythmias during the first 8 months following implantation, but then detected the sudden onset of a persistent AT/AF episode that lasted for more than 2 years. Eight days following the onset of this arrhythmic episode, the patient suffered an ischemic stroke. While this patient's implantable device did not have the capability to automatically notify the physician or patient as to the presence of AT/AF, many modern implantable devices are able to generate a wireless notification in response to prolonged AT/AF episodes. In this particular example, there may have been sufficient time (8 days) to implement a treatment strategy to potentially prevent this event had the AT/AF been known.

Discontinuation of Anticoagulation

Less is known about the ability to discontinue anticoagulation following a successful rhythm control intervention. With recent advances in the field of AF ablation, more evidence is emerging that it may be safe to discontinue oral anticoagulation in low to moderate risk patients who have successfully had their rhythm controlled by ablative techniques.[48,49] However, as shown in Figure 59.5, AF episodes may recur after many months or even years following an apparently successful AF ablation. Consequently, it may be important to continuously monitor a patient's cardiac rhythm so that action can be taken in the event of asymptomatic AT/AF recurrences. As previously mentioned, implantable devices can be configured to automatically send a notification when AT/AF of a certain duration is detected in these patients, thereby permitting safer discontinuation of anticoagulation therapy. A study is underway in CRT-D patients to investigate the use of continuous ambulatory monitoring to prospectively guide the initiation and withdrawal of anticoagulation therapy compared to conventional clinical management.[50] Furthermore, new anticoagulation medications such as dabigatran, which offer the promise of easier administration and titration than conventional warfarin, may permit a "pill-in-the-pocket" approach to stroke prevention in combination with continuous monitoring and their associated diagnostics. This could allow for improved stroke prevention during arrhythmic periods while reducing the risk of bleeds during extended periods of sinus rhythm.

One particularly challenging group to manage is those AF patients with a single $CHADS_2$ risk factor. The current AF guidelines[12] recommend either aspirin or oral anticoagulation for patients with AF and one stroke risk factor (Figure 59.15A). One study with implantable devices provided additional clarity regarding which patients with a $CHADS_2$ score of 1 may be able to safely discontinue oral anticoagulation.[20] The investigators found that stroke risk could be stratified into two groups based on a combination of stroke risk factors and AT/AF burden as measured via continuous monitoring (Figure 59.15B). Patients with a single stroke risk factor and a daily AT/AF burden below 24 hours on all days were part of the low-risk cohort (shown in green) while patients with a single risk factor and AT/AF that persisted for 24 hours on a single day were part of the high-risk cohort (shown in red). While a prospective, randomized study would be necessary to confirm these preliminary findings, the study suggests that continuous AT/AF burden data may be a useful tool for guiding oral anticoagulation among the sizable population of AF patients with a single stroke risk factor. Furthermore, several studies have shown that detection of patients with AT/AF >24 hours on a single day is best accomplished with continuous monitoring.[19,20]

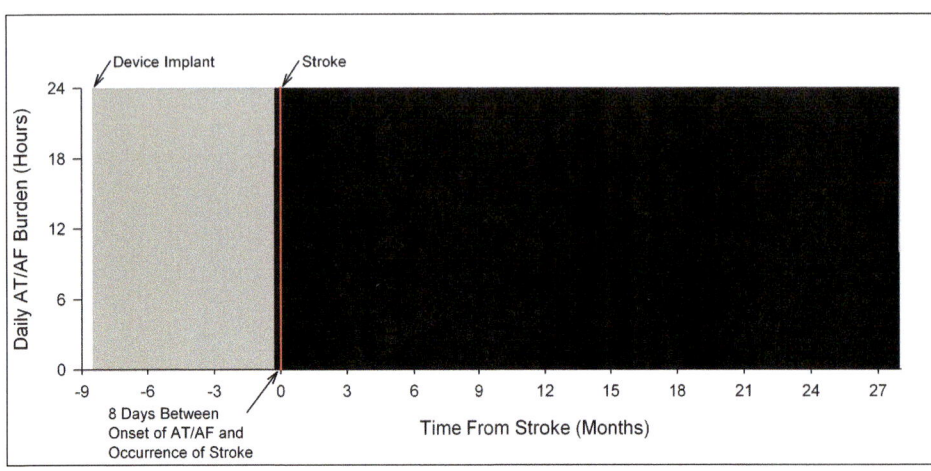

Figure 59.14 A patient with no known history of AF but significant stroke risk factors suffered an ischemic stroke 8 days after the onset of a persistent AT/AF episode.

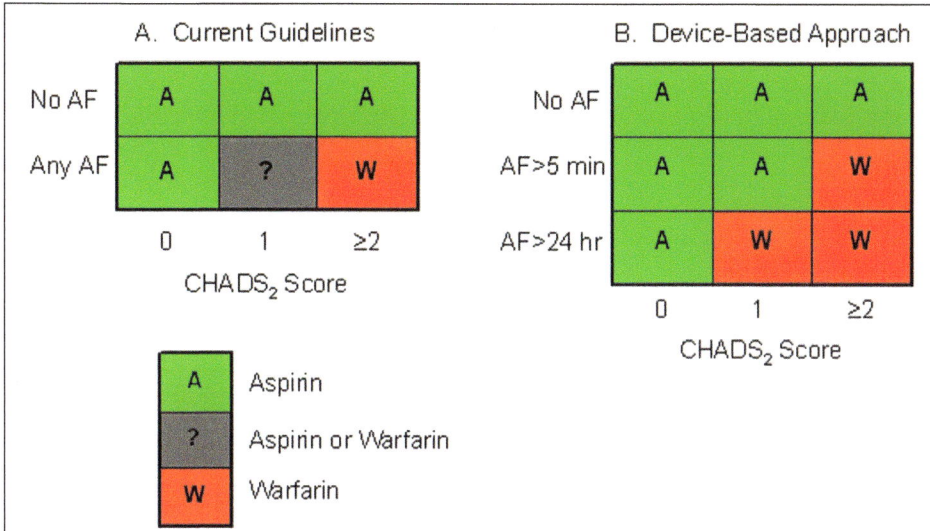

Figure 59.15 Current guidelines are ambiguous regarding the use of oral anticoagulation in patients with AF and a $CHADS_2$ score of 1 (**Panel A**). Continuous monitoring data from implantable devices suggests that AT/AF burden could be incorporated to help stratify $CHADS_2$ patients into groups with low and high risk.

Remote Monitoring of Devices

While the ability to interrogate an implantable device and view its diagnostic information during an office visit is important, having more timely or remote access to this data may be valuable in improving patient care. Device manufacturers now provide the ability for patients to transmit device data remotely from their home. This capability is useful for patients who would otherwise need to travel great distances to reach their doctor's office. It also allows physicians to extend the interval between traditional office visits by alternating in-clinic visits with remote data transmissions. Some newer devices have the ability to automatically transmit device data when certain prespecified conditions within the device are satisfied. Several studies have been conducted to compare different follow-up strategies and to determine the clinical impact of having access to this diagnostic information in a more timely fashion.

The PREFER study was designed to compare remote pacemaker interrogations to transtelephonic monitoring (TTM) for the earlier diagnosis of clinically actionable events.[51] Patients in the study were followed for a duration of 12 months. Patients randomized to the remote interrogation arm transmitted their device data via the Medtronic CareLink® system every 3 months and were seen in the office at 12 months. Patients randomized to the control arm performed a TTM transmission at 2-month intervals and were seen in the office at 6 and 12 months. Clinically actionable events related to AT/AF included episodes that lasted longer than 48 hours, new onset of AT/AF in patients without a prior history of AT/AF, and a ventricular rate during AT/AF > 100 bpm in conjunction with at least 20% arrhythmia burden on a single day. The median time to the first clinically actionable event was significantly shorter in the remote transmission arm compared to the control arm (4.9 vs 6.3 months, $P < 0.001$).[52] In the control arm, only 2% of clinically actionable events were detected via TTM while in the remote arm, 66% of clinically actionable events were detected via remote device transmissions. The rate of AT/AF related events identified (AT/AF > 48 hours, ventricular rate during AT/AF > 100 bpm, new onset AT/AF) was almost twice as high in the remote versus control arm.

The CONNECT study was designed to demonstrate that remote monitoring with automatic clinician notifications reduces the time from a clinical event to a clinical decision compared to standard in-office care.[53] Patients ($n = 1997$) were randomized to either an in-office arm where patients were seen in the office at 1, 3, 6, 9, 12, and 15 months or a remote arm where the 3-, 6-, 9-, and 12-month office visits were replaced with remote device data transmissions. In addition, the remote arm automatically transmitted data when certain alert conditions within the device were satisfied. The investigators reported that the time from a clinical event to a clinical decision was significantly shorter in the remote arm (median 4.6 days) versus the control arm (median 22 days), ($P < 0.001$).[54] While there was no difference in the overall rate of hospitalizations between the two arms, the average hospitalization duration was significantly reduced by 18% in the remote arm compared to the control arm (3.3 vs 4.0 days, $P = 0.002$). The estimated cost savings due to this reduction in the duration of hospitalization was $1793 per event.

Syncope

Syncope is a sudden transient loss of consciousness secondary to temporary reduction in cerebral blood flow. Syncope is a common clinical presentation that account for 5% of emergency department visits and 2% of hospitalizations.[55] Cardiac arrhythmias (both brady- and tachyarrhythmias) are potentially lethal and are the second most common cause of syncope, especially in patients with underlying cardiovascular disease. Up to one-third of patients presenting with syncope secondary to unmanaged ventricular arrhythmias experience sudden cardiac death within 1 year.[56] Establishing the cause of syncope is still a challenging problem. Recording the heart rhythm during a symptomatic recurrence often provides important evidence that can establish or exclude an arrhythmic etiology. Electrocardiographic recordings are often used for this purpose but are difficult to obtain with many existing methods.

A standard 12-lead ECG establishes diagnosis in only 5% of patients. Examples of diagnostic electrocardiogram findings are prolongation of QT interval, ventricular pre-excitation, evidence of high-grade atrioventricular block, and acute myocardial infarction.

The signal-averaged electrocardiogram (SAECG) is used for detection of low-amplitude signals (late potentials) in the terminal portion of QRS complex, which suggest presence of substrate and inducibility of ventricular arrhythmias. Since it is an indirect marker, it is currently not used in the routine evaluation of patients with syncope.

Inpatient telemetry and ambulatory ECG monitoring are the conventional techniques used in patients with syncope. These techniques allow only for brief periods of monitoring in the longitudinal care of these patients and have a low diagnostic yield ranging from 5% to 20%.[57] This is due to the infrequent and unpredictable nature of syncopal events. Holter monitoring is most likely to provide diagnostic information when used in the occasional patient with frequent or daily episodes of syncope. Advances in implantable device technology and implantation techniques now allow for prolonged and continuous ECG monitoring using event or loop recorders.

External Event and Loop Recorders

Event monitors are currently indicated in the evaluation of patients with recurrent episodes of syncope. Event monitors are small, portable devices that are carried or worn continuously by the patient and can be activated by the patient to record electrocardiographic rhythm strips. The tracings can be stored and transmitted over telephone lines at a later time. Patient-activated external loop recorders do not yield a symptom–rhythm correlation in over two-thirds of patients, either because of device malfunction, patient noncompliance, or inability to activate the recorder. In the evaluation of patients with syncope, continuous loop event monitors are preferred as they can capture retrospective and prospective electrocardiographic recordings. Usually, these devices are often programmed with 4 minutes of retrospective memory and 1 minute of prospective memory on activation. When used in selected patient populations, a diagnostic yield as high as 25% has been seen.[58] However, there is a clear relationship between the duration of monitoring and the diagnostic yield.

Implantable Loop Recorders

In patients with extremely infrequent syncopal episodes, an implantable event monitor is most useful. The implantable loop recorder has become the ideal diagnostic tool for long-term monitoring of patients with unexplained syncope. The implantable loop recorder (ILR), eg, Reveal® (Medtronic, Minneapolis, MN) or Confirm™ (St. Jude Medical, St. Paul, MN), is a small, lightweight device with two electrodes on the surface of the device, which is placed subcutaneously under local anesthesia and has a battery life of 18 to 36 months (Figure 59.16). The device can be configured to trigger automatically according to programmed detection criteria as well as with a handheld patient activator to activate ECG recording as a result of a symptomatic episode. It has the ability to record the current and preceding rhythm for up to 40 minutes after a spontaneous event. Klein et al demonstrated its clinical utility when they were able to obtain a diagnosis in 21 of 24 unexplained syncope patients (88%) within 2 years after implantation of a loop recorder.[59,60] They compared prolonged monitoring using an implantable loop recorder with "conventional testing" using an external loop recorder, tilt, and electrophysiological testing in 60 patients for 1 year. Prolonged monitoring had significantly greater diagnostic yield compared to conventional testing (55% vs 19%, $P = 0.0014$).[61] In another study, loop recorders had a much higher diagnostic yield compared to Holter monitoring (63% vs 24%; $P < 0.0001$) for the mechanism of syncope.[62]

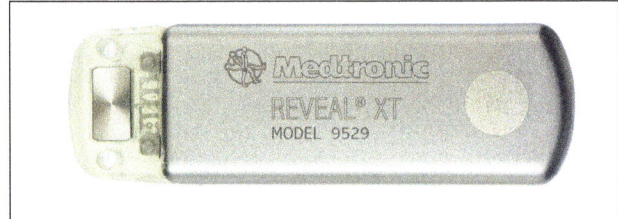

Figure 59.16 Implantable loop recorders are capable of detecting both syncope and atrial arrhythmias. *Source:* Reproduced with permission of Medtronic, Inc.

The auto-activation feature to capture arrhythmias without relying on patient compliance or perception of symptoms has the greatest diagnostic yield. However, this feature can be limited by the detection of inaccurate arrhythmias and can also fail to record arrhythmic events. New features included in these devices have shown to reduce false detection of asystole, bradyarrhythmia, or tachyarrhythmia by 85.2% ($P < 0.001$), with a small reduction in the detection of appropriate episodes (1.7%, $P < 0.001$).[63]

The specific improvements include:

- *R-wave sensing filter:* The sensing filter was modified with a wider frequency band to improve sensing of subcutaneous R waves and an additional filter was added to reject power line noise.

- *R-wave sensing threshold:* The original R-wave sensing scheme employed a fixed sensing threshold that operated on the ECG after bandpass filtering and rectification. This threshold was manually adjusted for each patient, in response to ECG amplitudes and recorded episodes, in an effort to sense all R waves while avoiding oversensing. The subcutaneous bipole of ILRs is susceptible to large R-wave amplitude reduction (possibly related to small changes in device position), large amplitude T waves (at times nearing the R-wave amplitude), and myopotential and other noise interference. Because of these features of subcutaneous ECGs, a fixed threshold sensing algorithm could be more susceptible to the storage of false arrhythmias due to either undersensing or oversensing. The new sensing algorithm has a threshold that adapts to the amplitude of the R wave and decays over time, in a manner that was previously optimized on a separate database of subcutaneous bipole signals. Briefly, following a sensed R wave, the threshold rapidly adapts to R-wave amplitude changes while avoiding oversensing of P waves, T waves, and small amplitude noise during asystole. Specifically, the threshold is first set to a percentage of the previously sensed R-wave amplitude and then decays to the minimum sensitivity setting.

- *Noise detection:* Two noise detectors were implemented to reject periods of noise. Each interval between sensed R waves is classified as either noisy or non-noisy. Noisy intervals are further classified by the type of noise detected: high-frequency noise (intervals containing two or more refractory sensed events) and amplifier saturation. This last situation, also referred to as "transient loss of signal," commonly causes false asystole detection in the original ILR.

- *Arrhythmia detection:* The tachycardia and bradycardia arrhythmia detection algorithms were improved to account for periods of noise. Detection of a noisy interval causes the tachycardia and bradycardia interval counters to decrement, requiring more evidence to detect an event in the presence of noise. Additionally, the tachyarrhythmia detector was improved to be similar to current ICD tachycardia rate detectors. The tachyarrhythmia detector includes two zones: a consecutive tachycardia interval counter (ie, 16 short intervals in a row required for detection) and a probabilistic fast tachycardia interval counter (ie, at least 12 of the most recent 16 intervals must be short for detection), with a different programmable rate boundary for each (the original algorithm had only a consecutive counter).

The diagnostic value of the implantable event recorder is now well established. Implantable loop recorders have also demonstrated "cost benefit per diagnosis" compared to conventional monitoring for recurrent unexplained syncope in select patients.[64]

Current guidelines recommend its use in unexplained and recurrent syncope.[65] It is also appropriate to use them in the initial phase of a syncope work-up, instead of completion of conventional investigations, especially in patients with clinical or electrocardiographic features suggestive of an arrhythmic syncope.

Limitations

The major limitations of implantable loop recorders are the need for a surgical implant and a small risk of infection. The benefit of loop recorders is population specific and therefore should be used in selected patients. The monitored findings are considered diagnostic, although they may not always be mechanistically related to the index syncopal event. However, studies have shown that symptoms resolved in all the patients treated on the basis of the loop recorder findings.

Heart Failure

Long-term management of patients with congestive heart failure (CHF) is a growing burden on healthcare systems. In addition, signs and symptoms within this population are often poorly correlated with actual disease status.[66,67] Swan-Ganz catheterization and echocardiography are costly and not well suited for repeated serial measurement. Recently, considerable investigation has focused on the development of alternative methods of assessing heart failure disease status. Implantable hemodynamic sensors offer a potential surrogate for serial invasive catheterizations in tailoring and titrating medical therapy. Furthermore, continuous monitoring of hemodynamic measurements might provide unique insight regarding pathophysiological mechanisms and chronic responses to therapeutic regimens.

Pressure Monitoring Systems

Right-sided Pressure Monitoring

A totally implantable hemodynamic monitor (IHM) system consists of a pacemaker-like device that processes and stores information and a transvenous lead incorporating a high-fidelity pressure sensor near its tip (Figure 59.17A).[68] The implantation procedure is similar to that of a single chamber pacemaker system. The pressure sensing lead is positioned in the right ventricular outflow tract or high right ventricular septum in an area of high blood flow. In addition to right ventricular systolic and diastolic pressure and estimated pulmonary arterial diastolic pressure (ePAD), the IHM also measures and stores peak positive and negative dP/dt, heart rate, patient activity, right ventricular preejection and systolic time intervals, and body temperature. A strong correlation ($r = 0.84$) has been demonstrated between actual pulmonary artery pressures and the ePAD estimates under a variety of physiologic conditions.[69-72] The implantable system continuously monitors and stores hemodynamic information that can be accessed remotely via the Internet. The web interface automatically processes and concatenates new data received from the device and displays visual trends over time (Figure 59.17B).

Multiple clinical studies have demonstrated both the safety and accuracy of the implantable hemodynamic monitoring system. The COMPASS-HF (Chronicle Offers Management to Patients with Advanced Signs and Symptoms of Heart Failure) trial randomized 274 NYHA Class III-IV patients to Chronicle-guided management group ($n = 134$) or control group ($n = 140$) and followed them for 6 months.[73,74] The study demonstrated that the IHM was safe and able to reduce the rate of heart failure–related events. However, the observed 21% reduction in heart failure events was not statistically significant.

Retrospective analyses from COMPASS-HF provided new insights into the pathophysiology of the transition from stable, compensated HF to the decompensated state in subjects with left ventricular ejection fraction (LVEF) less than 35% and among HF patients with preserved LVEF. The currently ongoing Reducing Events in Patients with Chronic Heart Failure (REDUCEhf) trial will prospectively test the hypothesis that the ambulatory hemodynamic monitoring can indeed reduce the rate of heart failure–related hospitalization.[75]

Left-sided Pressure Monitoring

In addition to right-sided cardiac pressure monitoring, an implantable device that measures left atrial pressure directly is currently being tested in clinical trials.[76] The implanted system consists of a hand-held patient activator monitor that stimulates a passive subcutaneous antenna coil. A lead connects the coil to the sensor module that is anchored in the left atrium from the right side via the fossa ovalis using a femoral venous approach. An initial clinical trial of 8 patients determined that "monitoring of direct LAP with a new implantable device was well tolerated, feasible, and accurate at a short-term follow-up."[77]

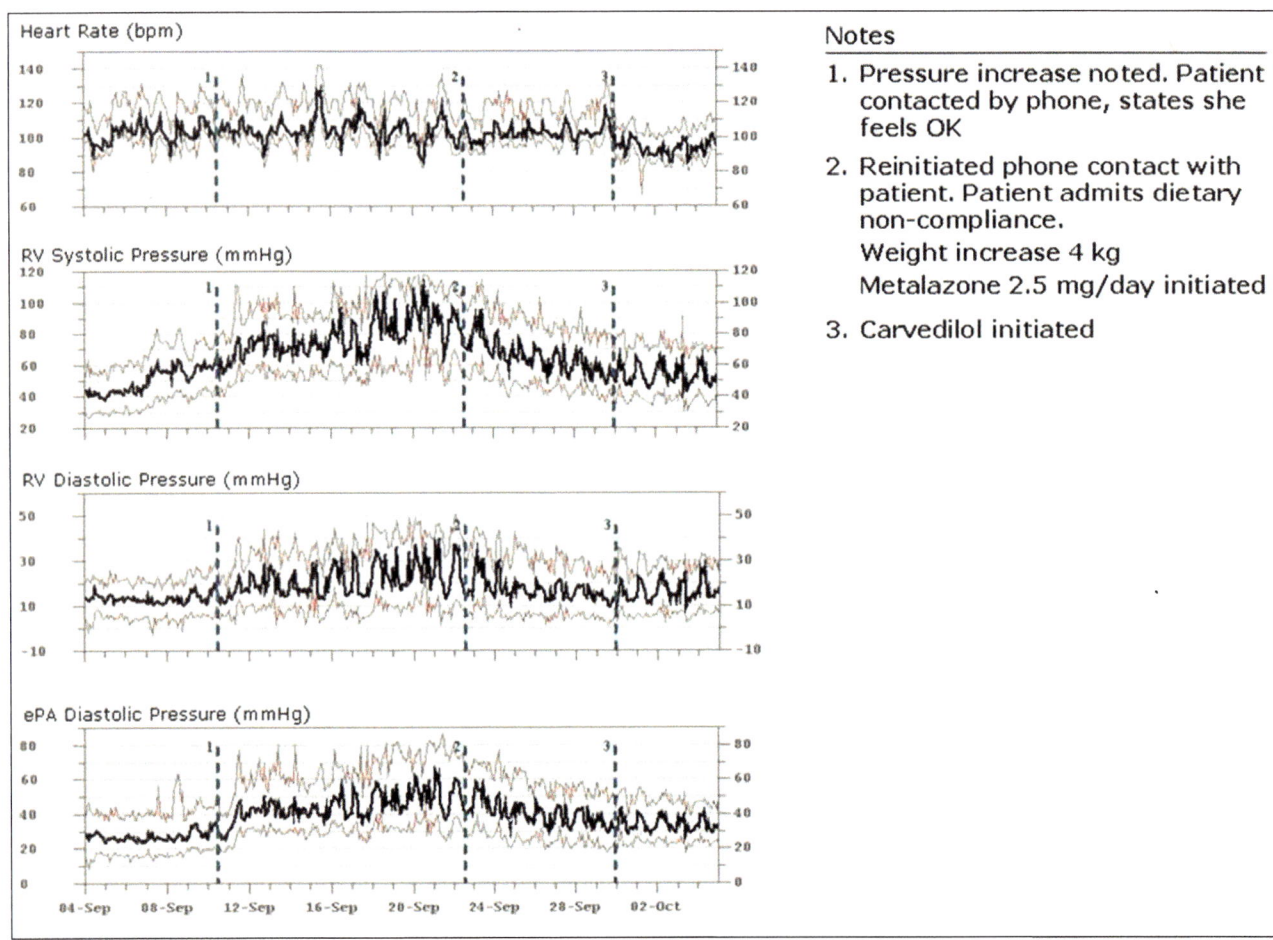

Figure 59.17 The trends show the daily median (**black line**) and the daily ranges (**pink lines**) of various pressure-derived parameters over 1 month when the patient admitted nonadherence to dietary restrictions. Clinical notes corroborate the associated pressure changes.

A larger randomized clinical trial is underway at the time of this writing.

Intrathoracic Impedance Monitoring

The correlation between changes in biological impedance and physiologic parameters, such as respiration rate and cardiac hemodynamics, has been the subject of scientific investigation for decades.[78-80] Recently, the theories behind impedance monitoring of hemodynamic events has been applied to implantable devices. The recent MidHeft trial[81] provided the first clinical evidence that daily monitoring of intrathoracic impedance measured between the right ventricular defibrillation coil and the devise case (Figure 59.18) could provide a clinically useful tool for monitoring the onset of acute heart failure decompensation. Device-recorded daily impedance data from this nonrandomized double-blinded prospective trial ($n = 33$) was used to develop and validate an algorithm to detect acute pulmonary fluid accumulation based on day-to-day changes in the actual recorded daily intrathoracic impedance. The algorithm automatically calculates a dynamic reference impedance based upon trends in the measured daily intrathoracic impedance. Differences between the measured daily impedance and the calculated reference impedance are used to increment or reset a "fluid index" (Figure 59.19). Results from the trial validation set indicated that the fluid index crossed a predetermined fluid index threshold (60 ohm-days) prior to hospitalization in over 77% of the events. The changes in the calculated fluid index occurred 15 days prior to symptom onset, on average. The rate of fluid index threshold crossings that were not immediately associated with hospitalization was 1.5 events per patient per year.[81]

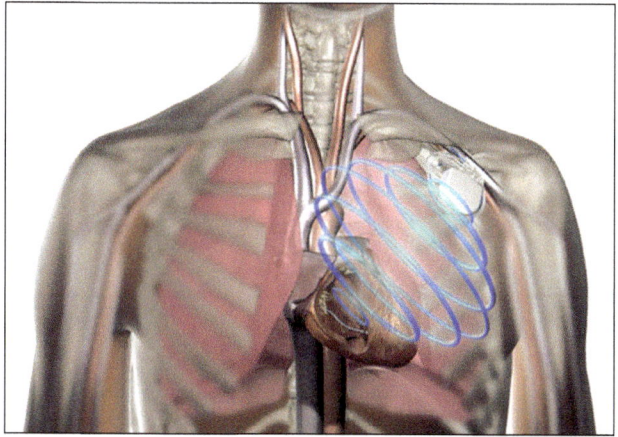

Figure 59.18 Cartoon representation of intrathoracic impedance measurement: A low amplitude constant current pulse is transmitted from the right ventricular therapy lead to the device case and the resultant voltage and impedance is determined. *Source:* Reproduced with permission of Medtronic, Inc.

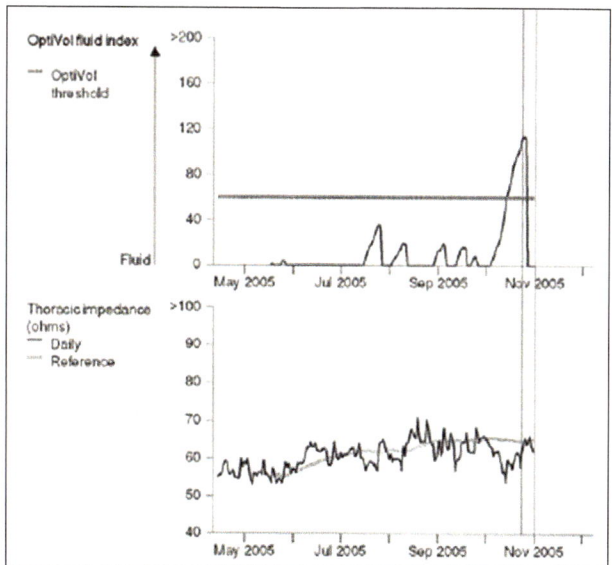

Figure 59.19 Sample implantable device patient diagnostic report including intrathoracic impedance fluid index and programmable threshold as well as the raw recorded daily and calculated reference impedance. Decreases in the trend of the measured daily impedance are reflected by consistent increases in the calculated fluid index. Fluid index values greater than the preprogrammed threshold indicate potentially worsening heart failure due to thoracic fluid accumulation.

Several recent investigations have further validated the clinical utility of chronic heart failure monitoring via intrathoracic impedance. Vollmann and colleagues performed a nonrandomized, multicenter investigation of 372 CRT-D patients with intrathoracic impedance monitoring.[82] Most subjects were also alerted to fluid index threshold crossings by an audible alert tone transmitted by the device. The results indicated an adjusted sensitivity of 60% and positive predictive value of 60% for various clinically relevant events associated with heart failure. In another study, Ypenburg and colleagues followed 115 CRT-D subjects with intrathoracic impedance monitoring over 9 months.[83] The sensitivity and specificity of the fluid index reportedly depended strongly on the programmed detection threshold. The authors concluded that optimal algorithm performance may require individualized optimization of the threshold value for the particular patient. Small and colleagues also recently investigated intrathoracic impedance monitoring in 326 US CRT-D patients with no audible alert, since the alert is currently unavailable within the United States.[84] The analysis included univariate and multivariate linear regression of changes in the fluid index as well as other device-recorded diagnostic parameters. The results indicated that each intrathoracic impedance fluid index threshold crossing was associated with a 35% increased probability of a heart failure hospitalization within the same year as the crossing (Figure 59.20). Additional trials have also shown that acute changes in intrathoracic impedance are correlated with both weight[85] and B-type natriuretic peptide (BNP) levels.[86,87] Taken as a whole, these trials confirmed that intrathoracic impedance monitoring can provide a useful clinical tool to help manage patients with congestive heart failure.

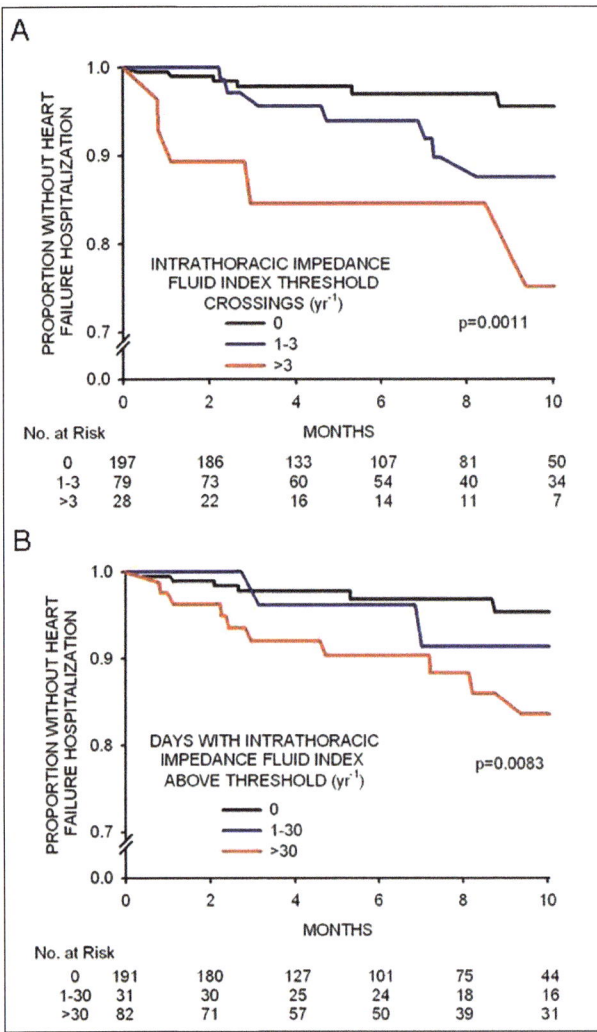

Figure 59.20 Kaplan-Meier survival analysis of time to first HF hospitalization for groups of patients with similar frequency of thoracic impedance fluid index threshold crossings. Patients with more frequent crossings and patients with longer duration crossings over the previous 4 months were significantly more likely to be hospitalized for heart failure over the subsequent months. *Source:* Small R, Wickemeyer W, Germany R, et al.[84] Used with permission.

Peak Endocardial Acceleration

The relative motion of the right ventricular wall, including the septum, can be detected by measuring the peak endocardial acceleration (PEA) using a sensor integrated into a ventricular pacing lead.[88-90] Bordachar et al have correlated this index with LV dP/dT.[88] A recent multicenter observational trial of 15 patients concluded that increases in PEA amplitude were associated with pharmacological inotropic stimulation and were paralleled by changes in RV dP/dt_{max}, suggesting that PEA is an index of myocardial contractility.[89] Indeed, algorithms have been developed to use closed-loop feedback from a lead-based accelerometer to control device therapies including pacing rate and CRT therapy. However, there is some debate whether the PEA signal is independent of heart sounds,[91] since these two signals are strongly temporally correlated. Likewise, the inclusion of additional sensors on ventricular pacing leads may have an uncertain impact on long-term pacing lead reliability.

Heart Rate Variability/Day Night Heart Rate

Most implantable devices are able to monitor both paced and intrinsic ventricular cycle lengths, and hence changes in both day and night heart rates as well as heart rate variability. Such diagnostic data may provide relative insight into the function of the autonomic nervous system. Recently, Adamson and colleagues reported reductions in device-measured indices of heart rate variability prior to episodes of acute heart failure decompensation.[92] Similarly, the OFISSER clinical trial results demonstrated increased night heart rates associated with acute heart failure decompensation in patients with CRT-D therapy.[84] However, heart rate–based diagnostic parameters have important limitations. Heart rate variability parameters assume that the rate is controlled by the sinus node. Thus, if the subject is in atrial fibrillation, or if the device is controlling the atrial rate by frequent atrial pacing, then the diagnostic information is not available. This scenario may represent a significant proportion of time for some patients with implantable devices, especially those who are pacemaker dependent.

Clinical Adoption and Remote Monitoring

Many devices may also automatically transmit all sensor-derived parameter trends from the patient's home directly to the clinic via a bedside monitoring/telemetry device. This device may be programmed by the clinic to transmit automatically based on preset schedule. Alternatively, diagnostic data transmission can also be triggered based on detected clinical events. For example, some devices can be programmed to alert the clinic directly if the patient experiences new onset atrial tachyarrhythmias or if the ventricular rate during a sustained atrial tachyarrhythmia exceeds a preprogrammed threshold. Such remote monitoring "care alerts" may be quite useful to help monitor rate and rhythm control strategies. Also, remote monitoring of heart failure parameters is recommended in at least one published guideline.[93] Such remote monitoring capabilities also offer the potential to transmit nondevice recorded information automatically, such as weight, blood pressure, and associated symptoms back to the managing clinic.

Integrated Diagnostics

The availability of useful physiologic clinical parameters derived from implantable device-based sensors is likely to increase. Future devices may include additional sensors to track respiration rate, minute ventilation, sleep apnea, tissue perfusion, cardiac output, acute ischemia, electrical alternans, and heart rate turbulence. Indeed, some recently released devices already contain some of these fascinating capabilities. The development of practical chemical sensors is also feasible. For example, some external glucose pumps for the chronic management of diabetes also can connect wirelessly to continuous glucose monitoring sensors placed subcutaneously to monitor changes in blood glucose.[94] The ability of such chemical sensors to augment other device monitoring capabilities for heart failure or other risks will require additional investigation.

Future Directions

With the number of patients with cardiac arrhythmias expected to rise dramatically faster than the number of physicians caring for them, new and creative ways of monitoring these patients in the future will be required. Remote device monitoring may be one tool to allow physicians to more efficiently follow their device patients. Another significant change in device-based monitoring for cardiac arrhythmias has been the advent of subcutaneous devices implanted solely for the purpose of monitoring arrhythmia status. While these devices appear to be promising in terms of their ability to identify patients with previously undiagnosed AF and aid in the management of patients known to have AF, clinical trials will be necessary to demonstrate their value in improving clinical outcomes for these patients. Miniaturization of these "monitoring-only" devices may also permit nonelectrophysiologists to implant and follow patients who have cardiac arrhythmias but who do not have a traditional indication for a pacemaker, ICD, or CRT device. This could help by distributing the ever-increasing number of device patients among a wider group of physicians.

In the future, it is also likely that implantable devices will have even more memory and capacity to store arrhythmia data. The challenge for device manufacturers will be to condense these large volumes of data into simple and useful information that can help improve both patient outcomes and efficiency of care.

References

1. Miyasaka Y, Barnes ME, Gersh BJ, et al. Secular trends in incidence of atrial fibrillation in Olmsted County, Minnesota, 1980 to 2000, and implications on the projections for future prevalence. *Circulation*. 2006;114:119-125.
2. Strickberger SA, Ip J, Saksena S, et al. Relationship between atrial tachycardias and symptoms. *Heart Rhythm*. 2005;2:125-131.
3. Page RL, Wilkinson WE, Clair WK, et al. Asymptomatic arrhythmias in patients with symptomatic paroxysmal atrial fibrillation and paroxysmal supraventricular tachycardia. *Circulation*. 1994;89:224-227.
4. Hindricks G, Piorkowski C, Tanner H, et al. Perception of atrial fibrillation before and after radiofrequency catheter ablation: relevance of asymptomatic arrhythmia recurrence. *Circulation*. 2005;112:307-313.
5. Israel CW, Grönefeld G, Ehrlich JR, et al. Long-term risk of recurrent atrial fibrillation as documented by an implantable monitoring device: implications for optimal patient care. *J Am Coll Cardiol*. 2004;43:47-52.
6. Hart RG, Halperin JL. Atrial fibrillation and thromboembolism: a decade of progress in stroke prevention. *Ann Intern Med*. 1999;(131):688-695.
7. Bialy D, Lehmann MH, Schumacher DN, et al. Hospitalization for arrhythmias in the United States: importance of atrial fibrillation. *J Am Coll Cardiol*. 1992;19:41A.
8. Kannel WB, Abbott RD, Savage DD, McNamara PM. Coronary heart disease and atrial fibrillation: the Framingham Study. *Am Heart J*. 1983;106:389-396.
9. Wyse DG, Waldo AL, DiMarco JP, et al. A comparison of rate control and rhythm control in patients with atrial fibrillation. *N Engl J Med*. 2002;347:1825-1833.
10. Vasamreddy CR, Dalal D, Dong J, et al. Symptomatic and asymptomatic atrial fibrillation in patients undergoing radiofrequency catheter ablation. *J Cardiovasc Electrophysiol*. 2006;17:134-139.
11. Quirino G, Giammaria M, Corbucci G, et al. Diagnosis of paroxysmal atrial fibrillation in patients with implanted pacemakers: relationship to symptoms and other variables. *Pacing Clin Electrophysiol*. 2009;32:91-98.
12. Fuster V, Rydén LE, Cannom DS, et al. 2011 ACCF/AHA/HRS focused updates incorporated into the ACC/AHA/ESC 2006 guidelines for the management of patients with atrial fibrillation: a report of the American College of Cardiology Foundation/American Heart Association Task Force on practice guidelines. *Circulation*. 2011;123:e269-e367.
13. Savelieva I, Camm AJ. Clinical relevance of silent atrial fibrillation: prevalence, prognosis, quality of life, and management. *J Interv Card Electrophysiol*. 2000;4:369-382.
14. Rothman SA, Laughlin JC, Seltzer J, et al. The diagnosis of cardiac arrhythmias: a prospective multi-center randomized study comparing mobile cardiac outpatient telemetry versus standard loop event monitoring. *J Cardiovasc Electrophysiol*. 2007;18:241-247.
15. Purerfellner H, Gillis AM, Holbrook R, Hettrick DA. Accuracy of atrial tachyarrhythmia detection in implantable devices with arrhythmia therapies. *Pacing Clin Electrophysiol*. 2004;27:983-992.
16. Israel CW, Hugl B, Unterberg C, et al. Pace-termination and pacing for prevention of atrial tachyarrhythmias: results from a multicenter study with an implantable device for atrial therapy. *J Cardiovasc Electrophysiol*. 2001;12:1121-1128.
17. Sarkar S, Ritscher D, Mehra R. A detector for a chronic implantable atrial tachyarrhythmia monitor. *IEEE Trans Biomed Eng*. 2008;55:1219-1224.
18. Hindricks G, Pokushalov E, Urban L, et al. Performance of a new leadless implantable cardiac monitor in detecting and quantifying atrial fibrillation: Results of the XPECT trial. *Circ Arrhythm Electrophysiol*. 2010;3:141-147.

19. Ziegler PD, Koehler JL, Mehra R. Comparison of continuous versus intermittent monitoring of atrial arrhythmias. *Heart Rhythm.* 2006;3:1445-1452.
20. Botto GL, Padeletti L, Santini M, et al. Presence and duration of atrial fibrillation detected by continuous monitoring: crucial implications for the risk of thromboembolic events. *J Cardiovasc Electrophysiol.* 2009;20:241-248.
21. Ziegler PD, Koehler J, Mongeon L, et al. Prevalence of paroxysmal, persistent, and chronic atrial fibrillation in the ICD versus CRT-D population: Continuous monitoring data from 141,231 patients in the CareLink database. *Heart Rhythm.* 2009;6(5):S193.
22. Borek P, Koehler J, Ziegler P, et al. Impact of AF on mortality in 44,104 patients with CRT-D. *Heart Rhythm.* 2010;7(5):S26.
23. Madan N, Saksena S. Long-term rhythm control of drug-refractory atrial fibrillation with "hybrid therapy" incorporating dual-site right atrial pacing, antiarrhythmic drugs, and right atrial ablation. *Am J Cardiol.* 2004;93(5):569-575.
24. Rao HB, Saksena S. Impact of "hybrid therapy" on long-term rhythm control and arrhythmia related hospitalizations in patients with drug-refractory persistent and permanent atrial fibrillation. *J Interv Card Electrophysiol.* 2007;18(2):127-136.
25. Saksena S, Slee A, Saad M, Nagarakanti R. Atrial Fibrillation "Burden" rather than a single arrhythmia recurrence identifies risk of adverse cardiovascular events on antiarrhythmic drugs: Further insights from the AFFIRM trial. *J Am Coll Cardiol.* 2015;65(10):A91.
26. Botto GL, Santini M, Padeletti L, et al. Temporal variability of atrial fibrillation in pacemaker recipients for bradycardia: implications for crossover designed trials, study sample size, and identification of responder patients by means of arrhythmia burden. *J Cardiovasc Electrophysiol.* 2007;18(3):250-257.
27. Saksena S, Hettrick D, Koehler J, et al. Progression of paroxysmal atrial fibrillation to persistent atrial fibrillation in patients with bradyarrhythmias. *Am Heart J.* 2007;154(5):884-892.
28. Saksena S, Skadsberg N, Rao H, Filipecki A. Biatrial and 3-Dimensional Mapping of spontaneus atrial arrhythmias in patients with refractory atrial fibrillation. *J Cardiovasc Electrophysiol.* 2005;16(5):494-504.
29. Nagarakanti R, Saksena S, Hettrick D, et al. Progression of new onset to established persistent atrial fibrillation: an implantable device-based analysis with implications for clinical classification of persistent atrial fibrillation. *J Interv Card Electrophysiol.* 2011;32(1):7-15.
30. Martinek M, Aichinger J, Nesser HJ, et al. New insights into long-term follow-up of atrial fibrillation ablation: full disclosure by an implantable pacemaker device. *J Cardiovasc Electrophysiol.* 2007;18:818-823.
31. Hanke T, Charitos EI, Stierle U, et al. Twenty-four-hour Holter monitor follow-up does not provide accurate heart rhythm status after surgical atrial fibrillation ablation therapy: up to 12 months experience with a novel permanently implantable heart rhythm monitor device. *Circulation.* 2009;120: S177-S184.
32. Arya A, Silberbauer J, Teichman SL, et al. A preliminary assessment of the effects of ATI-2042 in subjects with paroxysmal atrial fibrillation using implanted pacemaker methodology. *Europace.* 2009;11:458-464.
33. Ezekowitz MD, Nagarakanti R, Lubinski A, et al. A randomized trial of budiodarone in paroxysmal atrial fibrillation. *J Interv Card Electrophysiol.* 2012;34:1-9.
34. Ziegler PD, Koehler J, Mongeon L, et al. Poor ventricular rate control in the persistent versus paroxysmal atrial fibrillation population: Continuous monitoring data from 141,231 patients in the CareLink database. *Heart Rhythm.* 2009;6(5):S461.
35. Van Gelder IC, Groenveld HF, Crijns HJ, et al. Lenient versus strict rate control in patients with atrial fibrillation. *N Engl J Med.* 2010;362:1363-1373.
36. Willems R, Morck ML, Exner DV, et al. Ventricular high-rate episodes in pacemaker diagnostics identify a high-risk subgroup of patients with tachy-brady syndrome. *Heart Rhythm.* 2004;1:414-421.
37. Knight BP, Desai A, Coman J, et al. Long-term retention of cardiac resynchronization therapy. *J Am Coll Cardiol.* 2004;44:72-77.
38. Ousdigian K, Heywood JT, Koehler J, et al. Reduced bi-ventricular pacing is associated with decreased survival in 9,360 CRT-D patients with AF. *Heart Rhythm.* 2010;7(5):S449.
39. Jabaudon D, Sztajzel J, Sievert K, et al. Usefulness of ambulatory 7-day ECG monitoring for the detection of atrial fibrillation and flutter after acute stroke and transient ischemic attack. *Stroke.* 2004;35:1647-1651.
40. Bansil S, Karim H. Detection of atrial fibrillation in patients with acute stroke. *J Stroke Cerebrovasc Dis.* 2004;13:12-15.
41. Tayal AH, Tian M, Kelly KM, et al. Atrial fibrillation detected by mobile cardiac outpatient telemetry in cryptogenic TIA or stroke. *Neurology.* 2008;71:1696-1701.
42. Ziegler PD, Glotzer TV, Daoud EG, et al. Incidence of newly detected atrial arrhythmias via implantable devices in patients with history of thromboembolic events. *Stroke.* 2010;41:256-260.
43. Sinha AM, Diener HC, Morillo CA, et al. Cryptogenic stroke and underlying atrial fibrillation (CRYSTAL AF): Design and rationale. *Am Heart J.* 2010;160:36-41.
44. Kamel H, Johnson DR, Hegde M, et al. Detection of atrial fibrillation after stroke and the risk of recurrent stroke. *J Stroke Cerebrovasc Dis.* 2012;21:726-731.
45. Glotzer TV, Hellkamp AS, Zimmerman J, et al. Atrial high rate episodes detected by pacemaker diagnostics predict death and stroke: report of the Atrial Diagnostics Ancillary Study of the MOde Selection Trial (MOST). *Circulation.* 2003;107: 1614-1619.
46. Capucci A, Santini M, Padeletti L, et al. Monitored atrial fibrillation duration predicts arterial embolic events in patients suffering from bradycardia and atrial fibrillation implanted with antitachycardia pacemakers. *J Am Coll Cardiol.* 2005;46:1913-1920.
47. Glotzer TV, Daoud EG, Wyse DG, et al. The relationship between daily atrial tachyarrhythmia burden from implantable device diagnostics and stroke risk: The TRENDS Study. *Circ Arrhythm Electrophysiol.* 2009;2:474-480.
48. Themistoclakis S, Corrado A, Marchlinski FE, et al. The risk of thromboembolism and need for oral anticoagulation after successful atrial fibrillation ablation. *J Am Coll Cardiol.* 2010;55:735-743.
49. Nademanee K, Schwab MC, Kosar EM, et al. Clinical outcomes of catheter substrate ablation for high-risk patients with atrial fibrillation. *J Am Coll Cardiol.* 2008;51:843-849.
50. Ip J, Waldo AL, Lip GY, et al. Multicenter randomized study of anticoagulation guided by remote rhythm monitoring in patients with implantable cardioverter-defibrillator and CRT-D devices: Rationale, design, and clinical characteristics of the initially enrolled cohort The IMPACT study. *Am Heart J.* 2009;158:364-370.
51. Chen J, Wilkoff BL, Choucair W, et al. Design of the Pacemaker REmote Follow-up Evaluation and Review (PREFER) trial to assess the clinical value of the remote pacemaker interrogation in the management of pacemaker patients. *Trials.* 2008;9:18-23.

52. Crossley GH, Chen J, Choucair W, et al. Clinical benefits of remote versus transtelephonic monitoring of implanted pacemakers. *J Am Coll Cardiol.* 2009;54:2012-2019.
53. Crossley G, Boyle A, Vitense H, et al. Trial design of the clinical evaluation of remote notification to reduce time to clinical decision: the Clinical evaluation Of remote NotificatioN to rEduCe Time to clinical decision (CONNECT) study. *Am Heart J.* 2008;156:840-846.
54. Crossley GH, Boyle A, Vitense H, et al. The CONNECT (Clinical Evaluation of Remote Notification to Reduce Time to Clinical Decision) trial: the value of wireless remote monitoring with automatic clinician alerts. *J Am Coll Cardiol.* 2011;57:1181-1189.
55. Day SC, Cook EF, Funkenstein H, Goldman L. Evaluation and outcome of emergency room patients with transient loss of consciousness. *Am J Med.* 1982;73:15-23.
56. Kapoor WN, Karpf M, Wieand S, et al. A prospective evaluation and follow-up of patients with syncope. *N Engl J Med.* 1983;309:197-204.
57. Gibson TC, Heitzman MR. Diagnostic efficacy of 24-hour electrocardiographic monitoring for syncope. *Am J Cardiol.* 1984;53:1013-1017.
58. Linzer M, Pritchett EL, Pontinen M, et al. Incremental diagnostic yield of loop electrocardiographic recorders in unexplained syncope. *Am J Cardiol.* 1990;66:214-219.
59. Murdock CJ, Klein GJ, Yee R, et al. Feasibility of long-term electrocardiographic monitoring with an implanted device for syncope diagnosis. *Pacing Clin Electrophysiol.* 1990;13:1374-1378.
60. Krahn AD, Klein GJ, Yee R. Recurrent syncope: Experience with an implantable loop recorder. *Cardiol Clin.* 1997;15:313-326.
61. Krahn AD, Klein GJ, Yee R, Skanes AC. Randomized assessment of syncope trial: conventional diagnostic testing versus a prolonged monitoring strategy. *Circulation.* 2001;104:46-51.
62. Sivakumaran S, Krahn AD, Klein GJ, et al. A prospective randomized comparison of loop recorders versus Holter monitors in patients with syncope or presyncope. *Am J Med.* 2003;115:1-5.
63. Brignole M, Bellardine Black CL, Thomsen PE, et al. Improved arrhythmia detection in implantable loop recorders. *J Cardiovasc Electrophysiol.* 2008;19:928-934.
64. Krahn AD, Klein GJ, Yee R, et al. Cost implications of testing strategy in patients with syncope. *J Am Coll Cardiol.* 2003;42:495-501.
65. Guidelines for the diagnosis and management of syncope (version 2009): the Task Force for the Diagnosis and Management of Syncope of the European Society of Cardiology (ESC). *Eur Heart J.* 2009;30:2631-2671.
66. Wilson JR, Hanamanthu S, Chomsky DB, Davis SF. Relationship between exertional symptoms and functional capacity in patients with heart failure. *J Am Coll Cardiol.* 1999;33:1943-1947.
67. Androne AS, Hryniewicz K, Hudaihed A, et al. Relation of unrecognized hypervolemia in chronic heart failure to clinical status, hemodynamics, and patient outcomes. *Am J Cardiol.* 2004;93:1254-1259.
68. Bennett T, Kjellstrom, B, Taepke R, Ryden, L. Development of implantable devices for continuous ambulatory monitoring of central hemodynamic values in heart failure patients. *Pacing Clin Electrophysiol.* 2005;28:573-584.
69. Adamson PB, Magalski A, Braunschweig F, et al. Ongoing right ventricular hemodynamics in heart failure: clinical value of measurements derived from an implantable monitoring system. *J Am Coll Cardiol.* 2003;41:565-571.
70. Ohlsson A, Kubo SH, Steinhaus D, et al. Continuous ambulatory monitoring of absolute right ventricular pressure and mixed venous oxygen saturation in patients with heart failure using an implantable haemodynamic monitor: results of a 1 year multicentre feasibility study. *Eur Heart J.* 2001;22:942-954.
71. Reynolds DW, Bartelt N, Taepke R, Bennett TD. Measurement of pulmonary artery diastolic pressure from the right ventricle. *J Am Coll Cardiol.* 1995;25:1176-1182.
72. Steinhaus DM, Lemery R, Bresnehan DR, et al. Initial experience with an implantable hemodynamic monitor. *Circulation* 1996; 93:745-752.
73. Bourge RC, Abraham WT, Adamson PB, et al. Randomized controlled trial of an implantable continuous hemodynamic monitor in patients with advanced heart failure: The COMPASS-HF Study. *J Am Coll Cardiol.* 2008;51:1073-1079.
74. Zile MR, Bourge RC, Bennett TD, et al. Application of implantable hemodynamic monitoring in the management of patients with diastolic heart failure: a sub-study of the COMPASS-HF Trial. *J Card Fail.* 2008;14:816-823.
75. Adamson PB, Conti JB, Smith AL, et al. Reducing events in patients with chronic heart failure (REDUCEhf) study design: continuous hemodynamic monitoring with an implantable defibrillator. *Clin Cardiol.* 2007;30:567-575.
76. Walton AS, Krum H. The Heartpod implantable heart failure therapy system. *Heart Lung Circ.* 2005;14 Suppl 2:S31-33.
77. Ritzema J, Melton IC, Richards AM, et al. Direct left atrial pressure monitoring in ambulatory heart failure patients: initial experience with a new permanent implantable device. *Circulation.* 2007;18;116:2952-2959.
78. Baan J, Jong TT, Kerkhof PL, et al. Continuous stroke volume and cardiac output from intra-ventricular dimensions obtained with impedance catheter. *Cardiovasc Res.* 1981;15:328-334.
79. Ellenbogen KA, Wood MA, Shepard RK, et al. Detection and management of an implantable cardioverter defibrillator lead failure: incidence and clinical implications. *J Am Coll Cardiol.* 2003;41:73-80.
80. Cole CR, Jensen DN, Cho Y, et al. Correlation of impedance minute ventilation with measured minute ventilation in a rate responsive pacemaker. *Pacing Clin Electrophysiol.* 2001;24:989-993.
81. Yu CM, Wang L, Chau E, et al. Intrathoracic impedance monitoring in patients with heart failure: correlation with fluid status and feasibility of early warning preceding hospitalization. *Circulation.* 2005;112:841-848.
82. Vollmann D, Nägele H, Schauerte P, et al. European InSync Sentry Observational Study Investigators. Clinical utility of intrathoracic impedance monitoring to alert patients with an implanted device of deteriorating chronic heart failure. *Eur Heart J.* 2007;28:1835-1840.
83. Ypenburg C, Bax JJ, van der Wall EE, et al. Intrathoracic impedance monitoring to predict decompensated heart failure. *Am J Cardiol.* 2007;99:554-557.
84. Small R, Wickemeyer W, Germany R, et al. Changes in intrathoracic impedance are associated with subsequent risk of hospitalizations for acute decompensated heart failure: clinical utility of implanted device monitoring without a patient alert. *J Card Fail.* 2009;15(6):475-481.
85. Andriulli J, Crossley G, McKenzie J, et al. Acute weight increases are associated with decreased intrathoracic impedance in heart failure patients: initial results of the IMPEDE HF Trial. *J Card Fail.* 2008;14:S70 (abstract).
86. Lüthje L, Vollmann D, Drescher T, et al. Intrathoracic impedance monitoring to detect chronic heart failure deterioration: relationship to changes in NT-proBNP. *Eur J Heart Fail.* 2007;9:716-722.

87. Matsushita K, Ishikawa T, Sumita S, et al. Daily shock impedance measured by implantable cardioverter defibrillator is useful in the management of congestive heart failure. *Circ J.* 2006;70:1462-1465.
88. Bordachar P, Labrousse L, Ploux S, et al. Validation of a new noninvasive device for the monitoring of peak endocardial acceleration in pigs: implications for optimization of pacing site and configuration. *J Cardiovasc Electrophysiol.* 2008;19:725-729.
89. Rickards AF, Bombardini T, Corbucci G, Plicchi G. An implantable intracardiac accelerometer for monitoring myocardial contractility. The Multicenter PEA Study Group. *Pacing Clin Electrophysiol.* 1996;19:2066-2071.
90. Vogel M, Schmidt MR, Kristiansen SB, et al. Validation of myocardial acceleration during isovolumic contraction as a novel noninvasive index of right ventricular contractility: comparison with ventricular pressure-volume relations in an animal model. *Circulation.* 2002;105:1693-1699.
91. Tassin A, Kobeissi A, Vitali L, et al. Relationship between amplitude and timing of heart sounds and endocardial acceleration. *Pacing Clin Electrophysiol.* 2009;32:S101-S104.
92. Adamson PB, Smith AL, Abraham WT, et al. InSync III Model 8042 and Attain OTW Lead Model 4193 Clinical Trial Investigators. Continuous autonomic assessment in patients with symptomatic heart failure: prognostic value of heart rate variability measured by an implanted cardiac resynchronization device. *Circulation.* 2004;110:2389-2394.
93. Wilkoff BL, Auricchio A, Brugada J, et al. HRS/EHRA Expert Consensus on the Monitoring of Cardiovascular Implantable Electronic Devices (CIEDs): description of techniques, indications, personnel, frequency and ethical considerations: developed in partnership with the Heart Rhythm Society (HRS) and the European Heart Rhythm Association (EHRA); and in collaboration with the American College of Cardiology (ACC), the American Heart Association (AHA), the European Society of Cardiology (ESC), the Heart Failure Association of ESC (HFA), and the Heart Failure Society of America (HFSA). Endorsed by the Heart Rhythm Society, the European Heart Rhythm Association (a registered branch of the ESC), the American College of Cardiology, the American Heart Association. *Europace.* 2008;10:707-725.
94. Steil GM, Rebrin K, Mastrototaro J, et al. Determination of plasma glucose during rapid glucose excursions with a subcutaneous glucose sensor. *Diabetes Technol Ther.* 2003;5:27-31.

CHAPTER 60

Indications and Outcomes of Lead Extraction and Replacement Procedures for Pacemaker and Defibrillator Systems

Steven P. Kutalek, MD

Introduction

The ability to remove a lead system is critical to the management of cardiac implantable device patients. Since its inception in the late 1980s, pacemaker and implantable cardioverter-defibrillator (ICD) lead extraction has experienced a gradual rise in acceptance as a viable technique for device removal and revision, with a multiplicity of indications. The major concern over safety of the procedure has been addressed in numerous retrospective registries and in prospective clinical databases examining specific extraction indications.[1-6]

The prior chapter on surgical aspects of device implantation (Chapter 53) has addressed some specific issues of tools and techniques. This chapter will describe safety implications of the procedures, minimization of risk, and training to perform the procedure effectively and to the patient's best benefit.

Safety of Lead Extraction

The safe performance of this procedure requires a sound understanding of the indications for its use, the factors that increase and minimize risk, and the proper utilization of extraction tools to guarantee a safe procedure.

Indications

Indications for lead extraction have changed over the years since inception of this invasive procedure. Designed originally as an alternative to open-chest surgical removal of lead systems, reasons to perform lead extraction have changed with the evolution of implantable systems' technology. For example, unipolar leads with heavy outer insulators have the durability to remain functional for long periods of time because of the lack of an inner insulation sleeve, though they have their own drawbacks with respect to myopotential sensing. The heavy insulation could make them more durable for removal, but most are nonisodiametric (ie, having a larger diameter lead tip than lead body) making them more difficult to remove. Being polyurethane, their insulations have a tendency to degrade, and their conductors do not have the durability of newer lead systems. These issues make lead breakdown more likely during extraction, especially of older leads, which may require more complex tools, longer procedure times, and increased risk. All this is added to the longer duration of implant, which increases vascular fibrosis around the lead.

Such an example indicates the need to understand precisely the type of lead being approached in an extraction procedure. It also demonstrates the requirement for adaptation and individualization of technique to the specific lead(s) to be removed.

In the original series, indications for lead extraction were equally divided among infection and device malfunction. Characteristic device malfunction predominantly involved breakdown of inner insulation between the two coaxial coils of early generation polyurethane bipolar pacing leads. This would be manifest by low pacing impedance in the bipolar mode. A large number of leads of the Medtronic 4004 series were affected, and many removed, for this indication. Occasionally, conductor fracture would also occur.[1,2]

As a tribute to technologic advances made through lead development, the incidence of inner insulation breakdown has been markedly reduced, decreasing the need for lead extraction for this indication. Most inner insulations are now constructed of silicone. Likewise, coradial lead designs with individually insulated conductors demonstrate a reduced incidence of lead malfunction.

Nevertheless, lead malfunction may still occur, especially in the form of exit block at the tip of the lead, conductor fracture, and insulation breach. Young patients are more likely to fracture pacing leads due to their very active lifestyles, yet these leads tend to fibrose more heavily in a young patient with a vigorous healing response. This makes lead extraction more risky, but the risk is offset by the healthy vascular tissue of a young patient.[7,8]

Lead malfunction has taken a more central role in the need for lead extraction with the continued downsizing of ICD leads. Thinner insulation and conductor cables in the Fidelis™ (Medtronic, Minneapolis, MN) and Riata™ (St. Jude Medical, St. Paul, MN) high-energy lead families have led to FDA recalls for both, and evident electrical malfunction with either system constitutes an outright indication for lead extraction. The very nature of these leads, being ICD leads versus pacing leads, increases the risk of lead extraction in these patients, especially if a superior vena cava (SVC) coil is present to fibrose against the wall of the central veins. Removal of the Fidelis lead can be accomplished with minimal extraction risk, a tribute to advancements in extraction tools and the experience and diligence of the operators engaged in maintaining proficiency and safety during the procedure.[9-12] (▶ Video 60.1, ▶ Video 60.2, ▶ Video 60.3, ▶ Video 60.4, ▶ Video 60.5, ▶ Video 60.6, and ▶ Video 60.7 depict a typical laser lead extraction of an ICD system.)

In all series, infection makes up a large proportion of the indications for lead removal. The possibility of infection has been present since the inception of implantable devices, as a foreign body is inserted through a cutaneous access site into the bloodstream. Skin pathogens and blood-borne organisms may lead to a spectrum of infections, from localized pocket erosion or draining fistulae, to systemic infections with or without endocarditis and intracardiac vegetations. In our series over the past 11 years, the incidence of infection as a primary indication for lead extraction has increased from 40% to 60% for the past 3 years (Figure 60.1).[7]

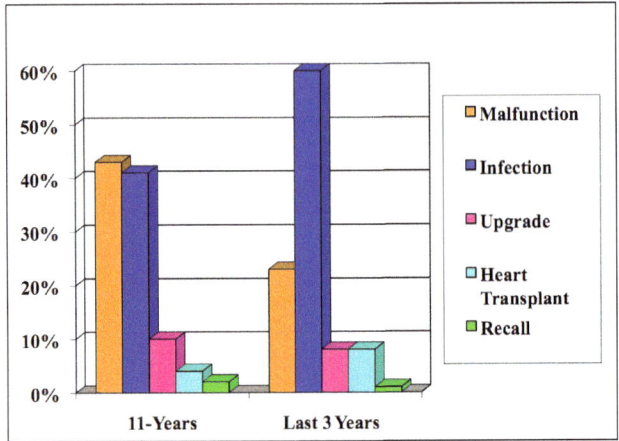

Figure 60.1 Graphic depiction of the change in indications for pacemaker and ICD lead extraction at the Drexel University College of Medicine. The graph on the left depicts the prior 11 years of experience, compared with the prior 3 years of experience on the right graph.

Despite the increased incidence of infections in implantable device patients, infection still affects a minority of those who receive these devices; in most series on the order of 1% to 2%, though higher numbers have been reported. There are other reasons, though, that infections have taken a front row seat in the indication for lead extraction. There are new indications for ICD implantation in younger patients who will live longer and have repeated device replacements. The need for device upgrade has increased with new indications for biventricular pacing and with improved survival on medical treatment for congestive heart failure. It is clear that device replacement carries a higher risk of infection, and other morbidities, than does initial device implantation.[13] Patients with implantable left ventricular assist devices receive defibrillators to terminate ventricular tachyarrhythmias to avoid right-sided failure; the two devices and multiple manipulations increase infection risk. Patients with diabetes and those on dialysis routinely receive implantable devices, despite a clear increase in the infection risk in these individuals.

Extracting leads in infected patients overall is not more difficult than removing leads for other indications. With acute infections, the development of a *Staph* biofilm over the lead body appears to reduce the fibrotic potential surrounding the lead. The presence of such biofilms and the inability to cure *Staph* infections without lead removal has been known for some time (Figure 60.2).[14]

With longer duration implants and chronic infections not directly related to the implant procedure, or in infected patients with previously indwelling chronic leads, the difficulty of extraction is similar to that for other leads with the same implant duration. Only in patients with large intracardiac vegetations is the risk of periprocedural morbidity increased. Mortality rates appear to be unaffected by the presence of a vegetation less than 3 cm in diameter, though subsegmental pulmonary emboli may occur. The overall mortality in these patients with active

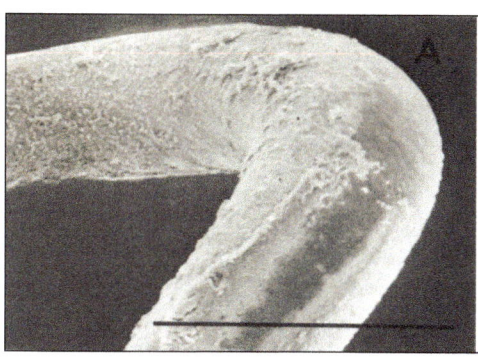 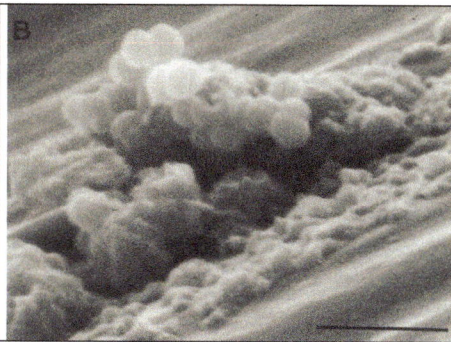

Figure 60.2 Scanning electron micrograph of a *Staphylococcus* biofilm adherent to a pacemaker lead body. **Panel A:** shows lower magnification; **Panel B:** shows higher magnification. Note the publication date of 1984. *Source:* Marrie TJ, Costerton W.[14] Used with permission.

endocarditis is related to infection burden, and not to the lead extraction procedure itself. Thirty-day postoperative mortality following lead extraction in patients with intracardiac vegetations approaches 30%.[15]

In some instances, lead extraction may be indicated for ancillary reasons, such as a retained SVC coil in patients who receive orthotropic heart transplantation in whom the leads are not removed entirely during the index operation. In these patients, as in others who have had prior thoracic surgery, the risk of lead extraction appears reduced, likely due to enhanced intrathoracic fibrosis strengthening the venous walls and making pericardial tamponade and perforation less likely.[2]

With other class IIa and IIb indications for lead extraction in patients with occluded vessels and with retained functional or nonfunctional leads, lead extraction risk follows that of the typical extraction patient. The Heart Rhythm Society (HRS) consensus document describes current accepted indications for lead extraction.[16] The potential risks of abandoned leads have been well addressed.[17-19] (▶ Video 60.8, ▶ Video 60.9, ▶ Video 60.10, ▶ Video 60.11, and ▶ Video 60.12 depict the use of ancillary tools for extraction of lead remnants.)

Risk Profiles

Large-scale registry data and the LEXICON trial delineate risk profiles of patients who undergo the procedure. In general, the risk of lead extraction has been reduced in the more than two decades since its inception. This is due in large part to two major factors: (1) improvements in lead extraction tools and (2) a vastly more experienced community of extracting physicians.

Risk is greatest in the elderly female with multiple leads. The presence of a SVC coil increases procedural risk. Low body surface area below 25 cm²/kg increases risk. Greater lead implant duration increases risk, and fibrosis, though not necessarily risk, is increased in younger patients with ICDs. Younger patients tend to scar more heavily than the elderly, although elderly patients have more friable blood vessels. Overall hospital course is greatly influenced by comorbidities, such as renal failure, bleeding diatheses, severe congestive heart failure or pulmonary disease, diabetes, the presence of vegetations, and prolonged systemic infection.[2-6,14,20]

ICD lead design has played a role in reduction of risk as well. Earlier ICD leads were constructed with exposed bare-wire loops or heavily indented, large-gauge wire coils as the high-energy electrodes. These leads are still extant in some patients, and they clearly constitute a greater risk for lead extraction than do modern ICD designs. These newer technologies incorporate silicone backfilling into the ICD coils or GORE-TEX® coating of the coils to prevent tissue ingrowth, as well as isodiametric design. Implanting ICD leads without a SVC coil also reduces the risk of subsequent extraction, in that there is less fibrosis in an area where perforation could cause major intrathoracic hemorrhage.

In this sense, the plan for lead extraction begins with the initial implant of the device. This is very important for young patients who receive implantable cardiac device, in that they are likely to fracture leads (sometimes more than once) due to their high degree of mobility. Careful attention to the types of leads placed and the implant procedure can markedly reduce the need for, and risk of, future lead extraction. Young patients deserve single-coil ICD leads, in which defibrillation thresholds vary little from leads with two high-energy coils. Access via axillary vein puncture rather than a subclavian approach reduces the likelihood of lead fracture and prevents bony growth around the lead in the subclavian area; both improve the chances for a successful lead extraction if required in the future.

The LEXICON trial, a registry of laser lead extraction, indicated that low body surface area was correlated with higher extraction risk. These patients have more friable blood vessels and smaller vessels overall, though the size and aggressiveness of the tools does not differ from those extraction tools used for larger individuals.[6]

Training and Experience

The LEXICON trial also demonstrated that experience with extraction tools reduces risk, with the lowest risk occurring in the centers in which the laser was utilized frequently. Overall, morbidity was 1.4%, with a reduced morbidity rate of 0.78% in high-volume centers; mortality rate was 0.27%. This theme is recurrent in the extraction literature. Though the procedure incorporates some of the skills inherent in device implantation and interventional cardiology, performing a safe extraction can only be done after appropriate training and experience. There are clear-cut breakpoints at which the risk of extraction goes down; risk is lower with extraction experience after 30 cases, and again after 300 cases.[3,6,16,21]

The HRS consensus document delineates requirements for fellowship training for lead extraction, ie, a minimum of 40 leads extracted as the primary operator, with experience with a variety of extraction tools.[16] Training requirements for those physicians already in practice are not distinctly specified; what is clear, however, is that adequate exposure and training, with mentorship, are crucial to a safe extraction environment. New and experienced extractors should maintain a database of their own procedures and complications. They should be active in continuing medical education for the procedure and become facile with new techniques and new equipment as they enter the clinical realm.

Through prospective database tracking, operators maintain a continuing understanding of their own risk profile and that of their institution. In-services and reviews of safe techniques and emergency drills add to the confidence of the extraction team that they will be able to safely handle the most serious of complications. Training involves the entire team, as everyone's abilities add to the safety of the procedure.

As in other areas of cardiovascular education, simulator training for laser extraction provides a safe method to work through various case scenarios. The operator and trainee are able to obtain a realistic experience, manage "complications," and gain a real understanding of the forces of pull and push (pull should always be greater than push) required to remove leads with extraction tools.

Each procedure provides a challenge in its own way. Depending on the clinical situation, the operator may be required to deal with heavily calcified scar tissue, vascular bleeding, adherence of leads to one another, broken leads, vegetations, or other unusual situations. In an unanticipated scenario, the operator should contact a mentor or trusted extraction colleague for advice. Open discussion plays such an important role in this field; this is the result of rapidly changing indications, the large variety of leads implanted, the expansive breadth of patient illnesses associated with device implantation and extraction, and changes in device status, such as new lead recalls or unanticipated fractures.

The Operating Site

The place where lead extraction is performed, ie, in the operating room or in the electrophysiology (EP) laboratory, is much less important than the preparation of the team for a life-threatening emergency. This intimately involves the cardiothoracic surgical team. In no instance should a lead extraction program be initiated in a center without cardiothoracic surgical on-site support. The advantage of superb fluoroscopy in the EP laboratory needs to be weighed against the availability of necessary surgical supplies, appropriate anesthesia facilities and equipment, and the ability to rapidly obtain cardiopulmonary bypass capability if needed. A cardiothoracic surgical suite obviates these needs, but may have the disadvantage of poor, and sometimes quite, inadequate visualization of leads, especially thin pacing leads, lead remnants, and some of the extraction sheaths themselves.

Hybrid operating rooms combine the best of both worlds. Designed around fixed high-gain fluoroscopic imaging units, these rooms can be designed to accommodate the needs of the extraction team and be rapidly and seamlessly converted to a full cardiothoracic operating facility. Building and equipping a hybrid room is expensive, but the savings in safety and efficiency make this an attractive alternative.

Complication Rates

The earliest published large series of complication rates for lead extraction involved a small cadre of extraction specialists who contributed their data to multicenter registries to track success and complication rates across a broad spectrum of patients. There was a learning curve for each of the operators, and the tools involved were the most basic, yet effective, mechanical Byrd dilator sheaths along with mechanical femoral extraction tools. The nature of the complications observed was similar to those that exist today (Table 60.1).

Table 60.1 Lead extraction complications from the MAUDE Database

Extraction Device	n	Events (n)	
		Death	Injury
Laser sheath	45	25	20
Mechanical sheath	32	12	20
Electrosurgical dissection sheath	2	2	0
Unspecified extraction device	26	18	8
TOTAL	105	57	48

Source: Adapted from Lead extraction devices associated with reported deaths and serious injuries in the FDA MAUDE Database: 1995–2008. Hauser RG, et al. *Europace.* 2010;12(3):395-401.

Overall complication rates in these early databases involved both morbidity and mortality. There was some variability among centers depending on their experience and the complexity of their procedures. Increased difficulty with extraction and higher complication rates were observed in the early years, in patients with more numerous leads, with ICD leads as opposed to pacing leads, and in elderly females. Total complications ranged from 1.6% to 1.9%, with mortality rates of 0.4% to 0.8%. Other smaller series had complication rates as high as 10%, with mortality rates up to 5%.[1,2]

The advent of laser technology applications to lead extraction met with similar complication rates compared to the use of nonpowered mechanical extraction sheaths. The first multicenter experience with laser extraction compared its efficacy for lead removal with mechanical dilator sheaths. The PLEXUS trial in 1999 showed the laser was more effective overall for removal of leads (94% for laser vs 64% for mechanical, $P = 0.001$). Because of the design of the trial, however, investigators were not obligated to remain with one technology once randomized, and there were frequent crossovers from mechanical to laser sheaths to facilitate ease of extraction. Overall complication rates were 2%, with mortality of 0.65% for laser extraction.[3]

Subsequent trials show comparable or lower complication rates. Byrd and coauthors published in 2002 overall success rates of 93% for laser lead extraction in a multicenter compilation of 1,684 patients from 89 centers. Morbidity was 1.9%, with a total mortality rate of 0.6%.[4]

The laser-powered sheath itself was subsequently modified to incorporate a 15° bevel at the tip (instead of a flat tip) with a softer distal end of the sheath. The tip bevel allows the operator to position the early cutting surface of the sheath to the inside of the curve when passing it around the major curves in the great veins, especially from the brachiocephalic vein to the SVC (Figure 60.3). This is the area of greatest risk for extraction, as the vessels, if torn, bleed profusely into the right pleural space from above the pericardial reflection.

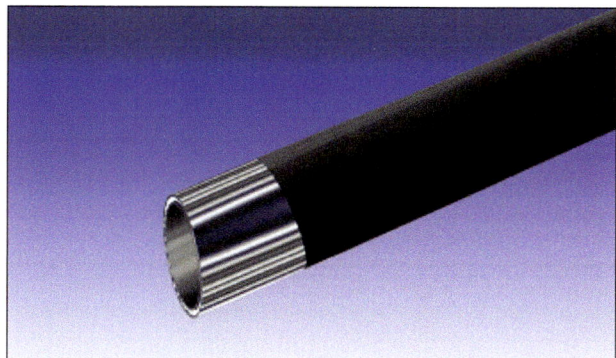

Figure 60.3 The addition of a beveled tip to the laser sheath has made it possible to direct energy placement while advancing the sheath to the inside of a major vessel rather than against the vessel wall. *Source:* Spectranetics Corp. Used with permission.

The most recently published compilation of laser extraction data comes from the LEXICON trial, a multicenter review of 1,449 patients from 13 centers. With the changes in laser technology and increased experience among extractors and extraction centers, morbidity rates decreased to 1.4% and were as low as 0.78% in the highest volume centers. The overall mortality rate for laser extraction was reduced to 0.27%.[6]

Is it possible to sustain such low complication rates? In a positive sense, the experience of the extraction community has increased tremendously in the more than two decades that the procedure has been in use. Operators have a better understanding of patient risk profiles and of the interaction of their own capabilities with the patient scenario. Additionally, lead technology has improved. Both pacemaker and ICD leads have become more durable. Both are now isodiametric and primarily silicone-based, with greater tensile strength and more durable materials that are less likely to disintegrate with lead removal. Silicone backfill in ICD high-energy coils or GORE-TEX coating over the coils (Figure 60.4) appears to improve the extractability of these complex leads. Finally, the need for a team approach to maintain safety is clear. With all these factors, it is possible to maintain a relatively low complication rate for lead extraction.[22]

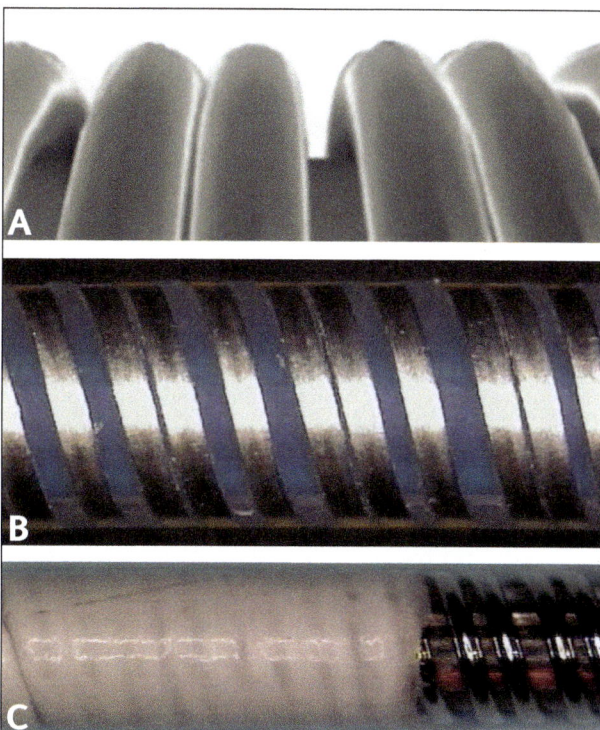

Figure 60.4 A variety of leads now have silicone back-filling applied between the high-energy coils or a GORE-TEX coating over the coils. **Panel A:** An older nonbackfilled lead showing bare high-energy wires into which fibrous scar can readily grow. **Panel B:** A flat wire ICD high-energy coil with silicone back-filling (St. Jude Medical). **Panel C:** The end of a GORE-TEX coating on a high-energy coil. The current lead version has a small area of uncovered wires where tissue may adhere. *Source:* Panel A and Panel B: Image courtesy of The Spectranetics Corporation. Adapted from SJM Design Advantage Publication, Distributed October 2007. **Panel C:** Boston Scientific Corp. Used with permission.

In a negative sense, some leads are becoming more difficult to remove because of longer implant durations in patients who are living longer with their devices. Implantation of systems into younger patients, who tend to scar more heavily than the elderly, adds to the degree of fibrosis around the leads. Longer implant duration also contributes to the tendency to have more leads capped and additional leads implanted, just based on the fact that extraction centers are not ubiquitous and not all patients are referred for the procedure when it could be offered to them.

Protocols

Laboratory Preparation

As noted previously, there are no data that suggest that performing lead extraction in an operating room reduces risk compared with performing it in an electrophysiology laboratory. What is critical, though, is open communication between all members of the extraction team. This includes the performing physician, surgical assistants, nurses, anesthesia, and the surgical backup team. There are certain items that cannot be overlooked in preparation for the procedure. These include gathering a full understanding of the types of leads and implant durations that are to be considered; it is not unknown to discover a "surprise" when the fluoroscopy is turned on, and that moment is not the right time to make alternate plans for the procedure because of previously unknown leads.

More important are the preparation of safety features in the laboratory or operating room and the coordination of various staff members. Each participant has a role to play, and these must be delineated in advance. The phone numbers of the cardiothoracic surgeon backing up the procedure and the cardiothoracic pump team should be posted in direct view of the operating team. Echocardiography equipment should be in the room, or the operator should have placed a transesophageal or intracardiac echocardiography probe. Cross-matched blood must be available in the room or in a readily accessible blood bank in close proximity to the operating suite.

All team members need to be aware of the potential complications and their specific roles should complications arise. When a sternotomy or thoracotomy needs to be performed for a perforation of the SVC or the RA/SVC junction, opening the chest in less than 10 minutes improves survival. Table 60.2 outlines a preparation checklist that should be adapted to the laboratory.

The team members may decide to perform a mock drill, whereby they stage a complication, such as cardiac tamponade or SVC perforation, which requires emergent intervention. This is the best way to ensure that the entire team is prepared. Are thoracotomy trays in the lab and sterile? Are sternal saws and batteries operating? Does the surgeon on call actually arrive in the room within a few minutes? Has a member of the team actually spoken with the surgeon before the case to make the surgeon aware that assistance may be needed? Based on the results of the mock drill, the team can adapt to improve performance in the event a true emergency occurs.

Table 60.2 Preoperative checklist for lead extraction

Patient	• Number and types of leads identified
	• Lead implant dates
	• Pacemaker dependence known
	• LVEF and cardiac condition known
	• Contraindications and potential comorbidities known
	• Family or significant other aware of procedure and risks
Personnel	• All team members have been assigned a role
	• Anesthesia in the room during the removal of leads
	• Cardiothoracic surgeon identified and briefed on the case
	• Relevant phone numbers posted in the lab/operating suite
	• Cardiothoracic surgical pump team standing by
Equipment	• Fluoroscopic and image recording equipment operating
	• Temporary pacing box in the lab with fresh batteries
	• Pericardiocentesis needle/tray immediately accessible
	• Thoracotomy trays (two) in room
	• Two sternal saws in room, two blades, and batteries charged
	• Resuscitation equipment in room
	• Blood immediately available
Monitoring	• ECG, pulse oximetry, end tidal CO2, blood pressure, temperature
	• Echocardiography machine in room (preferred: transesophageal or intracardiac echocardiographic probe inserted)
	• Preoperative cine recording of pleural spaces and cardiac silhouette motion

Temporary Pacing

Prior to the procedure, interrogate the device to check the patient's underlying rhythm. With *any* question as to the stability of the patient's native rhythm, place a temporary transvenous pacing electrode from the femoral vein to the right ventricular apex for backup during the procedure. Bradycardia can be exacerbated by vagal stimulus with traction on the leads in the great vessels and the heart.

In dependent patients where devices are explanted due to infection, longer-term temporary pacing is required. We prefer to place a temporary transvenous pacemaker electrode via the right internal jugular vein directly to the low right ventricular septum. This lead is a standard bipolar screw-in pacemaker lead with an IS-1 header. After adequate lead is allowed for deep inspiration, the lead is secured to skin with 2 nonabsorbable sutures around the anchoring sleeve. The patient's explanted device (or an alternate) may then be attached to the lead, and the entire system is secured to the skin surface with a suture and transparent plastic dressing. This approach has the advantage of allowing the patient to be mobile and ambulatory in the room, awaiting reimplantation on the side opposite to the infected explant site.

Echocardiography

Preoperative echocardiography delineates overall cardiac function and the absence (or presence) of pericardial fluid. Postoperative transesophageal echocardiography defines the presence or absence of vegetations at the right atrium or tricuspid valve, or of residual scar tissue within the SVC as a remnant of the extraction procedure.

A greater number of extractors now perform real-time echocardiography during the extraction procedure, either transesophageal or intracardiac. This likely improves safety of the procedure. The probe is used to evaluate for the presence, location, and size of vegetations at the beginning and end of the procedure. It can then be "parked" to allow continuous observation of the pericardial space. For any hypotensive episode, the operator has an immediate reference to see whether the patient is developing a pericardial effusion or whether the event was merely vagal. Fluoroscopy confirms whether there is intrathoracic bleeding with the development of a new pleural effusion. The advantages of intracardiac echocardiography advanced via a femoral vein are (1) it does not require continuous intubation of the patient for those operators who use conscious sedation and (2) it gives direct visualization of the right atrium, tricuspid valve, and transvenous leads on the right side of the heart.

Vegetations

About 10% of patients who present with infected CIEDs have intracardiac vegetations, often adherent to the lead itself in the right atrium or at the tricuspid valve, or adherent to the right atrium or tricuspid valve itself (Figure 60.5). Multiple publications have documented the safety of extracting leads transvenously despite the presence of intracardiac vegetations. Although pulmonary emboli can occur, they are routinely subsegmental and do not cause mortality or significant morbidity (Figure 60.6).[15]

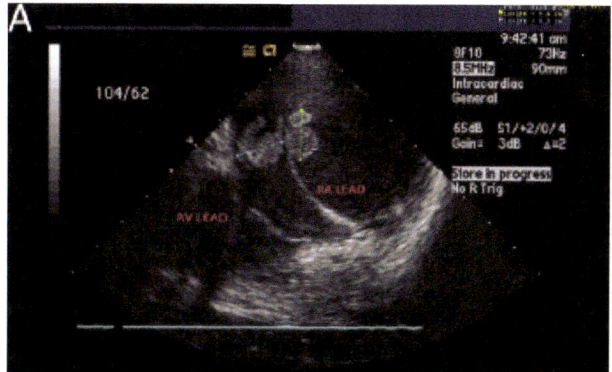

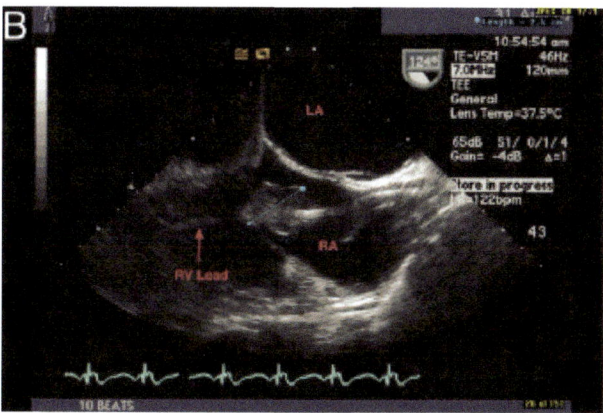

Figure 60.5 Intracardiac and transesophageal echocardiograms demonstrating a vegetation. **Panel A:** Intracardiac echocardiogram (ICE) shows vegetations attached to both right ventricle (RV) and right atrium (RA) leads. **Panel B:** Transesophageal echocardiogram (TEE) of lead vegetation attached to the RV lead as it crosses the tricuspid valve. The approximate diameter is 2.4 cm. LA = left atrium. *Source:* Grammes JA, Schulze CM, Al-Bataineh M, et al.[15] Used with permission.

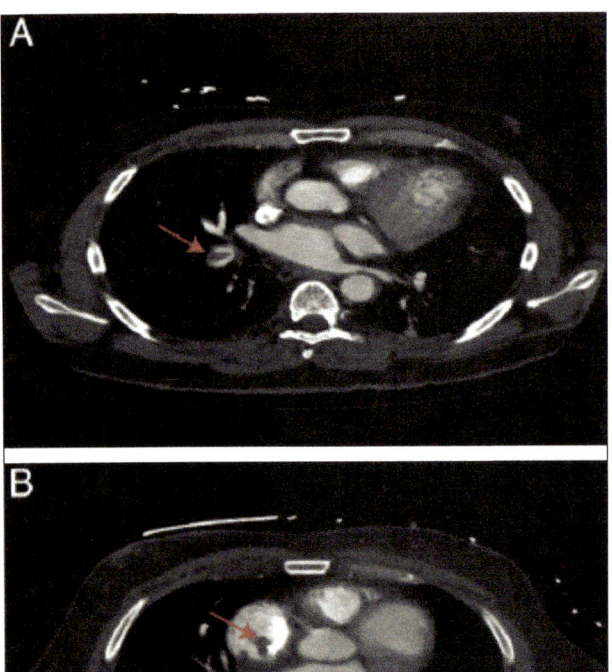

Figure 60.6 Computed tomography (CT) angiogram of documented subsegmental pulmonary emboli in an extraction patient who had a vegetation attached to the lead. There were no long-term sequelae in this patient. High-resolution CT angiography indicates (**Panel A**) a filling defect in the right middle pulmonary artery (**red arrow**), consistent with septic pulmonary embolism, and (**Panel B**) a filling defect in the right atrium (**red arrow**) at the junction with the SVC, consistent with retained vegetation. *Source:* Grammes JA, Schulze CM, Al-Bataineh M, et al.[15] Used with permission.

The size of vegetation that can be tackled with transvenous lead extraction remains unclear. Embolization of a piece of a 3-cm vegetation that is only 0.5 cm thick is less likely to occlude a major pulmonary artery than embolization of a spherical 3-cm mass. We recommend an alternative approach for such a large spherical vegetation; this may include surgical removal via a limited right thoracotomy, or continued intravenous antibiotic treatment to shrink the vegetation before lead extraction.

In infected patients with intracardiac vegetations, device reimplantation may occur after sterilization of the bloodstream, ie, negative blood cultures, and when right atrium and tricuspid valve vegetations are no longer present. The opposite side is preferred, but in some patients with bilateral infection or contraindications to the use of the opposite side, a lateral subpectoral approach may be used to enter a deep, separate fascial plane (Figure 60.7).[23] If vegetations remain, an epicardial approach may be required in dependent patients.

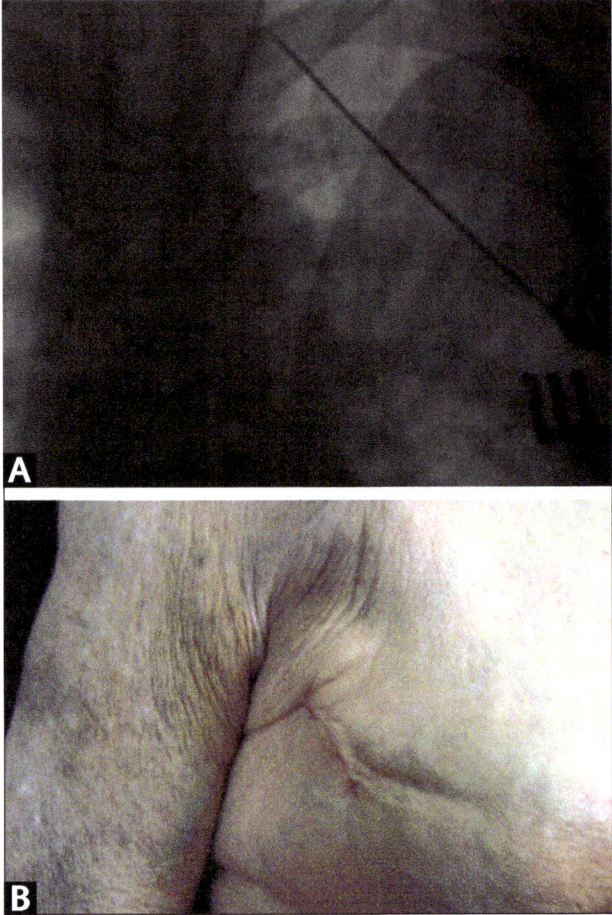

Figure 60.7 **Panel A:** Access to the axillary vein from a lateral subpectoral approach. The needle is inserted toward the axillary vein under fluoroscopic guidance, after the pectoralis major muscle is lifted from the lateral border from an incision that is vertical just posterior to the anterior axillary line. **Panel B:** A patient with a recent lateral subpectoral device implantation. The incision is in a vertical orientation near the anterior axillary line.

In some patients, dense fibrotic scar tissue remains as a byproduct of the extraction, visualized as stranding along the course of the explanted lead, especially in the SVC or in the right atrium. These casts have a "railroad track" appearance, as they represent the residual scar tubes from which the lead was removed (Figure 60.8). The presence of such residual casts does not increase the risk of thrombosis or the perpetuation of infection, and reimplantation does not need to be delayed.

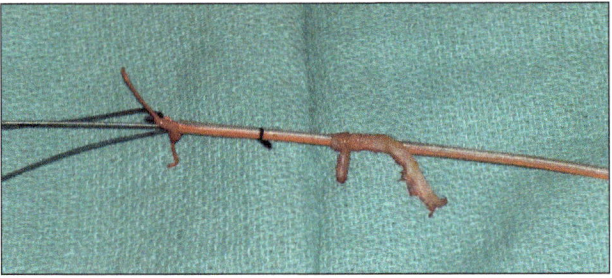

Figure 60.8 Depiction of a fibrous cast that had surrounded a pacing lead that was removed by extraction.

Thoracic Surgical Approach

The cardiothoracic surgeon must know immediately how to enter the chest for any given form of complication that may occur from lead extraction. The surgical approach depends on the location of vascular or cardiac injury. Additionally, the team must be prepared and drilled to ensure a rapid response to any emergency (Table 60.3).

Table 60.3 Approach to resuscitation

	Document the Problem
Fluoroscopy	• Reduced cardiac silhouette motion
	• New or expanding right pleural effusion
SVC venography	• If time, document location of laceration
Echocardiography	• Pericardial effusion, new or expanding
	Interventional Approach
Immediate	• Maintain airway
	• IV fluid resuscitation
	• IV albumin
	• Paced red blood cells (or whole blood) as needed
	• Activate ACLS protocol
	• **Call for help**
Tamponade	• Needle or operative drainage of effusion
	• Sternotomy required if intrapericardial SVC laceration
	• Subxyphoid operative access for right ventricular laceration
	• Sternotomy access for right atrial laceration
New or expanding right pleural effusion	• SVC/RA junction – sternotomy or right thoracotomy
	• High SVC or brachiocephalic vein – high right thoracotomy

Pericardial Tamponade

Pericardial tamponade may be recognized by hypotension, sinus tachycardia, reduced cardiac silhouette motion, and a double density at the cardiac apex under fluoroscopic imaging due to the presence of pericardial fluid. The situation needs to be recognized immediately; the anesthesiologist should not independently treat the patient with pressor agents for hypotension without advising the operator of the reduction in blood pressure, as hypotension may be indicative of vascular or cardiac injury requiring immediate intervention.

Every extractor should be skilled in pericardiocentesis. A needle or pericardiocentesis kit allows subxyphoid access with a 16- or 14-gauge needle, followed by confirmation with a guidewire or dye injection into the pericardial space. An indwelling intracardiac echocardiographic probe may assist with access, and also with diagnosis of a significant pericardial effusion.

If bleeding persists, cardiothoracic surgery needs to access the pericardial space. When the culprit lead was in the right ventricular apex, a subxiphoid surgical approach to the pericardium will allow access to the right ventricular perforation to enable it to be oversewn if necessary. For an RA perforation or uncertain location of the cardiac laceration, sternotomy is indicated. Cardiac tamponade that occurs with extraction tools in the SVC may indicate a tear in the intrapericardial portion of the SVC and requires sternotomy for repair.

Vascular Tears

Vascular tears in the SVC or the RA/SVC junction may require a right thoracotomy approach. The higher the perforation in the SVC, or if located in the brachiocephalic vein, the more difficult the surgical access to the perforated great vessel. A high thoracotomy may be required for high-level lacerations. When the location of the laceration is unclear, sternotomy will usually allow access to the bleeding source. The extrapericardial SVC will bleed into the thorax, while the intrapericardial portion will bleed into the pericardium to cause tamponade.

An SVC laceration 1 cm in size may bleed up to a liter of blood per minute into the thoracic cavity. Thus, speed in entering the chest is critical; there can be no delay in access. The chest should have been prepared at the onset of the procedure. Brief discussion with the operator should indicate to the surgeon the correct approach. Blood is hung immediately.

In the couple of minutes of assessment, the operator may inject dye into the SVC to localize the site of bleeding. In no instance, however, should entrance into the chest via thoracotomy or sternotomy be delayed to try to do a venogram.

Clearly, team effort is essential.

Extraction Safety Issues with Specific Lead Types

Coronary Sinus Leads

Extraction of coronary sinus leads provides no specific difficulty with respect to removing the lead from the coronary sinus proper. Our institution has removed over 150 coronary sinus leads through extraction, often in conjunction with the removal of other leads in the same patients (Video 60.1 and Video 60.2).

The great majority of these leads are passive fixation. These are easily removed from the coronary sinus proper, with no adherence to venous tissue within the coronary sinus itself. It appears, however, that 10% to 12% of these leads require the use of extraction tools after the tip of the lead has been removed from the coronary sinus proper. Our data show that one-third of these leads become lodged at the tricuspid valve/coronary sinus ostium, one-third in the SVC, and one-third in the brachiocephalic vein. In this percentage of leads, the use of extraction tools is required; thus, all the precautions for lead extraction need to be followed.[24]

An active fixation lead may not be removed with such ease. The Medtronic SarFix (Medtronic, Inc.) lead has deployable fins that hold with vigor in the branches of the coronary sinus. Several reports document the difficulty that can occur while removing this lead. The fins do not generally fully retract, making the extraction of the lead quite complex. Use of extraction tools within the coronary sinus or surgical removal may be required.[25]

Medtronic Fidelis Lead

The fracture incidence of this lead continues to increase (Figure 60.9). Over 20% of these leads have demonstrated a tendency to fracture over 8 years, and the incidence is highest (up to 16% in 5 years) in the youngest individuals, especially in those less than 40 years old. The fracture incidence is also increased in women and in patients with hypertrophic cardiomyopathy, arrhythmogenic right ventricular dysplasia, and genetic channelopathies with an arrhythmia substrate.[26] Moreover, the presence of a rate-sensing fracture predicts a high-energy malfunction in greater than 22% of patients over the ensuing 21 months. This requires that a new high-energy lead be placed, not just a rate sensing lead. In many of these patients, the decision is made to extract the preexisting Fidelis lead at the same procedure at which the new ICD lead is placed.[26,27]

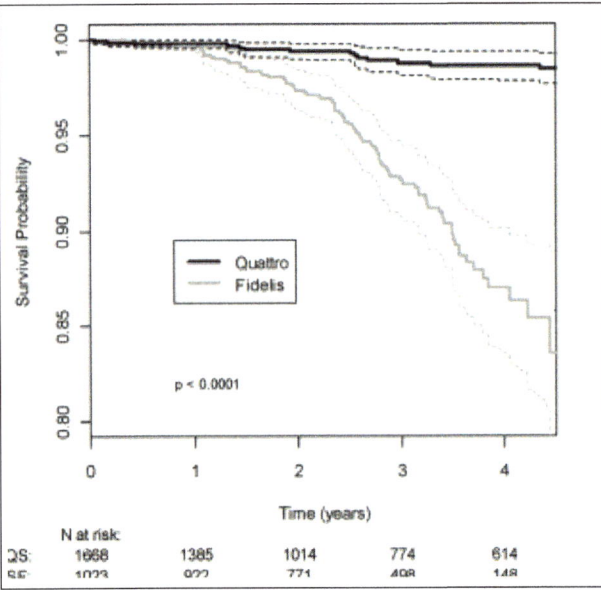

Figure 60.9 Graphical depiction of the failure curves of the Fidelis lead compared with the Quattro lead. The rate of failure is significantly higher for the Fidelis lead over 5 years. *Source:* Hauser RG, Maisel WH, Friedman PA, Kallinen LM, Mugglin AS, Kumar K.[26] Used with permission.

With the strong cable properties of internal components, despite malfunction of the lead, the lead can be removed in a relatively straightforward manner using standard extraction equipment. The operator should place a locking stylet down the lead, tie a heavy suture to the high-energy wires, and tie another heavy suture to the lead insulation. Standard extraction sheaths may then be used to remove the lead.[28-30]

As with all removed device material, though especially in light of its recall, the removed lead should be retained and sent to the manufacturer for analysis.

St. Jude Medical Riata Lead

Fluoroscopic imaging has demonstrated exteriorization of cables from the inside out in some of these leads that have pure silicone insulation. Some of the leads with exteriorized cables, and some with no exteriorized cables, malfunction electrically. The electrical malfunction involves primarily electrical noise sensing, which can lead to inhibition of pacing output, as well as low high-voltage impedance (Figure 60.10). Exteriorized cables are each individually insulated; thus, the malfunction that can occur in patients with exteriorized cables may or may not be related to these cables. Return of removed leads is, again, essential to better understand these failure mechanisms.

Removal of the Riata lead is not as straightforward as removal of a Fidelis lead. The original Riata leads were manufactured with high-energy coils that had no silicone back-filling, but were instead bare wire coils. These coils are prone to a great degree of tissue in-growth and fibrosis; this makes extraction of the lead more difficult. Additionally, exteriorized cables can bunch up in front of the extraction sheath. The high-energy coils, being loose, may also "snowplow" in front of the extraction sheath. Because of these specific lead properties, most extractors recommend upsizing the extraction sheath by one level; if using a laser sheath for extraction, an outer sheath should also be used. The outer sheath can be placed over the coils or exteriorized cables if they do provide any difficulty with passing the inner sheath (Figures 60.11 and 60.12).[31-33]

This lead provides an excellent example of specific characteristics in construction that make it so important to understand the nuances of each lead model that the extractor approaches.

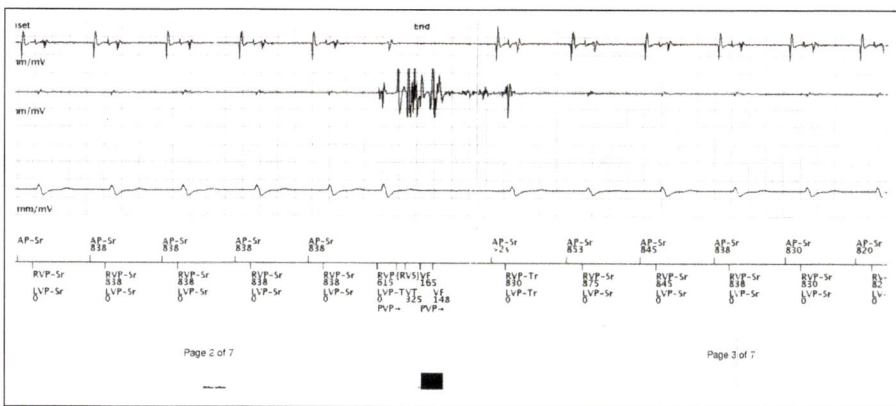

Figure 60.10 Noise sensing depicted on intracardiac electrogram recordings from a fractured Riata lead. The three electrogram channels depict the right atrial, near-field right ventricular, and far-field ventricular electrograms. High-frequency noise sensing from the right ventricular lead detected in the VT and VF zones causes inhibition of pacing output in this dependent patient.

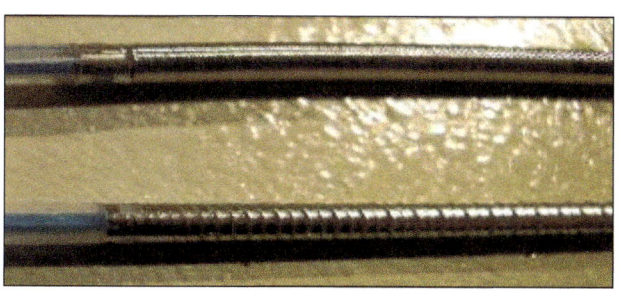

Figure 60.11 Comparative photographs of an early generation Riata ICD lead with bare wire coils, compared with a later Riata-ST lead with silicone back-fill between the high-energy coils. The upper lead demonstrates round wires from the Riata 1580/1581 series of leads, while the lower lead demonstrates flat wire technology from the Riata 7000/7001 series of leads. *Source:* St. Jude Medical. Used with permission.

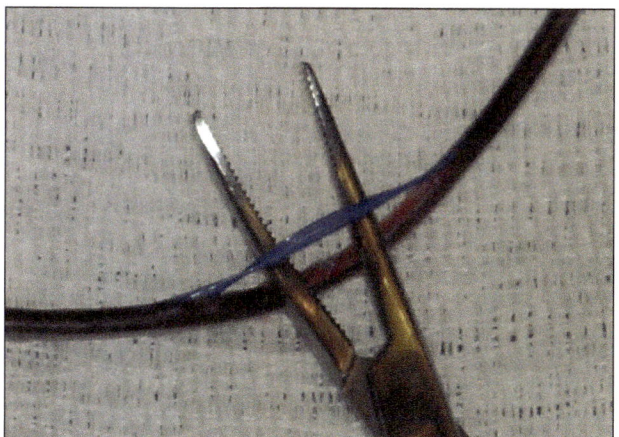

Figure 60.12 Exteriorized cables form a Riata lead removed by extraction. Note that the high-energy wires are individually coated with insulation material.

"Fine Points" and Conclusion

Although the risk of lead extraction has been substantially reduced over the years using the techniques and laboratory preparations described, there remains a potential for life-threatening complications to occur. Laboratory preparation and a cohesive team approach are essential to prevent a morbidity from becoming a mortality. Because of the potential for risk, the operator should (1) maintain adherence to guidelines for indications and training and (2) not perform procedures deemed outside the limits of her/his ability. We always involve the significant other, close family member, or POA in the preoperative discussion of the procedure and risks with the patient.

Finally, the need for continuing education cannot be overemphasized. Even experienced extractors learn from every procedure; the most important lesson is that no two patients and leads are the same. There are, however, guiding principles, and there are experienced operators who are willing and enthusiastic about sharing their experience and knowledge. A preoperative discussion with such an individual and a sincere evaluation of one's own abilities can make the difference to lead to a successful and safe result.

References

1. Smith HJ, Fearnot NE, Byrd CL, Wilkoff BL, Love CJ, Sellers TD. Five years' experience with intravascular lead extraction. *Pacing Clin Electrophysiol*. 1994;17:2016-2020.
2. Byrd CL, Wilkoff BL, Love CJ, Sellers TD, Turk KT, Reeves R, et al. Intravascular extraction of problematic or infected permanent pacemaker leads: 1994–1996. *Pacing Clin Electrophysiol*. 1999;22:1348-1357.
3. Wilkoff BL, Byrd CL, Love CJ, Hayes DL, Sellers TD, Schaerf R, et al. Pacemaker lead extraction with the laser sheath: results of the pacing lead extraction with the excimer sheath (PLEXES) trial. *J Am Coll Cardiol*. 1999;33:1671-1676.
4. Byrd CL, Wilkoff BL, Love CJ, Sellers TD, Reiser C. Clinical study of the laser sheath for lead extraction: the total experience in the United States. *Pacing Clin Electrophysiol*. 2002;25:804-808.
5. Henrikson CA, Brinker JA. How to prevent, recognize and manage complications of lead extraction. Part III: procedural factors. *Heart Rhythm*. 2008;5:1352-1354.
6. Wazni O, Epstein LM, Carrillo RG, Love C, Adler SW, Riggio DW, et al. Lead extraction in the contemporary setting: the LExICon study: an observational retrospective study of consecutive laser lead extractions. *J Am Coll Cardiol*. 2010;55(6):579-586.
7. Kutalek SP. Pacemaker and defibrillator lead extraction. *Curr Opin Cardiol*. 2004;19(1):19-22.
8. Love CJ. Lead extraction. *Heart Rhythm*. 2007;4:1238-1243.

9. Hauser RG, Kallinen LM, Almquist AK, Gornick CC, Katsiyiannis WT. Early failure of a small-diameter high-voltage implantable cardioverter–defibrillator lead. *Heart Rhythm*. 2007;4:892-896.
10. Hauser RG, Hayes DL. Increasing hazard of Sprint Fidelis implantable cardioverter lead failure. *Heart Rhythm*. 2009;6:605-610.
11. Samsel T. Sprint Fidelis Lead Performance Update. 13 March 2009. http://www.medtronic.com/product-advisories/physician/sprint-fidelis/PHYSLETTER-2009-03-13.htm. Accessed March 30, 2009.
12. Melanie M, Love CJ, Fischer A, Carrillo RG, Garisto JD, Bongiorni MG, et al. Multicenter experience with extraction of the sprint fidelis implantable cardioverter-defibrillator lead. *J Am Coll Cardiol*. 2010; 56:646-650.
13. Poole JE, Gleva MJ, Mela T, Chung MK, Uslan DZ, Borge R, et al, for the REPLACE Registry Investigators. Complication rates associated with pacemaker or implantable cardioverter-defibrillator generator replacements and upgrade procedures: results from the REPLACE Registry. *Circulation*. 2010;122:1553-1561.
14. Marrie TJ, Costerton W. Morphology of bacterial attachment to cardiac pacemaker leads and power packs. *J Clinical Microbiol*. 1984;19:911-914.
15. Grammes JA, Schulze CM, Al-Bataineh M, et al. Percutaneous pacemaker and implantable cardioverter-defibrillator lead extraction in 100 patients with intracardiac vegetations defined by transesophageal echocardiogram. *J Am Coll Cardiol*. 2010;55:886-894.
16. Wilkoff BL, Love CJ, Byrd CL, Bongiorni MG, Carrillo RG, Crossley GH, et al. Transvenous lead extraction: Heart Rhythm Society expert consensus on facilities, training, indications, and patient management. *Heart Rhythm*. 2009,6:1085-1104.
17. de Cock CC, et al. Long-term outcome of patients with multiple (> or = 3) noninfected leads: a clinical and echocardiographic study. *Pacing Clin Electrophysiol*. 2000;23:423-426.
18. Suga C, Hayes DL, Hyberger LK, Lloyd MA. Is there an adverse outcome from abandoned pacing leads? *J Interv Card Electrophysiol*. 2000;4:493-499.
19. Bohm, Adam, et al. Complications due to abandoned noninfected pacemaker leads. *Pacing Clin Electrophysiol*. 2001;24:1721-1724.
20. Hauser RG, Kallinen L. Deaths associated with implantable cardioverter defibrillator failure and deactivation reported in the United States Food and Drug Administration Manufacturer and User Facility Device Experience Database. *Heart Rhythm*. 2004;1:399-405.
21. Bracke FA, Meijer A, Van Gelder B. Learning curve characteristics of pacing lead extraction with a laser sheath. *Pacing Clin Electrophysiol*. 1996;21:2309-2313.
22. Jones SO, Eckart RE, Albert CM, Epstein LM. Large, single-center, single-operator experience with transvenous lead extraction: outcomes and changing indications. *Heart Rhythm*. 2008;5:520-525.
23. Al-Bataineh M, Sajadi S, Fontaine JM, Kutalek S. Axillary subpectoral approach for pacemaker or defibrillator implantation in patients with ipsilateral prepectoral infection and limited venous access. *J Interv Card Electrophysiol*. 2010:27(2):137-142.
24. Kasravi B, Tobias S, Barnes MJ, Messenger JC. Coronary sinus lead extraction in the era of cardiac resynchronization therapy: single center experience. *Pacing Clin Electrophysiol*. 2005;28:51-53.
25. Maytin M, Carrillo RG, Baltodano P, Schaerf RH, Bongiorni MG, et al. Multicenter experience with transvenous lead extraction of active fixation coronary sinus leads. *Pacing Clin Electrophysiol*. 2012;35:1-7.
26. Hauser RG, Maisel WH, Friedman PA, Kallinen LM, Mugglin AS, Kumar K, et al. Longevity of Sprint Fidelis implantable cardioverter-defibrillator leads and risk factors for failure—implications for patient management. *Circulation*. 2011;123:358-363.
27. Urgent Medical Device Information - Sprint Fidelis® Lead Patient Management Recommendations, October 15, 2007. Medtronic physician advisory letter.
28. Neuzil P, Taborsky M, Rezek Z, Volpalka R, Sediva L, Niederle P, et al. Pacemaker and ICD lead extraction with electrosurgical dissection sheaths and standard transvenous extraction systems: results of a randomized trial. *Europace*. 2007;9:98-104.
29. Saad EB, Saliba WI, Schweikert RA, Al-Khadra AS, Abdul Karim A, Niebauer MJ, et al. Nonthoracotomy implantable defibrillator lead extraction: results and comparison with extraction of pacemaker leads. *Pacing Clin Electrophysiol*. 2003;26:1944-1950.
30. Kennergren C, Bucknall CA, Butter C, Charles R, Fuhrer J, Grosfeld M, et al. Laser assisted lead extraction: the European experience. *Europace*. 2007;9:651-656.
31. Krebsbach A, Aljumaid F, Henrikson CA, Calkins H, Berger RD, Cheng A. Premature failure of a Riata defibrillator lead without impedance change or inappropriate sensing: A case report and review of the literature. *J Cardiovasc Electrophysiol*. 2011;Vol:1-3.
32. Jalal Z, Derval N, Ploux S, Bordachar P. Unusual failure of a multilumen, small-diameter implantable cardioverter-defibrillator lead. *Heart Rhythm*. 2010;7:1166-1167.
33. Durata™ Lead Design Advantage, SJM white paper no. 60018312 US, http://www.sjmprofessional.com/Products/US/ICD-Systems/Durata-Defibrillation-Lead.aspx.

Video Legends

Video 60.1 Initial AP cine demonstrating three bipolar leads in typical locations. Note that the leads appear to move as one unit through the left brachiocephalic vein, where there is lead-to-lead binding.

Video 60.2 A typical coronary sinus lead extraction is depicted. The lead is removed with direct traction, with no evidence of binding; 90% of coronary sinus leads are removed in this way, with 10% requiring the use of extraction tools.

Video 60.3 After the atrial lead is removed, the laser is gently advanced over the high-energy lead. The bevel of the laser is turned toward the inside of the curve throughout its course over the lead. The ICD coil begins to slightly uncoil with the required tension on the lead to maintain a stable rail.

Video 60.4 With heavy binding in the subclavian area, the outer sheath (Teflon®) is advanced over the laser to break up heavy fibrosis, to expand the lumen, and to reduce binding of the laser with surrounding scar tissue. The outer sheath is advanced just past the laser, with the bevel toward the inside of the curve.

Video 60.5 The laser continues slow advancement over the proximal high-energy coil. The coil gradually unwinds, due to the appropriate tension on the lead to maintain a stable rail. The laser bevel is oriented toward the inside of the curve.

Video 60.6 With heavy binding in the SVC, the outer sheath is advanced to break up the binding site. The bevel is oriented toward the inside of the curve, and there is substantial traction on the lead to pull it away from the SVC wall.

Chapter 60: Lead Extraction and Replacement Procedures for Pacemaker and Defibrillator Systems

Video 60.7 Use of the inner and outer sheaths together breaks up the last fibrotic area, and the lead is removed in its entirety. Bevel orientation and traction are maintained.

Video 60.8 Two FineLine coradial leads. The coils on one lead are stretched, not allowing a locking stylet to pass. The other lead is completely fractured and intravascular, precluding a superior approach for removal.

Video 60.9 The stretched ventricular lead has been removed to the level of the clavicle. It binds here due to calcification around the entry site. A metal dilator is unable to pass the calcification, and the lead ultimately breaks off here.

Video 60.10 A needle's eye snare is used femorally to remove the remnant atrial lead in its entirety.

Video 60.11 The remnant ventricular lead segment is grasped with a large snare, also from the femoral approach.

Video 60.12 The ventricular lead remnant is pulled into the femoral extraction sheath.

SECTION 3

CLINICAL INDICATIONS AND EVIDENCE-BASED OUTCOMES STANDARDS IN INTERVENTIONAL ELECTROPHYSIOLOGY

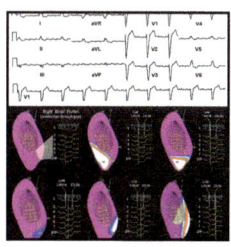
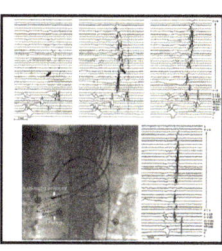
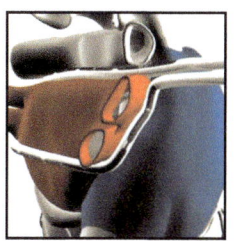
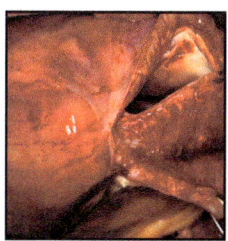

CHAPTER 61

Catheter Ablation of AV Junction and Paroxysmal SVT

Sanjaya Gupta, MD; Karl J. Ilg, MD; Hakan Oral, MD

Introduction

Over the last 3 decades, radiofrequency catheter ablation (RFA) evolved to become a primary treatment modality for the vast majority of paroxysmal supraventricular arrhythmias (PSVT).[1] RFA of the atrioventricular (AV) junction has also been effectively used to achieve ventricular rate control in patients with atrial fibrillation (AF) refractory to pharmacological therapy. Current indications and evidence-based outcomes of RFA of AV junction and supraventricular tachycardias will be reviewed in this chapter.

Catheter Ablation of the AV Junction

Clinical Indications

Ablation of the AV junction with concomitant implantation of a permanent pacemaker to achieve ventricular rate control in patients with AF and rapid ventricular response rates that have been refractory to pharmacological therapy is a time-honored electrophysiology procedure. However, AV junction ablation is being performed less frequently today than before due to recent advances in treatment of AF. Still, this approach remains indicated for patients with AF who have failed pharmacological means for rate/rhythm control, and/or catheter or surgical ablation procedures to eliminate AF.[2] The obvious disadvantage of this approach is that the patient is left in AF and does not benefit from a reduction in risk of stroke or restoration of AV synchrony that would result from restoration of sinus rhythm. In addition, the patient is rendered pacemaker-dependent for the remainder of his or her lifetime. Furthermore, patients with rapid ventricular rates must be monitored for 48 hours after AV junction ablation and paced at a relatively fast rate (80–90 bpm/min) for several weeks to minimize the risk of bradycardia-dependent proarrhythmia.

The most compelling indication for AV junction ablation and pacemaker implantation is for patients with evidence of a tachycardia-mediated cardiomyopathy as a result of AF with a poorly controlled ventricular response. For these patients, consideration should be given to implantation of a biventricular pacemaker or ICD to avoid further deterioration of cardiac function caused by a high burden of right ventricle–only pacing.[2]

Another related indication for catheter ablation of the AV junction is for patients who have a biventricular pacemaker or defibrillator implanted and are unable to achieve adequate biventricular pacing due to poorly controlled AF.[2]

Table 61.1 Clinical indications for catheter ablation of AV junction

Class	Level of Evidence	
IIa	B	To achieve ventricular rate control in patients with atrial fibrillation that is refractory to pharmacologic therapy
IIb	B	When rate cannot be controlled with pharmacologic therapy, or tachycardia-mediated cardiomyopathy is suspected
III	C	Catheter ablation of the AV node should not be performed without a prior trial of medication to control the ventricular rate

Source: Adapted from Blomstrom-Lundqvist C, et al.[19]

Evidence-based Outcomes of Catheter Ablation of AV Junction

A meta-analysis of 21 studies that included 1,181 patients with AF who underwent catheter ablation of the AV junction and pacemaker implantation demonstrated that the majority of patients had an improvement in symptoms, quality of life, and healthcare utilization as compared to patients with symptomatic AF refractory to medical treatment.[3] Objective improvement in cardiac function has been reported after AV junction ablation in patients with AF and a left ventricular ejection fraction < 40%. The mean ejection fraction improved from 26% ± 8% to 34% ± 13%, and 29% of the patients had complete normalization of their ejection fraction.[4] One-year mortality after catheter ablation of the AV junction and pacemaker implantation has been reported as 6.3%, including 2.0% risk of sudden cardiac death. While a causal link has been difficult to prove, it is thought that this may be due to an increased risk of torsades de pointes caused by sudden loss of atrial control of ventricular rate, and relative bradycardia that develops after prolonged tachycardia. Patients are monitored for at least 24 hours after AV junction ablation and ventricular pacing ≥ 85 beats per minute for ≥ 4 weeks after AV junction has been suggested to mitigate the risk of proarrhythmia after AV junction ablation.[5] In another study, no difference in long-term survival was found.[6]

Survival rates have been compared between patients with AF who underwent AV junction ablation, patients who had pulmonary vein antrum isolation (PVAI), and patients who were managed with antiarrhythmic drugs and direct-current cardioversion. One thousand patients were followed over a seven-year period, of which 34.5% had PVAI, 15.7% had AV junction ablation, and 49.8% were managed with antiarrhythmic drugs and direct current cardioversion. During follow-up, mortality was 2.1% in the PVAI group, 16.5% in the antiarrhythmic group, and 25.7% in the AV junction ablation group.[7]

The role of biventricular pacing after AV junction in patients with AF, regardless of the left ventricular ejection fraction, was investigated in the Post AV Node Ablation Evaluation (PAVE) study.[8] In this study, 184 patients with permanent AF underwent AV junction ablation and then were randomized to receive either biventricular pacing or standard right ventricular (RV) apical pacing. After 6 months, patients in the biventricular pacing group had a longer 6-minute walk distance, greater peak oxygen consumption, and higher quality-of-life indices as compared to the patients who had standard RV pacing. Furthermore, the RV apical pacing group had a further decline in left ventricular (LV) function, while patients in the biventricular pacing group had a stable ejection fraction after 6 months. A subgroup analysis of this study demonstrated that patients who received a biventricular pacemaker and had an initial LV ejection fraction of ≤45% or who had NYHA class II/III symptoms prior to AV junction ablation had a greater improvement in 6-minute walk distance as compared to biventricular pacemaker patients who had only NYHA class I symptoms or had normal systolic function.

In 154 patients with AF who underwent CRT-D implantation, ventricular rate control was achieved by AV junction ablation in 45 (29%) and pharmacologically in 109 (71%).[9] While ejection fraction improved in both groups, patients who underwent AV node ablation had a greater improvement in NYHA class than patients who were treated pharmacologically. In this study, AV node ablation was associated with an improvement in survival (96.0% vs 76.5%, $P = 0.008$). AV node ablation was identified as an independent predictor of improved survival and lower probability of heart transplantation and left ventricular assist device implantation.

These studies suggest that biventricular device implantation after ablation of the AV junction should be considered in patients with AF who have a reduced left ventricular ejection fraction and/or who have NYHA class II/III symptoms. If patients who had previously undergone AV junction ablation and had received RV pacing develop symptomatic heart failure or deterioration of left ventricular function, upgrade to a biventricular pacemaker should be strongly considered. However, in patients with AF who have a normal ejection fraction at the time of catheter ablation of the AV node, standard pacemaker implantation is appropriate.[2,6]

Catheter Ablation of Paroxysmal Supraventricular Tachycardia

General Overview

Catheter ablation is often the treatment of choice for the three most common types of PSVT: atrioventricular nodal reciprocating tachycardia (AVNRT), atrioventricular reciprocating tachycardia (AVRT), and atrial tachycardia (AT). AVNRT is the most common of these three arrhythmias. However, the prevalence of AT and atrial flutter has been on the rise as a consequence of previous left-atrial ablation procedures performed to eliminate AF.

There have been a number of published case series that reported the safety and efficacy of catheter ablation for PSVT. However, large-scale randomized trials have been scarce. In a prior study that reported a 14-year experience in 5,330 patients, the overall success rate was 81% for AT, 92% for accessory pathways or atrial flutter, and 99% for AVNRT or AV node ablation. The mean age of the patients was 50 ± 18 years, and 66% were women. There was no difference in outcomes of patients younger or older than age 75. The prevalence of complications of catheter ablation of paroxysmal SVT was 1.4%, including 11 major events such as myocardial infarction, pulmonary embolism (3 patients), and permanent pacemaker implantation (7 patients).[10]

Catheter Ablation of Atrioventricular Nodal Reciprocating Tachycardia

Clinical Indications

Catheter ablation has become a first-line therapy for most patients with AVNRT, primarily due to the long-term need and modest efficacy of pharmacologic therapy, and the very favorable efficacy and safety profile of catheter ablation. Nevertheless, the decision to perform a slow pathway catheter ablation for AVNRT must be individualized for each patient based on clinical judgment and individual patient preference. The most common indications for catheter ablation are recurrent symptomatic AVNRT, poorly tolerated AVNRT with hemodynamic compromise, and recurrent AVNRT that is refractory to medical management in patients who desire complete suppression of the arrhythmia. In addition, certain patients, such as pilots or commercial drivers, may be required to demonstrate complete freedom from arrhythmia to maintain employment.

Table 61.2 Clinical indications for catheter ablation for AVNRT

Class	Level of Evidence	
I	B	Poorly tolerated AVNRT with hemodynamic compromise
I	B	Recurrent symptomatic AVNRT
I	B	AVNRT with infrequent or single episode in patients who desire complete control of arrhythmia
I	B	Infrequent, well-tolerated AVNRT
I	B	Documented PSVT with only dual AV nodal pathways or single echo beats demonstrated during electrophysiological study and no other identified cause of arrhythmia

Source: Adapted from Blomstrom-Lundqvist C, et al.[19]

Slow pathway catheter ablation is typically performed in patients with documented supraventricular tachycardia with inducible AVNRT during an electrophysiology study. However, not all patients with PSVT have an inducible tachycardia during an electrophysiology study. For these patients, if they have a clinically documented narrow complex tachycardia and evidence of dual AV node physiology during an electrophysiology study, it is reasonable to perform slow pathway modification, even in the absence of an inducible tachycardia.[1] In this circumstance, the usual procedural endpoint of noninducibility of the clinical tachycardia cannot be achieved, so the attainment of accelerated junctional rhythm is used as a surrogate endpoint. Complete elimination of slow pathway conduction, if feasible, also indicates a procedural endpoint. However, it should be noted that elimination of slow pathway conduction should not be considered the ultimate procedural endpoint, as clinically successful outcomes are achieved even in patients who have residual single AV nodal echo beats. Aggressive attempts to completely eliminate residual slow conduction may unnecessarily increase the risk of inadvertent complete heart block.

Evidence-based Outcomes

The most common outcome for successful AVNRT ablation is noninducibility of the clinical tachycardia. However, many patients without inducible tachycardia may still have evidence of residual slow pathway activity. A retrospective study examined the results of 55 patients who underwent slow pathway catheter ablation for AVNRT. Forty-two percent of these patients had evidence of persistent dual AV nodal physiology, while 58% of these patients had complete elimination of slow pathway conduction. During 12 ± 8 months of follow-up, recurrence of AVNRT was seen in 9% of patients with residual slow pathway conduction and 16% of patients without residual slow pathway conduction. This difference was not statistically significant. Interestingly, a site of ablation that was at or below the coronary sinus os was associated with a higher recurrence rate than ablation sites located more medially and anteriorly.[11]

Slow pathway ablation for AVNRT was successful in 96.1% and the only significant complication was 1% incidence of second- or third-degree AV block, according to a NASPE prospective catheter ablation registry.[12] Similar success rates are seen in patients with documented PSVT without inducible tachycardia during an electrophysiology study but with evidence of dual AV node physiology who undergo empiric slow pathway ablation. One study examined the outcomes of 7 consecutive patients with documented PSVT who were noninducible in the electrophysiology laboratory despite the use of isoproterenol and atropine. All patients had evidence of dual AV node physiology or inducible AV nodal echo beats during the electrophysiology study. All 7 patients underwent catheter ablation of the slow pathway using an anatomic and electrogram-guided approach. During a follow-up of 15 ± 10 months, no patient had a recurrence of SVT.[13] In a follow-up to this study, another study examined 27 patients with documented PSVT but noninducible tachycardia who were randomized to catheter ablation or no ablation. During 23 ± 13 months of follow-up, none of 16 patients who were randomized to empiric slow pathway ablation had a recurrence of tachycardia. In contrast, 7 out of 11 patients randomized to no ablation had a recurrence of PSVT.[14] Therefore, both of these studies support the practice of empiric slow pathway ablation in patients with clinically documented evidence of PSVT and evidence of dual AV node physiology without inducible tachycardia on electrophysiology study.

While most centers perform slow pathway ablation for AVNRT, it is possible to also perform fast pathway ablation instead. One study described a stepwise anatomic and electrogram-guided strategy for fast pathway ablation in 53 patients. After 3.4 ± 3.1 radiofrequency pulses, AVNRT was noninducible in 96% of patients, and there was no incidence of complete AV block. At 12 ± 7 months, 6% of patients developed recurrent AVNRT.[15]

Catheter Ablation of Atrioventricular Reciprocating Tachycardia

Clinical Indications

Patients with a manifest accessory pathway have evidence of preexcitation on their electrocardiogram and are classified as having Wolff-Parkinson-White (WPW) pattern. Patients who have electrocardiographic evidence of preexcitation as well as symptomatic palpitations, syncope, or documented tachycardia are considered to have WPW syndrome. All patients who have WPW syndrome should be referred for catheter ablation. If patients have evidence of AF or have sustained a sudden cardiac arrest, catheter ablation should also be considered urgently.

Management of patients with asymptomatic WPW pattern is controversial and must be individualized for each patient. One large prospective long-term study included 212 patients with asymptomatic preexcitation who underwent a baseline electrophysiology study and were followed up for 38 ± 16 months. Among the 212 patients, 33 eventually developed symptoms, including 3 patients with ventricular fibrillation and 1 patient who died. A repeat electrophysiologic study was performed in 162 patients, and 47/162 had an inducible tachycardia. A clinical supraventricular tachycardia later recurred in 3.4% of patients who were noninducible and in 62% of the patients who were inducible during electrophysiologic testing. Patients who were younger, who had shorter antegrade accessory pathway refractory periods, and who had multiple accessory pathways were more likely to develop supraventricular tachycardia.[16] Despite the results of this study, the role of an electrophysiology study and catheter ablation in asymptomatic patients remains to be more clearly defined. However, in certain asymptomatic patients such as airline pilots or commercial drivers, catheter ablation can be considered to mitigate the risk of recurrent supraventricular tachycardia.

Table 61.3 Clinical Indications for catheter ablation for AVRT

Class	Level of Evidence	
I	B	WPW syndrome (preexcited and symptomatic arrhythmias), well tolerated
I	B	WPW syndrome (with AF and rapid conduction or poorly tolerated AVRT)
I	B	AVRT, poorly tolerated (no preexcitation)
IIa	B	Single or infrequent AVRT episode(s) (no preexcitation)
IIa	B	Preexcitation, asymptomatic

Source: Adapted from Blomstrom-Lundqvist C, et al.[19]

Evidence-based Outcomes

The reported success rate of catheter ablation of atrioventricular reciprocating tachycardia is approximately 96% according to published series.[17] The success rate for left free wall accessory pathways is thought to be higher than at other locations. Recurrence after successful ablation can be observed in up to 5% of the patients and is often thought to be caused by tissue edema or mechanical stunning during catheter manipulation. As the inflammation resolves, conduction over the accessory pathway may recover. A repeat ablation procedure at the same location as the initial ablation is typically successful in these cases. Occasionally, a second accessory pathway is present; there appears to be an association between posteroseptal and right-sided accessory pathways.[18] Therefore, it is prudent to map the entire tricuspid annulus when performing right-sided ablation procedures.

Complications are rare during catheter ablation of accessory pathways and have been reported as 4.4% for overall complications and 0.8% to 2.0% for significant complications including death.[19] The most common major complications are cardiac tamponade (incidence 0.13% to 1.1%) and complete AV block (incidence 0.17% to 1.0%). Complete AV block is a complication that may occur during ablation of septal accessory pathways close to the AV junction.

It should be noted that a majority of published series are based on the early experience on catheter ablation. With the current experience and technology, the risk of significant complications during catheter ablation of supraventricular arrhythmias is expected to be < 1% to 2% and primarily includes myocardial perforation and pericardial tamponade, inadvertent injury to the AV node only if the target site is close to the node, vascular injury, thromboembolic events particularly for the arterial procedures, and pneumo- or hemothorax if subclavian or internal jugular venous access is sought.

Catheter Ablation of Atrial Tachycardia

Clinical Indications

The most common indication for catheter ablation of AT is for recurrent symptomatic or hemodynamically unstable arrhythmias. Catheter ablation is also a first-line therapy for incessant ATs, regardless of whether they are symptomatic, particularly if they are associated with a tachycardia-mediated cardiomyopathy, which has been reported to complicate 10% of cases of atrial tachycardia.[20] Catheter ablation is not usually indicated for ATs that are nonsustained, particularly if they are asymptomatic.[19]

Table 61.4 Clinical indications for catheter ablation for AT

Class	Level of Evidence	
I	B	Recurrent symptomatic AT
I	B	Asymptomatic or symptomatic incessant AT
III	C	Nonsustained and asymptomatic

Source: Adapted from Blomstrom-Lundqvist C, et al.[19]

Evidence-based Outcomes

Atrial tachycardias originate from the left atrium in 18%; they are multifocal in 10%; and the remaining majority originates from the right atrium. The success rate for catheter ablation of focal AT has been reported as 86% with a recurrence rate of 8%.[19] The incidence of complications is 1% to 2% and includes cardiac perforation, phrenic nerve damage, sinus node dysfunction, and AV block.[19] In patients with a tachycardia-mediated cardiomyopathy, successful ablation has been reported to restore LV function within 3 months in 97% of patients.[20]

In another study that included 105 patients with AT, the success rate after catheter ablation was 77% regardless of the site of origin.[21] Ablation of ATs that were paroxysmal was more successful (88%) than ATs that were permanent (71%) or incessant (41%). The mean local endocardial activation time (recorded from local electrogram to surface P wave) was −47 ± 17 ms at successful and −29 ± 21 ms at unsuccessful sites. Age, gender, tachycardia cycle length, presence of cardiomyopathy and temperature achieved during ablation were not predictive of procedural success.

For left ATs, pulmonary veins are a common site of origin, with the superior veins being more frequently involved than the inferior veins. The majority (93%) are ostial in location. In a prior study that included 27 patients, RFA was successful in 96%.[22] Over the last decade, left ATs have become more prevalent as a result of prior extensive left atrial ablation for AF or atypical atrial flutter. The majority (88%) of these ATs have a reentrant mechanism, and the remainder are focal in origin. Catheter ablation has been reported to eliminate 85% of these tachycardias, and the most common target sites were the mitral isthmus, the roof, and the septum. The critical isthmus was around a previous ablation line, suggesting slow conduction along a gap due to incomplete ablation as the mechanism. It is likely that the incidence of these arrhythmias can be reduced by limiting the number of linear lesions and/or demonstration of complete linear block.[23]

The incidence and electrophysiologic characteristics of multifocal ATs were reported in 250 patients with an AT who were referred for catheter ablation.[24] In 17.6% of the patients, ≥2 foci were identified. Patients with multifocal AT were more likely to have a cardiovascular comorbidity, and the ATs were more likely to have a left atrial origin and a shorter cycle length, as compared to patients with a unifocal AT. Multifocal AT was predictive of failed ablation.

Focal ATs have been reported to infrequently originate from unusual sites, such as the superior vena cava (SVC), the appendages, or the coronary sinus. Focal catheter ablation at these sites was associated with long-term freedom from recurrent arrhythmias.[22,25-27]

Permanent Junctional Reciprocating Tachycardia

Permanent junctional reciprocating tachycardia (PJRT) is an uncommon arrhythmia that is characterized by episodes of narrow, complex tachycardia alternating with normal sinus rhythm. It is typically incessant and often recognized during infancy, although patients may not present until adulthood. The tachycardia has an RP interval that is greater than the PR interval, and the P waves are typically inverted in leads II, III, aVF, and V_4–V_6. Antegrade conduction is over the AV node, whereas retrograde ventricular-atrial conduction occurs over an accessory pathway with slow and decremental conduction. Catheter-based ablation is focused on identifying the earliest retrograde atrial activation during tachycardia.[28]

In a prior report, 32 patients with PJRT who had 33 accessory pathways were studied. The pathway location was posterior septal in 76% of patients, midseptal in 4% of patients, right posterior in 3% of patients, left posterior in 3% of patients, and left lateral in 3% of patients. If the retrograde P wave was positive in lead I, it suggested that the ablation could be performed from the right side, while a negative retrograde P wave in lead I did not exclude this approach.[28] Tachycardia recurred in 13% of the patients, and all but one of these patients had a successful ablation with a second procedure. All patients with a concomitantly depressed left ventricular function demonstrated improvement in ejection fraction after ablation.[28]

Other Supraventricular Arrhythmias

Sinus node reentry tachycardia is a relatively rare supraventricular arrhythmia; estimates of incidence vary. Catheter ablation is only indicated for patients with frequent, poorly tolerated, or symptomatic arrhythmias despite drug therapy and is generally successful.

Idiopathic automatic junctional tachycardia is rare in the adult population and responds poorly to pharmacological therapy. Catheter ablation is indicated for incessant arrhythmias, particularly if associated with a tachycardia-mediated cardiomyopathy. The target of ablation therapy is successful in 91% of patients in a small series. However, the risk of AV block during this procedure has been estimated as high as 5% to 10%.[19] The anatomic location of the target site for ablation of junctional tachycardia can be determined by mapping the point of earliest retrograde atrial activation, if mapping is performed during tachycardia. In one small series of 5 patients, this location was reported to occur high in the triangle of Koch in 4 patients and low in 1 patient.[29]

Clinical Indications and Evidence-based Outcomes for Catheter-based Cryoablation

While RFA is still the mainstay of treatment for PSVT and AV junction ablation, cryoablation was developed to allow potential equivalent efficacy with a lower risk of inadvertent AV block. Therefore, the most common clinical indication for cryoablation is usually targeting a focus that is suspected to be too close to the AV node. An initial multicenter trial evaluated the safety and efficacy of cryoablation for treatment of PSVT as well as AV junction ablation in 166 patients. The acute procedural success was 91% overall, with a success rate of 91% for AVNRT, 69% for AVRT, and 67% for AV junction ablation. There was no incidence of AV block requiring pacemaker implantation in the AVNRT or AVRT patients.[30]

Cryoablation is utilized more frequently in pediatric electrophysiology laboratories. Several studies have examined the safety and efficacy of cryotherapy in children and young adults. One study examined the use of cryoablation in 35 young patients (mean age 15.6 years) for accessory pathways located near normal conduction tissue or within the coronary venous system. Acute procedural success was obtained in 78% of accessory pathways with no incidence of complications, other than PR prolongation in one patient and right bundle branch block in another. After a follow-up period of 207 days, there was a 45% recurrence rate, and likelihood of recurrence was associated with younger age and midseptal accessory pathway location. As compared to RFA at the same institution, the authors concluded that cryotherapy offered similar initial success rates and lower incidence of complications, but a higher recurrence rate.[31]

Another study examined the use of cryotherapy in 29 young patients (mean age 13 years) for left-sided accessory pathways. Acute procedural success rate for patients receiving cryotherapy was 97% with a recurrence rate of 4.2%. In contrast, patients receiving RFA for left-sided pathways at the same institution had an acute procedural success rate of 100% and a recurrence rate of 14%.[32] These studies suggest that cryotherapy is a safe and effective alternative to radiofrequency ablation for the treatment of PSVT in a younger patient and has a lower incidence of permanent conduction abnormalities. However, cryotherapy appears to have a higher incidence of recurrence.

Recently, a large, prospective, randomized controlled trial compared cryoablation and radiofrequency ablation for treatment of AVNRT in adults.[33] In this study, 509 patients with AVNRT were randomized to slow pathway ablation using either cryoablation or RFA. The endpoint of immediate procedural success was equivalent between the two groups (96.8% versus 98.4%). The incidence of permanent AV block as a complication of ablation did not differ between the two groups (0% vs 0.4%). However, recurrence of AVNRT was significantly higher among the patients who underwent cryoablation than those who had RFA (9.4% versus 4.4%, $P = 0.029$). Furthermore, procedural duration was longer in the cyroablation group (138 ± 54 minutes versus 123 ± 48 minutes, $P = 0.029$), and there was a higher incidence of equipment problems in the cryoablation group.

Summary

Radiofrequency catheter ablation of the AV junction in conjunction with pacemaker implantation is a safe and effective therapy in patients with permanent AF and rapid ventricular response rates that is refractory to medical or ablative therapy. While this therapy does not reduce the risk of stroke and may be associated with proarrhythmia early after the ablation, patients often experience an improvement in symptoms and cardiac function. Similarly, in patients with AF who receive a suboptimal amount of biventricular pacing, AV junction ablation can be helpful to facilitate biventricular pacing.

Radiofrequency catheter ablation is a first-line therapy for paroxysmal SVT. Success rates vary according to the subtype of arrhythmia and location of the pathway. Complications of catheter ablation are rare, and the most common complication is permanent AV block requiring pacemaker implantation.

References

1. Morady F. Catheter ablation of supraventricular arrhythmias: state of the art. *J Cardiovasc Electrophysiol*. 2004;15(1):124-139.
2. Fuster V, et al. 2011 ACCF/AHA/HRS Focused Updates Incorporated into the ACC/AHA/ESC 2006 Guidelines for

the Management of Patients with Atrial Fibrillation: A Report of the American College of Cardiology Foundation/American Heart Association Task Force on Practice Guidelines Developed in partnership with the European Society of Cardiology and in collaboration with the European Heart Rhythm Association and the Heart Rhythm Society. *J Am Coll Cardiol.* 2011;57(11):e101-198.
3. Wood MA, et al. Clinical outcomes after ablation and pacing therapy for atrial fibrillation: a meta-analysis. *Circulation.* 2000;101(10):1138-1144.
4. Ozcan C, et al. Significant effects of atrioventricular node ablation and pacemaker implantation on left ventricular function and long-term survival in patients with atrial fibrillation and left ventricular dysfunction. *Am J Cardiol.* 2003;92(1):33-37.
5. Nowinski K, et al. Transient proarrhythmic state following atrioventricular junctional radiofrequency ablation. *Pacing Clin Electrophysiol.* 2002;25(3):291-299.
6. Ozcan C, et al. Long-term survival after ablation of the atrioventricular node and implantation of a permanent pacemaker in patients with atrial fibrillation. *N Engl J Med.* 2001;344(14):1043-1051.
7. Sonne K, et al. Pulmonary vein antrum isolation, atrioventricular junction ablation, and antiarrhythmic drugs combined with direct current cardioversion: survival rates at 7 years follow-up. *J Interv Card Electrophysiol.* 2009;26(2):121-126.
8. Doshi RN, et al. Left ventricular-based cardiac stimulation post AV nodal ablation evaluation (the PAVE study). *J Cardiovasc Electrophysiol.* 2005;16(11):1160-1165.
9. Dong K, et al. Atrioventricular nodal ablation predicts survival benefit in patients with atrial fibrillation receiving cardiac resynchronization therapy. *Heart Rhythm.* 2010;7(9):1240-1245.
10. O'Hara GE, et al. Catheter ablation for cardiac arrhythmias: a 14-year experience with 5330 consecutive patients at the Quebec Heart Institute, Laval Hospital. *Can J Cardiol.* 2007;23(Suppl B):67B-70B.
11. Manolis AS, Wang PJ, Estes NA III. Radiofrequency ablation of slow pathway in patients with atrioventricular nodal reentrant tachycardia. Do arrhythmia recurrences correlate with persistent slow pathway conduction or site of successful ablation? *Circulation.* 1994;90(6):2815-2819.
12. Scheinman MM, Huang S. The 1998 NASPE prospective catheter ablation registry. *Pacing Clin Electrophysiol.* 2000;23(6):1020-1028.
13. Bogun F, et al. Slow pathway ablation in patients with documented but noninducible paroxysmal supraventricular tachycardia. *J Am Coll Cardiol.* 1996;28(4):1000-1004.
14. Lin JL, et al. Clinical and electrophysiologic characteristics and long-term efficacy of slow-pathway catheter ablation in patients with spontaneous supraventricular tachycardia and dual atrioventricular node pathways without inducible tachycardia. *J Am Coll Cardiol.* 1998;31(4):855-860.
15. Kottkamp H, et al. An anatomically and electrogram-guided stepwise approach for effective and safe catheter ablation of the fast pathway for elimination of atrioventricular node reentrant tachycardia. *J Am Coll Cardiol.* 1995;25(5):974-981.
16. Pappone C, et al. Usefulness of invasive electrophysiologic testing to stratify the risk of arrhythmic events in asymptomatic patients with Wolff-Parkinson-White pattern: results from a large prospective long-term follow-up study. *J Am Coll Cardiol.* 2003;41(2):239-244.
17. Calkins H, et al. Catheter ablation of accessory pathways, atrioventricular nodal reentrant tachycardia, and the atrioventricular junction: final results of a prospective, multicenter clinical trial. The Atakr Multicenter Investigators Group. *Circulation.* 1999;99(2):262-270.
18. Morady F, et al. Coexistent posteroseptal and right-sided atrioventricular bypass tracts. *J Am Coll Cardiol.* 1985;5(3):640-646.
19. Blomstrom-Lundqvist C, et al. ACC/AHA/ESC Guidelines for the Management of Patients with Supraventricular Arrhythmias—Executive Summary. A Report of the American College of Cardiology/American Heart Association Task Force on Practice Guidelines and the European Society of Cardiology Committee for Practice Guidelines (Writing Committee to Develop Guidelines for the Management of Patients with Supraventricular Arrhythmias) developed in collaboration with NASPE-Heart Rhythm Society. *J Am Coll Cardiol.* 2003;42(8):1493-1531.
20. Medi C, et al. Tachycardia-mediated cardiomyopathy secondary to focal atrial tachycardia: long-term outcome after catheter ablation. *J Am Coll Cardiol.* 2009;53(19):1791-1797.
21. Anguera I, et al. Outcomes after radiofrequency catheter ablation of atrial tachycardia. *Am J Cardiol.* 2001;87(7):886-890.
22. Kistler PM, et al. Focal atrial tachycardia from the ostium of the coronary sinus: electrocardiographic and electrophysiological characterization and radiofrequency ablation. *J Am Coll Cardiol.* 2005;45(9):1488-1493.
23. Chae S, et al. Atrial tachycardia after circumferential pulmonary vein ablation of atrial fibrillation: mechanistic insights, results of catheter ablation, and risk factors for recurrence. *J Am Coll Cardiol.* 2007;50(18):1781-1787.
24. Hu YF, et al. Electrophysiologic characteristics and catheter ablation of focal atrial tachycardia with more than one focus. *Heart Rhythm.* 2009;6(2):198-203.
25. Roberts-Thomson KC, et al. Focal atrial tachycardias arising from the right atrial appendage: electrocardiographic and electrophysiologic characteristics and radiofrequency ablation. *J Cardiovasc Electrophysiol.* 2007;18(4):367-372.
26. Wang YL, et al. Focal atrial tachycardia originating from the left atrial appendage: electrocardiographic and electrophysiologic characterization and long-term outcomes of radiofrequency ablation. *J Cardiovasc Electrophysiol.* 2007;18(5):459-464.
27. Zhang T, et al. Focal atrial tachycardia arising from the right atrial appendage: electrophysiologic and electrocardiographic characteristics and catheter ablation. *Int J Clin Pract.* 2009;63(3):417-424.
28. Gaita F, et al. Catheter ablation of permanent junctional reciprocating tachycardia with radiofrequency current. *J Am Coll Cardiol.* 1995;25(3):648-654.
29. Law IH, et al. Transcatheter cryothermal ablation of junctional ectopic tachycardia in the normal heart. *Heart Rhythm.* 2006;3(8):903-907.
30. Friedman PL, et al. Catheter cryoablation of supraventricular tachycardia: results of the multicenter prospective "frosty" trial. *Heart Rhythm.* 2004;1(2):129-138.
31. Bar-Cohen Y, et al. Cryoablation for accessory pathways located near normal conduction tissues or within the coronary venous system in children and young adults. *Heart Rhythm.* 2006;3(3):253-258.
32. Gist KM, et al. Acute success of cryoablation of left-sided accessory pathways: a single institution study. *J Cardiovasc Electrophysiol.* 2009;20(6):637-642.
33. Deisenhofer I, et al. Cryoablation versus radiofrequency energy for the ablation of atrioventricular nodal reentrant tachycardia (the CYRANO Study): results from a large multicenter prospective randomized trial. *Circulation.* 2010;122(22):2239-2245.

CHAPTER 62

Catheter Ablation of Atrial Flutter and Fibrillation

Jasbir S. Sra, MD; Sanjeev Saksena, MBBS, MD

Introduction

Atrial fibrillation (AF) and atrial flutter (AFL) are the two most common arrhythmias targeted for catheter ablation.[1-32] Both cavotricuspid isthmus (CTI)–dependent typical AFL and atypical flutters originating from other locations in the right and left atrium can be targeted.[1-6] Atypical left AFLs are usually seen after AF ablation.[4-6] Unlike the typical counterclockwise patterns of CTI flutters, in many instances, there may not be predetermined anatomical boundaries delineating the circuits of left atrial flutters. Similarly, after extensive ablation in the left atrium, characteristics of CTI flutter post–AF ablation may be different from the usual sawtooth appearance seen in typical counterclockwise CTI flutter.[10] Activation mapping and entrainment mapping are useful in delineating these circuits for successful ablation.

Targeting focal ablation in the pulmonary veins has proved suboptimal. The ablation procedure has progressed, by necessity, to ostial ablation and/or electrical isolation of all pulmonary veins to address the triggering foci seen in more than 90% of paroxysmal AF cases, with two or more pulmonary veins involved 70% of the time.[8-20] In some patients, non-pulmonary vein sites such as the superior vena cava (SVC), the coronary sinus, the ligament of Marshall, and nonvenous sites such as the crista terminalis and posterior left atrium may initiate paroxysms of AF and may need to be targeted.[13-15]

However, over long-term follow-up, only 20% of patients with long-standing persistent AF return to sinus rhythm after pulmonary vein isolation alone.[17-22] Methods to improve efficacy of AF ablation include circumferential ablation, linear ablation connecting the superior pulmonary veins, mitral isthmus ablation, and targeting electrograms such as complex fractionated electrograms (CFAEs)—electrograms with continuous activity and significant gradient between the proximal and distal electrodes of the ablating catheter.[18-22]

Although major advances have been made in the field of catheter ablation of AF, compared to ablation of other supraventricular tachycardias such as CTI flutter, there remain significant limitations, and improvements in the effectiveness of current techniques have been relatively modest. This chapter provides an overview of clinical indications and evidence-based outcomes in patients undergoing ablation for AFL and AF.

Atrial Flutter Ablation

Typical Right Atrial Flutter

Typical AFL involves right atrial macroreentry where, in addition to the circuit propagating anteriorly and superiorly along the septum and descending down the lateral aspect of the right atrium, the impulse propagates between the inferior vena cava (IVC) and the tricuspid annulus through the CTI. In addition, the Eustachian valve and ridge forms a line of conduction block between the IVC and crista terminalis, forming a second septal isthmus between the tricuspid annulus and the coronary sinus ostium.[1,2]

The endpoint of AFL ablation is termination of AFL and demonstration of bidirectional conduction block (Figure 62.1). The second line of conduction block

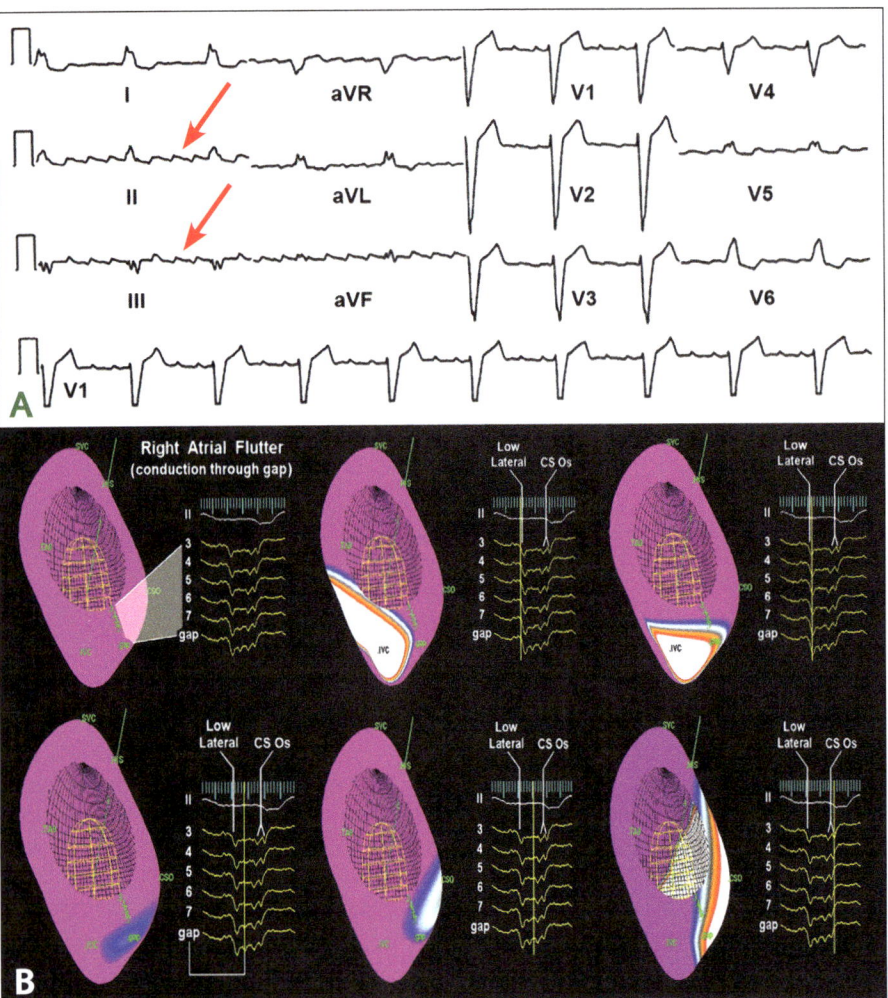

Figure 62.1 **Panel A:** ECG during counterclockwise cavotricuspid isthmus (CTI)–dependent flutter. Note the classic sawtooth appearance (**arrow**) of the flutter waves in the inferior leads. **Panel B:** ESI map showing conduction pattern of the counterclockwise atrial flutter with conduction through the cavotricuspid isthmus.

created by the Eustachian valve and ridge extending between the IVC and the coronary sinus ostium forces the AFL circuit to propagate between the coronary sinus ostium and the tricuspid annulus, forming a narrower isthmus. Thus, an ablation line extending from the tricuspid annulus to the coronary sinus ostium and on to the IVC can eliminate AFL.

In some patients, AFL ablation may be difficult. The sub-Eustachian right atrial pouch should be considered a potential target if there is increase in impedance during ablation. Any decrease in power during ablation accompanied by failure to successfully ablate AFL should alert one to this condition.[3] Computed tomography (CT) imaging can help make the diagnosis. Ablation can be performed more laterally in these patients.

Chronic success rate of ablation of CTI-dependent AFL ranges from 90% to 100%.[25-32] In one randomized study in which patients were treated with antiarrhythmic drugs and/or catheter ablation, at a mean follow-up of 21 months, 63% of the patients treated with antiarrhythmic drugs alone required one or more hospitalizations compared with 22% of those treated with catheter ablation.

It has also been shown that 15% to 20% of patients with AF treated with antiarrhythmic drugs develop AFL.

CTI ablation is the treatment of choice as it facilitates the management of AF with drugs. The recurrence of AF is much higher if AF is the predominant rhythm prior to AFL ablation.

CTI-dependent AFL after AF Ablation

The electrocardiographic (ECG) pattern of CTI flutter can change significantly following left atrial ablation of AF and should not be ignored in patients presenting with AFL after AF ablation. In one study, ECG pattern waves were upright in 12 of 15 patients with counterclockwise CTI-dependent flutter, suggesting that left atrial activation contributes little to the genesis of flutter waves following extensive left atrial ablation. Entrainment mapping of the CTI is helpful in identifying the circuit precisely.[18,19]

Atypical Right Atrial Flutter

Most common variants of atypical right atrial flutter (RAFL) include lower loop reentry (LLR), upper loop reentry, or scar-related AFL[4-6] (Figure 62.2). One study systematically evaluated nonisthmus-dependent RAFL in

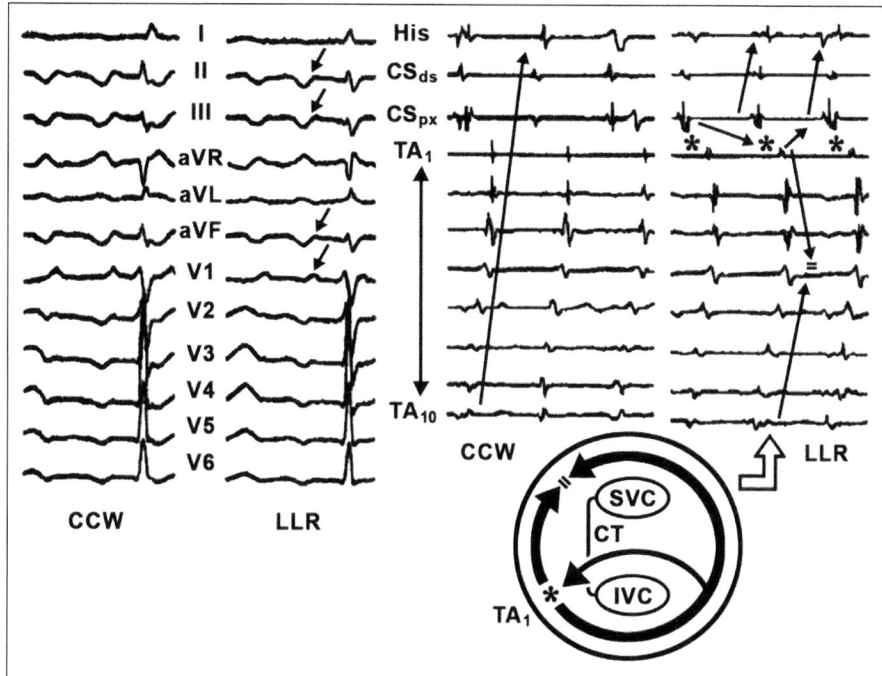

Figure 62.2 Sustained, spontaneous atrial flutters (AFLs) with two different cycle lengths (CLs) from same patient. Tracings on left show 12-lead ECG in a patient with counterclockwise (CCW) AFL with cycle length of 285 ms. Adjacent 12-lead ECG was recorded during lower loop reentry (LLR). **Arrows (left-hand panel)** point to decrease in inferior forces with LLR and slight changes in V_1 (**arrow**). Tracings on right show intracardiac recordings during both CCW and LLR. Schema below shows LLR with early break (**marked by asterisk**) in the region of the low lateral right atrium (RA) (TA_1). Conversion of CCW to LLR is associated with increase in transisthmus conduction time (TA_1-CS_{PX}). Shortening of tachycardia cycle length with LLR is responsible for increase in isthmus conduction time. **Arrows (right-hand panel)** point to activation wavefront, and = refers to areas of collision. CS_{ds} = distal coronary sinus; CS_{px} = proximal coronary sinus; CT = crista terminalis; IVC = inferior vena cava; SVC = superior vena cava. *Source:* Used with permission from Bochoeyer A, Yang Y, Cheng J, et al.[4]

372 patients. Of the 26 patients with atypical AFL, 13 had LLR. In these patients, surface ECG was similar to that of counterclockwise CTI except for decreased amplitude of the terminal forces in the inferior leads. This type of atypical AFL resulted from a breakthrough site across the CT during typical counterclockwise CTI-dependent AFL. Bidirectional block in the CTI can eliminate LLR. In several other patterns, the wavefront breaks at a more superior portion of the tricuspid annulus. ECG morphology may or may not change in these examples, depending on whether the breakthrough is lower or higher, and the pattern of left atrial activation may determine whether there is advancement of the His atrial recording compared to the coronary sinus.

In 7 of the 8 episodes of upper loop reentry in the study, the ECG mimicked clockwise CTI-dependent AFL. This type of AFL is characterized by early breakthrough in the lateral annulus and collision of the activation front over the crista terminalis.

Macroreentrant circuits around the scar tissue should be considered in patients with prior cardiac surgery. Detailed mapping is needed to identify sites of conduction block, join these sites, and successfully ablate these difficult flutters.

Atypical Left Atrial Flutter

Although atypical left atrial flutters (LAFLs) have been described postsurgery, the most common LAFLs seen are postablation of long-lasting persistent AF.[6,18,19] Ten percent of patients with recurrence of atrial arrhythmias postablation have atrial tachycardia or AFL, and most of these have left AFL. Left AFL is usually characterized by a positive deflection in V1 and low voltage deflections in limb leads. These flutters can occur in the mitral isthmus area, between the mitral annulus and left inferior pulmonary vein (LIPV), around the pulmonary veins, along the roof area connecting the superior pulmonary veins, anterior mitral annulus, and left atrial septum (Figures 62.3, 62.4, 62.5, and 62.6). The usual cause of these flutters is incomplete lines without validation of conduction blocks.

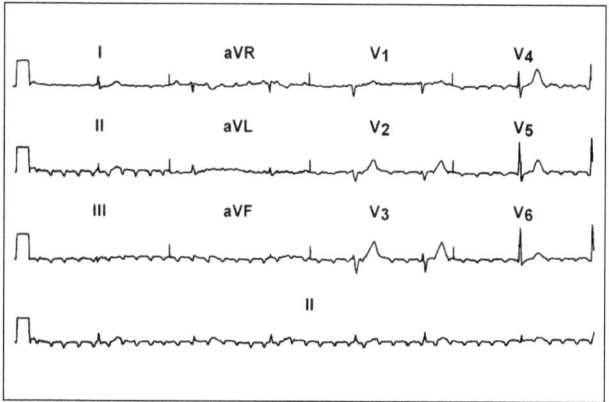

Figure 62.3 Atypical left atrial flutter. ECG of a patient with atrial flutter following AF ablation. P-wave morphology suggests atypical left atrial flutter.

Activation and entrainment mapping is used in an attempt to delineate the flutter circuit. However, in the presence of significant scarring from prior AF ablation, activation mapping may point to the wrong location of the reentrant circuit. High capture thresholds may also limit the accuracy of entrainment mapping over large areas previously ablated. Another challenging aspect is the presence of multiple simultaneous circuits. Recognition and ablation of the critical isthmus in these situations may be difficult. Despite these limitations, catheter ablation remains the treatment of choice in these patients.

Identification of reentrant circuits involving previously ablated but incomplete lines requires detailed mapping of these sites, which can be identified by low-amplitude fractionated signals. Identification of these gaps during the arrhythmia, however, is sometimes difficult and may require mapping during sinus rhythm.

Atrial Fibrillation Ablation

Atrial fibrillation is a common arrhythmia. Although significant work remains, recent advances in the understanding of the mechanism of AF have led to the development of some elegant catheter mapping techniques for AF ablation.[20-48] The 2006 Revised ACC/AHA/ESC AF Management Guidelines recommend catheter ablation as

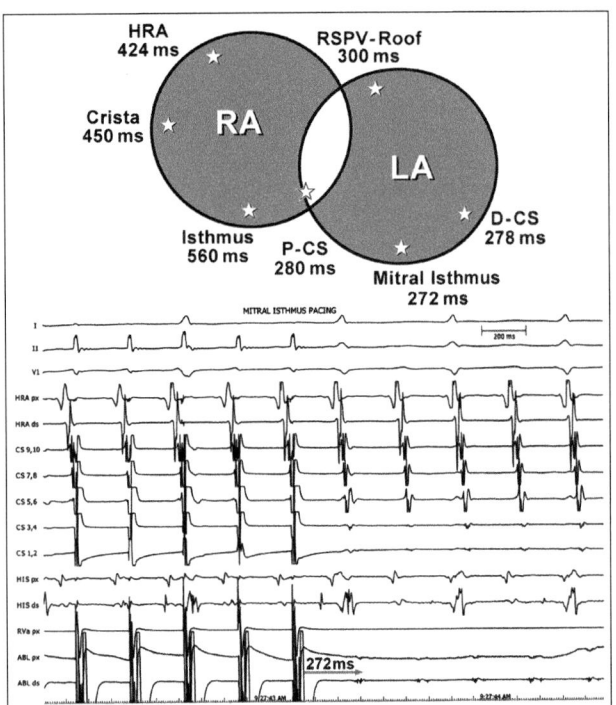

Figure 62.4 Entrainment mapping of atrial flutter. **Top panel** depicts entrainment mapping from different sites in the right and left atrium. Best entrainment is shown in the mitral isthmus location as depicted in the **bottom panel**.

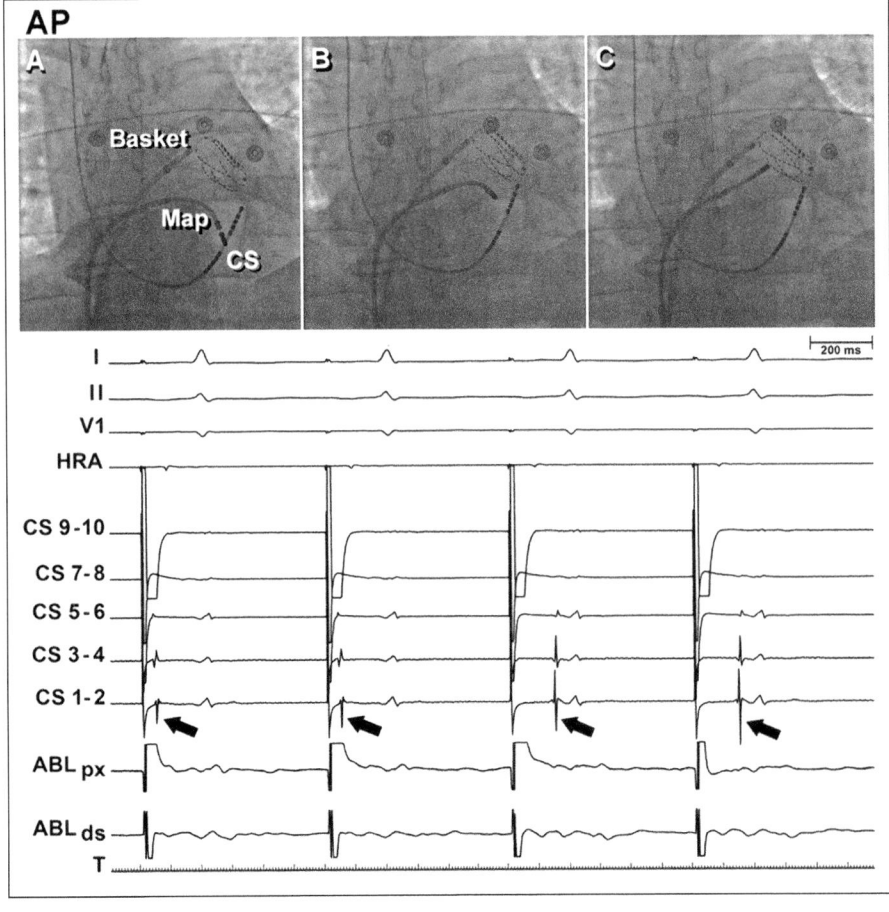

Figure 62.5 Mitral isthmus ablation. **Top panel:** Anteroposterior fluoroscopic views are shown. The mapping and ablation catheter is gradually moved from the mitral annulus posteriorly (**panel A**), as depicted by the location of the coronary sinus catheter (CS), to the left inferior pulmonary vein, outlined by the multielectrode basket catheter (mid-isthmus in **panel B**, left inferior pulmonary vein in **panel C**). **Bottom panel:** During ablation in the coronary sinus and proximal coronary sinus pacing, from CS 9,10, the pacing spike to the atrial electrogram on the distal coronary sinus is short, suggesting continued conduction across the coronary sinus. During continued ablation, there is sudden prolongation of pacing to the distal coronary sinus electrogram, suggesting achievement of complete block across the coronary sinus. Source: Sra J, Akhtar M. Mapping techniques for atrial fibrillation ablation. Curr Probl Cardiol. 2007;32:663-768. With permission from Elsevier.

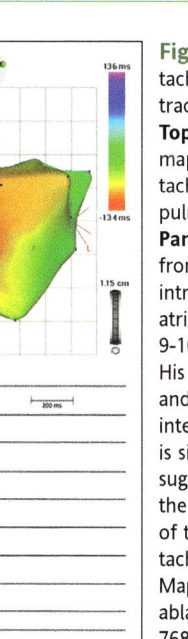

Figure 62.6 Right superior vein tachycardia. **Top left panel** depicts ECG tracings of organized atrial arrhythmia. **Top right panel:** Electroanatomic map depicts figure-of-eight reentrant tachycardia around the right superior pulmonary vein (RSPV). **Bottom panel: Panel A:** Intracardiac recordings from surface ECG leads I, II, and V_1, intracardiac recordings from high right atrium, proximal coronary sinus (CS 9-10) to distal coronary sinus (CS 1-2), His (HIS), and ablation proximal (ABLpx) and distal (ABLds). **Panel B:** Postpacing interval from the ablation catheter is similar to tachycardia cycle length, suggesting that the catheter is close to the tachycardia circuit. **Panel C:** Ablation of this site leads to termination of the tachycardia. *Source:* Sra J, Akhtar M. Mapping techniques for atrial fibrillation ablation. *Curr Probl Cardiol.* 2007;32:663-768. With permission from Elsevier.

a reasonable alternative to pharmacological therapy to prevent recurrent AF in symptomatic patients with little or no left atrial enlargement (class 2A recommendation, level of evidence C). Furthermore, the maintenance of the sinus rhythm treatment algorithm lists catheter ablation as second-line therapy for all categories of patients.[33] The HRS/EHRA/ECAS Expert Consensus Statement[33,34] on Catheter and Surgical Ablation of Atrial Fibrillation: Recommendations for Personnel, Policy, Procedures, and Follow-Up include a directive regarding symptomatic AF refractory or intolerant to at least one class 1 or 3 antiarrhythmic medication. It states: "In rare clinical situations, it may be appropriate to perform AF ablation as first line therapy, for example, in selected symptomatic patients with heart failure and/or reduced ejection fraction."

Catheter Mapping and Ablation for AF

The pulmonary veins, left atrium, right atrium, coronary sinus, and SVC have all been targeted in some form during AF ablation.

Autopsy studies and three-dimensional (3D) imaging have identified significant variations of pulmonary vein anatomy.[35] The ostium of the pulmonary veins has a funnel-shaped transition, which is predominantly seen in the left pulmonary veins. The orifice of the LIPV is closer to the mitral annulus than the orifice of the right inferior pulmonary vein (RIPV). A thin ridge usually separates the left superior pulmonary vein (LSPV) and the left atrial appendage (LAA).

The left atrial myocardium extends into the pulmonary veins, more so into the superior pulmonary veins. This extension is referred to as the "myocardial sleeves." An important anatomic feature is that these myocardial sleeves are located on the outer side of the venous adventitial (epicardial) side of the pulmonary vein, separated from the smooth layer of the vein by fibrofatty tissue.[24] These anatomical features have clinical implications as aggressive ablation can lead to intimal smooth muscle proliferation, resulting in pulmonary vein stenosis.[24-37]

Initial observations by Haïssaguerre and colleagues showed the importance of the role of spontaneous ectopic foci arising from in and around the pulmonary veins in triggering paroxysms of AF (Figure 62.7).[8]

In addition to the possibility that spontaneous ectopic beats originating from the pulmonary veins initiate paroxysms of AF, sustained rapid discharges from these foci may drive AF, true focal AF. Thus, the pulmonary vein is both a trigger and substrate for AF. The following section deals with the techniques of electrophysiologic-guided catheter ablation of AF.

Ablation of Pulmonary Vein Triggers

Initial catheter techniques used in AF ablation targeted the pulmonary vein triggers.[8,9,11] In this technique, catheters were sequentially placed in different pulmonary veins to record spontaneous ectopy as more than 90% of the ectopy triggering AF originates in the pulmonary veins. Arrhythmogenic pulmonary veins were defined as pulmonary veins giving rise to spontaneous discharges. Earliest local activity was usually mapped to within the main pulmonary vein (2 to 4 cm) or one of its branches, and depolarization was marked by a pulmonary vein potential preceding the onset of atrial activation by 35 to 45 ms.

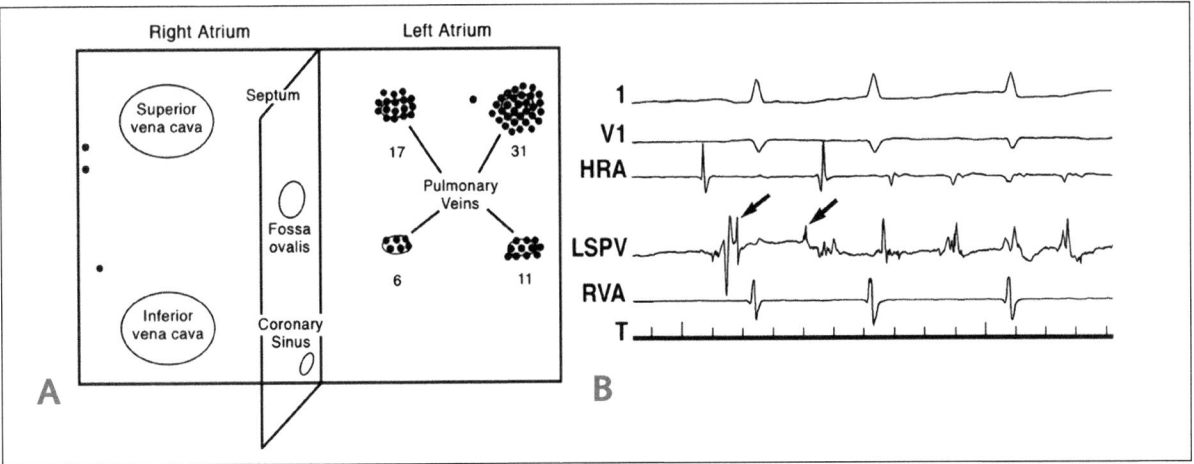

Figure 62.7 Spontaneous initiation of atrial fibrillation by ectopic beats originating in the pulmonary veins. **Panel A:** Diagram of the sites of 69 foci triggering atrial fibrillation in 45 patients. Note the clustering in the pulmonary veins, particularly in both superior pulmonary veins. Numbers indicate the distribution of foci in the pulmonary veins. *Source:* Copyright © 1998 Massachusetts Medical Society. All rights reserved. Reproduced with permission.[8] **Panel B:** Initiation of atrial fibrillation. Tracings from top to bottom are surface ECG leads 1, V$_1$, intracardiac recording from high right atrium (HRA), recording from a catheter placed inside the left superior pulmonary vein (LSPV), right ventricle, and time lines (T). First beat is normal sinus rhythm as shown by activation sequence showing early HRA followed by LSPV. Left atrial pulmonary vein conduction is shown by later activation in the pulmonary vein. A premature ectopic beat originating from the LSPV, as shown by reversal of activation (**arrow**), initiates atrial fibrillation. *Source:* Sra J, Akhtar M. Mapping techniques for atrial fibrillation ablation. *Curr Probl Cardiol.* 2007;32:663-768. With permission from Elsevier.

Use of this technique resulted in a 62% success rate in patients who remained free of AF over an 8 ± 6-month follow-up period. However, 70% of these patients required multiple procedures.

In a subsequent study of 225 patients, 96% of the triggering foci originated in the pulmonary veins, and 74% of the patients had more than one arrhythmogenic pulmonary vein (mean 2.1 pulmonary veins per patient).[12] In some instances, this technique is limited by the absence of spontaneous ectopy even after provoking measures are implemented. Furthermore, there is inadequate procedural endpoint, and ablation inside the pulmonary vein increases the risk of pulmonary vein stenosis. For these reasons, and because multiple foci may be located within a single pulmonary vein, the focal ablation has progressed to ostial ablation and electrical isolation of all pulmonary veins.

Catheter Techniques for Electrical Isolation of Pulmonary Veins

The technique of electrical isolation is designed to completely eliminate the electrical connections between the pulmonary veins and the left atrium.

Pulmonary vein mapping has been greatly facilitated by the introduction of circumferential mapping of the pulmonary vein ostia using multielectrode circular catheters.[13-15] Now it is possible to determine electrical activity within and between the pulmonary veins and the left atrium. Electrical conduction into the pulmonary veins is not homogeneous, which is consistent with the presence of discrete rather than fully circumferential left atrium–pulmonary vein connections.

As left atrium–pulmonary vein proximity can cause fusion of potentials (Figure 62.8), pacing from the distal coronary sinus and, at times, from the LAA can be helpful in differentiating pulmonary vein potentials from the adjacent left atrium. Double- and triple-component electrograms can also be seen in the anterior part of the right superior pulmonary vein (RSPV) initial component, coinciding with the onset of the P waves from the adjacent SVC, and the latter component, coinciding with the activation of the upper interatrial septum.

Left atrium–pulmonary vein (LAPV) connections may be predominantly located at the bottom of the superior pulmonary veins (85% prevalence). An additional useful criterion for locating LAPV connections is polarity reversal, defined as opposite polarity across adjacent bipolar electrograms. Use of polarity-reversal criterion may result in shorter radiofrequency (RF) application time needed to electrically disconnect the pulmonary veins.

Catheter mapping and ablation can be performed even as patients are in AF. In this situation, the most disorganized electrograms, depicting the shortest cycle lengths, can be targeted first. This type of approach may require that more lesions be administered to achieve electrical disconnection of the pulmonary veins, as there is usually overlapping of near-field and far-field activity. Verifying complete electrical disconnection during normal sinus rhythm is ideal. According to the HRS consensus document, ablation strategies that target the pulmonary veins and/or pulmonary vein antrum are the cornerstone for most AF ablation procedures. If the pulmonary veins are targeted, complete electrical isolation should be the goal. For surgical pulmonary vein isolation, entrance and/or exit block should be demonstrated. Careful identification

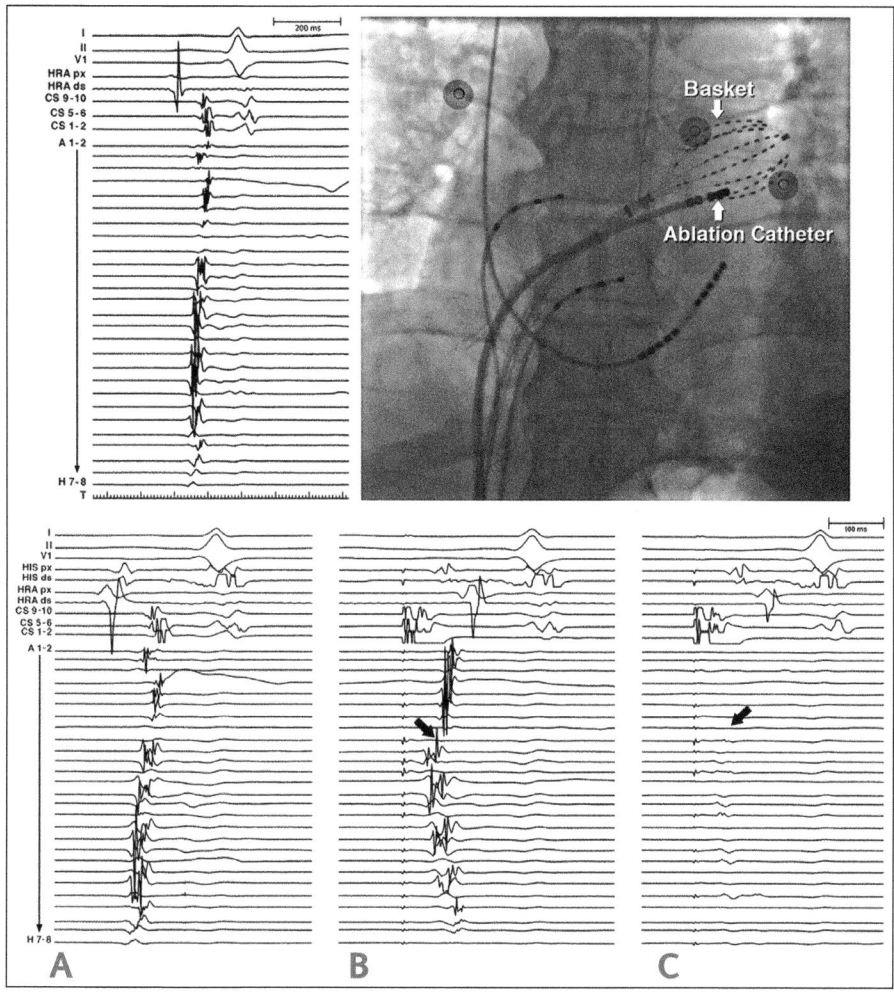

Figure 62.8 **Top panel** shows fused potentials in the LSPV during sinus rhythm. **Bottom panel**, A to C, depicts differentiation and ablation of far-field potentials in the LSPV. Tracings are as before. **Panel A:** Fused potentials in the LSPV. **Panel B:** Distal coronary sinus pacing separates the left atrial and pulmonary vein potentials (**arrow**). **Panel C:** Ablation at the pulmonary vein ostium eliminates the potentials. *Source:* Sra J, Akhtar M. Mapping techniques for atrial fibrillation ablation. *Curr Probl Cardiol.* 2007;32:663-768. With permission from Elsevier.

of the pulmonary vein ostia is mandatory to avoid ablation within the pulmonary veins.

Efficacy and Safety of Catheter-based Pulmonary Vein Isolation

As many as 40% to 50% of patients with AF experience recurrence within days of the ablation.[13-17] Long-term success rates have been observed to be lower in patients with early recurrence versus those who remained free of AF postprocedure without the need for antiarrhythmic drugs (31% vs 85%). It has been postulated that this early recurrence is due to the transient stimulatory effect of RF energy on the atrial myocardium or the autonomic nervous system. Administering RF lesions of longer duration and applying deeper lesions, using some of the currently available technologies such as the irrigated-tip catheter, can help reduce the early recurrence of AF.

Long-term success rates with the catheter-guided pulmonary vein isolation approach have been reported to be in the range of 22% to 85%. Variability in success rates probably relates to different criteria used in patient selection, varying definitions of procedural success, the total number of ablations attempted, the type of AF, and the use of antiarrhythmic medications. Delayed cure can occur in 20% to 30% of the patients who experience early recurrence of AF. It has been shown that the majority of recurrences occur due to the presence of residual or relapsed pulmonary vein potentials left over from previously isolated pulmonary veins, nontargeted pulmonary veins, and, sometimes, non-pulmonary vein foci. In one study, 54% of recurrences occurred due to relapse in previously isolated pulmonary veins, 32% from nontargeted pulmonary veins, and 14% from non-pulmonary vein foci.

Pulmonary vein stenosis, as a complication of ablation in the pulmonary vein, is of special concern.[36] The incidence of this complication is reported to be about 1.7%. As most patients with pulmonary vein narrowing are asymptomatic, however, incidence actually may be higher. Use of mapping and 3D imaging techniques such as CT or magnetic resonance (MR), which can depict narrowing of the pulmonary veins much more accurately,[26,35,36] may help determine just how common pulmonary vein stenosis really is. In symptomatic patients, pulmonary vein dilatation and stenting may be needed. Other serious complications include thromboembolism, cardiac tamponade, and left atrial-esophageal fistula, usually seen after extensive posterior lesions have been administered. Incidence of these complications is usually less than 1%.[17]

Catheter Mapping and Ablation of Non-pulmonary Vein Sites

According to the HRS consensus document, if a focal trigger is identified outside a pulmonary vein at the time of an AF ablation, it should be targeted, if possible. Non-pulmonary vein triggers initiating AF can be identified in up to one-third of unselected patients referred for catheter ablation. Supraventricular tachycardias such as AV nodal reentry or accessory pathway-mediated atrioventricular reciprocating tachycardia may also be identified in up to 4% of unselected patients referred for AF ablation and may serve as a trigger. Non-pulmonary vein triggers can be provoked in patients with both paroxysmal and more persistent forms of AF.

In selected patients, elimination of only the non-pulmonary vein triggers has resulted in elimination of AF. The sites of origin for non-pulmonary vein atrial triggers include the posterior wall of the left atrium, the superior vena cave, crista terminalis, fossa ovalis, coronary sinus behind the Eustachian ridge, along the ligament of Marshall, and adjacent to the AV valve annuli.[9] Furthermore, reentrant circuits maintaining AF may be located within the right and left atria. Provocative maneuvers such as the administration of isoproterenol in incremental doses of up to 20 g/min, and/or cardioversion of induced and spontaneous AF, can aid in identification of pulmonary vein and non-pulmonary vein triggers.

Only 20% of patients with long-standing AF undergoing pulmonary vein isolation alone are in sinus rhythm during long-term follow-up. In patients with long-standing persistent AF, and in more than 50% of patients with paroxysmal AF, pulmonary vein isolation alone is insufficient to maintain sinus rhythm. Improved mapping techniques for non-pulmonary vein foci and modification of the substrate itself may be required to further improve long-term outcome.

As described before, non-pulmonary vein foci, which may initiate paroxysms of AF, may arise from the SVC, the coronary sinus, the ligament of Marshall, and nonvenous sites such as the crista terminalis and the posterior left atrium.[9,11,12] In 20% to 30% of patients, it may be difficult to identify these locations.

It has been shown that ablation of these foci can result in termination of AF and long-term prevention of AF.[9] Electrophysiologic characteristics involved in the initiation of AF in the SVC are somewhat different from those involved in initiation of AF in the pulmonary veins. In the SVC, a rapid run of ectopic beats (normally more than 3) usually initiates AF.

As with the pulmonary vein, the ablation strategy for the SVC is total electrical disconnection if possible. However, ablation of the SVC should be reserved for a select group of patients where there is clear association of SVC with the initiation of AF as there is a risk of SVC stenosis, the development of SVC syndrome, sinus node modification, and phrenic nerve injury.

The ligament of Marshall contains muscle bundles and the vein of Marshall. The ligament of Marshall is known to play a role in the initiation of AF in a subset of patients. Several catheter techniques have been developed to study ligament of Marshall activity. A small 1.5-Fr catheter may be directly cannulated into the ligament of Marshall via the coronary sinus. The ligament of Marshall has three structures, the muscle tract or Marshall bundle, the vein of Marshall, and the autonomic nerves. The vein of Marshall drains into the coronary sinus. The Marshall bundle is directly connected to the coronary sinus musculature. The Marshall bundle potentials, starting from the coronary sinus to the left pulmonary veins, can be recorded in about 50% of patients.

Coronary Sinus Ablation

Coronary sinus ablation may be required in more than 60% of patients with persistent AF in order to achieve complete block of mitral isthmus conduction. As shown before, atypical AFL, especially after AF ablation, can sometimes originate from the coronary sinus. Overall, coronary sinus ablation is quite safe if performed carefully. In a consecutive series of 33 patients with persistent AF, 7.4 ± 6.7 lesions (average duration 25 ± 7 seconds per lesion) were required to create conduction block. In three of these patients, AF terminated only after coronary sinus ablation was performed (Figure 62.9). No complications were noted in any of these patients.

Linear Lesions

It is desirable to supplement pulmonary vein isolation with appropriate additional lesions, especially in patients with long-standing persistent AF, as significant recurrence of AF post-initial pulmonary vein isolation alone remains a persistent limitation of currently available ablation techniques. Several combinations of linear lesions have been evaluated in search of an ideal configuration to ablate patients with AF. These include isolated left and right atrial lesions and a combination of the two. In addition to a RAFL line, commonly used linear lesions include a mitral isthmus line, a connecting line between the superior pulmonary veins, a left septal line, and a posterior mitral line.

The mitral isthmus encompasses a narrow region between the LIPV and the mitral annulus. As a short, well-defined target area, it is an attractive but difficult area to ablate. A linear lesion is created by placing an ablation catheter at the mitral annulus and dragging it to the ostium of the LIPV. Conduction block is confirmed by progressive delay in conduction across the ablation line during pacing from the coronary sinus. Bidirectional block can be confirmed by pacing from either side of the line of block. However, in more than 60% of patients undergoing ablation of the mitral isthmus, persistent isthmus conduction can occur due to epicardial conduction

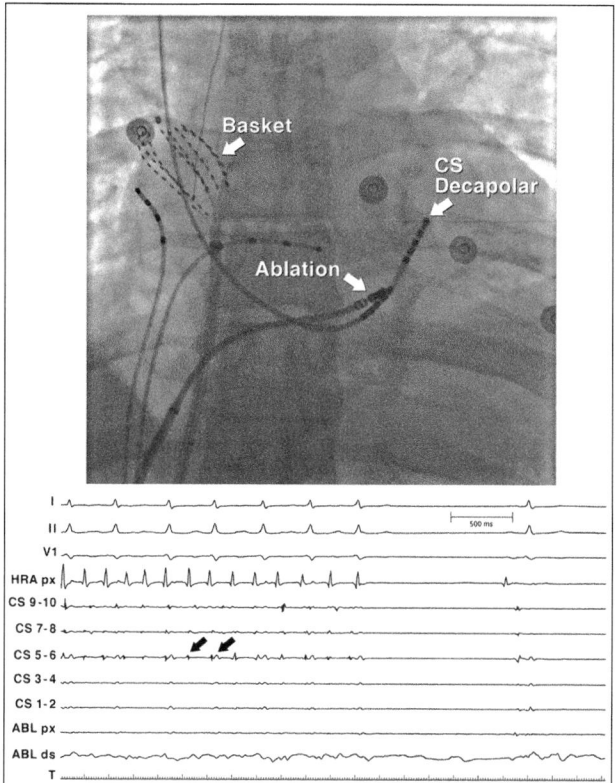

Figure 62.9 Coronary sinus (CS) as a source of atrial fibrillation. **Top panel** depicts catheter location in the coronary sinus. **Bottom panel** depicts tracings, from top to bottom: surface ECG leads I, II, V_1 intracardiac recordings from high right atrium (HRApx), proximal coronary sinus (CS 9,10) to distal coronary sinus (CS 1,2), and proximal (ABLpx) and distal (ABLds) recordings. Following isolation of pulmonary veins and left atrial ablation, atrial fibrillation continues. Ablation of CS 5,6 terminates atrial fibrillation. *Source:* Sra J, Akhtar M. Mapping techniques for atrial fibrillation ablation. *Curr Probl Cardiol.* 2007;32:663-768. With permission from Elsevier.

through the coronary sinus. In these patients, RF catheter ablation within the coronary sinus is usually required to achieve complete conduction block. Despite the conduction block, there is no change in the atrial activation sequence during sinus rhythm. There is a higher risk of cardiac tamponade, which can be reduced by using lower power, especially in the coronary sinus. Use of the 3D mapping and catheter tracking systems described earlier can facilitate the creation of this line.

As mitral isthmus ablation is somewhat complicated, and as epicardial ablation is necessary in many instances to achieve complete block, it is usually reserved for patients with persistent AF or those with perimitral flutter.[18]

Due to possible higher risk of left atrium–esophageal fistula during posterior linear ablation, attempts have been made to connect the superior pulmonary veins at the root of the left atrium. Ablation is usually performed at the most cranial part of the roof (Figure 62.10). Complete block across the line can be confirmed by demonstrating continuous double potentials and an activation detour during LAA pacing, propagating around the pulmonary veins to activate the posterior wall caudocranially. In a prospective study of 90 patients with paroxysmal AF, 87% of the roofline group and 69% of the group undergoing pulmonary vein isolation alone had no recurrence of AF at 15 ± 4 months ($P = 0.04$).[19] The clinical benefit of this mapping and ablation technique may be similar to other linear ablation lines, such as the posterior line, but it can be accomplished in a shorter period of time.

A left septal and posterior mitral line lesion set is usually reserved for patients undergoing long-standing persistent AF ablation. The catheter is looped in the left atrium to the right pulmonary veins. This positions the catheter on the septum anterior to the pulmonary veins. The catheter is gradually withdrawn, initially along the left septum anterior to the pulmonary veins, then to the posterior mitral annulus and on to the lateral left atrium. As the location of the mitral annulus can be as much as 1 cm away from the coronary sinus, additional lesions are usually required in the coronary sinus to eliminate potentials.

Because left atrial linear ablation is technically challenging and incomplete lines may be proarrhythmic, it is important to identify patients who will benefit from additional substrate modification.

Circumferential Left Atrial Ablation

Another technique involves circumferential left atrial ablation using an anatomic approach[20] (Figure 62.11). Several studies have reported the technical success of this approach. In this technique, a 3D map of the left atrium is created using Carto Mapping System (Biosense Webster, Diamond Bar, CA) or EnSite NavX System (Endocardial Solutions, St. Jude Medical, St. Paul, MN), then encircling the left and right pulmonary veins 1–2 cm from the ostia of the pulmonary veins achieves left atrial circumferential ablation. As there is a narrow rim of atrial tissue between the LAA and the left pulmonary veins anteriorly on the left side, ablation is usually performed on the left pulmonary veins. In addition to the technique, originally described by Pappone, this approach generally involves the creation of connecting lines posteriorly or at the roof of the pulmonary veins along with mitral isthmus ablation. The completeness of conduction block across these lines is usually assessed. In a study of 80 patients with paroxysmal AF, 40 patients were randomized for circumferential left atrial ablation and 40 for segmental pulmonary vein isolation. The mean procedure and fluoroscopy times were 156 ± 45 and 50 ± 17 minutes vs 149 ± 33 and 39 ± 12 minutes ($P = \text{NS}$). At 6 months, 67% of patients who underwent segmental pulmonary vein isolation and 80% of patients who underwent circumferential left atrial ablation were free of AF.[14]

During a longer-term follow-up, however, as much as 20% of these patients may develop atypical AFLs, thus negating the initial benefits of this approach. This could presumably be due to incomplete lines. In a subsequent study of 64 AF patients (45% in paroxysmal AF), use of

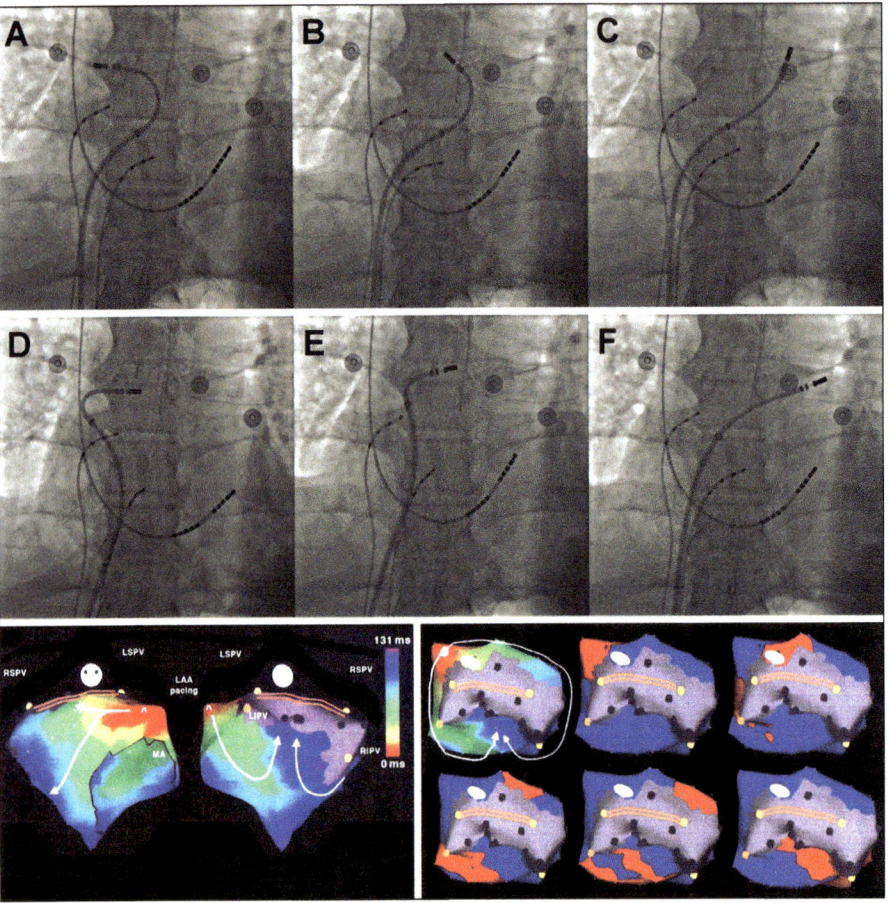

Figure 62.10 Creation of a roof line connecting the superior pulmonary veins (PV). **Top panel** (A–C) depicts looping the catheter in the RSPV. The catheter is gradually opened toward the LSPV. **Middle panel** shows looping of catheter away from the RSPV. The catheter is then gradually pushed toward the LSPV. **Bottom panel:** Demonstration of conduction block across the roof line on 3D mapping. **Left lower panel** shows anteroposterior and right posterosuperior 3D Carto activation map during pacing from LAA. White lines represent areas of block. Lower-line block is due to mitral isthmus ablation. *Sources:* Sra J, Akhtar M. Mapping techniques for atrial fibrillation ablation. *Curr Probl Cardiol.* 2007;32:663-768. With permission from Elsevier. Hocini et al. Creation of roof line in paroxysmal atrial fibrillation: a prospective randomized study. *Circulation.* 2005;112:3688-3696. Reproduced with permission.

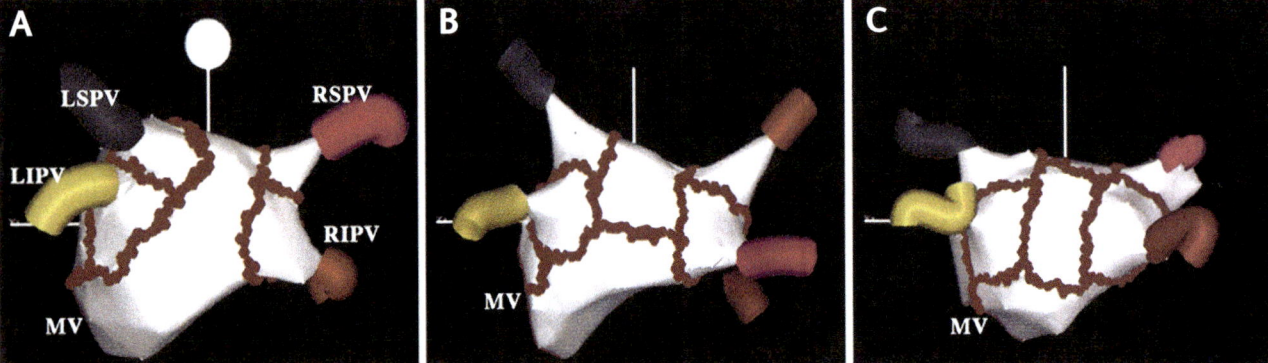

Figure 62.11 Electroanatomic left atrium (LA) map (posteroanterior view). Note the lesion set. Circular radiofrequency lesions deployed around each pulmonary vein (PV) constitute the basic ablation schema (**Panel A**). Additional linear lesions have been added in this patient in order to prevent left atrial incisional tachycardia (linear lesion connects the RIPV and the mitral annulus—**Panel B**) and in an attempt to reduce the electrically active atrial tissue at the posterior left atrial wall (additional linear lesions between the RIPV and LIPV and between pairs of superior and inferior pulmonary veins—**Panel C**). *Source:* Pappone C, Augello G, Rosanio S. Catheter ablation of pulmonary vein atrial fibrillation: circumferential ablation. In: Chen SA, Haïssaguerre M, Zipes DP, editors, *Thoracic Vein Arrhythmias*. Malden, MA: Blackwell-Futura; 2004. Reproduced with permission.

this approach achieved complete pulmonary vein isolation in only 12% to 29% of patients. As compared to the prior study, during a longer-term follow-up of 13 ± 1 months, single-procedure success rate was 45%, incomplete pulmonary vein isolation being a predictor of failure. Over time, this approach has evolved to include the use of more proximal lesions and more ablation energy at sites eliciting vagal responses.

AF Ablation of Long-lasting Persistent AF

As the technique of pulmonary vein isolation alone has a poor outcome in patients with persistent AF of long duration, a variety of techniques have been proposed recently to improve ablation efficacy in these patients. Circumferential pulmonary vein isolation using other strategic lines (described above) is one such approach. In one recent study, 60 patients with persistent AF (17 ± 27 months) were randomized for various ablation techniques. Ablation was performed in a randomized sequence at different left atrial regions and included various combinations of the following ablation techniques: isolation of the pulmonary veins; isolation of other thoracic veins; atrial tissue ablation targeting all regions with rapid or heterogeneous activation guided by activation mapping; linear lesions at the roof connecting the pulmonary veins; and mitral isthmus and septal ablation as described before.

Following ablation at these sites, AF was terminated in 52 (87%) patients.[21] Mapping revealed that AF was terminated directly in 7 patients or via ablation of 1-to-6 intermediate atrial tachycardias (ATs) in 45 patients. Thirty-eight ATs were focal, originating predominantly from the anterior left atrium, LAPV junction, and coronary sinus. Forty-nine tachycardias were macroreentrant, involving the mitral or cavotricuspid isthmus, or the left atrial roof. Three months after ablation, sustained AT was documented in 24 patients. In 23 of those patients, mapping showed a single AT in 7 patients, while multiple ATs were observed in 16 patients. Macroreentry was confirmed to be caused by gaps in the ablation lines, while focal AT originated from discrete sites or isthmuses near the LAA, coronary sinus, pulmonary veins, or fossa ovalis. After repeat ablation of these sites over the next 11 ± 6 months, 57 (95%) patients were in sinus rhythm. However, ablation of persistent AF and identifying sources of recurrence after the initial procedure is a cumbersome and tedious process.

Ablation of Complex Fractionated Electrograms

Intraoperative mapping of AF has shown that CFAEs are mostly found in areas of slow conduction or at points where the wavelets turn around at the end of the arcs of functional block. Such CFAEs have relatively short cycle lengths and heterogeneous spatial and temporal distribution. Recent studies have attempted to target these CFAEs and other electrograms in order to terminate and prevent recurrence of AF (Figure 62.12).[22]

In the 2004 study[22] of 121 patients with AF (57 paroxysmal), CFAEs were found in 7 of the 9 regions of both atria, but were mainly confined to the interatrial septum, the pulmonary veins, the roof of the left atrium, the left posteroseptal mitral annulus, and the coronary sinus ostium. The fibrillation cycle length along both sides of the septum was ≤120 ms, in contrast with the 235 to 280 ms length at the LAA and RAA. According to this report, at 1-year follow up, 92 (76%) of the 121 patients were free of arrhythmia.

However, other studies have not corroborated these findings, and it has also been demonstrated that these electrograms may be dynamic at times. Attempts have been made to identify and ablate other electrograms, such as continuous activity, electrograms showing significant gradient, and those with fractionation,[37] as well as ablation of autonomic ganglion, which can be difficult.[38,39]

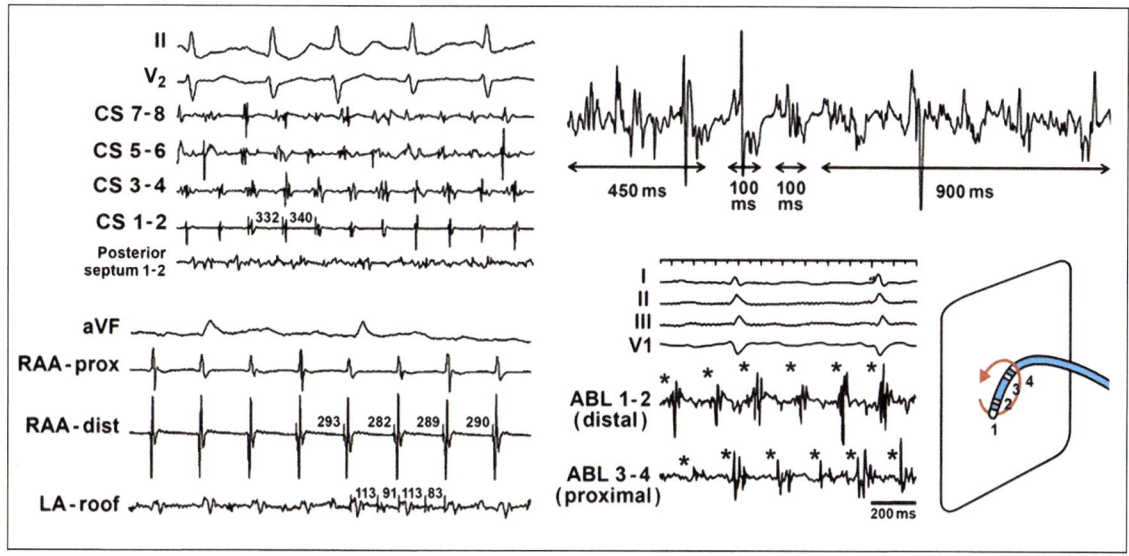

Figure 62.12 **Top left panel:** Example of complex fractionated atrial electrograms (CFAE) with continuous prolonged activation complex over the posterior septal area. **Bottom left panel** shows another type of CFAE at the left atrium-roof, where electrograms exhibit a very short cycle length compared with the rest of the atria (CS = coronary sinus). *Source:* Reproduced with permission from the American College of Cardiology.[22] **Top right panel:** Continuous activities with duration of 450 ms and 900 ms are interrupted by an isoelectric line of >50 ms. Duration of continuous activity in this observation window is 90%. **Bottom right panel:** Temporal gradient of at least 70 ms between the distal and proximal bipoles is shown. *Sources:* Yoshihide T, O'Neill M, Hocini M, et al. Characterization of electrograms associated with termination of chronic atrial fibrillation by catheter ablation. *J Am Coll Cardiol.* 2008;51:1003-1010. Reproduced with permission from the American College of Cardiology; Nademanee K, McKenzie J, Kosar E, et al. A new approach for catheter ablation of atrial fibrillation: mapping of the electrophysiologic substrate. *J Am Coll Cardiol.* 2004; 43:2044-2053. Reproduced with permission from the American College of Cardiology.

Newer Technologies for Catheter Ablation of Pulmonary Veins and Left Atrium

Several new technologies and energy sources have been developed to improve the efficacy of AF ablation.[40-48] Newer energy sources under evaluation to aid in isolating the pulmonary veins include radiofrequency, cryothermy, ultrasound, laser, and microwave. The merits and limitations of these power sources are depicted in Table 62.1. Apart from microwave energy used in the surgical ablation of AF, these energy sources are still in the clinical trial stage.

Radiofrequency is commonly used for AF ablation. Several studies have shown that RF energy can produce precise and effective lesions. Excessive temperatures at the tissue-catheter interface can cause coagulation formation, carbonization, and steam popping due to pockets of vapor being produced under pressure. This can result in crater formation or, rarely, myocardial rupture. These limitations prohibit the use of excessive temperatures and, therefore, limit the depth of lesion possible using RF energy.

One important advancement in achieving deeper lesions in the left atrium has been the introduction of irrigated-tip electrodes. Changing the temperature by irrigating the tip of the catheter prevents overheating of the endocardium while allowing sufficient energy delivery to achieve a deeper lesion. These catheters infuse saline throughout the electrode tip, thus slowing surface heating. Studies have shown that catheters with cooling mechanisms can create significantly deeper lesions than nonirrigated catheters.

There has been a number of recent studies related to cryoablation as well. In one study, 50 patients (age 59 ± 9 years, ejection fraction 0.59 ± 0.06, left atrial size 41 ± 5 mm) with paroxysmal AF were studied. Twenty-five patients underwent PVI using a 28-mm cryoballoon. A control group of 25 patients underwent PVI using an open-irrigation RF ablation catheter. Myocardial injury was determined by measuring troponin T (TnT). Pulmonary vein reconnection patterns were studied in case of repeat procedures. Procedure duration was 166 ± 32 minutes in the cryoballoon group versus 197 ± 52 minutes in the RF group ($P = 0.014$), with similar ablation times (cryoballoon: 45 minutes [interquartile range 40 to 52.5 minutes]; RF: 47 minutes [interquartile range 44 to 65 minutes], $P = 0.17$). Postprocedural TnT in the RF group was 1.29 ± 0.41 µg/L versus 0.76 ± 0.55 µg/L in the cryoballoon group ($P = 0.002$). In 12 patients who underwent repeat ablation, 74% of pulmonary vein reconnection sites were inferiorly located in the cryoballoon group compared to 17% in the RF group ($P = 0.0004$). With 1.2 ± 0.4 and 1.3 ± 0.6 procedures per patient, 88% of patients in the cryoballoon group and 92% in the RF group were in stable sinus rhythm after follow-up of 12 ± 3 months ($P = NS$).

In another study with AFL, a total of 191 patients were randomized to RF ablation or cryoablation of the CTI using an 8-mm-tip catheter. At 3 months, persistent bidirectional block could be confirmed in 85% of the RF group versus 65.6% of the cryoablation group. Persistence of bidirectional block in patients treated with cryoablation reinvestigated after 3 months is inferior to that of patients

Table 62.1 Energy sources other than cryothermal for catheter ablation

Energy Source	Frequency or Wavelength	Mechanism of Heating	Relation of Heating to Distance (r) from Source	Tissue Contact Needed	Advantages	Disadvantages
Radiofrequency	300–700 kHz	Resistive	$1/r^4$	Yes	Easy, inexpensive, vast clinical experience	Limited lesion size, charring with nonirrigated tip
Microwave	915–2,450 MHz	Dielectric	$1/r^2$	No	Penetrates scar and fat, large lesions, linear catheters possible, no clinical experience	Complex catheter design, energy titration
Laser	300–2,000 nm	Photon absorption	Complex exponential decline	No	Large lesions, can spare endocardium, linear catheters possible, no clinical experience	Difficulty controlling depth, complex effects with tissue properties and distance from source
Ultrasound	500 kHz to 20 MHz	Mechanical stress and strain	Varies with focal length	No	Can be focused for encircling lesions and focal lesions far from source, limited clinical experience	Difficulty controlling depth, highly directional

Source: From Doshi SK, Keane D. Catheter ultrasound, microwave and laser: biophysics and applications. In: Huang SKS, Wood MA, eds. *Catheter Ablation of Cardiac Arrhythmias*. Philadelphia, PA: Saunders-Elsevier, 2006:69-82. Reproduced with permission.

treated with RF ablation, as evidenced by the higher recurrence rate of common AFL seen in this study.

There have also been a number of recent developments in the area of remote navigation of mapping and ablation catheters, and real-time visualization of these catheters.[49,50] A remote magnetic navigation system (NIOBE®, Stereotaxis, Inc., St. Louis, MO) consists of two focused-field magnets of a neodymium–iron boron compound that are computer controlled and located on either side of the body.

The Hansen robotic system (Sensei™ Robotic Catheter System, Hansen Medical Inc., Mountain View, CA) consists of a robotic catheter control system. A steerable sheath is used to navigate within the cardiac chambers. This system can also be maneuvered remotely, at the patient's bedside, with a slave system that steers the catheter control system. A standard catheter is placed through the sheath to perform mapping and ablation. The advantage of this system is that it is an open system through which any catheter can be used. It is relatively mobile and can be moved between labs. Another mechanically driven robotic navigation system is the Amigo™ Remote Catheter System and the Amigo remote controller (Catheter Robotics, Inc, Mount Olive, NJ). This system is an open architecture system and allows for several catheter families to be utilized in conjunction with the device.

It is portable and allows for radiation reduction to the operator. It can be easily moved between laboratories, does not require special catheters or sheaths, and maintains the tactile feel of the catheter being used.[51]

Fluoroscopy does not provide adequate anatomic visualization of the left atrium and the pulmonary veins due to its poor soft-tissue contrast and the two-dimensional (2D) projective nature of the formed image. Integration of images has been used to incorporate within a single view the varied information captured by different imaging modalities. Intrasubject intermodal registration using 2D fluoroscopy and 3D preprocedural CT, MR, and ultrasound-based systems is an area of current focus (Figure 62.13).

Current Terminology and Definitions for Catheter Ablation in Atrial Fibrillation

Recent efforts have attempted to standardize the terminology and definitions applicable to interventions such as catheter and surgical ablation in atrial fibrillation. In the 2012 intersociety document, the following areas were addressed.

Types of atrial fibrillation patients being submitted for catheter ablation were defined in Table 62.2.

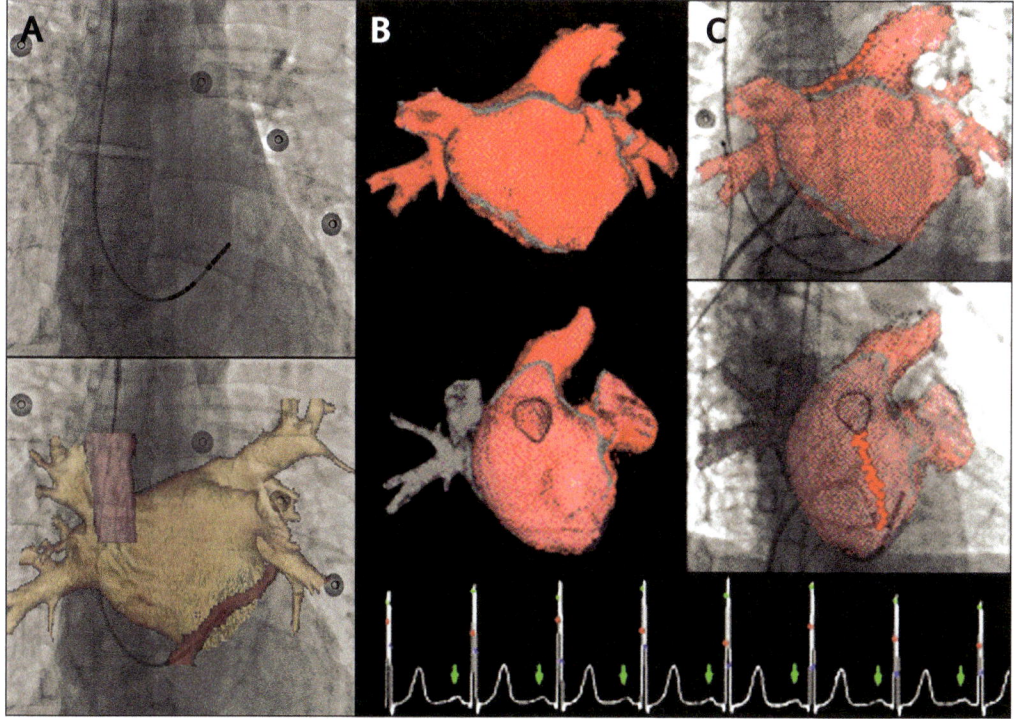

Figure 62.13 3D to 2D registration process. Fluoroscopy image of coronary sinus (CS) catheter is shown in **upper left panel A**. A transformation links the superior vena cava (SVC) and the coronary sinus on the segmented CT (anterior and posterior CT views of the left atirum are shown in **panel B**) image and the coronary sinus catheter on the fluoroscopy image, and is used to register the 3D image of the left atrium with the fluoroscopy image (**bottom left panel A**). **Right panel C** shows mitral isthmus and roof lines created using CT fluoro registered images. *Source:* Sra J, Akhtar M. Mapping techniques for atrial fibrillation ablation. *Curr Probl Cardiol.* 2007;32:663-768. With permission from Elsevier.

Table 62.2 Types of classification of atrial fibrillation**

Atrial Fibrillation Episode	An atrial fibrillation episode is defined as AF that is documented by ECG monitoring and has a duration of at least 30 seconds, or if less than 30 seconds, is present continuously throughout the ECG monitoring tracing. The presence of subsequent episodes of AF requires that sinus rhythm be documented by ECG monitoring between AF episodes.
Paroxysmal AF*	Paroxysmal AF is defined as recurrent AF (≥ 2 episodes) that terminates spontaneously within 7 days. Episodes of AF of ≤ 48 hours' duration that are terminated with electrical or pharmacologic cardioversion should also be classified as paroxysmal AF episodes.
Persistent AF*	Persistent AF is defined as continuous AF that is sustained beyond 7 days. Episodes of AF in which a decision is made to electrically or pharmacologically cardiovert the patient after ≥ 48 hours of AF, but prior to 7 days, should also be classified as persistent AF episodes.
Longstanding Persistent AF	Longstanding persistent AF is defined as continuous AF of greater than 12 months' duration.
Permanent AF	The term permanent AF is not appropriate in the context of patients undergoing catheter or surgical ablation of AF, as it refers to a group of patients for which a decision has been made not to restore or maintain sinus rhythm by any means, including catheter or surgical ablation. If a patient previously classified as having permanent AF is to undergo catheter or surgical ablation, the AF should be reclassified.

It is recognized that patients may have both paroxysmal and persistent AF. A patient's AF type should be defined as the most frequent type of AF experienced within six months of an ablation procedure. Continuous AF is AF that is documented to be present on all ECG monitoring performed during a defined period of time.
** We recommend that the term "chronic AF" not be used in the context of patients undergoing ablation of AF as it is ambiguous, and there is no standardized definition of this term.
Source: Reproduced with permission from Calkins J, Brugada J, Packer D, et al.[34]

The term chronic atrial fibrillation is now eliminated. The definitions for procedural outcomes for catheter and surgical ablation in AF patients were standardized (Table 62.3).

The key elements of a standalone catheter ablation procedure for AF were defined as follows (Table 62.4):

Recommendation as to periprocedural anticoagulation were also formulated (Table 62.5).

Table 62.3 Definitions for use when reporting outcomes of AF ablation and in clinical trials of catheter or surgical ablation of AF

Acute Procedural Success	Acute procedural success is defined as electrical isolation of all pulmonary veins. A minimal assessment of electrical isolation of the PVs should consist of an assessment of entrance block. If other methods are used to assess PV isolation, including exit block and/or the use of provocative agents such as adenosine or isoproterenol, they should be pre-specified. Furthermore, it is recommended that the wait time used to screen for early recurrence of PV conduction once initial electrical isolation is documented be specified in all prospective clinical trials.
One Year Success*	One-year success is defined as freedom from AF/AFL/AT off antiarrhythmic drug therapy as assessed from the end of the 3-month blanking period to 12 months following the ablation procedure.
Clinical/ Partial Success*	Clinical/partial success is defined as a 75% or greater reduction in the number of AF episodes, the duration of AF episodes, or the % time a patient is in AF as assessed with a device capable of measuring AF burden in the presence or absence of previously ineffective antiarrhythmic drug therapy.
Long-Term Success*	Long-term success is defined as freedom from AF/AFL/AT recurrences following the 3-month blanking period through a minimum of 36 months' of follow-up from the date of the ablation procedure in the absence of class I and III AAD therapy.
Recurrent AF	Recurrent AF/AFL/AT is defined as AF/AFL/AT of at least 30 seconds' duration that is documented by an ECG or device recording system and occurs following catheter ablation. Recurrent AF/AFL/AT may occur within or following the post ablation blanking period. Recurrent AF/AFL/AT that occurs within the postablation-blanking period is not considered a failure of AF ablation.
Early Recurrence of AF	Early recurrence of AF is defined as a recurrence of atrial fibrillation within three months of ablation. Episodes of atrial tachycardia or atrial flutter should also be classified as a "recurrence."
Recurrence of AF	Recurrence of AF post ablation is defined as a recurrence of atrial fibrillation more than 3 months following AF ablation. Episodes of atrial tachycardia or atrial flutter should also be classified as a "recurrence."
Late Recurrence of AF	Late recurrence of AF is defined as a recurrence of atrial fibrillation 12 months or more after AF ablation. Episodes of atrial tachycardia or atrial flutter should also be classified as a "recurrence."
Blanking Period	A blanking period of three months should be employed after ablation when reporting efficacy outcomes. Thus, early recurrences of AF/AFL/AT within the first 3 months should not be classified as treatment failure. If a blanking period of less than 3 months is acceptable and if is chosen, it should be pre- specified and included in the methods section.

Detectable AF	Detectable AF is defined as AF of at least 30 seconds' duration when assessed with ECG monitoring. If other monitoring systems are used, including implantable pacemakers, implantable defibrillators, and subcutaneous ECG monitoring devices, the definition of detectable AF needs to be pre-specified in the clinical trial based on the sensitivity and specificity of AF detection with the particular device. We recommend that episodes of atrial flutter and atrial tachycardia be included within the broader definition of a detectable AF/AFL/AT episode.	
Entrance Block	Entrance block is defined as the absence, or if present, the dissociation, of electrical activity within the PV antrum. Entrance block is most commonly evaluated using a circular multielectrode mapping catheter positioned at the PV antrum. Entrance block also can be assessed using detailed point-by-point mapping of the PV antrum guided by an electroanatomic mapping system. The particular method used to assess entrance block should be specified in all clinical trials. Entrance block of the left PVs should be assessed during distal coronary sinus or left atrial appendage pacing in order to distinguish far-field atrial potentials from PV potentials.	
Enrolled Subject	An enrolled subject is defined as a subject who has signed written informed consent to participate in the trial in question.	

When reporting outcomes of AF ablation, the development of atrial tachycardia or atrial flutter should be included in the broad definition of recurrence following AF ablation. All studies should report freedom from AF, atrial tachycardia, and atrial flutter. These endpoints can also be reported separately. All studies should also clearly specify the type and frequency of ECG monitoring as well as the degree of compliance with the prespecified monitoring protocol.
Source: Reproduced with permission from Calkins J, Brugada J, Packer D, et al.[34]

Table 62.4 Ablation technique recommendations

- Ablation strategies that target the PVs and/or PV antrum are the cornerstone for most AF ablation procedures.
- If the PVs are targeted, electrical isolation should be the goal.
- Achievement of electrical isolation requires, at a minimum, assessment and demonstration of entrance block into the PV.
- Monitoring for PV reconduction for 20 minutes following initial PV isolation should be considered.
- For surgical PV isolation, entrance and/or exit block should be demonstrated.
- Careful identification of the PV ostia is mandatory to avoid ablation within the PVs.
- If a focal trigger is identified outside a PV at the time of an AF ablation procedure, ablation of that focal trigger should be considered.
- If additional linear lesions are applied, operators should consider using mapping and pacing maneuvers to assess for line completeness.
- Ablation of the cavotricuspid isthmus is recommended in patients with a history of typical atrial flutter or inducible cavotricuspid isthmus dependent atrial flutter.
- If patients with longstanding persistent AF are approached, operators should consider more extensive ablation based on linear lesions or complex fractionated electrograms.
- It is recommended that RF power be reduced when creating lesions along the posterior wall near the esophagus.

Source: Reproduced with permission from Calkins J, Brugada J, Packer D, et al.[34]

Table 62.5 Anticoagulation strategies: Pre, during, and post ablation

Pre Ablation	• Anticoagulation guidelines that pertain to cardioversion of AF be adhered to in patients who present for an AF ablation in atrial fibrillation at the time of the procedure. In other words, if the patient has been in AF for 48 hours or longer or for an unknown duration, we require three weeks of systemic anticoagulation at a therapeutic level prior to the procedure, and if this is not the case, we advise that a TEE be performed to screen for thrombus. Furthermore, each of these patients will be anticoagulated systemically for two months post ablation. • Prior to undergoing an AF ablation procedure a TEE should be performed in all patients with atrial fibrillation more than 48 hours in duration or of an unknown duration if adequate systemic anticoagulation has not been maintained for at least 3 weeks prior to the ablation procedure. • Performance of a TEE in patients who are in sinus rhythm at the time of ablation or patients with AF who are in AF but have been in AF for 48 hours or less prior to AF ablation may be considered but is not mandatory. • The presence of a left atrial thrombus is a contraindication to catheter ablation of AF. • Performance of catheter ablation of AF on a patient who is therapeutically anticoagulated with warfarin should be considered.
During Ablation	• Heparin should be administered prior to or immediately following transseptal puncture during AF ablation procedures and adjusted to achieve and maintain an ACT of 300 to 400 seconds. • Performance of AF ablation in a patient systemically anticoagulated with warfarin does not alter the need for intravenous heparin to maintain a therapeutic ACT during the procedure. • Administration of protamine following ablation to reverse heparin should be considered.

Post Ablation	• In patients who are not therapeutically anticoagulated with warfarin at the time of AF ablation, low-molecular-weight heparin or intravenous heparin should be used as a bridge to resumption of systemic anticoagulation with warfarin following AF ablation. • Initiation of a direct thrombin or Factor Xa inhibitor after ablation may be considered as an alternative post procedure anticoagulation strategy. • Because of the increased risk of post procedure bleeding on full dose low-molecular-weight heparin (1 mg/kg bid) a reduction of the dose to 0.5 mg/kg should be considered. • Systemic anticoagulation with warfarin or a direct thrombin or Factor Xa inhibitor is recommended for at least two months following an AF ablation procedure. • Decisions regarding the continuation of systemic anticoagulation agents more than two months following ablation should be based on the patient's risk factors for stroke and not on the presence or type of AF. • Discontinuation of systemic anticoagulation therapy post ablation is not recommended in patients who are at high risk of stroke as estimated by currently recommended schemes ($CHADS_2$ or $CHA_2DS\ VASc$)[e3]. • Patients in whom discontinuation of systemic anticoagulation is being considered should consider undergoing continuous ECG monitoring to screen for asymptomatic AF/AFL/AT.

Source: Reproduced with permission from Calkins J, Brugada J, Packer D, et al.[34]

The development of novel oral anticoagulants has sparked a great deal of discussion as to the optimal periprocedural use of these drugs. A variety of single center reports have emerged for dabigatran have suggested that it is comparable to warfarin in safety especially if held for 24 hours before a catheter ablation procedure.[52-55] More recent data suggests that there is an impact on anticoagulation during the ablation procedure. Snipelisky et al first reported increased intra-procedural variability in activated clotting time and this has been further investigated.[52] Bassiouny et al noted that dabigatran resulted in earlier achievement of therapeutic ACT levels suggesting facilitation.[56] Early data on rivaroxaban is now emerging and suggests similar benefit.[57] However, the lack of randomized controlled trials has been an important issue.[58] These have now been initiated. The first such trial design, VENTURE-AF< has been reported for rivaroxaban, and is now in progress at the time of publication of this chapter.

Evidence-based Guidelines for Catheter Ablation in Atrial Fibrillation

Recent guidelines have also redefined the role of catheter ablation procedures in different types of atrial fibrillation and in relation to alternative therapies such as antiarrhythmic drugs in more detail and with reference to co-morbidities (Figure 62.14). The classification of evidence-based guidelines and their evidence base is described in detail in the next chapter.

In the 2012 intersociety guidelines from the electrophysiology societies, the recommendations for catheter and surgical ablation in different types of atrial fibrillation are summarized in Table 62.6.

Catheter ablation is considered a class 1 indication for paroxysmal AF refractory to al lest one class 1 or 3 antiarrhythmic drug. It is a class 2A indication in recent onset persistent AF with a strong level of evidence and class 2B indication in long standing persistent AF with a lower level of evidence. As a first line option, this is limited to a class 2A option for paroxysmal AF in patients unwilling or unable to take antiarrhythmic drugs.

In the 2014 ACC-AHA-HRS guidelines, a more global perspective relative to other therapies is offered.

Catheter ablation indications are specified relative to the presence or absence of structural heart disease. It can be a first line therapy in the absence of structural heart disease and after antiarrhythmic drug trial(s) in structural heart disease. This is relevant to patients with coronary heart disease and heart failure with AF.

Table 62.6 Indications for catheter ablation of AF

Symptomatic AF refractory or intolerant to at least one Class 1 or 3 antiarrhythmic medication	Class	Level
Paroxysmal: Catheter ablation is recommended*	I	A
Persistent: Catheter ablation is reasonable	IIa	B
Longstanding Persistent: Catheter ablation may be considered	IIb	B
Symptomatic AF prior to initiation of antiarrhythmic drug therapy with a Class 1 or 3 antiarrhythmic agent	**Class**	**Level**
Paroxysmal: Catheter ablation is reasonable	IIa	B
Persistent: Catheter ablation may be considered	IIb	C
Longstanding Persistent: Catheter ablation may be considered	IIb	C

*CATHETER ablation of symptomatic paroxysmal AF is considered a Class 1 indication only when performed by an electrophysiologist who has received appropriate training and is performing the procedure in an experienced center.
Source: Reproduced with permission from Calkins J, Brugada J, Packer D, et al.[34]

Thus, the role of catheter ablation in the management of AF is expanding and is supported by increasing levels of evidence in clinical practice.

Catheter ablation of type 1 atrial flutter is now considered a class 1 indication and a first line of therapy option based on co-morbid status. In general, catheter ablation of type 2 atrial flutter is performed in patients refractory to antiarrhythmic drug therapy and is influenced by co-morbidities. In clinical trials, ablation of type 1 atrial flutter was associated with superior outcomes compared to antiarrhythmic drug therapy.[61-63] In a definitive report by Natale et al, a comparative trial of antiarhthymic drugs versus catheter ablation showed a clear benefit of the latter.[63] After a mean follow-up of 21 months, 11 of 30 patients (36%) receiving drugs were in sinus rhythm, versus 25 of 31 (80%) patients who underwent RF ablation ($p < 0.01$). Of the patients receiving drugs, 63% required one or more rehospitalizations, whereas post-RF ablation, only 22% of patients were rehospitalized ($p < 0.01$). Observational data suggest benefit of type 2 atrial flutter ablation in a variety of disease states and iatrogenic conditions. Scar related flutter is postoperative patients or septal defects have had favorable outcomes in observational clinical studies.[64,65] No randomized clinical trials are currently available to formulate practice guidelines.

Catheter ablation of atrial flutter elicited after drug therapy or drug infusion in patients with atrial fibrillation has been advocated by some centers.[66,67] However, long-term results of catheter ablation of type 1atrial flutter in drug treated patients with atrial fibrillation has been unsuccessful as stand alone therapy. Long term outcomes show invariable recurrence when used alone or with antiarrhythmic drugs as hybrid therapy.[68] Thus, this approach is not advocated at this time.

Summary

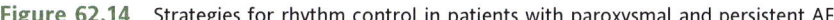

Significant advances in understanding the mechanisms of AF initiation, sustainment, and catheter mapping have led to increased efficacy in AF ablation. Improvements in technologies such as different energy sources, 3D imaging, navigation and image integration, and computer processing of the vast amount of data is making the clinical availability of these techniques a reality. Ablation of AF is rapidly expanding and, like other supraventricular arrhythmias, may become the treatment of choice in many patients.

Figure 62.14 Strategies for rhythm control in patients with paroxysmal and persistent AF.

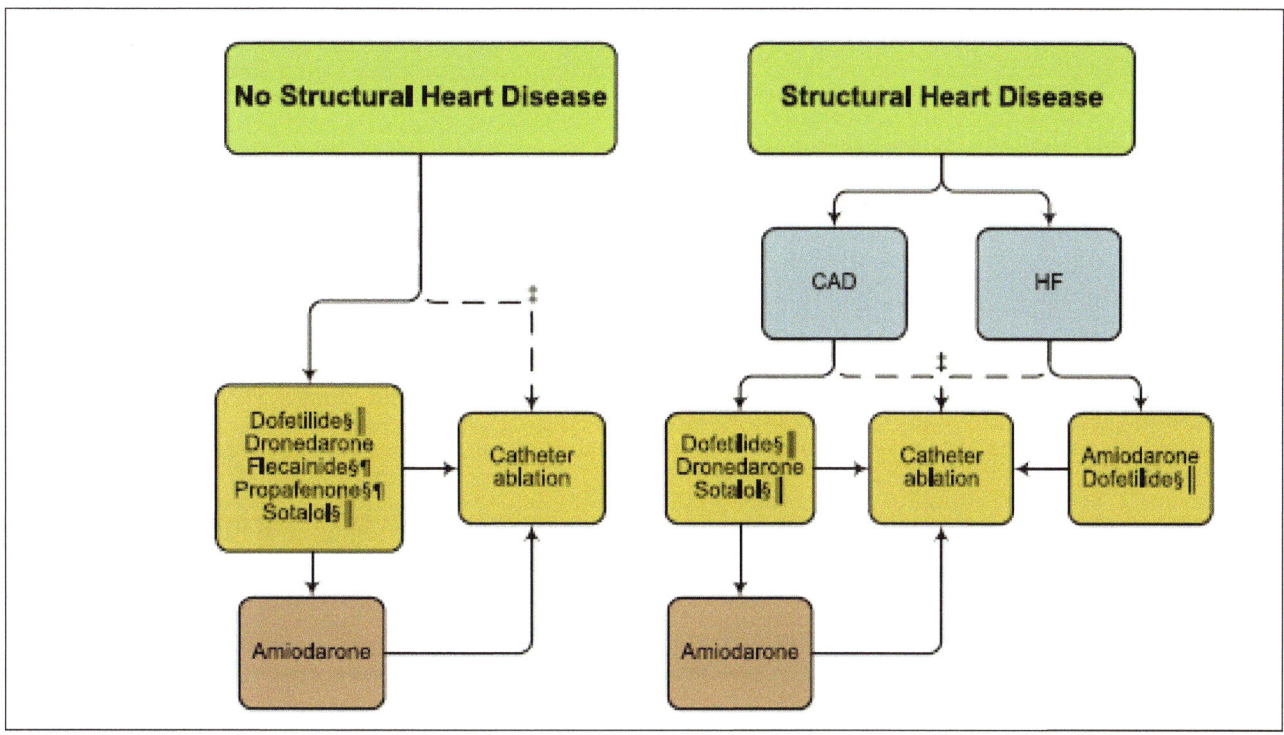

*Catheter ablation is only recommended as first-line therapy for patients with paroxysmal AF (class IIa recommendation).
†Drugs are listed alphabetically.
‡Depending on patient preference when performed in experienced centers.
§Not recommended with severe LVH (wall thickness > 1.5 cm).
¶Should be used with caution in patients at risk for torsades de pointes ventricular tachycardia. Should be combined with AV nodal blocking agents. AF indicates atrial fibrillation; AV, atrioventricular; CAD, coronary artery disease; HF, heart failure; LVH, left ventricular hypertrophy.
Source: Reprinted with permission of *J Am Coll Cardiol.* 2014;64(21):2246-2280.

However, due to the extensive cost of these procedures and the availability of a wide array of systems, it is imperative that future studies focus on validating efficacy and safety in particular patient-specific situations.

It is important to note that this statement summarizes the opinion of the Task Force members based on their experience and a review of the literature. It is thought that the consensus document can improve patient care by providing a foundation for those involved with ablation of AF. It is recognized that this field continues to evolve rapidly and that this document will need to be updated.

Acknowledgments

The authors gratefully acknowledge the help of Barbara Danek, Joe Grundle, and Katie Klein in the editorial preparation of this manuscript and Brian Miller, Brian Schurrer, and David Krum in helping with the manuscript and in preparing the illustrations.

References

1. Shah DC, Jaïs P, Haïssaguerre M, et al. Three-dimensional mapping of the common atrial flutter circuit in the right atrium. *Circulation*. 1997;96:3904-3912.
2. Nakagawa H, Lazzara R, Khastgir T, et al. Role of the tricuspid annulus and the Eustachian valve/ridge on atrial flutter. Relevance to catheter ablation of the septal isthmus and a new technique for rapid identification of ablation success. *Circulation*. 1996;94:407-424.
3. Sorgente A, Moccetti T. Abnormal right atrial pouch in a patient with heart failure and cavotricuspid isthmus-dependent atrial flutter. *Heart Rhythm*. 2011;8(4):639-640.
4. Bochoeyer A, Yang Y, Cheng J, et al. Surface electrocardiographic characteristics of right and left atrial flutter. *Circulation*. 2003;108:60-66.
5. Yang Y, Cheng J, Bochoeyer A, et al. Atypical right atrial flutter patterns. *Circulation*. 2001;103:3092-3098.
6. Jaïs P, Hocini M, Sanders P, et al. An approach to noncavotricuspid isthmus dependent flutter. *J Cardiovasc Electrophysiol*. 2005;16:666-673.
7. Kannel WB, Abbott RD, Savage DD, McNamara PM. Epidemiologic features of chronic atrial fibrillation: the Framingham study. *N Engl J Med*. 1982;306:1018-1022.
8. Haïssaguerre M, Jaïs P, Shah DC, et al. Spontaneous initiation of atrial fibrillation by ectopic beats originating in the pulmonary veins. *N Engl J Med*. 1998;339:659-666.
9. Lin WS, Tai CT, Hsieh MH, et al. Catheter ablation of paroxysmal atrial fibrillation initiated by non-pulmonary vein ectopy. *Circulation*. 2003;107:3176-3183.
10. Chugh A, Oral H, Good E, et al. Catheter ablation of atypical atrial flutter and atrial tachycardia within the coronary sinus after left atrial ablation for atrial fibrillation. *J Am Coll Cardiol*. 2005;46:83-91.
11. Jaïs P, Haïssaguerre M, Shah DC, et al. A focal source of atrial fibrillation treated by discrete radiofrequency ablation. *Circulation*. 1997;95:572-576.
12. Haïssaguerre M, Shah DC, Jaïs P, et al. Mapping guided ablation of pulmonary veins to cure atrial fibrillation. *Am J Cardiol*. 2000;105:86:9K-19K.
13. Oral H, Knight BP, Tada H, et al. Pulmonary vein isolation for paroxysmal and persistent atrial fibrillation. *Circulation*. 2002;105:1077-1081.
14. Oral H, Knight BP, Ozaydin M, et al. Clinical significance of early recurrences of atrial fibrillation after pulmonary vein isolation. *J Am Coll Cardiol*. 2002;40:100-104.
15. Ouyang F, Antz M, Ernst S, et al. Recovered pulmonary vein conduction as a dominant factor for recurrent atrial tachyarrhythmias after complete circular isolation of the pulmonary veins: lessons from double Lasso technique. *Circulation*. 2005;111:127-135.
16. Gerstenfeld EP, Callans DJ, Dixit S, et al. Mechanisms of organized left atrial tachycardias occurring after pulmonary vein isolation. *Circulation*. 2004;110:1351-1357.
17. Cappato R, Calkins H, Chen SA, et al. Worldwide survey on the methods, efficacy, and safety of catheter ablation for human atrial fibrillation. *Circulation*. 2005;111:1100-1105.
18. Jaïs P, Hocini M, Hsu LF, et al. Technique and results of linear ablation at the mitral isthmus. *Circulation*. 2004;110:2996-3002.
19. Hocini M, Jaïs P, Sanders P, et al. Techniques, evaluation, and consequences of linear block at the left atrial roof in paroxysmal atrial fibrillation: a prospective randomized study. *Circulation*. 2005;112:3688-3696.
20. Pappone C, Rosanio S, Oreto G, et al. Circumferential radiofrequency ablation of pulmonary vein ostia: a new anatomic approach for curing atrial fibrillation. *Circulation*. 2000;102:2619-2628.
21. Haïssaguerre M, Hocini M, Sanders P, et al. Catheter ablation of long-lasting persistent atrial fibrillation: clinical outcome and mechanisms of subsequent arrhythmias. *J Cardiovasc Electrophysiol*. 2005;16:1138-1147.
22. Nademanee K, McKenzie J, Kosar E, et al. A new approach for catheter ablation of atrial fibrillation: mapping of the electrophysiologic substrate. *J Am Coll Cardiol*. 2004;43:2044-2053.
23. Pappone C, Rosanio S, Augello G, et al. Mortality, morbidity, and quality of life after circumferential pulmonary vein ablation for atrial fibrillation: outcomes from a controlled nonrandomized long-term study. *J Am Coll Cardiol*. 2003;42:185-197.
24. Saito T, Waki K, Becker AE. Left atrial myocardial extension onto pulmonary veins in humans: anatomic observations relevant for atrial arrhythmias. *J Cardiovasc Electrophysiol*. 2000;11:888-894.
25. Willems S, Weiss C, Ventura R, et al. Catheter ablation of atrial flutter guided by electroanatomic mapping (CARTO): a randomized comparison to the conventional approach. *J Cardiovasc Electrophysiol*. 2000;11:1223-1230.
26. Kottkamp H, Hugl B, Krauss B, et al. Electromagnetic versus fluoroscopic mapping of the inferior isthmus for ablation of typical atrial flutter: a prospective randomized study. *Circulation*. 2000;102:2082-2086.
27. Natale A, Newby KH, Pisano E, et al. Prospective randomized comparison of antiarrhythmic therapy versus first-line radiofrequency ablation in patients with atrial flutter. *J Am Coll Cardiol*. 2000;35:1898-1904.
28. Schumacher B, Jung W, Lewalter T, et al. Radiofrequency ablation of atrial flutter due to administration of class IC antiarrhythmic drugs for atrial fibrillation. *Am J Cardiol*. 1999;83:710-713.
29. Tai CT, Chiang CE, Lee SH, et al. Persistent atrial flutter in patients treated for atrial fibrillation with amiodarone and propafenone: electrophysiologic characteristics, radiofrequency catheter ablation, and risk prediction. *J Cardiovasc Electrophysiol*. 1999;10:1180-1187.

30. Nabar A, Rodriguez LM, Timmermans C, et al. Radiofrequency ablation of "class IC atrial flutter" in patients with resistant atrial fibrillation. *Am J Cardiol.* 1999;83:785-787.
31. Reithmann C, Hoffmann E, Spitzlberger G, et al. Catheter ablation of atrial flutter due to amiodarone therapy for paroxysmal atrial fibrillation. *Eur Heart J.* 2000;21:565-572.
32. Triedman JK, Alexander ME, Berul CI, et al. Electroanatomic mapping of entrained and exit zones in patients with repaired congenital heart disease and intra-atrial re-entrant tachycardia. *Circulation.* 2001;103:2060-2065.
33. Blomstrom CL, Scheinmann M, Aliot EM, et al. ACC/AHA guidelines for the management of patients with supraventricular arrhythmias. *J Am Coll Cardiol.* 2003;42:1493-1531.
34. Calkins H, Brugada J, Packer D, et al. HRS/EHRA/ECAS expert consensus statement on catheter and surgical ablation of atrial fibrillation: recommendations for personnel, policy, procedures and follow up. *Heart Rhythm.* 2007;4:816-860.
35. Kato R, Lickfett L, Meininger G, et al. Pulmonary vein anatomy in patients undergoing catheter ablation of atrial fibrillation: lessons learned by use of magnetic resonance imaging. *Circulation.* 2003;107:2004-2010.
36. Packer DL, Keelan P, Munger TM, et al. Clinical presentation, investigation, and management of pulmonary vein stenosis complicating ablation for atrial fibrillation. *Circulation.* 2005;111:546-554.
37. Takahashi Y, O'Neill M, Hocini M, et al. Characterization of electrograms associated with termination of chronic atrial fibrillation by catheter ablation. *J Am Coll Cardiol.* 2008; 51:1003-1010.
38. Armour JA, Murphy DA, Yuan BX, MacDonald S, Hopkins DA. Gross and microscopic anatomy of the human intrinsic cardiac nervous system. *Anat Rec.* 1997;247:289-298.
39. Scanavacca M, Pisani CF, Hachul D, et al. Selective atrial vagal denervation guided by evoked vagal reflex to treat patients with paroxysmal atrial fibrillation. *Circulation.* 2006;114:876-885.
40. Ben-Haim SA, Osadchy D, Schuster I, Gepstein L, Hayam G, Josephson ME. Nonfluoroscopic, in vivo navigation and mapping technology. *Nat Med.* 1996;2:1393-1395.
41. Peters NS, Jackman WM, Schilling RJ, Beatty G, Davies DW. Images in cardiovascular medicine. Human left ventricular endocardial activation mapping using a novel noncontact catheter. *Circulation.* 1997;95:1658-1660.
42. Sra J, Hauck J, Krum D, Schweitzer J. Three-dimensional right atrial geometry construction and catheter tracking using cutaneous patches. *J Cardiovasc Electrophysiol.* 2003;14:897.
43. Cummings JE, Pacifico A, Drago JL, Kilicaslan F, Natale A. Alternative energy sources for the ablation of arrhythmias. *Pacing Clin Electrophysiol.* 2005;28:434-443.
44. Macle L, Jaïs P, Weerasooriya R, et al. Irrigated-tip catheter ablation of pulmonary veins for treatment of atrial fibrillation. *J Cardiovasc Electrophysiol.* 2002;13:1067-1073.
45. Faddis MN, Blume W, Finney J, et al. Novel, magnetically guided catheter for endocardial mapping and radiofrequency catheter ablation. *Circulation.* 2002;106:2980-2985.
46. Thornton AS, Jordaens LJ. Advances in the approaches to ablation of complex arrhythmias. *J Cardiovasc Electrophysiol.* 2007;18:S2-S10.
47. Kühne M, Suter Y, Altmann D, et al. Cryoballoon versus radiofrequency catheter ablation of paroxysmal atrial fibrillation: biomarkers of myocardial injury, recurrence rates, and pulmonary vein reconnection patterns. *Heart Rhythm.* December 2010;7(12):177.
48. Kuniss M, Vogtmann T, Ventura R, et al. Prospective randomized comparison of durability of bidirectional conduction block in the cavotricuspid isthmus in patients after ablation of common atrial flutter using cryothermy and radiofrequency energy: the CRYOTIP study. *Heart Rhythm.* December 2009;6(12):1699-1705. Epub September 11, 2009.
49. Al Ahmad A, Grossman JD, Wang PJ. Early experience with a computerized robotically controlled catheter system. *J Interv Card Electrophysiol.* 2005;12:199-202.
50. Sra J, Ratnakumar S. Cardiac image registration of the left atrium and pulmonary veins. *Heart Rhythm.* 2008;85:609-617.
51. Khan EM, Frumkin W, Ng G, et al. First experience with a novel remote robotic catheter system: Amigo™ mapping trial. *J Interv Card Electrophysiol.* 2013;37:121-129.
52. Snipelisky D, Kauffman C, Prussak KA, et al. A comparison of bleeding complications post-ablation between warfarin and dabigatran. *J Intervent Card Electrophysiol.* 2012;35(1):29-33. DOI: 10.1007/s10840-012-9708.
53. Imamura K, Yoshida A, Takei A, et al. Dabigatran in the peri-procedural period for radiofrequency ablation of atrial fibrillation: efficacy, safety, and impact on duration of hospital stay. *J Interventional Cardiac Electrophysiol.* 2013;37:223-231.
54. Kaiser D, Streur MM, Nagarakanti R, et al. Continuous warfarin versus periprocedural dabigatran to reduce stroke and systemic embolism in patients undergoing catheter ablation for atrial fibrillation or left atrial flutter Journal 2013, Volume 37, Issue 3, 241-247.
55. Kim JS1, She F, Jongnarangsin K, et al. Dabigatran vs. warfarin for radiofrequency catheter ablation of atrial fibrillation. *Heart Rhythm.* 2013;10(4):483-489.
56. Bassiouny M, Saliba W, Rickard J, et al. Use of Dabigatran for Peri-Procedural Anticoagulation in Patients Undergoing Catheter Ablation for Atrial Fibrillation. *Circ Arrhthym Electrophysiol.* 2013:6:460-466.
57. Providência R, Marijon R, Albenque J-P, et al. Rivaroxaban and dabigatran in patients undergoing catheter ablation of atrial fibrillation. Europace online DOI: http://dx.doi.org/10.1093/europace/euu007
58. Noheria A, Asirvatham S. Periprocedural dabigatran anticoagulation for atrial fibrillation ablation: do we have enough information to make a rational decision. *J Interv Card Electr.* 2013;37(3):209-211.
59. Naccarelli GV, Cappato R, Hohnloser S et al: Rationale and design of VENTURE-AF: a randomized, open-label, active-controlled multicenter study to evaluate the safety of rivaroxaban and vitamin K antagonists in subjects undergoing catheter ablation for atrial fibrillation. *J Interv Card Electr.* 2014;41,107-116.
60. January C, WannS, Alpert JS, et al for the ACC-AHA-HRS Task Force: 2014 AHA/ACC/HRS Guideline for the Management of Patients With Atrial Fibrillation: Executive Summary. *JACC.* 2014;64:2246-2280.
61. Schumacher B, Pfeiffer D, Tebbenjohanns J, Lewalter T, Jung W, Luderitz B. Acute and long-term effects of consecutive radiofrequency applications on conduction properties of the subeustachian isthmus in type I atrial flutter. *J Cardiovasc Electrophysiol.* 1998;9:152-163.
62. Tai CT, Chen SA, Chiang CE, Lee SH, Wen ZC, Huang JL, et al. Long-term outcome of radiofrequency catheter ablation for typical atrial flutter: risk prediction of recurrent arrhythmias. *J Cardiovasc Electr.* 1998;9:115-21.
63. Natale A, Newby KH, Pisanó E, Leonelli F, et al. Prospective randomized comparison of antiarrhythmic therapy versus first-line radiofrequency ablation in patients with atrial flutter. *J Am Coll Cardiol.* 2000;35(7):1898-1904.
64. Jaïs P, Shah DC, Haïssaguerre M, Hocini M, Peng JT, Takahashi A, et al. Mapping and ablation of left atrial flutters. *Circulation.* 2000;101:2928-2934.

65. Coffey JO, d'Avila A, Dukkipati S et al. Catheter ablation of scar-related atypical atrial Flutter. *Europace*. 2013;15, 414-419.
66. Stabile G, De Simone A, Turco, P, et al. Response to flecainide infusion predicts long-term success of hybrid pharmacologic and ablation therapy in patients with atrial fibrillation. *J Am Coll Cardiol*. 2001;37,1639-1644.
67. Turco P, De Simone A, La Rocca V, et al. Long-term results of hybrid therapy in patients with atrial fibrillation who develop atrial flutter during flecainide infusion. *PACE*. 2005;28 (Suppl 1), S124-S127.
68. Anastasio N, Frankel DS, Deyell M, et al. Nearly uniform failure of atrial flutter ablation and continuation of antiarrhythmic agents (hybrid therapy) for the long-term control of atrial fibrillation. *J Interv Cardiac Electr*. 2012;35:57-61.

CHAPTER 63

Ventricular Tachycardia and Ventricular Fibrillation

Indrajit Choudhuri, MD; Masood Akhtar, MD

Organization, Scope, and Rationale

This chapter will address the interventional management of ventricular tachyarrhythmias (VTA), focusing on indications and outcomes. This should serve as a source to guide clinically appropriate interventional therapy of VTA, whether ventricular tachycardia (VT) or ventricular fibrillation (VF). This content is not an independent review of the topic, as it has been extensively evaluated by expert panels over the past decade, but rather summarizes the most recent and updated pertinent clinical guidelines and consensus.[1-5] Ventricular fibrillation is handled in this context, as there is scant data to guide therapy for VF as distinct from VT.

Interventional management of VTA primarily relates to ablative and device therapy, which generally includes implantable cardioverter-defibrillators (ICD), but rarely permanent pacemakers (PPMs), as well as the role of invasive electrophysiology (EP) study in guiding therapy. While ICD therapy for management of VTA and prevention of sudden cardiac death (SCD) has been studied extensively, as has the role of EP study, the data for catheter ablation is relatively new as techniques evolve and relevant follow-up duration for reporting is achieved. For consistency and meaningful evaluation of outcomes, clinical characteristics, specific VT morphologies (Table 63.1), and reporting standards with respect to catheter ablation must be defined.[4]

When considering management of patients with VTA and SCD, decisions regarding interventional EP therapy hinge on the presence of structural or electrical heart disease and the resulting elevated sudden death risk, and whether ICD therapy is indicated, with the caveat that consideration of ICD therapy is applicable only to patients who receive optimal medical therapy and have a reasonable expectation of survival with good functional status for more than 1 year. EP testing is often invaluable in providing additional diagnostic data and guiding therapy. In patients with structural heart disease, ablation is generally reserved for those in whom primary ICD therapy has already been prescribed, recurrent ventricular arrhythmias provoke repeated ICD therapies, or ICD therapy is ineffective. VT ablation may also be considered as primary therapy in specific situations, either in conjunction with the ICD or in situations where ICD therapy is inappropriate. In patients with normal hearts (that is, with no ostensible cardiac abnormalities) who present with unstable arrhythmias, ablation can be considered the primary therapeutic option, though an ICD should be strongly considered as well. In general, catheter ablation of VT should be considered early in the treatment of patients with recurrent VT, irrespective of the cardiac substrate.[2]

In the following sections, a focus on VT ablation training requirements is presented first. The remaining indications are presented by disease state, with interventional EP management for secondary prevention of sudden death and structural heart disease presented first, as this is the most common and hence most clinically relevant population presenting with unstable VT/VF and SCD. Primary electrical disorders are presented next—although the rarest of clinical entities, they do represent a form of heart disease and are discussed separately from truly normal hearts. VTA in normal hearts are discussed with a shift in the focus of interventional EP therapy from ICD to VT ablation as first-line therapy. Additional sections are offered discussing interventional EP therapy for VT in special populations including pediatric and congenital heart disease patients as well as a brief section on polymorphic VT/VF.

Table 63.1 Definitions

Clinical Characteristics

Clinical ventricular tachycardia (VT) is VT that has occurred spontaneously based on analysis of 12-lead electrocardiographic (ECG) QRS morphology and rate. There are many potential problems and assumptions with this designation as it is applied to inducible VT in the electrophysiology laboratory.

Hemodynamically unstable VT causes hemodynamic compromise requiring prompt termination.

Idiopathic VT is a term that has been used to indicate VT that is known to occur in the absence of clinically apparent structural heart disease.

Idioventricular rhythm is three or more consecutive beats at a rate of < 100/min that originate from the ventricles independent of atrial or atrioventricular (AV) nodal conduction.

Incessant VT is continuous sustained VT that recurs promptly despite repeated intervention for termination over several hours.

Nonclinical VT is a term that has been used to indicate a VT induced by programmed ventricular stimulation that has not been documented previously. This term is problematic because some VTs that have not been previously observed will occur spontaneously. It is recommended that this term be avoided. Induced VTs with a QRS morphology that has not been previously observed should be referred to as "undocumented VT morphology."

Nonsustained VT terminates spontaneously within 30 seconds.

Presumptive clinical VT is similar to a spontaneous VT based on rate and ECG or electrogram data available from implantable cardioverter-defibrillator (ICD) interrogation, but without the 12-lead ECG documentation of either the induced or spontaneous VT.

Repetitive monomorphic VT is continuously repeating episodes of self-terminating nonsustained VT.

Sustained VT is a continuous VT for ≥ 30 seconds or that requires an intervention for termination (such as cardioversion).

Ventricular tachycardia is a tachycardia (rate > 100/min) with three or more consecutive beats that originate from the ventricles independent of atrial or AV nodal conduction.

VT storm is considered three or more separate episodes of sustained VT within 24 hours, each requiring termination by an intervention.

VT Morphologies

Monomorphic VT has a similar QRS configuration from beat to beat. Some variability in QRS morphology at initiation is not uncommon, followed by stabilization of the QRS morphology.

Multiple monomorphic VTs refers to more than one morphologically distinct monomorphic VT, occurring as different episodes or induced at different times.

Polymorphic VT has a continuously changing QRS configuration from beat to beat indicating a changing ventricular activation sequence.

Pleomorphic VT has more than one morphologically distinct QRS complex occurring during the same episode of VT, but the QRS is not continuously changing.

Right and left bundle branch block-like VT configurations are terms used to describe the dominant deflection in V_1, with a dominant R wave described as "right bundle branch block-like" and a dominant S wave as "left bundle branch block-like" configurations. This terminology is potentially misleading as the VT may not show features characteristic of the same bundle branch block-like morphology in other leads.

Unmappable VT does not allow interrogation of multiple sites to define the activation sequence or perform entrainment mapping; this may be due to hemodynamic intolerance that necessitates immediate VT termination, spontaneous or pacing-induced transition to other morphologies of VT, or repeated termination during mapping.

Ventricular flutter is a term that has been applied to rapid VT that has a sinusoidal QRS configuration that prevents identification of the QRS morphology. It is preferable to avoid this term, in favor of monomorphic VT with indeterminate QRS morphology.

Mechanisms

Scar-related reentry describes arrhythmias that have characteristics of reentry and originate from an area of myocardial scar identified from electrogram characteristics or myocardial imaging. Large reentry circuits that can be defined over several centimeters are commonly referred to as "macroreentry."

Focal VT has a point source of earliest ventricular activation with a spread of activation away in all directions from that site. The mechanism can be automaticity, triggered activity, or microreentry.

Source: Reproduced from Aliot et al,[4] with permission from Elsevier.

	CLASS I Benefit >>> Risk Procedure/Treatment SHOULD be performed/administered	CLASS IIa Benefit >> Risk Additional studies with focused objectives needed IT IS REASONABLE to perform procedure/administer treatment	CLASS IIb Benefit ≥ Risk Additional studies with broad objectives needed; additional registry data would be helpful Procedure/Treatment MAY BE CONSIDERED	CLASS III Risk ≥ Benefit Procedure/Treatment should NOT be performed/administered SINCE IT IS NOT HELPFUL AND MAY BE HARMFUL
LEVEL A Multiple populations evaluated* Data derived from multiple randomized clinical trials or meta-analyses	■ Recommendation that procedure or treatment is useful/effective ■ Sufficient evidence from multiple randomized trials or meta-analyses	■ Recommendation in favor of treatment or procedure being useful/effective ■ Some conflicting evidence from multiple randomized trials or meta-analyses	■ Recommendation's usefulness/efficacy less well established ■ Greater conflicting evidence from multiple randomized trials or meta-analyses	■ Recommendation that procedure or treatment is not useful/effective and may be harmful ■ Sufficient evidence from multiple randomized trials or meta-analyses
LEVEL B Limited populations evaluated* Data derived from a single randomized trial or nonrandomized studies	■ Recommendation that procedure or treatment is useful/effective ■ Evidence from single randomized trial or nonrandomized studies	■ Recommendation in favor of treatment or procedure being useful/effective ■ Some conflicting evidence from single randomized trial or nonrandomized studies	■ Recommendation's usefulness/efficacy less well established ■ Greater conflicting evidence from single randomized trial or nonrandomized studies	■ Recommendation that procedure or treatment is not useful/effective and may be harmful ■ Evidence from single randomized trial or nonrandomized studies
LEVEL C Very limited populations evaluated* Only consensus opinion of experts, case studies, or standard of care	■ Recommendation that procedure or treatment is useful/effective ■ Only expert opinion, case studies, or standard of care	■ Recommendation in favor of treatment or procedure being useful/effective ■ Only diverging expert opinion, case studies, or standard of care	■ Recommendation's usefulness/efficacy less well established ■ Only diverging expert opinion, case studies, or standard of care	■ Recommendation that procedure or treatment is not useful/effective and may be harmful ■ Only expert opinion, case studies, or standard of care
Suggested phrases for writing recommendations†	should is recommended is indicated is useful/effective/beneficial	is reasonable can be useful/effective/beneficial is probably recommended or indicated	may/might be considered may/might be reasonable usefulness/effectiveness is unknown/unclear/uncertain or not well established	is not recommended is not indicated should not is not useful/effective/beneficial may be harmful

Estimate of certainty (precision) of treatment effect — vertical axis. Size of treatment effect — horizontal axis.

*Data available from clinical trials or registries about the usefulness/efficacy in different subpopulations, such as gender, age, history of diabetes, history of prior myocardial infarction, history of heart failure, and prior aspirin use. A recommendation with Level of Evidence B or C does not imply that the recommendation is weak. Many important clinical questions addressed in the guidelines do not lend themselves to clinical trials. Even though randomized trials are not available, there may be a very clear clinical consensus that a particular test or therapy is useful or effective.

†In 2003, the ACC/AHA Task Force on Practice Guidelines developed a list of suggested phrases to use when writing recommendations. All guideline recommendations have been written in full sentences that express a complete thought, such that a recommendation, even if separated and presented apart from the rest of the document (including headings above sets of recommendations), would still convey the full intent of the recommendation. It is hoped that this will increase readers' comprehension of the guidelines and will allow queries at the individual recommendation level.

Figure 63.1 Applying classification of recommendations and level of evidence. *Source:* Epstein et al,[1] with permission from Wolters Kluwer Health.

Classification of Recommendations

The recommendations for indications contained herein pertain to the *interventional* management of patients with ventricular arrhythmias and prevention of SCD, and recapitulate the pertinent clinical evidence and expert opinion reviewed in five documents: (1) 2008 Guidelines for Device-Based Therapy of Cardiac Rhythm Abnormalities, (2) 2006 Guidelines for Management of Patients with Ventricular Arrhythmias and the Prevention of Sudden Cardiac Death, (3) COCATS Task Force 6, (4) the consensus document on VT ablation, and (5) evaluation of syncope guidelines,[1-5] and is supplemented by additional sources. Together they comprise data gathered through review of more than 500 primary and secondary source documents, resulting in the classification of recommendations and level of evidence as expressed in the ACC/AHA/ESC format (Figure 63.1, Table 63.2).

Table 63.2 Guidelines for classification of recommendations and level of evidence

Classification of Recommendations

- Class I: Conditions for which there is evidence and/or general agreement that a given procedure or treatment is beneficial, useful, and effective.
- Class II: Conditions for which there is conflicting evidence and/or divergence of opinion about the usefulness/efficacy of a procedure or treatment.
- Class IIa: Weight of evidence/opinion is in favor of usefulness/efficacy.
- Class IIb: Usefulness/efficacy is less well established by evidence/opinion.
- Class III: Conditions for which there is evidence and/or general agreement that a procedure/treatment is not useful/effective and in some cases may be harmful.

Level of Evidence

- Level of Evidence A: Data derived from multiple randomized clinical trials or meta-analyses.
- Level of Evidence B: Data derived from a single randomized trial or nonrandomized studies.
- Level of Evidence C: Only consensus opinion of experts, case studies, or standard-of-care.

Standards and Requirements for Meaningful Application of Interventional Electrophysiologic Therapy for VTA

Training Requirements in Clinical Cardiac Electrophysiology

Clinical cardiac electrophysiology training includes a minimum of 4 years of training in clinical cardiology and EP. Current Accreditation Council for Graduate Medical Education requirements specify a 3-year training program in general cardiology, consisting of a core 24-month clinical program and an additional 12 months, which may involve research and/or elective time in EP. A dedicated 4th year of training in clinical cardiac EP is required.[3]

To complete Level 3 certification in cardiac EP procedures, in addition to Level 1 and 2 requirements, trainees should perform at least 150 EP procedures as the designated primary operator and analyze 100–150 initial diagnostic studies covering the breadth of arrhythmias, with a minimum of 50–75 for supraventricular arrhythmias. The trainee must also have been a primary operator during more than 25 EP evaluations of implantable antiarrhythmic devices.[3]

Trainees must demonstrate proficiency with surgical asepsis principles, implantation techniques, and management of implant-related complications, and participate as the primary operator (under direct supervision) in at least 25 ICD, 25 dual-chamber pacemakers or defibrillators, and 25 cardiac resynchronization therapy (CRT) device implant procedures. Furthermore, 30 cardiac implantable electronic device (CIED) revisions or replacements, including at least 10 ICD revisions as the primary operator, are a requisite for Level 3 qualification. Specialists intending to provide expert care in ICD and cardiac resynchronization management must achieve Level 3 proficiency in EP and CIED implant techniques during their general cardiology and advanced training, and must also perform a minimum of at least 200 ICD and permanent pacemaker (PPM) interrogations. Training must include stimulation-threshold testing and device programming. An extensive knowledge of ICD indications, contraindications, and management of complications is mandatory, as is the ability to determine defibrillation thresholds and manage high defibrillation thresholds, an understanding of drug and pacemaker/ICD interactions, and a thorough knowledge of ICD programming. Trainees must also have extensive knowledge of left ventricular lead indications and contraindications, and management of biventricular malfunctions and interactions, as well as postoperative complications (Table 63.3).[3]

Table 63.3 Core cardiac arrhythmia and electrophysiology curriculum training

Level	Minimum Number of Procedures	Cumulative Duration of Training (months)
1	10 temporary pacemakers	2
	10 cardioversions	
2	100 CIED interrogations/programming	6
3	150+ EP cases	12–24
	75 ablations	
	30–50 atrial fibrillation ablations	
	10+ transseptal procedures	
	75 CIED (25 ICD, 25 dual-chamber devices, 25 CRT devices)	
	30 CIED revisions/replacements	
	200 CIED interrogations/programming (100 ICDs, 100 pacemakers)	

CIED = cardiac implantable electrical device; CRT = cardiac resynchronization therapy; EP = electrophysiology; ICD = implantable cardioverter-defibrillator.
Source: Reproduced from Naccarelli et al,[3] with permission from Elsevier.

Catheter Ablation of VTA: Facility Standards

Catheter mapping and ablation in patients with ventricular arrhythmias is challenging and requires advanced technical skills and dexterity. VT ablation procedures should be performed in experienced centers that have a dedicated EP program adequately equipped to offer appropriate patient assessment and selection, treatment strategies, and follow-up after ablation (Table 63.4).

Only fully trained cardiac electrophysiologists should perform ablation for ventricular arrhythmias, and training and operator skills must continue to advance and evolve with strategies, methods, and technology. Physicians entering training programs that include VT ablation must be familiar with current cardiopulmonary resuscitation (CPR) techniques.[4] Trainees must already be comfortable with ablation techniques for supraventricular tachycardias and should comply with the requirements specified in the American College of Cardiology (ACC)/American Heart Association (AHA) 2006 Update of the Clinical Competence Statement on Invasive Electrophysiology Studies, Catheter Ablation and Cardioversion.

Table 63.4 Specialized training for VT ablation

Specialized Training for VT Ablation Must Address:
1. Selection of patients who may benefit from an ablation procedure.
2. Thorough knowledge of the anatomy of the ventricles, the valvular apparatus, and coronary vasculature.
3. Knowledge of different mechanisms that potentially cause ventricular arrhythmias.
4. Knowledge of other treatment modalities (including antiarrhythmic drugs, implantable defibrillators, and surgery).
5. Cardiac hemodynamics and the potential deleterious hemodynamic effects of ventricular arrhythmias.
6. Recognition, prevention, and management of complications.
7. Current strategies, methods, and technology for VT ablation procedures, including state-of-the-art imaging techniques.
8. How to perform structured patient screening, selection, treatment, and follow-up.
9. Technical skills.

Source: Reproduced from Aliot et al,[4] with permission from Elsevier.

VT ablation should be performed only at institutions meeting certain minimum requirements, including availability of a dedicated, adequately equipped EP suite fitted with appropriate tools and technology for complex arrhythmia mapping and ablation as well as personnel trained in CPR and experienced in monitoring and assisting ablation procedures. The facility also must have available anesthesiology services, interventional cardiology, and onsite immediate cardiac surgery capability.[4]

Specific Recommendations for Interventional EP Therapy for VTA

Patients with Structural Heart Disease

Secondary Prevention of Sudden Cardiac Death

Secondary prevention refers to prevention of SCD in patients who survived cardiac arrest or sustained VT. Patients with cardiac conditions associated with a high risk of SCD who have unexplained syncope, likely due to ventricular arrhythmias, are also considered to carry a secondary indication. Accordingly, in patients with unexplained syncope in whom clinically relevant VT/VF is induced at EP study, the induced arrhythmia is assumed to underlie syncope, and such patients should be considered candidates for ICD therapy. Of note, while SCD related to VF or unstable VT is rare in patients without structural heart disease, an unstable presentation warrants ICD therapy whether heart disease is present or not and irrespective of whether ablation is performed, except in specific instances, such as rapid conduction of atrial fibrillation (AF) over an accessory pathway, in which durable success can be anticipated. Accordingly, current data supporting ICD therapy in patients with structural heart disease and prior SCD from VF/unstable VT is presented (Table 63.5). It may seem a philosophical question whether patients already prescribed ICD therapy remain at risk for SCD from ventricular arrhythmias; however, syncope (and rarely, sudden death) can still occur if ICD therapy is delayed or ineffective. Hence, VT ablation in patients with structural heart disease is also presented in this section.[1,2,4,5]

ICD Trials

Trials of ICD therapy in patients resuscitated from cardiac arrest demonstrate survival benefits with ICD compared to EP-guided drug therapy using class I agents, sotalol, and empirical amiodarone. In the largest of these,[6] unadjusted survival estimates were 89.3% versus 2.3% at 1 year, 81.6% versus 74.7% at 2 years, and 75.4% versus 64.1% at 3 years ($P = 0.02$) for the ICD group and the antiarrhythmic drug group, respectively. Relative risk reduction with ICD therapy was 39% (95% confidence interval [CI]: 19%–59%) at 1 year, 27% (95% CI: 6%–48%) at 2 years, and 31% (95% CI: 10%–52%) at 3 years, and this has been confirmed in subsequent trials. Large prospective secondary prevention trials—Antiarrhythmics Versus Implantable Defibrillators (AVID),[6] Cardiac Arrest Study Hamburg (CASH),[7] and Canadian Implantable Defibrillator Study (CIDS)[8]—have demonstrated a 50% relative risk reduction in arrhythmic death and a 25% relative risk reduction in all-cause mortality with ICD therapy. In general for secondary prevention of SCD, there are ample and robust data showing a consistent effect of improved survival with ICD therapy compared with antiarrhythmic drug therapy (Table 63.6).[1]

Coronary Artery Disease

Patients with coronary artery disease (CAD) represent the majority of patients receiving ICDs in trials of secondary prevention of sudden death. Between 73% and 83% of patients enrolled in the AVID, CASH, and CIDS trials had underlying CAD,[6-8] and evidence strongly supports a survival benefit in such patients with an ICD compared with other therapeutic options. The mean left ventricular ejection fraction (LVEF) ranged from 32% to 45% in these

Table 63.5 Major ICD trials for prevention of sudden cardiac death

Trial	Year	Patients (n)	Inclusion Criteria: LVEF % Less Than or Equal to	Other Inclusion Criteria	Hazard Ratio*	95% Confidence Interval	P Value
MADIT I	1996	196	35	NSVT and positive EP	0.46	0.26-0.82	0.009
MADIT II	2002	1,232	30	Prior myocardial infarction	0.69	0.51-0.93	0.016
CABG-Patch	1997	900	36	Positive SAECG and CABG	1.07	0.81-1.42	0.64
DEFINITE	2004	485	35	NICM, PVCs, or NSVT	0.65	0.40-1.06	0.08
DINAMIT	2004	674	35	6 to 40 days after myocardial infarction and impaired HRV	1.08	0.76-1.55	0.66
SCD-HeFT	2005	1,676	35	Prior myocardial infarction or NICM	0.77	0.62-0.96	0.007
AVID	1997	1,016	40	Prior cardiac arrest	0.62	0.43-0.82	<0.02
CASH†	2000	191	M: 45 ± 18 at baseline	Prior cardiac arrest	0.77	1.112‡	0.081§
CIDS	2000	659	35	Prior cardiac arrest, syncope	0.82	0.60-1.10	NS

*HAZARD ratios for death due to any cause in the ICD group compared with the non-ICD group.
†Includes only ICD and amiodarone patients from CASH.
‡Upper bound of 97.5% confidence interval.
§One-tailed.

AVID = Antiarrhythmics Versus Implantable Defibrillators; CABG = coronary artery bypass graft surgery; CASH = Cardiac Arrest Study Hamburg; CIDS = Canadian Implantable Defibrillator Study; DEFINITE = Defibrillators in Nonischemic Cardiomyopathy Treatment Evaluation; DINAMIT = Defibrillator in Acute Myocardial Infarction Trial; EP = electrophysiological study; HRV = heart rate variability; LVEF = left ventricular ejection fraction; MADIT I = Multicenter Automatic Defibrillator Implantation Trial I; MADIT II = Multicenter Automatic Defibrillator Implantation Trial II; myocardial infarction = myocardial infarction; NICM = nonischemic cardiomyopathy; NS = not statistically significant; NSVT = nonsustained ventricular tachycardia; PVCs = premature ventricular complexes; SAECG = signal-averaged electrocardiogram; and SCD-HeFT = Sudden Cardiac Death in Heart Failure Trial. *Source:* Reproduced from Epstein et al,[1] with permission from Wolters Kluwer Health.

Table 63.6 Recommendations for ICD therapy for secondary prevention of ventricular tachyarrhythmias and sudden cardiac death in structural heart disease

Class I

1. ICD therapy is indicated in patients who are survivors of cardiac arrest due to VF or hemodynamically unstable sustained VT after evaluation to define the cause of the event and to exclude any completely reversible causes (Level of Evidence: A).
2. ICD therapy is indicated in patients with structural heart disease and spontaneous sustained VT, whether hemodynamically stable or unstable (Level of Evidence: B).
3. ICD therapy is indicated in patients with syncope of undetermined origin with clinically relevant, hemodynamically significant sustained VT or VF induced at EP study (Level of Evidence: B).

Class IIa

1. ICD implantation is reasonable for patients with unexplained syncope, significant left ventricular dysfunction, and NIDCM (Level of Evidence: C).
2. ICD implantation is reasonable for patients with sustained VT and normal or near-normal ventricular function with or without structural heart disease (Level of Evidence: C).
3. ICD therapy is reasonable in patients who have recurrent stable VT, a normal or near-normal LVEF, and optimally treated heart failure (Level of Evidence: C).

EP = electrophysiology; ICD = implantable cardioverter-defibrillator; LVEF = left ventricular ejection fraction; NIDCM = nonischemic dilated cardiomyopathy; VF = ventricular fibrillation; VT = ventricular tachycardia. *Source:* Data collected from references 1–5.

trials with left ventricular dysfunction attributed largely to prior myocardial infarction, and multiple analyses have demonstrated that patients with left ventricular dysfunction may experience greater survival benefit with an ICD compared with drug therapy, though optimum medical treatment should be prescribed in all patients.[1] Patients experiencing cardiac arrest due to VF that occurs more than 48 hours after myocardial infarction may be at risk for recurrent cardiac arrest, and such patients should be evaluated and optimally treated for ischemia. If ischemia immediately preceding the onset of VF is implicated without evidence of prior myocardial infarction, complete coronary revascularization should be the primary goal as opposed to patients with evidence of myocardial infarction in whom target vessel revascularization may be adequate. If coronary revascularization is not possible and there is evidence of significant left ventricular dysfunction, patients resuscitated from VF should be considered candidates for ICD therapy if there is reasonable neurocognitive recovery and expected survival of more than 1 year.[1]

Cardiac biomarkers may be released not only in acute coronary syndrome but also heart failure, renal failure, the ventricular arrhythmia itself, and possibly even repeated defibrillation shocks, and can sometimes confound the evaluation of such patients. Patients with CAD who present with sustained monomorphic VT or VF and low-level elevations of cardiac biomarkers should be treated similarly to patients who have sustained VT and no documented rise in biomarkers because prolonged episodes of sustained monomorphic VT or VF may impose myocardial metabolic demands that exceed supply in patients with CAD. In this case, the result would be myocyte injury/necrosis and release of cardiac troponin. Evaluation for ischemia should be undertaken; however, it should not be assumed that a new myocardial infarction was the cause of sustained VT or biomarker elevation. In the absence of data to support acute myocardial infarction, such patients may be considered at risk for recurrent sustained VT or VF and should be treated as patients without biomarker release.[1]

Nonischemic Dilated Cardiomyopathy

Patients with nonischemic dilated cardiomyopathy (NIDCM) and prior episodes of VF or sustained VT are at high risk for recurrent VTA and cardiac arrest. Empirical antiarrhythmic therapy or drug therapy guided by EP testing does not improve survival.[1] ICD therapy has been shown to be superior to amiodarone for secondary prevention of VT and VF,[7-9] and NIDCM subgroups benefited similarly or more than ischemic heart failure groups.[6-8] On this basis, consideration for ICD therapy is appropriate and preferred in patients with NIDCM who are resuscitated from cardiac arrest caused by VF or VT.[1]

Hypertrophic Cardiomyopathy

Hypertrophic cardiomyopathy is the most common cause of cardiac arrest in individuals younger than 40 years, affecting approximately 1 of every 500 persons in the general population. Sudden death may be its first manifestation, but hypertrophic cardiomyopathy should be particularly suspected in young individuals suffering cardiac arrest during exertion, as exercise increases the risk of life-threatening VTA. A history of prior cardiac arrest portends a substantial risk of future events. Although no randomized data are available, in patients with cardiac arrest and sustained VT or VF, a high percentage of patients receive appropriate ICD discharge during follow-up at a rate of 11% per year.[1] Hence, the ICD is the preferred therapy for patients with hypertrophic cardiomyopathy resuscitated from prior cardiac arrest.[1]

Arrhythmogenic Right Ventricular Dysplasia/Cardiomyopathy

Arrhythmogenic right ventricular dysplasia/cardiomyopathy (ARVD/C) is a genetic condition characterized by fibrofatty infiltration of the right ventricle and, less commonly, the left ventricle. It usually manifests clinically with sustained monomorphic VT of left bundle branch block morphology in young individuals during exercise. Indicators of high risk include prior cardiac arrest, unexplained syncope, syncope due to VT, and presentation with polymorphic VT (PMVT), and constitute a secondary prevention indication. No prospective trials of pharmacological therapy versus ICD therapy for secondary prevention of SCD have been conducted in patients with ARVD/C; however, observational reports consistently demonstrate a high frequency of appropriate ICD use for life-threatening ventricular arrhythmias and a very low rate of arrhythmic death in patients treated with ICD.[1]

EP Evaluation of Patients with Structural Heart Disease Presenting with Wide QRS Tachycardia or Unstable VTA

In patients presenting with wide QRS tachycardia, the diagnosis of VT should be suspected in patients with structural heart disease (positive predictive value 95%) and electrocardiographic (ECG) evidence of prior myocardial infarction (positive predictive value 98%); the correct diagnosis may be made in most patients from the surface ECG when appropriate morphologic criteria are collectively applied. Yet the misdiagnosis of wide QRS tachycardia is common and may have serious implications for the patient, including mismanagement and death. EP testing has proven invaluable in distinguishing the various etiologies and origin of wide QRS tachycardia. With few exceptions, patients with wide QRS tachycardia in whom the nature of the arrhythmic problem is not known or the direction of therapy is not clear should undergo EP study.[10,11]

In patients suffering cardiac arrest, if the onset of arrhythmia is documented, VF is often identified as the initial cause. Patients dying suddenly often have underlying structural heart disease (usually CAD or primary myocardial disease) and are prone to VT/VF due to electrical instability. Hence, both the nature and extent of organic heart disease as well as vulnerability to recurrent VT/VF should be investigated (Table 63.7). EP study is considered a routine part of the overall patient assessment in this group of individuals.[12]

EP studies in survivors of VT/VF are desirable for a variety of reasons. First, in our experience, almost 40% of patients with monomorphic VT in association with idiopathic dilated cardiomyopathy (DCM) and valvular heart disease have bundle branch reentry as the underlying mechanism. This is preferably managed with bundle branch ablation, which is curative, rather than with ICD alone.[11] Second, several VT morphologies or other arrhythmias may be identified in addition to the presenting/clinical VT. Rapid supraventricular tachycardia may require separate attention to prevent unnecessary ICD shocks, either through antiarrhythmic therapy or ablation. The coexistence of sick sinus or conduction system disease may be aggravated by antiarrhythmic therapy and necessitate pacing. Awareness preoperatively would contribute to appropriate device selection. Finally, in rare instances, supraventricular arrhythmia may trigger VT/VF. This may happen in patients with severe CAD, congestive heart failure, or Wolff–Parkinson–White (WPW) syndrome, to name a few scenarios. Elimination of the underlying triggers should be the primary therapeutic approach with the need for an ICD a secondary concern.

Table 63.7 Recommendations for EP testing for secondary prevention of ventricular tachyarrhythmias and sudden cardiac death in structural heart disease

Class I

1. EP testing is recommended for diagnostic evaluation of patients with remote myocardial infarction or NIDCM with symptoms suggestive of ventricular tachyarrhythmias including palpitations, presyncope, and syncope (Level of Evidence: B).
2. EP testing is recommended in patients with syncope of unknown cause with impaired left ventricular function or structural heart disease (Level of Evidence: B).
3. EP testing is useful in patients with coronary artery disease for the diagnostic evaluation of wide QRS complex tachycardias of unclear mechanism (Level of Evidence: C).
4. EP testing is useful to diagnose bundle branch reentrant tachycardia and to guide ablation in patients with NIDCM (Level of Evidence: C).
5. EP testing is useful for diagnostic evaluation in patients with NIDCM with sustained palpitations, wide QRS complex tachycardia, presyncope, or syncope. (Level of Evidence: C).

EP = electrophysiology; NIDCM = nonischemic dilated cardiomyopathy.
Source: Data collected from references 1–5.

EP Testing in Patients with Structural Heart Disease Presenting with Unexplained Syncope

Syncope in patients with structural heart disease, particularly in the setting of significant left ventricular dysfunction, is ominous due to its association with high recurrence and death rates.[1,2] The goal of evaluating syncope in such patients is to establish risk of sudden death and potential causes.[5] EP testing may achieve a diagnostic yield of 50% in CAD patients but is not sensitive in patients with NIDCM. In patients with syncope of undetermined origin in whom clinically relevant VT/VF is induced at EP study, the induced arrhythmia may be expected to explain syncope, and such patients should be considered candidates for ICD therapy.[1,2] Alternatively, induction of polymorphic VT or VF with aggressive stimulation techniques is not specific and must be considered in a clinical context.[11,12]

Coronary Artery Disease

In CAD patients who develop syncope, the risk of death varies directly with degree of left ventricular dysfunction. Such patients should undergo EP testing after excluding other potential reversible causes, particularly ischemia.[5] EP testing for sudden death risk stratification is useful in patients with left ventricular dysfunction (LVEF < 40%) due to prior myocardial infarction; though independent of LVEF, patients with CAD and syncope who have inducible monomorphic VT should be prescribed ICD therapy. Inducible VT is less likely in patients with relatively preserved left ventricular function (LVEF ≥ 35%), but despite the low yield, EP testing remains appropriate given the dire consequences (Table 63.7). Furthermore, considering that patients with moderate or worse left ventricular dysfunction (LVEF ≤ 35%) receive substantial survival benefits from ICD therapy without EP testing, patients with syncope and severe ischemic cardiomyopathy are appropriate candidates for ICD therapy irrespective of the results of EP testing.[1,2,5]

Nonischemic Dilated Cardiomyopathy

In patients with NIDCM, syncope is associated with increased mortality.[5] The likely reason is that syncope occurs due to self-terminating ventricular arrhythmias that can lead to sudden death if sustained or incessant. In patients with NIDCM and clinical presentation suspicious for ventricular arrhythmias, including syncope, near-syncope, and wide QRS tachycardia, EP study should be performed (Table 63.7), though programmed ventricular stimulation in patients with NIDCM generally has poor sensitivity and negative predictive value[1,2,5] compared to patients with CAD. Studies including NIDCM patients presenting with syncope have demonstrated a 45% 1-year mortality in patients with advanced heart failure[13] regardless of the cause of syncope, and in patients undergoing EP testing, the appropriate shock rate was 50% by 2 years, similar to NIDCM patients who presented with cardiac arrest.[14] Furthermore, a disproportionately high number of appropriate ICD shocks has been seen in patients with NIDCM presenting with syncope and *negative EP testing*.[15] As NIDCM patients *without syncope* are known to benefit from ICD therapy[16,17] and syncope is felt to further increase the risk of sudden death due to VTA, ICD therapy is appropriate in patients with NIDCM presenting with syncope.[5]

Role of VT Ablation in Structural Heart Disease

VT is a common complication of structural heart disease and carries significant risk for mortality in patients with low LVEF. In those with extensive structural abnormalities, especially prior myocardial infarction but also in patients with diffuse scarring, multiple morphologies of VT are often present. Hence, ablation of a single VT morphology can provide palliation but not eliminate the need for device or antiarrhythmic therapy. VT can originate in or involve extensive areas of the myocardium, and irrigated radiofrequency ablation improves outcomes.[18] Mapping techniques have been developed that distinguish bystander regions from critical components of the VT circuits.[18-21] Three-dimensional mapping systems permit anatomical reconstructions and correlation of EP characteristics with anatomy and permit mapping during sinus rhythm, thereby facilitating ablation in patients who do not tolerate VT well. Use of these techniques may result in better long-term success rates.[2,4]

In general, patient outcome is reasonably good after VT ablation, and procedural mortality and morbidity are acceptable. Ablation usually reduces the frequency of VT episodes. The use of mapping systems to guide radiofrequency delivery and maintain lesions in low-voltage regions is recommended to reduce risk of damage to functioning myocardium. In general, it is felt that ablation should be considered relatively early, before multiple recurrences of VT and repeated courses of drug therapy (Table 63.8).[4,18]

Table 63.8 Recommendations for ablation and adjunctive therapies for management of ventricular tachycardia and prevention of sudden cardiac death

Class I

1. Ablation is indicated as adjunctive therapy in patients with an ICD who are receiving multiple shocks as a result of sustained VT that is not manageable by reprogramming or changing drug therapy or who do not wish long-term drug therapy (Level of Evidence: C).
2. Ablation is indicated in patients with bundle branch reentrant VT (Level of Evidence: C).

Class IIa

1. Catheter ablation can be useful for patients with implanted ICDs who experience incessant or frequently recurring VT (Level of Evidence: B).
2. In patients experiencing inappropriate ICD therapy, EP evaluation can be useful for diagnostic and therapeutic purposes (Level of Evidence: C).

EP = electrophysiology; ICD = implantable cardioverter-defibrillator; VT = ventricular tachycardia. *Source:* Data collected from references 1–5.

Considerations in Patients with ICDs

Patients undergoing catheter ablation of VT usually have a previously implanted ICD or will undergo device implantation after ablation. Radiofrequency ablation may affect both the myocardial VT substrate and ICD pacing and sensing. Stimulation thresholds and intracardiac electrogram amplitudes should be measured before and after ablation to ensure appropriate device function. As radiofrequency current can result in an increase in myocardial stimulation threshold of a previously implanted lead, the stimulus amplitude should be programmed to anticipate a rise in pacing threshold. If electrogram amplitude has decreased substantially, and particularly if it is under 3 mV, VF induction may be indicated to ensure effective sensing by the ICD.[4]

In general, the results of catheter ablation of VT should have little influence on the indications for ICD implantation. Most patients who have VT related to structural heart disease will continue to have a standard indication for ICD therapy for primary prevention. The VT recurrence rate remains substantial even when all VTs have been rendered noninducible, so secondary prophylaxis remains indicated.[4]

Outcomes of VT Ablation in Patients with Prior Myocardial Infarction

Patient series reported from single centers vary with respect to disease severity, VT characteristics and associated hemodynamic tolerability, mapping and ablation techniques, and ablation endpoints. Of 802 patients from 19 centers reported in the past decade, at least one VT was ablated in 72% to 96% of patients, and all inducible VTs were ablated in 38% to 72% of patients,[4] with associated procedure-related mortality of 0.5%. In studies reporting mean follow-up longer than 1 year, 50% to 88% of patients were free of VT, with the necessity to continue antiarrhythmic therapy ranging from 30% to 100%. Mortality during follow-up ranged from 0% to 32%.[4]

The Multicenter Thermocool Ventricular Tachycardia Ablation Trial[22] enrolled patients with recurrent VT (median of 11 episodes in the previous 6 months) for ablation with open-irrigation radiofrequency guided by electroanatomic mapping using substrate and/or entrainment mapping. In the 231 patients enrolled, median LVEF was 25%, median age was 68 years, 62% had clinical heart failure, 70% had failed amiodarone, and 94% had an ICD. Multiple VTs were inducible (median of 3 inducible VTs per patient) and VT was unmappable in 69% of patients. Ablation abolished at least 1 VT in 81% of patients, and all VTs were rendered noninducible in 49% of patients. Accordingly, recurrent VT during 6 months of follow-up occurred in 51%, but the frequency of VT was markedly reduced in a large number of patients. In patients with ICD for at least 6 months before and after ablation, the median number of VT episodes was reduced from 11 to 0, and 67% of patients had a >75% reduction in VT occurrences. The 1-year mortality was 15%, with two-thirds of deaths due to a relatively equal proportion of either VTA or heart failure. No strokes or thromboembolic events occurred, and procedure-related mortality was 3%, with 6 deaths related to uncontrollable VT and 1 due to tamponade with myocardial infarction.[4,22]

A similar study, the Euro-VT-Study,[23] performed open-irrigated catheter ablation guided by electroanatomic mapping in 63 patients from 8 centers. Patients had a median of 17 VT episodes in the 6 months prior to ablation with an average of 3 inducible VT. Most (two-thirds) had unmappable VT. At least 1 VT was ablated in 81% of patients; all inducible VTs were abolished in ~50%

of patients. Procedure-related mortality was 2.7%, and during 6 months of follow-up, 51% of patients remained free of VT.[4,23]

The Substrate Mapping and Ablation in Sinus Rhythm to Halt Ventricular Tachycardia (SMASH-VT) multicenter study[24] enrolled 128 patients with prior myocardial infarction (average age 67 ± 9 years; LVEF 30%–32%) who were receiving an initial ICD for secondary prevention of VF, unstable VT, or syncope with inducible VT. In SMASH-VT, 102 patients were randomized to substrate-based ablation or no ablation. No procedure-related deaths occurred. During mean follow-up of 23 months, 33% of the control group, but only 12% of the ablation group, received appropriate ICD therapy for VT or VF. There was a nonsignificant trend toward improved mortality in the ablation arm (9% vs 17%, $P = 0.29$). Prophylactic VT ablation in patients with ICDs implanted for primary or secondary prevention is investigational, and further trials are needed to assess this approach.[4,24]

Catheter ablation can be immediately lifesaving for patients with VT storm or incessant VT.[4] Electrical storm can be controlled acutely in more than 90% of patients. During follow-up, 74% to 92% remained free of incessant VT or VT storm, although single episodes of VT recurred in approximately a third of patients. It is relevant that these results suggest that successful catheter ablation of VT storm is not only feasible but may impact prognosis, as VT storm recurrence is associated with higher mortality.[4,18,25,26]

Outcomes of VT Ablation in Nonischemic Cardiomyopathy

Studies of catheter ablation of myocardial VT are from small single-center series.[27-29] In 19 patients with recurrent sustained monomorphic VT (SMVT) due to DCM, endocardial ablation abolished all inducible VT in 14 patients.[29] After 22 months of follow-up, 5 patients were alive without VT recurrence. In a different series of 22 patients, epicardial mapping and ablation was employed if endocardial ablation failed.[28] Scar-related reentry circuits were identified in the endocardium in 12 patients and in the epicardium in all 7 who underwent epicardial mapping after failed endocardial ablation. All VTs were eliminated in 12 of 22 patients, and at least 1 VT was ablated in an additional 4 patients. During mean follow-up of 11 months (334 days), VT recurred in 46% of patients, 1 patient died of heart failure, and cardiac transplantation was performed in 2 patients. As for ischemic heart disease, ablation can be lifesaving in patients with incessant VT or VT storm.[2,4]

Outcomes of VT Ablation in Bundle Branch Reentrant VT

Bundle branch reentrant VT is often associated with cardiomyopathy and should be sought in patients with DCM presenting with VT. Catheter ablation of the bundle branches is indicated and is curative of VT in 100% but not of the underlying structural abnormality; therefore, adjunct device therapy should be strongly considered. In patients with clinical heart failure and left ventricular dysfunction, particularly LVEF < 35%, a biventricular ICD should be considered. The right bundle branch is the preferred ablation target, even in patients with baseline left bundle branch block, but backup bradycardia pacing may be required in up to 30% of patients.[2]

Outcomes of VT Ablation in Right Ventricular Dysplasia/Cardiomyopathy

The belief that ARVD/C is a degenerative disorder has greatly influenced treatment plans, specifically leading to the concept that catheter ablation is not curative and is inherently limited as a long-term strategy.[30] Hence catheter ablation of VT in ARVD/C patients is not currently supported by the guidelines as a first-line therapy.

Indeed, the short- and long-term success rates of substrate mapping were evaluated by Verma et al in 22 patients with ARVD/C, using a substrate-based endocardial ablation technique that delivered either linear lesions to connect scar/abnormal myocardium to a valve continuity or other scar, or encircled the scar/abnormal region.[31] Acute procedural success, defined as noninducibility of VT, was achieved in 82% of patients, though VT recurred in 23%, 27%, and 47% of patients after 1, 2, and 3 years of follow-up, respectively.[18] In a study of 24 patients with ARVD/C undergoing 48 endocardial VT ablations, the VT recurrence rate was 85% over a follow-up period of 32 ± 36 months, despite elimination of all clinical VTs in 77% of procedures. The VT recurrence-free survival rate was only 25% at 14 months. These results may reflect, in part, the important procedural limitation that electroanatomic mapping was used in only 10% of procedures, subjecting 90% of patients to a nonsubstrate-based approach that may be less effective, particularly in this population.[18] Furthermore, the approach was limited to an endocardial examination of the myocardium.

In more recent studies, however, it has been demonstrated that disease progression is not uniform and that the occurrence of VT may not be related only to endocardial scar burden. In a small series of patients with ARVD/C presenting for repeat EP study and VT ablation, the majority (9 of 11) did *not* exhibit endocardial disease progression, yet they developed recurrent VT.[30] This suggests that if the endocardial substrate truly remained stable, then recurrent VT may not be due to endocardial disease progression. This implicates the epicardial substrate as potentially relevant to the natural course of patients with ARVC/D, and in the absence of endocardial scar enlargement, efforts to control scar-based VT with ablation seem to have an improved outcome when a combined endocardial and epicardial approach is employed.[32,33]

When combined epicardial-endocardial ablation was performed in patients with recurrent VT after endocardial ablation, 10 of 13 patients (77%) were free of sustained VT during a mean follow-up of 18.3 ± 12.7 months from the last ablation procedure.[32] Similarly, in a prospective evaluation of endocardial ablation compared to endocardial-epicardial ablation in patients with ARVD/C, over a follow-up of at least 3 years, freedom from VT or appropriate ICD therapy was 52.2% (12 of 23) in the group undergoing endocardial ablation only, and 84.6% (22 of 26) in the group undergoing the combined endocardial-epicardial ablative procedure. Also, 5 patients who only received endocardial ablation (5 of 23, 21.7%) and 18 patients who received endocardial and epicardial ablation (18 of 26, 69.2%) were off antiarrhythmic drugs ($P < 0.001$).[33]

Ventricular thinning may increase the risk of perforation, and therefore some authorities advocate avoidance of irrigated-tip ablation, particularly at the right ventricular apex. At the same time, irrigated-tip ablation in the thin-walled dysplastic myocardium may improve ability to achieve complete transmurality, potentially contributing to acute success. Emphasis on rigorous application of the Task Force criteria is critical in identifying appropriate patients.

Although the high early recurrence rate suggested by some studies calls into question the role of early catheter ablation as an effective antiarrhythmic strategy,[18] it also should suggest that lack of scar progression endocardially does not imply stable disease, such that incorporating an epicardial ablation strategy may provide durable suppression of VT.

Primary Prevention of Sudden Cardiac Death

Primary prevention refers to the prevention of SCD in individuals *without* a history of cardiac arrest or sustained VT *but at increased risk,* and includes those with structural and/or primary electrical disease of the heart. Clinical trials have evaluated the risks and benefits of ICD therapy in primary prevention of SCD and have demonstrated improved survival in multiple patient populations with structural heart disease, including those with left ventricular dysfunction and prior myocardial infarction, as well as heart failure due to either CAD or NIDCM. (Primary and secondary prevention trials are summarized in Table 63.5). Prospective registry data are less robust but still useful for risk stratification, and also recommend ICD implantation in other populations, including select patients with structural heart disease such as hypertrophic cardiomyopathy and ARVD/C as well as those with primary electrical disease such as long QT syndrome (long QT syndromes). In other less common structural and electrical disorders (eg, cardiac sarcoidosis, left ventricular noncompaction, Brugada syndrome, catecholaminergic polymorphic VT [CPVT], and short QT syndrome), clinical reports and retrospectively analyzed series provide less rigorous evidence in support of current recommendations for ICD use but constitute the best available evidence in these conditions. While ICD is the mainstay for sudden death prevention in these varied populations, EP study can play a role in determining anticipated risk on which the decision to prescribe ICD therapy hinges. In addition, EP study may be useful in determining the role of ablation in specific primary prevention situations (Tables 63.9 and 63.10).[1,2]

ICD Trials and Role of EP Study in Structural Heart Disease

Coronary Artery Disease

ICD Trials

Substantial clinical trial data has provided evidence supporting use of ICDs in patients with chronic ischemic heart disease, particularly those with prior myocardial infarction and left ventricular dysfunction. Clinical characteristics portending high risk have emerged from these studies, including history of myocardial infarction, spontaneous nonsustained VT (NSVT), inducible VT at EP study, and depressed LVEF (≤35% in Multicenter Automatic Defibrillator Implantation Trial [MADIT][34] or ≤40% in Multicenter Unsustained Tachycardia Trial [MUSTT]).[35] MADIT showed a major relative risk reduction of 54% with ICD. MUSTT was not specifically a trial of ICD therapy because it compared no therapy with EP-guided therapy, but in the group randomized to EP-guided therapy, benefit was seen only among those who received an ICD. In MADIT II,[36] which enrolled 1,232 patients with ischemic cardiomyopathy and LVEF ≤30% without requiring spontaneous or induced arrhythmias, an absolute all-cause mortality reduction of 5.8% (20% control group, 14.2% ICD group) was attributed to ICD therapy (relative risk 31%; $P = 0.016$). The Sudden Cardiac Death in Heart Failure Trial (SCD-HeFT) included patients with NYHA class II or III symptoms due to both ischemic and nonischemic cardiomyopathies and LVEF ≤35%.[16] In patients with ischemic heart disease, the 5-year event rates were 43.2% in the placebo arm and 35.9% in the ICD arm (hazard ratio 0.79; $P = 0.05$) and supported the overall conclusion that ICD therapy in high-risk individuals with CAD results in a net risk reduction for total mortality of between 20% and 30%.[1]

Table 63.9 Recommendations for primary prevention of sudden cardiac death in patients with structural heart disease

Class I

1. ICD therapy is indicated in patients with LVEF < 35% due to prior myocardial infarction who are at least 40 days post–myocardial infarction and categorized as NYHA functional class II or III (Level of Evidence: A).
2. ICD therapy is indicated in patients with nonischemic NIDCM who have an LVEF ≤ 35% and who are categorized as NYHA functional class II or III (Level of Evidence: B).
3. ICD therapy is indicated in patients with left ventricular dysfunction due to prior myocardial infarction who are at least 40 days post-myocardial infarction, have an LVEF < 30%, and are categorized as NYHA functional class I (Level of Evidence: A).
4. ICD therapy is indicated in patients with NSVT due to prior myocardial infarction, LVEF < 40%, and inducible VF or sustained VT at EP study (Level of Evidence: B).

Class IIa

1. ICD implantation is reasonable for patients with unexplained syncope, significant left ventricular dysfunction, and NIDCM (Level of Evidence: C).
2. ICD implantation is reasonable for patients with hypertrophic cardiomyopathy who have 1 or more major risk factors for SCD (Level of Evidence: C).
3. ICD implantation is reasonable for the prevention of SCD in patients with ARVD/C who have 1 or more risk factors for SCD (Level of Evidence: C).
4. ICD implantation is reasonable for nonhospitalized patients awaiting transplantation (Level of Evidence: C).
5. ICD implantation is reasonable for patients with cardiac sarcoidosis, giant cell myocarditis, or Chagas disease (Level of Evidence: C).

Class IIb

1. ICD therapy may be considered in patients with nonischemic heart disease who have LVEF ≤ 35% and are categorized as NYHA class I (Level of Evidence: C).
2. ICD therapy may be considered in patients with syncope and advanced structural heart disease in whom thorough invasive and noninvasive investigations have failed to define a cause (Level of Evidence: C).
3. ICD therapy may be considered in patients with a familial cardiomyopathy associated with SCD (Level of Evidence: C).
4. ICD therapy may be considered in patients with left ventricular noncompaction (Level of Evidence: C).

Class III

1. ICD therapy is not indicated for patients who do not have a reasonable expectation of survival with an acceptable NYHA functional status for at least 1 year, even if they meet ICD implantation criteria specified in the class I, IIa, and IIb recommendations above (Level of Evidence: C).
2. ICD therapy is not indicated for patients with incessant VT or VF (Level of Evidence: C).
3. ICD therapy is not indicated in patients with significant psychiatric illnesses that may be aggravated by device implantation or that may preclude systematic follow-up (Level of Evidence: C).
4. ICD therapy is not indicated for NYHA class IV patients with drug-refractory congestive heart failure who are not candidates for cardiac transplantation or CRT-defibrillator (Level of Evidence: C).
5. ICD therapy is not indicated for syncope of undetermined cause in a patient without inducible ventricular tachyarrhythmias and without structural heart disease (Level of Evidence: C).
6. ICD therapy is not indicated when VF or VT is amenable to surgical or catheter ablation (eg, atrial arrhythmias associated with Wolff-Parkinson-White syndrome, right ventricular or left ventricular outflow tract VT, idiopathic VT, or fascicular VT in the absence of structural heart disease) (Level of Evidence: C).
7. ICD therapy is not indicated for patients with ventricular tachyarrhythmias due to a completely reversible disorder in the absence of structural heart disease (eg, electrolyte imbalance, drugs, or trauma) (Level of Evidence: B).

ARVD/C = arrhythmogenic right ventricular dysplasia/cardiomyopathy; CRT = cardiac resynchronization therapy; EP = electrophysiology; ICD = implantable cardioverter-defibrillator; LVEF = left ventricular ejection fraction; myocardial infarction = myocardial infarction; NIDCM = nonischemic dilated cardiomyopathy; NSVT = nonsustained VT; NYHA = New York Heart Association; SCD = sudden cardiac death; VF = ventricular fibrillation; VT = ventricular tachycardia.
Source: Data collected from references 1–5.

Alternatively, two trials considering two specific clinical scenarios—either at the time of surgical revascularization or within 40 days of an acute myocardial infarction—failed to show improved all-cause survival with ICD therapy. In the Coronary Artery Bypass Graft-Patch (CABG-Patch) trial,[37] routine ICD therapy did not improve survival in patients with CAD undergoing bypass surgery felt to be at high risk of SCD on the basis of an abnormal signal-averaged ECG and moderate left ventricular dysfunction (LVEF ≤ 35%). Similar data about the effects of percutaneous revascularization are not available, though these findings have been extrapolated to patients undergoing percutaneous coronary intervention (PCI). In the Defibrillator in Acute Myocardial Infarction Trial (DINAMIT),[38] 674 patients with a recent myocardial infarction (within 6–40 days), reduced left ventricular function (LVEF ≤ 35%), and impaired cardiac autonomic function (depressed heart rate variability or elevated average heart rate) were randomized to either ICD therapy or no ICD therapy. Arrhythmic death was reduced in the

Table 63.10 Recommendations for EP testing and ablation for primary prevention of ventricular tachyarrhythmias and sudden cardiac death

Class IIa
1. EP testing is reasonable for risk stratification in patients with remote myocardial infarction, NSVT, and LVEF ≤ 40% (Level of Evidence: B).

Class IIb
1. EP testing may be considered for risk assessment for SCD in patients with hypertrophic cardiomyopathy (Level of Evidence: C).
2. EP testing might be useful for risk assessment of SCD in patients with ARVD/C (Level of Evidence: C).
3. Ablation of asymptomatic PVCs may be considered when the PVCs are very frequent to avoid or treat tachycardia-induced cardiomyopathy (Level of Evidence: C).

Class III
1. Ablation of asymptomatic, relatively infrequent PVCs is not indicated (Level of Evidence: C).

ARVD/C = arrhythmogenic right ventricular dysplasia/cardiomyopathy; EP = electrophysiology; LVEF = left ventricular ejection fraction; NSVT = nonsustained ventricular tachycardia; PVCs = premature ventricular complexes; SCD = sudden cardiac death. *Source:* Data collected from references 1–5.

ICD group; total mortality was unaffected (18.7% vs 17.0%; hazard ratio for death in the ICD group 1.08; $P = 0.66$), attributed to competing mechanisms of mortality in the immediate peri-infarction period.[1]

EP Testing

In patients with CAD, asymptomatic NSVT, and LVEF < 40%, inducibility of sustained VT ranges between 20% and 40% and confers a worse prognosis. In a MUSTT substudy, ECG characteristics of NSVT (rate, duration, frequency, occurrence in-hospital vs out-of-hospital) did not correlate with inducibility, but survival was worse for in-hospital compared to out-of-hospital NSVT, suggesting that different risk stratification criteria may be necessary in asymptomatic ambulatory patients. In a MADIT II substudy, inducibility was 36%. Slower heart rate, lower LVEF, and a longer interval between myocardial infarction and an EP study correlated with higher inducibility and identified patients at high risk of subsequent VT. The absence of inducibility indicates a low risk with MADIT-like patients, with the caveat that these patients had a high rate of percutaneous revascularization, suggesting the associated benefit of target vessel revascularization. However, in CAD patients with severely reduced LVEF (< 30%), noninducibility does not necessarily portend a good prognosis, and persistent inducibility while receiving antiarrhythmic drugs predicts a worse prognosis. Patients in whom amiodarone–suppressed VT inducibility or slowed VT to a mean cycle length > 400 ms still had 30% higher mortality compared with patients who had an ICD placed due to lack of response to amiodarone. EP-guided antiarrhythmic drug testing in patients with NSVT who had induced sustained VT conferred no benefit.[1,2] In general, EP testing is valuable in distinguishing patients at high risk from those with lower risk for SCD in a population with clinical markers of sudden death risk.

Nonischemic Dilated Cardiomyopathy

ICD Trials

Evidence supporting ICD therapy for primary prevention in the NIDCM population is less robust than in patients with CAD due to underpowered trials and lower prevalence of the disease. In addition, primary prevention trials assessing ICD therapy in this population have not generally included asymptomatic patients with NYHA class I heart failure; therefore, the efficacy of ICDs in this population is not fully known. Because mortality may be low in this subgroup, the benefit of ICD therapy is moderate at best.[1,2]

The Defibrillators in Nonischemic Cardiomyopathy Treatment Evaluation (DEFINITE) trial[17] randomized 458 patients with NIDCM and NYHA class I to III heart failure, LVEF ≤ 35%, and more than 10 premature ventricular complexes (PVCs) per hour or NSVT, to optimal medical therapy with or without an ICD. All-cause mortality after 2 years was 14.1% in the standard therapy group versus 7.9% among those receiving an ICD, constituting a 35% relative risk reduction and strong trend toward reduction of mortality with ICD therapy, though statistical significance was not reached ($P = 0.06$). The results were consistent and comparable to those of similar trials.[1,2,17,39]

SCD-HeFT is the largest heart failure device trial conducted to date and compared amiodarone, ICD, and optimal medical therapy in 2,521 patients with CAD or NIDCM with NYHA class II or III heart failure, and LVEF ≤ 35%.[16] Over median follow-up of 45.5 months, total mortality in the medical group was 7.2% per year, with a relative risk reduction of 23% in the ICD group versus placebo (95% CI: 0.62–0.96; $P = 0.007$). Both the group with left ventricular dysfunction due to prior myocardial infarction and the nonischemic group saw comparable benefit, though absolute mortality was lower in the nonischemic group. The impact of amiodarone was mortality neutral compared to placebo.[1,2]

Heart Failure in Nonischemic Cardiomyopathy

The Comparison of Medical Therapy, Pacing and Defibrillation in Heart Failure (COMPANION) trial randomized patients with NYHA class III or IV heart failure, ischemic or nonischemic DCM, and QRS duration greater than 120 ms to receive optimal medical therapy alone or in combination with CRT with or without defibrillation capacity.[1,40] Of the 1,520 patients randomized, 903 were assigned to either the medical therapy or defibrillator arms, and 397 (44%) had

DCM. Cardiac resynchronization with an ICD significantly reduced all-cause mortality compared with pharmacological therapy alone in patients with DCM (hazard ratio for all-cause death: 0.50, 95% CI: 0.29–0.88; $P = 0.015$).[1,40]

Advanced Heart Failure Awaiting Cardiac Transplant

The high rate of sudden death in those anticipating cardiac transplant merits ICD implantation in most candidates with heart failure who are awaiting transplantation out of the hospital. The ICD has been highly effective as a bridge to transplantation for these individuals both with and without a prior history of life-threatening arrhythmias.

NYHA class IV heart failure is a heterogenous and dynamic state in which the absolute incidence of SCD increases but the proportion due to VTA declines, and therefore heart failure deaths account for a greater proportion of overall mortality. In other words, the ICD is more protective in those *less* sick. Once patients have persistent or frequently recurrent class IV heart failure symptoms on optimal therapy, life expectancy is less than 12 months, and an ICD is not indicated. In patients discharged on chronic inotropic infusion therapy for symptom palliation, despite an anticipated improvement in symptoms and the proarrhythmic potential of inotropic agents, these patients should not be prescribed ICD therapy unless awaiting transplantation.[1]

EP Testing

For patients with DCM, EP testing plays a minor role in evaluation and management of VT. This is related to low inducibility and reproducibility of EP study, and the poor predictive value of induced VT. Despite this, risk stratification may decrease the number of individuals required to undergo ICD implantation to save a life in this population. In patients with DCM who present with syncope in the absence of reversible or determinable causes, an ICD is indicated.[2]

Timing of ICD Therapy in NIDCM

A key issue in SCD prevention is time duration of medical therapy before prescribing ICD therapy. Two studies have evaluated time dependence of SCD risk relative to the timing of diagnosis of NIDCM. An analysis of the DEFINITE study demonstrated that those with recently diagnosed cardiomyopathy do not benefit less from an ICD than those with more remote diagnosis. Another analysis determined that patients with NIDCM experienced equivalent occurrences of treated and potentially lethal arrhythmias irrespective of diagnosis duration. On the basis of these data, ICD therapy should be considered in such patients provided that a reversible cause of transient left ventricular dysfunction has been excluded, particularly as the use of a time qualifier relative to the time of diagnosis of NIDCM may not reliably discriminate patients at high risk for SCD.[1]

Hypertrophic Cardiomyopathy

The first manifestation of hypertrophic cardiomyopathy may be SCD related to ventricular arrhythmia, thought to be triggered by myocardial ischemia, outflow obstruction, or AF, though less frequently due to bradycardia. The consensus document on hypertrophic cardiomyopathy from the ACC and the European Society of Cardiology has categorized major risk factors for SCD and includes prior cardiac arrest, spontaneous sustained VT, spontaneous NSVT, family history of SCD, syncope, left ventricular thickness ≥ 30 mm, and an abnormal blood pressure response to exercise. This consensus document also noted possible risk factors including AF, myocardial ischemia, left ventricular outflow obstruction, high-risk gene mutations, and intense physical exertion.[1]

Prior analyses indicate that in a high-risk hypertrophic cardiomyopathy cohort, ICD interventions were frequent and were highly effective in restoring normal sinus rhythm, and an important proportion of ICD discharges occurred in primary prevention patients who underwent ICD implantation for a single risk factor. Therefore, a single marker of high risk for sudden death may be sufficient to justify prophylactic ICD implantation in select patients.[1]

In a nonrandomized study, a subgroup of hypertrophic cardiomyopathy patients underwent ICD implantation for primary prophylaxis on the basis of perceived high risk for SCD (syncope, family history of SCD, NSVT, inducible VT, or septal thickness ≥ 30 mm) resulting in a lower rate of appropriate discharge of 5% per year. The ICD is *not* indicated in the majority of asymptomatic patients with hypertrophic cardiomyopathy, who will have a relatively benign course, and its role should be individualized in the patient considered to be at high risk for SCD.

Precise risk stratification has not been validated, and the value of EP testing in hypertrophic cardiomyopathy has been controversial at best but may be considered. Patients with multiple risk factors (especially severe septal hypertrophy, ≥ 30 mm) and those with SCD in close relatives (especially multiple relatives) appear to be at sufficiently high risk to merit consideration of ICD therapy.[1]

Arrhythmogenic Right Ventricular Dysplasia/Cardiomyopathy

The ICD has assumed a larger role in therapy of ARVD/C on the basis of the available clinical data from observational studies. Risk factors for life-threatening ventricular arrhythmias include induction of VT during EP testing, detection of NSVT on noninvasive monitoring, male gender, severe right ventricular dilation, extensive right ventricle involvement, young age at presentation (< 5 years), and left ventricular involvement. Patients with

ARVD/C genotypes associated with high risk for SCD, such as at locus 1q42-43 associated with right ventricular apex aneurysm and PMVT, should be considered for ICD therapy. In available clinical series evaluating ICD therapy in ARVD/C patients, SCD is rare, whereas appropriate ICD shocks are common.[1]

Role of EP Testing in ARVD/C

As mentioned above, induction of VTA during EP testing indicates increased risk for SCD. However, the overall prognostic role of EP testing in ARVD/C patients is not known. The response to EP testing may be influenced by disease severity, and progression of disease must be considered as well because the pathologic process of fibrofatty infiltration and replacement is expected to progress and will present future risk for SCD, even in patients in whom VT is noninducible.[2]

Isolated Noncompaction of the Left Ventricle

Noncompaction of the left ventricle is a rare congenital cardiomyopathy characterized anatomically by prominent trabeculae and deep intertrabecular recesses in the left ventricle without other major congenital cardiac malfunction that may occur truly in isolation or in association with other noncardiac congenital syndromes. The anatomic abnormalities likely occur due to arrest of normal embryogenesis of the ventricular endocardium and epicardium, preventing normal compaction of the loose myocardial meshwork and thereby posing substrate for slowed conduction, wavefront breakup, and clinical VTA. Ventricular arrhythmias are common in noncompaction, and SCD is the most common cause of mortality and can occur at any age. No specific risk stratification techniques have been validated in left ventricular noncompaction. Although there are no prospective trials or registry data, sufficient observational data exist to indicate that ICD therapy is a reasonable clinical strategy to reduce SCD risk.[1]

Rarer Cardiomyopathies (Familial Cardiomyopathy, Chagas Disease, Cardiac Sarcoid, Cardiomyopathy of Giant Cell Myocarditis)

In the absence of randomized trial data, clinical experience has demonstrated the sudden death risk associated with these rarer forms of left ventricular dysfunction. Chagasic and sarcoid cardiomyopathy are underrecognized, and there are only a few case reports and series describing experience with VT ablation in these patients. The indications are extrapolated from the broader experience with ischemic heart disease, and though the approach to ablation is as described for scar-related VT, specific considerations are notable.

Both disease entities produce a nonischemic cardiomyopathy due to an infiltrative scarring process that may lead to less-than-well-defined scar borders, as in ventricular dysplasia. As such, the distribution of scarring and interwoven conducting tissue may be expected to complicate ablation. VT ablation can acutely reduce VT burden, though in Koplan's experience with ablation of sarcoid-related VT, recurrence was seen in 75% within 6 months.[41] Over longer follow-up (up to 7 years), 50% of patients were completely free of VT after ablation and with use of antiarrhythmic and immunosuppressive agents, although the other 50% required cardiac transplantation for recurrent and uncontrollable VT.

The experience with ablation of Chagasic VT suggests several important findings. The inferolateral left ventricle is involved in 80% of patients, though an endocardial approach alone is likely to be unsatisfactory as, despite activation mapping meeting several diagnostic criteria, the VT isthmus may be identified and ablated in only up to 30% of VTs.[42] Sosa et al have demonstrated that epicardial circuits are highly prevalent within the inferolateral left ventricle[43] and epicardial mapping and ablation may facilitate ablation.[44]

Idiopathic giant cell myocarditis is an uncommon but important cause of cardiomyopathy, as it typically affects young individuals and is usually fatal if untreated.[45-50] Patients may develop heart block, requiring temporary or permanent pacemakers; hence implantation of an ICD[45] with or without CRT may be considered.

In patients proved to have cardiomyopathy that is familial or related to Chagas disease, sarcoidosis or giant cell myocarditis, ICD therapy should be considered.[1]

Polymorphic VT/VF and Primary Electrical Disorders

Polymorphic Ventricular Tachycardia and Ventricular Fibrillation

Polymorphic VT and VF may present as an arrhythmia storm and, in this uncommon instance, may be considered for catheter ablation. The prevalence of VT/VF storms in ICD patients is ~20%, whereas idiopathic VF is estimated to represent 5% to 10% of SCD cases. Beta-adrenergic blockers, various class I and III antiarrhythmic drugs, and even general anesthesia can be effective. Catheter ablation can play a crucial role when drugs fail, and has been described in patients with post–myocardial infarction VT, Brugada syndrome, long QT syndromes, right ventricular outflow tract (RVOT) ectopy, and normal hearts, that is, idiopathic VF.[4]

Following myocardial infarction, afterdepolarizations and triggered activity from Purkinje fibers in the infarct region may cause ventricular extrasystoles that initiate

PMVT/VF. In Brugada and long QT syndromes and some rare idiopathic VF patients, closely coupled monomorphic ectopic beats from the left or right ventricular Purkinje network or from the RVOT may lead to PMVT/VF. Patients with idiopathic VF typically have isolated premature ventricular beats that may represent the trigger, best appreciated immediately following resuscitation.[4]

Catheter ablation is recommended in select patients for recurrent PMVT/VF that is refractory to antiarrhythmic therapy when there is a suspected trigger that can be targeted for ablation (Table 63.11). This is a challenging procedure and should be performed only in experienced centers. Success is facilitated by very frequent ventricular ectopy to facilitate mapping, often necessitating that the procedure be performed emergently when the arrhythmia is active.[4]

Table 63.11 Recommendations for ablation of idiopathic ventricular fibrillation

Class IIb
1. Ablation of Purkinje fiber potentials may be considered in patients with ventricular arrhythmia storm consistently provoked by PVCs of similar morphology (Level of Evidence: C).

PVCs = premature ventricular complexes.

Genetic Arrhythmia Syndromes: Primary Electrical Disease

The primary electrical disorders are a group of disease processes affecting myocyte membrane ion channels that predispose to various arrhythmias including VT and VF. Each of these entities has been previously classified into the larger pathologic category of "idiopathic VF," although one by one, as the EP and molecular mechanisms have been elucidated, they have been given their own moniker in accordance with pathophysiologic findings or their "champions," as in the case of Brugada syndrome. These inherited arrhythmia syndromes include long and short QT syndromes, Brugada syndrome, and CPVT, and typically occur in the absence of structural heart disease but predispose to cardiac arrest. Because these are primary electrical disorders, most patients have no evidence of structural heart disease or left ventricular dysfunction, and long-term prognosis is excellent if arrhythmia is controlled and/or cardiac arrest can be prevented. Those with prior cardiac arrest or syncope are at very high risk for recurrent events, and ICD is the preferred therapy. The ICD may also be considered for primary prevention in patients with a family history of premature mortality, particularly if due to the inherited arrhythmia disorder. EP testing is generally not of clinical utility in these conditions.[1]

Long QT Syndrome

The long QT syndromes are a complex spectrum of molecularly distinct but phenotypically similar ion channel disorders characterized by delayed ventricular repolarization, which places patients at risk for developing PMVT in the setting of a prolonged QT interval. Long-term treatment with β-blockers, permanent pacing, or left cervicothoracic sympathectomy are helpful, but ICD implantation is recommended for patients with recurrent syncope despite drug therapy, sustained VTA, or cardiac arrest. ICD may be considered for primary prevention of SCD when there is a strong family history of SCD or when avoidance of medical therapy is desired (Table 63.12).[1] EP testing has not proved useful in long QT syndromes.[2]

Table 63.12 Recommendations for interventional EP therapy in long QT syndrome

Class I
1. Implantation of an ICD along with use of β-blockers is recommended for long QT syndrome patients with previous cardiac arrest and who have reasonable expectation of survival with a good functional status for more than 1 year (Level of Evidence: A).

Class IIa
1. Implantation of an ICD with continued use of β-blockers can be effective to reduce SCD in long QT syndrome patients experiencing syncope and/or ventricular tachycardia while receiving β-blockers and who have reasonable expectation of survival with a good functional status for more than 1 year (Level of Evidence: B).

Class IIb
1. Implantation of an ICD with the use of β-blockers may be considered for prophylaxis of SCD for patients in categories possibly associated with higher risk of cardiac arrest such as LQT2 and LQT3 and who have reasonable expectation of survival with a good functional status for more than 1 year (Level of Evidence: B).

ICD = implantable cardioverter-defibrillator; LQT = long QT syndrome; SCD = sudden cardiac death. *Source:* Data collected from references 1–5.

Brugada Syndrome

Brugada syndrome is characterized by ST-segment elevation in the right precordial leads, and is associated with high risk of SCD. Although the Brugada-pattern ECG most commonly shows J-point segment elevation in leads V_1 to V_3 with an elevated but steeply negative ST segment giving the appearance of atypical right bundle branch block with T-wave inversion and associated prolonged QT interval, the ECG pattern can be intermittent.[1]

ICD therapy is the only prophylactic measure that prevents SCD, though emerging evidence suggests a role for quinidine.[51] Therefore, clinical risk stratification for SCD is of particular importance. In some studies,[2,52,53] EP testing has been shown to have a low positive predictive value (23%), though over 3 years of follow-up it had a high negative predictive value (93%). However, Priori et al reported that EP testing does not predict subsequent cardiac arrest and advocated noninvasive risk stratification based on ECG and symptoms.[2,54] The role of EP testing for risk stratification in Brugada syndrome is debated and requires further evaluation and validation,[1] and will probably remain undefined until prospective data are obtained in patients studied with a uniform protocol in a large population with adequate follow-up (Table 63.13).[2]

Table 63.13 Recommendations for interventional electrophysiology therapy in Brugada syndrome

Class I

1. An ICD is indicated for Brugada syndrome patients with previous cardiac arrest receiving chronic optimal medical therapy and who have reasonable expectation of survival with a good functional status for more than 1 year (Level of Evidence: C).

Class IIa

1. An ICD is reasonable for Brugada syndrome patients with spontaneous ST-segment elevation in V1, V2, or V3 who have had syncope with or without mutations demonstrated in the *SCN5A* gene and who have reasonable expectation of survival with a good functional status for more than 1 year (Level of Evidence: C).
2. An ICD is reasonable for Brugada syndrome patients with documented VT that has not resulted in cardiac arrest and who have reasonable expectation of survival with a good functional status for more than 1 year (Level of Evidence: C).

Class IIb

1. EP testing may be considered for risk stratification in asymptomatic Brugada syndrome patients with spontaneous ST elevation with or without a mutation in the *SCN5A* gene (Level of Evidence: C).

ICD = implantable cardioverter-defibrillator; VT = ventricular tachycardia. *Source:* Data collected from references 1–5.

Catecholaminergic Polymorphic Ventricular Tachycardia

CPVT is characterized by ventricular arrhythmias that develop in association with physical or emotional stress. The resting ECG shows no diagnostic abnormalities at rest, and structural heart disease is universally absent. Risk stratification for SCD in CPVT has not been investigated given the relatively small number of patients reported, but most clinical descriptions indicate that β-blockers may be effective in preventing VT. Patients with VF are considered at higher risk and are usually treated with ICD in addition to β-blocker therapy. Recurrence of sustained VT, hemodynamically untolerated VT, or syncope attributable to VTA despite β-blockers are similarly considered markers of higher risk, and ICD therapy is reasonable. Furthermore, EP testing is not useful in the management of patients with CPVT since the arrhythmia is usually not inducible with programmed ventricular stimulation (Table 63.14).[1]

Pediatric and Congenital Heart Disease Patients

The indications for ICD therapy in pediatric patients and those with congenital heart disease have been derived

Table 63.14 Recommendations for interventional electrophysiology therapy in catecholaminergic ventricular tachycardia

Class I

1. Implantation of an ICD with use of β-blockers is indicated for patients with CPVT who are survivors of cardiac arrest and who have reasonable expectation of survival with a good functional status for more than 1 year (Level of Evidence: C).

Class IIa

1. Implantation of an ICD with the use of β-blockers can be effective for affected patients with CPVT with syncope and/or documented sustained ventricular tachycardia while receiving β-blockers and who have reasonable expectation of survival with a good functional status for more than 1 year (Level of Evidence: C).

CPVT = catecholaminergic ventricular tachycardia; ICD = implantable cardioverter-defibrillator. *Source:* Data collected from references 1–5.

primarily from randomized clinical trials in adults; thus, the indications for ICD therapy in pediatric patients resuscitated from or at high risk for SCD are similar to those for adults. Nonrandomized studies in children also support the class I recommendation that young patients resuscitated from SCD should undergo ICD implantation after excluding potentially reversible causes. Expectedly, sustained VT and unexplained syncope with inducible sustained or unstable VT in patients with congenital heart disease are also considered class I ICD indications. Catheter ablation or surgical therapies may provide an alternative or adjunctive therapy to the ICD in patients with congenital heart disease and recurrent VT.[1]

ICD recommendations for primary prevention of SCD in young patients are based on limited clinical experience and extrapolation of data from adult studies, as for secondary prevention indications. No randomized clinical trials have been performed to date given the relative infrequency of SCD in young patients, though congenital long QT syndromes and hypertrophic cardiomyopathy are contributors to risk in this population. With regard to primary prevention of SCD in patients with congenital heart disease, the heterogeneity of structural defects precludes generalization of risk stratification. SCD is reported in 1.2% to 3.0% of patients per decade after surgical treatment of tetralogy of Fallot, with risk factors including ventricular dysfunction, QRS duration, and atrial and ventricular arrhythmias. Elevated SCD risk has also been associated with transposition of the great arteries and congenital aortic stenosis. One other potential ICD indication is the patient with congenital coronary anomalies or coronary aneurysms or stenoses after Kawasaki disease, in which an ischemic substrate for malignant arrhythmias may be present.[1]

The lack of prospective and randomized clinical trials precludes exact recommendations regarding risk stratification and indications for ICD therapy for primary prevention of SCD in patients with postoperative congenital heart disease and ventricular dysfunction. This is complicated by the fact that right (pulmonary) ventricular dysfunction is more common than left (systemic) ventricular dysfunction, and that a variety of atrial arrhythmias and conduction blocks may independently predispose to arrhythmias or syncope.

In pediatric patients with DCM or other causes of impaired ventricular function who experience syncope or sustained ventricular arrhythmias, an ICD (with or without CRT) may be preferable to antiarrhythmic drugs due to potential for drug-induced proarrhythmia and myocardial depression. ICDs may also be considered a bridge to orthotopic heart transplantation in pediatric patients, particularly given the longer times to donor procurement in younger patients (Table 63.15).[1]

Table 63.15 Recommendations for ICD therapy in pediatric patients and patients with congenital heart disease

Class I

1. ICD implantation is indicated in the survivor of cardiac arrest after evaluation to define the cause of the event and to exclude any reversible causes (Level of Evidence: B).

2. ICD implantation is indicated for patients with symptomatic sustained ventricular tachycardia in association with congenital heart disease who have undergone hemodynamic and EP evaluation. Catheter ablation or surgical repair may offer possible alternatives in carefully selected patients (Level of Evidence: C).

Class IIa

1. ICD implantation is reasonable for patients with congenital heart disease with recurrent syncope of undetermined origin in the presence of either ventricular dysfunction or inducible ventricular arrhythmias at EP study (Level of Evidence: B).

Class IIb

1. ICD implantation may be considered for patients with recurrent syncope associated with complex congenital heart disease and advanced systemic ventricular dysfunction when thorough invasive and noninvasive investigations have failed to define a cause (Level of Evidence: C).

EP = electrophysiology; ICD = implantable cardioverter-defibrillator. *Source:* Data collected from references 1–5.

Outcomes of VT Ablation after Surgical Repair of Congenital Heart Disease

Sudden cardiac death remains the most common cause of late mortality in the setting of surgically corrected congenital heart disease. Ventricular scars from ventriculotomy or patches create the substrate for scar-related reentry. Focal VT has been reported as well. Myocardial hypertrophy occurs in a variety of malformations and also likely contributes to arrhythmia risk. The prevalence of VT after repair of tetralogy of Fallot ranges between 3% and 14%, with a risk for SCD estimated at 1.2% to 3.0% per decade, as stated earlier.[4]

The approach to catheter ablation of VT after surgical repair of congenital heart disease is as described for scar-related VT. Physicians undertaking these procedures should be familiar with the specific anatomic complexities and details of the surgical repair that pose a major challenge. Imaging with angiography and echocardiography and integration of magnetic resonance or computed tomography images to enhance the anatomic definition may be helpful. Identification of the region of scar and a substrate mapping approach to identify channels have been described.[4] Important considerations in this population are the altered and often distorted anatomy, presence of foreign material patches and conduit anastomoses creating obstacles to ablation, potential for VT to arise from sensitive areas including the His region and in close proximity to coronaries, and the need for large (8 mm) and irrigated-tip ablation catheters to achieve effective lesions due to underlying myocardial thickening from long-standing pressure and volume load.[18]

VT with left bundle branch block morphology, reflecting right ventricular or septal exit, is observed in more than 50% of cases. That the tachycardia is documented to originate so frequently at the site of surgical correction implicates the surgical procedure itself in the genesis of these ventricular arrhythmias. During catheter-based or intraoperative endocardial activation mapping, the site of earliest activation is usually found at the RVOT at the healed ventriculotomy site or close to the ventricular septal defect patch.[18]

In various series, the acute efficacy of radiofrequency ablation guided by conventional mapping techniques has been reported at 80% to 100% in patients with mappable VT. However, ~50% of patients who are candidates for VT ablation have unmappable VT, high-risk sites of involvement, and anatomic obstacles precluding effective ablation, contributing to VT ablation recurrence rates as high as 40%. In one report evaluating unstable VT after surgical repair of tetralogy of Fallot, the EnSite Array (St. Jude Medical Inc., St. Paul, MN) permitted mapping and ablation, rendering 100% of attempted patients acutely noninducible (80% of all patients), though 25% experienced recurrence. In these small series, no serious complications were reported.[18]

Role of Pacing in Prevention of Ventricular Arrhythmias

Cardiac pacing can *treat* ventricular arrhythmias. Antitachycardia pacing (ATP) has been employed as "pain-free" therapy in ICDs to prevent ICD shocks by overdriving VT and rendering the myocardial tissue/circuit refractory, with approximately 90% overall efficacy in treating monomorphic VT.[55] While specific guidelines regarding ICD programming are not available, and device programming is left to the discretion of the treating physician, ATP is often routinely made available at the time of ICD implant whether for primary or secondary prevention. Permanent antitachycardia pacemakers previously were utilized to terminate supraventricular tachycardias through atrial pacing. Permanent ATP as monotherapy for VT is not appropriate given that ATP algorithms are available in tiered-therapy ICDs capable of cardioversion and defibrillation in cases when ATP is ineffective or causes acceleration of the treated tachycardia. Implantation of a PPM for treatment of VTA is not appropriate.[1]

Alternatively, pacing can be used to *prevent* VTA as well. This situation arises in patients with pause-dependent QT prolongation and polymorphic VT in whom pacing can regularize and stabilize action potential duration and prevent significant ventricular pauses, as well as in patients with cardiomyopathy or at increased risk of developing progressive left ventricular dysfunction (eg, chronic right ventricular pacing after AV junction ablation) in whom biventricular pacing may avoid such consequences.[1]

Long QT Syndrome

The use of cardiac pacing with beta blockade for prevention of symptoms in patients with congenital long QT syndromes is supported by observational studies. The primary benefit of pacemaker therapy may be in maintaining adequate heart rate to abbreviate the QT interval in patients with sinus bradycardia or advanced AV block in association with congenital long QT syndromes, particularly with a sodium channelopathy, as well as avoidance of pause-dependent initiation of VTA (Table 63.16). Although pacemaker implantation may reduce the incidence of symptoms in these patients, the long-term survival benefit remains to be determined.[1]

Table 63.16 Recommendations for pacing to prevent ventricular tachyarrhythmias

Class I
1. Permanent pacing is indicated for sustained pause-dependent VT, with or without QT prolongation (Level of Evidence: C).
Class IIa
1. Permanent pacing is reasonable for high-risk patients with congenital long QT syndrome (Level of Evidence: C).
Class III
1. Permanent pacing is not indicated for frequent or complex ventricular ectopic activity without sustained VT in the absence of the long QT syndrome (Level of Evidence: C).
2. Permanent pacing is not indicated for torsades de pointes VT due to reversible causes (Level of Evidence: A).

VT = ventricular tachycardia. *Source:* Data collected from references 1–5.

Role of Biventricular Pacemakers in Prevention of Ventricular Arrhythmias

Regardless of the duration of native QRS complex, patients with left ventricular dysfunction who have a conventional indication for pacing and in whom ventricular pacing is expected to predominate may benefit from biventricular pacing. A prospective randomized trial[56] in patients with LVEF ≤ 40% and a conventional indication for pacing showed that biventricular pacing was associated with improved LVEF and functional class compared with right ventricular pacing. This effect on left ventricular function is believed to secondarily mitigate arrhythmic risk. It has also been demonstrated that left ventricular dysfunction in the setting of chronic right ventricular pacing, and possibly as a result of right ventricular pacing,[57] can be improved with upgrade to biventricular pacing.[1] Among patients undergoing AV junction ablation for chronic AF, the Left Ventricular-Based Cardiac Stimulation Post AV Nodal Ablation Evaluation (PAVE) trial prospectively randomized patients between right ventricular apical pacing and biventricular pacing,[58] and demonstrated that patients with right ventricular apical pacing had deterioration in LVEF that was avoided in patients biventricularly paced. These advantages of biventricular pacing were seen predominantly among patients with reduced LVEF or heart failure at baseline. Other studies have shown that among AF patients who experience heart failure after AV junction ablation and right ventricular pacing, an upgrade to biventricular pacing results in improved symptoms and improved left ventricular function.[1] In one study[59] of patients with NYHA class III through IV heart failure, an LVEF ≤ 35%, and a QRS complex ≥ 160 ms (or at least 120 ms in the presence of other evidence of ventricular dyssynchrony), sudden death was also significantly reduced with biventricular pacing. In addition, there is a role for CRT alone in some patients, especially those who wish to enhance their quality of life without defibrillation (CRT-P) due to either patient preference or existing contraindication to defibrillation capability. Notably, there is an important survival benefit, presumably due to the direct antiarrhythmic effect of successful CRT (Table 63.17).[1]

Interventional EP Management of VTA in Patients with Normal Hearts

While patients without ostensible heart disease account for a small percentage of patients with VT, they are of particular interest as ablation may be curative. VT in people with structurally *and* electrically normal hearts (ie, idiopathic VT) typically presents a single morphology arising from the right ventricle with a left bundle branch block inferior-axis morphology or from the left ventricle with a right bundle branch block morphology and, in general, are associated with a good prognosis, so ICD therapy is usually not indicated. Interventional EP management of VT in this setting revolves around catheter ablation and the role of EP testing to guide and evaluate efficacy of ablation,[2] and in appropriate patients, ablation should be offered.

Table 63.17 Recommendations for CRT in patients with severe systolic heart failure

Class I

1. For patients who have LVEF ≤35%, a QRS duration ≥ 0.12 seconds, and sinus rhythm, CRT with or without an ICD is indicated for the treatment of NYHA functional class III or ambulatory class IV heart failure symptoms with optimal recommended medical therapy (Level of Evidence: A).

Class IIa

1. For patients who have LVEF ≤35%, a QRS duration ≥ 0.12 seconds, and AF, CRT with or without an ICD is reasonable for the treatment of NYHA functional class III or ambulatory class IV heart failure symptoms with optimal recommended medical therapy (Level of Evidence: B).
2. For patients with LVEF ≤35% with NYHA functional class III or ambulatory class IV symptoms who are receiving optimal recommended medical therapy and who have frequent dependence on ventricular pacing, CRT is reasonable (Level of Evidence: C).

Class IIb

1. For patients with LVEF ≤35% with NYHA class I or II symptoms who are receiving optimal recommended medical therapy and who are undergoing implantation of a PPM and/or ICD with anticipated frequent ventricular pacing, CRT may be considered (Level of Evidence: C).

Class III

1. CRT is not indicated for asymptomatic patients with reduced LVEF in the absence of other indications for pacing (Level of Evidence: B).
2. CRT is not indicated for patients whose functional status and life expectancy are limited predominantly by chronic noncardiac conditions (Level of Evidence: C).

AF = atrial fibrillation; CRT = cardiac resynchronization therapy; ICD = implantable cardioverter-defibrillator; LVEF = left ventricular ejection fraction; NYHA = New York Heart Association; PPM = permanent pacemaker. *Source:* Data collected from references 1–5.

In series using the CARTO Mapping System (Biosense Webster, Diamond Bar, CA) and a combination of activation and pacemapping, acute success of ablation ranged from 83% to 100%, with recurrence rates of 0% to 19%. However, when sustained VT permitted adequate study, success rates in excess of 90% were achieved with recurrence rates of less than 5%[60] after acutely successful ablation.[4] Comparable ablation results have been reported using a multielectrode ablation catheter[61] and noncontact balloon-array mapping of mappable and unmappable RVOT VT.[62,63] Failure is usually due to inability to induce the arrhythmia for mapping, thereby limiting the diagnostic evaluation. In idiopathic left ventricular tachycardia ("verapamil-sensitive"), the overall success rate of ablation in reported series is ~95%.[4]

Role of Ablation of Premature Ventricular Complexes

PVCs can result in a reversible form of cardiomyopathy due to abnormal and irregular cadence of ventricular activation. The threshold PVC burden beyond which left ventricular dysfunction develops is not known but usually exceeds 20% in such patients, but may be as few as 5% PVCs in 24 hours.[4] The minimum duration of PVCs required to induce left ventricular dysfunction is also not clear, particularly as PVCs may not provoke symptoms and, hence, may not be detected. Catheter ablation of PVCs is recommended in patients with frequent PVCs or NSVT when they are highly symptomatic, refractory to drugs or avoidance of medical therapy is desired, or when they are presumed to have caused or to prevent left ventricular dysfunction if a predominant morphology can be identified (Table 63.18).[4]

Table 63.18 Ablation recommendations for patients with normal hearts or left ventricular dysfunction due to ventricular ectopy

Class I

1. Ablation is indicated in patients who are otherwise at low risk for SCD and have sustained predominantly monomorphic VT that is drug resistant, who are drug intolerant, or who do not wish long-term drug therapy (Level of Evidence: C).

Class IIa

1. Ablation can be useful therapy in patients who are otherwise at low risk for SCD and have symptomatic nonsustained monomorphic VT that is drug resistant, who are drug intolerant, or who do not wish long-term drug therapy (Level of Evidence: C).
2. Ablation can be useful therapy in patients who are otherwise at low risk for SCD and have frequent symptomatic, predominantly monomorphic PVCs that are drug resistant, who are drug intolerant, or who do not wish long-term drug therapy (Level of Evidence: C).

Class IIb

1. Ablation of asymptomatic PVCs may be considered when the PVCs are very frequent to avoid or treat tachycardia-induced cardiomyopathy (Level of Evidence: C).

Class III

1. Ablation of asymptomatic, relatively infrequent PVCs is not indicated (Level of Evidence: C).

PVCs = premature ventricular complexes; SCD = sudden cardiac death; VT = ventricular tachycardia. *Source:* Data collected from references 1–5.

Conclusions

The management of VT/VF remains an important objective in prevention of sudden death. As the field of interventional EP evolves, so will recommendations for indicated interventions. The ICD will likely remain the mainstay for years to come, although medical therapy will also continue to improve outcomes in patients at risk of sudden death, and trials evaluating the ICD against more novel therapies will continue to be required. Furthermore, VT ablation is increasingly performed, and as its role approaches first-line therapy in a number of disease states, it will also contribute to improved efficacy in preventing sudden death.

Acknowledgments

The authors gratefully acknowledge the help of Barbara Danek, Joe Grundle, and Katie Klein in the editorial preparation of this manuscript and Brian Miller and Brian Schurrer for their help with the figures.

References

1. Epstein AE, DiMarco JP, Ellenbogen KA, et al. ACC/AHA/HRS 2008 Guidelines for Device-Based Therapy of Cardiac Rhythm Abnormalities: a report of the American College of Cardiology/American Heart Association Task Force on Practice Guidelines (Writing Committee to Revise the ACC/AHA/NASPE 2002 Guideline Update for Implantation of Cardiac Pacemakers and Antiarrhythmia Devices): developed in collaboration with the American Association for Thoracic Surgery and Society of Thoracic Surgeons. *Circulation*. 2008;117:e350-408.
2. European Heart Rhythm Association; Heart Rhythm Society; Zipes DP, et al. ACC/AHA/ESC 2006 Guidelines for Management of Patients with Ventricular Arrhythmias and the Prevention of Sudden Cardiac Death. A report of the American College of Cardiology/American Heart Association Task Force and the European Society of Cardiology Committee for Practice Guidelines (Writing Committee to Develop Guidelines for Management of Patients with Ventricular Arrhythmias and the Prevention of Sudden Cardiac Death). *J Am Coll Cardiol*. 2006;48:e247-e346.
3. Naccarelli GV, Conti JB, DiMarco JP, Tracy CM; Heart Rhythm Society. Task Force 6: training in specialized electrophysiology, cardiac pacing, and arrhythmia management endorsed by the Heart Rhythm Society. *J Am Coll Cardiol*. 2008;51:374-380.
4. Aliot EM, Stevenson WG, Almendral-Garrote JM, et al. EHRA/HRS Expert Consensus on Catheter Ablation of Ventricular Arrhythmias: developed in a partnership with the European Heart Rhythm Association (EHRA), a Registered Branch of the European Society of Cardiology (ESC), and the Heart Rhythm Society (HRS); in collaboration with the American College of Cardiology (ACC) and the American Heart Association (AHA). *Heart Rhythm*. 2009;6:886-933.
5. Strickberger SA, Benson DW, Biaggioni I, et al. AHA/ACCF Scientific Statement on the evaluation of syncope: from the American Heart Association Councils on Clinical Cardiology, Cardiovascular Nursing, Cardiovascular Disease in the Young, and Stroke, and the Quality of Care and Outcomes Research Interdisciplinary Working Group; and the American College of Cardiology Foundation: in collaboration with the Heart Rhythm Society: endorsed by the American Autonomic Society. *Circulation*. 2006;113:316-327.
6. The Antiarrhythmics Versus Implantable Defibrillators (AVID) Investigators. A comparison of antiarrhythmic-drug therapy with implantable defibrillators in patients resuscitated from near-fatal ventricular arrhythmias. *N Engl J Med*. 1997;337:1576-1583.
7. Kuck KH, Cappato R, Siebels J, Ruppel R. Randomized comparison of antiarrhythmic drug therapy with implantable defibrillators in patients resuscitated from cardiac arrest: the Cardiac Arrest Study Hamburg (CASH). *Circulation*. 2000;102:748-754.
8. Connolly SJ, Gent M, Roberts RS, et al. Canadian implantable defibrillator study (CIDS): a randomized trial of the implantable cardioverter defibrillator against amiodarone. *Circulation*. 2000;101:1297-1302.
9. Powell AC, Fuchs T, Finkelstein DM, et al. Influence of implantable cardioverter-defibrillators on the long-term prognosis of survivors of out-of-hospital cardiac arrest. *Circulation*. 1993;88:1083-1092.
10. Akhtar M, Shenasa M, Jazayeri M, Caceres J, Tchou PJ. Wide QRS complex tachycardia. Reappraisal of a common clinical problem. *Ann Intern Med*. 1988;109:905-912.
11. Akhtar M. Techniques of electrophysiologic evaluation. In: Fuster V, O'Rourke RA, Walsh RA, Poole-Wilson P, eds. *Hurst's the Heart*, 12th ed. New York, NY: McGraw-Hill 2007:1064-1076.
12. Choudhuri I, Akhtar M. Electrophysiologic studies. In: Chatterjee K, Anderson M, Heistad D, Kerber R, eds. *Cardiology: An Illustrated Text Book*. New Delhi, India: Jay Pee Brothers Medical Publishers Ltd., 2012, pp. 686-697.
13. Middlekauff HR, Stevenson WG, Stevenson LW, Saxon LA. Syncope in advanced heart failure: high rise of sudden death regardless of origin of syncope. *J Am Coll Cardiol*. 1993;21:110-116.
14. Knight BP, Goyal R, Pelosi F, et al. Outcome of patients with nonischemic dilated cardiomyopathy and unexplained syncope treated with an implantable defibrillator. *J Am Coll Cardiol*. 1999;33:1964-1970.
15. Russo AM, Verdino R, Schorr C, et al. Occurrence of implantable defibrillator events in patients with syncope and nonischemic dilated cardiomyopathy. *Am J Cardiol*. 2001;88:1444-1446.
16. Mark DB, Nelson CL, Anstrom KJ, et al. Cost-effectiveness of defibrillator therapy or amiodarone in chronic stable heart failure: results from the Sudden Cardiac Death in Heart Failure Trial (SCD-HeFT). *Circulation*. 2006;114:135-142.
17. Kadish A, Dyer A, Daubert JP, et al. Prophylactic defibrillator implantation in patients with nonischemic dilated cardiomyopathy. *N Engl J Med*. 2004;350:2151-2158.
18. Choudhuri I, Sra J, Akhtar M. Catheter ablation of ventricular tachycardia: current techniques and new technologies. In: Camm AJ, Saksena S, eds. *Electrophysiologic Disorders of the Heart*, 2nd ed. Philadelphia: Saunders (Elsevier); 2012, pp. 1361-1396.
19. Stevenson WG, Friedman PL, Sager PT, et al. Exploring postinfarction reentrant ventricular tachycardia with entrainment mapping. *J Am Coll Cardiol*. 1997;29:1180-1189.
20. Stevenson WG, Khan H, Sager P, et al. Identification of reentry circuit sites during catheter mapping and radiofrequency ablation of ventricular tachycardia late after myocardial infarction. *Circulation*. 1993;88:1647-1670.
21. El-Shalakany A, Hadjis T, Papageorgiou P, et al. Entrainment/mapping criteria for the prediction of termination of ventricular tachycardia by single radiofrequency lesion in patients with coronary artery disease. *Circulation*. 1999;99:2283-2289.
22. Stevenson WG, Wilber DJ, Natale A, et al. Irrigated radiofrequency catheter ablation guided by electroanatomic mapping for recurrent ventricular tachycardia after myocardial infarction: the multicenter thermocool ventricular tachycardia ablation trial. *Circulation*. 2008;118:2773-2782.
23. Tanner H, Hindricks G, Volkmer M, et al. Catheter ablation of recurrent scar-related ventricular tachycardia using electroanatomical mapping and irrigated ablation technology: results of the prospective multicenter Euro-VT-Study. *J Cardiovasc Electrophysiol*. 2010;21:47-53.
24. Reddy VY, Reynolds MR, Neuzil P, et al. Prophylactic catheter ablation for the prevention of defibrillator therapy. *N Engl J Med*. 2007;357:2657-2665.

25. Exner DV, Pinski SL, Wyse DG, et al. Electrical storm presages nonsudden death: the Antiarrhythmics Versus Implantable Defibrillators (AVID) trial. *Circulation*. 2001;103: 2066-2071.
26. Carbucicchio C, Santamaria M, Trevisi N, et al. Catheter ablation for the treatment of electrical storm in patients with implantable cardioverter-defibrillators: short- and long-term outcomes in a prospective single-center study. *Circulation*. 2008;117:462-469.
27. Delacretaz E, Stevenson WG, Ellison KE, Maisel WH, Friedman PL. Mapping and radiofrequency catheter ablation of the three types of sustained monomorphic ventricular tachycardia in nonischemic heart disease. *J Cardiovasc Electrophysiol*. 2000;11:11-17.
28. Soejima K, Stevenson WG, Sapp JL, Selwyn AP, Couper G, Epstein LM. Endocardial and epicardial radiofrequency ablation of ventricular tachycardia associated with dilated cardiomyopathy: the importance of low-voltage scars. *J Am Coll Cardiol*. 2004;43:1834-1842.
29. Nazarian S, Bluemke DA, Lardo AC, et al. Magnetic resonance assessment of the substrate for inducible ventricular tachycardia in nonischemic cardiomyopathy. *Circulation*. 2005;112:2821-2825.
30. Riley MP, Zado E, Bala R, et al. Lack of uniform progression of endocardial scar in patients with arrhythmogenic right ventricular dysplasia/cardiomyopathy and ventricular tachycardia. *Circ Arrhythm Electrophysiol*. 2010;3:332-338.
31. Verma A, Kilicaslan F, Schweikert RA, et al. Short- and long-term success of substrate-based mapping and ablation of ventricular tachycardia in arrhythmogenic right ventricular dysplasia. *Circulation*. 2005;111:3209-3216.
32. Garcia FC, Bazan V, Zado ES, Ren JF, Marchlinski FE. Epicardial substrate and outcome with epicardial ablation of ventricular tachycardia in arrhythmogenic right ventricular cardiomyopathy/dysplasia. *Circulation*. 2009;120:366-375.
33. Bai R, Di Biase L, Shivkumar K, et al. Ablation of ventricular arrhythmias in arrhythmogenic right ventricular dysplasia/cardiomyopathy: arrhythmia-free survival after endo-epicardial substrate based mapping and ablation. *Circ Arrhythm Electrophysiol*. 2011;4:478-485.
34. Moss AJ, Hall WJ, Cannom DS, et al. Improved survival with an implanted defibrillator in patients with coronary disease at high risk for ventricular arrhythmia. Multicenter Automatic Defibrillator Implantation Trial Investigators. *N Engl J Med*. 1996;335:1933-1940.
35. Buxton AE, Lee KL, Fisher JD, Josephson ME, Prystowsky EN, Hafley G. A randomized study of the prevention of sudden death in patients with coronary artery disease. Multicenter Unsustained Tachycardia Trial Investigators. *N Engl J Med*. 1999;341:1882-1890.
36. Moss AJ, Zareba W, Hall WJ, et al. Prophylactic implantation of a defibrillator in patients with myocardial infarction and reduced ejection fraction. *N Engl J Med*. 2002;346:877-883.
37. Bigger JT Jr. Prophylactic use of implanted cardiac defibrillators in patients at high risk for ventricular arrhythmias after coronary-artery bypass graft surgery. Coronary Artery Bypass Graft (CABG) Patch Trial Investigators. *N Engl J Med*. 1997;337:1569-1575.
38. Hohnloser SH, Kuck KH, Dorian P, et al. Prophylactic use of an implantable cardioverter-defibrillator after acute myocardial infarction. *N Engl J Med*. 2004;351:2481-2488.
39. Grimm W, Alter P, Maisch B. Arrhythmia risk stratification with regard to prophylactic implantable defibrillator therapy in patients with dilated cardiomyopathy. Results of MACAS, DEFINITE, and SCD-HeFT. *Herz*. 2004;29:348-352.
40. Bristow MR, Saxon LA, Boehmer J, et al. Cardiac-resynchronization therapy with or without an implantable defibrillator in advanced chronic heart failure. *N Engl J Med*. 2004;350:2140-2150.
41. Koplan BA1, Soejima K, Baughman K, Epstein LM, Stevenson WG. Refractory ventricular tachycardia secondary to cardiac sarcoid: electrophysiologic characteristics, mapping, and ablation. *Heart Rhythm*. 2006;3:924-929.
42. Sarabanda AV, Sosa E, Simões MV, Figueiredo GL, Pintya AO, Marin-Neto JA. Ventricular tachycardia in Chagas' disease: a comparison of clinical, angiographic, electrophysiologic and myocardial perfusion disturbances between patients presenting with either sustained or nonsustained forms. *Int J Cardiol*. 2005;102:9-19.
43. Sosa E, Scanavacca M, D'Avila A, et al. Endocardial and epicardial ablation guided by nonsurgical transthoracic epicardial mapping to treat recurrent ventricular tachycardia. *J Cardiovasc Electrophysiol*. 1998;9:229-239.
44. Sosa E, Scanavacca M, D'Avila A, Bellotti G, Pilleggi F. Radiofrequency catheter ablation of ventricular tachycardia guided by nonsurgical epicardial mapping in chronic Chagasic heart disease. *Pacing Clin Electrophysiol*. 1999;22:128-130.
45. Cooper LT, Okura Y. Idiopathic giant cell myocarditis. *Curr Treat Options Cardiovasc Med*. 2001;3:463-467.
46. Cooper LT Jr. Giant cell myocarditis: diagnosis and treatment. *Herz*. 2000;25:291-298.
47. Cooper LT Jr, Berry GJ, Shabetai R. Idiopathic giant-cell myocarditis—natural history and treatment. Multicenter Giant Cell Myocarditis Study Group Investigators. *N Engl J Med*. 1997;336:1860-1866.
48. Marelli D, Kermani R, Bresson J, et al. Support with the BVS 5000 assist device during treatment of acute giant-cell myocarditis. *Tex Heart Inst J*. 2003;30:50-56.
49. Brilakis ES, Olson LJ, Berry GJ, et al. Survival outcomes of patients with giant cell myocarditis bridged by ventricular assist devices. *ASAIO J*. 2000;46:569-572.
50. Hanawa H, Izumi T, Saito Y, et al. Recovery from complete atrioventricular block caused by idiopathic giant cell myocarditis after corticosteroid therapy. *Jpn Circ J*. 1998;62:211-214.
51. Belhassen B, Glick A, Viskin S. Excellent long-term reproducibility of the electrophysiologic efficacy of quinidine in patients with idiopathic ventricular fibrillation and Brugada syndrome. *Pacing Clin Electrophysiol*. 2009;32:294-301.
52. Hermida JS, Lemoine JL, Aoun FB, Jarry G, Rey JL, Quiret JC. Prevalence of the Brugada syndrome in an apparently healthy population. *Am J Cardiol*. 2000;86:91-94.
53. Brugada P, Brugada J. Right bundle branch block, persistent ST segment elevation and sudden cardiac death: a distinct clinical and electrocardiographic syndrome. A multicenter report. *J Am Coll Cardiol*. 1992;20:1391-1396.
54. Priori SG, Aliot E, Blomstrom-Lundqvist C, et al. Task Force on Sudden Cardiac Death of the European Society of Cardiology. *Eur Heart J*. 2001;22:1374-1450.
55. Wathen MS, Sweeney MO, DeGroot PJ, et al. Shock reduction using antitachycardia pacing for spontaneous rapid ventricular tachycardia in patients with coronary artery disease. *Circulation*. 2001;104:796-801.
56. Kindermann M, Hennen B, Jung J, Geisel J, Böhm M, Fröhlig G. Biventricular versus conventional right ventricular stimulation for patients with standard pacing indication and left ventricular dysfunction: the Homburg Biventricular Pacing Evaluation (HOBIPACE). *J Am Coll Cardiol*. 2006;47:1927-1937.
57. Wilkoff BL, Cook JR, Epstein AE, et al. Dual-chamber pacing or ventricular backup pacing in patients with an implantable

defibrillator: the Dual Chamber and VVI Implantable Defibrillator (DAVID) trial. *JAMA.* 2002;288:3115-3123.
58. Doshi RN, Daoud EG, Fellows C, et al. Left ventricular-based cardiac stimulation post AV nodal ablation evaluation (the PAVE study). *J Cardiovasc Electrophysiol.* 2005;16:1160-1165.
59. Cleland JG, Daubert JC, Erdmann E, et al. The effect of cardiac resynchronization on morbidity and mortality in heart failure. *N Engl J Med.* 2005;352:1539-1549.
60. Bala R, Marchlinski FE. Electrocardiographic recognition and ablation of outflow tract ventricular tachycardia. *Heart Rhythm.* 2007;4:366-370.
61. Azegami K, Wilber DJ, Arruda M, Lin AC, Denman RA. Spatial resolution of pacemapping and activation mapping in patients with idiopathic right ventricular outflow tract tachycardia. *J Cardiovasc Electrophysiol.* 2005;16:823-829.
62. Gerstenfeld EP, Dixit S, Callans DJ, Rajawat Y, Rho R, Marchlinski FE. Quantitative comparison of spontaneous and paced 12-lead electrocardiogram during right ventricular outflow tract ventricular tachycardia. *J Am Coll Cardiol.* 2003;41:2046-2053.
63. Aiba T, Shimizu W, Taguchi A, et al. Clinical usefulness of a multielectrode basket catheter for idiopathic ventricular tachycardia originating from right ventricular outflow tract. *J Cardiovasc Electrophysiol.* 2001;12:511-517.

CHAPTER 64

Permanent Pacing: Clinical Indications and Evidence-based Outcomes Standards in Interventional Electrophysiology

Jaimie Manlucu, MD; Bhavanesh Makanjee, MD;
Andrew D. Krahn, MD; Raymond Yee, MD

Introduction

Permanent cardiac pacemakers were first introduced in the late 1950s as lifesaving treatment for atrioventricular block (AVB), particularly after cardiac surgery. More than five decades later, pacemaker therapy has expanded to include a number of clinical conditions manifesting as significant bradycardia and has found a new role in the treatment of drug-refractory heart failure. At the same time, medicine was also evolving; clinical practice was increasingly driven by scientific evidence derived from randomized clinical trials. This culminated in the first consensus practice guidelines for cardiac pacing published by the American College of Cardiology (ACC) and the American Heart Association (AHA) in 1984. The most recent update included participation by the Heart Rhythm Society (formerly NASPE) in 2008.[1] The European Society of Cardiology (ESC) in collaboration with the European Heart Rhythm Association last updated their guidelines in 2007.[2]

Professional societies have followed a process whereby consensus pacemaker indications are developed by an expert panel after gathering and reviewing all published evidence. Highest value is assigned to randomized clinical trials designed with adequate power to evaluate clinically relevant endpoints. Scientific evidence is assigned the highest grading when derived from two or more randomized clinical trials (Level A). In their absence, meta-analyses of available studies, database registries, and nonrandomized studies of various sizes are reviewed (Level B). Where clinical studies are lacking, the consensus opinion of experts may form the sole basis of recommendations (Level C).

After considering these levels, the expert panel renders recommendations about indications for pacemaker therapy under 3 categories:

Class I: Device implantation is recommended and should be performed for a particular condition.

Class II: Device implantation may be considered for a particular condition, but the evidence is less compelling. Recommendations in this class are often subdivided into class IIa, where the prevailing opinion is more favorable, or class IIb if expert opinion is quite divided.

Class III: Device implantation should not be performed because evidence indicates it is not beneficial or may be harmful.

It is worthwhile emphasizing that the strength of any recommendation (class I or II) does not always correlate with the quality of evidence, and this particularly true in regard to clinical bradycardias, which are mostly based on Level C evidence. Because pacemaker therapy has been the entrenched standard of medical care for bradycardias and viable alternative therapies do not exist, it is unlikely that randomized clinical studies will ever be conducted for primary electrical disease manifesting as AV block or sinus node dysfunction. In addition, it is important to remember that consensus guidelines are meant as a good reference point to aid medical decision making. They are not a substitute for good medical judgment. While physicians in North America and Europe are guided by the practice guidelines emanating from their respective professional bodies, practice in other geographic regions may vary because of resource availability, cultural differences, and other factors. It is beyond the scope of this chapter to discuss geographical practice differences.

There are 3 fundamental reasons for considering permanent pacemaker implantation: (1) significant documented bradycardias or conditions associated with a high risk of progression to significant bradycardias, (2) pacing to provide hemodynamic benefit in cardiomyopathies, and (3) pacing to prevent or terminate reentrant supraventricular tachycardias. This chapter will summarize accepted pacing indications and highlight areas of controversy or uncertainty.

Bradycardias

A bradycardia is defined as any cardiac rhythm ≤ 50 to 60 beats per minute regardless of setting, mechanism, or associated symptoms. This has engendered the mistaken notion that all bradycardias are detrimental and require treatment with a permanent pacemaker. However, bradycardias arise in a number of clinical situations and have a diverse range of causes. Bradycardias can be broadly divided into those that arise from inadequate or failed initiation (typically sinus node disease), and failure of conduction (typically AV node disease). These manifest most commonly with intermittent paroxysmal bradycardia leading to pauses, or sudden deceleration presenting with syncope or presyncope. Less commonly, chronotropic incompetence can present with exercise intolerance. Many bradycardias are asymptomatic and have a benign course or prognosis, making treatment unnecessary. A bradycardia warranting pacemaker therapy is one that causes hemodynamic instability and symptoms or is associated with increased risk of morbidity or mortality.

Atrioventricular Block

Pacemakers were first introduced for treatment of patients with atrioventricular (AV) block following cardiac surgery. To this day, it remains one of the most common indications for pacemaker implantation. It may be persistent (fixed), transient, or intermittent, but the distinction depends on the duration of continuous monitoring. As discussed earlier, disturbances of AV conduction can be the result of either physiologic or pathologic processes. Physiologic influences such as fluctuations in autonomic tone can cause transient AV block, whereas persistent or more severe degrees of AV block are more likely to result from pathologic processes. Pathologic AV block requiring permanent pacing has a diverse range of causes and manifestations.

ECG Manifestations of AV Block

AV block involves any impairment of atrial impulse conduction to the ventricles and is divided into three degrees of severity based on ECG features: first-, second-, and third-degree AV block. First-degree AV block is a misnomer; there is no actual block of atrial impulses but simply a slowing in AV conduction. This manifests as a prolongation of the PR interval to more than 200 ms (see Figure 64.1A).

Second-degree heart block is characterized by intermittent failure of impulse conduction resulting in P waves not followed by QRS complexes ("blocked"). This is further divided into several subtypes based on the ECG pattern of AV block, underlying pathophysiology, and prognosis. Mobitz type I ("Wenckebach") block most often involves block at the AV node level but can rarely occur with infranodal disease. The electrocardiographic hallmark is progressive PR interval prolongation on successive beats preceding a single nonconducted P wave (Wenckebach periodicity). The corollary is that the first conducted P wave after the block will usually display a shorter PR interval than the cycle preceding the blocked P wave (see Figure 64.1B). Because the block is usually in the AV node and the distal conduction system is not affected, the QRS of conducted beats and any escape pacemaker rhythm is usually narrow. However, it is not unusual to see patients with second-degree AV block who also have concomitant more distal conduction system disease so that the width of the intrinsic or escape QRS complex cannot be relied on solely to indicate the level of AV block. Mobitz type I block usually resolves with exercise or improves with maneuvers that reduce vagal tone and typically has a benign prognosis.

Mobitz type II block involves a single blocked P wave without any preceding or ensuing variations in PR interval (see Figure 64.1C). Mobitz II block has a higher likelihood of being the result of infranodal conduction disease. There is often evidence of more diffuse distal conduction system disease with wide QRS complexes, but the absence of such does not preclude infranodal block. Exercise or other maneuvers to increase the sinus rate will usually worsen AV block in contrast to block at the AV node level. Progression to complete heart block is common, and may be sudden and unpredictable. The escape rhythm is unreliable so that asystole with syncope or sudden death are possible.

When alternating P waves are blocked (2:1 AV block), it is not possible to identify any PR interval pattern preceding and following the blocked P waves (see Figure 64.1D). This form of second-degree AV block is in a distinct category. Pharmacologic or physiologic maneuvers to modulate vagal tone and sinus node rate can help distinguish the level of block. A definitive diagnosis is crucial since disease affecting the distal conduction system is prognostically more serious.

Third-degree or complete AV block is defined by a complete absence of AV conduction. Electrocardiographically, this manifests as an atrial rhythm that is completely dissociated from a slower, regular ventricular rhythm (see Figure 64.1E). The block can involve any level of the conduction system with the ventricular rate driven by an escape pacemaker distal to the level of block (ie, the AV node, His-Purkinje, or ventricular myocardium). By definition, a narrow QRS escape rhythm implies that the level of block is AV nodal. In the absence of a bundle branch block, an escape originating from the junction (AV node) will generate a narrow QRS, with a regular rate of 40–60 bpm. An escape rhythm arising distal to the His bundle will invariably generate a wide QRS rhythm less than 40 bpm. When symptomatic advanced AV block is combined with bifascicular or alternating bundle branch block, there is a higher associated mortality and incidence of sudden death.

The term "high-grade AVB" is often used in the literature. This somewhat vague term is usually employed to describe patterns of AVB that span the continuum between second- and third-degree AVB. For instance, when two or more consecutive P-wave cycles are blocked followed by resumption of conduction, high-grade AV block is applied while some would call it intermittent third-degree AVB (see Figure 64.1F).

Etiology and Pathophysiology

The causes of pathologic AV block are diverse. Most AV block is attributed to premature degeneration of the conduction system due to age-related changes. However, multiple secondary causes of AV block also exist. For example, genetic abnormalities can lead to cardiac conduction system disease. This can be isolated or affect multiple target organ systems. Examples of the latter include several muscular dystrophies or neuromuscular disorders. Other secondary causes of AV block include collagen disorders, inflammatory injury (Lyme disease), infections (Chagas disease), ischemia, and trauma to the conduction system. Drugs affecting the AV node (eg, cardiac glycosides, nondihydropyridine calcium channel blockers, β-blockers, and some antiarrhythmic agents like amiodarone and dronedarone) and certain metabolic disturbances (electrolyte imbalances, hypothyroidism, and hypothermia) are also important potential causes.

The origin of the escape pacemaker has significant clinical implications. A junctional escape rhythm tends to be stable and reliable. Conversely, wide escape rhythms arising from the distal conduction system or ventricular myocardium tend to be slower, unreliable, and prone to sudden cessation. Another potentially life-threatening complication of heart block is bradycardia-dependent torsades de pointes. In a subset of patients, the QT interval may prolong in response to bradycardia. This makes them susceptible to PVC-induced long-short RR intervals that initiate polymorphic VT, which can degenerate to ventricular fibrillation. Therefore, early intervention is also warranted in these patients.

Clinical Presentation

Whether a patient experiences symptoms with AV block depends on factors such as the duration of the AV block, the hemodynamic consequences of the AV block, and the rate and cadence of the ventricular rhythm. First-degree AV block rarely causes symptoms. However, with marked PR prolongation, the extended late diastolic filling period can lead to AV valve regurgitation and contribute to symptoms related to left heart failure. In the occasional patient, single isolated blocked sinus cycles (as occurs with second-degree AV block) can cause palpitations due to pulse irregularity. With Mobitz type I AVB, the asystolic interval is usually too short to cause symptoms related to cerebral underperfusion such as lightheadedness, presyncope, or syncope. Such symptoms are more likely to be encountered with Mobitz type II AVB or complete AVB, where the escape pacemaker automaticity is unreliable and may fail to abbreviate the asystolic period. If the AV block restricts the ventricular chronotropic response to exertion, patients may complain of fatigue or exertional intolerance. In evaluating the individual patient who presents with a bradycardia, there are two important issues to consider. The first is an assessment of the etiology of the bradycardia and to identify any reversible causes. Second, a clinician must determine whether the bradycardia is plausibly responsible for a patient's symptoms and whether those symptoms are commensurate with the bradycardia. Since one of the main goals of pacemaker therapy is to resolve a patient's presenting symptoms, it is important to have reasonable confidence that the symptoms are actually due to the bradycardia.

Pacemaker Indications in Acquired AV Block

Since there is no viable alternative treatment for symptomatic AV block, randomized clinical trials comparing pacemakers to medical therapy have not been, and likely will never be, performed. As a result, clinical evidence supporting pacemaker indications in AV block are based primarily on cohort studies and the consensus of expert opinion.

A permanent pacemaker is recommended (class I indication) for any patient with documented acquired Mobitz

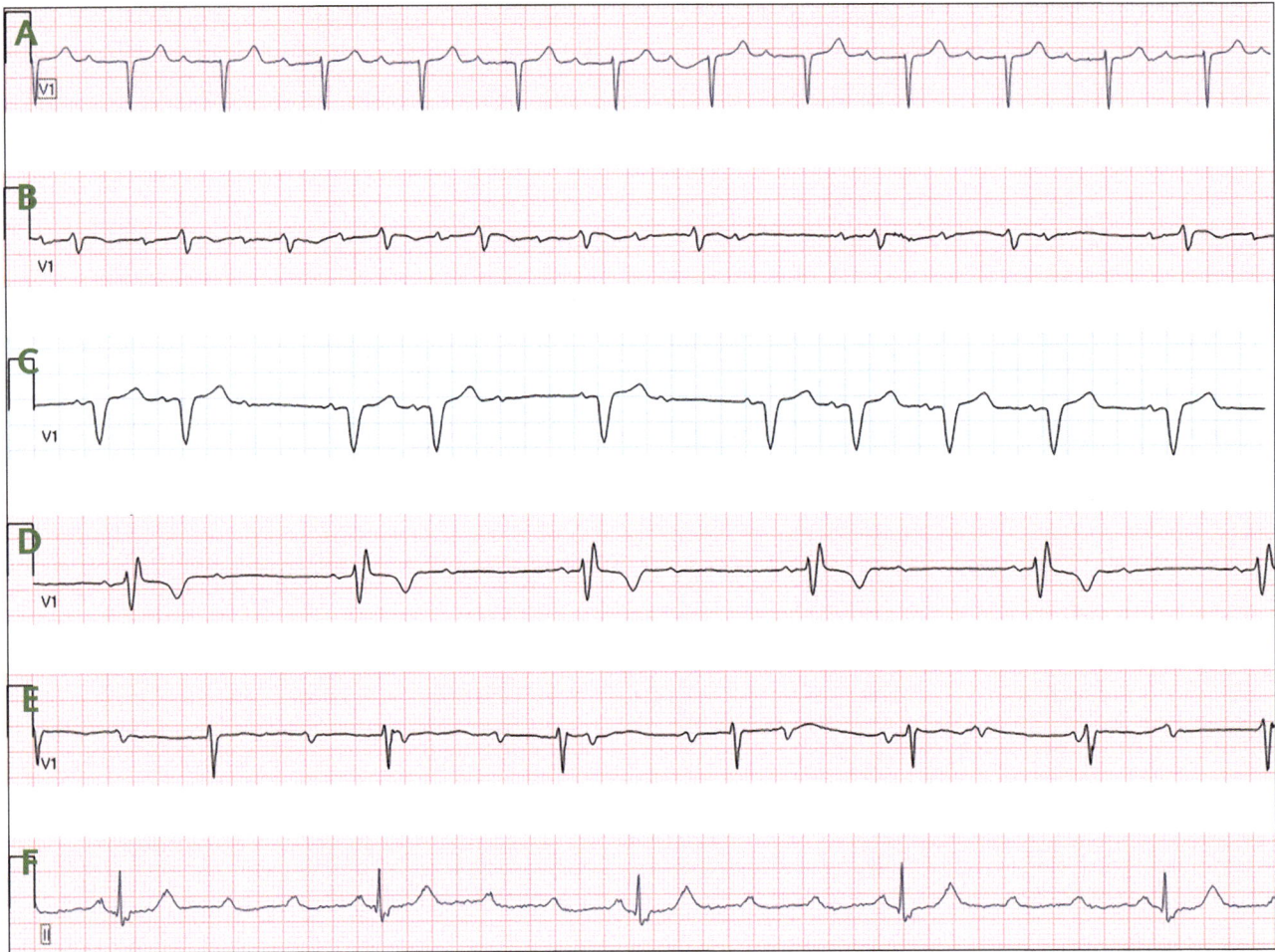

Figure 64.1 Electrocardiographic examples of AV block. (**A**) 1st degree AV block: AV with a fixed long PR interval; (**B**) 2nd degree AV block (Mobitz Type I): progressive PR interval prolongation preceding a single nonconducted P wave; (**C**) 2nd degree AV block (Mobitz Type II): intermittent loss of AV conduction without variations in the PR interval; (**D**) 2:1 AV block: every other P wave is not conducted (differentiating Mobitz Type I from Mobitz Type II not possible without physiologic or pharmacologic maneuvers); (**E**) Complete heart block: an atrial rhythm completely dissociated from a slower, regular ventricular rate; (**F**) High-grade AV block: sinus rhythm with 4:1 AV conduction (only every 4th P wave is conducted).

type II second-degree or third-degree AV block under any of the following circumstances:

1. *AV block that is not reversible.* This includes patients in whom necessary drug therapy contributes to AV block. Patients undergoing AV junctional catheter ablation or who develop AV block as a complication of cardiac surgery also warrant permanent pacing. In the setting of myocardial infarction, pacemakers are recommended if AV block persists and is felt to be infranodal, or is transient and the level of block is uncertain. In the setting of cardiac sarcoid, the occurrence of even transient high-grade AV block should prompt device implantation.

2. *AV block that causes significant symptoms or hemodynamic instability.* Significant symptoms include syncope, presyncope, exercise intolerance, symptoms due to bradycardia-related hypotension, or symptomatic congestive heart failure. Some systemic symptoms such as weakness, fatigue, dizziness, functional decline, and dyspnea are fairly nonspecific and should prompt further investigations to establish symptom–rhythm correlation prior to considering pacemaker implantation.

3. *Asymptomatic AV block if the escape pacemaker rhythm is unreliable.* This includes any patients with Mobitz type II AV block or third-degree AV block with asystolic pauses > 3 seconds (> 5 seconds if the atrial rhythm is atrial fibrillation), an escape rate < 40 bpm, or an infranodal escape rhythm.

4. *AV block in which the escape rhythm is > 40 bpm but the patient has evidence of left ventricle dysfunction or cardiomegaly.* In such circumstances, pacemakers appear to improve outcome and are recommended. Where second- or third-degree AVB occurs during exercise and is not thought to be secondary to myocardial ischemia, distal conduction system disease is likely and permanent pacing is also indicated. Patients with second- or third-degree AV block in

the setting of heritable neuromuscular diseases also warrant a permanent pacemaker, even if symptoms are lacking.

Permanent pacing is clearly **not** indicated (class III indication) under the following circumstances:

1. Asymptomatic first-degree AV block or Mobitz type I second-degree block.

2. AV block that is expected to resolve and not recur once a reversible cause has been addressed. A common example of this would be Mobitz type I second- or third-degree AV block with a narrow QRS escape rhythm following acute inferior wall myocardial infarction that resolves completely after a number of days.

Between the class I and class III recommendations, there are a number of situations where the value of permanent pacemakers is more controversial but may be considered (class II indications) in patients who have experienced second- or third-degree AV block. These include:

1. Patients who are asymptomatic and are found during electrophysiology study to have infranodal second-degree AV block;

2. Patients with third-degree AV block and a stable junctional escape rhythm (>40 bpm) without hemodynamic instability or compromise;

3. Patients with heritable neuromuscular disease and asymptomatic first- or second-degree Mobitz type I AV block; and

4. Patients with first-degree AV block that causes symptoms similar to pacemaker syndrome.

Congenital AV Block

Congenital third-degree AV block may exist as an isolated electrical abnormality or may be associated with congenital heart disease, such as endocardial cushion defects or congenitally corrected transposition of the great arteries (L-TGA). In isolated congenital AV block, a pacemaker is usually not needed at the time of initial diagnosis because the escape rhythm usually arises from the junctional tissue and remains stable for a number of years. However, permanent pacing is warranted once signs or symptoms suggest that the junctional escape rhythm is no longer reliable or is insufficient to maintain a stable hemodynamic state. Studies have shown improved longevity and the prevention of syncopal episodes even in this asymptomatic group.[3,4] Similar to those with acquired AV block, ominous warning signs warranting expeditious pacemaker implantation include presyncope or syncope; the occurrence of symptoms related to chronotropic incompetence (fatigue, exercise intolerance) or symptoms secondary to evolving heart failure or low cardiac output; the development of a wide QRS escape rhythm; a low resting junctional escape rate or failure to increase the junctional escape rate appropriately during exercise; evidence of left ventricular dysfunction or enlargement; complex ventricular ectopy at rest or during exertion; and development of QT interval prolongation and torsades de pointes.

Distal Conduction System Disease Without Previous AV Block

There are a variety of circumstances where AV block has not been documented but the patient has evidence of conduction system disease. The most common example would be bifascicular block or so-called trifascicular block (bifascicular block with concomitant first-degree AV block). Isolated fascicular block without symptoms or AV block does not require permanent pacing. However, a pacemaker is recommended (class I) when the patient has alternating right and left bundle branch block regardless of underlying cause (including myocardial infarction) or bifascicular block associated with intermittent Mobitz II or third-degree AV block.

Situations where pacing may be considered (class II) include patients experiencing unexplained syncope, with underlying conduction system disease without evidence of AV block (ie, bundle branch block) if other likely causes have been excluded. Limited evidence suggests that the moderate likelihood of progression to AV block makes "empiric" pacing reasonable, recognizing the small risk that an alternate cause of syncope will not be addressed by a pacemaker. Given the strong likelihood of progression and risk of sudden death, pacing should be strongly considered in patients with a heritable neuromuscular disorder (myotonic and muscular dystrophies) and distal conduction system disease. Likewise, pacing should be considered in asymptomatic patients with electrophysiologic evidence of infranodal disease (HV interval ≥ 100 ms).

Sinus Node Dysfunction

Sinus node dysfunction (SND) is primarily a disease of the elderly. It is best approached as a syndrome with a broad spectrum of causes whose common manifestation is disturbance of sinus node impulse formation and propagation.

ECG Manifestations of SND

SND includes persistent and inappropriate sinus bradycardia, paroxysmal sinus pauses or arrest, and tachycardia-bradycardia syndrome ("tachy-brady syndrome"). While sinus pauses are defined as an absence of sinus P waves for less than 3 seconds, sinus arrest refers to pauses greater than 3 seconds. In tachy-brady syndrome, the tachycardia may alternate with the bradycardia or be simultaneous. Alternating tachycardia-bradycardia usually involves paroxysmal atrial fibrillation or flutter with a rapid ventricular response as the tachycardia. When the atrial fibrillation terminates, the patient experiences a delay in resumption of sinus rhythm (postconversion arrest or asystole), significant sinus bradycardia, or any combination thereof. This is commonly referred to as "sick sinus syndrome." While the term tachy-brady syndrome is often applied to any patient with atrial fibrillation who happens to also have some degree of sinus bradycardia, even if it is appropriately slow, we would advise reserving the diagnosis for those patients whose bradycardia is symptomatic and/or extreme. The simultaneous form of tachycardia-bradycardia usually involves atrial fibrillation with a slow ventricular response rate due to concomitant AV nodal conduction problems. The associated tachyarrhythmia is thought to reflect underlying abnormalities in atrial tissue, creating a predisposition for both bradycardias and tachycardias.[5] Whether the simultaneous form of tachycardia-bradycardia truly represents sinus node dysfunction is somewhat controversial. Electrocardiographic examples of SND are displayed in Figure 64.2.

Etiology and Pathophysiology

The underlying pathology in many cases is unknown and assumed to be due to progressive deterioration of the sinus node and juxtanodal atrial tissue. Certainly any number of disease processes can degrade sinus node automaticity or perinodal conduction. The sinus node can be damaged by ischemic injury, surgical trauma, and infiltrative diseases (amyloidosis, hemochromatosis, sarcoidosis). Sinus node function can also be affected by metabolic derangements such as thyroid disease or drugs. Even at low doses, drugs may have an exaggerated depressant effect on sinus node function in patients with early or subclinical SND. Not infrequently, SND can be provoked or aggravated by antiarrhythmic drug therapy, which creates a therapeutic dilemma.

It is also important to recognize that the sinus node complex is modulated by the autonomic nervous system and that marked fluctuations in autonomic tone can yield electrocardiographic manifestations that mimic SND. During episodes of neurally mediated syncope, sinus pauses or arrest lasting more than 20 to 30 seconds can occur. Similarly, sleep apnea may cause marked nocturnal sinus bradycardia or arrest. These are important entities to distinguish from primary SND.

Clinical Presentation

Like AV block, SND can provoke a spectrum of symptoms depending on the particular electrocardiographic manifestation. Those with persistent sinus bradycardia or chronotropic incompetence may complain of fatigue or exertional limitations. Depending on the duration of asystole, sinus arrest or alternating tachycardia-bradycardia might provoke episodes of lightheadedness, presyncope, or syncope. Tachy-brady syndrome commonly causes complaints of palpitations, as well as syncope or presyncope when tachycardia terminates. Because these symptoms are not specific to SND, symptom–rhythm correlation is imperative. Unlike AV block, the natural history of SND is more benign, and the incidence of sudden death is low. Therefore, although pacing is the only effective therapy for SND, it does not appear to impact patient survival.[6-8]

Pacemaker Indications in Sinus Node Dysfunction

Both North American and European guidelines recommend pacemaker implantation in patients with (1) symptomatic SND, (2) SND precipitated or aggravated by necessary drug therapy, (3) recurrent syncope due to carotid sinus hypersensitivity, and/or (4) provocable asystolic pauses of > 3 seconds. Where correlation between symptoms and ECG manifestations are more tenuous, a permanent pacemaker may still be considered based on strong suspicion. Permanent pacing may also be considered if electrophysiologic testing is performed for unexplained syncope and corrected sinus node recovery times are blatantly abnormal. Permanent pacing is not

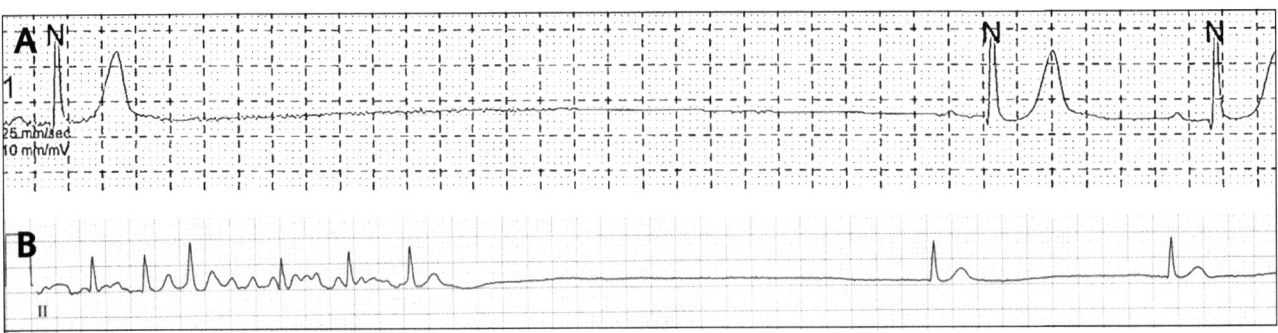

Figure 64.2 Electrocardiographic examples of sinus node dysfunction. Sinus arrest (**Panel A**): sinus bradycardia with a sinus pause > 3 seconds. Sick sinus syndrome (**Panel B**): long pause without sinus activity following conversion of atrial fibrillation.

indicated for SND if the patient is asymptomatic, where symptoms do not correlate with the ECG findings or when SND is expected to resolve and not recur. The various indications for permanent pacemaker implantation for both AV block and sinus node dysfunction are summarized in flowchart format in Figure 64.3.

Pacing Mode Selection for Bradycardia

To understand the debate about the most appropriate pacing modality, it is necessary to appreciate the evolution of pacemaker technology. The first pacemakers to be developed were single-lead devices that paced a single-chamber (atrium or ventricle), depending on the lead implant site. They paced the heart asynchronously (AOO or VOO); demand pacemakers (AAI or VVI) that inhibited pacing output during intrinsic rhythm came later. Eventually, dual-lead generators were introduced, making synchronized, sequential dual-chamber pacing (DDD) possible. A technological variant of the dual-chamber pacemaker is the single lead with pairs of atrial and ventricular electrodes that allowed sensing of intrinsic atrial activity with tracked ventricular pacing (single-pass VDD device). Finally, the maturation of pacemaker software made reprogramming of the pacing mode after device implant possible so that even a dual-chamber pacemaker could be programmed to a single-chamber pacing mode (eg, VVIR). The major decision to be made once a permanent pacemaker is deemed indicated is the type of device hardware to be implanted. Single-chamber devices have the advantage of less hardware to implant, lower cost, greater battery longevity, and simpler device management than dual-chamber devices. Conversely, dual-chamber devices offer inherently more physiologic pacing in exchange for the cost, complexity, and often a higher burden of right ventricular pacing than single-chamber atrial pacemakers. The central and long-standing issue has been whether DDD pacing mode confers improved patient outcomes that justify the limitations and costs. Unfortunately, the accumulated scientific evidence to date does not allow for simple decision making in patients with AVB or sinus node dysfunction.

With regard to patients with advanced AVB, initial small, retrospective studies comparing dual- versus single-chamber ventricular pacing yielded conflicting results.[9-11] Subsequent randomized clinical trials have brought some clarity to the issue. Small studies that included a portion of AVB patients observed no difference in mortality or clinical outcomes.[12,13] The Canadian Trial of Physiologic Pacing (CTOPP) enrolled 2,568 bradycardia patients, 52% of whom had isolated AV block and an additional 8% who had combined AV block and SND.[14] CTOPP reported no difference in the primary combined outcome of stroke or cardiovascular mortality in the overall study population. Importantly, subgroup analysis showed no differential response in AVB patients compared to those with SND as the pacemaker indication.

The United Kingdom Pacing and Cardiovascular Events (UKPACE) Trial compared VVI/R versus DDD pacing in elderly patients (mean age 80 years) with isolated second- or third-degree AV block.[15] The median follow-up was 4.6 years for death and 3 years for other cardiovascular events. Pacing mode hardware had no significant influence on the primary outcome of all-cause mortality or any of the secondary endpoints (cardiovascular mortality, stroke, atrial fibrillation, heart failure, angina, or myocardial infarction) although VVI pacing was associated with an increased

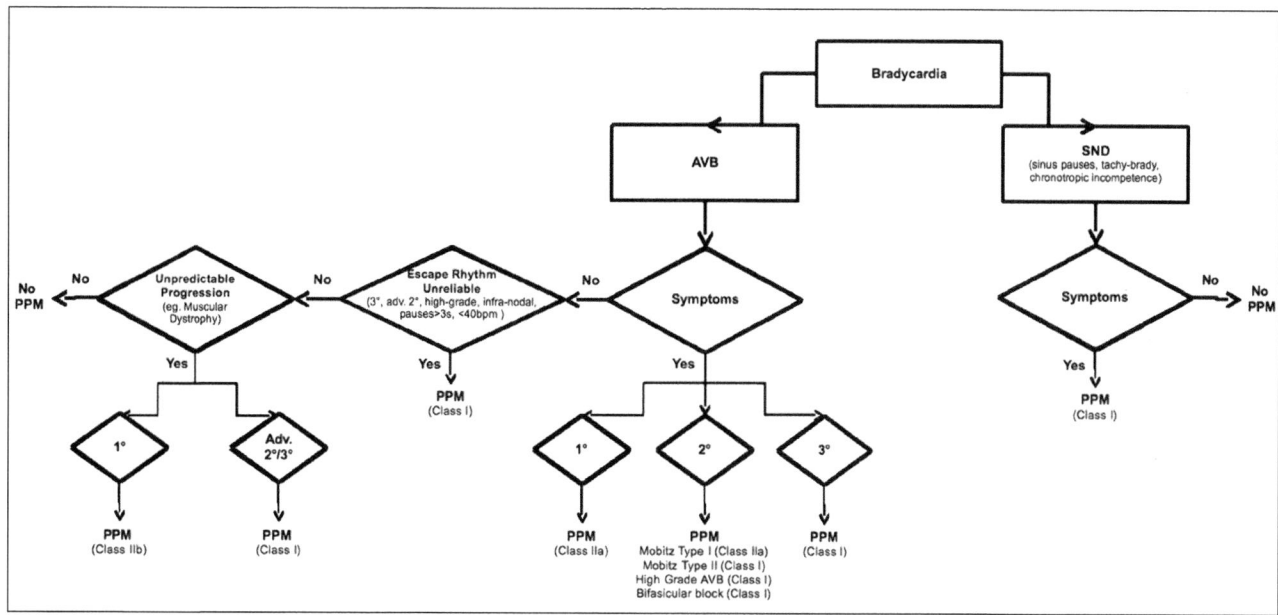

Figure 64.3 Indications for permanent pacemaker implantation. Summary of current guideline indications for permanent pacemaker implantation for AV block and sinus node dysfunction.

combined event rate of stroke, transient ischemic attack, or thromboembolism. However, event rates were similar with VVIR compared with DDD pacing. A subsequent meta-analysis of 7 trials found that atrial-based pacing did reduce the incidence of atrial fibrillation but not the composite outcome of stroke or cardiovascular death or overall mortality.[16] Thus, there is little evidence that dual-chamber pacing has compelling benefits for AVB patients over single-chamber ventricular pacing mode.

For patients with isolated SND, there are three possible pacing modality options: single-chamber atrial (AAI/R), single-chamber ventricular (VVI/R), or dual-chamber pacing mode (DDD/R). Single-chamber atrial pacing would preserve AV synchrony while avoiding the detrimental hemodynamic effects of ventricular pacing. However, AAI(R) pacing would not benefit those with substantial atrial fibrillation burden or adequately treat those who develop AV block, which occurs at a rate of 0.6% to 3% per year in those with SND.[17,18] Conversely, ventricular pacing would certainly provide backup pacing and address future AVB, but would not maintain AV synchrony.

Several large randomized clinical trials have examined pacing mode in SND patients. The Mode Selection trial in Sinus-Node Dysfunction (MOST) study directly compared VVIR versus DDDR mode.[19] All enrolled patients received dual-chamber pacemakers and were then programmed to DDDR (n = 1,014) or VVIR (n = 996). Over a median follow-up of 3 years, no difference was found in the combined endpoint of all-cause mortality, cardiovascular death, or nonfatal stroke. However, the rate of atrial fibrillation and heart failure hospitalization were lower in the DDDR group. In both arms, their incidence correlated directly with the cumulative amount of ventricular pacing.[20] These findings were virtually identical to those of the CTOPP trial involving both SND and AVB patients.

Early small randomized trials suggested that AAI/R pacing was superior to DDD, presumably because right ventricular pacing was avoided.[21,22] AAIR and DDDR were compared in the recently concluded Danish Multicenter Randomized Trial on Single Lead Atrial Pacing versus Dual-chamber Pacing in Sick Sinus Syndrome (DANPACE) trial.[23] In accordance with previous studies, there was no difference in death from any cause detected between the two groups. However, there was a 2-fold higher incidence of reoperation in the AAI group (1.7% per year) attributable to the need for a ventricular pacing lead. Unexpectedly, paroxysmal atrial fibrillation occurred more commonly with AAI/R, although the risk of chronic atrial fibrillation during the limited follow-up period was not increased.

Thus, there is no compelling evidence that the physiologic benefits of DDD or AAI/R modes translate directly into better patient outcome, making VVIR mode a reasonable option in many SND patients. Although the higher incidence of AF with VVI mode is of some concern, what has emerged as a central priority in pacemaker therapy is the imperative to avoid unnecessary ventricular pacing.[20,24] To a great extent, advances in pacing technology have rendered single-chamber atrial pacing an anachronism. Dual-chamber pacemakers now contain advanced pacing algorithms that effectively pace patients in AAI mode but are able to rapidly convert to DDD mode in the event of AVB. Therefore, the decision to implant single-chamber ventricular or dual-chamber hardware should still be decided on an individual basis, taking into account each patient's particular medical circumstances and the likelihood that dual-chamber pacing will improve quality of life.

The dilemma for clinicians is that DDD pacemakers have a sound physiological and hemodynamic rationale, but no impact on patient population outcome measures. This does not mean that DDD pacemakers make no difference in individual patients, but simply that there is no evidence that they need to be implanted in everyone. Most physicians would agree that some patients should preferentially receive a DDD pacemaker, but the criteria identifying those patients may differ among physicians. One approach would be to consider every bradycardia patient a potential candidate for dual-chamber pacing and then look for clinical factors that would either limit the extent of benefit they may derive or, conversely, factors that might make DDD pacing compelling for hemodynamic reasons. For example, a patient with permanent atrial fibrillation or a serious medical illness limiting his or her quantity or quality of life (for instance, dementia or severe chronic lung disease) would not benefit, and a VVI/R pacemaker would suffice. Similarly, in patients with intermittent bradycardia, where pacing would be infrequent and short-lived, loss of AV synchrony from backup VVI pacemaker may have negligible negative consequences. On the other hand, patients who would suffer severe hemodynamic deterioration with loss of AV synchrony (such as hypertrophic cardiomyopathy) should receive a DDD pacemaker.

For the SND patient who has a reasonable life expectancy and is enjoying a reasonable quality of life, one should strongly consider a dual-chamber device that possesses AVI pacing mode (automatic switching between AAI and DDD modes) to minimize ventricular pacing. AVI mode is preferred over algorithms that simply increase the AV delay. Where keeping the amount of intravascular lead hardware to a minimum is a priority, a single-chamber atrial pacemaker might be considered especially if sinus arrest is intermittent and infrequent. If the patient has atrial fibrillation, a pacemaker that includes a ventricular lead (DDDR or VVIR) would be indicated. For the patient with SND and pronounced first-degree AVB who have significant left ventricle dysfunction where the likelihood of ventricular pacing is high, one should consider cardiac resynchronization therapy (see section on Cardiomyopathies).

Among patients with AV block, most should at least be considered for a dual-chamber system (DDDR or

VDDDR) because of the hemodynamic benefits of maintaining AV synchrony. Clinical factors that might favor consideration of a VVI/R pacemaker instead include advanced patient age, comorbid disease that limits patient prognosis or functional capacity, left ventricular systolic dysfunction, and expected burden of pacing. The patient with significant left ventricular systolic dysfunction requires careful consideration. A DDDR system may be important in maintaining optimal left ventricle filling and systolic performance. We await the results of several important ongoing clinical trials to determine whether these patents should be considered for a CRT device instead.

Neurocardiogenic Syncope and Sleep Apnea

Neurocardiogenic syncope and sleep apnea constitute an unusual collection of medical disorders that manifest as bradycardia, for which pacemaker therapy has been considered. Where they differ from the previously discussed bradycardias is that, in these disorders, there is no inherent abnormality of the cardiac conduction system. Rather, the bradycardia is primarily due to fluctuations in autonomic tone. The rationale for permanent pacing in this circumstance is that, regardless of pathophysiologic mechanism, bradycardia is the immediate cause of symptoms and it cannot be reliably prevented.

Neurocardiogenic Syncope

Neurocardiogenic syncope encompasses a number of entities, including carotid sinus hypersensitivity, vasovagal syncope, micturition syncope, and glossopharyngeal syncope. Bradycardia in these syndromes is due to activation of an autonomic reflex by a variety of triggers. The net result is varying degrees of vasodilation (vasodepressor component) and bradycardia (cardio-inhibitory component) that contribute to hypotension and cerebral hypo-perfusion.

Vasovagal syncope is a benign disorder that predominantly afflicts young patients with structurally normal hearts. The efficacy of pacing in vasovagal syncope has been the subject of 5 multicenter randomized controlled studies. A potential benefit for pacing was initially suggested in 3 nonblinded trials. However, 2 subsequent blinded trials (Vasovagal Pacemaker Study II [VPS-II] and Vasovagal Syncope and Pacing Trial [SYNPACE]) failed to demonstrate any significant benefit of dual-chamber pacing.[25-29] A meta-analysis of these studies suggested that 84% of the apparent benefit of pacing was due to an expectation effect (placebo).[30] Pacing therapy is therefore not generally recommended but may be considered (class II) in specific cases. Examples include the patient who has significant morbidity from recurrent syncope, particularly those with minimal prodrome or those patients who manifest profound prolonged asystolic pauses (for example, 20 seconds or more) during spontaneous episodes. Results from the ISSUE3 Trial, which is currently enrolling vasovagal syncope patients with loop recorder documented pauses of ≥6 seconds duration, should be helpful in clarifying the role of pacing therapy. Intuitively, patients who have a predominant vasodilatory response as a cause for their syncope will not benefit from pacing. If pacing therapy is contemplated, DDD/R pacemakers should be used to maintain optimal hemodynamics during episodes.

Obstructive Sleep Apnea (OSA)

Obstructive sleep apnea is associated with a variety of brady- and tachyarrhythmias. Sinus bradycardia and asystole are the most common rhythm disturbances, with sinus pauses that can last up to 10 seconds. These occur predominantly during sleep and can persist into waking hours. OSA-related bradycardia appears to be provoked by enhanced vagal tone during periods of hypopnea, termed cyclic variation of the heart rate. The clinical significance of these pauses and whether pacing is indicated if bradycardia is present during waking hours remain unclear. Preliminary studies in patients with OSA and pacemakers suggested a prominent beneficial effect on sleep apnea, but follow-up studies including crossover studies have not borne out the index observation.[31] Sleep-disordered breathing in the systolic heart failure population is associated with increased mortality. There is limited evidence that biventricular pacing may improve outcomes in this population. In a study, examining a population with central sleep apnea and systolic heart failure, cardiac resynchronization therapy was associated with a reduction in apneic episodes and improved sleep quality.[32] The improvement in sleep-disordered breathing is thought to be due to CRT's positive effects on left ventricular function and hemodynamics. The resulting decline in left ventricle filling and pulmonary pressures reduce the hyperventilation and hypocapneic reflexes that perpetuate central sleep apnea.

Falls in the Elderly

The pathophysiology of recurrent falls and syncope in the elderly population is complex and multifactorial. Due to poor event recall and a high proportion of unwitnessed events, a cause is often not found.[33] However, due to the high prevalence of cardioinhibitory carotid sinus hypersensitivity (CICSH) in the elderly with unexplained falls,[34] a number of studies have been performed examining the potential role of permanent pacing in the prevention of unexplained falls. The SAFE PACE trial randomized elderly patients presenting with nonaccidental falls to dual-chamber pacing (with rate drop response) or control in an unblinded fashion. After a year of follow-up, the paced patients were significantly less likely to fall than were controls.[35] Despite these promising results, a subsequent blinded trial randomizing patients to either rate-responsive dual-chamber pacing or an implantable loop recorder was unable to show a benefit with pacing.[36] A double-blind, randomized crossover trial examining the effect of dual-chamber pacing with rate drop response programming (DDD/RDR) over placebo (ODO programming) in a similar population was also negative.[37] Based on this data, current guidelines suggest that permanent pacing is a reasonable consideration (class IIa recommendation; Level of Evidence C) for those presenting with syncope with unclear cause and a hypersensitive cardioinhibitory response of greater than 3 seconds.[38] The clinical trials evaluating the effect of pacing in the elderly population presenting with falls are summarized in Table 64.1.

Cardiomyopathies

Dilated Cardiomyopathy and Cardiac Resynchronization Therapy (CRT)

Patients with dilated cardiomyopathy from any cause may develop disturbances in ventricular electrical activation. The resulting QRS prolongation is associated with increased morbidity and mortality.[39,40] It is now appreciated that these electrical delays (whether intrinsic or pacing-induced) create mechanical inter- and intraventricular dyssynchrony that contribute to functional mitral regurgitation, impaired diastolic filling, and worsened left ventricular systolic performance.[41] Pacing right and left ventricles synchronously (referred to as biventricular pacing or cardiac resynchronization therapy) circumvents the disordered electrical activation and restores some measure of mechanical synchrony. These hemodynamic improvements have been repeatedly shown to translate to improved heart failure symptoms, functional capacity, NYHA heart failure class, quality of life scores, and reduced heart failure hospitalization. One meta-analysis reported a 29% reduction in heart failure hospitalizations and a 51% relative reduction mortality.[42] The left ventricular lead is usually implanted in a coronary vein via the coronary sinus, but this cannot be accomplished in up to 5% to 10% of patients. In addition, one-third or more of patients have minimal or no response to CRT. The reasons for this remain unknown.

Clinical Trial Evidence

CRT has been shown to reduce total mortality in patients with dilated cardiomyopathy (ischemic or nonischemic), LVEF ≤35%, wide QRS, and NYHA class II–IV heart failure symptoms despite optimal medical therapy. The CARE-HF study employed a primary endpoint that was a composite of all-cause death or hospitalization for cardiovascular events in patients with NYHA II–IV symptoms.[43] A 36% relative reduction in mortality and a 46% reduction in the primary composite endpoint were observed with CRT and confirmed one finding of the COMPANION trial.[44]

Encouraged by the clinical benefit of CRT in moderate to severe heart failure, several clinical studies were executed to evaluate its value in milder heart failure patients. The REVERSE trial enrolled 610 wide QRS patients with milder heart failure symptoms (NYHA I–II) and an LVEF of ≤40%. All patients received a CRT device (CRT-P or CRT-D) but were randomized to have the device ON or OFF for a minimum of 12 months. Patients enrolled in European centers were followed for 24 months. The primary endpoint was the number of patients with worsened clinical composite response (based on NYHA status, heart failure symptoms, hospitalization, death). For the entire study population, no statistically significant reduction in the rate of worsened clinical composite response with CRT ON was reported. However, there was echocardiographic evidence of left ventricular reverse remodeling with CRT ON.[45] In the European cohort of 262 patients, worsening

Table 64.1 Trials examining permanent pacing in elderly patients presenting with unexplained falls

	Year	n	Mean Age (years)	Trial Design	Intervention	Result	Mean Follow-up
Kenney et al[35] (SAFE PACE)	2001	175	73 ± 10	RCT Unblinded	DDD/RDR vs no intervention	DDD/RDR reduced falls (OR = 0.42; 95% CI 0.23 to 0.75)	1 year
Ryan et al[36] (SAFE PACE 2)	2010	141	78 ± 7	RCT Double Blind	DDD/RDR vs ILR	No difference (RR = 0.79; 95% CI 0.41 to 1.50)	2 years
Parry et al[37]	2009	34	77 ± 9	RCT Double Blind Crossover	DDD/RDR vs ODO	No difference (RR = 0.82 with a 95% CI of 0.62 to 1.10)	1 year

CI = confidence interval; DDD/RDR = dual-chamber pacing with rate drop response; ILR = implantable loop recorder; ODO = dual-chamber sensing only (no pacing); OR = odds ratio; RCT = randomized controlled trial.

clinical composite response was significantly reduced with CRT compared to control patients (19% vs 34%).[46] MADIT-CRT randomized patients with NYHA I or II heart failure (in sinus rhythm, LVEF ≤30%, QRS duration ≥130 ms) in 3:2 ratio to CRT-D or ICD alone. Over an average follow-up period of 2.4 years, CRT-D was associated with a 34% relative reduction in primary endpoint compared with ICD therapy alone. This was driven by the reduction in heart failure events. MADIT-CRT failed to show any significant difference in mortality.[47]

The RAFT study is the most recently completed trial.[48] Patients enrolled were similar to MADIT-CRT except that they included a large number of NYHA class II patients (81%), a number of AF patients with a controlled ventricular response, and some who were pacemaker dependent. Patients were randomized in 1:1 ratio to CRT-D or ICD alone. Over a mean follow-up period of 40 months, CRT-D reduced the primary endpoint by 25% (33% vs 40%, $P = 0.001$) compared to ICD alone. Equally as important, there was a 25% relative reduction in all-cause mortality in patients receiving CRT, over and above the mortality benefit provided by an ICD.

Because only two-thirds of patients will respond to resynchronization therapy, studies evaluating the mechanisms underlying "nonresponse" continue to grow. Many studies have focused on identifying the optimal patient characteristics for CRT candidacy. For instance, clinical benefit has not been clearly demonstrated in patients with narrow QRS (< 120 ms) despite echocardiographic evidence of mechanical dyssynchrony.[49] Moreover, subgroup analysis of large randomized studies such as MADIT-CRT and RAFT suggest that certain populations, such as those with right bundle branch block, a QRS duration < 150 ms, or atrial fibrillation (AF), may not benefit as much from CRT.[44,48] Identifying the patients in these subgroups who may or may not benefit from CRT remains the challenge.

CRT in Patients with Atrial Fibrillation

There are several factors that may contribute to the suboptimal response to CRT in the AF population. Inadequate rate control is a common culprit. AF with rapid ventricular response results in frequent fusion or pseudofusion beats, which compromises the degree of resynchronization. There has been some evidence that adjunctive AV node ablation may be superior to drug therapy alone in facilitating structural and clinical response to CRT in patients with permanent AF. In a series of 673 patients receiving CRT for conventional indications (LVEF ≤35%, NYHA class ≥II, and QRSd ≥120 ms), those who underwent AV node ablation had the most improvement in left ventricular function and functional capacity.[50] Interestingly, this study also suggests that adjunctive AV node ablation may even allow AF patients to benefit from resynchronization therapy to the same degree as those with sinus rhythm. A similar observation was made in retrospective studies.[50,51] Prospective randomized trials are required to validate this finding.

CRT in Patients Requiring Chronic Right Ventricular Pacing

Due to the well-established detrimental effects of chronic right ventricular pacing, the effect of CRT on those who develop left ventricular dysfunction due to chronic right ventricular pacing has also been studied. The Homburg Biventricular Pacing Evaluation (HOBIPACE) trial was a randomized crossover study in which 30 patients (left ventricular end-diastolic diameter ≥60 mm and LVEF ≤40%) were subjected to 3 months each of right ventricular pacing and CRT. In comparison to right ventricular pacing alone, CRT was associated with reverse remodeling, improvement in heart failure symptoms, and improved LVEF.[52] Similar observations were made when 60 chronically right ventricular–paced patients were upgraded to a biventricular pacing system.[53] Although these studies are encouraging, their results need to be confirmed in larger randomized trials. The BLOCK-HF trial randomized 691 patients with atrioventricular block and left ventricular systolic dysfunction defined at ejection fraction < 50%, and NYHA class I, II, or III heart failure symptoms. Those who were randomly assigned to biventricular pacing had significantly better outcomes with respect to survival, heart failure hosptialization, and urgent heart failure visits with cardiac resynchronization therapy usage in both pacemaker and defibrillator recipients. This trial provides compelling evidence that those with a high burden of pacing do benefit from resynchronization therapy.[54]

Indications for CRT Device Implantation

According to the recently updated 2012 ACCF/AHA/HRS guidelines,[55] CRT device therapy carries a class I indication in patients with ischemic or nonischemic dilated cardiomyopathy with an LVEF ≤35% who have a left bundle branch block ≥150 ms (≥130 ms per the 2013 Canadian Cardiovascular Society guidelines[56]) and are NYHA functional class II or III or ambulatory class IV heart failure despite optimal medical therapy. Those with dilated cardiomyopathy who have well-controlled atrial fibrillation or require ventricular pacing for bradycardia have a class II indication for a CRT device. Suffice it to say that indications are in a state of flux in view of evolving clinical trial evidence. What to do with those with chronic AF, RBBB, or nonspecific intraventricular conduction delay QRS durations between 120 and 150 ms or existing right ventricular pacemakers will likely remain controversial until more scientific evidence accumulates. For the time being, it may be wiser to consider the patient's medical profile in its entirety rather than excluding patients from CRT therapy based on any one of these parameters. Moreover, there is building evidence that factors such as myocardial scar burden, the location of scar with respect to the area of mechanical dyssynchrony, LV lead position, right heart function, and renal dysfunction may be important factors in the likelihood of CRT response. Recent evidence also suggests that imaging-guided targeted LV lead placement may also improve response rates.[57]

Hypertrophic Obstructive Cardiomyopathy

Initial nonrandomized data suggested that the implantation of dual-chamber pacemakers reduced symptoms and left ventricular outflow tract gradient in patients with hypertrophic obstructive cardiomyopathy.[58] The putative mechanism was pacing-induced intraventricular dyssynchrony and remodeling. Unfortunately, 3 subsequent randomized controlled trials with appropriate blinding found that symptomatic improvement did not correlate with a reduction in gradient, suggesting that this was largely due to a placebo effect.[57-59] Therefore, current data and guidelines do not support routine pacemaker implantation in patients with symptomatic outflow tract obstruction. Pacing should be reserved for those who develop complete heart block following alcohol septal ablation or surgical myomectomy. Maintenance of AV synchrony with a DDD/R pacemaker is advised because of the significant diastolic dysfunction. In patients with hypertrophic cardiomyopathy and risk factors for sudden cardiac death, an implantable cardioverter-defibrillator should be strongly considered.

The current class I and class II guideline indications for permanent pacemaker implantation are summarized in Tables 64.2 and 64.3.

Pacing for Tachycardias

At one time, pacemaker therapy for chronic control of certain supraventricular tachycardias (SVT) was a serious consideration. The advent of catheter ablation to cure patients with various SVTs has rendered permanent pacemakers a historical curiosity with no real relevance to most patients today. However, in patients with tachyarrhythmias, chronic pacing might be considered in two particular scenarios. The first is the patient who develops malignant ventricular arrhythmias in the context of QT prolongation syndromes, wherein bradycardia may be an important component. The other situation is antitachycardia pacing, either as a component of defibrillator therapy to terminate reentrant ventricular arrhythmias, or (less commonly) as a feature of certain pacemaker platforms designed to interrupt or prevent atrial arrhythmias.

Long QT syndrome (LQTS) is a heritable arrhythmogenic condition associated with risk of syncope and sudden death due to torsades de pointes. Arrhythmic risk varies significantly between affected individuals and is

Table 64.2 Class I indications for permanent pacemaker implantation

Condition	Class I Indications
Sinus Node Dysfunction	Symptomatic bradycardia* due to chronotropic incompetence or pauses
AV Block	Symptomatic second-degree or third-degree AV block*§
	Asymptomatic
	• pauses > 3 s (> 5 s in AF), an escape rate < 40 bpm, or an infranodal escape
	• advanced AV block with neuromuscular disease
	• third-degree AV block if
	• infranodal escape or
	• LV dysfunction/cardiomegally
	• exercise-induced second-degree or third-degree AV block
	• bifascicular block with
	• advanced second-degree or third-degree AV block
	• alternating bundle branch block
Cardiac Resynchronization Therapy	NYHA II-IV, LVEF < 35%, sinus rhythm and LBBB > 150 ms on GDMT
Neurocardiogenic Syncope	Recurrent syncope due to hypersensitive carotid sinus syndrome and asystole > 3 s
Pacing to Prevent Tachycardia	Sustained pause-dependent VT (with or without long QT)

* spontaneous or due to necessary drug therapy
§ following cardiac surgery, ablation, or MI
LVEF = left ventricular ejection fraction; s = seconds; LBBB = left bundle branch block; GDMT = guideline-directed medical therapy.

dependent on a variety of factors, including the specific LQT mutation, its interaction with a patient's particular genetic milieu, and potential triggers such as drugs and metabolic imbalances. Cardiac pacing is a reasonable consideration in those who continue to have syncope or ventricular arrhythmias despite β-blocker therapy. Pacing is thought to be particularly effective for those in whom dispersion of repolarization is aggravated by bradycardia, which promotes pause-dependent arrhythmias. Pacing at a rate that reduces the QTc has been shown to be reasonably effective.[59,60] The most recent ACC/AHA joint guidelines give pacing in LQTS a class IIa recommendation. However, the relatively high mortality in patients who remain symptomatic despite β-blockers warrants consideration of ICD implantation instead.

Painless termination of reentrant ventricular arrhythmias in the form of antitachycardia pacing algorithms has become an essential component of defibrillator therapy. Programmed electrical stimulation and rapid burst pacing of an appropriately detected arrhythmia has been shown to successfully treat ventricular arrhythmias avoiding the need for ICD shocks.[61]

Table 64.3 Class II indications for permanent pacemaker implantation

Condition	Class II Indications
Sinus Node Dysfunction	HR < 40 bpm and symptoms suspected to be from SND
	Syncope of unknown cause with evidence of SND on EPS
AV Block	Asymptomatic • third-degree AVB (HR > 40 bpm) • advanced second-degree AV block with narrow QRS • second-degree AVB found to be intra- or infranodal at EPS
	Symptomatic AV block of any level (first degree or second degree)
	Neuromuscular disease and • AV block of any degree • bifascicular block
	AV block due to drug use/toxicity that is likely to recur even after drug withdrawal
	Bifascicular block and • syncope of unclear etiology • EPS showing HV interval ≥ 100 ms or pacing induced infra-His block
Cardiac Resynchronization Therapy	NYHA II-IV, LVEF < 35%, on GDMT and: 1) non-LBBB conduction delay with QRS width >150 ms or 2) patients with well-controlled AF who are otherwise CRT candidates or 3) pacemaker-dependent
Neurocardiogenic Syncope	Syncope of unclear etiology and hypersensitive carotid sinus cardioinhibitory response of > 3 s
	Significantly symptomatic neurocardiogenic syncope with spontaneous or tilt-table-provoked bradycardia
Pacing to Prevent Tachycardia	High-risk congenital LQT
	To prevent symptomatic, drug refractory recurrent AF and coexisting SND
Hypertrophic Obstructive Cardiomyopathy	Symptomatic outflow tract obstruction

AF = atrial fibrillation; EPS = electrophysiology study; LVEF = left ventricular ejection fraction; s = seconds; SND = sinus node dysfunction.

Pacemakers with atrial antitachycardia algorithms capable of terminating supraventricular tachycardias are also available. These specialized platforms are armed with the ability to automatically respond with programmed stimulation following appropriate arrhythmia detection and/or activation by an external device. However, due to various factors, the efficacy of these algorithms is difficult to assess, and has not been reliably duplicated in randomized trials. While the most recent practice guidelines suggest that they are a reasonable consideration (class IIa recommendation) in those with symptomatic paroxysmal supraventricular tachycardia, the reality is that devices are rarely used in this situation and are reserved solely for the rare patient refractory to medical therapy and catheter ablation.[38]

Algorithms designed to prevent atrial fibrillation with atrial overdrive pacing have also been studied. However, data is limited and inconsistent. The Atrial Dynamic Overdrive Pacing Trial evaluated the safety and efficacy of an AF suppression algorithm relative to DDDR pacing alone in sinus node dysfunction patients, with concomitant AF an indication for permanent pacing.[62] The algorithm was intended to atrial pace slightly faster than the intrinsic sinus rate while allowing for normal diurnal variation in heart rate. This algorithm reportedly decreased symptomatic AF burden by 25% relative to controls. However, the absolute difference was small (2.5% vs 1.87%), and there was no significant difference in mean number of AF episodes, total hospitalizations, quality of life scores, adverse events, or mortality.

Therefore, based on the current body of evidence, permanent pacing for the prevention of symptomatic recurrent atrial fibrillation in the presence of sinus node dysfunction currently carries a class IIb recommendation.[38] Permanent pacing to prevent atrial fibrillation in the absence of an independent indication for pacing is not recommended.[38] Consistent data supporting alternative single-site atrial pacing, multisite atrial pacing, and biatrial pacing to prevent atrial fibrillation is also lacking, but continues to be explored.

Conclusion

Since the implantation of the first pacemaker in the mid-20th century, an impressive body of evidence has emerged supporting their effectiveness in treating bradycardia-related symptoms, morbidity, and mortality. Over the last 50 years, pacemakers have evolved into smaller and increasingly more sophisticated devices. Advancements in technology and progress in our understanding of their utility in various conditions continue to improve our ability to identify those who will benefit most from pacing. Given the human resources and financial cost involved in pacemaker implantation and follow-up, guideline recommendations based on evidence are crucial in ensuring their appropriate allocation and application. Although guidelines and clinical trials provide a broad framework for clinical practice, astute clinical judgment will always be required when considering the individual patient.

References

1. Epstein AE, DiMarco JP, Ellenbogen KA, et al. ACC/AHA/HRS 2008 guidelines for device-based therapy of cardiac rhythm abnormalities: a report of the American College of Cardiology/American Heart Association Task Force on Practice Guidelines (Writing Committee to Revise the ACC/AHA/NASPE 2002 Guideline Update for Implantation of Cardiac Pacemakers and Antiarrhythmia Devices) developed in collaboration with the American Association for Thoracic Surgery and Society of Thoracic Surgeons. *J Am Coll Cardiol.* May 27 2008;51(21):e1-62.
2. Vardas PE, Auricchio A, Blanc JJ, et al. Guidelines for cardiac pacing and cardiac resynchronization therapy: the Task Force for Cardiac Pacing and Cardiac Resynchronization Therapy of the European Society of Cardiology. Developed in collaboration with the European Heart Rhythm Association. *Eur Heart J.* Sep 2007;28(18):2256-2295.
3. Michaelsson M, Jonzon A, Riesenfeld T. Isolated congenital complete atrioventricular block in adult life. A prospective study. *Circulation.* Aug 1 1995;92(3):442-449.
4. Sholler GF, Walsh EP. Congenital complete heart block in patients without anatomic cardiac defects. *Am Heart J.* Dec 1989;118(6):1193-1198.
5. Mond HG, Irwin M, Ector H, Proclemer A. The world survey of cardiac pacing and cardioverter-defibrillators: calendar year 2005, an International Cardiac Pacing and Electrophysiology Society (ICPES) project. *Pacing Clin Electrophysiol.* Sep 2008;31(9):1202-1212.
6. Simon AB, Zloto AE. Symptomatic sinus node disease: natural history after permanent ventricular pacing. *Pacing Clin Electrophysiol.* May 1979;2(3):305-314.
7. Alt E, Volker R, Wirtzfeld A, Ulm K. Survival and follow-up after pacemaker implantation: a comparison of patients with sick sinus syndrome, complete heart block, and atrial fibrillation. *Pacing Clin Electrophysiol.* Nov 1985;8(6):849-855.
8. Menozzi C, Brignole M, Alboni P, et al. The natural course of untreated sick sinus syndrome and identification of the variables predictive of unfavorable outcome. *Am J Cardiol.* Nov 15 1998;82(10):1205-1209.
9. Alpert MA, Curtis JJ, Sanfelippo JF, et al. Comparative survival after permanent ventricular and dual chamber pacing for patients with chronic high degree atrioventricular block with and without preexistent congestive heart failure. *J Am Coll Cardiol.* Apr 1986;7(4):925-932.
10. Linde-Edelstam C, Gullberg B, Norlander R, Pehrsson SK, Rosenqvist M, Ryden L. Longevity in patients with high degree atrioventricular block paced in the atrial synchronous or the fixed rate ventricular inhibited mode. *Pacing Clin Electrophysiol.* Mar 1992;15(3):304-313.
11. Zanini R, Facchinetti A, Gallo G, et al. Survival rates after pacemaker implantation: a study of patients paced for sick sinus syndrome and atrioventricular block. *Pacing Clin Electrophysiol.* Jul 1989;12(7 Pt 1):1065-1069.
12. Mattioli AV, Vivoli D, Mattioli G. Influence of pacing modalities on the incidence of atrial fibrillation in patients without prior atrial fibrillation. A prospective study. *Eur Heart J.* Feb 1998;19(2):282-286.
13. Lamas GA, Orav EJ, Stambler BS, et al. Quality of life and clinical outcomes in elderly patients treated with ventricular pacing as compared with dual-chamber pacing. Pacemaker Selection in the Elderly Investigators. *N Engl J Med.* Apr 16 1998;338(16):1097-1104.
14. Connolly SJ, Kerr CR, Gent M, et al. Effects of physiologic pacing versus ventricular pacing on the risk of stroke and death due to cardiovascular causes. Canadian Trial of Physiologic Pacing Investigators. *N Engl J Med.* May 11 2000;342(19):1385-1391.
15. Toff WD, Camm AJ, Skehan JD. Single-chamber versus dual-chamber pacing for high-grade atrioventricular block. *N Engl J Med.* Jul 14 2005;353(2):145-155.
16. Healey JS, Toff WD, Lamas GA, et al. Cardiovascular outcomes with atrial-based pacing compared with ventricular pacing: meta-analysis of randomized trials, using individual patient data. *Circulation.* Jul 4 2006;114(1):11-17.
17. Andersen HR, Nielsen JC, Thomsen PE, et al. Atrioventricular conduction during long-term follow-up of patients with sick sinus syndrome. *Circulation.* Sep 29 1998;98(13):1315-1321.
18. Brandt J, Anderson H, Fahraeus T, Schuller H. Natural history of sinus node disease treated with atrial pacing in 213 patients: implications for selection of stimulation mode. *J Am Coll Cardiol.* Sep 1992;20(3):633-639.
19. Lamas GA, Lee KL, Sweeney MO, et al. Ventricular pacing or dual-chamber pacing for sinus-node dysfunction. *N Engl J Med.* Jun 13 2002;346(24):1854-1862.
20. Sweeney MO, Hellkamp AS, Ellenbogen KA, et al. Adverse effect of ventricular pacing on heart failure and atrial fibrillation among patients with normal baseline QRS duration in a clinical trial of pacemaker therapy for sinus node dysfunction. *Circulation.* Jun 17 2003;107(23):2932-2937.
21. Andersen HR, Thuesen L, Bagger JP, Vesterlund T, Thomsen PE. Prospective randomised trial of atrial versus ventricular pacing in sick-sinus syndrome. *Lancet.* Dec 3 1994;344 (8936):1523-1528.
22. Nielsen JC, Andersen HR, Thomsen PE, et al. Heart failure and echocardiographic changes during long-term follow-up of patients with sick sinus syndrome randomized to single-chamber atrial or ventricular pacing. *Circulation.* Mar 17 1998;97(10):987-995.
23. Nielsen JC, Thomsen PE, Hojberg S, et al. A comparison of single-lead atrial pacing with dual-chamber pacing in sick sinus syndrome. *Eur Heart J.* Mar 2011;32(6):686-696.
24. Wilkoff BL, Cook JR, Epstein AE, et al. Dual-chamber pacing or ventricular backup pacing in patients with an implantable defibrillator: the Dual Chamber and VVI Implantable Defibrillator (DAVID) Trial. *JAMA.* Dec 25 2002;288(24):3115-3123.
25. Sutton R, Brignole M, Menozzi C, et al. Dual-chamber pacing in the treatment of neurally mediated tilt-positive cardioinhibitory syncope: pacemaker versus no therapy: a multicenter randomized study. The Vasovagal Syncope International Study (VASIS) Investigators. *Circulation.* Jul 18 2000;102(3):294-299.
26. Connolly SJ, Sheldon R, Roberts RS, Gent M. The North American Vasovagal Pacemaker Study (VPS). A randomized trial of permanent cardiac pacing for the prevention of vasovagal syncope. *J Am Coll Cardiol.* Jan 1999;33(1):16-20.
27. Ammirati F, Colivicchi F, Santini M. Permanent cardiac pacing versus medical treatment for the prevention of recurrent vasovagal syncope: a multicenter, randomized, controlled trial. *Circulation.* Jul 3 2001;104(1):52-57.
28. Connolly SJ, Sheldon R, Thorpe KE, et al. Pacemaker therapy for prevention of syncope in patients with recurrent severe vasovagal syncope: Second Vasovagal Pacemaker Study (VPS II): a randomized trial. *JAMA.* May 7 2003;289 (17): 2224-2229.
29. Raviele A, Giada F, Menozzi C, et al. A randomized, double-blind, placebo-controlled study of permanent cardiac pacing for the treatment of recurrent tilt-induced vasovagal syncope. The vasovagal syncope and pacing trial (SYNPACE). *Eur Heart J.* Oct 2004;25(19):1741-1748.

30. Sud S, Massel D, Klein GJ, et al. The expectation effect and cardiac pacing for refractory vasovagal syncope. *Am J Med.* Jan 2007;120(1):54-62.
31. Krahn AD, Yee R, Erickson MK, et al. Physiologic pacing in patients with obstructive sleep apnea: a prospective, randomized crossover trial. *J Am Coll Cardiol.* Jan 17 2006;47(2):379-383.
32. Sinha AM, Skobel EC, Breithardt OA, et al. Cardiac resynchronization therapy improves central sleep apnea and Cheyne-Stokes respiration in patients with chronic heart failure. *J Am Coll Cardiol.* Jul 7 2004;44(1):68-71.
33. Kenny RA. Syncope in the elderly: diagnosis, evaluation, and treatment. *J Cardio Electrophysiol.* Sep 2003;14(9 Suppl):S74-77.
34. Richardson DA, Bexton RS, Shaw FE, Kenny RA. Prevalence of cardioinhibitory carotid sinus hypersensitivity in patients 50 years or over presenting to the accident and emergency department with "unexplained" or "recurrent" falls. *Pacing Clin Electrophysiol.* Mar 1997;20(3 Pt 2):820-823.
35. Kenny RA, Richardson DA, Steen N, Bexton RS, Shaw FE, Bond J. Carotid sinus syndrome: a modifiable risk factor for nonaccidental falls in older adults (SAFE PACE). *J Am Coll Cardiol.* Nov 1 2001;38(5):1491-1496.
36. Ryan DJ, Nick S, Colette SM, Roseanne K. Carotid sinus syndrome, should we pace? A multicentre, randomised control trial (SAFEPACE 2). *Heart.* Mar 2010;96(5):347-351.
37. Parry SW, Steen N, Bexton RS, Tynan M, Kenny RA. Pacing in elderly recurrent fallers with carotid sinus hypersensitivity: a randomised, double-blind, placebo controlled crossover trial. *Heart.* Mar 2009;95(5):405-409.
38. Epstein AE, DiMarco JP, Ellenbogen KA, et al. ACC/AHA/HRS 2008 Guidelines for Device-Based Therapy of Cardiac Rhythm Abnormalities: a report of the American College of Cardiology/American Heart Association Task Force on Practice Guidelines (Writing Committee to Revise the ACC/AHA/NASPE 2002 Guideline Update for Implantation of Cardiac Pacemakers and Antiarrhythmia Devices): developed in collaboration with the American Association for Thoracic Surgery and Society of Thoracic Surgeons. *Circulation.* May 27 2008;117(21):e350-408.
39. Baldasseroni S, Opasich C, Gorini M, et al. Left bundle-branch block is associated with increased 1-year sudden and total mortality rate in 5517 outpatients with congestive heart failure: a report from the Italian network on congestive heart failure. *Am Heart J.* Mar 2002;143(3):398-405.
40. Shamim W, Francis DP, Yousufuddin M, et al. Intraventricular conduction delay: a prognostic marker in chronic heart failure. *Int J Cardiol.* Jul 31 1999;70(2):171-178.
41. Xiao HB, Brecker SJ, Gibson DG. Effects of abnormal activation on the time course of the left ventricular pressure pulse in dilated cardiomyopathy. *Br Heart J.* Oct 1992;68(4):403-407.
42. Bradley DJ, Bradley EA, Baughman KL, et al. Cardiac resynchronization and death from progressive heart failure: a meta-analysis of randomized controlled trials. *JAMA.* Feb 12 2003;289(6):730-740.
43. Cleland JG, Daubert JC, Erdmann E, et al. The effect of cardiac resynchronization on morbidity and mortality in heart failure. *N Engl J Med.* Apr 14 2005;352(15):1539-1549.
44. Bristow MR, Saxon LA, Boehmer J, et al. Cardiac-resynchronization therapy with or without an implantable defibrillator in advanced chronic heart failure. *N Engl J Med.* May 20 2004;350(21):2140-2150.
45. Linde C, Abraham WT, Gold MR, St John Sutton M, Ghio S, Daubert C. Randomized trial of cardiac resynchronization in mildly symptomatic heart failure patients and in asymptomatic patients with left ventricular dysfunction and previous heart failure symptoms. *J Am Coll Cardiol.* Dec 2 2008;52(23):1834-1843.
46. Daubert C, Gold MR, Abraham WT, et al. Prevention of disease progression by cardiac resynchronization therapy in patients with asymptomatic or mildly symptomatic left ventricular dysfunction: insights from the European cohort of the REVERSE (Resynchronization Reverses Remodeling in Systolic Left Ventricular Dysfunction) trial. *J Am Coll Cardiol.* Nov 10 2009;54(20):1837-1846.
47. Moss AJ, Hall WJ, Cannom DS, et al. Cardiac-resynchronization therapy for the prevention of heart-failure events. *New Eng J Med.* Oct 1 2009;361(14):1329-1338.
48. Tang AS, Wells GA, Talajic M, et al. Cardiac-resynchronization therapy for mild-to-moderate heart failure. *N Engl J Med.* Dec 16 2010;363(25):2385-2395.
49. Beshai JF, Grimm RA, Nagueh SF, et al. Cardiac-resynchronization therapy in heart failure with narrow QRS complexes. *N Engl J Med.* Dec 13 2007;357(24):2461-2471.
50. Gasparini M, Auricchio A, Regoli F, et al. Four-year efficacy of cardiac resynchronization therapy on exercise tolerance and disease progression: the importance of performing atrioventricular junction ablation in patients with atrial fibrillation. *J Am Coll Cardiol.* Aug 15 2006;48(4):734-743.
51. Ferreira AM, Adragao P, Cavaco DM, et al. Benefit of cardiac resynchronization therapy in atrial fibrillation patients vs. patients in sinus rhythm: the role of atrioventricular junction ablation. *Europace.* Jul 2008;10(7):809-815.
52. Kindermann M, Hennen B, Jung J, Geisel J, Bohm M, Frohlig G. Biventricular versus conventional right ventricular stimulation for patients with standard pacing indication and left ventricular dysfunction: the Homburg Biventricular Pacing Evaluation (HOBIPACE). *J Am Coll Cardiol.* May 16 2006;47(10):1927-1937.
53. Baker CM, Christopher TJ, Smith PF, Langberg JJ, Delurgio DB, Leon AR. Addition of a left ventricular lead to conventional pacing systems in patients with congestive heart failure: feasibility, safety, and early results in 60 consecutive patients. *Pacing Clin Electrophysiol.* Aug 2002;25(8):1166-1171.
54. Curtis AB, Worley SJ, Adamson PE et al. Biventricular pacing for atrioventricular block and systolic heart failure. *New Eng J Med.* 2013;368:1587-1593.
55. Tracy CM, Epstein AE, Darbar D, et al. 2012 ACCF/AHA/HRS focused update of the 2008 guidelines for device-based therapy of cardiac rhythm abnormalities: a report of the American College of Cardiology Foundation/American Heart Association Task Force on Practice Guidelines and the Heart Rhythm Society [corrected]. *Circulation.* Oct 2 2012;126(14):1784-1800.
56. Exner DV, Birnie DH, Moe G, et al. Canadian Cardiovascular Society guidelines on the use of cardiac resynchronization therapy: evidence and patient selection. *Can J Cardiol.* Feb 2013;29(2):182-195.
57. Khan FZ, Virdee MS, Palmer CR, et al. Targeted left ventricular lead placement to guide cardiac resynchronization therapy: the TARGET study: a randomized, controlled trial. *J Am Coll Cardiol.* Apr 24 2012;59(17):1509-1518.
58. McDonald K, McWilliams E, O'Keeffe B, Maurer B. Functional assessment of patients treated with permanent dual chamber pacing as a primary treatment for hypertrophic cardiomyopathy. *Eur Heart J.* Aug 1988;9(8):893-898.
59. Viskin S. Cardiac pacing in the long QT syndrome: review of available data and practical recommendations. *J Cardiovasc Electrophysiol.* May 2000;11(5):593-600.
60. Dorostkar PC, Eldar M, Belhassen B, Scheinman MM. Long-term follow-up of patients with long-QT syndrome treated with β-blockers and continuous pacing. *Circulation.* Dec 14 1999;100(24):2431-2436.

61. Wathen MS, DeGroot PJ, Sweeney MO, et al. Prospective randomized multicenter trial of empirical antitachycardia pacing versus shocks for spontaneous rapid ventricular tachycardia in patients with implantable cardioverter-defibrillators: Pacing Fast Ventricular Tachycardia Reduces Shock Therapies (PainFREE Rx II) trial results. *Circulation*. Oct 26 2004;110(17):2591-2596.

62. Carlson MD, Ip J, Messenger J, et al. A new pacemaker algorithm for the treatment of atrial fibrillation: results of the Atrial Dynamic Overdrive Pacing Trial (ADOPT). *J Am Coll Cardiol*. Aug 20 2003;42(4):627-633.

CHAPTER 65

Clinical Indications and Evidence-based Outcomes Standards in Interventional Electrophysiology: Implantable Cardioverter-defibrillator Therapy

Bharat K. Kantharia, MD; Arti N. Shah, MD; Sanjeev Saksena, MBBS, MD

Introduction

Sudden cardiac death (SCD) is a major public health issue worldwide. SCD is defined as death from an unexpected circulatory arrest, usually due to a cardiac arrhythmia, occurring within an hour of the onset of symptoms. The worldwide incidence of SCD is very high. In the United States, the estimated annual incidence is approximately 300,000.[1] Similar population-incidence of 1/1,000 per year has been observed in Europe and Japan.[2,3] The very nature of cardiac death that occurs suddenly leaves physical morbidities and devastating psychosocial effects on those patients who are successfully revived and their family members. (The term sudden cardiac arrest [SCA] is used when medical intervention (eg, defibrillation) reverses the event.[4])

The implantable cardioverter-defibrillator (ICD) was invented by Mirowski and his colleagues in 1980.[5] With many technological advancement and implantation techniques such as implementation of a nonthoracotomy insertion technique by Saksena et al,[6] ICD insertion has become a widely employed procedure. ICD therapy has been shown in multiple clinical trials to effectively reduce incidence of SCD resulting from malignant ventricular tachycardia (VT) and ventricular fibrillation (VF). These arrhythmias are seen in a variety of cardiac disease states. In addition to patients with coronary artery disease, dilated cardiomyopathy, and heart failure, a significant number of patients with other substrates, such as genetic channelopathies, the long QT syndromes (LQTS), Brugada syndrome, and hypertrophic cardiomyopathy (HCM), also require ICDs to prevent SCD. In this chapter, we discuss the evidence-based clinical indications and outcomes standards for the ICD therapy.

Basis for Guidelines for ICD Therapies

Advancements in ICD technology in the last two decades allow the currently available ICDs to be implanted transvenously without major surgery under local anesthesia, and provide sophisticated atrial and ventricular pacing including cardiac resynchronization therapy (CRT) as well antitachycardia therapies. Although presently in the early phase of development, an entirely subcutaneous ICD system is also now available that overcomes some of the problems associated with transvenous leads in the current conventional ICDs.[7] In spite of these advancements, it is important to bear in mind that the primary role of ICDs is to successfully treat VF with defibrillation shocks, and VT with overdrive antitachycardia pacing (ATP) and internal cardioversion shocks.

It is also necessary to consider ICD indications in terms of secondary and primary prevention of SCD. The survivors of SCD and out-of-hospital cardiac arrest are at significantly higher risks for future episodes of malignant VT and VF, and would benefit from ICD therapy for "secondary" prevention. On the other hand, many patients with cardiovascular diseases who have not yet experienced life-threatening cardiac arrhythmias nevertheless may be considered to be at significantly higher risk for SCD. In such high-risk patients, ICDs may be implanted preemptively for "primary" prophylaxis of SCD.

ICD therapy implementation has been supported by results derived from many large clinical trials, some of which are included in Table 65.1. Major professional organizations have adopted guidelines for the use of ICDs. Early guidelines established by a joint task force by the American College of Cardiology (ACC) and the American Heart Association (AHA) in 1984 and the North American Society of Pacing and Electrophysiology (1990) have been merged, revised, and updated many times in collaboration with the American Association for Thoracic Surgery, Society of Thoracic Surgeons.[1,8-10] More recently, the American College of Cardiology Foundation (ACCF), in collaboration with the Heart Rhythm Society (HRS), published an appropriate use criteria (AUC) document for indication of ICD and CRT implantation for a broad spectrum of clinical scenarios.[11]

Based on the strength of evidence ranked as Level A (data derived from multiple randomized clinical trials that involved a large number of individuals), Level B (data derived either from a limited number of trials that involved a comparatively small number of patients or from well-designed data analyses of nonrandomized studies or observational data registries), and Level C (the primary source of the recommendation from the consensus of experts), the indications have been divided into the following classes:

- Class I – ICD recommended and should be implanted.
- Class IIa – ICD could be useful and beneficial, and probably recommended and indicated.
- Class IIb – ICD might be considered but its usefulness and effectiveness not well established.
- Class III – ICD is not recommended, and in some cases its use may be harmful.

While considering evidence-based practice principles that need to be applied to a large population such as the one in whom ICD therapy may be considered, one also needs to comprehend statistical analyses and findings of large trials and their meta-analyses. For example, the terms "absolute risk reduction" and "relative risk reduction" may not be used interchangeably, but are rather complementary to each other. In case of ICD therapy for prevention of SCD, the "absolute risk reduction" would be the difference in the event or the endpoint rates between the control (no ICD) and intervention (ICD) groups. The "relative risk reduction" is the percentage reduction in the event or the endpoint rates. Another parameter that is commonly used is the number needed to treat (NNT), which is the reciprocal of the absolute risk reduction. Thus, although based on the principles of statistics, there are inherent clinical limitations to such recommendations, and they remain guidelines for clinical practice. When applying these guidelines in clinical practice, physicians should apply their best clinical judgment in making decisions about ICD therapy based on circumstances of individual cases.[12]

Secondary Prevention

Regardless of the nature of the cardiac disease and underlying arrhythmia substrate, evidence from multiple randomized trials support ICD implantation for secondary prevention of SCD and arrhythmic cardiac arrest. Among many ICD trials for secondary prevention, the findings from 3 major trials—the Antiarrhythmics Versus Implantable Defibrillators (AVID),[13] the Canadian Implantable Defibrillator Study (CIDS),[14] and the Cardiac Arrest Study Hamburg (CASH)[15]—are noteworthy. In AVID, a multicenter randomized trial, 1,016 enrolled patients who were resuscitated from near-fatal VF, or had experienced sustained symptomatic VT with or without syncope, and had left ventricular dysfunction with ejection fraction (EF) of ≤ 40%, were randomized to an ICD or drug therapy (mainly amiodarone). The trial showed a greater survival with ICD than without—89.3% vs 82.3% at 1 year, 81.6% vs 74.7% at 2 years, and 75.4% vs 64.1% at 3 years, with an overall 31% relative reduction in primary endpoint of all-cause mortality ($P < 0.02$) with ICD therapy. In the CIDS trial, 659 patients with resuscitated VF or VT or with syncope were randomized to treatment with an ICD or amiodarone. Although the CIDS trial showed a 20% reduction in the risk of all-cause mortality and a 33% reduction in the risk of SCD in the ICD group, the differences for these endpoints were not statistically significant ($P = 0.14$ and $P = 0.09$, respectively). Compared to AVID and CIDS, CASH was a relatively small trial and comprised 288 patients who were randomized to ICD or antiarrhythmic drug therapy (amiodarone, metoprolol, or propafenone; note that the propafenone arm was stopped early in the trial). These patients also had relatively preserved LV function with higher EF compared to the patients in the AVID and

Table 65.1 Trials of ICD therapy for prevention of sudden cardiac death

Trial	Publication Year	N	Prevention	Criteria	Results
MADIT	1996	196	Primary	LVEF ≤35%, prior MI, asymptomatic NSVT, NYHA class I–III, inducible VT refractory to intravenous procainamide on EP study	54% reduction in total mortality with ICD therapy
CABG-Patch	1997	900	Primary	LVEF ≤35%, patients scheduled for CABG, positive SAECG results	No reduction in total mortality with ICD therapy
MUSTT	1999	704	Primary	LVEF ≤40%, CAD, NSVT, inducible VT on EP study	51% reduction of total mortality with ICD therapy
MADIT II	2002	1,232	Primary	LVEF ≤30%, prior MI	31% reduction of all-cause mortality with ICD
DEFINITE	2004	229	Primary	LVEF ≤36%, nonischemic dilated cardiomyopathy, NSVT or PVCs at Holter monitoring	ICD reduced rate of death from any cause (7.9% vs 14% at 2 years)
DINAMIT	2004	674	Primary	LVEF ≤35%, recent MI (within 4–40 days), impaired cardiac autonomic modulation (HR variability)	No reduction in death from any cause with ICD therapy ($P = 0.66$) Reduction of arrhythmic deaths with ICD ($P = 0.009$)
COMPANION	2004	1,520	Primary	NYHA class III–IV due to ischemic and nonischemic cardiomyopathy, QRS ≥ 120 ms	CRT with pacemaker and ICD was associated with a 36% reduction of risk of death from any cause
SCDHeFT	2005	2,521	Primary	LVEF ≤35%, NHYA class II–III (ischemic and nonischemic)	23% reduction of overall mortality with ICD
IRIS	2009	898	Primary	5 to 31 days after acute MI, LVEF ≤40% and a heart rate of 90 or more bpm on the first available ECG, nonsustained VT during Holter monitoring or both	No overall mortality reduction in the ICD group (HR, 1.04; 95% CI, 0.81 to 1.35; $P = 0.78$)
CAT	2002	104	Primary	nonischemic cardiomyopathy, LVEF ≤30%, asymptomatic nonsustained VT, and NYHA class II/III heart failure	No reduction in total mortality with ICD therapy
AMIOVIRT	2003	103	Primary	nonischemic cardiomyopathy, LVEF ≤35%, asymptomatic nonsustained VT, and NYHA class I–III heart failure	No reduction in total mortality with ICD therapy
AVID	1997	1,016	Secondary	Survived VT/VF cardiac arrest or VT with syncope or VT with LVEF ≤40%	31% reduction of mortality with ICD at 3 years
CASH	2000	288	Secondary	Cardiac arrest due to VF or VT	23% reduction of all-cause mortality with ICD
CIDS	2000	659	Secondary	Cardiac arrest due to VF or sustained VT and syncope or poor tolerated VT and LVEF < 40% or syncope and inducible or monitored VT	20% reduction of all-cause mortality with ICD

AMIOVIRT = Amiodarone versus Implantable Cardioverter-Defibrillator Randomized Trial; AVID = Antiarrhythmics Versus Implantable Defibrillators; CASH = Cardiac Arrest Study Hamburg; CAT = Cardiomyopathy Trial; CAD = coronary artery disease; CABG = coronary bypass graft; CABG-Patch = Coronary Artery Bypass Graft-Patch; CIDS = Canadian Implantable Defibrillator Study; CRT = cardiac resynchronization therapy; COMPANION = Comparison of Medical Therapy, Pacing, and Defibrillation in Heart Failure Trial; DEFINITE = Defibrillators in Non-Ischemic Cardiomyopathy Treatment Evaluation; DINAMIT = Defibrillators in Acute Myocardial Infarction Trial; EP = electrophysiology; HR = heart rate; IRIS = Immediate Risk Stratification Improves Survival trial; ICD = implantable cardioverter-defibrillator; LVEF = left ventricular ejection fraction; MADIT = Multicenter Automatic Defibrillator Implantation Trials; MUSTT = Multicenter Unsustained Tachycardia Trial; MI = myocardial infarction; NSVT = nonsustained ventricular tachycardia; NYHA = New York Heart Association; PVCs = premature ventricular contractions; SAECG = signal-averaged electrocardiogram; SCDHeFT = Sudden Cardiac Death in Heart Failure Trial; VT = ventricular tachycardia; VF = ventricular fibrillation.

CIDS trials. The CASH trial also showed a 23% reduction in total mortality (statistically nonsignificant, $P = 0.2$) with ICD therapy as compared with antiarrhythmic therapy with amiodarone or metoprolol. A meta-analysis of the AVID, CIDS, and CASH trials of secondary prevention demonstrated a significant 28% ($P = 0.006$) reduction in the risk of SCD with an ICD almost entirely due to reduction in arrhythmic death, and particularly in patients with left ventricular dysfunction (LVEF < 35%).[16] Lee et al,[17] using the MEDLINE, EMBASE, and Cochrane Library electronic databases, performed additional meta-analyses of available trials to compare the effectiveness of the ICD and medical strategies for prevention of arrhythmic events and death. When another secondary prevention trial by Wever et al[18] was included in the meta-analysis, the results showed significant reduction in mortality ($P = 0.0002$) with ICDs (the overall pooled relative risk (RR) = 0.75 with a 95% confidence interval (CI) = 0.64 to 0.87. The absolute reduction in all-cause mortality in secondary prevention was 7% (95% CI, 4% to 11%; number needed to treat, NNT: 15). The survival benefit with the ICD was robust in sensitivity analysis and not heavily influenced by any of the trials individually. Although the majority of patients in these studies had ischemic substrate due to coronary artery disease, subgroups of patients with nonischemic dilated cardiomyopathy in these studies also demonstrated beneficial effects of ICDs. Thus, ICD is indicated in a survivor of SCD irrespective of the substrate unless definite reversible cause may be identified as the sole etiology of cardiac arrest.

Invasive electrophysiological (EP) study plays an insignificant role in terms of determining ICD implantation for secondary prevention. Among patients who survive cardiac arrest with or without documented VT/VF, less than 50% have inducible sustained VT/VF by EP study.[19] In the Midlands Trial of Empirical Amiodarone versus Electrophysiology-guided Interventions and Implantable Cardioverter-defibrillators (MAVERIC) study comprising 214 survivors of SCD randomized to empirical amiodarone versus prospective selection of patients to receive ICDs by EP study, no significant differences in survival or arrhythmia recurrence existed between the two treatment arms after 6 years. However, ICD recipients had a lower mortality than non-ICD recipients, regardless of allocated treatment (hazard ratio [HR] = 0.54, $P = 0.0391$).[20] Survivors of SCD in whom no ventricular tachyarrhythmias could be induced at EP study remain at risk for recurrence of ventricular tachyarrhythmias. In a randomized study by Crandall et al of 194 consecutive patients in whom VT/VF could not be induced, 91 received ICD and 95 did not. Patients treated with an ICD had an improvement in SCD-free survival ($P = 0.04$).[21] On this basis, routine EP study has no role in the management of such patients, who should be offered empirical ICD therapy according to the results of other secondary prevention ICD trials.

Primary Prevention

Despite the fact that incidence of SCD is lowest (< 1% per year) in people with no prior event, it is this general population in whom the majority of SCD occurs.[22] On the other hand, in the very-high-risk group comprised of patients with a history of myocardial infarction and severe left ventricular dysfunction, most deaths are not sudden. Therefore, ICD implantation as a primary prophylaxis measure should be performed after appropriate risk stratification and with a balanced strategy such that the individuals at risk receive the most benefit from ICDs in terms of prevention of SCD. In that context, besides invasive EP study, several noninvasive risk-stratifying methods such as diminished left ventricular ejection fraction (LVEF), exercise-related heart failure and ventricular arrhythmias, prolonged QRS duration, QT interval and dispersion, ambulatory Holter recordings of ventricular ectopy and nonsustained VT, abnormal signal-averaged ECGs, T-wave alternans, heart rate variability, and baroreceptor sensitivity may be utilized.[23] From the arrhythmia substrate point of view, the "primary prevention" ICD trials have been focused to the coronary artery disease, dilated cardiomyopathy, and congestive heart failure subgroups.

Among the major "primary prevention" trials, the patient populations studied were: (1) ischemic cardiomyopathy, LVEF ≤ 35%, asymptomatic nonsustained VT, inducible and nonsuppressible VT for the Multicenter Automatic Defibrillator Implantation Trial (MADIT-I)[24]; (2) ischemic cardiomyopathy, LVEF ≤ 40%, nonsustained VT, inducible VT for the Multicenter Unsustained Tachycardia Trial (MUSTT)[25]; (3) ischemic cardiomyopathy, LVEF ≤ 30% for the MADIT-II[26] trial; (4) ischemic and nonischemic cardiomyopathy, LVEF ≤ 35%, New York Heart Association (NYHA) heart failure class II–III for the Sudden Cardiac Death in Heart Failure Trial (SCDHeFT)[27]; (5) nonischemic cardiomyopathy, LVEF ≤ 30%, asymptomatic nonsustained VT, and NYHA class II/III heart failure, in the Cardiomyopathy Trial (CAT)[28]; (6) nonischemic cardiomyopathy, LVEF ≤ 36%, and premature ventricular complexes or nonsustained VT in the Defibrillators in Non-Ischemic Cardiomyopathy Treatment Evaluation (DEFINITE) study[29]; and (7) nonischemic cardiomyopathy, LVEF ≤ 35%, asymptomatic nonsustained VT, and NYHA class I–III heart failure in the Amiodarone Versus Implantable Cardioverter-Defibrillator Randomized Trial (AMIOVIRT).[30] With the exception of CAT and AMIOVERT, major primary prevention ICD trials showed a significant benefit of ICD therapy. The MADIT-I, MUSTT, MADIT-II, and SCDHeFT trials demonstrated reduction in mortality with ICDs by 19% over 2 years, 31% over 5 years, 6% over 2 years, and 7% over 5 years, respectively. In the DEFINITE trial, a significant reduction (80%) in sudden arrhythmic cardiac death and a 35% reduction in all-cause mortality (although not statistically significant) over 2 years with ICD therapy in patients with nonischemic cardiomyopathy patients were observed.[29] The MADIT-I and MUSTT trials, both of which included inducible VT during invasive EP study as a required inclusion criterion in addition to LVEF ≤35% and ≤40%, respectively, showed much higher reduction in primary endpoint of all-cause mortality by 56% and 76% relative risk reduction in MADIT-II trial, which enrolled patients only on the basis of LV dysfunction, that is, LVEF < 30%, a significant relative risk reduction of 31% in all-cause mortality observed with ICD therapy. This further underscores the fact that, like "secondary prevention," barring patients who fit the profile of MUSTT patients who have LVEF of 35%–40% and spontaneous nonsustained VT, routine EP study has no major role in the management of the specific subset of patients at risk of SCD, and these patients should be offered empirical ICD therapy.

The role of ICDs for primary prevention of mortality among the patients with congestive heart failure (CHF) is best derived from the SCDHeFT trial.[27] In this large, randomized study, 2,521 patients with NYHA class II or III and EF < 35% were enrolled. They were randomized to optimized heart failure therapy; optimized heart failure therapy with the addition of amiodarone; or medical treatment with the addition of a shock-only single-lead ICD. With a single-lead ICD, it is not possible to correct atrioventricular or intraventricular dyssynchrony and provide cardiac resynchronization therapy (CRT). At 5 years' follow-up, there was 23% relative reduction in primary endpoint of all-cause mortality observed in the ICD group independent of the etiology of heart failure (ischemic or nonischemic), while the mortality rates were similar in the placebo and amiodarone groups.

In patients with severe CHF needing cardiac resynchronization therapy (CRT), the Comparison of Medical Therapy, Pacing, and Defibrillation in Heart Failure (COMPANION)[31] trial showed lower (36%) relative reduction in all-cause mortality with CRT-D (ICD combined with CRT) when compared with optimized medical therapy. The COMPANION trial was a multicenter trial evaluating the effect of CRT on mortality, morbidity, and exercise performance in symptomatic heart failure patients without ICD indications. The COMPANION trial was a randomized three-arm trial of patients in NYHA class III or IV with an LVEF of ≤35 % and a prolonged QRS duration (>120 ms) and LV dilation (LV end-diastolic diameter >60 mm). The objectives of the study were to determine whether optimal pharmacologic therapy used with CRT alone or CRT in combination with ICD was superior to optimal pharmacologic treatment alone in reducing combined all-cause mortality, hospitalizations, and cardiac morbidity and in improving functional capacity of cardiac performance and quality of life. This trial showed that CRT reduced the composite endpoint of death or hospitalization for major cardiovascular events by 12%. However, significant mortality was achieved only in the CRT–ICD arm. In the Multicenter Longitudinal Observational Study (MILOS),[32] which included 1,303 patients treated with CRT alone (CRT-P) or with ICD backup (ie, CRT-D), the cumulative event-free survivals were 92% and 56% at 1 and 5 years, respectively, and the cumulative incidence of death from heart failure and that of sudden death were 25.1% and 9.5%, respectively.[32] It was the ICD part of the system, (ie, CRT-D) that was associated with 20% decrease in mortality, and the protective effect against sudden cardiac death was highly significant ($P < 0.002$).[32]

Cardiac resynchronization therapy with ICD (CRT-D) has also been shown to decrease the risk of heart failure events, even in patients with minimal heart failure symptoms (NYHA class I or II) but with low LVEF (≤30%) and wide QRS complexes (QRS duration ≥130 ms), as shown in the Multicenter Automatic Defibrillator Implantation Trial with Cardiac Resynchronization Therapy (MADIT-CRT) trial.[33] In this trial, during an average follow-up of 2.4 years, the primary endpoint of death from any cause or a nonfatal heart failure event occurred in 187 of 1,089 patients in the CRT–ICD group (17.2%) and 185 of 731 patients in the ICD-only group (25.3%) (HR in the CRT–ICD group, 0.66; 95% CI, 0.52 to 0.84; $P = 0.001$). The benefit did not differ significantly between patients with ischemic cardiomyopathy and those with nonischemic cardiomyopathy.

The Resynchronization–Defibrillation for Ambulatory Heart Failure Trial (RAFT)[34] was another multicenter, double-blind, randomized, controlled study that enrolled 1,798 patients with NYHA class II or III heart failure, an LVEF of ≤30%, and an intrinsic QRS duration of ≥120 ms or a paced QRS duration of ≥200 ms to receive either CRT-D or an ICD alone. The primary outcome of death from any cause or hospitalization for heart failure occurred in 33.2% of the CRT-D group and 40.3% of the ICD group (HR in the CRT-D group, 0.75; 95% CI, 0.64 to 0.87; $P < 0.001$). However, at 30 days after device implantation, more adverse events—including hemothorax or pneumothorax, device-pocket hematoma requiring intervention, device-pocket infection, device-pocket problems requiring revision lead dislodgement, and coronary sinus dissection—were observed in the CRT-D group.

As opposed to the above trials, which showed the beneficial role of the ICDs, results of the Coronary Artery Bypass Graft-Patch (CABG Patch) trial,[35] the Defibrillators in Acute Myocardial Infarction Trial (DINAMIT) study,[36] and the Immediate Risk Stratification Improves Survival (IRIS) trial[37] were unfavorable for the ICDs in their "primary prevention" role. In these studies, ICDs were implanted at the time of CABG surgery (CABG Patch) or early in the course of acute myocardial infarction (DINAMIT and IRIS). In the CABG Patch trial, 900 patients who had abnormal signal-averaged ECGs and LVEF < 36% were randomly assigned to ICD implantation or no ICD concomitant to CABG surgery. No difference in the primary endpoint of overall mortality at mean follow-up of 32 (±16) months was found. The disparity of the outcome in the CABG Patch trial may be attributed to the fact that cardiac revascularization performed at the time of ICD implantation might have modified the patients' risk profile to a lower risk category. Secondly, the CABG Patch trial used signal-averaged ECGs, a rather weaker risk predictor than inducible VT (MADIT-I and MUSTT trials). In the DINAMIT study, patients who had impaired cardiac autonomic function (manifested as depressed heart rate variability or an elevated average 24-hour heart rate on Holter monitoring) in addition to LVEF ≤35% 6 to 40 days after a myocardial infarction were randomized to receive ICD or no ICD. The DINAMIT study showed that successful prevention of arrhythmic death with ICDs (HR, 0.42; 95% CI, 0.22 to 0.83; P = 0.009) was counterbalanced by excess death from nonarrhythmic etiologies (HR, 1.75; 95% CI, 1.11 to 2.76; P = 0.02) seen more commonly in the setting of acute ischemia.

In the IRIS study, patients were enrolled 5 to 31 days after acute myocardial infarction if they had LVEF ≤40% and a heart rate of ≥90 bpm on the first available ECG, nonsustained VT during Holter monitoring or both. With these criteria that included different risk-stratifying markers than the DINAMIT study, the study cohort comprised a larger population at risk. However, the results of the IRIS study were almost identical to the DINAMIT study such that the overall mortality was not reduced in the ICD group (HR, 1.04; 95% CI, 0.81 to 1.35; P = 0.78). Although there were fewer sudden cardiac deaths in the ICD group than in the control group (HR, 0.55; 95% CI, 0.31 to 1.00; P = 0.049), the number of nonsudden cardiac deaths was higher (HR, 1.92; 95% CI, 1.29 to 2.84; P = 0.001). The outcome data from the CABG Patch, DINAMIT, and IRIS studies indicate that implantation of ICDs should not be performed within 30 days after CABG surgery or within 40 days after acute myocardial infarction.

The question of whether the results of numbers of randomized clinical trials conducted to assess the role of ICD for primary prevention of SCD are similar when applied in clinical practice was partly answered in a retrospective analysis of National Cardiovascular Data Registry data of patients who received ICD, meeting two of the primary prevention trials, namely, the MADIT-II and SCDHeFT criteria.[38] In the matched cohorts, there was no significant difference in survival between the registry and trial patients (2-year mortality rates: 13.9% and 15.6%, respectively; adjusted ICD Registry vs trial HR, 1.06; 95% CI, 0.85 to 1.31; P = 0.62 for comparison with MADIT-II and 3-year mortality rates: 17.3% and 17.4%, respectively; adjusted registry vs trial HR, 1.16; 95% CI, 0.97–1.38; P = 0.11 for comparison with SCDHeFT).[38] With appropriate programming of ICDs—for example, therapies for tachyarrhythmias of 200 bpm or higher and a prolonged delay in therapy at 170 bpm or higher—a reduction in inappropriate therapies and in all-cause mortality is accomplished, as shown by the Multicenter Automatic Defibrillator Implantation Trial–Reduce Inappropriate Therapy (MADIT-RIT) study.[39] Thus, there are ample supportive studies and trials for evidence-based practice of ICDs as primary prevention measures against SCD.

Role of ICDs in Other Specific Arrhythmogenic Substrates

When data on the secondary and primary prevention trials are pooled and meta-analyses of these trials are performed,[16,40,41] it becomes evident that ICDs are associated with nearly 57% reduction in the risk of an arrhythmic death and a nearly 30% decrease in risk of all-cause mortality as compared with medical therapy alone. However, given the strict designs of these trials, the results of these trials may neither be easily extrapolated to other disease substrates, such as hypertrophic cardiomyopathy (HCM), arrhythmogenic right ventricular dysplasia, or genetic channelopathies including long QT syndromes (LQTS) and Brugada syndrome, nor to the subgroups such as the pediatric age group, very old (> 80 years) patients, patients who are morbidly obese, or those who have significant comorbidities like end-stage renal failure requiring hemodialysis.

Hypertrophic Cardiomyopathy

Hypertrophic cardiomyopathy (HCM) is a common inherited disorder with an estimated prevalence of 1 in 500 in the general population, and is associated with the risk for sudden death, especially in young people.[42-45] In HCM, the substrate for VT and VF is caused by the characteristic structural abnormalities of interstitial fibrosis, myocardial disarray, and ventricular hypertrophy that result from various mutations of the genes encoding myocardial contractile proteins. The role of ICDs for secondary and primary prevention of SCD in patients with HCM has essentially been studied in the form of observational and registry data.[46-49] Although these studies provide consensus on the use of ICD in patients who survive cardiac arrest and/or have spontaneous sustained VT, the role of ICDs for primary prevention of SCD in patients with HCM required further clarification, especially in light of the fact that serious device-related complications, including lead malfunction, high defibrillation thresholds, and inappropriate shocks, are observed more commonly in young patients with HCM. To the specific question of appropriateness of ICDs, the results of a large multicenter registry study that enrolled 506 patients with HCM are interesting.[50] In this study, appropriate ICD intervention for VT/VF was observed in 103 patients (20%). The intervention rates were 10.6% per year (5-year cumulative probability, 39% [SD, 5%]) and 3.6% per year (5-year probability, 17% [SD, 2%]) for secondary and primary prevention, respectively. For primary prevention, 18 of the 51 patients with appropriate ICD interventions (35%) had undergone implantation for only a single risk factor. Furthermore, the likelihood of appropriate discharge was similar in patients with 1, 2, 3, or more risk markers.[50] Therefore, in line with ACC/AHA/ESC 2006 guidelines for management of patients with ventricular arrhythmias and the prevention of SCD,[51] and the joint 2011 American College of Cardiology Foundation (ACCF) and the AHA guidelines for the diagnosis and treatment of HCM,[45] presence of certain factors (Table 65.2) indicating that high risk for SCD may be sufficient to justify prophylactic ICD in patients with HCM.[52]

Table 65.2 Risk factors for sudden cardiac death in hypertrophic cardiomyopathy

Major

1. Prior aborted SCD
2. Family history of HCM-related SCDs
3. Episode of unexplained, recent syncope
4. Massive left ventricular hypertrophy (thickness > 30 mm)
5. Nonsustained VT on serial ambulatory 24-hour (Holter) ECGs
6. Hypotensive or attenuated blood pressure response to exercise

Possible and Potential Arbitrators

1. Atrial fibrillation
2. Myocardial ischemia
3. Left ventricular outflow obstruction
4. High-risk mutation
5. Intense (competitive) physical exertion
6. End-stage phase
7. Left ventricular apical aneurysm
8. Extensive delayed enhancement on MRI scan
9. Alcohol septal ablation

HCM = hypertrophic cardiomyopathy, MRI = magnetic resonance imaging, SCD = sudden cardiac death, VT = ventricular tachycardia.

Arrhythmogenic Right Ventricular Dysplasia/Cardiomyopathy

Arrhythmogenic right ventricular dysplasia/cardiomyopathy (ARVD/C) is a genetic cardiomyopathy that is characterized by loss of right ventricular myocyte with fibrofatty replacement and is associated with an increased risk of sudden death from ventricular arrhythmias.[53-55] Several major studies have defined the role of ICDs in ARVD/C for prevention of SCD, especially in those who had had prior VT/VF.[56-59] In these studies, over a follow-up period of 3 to 7 years, 48%–70% of patients received an appropriate ICD therapy. Predictive variables associated with appropriate ICD therapies included prior VT/VF, younger age, left ventricular dysfunction, inducible VT at electrophysiologic study, male gender, and diffuse RV involvement. Most importantly, there was no difference in the rate of ICD therapy in the primary and secondary prevention groups. More recently, well-established registry data of the Johns Hopkins Right Ventricular Dysplasia Program confirmed a high (66%) appropriate ICD intervention in patients with ARVD/C, especially in those patients with diffuse right ventricular involvement and prior ventricular arrhythmias.[60] This study also showed that those patients who met the task force criteria of definite ARVD/C had a higher likelihood of receiving an appropriate ICD therapy compared with patients who have only probable ARVD/C (73% vs 33%). Furthermore, no patients with probable ARVD/C and a negative electrophysiologic study experienced an appropriate ICD discharge, suggesting that it may be possible to identify low-risk subgroups of ARVD/C patients. And lastly, there was no difference in the incidence of life-threatening VT/VF between the primary and secondary prevention groups.[60]

Brugada Syndrome

Brugada syndrome, a genetic disorder involving mutation of cardiac sodium channel gene, is clinically characterized by distinct ECG manifestations of ST-segment elevation in the right precordial leads and is associated with a high risk for SCD in young and otherwise healthy adults, and less frequently in children and infants.[61] While ICD implantation for secondary prevention of SCD is indicated for patients who experienced cardiac arrest or syncope from polymorphic VT, risk stratifications for patients with Brugada pattern ECG and syndrome for ICD implantation for primary prevention remain difficult, especially in light of the fact that most individuals with this condition are asymptomatic and VF and SCD usually occur at rest and at night. In a study performed by Brugada et al[62] of a large cohort of patients with Brugada syndrome without previous cardiac arrest, inducibility of a sustained ventricular arrhythmia by programmed ventricular stimulation during EP study (HR, 5.88; 95% CI, 2.0–16.7, $P = 0.0001$) and a history of syncope (HR, 2.50; 95% CI, 1.2–5.3; $P = 0.017$) were identified as the predictors of SCD and VF during mean follow-up of 24 ± 32 months by multivariate analysis. Logistic regression analysis showed that a patient with a spontaneously abnormal ECG, a previous history of syncope, and inducible sustained ventricular arrhythmias had a probability of 27.2% of encountering a lethal arrhythmic event during follow-up.[62] However, such strong association of inducibility of VT by programmed ventricular stimulation was not observed in other studies,[63,64] and it was further observed that the stimulation protocol markedly influences the extent of inducibility of VT.[65] In the PRELUDE (PRogrammed ELectrical stimUlation preDictive valuE) prospective registry that enrolled patients with a spontaneous or drug-induced type I ECG and without history of cardiac arrest, inducibility of VT/VF by programmed electrical stimulation was unable to identify high-risk patients. Instead, it was the history of syncope and spontaneous type I ECG (HR = 4.20), ventricular refractory period < 200 ms (HR = 3.91), and QRS fragmentation (HR = 4.94) that were significant predictors of arrhythmias.[66]

Furthermore, a meta-analysis of 30 prospective studies with data on 1,545 patients with Brugada ECG pattern performed by Gehi et al[67] showed that there was significant heterogeneity among the studies that looked at inducibility of VT by programmed ventricular stimulation as predictive of VF and SCD in these patient populations, the relative risk (RR) for events (SCD, syncope, or ICD shocks) in patients inducible compared with noninducible at EPS remained nonsignificant ($P = 0.64$) at 0.89 (95% CI, 0.53–1.48). This study also showed that the RR of an event was increased ($P < 0.001$) among patients with a history of syncope or SCD (RR = 3.24 [95% CI, 2.13, 4.93]), men compared with women (RR = 3.47 [95% CI, 1.58, 7.63]), and patients with a spontaneous compared with sodium channel blocker–induced Type I Brugada ECG (RR = 4.65 [95% CI, 2.25, 9.58]). The RR of events was not significantly increased in patients with a family history of SCD ($P = 0.97$) or a mutation of the *SCN5A* gene ($P = 0.18$).[67] A smaller study by Steven et al[68] on a long-term (7.9 ± 3.6 years) follow-up in 33 patients with Brugada syndrome treated with ICDs further underscores the problem with risk stratification in patients with Brugada syndrome. In this study, no patients without prior cardiac arrest had sustained arrhythmic episodes during their follow-up. On the other hand, ICD-related adverse effects occurred in 33% of patients, including inappropriate shocks in 15% of the patients.[68] As per the Consensus Report,[61] the following considerations should be given when ICD implantation is recommended for patients with Brugada syndrome:

1. Symptomatic patients displaying the type 1 Brugada ECG (either spontaneously or after sodium channel blockade) who present with aborted SCD should receive an ICD.

2. Patients presenting with symptoms such as syncope, seizure, or nocturnal agonal respiration should undergo ICD implantation after noncardiac causes of these symptoms have been carefully ruled out.

3. Asymptomatic patients displaying a type 1 Brugada ECG (either spontaneously or after sodium channel blockade) should undergo EP study if a family history of SCD is suspected to be the result of Brugada syndrome. Invasive EP study is justified when family history is negative for sudden cardiac death if the type 1 ECG occurs spontaneously. If inducible for ventricular arrhythmia, then the patient should receive an ICD.

4. Asymptomatic patients who have no family history and who develop a type 1 ECG only after sodium channel blockade should be closely followed up.

Long QT Syndrome

The long QT syndrome (LQTS) is a group of inherited disorders of cardiac ion channels and is characterized by prolonged ventricular repolarization (QT interval) and ventricular tachyarrhythmias, which may manifest as syncope or SCD. In a large study by Schwartz et al[69] that involved 670 LQTS patients of known genotype (LQTS 1, 2, and 3) and demonstrated genotype–phenotype correlation, it was found that in spite of optimal medical therapy with β-blockers, 19% of patents, predominantly in LQT2 and LQT3 genotype, had recurrences of cardiac arrest and SCD and would have conceivably benefited from ICD therapy. Accordingly, risk stratification scheme was developed to categorize patients into low- (< 30%), intermediate- (30%–50%), and high- (> 50%) risk groups based on their genotype, sex, and duration of corrected QT interval.[70] Based on a search on ICD manufacturer's database alone, in a study by Groh et al[71] in 1996 that identified 35 patients who had received ICDs for LQTS, 60% of the patients had at least 1 appropriate cardioverter-defibrillator discharge during a mean follow-up of 31 months. In a study by Zareba et al,[72] clinical characteristics and outcome data of 125 patients implanted with ICDs were compared with LQTS patients who had similar risk indications but were not treated with ICDs. In this study, total mortality as an endpoint was lower at 1.3% mortality over an average follow-up of 3 years in patients treated with ICDs compared to 16% in non-ICD patients during mean 8-year follow-up.[72] In another small single-center study, only corrected QT interval (> 500 ms) and prior survived cardiac arrest were identified by a logistic regression analysis as prognostic factors for future ICD shocks; multiple shocks could be reduced by β-blockers, after increasing antibradycardia pacing rate, or starting the rate-smoothing algorithm.[73] Data from the International LQTS Registry, published in 2008, showed that while none of the patients implanted with an ICD who had experienced cardiac arrest previously had recurrence of cardiac arrest after ICD implantation during a follow-up period of 3.5 ± 3.4 years, appropriate ICD discharge occurred in 15% of all patients who received ICD implantation.[74] More recently, Schwartz et al[75] reported data from the European Long-QT Syndrome Implantable Cardioverter-Defibrillator (LQTS ICD) Registry. This registry is modestly large, but with overrepresentation of women and LQT3 patients, its data is somewhat skewed. Furthermore, although virtually no patients before ICD implantations were symptomatic among LQT1 and LQT2 patients, only 45% of patients with LQT3 were asymptomatic prior to ICD implantation. Among the total cohort of the study, only 44% had cardiac arrest before ICD implantation, and 41% of patients received an ICD without prior pharmacological therapy. During follow-up, 4.6 ± 3.2 years, 28% of patients received at least 1 appropriate shock, and adverse events occurred in 25% of patients in the study. Appropriate ICD therapies were predicted by age < 20 years at implantation (HR, 2.3; 95% CI, 1.38–3.8), a QTc > 500 ms (HR, 1.41; 95% CI, 1.03–1.92), prior cardiac arrest (HR, 1.81; 95% CI, 1.09–3.0), and cardiac events despite therapy (HR, 1.81; 95% CI, 1.08–3.0). Appropriate shocks occurred in no patients with none of these factors and in 70% of those with all factors within 7 years. Neither gender nor a positive family history for SCD showed an association with the probability of ICD therapy during follow-up. Importantly, no significant difference was observed among the 3 main genetic subtypes, whereas the double-mutation carriers had a significantly higher rate of appropriate ICD therapy compared with LQT2 and LQT3. Based on the findings of the study, the investigators proposed a score system based on the number of these risk factors called M-FACT, with scoring as follows:

- M = –1 point for cardiac event–free on therapy for > 10 years.
- F = QTc interval: 0 points for ≤ 500 ms, 1 point for > 500 and ≤ 550 ms, and 2 points for > 550 ms.
- A = age at implantation: 0 points for > 20 years, 1 point for ≤ 20 years.
- C = cardiac arrest: 0 points for no prior cardiac arrest, 1 point for prior cardiac arrest.
- T = events on therapy: 0 points for no events, 1 point for no events.

The 7-year cumulative survival to a first appropriate ICD shock progressively decreases from 100% for patients with no risk factors to 30% for patients with ≥ 4 point score.

Effects of Comorbidities and Other Variables on the Outcome of ICD Therapy

Although ICDs have been shown to be highly effective for primary and secondary prevention of SCD from VT/VF, their implantation indication in a given case needs a fair assessment on an individual basis taking into consideration the presence of comorbidities and other variables, such as the patient's age and gender, that may contribute to the clinical outcome of ICD therapy. Among the comorbidities, diabetes mellitus and renal failure merit special mention.

Among the predictors of early (1-year) mortality in ICD recipients, in a large cohort consisting of 1,703 patients in the Synergistic Effects of Risk Factors for Sudden Cardiac Death (SERF) study, diabetes mellitus independently predicted mortality with HR of 1.68 (95% CI, 1.18).[76] Diabetes mellitus was also found to be a multivariate risk predictor of all-cause mortality with HR of 1.36 (95% CI, 1.07–1.74) during a long-term follow-up of up to 9 years in patients randomized to ICD therapy enrolled in the MADIT-II study.[77]

For chronic renal failure, not only the mere presence of renal failure but also the degree of renal impairment play a significant role in the clinical outcome in patients with ICDs, as was shown in the MADIT-II study.[78] For each 10-U reduction in the estimated glomerular filtration rate (eGFR), the risk of all-cause mortality and SCD was shown to increase by 16% ($P = 0.005$) and 17% ($P = 0.03$), respectively. Importantly, although ICD therapy was beneficial with overall risk reduction for all-cause mortality by 32% and for SCD by 66% in patients with moderate renal failure, eGFR ≥ 35 mL/min/1.73 m², ICDs were not effective to prevent all-cause mortality or SCD in patients with severe renal failure with an eGFR < 35 mL/min/1.73 m².[78] Poor outcome including higher mortality, incremental HR from 1.0 to 10.15, in patients with mild to severe renal failure respectively, especially in patients requiring hemodialysis, has been shown in other studies as well.[79-82] Although strongly associated with appropriate ICD therapy (HR, 2.30; 95% CI, 1.17–4.54), end-stage renal failure requiring hemodialysis is also independently associated with higher total in-hospital complications (HR, 1.38; 95% CI, 1.23–1.54).[83-84] It is therefore prudent that clinicians assess the risk/benefit ratio of ICD therapy on an individual basis for patients with severe renal failure on hemodialysis who are sicker and may have much comorbidity that may further contribute to poor health and higher mortality.

In some patients, their advanced age may pose a clinical and ethical dilemma regarding indications for ICD therapy, especially in view of the fact that virtually all major large randomized trials had excluded very old patients from the trials. Whatever little data that are available are derived from meta-analysis of few trials and registries. In a meta-analysis performed by Santangeli et al[85]; from a total of 5,783 patients enrolled in 5 major trials, MADIT-II, DEFINITE, DINAMIT, SCDHeFT, and IRIS, 44% of patients were elderly. The definition of "elderly" was not uniform; the definition included patients 65 years or older in DEFINITE, SCDHeFT, and IRIS, and 60 years or older in MADIT-II and DINAMIT. Two trials, DINAMIT and IRIS, enrolled patients early after acute myocardial infarction, and these were excluded from the primary analysis. Analysis of DEFINITE, MADIT-II, and SCDHeFT trials showed that in the elderly prophylactic ICD therapy was associated with a small reduction in all-cause mortality compared with medical therapy

(HR, 0.75; 95% CI, 0.61 to 0.91). The benefit of ICDs, however, was not confirmed when MADIT-II patients older than 70 years were excluded or when data from DINAMIT and IRIS were included. The observed survival benefit in older patients was smaller though still statistically significant.[85] Tsai et al[86] analyzed data obtained from the National Cardiovascular Data Registry (NCDR®)-ICD Registry™, which is an ongoing registry begun in 2006 in response to a mandate from the Centers for Medicare and Medicaid Services (CMS). Analysis of data from 44,805 participants—14,518 between the ages of 65–74 years and 15,375 of 75 years or above—showed that although age was associated with a high risk of nonarrhythmic death (6% for < 65 years, 8% for 65–74 years, 10% for ≥ 75 years), this association was markedly attenuated after adjusting for comorbid conditions and nonelective timing of ICD implantation (HR, 1.12; 95% CI, 1.10–1.14 per 5-year increment).[86] Given their advanced age and frequent comorbidities, it is difficult to assess effectiveness of ICDs in the very elderly patients, for example, octogenarians, nonagenarians, and even centenarians.[87-89] Among the predictors of survival in this unique patient population, although age and renal function remain the main determinants of survival in octogenarians and nonagenarians with left ventricular dysfunction (ie, EF ≤ 35%), after adjusting for age, EF, glomerular filtration rate (GFR), and other comorbidity indices, ICDs have not shown to confer any survival benefit (HR, 0.71; 95% CI, 0.42 to 1.20).[87] In a retrospective analysis of data from 225 octogenarian patients with ICDs, Ertel et al[88] found that the actuarial 1-year mortality of octogenarian ICD recipients with severe left ventricular dysfunction (EF ≤ 20%) was 38.2% versus 13.1% in patients > 80 years with an EF > 20% and 10.6% in patients < 80 years with an EF ≤ 20% (P < 0.001 for both).[88] Tsai et al,[87] in their analysis of the NCDR-ICD Registry data, also found increased odds of any adverse event or death among 75- to 79-year-olds (HR, 1.14; 95% CI, 1.03 to 1.25), 80- to 84-year-olds (HR, 1.22; 95% CI, 1.10 to 1.36), and patients 85 years and older (HR, 1.15; 95% CI, 1.01 to 1.32), compared with patients under 65 years old.[90]

Several studies, including the subgroup analyses of large trials such as MADIT-II, SCDHeFT, and the INTRINSIC RV (Inhibition of Unnecessary RV Pacing with AV Search Hysteresis in ICDs) have shown similar mortality and ICD effectiveness in women and men.[91-94] Thus, there should be no gender bias for ICD therapy.

Conclusions

Since their initial introduction into clinical practice, the indications for implantation of ICDs have expanded. There is ample evidence, as discussed, to this date to indicate that ICDs are useful for both secondary and primary prevention of SCD due to VT and VF for both ischemic and nonischemic substrate. However, beyond this principle role, due to tremendous advances made in the ICD technology, modern ICDs have capabilities also to provide multi-chamber cardiac pacing and cardiac resynchronization therapy; and capabilities to store retrievable data related to battery and lead performances, pacing and sensing parameters, patients' arrhythmia burden, activity level, autonomic function, and heart failure status etc. Recently, major device manufacturers have introduced their unique versions of "remote monitoring" technology that allows home transmitters to interrogate devices, download, and transmit collected and stored data via the Internet to a protected network. In the era of practicing evidence-based clinical medicine, we would certainly require more scientific clinical trials, registries, and observations to further evaluate and validate not only new hypotheses and new technologies but also long-term applicability of ICD therapy safely and effectively.

References

1. Zipes DP, Camm AJ, Borggrefe M, et al. ACC/AHA/ESC 2006 guidelines for management of patients with ventricular arrhythmias and the prevention of sudden cardiac death: a report of the American College of Cardiology/American Heart Association Task Force and the European Society of Cardiology Committee for Practice Guidelines (Writing Committee to Develop Guidelines for Management of Patients With Ventricular Arrhythmias and the Prevention of Sudden Cardiac Death). *J Am Coll Cardiol*. 2006;48:e247-e346.
2. Myerburg RJ, Kessler KM, Castellanos A. Sudden cardiac death. Structure, function, and time-dependence of risk. *Circulation*. 1992;85(suppl 1):I2-I10.
3. Kawamura T, Kondo H, Hirai M, et al. Sudden death in the working population; a collaborative study in Central Japan. *Eur Heart J*. 1999;20(5):338-343.
4. Priori SG, Aliot E, Blomstrom-Lundqvist C, et al. Task Force on Sudden Cardiac Death of the European Society of Cardiology. *Eur Heart J*. 2001;22:1374-1450.
5. Mirowski M, Reid PR, Mower MM, et al. Termination of malignant ventricular arrhythmias with an implanted automatic defibrillator in human beings. *N Engl J Med*. 1980;303(6):322-324.
6. Saksena S, Parsonnet V. Implantation of an implantable cardioverter/defibrillator without thoracotomy using a triple electrode system. *J Am Med Assoc*. 1988;259:69-72.
7. Bardy GH, Smith WM, Hood MA, et al. An entirely subcutaneous implantable cardioverter-defibrillator. *N Engl J Med*. 2010;363(1):36-44.
8. Frye RL, Collins JJ, DeSanctis RW, et al. Guidelines for permanent cardiac pacemaker implantation, May 1984: A report of the Joint American College of Cardiology/American Heart Association Task Force on Assessment of Cardiovascular Procedures (Subcommittee on Pacemaker Implantation). *Circulation*. 1984;70:331A-339A.
9. Epstein AE, DiMarco JP, Ellenbogen KA, et al. American College of Cardiology/American Heart Association Task Force on Practice Guidelines (Writing Committee to Revise the ACC/AHA/NASPE 2002 Guideline Update for Implantation of Cardiac Pacemakers and Antiarrhythmia Devices); American Association for Thoracic Surgery; Society

of Thoracic Surgeons. *J Am Coll Cardiol.* 2008;51(21):e1-e62/ *Circulation.* 2008;117:e350-e408.
10. Epstein AE, DiMarco JP, Ellenbogen KA, et al. 2012 ACCF/AHA/HRS focused update incorporated into the ACCF/AHA/HRS 2008 guidelines for device-based therapy of cardiac rhythm abnormalities: a report of the American College of Cardiology Foundation/American Heart Association Task Force on Practice Guidelines and the Heart Rhythm Society. *J Am Coll Cardiol.* 2013;61:e6-e75.
11. Russo AM, Stainback RF, Bailey SR, et al. ACCF/HRS/AHA/ASE/HFSA/SCAI/SCCT/SCMR 2013 appropriate use criteria for implantable cardioverter-defibrillators and cardiac resynchronization therapy: a report of the American College of Cardiology Foundation Appropriate Use Criteria Task Force, Heart Rhythm Society, American Heart Association, American Society of Echocardiography, Heart Failure Society of America, Society for Cardiovascular Angiography and Interventions, Society of Cardiovascular Computed Tomography, and Society for Cardiovascular Magnetic Resonance. *J Am Coll Cardiol.* 2013;61:1318-1368.
12. Myerburg RJ, Reddy V, Castellanos A. Indications for implantable cardioverter-defibrillators based on evidence and judgment. *J Am Coll Cardiol.* 2009;54(9):747-763.
13. The AVID investigators. A comparison of antiarrhythmic drug therapy with implantable defibrillators in patients resuscitated from near fatal ventricular arrhythmias. *N Engl J Med.* 1997;337:1576-1583.
14. Connolly SJ, Gent M, Roberts RS, et al. Canadian Implantable Defibrillator Study (CIDS): a randomized trial of the implantable cardioverter-defibrillator against amiodarone. *Circulation.* 2000;101:1297-1302.
15. Kuck KH, Cappato R, Siebels J, Rüppel R. Randomized comparison of antiarrhythmic drug therapy with implantable defibrillators in patients resuscitated from cardiac arrest: the Cardiac Arrest Study Hamburg (CASH). *Circulation.* 2000;102:748-754.
16. Connolly SJ, Hallstrom AP, Cappato R, et al. Meta-analysis of the implantable cardioverter defibrillator secondary prevention trials: AVID, CASH and CIDS studies. *Eur Heart J.* 2000;21:2071-2078.
17. Lee DS, Green LD, Liu PP, et al. Effectiveness of implantable defibrillators for preventing arrhythmic events and death: a meta-analysis. *J Am Coll Cardiol.* 2003;41:1573-1582.
18. Wever EF, Hauer RN, van Capelle FL, et al. Randomized study of implantable defibrillator as first-choice therapy versus conventional strategy in postinfarct sudden death survivors. *Circulation.* 1995;91:2195-2203.
19. Becker R, Melkumov M, Senges-Becker JC, et al. Are electrophysiological studies needed prior to defibrillator implantation? *Pacing Clin Electrophysiol.* 2003;26(8):1715-1721.
20. Lau EW, Griffith MJ, Pathmanathan RK, et al. The Midlands Trial of Empirical Amiodarone versus Electrophysiology-guided Interventions and Implantable Cardioverter-defibrillators (MAVERIC): a multi-centre prospective randomised clinical trial on the secondary prevention of sudden cardiac death. *Europace.* 2004;6(4):257-266.
21. Crandall BG, Morris CD, Cutler JE, et al. Implantable cardioverter-defibrillator therapy in survivors of out-of-hospital sudden cardiac death without inducible arrhythmias. *J Am Coll Cardiol.* 1993;21(5):1186-1192.
22. Myerburg RJ, Kessler KM, Castellanos A. SCD. Structure, function, and time dependence of risk. *Circulation.* 1992;85:I2-I10.
23. Goldberger JJ, Cain ME, Hohnloser SH, et al. American Heart Association/American College of Cardiology Foundation/Heart Rhythm Society scientific statement on noninvasive risk stratification techniques for identifying patients at risk for sudden cardiac death: a scientific statement from the American Heart Association Council on Clinical Cardiology Committee on Electrocardiography and Arrhythmias and Council on Epidemiology and Prevention. *Circulation.* 2008;118: 1497-1518.
24. Moss AJ, Hall WJ, Cannom DS, et al, for the Multicenter Automatic Defibrillator Implantation Trial Investigators. Improved survival with an implanted defibrillator in patients with coronary disease at high risk for ventricular arrhythmia. *N Engl J Med.* 1996;335:1933-1940.
25. Buxton AE, Lee KL, Fisher JD, Josephson ME, Prystowsky EN, Hafley G. A randomized study of the prevention of sudden death in patients with coronary artery disease. *N Engl J Med.* 1999;341:1882-1890.
26. Moss AJ, Zareba W, Hall WJ, et al, Multicenter Automatic Defibrillator Implantation Trial II Investigators. Prophylactic implantation of a defibrillator in patients with myocardial infarction and reduced ejection fraction. *N Engl J Med.* 2002;346:877-888.
27. Bardy GH, Lee KL, Mark DB, et al, Sudden Cardiac Death in Heart Failure Trial (SCD-HeFT) Investigators. Amiodarone or an implantable cardioverter-defibrillator for congestive heart failure. *N Engl J Med.* 2005;352(3): 225-237.
28. Bansch D, Antz M, Boczor S, et al. Primary prevention of sudden cardiac death in idiopathic dilated cardiomyopathy: the Cardiomyopathy Trial (CAT). *Circulation.* 2002;105: 1453-1458.
29. Kadish A, Dyer A, Daubert JP, et al. Prophylactic defibrillator implantation in patients with nonischemic dilated cardiomyopathy. *N Engl J Med.* 2004;350:2151-2158.
30. Strickberger SA, Hummel JD, Bartlett TG, et al, AMIOVIRT Investigators. Amiodarone versus implantable cardioverter-defibrillator: randomized trial in patients with nonischemic dilated cardiomyopathy and asymptomatic nonsustained ventricular tachycardia AMIOVIRT. *J Am Coll Cardiol.* 2003;41:1707-1712.
31. Bristow MR, Saxon LA, Boehmer J, et al, Comparison of Medical Therapy, Pacing, and Defibrillation in Heart Failure (COMPANION) Investigators. Cardiac resynchronization therapy with or without an implantable defibrillator in advanced chronic heart failure. *N Engl J Med.* 2004;350: 2140-2150.
32. Auricchio A, Metra M, Gasparini M, Lamp B, Klersy C, Curnis A, Fantoni C, et al, for the Multicenter Longitudinal Observational Study (MILOS) Group. Long-term survival of patients with heart failure and ventricular conduction delay treated with cardiac resynchronization therapy. *Am J Cardiol.* 2007;99:232-238.
33. Moss AJ, Hall WJ, Cannom DS, et al, MADIT-CRT Trial Investigators. Cardiac-resynchronization therapy for the prevention of heart-failure events. *N Engl J Med.* 2009;361: 1329-1338.
34. Tang AS, Wells GA, Talajic M, et al, Resynchronization-Defibrillation for Ambulatory Heart Failure Trial Investigators. Cardiac-resynchronization therapy for mild-to-moderate heart failure. *N Engl J Med.* 2010;363(25):2385-2395.
35. Bigger JT, for the Coronary Artery Bypass Graft (CABG) Patch Trial Investigators. Prophylactic use of implanted cardiac defibrillators in patients at high risk for ventricular arrhythmias after coronary artery bypass graft surgery. *N Engl J Med.* 1997;337:1569-1575.
36. Hohnloser SH, Kuck KH, Dorian P, et al, DINAMIT Investigators. Prophylactic use of an implantable cardioverter-defibrillator after acute myocardial infarction. *N Engl J Med.* 2004;351:2481-2488.

37. Steinbeck G, Andresen D, Seidl K, et al, IRIS Investigators. Defibrillator implantation early after myocardial infarction. *N Engl J Med*. 2009;361(15):1427-1436.
38. Al-Khatib SM, Hellkamp A, Bardy GH, et al. Survival of patients receiving a primary prevention implantable cardioverter-defibrillator in clinical practice vs clinical trials. *JAMA*. 2013;309(1):55-62.
39. Moss AJ, Schuger C, Beck CA, et al, MADIT-RIT Trial Investigators. Reduction in inappropriate therapy and mortality through ICD programming. *N Engl J Med*. 2012;367(24):2275-2283.
40. Ezekowitz JA, Armstrong PW, McAlister FA. Implantable cardioverter defibrillators in primary and secondary prevention: a systematic review of randomized, controlled trials. *Ann Intern Med*. 2003;138:445-452.
41. Nanthakumar K, Epstein AE, Kay GN, Plumb VJ, Lee DS. Prophylactic implantable cardioverter-defibrillator therapy in patients with left ventricular systolic dysfunction: a pooled analysis of 10 primary prevention trials. *J Am Coll Cardiol*. 2004;44:2166-2172.
42. Maron BJ, Olivotto I, Spirito P, et al. Epidemiology of hypertrophic cardiomyopathy-related death: revisited in a large non-referral-based patient population. *Circulation*. 2000;102(8):858-864.
43. Maron BJ. Hypertrophic cardiomyopathy: a systematic review. *JAMA*. 2002;287:1308-1320.
44. Maron BJ, McKenna WJ, Danielson GK, et al. American College of Cardiology/European Society of Cardiology Clinical Expert Consensus Document on Hypertrophic Cardiomyopathy. A report of the American College of Cardiology Task Force on Clinical Expert Consensus Documents and the European Society of Cardiology Committee for Practice Guidelines Committee to Develop an Expert Consensus Document on Hypertrophic Cardiomyopathy. *J Am Coll Cardiol*. 2003;42:1687-1713.
45. Gersh BJ, Maron BJ, Bonow RO, et al. 2011 ACCF/AHA guideline for the diagnosis and treatment of hypertrophic cardiomyopathy: a report of the American College of Cardiology Foundation/American Heart Association Task Force on Practice Guidelines. *J Am Coll Cardiol*. 2011;58:e212-e260.
46. Elliott PM, Sharma S, Varnava A, Poloniecki J, Rowland E, McKenna WJ. Survival after cardiac arrest or sustained ventricular tachycardia in patients with hypertrophic cardiomyopathy. *J Am Coll Cardiol*. 1999;33(6):1596-1601.
47. Maron BJ, Shen WK, Link MS, et al. Efficacy of implantable cardioverter-defibrillators for the prevention of sudden death in patients with hypertrophic cardiomyopathy. *N Engl J Med*. 2000;342:365-373.
48. Begley DA, Mohiddin SA, Tripodi D, Winkler JB, Fananapazir L. Efficacy of implantable cardioverter defibrillator therapy for primary and secondary prevention of sudden cardiac death in hypertrophic cardiomyopathy. *Pacing Clin Electrophysiol*. 2003;26(9):1887-1896.
49. Proclemer A, Ghidina M, Facchin D, Rebellato L, Corrado D, Gasparini M, Gregori D. Use of implantable cardioverter-defibrillator in inherited arrhythmogenic diseases: data from Italian ICD Registry for the years 2001–6. *Pacing Clin Electrophysiol*. 2009;32(4):434-445.
50. Maron BJ, Spirito P, Shen WK, et al. Implantable cardioverter-defibrillators and prevention of sudden cardiac death in hypertrophic cardiomyopathy. *JAMA*. 2007;298(4):405-412.
51. Zipes DP, Camm AJ, Borggrefe M, et al. ACC/AHA/ESC 2006 guidelines for management of patients with ventricular arrhythmias and the prevention of sudden cardiac death—executive summary: a report of the American College of Cardiology/American Heart Association Task Force and the European Society of Cardiology Committee for Practice Guidelines (Writing Committee to Develop Guidelines for Management of Patients with Ventricular Arrhythmias and the Prevention of Sudden Cardiac Death). *Eur Heart J*. 2006;27:2099-2140.
52. Maron BJ. Risk stratification and role of implantable defibrillators for prevention of sudden death in patients with hypertrophic cardiomyopathy. *Circ J*. 2010;74:2271-2282.
53. Marcus F, Fontaine G, Guiraudon G, Frank R, Laurenceau JL, Malergue C, Grosgogeat Y. Right ventricular dysplasia: a report of 24 adult cases. *Circulation*. 1982;65:384-398.
54. Marcus F, McKenna W, Sherrill D, et al. Diagnosis of arrhythmogenic right ventricular cardiomyopathy/dysplasia: proposed modification of the Task Force Criteria. *Circulation*. 2010;121:1533-1541.
55. Patel HC, Calkins H. Arrhythmogenic right ventricular dysplasia. *Curr Treat Options Cardiovasc Med*. 2010;12(6):598-613.
56. Corrado D, Leoni L, Link MS, et al. Implantable cardioverter-defibrillator therapy for prevention of sudden death in patients with arrhythmogenic right ventricular cardiomyopathy/dysplasia. *Circulation*. 2003;108:3084-3091.
57. Wichter T, Paul M, Wollmann C, et al. Implantable cardioverter/defibrillator therapy in arrhythmogenic right ventricular cardiomyopathy: single-center experience of long-term follow-up and complications in 60 patients. *Circulation*. 2004;109:1503-1508.
58. Roguin A, Bomma CS, Nasir K, et al. Implantable cardioverter-defibrillators in patients with arrhythmogenic right ventricular dysplasia/cardiomyopathy. *J Am Coll Cardiol*. 2004;43:1843-1852.
59. Hodgkinson KA, Parfrey PS, Bassett AS, et al. The impact of implantable cardioverter-defibrillator therapy on survival in autosomal-dominant arrhythmogenic right ventricular cardiomyopathy (ARVD5). *J Am Coll Cardiol*. 2005;45:400-408.
60. Piccini JP, Dalal D, Roguin A, et al. Predictors of appropriate implantable defibrillator therapies in patients with arrhythmogenic right ventricular dysplasia. *Heart Rhythm*. 2005;2:1188-1194.
61. Antzelevitch C, Brugada P, Borggrefe M, et al. Brugada syndrome: report of the second consensus conference: endorsed by the Heart Rhythm Society and the European Heart Rhythm Association. *Circulation*. 2005;111:659-670.
62. Brugada J, Brugada R, Brugada P. Determinants of sudden cardiac death in individuals with the electrocardiographic pattern of Brugada syndrome and no previous cardiac arrest. *Circulation*. 2003;108:3092-3096.
63. Priori SG, Napolitano C, Gasparini M, et al. Natural history of Brugada syndrome: insights for risk stratification and management. *Circulation*. 2002;105:1342-1347.
64. Kanda M, Shimizu W, Matsuo K, et al. Electrophysiologic characteristics and implications of induced ventricular fibrillation in symptomatic patients with Brugada syndrome. *J Am Coll Cardiol*. 2002;39:1799-1805.
65. Eckardt L, Kirchhof P, Schulze-Bahr E, et al. Electrophysiologic investigation in Brugada syndrome; yield of programmed ventricular stimulation at two ventricular sites with up to three premature beats. *Eur Heart J*. 2002;23:1394-1401.
66. Priori SG, Gasparini M, Napolitano C, et al. Risk stratification in Brugada syndrome: results of the PRELUDE (PRogrammed ELectrical stimUlation preDictive valuE) registry. *J Am Coll Cardiol*. 2012;59(1):37-45.
67. Gehi AK, Duong TD, Metz LD, Gomes JA, Mehta D. Risk stratification of individuals with the Brugada electrocardiogram: a meta-analysis. *J Cardiovasc Electrophysiol*. 2006;17(6):577-583.

68. Steven D, Roberts-Thomson KC, Inada K, et al. Long-term follow-up in patients with presumptive Brugada syndrome treated with implanted defibrillators. *J Cardiovasc Electrophysiol.* 2011;(10):1115-1119.
69. Schwartz PJ, Priori SG, Spazzolini C, et al. Genotype-phenotype correlation in the long-QT syndrome: gene-specific triggers for life-threatening arrhythmias. *Circulation.* 2001;103:89-95.
70. Priori SG, Schwartz PJ, Napolitano C, et al. Risk stratification in the long-QT syndrome. *N Engl J Med.* 2003;348:1866-1874.
71. Groh WJ, Silka MJ, Oliver RP, Halperin BD, McAnuhy JH, Kron J. Use of implantable cardioverter-defibrillators in the congenital long QT syndrome. *Am J Cardiol.* 1996;78:703-706.
72. Zareba W, Moss AJ, Daubert JP, Hall WJ, Robinson JL, Andrews M. Implantable cardioverter defibrillator in high-risk long QT syndrome patients. *J Cardiovasc Electrophysiol.* 2003;14(4):337-341.
73. Mönnig G, Köbe J, Löher A, et al. Implantable cardioverter-defibrillator therapy in patients with congenital long-QT syndrome: a long-term follow-up. *Heart Rhythm.* 2005;2(5):497-504.
74. Goldenberg I, Moss AJ, Bradley J, et al. Long-QT syndrome after age 40. *Circulation.* 2008;117(17):2192-2201.
75. Schwartz PJ, Spazzolini C, Priori SG, et al. Who are the long-QT syndrome patients who receive an implantable cardioverter-defibrillator and what happens to them? Data from the European Long-QT Syndrome Implantable Cardioverter-Defibrillator (LQTS ICD) Registry. *Circulation.* 2010;122(13):1272-1282.
76. Stein KM, Mittal S, Gilliam FR, et al. Predictors of early mortality in implantable cardioverter-defibrillator recipients. *Europace.* 2009;11(6):734-740.
77. Cygankiewicz I, Gillespie J, Zareba W, et al, MADIT II Investigators. Predictors of long-term mortality in Multicenter Automatic Defibrillator Implantation Trial II (MADIT II) patients with implantable cardioverter-defibrillators. *Heart Rhythm.* 2009;6(4):468-473.
78. Goldenberg I, Moss AJ, McNitt S, et al, Multicenter Automatic Defibrillator Implantation Trial-II Investigators. Relations among renal function, risk of sudden cardiac death, and benefit of the implanted cardiac defibrillator in patients with ischemic left ventricular dysfunction. *Am J Cardiol.* 2006;98:485-490.
79. Hager CS, Jain S, Blackwell J, Culp B, Song J, Chiles CD. Effect of renal function on survival after implantable cardioverter defibrillator placement. *Am J Cardiol.* 2010;106(9):1297-1300.
80. Eckart RE, Gula LJ, Reynolds MR, Shry EA, Maisel WH. Mortality following defibrillator implantation in patients with renal insufficiency. *J Cardiovasc Electrophysiol.* 2006;17(9):940-943.
81. Sakhuja R, Keebler M, Lai TS, et al. Meta-analysis of mortality in dialysis patients with an implantable cardioverter defibrillator. *Am J Cardiol.* 2009;103(5):735-741.
82. Khan F, Adelstein E, Saba S. Implantable cardioverter defibrillators confer survival benefit in patients with renal insufficiency but not in dialysis-dependent patients. *J Interv Card Electrophysiol.* 2010;28(2):117-123.
83. Robin J, Weinberg K, Tiongson J, et al. Renal dialysis as a risk factor for appropriate therapies and mortality in implantable cardioverter-defibrillator recipients. *Heart Rhythm.* 2006;3(10):1196-1201.
84. Aggarwal A, Wang Y, Rumsfeld JS, Curtis JP, Heidenreich PA, National Cardiovascular Data Registry. Clinical characteristics and in-hospital outcome of patients with end-stage renal disease on dialysis referred for implantable cardioverter-defibrillator implantation. *Heart Rhythm.* 2009;6(11):1565-1571.
85. Santangeli P, Di Biase L, Dello Russo A, et al. Meta-analysis: age and effectiveness of prophylactic implantable cardioverter-defibrillators. *Ann Intern Med.* 2010;153(9):592-599. Erratum in *Ann Intern Med.* 2011;154(11):780.
86. Tsai V, Goldstein MK, Hsia HH, Wang Y, Curtis J, Heidenreich PA, on behalf of the National Cardiovascular Data Registry. Age differences in primary prevention implantable cardioverter-defibrillator use in U.S. individuals. *J Am Geriatr Soc.* 2011;59(9):1589-1595.
87. Mezu U, Adelstein E, Jain S, Saba S. Effectiveness of implantable defibrillators in octogenarians and nonagenarians for primary prevention of sudden cardiac death. *Am J Cardiol.* 2011;108(5):718-722.
88. Ertel D, Phatak K, Makati K, et al. Predictors of early mortality in patients age 80 and older receiving implantable defibrillators. *Pacing Clin Electrophysiol.* 2010;33(8):981-987.
89. Shah A, Kantharia B. Safety and efficacy of permanent pacemaker and implantable cardioverter defibrillator therapy in the nonagenarians and centenarians. *Europace.* 2011;13(Suppl 3):1375-1385. doi: 10.1093/Europace/Eur 23/.
90. Tsai V, Goldstein MK, Hsia HH, Wang Y, Curtis J, Heidenreich PA, on behalf of the National Cardiovascular Data's ICD Registry. Influence of age on perioperative complications among patients undergoing implantable cardioverter-defibrillators for primary prevention in the United States. *Circ Cardiovasc Qual Outcomes.* 2011;4(5):549-556.
91. Chen HA, Hsia HH, Vagelos R, Fowler M, Wang P, Al-Ahmad A. The effect of gender on mortality or appropriate shock in patients with nonischemic cardiomyopathy who have implantable cardioverter-defibrillators. *Pacing Clin Electrophysiol.* 2007;30(3):390-394.
92. Zareba W, Moss AJ, Jackson Hall W, et al, MADIT II Investigators. Clinical course and implantable cardioverter defibrillator therapy in postinfarction women with severe left ventricular dysfunction. *J Cardiovasc Electrophysiol.* 2005;16(12):1265-1270.
93. Russo AM, Poole JE, Mark DB, Anderson J, et al. Primary prevention with defibrillator therapy in women: results from the Sudden Cardiac Death in Heart Failure Trial. *J Cardiovasc Electrophysiol.* 2008;19(7):720-724.
94. Russo AM, Day JD, Stolen K, et al. Implantable cardioverter defibrillators: do women fare worse than men? Gender comparison in the INTRINSIC RV trial. *J Cardiovasc Electrophysiol.* 2009;20(9):973-978.

CHAPTER 66A

Indications for Surgical Ablation of Tachyarrhythmias: Atrial Fibrillation/Atrial Flutter

David C. Kress, MD

Introduction

Surgical therapy of atrial fibrillation (AF) and atrial flutter has evolved from a cut-and-sew era in which the only ablative energy available was nitrous oxide cryoablation with primitive hand-pieces. There are now multiple ablative energy sources available, each with specialized delivery tools. Placement of transmural contiguous linear lesions based on directly visualized anatomic landmarks can be easily accomplished with surgical techniques and can be decisive in the ablation of atrial arrhythmias.

Surgical lesion patterns also have evolved from the original Maze 3. This is due in part to a better understanding of the fundamental role of pulmonary vein triggers in the development of paroxysmal atrial fibrillation (PAF). Subsequent investigators have attempted to deconstruct the Maze 3 into component lesions that address specific failure mechanisms, such as left atrial macroreentry flutters, while incorporating pulmonary vein isolation. This appreciation of essential versus nonessential lesions has led to the development of minimally invasive surgical procedures in selected patients, and allowed optimal deployment of surgical ablation tools in open chest procedures. Results from several large series that vary with respect to surgical technique, percentage of patients with PAF, whether ambulatory monitoring was used in follow-up, and freedom from AF or antiarrhythmic drugs are summarized in Table 66A.1.[1-9]

In 2007, an HRS/EHRA/ECAS Expert Consensus Statement[10] summarized the indications for surgical ablation of AF:

1. Symptomatic AF patients undergoing other cardiac surgical procedures.

2. Selected asymptomatic AF patients undergoing cardiac surgery in whom the ablation can be performed with minimal risk.

3. Stand-alone AF surgery should be considered for symptomatic AF patients who prefer a surgical approach, have failed one or more attempts at catheter ablation, or are not candidates for catheter ablation.

The referral of patients for stand-alone AF surgery in lieu of catheter ablation for symptomatic, medically refractory AF was left to the discretion of the physician and patient based on "each institution's experience with catheter ablation and surgical ablation of AF, the relative outcomes and risks of each in the individual patient, and patient preference."[10] This was based on the lack of head-to-head comparisons of the outcomes of catheter and sole-therapy surgical ablation.

This chapter distinguishes the key features of different available surgical approaches in order to highlight their specific strengths and weaknesses. The indications for the use of these procedures are better understood in this context. We then go back to the elements of the consensus statement to address which surgical procedures are likely

Table 66A.1 Representative surgical series of Maze 3 or other derived procedures for the treatment of atrial fibrillation

Author	No. of Patients	Method	Lesion Set	% Paroxysmal	% Concomitant	Ambulatory Monitoring	Freedom from AF	% Off AADs
Nasso[1] (2011)	104	Epicardial RF	Box	N/A	0	24 hour if AADs stopped	89% at 17 mo	51% at 17 mo
Cox[2] (1996)	118	Cut and sew	Maze 3	N/A	N/A	No	98% from 3 to 102 mo	N/A
Gammie[3] (2009)	119	Argon cryo	Maze 3	35	89	Yes in 75%	60% at 38 mo	N/A
Ballaux[4] (2006)	203	Cut and sew	Maze 3	70	32	Yes in half	80% (lone AF) and 65% (concomitant) at 48 mo	76% (lone AF) and 63% (concomitant) at 48 mo
Damiano[5] (2011)	282	Bipolar RF/cryo	Maze 4	42	66	Since 2006	89% at 12 mo	78% at 12 mo
Geidel[6] (2011)	325	Monopolar/ bipolar RF	PV isolation, connecting lesion	0	100	24 hour, early and late follow-up	71% at 60 mo	22% at 3 years
Stulak[7] (2007)	335	Cut and sew	Maze 3	48	82	No	70% (concomitant) at median 33 mo	N/A
Kim[8] (2010)	435	Microwave/ cryo	Maze 3	10.3	100	Yes if symptoms	70% at 84 mo	77%-81% at 5 years
Barnett[9] (2006)	1,801	Meta-analysis, 69 studies	Biatrial 94%, left atrial 6%	N/A	N/A	No	85% at 36 mo	N/A

AF = atrial fibrillation; AADs = antiarrhythmic drugs; cryo = cryoablation; mo = month; N/A = not available; PV = pulmonary vein; RF = radiofrequency. Source: References 1–9.

to fulfill requirements such as success with concomitant valve surgery, minimize risk, or have success for failed catheter ablation. Surgery for atrial flutter is separately addressed. Note that in the section on the treatment of failed catheter ablation there is a discussion of patients with postablation left atrial flutters.

Surgical Procedures

Lesion Patterns

Biatrial Lesion

Lesion patterns in surgery are created with attention to visual anatomical landmarks. The prototypical biatrial lesion pattern is the Maze 3 (Figure 66A.1), which was developed by Cox and Schuessler.[11,12] This operation was designed as a cut-and-sew procedure with adjunctive cryoablation. The key elements of the Maze 3 are bilateral pulmonary vein isolation, a mitral isthmus lesion, posterior left atrial connecting lesions, left atrial appendectomy, and a right atrial cavotricuspid isthmus lesion.

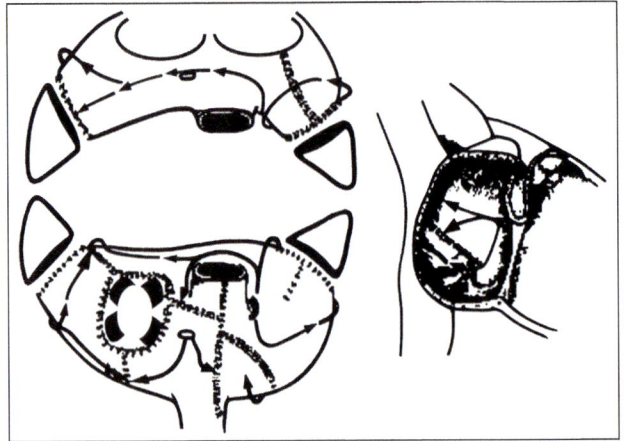

Figure 66A.1 The Maze 3 lesion pattern. Source: From Cox J.[12] Modified with permission from Elsevier.

These building block lesions can be found in the Maze 4 (Figure 66A.2),[13] in the Radial Procedure (Figure 66A.3),[14,15] and in some left atrial lesion patterns (Figure 66A.4)[16,17] that are paired with a cavotricuspid isthmus ablation.

Chapter 66A: Indications for Surgical Ablation of Tachyarrhythmias: Atrial Fibrillation/Atrial Flutter

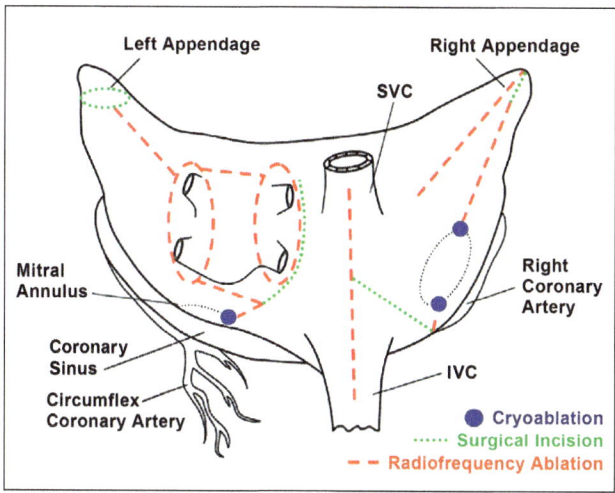

Figure 66A.2 The Maze 4 lesion pattern. *Source:* From Lall SC, et al.[13] Reproduced with permission from Elsevier.

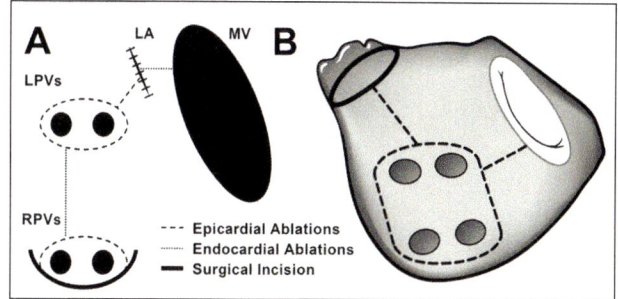

Figure 66A.4 **Panel A:** Benussi lesion pattern. Isolates and connects pulmonary veins, connects to mitral valve, and connects to and removes the left atrial appendage (LAA). *Source:* From Benussi S, et al.[16] Reproduced with permission from Oxford University Press. **Panel B:** Gillinov lesion pattern. Bilateral pulmonary vein isolation with box lesion, mitral valve isthmus lesion, and connecting lesion to LAA, which is excised. *Source:* From Gillinov AM.[17] Reproduced with permission from Wolters Kluwer Health.

Stand-alone Lesion Sets: There are two stand-alone lesion sets that have been used for epicardial ablation:

1. Bilateral pulmonary vein isolation with (Figure 66A.5)[18,19] or without (Figure 66A.6)[20] nonisthmus connecting lesions. Ganglionated plexus identification and ablation is also performed at some surgical centers as an adjunct to epicardial ablation.[21,22]

2. A "box lesion" (Figure 66A.7) that runs anterior to the four pulmonary veins.[23,24]

These approaches represent two different ways to isolate muscle sleeve triggers located in the pulmonary veins. Each has limitations that may lead to treatment failures.

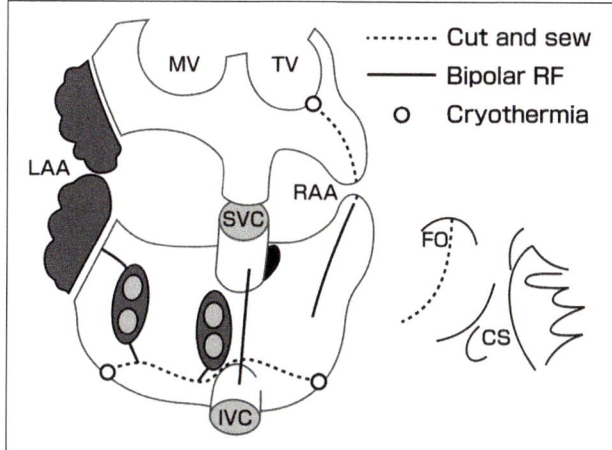

Figure 66A.3 The Radial Procedure lesion pattern. *Source:* From Nitta T.[15] Reproduced with permission from Elsevier.

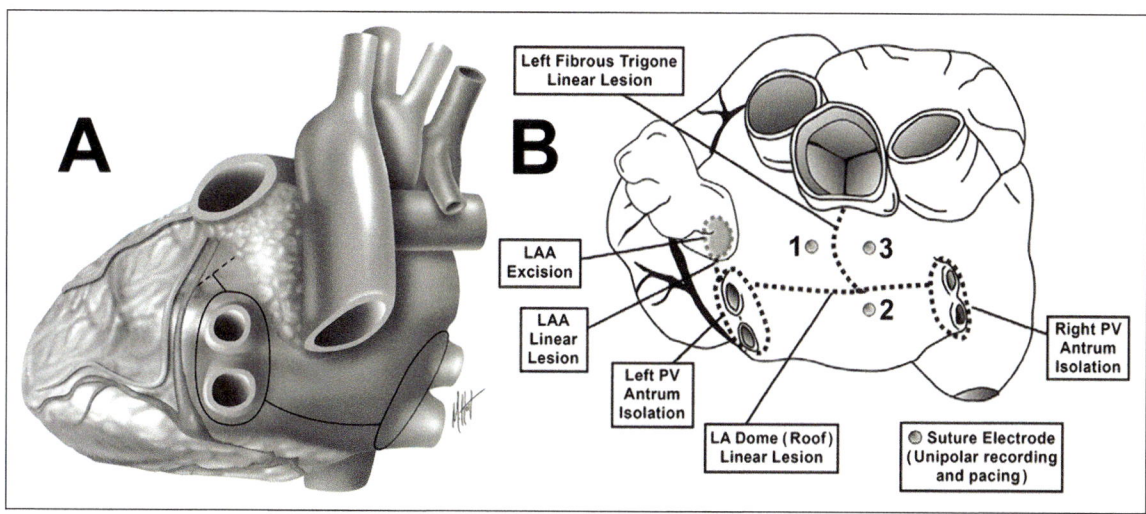

Figure 66A.5 **Panel A:** Kress lesion pattern. Isolates and connects pulmonary veins and LAA, which is removed. Originally performed via sternotomy using microwave ablation. *Source:* From Kress DC.[18] Reproduced with permission from Elsevier. **Panel B:** Edgerton lesion pattern. Similar to A, but adds a lesion to the mitral valve annulus at the left fibrous trigone using a right-sided transverse sinus approach. *Source:* From Edgerton JR, et al.[19] Reproduced with permission from Elsevier.

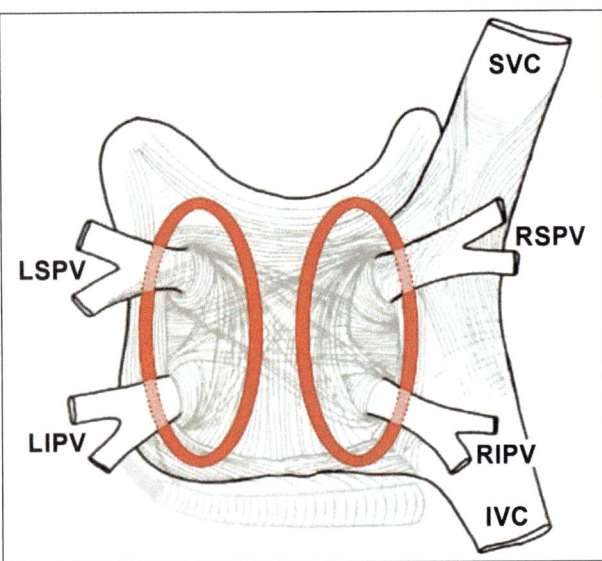

Figure 66A.6 Bilateral pulmonary vein isolation, currently performed with bipolar radiofrequency ablation clamps via bilateral thoracic port access. *Source:* From Calkins H, et al.[10] Reproduced with permission from Elsevier.

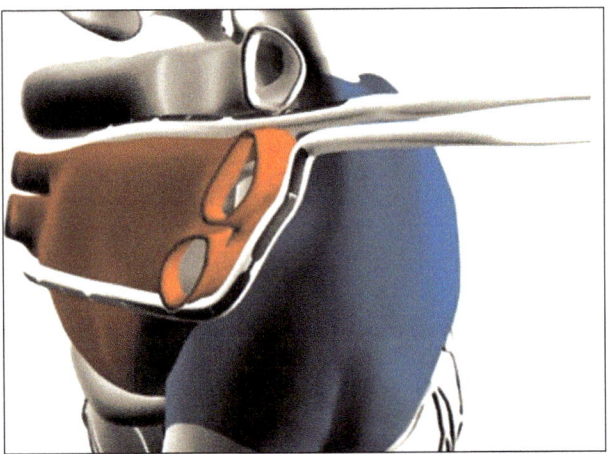

Figure 66A.7 Box lesion, which surrounds the left atrium anterior to all four pulmonary veins. *Source:* From Saltman AE, et al.[23] Reproduced with permission from Forum Multimedia Publishing.

Unusual trigger locations, such as in the posterior left atrium or superior vena cava, may be unrecognized and not effectively isolated by simple pulmonary vein isolation. With respect to the box lesion, it can in theory isolate triggers located in the posterior left atrium along with the pulmonary veins, but in practice it is quite difficult to achieve reproducible transmurality[25] or freedom from AF.[24] This can be due to thick insulating fat in folds of the left atrium and in the transverse sinus,[26] an overriding right atrium in Waterston's groove, and inadequate power to overcome cooling from the intra-atrial blood flow. Even a small gap in the box lesion can lead to treatment failure. Extra-long ablation catheters using either microwave or diode lasers have been developed for a right or bilateral thoracoscopy-based procedure to create the box lesion, but these are currently no longer available.

Energy Sources

In selecting a particular lesion pattern and surgical approach, it cannot be emphasized enough that every effort should be made to replace cut-and-sew lesions with ablative lesions that are transmural. Due to the sometimes transient nature of exit-block or entrance-block, reliance on energy sources that have good histologic evidence of chronic transmurality whenever possible is prudent. Endocardial lesions made with cryoablation in a dry surgical field and lesions made with bipolar radiofrequency ablation clamps meet this criterion,[27,28] and therefore procedures that create lesion patterns with these tools are preferred, particularly during sternotomy.

Three general principles can be stated regarding achievement of transmurality during surgical ablation, which are helpful in determining which energy source to use:

1. Epicardial ablation on a blood-filled atrium takes more energy than endocardial ablation in a bloodless field.[26]

2. Epicardial ablation performed off pump takes more energy than on pump due to greater convective cooling of the atrium during circulation.[18]

3. Cryoablation is more effective in a bloodless field than when applied epicardially on the atrial wall[29] (▶ Video 66A.1).

Drag lesions can be performed with radiofrequency pens to create lines, such as isthmus lesions, that are not easily or safely accessible by ablation clamps. However, real-time transmurality is difficult to ensure and has led many surgeons to use cryoablation in these circumstances. Pulmonary vein isolation can be assessed with epicardial confirmation of either entrance- or exit-block in the case of bilateral pulmonary vein isolation.[30] In some cases, delayed conduction during epicardial pacing can assess completeness of surgical connecting lesions.[19] Other studies, however, have shown a lack of correlation between acute electrical isolation and chronic transmurality.[29,31] In general, any intraoperative reliance on electrophysiologic assessment of transmurality should not substitute for sound adherence to visual landmarks and avoidance of ablative techniques that are unlikely to produce histologic full-thickness lesions.

Surgical Approaches

Sternotomy

Sternotomy (▶ Video 66A.2) is typically reserved for patients undergoing concomitant cardiac procedures that already require sternotomy. Stand-alone ablation via sternotomy is still indicated in patients for whom a biatrial lesion pattern on bypass is essential but has been supplanted in some centers by port access right thoracotomy cryoablation procedures on bypass.[32]

Minithoracotomy/Thoracoscopy

Thoracic approaches have fallen into 3 types:

1. Bilateral port access to use bipolar radiofrequency ablation clamps to perform stand-alone bilateral pulmonary vein isolation (▶ Video 66A.3, ▶ Video 66A.4, and ▶ Video 66A.5).

2. Thoracoscopic or port access to create the stand-alone box lesion anterior to the 4 pulmonary veins.[23,24]

3. Right port access to perform cryoablation, either stand-alone[32] or during minimally invasive mitral valve surgery.

A disadvantage of the purely right-sided access for AF ablation is that the left atrial appendage (LAA) can only be closed by an over-sew from the inside of the left atrium. An LAA recanalization rate of 36% has been reported with endocardial over-sew in one study.[33]

Midline Pericardioscopy

Pericardioscopy adopts a novel entry site into the pericardial space through the central tendon of the diaphragm (▶ Video 66A.6). Laparoscopic access is above the left lobe of the liver via a 2 cm subxyphoid incision. The pericardioscope can access the posterior and lateral left atrium, and a specially designed saline-irrigated radiofrequency ablation probe can then deliver epicardial lesions to surfaces not covered by pericardial reflections (Figure 66A.8).[34]

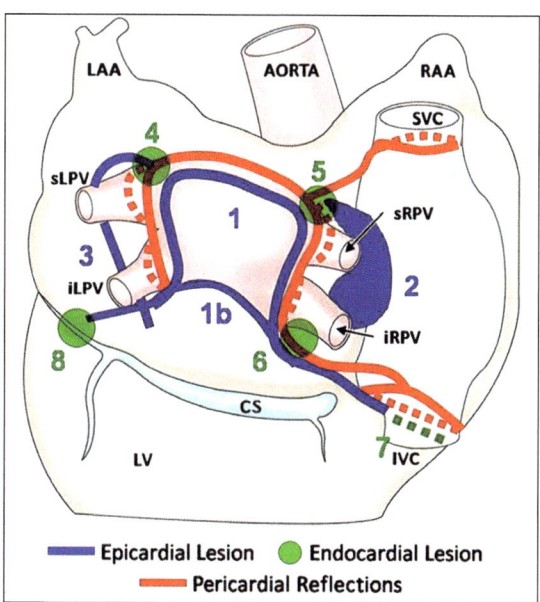

Figure 66A.8 Hybrid lesion pattern that uses pericardioscopic access to deliver epicardial lesions and catheter ablation for endocardial lesions. *Source:* Modified with permission from nContact, Inc. (Morrisville, NC).[34]

Lesion transmurality is assessed at the time of percutaneous ablation using electroanatomical mapping or catheter-based activation mapping. Complete pulmonary vein isolation requires either same setting or prior percutaneous ablation of regions not accessible by the pericardioscope. The LAA is not accessible via this approach

Patient-specific Recommendations

Symptomatic AF Patients Undergoing Other Cardiac Surgical Procedure

Patients already undergoing a mitral valve procedure should undergo preferably a biatrial lesion pattern that accomplishes pulmonary vein isolation, posterior left atrial isolation, LAA removal or exclusion, and both left and right atrial isthmus lesions. Catheter ablation once the patient has had a mitral valve prosthesis placed is contraindicated, another reason to place a comprehensive left atrial pattern in these patients. A recent meta-analysis of 5,885 patients undergoing either left atrial or biatrial procedures showed similar survival, but a superior freedom from atrial fibrillation of approximately 10% at all time points up to 3 years in patients who underwent a biatrial procedure.[9] Excessive left atrial size reduces efficacy, and left atrial reduction has been shown to improve freedom from AF at 1 year by 30% in patients with left atrial diameters greater than 6 cm.[35]

Patients undergoing procedures in which the left atrium will not otherwise be opened require individualization and surgical judgment that take into account how symptomatic they are; whether the AF is paroxysmal, persistent, or long-standing persistent; and whether an on-pump or off-pump procedure is otherwise contemplated. For example, a patient undergoing off-pump coronary artery bypass grafting who has symptomatic PAF may be an excellent candidate for bilateral pulmonary vein isolation and LAA occlusion or removal.

Asymptomatic AF Patients Undergoing Cardiac Surgery

Surgical AF procedures in these patients should be as risk free as possible and at a minimum remove or occlude the LAA. In a patient with long-standing persistent AF undergoing a mitral valve procedure, addition of biatrial lesions should have minimal additional risk.

On the other hand, conversion of an off-pump procedure to an on-pump procedure solely to perform a biatrial pattern probably poses more risk than bilateral pulmonary vein isolation and LAA occlusion or removal. Subsequent catheter ablation can be performed for additional left and right atrial lesions should the patient become symptomatic.

Stand-alone AF Surgery

Stand-alone AF surgery should be offered following a multidisciplinary evaluation by both an EP surgeon and an electrophysiologist who either performs catheter ablation or is familiar with the availability and results of catheter ablation in the patient's community. The actual success rates and complication rates with each procedure ideally would guide the patient's decision-making process; however, in the real world, it should be recognized that few centers have sufficiently large patient volumes and long-term follow-up in both catheter and surgical ablation to accomplish this without reference to published literature.

Symptomatic AF Patients Who Prefer a Surgical Approach or Are Not Candidates for Catheter Ablation

PAF is best approached at this time with bilateral pulmonary vein isolation, with or without epicardial connecting lesions, and with or without ganglionated plexus ablation. A bilateral thoracoscopic or port access approach also will allow LAA exclusion or excision in the majority of these patients. Until an epicardial ablation catheter is developed that can reliably create the box lesion without gaps or nontransmural areas, its use should be avoided in this setting.[24]

Symptomatic AF Patients Who Have Failed One or More Attempts at Catheter Ablation

Catheter ablation can lead to left atrial flutters and focal left atrial tachycardias refractory to repeat attempts at catheter ablation.[36,37] Simple pulmonary vein isolation is unlikely to terminate such rhythms, and unfortunately, atrioventricular nodal ablation with pacemaker placement is often advised to avoid a formal sternotomy and biatrial lesion pattern.

In symptomatic patients who wish to try to maintain atrial contractility and avoid lifelong warfarin, a stand-alone biatrial surgical ablation procedure is reasonable, even if it requires a sternotomy. Complete isolation of the posterior left atrium with the equivalent of a box lesion should be included to eliminate possible triggers in this location.

Hybrid ablation that combines epicardial with endocardial left atrial lesions may be successful despite previous failure with catheter ablation alone and may represent an intermediate solution for such patients to avoid AV nodal ablation or a sternotomy surgical ablation.

Atrial Flutter

Right atrial flutter in patients undergoing cardiopulmonary bypass can and should be ablated with a cavotricuspid isthmus lesion. This is usually accomplished with cryoablation due to its deep penetration in the complicated region around the coronary sinus, Eustachian valve, and medial inferior vena cava.

An alternative method is a lesion running between each cava, and a crossing lesion up the mid-right atrium to the AV groove. These can be quickly applied with a bipolar radiofrequency clamp and a radiofrequency drag lesion or cryoablation lesion used to continue this lesion to the anterior tricuspid valve leaflet. This is part of the Maze 4 lesion pattern.

Patients with AF who have atrial flutter episodes should be managed based on the indications for surgical treatment of AF. The standard Maze 4, the Radial Incision Approach, or other biatrial patterns that have a mitral valve isthmus and cavotricuspid isthmus lesion should be adequate. If the atrial flutter is thought to arise solely from the right atrium, and it is desired to avoid cardiopulmonary bypass, an epicardial surgical ablation with subsequent right atrial catheter ablation can be performed as an alternative.

Atrial flutters arising from failed catheter ablation are usually left atrial in location and are discussed in the previous section.

Special Issues

Management of the Left Atrial Appendage

There is compelling data that the LAA should be removed or closed whenever feasible in patients with AF undergoing a cardiac surgical procedure. Some patients are better served by leaving the LAA alone: those for whom (1) the potential for bleeding adds procedural risk, (2) the likelihood of incomplete closure or removal leaves a cul-de-sac with continued thromboembolism risk, or (3) recanalization of an endocardial over-sew seems likely.

New-onset Paroxysmal AF

New-onset PAF is sometimes the precipitating event that brings the patient with congestive heart failure or acute myocardial infarction into the emergency room, and subsequent evaluation then discloses a surgical condition involving valvular disease, coronary artery disease, or both. These patients therefore fall into the symptomatic group undergoing other cardiac procedures, with the distinction that the underlying cardiac disorder is also responsible for the symptoms.

Surgical treatment ranges from simple atrial appendage exclusion or removal to bilateral pulmonary vein isolation or even a biatrial lesion pattern in patients undergoing a valve procedure. Risk minimization is an important consideration, as the correction of the underlying cardiac disorder and antiarrhythmic drug therapy might otherwise make these patients asymptomatic with AF in the future.

Chronic AF in Patients Who Had Prior AV Nodal Ablation and Have a Permanent Pacemaker

In patients with normal left ventricular function, simple LAA exclusion or ligation is reasonable. The main goal in these patients is to discontinue anticoagulation. In patients who may benefit from a restoration of atrial contraction, such as those with diastolic dysfunction, a biatrial lesion pattern during another cardiac procedure may restore atrial capture and contractility and allow dual-chamber pacing. The decision is best made in conjunction with the referring cardiologist.

Hybrid Surgical/Catheter Ablation

This surgical approach shares indications with standard percutaneous AF ablation as a method to reduce the overall procedure time, improve lesion transmurality, and aid in eliminating atrial tachyarrhythmias arising from prior left atrial ablation. It is contraindicated in patients with prior cardiac procedure or history of pericarditis. Patients with extensive prior upper abdominal surgery have a relative contraindication, and consultation with a general surgeon can help clarify the options to achieve the required diaphragmatic access.

References

1. Nasso G, Bonifazi R, Del Prete A, et al. Long-term results of ablation for isolated atrial fibrillation through a right minithoracotomy: toward a rational revision of treatment protocols. *J Thorac Cardiovasc Surg*. 2011;142:e41-e46.
2. Cox JL, Schuessler RB, Lappas DG, Boineau JP. An 8 1/2-year clinical experience with surgery for atrial fibrillation. *Ann Surg*. 1996;224:267-275.
3. Gammie JS, Didolkar P, Krowsoski LS, et al. Intermediate-term outcomes of surgical atrial fibrillation correction with the CryoMaze procedure. *Ann Thorac Surg*. 2009;87:1452-1459.
4. Ballaux PK, Geuzebroek GS, van Hemel NM, et al. Freedom from atrial arrhythmias after classic Maze III surgery: a 10-year experience. *J Thorac Cardiovasc Surg*. 2006;132:1433-1440.
5. Damiano RJ Jr, Schwartz FH, Bailey MS, et al. The Cox maze IV procedure: predictors of late recurrence. *J Thorac Cardiovasc Surg*. 2011;141:1113-1121.
6. Geidel S, Krause K, Boczor S, et al. Ablation surgery in patients with persistent atrial fibrillation: an 8-year clinical experience. *J Thorac Cardiovasc Surg*. 2011;141:377-382.
7. Stulak JM, Sundt TM III, Dearani JA, et al. Ten-year experience with the Cox-Maze procedure for atrial fibrillation: how do we define success? *Ann Thorac Surg*. 2007;83:1319-1324.
8. Kim JB, Yun TJ, Chung CH, et al. Long-term outcome of modified maze procedure combined with mitral valve surgery: analysis of outcomes according to type of mitral valve surgery. *J Thorac Cardiovasc Surg*. 2010;139:111-117.
9. Barnett SD, Ad N. Surgical ablation as treatment for the elimination of atrial fibrillation: a meta-analysis. *J Thorac Cardiovasc Surg*. 2006;131:1029-1035.
10. Calkins H, Brugada J, Packer DL, et al. HRS/EHRA/ECAS Expert consensus statement on catheter and surgical ablation of atrial fibrillation: recommendations for personnel, policy, procedures and follow-up. A report of the Heart Rhythm Society (HRS) Task Force on Catheter and Surgical Ablation of Atrial Fibrillation. Developed in partnership with the European Heart Rhythm Association (EHRA) and the European Cardiac Arrhythmia Society (ECAS): in collaboration with the American College of Cardiology (ACC), American Heart Association (AHA) and the Society of Thoracic Surgeons (STS). *Heart Rhythm*. 2007;4:816-861.
11. Cox J, Schuessler R, D'Agostino H, et al. The surgical treatment of atrial fibrillation. III. Development of a definitive surgical procedure. *J Thorac Cardiovasc Surg*. 1991;101(4):569-583.
12. Cox JL. Evolving applications of the Maze procedure for atrial fibrillation (invited editorial). *Ann Thor Surg*. 1993;55:578-580.
13. Lall SC, Melby SJ, Rochus K, et al. The effect of ablation technology on surgical outcomes after the Cox-Maze procedure: a propensity analysis. *J Thorac Cardiovasc Surg*. 2007;133:389-396.
14. Nitta T, Lee R, Watanabe H, et al. Radial approach: a new concept in surgical treatment for atrial fibrillation. II. Electrophysiologic effects and atrial contribution to ventricular filling. *Ann Thorac Surg*. 1999;67:36-50.
15. Nitta T. The radial procedure for atrial fibrillation. *Operative Tech Cardiothorac Surg*. 2004;9(1):83-95.
16. Benussi S, Pappone C, Nascimbene S, et al. A simple way to treat chronic atrial fibrillation during mitral valve surgery: the epicardial radiofrequency approach. *Eur J Cardiothorac Surg*. 2000;17:524-529.
17. Gillinov AM. Advances in surgical treatment of atrial fibrillation. *Stroke*. 2007;38:618-623.
18. Kress DC, Tector AJ, Downey FX, McDonald MM. Off pump microwave ablation of atrial fibrillation during mitral valve surgery. *Operative Tech Cardiothorac Surg*. 2004;9(1):43-58.
19. Edgerton JR, Jackman WM, Mack MJ. A new epicardial lesion set for minimal access left atrial Maze: the Dallas lesion set. *Ann Thorac Surg*. 2009;88:1655-1657.
20. Wolf RK, Schneeberger EW, Osterday R, et al. Video-assisted bilateral pulmonary vein isolation and left atrial appendage exclusion for atrial fibrillation. *J Thorac Cardiovasc Surg*. 2005;130:797-802.
21. Mehall JR, Kohut RM, Schneeberger EW, Taketani T, Merrill WH, Wolf RK. Intraoperative epicardial electrophysiologic mapping and isolation of autonomic ganglionic plexi. *Ann Thorac Surg*. 2007;83:538-541.
22. Doll N, Pritzwald-Stegmann P, Czesla M, et al. Ablation of ganglionic plexi during combined surgery for atrial fibrillation. *Ann Thorac Surg*. 2008;86:1659-1663.
23. Saltman AE, Rosenthal LS, Francalancia N, Lahey SJ. A completely endoscopic approach to microwave ablation for atrial fibrillation. *Heart Surg Forum*. 2003;6:E38-E41.
24. Pruitt JC, Lazzara RR, Ebra G. Minimally invasive surgical ablation of atrial fibrillation: the thoracoscopic box lesion approach. *J Interv Card Electrophysiol*. 2007;20:83-87.
25. Gaynor SL, Byrd GD, Diodato MD, et al. Microwave ablation for atrial fibrillation: dose-response curves in the cardioplegia-arrested and beating heart. *Ann Thorac Surg*. 2006;81:72-77.
26. Thomas SP, Guy DJ, Boyd AC, Eipper VE, Ross DL, Chard RB. Comparison of epicardial and endocardial linear ablation using handheld probes. *Ann Thorac Surg* 2003;75:543-548.
27. Prasad SM, Maniar HS, Diodato MD, Schuessler RB, Damiano RJ Jr. Physiological consequences of bipolar radio-frequency energy on the atria and pulmonary veins: a chronic animal study. *Ann Thorac Surg*. 2003;76:836-842.

28. Melby SJ, Gaynor SL, Lubahn JG, et al. Efficacy and safety of right and left atrial ablations on the beating heart with irrigated bipolar radiofrequency energy: a long-term animal study. *J Thorac Cardiovasc Surg*. 2006;132:853-860.
29. Milla F, Skubas N, Briggs WM, et al. Epicardial beating heart cryoablation using a novel argon-based cryoclamp and linear probe. *J Thorac Cardiovasc Surg*. 2006;131:403-411.
30. Ahlberg SE, Hong J, Stewart MT, Francischelli DE, Kress DC. Exit vs. entrance block testing for cardiac lesion assessment. *Conf Proc IEEE Eng Med Biol Soc*. 2009;2009: 3282-3285.
31. van Brakel TJ, Bolotin G, Kenneth J. Salleng KJ, et al. Evaluation of epicardial microwave ablation lesions: histology versus electrophysiology. *Ann Thorac Surg*. 2004;78:1397-1402.
32. Moten SC, Rodriguez E, Cook RC, Nifong LW, Chitwood WR Jr. New ablation techniques for atrial fibrillation and the minimally invasive cryo-Maze procedure in patients with lone atrial fibrillation. *Heart, Lung and Circulation*. 2007;16: S88-S93.
33. Katz ES, Tsiamtsiouris T, Applebaum RM, Schwartzbard A, Tunick PA, Kronzon I. Surgical left atrial appendage ligation is frequently incomplete: a transesophageal echocardiographic study. *J Am Coll Cardiol*. 2000;36:468-471.
34. Kiser AC, Landers M, Horton R, et al. The convergent procedure: a multidisciplinary atrial fibrillation treatment. *Heart Surg Forum*. 2010;13(5):E317-E321.
35. Marui A, Nishina T, Tambara K, et al. A novel atrial volume reduction technique to enhance the Cox Maze procedure: initial results. *J Thorac Cardiovasc Surg*. 2006;132:1047-1053.
36. Haïssaguerre M, Hocini M, Sanders P, et al. Catheter ablation of long-lasting persistent atrial fibrillation: clinical outcome and mechanisms of subsequent arrhythmias. *J Cardiovasc Electrophysiol*. 2005;16:1138-1147.
37. Knecht S, Veenhuyzen G, O'Neill MD, et al. Atrial tachycardias encountered in the context of catheter ablation for atrial fibrillation. Part II: mapping and ablation. *PACE*. 2009;32:528-538.

Video Legends

Video 66A.1 Typical right atrial argon cryothermia lesions as part of biatrial ablation procedure.

Video 66A.2 Sternotomy exposure of the left pulmonary veins off bypass.

Video 66A.3 Port access right pulmonary vein isolation using dry bipolar radiofrequency clamp.

Video 66A.4 Port access left pulmonary vein isolation using dry bipolar radiofrequency clamp.

Video 66A.5 Port access left atrial appendectomy with pericardium reinforced stapler.

Video 66A.6 Synopsis of pericardioscopic procedure.

CHAPTER 66B

Indications for Surgical Ablation of Tachyarrhythmias: Ventricular Tachycardia

Lindsey L. Saint, MD; Jason O. Robertson, MD, MS;
Ralph J. Damiano, Jr., MD

Introduction

The success of catheter-based ablation and implantable cardioverter-defibrillators (ICDs) has significantly diminished referrals for the surgical treatment of drug-refractory ventricular tachycardia (VT). Thus, many physicians have overlooked the fact that surgery continues to play a role in select patients. There is a new generation of electrophysiologists and cardiac surgeons who are practicing in the current era and are unfamiliar with VT surgery. The following chapter will discuss both the historical and present indications for the surgical treatment of VT, as well as the efficacy of current procedures when used in select patients in the ICD era.

History of Ventricular Tachycardia Surgery

Before the electrophysiological mechanisms behind VT were fully understood, a variety of surgical interventions were tried empirically in order to diminish the morbidity and mortality associated with this lethal tachyarrhythmia. One such treatment was spurred by the early recognition that ventricular tachyarrhythmias are influenced by autonomic activity, with enhanced sympathetic tone making ventricular tachyarrhythmias more likely to occur and diminished sympathetic tone decreasing this tendency.[1] These observations were confirmed by work in the laboratory, which demonstrated that animals that had undergone cardiac denervation via cervicothoracic sympathectomy had a reduced incidence of both ventricular tachyarrhythmias and death following experimentally induced myocardial infarction.[2] Later, it was found that providing sympathetic extrastimulation after an experimentally induced myocardial infarction increased the rate of ventricular arrhythmias in laboratory animals.[3]

As a result of these experimental findings, surgical thoracic sympathectomy was introduced clinically in the early 1960s to treat patients with medically refractory VT.[4] This approach was met with only moderate success. In a review of the literature published before 1978, 12 patients were reported to have undergone surgical thoracic sympathectomy as treatment for recurrent ventricular arrhythmias associated with coronary artery disease.[5] Of these patients, there were 3 operative mortalities (25%), and 2 failures of surgical management (17%). Only a modest 58% of patients experienced relief from persistent ventricular tachyarrhythmias.

By the late 1960s, it had become clear that myocardial ischemia initiated many, but not all, ventricular arrhythmias. Although surgical approaches were not yet based on electrophysiologic data and were therefore still indirect by nature, subclassification of ventricular arrhythmias into nonischemic and ischemic etiologies became possible. By distinguishing these two clinical entities, distinct indications for surgical VT ablation were formed based on differences in the clinical presentations and anatomic substrates of these subgroups.

Ischemic Ventricular Tachycardias

In the late 1960s, it became apparent that myocardial ischemia initiated many ventricular arrhythmias. In fact, the most common ventricular arrhythmias were found to be those associated with ischemic heart disease, often in relation to areas of infarction and scar.[6] Before the introduction of electrophysiologic mapping equipment, this discovery led to the development of two indirect surgical approaches that were meant to address the ischemic pathophysiology associated with these arrhythmias: infarctectomy and coronary artery bypass grafting.[7,8] Unfortunately, these initial procedures had high mortality rates, and relatively poor long-term success.[9] A review of the early literature reveals that, prior to 1978, 167 patients underwent coronary arterial bypass grafting, aneurysmectomy/infarctectomy, or aortocoronary bypass plus aneurysmectomy.[5] The intraoperative mortality rate was 26%, and another 16% of patients experienced recurrent intractable ventricular tachyarrhythmias. The overall success rate was a modest 58%.

Hastened by the disappointing results of the indirect surgical approaches to refractory ischemic ventricular tachyarrhythmias, advances in technology during the 1970s expanded the understanding of the mechanism behind the phenomenon. Wellens and others introduced intraoperative cardiac mapping techniques that not only identified myocardial activation during dysrhythmias, but also demonstrated that VT was a reentrant arrhythmia, capable of being initiated in the electrophysiology lab.[10,11] Based on these findings, the first directed surgical treatment of refractory VT was reported in 1975.[12] Epicardial mapping was used to localize the site of earliest epicardial activity to the margin of an aneurysm in a patient with refractory VT following two myocardial infarctions. Subsequent resection of this area abolished the patient's arrhythmia. Using epicardial, endocardial, and intramural mapping, Wittig and Boineau demonstrated success first in animals, and later in patients, with intraoperative localization of the arrhythmogenic focus and subsequent resection of the offending substrate.[13] Although these early procedures showed promise, their results were somewhat unpredictable. Additionally, it was discovered that VT often arose from the border zone between infarcted and normal myocardium and that the reentrant circuit was often subendocardial in origin.[14-18] These findings spurred the development of two new techniques: the encircling endocardial ventriculotomy and endocardial resection procedures.

The encircling endocardial ventriculotomy was introduced in 1978 by Guiraudon et al, on the basis that microreentrant circuits in the border zone of infarcted tissue were responsible for VT.[19] A near-transmural incision was made from the endocardial surface of the left ventricle down to the epicardial surface, encompassing all of the endocardial fibrosis separating pathologic from normal myocardium. By design, the procedure either abolished the reentrant loop present between the normal and infarcted tissue, or effectively isolated the entire border zone from the normal myocardium. The technique was met with clinical success, with early reports showing a relatively low operative mortality of 14% and an overall success rate of 84%.[5] However, the procedure also demonstrated a high morbidity, with most late deaths due to significant ventricular dysfunction and subsequent low-output syndrome.[20]

The endomyocardial resection procedure, guided by epicardial and endocardial mapping at the time of surgery, was introduced by Josephson et al in 1979.[21] The location of the arrhythmogenic substrate was found by endocardial mapping while the patient was in VT. After it was identified, the thin layer of surviving muscle strands that exists between the fibrotic endocardium and underlying fibrotic myocardium was identified and resected along a plane. The procedure was based on the supposition that the remaining living myocardial cells provided a substrate that served to propagate the arrhythmia. Initial data were good, with only one operative mortality, and 11 of 12 patients were free from recurrent VT at 1 year.[22] In 1982, Moran et al modified the procedure, advocating for an extended resection of all visible scar, thus obviating the need for intraoperative mapping.[23] These new procedures resulted in operative mortalities between 5% and 23% and some studies showing a postoperative inducibility of ventricular tachyarrhythmia rate as low as 2%.[24-29] Iterations of the endomyocardial resection procedure are still practiced today and will be discussed later in the chapter.

Nonischemic Ventricular Tachycardias

Nonischemic VTs occur in the absence of coronary artery disease. Although a somewhat obscure group of conditions, these arrhythmias are generally found to originate in the right ventricle and are likely to be resistant to medical therapy.[6] Before the advent of ICDs and the increased availability of cardiac transplantation, nonischemic VTs provided a variety of rare indications for surgical ablation.

The most common cause of nonischemic VT was first described by Fontaine and associates in 1979.[30] *Arrhythmogenic right ventricular dysplasia* is a congenital cardiomyopathy syndrome characterized by the transmural infiltration of adipose tissue. This unique pathology results in ventricular wall weakness and aneurysmal bulging of three areas of the right ventricle: the infundibulum, apex, and posterior basilar region. Furthermore, hypertrophic muscular bands in the infundibulum and anterior right ventricular wall result in pseudodiverticula, creating the "feathering" appearance of the right ventricular outflow tract that is characteristic of this syndrome.[31] Ventriculography performed in these patients demonstrates diffuse dilatation of the right ventricle, as well as significantly reduced right ventricular contractility and a delay in right ventricular emptying. Clinically, these patients suffer from intractable VT originating from one or all of the pathologic areas of the right ventricle, causing a pattern consistent with a left bundle branch block on ECG.

Surgery for VT associated with *arrhythmogenic right ventricular dysplasia* was rarely indicated in patients with medically refractory VT who were at significant risk for sudden cardiac death. Intraoperative mapping data frequently demonstrated involvement of the entire right ventricular free wall, causing the condition to commonly present with multiple morphologic types of VT.[32] In order to address the electrophysiological pathology of the condition, a drastic but successful procedure was developed. The right ventricular disconnection procedure surgically isolated the arrhythmogenic right ventricular free wall, leaving the rest of the heart in sinus rhythm.[33] One such patient from our experience was a 16-year-old boy who had undergone more than 250 episodes of full cardiopulmonary resuscitation and placement of one of the first implantable automatic defibrillators by the time of surgery in 1982. The patient was still alive and well at time of final follow-up 17 years later.[33] Although modern interventional advancements have made this procedure obsolete, the physiology learned from this operation has contributed to the development of mechanical left and/or right heart assist devices as well as the popular contemporary practice of biventricular pacing for heart failure.

Another indication for the surgical ablation of a nonischemic VT historically was the presence of familial or idiopathic *prolonged QT interval syndrome*. This syndrome is often associated with other congenital abnormalities, such as deafness, episodic paralysis, and dysmorphic features.[34,35] The hallmark of this syndrome is the variation in T-wave morphology that frequently precedes a unique polymorphic type of VT, known as torsades de pointes. In this type of VT, the polarity of the signals on electrocardiogram are inconsistent, producing a characteristic illusion of a "twisting of the points" of the QRS complex around an isoelectric baseline. Frequently in these patients, torsades de pointes is initiated by medications that prolong the QT interval, supporting the hypothesis that this arrhythmia is secondary to an abnormality in myocardial repolarization, rather than depolarization, as in many other ventricular arrhythmias. Due to the distinct electropathophysiology associated with this syndrome, patients are particularly susceptible to alterations in autonomic tone, putting them at appreciable risk of torsades de pointes with increased exertion.

Due to its proclivity to cause sudden cardiac death in otherwise healthy patients with *prolonged QT interval syndrome*, interventions to control cardiac sympathetic innervation were devised. Although medical therapy with β-blockers was always the mainstay of therapy in this patient population, surgical interventions were developed to prevent torsades de pointes in those patients who did not respond to medical management.[36] Left cervicothoracic sympathectomy with ablation of the lower half of the left stellate ganglion and the 2nd through 4th left thoracic sympathetic ganglia was performed in order to antagonize the effects of sympathetic activity on the heart. Although this operation effectively interrupted the major source of norepinephrine released in the heart, and thus produced significant cardiac denervation, it also resulted in Horner's Syndrome in some patients.[37] Moreover, in long-term studies, the procedure was found to be less than 50% effective at preventing recurrence of symptoms such as syncope, aborted cardiac arrest, and sudden death in high-risk patients when used as an isolated therapeutic modality.[38] With the development of improved pharmacologic interventions and the advent of ICDs, few indications for surgical ablation as a treatment for high-risk patients with *prolonged QT interval syndrome* still exist. Today, left cervicothoracic sympathectomy for this condition is primarily a historical procedure, considered only rarely as adjunctive treatment in patients with recurrent severe symptoms despite optimal β-blocker therapy and an ICD, or in patients with recurrent severe symptoms that cannot tolerate β-blockers.[38,39]

Current Techniques and Results in Ventricular Tachycardia Surgery

Implantable defibrillators and catheter ablation have significantly decreased the role of surgery in the treatment of VT. At our institution, the number of patients receiving surgery for VT fell by almost 90% in the years 1996-2006 when compared to the previous decade (Figure 66B.1).

However, ICDs fail to treat the underlying arrhythmogenic substrate, and the efficacy of catheter ablation is not uniform for all patients.[40] Additionally, although rarely, acute surgical intervention may be required following a complication during catheter ablation of VT, highlighting the need for an understanding of the intraoperative management of the arrhythmia and the subsequent treatment options available to the patient.[41] Whereas approaching the arrhythmia in the operating room after establishing hemodynamic stability is advisable in the acute setting, it is important to realize that dense adhesions after surgical repair of a complication may preclude repeating the ablation procedure via a percutaneous epicardial approach in the future. Therefore, it is important to understand both the present indications for surgery and the current surgical options available to patients, and to recognize that a low operative mortality and good late results can be expected in properly selected patients. This is largely a result of the fact that high-risk patients are no longer considered surgical candidates since alternative interventional or palliative therapies exist. Moreover, adjunctive ICD therapy is liberally utilized, further reducing late risk.

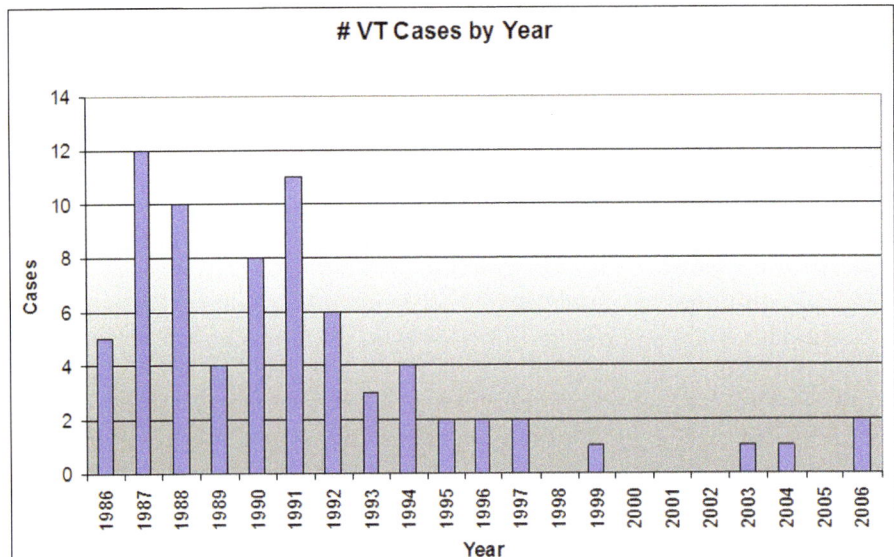

Figure 66B.1 Declining numbers of operations for VT surgery performed at Washington University between 1986 and 2006.

Revascularization

Ischemia is a common cause for arrhythmias leading to sudden cardiac death in patients with coronary artery disease. Ischemic injury to subendocardial and subepicardial tissue leads to areas of slow and disorganized conduction that may promote ventricular fibrillation (VF). It has been demonstrated that reentry originates in the border zone between normal and infarcted tissue.[14-18] In patients where ischemia is one of the main causes of lethal arrhythmias, revascularization has therefore been considered a rational therapy to prevent sudden cardiac death (SCD). In practice, however, the influence of coronary revascularization in patients with coronary artery disease (CAD) and malignant ventricular arrhythmias has produced mixed results. Success with this strategy depends largely on proper selection of patients and appropriate use of adjunctive ICD therapy.

While a majority of survivors of near-fatal ventricular arrhythmias have significant CAD,[42] only a minority have an acute coronary occlusion at the time of the event.[43] The role of reversible myocardial ischemia in provoking cardiac arrest in the remaining patients remains unclear, and it is accepted that additional antiarrhythmic procedures may be required, as the arrhythmias may not be suppressed by coronary artery bypass grafting (CABG) alone. It is understood that revascularization cannot reverse areas of myocardial scarring, and many patients, such as those with diabetes, have small vessel disease that is not amenable to bypass surgery. However, there is a distinct subgroup of patients in whom revascularization alone may treat inducible ventricular arrhythmias.

There is ample evidence from the electrophysiology laboratory to suggest that CABG can alter the arrhythmogenic substrate in selected patients with ventricular arrhythmias.[44,45] Several groups have demonstrated that between 40% and 60% of patients with CAD who presented with VT or VF and underwent CABG had no inducible ventricular arrhythmias postoperatively.[46-48]

Identifying markers for which patients will respond to revascularization has been difficult. One study by Kelly et al examined the effects of several clinical, angiographic, and electrophysiologic variables on inducible arrhythmias, arrhythmia recurrence, and long-term survival in a selected subgroup of 50 survivors of cardiac arrest who underwent CABG.[47] Their group found that the only significant predictor of ventricular arrhythmia suppression by CABG was preoperative inducible VF in contrast to inducible VT. Postoperatively, VF was not present in any of the patients who had manifested the arrhythmia on the preoperative electrophysiologic study, whereas inducible VT persisted in 80% of patients in whom preoperative programmed cardiac stimulation resulted in monomorphic VT. Reduced left ventricular ejection fraction (LVEF) narrowly missed statistical significance as a predictor of failure. These findings suggest that there may be a causal relationship between reversible ischemia and induced VF. However, reversible ischemia appears to have less of an effect on inducible monomorphic VT, which may be due to the presence of persistent myocardial scarring and arrhythmogenic milieu that are not substantially altered by revascularization alone.

In retrospective clinical analyses, the magnitude of benefit attributed to revascularization has varied from study to study.[49-51] The Antiarrhythmics Versus Implantable Defibrillators (AVID) registry included 3,117 patients with life-threatening ventricular arrhythmias, of whom 77% had documented CAD and 17% underwent CABG after the index event.[50] This study demonstrated that patients who underwent a revascularization procedure had improved survival at a mean follow-up period of 24.2 ± 13.5 months. Crude death rates were 21.4% ± 4.8% in the revascularization group and 29.4% ± 2.0% in the medically treated group (hazard ratio = 0.67, $P = 0.002$). The patients who underwent revascularization were more likely to have had VF and higher ejection fractions than those who were not revascularized. The AVID registry also showed that ICD implantation offered a similar survival advantage for patients with CAD regardless of whether they receive or do not receive coronary revascularization after an index life-threatening arrhythmia.

Similarly, our group demonstrated a significant survival advantage with ICD implantation following CABG for patients with LVEF ≤25% and perioperative ventricular tachyarrhythmias.[52] Survival at 1, 3, and 5 years was 88%, 79%, and 67% for the CABG-only group compared to 94%, 89%, and 83% for the CABG+ICD group, respectively ($P < 0.05$). Sudden cardiac death accounts for approximately 20% of deaths in patients with an LVEF < 30%,[53,54] and that percentage increased to 35% in patients with arrhythmias and recent myocardial infarction.[54] Therefore, a survival advantage with ICD implantation can be seen as early as 1 year postoperatively.

The Coronary Artery Bypass Graft (CABG)-Patch trial looked at the utility of ICD implantation for primary prevention of sudden cardiac death in patients requiring CABG that have increased risk for SCD.[55] In this particular study, no significant improvement in survival was demonstrated with CABG+ICD insertion over CABG alone. While randomized, the patients had no history of previous ventricular tachyarrhythmias and were determined to be at risk for SCD based on an abnormal signal-averaged electrocardiogram (SAECG) and preoperative, severely depressed LVEF. By design, the CABG-Patch trial utilized predictors of risk that could have been improved by surgical revascularization; thus, the risk factors for SCD were unstable in this population and weaker than those used in some other studies.[56] Nevertheless, the CABG+ICD group did have fewer arrhythmic deaths than the CABG alone group.

While the benefit of ICD implantation is not contested, not every patient with malignant ventricular arrhythmias undergoing CABG requires ICD implantation at the time of surgery.[57-59] Instead, pathophysiologic considerations should be weighed in conjunction with postoperative electrophysiologic studies, which are sensitive in detecting failure of CABG alone to cure the arrhythmia.[59] Studies have shown no difference between single- and two-staged approaches toward CABG and ICD implantation in terms of perioperative or long-term mortality, cost, length of hospital stay, and complications. Of course, sparing a patient unnecessary ICD implantation obviates the need for mandatory ICD follow-up and periodic generator replacements and may spare the patient unnecessary costs and anxiety that sometimes come from fear of an inappropriate shock.

In conclusion, patients with significant CAD, no ventricular dilatation or aneurysm, and documented exercise- or ischemia-induced ventricular arrhythmias are candidates for CABG ± ICD insertion. Postoperative exercise testing, pathophysiologic considerations such as severely reduced LVEF, and electrophysiological studies are used to determine whether ICD implantation is warranted.

Endocardial Resection and Cryoablation

Endocardial resection has been the most commonly performed operation for VT.[21,22,60] From a technical standpoint, this procedure entails the resection of all endocardial scar (Figure 66B.2). It is intended for use after a myocardial infarction, and it is often combined with more complex reconstructive operative techniques.

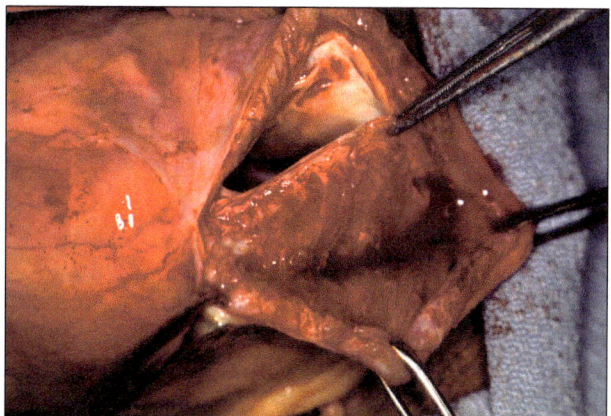

Figure 66B.2 Intraoperative photo demonstrating the surgical technique utilized during an endocardial resection procedure.

Two general approaches have become prevalent in VT surgery: (1) local ablation or resection of arrhythmogenic foci after precise intraoperative mapping[61] and (2) more extensive ablation or resection without mapping.[60-66] While intraoperative cardiac mapping has yielded a wealth of information on the mechanisms of ventricular arrhythmias, it is uncommonly used in current practice. Studies have demonstrated that 20% to 40% of patients who undergo subendocardial resection for VT cannot be mapped intraoperatively because their VT is either noninducible or nonmappable, or because of intraoperative hemodynamic instability.[66,67] Visually directed extended endocardial resection in patients with VT and prior myocardial infarction has had favorable long-term outcomes.[65,68] Nath et al compared 29 patients undergoing endocardial resection for VT that could not be induced or mapped in the operating room with 85 patients who underwent a map-guided endocardial resection.[65] They found that the rate of postoperative clinical VT recurrence or inducibility was the same in both groups, and, likely due to differences in patient clinical characteristics, long-term actuarial survival trended toward improvement in the visually directed group. It is understood that multiple arrhythmogenic sites may be present in a given patient but not necessarily captured with intraoperative mapping, and so more extensive resection of identifiable scar has in some instances resulted in better arrhythmia control.[64]

At our center, we prefer a non-map-guided approach with resection of all visible scar, but anatomic characteristics, such as extensive ventricular involvement and location near the posterior papillary muscle, may limit complete resection. In these instances, cryoablation has been used either adjunctively or as the sole therapy. Encircling endocardial cryoablation, consisting of a circumferential cryoablation of the infarct scar, can achieve excellent results and be curative in selected VT patients.[40,63,64,66] The procedure is relatively simple and reproducible at most surgical centers, and while preoperative cardiac mapping is useful in defining a surgical plan, intraoperative mapping is not necessary for the success of this procedure.[63,64,66]

From a technical standpoint, our group prefers a nitrous oxide–based cryoprobe in these circumstances. Nitrous oxide gas, which can reach a minimum temperature of –89.5°C at one atmosphere of pressure, is applied to the target tissues for 2 to 3 minutes in order to cause transmural myocardial cell death, which has been shown to occur at a temperature of –20°C. Heat is removed from the tissue as a function of the temperature difference between the probe and the target tissue, the specific heat of the gas used for cooling, and the mass transfer rate of the gas in the probe. Although surgery for VT originating in the outflow tract region near the coronaries has largely been replaced by catheter ablation procedures, it is important to avoid the coronary arteries when performing focal surgical cryoablation in this region.[41,69] The damage caused by direct cryoablation to coronary artery tissue has been well documented, and leads to atheroma-like plaque formation and intimal hyperplasia in the majority of cases.[70]

Since the use of ICDs has become more widespread, results of endocardial resection with curative intent have been compared to palliation with ICD insertion in patients with ventricular tachyarrhythmias in ischemic heart disease.[71] Candidates for endocardial resection all had reproducible VT and were generally suffering from sequelae of a postinfarctional scar or aneurysm but had preserved contractility of the remaining myocardium. In contrast, the ICD patient group was more likely to have diffusely diseased myocardium from multiple previous myocardial infarctions, and 2/3 of the ICD patients had underlying arrhythmias that included VF. Fieguth et al[71] found that long-term outcomes in these two groups were comparable, with freedom from sudden cardiac death in 90% of patients and freedom from cardiac death in 74% of patients after 5 years. Patients who had ICDs implanted, however, had a significantly reduced quality of life with a linearized incidence of 10.3 shocks/year. Overall, 73% of ICD patients received shocks.

Whatever technique is chosen for direct VT surgery, correction of additional abnormalities is necessary in order to obtain good long-term results.[62] CABG,[63] mitral valve repair or replacement, and left ventricular remodeling via either endoaneurysmorrhaphy[72] or the Dor procedure[62] are necessary for improved long-term electrical stability and hemodynamics.

In our experience, endocardial resection procedures have had a successful, though declining, role in the surgical management of VT. Since 1986, 74 patients have undergone an endocardial resection procedure with adjunctive cryotherapy for ventricular arrhythmias at Barnes-Jewish Hospital (Table 66B.1). A majority of the patients were male, with a mean age of 57 ± 14 years. Twenty-two percent of patients were in NYHA class III or IV heart failure, and the mean LVEF was 34% ± 9%. Ninety-two percent of patients underwent endocardial resection with a concomitant procedure, including left ventricular aneurysm repair alone (26%), CABG alone (5%), CABG plus left ventricular aneurysm repair (46%), and left ventricular aneurysm repair plus another cardiac procedure (15%). The overall 30-day operative mortality was 15% with no operative mortality documented during the last 10 years (Table 66B.2). Late follow-up was completed in 89% of patients and showed survival of 74% at 1 year and 65% at 5 years (Figure 66B.3). As previously alluded to, 88% of cases were performed during the first decade of our experience (1986–1996), reflecting the diminishing referral of patients for VT surgery.

Table 66B.1 Baseline characteristics: Washington University experience

Variable	# (n = 74)
Age (years)	57 ± 14 (12–76)
Gender (male)	60 (81%)
NYHA Class III or IV	16 (22%)
Mean LVEF (%)	34 ± 9
Hypertension	32 (43%)
Myocardial Infarction	65 (88%)
Cardiac Arrest	17 (23%)

Table 66B.2 Outcomes: Washington University Experience

Variable	1986–1994 (n = 63)	1995–2006 (n = 11)
Mean Cross Clamp Time (minutes)	44 ± 36	98 ± 29
Operative Mortality (≤30 days)	11 (17%)	0 (0%)
IABP Placement	15 (24%)	4 (36%)
Median ICU Length of Stay (days)	4 (1–80)	3 (1–7)
Median Hospital Length of Stay (days)	13 (6–80)	11 (6–34)

IABP = Intra-aortic balloon pump; NYHA = New York Heart Association.

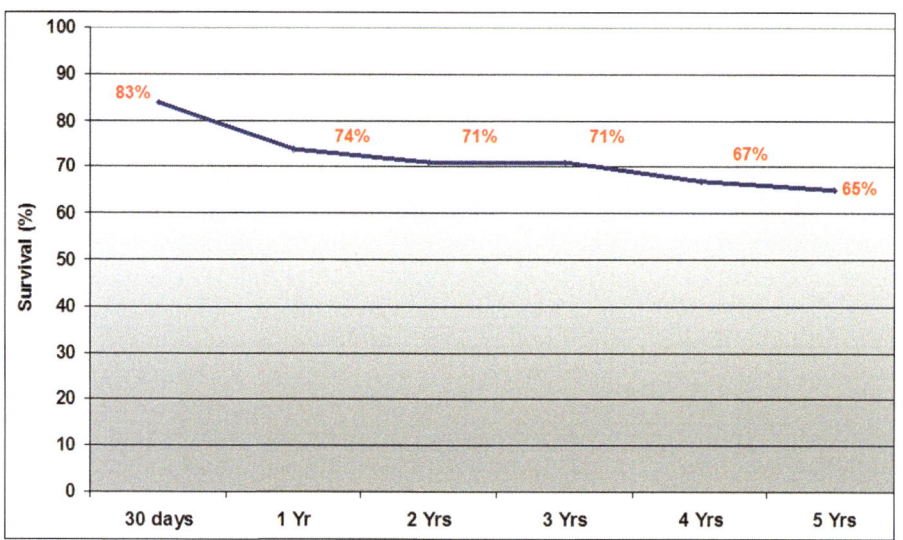

Figure 66B.3 Long-term mortality after surgery for VT at Washington University between 1986 and 2006.

Surgical Ventricular Restoration

In 1985, Vincent Dor described a surgical technique called the endoventricular circular patch plasty that was intended to improve geometric reconstruction as compared with the standard linear repair in left ventricular aneurysm surgery. Surgical ventricular restoration (SVR) is a somewhat broader term that arose from surgical repair of ventricular aneurysms and has now come to be applied to a group of surgical procedures designed to correct the effects of postinfarction ventricular remodeling. It is also sometimes referred to as surgical ventricular remodeling or reconstruction, surgical anterior ventricular endocardial reconstruction (SAVER), or the Dor procedure. SVR is specifically intended to reduce the size and sphericity of the left ventricle by excluding akinetic and dyskinetic areas. These techniques are best suited for discrete aneurysms. Diffuse hypokinetic or akinetic areas are considered a less optimal substrate for surgery.[73]

Candidates for SVR are typically patients who have had a remote anterior or anteroseptal myocardial infarction, significant ventricular enlargement with a large area of akinesis or dyskinesis of nonviable myocardium, a clinical picture consistent with heart failure (LVEF < 40%), retained function of the basilar and lateral portions of the heart, and good right ventricular function. These patients should also be candidates for repair of any other concomitant cardiac disease. Dor currently emphasizes the importance of complete revascularization, repair of any mitral pathology, and endocardial resection with cryoablation at the time of operative SVR.

The patient population described typically suffers from associated ventricular arrhythmias for several reasons. First, as previously mentioned, electrical dyssynchrony results from postinfarction remodeling, and triggers for ventricular arrhythmias typically occur at the scar border zone in patients with ischemic cardiomyopathy.[16,18] Second, increased ventricular volume causes high wall stress and stretch, and stretch has been shown to be arrhythmogenic.[74] Third, left ventricular aneurysms represent an independent risk factor for SCD after MI.[75] SVR addresses each of these issues by removing the anatomic substrate during resection of the postinfarct scar and/or aneurysm, accomplishing volume reduction and mechanical resynchronization and relieving ischemia through complete revascularization and reduction in myocardial wall tension and oxygen demand.

Results with this approach have been excellent. In 1994, Dor et al reported on 106 patients with ischemic ventricular arrhythmias that underwent reconstruction for postinfarction left ventricular aneurysm and visually directed endocardiectomy plus or minus cryoablation and coronary revascularization.[62] At a mean follow-up of 21.3 months, only 10.8% of patients had inducible VT and no spontaneous VT was documented. In 2004, Mickleborough[79] reported her long-term outcomes following ventricular reconstruction and coronary revascularization in 285 patients with akinesia or dyskinesia associated with relative wall thinning, including 32 patients who required posterior repairs. Forty-one percent of these patients had concomitant operations for VT. Nine patients (3.2%) required an ICD for VT, and excluding those, freedom from VT and sudden cardiac death at 1, 5, and 10 years was 99%, 97%, and 94%, respectively. In another study by Sartipy and colleagues, 53 patients with left ventricular aneurysm and inducible VT underwent SVR, including visually directed endocardial resection and cryoablation.[76] At a mean follow-up of 3.7 ± 2.0 years, the freedom from spontaneous VT was 90%, and 5 of 35 patients who underwent a postoperative EP study had inducible VT. Thus, success has been highly reproducible.

In another study, Sartipy further demonstrated that quality of life, as assessed by the physical component summary score of the Medical Outcome Study 36-Item Short Form, improved significantly by 6 months after the Dor procedure.[76] There was a clinically relevant improvement in both physical (+25%, $P < 0.001$) and mental (+37%, $P = 0.003$) aspects of quality of life at late follow-up. This is likely due in part to the fact that the Dor procedure restores left ventricular geometry, resulting in a mean ejection fraction increase between 10% and 15% and significant alleviation of symptoms.[77-79] These data are reinforced by the international RESTORE group, which examined SVR in a registry of 1,198 postinfarction patients between 1998 and 2003.[80] They found that 5-year overall freedom from hospital readmission for CHF was 78%. Moreover, 67% of patients had preoperative NYHA class III or IV symptoms, whereas 85% of patients were NYHA functional class I or II postoperatively.

Nevertheless, the efficacy of left ventricular restoration alone has been controversial. Matthias Bechtel and associates reported a series of 147 patients who underwent left ventricular aneurysm repair without concomitant antiarrhythmic surgery.[81] Among 19 late deaths, 7 (37%) were sudden deaths, which were significantly associated with postoperative ventricular tachyarrhythmias. Similarly, the Cleveland Clinic experience illustrated disappointing results with left ventricular reconstruction without endocardial resection and with a low incidence of cryoablation (13% of patients).[82] In their series, 42% (48/113) of patients who had a postoperative electrophysiology study had inducible VT. Those patients with ICDs had a 15% incidence of either SCD or appropriate shocks, and two-thirds of postoperative arrhythmias occurred within the first 90 days following surgery. As a result, they recommend a strategy of early postoperative electrophysiology testing, ICD implantation, or both following left ventricular reconstruction, which in their series drove the overall incidence of sudden death below 1%.

DiDonato and Dor attribute these poor results to differences in surgical technique, primarily the failure to perform endocardial resection, with or without cryoablation, at the border of the transitional zone. They also noted that the stimulation protocol at the Cleveland Clinic was more aggressive than their own, and that the Clinic had not measured the volume reduction achieved or performed a preoperative EP study, thereby failing to demonstrate either the adequacy of the surgery or the preoperative ventricular arrhythmia border. In 2004, DiDonato demonstrated in 382 patients that left ventricular restoration with endocardial resection and cryoablation reduced the incidence of inducible VT from 41% to 8%, suggesting that many patients may not require a postoperative ICD.[83] The argument based on the MADIT II trial[84] that patients with CAD and an ejection fraction less than 30% benefit from ICD implantation irrespective of EP testing is countered with the fact that SVR results in a significant improvement in EF. Patients who would have fit MADIT II criteria before SVR might no longer be ICD candidates. DiDonato notes that only 7% of 464 patients in one series had a postoperative EF < 30%, and their overall rate of ICD implantation in their entire population of 1,448 survivors is only 5%.[85] Their group, therefore, recommends waiting for pump function to improve before considering implantation of an ICD, which is effective as long as arrhythmic events do not occur early after surgery. In our experience at Washington University, all patients undergo postoperative electrophysiologic testing and/or implantation of an ICD following the Dor procedure if they have had a history of ventricular arrhythmias or inducible VT preoperatively in order to prevent deaths from early arrhythmias.

Most recently, the STICH trial has reported the conclusion that adding SVR to reduce ventricular volume to CABG does not improve symptoms or exercise tolerance and fails to lower death rate or cardiac rehospitalization when compared to CABG alone.[86] This trial is considered flawed and many consider the results invalid. Foremost, the left ventricular volume was reduced by only 19% in the STICH trial, reflecting an inadequate repair as determined by the Surgery Therapy Committee, whose "acceptable STICH procedure" guideline required a 30% reduction at the 4-month postoperative cardiac MRI.[87] Previous studies have reported an average reduction of end-systolic volume index (ESVI) of 40% with a range between 30% and 58%, suggesting that the STICH SVR procedure may have involved an inadequately small left ventricular plication or limited intracavitary reconstruction.[87] Moreover, this trial enrolled 13% of patients who had never had an MI and changed criteria such that enrollment required documented left ventricular anterior wall dysfunction rather than demonstration of scar. This could have captured patients with hibernating myocardium that would recover following CABG alone. There were additional observations that the NYHA functional class was lower in the STICH trial than in previous reports and criticisms regarding surgeon qualifications, among others. Dor subsequently published the results of 117 patients who would have been ineligible for the STICH trial and demonstrated durable improvement in left ventricular function.[88] Therefore, caution should be exercised so as not to extrapolate the results of the STICH trial and inappropriately deny appropriate patients an effective treatment for ischemic cardiomyopathies.

Present Indications

A key advantage of treating VT with surgery, as opposed to catheter ablation, is that the associated left ventricular pathology may be addressed simultaneously. The surgical approach should be individualized to each patient based on the etiology of VT, the arrhythmogenic substrate, and any underlying cardiac disease. When available, it may be guided by preoperative electrophysiological and electroanatomic mapping. Surgery is currently indicated in the following circumstances:

1. In patients with ischemic ventricular tachyarrhythmias requiring revascularization with poor left ventricular function and no significant wall thinning, CABG and ICD placement is the recommended treatment. If significant wall thinning or a discrete aneurysm is present, ventricular remodeling, extended endocardial resection, and cryoablation should be performed.

2. Surgery for VT should be considered for patients who have failed medical management and are suffering from frequent ICD discharges that are poorly tolerated, assuming that the patients have an amenable anatomic substrate.[89,90] In the presence of frequent ICD shocks with a discrete left ventricular aneurysm and/or wall thinning, ventricular remodeling, extended endocardial resection, and cryoablation should be considered.

3. In patients with end-stage cardiomyopathy resulting in incessant VT that cannot be otherwise managed, palliation with a cardiac assist device may be used either as a bridge to transplant or as destination therapy.[91-93]

It is critical to note that patients referred for surgery for left ventricular dysfunction and congestive heart failure should be offered a concomitant procedure to treat VT when indicated. Several surgical procedures, such as CABG, left ventricular reconstruction or remodeling, and mitral valve repair can have a significant impact on late survival.[80,83] Moreover, since surgery is highly successful in preventing recurrent VT, these patients experience fewer ICD shocks and have a much improved quality of life.[80,83]

Conclusions

In conclusion, surgical ablation was an important therapy for drug-refractory VT before the widespread use of ICDs and catheter-based ablation. Although these other treatment modalities have decreased referrals for surgical ablation, surgery remains a valuable therapeutic option for certain subgroups of patients.

References

1. Moore EN, Spear JF. Ventricular fibrillation threshold; its physiological and pharmacological importance. *Arch Intern Med.* 1975;135:446-453.
2. Harris AS, Estandia A, Tillotson RF. Ventricular ectopic rhythms and ventricular fibrillation following cardiac sympathectomy and coronary occlusion. *Am J Physiol.* 1951;165:505-512.
3. Harris A. Genesis of ventricular tachycardia and fibrillation following coronary occlusion. In: Dreifus LS, Likoff W, ed. *Mechanisms and Therapy of Cardiac Arrhythmias.* New York, NY: Grune and Stratton; 1966:293.
4. Estes EH Jr, Izlar HL Jr. Recurrent ventricular tachycardia. A case successfully treated by bilateral cardiac sympathectomy. *Am J Med.* 1961;31:493-497.
5. Boineau JP, Cox JL. Rationale for a direct surgical approach to control ventricular arrhythmias: relation of specific intraoperative techniques to mechanism and location of arrhythmic circuit. *Am J Cardiol.* 1982;49:381-396.
6. Cox J. Cardiac arrhythmia surgery. In: Wells S, ed. *Current Problems in Surgery.* Chicago, IL: Year Book Medical Publishers, Inc; 1989:278.
7. Ecker RR, Mullins CB, Grammer JC, Rea WJ, Atkins JM. Control of intractable ventricular tachycardia by coronary revascularization. *Circulation.* 1971;44:666-670.
8. Heimbecker RO, Lemire G, Chen C. Surgery for massive myocardial infarction. An experimental study of emergency infarctectomy with a preliminary report on the clinical application. *Circulation.* 1968;37:II3-11.
9. Ungerleider RM, Holman WL, Stanley TE III, et al. Encircling endocardial ventriculotomy for refractory ischemic ventricular tachycardia. I. Electrophysiological effects. *J Thorac Cardiovasc Surg.* 1982;83:840-849.
10. Wellens HJ, Schuilenburg RM, Durrer D. Electrical stimulation of the heart in patients with ventricular tachycardia. *Circulation.* 1972;46:216-226.
11. Josephson ME, Horowitz LN, Farshidi A, Spear JF, Kastor JA, Moore EN. Recurrent sustained ventricular tachycardia. 2. Endocardial mapping. *Circulation.* 1978;57:440-447.
12. Gallagher JJ, Oldham HN, Wallace AG, Peter RH, Kasell J. Ventricular aneurysm with ventricular tachycardia. Report of a case with epicardial mapping and successful resection. *Am J Cardiol.* 1975;35:696-700.
13. Wittig JH, Boineau JP. Surgical treatment of ventricular arrhythmias using epicardial, transmural, and endocardial mapping. *Ann Thorac Surg.* 1975;20:117-126.
14. Cox JL, McLaughlin VW, Flowers NC, Horan LG. The ischemic zone surrounding acute myocardial infarction. Its morphology as detected by dehydrogenase staining. *Am Heart J.* 1968;76:650-659.
15. Dillon SM, Allessie MA, Ursell PC, Wit AL. Influences of anisotropic tissue structure on reentrant circuits in the epicardial border zone of subacute canine infarcts. *Circ Res.* 1988;63:182-206.
16. Fenoglio JJ Jr, Pham TD, Harken AH, Horowitz LN, Josephson ME, Wit AL. Recurrent sustained ventricular tachycardia: structure and ultrastructure of subendocardial regions in which tachycardia originates. *Circulation.* 1983;68:518-533.
17. Gardner PI, Ursell PC, Fenoglio JJ Jr, Wit AL. Electrophysiologic and anatomic basis for fractionated electrograms recorded from healed myocardial infarcts. *Circulation.* 1985;72:596-611.
18. Scherlag BJ, el-Sherif N, Hope R, Lazzara R. Characterization and localization of ventricular arrhythmias resulting from myocardial ischemia and infarction. *Circ Res.* 1974;35:372-383.
19. Guiraudon G, Fontaine G, Frank R, Escande G, Etievent P, Cabrol C. Encircling endocardial ventriculotomy: a new surgical treatment for life-threatening ventricular tachycardias resistant to medical treatment following myocardial infarction. *Ann Thorac Surg.* 1978;26:438-444.
20. Guiraudon G, Fontaine G, Frank R, Cabrol C, Grosgogeat Y. [Encircling endocardial ventriculotomy in the treatment of recurrent ventricular tachycardia after myocardial infarction]. *Arch Mal Coeur Vaiss.* 1982;75:1013-1021.
21. Josephson ME, Harken AH, Horowitz LN. Endocardial excision: A new surgical technique for the treatment of recurrent ventricular tachycardia. *Circulation.* 1979;60:1430-1439.

22. Harken AH, Josephson ME, Horowitz LN. Surgical endocardial resection for the treatment of malignant ventricular tachycardia. *Ann Surg.* 1979;190:456-460.
23. Moran JM, Kehoe RF, Loeb JM, Lichtenthal PR, Sanders JH Jr, Michaelis LL. Extended endocardial resection for the treatment of ventricular tachycardia and ventricular fibrillation. *Ann Thorac Surg.* 1982;34:538-552.
24. Hargrove WC, Miller JM. Endocardial ablation for ischemic ventricular tachycardia. *Cardiac Surg.* 1990;4:247-253.
25. McGiffin DC, Kirklin JK, Plumb VJ, et al. Relief of life-threatening ventricular tachycardia and survival after direct operations. *Circulation.* 1987;76:V93-V103.
26. Swerdlow CD, Mason JW, Stinson EB, Oyer PE, Winkle RA, Derby GC. Results of operations for ventricular tachycardia in 105 patients. *J Thorac Cardiovasc Surg.* 1986;92:105-113.
27. Moran JM, Kehoe RF, Loeb JM, Sanders JH Jr, Tommaso CL, Michaelis LL. Operative therapy of malignant ventricular rhythm disturbances. *Ann Surg.* 1983;198:479-486.
28. Kron IL, Lerman BB, Nolan SP, Flanagan TL, Haines DE, DiMarco JP. Sequential endocardial resection for the surgical treatment of refractory ventricular tachycardia. *J Thorac Cardiovasc Surg.* 1987;94:843-847.
29. Ferguson TB Jr, Smith JM, Cox JL, Cain ME, Lindsay BD. Direct operation versus ICD therapy for ischemic ventricular tachycardia. *Ann Thorac Surg.* 1994;58:1291-1296.
30. Fontaine G, Guiraudon G, Frank R. Management of chronic ventricular tachycardia. In: Narula O, ed. *Innovations in Diagnosis and Management of Cardiac Arrhythmias.* Baltimore, MD: Williams & Wilkins Co; 1979.
31. Fontaine G, Fontaliran F, Linares-Cruz E. The arrhythmogenic right ventricle. In: Iwa T, Fontaine G, ed. *Cardiac Arrhythmias: Recent Progress in Investigation and Management.* Amsterdam, the Netherlands: Elsevier; 1988.
32. Cox J, Ferguson T. Surgery for ventricular tachyarrhythmias. In: Wells S, ed. *Current Problems in Surgery: Cardiac Arrhythmia Surgery.* Chicago, IL: Year Book Medical Publishers Inc; 1989.
33. Cox JL. Cardiac surgery for arrhythmias. *J Cardiovasc Electrophysiol.* 2004;15:250-262.
34. Duggal P, Vesely MR, Wattanasirichaigoon D, Villafane J, Kaushik V, Beggs AH. Mutation of the gene for risk associated with both Jervell and Lange-Nielsen and Romano-Ward forms of long-QT syndrome. *Circulation.* 1998;97:142-146.
35. Tristani-Firouzi M, Jensen JL, Donaldson MR, et al. Functional and clinical characterization of KCNJ2 mutations associated with LQT7 (Andersen syndrome). *J Clin Invest.* 2002;110:381-388.
36. Schwartz PJ, Periti M, Malliani A. The long Q-T syndrome. *Am Heart J.* 1975;89:378-390.
37. Ouriel K, Moss AJ. Long QT syndrome: an indication for cervicothoracic sympathectomy. *Cardiovasc Surg.* 1995;3:475-478.
38. Schwartz PJ, Priori SG, Cerrone M, et al. Left cardiac sympathetic denervation in the management of high-risk patients affected by the long-QT syndrome. *Circulation.* 2004;109:1826-1833.
39. Zipes DP, Camm AJ, Borggrefe M, et al. ACC/AHA/2006 guidelines for management of patients with ventricular arrhythmias and the prevention of sudden cardiac death—executive summary: a report of the American College of Cardiology/American Heart Association task force and the European Society of Cardiology committee for practice guidelines (writing committee to develop guidelines for management of patients with ventricular arrhythmias and the prevention of sudden cardiac death) developed in collaboration with the European Heart Rhythm Association and the Heart Rhythm Society. *Eur Heart J.* 2006;27:2099-2140.
40. Anter E, Hutchinson MD, Deo R, et al. Surgical ablation of refractory ventricular tachycardia in patients with nonischemic cardiomyopathy. *Circulation.* 2011;4:494-500.
41. Aliot EM, Stevenson WG, Almendral-Garrote JM, et al. EHRA/HRS expert consensus on catheter ablation of ventricular arrhythmias: developed in a partnership with the European Heart Rhythm Association (EHRA), a registered branch of the European Society of Cardiology (ESC), and the Heart Rhythm Society (HRS); in collaboration with the American College of Cardiology (ACC) and the American Heart Association (AHA). *Heart Rhythm.* 2009;6:886-933.
42. Weaver WD, Lorch GS, Alvarez HA, Cobb LA. Angiographic findings and prognostic indicators in patients resuscitated from sudden cardiac death. *Circulation.* 1976;54:895-900.
43. Davies MJ, Thomas A. Thrombosis and acute coronary-artery lesions in sudden cardiac ischemic death. *N Engl J Med.* 1984;310:1137-1140.
44. Can L, Kayikcioglu M, Halil H, et al. The effect of myocardial surgical revascularization on left ventricular late potentials. *Ann Noninvasive Electrocardiol.* 2001;6:84-91.
45. Takami Y, Ina H. Quantitative improvement in signal-averaged electrocardiography after coronary artery bypass grafting. *Circulation.* 2003;67:146-148.
46. Garan H, Ruskin JN, DiMarco JP, et al. Electrophysiologic studies before and after myocardial revascularization in patients with life-threatening ventricular arrhythmias. *Am J Cardiol.* 1983;51:519-524.
47. Kelly P, Ruskin JN, Vlahakes GJ, Buckley MJ Jr, Freeman CS, Garan H. Surgical coronary revascularization in survivors of prehospital cardiac arrest: its effect on inducible ventricular arrhythmias and long-term survival. *J Am Coll Cardiol.* 1990;15:267-273.
48. Manolis AS, Rastegar H, Estes NA III. Effects of coronary artery bypass grafting on ventricular arrhythmias: results with electrophysiological testing and long-term follow-up. *Pacing Clin Electrophysiol.* 1993;16:984-991.
49. Brockes C, Rahn-Schonbeck M, Duru F, Candinas R, Seifert B, Turina M. ICD implantation with and without combined myocardial revascularisation—incidence of ICD therapy and late survival. *Thorac Cardiovasc Surg.* 2002;50:333-336.
50. Cook JR, Rizo-Patron C, Curtis AB, et al. Effect of surgical revascularization in patients with coronary artery disease and ventricular tachycardia or fibrillation in the Antiarrhythmics Versus Implantable Defibrillators (AVID) registry. *Am Heart J.* 2002;143:821-826.
51. Trappe HJ, Klein H, Wahlers T, et al. Risk and benefit of additional aortocoronary bypass grafting in patients undergoing cardioverter-defibrillator implantation. *Am Heart J.* 1994;127:75-82.
52. Al-Dadah AS, Voeller RK, Rahgozar P, et al. Implantable cardioverter-defibrillators improve survival after coronary artery bypass grafting in patients with severely impaired left ventricular function. *J Cardiothor Surg.* 2007;2:6.
53. Buxton AE, Lee KL, Fisher JD, Josephson ME, Prystowsky EN, Hafley G. A randomized study of the prevention of sudden death in patients with coronary artery disease. Multicenter Unsustained Tachycardia Trial investigators. *N Engl J Med.* 1999;341:1882-1890.
54. Moss AJ, Hall WJ, Cannom DS, et al. Improved survival with an implanted defibrillator in patients with coronary disease at high risk for ventricular arrhythmia. Multicenter Automatic Defibrillator Implantation Trial investigators. *N Engl J Med.* 1996;335:1933-1940.
55. Bigger JT Jr. Prophylactic use of implanted cardiac defibrillators in patients at high risk for ventricular arrhythmias after coronary-artery bypass graft surgery. Coronary Artery Bypass

Graft (CABG) Patch Trial investigators. *N Engl J Med.* 1997;337:1569-1575.
56. Block M, Breithardt G. The implantable cardioverter defibrillator and primary prevention of sudden death: the Multicenter Automatic Defibrillator Implantation Trial and the Coronary Artery Bypass Graft (CABG)-Patch Trial. *Am J Cardiol.* 1999;83:74D-78D.
57. Cernaianu AC, Cilley JH Jr, Libby JA, Volosin R, DelRossi AJ. Implantation of a cardioverter-defibrillator after coronary artery bypass surgery. *ASAIO J.* 1992;38:M257-260.
58. Lee JH, Folsom DL, Biblo LA, et al. Combined internal cardioverter-defibrillator implantation and myocardial revascularization for ischemic ventricular arrhythmias: optimal cost-effective strategy. *Cardiovasc Surg.* 1995;3:393-397.
59. Pinski SL, Mick MJ, Arnold AZ, et al. Retrospective analysis of patients undergoing one- or two-stage strategies for myocardial revascularization and implantable cardioverter defibrillator implantation. *Pacing Clin Electrophysiol.* 1991;14:1138-1147.
60. Harken AH, Horowitz LN, Josephson ME. Comparison of standard aneurysmectomy and aneurysmectomy with directed endocardial resection for the treatment of recurrent sustained ventricular tachycardia. *J Thorac Cardiovasc Surg.* 1980;80:527-534.
61. Ostermeyer J, Kirklin JK, Borggrefe M, Cox JL, Breithardt G, Bircks W. Ten years electrophysiologically guided direct operations for malignant ischemic ventricular tachycardia—results. *Thorac Cardiovasc Surg.* 1989;37:20-27.
62. Dor V, Sabatier M, Montiglio F, Rossi P, Toso A, Di Donato M. Results of nonguided subtotal endocardiectomy associated with left ventricular reconstruction in patients with ischemic ventricular arrhythmias. *J Thorac Cardiovasc Surg.* 1994;107:1301-1307; discussion 1307-1308.
63. Frapier JM, Hubaut JJ, Pasquie JL, Chaptal PA. Large encircling cryoablation without mapping for ventricular tachycardia after anterior myocardial infarction: long-term outcome. *J Thorac Cardiovasc Surg.* 1998;116:578-583.
64. Guiraudon GM, Thakur RK, Klein GJ, Yee R, Guiraudon CM, Sharma A. Encircling endocardial cryoablation for ventricular tachycardia after myocardial infarction: experience with 33 patients. *Am Heart J.* 1994;128:982-989.
65. Nath S, Haines DE, Kron IL, DiMarco JP. The long-term outcome of visually directed subendocardial resection in patients without inducible or mappable ventricular tachycardia at the time of surgery. *J Cardiovasc Electrophysiol.* 1994;5:399-407.
66. Thakur RK, Guiraudon GM, Klein GJ, Yee R, Guiraudon CM. Intraoperative mapping is not necessary for VT surgery. *Pacing Clin Electrophysiol.* 1994;17:2156-2162.
67. Chen WY, Lai ST, Shih CC. Endoaneurysmorrhaphy and cryoablation for postinfarction left ventricular aneurysm with ventricular tachycardia. *J Chin Med Assoc.* 2007;70:117-120.
68. Kron IL, Lerman BB, DiMarco JP. Extended subendocardial resection. A surgical approach to ventricular tachyarrhythmias that cannot be mapped intraoperatively. *J Thorac Cardiovasc Surg.* 1985;90:586-591.
69. Tada H. Catheter ablation of tachyarrhythmias from the aortic sinuses of Valsalva—when and how? *Circulation.* 2012;76:791-800.
70. Holman WL, Ikeshita M, Ungerleider RM, Smith PK, Ideker RE, Cox JL. Cryosurgery for cardiac arrhythmias: acute and chronic effects on coronary arteries. *Am J Cardiol.* 1983;51:149-155.
71. Fieguth HG, Trappe HJ, Wahlers T, Siclari F, Frank G, Borst HG. Surgical interventions in ischemic ventricular tachyarrhythmias—endocardial resection or implanted cardioverter/defibrillator. *Eur J Cardiothorac Surg.* 1994;8:400-403.
72. Cooley DA, Frazier OH, Duncan JM, Reul GJ, Krajcer Z. Intracavitary repair of ventricular aneurysm and regional dyskinesia. *Ann Surg.* 1992;215:417-423; discussion 423-424.
73. Wellens F, Geelen P, Demirsoy E, et al. Surgical treatment of tachyarrhythmias due to postinfarction left ventricular aneurysm with endoaneurysmorrhaphy and cryoablation. *Eur J Cardiothorac Surg.* 2002;22:771-776.
74. Koilpillai C, Quinones MA, Greenberg B, et al. Relation of ventricular size and function to heart failure status and ventricular dysrhythmia in patients with severe left ventricular dysfunction. *Am J Cardiol.* 1996;77:606-611.
75. Hassapoyannes CA, Stuck LM, Hornung CA, Berbin MC, Flowers NC. Effect of left ventricular aneurysm on risk of sudden and nonsudden cardiac death. *Am J Cardiol.* 1991;67:454-459.
76. Sartipy U, Albage A, Lindblom D. Improved health-related quality of life and functional status after surgical ventricular restoration. *Ann Thorac Surg.* 2007;83:1381-1387.
77. Isomura T. Surgical left ventricular reconstruction. *Gen Thorac Cardiovasc Surg.* 2011;59:315-325.
78. Maxey TS, Reece TB, Ellman PI, et al. Coronary artery bypass with ventricular restoration is superior to coronary artery bypass alone in patients with ischemic cardiomyopathy. *J Thorac Cardiovasc Surg.* 2004;127:428-434.
79. Mickleborough LL, Merchant N, Ivanov J, Rao V, Carson S. Left ventricular reconstruction: early and late results. *J Thorac Cardiovasc Surg.* 2004;128:27-37.
80. Athanasuleas CL, Buckberg GD, Stanley AW, et al. Surgical ventricular restoration: the RESTORE Group experience. *Heart Fail Rev.* 2004;9:287-297.
81. Matthias Bechtel JF, Tölg R, Graf B, et al. High incidence of sudden death late after anterior LV-aneurysm repair. *Eur J Cardiothorac Surg.* 2004;25:807-811.
82. O'Neill JO, Starling RC, Khaykin Y, et al. Residual high incidence of ventricular arrhythmias after left ventricular reconstructive surgery. *J Thorac Cardiovasc Surg.* 2005;130:1250-1256.
83. DiDonato M, Sabatier M, Dor V, Buckberg G. Ventricular arrhythmias after LV remodelling: surgical ventricular restoration or ICD? *Heart Fail Rev.* 2004;9:299-306; discussion 347-351.
84. Moss AJ, Zareba W, Hall WJ, et al. Prophylactic implantation of a defibrillator in patients with myocardial infarction and reduced ejection fraction. *N Engl J Med.* 2002;346:877-883.
85. Di Donato M, Sabatier M, Menicanti L, Dor V. Incidence of ventricular arrhythmias after left ventricular reconstructive surgery. *J Thorac Cardiovasc Surg.* 2007;133:289-291; discussion 292-293.
86. Jones RH, Velazquez EJ, Michler RE, et al. Coronary bypass surgery with or without surgical ventricular reconstruction. *N Engl J Med.* 2009;360:1705-1717.
87. Buckberg GD, Athanasuleas CL. The STICH Trial: misguided conclusions. *J Thorac Cardiovasc Surg.* 2009;138:1060-1064 e1062.
88. Dor V, Civaia F, Alexandrescu C, Sabatier M, Montiglio F. Favorable effects of left ventricular reconstruction in patients excluded from the Surgical Treatments for Ischemic Heart Failure (STICH) Trial. *J Thorac Cardiovasc Surg.* 2011;141:905-916, 916 e901-904.
89. Godemann F, Butter C, Lampe F, et al. Panic disorders and agoraphobia: side effects of treatment with an implantable cardioverter/defibrillator. *Clin Cardiol.* 2004;27:321-326.
90. Wallace RL, Sears SF Jr, Lewis TS, Griffis JT, Curtis A, Conti JB. Predictors of quality of life in long-term recipients of implantable cardioverter defibrillators. *J Cardiopulm Rehabil.* 2002;22:278-281.

91. Fasseas P, Kutalek SP, Samuels FL, Holmes EC, Samuels LE. Ventricular assist device support for management of sustained ventricular arrhythmias. *Tex Heart Inst J*. 2002;29:33-36.
92. Kulick DM, Bolman RM III, Salerno CT, Bank AJ, Park SJ. Management of recurrent ventricular tachycardia with ventricular assist device placement. *Ann Thorac Surg*. 1998;66:571-573.
93. Ziv O, Dizon J, Thosani A, Naka Y, Magnano AR, Garan H. Effects of left ventricular assist device therapy on ventricular arrhythmias. *J Am Coll Cardiol*. 2005;45:1428-1434.

SECTION 4

NEW DIRECTIONS FOR INTERVENTIONAL THERAPY

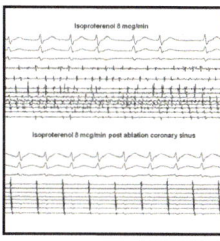 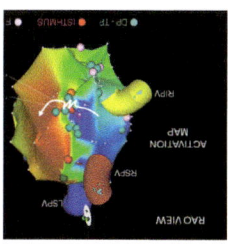 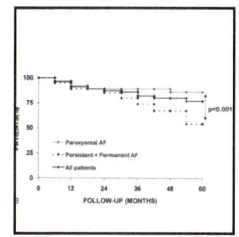 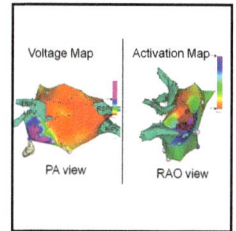

CHAPTER 67

Hybrid Device, Ablation, and Drug Therapy in Atrial Fibrillation

Sanjeev Saksena, MBBS, MD

Introduction

The clinical practice of using combinations of antiarrhythmic therapies for arrhythmia management has been applied for more than three decades, largely on an empiric clinical basis. Initially driven by the development of individual therapies for specific rhythm disorders, the coexistence of multiple arrhythmias in a single individual led to the application of combination therapies. The earliest examples would include the use of pacing for bradyarrhythmias and antiarrhythmic drugs or catheter ablation for atrial tachyarrhythmias (AT) in the afflicted patient with bradycardia–tachycardia syndrome. Other combinations followed, with the most recent including various combinations of pharmacologic therapies with each other, eg, differing antiarrhythmic drug classes or antiarrhythmics with other nonarrhythmic drug classes, or with nonpharmacologic therapies. Reports of patient outcomes and therapy management in this clinical scenario with antiarrhythmic drugs have suggested potential for synergy in efficacy with reduced adverse effects compared to monotherapy.

Conceptual Basis for Hybrid Approaches

The underlying tenets for a "hybrid" approach lie in the belief that therapies have adjunctive beneficial therapeutic effects. Cumulative benefits of multiple interventions in a single patient population can have varying outcomes. Califf and DeMets examined this issue conceptually in their analysis of two interventions that could reduce risk in the setting of clinical syndromes.[1] They noted that risk reduction with most cardiovascular therapies is modest, relative risk reduction of more than 25% is rare, and absolute risk reduction is even more modest. In a theoretical projection of outcomes, the end result could be positive, neutral, or negative. If positive, it could be additive, where the positive effects are the sum of the benefits of individual therapies; subadditive, where the sum is less than individual benefits; or synergistic, enhancing the individual outcomes. The current approach to reducing mortality in the clinical syndrome of congestive heart failure supports these concepts and also provides insights to hybrid approaches. It employs three different drug classes (β-blockers, vasodilators, and diuretics) and two types of device therapy (cardiac resynchronization pacing and defibrillation) with catheter ablation interventions being restricted to some specific disease states and clinical scenarios. This provides important insights into methodology for achieving successful outcomes with a combination, staged hybrid therapy approach. The mechanisms of action and benefit of individual drug classes vary greatly, and cardiac resynchronization and defibrillation also have totally different mechanisms of beneficial effects as interventions. Nonuniform applicability of these drugs in heart failure subpopulations is also evident. For example, cardiac resynchronization is not suitable in the absence of ventricular conduction delay.

Thus, while the concept of hybrid therapy is likely to also have potential for additive benefits, it is likely that differing hybrid approaches employing additive interventions in atrial fibrillation (AF) may also have outcomes specific to the approach employed and the AF subpopulation involved. Santangeli has highlighted the demographic distribution of AF patients[2] and the subgroup likely to be suitable for left atrial or pulmonary vein isolation catheter ablation interventions. Note that the vast majority of AF patients do not reside in the identified subpopulation; they are largely elderly and likely to have significant comorbidities and specific risks with each therapy used. For example, the use of flecainide in the presence of prior myocardial infarction would be of concern, but sotalol or amiodarone would be appropriate. In AF, available interventions for rhythm control include antiarrhythmic drugs, catheter ablation, and implantable device therapy. While antiarrhythmic drugs have had the broadest and longest experience in clinical practice, device and ablative approaches have been used to a varying degree in specific AF subpopulations.

An early example of hybrid antiarrhythmic drug therapy was the combination of mexiletine and quinidine in the treatment of ventricular arrhythmias. A more recent advance focuses on the combined use of amiodarone with ranolazine in AF.[3] The former was explored as a method to reduce the frequent intolerance to each drug when higher-dose therapy was pursued for each agent alone, while potentially enlisting benefits of two antiarrhythmic drug classes. Clinical data suggest benefit when amiodarone was combined with an angiotensin converting enzyme inhibitor in prevention of AF recurrence after cardioversion, particularly in patients with hypertension.[4] While drug–drug combination therapy has been employed to a limited extent in clinical practice, the use of drug–device or drug–ablation combination has been much more widely executed in current day practice. Despite its wide clinical use, there is very limited discussion and published analysis of this subject. The purpose of this chapter is to provide a scientific framework for current practice, analyze existing techniques that are available for application, and compile available data for the interventional electrophysiologist and other clinical practitioners.

Antiarrhythmic Drug Combinations of AF

Antiarrhythmic drugs employed in current clinical practice are largely class 1C (flecainide and propafenone) and class 3 (sotalol, dronedarone, dofetilide, and amiodarone). The individual electrophysiologic effects of each agent have been well studied and include effects on triggering ectopic beats, slowed intra-atrial conduction, and in some instances, antiadrenergic effects. More detailed treatment of this subject can be found elsewhere. Class 2 and 4 agents are largely used for rate-control therapy.

Each drug has been studied in clinical trials. Efficacy of flecainide, sotalol, amiodarone, and propafenone has been demonstrated for arrhythmia-based endpoints such as time to first AF recurrence. Recurrence rates vary from 20% to 50% at 1 year, depending on the population studied and individual drug. Figure 67.1 shows recent comparative data from one such clinical trial, the Canadian Trial on Atrial Fibrillation. There is a significant impact on arrhythmia suppression, with significant attrition in the medium term. Attrition is most likely related to the arrhythmia/substrate disease progression (Figure 67.1) Amiodarone outperformed sotalol and propafenone with approximately 75% efficacy at 1 year versus just over 40% for the latter two drugs.

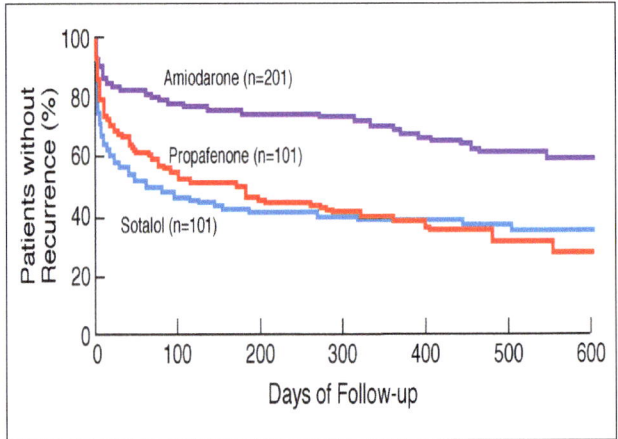

Figure 67.1 Antiarrhythmic drug efficacy in the Canadian trial on Atrial Fibrillation. The primary endpoint was time to first AF recurrence. Amiodarone was more effective than sotalol or propafenone in this study. *Source:* Modified from Roy D, et al. Amiodarone to prevent recurrence of atrial fibrillation. *N Engl J Med.* 2000 Mar 30;342(13):913-920.

Mortality and morbidity data for these drugs were first reported as pooled data, but in a recent analysis of the AFFIRM trial, individual outcomes have been reported (Figure 67.2A–C). The primary endpoint included a composite cardiovascular hospitalization and mortality outcome, and secondary endpoints of individual outcomes were evaluated as well.[5] Individually, these drugs had inferior outcomes compared to rate, largely due to cardiovascular hospitalizations, though a mortality risk was identified as a trend with amiodarone. Dofetilide also has been tested in arrhythmia endpoint and outcomes trials, with no negative impact on mortality, especially after myocardial infarction or in the presence of systolic left ventricular dysfunction.[6] Dronedarone has shown differing outcomes in differing AF subpopulations with improved outcomes compared to placebo in AF without significant heart failure and inferior outcomes to placebo in symptomatic heart failure and in permanent AF.[7-9] Amiodarone has shown particularly poor outcome in patients with concomitant thyroid disease in the AFFIRM trial.[5,10] The inferences from these data are that they define AF subpopulations that are unsuitable for each of these agents, even in a hybrid therapy prescription.

Mechanisms of efficacy of nonpharmacologic therapies are still being examined and defined. For rate control in AF, the use of atrioventricular junction ablation with demand ventricular pacing or DDD pacing has resulted in improvement in surrogate endpoints such as quality of life

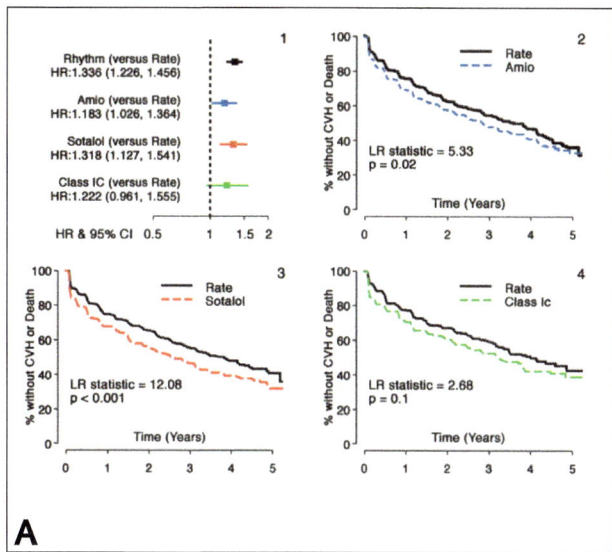

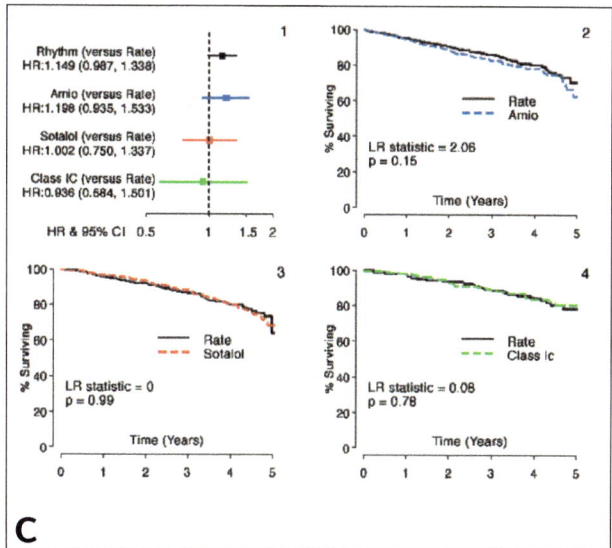

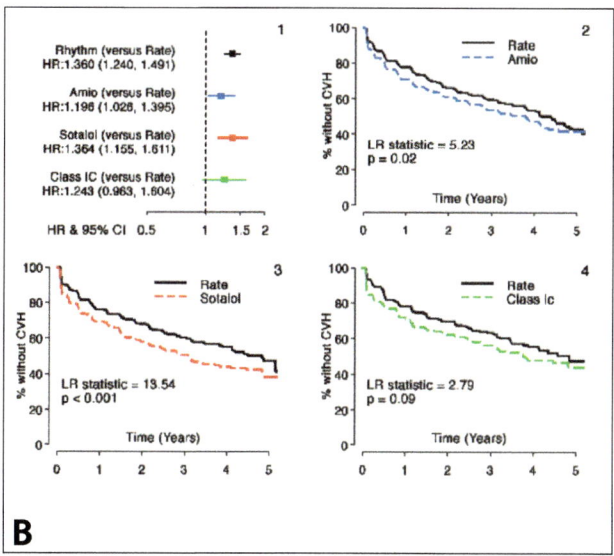

Figure 67.2 Clinical outcomes by individual antiarrhythmic drug in the AFFIRM study using propensity score matched cohorts of antiarrhythmic drug compared to rate control. **Panel A:** Survival free of composite endpoint of mortality and first cardiovascular hospitalization. **Panel B:** Survival. **Panel C:** Survival free of cardiovascular hospitalization. *Source:* Reproduced with permission from Saksena, et al. *J Am Coll Cardiol.* 2011;58:1975-1985.

and left ventricular ejection fraction in patients with impaired LV function and cardiovascular hospitalizations.[11] The use of biventricular pacing showed improved outcomes with respect to right ventricular pacing.[12] The impact of long-term right ventricular pacing on ventricular performance was reversed by this pacing mode.

Impact of Advances in the Mechanisms of Arrhythmias

Another aspect to the development of hybrid therapy approaches is an increasing understanding of the mechanisms of AF. These may occur at a fundamental cellular and subcellular level as well as interacting with structural heart disease in man. For example, it is now possible to target more than one ionic current in the action potential using either multichannel-blocking agents such as amiodarone or combination therapy such as ranolazine and dronedarone. In the latter instance, low concentrations of dronedarone (10 μmol/L) and ranolazine (5 μmol/L) have little potency individually in suppression of arrhythmogenic mechanisms in canine pulmonary vein, left atrial and left ventricular preparations.[13] Individually, induction of AF is prevented in 17% and 29% of experiments. Combined, the drugs suppressed AF in 90% of experimental preparations. Clinical studies of this approach are detailed later in this chapter.

Progression of an arrhythmia may have several components. Each of these elements may prevent effectiveness of antiarrhythmic therapy. AF is a prime example of this cascade. Experimental studies have demonstrated that rapid atrial pacing rates induce ionic changes that impair functional electrical properties of the atrium, resulting in shortened action potential durations and refractory periods, permitting AF induction in otherwise normal atria.[14] However, continued AF induces changes in both atrial contractility (referred to as the "second" factor) and structural remodeling (the "third" factor).[15] Changes in calcium loading of cells may mediate some of these changes.[16] The last element is surprisingly rapid. Experimental studies show canine atrial fibroblastic promotion by media from tachypaced atrial derived HL-1 cells.[17] Atrial fibrosis promotion is seen within 4 months, histologically confirming structural remodeling.[18] In animal models of heart failure, the development of such structural changes is associated with greater complexity in electrophysiologic propagation and multiple wavefronts.[19] Abnormal conduction patterns have been defined with spiral wave reentry and multiple wavelets during the development and established stages of AF in the animal model.[20] Debate centers on the level of organization of these during experimental and clinical AF.[21] High-density mapping methods in man suggest the presence of organized tachycardias (ATs) or "rotors" with spiral wave reentry propagation based on the signal acquisition or analytic method employed.[22,23] Electrogram analyses show evidence of rapid, fragmented electrograms, referred to as complex fragmented atrial electrograms (CFAE), that could reflect one or more of these underlying mechanisms.[24] Table 67.1 enumerates some of these diverse basic mechanisms translating into elements seen during clinical evaluation of the AF patient. Individually or in combination, they promote AF development and maintenance. In turn, interruption of more than one element of this arrhythmogenic cascade is likely necessary to achieve durable clinical benefit. This may be more readily achieved with a hybrid approach.

Table 67.2 shows options in targeting components of the pathophysiologic cascade supporting arrhythmias and their substrate in AF patients and the conceptual basis of synergistic hybrid therapy. Individually, they may impact only one or a few elements in this cascade. In combination using a hybrid approach, they could have a larger and more significant impact.

Table 67.1 Clinical arrhythmias and substrate findings in patients with AF

Triggers (high density)	• Premature atrial beats
	• Salvoes of atrial premature beats
	• Sinus bradycardia or tachycardia
	• Atrial tachycardia arising from atrial tissue in the great veins
	• Common right atrial flutter
Onset or transitional tachycardia (transient or prolonged)	• Common atrial flutter
	• Macroreentrant atrial tachycardia
	• Atypical atrial flutter
	• Paroxysmal supraventricular tachycardia
Perceptors (substrate potential to support >1 tachyarrhythmia)	• Intra-atrial conduction delay
	• Diseased and scarred atrial myocardium
	• Atrial hypertrophy and dilation

Source: Modified from Saksena S, Madan N.[25]

Table 67.2 AF therapies based on mechanisms

Triggers	• Premature atrial beats
	– Drug therapy for suppression
	– Focal ablation at origin or isolation/disarticulation of propagation pathways
	– Overdrive or novel pacing algorithm for suppression
	• Sinus bradycardia
	– Atrial-based pacing to prevent bradycardia
	• Sinus tachycardia
	– Drug therapy, eg, β-blockers
	• Atrial tachycardia arising from atrial tissue in the great veins
	– Drug therapy for prevention
	– Focal ablation or isolation
	– Overdrive or novel pacing algorithms for suppression
	• Common right atrial flutter
	– Drug therapy for conduction block
	– Cavotricuspid isthmus ablation for circuit interruption
	– Antitachycardia pacing for termination

Onset or transitional arrhythmia (transient or prolonged)	• Common atrial flutter
	  – Drug therapy for conduction block
	  – Cavotricuspid isthmus ablation for circuit interruption
	  – Antitachycardia pacing for termination
	• Macroreentrant atrial tachycardia
	  – Focal or linear atrial ablation of critical tissue
	  – Antitachycardia pacing for termination
	• Atypical atrial flutter
	  – Atrial ablation of slow conduction zone
	  – Antitachycardia pacing—50 Hz
	• Paroxysmal supraventricular tachycardia
	  – Atrial ablation
	  – Drug therapy
	  – Antitachycardia pacing

Perceptors (permanent potential)	• Intra-atrial conduction delay
	  – Dual-site right atrial or biatrial pacing for resynchronization
	  – Drug therapy to induce conduction block
	  – Diseased and scarred atrial myocardial substrate
	  – Linear atrial ablation to induce conduction block and compartmentalization
	• Atrial hypertrophy, distension, and dilation
	  – Drug therapy, eg, trandolapril, reduces atrial stretch, improves compliance, 5HT4 receptor blockers, atrial repolarization delaying agents (ADRA)
	  – Linear atrial ablation compartmentalizes atrial substrate to prevent multiple circuits
	  – Dual-site right atrial pacing improved atrial transport and reduces atrial dilation
	• Termination of sustained AF
	  – Antiarrhythmic drug
	  – Antitachycardia pacing
	  – Defibrillation shocks

Source: Reproduced with permission from Saksena S, Madan N.[25]

Primary versus Secondary Prevention of AF

Upstream therapies such as renin–angiotensin system inhibition have been proposed to prevent progression. In experimental studies, these have shown a reduction in atrial fibrosis, but when used individually in clinical studies, this benefit has not been validated. In contrast, a few small clinical studies may point to value when such therapies are used in combination with antiarrhythmic drugs.[3] Another approach is downstream intervention in combination with antiarrhythmic drugs. We have demonstrated that dual-site right atrial pacing and biatrial pacing can produce electrical resynchronization in diseased human atria in patients with AF.[26-29] In addition, more recent data suggest that there is hemodynamic improvement of left atrial and left ventricular mechanics with this approach.[30,31] The improvement in mechanics is a potential mechanism of the long-term maintenance of rhythm control in hybrid pacing and drug therapy of AF. The use of antiarrhythmic drugs with dual-site right atrial pacing has been shown to have benefit in patients with drug refractory paroxysmal AF in one randomized controlled study and in observational studies with both paroxysmal and persistent AF.

Finally, the use of pharmacologic and nonpharmacologic therapies in combination offers a powerful set of tools to address challenges in rhythm control. The value of combined use of antiarrhythmic drugs and catheter ablation in patients with prior implantable defibrillators has shown that reduction in arrhythmia event rates can be achieved by these methods. The use of catheter ablation in AF in combination with antiarrhythmic drugs or atrial pacing can also show similar benefit in arrhythmia recurrence prevention.

Types of Hybrid Therapy in AF

Table 67.3 enumerates the early approaches to hybrid therapies used in the treatment of AF.

Table 67.3 Hybrid approaches in treatment of AF

	Drug + Ablation				
Series	Ablation Technique	Patients	Mean Follow-up (Months)	% Rhythm Control	% PV Stenosis
Garg[16]	RA Maze	PAF	12	56(18)	No
Stabile[35]	Tricuspid isthmus	PAF + CAF	24	58(8)	No
Gerstenfeld[8]	PVA	PAF 71	6	31(23)	8.3 (Angio)
Natale[80]	PVA	PAF 211	4–10	71%–85%(81)	11.5 (CT)
Lanagaratnam[36]	PVI	PAF 71	29	83(21)	36 (CT)
Natale[47]	CUVA	PAF 30	12	80(47)	3 (CT)
	Drug + Device Therapy				
Series	Device Technique	Patients	Mean Follow-up (Months)	% Rhythm Control	% Complications
Metrix	Atrial ICD	186	9	84	6%
Jewel AF[41]	A-V ICD	537	11 ± 8	86	NA
Delfaut[42]	Dual RA pacing	30	12	80	6%
D'Allones[43]	Biatrial pacing	86	33	64	15%

Source: Reproduced with permission from Saksena S, Madan N.[25]

These reflect an early recognition of the need for combination therapy in AF. One avenue that is being explored is the use of 2 complementary antiarrhythmic drugs in combination. In the HARMONY trial reported in 2014, 134 patients with paroxysmal AF (burden from 2% to 70% during a 4-week run-in period) and no other antiarrhythmic use were randomized to 5 arms that included twice-daily treatment with one of two ranolazine/dronedarone combinations, either drug by itself or placebo (unpublished data, Late Breaking Clinical Trials, Heart Rhythm Society, 2014, available at www.hrsonline.org). Over 12 weeks, the AF burden fell by 45% ($P = 0.072$) for the 26 patients on the ranolazine 750 mg plus dronedarone 150 mg regimen, compared with the 26 patients on placebo; 27% of the group achieved an AF-burden reduction of at least 70%. The AF burden went down 59% ($P = 0.008$) for the 27 patients who took ranolazine 750 mg plus dronedarone 225 mg; 45% of them achieved reductions of at least 70%. Neither ranolazine 750 mg alone ($n = 26$) nor dronedarone 225 mg alone ($n = 26$) were associated with significant reductions in AF burden: only 17% and 9%, respectively, compared with placebo.

Antiarrhythmic Drugs and Catheter Ablation

Combination therapy using antiarrhythmic drugs with catheter ablation has been largely performed in supraventricular tachyarrhythmias and AF. In patients with ventricular tachycardia and ventricular fibrillation, these have been undertaken largely in patients with previously implanted defibrillators and have contrasted concomitant drug use with an ablative intervention. These are discussed in other chapters in this text.

Antiarrhythmic Drug Therapy and Catheter Ablation in Paroxysmal AF

The rationale for hybrid therapy is confirmed by prospective clinical studies that examine the efficacy of antiarrhythmic drugs and catheter ablation. In paroxysmal AF with little or no comorbidity, this question has been seriously examined. A variety of clinical trials have directly compared the efficacy of antiarrhythmic drugs to catheter ablation using pulmonary vein isolation procedures on the time to recurrence of AF. Initially performed for device approval clinical trials, they suggested a large clinical benefit of catheter ablation. In a recent review of 200 studies, Al-Khatib et al suggested a treatment effect as large as an odds ratio of 5.87 (CI 3.18-10.85).[32] However, recent studies in the form of randomized clinical trials for the two therapies have shown more limited benefit. In one recent trial, RAAFT-2, the primary outcome was time to first recurrence of AF or atrial tachycardia.[33] Sixty-one patients in the antiarrhythmic drug group (945 treated with a class Ic agent) and 66 in the radiofrequency ablation group (pulmonary vein isolation with or without additional lesions) were followed up for 24 months. The time to the first documented AT of more than 30 seconds (symptomatic or asymptomatic AF, atrial flutter, or atrial tachycardia), detected by either scheduled or unscheduled electrocardiogram, Halter, transtelephonic monitor, or rhythm strip, was examined. Forty-four patients (72.1%) in the antiarrhythmic group and in 36 patients (54.5%) in the ablation group experienced the primary efficacy outcome (hazard ratio [HR], 0.56 [95% CI, 0.35 – 0.90]; $P=0.02$). Secondary outcomes, eg, the first recurrence of symptomatic AF, atrial flutter, or atrial tachycardia, occurred in 59% in the drug group and 47% in the ablation group (HR, 0.56 [95% CI, 0.33 – 0.95]; $P = 0.03$). Four patients had cardiac tamponade in the ablation group. These data do suggest superiority of the ablation approach as the initial treatment in paroxysmal AF, with increased procedural risk. However, almost 50% of patients with ablative therapy had recurrent AF at 2 years. In contrast, large observational studies have documented enhanced success rates when ablative therapy is combined with antiarrhythmic drug therapy. However, a true prospective, randomized trial examining this hypothesis is still awaited.

Formal prospective, randomized clinical studies on the use of individual antiarrhythmic drugs in AF are sparse at this time. Observational data on concomitant use are available from surveys and single-center experiences.[34,35] In an early survey, Cappato and coworkers noted that the success rate of AF ablation procedures was significantly enhanced by the additional use of antiarrhythmic drugs after the procedure (Table 67.4).

Rhythm control with improvement both in symptoms and AF recurrence rates was achieved in 15.8% to 34% of patients, particularly if serial ablation procedures were not performed. Similar experiences have been reported by single-center studies. In an early publication, Cheema et al noted that the success rate of a single AF ablation procedure was 37% in paroxysmal AF and 20% in persistent AF.[36] Serial procedures improve efficacy, but significant recurrence rates persist even at 3 to 5 years. The use of antiarrhythmic drugs improved long-term efficacy by 15% in the Bordeaux experience.[37] In contrast, Stabile et al reported a success rate of 54% after a single procedure in the medium term when the patients were maintained postoperatively on an antiarrhythmic drug.[38] More recently, in the RASTA trial using a more extensive ablative procedure with additional trigger ablation or complex fractionated electrogram ablation in the left atrium, Dixit and colleagues reported success rates of 29% to 54% in a prospective study of the three ablative approaches. This increased significantly to 45% to 64% when antiarrhythmic drug therapy was not withdrawn ($P = 0.016$). The risk of complications with a single ablation procedure was 2% to 8% in this study.[39] These findings were confirmed in a large review of published studies. In a meta-analysis of published studies, Calkins et al analyzed 6936 patients undergoing ablation procedures in 63 studies.[40] They noted a single-procedure success rate reporting of 54% increasing to 77% when antiarrhythmic drugs were continued or not definitively withdrawn. Multiple-procedure success rates were 71%. A large prospective registry was reported by Arbelo et al for 72 European centers in 10 countries enrolling 1410 treatment-naive AF patients at first encounter.[41] The overall success of a single ablation procedure was 40.7%, was 43.7% in paroxysmal AF, and was 30.7% persistent AF. Forty-nine percent of patients were maintained long term on antiarrhythmic drug therapy at 12 months. This permitted 50% of patients to achieve symptom-free status.

These data support and define a role for hybrid therapy in AF using antiarrhythmic drugs after ablation procedures. After a single procedure, these agents improve outcomes with respect to arrhythmia recurrences and symptoms in the medium term. Long-term outcomes are unavailable. It is reasonable to conclude that the use of postoperative concomitant antiarrhythmic drug therapy is a competitive option to limit repeat ablation procedures and procedural complication risk.

Hybrid Atrial Flutter Ablation and Antiarrhythmic Drug Therapy

Cavotricuspid isthmus ablation alone in patients with atrial flutter alone or in combination with AF has been remarkably unsuccessful in AT control. A high recurrence rate of AF was documented even in early studies with medium-term follow-up. The additional use of

Table 67.4 Success rate of AF ablation procedures with and without AADs

# Ablations	Centers	# PTs	Ablation Success	Abl + AAD Success	Overall
1–30	35	547	29.8	30.1	59.9
31–60	15	639	33.3	34	67.5
61–90	12	923	36.9	33.7	70.6
91–120	7	728	33.6	30.4	81.6
121–150	4	56	44.3	28.8	62.4
151–180	4	671	52.7	29.7	74
181–230	4	607	62.5	22.7	75.4
231–300	3	830	63.8	28.4	91
> 300	7	3244	52	15.8	87.9

Source: Reproduced with permission from Cappato et al.[34]

antiarrhythmic drug therapy was advocated to improve outcomes.[42] The use of limited ablation, such as cavotricuspid isthmus ablation and antiarrhythmic drugs alone, was first advocated over two decades ago in patients with atrial flutter alone. Schumacher et al noted a reduction in AT recurrences with elimination in 36% in medium-term follow-up and reduction in AF event rates in those with recurrences.[42] Stabile et al suggested identification of these patients who benefit with IV flecainide infusions.[43] While short-term data suggested improvement in arrhythmia control, long-term evaluation has not substantiated its value. In recent reports, there has been recurrent ATs noted in the vast majority of these patients. Anastasio et al reported over 90% recurrence at 5 years of follow-up.[44] Others have noted high recurrence rates in all groups with atrial flutter and AF, with minimal additional benefit in patients presenting with atrial flutter alone.[45] In contrast, our group has reported more significant benefit when hybrid therapy incorporated a dual-site right atrial pacing therapy component. Thus, in drug-refractory patients with AF treated with combination therapy with device, drug, and CV isthmus ablation, Prakash et al reported recurrence rates of 25% at 18 months.[46] The incremental value of pacing techniques is discussed below.

Atrial Pacing and Antiarrhythmic Drug Therapy

A variety of atrial pacing modes have been evaluated for the prevention or suppression of AF, largely but not exclusively in patients with concomitant bradycardias. Initially performed largely as a monotherapy, variable outcomes were reported. A few seminal trials are detailed here. A much larger body of literature is available, and the reader is referred to reviews for more detailed treatment of the subject.

In patients with sick sinus syndrome, several clinical trials reported on the superiority of right atrial pacing over demand ventricular pacing in prevention of the subsequent development of AF. Andersen initially documented this observation in a moderate-size clinical trial, and this was subsequently confirmed in the larger MOST study.[47,48] However, it remained unclear as to whether this benefit was observed due to actual contribution of atrial rate support or due to deleterious effects of ventricular pacing and the role and extent of atrial pacing achieved. Ventricular pacing has been shown to have adverse hemodynamic effects with structural changes in the myocardium. Subsequent studies have clarified this issue. In the DAPPAF trial, patients with bradycardia and recurrent AF on antiarrhythmic drugs achieved no benefit with high right atrial pacing compared to support pacing for bradycardia prevention when evaluated using device diagnostics to detect time to the first AF recurrence as the primary endpoint.[49] Other single-site atrial pacing modes have been employed. Low septal right atrial pacing showed few benefits compared to high right atrial pacing in the ASPECT study using the same endpoint of time to first AF recurrence.[50] Antiarrhythmic drug therapy was variable in both trials and no benefit was seen with either single-site pacing modes in patients with or without background antiarrhythmic drug therapy. More recently, specialized algorithms have been used using more sensitive endpoints such as total device measured AF burden. Using one such algorithm, the ADOPT trial compared DDD pacing with and without the dynamic overdrive pacing algorithm in patients with sick sinus syndrome on background antiarrhythmic drug therapy.[51] Patients with the algorithm on achieved 93% consistent atrial pacing compared to 67% in control group without it. Both atrial pacing modes reduced AF burden during a 6-month follow-up period, but this effect was greater with the higher degree of pacing in the active treatment group (Figure 67.3). However, the absolute effect on AF burden was very modest with reductions of 1% to 2%. Whether this is clinically significant remains in doubt.

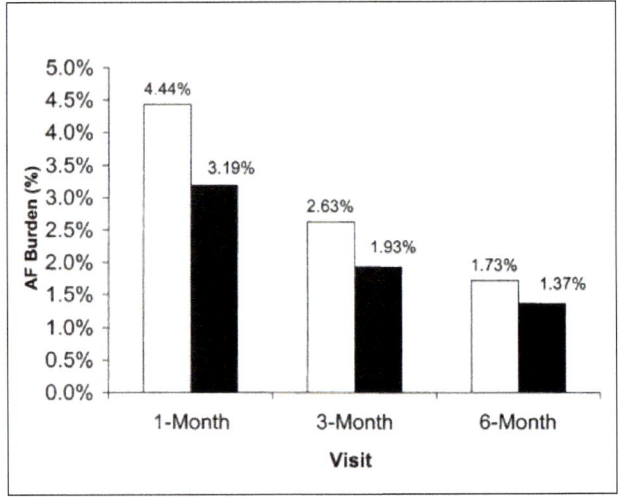

Figure 67.3 Reduction in episodes of symptomatic AF. AF declined in the population as a whole, and slightly more so in the treatment group. **Open bars,** control; **solid bars,** treatment. *Source:* Reproduced with permission from Carlson et al.[51]

More recently, the SAFE study examined the same algorithm with two single-site pacing modes, the high right atrium and the low septal right atrium, using this algorithm.[52] The time to development of persistent AF was similar regardless of pacing lead location or algorithm activation.[52] This suggests that the electrical therapy combinations studied had no clinical impact on the progression of AF. Importantly, background antiarrhythmic drug therapy was not a prerequisite for this patient population. In neither instance were clinically relevant endpoints achieved with single-site atrial pacing modes, particularly as stand-alone therapy. In a recent commentary, the current state of the art was summarized as a lack of evidence to support single-site atrial pacing for the primary or secondary prevention of AF in patients without bradycardia–tachycardia syndrome.[53] A greater body of evidence, for example the SAVE PACE study, supports the use of minimal ventricular pacing algorithms to reduce the rate of progression to persistent AF.[54] In this particular study, 17% of patients were also on background antiarrhythmic drug therapy. There was a significant reduction in the progression to persistent AF in the minimal ventricular pacing subgroup. These data support the use of these algorithms when programming dual-chamber pacemakers in patients with AF.

Multisite Atrial Pacing in Hybrid Therapy Algorithms

Conceptual Basis for Multisite Pacing

The early observations on clinical electrophysiologic changes in patients with AF noted loss of rate-adaptive atrial refractoriness behavior and prolongation of intra- and interatrial conduction intervals.[55] Early work on multisite atrial pacing utilized dual atrial pacing to reduce atrial conduction delay and atrial dispersion of refractoriness.[26,29] This was combined with overdrive atrial pacing, rate support, or pacing prevention algorithms to achieve continuous atrial pacing. This could theoretically suppress triggering ectopic beats and modify conduction and repolarization to prevent reentry due to dispersion of refractoriness or conduction delay. This could potentially prevent the initiation of AF and/or its maintenance.

Clinical Techniques for Multisite Atrial Pacing

Two techniques have been widely used. Use of two atrial leads placed in the high right atrium and either distal coronary sinus (biatrial pacing; Figure 67.4A) or coronary sinus ostium (dual-site right atrial pacing; Figure 67.4B) have been studied. Biatrial pacing, first proposed by Daubert, employed a high right atrial lead and a distal or

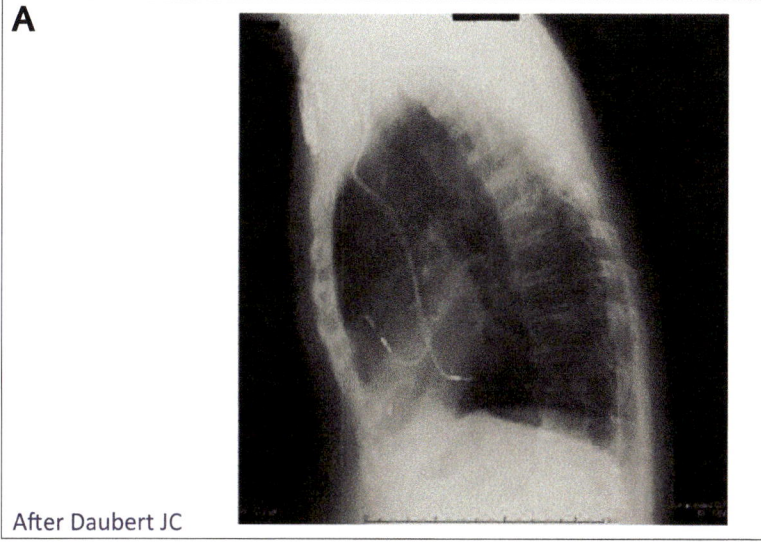

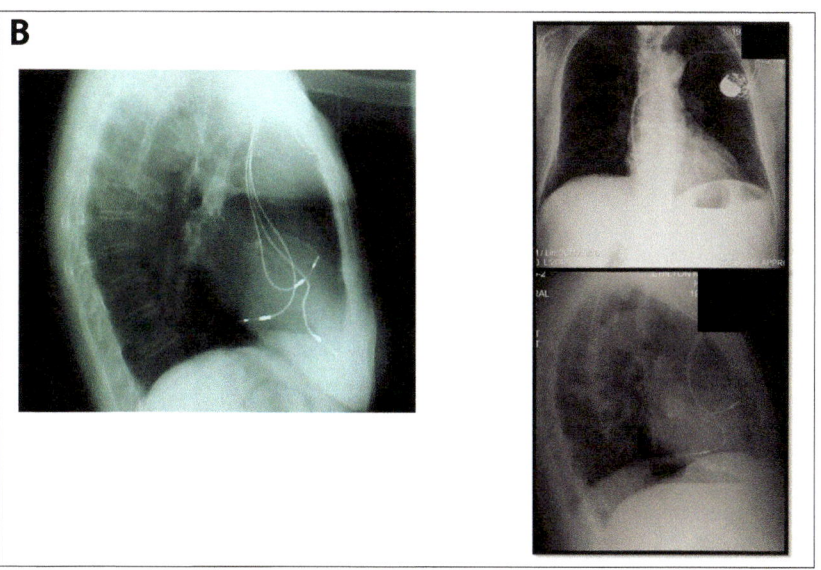

Figure 67.4 **Panel A:** Chest radiograph in lateral view and showing lead configuration in biatrial pacing system. Note the conventionally positioned high right lead and a passive fixation lead in the mid-coronary sinus. Sensing issues with ventricular electrograms and stability in this location require considerable technical expertise and attention at implant. **Panel B:** (**Left**) Lateral view of a chest radiograph showing a dual-site right atrial pacing system. The conventionally placed high right atrial lead and right ventricular apical lead are shown. The coronary sinus lead is fixed at the inferior margin of the ostium. The two atrial leads are cross-connected by a Y-connector to the atrial port of a conventional DDD pacemaker generator. (**Right**) Dual-site right atrial pacing system without a conventional ventricular lead in an 82-year-old patient with drug refractory paroxysmal AF, sick sinus syndrome, and intact atrioventricular conduction. Previously ineffective sotalol therapy was continued as background therapy. At 12 years of follow-up, AF burden was 0%.

mid–coronary sinus tined lead connected to the atrial and ventricular ports of a dual-chamber pacemaker programmed to the triggered mode.[56] In this mode, atrial electrogram sensing triggered the coronary sinus pacing stimulus. This inevitably imposed a delay between the right and left atrial activation timing, albeit short, often less than 20 ms.

In contrast, dual-site right atrial pacing, first proposed by us, was employed in patients with drug-refractory symptomatic AF or flutter and a documented primary or drug-induced bradycardia.[26] We implanted either a DDDR pacemaker generator with dual atrial leads and a right ventricular lead or a single-chamber pacemaker with the dual atrial leads alone (Figure 67.4B). The leads are typically inserted through the cephalic vein and subclavian access is used if the cephalic vein is not present or of sufficient caliber to permit three leads being passed. Introducer sheaths assist in lead placement and avoid rubbing and dislodgement. In the atrium we utilized a high right atrial electrode and an ostia coronary sinus placement of the left atrial lead.[26] A double-curve stylet (primary RA curve with short contrary sinus hook at tip) is used for placement of the coronary sinus ostial lead. The two pacing leads are fixed in the right atrium, one at the high right atrium and the other just outside the coronary sinus ostium. An active screw-in fixation lead is invariably used at the coronary sinus ostium. The atrial leads are connected via a Y-connector to the atrial output of the pacemaker. The cathode is the high right atrial lead and the coronary sinus lead is used as the anode. These leads are cross-connected using the distal electrodes with a Y-connector to the atrial port of a dual-chamber pacemaker generator. This enables simultaneous right and coronary sinus stimulation and a right ventricular lead implantation. The ventricular lead, if indicated, is positioned at the right ventricular apex and is connected to the ventricular output of the pacemaker. The pacemaker is programmed in the DDDR or AAIR mode, depending on native AV conduction, with a lower rate between 80 to 90 bpm; an individual rate response and the sensor threshold are selected to obtain continuous overdrive atrial pacing. Bipolar atrial pacing establishes dual-site RA pacing from both cathodal and anodal electrodes with a biphasic P-wave morphology with a negative terminal component in leads II, III, and aVF (Figure 67.5A). The atrial sensing

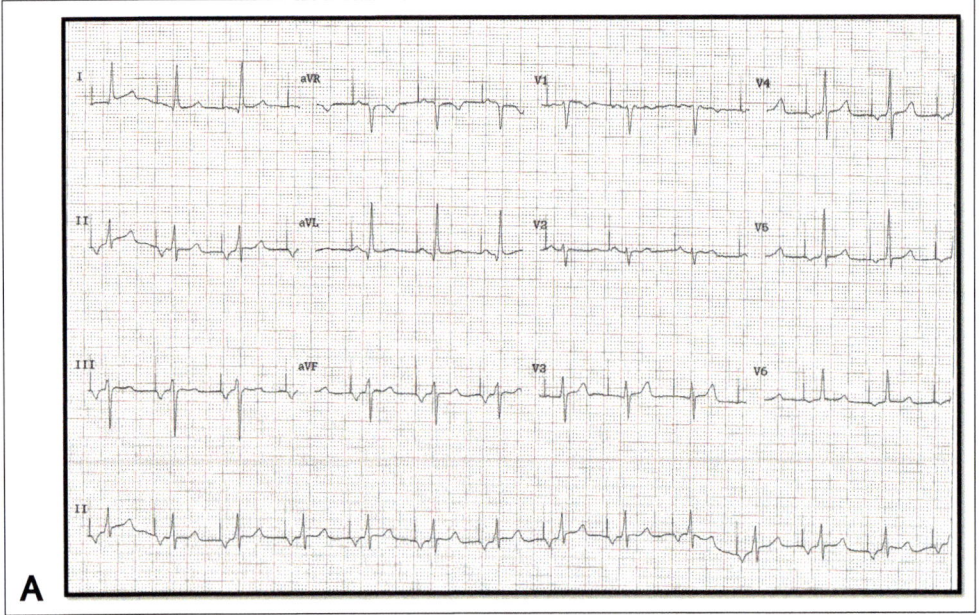

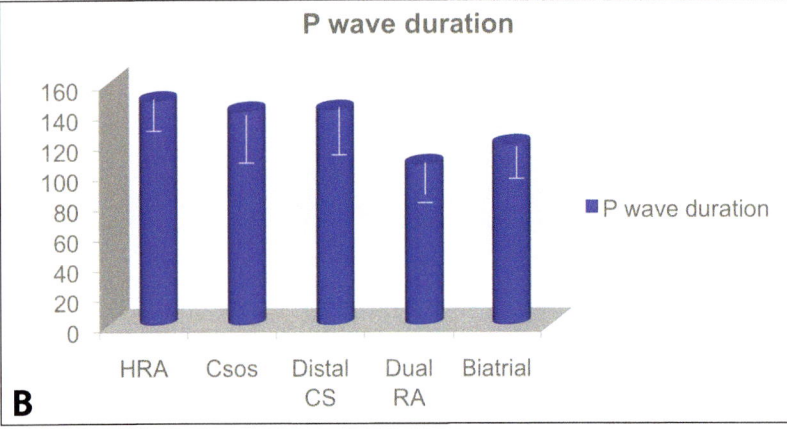

Figure 67.5 **Panel A:** 12-lead electrocardiogram in a patient during dual-site right atrial pacing. Note the biphasic P-wave morphology in V1 with a major terminal negative component in the inferior leads. **Panel B:** P-wave duration during different alternative site pacing modes compared to high right atrial pacing in a cohort of patients with AF. *Source:* Modified from Delfaut et al.[27]

threshold is usually set at 0.5 mV. Long AV delays in the DDDR mode or AAIR pacing are used whenever possible. Upon detection of an atrial high-rate event (> 175 bpm), the atrial electrogram intervals are stored in the pacemaker memory up to a maximum of 8 consecutive events. The pacemaker's data logs also store atrial electrograms for recorded AF or AT events. The percentage of atrial pacing is perioperatively reviewed to ensure that the objective of continuous atrial pacing is achieved. Continuous atrial overdrive pacing is considered acceptable if the percentage of paced atrial events are > 80% of all atrial events. If this percentage of atrial pacing is not reached, the pacemaker is reprogrammed to a more aggressive atrial pacing prescription and/or the drug regimen is modified by either increasing the dose or changing the drug.

Both methods have been investigated for their physiologic impact and clinical evaluation in patients with bradycardia and AF. This evaluation has included long-term observational data as well as medium-term randomized clinical trials. Only the dual-site RA pacing method has been employed in a systematic fashion in a hybrid therapy prescription for AF prevention or suppression in conjunction with antiarrhythmic drugs and catheter ablation. It has been used in populations mostly with, but occasionally without, concomitant bradycardia.

Physiologic Effects of Multisite Atrial Pacing

Electrophysiologic and Mechanical Abnormalities in Bradycardias and AF

Normal intra-atrial and interatrial conduction is altered in patients with AF. Intra-atrial conduction measured in the right atrium (RA) by P-wave onset to His bundle atrial electrogram (PA interval) normally ranges from 10 to 45 ms. Interatrial conduction to the left atrium (LA), P-wave onset to distal coronary sinus atrial electrogram, ranges from 40 to 130 ms.[57] Interestingly, in early studies, single-site RA pacing prolonged these intervals (RA up to 75 ms, LA up to 150 ms).[57] P-wave prolongation has also been associated with the development of AF in epidemiologic studies. This prolongation is most often due to concomitant intra-atrial and interatrial conduction delays. Severe prolongation can result in split atrial activation with two disparate electrograms especially in coronary sinus and septal atrial electrogram recordings.[58] Left atrial size increase correlates well with interatrial conduction delay increments.[59] Recently, Eicher has described atrial mechanical dyssynchrony with interatrial conduction delay.[60] Right and left atrial tissue Doppler imaging shows regional atrial dyssynchrony in the presence of such conduction delays, promoting less effective atrial emptying, further atrial dilatation, and progressive atrial remodeling. This has been noted in patients presenting with heart failure with preserved systolic function. Concomitant atrioventricular block, especially first-degree block, can result in presystolic mitral regurgitation due to delayed mitral valve closure.

Atrial Resynchronization with Atrial Pacing

Electrical Atrial Resynchronization

The impact of dual-site atrial pacing can be ascribed to three positive effects on atrial physiology and function. These include atrial electrical resynchronization, improvement of mechanical atrial function, and long-term atrial reverse remodeling. In contrast, single-site atrial pacing may or may not have some of these positive effects.

Atrial electrical resynchronization with pacing modes was first studied systematically by Prakash and coworkers.[29] Electrophysiologic effects of high right atrial, proximal and distal coronary sinus, dual-site right atrial, and biatrial pacing were studied in patients with AF. P-wave duration during pacing was significantly abbreviated by both dual-site RA and biatrial pacing ($P < 0.001$ vs high RA pacing, respectively) but not by any other single-site atrial pacing method (Figure 67.5B). Both dual-site atrial pacing modes also significantly abbreviated P-wave durations for closely coupled high RA premature beats ($P < 0.001$) in contrast to high RA pacing. During the basic pacing drive and for high RA extrastimuli, RA activation at the crista terminalis and atrial septum was comparable in sinus rhythm, high RA pacing, and in both dual-site atrial pacing methods, but was significantly delayed by coronary sinus ostial and distal coronary sinus pacing. In contrast, proximal coronary sinus activation was delayed with high RA pacing compared with all other pacing modes, and high RA extrastimuli encountered reduced conduction delay at this location with dual-site atrial pacing modes. LA activation was advanced superiorly by both single-site coronary sinus pacing methods and both dual-site atrial pacing techniques. Inferior and lateral LA activation was advanced by all pacing modes using a coronary sinus pacing site. However, earlier activation of LA sites occurred for high RA premature beats after both dual-site pacing methods ($P < 0.05$) compared with single-site pacing modes. Incremental conduction delay at different atrial regions for closely coupled high RA extrastimuli ranged from 33% to 120% during high RA pacing and was significantly attenuated at multiple RA and LA sites by dual-site RA and biatrial pacing. From these data, it is apparent that distinct global as well as regional electrophysiologic effects occur and likely mediate the variable antiarrhythmic and mechanical effects of different single-site atrial pacing sites as well as multisite atrial pacing methods. The surface 12-lead ECG shows a biphasic P wave in the inferior leads with a terminal negative component. This is also seen in lead V_1 (Figure 67.5A). Bachmann's bundle pacing in the high interatrial septum has reduced P-wave duration but is associated with continued delays in the activation of the free wall of the right and left atrium.[61]

Three-dimensional (3D) mapping of atrial activation has also been performed. ▶ Video 67.1, ▶ Video 67.2, and ▶ Video 67.3 show 3D activation of the right atrium using an EnSite (St. Jude Medical, Sylmar, CA) balloon array during single-site high right atrial pacing, (Video 67.1) low septal right atrial pacing at the coronary sinus ostium (Video 67.2), and dual-site right atrial pacing at both sites simultaneously (Video 67.3). Note the more rapid global right atrial activation with two wavefronts with lines of collision in the lateral and septal right atrium. Preferential left activation along the coronary sinus and left atrial septum has also been demonstrated in such studies. Septal pacing has been studied using 3D intracardiac echocardiography to validate pacing site.[62] Interatrial septal pacing resulted in a significant reduction of the P-wave duration as compared to sinus rhythm, but supra-fossa pacing showed greater reduction of the P-wave duration than IF pacing (59.4 ± 6.6 ms vs 30.2 ± 13.6 ms; $P < 0.004$).

The effects of multisite pacing on the electrophysiology and inducibility of AF in patients with AF has been studied in our laboratory.[63] In acute studies, there was a significant abbreviation of the P-wave duration to 103 ± 17 ms with dual-site pacing compared with sinus rhythm (120 ± 12 ms, $P = 0.005$) and high right atrial pacing (121 ± 17 ms, $P = 0.005$). This was also associated with a characteristic change in P-wave configuration with an inferior and leftward axis shift. The effective refractory period at the high right atrium remained unchanged with dual-site atrial pacing compared with single-site high right atrial pacing. In patients with inducible AF or atrial flutter who could be tested after dual-site atrial pacing, the acutely induced AT was suppressed in 9 of 16 patients (56%). The difference in the effective refractory period between the high right atrium and the coronary sinus ostium pacing sites was significantly greater (33 ± 12 ms) in patients with suppression of AT with dual-site atrial pacing compared with patients without suppression (15 ± 13 ms, $P = 0.001$). P-wave abbreviation did not correlate with arrhythmia suppression. These data suggest that electrical resynchronization of dispersion of atrial refractoriness assists in prevention of AF induction in these patients.

Mechanical Atrial Resynchronization

Atrial mechanical function has been assessed for both single-site and dual-site atrial pacing with Doppler flow, tissue Doppler imaging, and 3D echocardiography. The findings are fairly consistent. Biatrial pacing and dual-site right atrial pacing both improve left atrial filling as measured by mitral valve flow patterns using Doppler flow imaging.[64] Doi and coworkers systematically studied single and dual atrial pacing modes (Figure 67.6A). In their acute studies, they showed improved left atrial A-wave amplitude with biatrial and dual-site right atrial pacing.[64] Left atrial hemodynamics were also improved acutely with these modes with lower pulmonary capillary wedge pressures, left atrial pressure, and cardiac output.[65] These findings were later validated by Burri et al in patients with AF undergoing catheter ablation procedures.[66] Strain Doppler imaging has shown atrial dyssynchrony in patients with AF.[67] Matsumoto et al first showed improved septal and lateral left atrial strain and improved synchrony with biatrial rather than right atrial appendage pacing in 6 patients with brady–tachy syndrome and AF. Bachmann's bundle pacing and dual-site right atrial pacing also acutely showed improved interatrial dyssynchrony and intra-LA dyssynchrony with tissue Doppler imaging.[68] Three-dimensional echocardiography showed improved left atrial function after alternate-site pacing. Long-term maintenance of atrial filling improvement has been shown in the DAPPAF trial by Prakash, et al.[30] Increased A-wave amplitude was seen with dual-site right atrial pacing compared to high right atrial pacing or support pacing at a mean follow-up of 4.5 months (range 1–6 months) (Figure 67.6B). Long-term data are awaited for Bachmann bundle or biatrial pacing.

Atrial Reverse Remodeling

The impact of multisite atrial pacing on the remodeled atrium in patients with AF has been studied. Medium- and long-term data are available from studies of dual-site right atrial pacing.[30,31] Prakash and coworkers showed the high RA pacing in DDDR mode resulted in increased left ventricular (LV) end systolic volume (78 ± 42 mL vs 60 ± 31 mL, $P = 0.001$) and reduced LV ejection fraction ($44\% \pm 14\%$ vs $50\% \pm 11\%$, $P = 0.007$), while these parameters did not change during dual-site RA pacing during a mean follow-up period of 4.5 months. Dual-site RA pacing resulted in increased peak A-wave velocity (75 ± 19 cm/s vs 63 ± 23 cm/s, $P = 0.003$) and left atrial filling fraction compared to baseline (0.47 ± 0.15 vs 0.38 ± 0.13, $P = 0.005$). Dual-site RA pacing prevented the progressive dilatation of the left ventricle, reduction in left ventricular and right atrial ejection fraction during high RA DDDR pacing.

More recently, long-term data attesting to atrial reverse remodeling has been reported by Nagarakanti et al.[31] The long-term impact of dual-site RA pacing was studied in 34 patients with drug refractory AF with pacemakers with dual RA leads. Baseline echocardiographic indices were compared with last follow-up data, with a mean interval of 37 ± 25 (range 7–145) months. Mean LA diameter declined from 45 ± 5 mm at baseline to 42 ± 7 mm ($P = 0.003$). Mean LV ejection fraction was unchanged from $52\% \pm 9\%$ at baseline and $54\% \pm 6\%$ at last follow-up ($P = 0.3$). There was no significant change in LV dimensions with mean LV end diastolic diameter being 51 ± 6 mm at baseline and 53 ± 5 mm at last follow-up ($P = 0.3$). Mean LV end-systolic diameter also remained unchanged from 35 ± 6 mm at baseline to 33 ± 6 mm at last follow-up ($P = 0.47$). This data is conclusive evidence of atrial reverse remodeling after dual-site RA pacing.

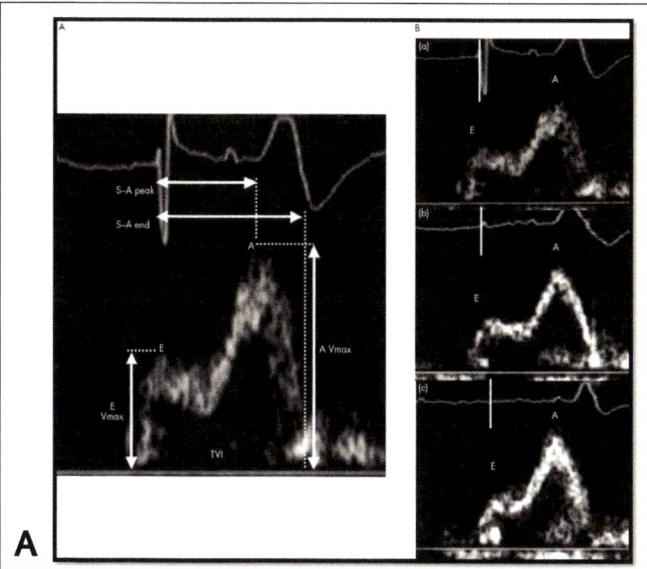
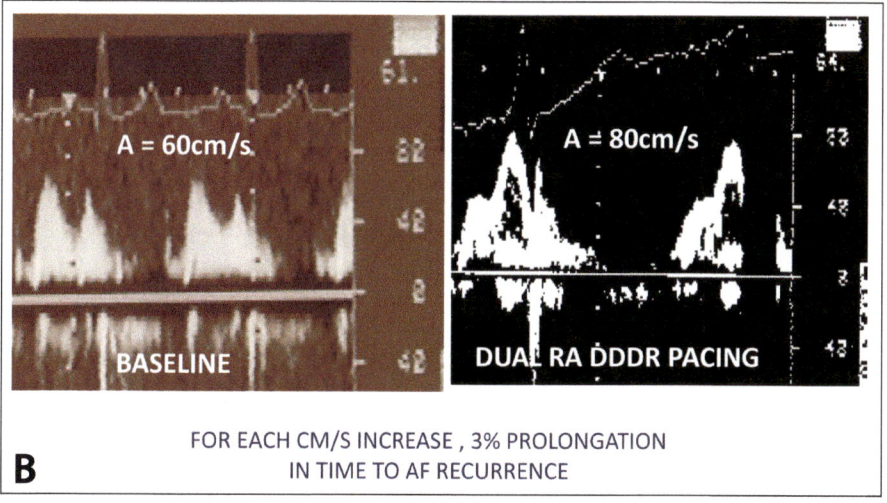

Figure 67.6 Panel A: The optimization of the atrioventricular (AV) delay defined as the time when the end of the atrial filling wave (A) on the transmitral flow coincided with the onset of the first heart sound (S1), using simultaneous heart-sound monitoring. **Dotted line** indicates the onset of the first heart sound. E represents the early filling wave; S2 is the second heart sound. (A) Sample of the echocardiographic measurements. (B) Representative patterns of transmitral Doppler flow during AV sequential pacing with the optimal AV delays. **White bars** indicate the atrial pacing spike. (a) High right atrial (HRA) pacing; (b) Coronary sinus (CS) pacing; (c) Biatrial (BiA) pacing. The BiA pacing produced the most increased peak velocity of the atrial filling wave (A V_{max}) and the shortest interval from the atrial pacing spike on the electrocardiogram to the peak of the atrial filling wave (S-A peak). E indicates V_{max} or peak velocity of the early filling wave; **TVI** is mitral flow time velocity integral. Source: Reproduced with permission from Takagi et al.[64] **Panel B:** Example of patient included in the medium-term analysis of dual-site right atrial pacing whose A-wave velocity and in turn atrial contribution of ventricular filling increased from 60 cm/s at baseline to 80 cm/s with dual-site right atrial pacing. Source: Reproduced with permission from Nagarakanti et al.[31]

Observational and Evidence-based Outcomes with Alternative and Multisite Atrial Pacing

Clinical experiences have been reported with multisite atrial pacing using both biatrial and dual-site RA pacing. Observational data on the feasibility of biatrial, dual-site RA pacing, Bachmann's bundle pacing, and low septal RA pacing initially suggested value in all these methods.[69-71] The overall data on alternate site and dual atrial pacing is now substantial but diverse. Both observational data and randomized clinical trials have been performed in the medium term, but long-term data is largely restricted to observational studies. Dual-site pacing has been performed as stand-alone therapy in many medium-term studies but as part of a hybrid therapy, staged treatment algorithm in long-term observational studies

Long-term biatrial pacing has reported rhythm control in 64% of patients at a mean follow-up of 33 months but has a high (> 20%) coronary sinus lead dislodgement rate.[69] Bachmann's bundle pacing was reported to prevent progression to persistent or permanent AF at 1 year.[70] Padeletti et al noted similar observations with low septal RA pacing.[71] Longer-term observational data provided a clearer picture of the freedom from recurrent AF and maintenance of sinus rhythm or atrial paced rhythm to achieve rhythm control. However, many of these studies allowed concomitant antiarrhythmic therapy and offer limited information on the value of pacing alone.

The Septal Pacing for Atrial Fibrillation Suppression Evaluation (SAFE) study was a definitive study of alternative single-site pacing in the primary prevention of AF and its progression in patients with sick sinus syndrome and AF requiring cardiac pacing.[53] Three hundred eighty-five patients were randomly assigned to RA appendage and RA septal pacing with an atrial overdrive pacing algorithm programmed ON or OFF. The study failed to demonstrate any reduction in persistent AF-free survival with either pacing site relative to the other regardless of the overdrive pacing algorithm use. The progression to persistent AF ranged from 20% to 30% in these arms over a 3-year period.

Stand-alone Multisite Atrial Pacing

The stand-alone efficacy of alternate site and dual atrial pacing has been assessed in short- and medium-term randomized clinical trials with variable endpoints in patients with bradycardia–tachycardia syndrome. Initial feasibility studies suggested improved rhythm control with atrial low septal lead placement combined with the continuous atrial pacing (CAP) algorithm over RA appendage pacing.[72] The paroxysmal AF episodes per month significantly decreased in the septal pacing group compared to the RA appendage pacing group in both CAP-OFF (0.2 ± 0.5 vs 2.1 ± 4.2, $P < 0.05$) and CAP-ON (0.2 ± 0.5 vs 1.9 ± 3.8, $P < 0.05$) conditions. Paroxysmal AF burden was significantly lower in the septal than in the RA appendage pacing group in CAP-OFF (47 ± 84 min/d vs 140 ± 217, $P < 0.05$) and in CAP-ON (41 ± 72 vs 193 ± 266, $P < 0.05$) conditions. However, a 3-month prospective, randomized crossover evaluation in the ASPECT study showed no changes in device-recorded AT/AF frequency or burden were observed with algorithms OFF versus ON or between patients randomized to septal versus nonseptal lead location.[50] There was a modest reduction in symptomatic AT/AF events. Biatrial pacing was tested with two other pacing modes in the SYNBIAPACE study.[73] This study consisted of an intrapatient comparison of three different pacing modes according to a dual crossover design over periods of 3 months: (1) "inhibited" or no atrial pacing, (2) standard DDD pacing (70 bpm) at a single high right atrial sit, and (3) biatrial synchronous pacing (DDTA, 70 bpm). The primary endpoint was the time of the first arrhythmia recurrence, as documented by the Holter functions of the pacemaker, including intracardiac ECG storage. Forty-three patients with no conventional indication for permanent pacing (mean age 64 years) completed the whole protocol. The mean P-wave duration before pacemaker implantation was 148 ± 31 ms; the study did not reveal any difference between the three pacing modes in both the time to first recurrence and the total time spent in arrhythmia.

Observational data on dual-site RA pacing was reported in patients on background antiarrhythmic therapy. However, a prospective randomized clinical trial, the Dual-site Atrial Pacing for Prevention of AF (DAPPAF) study, which compared support pacing, high RA pacing, and dual-site RA pacing, was performed without this stipulation to evaluate the pacing site configuration.[49] Pacemakers were programmed to overdrive pacing in the latter two active treatment arms. Six-month crossover treatment periods in all three modes were evaluated. There was no significant difference in time to first AF recurrence seen in the total patient population. However, as detailed later in this chapter, the subgroup with background antiarrhythmic therapy showed a significant prolongation of time to first AF recurrence as well as symptomatic AF events (Figure 67.7). It is reasonable to conclude that single- or dual-site atrial pacing as a stand-alone therapy offers no definitive clinical benefit with septal or dual atrial pacing modes in patients with brady–tachy syndrome. This is reflected in current evidence-based guidelines for treatment of such patients.[75]

Multisite Atrial Pacing in a Hybrid Therapy Algorithm

Hybrid therapy using antiarrhythmic drugs and atrial pacing has been tested to a significant extent with new pacing modes. Dual-site RA pacing alone has been tested systematically in a hybrid therapy algorithm in small and large observational trials with medium-term and long-term outcome data. Saksena et al reported the feasibility and benefit of dual-site RA pacing when added to background antiarrhythmic therapy in 1996, initially in a crossover comparison with high RA pacing with 3- and 6-month observation periods in patients with drug-refractory paroxysmal AF.[26] Atrial pacing resulted in a marked decline in AF recurrences ($P < 0.001$). During dual-site pacing with an optimal drug regimen, there was no AF recurrence in any patient, compared with 5 recurrences in 12 patients during single-site pacing ($P = 0.03$).

Longer-term outcome of the pilot patient group was reported by Delfaut and coworkers from our group in 1998.[27] During single- or dual-site RA pacing in patients with drug-refractory paroxysmal AF and bradycardia (primary or drug-induced), mean arrhythmia-free intervals increased from 9 ± 10 days in the control period preceding implant to 143 ± 110 days ($P < 0.0001$) in single-site RA pacing and 195 ± 96 days in dual-site RA pacing ($P < 0.005$ vs single-site pacing and $P < 0.0001$ vs control). Dual-site RA pacing with background, previously ineffective antiarrhythmic drug therapy significantly increased the proportion of patients free of AF recurrence (89%) as compared to single-site RA pacing (62%, $P = 0.02$) on the same drug therapy. Effective rhythm control was initially achieved in 86% of patients at institution of hybrid drug and dual-site RA pacing therapy. In long-term follow-up, 78% of patients at 1 year and 56% at 3 years remained free of symptomatic AF. The need for cardioversion was reduced after pacemaker implant and antithrombotic therapy was reduced ($P < 0.06$) without any thromboembolic event.

Subsequently, the long-term experience with 113 patients, with paroxysmal and persistent AF and bradyarrhythmias followed for up to 5 years (mean 30 months) was reported by Madan, et al.[28] These patients were elderly (mean age 69 ± 11 years, 57% men), who had sick sinus syndrome ($n = 59$), conduction system disease ($n = 14$), or drug-induced bradycardias ($n = 59$). They had failed a mean of 2.5 antiarrhythmic drugs. Figures 67.8A and 67.8B show maintenance of rhythm control (sinus rhythm or atrial pacing validated by device diagnostics), total survival, and freedom from any AF recurrence requiring cardioversion after hybrid therapy prescription. Five-year actuarial survival in this population exceeds 80%, with over 85% of patients maintaining rhythm

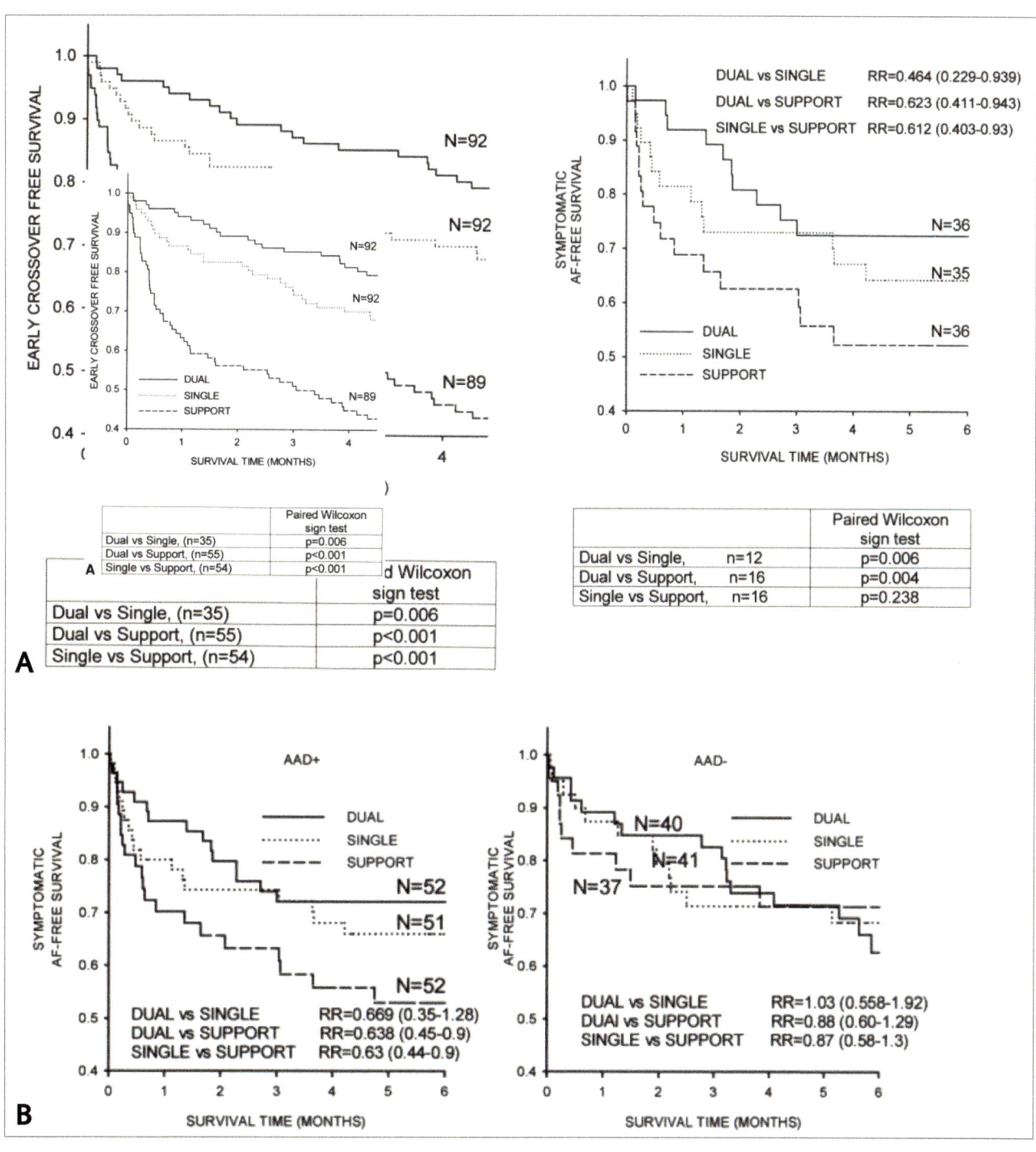

Figure 67.7 **Panel A: (Left)** Freedom from crossover within 4.5 months of entering randomized treatment phase for each pacing mode using an intention-to-treat analysis. The percentage of patients surviving in the pacing mode is tabulated on the Y-axis, and the follow-up duration in the mode on the X-axis. Dual right atrial (RA) pacing shows a higher proportion of patients able to remain in the randomized treatment mode as compared with other modes. As a result of crossovers, study endpoints, or adverse events, this resulted in a decreased AF recurrence rate (38.5% in the support mode and 33.7% in the high RA pacing mode). Dual, dual-site RA pacing; single, high RA pacing; support, demand pacing in atrium or ventricle at low support rate. **Right panel:** Freedom from all symptomatic AF in each randomized pacing mode in the entire study population using an intention-to-treat analysis. Dual RA pacing, but not high RA pacing, shows a trend to prolongation of time interval to AF recurrence. Despite reduced event rates in the other two arms due to crossover, in the entire study population, the time to first symptomatic recurrence of AF trended to be longer in the dual-site RA pacing mode than the support mode (Cox proportional hazards survival ratio 0.715, paired Wilcoxon p = 0.07). **Panel B:** Freedom from all symptomatic AF in each randomized pacing mode in study population, receiving concomitant class 1 or 3 antiarrhythmic drugs (AAD) **(left)** or without concomitant AAD therapy **(right)** using an intention-to-treat analysis. Dual right atrial (RA) pacing, but not high RA pacing, shows prolongation of time interval to AF recurrence as compared to support pacing and a trend to prolongation as compared with high RA pacing in drug-treated patients. There is no difference in outcome in patients on any randomized pacing mode without concomitant drug therapy. *Source:* Reproduced with permission from Saksena et al.[49]

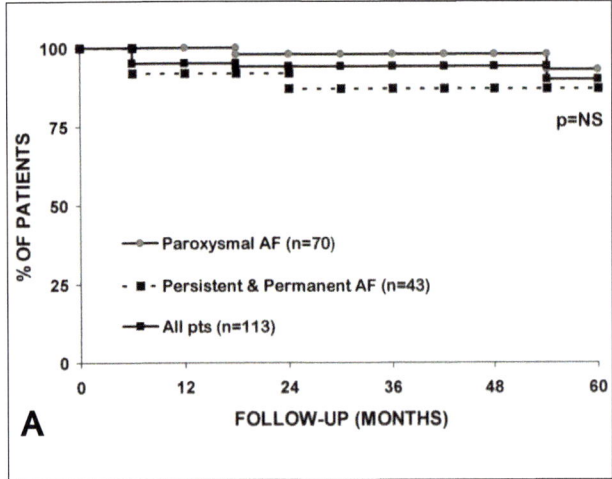 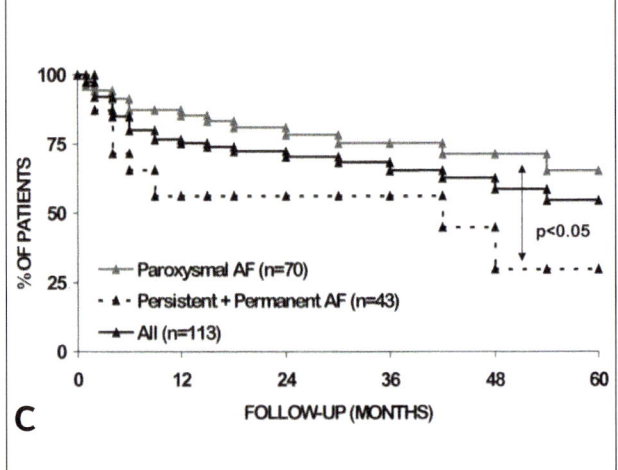
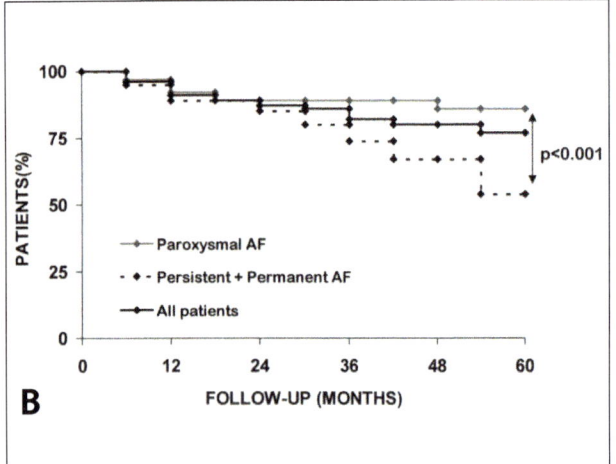 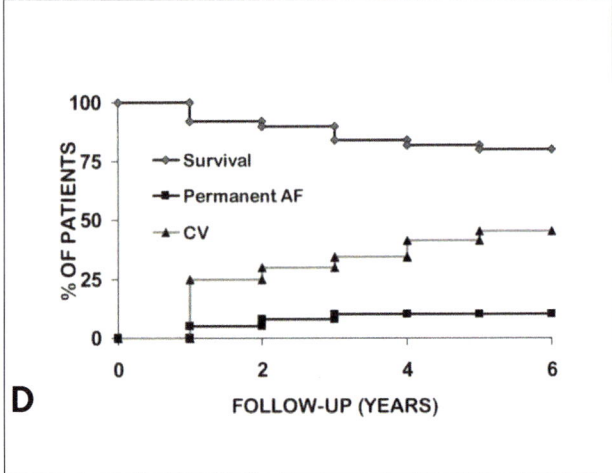

Figure 67.8 Comparison of AF subpopulations with paroxysmal AF with patients with persistent or permanent AF. The total population data are shown as a reference. (**A**) Long-term rhythm control; (**B**) Survival from all-cause mortality; (**C**) Freedom from symptomatic AF; and (**D**) Freedom from cardioversion therapy. X axis = percentage of patients; y axis = follow-up (expressed in months).

control. The hybrid therapy prescription included continued background antiarrhythmic drug therapy, continuous dual-site RA pacing (> 80% atrial pacing), and monitoring for early AF recurrences, many of which resolved spontaneously, as shown in Figure 67.9. Approximately 30% of patients required one or more cardioversions for early (25%) and late persistent AF recurrences during follow-up (mean cardioversions was 2 per cardioverted patient). Late recurrences are often prompted by coexisting conditions such as pulmonary infection, heart failure, etc., and may resolve with resolution of the primary triggering condition. In patients with delayed recurrences of persistent AF or atrial flutter without comorbidities, catheter ablation of atrial flutter or linear right atrial compartmentalization was performed. Linear ablation was performed in patients with ≥ 3 late recurrences of persistent AF in a given year. Thirty-two percent of patients required an ablative intervention in addition to pacing. Linear catheter ablation was employed more frequently in patients with persistent AF (Figure 67.9). Clinical outcomes from one series are shown in Figure 67.10.

More recently, we have employed dual-site RA pacing in patients with recurrences after pulmonary vein isolation procedures and bradycardias. The value of this approach is still under study.

Atrial Dual-site Pacing and Catheter Ablation with Background Antiarrhythmic Drug Therapy

With increasing experience, we have extended of the patient population for hybrid therapy to refractory AF patients with persistent and "permanent" AF that have been previously treated with multiple antiarrhythmic drugs or catheter ablation.[74-76] Hybrid prescriptions have now expanded to include previous or staged catheter ablation of concomitant type 1 atrial flutter (▶ Video 67.4) or linear RA compartmentalization (Figures 67.10, 67.11,

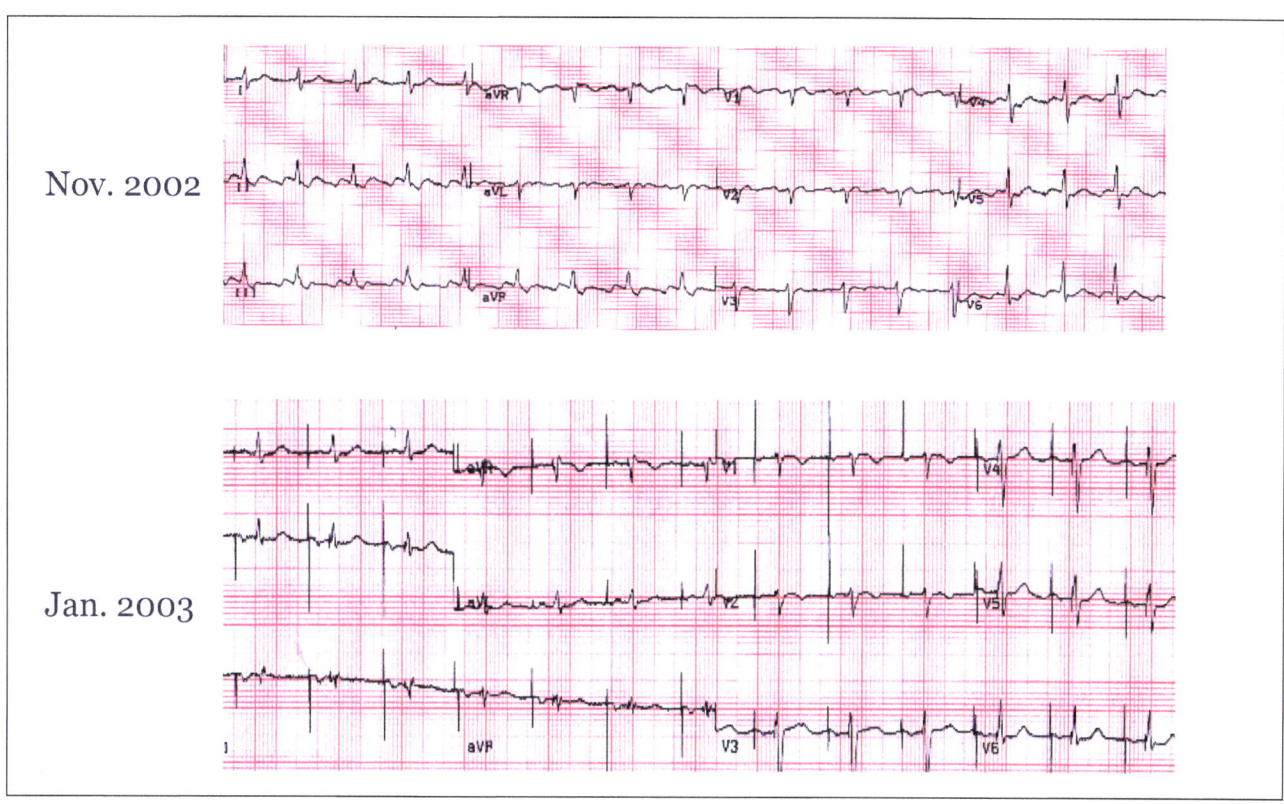

Figure 67.9 Evolution of rhythm control after hybrid therapy. An early recurrence of atrial flutter in this patient after dual-site atrial pacing and antiarrhythmic drug therapy (**top panel**) resolved spontaneously without cardioversion and was succeeded by long-term rhythm control (**bottom panel**) in the dual-site right atrial paced mode.

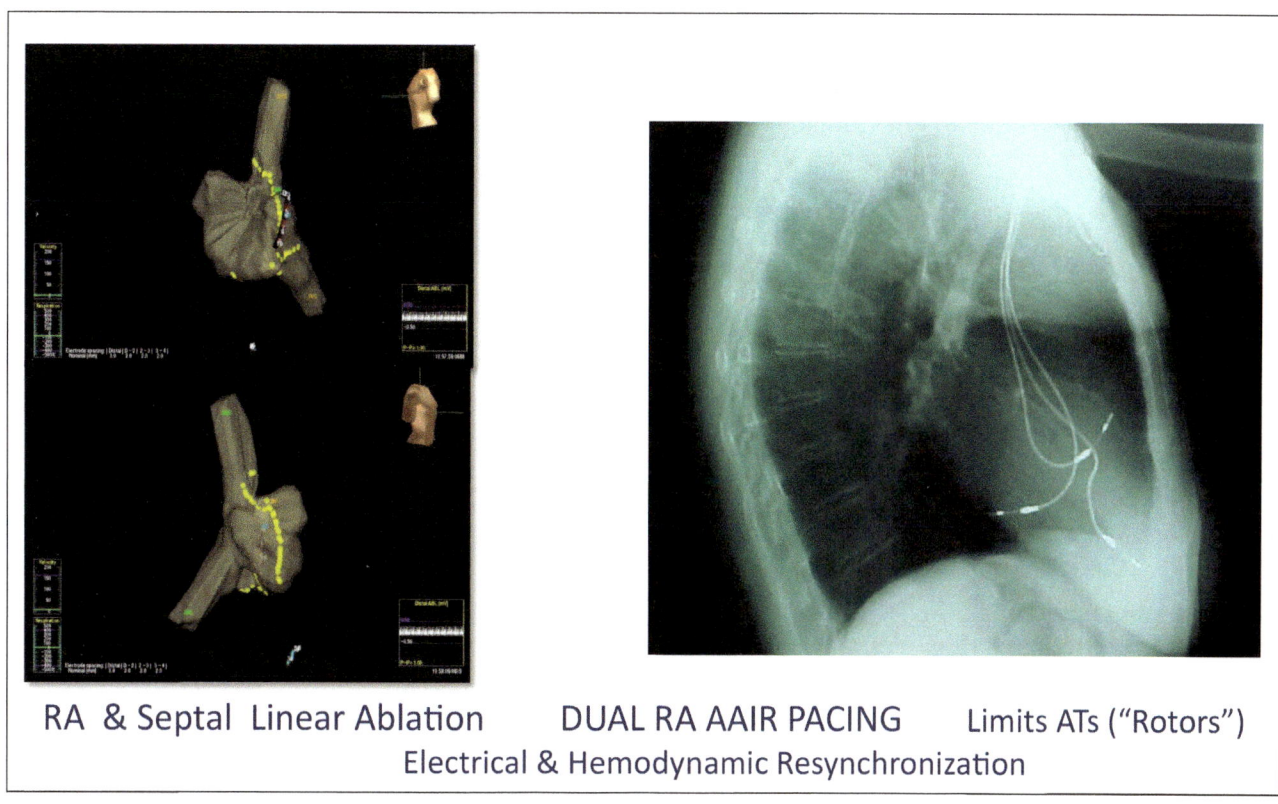

Figure 67.10 Hybrid therapy in a patient with persistent AF and drug-induced bradycardia. Right atrial compartmentalization is shown on a 3D NavX map on the left panel with the three lines to create compartments (see text for details). The dual-site atrial pacing system resynchronized the anterior and posterior compartments to suppress residual AT that could initiate or maintain AF.

and 67.12), particularly in patients with new-onset or established persistent AF. Linear ablation is performed using serial point radiofrequency lesions to construct a posterolateral intercaval line, septal lines from the superior vena cava to the fossa ovalis and coronary sinus ostium to the tricuspid valve annulus, and a cavotricuspid isthmus line (Figure 67.10, left panel). Completion of an anterior RA compartment and posterior RA and LA compartments is tested by pacing (Video 67.5A and Video 67.5B). A dual-site RA pacing system is inserted with the leads in the anterior and posterior compartments (Figure 67.10, right panel). Filipecki showed the initial value of this method with a reduction in P-wave duration with dual-site RA pacing after linear RA ablation.[74,75] There can be initial recurrences, which improve during the first year of follow-up due to sequential electrical atrial resynchronization and mechanical effects leading to reverse atrial remodeling (Figure 67.11). Progressive, often exponential reduction of AF burden is seen in the first 6 to 12 months of follow-up (Figure 67.12). This resulted in improved rhythm control. More recently, pulmonary vein isolation and LA compartmentalization have been employed with dual RA pacing systems. In patients requiring ICD therapy, dual-site RA pacing was used for AF suppression in this population. Table 67.5 shows some early experience with this approach.

Table 67.5 Studies of hybrid regimens for AF treatment

Series	Method	Patients	AF Type	Follow-up (months)	Rhythm Control
Saksena[11]	DAP + AAD ± ABL	118	Parox/Persist	1–54 (20 ± 14)	79%
Prakash[12]	DAP + AAD + TVI ABL	40	Parox AF ± A Flutter	5–56 (26 ± 14)	90% at 2 yrs
Saksena[43]	DAP + AAD ± ABL ± CV	113	Parox (70)	1–81 (30 ± 23)	92% at 3 yrs
Filipecki[45]	AP/ICD + RA Maze + AAD	25	Persist/Perm	6–49 (17 ± 10)	75% at 18 mos

Source: Modified from Saksena S, Madan N.[25]

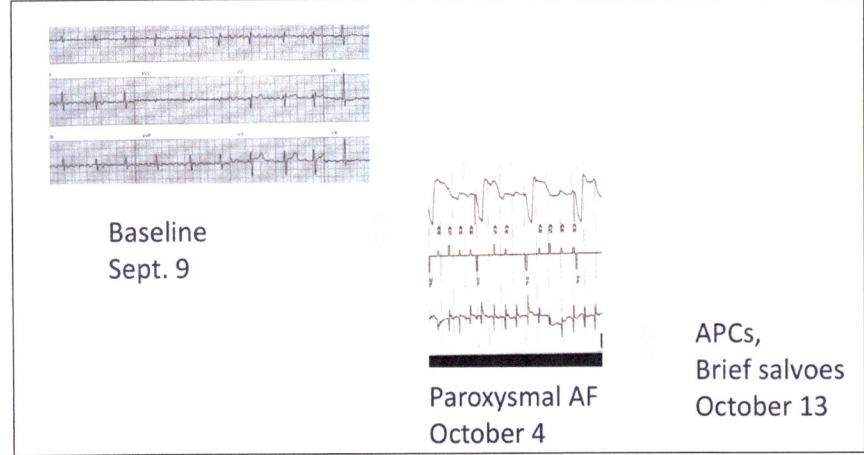

Figure 67.11 Spontaneous evolution of rhythm after right atrial compartmentalization ("Maze") and dual-site right atrial pacing in a patient with persistent AF. Note the persistent AF episode immediately on completion of hybrid therapy in September, spontaneously terminated without cardioversion by October 4; device diagnostics recorded runs of paroxysmal AF. Ten days later, only brief salvoes of atrial premature beats were noted on the diagnostics without sustained runs of atrial tachycardia or AF.

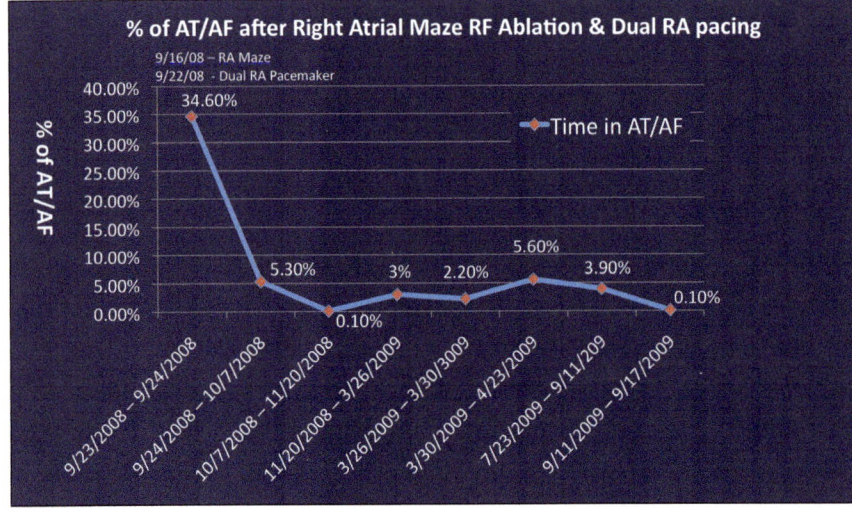

Figure 67.12 Plot of AF burden as measured by pacemaker diagnostics in a patient with persistent AF immediately on completion of hybrid ablation, drug and pacing therapy on September 22, 2008 and followed over the next 12 months. Note the initial rapid decline in burden followed by a gradual decline and stabilization at a very low level during long-term follow-up.

In a cohort of 47 patients with drug-refractory persistent AF with bradycardias, mean age 66 years, which included new-onset and established persistent AF, Rao and Saksena reported restoration of rhythm control in 83% of patients at 3-year follow-up (Figure 67.13).[76] More than 40% of patients had no recurrence of persistent AF after hybrid therapy and required no cardioversions (Figure 67.14). There was also a significant reduction in AF hospitalizations and cardioversion-related hospitalizations after hybrid therapy (Figure 67.15).

Use of multisite atrial pacing using dual-site RA pacing has been classified as a class 2B indication for preventive pacing for AF in the 1998 guidelines from the ACC/AHA and most recently as a class 2 indication in 2012. It is restricted to patients with bradycardias based on available data.[77,78]

Hybrid Therapy in AF with Heart Failure

Eicher and colleagues have reported on the role of atrial dyssynchrony in patients with heart failure.[60] They have noted that biatrial pacing has been effective in patients with heart failure with preserved ejection (HFpEF), particularly in patients with prolonged P-wave duration. A subgroup had AF. We have more recently employed dual-site RA pacing in 71 patients with heart failure refractory to antiarrhythmic drugs and/or catheter ablation in the RA or LA.[79] Dual-site RA pacing was added to background antiarrhythmic drug therapy and/or failed ablation. As in persistent AF patients, catheter ablation was performed in the RA or LA as indicated prior to or along with pacing. Thirty-six patients had HFpEF (median follow-up, 7.2 years) and 35 had heart failure with systolic dysfunction

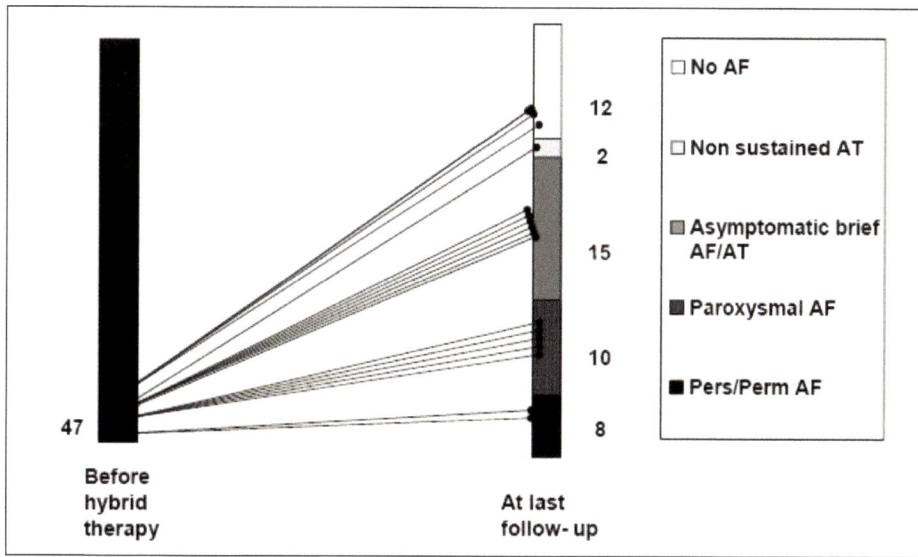

Figure 67.13 Device data logs at the start of hybrid ablation, drug, and pacing therapy (**left column**) and at study cutoff (**right column**). Most patients are in rhythm control with brief, self-terminating AT, asymptomatic brief AF/AT, asymptomatic paroxysmal AF, or atrial tachycardia of very brief duration (seconds to < 1 min). A minority has infrequent sustained and symptomatic paroxysmal AF. AT = atrial tachycardia; AF, atrial fibrillation; pers/perm, permanent/persistent; PAF, paroxysmal AF. Source: Reproduced with permission from Epstein et al.[76]

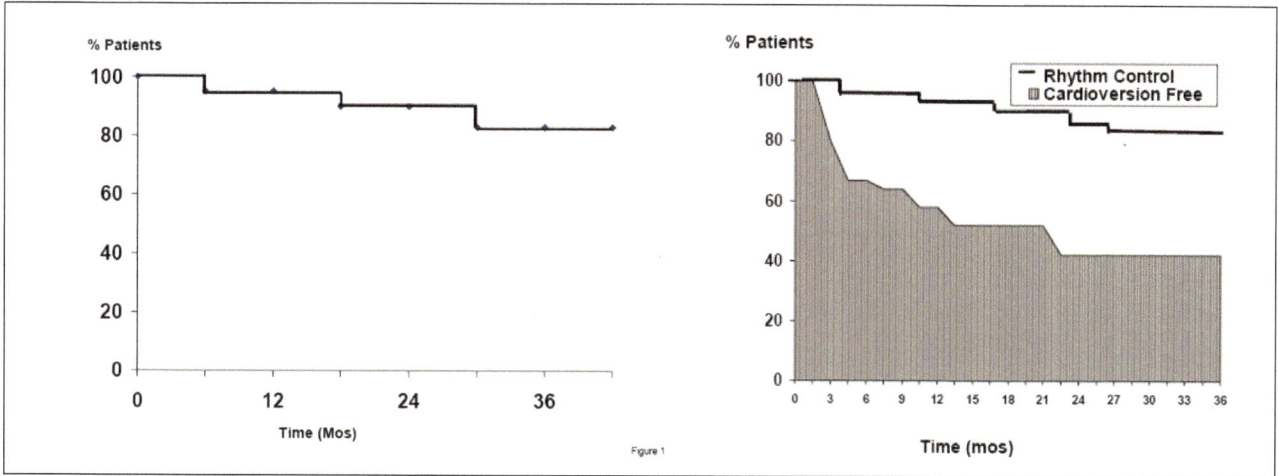

Figure 67.14 **Left panel:** Actuarial curve showing long-term freedom from persistent AF after hybrid pacing, drug and ablation therapy, which was 97%, 90%, and 83% at 6 months, 2 years, and 3 years, respectively. **Right panel:** Freedom from persistent AF (shown as rhythm control) and cardioversion (shown as cardioversion free) in the study group. Fifty-three percent of the patients experienced AF recurrences requiring cardioversion, which enabled maintenance for 83% of the patients free of AF. Source: Reproduced with permission from Epstein et al.[76]

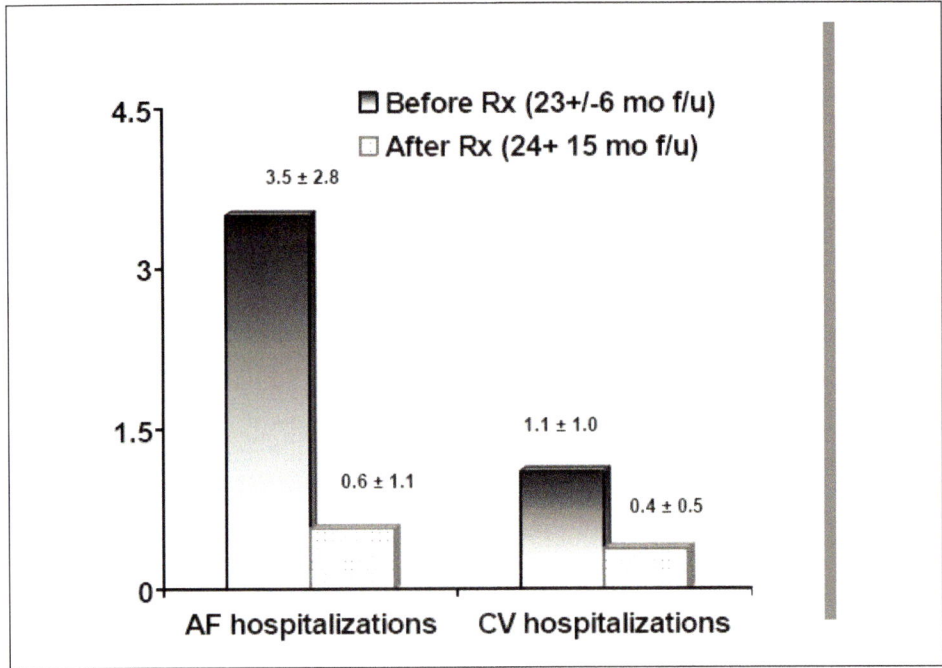

Figure 67.15 Mean AF hospitalizations and cardioversions per patient declined significantly following hybrid therapy. *Source:* Reproduced with permission from Epstein et al.[76]

(HFrEF) (median follow-up, 5.1 years). Eighty-nine percent of HFpEF patients and 85% of HFrEF patients were in rhythm control at last follow-up. Overall survival was 62% at 5 years, with higher survival in the HFpEF (78%) versus HFrEF (50%; $P = 0.02$).

Hybrid Therapy in Patients with AF without Bradycardias

Boccadamo and coworkers first reported the use of dual-site RA pacing in a pilot group of patients with AF without bradyarrhythmias with a mean age of 65 years.[79] All patients had comorbidities (hypertension in 12; dilated cardiomyopathy in 3). Persistent AF was present in 8 patients and paroxysmal AF in 7 patients; mean AF duration was 61 months (range 3–216 months, mean LA diameter was 39 mm (range 33–46 mm), and mean LV ejection fraction was 55% (range 18%–81%). Single-chamber atrial pacing was used in 10 patients, dual-chamber in 5 patients. The mean duration of follow-up was 24 ± 12 months (range 3–41). Twelve patients showed substantial improvement in AF events. During this period, the number of episodes of AF decreased from a mean of 13 ± 38 (range 1–150) to 0.4 ± 0.7 (range 0–2.3) per month ($P < 0.001$). In the subgroup of patients with persistent AF, the number of episodes decreased from a mean of 20.4 ± 52.4 (range 1–150) to 0.6 ± 0.9 (range 0–2.3) ($P < 0.001$). In patients with paroxysmal AF, the number of episodes decreased from 4.6 ± 3.5 (range 2–12) to 0.2 ± 0.5 (range 0–1.4) ($P < 0.001$). One patient (6.7%) developed permanent AF 16 months after the implant, with 2 remaining patients (13%) showing no improvement. After the pacemaker implant, the number of class 1 antiarrhythmic drugs fell from 18 to 6 ($P < 0.001$) and that of class 2 changed from 0 to 7 ($P < 0.001$). The use of class 3 and 4 did not change significantly.

We have analyzed our experience related to the presence or absence of primary bradycardias with respect to rhythm control. Figure 67.16 shows the long-term outcome of patients with refractory AF with or without primary bradycardias at presentation. Note that there is no difference in the degree of rhythm control achieved in both groups. Thus, patients without primary bradycardias achieved >80% long-term rhythm control with hybrid therapy.

There are several potential roles for hybrid therapy and atrial resynchronization (Table 67.6). These include primary prevention of AF in patients with sick sinus syndrome to prevent the development of AF or its progression. In secondary prevention, there are several possible target populations. These include brady–tachy syndrome, drug-refractory paroxysmal or persistent AF, and patients with ventricular arrhythmias requiring ICD therapy. In this latter group, dual-site RA pacing has been performed. New roles in heart failure populations, with and without systolic dysfunction, are being explored. They may include primary prevention or secondary prevention of AF as well as management of heart failure. Future clinical studies should elucidate these opportunities for application. Finally, the large majority of elderly patients with AF may have a therapeutic option beyond antiarrhythmic drugs alone with hybrid drug, device, and ablation therapy.

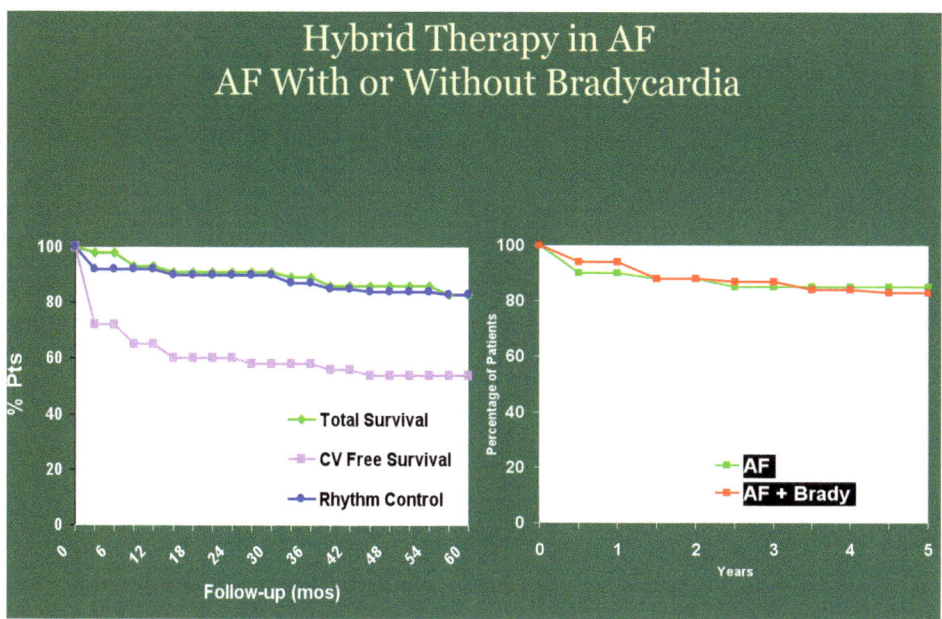

Figure 67.16 Long-term rhythm control in patients with and without primary bradycardia after hybrid therapy incorporating dual-site right atrial pacing. **Left panel:** Overall rhythm control, actuarial survival, and cardioversion free survival in 113 patients during long-term follow-up. **Right panel:** Long-term rhythm control based on the presence or absence of primary bradyarrhythmia warranting pacemaker insertion. *Source:* Derived from Saksena et al. *Heart Rhythm.* 2004;1:S271.

Table 67.6 Future roles of hybrid therapy

Potential patient populations for atrial resynchronization

Primary prevention of AF
- Stand-alone therapy:
  – Upstream therapy in sick sinus syndrome

Secondary prevention of AF
- In a treatment strategy for:
  – Bradycardia–tachycardia syndrome with AF
  – Symptomatic drug-refractory paroxysmal AF
  – Drug-refractory persistent AF
  – Congestive heart failure with drug-refractory AF
  – Ventricular arrhythmias requiring ICD therapy with refractory AF
- Novel therapeutic option for:
  – Elderly populations with symptomatic, drug-refractory paroxysmal or persistent AF and primary or secondary bradycardia

Conclusions

Hybrid therapy combining antiarrhythmic drugs, dual-site atrial pacing, and catheter ablation shows promise in patients with refractory to antiarrhythmic drugs, atrial pacing alone, or catheter ablation. Presence of concomitant bradycardias, either primary or drug-induced, is currently approved as a class 2 indication for dual-site atrial pacing. This avenue offers a particular advantage to elderly populations with refractory AF for whom antiarrhythmic drugs offer a limited and sole therapeutic option for rhythm control and demand ventricular or single-site atrial pacing is used solely to prevent bradyarrhythmias. In these patients, hybrid therapy with dual-site RA pacing or limited catheter ablation in the RA offers promise for rhythm control.

References

1. Califf RL, DeMets DM. Principles from clinical trials relevant to clinical practice: Part III. *Circulation.* 2002;106:1015-1021.
2. Santangeli P, Di Biase L, Natale A. Ablation versus drugs: what is the best first-line therapy for paroxysmal atrial fibrillation? Antiarrhythmic drugs are outmoded and catheter ablation should be the first-line option for all patients with paroxysmal atrial fibrillation: Pro. *Circ Arrhythm Electrophysiol.* 2014;7(4):739-746.
3. Fragakis N, Koskinas KC, Katritsis DG, Pagourelias ED, Zografos T, Geleris P. Comparison of effectiveness of ranolazine plus amiodarone versus amiodarone alone for conversion of recent-onset atrial fibrillation. *Am J Cardiol.* 2012;110(5):673-677.
4. Madrid AH, Bueno MG, Rebollo JM, et al. Use of irbesartan to maintain sinus rhythm in patients with long-lasting persistent atrial fibrillation: a prospective and randomized study. *Circulation.* 2002;106(3):331-336.
5. Saksena S, Slee A, Waldo AL, et al. Cardiovascular outcomes in the AFFIRM trial (Atrial Fibrillation Follow-Up Investigation of Rhythm Management): an assessment of individual antiarrhythmic drug therapies compared with rate control with propensity score-matched analyses. *J Am Coll Cardiol.* 2011;58:1975-1985.
6. Køber L, Bloch Thomsen PE, Møller M, et al; Danish Investigations of Arrhythmia and Mortality on Dofetilide (DIAMOND) Study Group. Effect of dofetilide in patients with recent myocardial infarction and left-ventricular dysfunction: a randomised trial. *Lancet.* 2000;356(9247):2052-2058.
7. Hohnloser SH, Crijns HJ, van Eickels M, et al; ATHENA Investigators. Effect of dronedarone on cardiovascular events in atrial fibrillation. *N Engl J Med.* 2009 Feb 12;360(7):668-678.
8. Køber L, Torp-Pedersen C, McMurray JJ, et al, for the Dronedarone Study Group. Increased mortality after dronedarone therapy for severe heart failure. *N Engl J Med.* 2008;358(25):2678-2687.
9. Connolly SJ, Camm AJ, Halperin JL, et al, for the PALLAS Investigators. Dronedarone in high-risk permanent atrial fibrillation. *N Engl J Med.* 2011;365(24):2268-2276.

10. Saksena S, Slee A, Liu T, Verma A, Rathod S. Impact of treatment strategies on clinical outcomes of atrial fibrillation patients with thyroid disease. *J Am Coll Cardiol.* 2010;55(10 Suppl 1):A6.E59.
11. Kay GN, Ellenbogen KA, Giudici M, et al. The Ablate and Pace Trial: a prospective study of catheter ablation of the AV conduction system and permanent pacemaker implantation for treatment of atrial fibrillation. APT Investigators. *J Interv Card Electrophysiol.* 1998;2(2):121-135.
12. Brignole M, Botto G, Mont L, et al. Cardiac resynchronization therapy in patients undergoing atrioventricular junction ablation for permanent atrial fibrillation: a randomized trial. *Eur Heart J.* 2011;32(19):2420-2429.
13. Burashnikov A, Sicouri S, Di Diego JM, Belardinelli L, Antzelevitch C. Synergistic effect of the combination of ranolazine and dronedarone to suppress atrial fibrillation. *J Am Coll Cardiol.* 2010;56(15):1216-1224.
14. Allessie M. The "second factor": a first step toward diagnosing the substrate of atrial fibrillation? *J Am Coll Cardiol.* 2009;53(14):1192-1193.
15. Schotten U, Duytschaever M, Ausma J, Eijsbouts S, Neuberger HR, Allessie M. Electrical and contractile remodeling during the first days of atrial fibrillation go hand in hand. *Circulation.* 2003;107(10):1433-1439.
16. Yue L, Feng J, Gaspo R, Li GR, Wang Z, Nattel S. Ionic remodeling underlying action potential changes in a canine model of atrial fibrillation. *Circ Res.* 1997;81(4):512-525.
17. Burstein B, Qi XY, Yeh YH, Calderone A, Nattel S. Atrial cardiomyocyte tachycardia alters cardiac fibroblast function: a novel consideration in atrial remodeling. *Cardiovasc Res.* 2007;76(3):442-452.
18. Ausma J, Wijffels M, Thoné F, Wouters L, Allessie M, Borgers M. Structural changes of atrial myocardium due to sustained atrial fibrillation in the goat. *Circulation.* 1997;96(9):3157-3156.
19. Danshi Li, Samir Fareh, Tack Ki Leung, Stanley Nattel, M. Promotion of atrial fibrillation by heart failure in dogs: atrial remodeling of a different sort. *Circulation.* 1999;100(1):87-95.
20. Gray RA, Pertsov AM, Jalife J. Spatial and temporal organization during cardiac fibrillation. *Nature.* 1998;392:75-78.
21. Allessie M, de Groot N. Rotors have not been demonstrated to be the drivers of atrial fibrillation. *J Physiol.* 2014;592(Pt 15):3167-3170.
22. Saksena S, Skadsberg N, Rao H, Filipecki A. Biatrial and 3-dimensional mapping of spontaneous atrial arrhythmias in patients with refractory atrial fibrillation. *J Cardiovasc Electrophysiol.* 2005;16(5):494-504.
23. Narayan SM, Krummen DE, Shivkumar K, Clopton P, Rappel W-J, Miller J. Treatment of atrial fibrillation by the ablation of localized sources: the Conventional Ablation for Atrial Fibrillation With or Without Focal Impulse and Rotor Modulation: CONFIRM Trial. *J Am Coll Cardiol.* 2012;60:628-636.
24. Nademanee K, McKenzie J, Kosar E, et al. A new approach for catheter ablation of atrial fibrillation: mapping of the electrophysiologic substrate. *J Am Coll Cardiol.* 2004;43(11):2044-2053.
25. Saksena S, Madan N. Hybrid therapy for atrial fibrillation: algorithms and outcome. *J Interv Card Electrophysiol.* 2003;9:235-247.
26. Saksena S, Prakash A, Hill M, et al. Prevention of recurrent atrial fibrillation with chronic dual-site right atrial pacing. *J Am Coll Cardiol.* 1996;28(3):687-694.
27. Delfaut P, Saksena S, Prakash A, Krol RB. Long-term outcome of patients with drug-refractory atrial flutter and fibrillation after single- and dual-site right atrial pacing for arrhythmia prevention. *J Am Coll Cardiol.* 1998;32(7):1900-1908.
28. Madan N, Saksena S. Long-term rhythm control of drug-refractory atrial fibrillation with "hybrid therapy" incorporating dual-site right atrial pacing, antiarrhythmic drugs, and right atrial ablation. *Am J Cardiol.* 2004;93(5):569-575.
29. Prakash A, Delfaut P, Krol RB, Saksena S. Regional right and left atrial activation patterns during single- and dual-site atrial pacing in patients with atrial fibrillation. *Am J Cardiol.* 1998;82,(10):1197-1204.
30. Prakash A, Saksena S, Ziegler P, et al. Dual site right atrial pacing can improve the impact of standard dual chamber pacing on atrial and ventricular mechanical function in patients with symptomatic atrial fibrillation: further observations from the Dual Site Atrial Pacing for Prevention of Atrial Fibrillation Trial. *J Interv Card Electrophysiol.* 2005;12(3):177-187.
31. Nagarakanti R, Slee A, Saksena S. Left atrial reverse remodeling and prevention of progression of atrial fibrillation with atrial resynchronization device therapy utilizing dual-site right atrial pacing in patients with atrial fibrillation refractory to antiarrhythmic drugs or catheter ablation. *J Interv Card Electrophysiol.* 2014;40(3):245-254.
32. Al-Khatib SM, Allen LaPointe NM, Chatterjee R, et al. Rate and rhythm-control therapies in patients with atrial fibrillation: a systematic review. *Ann Intern Med.* 2014;160(11):760-773.
33. Morillo CA, Verma A, Connolly SJ, et al.; RAAFT-2 Investigators. Radiofrequency ablation vs antiarrhythmic drugs as first-line treatment of paroxysmal atrial fibrillation (RAAFT-2): a randomized trial. *JAMA.* 2014;311(7):692-700.
34. Cappato R, Calkins H, Chen SA, et al. Worldwide survey on the methods, efficacy, and safety of catheter ablation for human atrial fibrillation. *Circulation.* 2005;111(9):1100-1105.
35. Cappato R, Calkins H, Chen SA, et al. Updated worldwide survey on the methods, efficacy, and safety of catheter ablation for human atrial fibrillation. *Circ Arrhythm Electrophysiol.* 2010;3(1):32-38.
36. Cheema A, Vasamreddy CR, Dalal D, et al. Long-term single procedure efficacy of catheter ablation of atrial fibrillation. *J Interv Card Electrophysiol.* 2006;15(3):145-155.
37. Scherr D, Khairy P, Miyazaki S, et al. Five-year outcome of catheter ablation of persistent atrial fibrillation using termination of atrial fibrillation as a procedural endpoint. *Circ Arrhythm Electrophysiol.* 2014. Pii:CIRCEP.114.001943. [Epub ahead of print]
38. Turco P, De Simone A, La Rocca V, et al. Long-term results of hybrid therapy in patients with atrial fibrillation who develop atrial flutter during flecainide infusion. *Pacing Clin Electrophysiol.* 2005;28 Suppl 1:S124-S127.
39. Dixit S, Marchlinski FE, Lin D, et al. Randomized ablation strategies for the treatment of persistent atrial fibrillation: RASTA study. *Circ Arrhythm Electrophysiol.* 2012;5(2):287-294.
40. Calkins H, Reynolds MR, Spector P, et al. Treatment of atrial fibrillation with antiarrhythmic drugs or radiofrequency ablation: two systematic literature reviews and meta-analyses *Circ Arrhythm Electrophysiol.* 2009;2:349-361.
41. Arbelo E, Brugada J, Hindricks G, et al. The atrial fibrillation ablation pilot study: a European survey on methodology and results of catheter ablation for atrial fibrillation. *Eur Heart J.* 2014;35:1466-1478.
42. Schumacher B, Jung W, Lewalter T, Vahlhaus C, Wolpert C. Radiofrequency ablation of atrial flutter due to administration of class IC antiarrhythmic drugs for atrial fibrillation. *Am J Cardiol.* 1999;83(5):710-713.
43. Stabile G, De Simone A, Turco P, et al. Response to flecainide infusion predicts long-term success of hybrid pharmacologic

and ablation therapy in patients with atrial fibrillation. *J Am Coll Cardiol.* 2001;37(6):1639-1644.
44. Anastasio N, Frankel DS, Deyell MW, et al. Nearly uniform failure of atrial flutter ablation and continuation of antiarrhythmic agents (hybrid therapy) for the long-term control of atrial fibrillation. *J Interv Card Electrophysiol.* 2012;35(1):57-61.
45. Garcia Seara J, Raposeiras Roubin S, Gude Sampedro F, et al. Failure of hybrid therapy for the prevention of long-term recurrence of atrial fibrillation. *Int J Cardiol.* 2014;176(1):74-79.
46. Prakash A, Saksena S, Krol RB, Filipecki A, Philip G. Catheter ablation of inducible atrial flutter, in combination with atrial pacing and antiarrhythmic drugs ("hybrid therapy") improves rhythm control in patients with refractory atrial fibrillation. *J Interv Card Electrophysiol.* 2002;6(2):165-172.
47. Andersen HR, Nielsen JC, Thomsen PEB, et al. Long-term follow-up of patients from a randomized trial of atrial versus ventricular pacing for sick sinus syndrome. *Lancet.* 1997;350:1210-1216.
48. Lamas GA, Lee K, Sweeney MO, et al. Ventricular pacing or dual-chamber pacing for sinus-node dysfunction. The Mode Selection Trial (MOST) in sinus node dysfunction. *J Am Coll Cardiol.* 2002;346:1854-1862.
49. Saksena S, Prakash A, Ziegler P, et al. for the DAPPAF investigators: The Dual-Site Atrial Pacing for Prevention of Atrial Fibrillation (DAPPAF) trial: improved suppression of recurrent atrial fibrillation with dual site atrial pacing and antiarrhythmic drug therapy. *J Am Coll Cardiol.* 2002;40:1140-1150.
50. Padeletti L, Purefellner H, Adler SW, for the Worldwide ASPECT Investigators. Combined efficacy of atrial septal lead placement and atrial pacing algorithms for prevention of paroxysmal atrial tachyarrhythmia. *J Cardiovasc Electrophysiol.* 2003;14:1189-1195.
51. Carlson M, Ip J, Messenger J, et al. A new pacemaker algorithm for the treatment of atrial fibrillation. Results of the Atrial Dynamic Overdrive Pacing (ADOPT) Trial. *J Am Coll Cardiol.* 2003;42(4):627-633.
52. Lau CP, Tachapong N, Wang C-C, et al.; SAFE study investigators. Prospective randomized study to assess the efficacy of site and rate of atrial pacing on long-term progression of atrial fibrillation in sick sinus syndrome: Septal Pacing for Atrial Fibrillation Suppression Evaluation (SAFE) Study. *Circulation.* 2013;128:687-693.
53. Lin AC, Knight BP. SAFE combinations fail to open the door to atrial fibrillation prevention. *Circulation.* 2013;128(7):679-680.
54. Sweeney MO, Bank AJ, Nash E, et al. for the Search AV Extension and Managed Ventricular Pacing for Promoting Atrioventricular Conduction (SAVE PACe) Trial. Minimizing ventricular pacing to reduce atrial fibrillation in sinus-node disease. *N Engl J Med.* 2007;357:1000-1008.
55. Attuel P, Childers R, Cauchemez B, Poveda J, Mugica J, Coumel P. Failure in the rate adaptation of the atrial refractory period: its relationship to vulnerability. *Int J Cardiol.* 1982;2(2):179-197.
56. Daubert C, Gras D, Berder V, Leclercq C, Mabo P. [Permanent atrial resynchronization by synchronous bi-atrial pacing in the preventive treatment of atrial flutter associated with high degree interatrial block]. *Arch Mal Coeur Vaiss.* 1994;87(11 Suppl):1535-1534.
57. Josephson MA, Seides S. *Clinical Cardiac Electrophysiology.* Philadelphia: Lea and Febiger, 1979.
58. Daubert JC, Pavin D, Jauvert G, Mabo P. Intra- and interatrial conduction delay: implications for cardiac pacing. *Pacing Clin Electrophysiol.* 2004;27(4):507-502.
59. Ariyarajah V, Mercado K, Apiyasawat S, et al. Correlation of left atrial size with P-wave duration in interatrial block. *Chest.* 2005;128: 2615-2618.
60. Laurent G, Eicher JC, Mathe A, et al. Permanent left atrial pacing therapy may improve symptoms in heart failure patients with preserved ejection fraction and atrial dyssynchrony: a pilot study prior to a national clinical research programme. *Eur J Heart Fail.* 2013;15(1):85-93.
61. Duytschaever M, Danse P, Eysbouts S, Allessie M. Is there an optimal pacing site to prevent atrial fibrillation? An experimental study in the chronically instrumented goat. *J Cardiovasc Electrophysiol.* 2002;13(12):1264-1271.
62. Szili-Torok T, Kimman GJ, Scholten MF, et al. Interatrial septum pacing guided by three-dimensional intracardiac echocardiography. *J Am Coll Cardiol.* 2002;40:2139-2143.
63. Prakash A, Saksena S, Hill M, et al. Acute effects of dual-site right atrial pacing in patients with spontaneous and inducible atrial flutter and fibrillation. *J Am Coll Cardiol.* 1997;29(5):1007-1014.
64. Doi A, Takagi M, Toda I, Yoshiyama M, Takeuchi K, Yoshikawa J. Acute hemodynamic benefits of biatrial atrioventricular sequential pacing: comparison with single atrial atrioventricular sequential pacing. *Heart.* 2004;90(4):411-448.
65. Takagi M, Doi A, Shirai N, et al. Acute improvement of atrial mechanical stunning after electrical cardioversion of persistent atrial fibrillation: comparison between biatrial and single atrial pacing. *Heart.* 2005;91(1):58-63.
66. Burri H, Bennani I, Domenichini G, et al. Biatrial pacing improves atrial haemodynamics and atrioventricular timing compared with pacing from the right atrial appendage. *Europace.* 2011;13(9):1262-1267.
67. Matsumoto A, Ishikawa T, Sumita S, et al. Assessment of atrial regional wall motion using strain Doppler imaging during biatrial pacing in the bradycardia-tachycardia syndrome. *Pacing Clin Electrophysiol.* 2006;29:220-225.
68. Dabrowska-Kugacka A, Lewicka-Noval E, Rucinksi P, et al. Atrial electromechanical sequence and contraction synchrony during single- and multisite atrial pacing in patients with brady-tachycardia syndrome. *Pacing Clin Electrophysiol.* 2009;32:591-603.
69. D'Allonnes GR, Pavin D, Leclerq C, et al. Long-term effects of bi-atrial synchronous pacing to prevent drug refractory atrial tachyarrhythmia: a nine-year experience. *J Cardiovasc Electrophysiol.* 2000;11:1081-1091.
70. Bailin SJ, Adler S, Guidici M. Prevention of chronic atrial fibrillation by pacing in the region of Bachmann bundle: results from a multicenter randomized trial. *J Cardiovasc Electrophysiol.* 2001;12:912-917.
71. Padeletti L, Pieragnoli P, Ciapetti C, et al. Randomized crossover comparison of right atrial appendage pacing versus interatrial septum pacing for prevention of paroxysmal atrial fibrillation in patients with sinus bradycardia. *Am Heart J.* 2001;142:1047-1055.
72. Ricci R, Santini M, Puglisi A, et al. Impact of consistent atrial pacing algorithm on premature atrial complexes number and paroxysmal atrial fibrillation recurrences in brady-tachy syndrome: a randomized prospective cross-over study. *J Interv Card Electrophysiol.* 2001;5:33-44.
73. Mabo P, Paul V, Jung W, et al. Biatrial synchronous pacing for atrial arrhythmia prevention: the SYNBIAPACE study. *Eur Heart J.* (abstr) 1999:20:4.
74. Filipecki A, Saksena S, Prakash A, Philip G. Improved rhythm control with overdrive atrial pacing and right linear right atrial ablation in patients with persistent and permanent atrial fibrillation. *Am J Cardiol.* 2002;6:165-172.

75. Rao HB, Saksena S. Impact of "hybrid therapy" on long-term rhythm control and arrhythmia related hospitalizations in patients with drug-refractory persistent and permanent atrial fibrillation. *J Interv Card Electrophysiol.* 2007;18:127-136.
76. Epstein AE, DiMarco JP, Ellenbogen KA, et al. American College of Cardiology/American Heart Association Task Force on Practice Guidelines (Writing Committee to Revise the ACC/AHA/NASPE 2002 Guideline Update for Implantation of Cardiac Pacemakers and Antiarrhythmia Devices); American Association for Thoracic Surgery; Society of Thoracic Surgeons. ACC/AHA/HRS 2008 guidelines for device-based therapy of cardiac rhythm abnormalities: a report of the American College of Cardiology/American Heart Association Task Force on Practice Guidelines (Writing Committee to Revise the ACC/AHA/NASPE 2002 Guideline Update for Implantation of Cardiac Pacemakers and Antiarrhythmia Devices) developed in collaboration with the American Association for Thoracic Surgery and Society of Thoracic Surgeons. *J Am Coll Cardiol.* 2008;51:e1-e62.
77. Epstein AE, DiMarco JP, Ellenbogen KA, et al. American College of Cardiology Foundation. ACC/AHA/HRS 2012 guidelines for device-based therapy of cardiac rhythm abnormalities: a report of the American College of Cardiology/American Heart Association Task Force on Practice Guidelines developed in collaboration with the American Association for Thoracic Surgery and Society of Thoracic Surgeons. Guidelines. *J Am Coll Cardiol.* 2013;22;61(3):e6-e75.
78. Saksena S, Saad M, Slee A, et al. Atrial resynchronization combined with "background" antiarrhythmic therapy improves survival in in patients with atrial fibrillation and heart failure with or without systolic left ventricular dysfunction. *J Interv Card Electrophysiol.* 2015 (in press).
79. Boccadamo R, Di Belardino N, Mammucari A, Boccadamo V. Dual site right atrial pacing in the prevention of symptomatic atrial fibrillation refractory to drug therapy and unrelated to sinus bradycardia. *J Interv Card Electrophysiol.* 2002;6(2):141-147.
80. Marrouche, et al. *J Am Coll Cardiol.* 2002;40:464-474.

Video Legends

Video 67.1   3D EnSite array balloon mapping of high right atrial pacing in a patient with refractory atrial flutter and atrial fibrillation before cavotricuspid isthmus ablation. Note that the left image shows a right lateral view and the right image shows a left anterior oblique view of the activation wavefront as it arises in the high lateral right atrium and propagates anteromedially and then inferiorly terminating at the inferior vena cava ostium in this patient.

Video 67.2   3D EnSite array balloon mapping of coronary sinus ostial pacing in a patient with refractory atrial flutter and AF before cavotricuspid isthmus ablation. Note that the left image shows a right lateral view and the right image shows a left anterior oblique view of the activation wavefront as it arises inferiorly at the posterior right atrium near the ostium. It propagates superiorly along the septum and posterior right atrium before emerging in the high atrium and anteriorly in this patient. Regional wall motion activation in the right atrium differs markedly from the high right atrial pacing wavefront.

Video 67.3   3D EnSite array balloon mapping of dual-site right atrial pacing in a patient with refractory atrial flutter and AF before cavotricuspid isthmus ablation. Note that the left image shows a right lateral view and the right image shows a left anterior oblique view. Two simultaneous wavefronts are seen, superiorly and inferiorly, which activate all regions of the right atrium much more rapidly and simultaneously than during any single-site pacing mode.

Video 67.4   3D EnSite array balloon mapping of dual-site right atrial pacing in a patient with refractory atrial flutter and AF. Cavotricuspid isthmus linear ablation lesions and failure of paced wavefront to cross the linear lesion created by ablation. The wavefront leading edge is shown by the motion of the red asterisk, and it reflects off the line and propagates posteriorly.

Video 67.5   3D EnSite array balloon mapping of propagation of atrial paced in a patient with refractory AF after right atrial compartmentalization. Linear lesions are created with radiofrequency ablation in the lateral right atrium (intercaval line), superior vena cava to fossa ovalis to coronary sinus ostium to tricuspid valve (septal line) and cavotricuspid isthmus line (isthmus) line.

A: The 3D map is shown in the anterior projection and propagation of a paced wavefront in the anterior compartment is shown. Note that the wavefront remains confined to the anterior right atrial compartment and reflects off the linear lesions.

B: The 3D map is shown in the posterocaudal projection and propagation of a paced wavefront in the posterior compartment is shown. Note that the wavefront arises at the coronary sinus ostial region and remains confined to the posteroseptal right atrial compartment and reflects off the linear lesions.

CHAPTER 68

Staged Therapy Approaches in Atrial Fibrillation

Mario D. Gonzalez, MD; Gerald V. Naccarelli, MD

Abstract

Atrial fibrillation (AF) is the most common cardiac arrhythmia requiring therapy and is associated with significant morbidity and mortality. The therapeutic strategies for treating AF include rate control, maintenance of sinus rhythm, and prevention of embolic events. Treatment of AF should also improve quality of life and survival. The effects of different therapeutic modalities on mortality have not been established. Treatment needs to be individualized to each patient and a given patient may require different therapies over time. When AF results in symptoms or in deterioration of left ventricular function, restoration and maintenance of sinus rhythm is required. This can be achieved with drugs and/or ablation therapy. Antiarrhythmic drugs unfortunately have a low success rate and may result in proarrhythmia, heart failure, or extra cardiac adverse effects. Catheter ablation is emerging as a superior alternative to drugs. Several studies have shown that catheter ablation is associated with better sinus rhythm maintenance than currently available antiarrhythmic drugs. However, it is an invasive procedure that can result in serious complications. Catheter ablation is only performed by a limited number of electrophysiologists who are not able to cope with the growing population of AF patients. Pharmacologic and ablative therapies should not be considered competing approaches but rather staged or complementary treatments in patients with AF. Ablation is usually considered when antiarrhythmic drugs fail to maintain AF and antiarrhythmic drugs are required before and following ablation. New antiarrhythmic drug strategies include more atrial selective agents, drugs similar to amiodarone but with less toxic profiles, or drugs with novel mechanisms of action such as gap junction facilitation of conduction.

Introduction

AF prevalence is increasing steadily and will more than double in the next 50 years.[1-3] Although the reasons for this increase in occurrence are not well known, the aging of the population and the increasing prevalence of hypertension, obesity, metabolic syndrome, and sleep apnea may explain this phenomenon. Treatment of this arrhythmia currently consumes 1% of the healthcare budget in developed countries.[4]

Despite our incomplete understating of the pathophysiology of AF, treatment has improved due to the recent development of new techniques in catheter ablation, new antiarrhythmic drugs, pacing, and anticoagulation. All therapies have limitations regarding efficacy and safety and frequently more than one therapeutic modality is used simultaneously or sequentially to treat patients with AF. Antiarrhythmic drugs are limited by frequent recurrences, adverse effects, and proarrhythmia. Catheter ablation has only moderate success, and the procedure must be repeated in approximately 25% of patients due to recurrence of conduction between the pulmonary veins and the left atrium, the presence of extra pulmonary foci, and/or abnormal atrial substrate. Repeat procedures are required more often in patients with persistent AF due to more extensive electrical abnormalities. Catheter ablation may be considered curative in patients in whom the substrate or the source of the arrhythmia is relatively localized, while in most patients the procedure should be considered palliative since the abnormal substrate is modified but not normalized. Hence, some patients—especially those with persistent AF—will require antiarrhythmic drugs to maintain sinus rhythm even after ablation has been performed. This cannot be considered a failure of the procedure since drugs are effective in many cases only after catheter ablation has been performed.

Catheter Ablation of AF

The groundbreaking discovery of Dr. Michel Haïssaguerre[5] accelerated the use of catheter ablation of AF. He recognized that in patients with paroxysmal AF, the arrhythmia is initiated by focal triggers emanating from the pulmonary veins. The initial strategy was aimed to eliminate these foci inside the veins but eventually resulted in unacceptable rates of pulmonary vein stenosis. The same author introduced a circular mapping catheter that records both atrial and pulmonary vein potentials at the ostium of these veins, which allows electrical isolation of the pulmonary veins from the left atrium by delivering radiofrequency ablation proximal to the ostium, without damaging these veins. Elimination of these triggers or isolation of the pulmonary veins prevents recurrence of paroxysmal AF in most patients. Eventually other sites were recognized, including the superior vena cava, the coronary sinus, and the atrial walls. The limitation has been that these early findings in patients with paroxysmal AF cannot be easily applied to patients with persistent AF who have more extensive abnormalities in the atrial substrate that predispose to the development and maintenance of AF.

At present, there is no uniform technique of AF ablation, but pulmonary vein isolation is the required first step in most patients with or without atrial substrate modification.[6] The procedure is tailored to each individual patient based on the clinical presentation, structural abnormalities, and the electrophysiologic findings during the procedure. Focal discharges from the walls of the left atrium, superior vena cava, and coronary sinus can also initiate AF (Figures 68.1 and 68.2). Elimination of these abnormal foci and substrate result in a success rate of approximately 75% in paroxysmal AF and 50% to 60% in persistent AF.[7] However, more than one procedure is required in many patients to achieve these results. This is especially true in patients with persistent AF. Recurrences after AF ablation can be explained due to resumption of conduction from the pulmonary veins into the left atrium,[8] persistence of focal sources (Figures 68.1 and 68.2), and/or an abnormal atrial substrate. By ablating within the left atrium, it is assumed that the abnormal substrate that initiates or supports AF will be eliminated. Ablation in the left atrium can be performed by creating lines of block between fixed anatomical obstacles, for example, between the left inferior pulmonary vein and the mitral annulus[9] (Figure 68.3) or by eliminating complex fractionated atrial electrograms recorded during AF[10] or during sinus rhythm[11-12] (Figure 68.4). The premise is that these complex electrograms represent an abnormal atrial substrate that maintains AF. Some, but not all, studies suggest that wider lesion sets are more efficacious than lesions closer to the ostia.[13,14] Extensive lesions increase the risk of embolic events, proarrhythmia, and esophageal injury. The esophagus is located very close to the posterior wall of the left atrium between the right and left pulmonary veins. Increasing numbers of left atrial esophageal fistulae have been reported.[15] This complication is rare, but it is almost always fatal. Although catheter ablation can eliminate AF in many patients, the procedure still has several limitations. AF cannot be eliminated in all patients; moreover, AF ablation requires extensive experience in transseptal catheterization,[16] detailed knowledge of left atrial anatomy and physiology, and the use of novel mapping and ablation techniques. Even in experienced centers, catheter ablation of AF can result in serious complications.[17] Finally, only a small percentage of world population with AF can undergo an ablation procedure due to the limited number of centers and experienced cardiac electrophysiologists.

Electrical isolation just proximal to the pulmonary vein ostia is effective in patients with paroxysmal AF but less successful in those with persistent AF[18] (Figure 68.5). This is not surprising since abnormalities in atrial conduction and refractoriness are usually present in patients with persistent AF.[19] Wide area circumferential ablation that involves atrial tissue proximal to the pulmonary veins is more successful in persistent AF.[20] Whichever approach is chosen, electrical isolation of the pulmonary veins has to be documented. Finally, mapping and ablation of complex fractionated electrograms (CFAEs) during AF, which possibly represent anisotropic reentry leading to rotors with high dominant frequency, can slow AF cycle length, convert to atrial tachycardia, or convert patients to sinus rhythm.[21] For more extensive atrial disease, the use of linear lesions may improve outcome or treat iatrogenic reentrant atrial tachycardias that occur after extensive ablation in the left atrium (Figure 68.6). By creating areas of complete block within the atria, the potential for macroreentrant atrial tachycardias is reduced or eliminated. However, this approach can paradoxically increase the risk of macroreentrant left atrial tachycardia development as slow conduction may develop when the lines are not

Chapter 68: Staged Therapy Approaches in Atrial Fibrillation

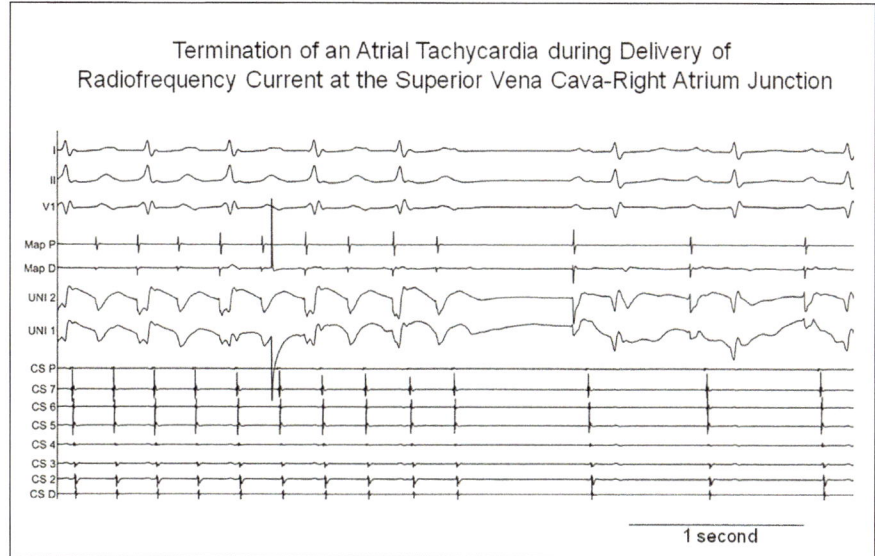

Figure 68.1 Focal source of atrial tachycardia originating at the superior vena cava-right atrial (SVC-RA) junction. Following electrical isolation of the pulmonary veins, AF could not be induced, but a regular tachycardia was induced during administration of isoproterenol 4 mcg/min. This tachycardia was eliminated by ablation at the SVC-RA junction.

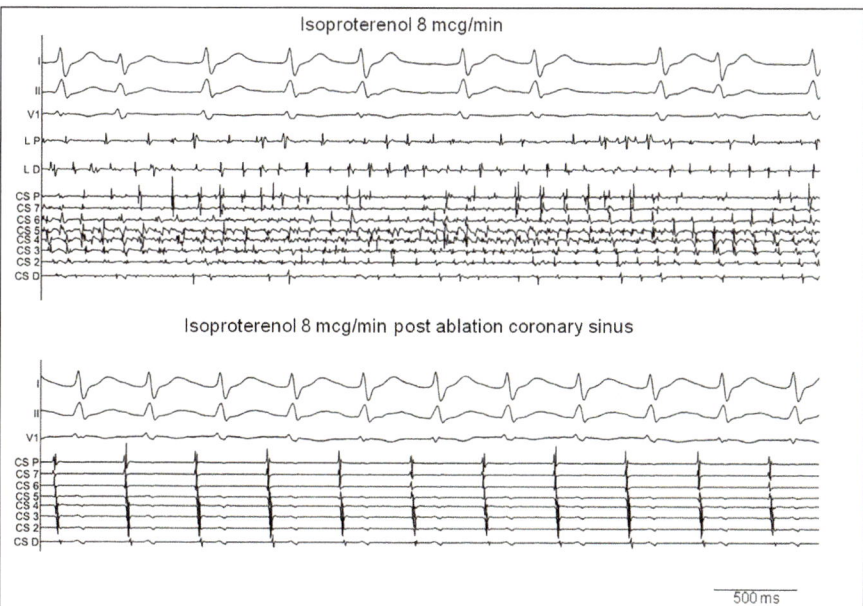

Figure 68.2 Focal source of AF originating from the coronary sinus musculature. The patient has had a previous pulmonary vein isolation procedure but had recurrence of AF. During administration of isoproterenol 8 mcg/min, rapid atrial activity was recorded in the coronary sinus (CS). Ablation in the CS prevented the reinduction of AF.

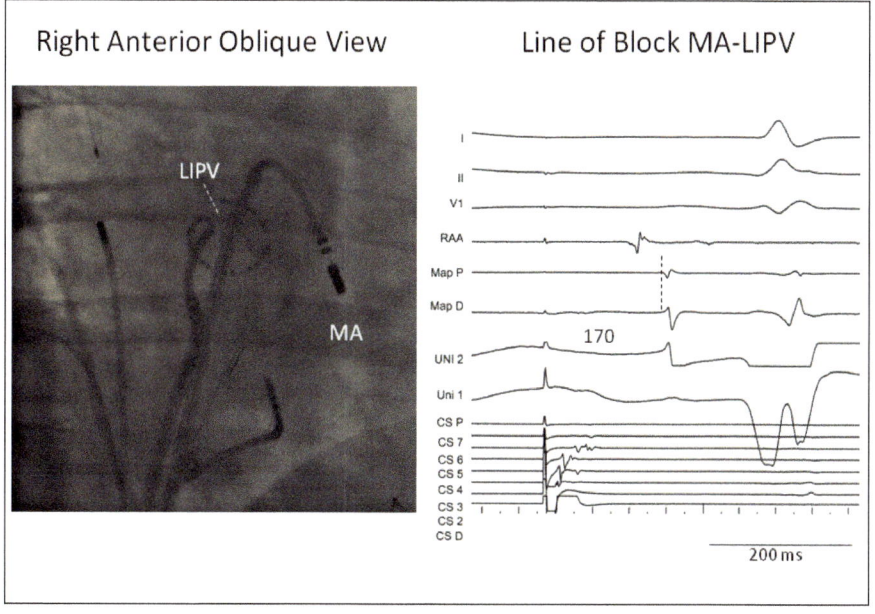

Figure 68.3 Demonstration of a complete line of block between the mitral annulus and the left inferior pulmonary vein (MA-LIPV). In the right anterior oblique view, the circular mapping catheter is positioned at the ostium of the LIPV. Following ablation, during pacing from the distal pair of electrodes of the coronary sinus catheter just inferior to the line of block, the mapping catheter located superior to the line of block records atrial activity 170 ms after the pacing stimulus. The proximal pair of electrodes is activated before the distal pair of electrodes, indicating a superior to inferior wavefront of activation.

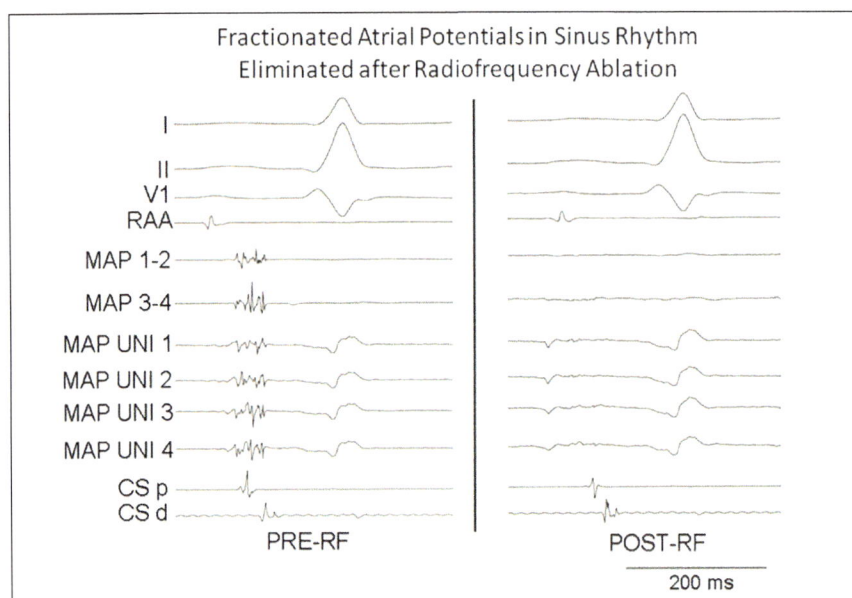

Figure 68.4 Complex fractionated atrial electrograms recorded during sinus rhythm. Bipolar electrograms (MAP 1-2 and MAP 3-4) and unipolar electrograms (MAP Uni 1, 2, 3, and 4) are shown along coronary sinus (CS) and right atrial appendage (RAA) electrograms and surface leads I, II, and V1. After catheter ablation (POST-RF), complex atrial potentials were eliminated.

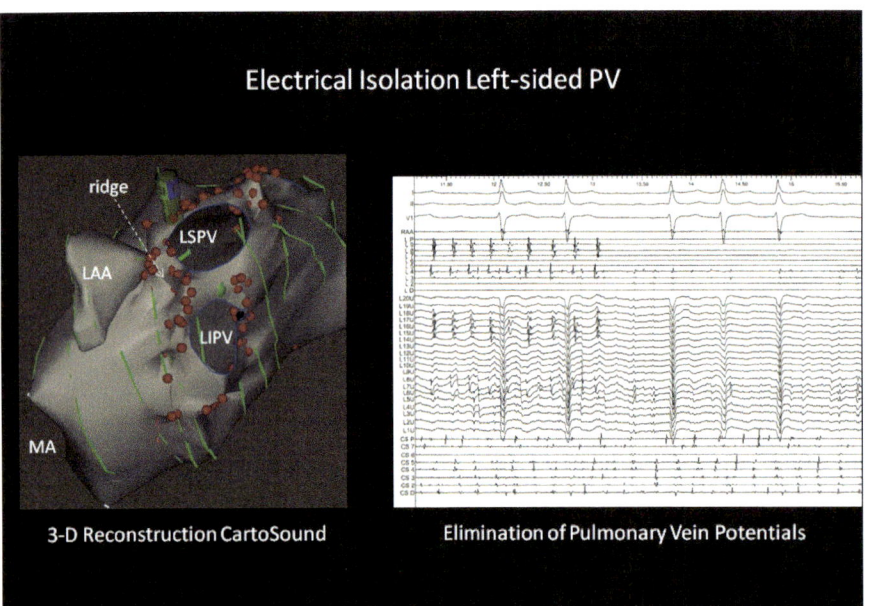

Figure 68.5 Electrical isolation of the left pulmonary veins (LPVs) during AF. Three-dimensional (3D) reconstruction of the left atrium and pulmonary veins (**left panel**) was obtained using intravascular echocardiography (CartoSound, Biosense Webster, Diamond Bar, CA). The pulmonary veins were removed to identify the pulmonary vein ostia and the ridge separating the left superior pulmonary vein (LSPV) from the left atrial appendage (LAA). Ablation was performed around the two LPVs. Ten bipolar and 20 unipolar electrograms were recorded at the ostium of the LSPV during ablation (**right panel**). Elimination of the pulmonary vein electrograms occurs when the vein is isolated from the left atrium.

complete. Patients with persistent AF who undergo pulmonary vein isolation followed by lines of block have a better chance to remain in sinus rhythm.[22] Finally, use of these various approaches in a step-wise fashion appear to be more successful than any one strategy alone.[23]

An important contribution of catheter ablation of AF is the fact that some patients with advanced congestive heart failure may drastically improve with maintenance of sinus rhythm following the procedure.[24]

Complications of Catheter Ablation

Catheter ablation of AF can be performed with low risk of complications. However, serious complications, including death, can occur and need to be discussed with the patient before the procedure. A published worldwide survey describes complications and mortality from 162 centers.[17,25,26] Mortality from this procedure occurs in 1/1,000 patients. The main causes of death include cardiac tamponade, stroke, and atrio-esophageal fistula.[27] Monitoring of intraluminal esophageal temperature has probably made the ablation procedure safer since the ablation is interrupted as soon a rise in the temperature occurs.[28] Cardiac tamponade can be reduced by careful access to the left atrium during transseptal puncture[16] and by gradual upward titration of radiofrequency energy during ablation. Stroke can be reduced by proper anticoagulation, adequate flushing of transseptal sheaths, and use of externally irrigated electrode catheters. Groin hematomas and pseudoaneurysms continue to be a problem. Careful venous access guided by ultrasound and management of anticoagulation pre- and postprocedure reduce these complications. The frequency of pulmonary vein stenosis as a result of catheter ablation has decreased over time. Initially when ablation was performed at the ostium or within the pulmonary veins up to 42% developed stenosis.[29] The incidence of pulmonary vein stenosis has decreased over time as ablation is now performed proximal to the vein and not inside this structure.[25] In addition, the use of low-power radiofrequency ablation and 3D reconstruction of the left atrium and the pulmonary veins using intracardiac echocardiography, computer tomography, magnetic resonance, and fast anatomical mapping have improved the safety of the procedure. The clinical manifestations of pulmonary vein stenosis depend on the number of pulmonary veins involved and the severity of the lesions.[30-32] Some patients are asymptomatic while others develop cough, dyspnea, chest pain, pulmonary infiltrates, and even hemoptysis. The induction of new arrhythmias by the procedure (proarrhythmias), such as macroreentrant atrial tachycardias, is another complication that occur mainly after extensive ablation procedures (Figure 68.6). Depending on the ablation approach, from 3% to as many as 40% of patients can develop micro- or macroreentrant tachycardias.[33-35] The most common macro-atrial tachycardia secondary to a previous ablation of AF is a reentry around the mitral annulus. Other reentrant loops involve the roof with activation proceeding between the right and left pulmonary veins (LPVs), between the right pulmonary veins (RPVs) and the paraseptal atrial wall (Figure 68.7),

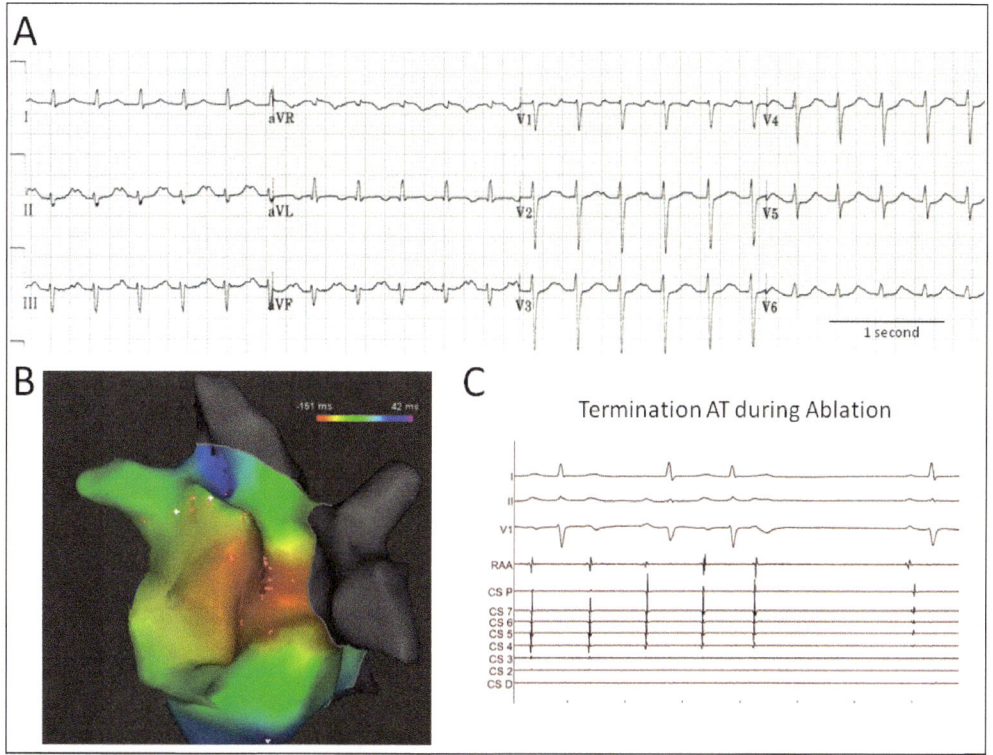

Figure 68.6 Incessant left atrial tachycardia occurring 1 year after catheter ablation of atrial fibrillation (**A**). 3D reconstruction of the left atrium and pulmonary veins (**B**) was obtained using fast, anatomical mapping. Earliest activation occurred at the ridge separating the left atrial appendage from the pulmonary veins. Radiofrequency ablation at the earliest site terminated the atrial tachycardia (**C**).

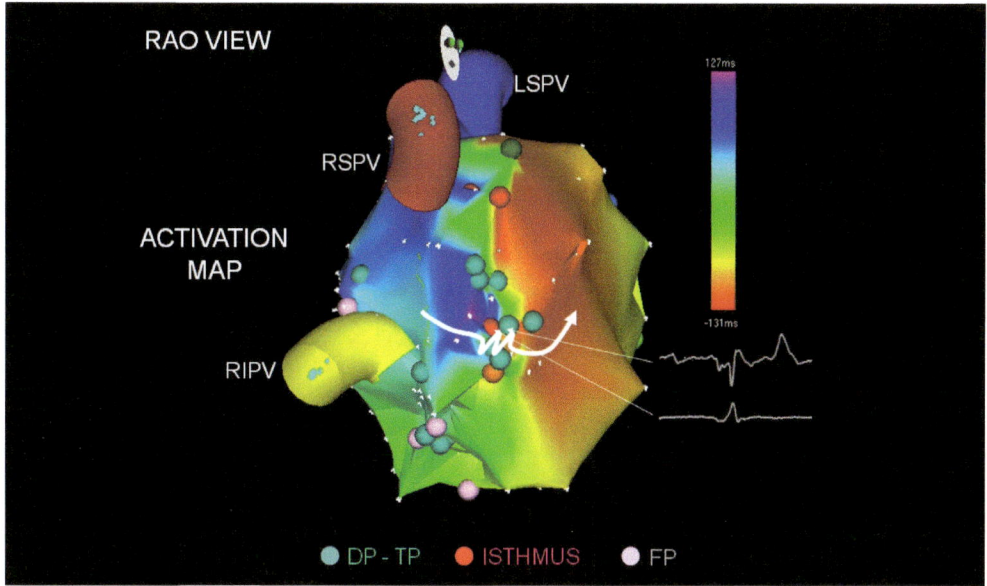

Figure 68.7 Incessant macroreentrant left atrial tachycardia occurring 6 months after catheter ablation of AF. Activation proceeded between the right-side pulmonary veins through an isthmus encompassed between lines of block represented by double potentials (DP).

and between the left pulmonary veins and the left atrial appendage. Antiarrhythmic agents are usually ineffective in controlling these arrhythmias. Mapping and ablation to eliminate regions of slow conduction along the critical isthmus terminates these tachycardias. Perforation leading to tamponade occurs in approximately 1% of cases.[25] This is usually treated by percutaneous pericardiocentesis but sometimes requires thoracotomy and creation of a pericardial window. Phrenic nerve injury leading to diaphragmatic paralysis or gastric emptying syndrome is reported at a rate of 0.1% to 0.48%. This is associated most commonly with ablation in the regions of the right superior pulmonary vein, left atrial appendage, and the SVC. Recovery is seen in approximately 66% of cases.[36] Fluoroscopic visualization of the movement of the diaphragm during ablation may reveal diaphragmatic stimulation or decreased movement that mandates rapid termination of radiofrequency energy delivery before permanent injury to the phrenic nerve occurs. Before delivery of radiofrequency current over the lateral aspects of the SVC–right atrial junction, pacing at high output may reveal phrenic nerve stimulation evidenced by diaphragmatic stimulation, indicating that ablation at that site may cause phrenic nerve paralysis. Cerebrovascular accidents and transient ischemic attacks are one of the most serious complications of AF ablation.[37] The risk of embolic events is approximately 1% and has decreased over time with the use of new imaging modalities and externally irrigated catheters.

Cryoballoon ablation has emerged as a new modality to isolate the pulmonary veins.[38] Cryoballoons provides circumferential isolation, eliminating the need for point-by-point delivery of radiofrequency energy with conventional catheters. Acute success rate is 98%, although isolation of the right inferior pulmonary vein presents a technical challenge since the balloon is not deflectable and needs to be advanced through a guidewire. Success is approximately 65% for patients with paroxysmal AF and 45% for persistent AF. The main concern is phrenic nerve paralysis that occurs in approximately 6% of patients when energy is applied at the ostium of the right superior pulmonary veins. Other complications are similar to other AF ablation procedures using radiofrequency energy including stroke, cardiac tamponade, and groin hematomas. Pulmonary vein stenosis can still occur. Atrio-esophageal fistulas have not yet been described using this energy source.

AF Recurrences and Repeat Procedures

Complete isolation of all four pulmonary veins is the main endpoint for current ablation procedures. Pulmonary vein reconnection is considered the most frequent cause of AF recurrence, but not the only cause. Early post ablation, atrial arrhythmias occur and do not necessarily imply failure of the procedure. Inflammatory changes induced by ablation appear to account for these arrhythmias. In fact, administration of corticosteroids may reduce these arrhythmias.[39] Recovery of pulmonary vein conduction unfortunately is a common occurrence. A well-designed study of patients undergoing pulmonary vein isolation who had a repeat procedure even in the absence of AF recurrence found that 80% of patients had partial recovery of pulmonary vein conduction at 4 months, even though AF recurrence occurred in only 32% of patients.[8] Therefore, not all patients who have reconnection of the pulmonary veins have recurrence of AF, but most patients with recurrence of the arrhythmia are found to have electrical reconnection of one or more veins. Silent AF is common after catheter ablation even in patients who are asymptomatic after the procedure. In other words, catheter ablation frequently improves quality of life even though AF is not totally suppressed. When analyzing event recordings after ablation,[40] the sensitivity of a patient detecting AF by symptoms is 75% and the specificity is 92%.

Catheter Ablation versus Antiarrhythmic Drugs

Until recently, catheter ablation was performed only after failure of medical therapy because the potential risks of the procedure. Several studies, however, have shown that ablation is more effective than antiarrhythmic agents in maintaining sinus rhythm and preventing AF recurrence. A recent multicenter randomized controlled trial in patients with paroxysmal AF, comparing antiarrhythmic drugs versus catheter ablation, demonstrated that 66% of patients in the catheter ablation group remained free of AF compared with only 16% in the group receiving antiarrhythmic drugs.[41] These patients were enrolled in the study after unsuccessful treatment with at least one antiarrhythmic drug, which may explain the poor effectiveness of these drugs in this population.

Five randomized studies comparing drugs versus ablation have been published recently. The Catheter Ablation or the Cure of Atrial Fibrillation (CACAF) trial[42] was a multicenter randomized study investigating the benefit of performing catheter ablation in addition to antiarrhythmic therapy in 137 patients with paroxysmal or persistent AF who were either intolerant or had failed 2 or more drugs. Patients were randomized to catheter ablation plus antiarrhythmic drugs or drugs only (control group). During 12 months of follow-up, 91.3% of control patients had AF recurrence as opposed to 44.1% of patients who underwent catheter ablation. Major complications occurred in 4.4% of patients who had catheter ablation. The number of hospitalizations during the follow-up period did not differ significantly between the 2 groups. A significant number of patients in the control group

(57%) eventually underwent catheter ablation, and 61% of them remained free of arrhythmias within a median follow-up of 18 months. The Atrial Fibrillation Ablation versus Antiarrhythmic Drugs (A4) trial[43] was a randomized multicenter study performed in 112 patients with symptomatic paroxysmal AF who had been treated unsuccessfully with at least one antiarrhythmic drug. After 1 year of follow-up, more patients in the ablation group than in the control group remained in sinus rhythm (75% vs 6%). Crossovers were permitted after 3 months of follow-up; in fact, 63% initially assigned to drug therapy underwent catheter ablation. Quality-of-life and exercise duration were superior in the ablation compared to the control group. Complications in the ablation group included cardiac tamponade ($n = 2$), hematomas ($n = 2$), and pulmonary vein stenosis ($n = 1$). Complications in the antiarrhythmic drug group included hyperthyroidism ($n = 1$) and cancer death ($n = 1$). No embolic events were observed in either group. The Ablation for Paroxysmal Atrial Fibrillation (APAF) trial[44] was a randomized study conducted in one center that included 198 patients with paroxysmal AF who had failed at least one antiarrhythmic agent. Patients were randomized to catheter ablation versus therapy with an antiarrhythmic drug they had not yet received. Crossover to ablation was allowed after 3 months of drug therapy. After a 12-month follow-up period, 86% of the patients in the ablation group were free of AF compared to 22% of those assigned to antiarrhythmic drugs. The number of hospitalizations was significantly lower in the ablation group. Maintenance of sinus rhythm after ablation was associated with significant decrease in left atrial size. No serious complications were observed in the ablation group. Side effects requiring drug discontinuation occurred in 23% of patients in the antiarrhythmic drug group. In 146 patients with chronic AF refractory to 2 or more antiarrhythmic agents, Oral et al[32] compared the benefit of catheter ablation versus amiodarone treatment in a randomized study performed at 2 centers. Patients randomized to amiodarone could undergo 2 cardioversions during the first 3 months and, if unsuccessful, could cross over to have an ablation. Intention-to-treat analysis showed a significantly higher number of patients in sinus rhythm at 12 months in the ablation than in the amiodarone group (74 vs 58%, $P < 0.05$). In the ablation group, restoration of sinus rhythm was associated with decrease in left atrial diameter, symptomatic improvement, and increase in left ventricular ejection fraction. Complications were limited to atypical atrial flutters in the ablation group (6%). The multicenter randomized Radiofrequency Ablation for Atrial Fibrillation (RAAFT) trial assessed catheter ablation as first-line therapy for patients with symptomatic AF.[45] The pilot phase of the trial randomized 70 patients with monthly AF episodes for at least 3 months who had not received prior antiarrhythmic or ablation therapy. At 12-month follow-up, the rate of symptomatic AF recurrence was significantly lower in the ablation than in the antiarrhythmic drug group (13% vs 63%). Similarly, there were fewer hospitalizations following ablation (9% vs 54%) associated with an improved quality of life. Complications in the ablation group included asymptomatic pulmonary vein stenosis in 1 patient.

In summary, several recent clinical trials have shown that catheter ablation when compared to currently available antiarrhythmic agents results in better rhythm control, quality of life, and reverse atrial and ventricular remodeling. However, AF ablation can result in serious complications. Mortality benefit for catheter ablation over antiarrhythmic therapy has not been shown yet. A multicenter trial of 3,000 patients in Europe and the United States (CABANA) is investigating specifically the impact of ablation on survival.

Antiarrhythmic Drugs

Antiarrhythmic drugs are usually the first line of therapy in patients with AF. This is due to the fact that they are readily available and perceived as a less intrusive treatment when compared with catheter ablation. However, since the possible toxic and proarrhythmic effects of these drugs are compounded over time, antiarrhythmic drugs can result in significant morbidity and mortality. Antiarrhythmic agents are moderately effective in preventing recurrences of AF, reducing its duration, and improving quality of life. However, these drugs are largely limited by their safety profile and poor tolerability as demonstrated in several clinical trials.[46-48]

Proarrhythmia can occur due to different mechanisms. First, drugs that prolong action potential duration and the dispersion of ventricular refractory periods may induce torsades de pointes[49] (Figure 68.8). This adverse effect is observed in patients receiving class III and IA agents that block potassium channels and therefore delay repolarization. The risk of torsades de pointes is increased in women as well as in patients with left ventricular hypertrophy, latent congenital long QT syndromes, bradycardia, hypokalemia, or hypomagnesemia.[50] Patients with underlying conduction system disease can develop advanced or complete AV block when sodium channel blockers are administered. In addition, the resulting bradycardia can induce torsades de pointes even in the absence of drugs that delay repolarization (Figure 68.9). Drugs that significantly slow conduction (Class IC) can convert AF into atrial flutter and result in 1:1 A-V conduction and syncope or death (Figure 68.10). Finally, as it is well known, in patients with structural heart disease, sodium channel blockers may induce ventricular tachycardia or ventricular fibrillation. Most antiarrhythmic drugs cannot be administered to patients with congestive heart failure because depression of sodium channel function reduces intracellular sodium, which in turn reduces calcium in the sarcoplasmic reticulum required for contraction. Amiodarone and dofetilide are used in these patients. However, since amiodarone is also a sodium channel blocker, it may compromise hemodynamic stability in patients with severe left ventricular function. Dronedarone can be used in patients with depressed contractility with the exception of patients with advanced heart failure or recent exacerbation. Similar to amiodarone, dronedarone prolongs depolarization. Probably due to its multichannel blocking effects and more uniform prolongation of ventricular depolarization, torsades de pointes are rare with these drugs[51] despite significant prolongation of the QT interval (Figure 68.11). Although dronedarone is not as effective as amiodarone in suppressing AF recurrences,[52] this drug reduces cardiovascular hospitalizations,[53] an endpoint not yet proven with other drugs or catheter ablation.

Patients undergoing catheter ablation frequently require antiarrhythmic agents before and after the procedure. Before ablation, antiarrhythmic agents are used to control disabling symptoms and also can be used to improve left ventricular function when tachycardia-induced cardiomyopathy is suspected.[54] Reversible left ventricular dysfunction is not only the result of rapid rates but also secondary to the irregular rhythm and lack of atrial contraction. Therefore, restoring sinus rhythm can improve left ventricular function and reduce atrial remodeling, which facilitates the ablation procedure.

Following ablation and especially during the first few weeks, patients frequently have AF or atrial tachycardias that do not necessarily imply failure of the procedure.[55] During this period of electrical instability, antiarrhythmic drugs are required to stabilize the substrate and reduce symptoms.

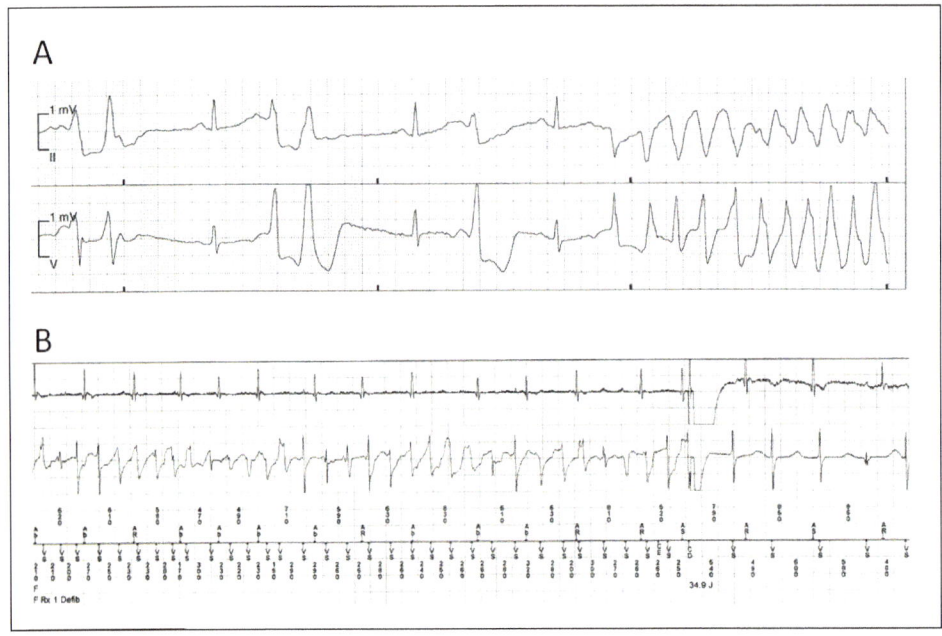

Figure 68.8 Sotalol given to a patient in order to control AF resulted in induced torsades de pointes (**Panel A**) and recurrent ICD shocks (**Panel B**).

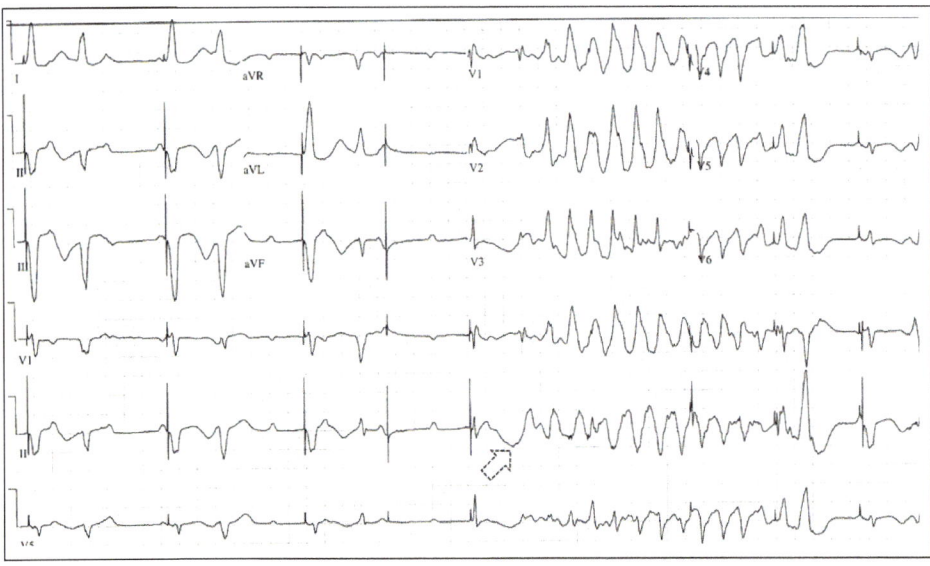

Figure 68.9 Bradycardia-induced torsades de pointes. A patient with a pacemaker at end of life was admitted with recurrent syncope and torsades de pointes secondary to the bradycardia. The arrhythmia subsided when a new generator was implanted.

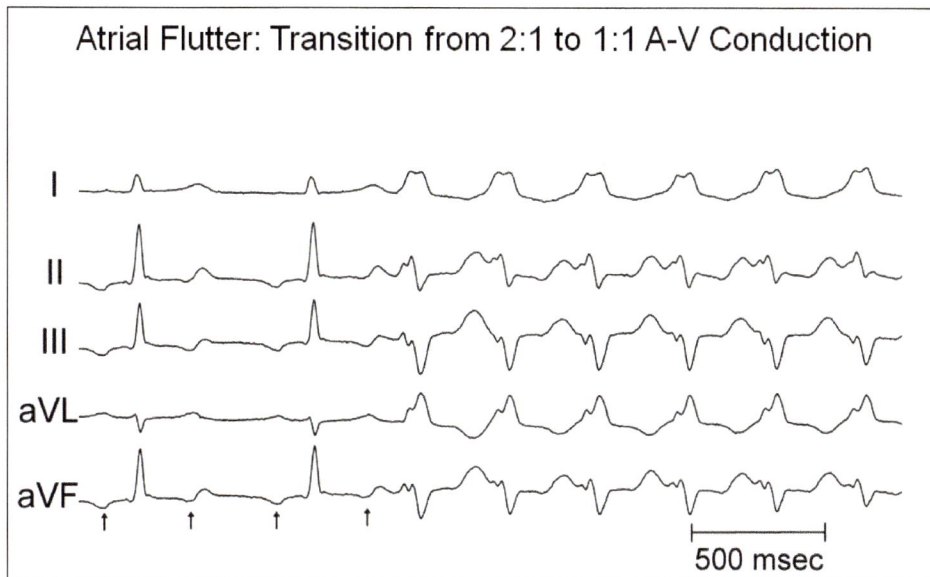

Figure 68.10 Transition from 2:1 to 1:1 A-V conduction during administration of flecainide in a patient with atrial flutter (**arrows**). During 1:1 A-V conduction, tachycardia-dependent left bundle branch block develops.

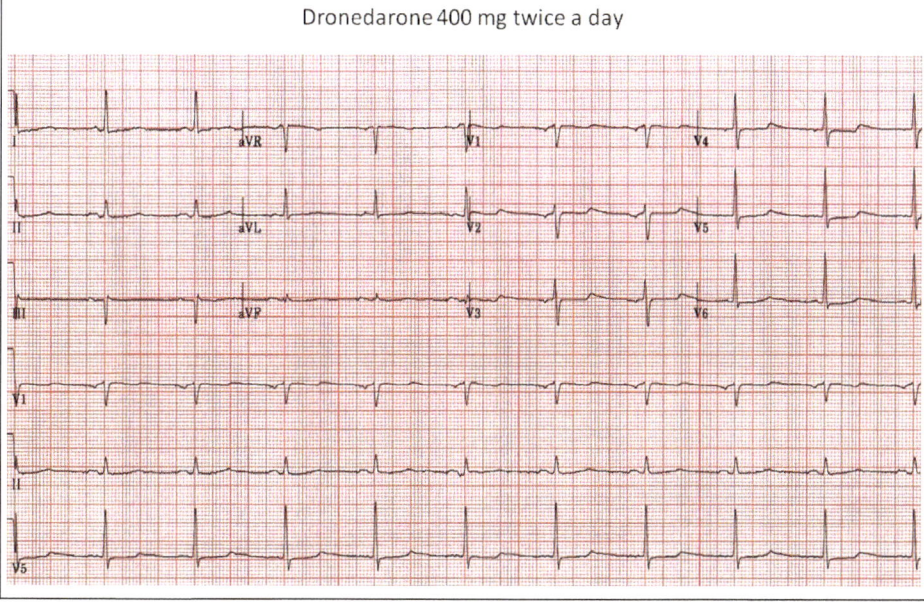

Figure 68.11 Prolongation of the QT interval in a patient taking dronedarone 400 mg twice daily. No arrhythmias have been documented.

Combined Use of Antiarrhythmic Agents and Catheter Ablation

Catheter ablation and antiarrhythmic drugs have limitations in their ability to control AF. A combined therapy can reduce complications and improve efficacy. Ablation therapy combined with antiarrhythmic drug therapy is superior to antiarrhythmic drug therapy alone in preventing atrial arrhythmia recurrences in patients with paroxysmal or persistent AF in whom antiarrhythmic drug therapy has initially failed. A multicenter randomized trial[56] analyzed the additive effect of catheter ablation therapy in preventing AF recurrences in patients with paroxysmal or persistent AF in whom antiarrhythmic drugs have failed. At 12 months of follow-up, 44% of patients in the ablation group have recurrences versus 91% in the control group.

Few studies have compared the effect of ablation therapy alone versus ablation plus drug therapy on freedom from AF. The Worldwide Survey on catheter ablation of AF found greater procedural success in patients on antiarrhythmic drugs in the early postablation period. Early recurrence in the first 2 months postablation is not uncommon and occurs in up to 35% of patients post pulmonary vein isolation within the first 2 weeks.[8] This unstable atrial substrate is usually transient and this period is considered a "blanking period" in ablation studies. Therefore, short-term adjunctive drug therapy is effective in reducing these early recurrences while the changes induced by the ablation procedure take place.[57] The role of long-term antiarrhythmic drugs post ablation has not been substantiated. A study comparing ablation versus ablation plus antiarrhythmic therapy found no change in the rate of AF recurrence,[57] although patients become less symptomatic while taking antiarrhythmic drugs.

Verma et al[58] have examined the effect of antiarrhythmic drugs following AF ablation. Patients able to maintain sinus rhythm with antiarrhythmic drugs after the procedure have more delay in conduction between the left atrium and the pulmonary veins than those who do not respond to antiarrhythmic agents. In other words, antiarrhythmic drugs are more effective when there is partial isolation of the pulmonary veins. This effect may be due to the fact that antiarrhythmic drugs can block conduction in partially depolarized tissues.

Catheter Ablation of Atrial Flutter in Patients Receiving Antiarrhythmic Drugs for AF

Isthmus-dependent atrial flutter develops in about 15% of patients on antiarrhythmic drugs for AF.[59] This occurs mainly with class IC drugs, which reduce conduction velocity and increase the wavelength, organizing the arrhythmia into the more stable rhythm.[60] Once atrial flutter develops on antiarrhythmic drugs, catheter ablation can be performed to eliminate atrial flutter, and the antiarrhythmic agents are continued to prevent recurrence of AF. The success of this approach was studied in patients with paroxysmal and persistent AF in whom flecainide infusion converted AF into atrial flutter.[60] At 5 years, 53% treated with flecainide and ablation remained free from atrial arrhythmias.

Antiarrhythmic Drugs and Pacing

Pacing by preventing bradycardia facilitates the use of the appropriate dose of antiarrhythmic drugs and AV nodal blocking agents that can reduce the recurrence of AF and slow the ventricular response when the arrhythmia recurs. Atrial pacing or dual chamber pacing is superior to ventricular pacing alone in the prevention of AF as right ventricular pacing has adverse hemodynamic effects resulting in a higher incidence of AF.[62-65] Atrial pacing, by preventing bradycardia and long pauses following premature atrial beats, reduces the frequency of AF. This occurs because patients prone to AF have paradoxical shortening of atrial action potentials at long cycle lengths. Bradycardia also induces a rate- and time-dependent electrical remodeling in ventricular myocardium that can result in torsades de pointes. Therefore, pacing can prevent torsades de pointes in patients receiving drugs that prolong ventricular repolarization and/or decrease heart rate. Successful long-term rhythm control using a hybrid approach has been shown in patients with refractory AF and indications for pacing.[66] The combination of dual-site atrial pacing, Class I/III antiarrhythmic drugs, and right atrial linear ablation maintained 89% of patients with paroxysmal AF and 74% of patients with persistent AF in sinus rhythm at 3 years. A recent multicenter randomized trial found that pulmonary-vein isolation is superior to atrioventricular-node ablation with biventricular pacing in patients with heart failure who had drug-refractory AF.[67]

Surgical Therapy

The first ablation therapy for AF was surgical and developed by Cox in 1989.[68] The replacement of the classic "cut and sew" Cox-Maze III procedure by ablation using radiofrequency, microwave, laser, and cryoablation energies have resulted in lower success rates.[69] In the majority of cases, the surgery is performed as an adjunct to other thoracic surgery such as coronary artery bypass grafting or valve surgery. More recently, minimally invasive procedures without the need for cardiopulmonary bypass are being developed.[70] Patients who fail surgical ablation can undergo catheter ablation thereafter. Recurrences of AF or the development of reentrant atrial tachycardias (Figure 68.12) can be explained by incomplete isolation of the pulmonary veins or creation of regions with slow conduction. In addition, triggers located outside the lines created by the surgical ablation can initiate the arrhythmia.[71]

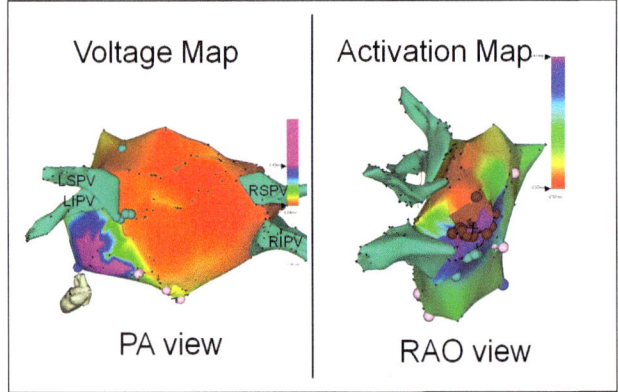

Figure 68.12 Incessant macroreentrant atrial tachycardia after microwave surgical ablation of AF. Voltage map of the left atrium (**left panel**) shows extensive scar in the posterior wall of the left atrium between the pulmonary veins. Activation map (**right panel**) shows inferior to superior activation anterior to the RPVs and the line of block that was created to terminate the atrial tachycardia.

Prolonged rhythm monitoring following radiofrequency ablation during concomitant cardiac surgery has recently been reported in the Surgical Atrial Fibrillation Suppression (SAFS) Study.[72] At 6 months, 75% of patients were in sinus rhythm according to a single ECG but only 62% of patients had no AF during 7-day Holter monitoring. All AF episodes in these patients were asymptomatic, which has important implications regarding anticoagulation therapy in these patients.

The Cox-Maze IV procedure, by using radiofrequency or cryo-energy instead of "cut and sew" lines, has shortened operative times.[73-74] This procedure has been used in patients with AF who do not require additional heart surgery. Perioperative mortality of 1% with 82% success rate at 12 months of follow-up was reported.[73-74]

Atrioventricular Junction Ablation and Pacing

Patients with advanced heart failure and who have rapid ventricular response despite maximal drug therapy may improve with implantation of a permanent pacemaker followed by radiofrequency AV junction ablation. This procedure is reserved for patients with advanced age or with otherwise poor prognosis and not candidates for catheter ablation of AF. Left ventricular function and quality of life can improve significantly.[75-76] Biventricular pacing should be considered to avoid the deleterious effects of long-term right ventricular pacing. However, before A-V junction ablation is considered, all other treatment options, including AF ablation, should be discussed with the patient.

Conclusions

At present, no single therapeutic modality is successful in the treatment and prevention of all forms of AF. Since the pathogenesis of AF is poorly understood, the management of this arrhythmia remains empirical and requires the selection of multiple drugs and procedures. New and safer antiarrhythmic drugs are being developed, making rhythm control more attainable. Adverse effects and proarrhythmia remain a clinical problem that is exacerbated in patients with organ dysfunction. Advances in catheter ablation techniques have made the procedure safer although serious complications still occur. Antiarrhythmic drugs, catheter ablation, surgical ablation, and pacing remain the cornerstone of AF therapy. These therapies frequently improve quality of life. However, limited information is available regarding the effect of these interventions on embolic complications and survival.

References

1. Miyasaka Y, Barnes ME, Gersh BJ, et al. Secular trends in incidence of atrial fibrillation in Olmsted County, Minnesota, 1980 to 2000, and implications on the projections for future prevalence. *Circulation*. 2006;114:119-125.
2. Benjamin EJ, Wolf PA, D'Agostino RB, et al. Impact of atrial fibrillation on the risk of death: the Framingham Heart Study. *Circulation*. 1998;98:946-952.
3. Go AS, Hylek EM, Phillips KA, et al. Prevalence of diagnosed atrial fibrillation in adults: national implications for rhythm management and stroke prevention: the AnTicoagulation and Risk Factors in Atrial Fibrillation (ATRIA) Study. *JAMA*. 2001;285:2370-2375.
4. Coyne KS, Paramore C, Grandy S, Mercader M, Reynolds M, Zimetbaum P. Assessing the direct costs of treating nonvalvular atrial fibrillation in the United States. *Value Health*. 2006;9:348-356.
5. Haïssaguerre M, Jaïs P, Shah DC, et al. Spontaneous initiation of atrial fibrillation by ectopic beats originating in the pulmonary veins. *N Engl J Med*. 1998;339:659-666.
6. Dixit S, Gerstenfeld EP, Ratcliffe SJ, et al. Single procedure efficacy of isolating all versus arrhythmogenic pulmonary veins on long-term control of atrial fibrillation: a prospective randomized study. *Heart Rhythm*. 2008;5:174-181.
7. Calkins H, Kuck KH, Cappato R, et al. HRS/EHRA/ECAS expert consensus on catheter and surgical ablation of atrial fibrillation: recommendations for personnel, policy, procedures and follow up. A report of the Heart Rhythm Society (HRS) Task Force on catheter and surgical ablation of atrial fibrillation. *Heart Rhythm*. 2012,9:634-696.
8. Cappato R, Negroni S, Pecora D, et al. Prospective assessment of late conduction recurrence across radiofrequency lesions producing electrical disconnection at the pulmonary vein ostium in patients with atrial fibrillation. *Circulation*. 2003;108:1599-1604.
9. Jaïs P, Hocini M, Hsu LF, et al. Technique and results of linear ablation at the mitral annulus. *Circulation*. 2004;110:2996-3002.
10. Nademanee K, Schwab MC, Kosar EM, et al. Clinical outcomes of catheter substrate ablation for high-risk patients with atrial fibrillation. *J Am Coll Cardiol*. 2008;51:843-849.
11. Banchs JE, Penny-Peterson E, Samii S, Wolbrette DL, Naccarelli GV, Gonzalez MD. Low incidence of reentrant atrial tachycardia after atrial fibrillation ablation using as a guide fractionated atrial potentials in sinus rhythm. *Rev Iberoam Electrofisiol*. 2009;1:27-33.
12. Pachon MJ, Pachon ME, Pachon MJ, et al. A new treatment for atrial fibrillation based on spectral analysis to guide the catheter RF-ablation. *Europace*. 2004;6:590-601.
13. Oral H, Scharf C, Chugh A, et al. Catheter ablation for paroxysmal atrial fibrillation: Segmental pulmonary vein ostial ablation versus left atrial ablation. *Circulation*. 2003;108:2355-2360.
14. Karch MR, Zrenner B, Deisenhofer I, et al. Freedom from atrial tachyarrhythmias after catheter ablation of atrial fibrillation. A randomized comparison between 2 current ablation strategies. *Circulation*. 2005;111:2875-2880.
15. Cummings JE, Schweikert RA, Saliba WI, et al. Brief communication: Atrial-esophageal fistulas after radiofrequency ablation. *Ann Intern Med*. 2006;144:572-574.
16. Gonzalez MD, Otomo K, Shah N, et al. Transseptal left heart catheterization for cardiac ablation procedures. *JICE*. 2001;5:89-95.
17. Cappato R, Calkins H, Chen SA, et al. Updated worldwide survey on the methods, efficacy, and safety of catheter ablation for human atrial fibrillation. *Circ Arrhythm Electrophysiol*. 2010;3:32-38.
18. Oral H, Knight BP, Tada H, et al. Pulmonary vein isolation for paroxysmal and persistent atrial fibrillation. *Circulation*. 2002:5;105(9):1077-1081.
19. Willems S, Klemm H, Rostock T, et al. Substrate modification combined with pulmonary vein isolation improves outcome of catheter ablation in patients with persistent atrial fibrillation: a prospective randomized comparison. *Eur Heart J*. 2006;23:2871-2878.
20. Elayi CS, Verma A, Di BL, et al. Ablation for longstanding permanent atrial fibrillation: results from a randomized study comparing three different strategies. *Heart Rhythm*. 2008;5:1658-1664.
21. Takahashi Y, O'Neill MD, Hocini M, et al. Characterization of electrograms associated with termination of chronic atrial fibrillation by catheter ablation. *J Am Coll Cardiol*. 2008;51:1003-1010.

22. Knecht S, Hocini M, Wright M, et al. Left atrial linear lesions are required for successful treatment of persistent atrial fibrillation. *Eur Heart J.* 2008;29:2359-2366.
23. O'Neill MD, Jaïs P, Takahashi Y, et al. The stepwise ablation approach for chronic atrial fibrillation—evidence for a cumulative effect. *J Interv Card Electrophysiol.* 2006;16:153-167.
24. Hsu LF, Jaïs P, Sanders P, et al. Catheter Ablation for Atrial Fibrillation in Congestive Heart Failure. *N Engl J Med.* 2004;351;23:2373-2383.
25. Cappato R, Calkins H, Chen SA, et al. Worldwide survey on the methods, efficacy, and safety of catheter ablation for human atrial fibrillation. *Circulation.* 2005;8;111:1100-1105.
26. Cappato R, Calkins H, Chen SA, et al. Prevalence and causes of fatal outcome in catheter ablation of atrial fibrillation. *J Am Coll Cardiol.* 2009;53:1798-1803.
27. Pappone C, Oral H, Santinelli V, et al. Atrio-esophageal fistula as a complication of percutaneous transcatheter ablation of atrial fibrillation. *Circulation.* 2004;109:2724-2726.
28. Redfearn DP, Trim GM, Skanes AC, et al. Esophageal temperature monitoring during radiofrequency ablation of atrial fibrillation. *J Cardiovasc Electrophysiol.* 2005;16:589-593.
29. Chen SA, Hsieh MH, Tai CT, et al. Initiation of atrial fibrillation by ectopic beats originating from the pulmonary veins: electrophysiologic characteristics, pharmacological response and effects of radiofrequency ablation. *Circulation.* 1999;100:1879-1886.
30. Saad EB, Rossillo A, Saad CP, et al. Pulmonary vein stenosis after radiofrequency ablation of atrial fibrillation (Functional characterization, evolution and influence of the ablation strategy). *Circulation.* 2003;108:3102-3107.
31. Prieto LR, Yu Kawai Y, Worley SE. Total pulmonary vein occlusion complicating pulmonary vein isolation: Diagnosis and treatment. *Heart Rhythm.* 2010;7:1233-1239.
32. Holmes DR Jr, Monahan KH, Packer D. Pulmonary vein stenosis complicating ablation for atrial fibrillation: clinical spectrum and interventional considerations. *JACC Cardiovasc Interv.* 2009;2:267-276.
33. Cummings JE, Schweikert R, Saliba W, et al. Left atrial flutter following pulmonary vein antrum isolation with radiofrequency energy: linear lesions or repeat isolation. *J Cardiovasc Electrophysiol.* 2005;16:293-297.
34. Deisenhofer I, Estner H, Zrenner B, et al. Left atrial tachycardia after circumferential pulmonary vein ablation for atrial fibrillation: incidence, electrophysiological characteristics, and results of radiofrequency ablation. *Europace.* 2006;8(8):573-582.
35. Karch MR, Zrenner B, Deisenhofer I, et al. Freedom from atrial tachyarrhythmias after catheter ablation of atrial fibrillation: A randomized comparison between two current ablation strategies. *Circulation.* 2005;111:2875-2880.
36. Sacher F, Monahan KH, Thomas SP, et al. Phrenic nerve injury after atrial fibrillation catheter ablation: characterization and outcome in a multicenter study. *J Am Coll Cardiol.* 2006;47:2498-2503.
37. Zhou L, Keane D, Reed G, Ruskin J. Thromboembolic complications of cardiac radiofrequency catheter ablation: a review of the reported incidence, pathogenesis and current research directions. *J Cardiovasc Electrophysiol.* 1999;10(4):611-620.
38. Andrade JG, Khairy P, Guerra PG, et al. Efficacy and safety of cryoablation for atrial fibrillation: A systematic review of published studies. *Heart Rhythm.* 2011;8:1444-1451.
39. Koyama T, Tada H, Sekiguchi Y, et al. Prevention of atrial fibrillation recurrence with corticosteroids after radiofrequency catheter ablation: a randomized controlled trial. *J Am Coll Cardiol.* 2010;56:1463-1472.
40. Neumann T, Erdogan A, Dill T, et al. Asymptomatic recurrences of atrial fibrillation after pulmonary vein isolation. *Europace.* 2006 Jul;8(7):495-498.
41. Wilber DJ, Pappone C, Neuzil P, et al. Comparison of antiarrhythmic drug therapy and radiofrequency catheter ablation in patients with paroxysmal atrial fibrillation: a randomized controlled trial. *JAMA.* 2010;303:333-340.
42. Stabile G, Bertaglia E, Senatore G, et al. Catheter ablation treatment in patients with drug-refractory atrial fibrillation: a prospective, multi-centre, randomized, controlled study (Catheter Ablation For The Cure Of Atrial Fibrillation Study). *Eur Heart J.* 2006;27:216-221.
43. Jaïs P, Cauchemez, B, Macle L, et al. Catheter ablation versus antiarrhythmic drugs for atrial fibrillation. The A4 Study. *Circulation.* 2008;118:2498-2505.
44. Pappone C, Augello G, Sala S, et al. A randomized trial of circumferential pulmonary vein ablation versus antiarrhythmic drug therapy in paroxysmal atrial fibrillation: the APAF Study. *J Am Coll Cardiol.* 2006;48:2340-2347.
45. Wazni OM, Marrouche NF, Martin DO, et al. Radiofrequency ablation versus antiarrhythmic drugs as first-line treatment of symptomatic atrial fibrillation: a randomized trial. *JAMA.* 2005;293:2634-2640.
46. Hohnloser SH, Kuck KH, Lilienthal J. Rhythm or rate control in atrial fibrillation—Pharmacological Intervention in Atrial Fibrillation (PIAF): a randomised trial. *Lancet.* 2000;356:1789-1794.
47. Van G, I, Hagens VE, Bosker HA, et al. A comparison of rate control and rhythm control in patients with recurrent persistent atrial fibrillation. *N Engl J Med.* 2002;347:1834-1840.
48. Wyse DG, Waldo AL, DiMarco JP, et al. A comparison of rate control and rhythm control in patients with atrial fibrillation. *N Engl J Med.* 2002;347:1825-1833.
49. Lazzara R. Antiarrhythmic drugs and torsade de pointes. *Eur Heart J.* 1993;14 Suppl H:88-92.
50. Wolbrette DL. Risk of proarrhythmia with class III antiarrhythmic agents: sex-based differences and other issues. *Am J Cardiol.* 91:39D-44D.
51. Sicouri S, Moro S, Litovsky SH, Elizari MV, Antzelevitch C. Chronic amiodarone reduces transmural dispersion of repolarization in the canine heart. *J Cardiovasc Electrophysiol.* 1997;8:1269-1279.
52. Le Heuzey JY, De Ferrari GM, Radzik D, Santini M, Zhu J, Davy JM. A short-term, randomized, double-blind, parallel-group study to evaluate the efficacy and safety of dronedarone versus amiodarone in patients with persistent atrial fibrillation: the DIONYSOS study. *J Cardiovasc Electrophysiol.* 2010;2:597-605.
53. Hohnloser SH, Crijns HJ, van Eickels M, et al. Effect of dronedarone on cardiovascular events in atrial fibrillation. *N Engl J Med.* 2009;360:668-678.
54. Grogan M, Smith HC, Gersh BJ, et al. Left ventricular dysfunction due to atrial fibrillation in patients initially believed to have idiopathic dilated cardiomyopathy. *Am J Cardiol.* 1992;69:1570-1573.
55. Roux JF, Zado E, Callans DJ, et al. Antiarrhythmics after ablation of atrial fibrillation (5A Study). *Circulation.* 2009;22;120:1036-1040.
56. Stabile G, Bertaglia E, Senatore G, et al. Catheter ablation treatment in patients with drug-refractory atrial fibrillation: a prospective, multicentre, randomized, controlled study (Catheter Ablation For The Cure Of Atrial Fibrillation Study). *Eur Heart J.* 2006;27:216-221.
57. Turco P, De SA, La RV, et al. Antiarrhythmic drug therapy after radiofrequency catheter ablation in patients with atrial fibrillation. *Pacing Clin Electrophysiol.* 2007;30:S112-S115.

58. Verma A, Kilicaslan F, Pisano E, et al. Response of atrial fibrillation to pulmonary vein antrum isolation is directly related to resumption and delay of pulmonary vein conduction. *Circulation*. 2005;112:627-635.
59. Reithmann C, Dorwarth U, Dugas M, et al. Risk factors for recurrence of atrial fibrillation in patients undergoing hybrid therapy for antiarrhythmic drug-induced atrial flutter. *Eur Heart J*. 2003;24:1264-1272.
60. Ortiz J, Niwano S, Abe H, et al. Mapping the conversion of atrial flutter to atrial fibrillation and atrial fibrillation to atrial flutter. Insights into mechanisms. *Circ Res*. 1994;74:882-894.
61. Turco P, De Simone A, La Rocca V, et al. Long-term results of hybrid therapy in patients with atrial fibrillation who develop atrial flutter during flecainide infusion. *Pacing Clin Electrophysiol*. 2005 Jan;28 Suppl 1:S124-S127.
62. Lamas GA, Lee KL, Sweeney MO, et al. Ventricular pacing or dual-chamber pacing for sinus-node dysfunction. *N Engl J Med*. 2002;346:1854-1862.
63. Silberbauer J, Sulke N. The role of pacing in rhythm control and management of atrial fibrillation. *J Interv Card Electrophysiol*. 2007;18:159-186.
64. Nielsen JC, Kristensen L, Andersen HR, Mortensen PT, Pedersen OL, Pedersen AK. A randomized comparison of atrial and dual-chamber pacing in 177 consecutive patients with sick sinus syndrome: echocardiographic and clinical outcome. *J Am Coll Cardiol*. 2003;42:614-623.
65. Kerr CR, Connolly SJ, Abdollah H, et al. Canadian Trial of Physiological Pacing: Effects of physiological pacing during long-term follow-up. *Circulation*. 2004 Jan 27;109(3):357-362.
66. Prakash A, Saksena S, Krol RB, Filipecki A, Philip G. Catheter ablation of inducible atrial flutter, in combination with atrial pacing and antiarrhythmic drugs ("hybrid therapy") improves rhythm control in patients with refractory atrial fibrillation. *J Interv Card Electrophysiol*. 2002;6:165-172.
67. Khan MN, Jaïs P, Cummings J, et al. Pulmonary-vein isolation for atrial fibrillation in patients with heart failure. *N Engl J Med*. 2008;359:1778-1785.
68. Cox JL, Schuessler RB, Cain ME, et al. Surgery for atrial fibrillation. *Semin Thorac Cardiovasc Surg*. 1989;1:67-73.
69. Stulak JM, Dearani JA, Sundt TM III, et al. Superiority of cut-and-sew technique for the Cox Maze procedure: comparison with radiofrequency ablation. *J Thorac Cardiovasc Surg*. 2007;133:1022-1027.
70. Matsutani N, Takase B, Ozeki Y, Maehara T, Lee R. Minimally invasive cardiothoracic surgery for atrial fibrillation: a combined Japan-US experience. *Circ J*. 2008;72:434-436.
71. McCarthy PM, Kruse J, Shalli S, et al. Where does atrial fibrillation surgery fail? Implications for increasing effectiveness of ablation. *Thorac Cardiovasc Surg*. 2010;139:860-867.
72. Veasey RA, Segal OR, Large JK, et al. The efficacy of intraoperative atrial radiofrequency ablation for atrial fibrillation during concomitant cardiac surgery-the Surgical Atrial Fibrillation Suppression (SAFS) Study. *J Interv Card Electrophysiol*. 2011;32(1):29-35.
73. Weimar T, Bailey MS, Watanabe Y, et al. The Cox-Maze IV procedure for lone atrial fibrillation: a single center experience in 100 consecutive patients. *J Interv Card Electrophysiol*. 2011;31(1):47-54.
74. Damiano RJ Jr, Schwartz FH, Bailey MS, et al. The Cox Maze IV procedure: predictors of late recurrence. *J Thorac Cardiovasc Surg*. 2011;141(1):113-121.
75. Lim KT, Davis MJ, Powell A, et al. Ablate and pace strategy for atrial fibrillation: long-term outcome of AIRCRAFT trial. *Europace*. 2007;9:498-505.
76. Tan ES, Rienstra M, Wiesfeld AC, Schoonderwoerd BA, Hobbel HH, Van Gelder IC. Long-term outcome of the atrioventricular node ablation and pacemaker implantation for symptomatic refractory atrial fibrillation. *Europace*. 2008;10:412-418.

CHAPTER 69

Hybrid Device, Ablation, and Drug Therapy in Ventricular Tachyarrhythmias

Carlo Lavalle, MD; Massimo Santini, MD

Introduction

Sustained ventricular arrhythmias—ventricular tachycardia (VT) and ventricular fibrillation (VF)—are important causes of morbidity and sudden cardiac death (SCD). Despite numerous efforts in recent years, anticipating and preventing SCD still remains an important "gamble" for modern cardiology. It remains one of the most important causes of death in the industrialized countries. Ventricular arrhythmias can occur in different physiopathological substrates. In most cases, ventricular arrhythmias occur in patients with structural heart disease, and in this particular setting such arrhythmias worsen the prognosis and may lead to sudden death. Coronary artery disease undoubtedly represents the most frequent cause of ventricular arrhythmias, and is responsible for 80% of the cases of sudden death.[1] In these patients, prevention and/or early interruption of ventricular tachyarrhythmias may improve prognosis and reduce mortality. Randomized clinical trials have shown that the implantable cardioverter-defibrillator (ICD) is the most effective therapy currently available to prevent sudden death by terminating ventricular arrhythmias.[2-4] Therefore, the ICD has become the standard therapy for primary and secondary prevention of sudden death in patients with left ventricular dysfunction.[5] However, it must be underlined that the ICD does not represent a cure of ventricular tachyarrhythmias and does not prevent VT/VF recurrence. It must be considered a sort of "palliative treatment" that interrupts the arrhythmic event; therefore, it still does not represent the optimal therapy of VT/VF.

Another point that must be kept in mind is the ICD shock is painful and may be associated with significant reduction of mental well-being and quality of life. About 50% of the patients with ICD are depressed, suffer from anxiety caused by the device, and require psychological support.[6-8] Although the ICD interrupts the VT/VF, many patients continue to have symptoms such as dizziness, palpitations, or syncope before receiving an ICD shock.[9] Furthermore, recurrent ventricular arrhythmias and shocks have been associated with increased heart failure and mortality.[10,11] In an analysis of the Multicenter Automatic Defibrillator Implantation Trial II (MADIT II) patients, an increased overall mortality was observed in patients who received appropriate and inappropriate shocks by the ICD. This could be in part explained by the progression of the underlying disease which could determine more frequent VT/VF but also atrial fibrillation (AF) episodes, often responsible of inappropriate shocks. The progression of the disease could be responsible for the increased mortality due to congestive heart failure. However, in the same study ventricular arrhythmias effectively treated with antitachycardia pacing (ATP) were not associated with adverse outcome.[12,13] There is concern that the ICD shocks themselves may cause direct myocardial injury and reduce survival.[14] The long-term prognostic significance of appropriate and inappropriate ICD shocks in the SCD-Heft population was also assessed in another study.[10] In accordance with the previous analysis, patients who receive shocks for an arrhythmia have a higher risk of death than those who do not receive ICD shocks. To better understand this observed association between ICD shocks and increased mortality and to have an idea of what happens to these patients in the real world, a recently published paper analyzed a large population of patients who received an ICD between 1996 and 2006 with a long-term follow-up, evaluating the occurrence of inappropriate ICD shocks. Furthermore, the authors tried to identify potential predictive parameters for inappropriate shocks and assess the impact of inappropriate shocks on long-term outcome. The study enrolled 1,544 patients, and during the follow-up, the occurrence of inappropriate ICD shocks and all-cause mortality was noted. During the follow-up, which lasted 41 ± 18 months, 13% of the patients experienced at least 1 inappropriate shock and the cumulative incidence progressively increased to 18% at 5-year follow-up. History of AF in patients who were younger than 70 years of age were found to be independent predictors of inappropriate shocks. Of note, experiencing a single inappropriate shock resulted in an increase in all-cause mortality, and mortality risk increased with every subsequent shock. Misdiagnosis of supraventricular arrhythmias was the leading cause of inappropriate shocks. One would expect that the evolving technology of ICDs with advanced detection algorithms would determine a reduction of inappropriate shocks, but this was not confirmed in this study.[15] This could be due to the evolving guidelines, which have expanded ICD indications to patients who have poorer cardiac condition with a higher risk and prevalence of AF, the strongest predictor of inappropriate shocks. This prospective study confirmed the findings of the subgroup analysis of the MADIT II and SCD-HeFT. The authors also concluded that a possible explanation of the increased mortality due to inappropriate shocks could be the myocardial damage determined by the ICD, which could lead to a further deterioration of left ventricular function. Various studies have supported this hypothesis, finding increased markers of myocardial damage after uncomplicated ICD testing at implantation.[16,17] Therefore, even if trials have demonstrated that ICD improves survival among patients at high risk of sudden death and its indications and use have greatly expanded, ICD shocks themselves may increase mortality. This further justifies the need to try to effectively suppress VT recurrences.

Arrhythmias may also occur in patients who do not have structural cardiomyopathy and who have apparently normal hearts but have genetically determined disorders of the cellular membrane ionic channels such as the Brugada syndrome, the long QT syndrome, the catecholaminergic polymorphic VT, and short QT syndrome. In this group, there are no structural heart abnormalities and the disorders are therefore considered primarily electrical in nature. In these patients, ventricular arrhythmias and sudden death often occur at a young age and are responsible for the sudden deaths in apparently normal hearts. The presence of syncope or documented ventricular arrhythmias (generally VF and torsades de pointes) is associated with poor prognosis. For all of these disorders, ICD implantation is definitely recommended for secondary prevention. Indications for primary prevention are still a matter of debate, and risk stratification has been proposed for each condition.

Finally, VTs may occur in structurally normal hearts. These idiopathic VTs are treated by catheter ablation, which alone represents an effective treatment.

In general, therapeutic options for the treatment of ventricular arrhythmias include antiarrhythmic drugs, ICDs, and catheter or surgical ablation. Although with different modalities, all these therapeutic options provide unique advantages for selected patients, but in most patients with life-threatening arrhythmias, the use of combined therapy is necessary with a hybrid approach. In considering which may be the most appropriate therapeutic approach(es) to treat ventricular arrhythmias, the underlying cardiac disease must be kept in mind. The prognostic significance of these arrhythmias is different if it occurs in individuals with or without cardiac disorders. The therapeutic approach of these arrhythmias is, therefore, individualized according to the underlying cardiomyopathy, severity of symptoms, and number of arrhythmic episodes.

Structural Heart Disease

As we have already discussed, even though ICD has proven to be superior to drug treatment in primary and secondary prevention of SCD, this therapy has some limitations. It does not represent a cure of VT/VF, since it does not prevent arrhythmic recurrences. It does not, therefore, represent the optimal therapy of VT/VF, especially in patients with frequent arrhythmia recurrence and high burden. In these patients, other treatment options, including drugs and catheter ablation, must be used in adjunct with ICD to reduce the number of shocks.

ICD and Drug Therapies

Benefits of Antiarrhythmic Drugs with ICD Therapy

Various studies have demonstrated that 16% to 70% of patients with ICD need to be initiated on antiarrhythmic drugs. The main goal of antiarrhythmic therapy in patients with ICD is to reduce appropriate device interventions, by interrupting recurrent VT/VF, and inappropriate shocks, by reducing frequency and by a better rate control of supraventricular arrhythmias (Table 69.1). We have already mentioned the impact that ICD shocks have on the psychological well-being of the patients; a reduction of device interventions leads to a better quality of life other than reducing the rate of ICD-related hospitalizations.[18] Further, prevention of supraventricular arrhythmias, in particular AF, can potentially also decrease the number of appropriate shocks; an association has been observed between persistent AF and occurrence of ventricular arrhythmias in ICD patients, with this supraventricular arrhythmia being a strong independent predictor of VT with respect to sinus rhythm.[19]

Another advantage of antiarrhythmic drugs is that they may increase the tachycardia cycle, which renders the arrhythmia hemodynamically better tolerated. Furthermore, the slower rate of the tachycardia facilitates successful termination by ATP, reducing the number of syncope episodes. Less device interventions likewise prolongs the battery life, which represents a further advantage.[18] Antiarrhythmic drugs are also of particular importance in the management of electrical storm, both in prevention and acute treatment.[20]

Drawbacks of Combining Antiarrhythmic Drugs with ICD

Nevertheless, antiarrhythmic drugs have a series of adverse effects that must be taken into account. First, they can interact negatively with ICD function, since they can increase defibrillation and pacing threshold and, therefore, interfere with the optimal function of the device. Threshold tests should be performed after initiation of antiarrhythmic drugs. Although slowing the rate of the VT may have advantages, if it slows down too much, it may fall below ICD detection such that VTs may escape device therapy. Therefore, if antiarrhythmic drugs are started after ICD implant, tests should be performed to define the tachycardia cycle length in order to ensure adequate tachycardia detection. Antiarrhythmic drugs also may reduce sinus rates and interfere with atrioventricular conduction, leading to an increase in bradycardia pacing therapy, reducing battery life, and worsening left ventricular function. Paradoxically, some antiarrhythmic drugs may determine an increase of tachyarrhythmic events, since they are potentially proarrhythmic. Extracardiac toxicity must also not be underestimated.[9,18]

Assessing Risk versus Benefit

All of these positive and negative points must be taken into consideration when initiating antiarrhythmic drug therapy (Table 69.1). For each patient, the risk of receiving ICD shock therapy should be assessed. ICD patients who receive their device for secondary prevention are at higher risk of receiving a therapeutic shock than primary prevention ICD patients. In primary prevention, worsening clinical conditions with hospitalization either for congestive heart failure or coronary event seem to be associated with a higher risk of ICD therapy, as observed in a subanalysis of the MADIT II.[21] A substudy of the AVID trial observed that patients receiving ICD as secondary prevention with VT as the index arrhythmia were more likely to receive appropriate therapy when compared to patients with VF as index arrhythmia.[22] These results were in accordance with those observed in another prospective cohort study that tried to identify predictors of subsequent ICD therapy after the first event; patients presenting with VT with an ejection fraction below 25% were at higher risk. Subsequent therapy occurred sooner after the first event and was unpredictable.[23] Risk factors for ICD shock therapy, and therefore possible indications to start drug therapy in adjunct to ICD, seem to be (1) ICD for secondary prevention, (2) having VT as the index arrhythmia, (3) recent appropriate ICD therapy, (4) a left ventricular ejection fraction < 25%, and (5) hospitalization for congestive heart failure or coronary event.

Table 69.1 Effects of antiarrhythmic drug therapy in ICD patients

Advantages	Disadvantages	Adverse effects
• Reduce VT recurrences and ICD shocks	• Increase defibrillation threshold	• Bradyarrhythmias that need pacing
• Reduce supraventricular arrhythmias and inappropriate ICD shocks	• Increase in pacing threshold	• Proarrhythmic effect
• Better rate control of supraventricular arrhythmias with reduction of inappropriate ICD shocks	• Interference in accurate arrhythmia detection due to slowing of the rate of the VT, which therefore is not correctly detected	• Impairment of myocardial function
		• Extracardiac toxicity
• Slowing of tachycardia leading to a higher success of ATP	• Decrease in amplitude of electrogram interfering with sensing	
• Slowing of tachycardia rate improving hemodynamic tolerance		
• Prolongation of ICD duration		
• Prevention of electrical storm		
• Improve quality of life		
• Reduce ICD-related hospitalization		

Timing and Efficacy of Adjunct Drug Therapy

Another question to be answered is when to start drug therapy in ICD recipients. Considering that after a VT, the second episode tends to occur sooner, antiarrhythmic drugs should be taken into consideration in patients receiving an ICD as secondary prevention. It is important to also consider the symptoms correlated with the arrhythmia and the type of therapy delivered by the device. If the arrhythmia is interrupted by ATP, modifications of this function can be considered before starting drug therapy.[18]

As for the choice of the drug to use in ICD patients, several large-scale trials have evaluated and compared the efficacy of various antiarrhythmic drugs. In a prospective multicenter trial, Pacifico et al enrolled 302 patients with ICD who were randomized to either sotalol or placebo. Sotalol was shown to reduce death from any cause, decrease the number of ICD shocks, and increase the time to delivery of first inappropriate shock, even though 27% of the patients stopped taking the drug because of adverse events.[24] The OPTIC study was a randomized controlled trial, which enrolled 412 patients with ICD implanted for inducible or spontaneously occurring VT/VF. The study compared amiodarone plus β-blocker to either sotalol or β-blocker alone. The combination of amiodarone plus β-blocker was more effective than β-blocker alone or sotalol in reducing both appropriate and inappropriate shocks. There was a trend toward a better efficacy of sotalol alone with respect to β-blocker alone, but the difference was not significant. However, the authors underline that the favored combination was associated with a higher risk of drug-related adverse events.[25]

Azimilide is a novel class III drug, still under investigation, which seems to be able to suppress both atrial and ventricular arrhythmias. The Shock Inhibition Evaluation with Azimilide (SHIELD) trial was a large, prospective, double-blind study that evaluated the efficacy of this drug in reducing all-cause shocks and arrhythmic events terminated by ATP.[26] The patients treated with both of the tested azimilide doses had reduced all-cause shocks and symptomatic arrhythmia terminated by ATP with respect to placebo. This novel antiarrhythmic drug also reduced all appropriate ICD interventions and increased the inter-event interval as compared to placebo. This suggests its potential for use in the treatment of electrical storm, since recurrent VT/VF events seem to be highly clustered, with most of the inter-event intervals < 1 day. This was confirmed by a subanalysis of the SHIELD trial, which demonstrated that azimilide reduces the risk of electrical storm in a dose-dependent manner.[27] A further point in favor of this drug is that it is well tolerated, with an incidence of adverse events similar to placebo.

As for the use of β-blockers in adjunct to ICD, although there are no placebo-controlled trials in ICD recipients, it must be remembered that β-blockers are fundamental in the treatment of postinfarction and heart failure patients and that in this population these drugs seem to reduce arrhythmia and SCD. An old pre-ICD meta-analysis suggested a greater benefit of β-blockers in preventing sudden death than all-cause mortality in postinfarction patients.[28] The Cardiac Insufficiency Bisoprolol Study II (CIBIS-II) trial was a multicenter double-blind, randomized placebo-controlled trial that evaluated the efficacy of bisoprolol in reducing all-cause mortality in chronic heart failure. The study demonstrated that this drug was able not only to significantly reduce all-cause mortality, but to significantly reduce sudden deaths.[29] β-blockers are, therefore, widely used in adjunct with ICD, especially in postinfarction and in heart failure patients. As we will see later, β-blockers represent first-line drug therapy in certain channelopathies.

Finally, The Cardiac Arrhythmia Suppression Trial (CAST) must be mentioned. This study was interrupted early because of an increased mortality in postinfarction patients with impaired left ventricular function treated with class IC drugs compared to those treated with placebo; therefore, this class of antiarrhythmic drugs does not seem to be safe or effective in preventing ventricular arrhythmias.[30] Another novel antiarrhythmic drug is currently under investigation: celivarone. Already under investigation for the treatment of AF, it is currently being tested in a randomized trial for the prevention of ICD interventions or death in ICD patients with LVEF ≤ 40%.

To date, the guidelines mention the use of drugs as adjuncts to ICD therapy but do not specifically recommend one with respect to another, with the exception of the genetic arrhythmia syndromes for which β-blockers are recommended. In the ACC/AHA/ESC 2006 guidelines, amiodarone, sotalol, and/or β-blockers are considered as adjuncts to ICD therapy in heart failure patients otherwise optimally treated. In patients with left ventricular dysfunction due to prior myocardial infarction, adjunctive therapies to ICD, including catheter ablation and pharmacological therapy with agents such as amiodarone or sotalol, are considered reasonable to improve symptoms due to frequent episodes of VT or VF.[31]

ATP Functionality and Adjunct Drug Therapy

Apart from guideline recommendations, important facts to keep in mind when initiating antiarrhythmic drugs are the possible side effects and the potential drug and device interactions, which must always be recognized and possibly anticipated. An important function of the ICD is the ATP, which offers the potential for painless termination of the VT. Before starting drug therapy, it is important to consider modification of this function. ATP has consistently been shown to be effective in terminating 85% to 90% of slow VT (> 320 ms) and 81%–89% of fast VT

(320–240 ms).[32] The ability to terminate sustained VT by overdrive pacing is influenced by the tachycardia cycle length, refractoriness at the stimulation site, conduction time from the stimulation site to the tachycardia origin, and duration of the excitable gap. In order to resolve the arrhythmia, the paced wavefront has to reach the VT origin and interact with it to enter the circuit. This is more difficult with shorter cycle lengths because the excitable gap is also shorter (Figures 69.1 and 69.2).[33]

The PainFREE trials (PainFREE Rx and PainFREE Rx II) carried out in the United States were specifically designed to evaluate whether empirical ATP would be as safe and effective in treating fast VT as shocks in a broad ICD population. The PainFREE Rx II trial demonstrated that ATP is highly effective in treating monomorphic VT, showing a relative shock reduction of 70% to 92%, depending mainly on cycle length, without any clinical difference in episode duration, arrhythmic syncope, acceleration, or sudden death while yielding improvement in quality of life.[34] European data are in close agreement with those reported by the Painfree Rx II study, as shown in the results by Santini et al.[35] The ADVANCE-D trial was a prospective, randomized study designed to evaluate the efficacy of two different sequences of ATP therapies (burst 15 pulses, 88% vs burst 8 pulses, 88%) during an episode of spontaneous fast VT. The primary endpoint was to compare the efficacy of the two ATP therapies. The study enrolled 925 patients in 60 centers in Europe. Patients were randomized to receive one of the two sequences of ATP as first-line therapy in case of fast VT. Overall, ADVANCE-D does not show strong evidence of the superiority of one specific ATP strategy. It does, however, definitively confirm that ATP therapy is highly effective and safe in treating fast VT in general population. Considering that recently published papers[10,12-13] have demonstrated that appropriate and inappropriate shocks are significant predictors of death, the importance and potential benefit of ATP in reducing shock therapy must be kept in mind. It may be claimed that ATP should always be programmed as first-option electrical therapy for fast VT. As for the influence of antiarrhythmic drugs on ATP, a study published by Bänsch et al identified class III drugs (amiodarone and sotalol) as independent risk predictors of VT that occur above the programmed tachycardia detection interval[36] and therefore may have a negative effect on ATP. On the other hand, in the ADVANCE-D trial the use of ACE-inhibitors seemed to improve ATP efficacy.[35] Previous studies have also shown that β-blockers interfere with parameters involved in the generation of tachycardia.[37] Kouakam et al further demonstrated that the lack of β-blocker use represented an independent risk factor for reduced success of ATP therapy.[38] A recently published paper specifically addressed the influence of β-blocker therapy on ATP effectiveness for monomorphic VT occurring in ICD patients. The authors concluded that β-blockers increase the effectiveness of ATP through a dose-dependent effect, and as a result they reduce the incidence of shocks due to VT.[39] In short, the effects of antiarrhythmic drugs can influence the number of therapies delivered by the ICD in several ways: not only by lowering the number of episodes of VTs but also by increasing the cycle length, leading to a slower arrhythmia

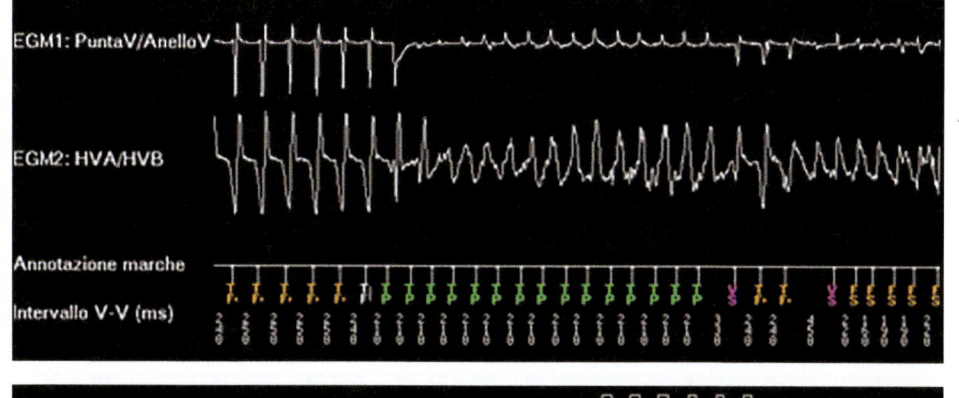

Figure 69.1 Example of stored electrogram showing a fast VT accelerated by ATP in VF.

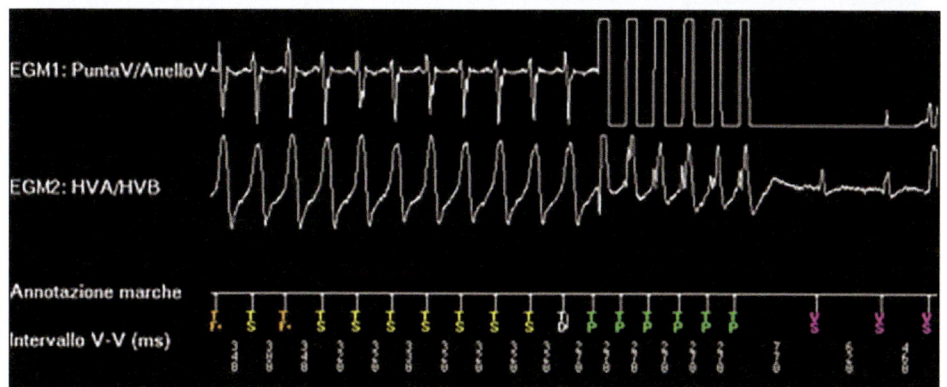

Figure 69.2 Example of stored electrogram showing a VT with lower cycle length successfully terminated by ATP.

amenable to ATP treatment, lowering the number of VT accelerations due to ATP (Figure 69.3). This benefit of antiarrhythmic drugs in preventing ICD shocks should be evaluated in each patient because of the increased capability and sophistication of modern-generation ICDs with reliable algorithms to prevent inappropriate and unnecessary shocks.

ICD and Catheter Ablation

As we have already considered, antiarrhythmic drugs are not always effective in preventing arrhythmic episodes and ICD shocks, and they may have serious adverse effects. An alternative approach to reduce VT/VF recurrence is VT ablation. VT ablation can be considered a curative approach to be used in adjunct to ICD. Catheter ablation of ventricular arrhythmias in patients with structural heart disease was introduced in the 1980s. Initially, the ablation procedure had some limitations; the most important was that only patients with stable and hemodynamically tolerated VT could be treated, since mapping was carried out during VT. Most patients with structural heart disease have different VTs inducible during electrophysiological study, indicating a complex arrhythmia substrate with multiple potential reentry circuits. In these patients, VTs often are unmappable because they are not hemodynamically tolerated, and the spontaneous episodes are promptly interrupted by the ICD so that an ECG tracing cannot be obtained. The second drawback was that it was not possible to obtain sufficiently deep lesions; in patients with prior myocardial infarction, scar-related VTs have often relatively wide reentry circuits that can extend deep in the myocardium. Third, some reentrant circuits were located in epicardial sites and were difficult to reach.

The introduction of electroanatomic mapping systems allowed electrophysiologists to define abnormal endocardium using detailed sinus rhythm voltage mapping. Marchlinski et al demonstrated that radiofrequency linear endocardial lesions extending from the dense scar to the normal myocardium or anatomic boundary are effective in controlling unmappable VT.[40] Another method of performing VT ablation during sinus rhythm was to use a noncontact mapping system. The advantage of this procedure was that it allowed the creation of an activation substrate map with only one beat of tachycardia, thereby rendering mappable unsustained or poorly tolerated arrhythmias. With a computerized mapping system utilizing a noncontact electrode balloon catheter to compute virtual electrograms simultaneously at multiple endocardial sites, accurate substrate maps were created, which were useful to guide ablation of unstable, unmappable, or unsustained VTs.[41] In this regard, late potentials may also be useful; signals in sinus rhythm arise from abnormal myocardium and suggest slow conduction pathways. They may, therefore, be appropriate targets for ablation during sinus rhythm in order to treat hemodynamically unstable or unmappable VTs. The results of Marchlinski et al suggested that ablation of such late potentials may result in successful elimination of the VT, but further investigation is warranted.[42]

Another limitation to VT ablation was that the circuits and reentry paths are often relatively large and located deep in the endocardium. The introduction of irrigated radiofrequency ablation electrodes partly overcame this problem.[43] Conventional endocardial radiofrequency ablation is not always able to prevent recurrence of the arrhythmia, and these failures could in part be explained by the presence of epicardial reentrant circuits. Percutaneous epicardial radiofrequency ablation has been introduced recently as an alternative approach for the treatment of recurrent VT.[44]

The progress in VT ablation techniques has therefore determined the expansion of the indications for VT

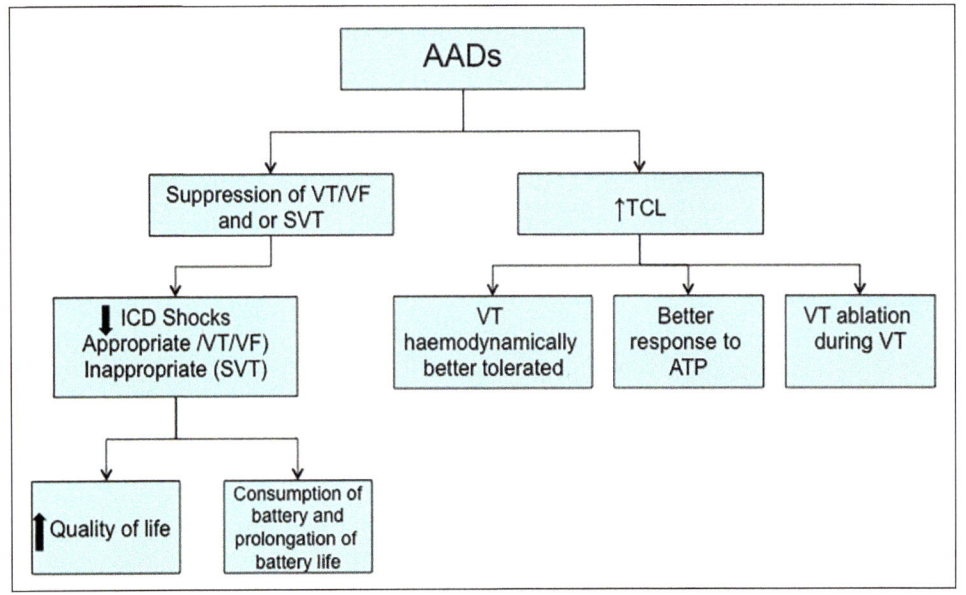

Figure 69.3 Reasons for treatment with AADs in ICD recipients.
AAD = antiarrhythmic drug; VT = ventricular tachycardia; VF = ventricular fibrillation; SVT = supraventricular tachycardia; TCL = tachycardia cycle length; ICD = implantable cardioverter-defilbrillator; ATP = antitachycardiapacing.

ablation in ICD patients. As previously described, the majority of VT occurs in patients with structural heart disease, predominately coronary heart disease, and ICD represents first-line therapy. Catheter ablation of VT in these patients has mostly been performed after multiple ICD interventions and after failure of one or multiple antiarrhythmic drugs. Ablation of the arrhythmia can be taken into consideration also in patients with incessant VT and/or electrical storm, which represents a life-threatening condition characterized by a high cardiac death rate (27%–54%).[45] Further, two recent trials have evaluated the possibility of VT ablation in patients who have not yet experienced an ICD shock. We can, therefore, distinguish three different groups of ICD patients in which catheter ablation can be taken into consideration: (1) patients with multiple ICD shocks, (2) patients with electrical storm or with incessant VT, and (3) patients with ICD but who have not yet experienced ICD shock.

Ablation in ICD Patients with Multiple ICD Shocks

Ablation of VT is mostly used as an adjunctive therapy in patients with structural heart disease and ICD experiencing multiple shocks, generally after failure of antiarrhythmic drugs. The feasibility and efficacy of VT ablation in these patients were evaluated in 3 multicenter studies.

The Cooled RFC Trial was a prospective multicenter study that enrolled 146 patients with structural heart disease, ICD implant, sustained monomorphic VT, and failure of at least 2 antiarrhythmic drugs. This trial was the first multicenter trial to evaluate the safety and efficacy of ablation of VT in structural heart disease using a cooled radiofrequency catheter.[46] The cooling of the ablation electrode by saline irrigation allowed an increase in the size of radiofrequency lesions as well as deeper ablation lesions. In this study, acute success (defined as elimination of mappable VT) was 75%. In 41% of the patients, no VT of any type was inducible after ablation. The 1-year recurrence rate by Kaplan-Meier method was 56%. Clinical success was observed in 81% of the patients, with a ≥ 75% reduction in the VT frequency in the 2 months after ablation compared to the 2 months before the procedure. The major complication rate in this study was 8%, which is in line with the data observed in other studies. The results of this study demonstrated that the ablation of sustained VT can be obtained with high initial success using cooled radiofrequency energy.

The largest study to date on catheter ablation in patients with prior myocardial infarction and recurrent VTs is the Multicenter THERMOCOOL Ventricular Tachycardia Ablation Trial.[43] This trial assessed the outcome of VT ablation using an irrigated radiofrequency catheter combined with an electroanatomic mapping system in patients with recurrent VT and prior myocardial infarction. Two-hundred and thirty-one patients were enrolled with prior myocardial infarction and sustained VT despite antiarrhythmic drug therapy. Patients without ICD were eligible after 2 episodes of sustained VT, but in the population studied > 90% had an ICD before ablation. In contrast to prior studies, patients with multiple and unmappable VT were included. The primary endpoint consisted in freedom from recurrent incessant VT or intermittent VT after 6 months of follow-up and was achieved in 53% of patients despite the fact that most of them had severely depressed ventricular function and drug-refractory VTs. In the majority of patients, there was a significant reduction of VT episodes. The authors concluded that catheter ablation is a reasonable option to reduce recurrent VT in patients with prior myocardial infarction and multiple and/or unmappable VTs, although mortality remained high (18% at 1 year).

In line with the preceding two U.S. studies, a prospective, multicenter, nonrandomized observational study was carried out in Europe, with the aim of assessing the efficacy and safety of electroanatomical mapping in combination with systematically used open-saline irrigated ablation technology for ablation of chronic recurrent mappable and unmappable VT in remote myocardial infarction.[47] The Euro-VT-Study enrolled 63 patients with prior myocardial infarction and episodes of symptomatic VT or incessant VT, refractory to medication and cardioversion. About two-thirds of the patients had received an ICD prior to ablation, and all had severely reduced ventricular function (mean LVEF, 30%). In the population studied, 63% of the patients had at least one clinically relevant unmappable VT. Acute success was obtained in 81% of the patients. During follow-up, 49%, including 19 of the initially successfully ablated patients, developed some type of VT recurrence. In 79% of patients with VT recurrence, a significant reduction of device therapy (ATP and shocks) was observed. One patient (1.5%) experienced a major adverse event during catheter ablation, whereas minor adverse events were observed in 5% of the patients. The authors concluded that ablation using an open-saline irrigated catheter guided by electroanatomic mapping was effective in treatment of mappable and unmappable VT in patients with remote myocardial infarction, with a high acute success rate and low rate of acute and subacute major adverse events. There was, however, as in all the preceding trials, a high recurrence rate, indicating that catheter ablation is largely adjunctive to drug and defibrillator therapy. On the other hand, catheter ablation of recurrent VT has proven to decrease ICD shocks and therefore improve quality of life. A limitation to all the studies of catheter ablation in ICD patients is that in almost all the studies, including single-center studies, antiarrhythmic drugs were not withdrawn systematically and, therefore, any beneficial effect of catheter ablation may be influenced by drug therapy. Furthermore, the efficacy of this therapeutic approach must be balanced with the safety profile of this procedure. Several single-center series have reported relatively high rates of complications due to the ablation procedure (cerebral and coronary embolism, cardiac tamponade, heart block, acute exacerbation of heart failure, and death) whereas the multicenter series have demonstrated differing complication rates. In the EURO-VT trial, there was no procedure-related mortality, the 1-year mortality rate was 8%, and there was only one major complication (1.6%); in the RFC and THERMOCOOL trials, the procedure-related mortality was 2.7% and 3%, respectively; the mortality rate at 1 year was 18% in both studies; and major complications occurred in 8% and 10% of the patients, respectively. Considering the high burden of illness of these patients, the relatively high complication rates are generally considered clinically acceptable. To better define the magnitude of benefit associated with catheter ablation of VT, in a recently published paper, Mallidi et al performed a meta-analysis combining all prospective randomized controlled trials and nonrandomized trials with control groups.[48] The purpose of the study was to define the relative risk of VT recurrence in patients undergoing catheter ablation as an adjunct to medical therapy versus medical therapy alone in a pooled analysis of controlled studies. Five studies were included, totaling 457 patients with structural heart disease. In 58% of the patients, adjunctive catheter ablation was performed, whereas in 42% only medical therapy was given. A statistically significant reduction of VT recurrences was noted in patients in which catheter ablation was carried out ($P < 0.001$) but there was no difference in mortality between the two groups. Two clinical trials are currently underway to directly compare catheter VT ablation to aggressive antiarrhythmic drug therapy. The Ventricular Tachycardia Ablation versus Enhanced Drug Therapy in Structural Heart Disease (VANISH) is a multicenter study enrolling patients with ischemic cardiomyopathy and appropriate ICD shocks, ATP, or ventricular storm despite at least one antiarrhythmic drug; they will be randomized to either catheter ablation or aggressive antiarrhythmic drug therapy. The Catheter Ablation versus Amiodarone for Shock Prophylaxis in Defibrillator Patients with Ventricular Tachycardia (CEASE-VT) includes patients with ischemic cardiomyopathy who are drug naïve and present with ICD shocks; the patients will be randomized to antiarrhythmic therapy or catheter ablation. The results of these studies will help define whether antiarrhythmic drugs or catheter ablation is the most effective therapeutic approach when patients with ischemic cardiomyopathy present with symptomatic ICD therapy. In the meantime, most clinicians refer these patients to ablation after at least one failure with antiarrhythmic drugs, weighing the relative risks and benefits of the two treatment options.[49]

Ablation in ICD Patients with Electrical Storm/Incessant VT

Incessant VT and/or electrical storm are life-threatening situations with poor short- and long-term prognoses. Slow incessant VT is either not detected by the ICD if the cycle length is below the programmed threshold of the device or otherwise can cause multiple ICD shocks. At times the only treatment option is catheter ablation, since the patients are often already taking antiarrhythmic drugs or, if not, antiarrhythmic therapy may further slow the conduction, obtaining a negative effect on arrhythmia cessation. In the setting of electrical storm, catheter ablation seems to be the treatment of choice, since it is able to interrupt the arrhythmic episodes either by eliminating the trigger for VT/VF (mostly ventricular premature beats) or by modifying the substrate.

There are few studies that evaluate the acute and long-term outcomes of this strategy. Carbucicchio et al carried out a single-center study to evaluate catheter ablation of electrical storm. They enrolled 95 patients with drug refractory electrical storm in whom catheter ablation was performed. The induction of any clinical VT by programmed electrical stimulation after the procedure and the in-hospital outcome assessed the short-term efficacy; the long-term analysis considered electrical storm recurrences, cardiac mortality, and VT recurrences. Electrical storm was acutely suppressed in all patients, and induction of any clinical VT by programmed electrical stimulation was prevented in 89% of the patients. At a median follow-up of 22 months, 92% of the patients were free of electrical storm and 66% were free of VT recurrences. No electrical storm recurrence was observed during follow-up in patients in whom either no VT could be induced or the clinical VT became noninducible. Cardiac mortality was observed in 11 patients during follow-up (12%) and was significantly higher in the group of patients with one or more clinical VTs still inducible after catheter ablation. The authors concluded that catheter ablation is not only effective in the short term, but in the long term may favorably affect cardiac mortality in subgroups of patients.[50]

The efficacy of catheter ablation in patients with electrical storm and structural heart disease was assessed in another recently published paper in which the authors enrolled 50 patients. In this study, catheter ablation was effective in suppression of the electrical storm in 84% of the patients. In 22 patients (44%) there was no inducible VT at the end of the procedure and in 20 patients only nonclinical VT were induced. During follow-up, 26 patients had recurrence of VT (52%) and 14 patients died (28%). Interestingly, noninducibility of VT at the end of the procedure was not predictive of electrical storm and/or VT recurrence and of mortality and this is in contrast with the results obtained by Carbucicchio et al. This may be explained by the lower number of subjects included in the study, the limited programmed electrical stimulation after the procedure due to hemodynamical instability of the patients, and the different population studied, which included subjects with polymorphic VT/VF. They concluded that catheter ablation is effective in acute suppression of electrical storm, and in the long term may prevent recurrence of any VT in about half of the treated patients. They also suggest that in some patients electrical storm is an epiphenomenon of progression of heart failure and even successful catheter ablation may not influence their long-term prognosis.[51]

Ablation in ICD Patients Before ICD Shocks

Catheter ablation has demonstrated to be effective in reducing shocks in patients with multiple ICD interventions. On the other hand, ICD shocks have shown to increase mortality. The true benefit of catheter ablation therefore is demonstrated only if ICD shocks are either completely or at least partially prevented. There are two trials that assessed the impact of prophylactic catheter ablation for prevention of defibrillator therapy. The Substrate Mapping and Ablation in Sinus Rhythm to Halt Ventricular Tachycardia (SMASH-VT) trial was a prospective, unblinded, randomized, controlled, multicenter study, which enrolled 128 patients. All subjects had a prior myocardial infarction and an ICD implanted either in secondary prevention (for VF, hemodymanically unstable VT, or syncope with inducible VT during electrophysiological study) or for primary prophylaxis but subsequently had received appropriate ICD therapy for a single event. These patients did not receive antiarrhythmic drugs. They were randomly assigned to defibrillator implantation alone or defibrillator implantation with adjunctive catheter ablation (64 patients in each group). The primary endpoint was survival free from any appropriate ICD therapy. During a 2-year follow-up, a 73% reduction of ICD shocks was observed in the group in which catheter ablation was performed with respect to patients with only ICD. Mortality was reduced in the group assigned to ablation as compared with the control group but the difference did not reach a statistical significance. This, however, seems to suggest that preventive catheter ablation may lead to improved survival.[52]

A retrospective analysis of this study was carried out to try to identify the predictive value of clinical and procedural variables on outcomes in this group of patients. Only the number of inducible VTs during the procedure was predictive of 2-year outcomes, whereas the persistent inducibility of nonclinical VT after catheter ablation did not influence long-term clinical success. This is in contrast with other studies in which the inducibility of nonclinical VT after catheter ablation has been associated with an increased likelihood of clinical recurrence. Which must be the clinical endpoint for VT ablation still remains an issue. The prevailing attitude is to target all the induced VT but the level of aggressiveness to achieve this must be taken into consideration.[53] Another trial assessed the prophylactic ablation of VT followed by implantation of an ICD in patients with prior myocardial infarction, first episode of stable VT, and reduced left ventricular function.[54] The Ventricular Tachycardia Ablation in Coronary Disease (VTACH) trial was a prospective, open, randomized, controlled, multicenter trial that enrolled 110 patients randomized to receive catheter ablation and then an ICD or ICD alone. The primary endpoint was time from defibrillator implantation to first recurrence of VT or VF, and the patients were followed up for at least 1 year. The secondary endpoints included survival free from severe clinical events (death, syncope, hospital admission for cardiac reason, and VT storm), number of appropriate ICD interventions (ATP and shocks), and quality of life. Time to recurrence of VT or VF was longer in the ablation group than in the control group, and according to the Kaplan-Meier analysis, at 2 years 47% of patients in the ablation group and 29% of controls were free from any VT or VF episode. Of note, in patients with LVEF of 30% or less, survival free from VT or VF did not differ between the treatment groups, whereas in patients with moderately impaired LVEF (> 30%) the difference was significant. The secondary endpoints of VT storm, syncope, or death did not differ between the groups, but fewer appropriate ICD interventions and hospital admissions for cardiac reasons were observed in the ablation group. The differences in quality of life favored the ablation group but did not reach significance, partly due to the low proportion of patients responding to the quality of life assessment. On the basis of these data, the authors conclude that prophylactic catheter ablation in patients with hemodynamically stable VT, previous myocardial infarction, and reduced left ventricular function should be strongly considered, before implantation of ICD, especially in patients with a LVEF of > 30%. The complication rate must be kept in mind if an interventional procedure is carried out prophylactically, but in the two studies that we have just considered, the incidence of ablation-related death was 0%; an incidence of 4.7% and of 3.8% of major complications was observed in the SMASH trial and in the VTACH trial, respectively. A lower incidence of procedure-related mortality and major complications was observed with respect to that seen in trials in which catheter ablation is carried out after multiple shocks.

In conclusion, catheter ablation reduces ICD shocks whether it is performed after multiple ICD shocks or prophylactically, and therefore the optimal timing of this procedure remains an open issue. Different studies have demonstrated that ICD shocks increase mortality, but there are no studies to date powered to test whether prevention or significant reduction of ICD interventions determines a reduction of total mortality. However, considering the favorable impact of catheter ablation on arrhythmia recurrence and ICD interventions, this therapeutic approach must be considered in adjunct to ICD therapy in patients with reduced left ventricular function. Further, it can be performed in patients with incessant VT and/or electrical storm in whom catheter ablation is a treatment able to acutely eliminate the arrhythmia and seems to improve prognosis. In most studies and in clinical practice, patients with ICD who undergo catheter ablation continue antiarrhythmic drugs; therefore, any beneficial effect may be a combination of both drugs and ablation therapy. The ongoing randomized studies to which we referred previously that directly compare catheter ablation and antiarrhythmic drug therapy may be of help in understanding the relative efficacy of these two therapeutic strategies.[55]

Microstructural Heart Disease

Brugada Syndrome

Brugada syndrome is a hereditary disease associated with alterations of the QRS morphology (right ventricular conduction delay and ST elevation in the right precordial leads), characterized by syncope and premature sudden death due to VF. The ECG manifestations of the syndrome are often dynamic or concealed and may be revealed by sodium channel blockers. ICD represents the most widely accepted therapeutic approach in these patients but the strategy for risk stratification is still a matter of debate.[56] ICD is certainly recommended in patients with aborted sudden death and in symptomatic patients. Asymptomatic patients displaying a Type 1 Brugada ECG (spontaneously or after sodium channel block) with inducible VT/VF should also be taken into consideration for ICD implant. For all the other patients, a close follow-up is recommended.[57]

With respect to the use of antiarrhythmic drugs in these patients, the literature consists mostly of case reports and relatively small series studies. None of the drugs have proven to completely prevent arrhythmias in Brugada patients. Currently, quinidine seems to be the treatment of choice for chronic therapy, even though it is currently indicated only in selected (severely symptomatic) patients and even this is considered as a class I recommendation.[58] Viskin et al are carrying out a prospective registry investigating the use of empiric quinidine therapy for asymptomatic Brugada,[59] and the QUIDAM study is an ongoing trial comparing quinidine to placebo in preventing ventricular arrhythmias in Brugada patients with ICD; there are, therefore, great expectations on this drug, either in adjunct to ICD or as an alternative in cases in which ICD is refused, unaffordable, or not feasible for any reason. Other drugs have been tested as antiarrhythmic treatment but either the results are controversial or the level of evidence is too low to date. Isoproterenol is the drug of choice in the acute treatment of malignant arrhythmias or electrical storm in these patients.

With respect to use of ablation procedures, Haïssaguerre et al first published a report in which they evaluated the possibility of ablating ventricular premature beats that trigger VT/VF in Brugada patients using noncontact mapping. In their experience, this strategy resulted in long-term freedom from VF.[60] Other authors have published similar experiences, but further investigations are required to confirm these data.[61] In conclusion, ICD to date remains the treatment of choice in these patients; drugs can be considered in case of recurrent ICD interventions, whereas more data are necessary to recommend catheter ablation.

Long QT Syndromes

The long QT syndromes (LQTS) represent a group of genetically transmitted disorders characterized by QT prolongation and by episodes of syncope and sudden death due to torsades de pointes. Physical stress and emotional stress are common triggers of syncope or sudden death, but occasionally these events may be triggered by loud noises or occur while the patient is at rest. The disease is caused by mutation of a gene encoding a cardiac ion channel important for ventricular repolarization. Numerous mutations have been identified, but the majority of patients can be classified in three different genetic subtypes (LQT1, LQT2, LQT3). Treatment decisions may be influenced by knowledge of the genetic basis of LQTS. Considering the relative rarity of the disease and the heterogeneity in the type and severity of its clinical presentation, there are no randomized trials and the guidelines refer to large registries that have followed patients over time. In addition to avoiding QT-prolonging drugs and high-intensity sports (class I recommendation), the standard treatment of LQTS involves the use of β-blockers. Observational studies have shown a superior survival among symptomatic patients who receive β-blockers as compared to those who did not.[62] The protective effect of β-blockers is related to their adrenergic blockade and is more effective in patients with LQT1 mutation, which fortunately represent the most common channel defect.[63] The use of β-blockers, therefore, represents a class I recommendation in all patients with diagnosis of LQTs. ICD in these patients is indicated as a class I recommendation after an aborted cardiac arrest in adjunct to β-blockers. ICD insertion is also indicated in patients who experience syncope and/or VT while receiving β-blocker therapy (class IIa recommendation) and as prophylaxis of SCD in association with β-blockers in patients considered at higher risk such as patients with LQT2 and LQT3 mutations, less responsive to β-blockers, and those with excessive QT prolongation (> 500 ms) (class IIb recommendation).[64] Pacing has been used in selected LQTS patients with sinus bradycardias and pause dependent torsades de pointes, but long-term follow-up has demonstrated an inappropriately high rate of SCD in these patients, so ICD backup is always recommended.[65] On the other hand, ICD allows adequate β-blocker therapy without the risk of inducing excessive bradycardia due to its pacing function. To date a single experience has been reported on VT ablation in LQTS patients. Haïssaguerre et al demonstrated the feasibility and efficacy of focal ablation of the triggers of VT/VF in their study, which included 4 patients with LQTS and 3 with Brugada, but further experience with this type of therapy is warranted.[60]

Catecholaminergic Polymorphic Ventricular Tachycardia

Cathecholaminergic polymorphic ventricular tachycardia (CPVT) presents with exercise or emotional stress-induced syncope and sudden cardiac death. Unfortunately, individuals with CPVT have normal resting ECGs, making diagnosis difficult. Clinical diagnosis is made based on symptoms, family history, and on the induction of the arrhythmia by exercise or isoproterenol infusion. Typically, the ventricular arrhythmia in this syndrome presents as a polymorphic tachycardia or bidirectional ventricular tachycardia, often preceded by ventricular ectopy, sometimes in a pattern of bigeminy, or supraventricular tachyarrhythmias. β-blockers have been proposed as the mainstay of CPVT therapy since early reports; they are also indicated in asymptomatic patients with a genetic diagnosis of CPVT.[64,66] Likewise, β-blockers are used in the treatment of sustained VT episodes in these patients.[67] However, although some authors have reported almost complete prevention from recurrence of cardiac events with β-blockers, others have reported an incomplete protection from exercise-induced arrhythmias.[66] Limited experience with amiodarone produced unfavorable results. Although there are no data on the value of an amiodarone plus β-blocker combination, this possibility may be considered in further studies. Several recent studies have demonstrated a favorable role of flecainide (class 1C drug) in prevention of arrhythmic recurrences in CPVT, suggesting a possible novel strategy.[68]

ICD implantation must also be taken into consideration in this genetic syndrome, always in adjunct with β-blockers. Implantation of an ICD with the use of β-blockers is indicated for patients with CPVT, survivors of cardiac arrest, or in patients who present with syncope and/or documented sustained VT while receiving β-blockers. When considering ICD implant in these young patients, one must keep in mind the risk of inappropriate shocks, so a careful programming of the device is needed. Catheter ablation of focus of onset was unsuccessful in both of the 2 patients in whom it was tried.

Arrhythmogenic Right Ventricular Cardiomyopathy

The arrhythmogenic right ventricular cardiomyopathy (ARVC) is a familial disease characterized by fibrofatty replacement in the myocardium and by ventricular arrhythmias. Palpitations, syncope, or aborted sudden death are the clinical manifestations. A VT with a left bundle branch block morphology must lead to suspicion of ARVC. Prevention of SCD is the most important management strategy in these patients. Evidence suggests that asymptomatic patients or healthy gene carriers do not require prophylactic treatment but should undergo a careful cardiac follow-up and should avoid physical exercise, which may trigger ventricular arrhythmia. In patients with hemodynamically stable arrhythmias, either β-blockers or class III antiarrhythmic drugs (sotalol or amiodarone) used alone or in combination are most effective.[69] ICD is indicated in patients with cardiac arrest, syncope or hemodynamically poorly tolerated VT despite medical therapy (class I). ICD is also indicated in primary prevention as a class IIa recommendation in those patients who have a severe right ventricular dysfunction or advanced disease with biventricular involvement in adjunct to optimal medical therapy. Prophylactic ICD implantation in patients with no clinical manifestation of the disease, but with a genetic diagnosis, is currently not recommended.[64] Radiofrequency ablation has been used in selected patients for the ablation of VT refractory to medical therapy, but relapses are frequent, and ablation does not prevent SCD.[70] However, in patients with ARVC who present with recurrent VTs and who are already ICD carriers, catheter ablation is effective and relatively easy and therefore should be taken into consideration for improving quality of life of these patients.

Structurally Normal Heart

Ventricular arrhythmias may occur also in structurally normal hearts. This group includes the idiopathic ventricular tachycardias: right ventricular outflow tract tachycardias, left ventricular outflow tract tachycardias, aortic cusp ventricular tachycardias, epicardial outflow tract ventricular tachycardias, mitral annulus ventricular tachycardia, and verapamil-sensitive intrafascicular reentrant tachycardia. They are all organized tachycardias with a good prognosis and are rarely associated with sudden death. If not controlled and recurrent they may, however, cause tachycardia-induced cardiomyopathy with depressed ventricular function. Therapy in this case is largely guided by symptoms, and the treatment of choice is transcatheter ablation, which generally resolves the problem.

Electrical Storm

The clustering of VT/VF within a short period of time, and more precisely, 3 or more episodes in 24 hours, has been defined as an electrical storm. In patients with ICDs, multiple shocks severely impair quality of life, increase hospitalization, and may cause premature ICD battery depletion. Such a situation may also evolve into an acute heart failure. Different authors have found that electrical storm is associated with higher mortality. In the AVID study, patients with electrical storm had a 2.4-fold increased risk of mortality overall, with even a higher risk in the 3 months following the event. The analysis also assessed that VT/VF unrelated to electrical storm was not independently associated with an increased risk of subsequent death. Among patients who received ICD in primary prevention, those with electrical storm had a 7.4-fold higher risk of death. Analysis of the various studies indicate that both in primary and secondary prevention ICD patients, electrical storm presages mortality, mostly due to nonsudden cardiac causes. This seems, therefore, to be related not so much to the potential arrhythmic instability as to the progression of cardiac dysfunction. Electrical storm could, in fact, represent an epiphenomenon of advanced structural heart disease in which the recurrent VT/VF and subsequent shocks may worsen left ventricular function and cause myocardial injury. Different studies have been carried out in order to investigate the incidence and prognosis of electrical storm; the results are variable, with incidence ranging from 10% to 28% in the studies involving secondary prevention ICD patients. In the MADIT II trial, the incidence was, in fact, significantly lower (about 4%). This great variability may be due to the difference in the populations examined and in the definition of electrical storm used.[71] In many cases, a trigger of electrical storm is not identified, and there are no conclusive data on what the risk factors for electrical storm are. A low LVEF, chronic renal failure, and ventricular tachycardia as the onset arrhythmia all seem to correlate with an increased risk of developing electrical storm. In primary prevention ICD patients, a combination of a very low LVEF (≤ 25%) with a wide QRS complex (≥ 120 ms) seems to be a prognostic factor for the occurrence of electrical storm.[72] As for the therapeutic approach, electrical storm represents a medical emergency (Figure 69.4); the

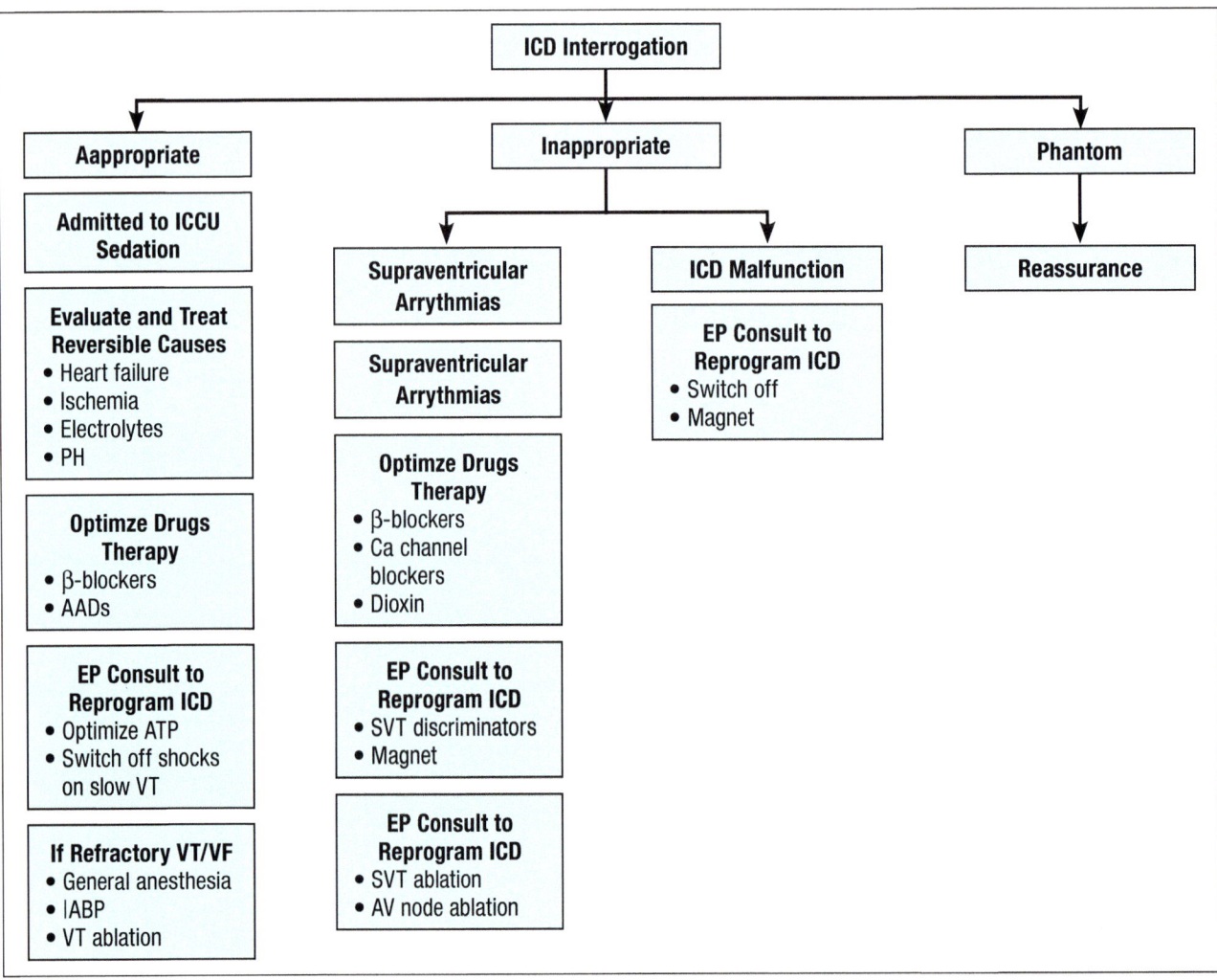

Figure 69.4 Management of electrical storm in ICD patients.

evaluation of the hemodynamic stability of the patients is of outmost importance. If triggers are identified, they must be rapidly corrected. Intravenous administration of β-blockers seem to have beneficial effects, possibly associated with sedatives, considering the potential triggering role of the emotional stress due to the multiple shocks. In the absence of prolonged QT or polymorphic ventricular tachycardia, amiodarone is generally the antiarrhythmic drug of choice, administered intravenously with β-blockers.[71] The SHIELD trial has shown that the antiarrhythmic experimental drug azimilide is effective in preventing electrical storm recurrence. Programming of the ICD is also important. Programming the device in order to deliver ATP for fast VT may reduce shocks.[71] Furthermore, Nordbeck et al recently published a paper in which the incidence of electrical storm was much lower in patients undergoing biventricular pacing with respect to those with pacing only in the left ventricle.[73] This was confirmed in a subanalysis of the Italian Insync ICD registry, in which electrical storm was less frequent in cardiac resynchronization therapy CRT patients.[74] Radiofrequency ablation to treat VT during electrical storm has shown to be effective and safe in patients refractory to medical therapy. A high rate of success was obtained in most of the reported cases, with a relatively low recurrence rate during the follow-up period.[50] Early intervention for electrical storm with catheter ablation therefore appears feasible.

References

1. Santini M, Lavalle C, Ricci PP. Primary and secondary prevention of sudden cardiac death: who should get an ICD? *Heart*. 2007;93(11):1478-1483.
2. Anderson JL, Hallstrom AP, Epstein AE et al. Design and results of the Antiarrhythmic vs. Implantable Defibrillators (AVID) registry. *Circulation*. 1999;99:1692-1699.
3. Moss AJ, Hall WJ, Cannon DS, et al, for the Multicenter Automatic Defibrillator Implantation Trial Investigators. Improved survival with an implanted defibrillator in patients with coronary disease at high risk for ventricular arrhythmia. *N Engl J Med*. 1996;335:1933-1940.
4. DiMarco JP. Implantable cardioverter-defibrillators. *N Engl J Med*. 2003; 349:1836-1847.
5. Epstein AE, DiMArco JP, Ellenbogen KA, et al. ACC/AHA/HRS 2008 Guidelines for Device-Based Therapy for Cardiac Rhythm Abnormalities: a report of the American College of Cardiology/American Heart Association Task Force on Practice Guidelines (Writing Committee to revise the ACC/AHA/NASPE 2002 Guideline Update For Implantation Of Cardiac Pacemakers And Antiarrhythmia Devices) developed in collaboration with the American Association for Thoracic Surgery and Society of Thoracic Surgeons. *Circulation*. 2008; 117:e350-e408.
6. McCready MJ, Exner DV. Quality of life and psychological impact of implantable cardioverter defibrillators: focus on randomized controlled trial data. *Cardiac Electrophysiol Rev*. 2003;7:63-70.
7. Kamphuis HCM, de Leeuw JRJ, Derksen R, et al. A 12 month quality of life assessment of cardiac arrest survivors treated with and without an implantable cardioverter defibrillator. *Europace*. 2002;4:417-425.
8. Singh S, Murawski MM. Implantable cardioverter defibrillator therapy and the need for concomitant antiarrhythmic drugs. *J Cardiovasc Pharm Therapeutics*. 2007;12(3):175-180.
9. Patel C, Yan GX, Kocovic D, Kowey PR. Ventricular tachycardia ablation versus drugs for preventing ICD shocks. *Circ Arrhythm Electrophysiol*. 2009;2:705-712.
10. Poole JE, Johnson GW, Hellkamp AS, et al. Prognostic importance of defibrillator shocks in patients with heart failure. *N Engl J Med*. 2008; 359:1009-1017.
11. Sweeney MO, Sherfesee L, DeGroot PJ, et al. Differences in effects of electrical therapy type for ventricular arrhythmias on mortality in implantable cardioverter defibrillator patients. *Heart Rhythm*. 2010;7:353-360.
12. Daubert JP, Zareba W, Cannom DS, et al. Inappropriate implantable cardioverter defibrillator shocks in MADIT II: frequency, mechanism, predictors and survival impact. *J Am Coll Cardiol*. 2008;51:1357-1365.
13. Goldenberg I, Moss AJ, Hall WJ, et al. Causes and consequences of heart failure after prophylactic implantation of a defibrillator in the multicenter automatic defibrillator implantation trial II. *Circulation*. 2006; 113:2810-2817.
14. Raitt MH. Implantable cardioverter-defibrillator shocks: a double-edged sword? *J Am Coll Cardiol*. 2008; 51:1366-1368.
15. Van Rees JB, Borleffs JW, de Bie MK, et al. Inappropriate implantable cardioverter defibrillator shocks. *J Am Coll Cardiol*. 2011;Vol 57(5):556-562.
16. Schluter T, Baum H, Plewan A, et al. Effects of implantable cardioverter defibrillator implantation and shock application on biochemical markers of myocardial damage. *Clin Chem*. 2001;47:459-463.
17. Hurst TM; Hinrichs M, Breidenbach C, et al. Detection of myocardial injury during transvenous implantation of automatic cardioverter defibrillators. *J Am Coll Cardiol*. 1999;34: 402-408.
18. Van Herendael H, Pinter A, Ahmad K et al. Role of antiarrhythmic drugs in patients with implantable cardioverter defibrillators. *Europace*. 2010;12:618-625.
19. Gronefeld GC, Mauss O, Li YG, et al. Association between atrial fibrillation and appropriate implantable cardioverter defibrillator therapy: results from a prospective study. *J Cardiovasc Electrophysiol*. 2000;11:1208-1214.
20. Huang DT, Traub D. Recurrent ventricular arrhythmia storms in the age of implantable cardioverter defibrillator therapy: a comprehensive review. *Progress Cardiovasc Disease*. 2008; 51(3):229-236.
21. Singh JP, Hall WJ, McNitt S, et al. Factors influencing appropriate firing of the implanted defibrillator for ventricular tachycardia/fibrillation: finding from the Multicenter Automatic Defibrillator Implantation Trial II (MADIT II). *J Am Coll Cardiol*. 2005;46: 1712-1720.
22. Raitt MH, Klein RC, Wyse DG, et al. Comparison of arrhythmia recurrence in patients presenting with ventricular fibrillation versus ventricular tachycardia in the Antiarrhythmic Versus Implantable Defibrillators (AVID) trial. *Am J Cardiol*. 2003;91:812-816.
23. Freedberg NA, Hill JN, Fogel RI, Prystowsky EN. Recurrence of symptomatic ventricular arrhythmias in patients with implantable cardioverter defibrillator after the first device therapy. *J Am Coll Cardiol*. 2001;37;1910-1915.
24. Pacifico A, Hohnloser SH, Williams JH, et al. Prevention of implantable-defibrillator shocks by treatment with sotalol. D,L-sotalol implantable cardioverter defibrillator study group. *N Engl J Med*. 1999;340:1855-1862.

25. Connolly SJ, Dorian P, Roberts RS, et al. Comparison of β-blockers, amiodarone plus β-blockers, or sotalol for prevention of shocks from implantable cardioverter defibrillators. *J Am Med Assoc.* 2006;295:165-171.
26. Dorian P, Borggrefe M, Al-Khalidi HR, et al. Placebo-controlled, randomized clinical trial of azimilide for prevention of ventricular tachyarrhymias in patients with an implantable cardioverter defibrillator. *Circulation.* 2004;110:3646-3654.
27. Hohnloser SH, Al-Khalidi HR, Pratt CM, et al. Electrical storm in patients with an implantable defibrillator: incidence, features and preventive therapy: insights from a randomized trial. *Eur Heart J.* 2006;27:3027-3032.
28. Yusuf S, Peto R, Lewis J, et al. Beta blockade during and after myocardial infarction: an overview of the randomized trials. *Prog Cardiovasc Dis.* 1985;27:335-371.
29. CIBIS-II Investigators and Committees. The Cardiac Insufficiency Bisoprolol Study II: a randomized trial. *Lancet.* 1999;353:9-13.
30. Echt DS, Liebson PR, Mitchell LB, et al. Mortality and morbidity in patients receiving encainide, flecainide or placebo: the Cardiac Arrhythmia Suppression Trial. *N Engl J Med.* 1991;324:781-788.
31. ACC/AHA/ESC 2006 guidelines for the management of patients with ventricular arrhythmias and the prevention of sudden cardiac death. *J Am Coll Cardiol.* 2006, 48(5):247-346.
32. Majid Haghjoo. Efficacy and safety of different antitachycardia pacing sites in the termination of ventricular tachycardia in patients with biventricular implantable cardioverter-defibrillator. *Europace.* 2011;13(4):509-513.
33. Josephson ME. *Clinical cardiac electrophysiology: techniques and interpretations.* 4th ed. Philadelphia: Lippincott, Williams and Wilkins; 2009; p 573.
34. Wathen M. Implantable cardioverter defibrillator shock reduction using new antitachycardia pacing therapies. *Am Heart J.* 2007;153,4:S44-S52.
35. Santini M, Lunati M, Defaye P, et al. Prospective multicenter randomized trial of fast ventricular tachycardia termination by prolonged versus conventional anti-tachyarrhythmia burst pacing in implantable cardioverter-defibrillator patients—ATP Delivery for Painless ICD Therapy (ADVANCE-D) Trial results. *J Interv Card Electrophysiol.* 2010;27(2):127-135.
36. Bänsch D, Castrucci M, Böcker D, et al. Ventricular tachycardias above the initially programmed tachycardia detection interval in patients with implantable cardioverter-defibrillators: Incidence, prediction and significance. *J Am Coll Cardiol.* 2000;36(2):557-565.
37. Wiesfeld AC, Crijns HJ, Tuininga YS, Lie KI. Beta adrenergic blockade in the treatment of sustained ventricular tachycardia or ventricular fibrillation. *Pacing Clin Electrophysiol.* 1996;19(7):1026-1035.
38. Kouakam C, Lauwerier B, Klug B, et al. Effect of elevated heart rate preceding the onset of ventricular tachycardia on antitachycardia pacing effectiveness in patients with implantable cardioverter defibrillators. *Am J Cardiol.* 2003; 92:26–32.
39. Jiménez-Candil J, Hernández J, Martín A, et al. Influence of beta-blocker therapy on antitachycardia pacing effectiveness for monomorphic ventricular tachycardias occurring in implantable cardioverter-defibrillator patients: a dose-dependent effect. *Europace.* 2010;12(9):1231-1238.
40. Marchlinski FE, Callens DJ, Gottlieb CD, Zado E. Linear ablation lesions for control of unmappable ventricular tachycardia in patients with ischemic and non ischemic cardiomyopathy. *Circulation.* 2000;101:1288-1296.
41. Della Bella P, Pappalardo A, Riva S, et al. Non-contact mapping to guide catheter ablation of untolerated ventricular tachycardia. *Eur Heart J.* 2002;23(9):742-752.
42. Hsia HH, Lin D, Sauer WH, Callens DJ, Marchlinski FE. Relationship of late potentials to the ventricular tachycardia circuit defined by entrainment. *J Interv Card Electrophysiol.* 2009;26(1): 21-29.
43. Stevenson WG, Wilber DJ, Natale A, et al. Irrigated radiofrequency catheter ablation guided by electroanatomic mapping for recurrent ventricular tachycardia after myocardial infarction: the Multicenter Thermocool Ventricular Tachycardia Ablation Trial. *Circulation.* 2008;118:2773-2782.
44. Sosa E, Scanavacca M, d'Avila A. Transthoracic epicardial catheter ablation to treat recurrent ventricular tachycardia. *Curr Cardiol Rep.* 2001;3(6):451-458.
45. Arya A, Haghjoo M, Dehghani MR, et al. Prevalence and predictors of electrical storm in patients with implantable cardioverter-defibrillator. *Am J Cardiol.* 2006; 97:389-392.
46. Calkins H, Epstein A, Packer D, et al. Catheter ablation of ventricular tachycardia in patients with structural heart disease using cooled radiofrequency energy. *J Am Coll Cardiol.* 2000;35(7):1905-1914.
47. Tanner H, Hindricks G, Volkmer M, et al. Catheter ablation of recurrent scar related ventricular tachycardia using electroanatomical mapping and irrigated ablation technology: results of the Prospective Multicenter Euro-VT-Study. *J Cardiovasc Electrophysiol.* 2010;21(1):47-53.
48. Mallidi J, Nadkarni GN, Berger RD, et al. Meta-analysis of catheter ablation as an adjunct to medical therapy for treatment of ventricular tachycardia in patients with structural heart disease *Heart Rhythm.* 2011;Vol 8(4):503-510.
49. El-Damaty A, Sapp JL. The role of catheter ablation for ventricular tachycardia in patients with ischemic heart disease. *Curr Opin Cardiol.* 2011;26:30-39.
50. Carbucicchio C, Santamaria M, Trevisi N, et al. Catheter Ablation for the Treatment of Electrical Storm in Patients with Implantable Cardioverter Defibrillators. *Circulation.* 2008;117:462-469.
51. Kozeluhova M, et al. Catheter ablation of electrical storm in patients with structural heart disease. *Europace.* 2011;13: 109-113.
52. Reddy VY, et al. Prophylactic Catheter Ablation for the Prevention of Defibrillator Therapy. (SMASH Trial) *N Engl J Med.* 2007;357:2657-2665.
53. Tung R, Josephson ME, Reddy V, Reynolds MR. Influence of Clinical and Procedural Predictors on Ventricular Tachycardia Ablation Outcomes: An Analysis from the Substrate Mapping and Ablation in Sinus Rhythm to Halt Ventricular Tachycardia Trial (SMASH-VT). *J Cardiovasc Electrophysiol.* 2010;21(7): 799-803.
54. Kuch KH, et al. Catheter ablation of stable ventricular tachycardia before defibrillator implantation in patients with coronary heart disease (VTACH): a multicenter randomised controlled trial. *Lancet.* 2010;375:31-40.
55. Kuck KH. Should catheter ablation be the preferred therapy for reducing ICD shocks? *Circ Arrhythm Electrophysiol.* 2009;2:713-720.
   Brugada J, Brugada R, Brugada P. Pharmacological and device approach to therapy of inherited cardiac diseases associated with cardiac arrhythmias and sudden death. *J Electrocardiol.* 2000;33 (Suppl):41-47.
56. Antzelevitch C, Brugada P, Borggrefe M, et al. Brugada syndrome. Report of the Second Consensus Conference. *Circulation.* 2005;111:659-670.
57. Postema PC, Wolpert C, Amin AS, et al. Drugs and Brugada Syndrome Patients: review of the literature, recommendations and up-to-date website. *Heart Rhythm.* 2009;6(9):1335-1341.

58. Viskin S, Wilde AAM, Tan HL, et al. Empiric quinidine therapy for asymptomatic Brugada Syndrome: time for a prospective registry. *Heart Rhythm.* 2009;6(3)401-404.
59. Haïssaguerre M, Extramiana F, Hocini M, et al. Mapping and ablation of ventricular fibrillation associated with long-QT and Brugada syndromes. *Circulation.* 2003;108:925-928.
60. Nakagawa E, Takagi M, Tatsumi H, et al. Successful radiofrequency catheter ablation for electrical storm of ventricular fibrillation in a patient with Brugada Syndrome. *Circ J.* 2008; 72: 1025-1029.
61. Hobbs JB, Peterson DR, Moss AJ, et al. Risk of aborted cardiac arrest or sudden cardiac death during adolescence in the long QT syndrome. *JAMA.* 2006;296:1249-1254.
62. Priori SG, Napolitano C, Schwartz PJ, et al. Association of long QT syndrome loci and cardiac events among patients treated with beta-blockers. *JAMA.* 2004;292:1341-1344.
63. ACC/AHA/ESC 2006. Guidelines for Management of Patients with Ventricular Arrhythmias and the Prevention of Sudden Cardiac Death. *J Am Coll Cardiol.* 2006;8(5):e247-e234.
64. Dorostkar PC, Eldar M, Belhassen B, Scheinman MM. Long-term follow-up of patients with long-QT syndrome treated with beta blockers. *Circulation.* 1999;100:2431-2436.
65. Napolitano C, Priori SG. Diagnosis and treatment of catecholaminergic polymorphic ventricular tachycardia. *Heart Rhythm.* 2007;4(5):675-667.
66. De Rosa G, Deloga AB, Piastra M, et al. Catecholaminergic polymorphic ventricular tachycardia: successful emergency treatment with intravenous propanolol. *Pediatr Emerg Care.* 2004;20:175-177.
67. Pott C, Dechering DG, Reinke F, et al. Successful treatment of catecholaminergic polymorphic ventricular tachycardia with flecainide: a case report and review of the current literature. *Europace.* 2011;13(6):897-901.
68. Basso C, Corrado D, Marcus FI, et al. Arrhythmogenic right ventricular cardiomyopathy. *Lancet.* 2009;373:1289-1300.
69. Fontaine G, Tonet J, Gallais Y, et al. Ventricular tachycardia catheter ablation in arrhythmogenic right ventricular dysplasia: a 16-year experience. *Curr Cardiol Rep.* 2000;2:498-506.
70. Huang DT, Traub D. Recurrent ventricular arrhythmia storms in the age of implantable cardioverter defibrillator therapy: a comprehensive review. *Progr Cardiovasc Disease.* 2008;51(3):229-236.
71. Arash A, Majid H, Mohammad R, et al. Prevalence and predictors of electrical storm in patients with implantable cardioverter defibrillator. *Am J Cardiol.* 2006;97:389-392.
72. Nordbeck P, Seidl B, Fey B, et al. Effects of cardiac resynchronization therapy on the incidence of electrical storm. *Int J Cardiol.* 2010; 143:330-336.
73. Gasparini M, Lunati M, Landolina M, et al. Electrical storm in patients with biventricular implantable cardioverter defibrillator: incidence, predictors and prognostic implications. *Am Heart J.* 2008;156:847-854.

INDEX

Page numbers followed by *f*, *t*, refer to figures, tables

A

AADs. *See* antiarrhythmic drugs
ablation
    See also type of
    anatomy and histopathology of interventions,187–202, 188*f*, 189*f*, 190*f*, 192*f*, 193*f*, 194*f*, 195*f*, 196*f*, 197*f*, 198*f*, 199*f*, 200*f*; 201*f*, 202*f*
Ablation for Paroxysmal Atrial Fibrillation (APAF) trial, 973
ACC. *See* American College of Cardiology
accessory pathways (APs)
    catheter ablation, 489–494, 496, 490*f*, 491*f*, 492*f*, 493*f*, 494*f*, 495*f*, 496*f*, 497*f*
    complications, 608
    diagnosis, 259
    epicardial anteroseptal, 499–501, 501*f*
    epicardial posteroseptal (coronary sinus myocardial-ventricular connections), 496, 497*f*, 498–499, 498*f*, 499*f*
    left midseptal, 499, 500*f*
    localization of, and mapping, 489–494, 496, 490*f*, 491*f*, 492*f*, 493*f*, 494*f*
    right and left appendage connections, 501–502
    unusual locations of, 497*f*
ACT. *See* activated clotting time
activated clotting time (ACT) test, 5
Acutronic Medical Systems, Monsoon Universal Jet Ventilator, 441, 442, 444, 447
adenosine, 9
    atrial fibrillation ablation and, 261, 333
    tachyarrhythmias and, 257–259
adenosine triphosphate, 9–10
ADOPT trial, 950
adrenaline and procainamide infusion worksheet, 254, 255*t*–256*t*
ADVANCE-D trial, 985
AE. *See* atrioesophageal
AF. *See* atrial fibrillation
AFCL. *See* atrial fibrillation cycle length
AFFIRM. *See* Atrial Fibrillation Follow-up Investigation of Rhythm Management
AFL. *See* atrial flutter
AHA. *See* American Heart Association
air embolism, 613
airway management, 434, 435–436, 453, 454*f*, 458–459
ALTITUDE study, 153, 155
American Association for Thoracic Surgery, 908
American College of Cardiology (ACC), 149, 465*t*, 869, 869*f*, 870*t*, 891, 908
    best practices, 731, 732*t*–733*t*
American Heart Association (AHA), 149, 465*t*, 869, 869*f*, 870*t*, 891, 908
American Society of Anesthesiologists (ASA), 434, 437, 447, 451, 453*t*, 458, 458*t*, 459
amiodarone, 477, 944, 944*f*, 974, 984, 988
Amiodarone versus Implantable Cardioverter-Defibrillator Randomized Trial (AMIOVIRT), 909*t*, 910
amionophylline, 261
AMIOVIRT. *See* Amiodarone versus Implantable Cardioverter-Defibrillator Randomized Trial
AMPLATZER device, 167, 168–169
amyloid heart disease, mapping triggers of PMVT/VF in, 400, 603
Anesthesia Quality Institute (AQI), 451
anesthesia/sedation
    administering, 433
    airway management, 434, 435–436, 453, 454*f*, 458–459
    for cardioversion, 278
    for catheter ablation, 278
    commonly used drugs, 279*t*, 456
    continuum of, and use of term "MAC," 434, 434*t*, 459
    for device implantation, 278, 455–456, 695
    documentation of, 458, 458*t*
    for electrophysiology procedures, 4
    goals of, 433, 434*f*
    hemodynamic effects of, 437*t*
    for high-frequency jet ventilation, 439, 441–448
    inhalation, 276, 438
    interaction of, 276, 456
    intravenous, 270–275
    intravenous, total, 439
    levels of, 454–455, 455*t*
    local, 268–270
    Mallampati classification, 434, 435*f*, 452–453
    monitoring, 277–278, 435, 458, 458*t*, 459
    muscle relaxants, 275, 446
    patient positioning, 438, 458
    for pediatric patients, 56, 56*t*, 407*t*, 409–410, 457
    personnel by procedure, recommended, 455, 455*t*
    physical status classification, 453, 453*t*
    preoperative preparation, 277
    preprocedure evaluation, 434–435, 435*f*, 452–457, 452*t*, 453*f*, 453*t*, 454*f*, 455*t*
    procedural, 457–458, 458*t*
    quality issues, 451, 458*t*
    recovery from, 460
    safety concerns, 438–439, 451
    types of, 276–277, 436–438, 455–456
angiography, coronary venous, 723–724, 724*f*
ANS. *See* autonomic nervous system
antiarrhythmic drugs (AADs)
    atrial antitachycardia pacing and, 984–986, 985*f*
    atrial fibrillation and, 973–974, 974*f*, 975*f*
    atrial fibrillation with catheter ablation and, 975–977, 976*f*
    atrial fibrillation with catheter ablation versus, 972–973
    atrial pacing and, 950–951, 950*f*
    Brugada syndrome, 990
    catheter ablation and, 948–950, 949*t*
    combinations, 944–945, 944*f*, 945*f*
    dual-site atrial pacing with catheter ablation and, 958–963, 959*f*, 960*t*, 960*f*, 961*f*, 962*f*, 963*f*
    implantable cardioverter-defibrillators and, 982–986, 983*t*, 985*f*, 986*f*
    limitations of, 973–974
    pacing and, 976
Antiarrhythmics Versus Implantable Defibrillators (AVID), 871, 872*t*, 908, 909*t*, 910, 932–933
anticoagulation
    monitoring, 810–812, 811*f*, 812*f*, 813*f*
    strategies, 861*t*–862*t*
antitachycardia pacing (ATP), 884–885
AP. *See* accessory pathways
APAF. *See* Ablation for Paroxysmal Atrial Fibrillation
apixaban, 706
apnea, 445, 459
AQI. *See* Anesthesia Quality Institute
arrhythmias
    See also epicardial ventricular arrhythmias; idiopathic annular ventricular arrhythmias; idiopathic ventricular arrhythmias; papillary muscle arrhythmias
    after surgery, image integration techniques for, 111, 111*f*
    atrial, 409–414, 412*f*, 803–813, 805*f*, 806*f*, 807*f*, 808*f*, 809*f*, 810*f*, 811*f*, 812*f*, 813*f*
    focal, 45

997

arrhythmias *(continued)*
    genetic syndromes, 882–883
    macroreentrant, 45
arrhythmogenic right ventricular cardiomyopathy (ARVC), 571
    catheter ablation, 581
    imaging, 123–124
    implantable cardioverter-defibrillators for, 991
arrhythmogenic right ventricular dysplasia/cardiomyopathy (ARVD/C)
    implantable cardioverter-defibrillators for, 873, 880–881, 913
    outcomes of ventricular tachycardia ablation, 876–877
Arruda algorithm, 17, 17*f*
ARVC. *See* arrhythmogenic right ventricular cardiomyopathy
ARVD/C. *See* arrhythmogenic right ventricular dysplasia/cardiomyopathy
ASA. *See* American Society of Anesthesiologists
ASPECT trial, 950, 956
ASPIRE trial, 583
ATP. *See* antitachycardia pacing; atrial antitachycardia pacing
atrial antitachycardia pacing (ATP), 143
    implantable cardioverter-defibrillators and, 984–986, 985*f*
atrial arrhythmias
    monitoring of, 803–813, 805*f*, 806*f*, 807*f*, 808*f*, 809*f*, 810*f*, 811*f*, 812*f*, 813*f*
    in pediatric patients with congenital heart disease, 409–414, 412*f*
Atrial Dynamic Overdrive Pacing trial, 903
atrial dyssynchrony, 718, 718*f*
atrial-esophageal fistula, 611–612
atrial fibrillation (AF)
    See also surgical ablation, for atrial fibrillation
    ablation, focal and map-guided, 527–537, 528*f*, 529*f*, 531*f*, 532*f*, 533*f*, 535*f*, 536*f*, 537*f*, 538*f*
    ablation, laser, 544–546, 544*f*, 545*f*, 546*t*
    ablation drugs, 261–262
    ablation procedures, 6–9, 667–675
    antiarrhythmic drugs and, 973–974, 974*f*, 975*f*
    antiarrhythmic drugs and atrial pacing, 950–951, 950*f*
    antiarrhythmic drugs and catheter ablation, 948–950, 949*t*
    anticoagulation strategies, 861*t*–862*t*
    cardiac resynchronization therapy, 901
    catheter ablation, 850–863, 852*t*, 853*t*, 855*f*, 856*f*, 857*f*, 858*t*, 859*f*, 860*t*, 861*t*, 862*t*, 863*f*, 968–972, 969*f*, 970*f*, 971*f*
    catheter ablation and antiarrhythmic drugs, 975–977, 976*f*
    catheter ablation and intracardiac echocardiography, 89, 89*f*
    catheter ablation versus antiarrhythmic drugs, 972–973
    circumferential left atrial ablation, 855–856, 856*f*
    complex fractionated atrial electrograms, 336–337, 534–535, 535*f*, 536*f*, 537*f*, 538*f*, 857, 857*f*, 968, 970*f*
    complications, 608–610, 608*t*, 609*t*, 610*t*
    computed tomography, magnetic resonance imaging, and 3D mapping systems for, 106–108, 107*f*
    coronary sinus ablation, 854, 855*f*
    cryoballoon ablation, 547–548, 547*f*, 972
    definitions and classification, 327–328, 328*f*, 859–860, 860*t*–862*t*
    dual-site atrial pacing with catheter ablation and antiarrhythmic drugs, 958–963, 959*f*, 960*t*, 960*f*, 961*f*, 962*f*, 963*f*
    echocardiography, 66–67
    electrical isolation of pulmonary veins, 852–853, 853*f*
    electrophysiological findings, 335–337, 335*t*
    electrophysiological techniques, 330–332, 331*f*, 332*f*, 333*f*
    energy sources, 858, 858*t*
    ganglionic plexi mapping and ablation, 337
    hybrid therapy in, types of, 947–948, 948*t*
    hybrid therapy in, with heart failure, 961–962
    hybrid therapy in, without bradycardias, 962
    indications for catheter ablation, 862*t*
    linear catheter ablation, 519–524
    linear lesions, 854–855, 856*f*
    long-lasting persistent, 856–857
    magnetic navigation, 245
    mapping, 851–856, 852*f*, 853*t*, 855*f*, 856*f*
    mapping (intraoperative), 51–52, 52*f*, 422–425, 423*f*, 424*f*, 425*f*
    mapping (3D), 106–108, 107*f*, 337–338, 338*f*, 339*f*, 340*f*, 341, 341*f*
    monitoring of, 803–813, 805*f*, 806*f*, 807*f*, 808*f*, 809*f*, 810*f*, 811*f*, 812*f*, 813*f*
    nests, 337, 536–537, 538*f*
    non-pulmonary vein triggers, 336, 854
    paroxysmal, 921, 926, 948–949
    pathophysiology, 328–329
    in pediatric patients, 57
    primary versus secondary prevention of, 947
    programmed stimulation, 333, 334*f*
    pulmonary vein triggers, 335–336, 851–852
    recurrences, 972, 976
    reentry theories, 329–330, 330*f*
    remote monitoring of patients with, 156
    remote navigation, 533, 859, 859*f*
    rhythm control strategies, 863*f*
    safety issues, 853
    spontaneous induction, 333, 334*f*, 335
Atrial Fibrillation Ablation vs. Antiarrhythmic Drugs trial, 973
Atrial Fibrillation Catheter Ablation Versus Surgical Ablation Treatment (FAST) trial, 643, 644, 645, 670
atrial fibrillation cycle length (AFCL), 523, 524
Atrial Fibrillation Follow-up Investigation of Rhythm Management (AFFIRM), 470, 806, 808, 944, 945*f*
atrial flutter (AFL)
    antiarrhythmic drugs and catheter ablation, 949–950
    atypical left, 849–850, 849*f*, 850*f*, 851*f*
    atypical right, 848–849, 849*f*
    catheter ablation, 508, 847–850, 848*f*, 849*f*, 850*f*, 851*f*
    cavotricuspid isthmus-dependent, 848, 949, 976
    complications, 512, 608
    dual loop right atrial tachycardias, 513
    echocardiography, 67
    electrocardiographic findings, 18–19, 19*f*, 20*f*
    left atrial macroreentry, 513–515, 514*f*, 515*f*
    left septal, 515
    mapping strategies, 505–506, 506*f*, 507*f*
    outcomes of ablation for cavotricuspid isthmus dependent, 511–512
    pacing maneuvers, 27, 28*t*, 29, 29*t*
    in pediatric patients, 56, 57
    right atrial free-wall reentry, 512, 513*f*
    right atrial septal reentry, 513
    surgical ablation, 926
    typical right, 847–848, 848*f*
    upper loop reentry, 512–513
atrial lead placement, 699
atrial pacing
    antiarrhythmic drugs and, 950–951, 950*f*
    dual-site, with catheter ablation and antiarrhythmic drugs, 958–963, 959*f*, 960*t*, 960*f*, 961*f*, 962*f*, 963*f*
    maneuvers, 29, 29*t*, 720–722, 721*f*, 722*f*
atrial pacing, multisite
    biatrial and dual-site right techniques, 951–953, 951*f*, 952*f*
    outcomes, 955–958, 957*f*, 958*f*
    physiologic effects of, 953–954, 955*f*
atrial resynchronization, 953–954, 953*f*, 955*f*
atrial reverse remodeling, 954
atrial septum, anatomy, 196, 196*f*
atrial tachycardias (ATs)
    See also focal artial tachycardias; macroreentrant atrial tachycardias
    catheter ablation, 843, 843*t*
    complications, 608, 610
    electrocardiographic findings, 14–16, 15*f*, 16*f*
    image integration techniques for, after atrial fibrillation ablation/surgery, 111
    mapping, intraoperative, 51, 422
    monitoring of, 803–813, 805*f*, 806*f*, 807*f*, 808*f*, 809*f*, 810*f*, 811*f*, 812*f*, 813*f*
    pacing maneuvers, 27, 28*t*, 29, 29*t*, 143
AtriCure, Inc.
    Bipolar Pen, 623, 623*f*
    Coolrail Linear Pen, 237, 237*f*, 238
    cryoICE, 234, 234*f*
    Isolator Multifunctional Pen, 237, 237*f*, 238
    Isolator Synergy clamp, 237, 237*f*
    Wolf Lumitip dissector with GlidePath Transfer Guide, 648–649, 648*f*
atrioesophageal (AE) fistula, 550, 670, 687
atrioventricular block, pacemaker indications for, 892–895, 894*f*, 897–899, 902*t*, 903*t*
atrioventricular bypass tracts, intraoperative mapping, 47, 48*f*, 49*f*
atrioventricular conduction system, identifying normal, 52–53
atrioventricular dyssynchrony, 718, 718*f*
atrioventricular groove, 194, 194*f*
atrioventricular junction (AVJ) ablation

cardiac resynchronization therapy and, 470–471
catheter ablation, 839–840, 839t
clinical efficacy, 467, 468t–469t
complications, 467, 607
confirmation of block, 466
follow-up, 470
heparin infusion, 466
left-sided approach, 465–466, 466f
limitations, 463
pacing mode, 467, 977
preparation for, 464
recommendations, 465t
right-sided approach, 464–465, 466f
strategies for ablation and pacing, 467
temperature control with energy, 466
atrioventricular nodal reentrant tachycardia (AVNRT)
atrioventricular nodal reciprocating tachycardia, 842
catheter ablation, 480–483, 481f, 841–842, 841t
complications, 607–608
continuous AV nodal function curves, 485
coronary sinus size and morphology, 478, 479f
cryoablation, 482
diagnosis, 480, 480f
differentiation between AVRT and, 29t, 303, 304f
drugs, 259, 260–261
dual nodal pathway, 302–303, 303f, 304f, 305, 305f, 306f, 307f, 479
eccentric retrograde coronary sinus activation, 483–484, 483f
electrocardiographic findings, 18, 18f, 19f
endpoints, 483, 483f
multiple nodal pathways, 484
pacing maneuvers, 27, 28t, 29, 29t
in pediatric patients, 56–57
preexisting prolonged PR interval, 485
atrioventricular node (AVN)
anatomy, 52, 192, 193f, 289–290, 290f, 478, 478f
block, types of, 291–292, 291f, 292f
clinical presentation of dysfunction, 292
common diseases associated with, 292–294
damage to, 52–53
dual physiology, 295–296, 296f
electrophysiology, 290, 294–296, 294f, 296f, 479, 480f
mapping, 296
refractoriness and decremental conduction, 295
role of, 290–291
atrioventricular reentrant tachycardia (AVRT)
anatomy of pathways, 305, 307, 308f
atrioventricular nodal reciprocating tachycardia, 842
catheter ablation, 842, 842t
differentiation between AVNRT and, 29t, 303, 304f
electrophysiological findings, 309, 310f
mapping, 296
pacing maneuvers, 27, 28t, 29, 29t
Atritech, Inc., Watchman LAA Closure Technology, 165, 167, 167f, 168
atropine, 9, 56t
for tachycardia ablation, 260–261
ATs. See atrial tachycardias
autonomic nervous system (ANS), atrial fibrillation substrate and, 660–661
autonomic testing of sinus node, 286–287
auto-PEEP, 442
AVID. See Antiarrhythmics Versus Implantable Defibrillators
AVJ. See atrioventricular junction
AVN. See atrioventricular node
AVNRT. See atrioventricular nodal reentrant tachycardia
AVRT. See atrioventricular reentrant tachycardia
azimilide, 984, 992

B

Bachmann's bundle, pacing from, 720
bacterial endocarditis, 550, 757
barbiturates, 272
battery technology, 141–142
Becker muscular dystrophy, 293
Belhassen's ventricular tachycardia, 13, 13f, 367
benzodiazepines, 270–272, 271f, 436, 456
best practices, 731, 732t–733t
β-blockers
arrhythmogenic right ventricular cardiomyopathy, 991
catecholaminergic polymorphic ventricular tachycardia and, 991
implantable cardioverter-defibrillators and, 984
long QT syndrome and, 990
biatrial pacing, 720
bifascicular block, 895
Biosense Webster
See also Carto
Lasso catheter, 332, 333f
NaviStar, 603, 604
PentaRay, 393, 599
ThermoCool, 600, 603, 604
Biotronik
Home Monitoring, 150
leads and delivery system, 138, 138f, 139f
bisoprolol, 984
biventricular devices and leads, 720
biventricular pacing (pacemakers), 772, 776, 776t, 777f, 810, 810f, 811f, 885, 900, 901
bleeding
implantation and, 711, 756–757
surgical ablation, 671, 686–687
BLOCK-HF trial, 901
Boston Scientific, 222
Latitude Patient Management System, 152
leads and delivery system, 138, 138f, 143
bradycardias
categories of, 892
diagnosing, 260
pacemakers for, 892–895, 894f, 897–899
breath stacking, 442
Brugada syndrome, 20, 21f
adrenaline/procainamide infusion worksheet, 255t–256t
antiarrhythmic drugs, 990
electrocardiograms, 252–254, 253f, 254f
hybrid procedures/therapy, 990
implantable cardioverter-defibrillators for, 882–883, 883t, 913–914, 990
polymorphic ventricular tachycardia and ventricular fibrillation in, 395–396, 396f, 601, 601f, 882–883
bundle branch reentrant ventricular tachycardia, 21, 21f, 876
bupivacaine, 269–270, 276

C

CABANA trial, 973
CABG. See coronary artery bypass grafting
CABG-Patch. See Coronary Artery Bypass Graft-Patch
CACAF. See Catheter Ablation or the Cure of Atrial Fibrillation
CAD. See coronary artery disease
calcium, 261
calcium-channel blockers, 477
Canadian Implantable Defibrillator Study (CIDS), 871, 872t, 908, 909t, 910
Canadian Trial of Physiologic Pacing (CTOPP), 897, 898
cardiac anatomy
atrial septum, 196, 196f
atrioventricular groove, 194, 194f
cavotricuspid isthmus, 190–191, 190f
chambers, relationships of, 188–189, 189f
coronary sinus and venous tributaries, 198, 198f
Eustachian and Thebesian valves, 190f, 191
internodal myocardium, 192–193
left atrial (mitral) isthmus, 195, 195f
left atrioventricular junction, 197
left atrium, 194–195, 195f
oval fossa, 191, 196–197, 197f
pulmonary veins, 195
pyramidal space, inferior, 193–194, 194f
relationship between heart and thoracic structures, 187–188, 188f
right atrium, 190, 190f
sinus node, 191, 192f
terminal crest, 190, 190f
triangle of Koch, atrioventricular node, and His bundle, 192, 193f
ventricles, 198–202, 199f, 200f, 201f, 202f
Cardiac Arrest Study Hamburg (CASH), 871, 872t, 908, 909t, 910
Cardiac Arrhythmia Suppression Trial (CAST), 984
cardiac contractility modulation (CCM), 144, 144f
cardiac implantable electronic devices, remote monitoring and. See cardiovascular/cardiac implantable electronic devices (CIEDs)
Cardiac Insufficiency Bisoprolo Study II (CIBIS-II), 984
cardiac magnetic resonance (CMR), 99
See also magnetic resonance imaging
cardiac perforation, 568
cardiac resynchronization therapy (CRT)
See also implantation techniques; leads
advantages and disadvantages, 767–768, 767f

atrial fibrillation, 901
atrioventricular interval optimization, 778–779, 778f
atrioventricular junction ablation and, 470–471
battery technology, 141–142
biventricular pacing loss, 776, 776t, 777f
delayed electrical activation, 775
echocardiography and, 68–69, 719–720, 720f
electromechanical dyssynchrony in congestive heart failure and, 717–720, 718f, 719f, 768–770, 770t
hemodynamic response, 775
implantation, optimizing, 772–776
indications for, 75–79, 717–718, 885, 886t, 900–902, 902t, 903t
left ventricular leads, 135–136, 139, 720–721, 723, 723f, 724–727, 725f, 772, 774–775, 774f
patient selection, optimizing, 768–772, 773t
postimplantation, optimizing, 776–779
response to, assessing, 776, 777f
super-responders versus nonresponders, 771–772, 771f, 776, 777f
trials, 768–769, 769t, 911
cardiac rhythm management (CRM) devices
discharge instructions, 754, 756
patient monitoring and evaluation, 754, 755f
postoperative care and complications, 753, 754, 754t, 756–759, 760t–761t, 762, 763f
cardiac tamponade, 611, 670, 970, 972
Cardima PATHFINDER catheter, 332
CardioFocus, Endoscopic Ablation System with Adaptive Contact, 544, 544f
cardioinhibitory carotid sinus hypersensitivity (CICSH), 899
cardiomyopathies
See also hypertrophic cardiomyopathy; ischemic cardiomyopathy; nonischemic cardiomyopathy; nonischemic dilated cardiomyopathy
arrhythmogenic right ventricular, 123–124, 571, 873, 880–881
Chagas disease, 124, 572, 581, 881
dilated, 900
idiopathic dilated, 571, 580–581
indications for implantable cardioverter-defibrillators, 75–79
noncompaction of left ventricle, 881
rare, 881
Cardiomyopathy Trial (CAT), 909t, 910
cardiovascular/cardiac implantable electronic devices (CIEDs)
See also device clinics; devices; implantation techniques
anesthesia for, 278
cardiac contractility modulation, 144, 144f
clinical cardiac training requirements, 870, 870t
electromechanic interference, 145–146
follow-up paradigm, 740–741, 740t, 741t, 742f, 743, 743t
limitations of current, 141
magnetic resonance imaging and, 121–122, 122f, 123f, 139–140, 145–146

programming and physiologic stimulation, 143–144, 144f
radiography, 783–802, 784f, 785f, 786f, 787f, 788f, 789f, 790f, 791f, 792f–793t, 793f, 794f, 795f, 796f, 797f, 798f, 799f, 800f, 801f
cardiovascular/cardiac implantable electronic devices, remote monitoring and, 144–145
atrial fibrillation and, 156
benefits of, 153–155
future for, 161
heart failure and, 156–157
legal issues, 158–159
reimbursement issues, 159–161
review of major studies on, 153–158
patient quality of life and acceptance, 157–158
safety alerts, 157
system integrity, 155–156
systems available, 149–152
cardioversion, anesthesia for, 278
CARTOMERGE Image Integration Software Module, 36, 36f, 101, 102, 104, 108
CARTOSOUND module, 36–37, 37f, 67, 107–108, 112, 530
CARTO System, 29, 35, 36–38, 36f, 37f, 38f, 103, 104, 105, 112, 337, 399, 400, 410, 413, 530, 855, 886
CARTO XP, 104, 112
CASH. *See* Cardiac Arrest Study Hamburg
CAST. *See* Cardiac Arrhythmia Suppression Trial
CAT. *See* Cardiomyopathy Trial
catecholaminergic polymorphic ventricular tachycardia (CPVT), 257, 258f, 883, 883t, 991
catheter ablation, 65
See also anesthesia/sedation; high-frequency jet ventilation (HFJV)
accessory pathways, 489–494, 496, 490f, 491f, 492f, 493f, 494f, 495f, 496f
anesthesia and airway management for, 434, 435–436, 453, 454f, 458–459
anesthesia for, 278
antiarrhythmic drugs and, 948–950, 949t, 975–977, 976f
antiarrhythmic drugs versus, 972–973
atrial fibrillation, 89, 89f, 850–863, 852f, 853t, 855f, 856f, 857f, 858t, 859f, 860t, 861t, 862t, 863f, 968–972, 969f, 970f, 971f
atrial flutter, 508, 847–850, 848f, 849f, 850f, 851f
atrial tachycardia, 843, 843t
atrioventricular junction, 839–840, 839t
atrioventricular nodal reentrant tachycardia, 480–483, 481f, 841–842, 841t
atrioventricular reentrant tachycardia, 842, 842t
catheter improvements, 209–212, 210f, 211f
complications, 607–614, 970–972, 971f
contact force, 212–213, 213f, 214f
definitions and classification, 327–328, 328f, 859–860, 860t–862t
dual-site atrial pacing with antiarrhythmic drugs and, 958–963, 959f, 960t, 960f, 961f, 962f, 963f
focal atrial tachycardias, 322

hybrid surgical ablation with, 927
idiopathic automatic junctional tachycardia, 844
idiopathic ventricular arrhythmia, 355, 356f
implantable cardioverter-defibrillators and, 986–990
inappropriate sinus tachycardia, 476–477, 476f
linear, 519–524, 521f, 522f, 523f
macroreentrant atrial tachycardias, 324
nonischemic cardiomyopathies, 580–581
paroxysmal supraventricular tachycardia, 840–841
permanent junctional reciprocating tachycardia, 843
sinus nodal reentrant tachycardia, 477, 844
sinus node, 475
ventricular tachycardia and ICE, 90–93, 90f, 91f, 92f, 93f
Catheter Ablation or the Cure of Atrial Fibrillation (CACAF) trial, 972–973
Catheter Ablation versus Amiodarone for Shock Prophylaxis in Defibrillator Patients with Ventricular Tachycardia (CEASE-VT), 988
catheter rigs, mapping and, 23–25, 23f, 24f, 25f, 25t
Catheter Robotics, Inc., Amigo Remote Catheter System, 859
catheters
See also intracardiac echocardiography
contact force, 212–213, 213f, 214f
electrophysiology procedures and, 6, 7f
large-tip, 209–210
linear, 222–223, 332
preformed multielectrode, 332
spot/focal, 222, 223f
tip cooling, 210–212, 210f, 211f
cavotricuspid isthmus (CTI)
anatomy, 190–191, 190f
atrial flutter, 848, 949, 976
conduction block, 509–511, 509f, 510f, 511f
dependent flutters and ablation, 508, 509f, 848
outcomes, 511–512
CCM. *See* cardiac contractility modulation
CEAPs. *See* clinically employed allied professionals
CEASE-VT. *See* Catheter Ablation versus Amiodarone for Shock Prophylaxis in Defibrillator Patients with Ventricular Tachycardia
celivarone, 984
CFAEs. *See* complex fractionated atrial electrograms
$CHADS_2$ score, 165
Chagas disease, 124, 572, 581, 881
chest x-rays. *See* radiography
CHF. *See* congestive heart failure
chlorhexidine, 459–460
chloroprocaine, 269
Chronicle Offers Management to Patients with Advanced Signs and Symptoms of Heart Failure (COMPASS-HF), 157, 816
chroprocaine, 268
CIBIS-II. *See* Cardiac Insufficiency Bisoprolo Study II

CICSH. *See* cardioinhibitory carotid sinus hypersensitivity
CIDS. *See* Canadian Implantable Defibrillator Study
CIEDs. *See* cardiovascular/cardiac implantable electronic devices
circumferential left atrial ablation, 855–856, 856f
circumferential pulmonary vein ablation (CPVA), linear catheter ablation in, 519–522, 521f, 522f
Clinical Evaluation of Remote Notification to Reduce Time to Clinical Decision (CONNECT), 153, 154, 160, 161, 813
clinically employed allied professionals (CEAPs), 739, 744
clopidogrel, 693
CMP. *See* Cox-Maze procedure
CMR. *See* cardiac magnetic resonance
COMPANION. *See* Comparison of Medical Therapy, Pacing and Defibrillation in Heart Failure
Comparison of Medical Therapy, Pacing and Defibrillation in Heart Failure (COMPANION) trial, 769t, 879, 900, 909t, 911
COMPAS trial, 153, 154, 160
COMPASS-HF. *See* Chronicle Offers Management to Patients with Advanced Signs and Symptoms of Heart Failure
complex fractionated atrial electrograms (CFAEs), 336–337, 534–535, 535f, 536f, 537f, 538f, 662, 674, 674f, 857, 857f, 968, 970f
computed tomography (CT), 65
    advantages of, 121, 799–800, 800f, 801f
    clinical applications, 106–113
    contrast-enhanced, 109, 109f
    image data acquisition and reconstruction, 98
    image display and storage, 98–99
    imaging process, 97–98, 119–120, 120f
    radiation exposure, 99
    registration with electroanatomic mapping systems, 103–105, 105f, 106f
    3D mapping systems with, 101, 530
congenital complete AV block, 292–293
congenital heart disease. *See* pediatric electrophysiology procedures and patients with congenital heart disease
congestive heart failure (CHF)
    cardiac resynchronization therapy and electromechanical dyssynchrony in, 717–720, 718f, 719f, 768–770, 770t
    monitoring, 815–819, 816f, 817f, 818f
CONNECT. *See* Clinical Evaluation of Remote Notification to Reduce Time to Clinical Decision
CONTAK trial, 769t
Cooled RFC Trial, 987, 988
coronary arteries, injury to, 612–613, 687
coronary artery bypass grafting (CABG), 932–933, 936
Coronary Artery Bypass Graft-Patch (CABG-Patch) trial, 872t, 878, 909t, 911–912, 933
coronary artery disease (CAD), 8, 346, 347, 572, 573
    implantable cardioverter-defibrillators trials, 871–873, 874, 877–879
coronary coil embolization, 583

coronary ischemia, 293
coronary sinus (CS)
    ablation, 854, 855f
    ablation, endocardial, 522
    ablation, epicardial, 523, 523f
    access, 723
    catheters, 6, 7f, 9f
    dissection and perforation, 727, 727f
    eccentric retrograde coronary sinus activation, 483–484, 483f
    injury, 687
    lead extraction, 831–832
    lead placement, 88, 723, 723f, 726t, 727, 727t
    myocardial-ventricular connections, 496, 497f, 498–499, 498f, 499f
    size and morphology, 478, 479f
    venous tributaries and, 198, 198f
coronary venous anatomy, 721–722, 721f, 722f, 772, 773f, 774
coronary venous angiography, 723–724, 724f
corrected sinus node recovery time (CSNRT), 287
Cox-Maze procedure (CMP), 233
    development of, 629, 653
Cox-Maze II procedure, 629
    cryosurgical with argon-based cryoprobes, 635–640, 636f, 637f, 637t, 638t, 638f, 639f
Cox-Maze III procedure (cut-and-sew)
    development of, 629–630, 630f, 668, 976
    difficulties with, 653, 654, 686
Cox-Maze IV procedure
    bipolar radiofrequency energy, 630
    clinical outcome, 631–632, 632f
    cryoablation, 630–631
    development of, 629, 629f, 668
    indications for, 632–633, 976–977
    postoperative management, 633
    preoperative management, 633
    surgical technique, 631, 631f
CPT. *See* Current Procedural Terminology
CPVA. *See* circumferential pulmonary vein ablation
CPVT. *See* catecholaminergic polymorphic ventricular tachycardia
CRM. *See* cardiac rhythm management
CRT. *See* cardiac resynchronization therapy
cryoablation
    atrioventricular nodal reentry tachycardia and, 482
    catheter systems, 546–547, 547f
    cavotricuspid isthmus and, 508
    clinical applications, 547
    Cox-Maze IV procedure, 630–631
    device characteristics, 234
    focal atrial tachycardias and, 322
    indications and outcomes, 844
    mapping and, 50, 50f, 51
    mechanism of, 234–235
    pediatric procedures, 409
    safety issues, 235, 409
    transmural lesions created by, 235
    ventricular tachycardia, 622–623, 623f, 933–934, 933f, 934t, 935f
cryoballoon, 223
    atrial fibrillation and, 547–548, 547f, 972
    clinical trials, 549t
    compared to radiofrequency, 549
    efficacy of, 548–549

    limitations and complications, 549–550
    pulmonary vein isolation and, 548, 548f
CryoCath Technologies, 222, 223, 546, 547f
cryoconsole, 223, 224f
CryoCor, 222
cryomapping, 311–312, 322, 408–409
cryosurgical Cox-Maze procedure, 635–640, 636f, 637f, 637t, 638t, 638f, 639f
cryosurgical probes, 223
cryotherapy
    atrial flutter, 508
    history of, 219–220, 220f
    lesion formation, pathophysiology of, 220–221, 220f
    lesion size, determinants of, 221, 235
    tissue and microcirculation, histological effects, 221, 221f, 234–235
cryothermal ablation
    advantages and disadvantages of, 221–222
    delivery systems, 222–224, 223f, 224f, 234
    physics of, 546
CS. *See* coronary sinus
CSNRT. *See* corrected sinus node recovery time
CT. *See* computed tomography
CTI. *See* cavotricuspid isthmus
CTOPP. *See* Canadian Trial of Physiologic Pacing
Current Procedural Terminology (CPT), coding system for reimbursement, 748–749, 749t–750t

D

dabigatran, 706
Dallas Lesion Set, 655–657, 655f
Danish Multicenter Randomized Trial on Single Lead Atrial Pacing, 898
DANPACE. *See* Dual-chamber Pacing in Sick Sinus Syndrome
DAPPAF. *See* Dual-site Atrial Pacing for Prevention of AF
DEEP. *See* dual endocardial and epicardial procedures
defibrillation
    See also cardiac implantable electronic devices; implantable cardioverter-defibrillators; implantation techniques
defibrillation threshold testing (DFT), 700–702, 701t
Defibrillator in Acute Myocardial Infarction Trial (DINAMIT), 872t, 878–879, 909t, 911, 912, 915, 916
Defibrillators in Nonischemic Cardiomyopathy Treatment Evaluation (DEFINITE) trial, 872t, 879, 880, 909t, 910, 915
DEFINITE. *See* Defibrillators in Nonischemic Cardiomyopathy Treatment Evaluation
degenerative diseases, 293
desflurane, 275f, 276, 438
device clinics
    care agreement, 735, 738f
    facility logistics and space, 734–735, 734f
    goals and purpose of, 734
    patients, responsibilities of, 735, 735t, 738f

personnel job description and
responsibilities, 735, 736*f*, 737*f*,
739–740
physicians, educational requirements,
735, 739
devices
See also cardiovascular/cardiac
implantable electronic devices; cardiac
rhythm management devices; device
clinics; implantable cardioverter-
defibrillators; implantation techniques
data management, 743, 745*f*, 762
ethical issues, 746–748
evaluation content, 741
evolution of, 731, 733, 733*f*
follow-up paradigm, 740–741, 740*t*,
741*t*, 742*f*, 743, 743*t*, 754, 756–759,
760*t*–761*t*, 762, 763*f*
patient education, 744, 746, 747*f*
recalls and safety alerts, 743–744, 744*t*,
746*f*
reimbursement, 748–749, 749*t*–750*t*
remote monitoring, 762
dexmedetomidine, 4, 271*f*, 274, 437, 437*t*, 456,
457, 458
DFT. *See* defibrillation threshold testing
diaphragmatic stimulation, 759
diazepam, 272, 279*t*
DICOM. *See* Digital Imaging and
Communications in Medicine
Digital Imaging and Communications in
Medicine (DICOM), 99
digoxin, 477
toxicity, electrocardiographic findings, 21
DINAMIT. *See* Defibrillator in Acute
Myocardial Infarction Trial
diode lasers, 228, 544
dofetilide, 702, 944, 974
dronedarone, 944, 948, 974, 975*f*
drugs
See also anesthesia/sedation; *name of*
antiarrhythmic drug combinations,
944–945, 944*f*, 945*f*
antiarrhythmic drugs and atrial pacing,
950–951, 950*f*
antiarrhythmic drugs and catheter
ablation, 948–950, 949*t*
context-sensitive half-life, 268
refractoriness, 464
for tachyarrhythmias, 257–259
for tachycardia ablation, 260–261
testing, 9, 249–262
Dual-chamber Pacing in Sick Sinus Syndrome
(DANPACE) trial, 898
dual endocardial and epicardial procedures
(DEEP), 667–675, 672*f*, 673*f*, 674*f*
Dual-site Atrial Pacing for Prevention of AF
(DAPPAF) trial, 950, 956
Duchenne muscular dystrophy, 293
dyssynchrony
atrial (inter and intra), 718, 718*f*
atrioventricular, 718, 718*f*
in congestive heart failure, 717–720, 718*f*,
719*f*, 768–770, 770*t*
left ventricular, 77–79, 78*f*, 79*f*, 719–720,
719*f*
ventricular (inter and intra), 718–719, 718*f*

E

EAM. *See* electroanatomic mapping
early repolarization syndrome, 396–397, 397*f*,
601
EBM. *See* evidence-based medicine
ECGs. *See* electrocardiograms
echocardiography
See also intracardiac echocardiography
atrial fibrillation and, 66–67
atrial flutter and, 67
cardiac resynchronization therapy and,
68–69, 719–720, 719*f*
dyssynchrony measures, 770*t*
lead extraction and, 829, 829*f*
left atrial function and size and, 66
left ventricular dyssynchrony, assessing,
719–720, 719*f*
reasons for, 65–66, 799
speckle tracking, 719
3D transesophageal, 66, 67–68, 71–80
ventricular tachycardias and, 68
Echocardiography Guided Cardiac
Resynchronization Therapy (EchoCRT)
study, 769–770
EchoCRT. *See* Echocardiography Guided
Cardiac Resynchronization Therapy
EGMs. *See* electrograms
EHRA. *See* European Heart Rhythm
Association
electrical storm/incessant ventricular
tachycardia, 988–989, 992–993, 992*f*
electroanatomic mapping (EAM), 24, 562
See also name of
advancements in, 35
Carto System, 29, 35, 36–38, 36*f*, 37*f*,
38*f*
EnSite Velocity Cardiac Mapping
System, 35, 39–40, 39*f*, 40*f*, 41*f*
focal atrial tachycardia and, 29, 30*f*,
321–322
intracardiac echocardiography and, 89
pediatric patients with congenital heart
disease, 409
radiation safety, 41, 42*f*
registration of computed tomography
and magnetic resonance imaging with,
103–105, 105*f*, 106*f*
sinus node and, 287–289, 288*f*, 289*f*
3D, 530
electrocardiograms (ECGs)
atrial flutter, 18, 19*f*, 20*f*
atrioventricular nodal reentry
tachycardia, 18, 19*f*
digoxin toxicity, 21
epicardial ventricular arrhythmias,
384–385, 384*f*
fascicular ventricular tachycardia, 13, 13*f*
hypertrophic cardiomyopathy, 21, 22*f*
idiopathic annular ventricular
arrhythmias, 379–383, 380*f*, 381*f*, 382*f*
left fascicular ventricular tachycardias,
371, 371*f*, 372*f*, 373–375, 373*f*, 375*f*
outflow tract ventricular tachycardia,
11–13, 12*f*, 13*f*, 360–361, 360*f*, 361*t*
papillary muscle arrhythmias, 377–378,
377*f*, 378*f*
premature ventricular complexes and
ventricular fibrillation, 20–21, 21*f*
repolarization abnormalities, 20
sinus node dysfunction, 895–896, 896*f*
sinus tachycardia and automatic atrial
tachycardia, 14–16, 15*f*, 16*f*
ventricular tachycardia with structural
heart disease, 14, 14*f*, 345–346, 346*f*
Wolff–Parkinson–White syndrome,
16–17, 17*f*, 18*f*
electrograms (EGMs)
atrial fibrillation and focal and map-
guided ablation, 527–537, 528*f*, 529*f*,
531*f*, 532*f*, 533*f*, 535*f*, 536*f*, 537*f*, 538*f*
complex fractionated atrial, 336–337,
534–535, 535*f*, 536*f*, 537*f*, 538*f*, 662,
674, 674*f*, 857, 857*f*
focal tachycardia, 29
fractionated, 110, 262, 320*f*, 322–323, 351
His bundle, 294–295, 294*f*
intracardiac, 23, 25, 26, 27, 28*f*, 28*t*,
144–145, 150, 154, 347, 349
location of intracardiac catheters in aortic
valve cusps, 557, 558*f*, 559–560, 559*f*,
560*f*
remote monitoring systems, 150, 151, 152
sinus node, 288, 288*f*
targets for AT ablation, 320*f*
ventricular tachycardia, 30
electrophysiology (EP) procedures
See also pediatric electrophysiology
procedures
anesthesia/sedation and, 4
catheters and, 6, 7*f*
clinical cardiac training requirements,
870, 870*t*
elements of a comprehensive study, 6–9,
8*f*, 9*f*
external defibrillators and, 4
imaging during, 6
informed consent for, 3, 55
patient history, need for, 3–4
provocative drug testing, 9
radiation exposure and, 5–6
recording systems and, 6
risks of, 3, 9
vascular access and, 5
Emery-Dreifuss muscular dystrophy, 293
endocardial leads, 142–143
endocardial mapping, 49, 49*f*, 427, 591, 592*f*
endocardial resection and cryoablation,
933–934, 933*f*, 934*t*, 935*f*
endocarditis, 550, 757
Endoscopic Ablation System with Adaptive
Contact, 544, 544*f*
endotracheal intubation, 436, 439, 458
end-tidal carbon dioxide, 277–278, 435, 436,
443, 445, 459
EnGuide, 410, 415
EnSite NavX, 104, 337, 338*f*, 410, 530, 855
EnSite Velocity Cardiac Mapping System, 35,
39–40, 39*f*, 40*f*, 41*f*, 104, 105
EnSite Versimo, 102
entrainment mapping
concealed, 26, 28*f*, 31
criteria of reentrant circuits, 26*t*
intraatrial reentry, 26, 27*f*, 28*f*
mid-diastolic potentials, 31
pacing maneuvers, 27, 28*t*, 29, 29*t*
pitfalls of, 27
post-pacing interval, 27, 27*f*, 31

ventricular tachycardia and, 30–31, 31*f*, 31*t*, 348, 349, 349*f*, 573–574, 573*t*, 574*t*, 575*f*
entrainment of gas, 443
EP. *See* electrophysiology
ephedrine, 456
epicardial coronary veins, mapping, 563–564
epicardial mapping
    ablation procedure, 593–596, 594*f*, 595*f*
    clues suggesting, 590–591, 590*t*, 591*f*
    complications, 596, 611
    obtaining access, 592–593, 593*f*
    type of heart disease and, 589–590, 590*f*
    ventricular tachycardia, 24, 24*f*, 25*f*, 50, 352, 427, 428*f*, 559*f*, 564, 579–580, 579*f*, 580*f*, 589–596, 589*f*, 590*f*, 591*f*, 592*f*, 593*f*, 594*f*, 595*f*
epicardial ventricular arrhythmias (EpiVA)
    anatomy and diagnosis, 383–384
    electrocardiograms, 384–385, 384*f*
    prognosis and follow-up, 386
epinephrine, 9, 56*t*
EpiVA. *See* epicardial ventricular arrhythmias
ESC. *See* European Society of Cardiology
esophageal injury, 550, 670, 687
esophageal thermal injury, 438–439
Estech
    Cobra Revolution bipolar clamp, 237, 237*f*
    Cobra, Adhere XL Probe and Cooled Surgical Probe, 236, 236*f*
ethanol ablation, 583
ethical issues, 746–748
Ethicon Endo-Surgery, Echelon Flex Endopath stapler, 649, 650*f*
etomidate, 271*f*, 273, 276, 277, 279*t*, 437, 437*t*
European Heart Rhythm Association (EHRA), 734, 735, 739, 741, 759, 891
European Society of Cardiology (ESC), 149, 465*t*, 869, 869*f*, 870*t*, 891
Euro-VT-Study, 875–876, 987, 988
Eustachian valve, anatomy, 190*f*, 191
evidence-based medicine (EBM), 731

F

falls in the elderly, pacemakers and, 899–900, 900*t*
fascicular block, bi- and tri-, 895
fascicular ventricular tachycardia
    See also left fascicular ventricular tachycardias
    cardiac conduction system damage, 567–568
    electrocardiographic findings, 13, 13*f*, 564–566
    reentry, 566
FAST. *See* Atrial Fibrillation Catheter Ablation Versus Surgical Ablation Treatment Trial
fentanyl, 4, 271*f*, 274–275, 276, 277, 279*t*, 437, 456, 457
fires, skin preparation and sterilization methods and, 459–460
flecainide, 944, 975*f*
fluid retention, 688
flumazenil, 272, 279*t*, 456
fluoroscopy, 65
    lead extraction and, 714

focal arrhythmias, 45
focal atrial tachycardias
    catheter ablation, 322
    characteristics, 315
    diagnosis, 316–317, 316*f*, 317*t*, 317*f*, 318*f*
    localization, 319–320, 319*f*, 320*f*
    mapping, 29, 30*f*, 320–322, 321*f*
    pathophysiology, 315–316
focal ventricular tachycardia, intraoperative mapping, 50–51, 50*f*, 51*f*
follow-up paradigm, 740–741, 740*t*, 741*t*, 742*f*, 743, 743*t*, 754, 756–759, 760*t*–761*t*, 762, 763*f*
Fontan procedure, 51, 410–412, 410*t*, 412*f*
FREEDOM trial, 778
FRI. *See* Functional Recovery Index
Functional Recovery Index (FRI), 460

G

Gallavardin phenomenon, 358, 359*f*
ganglionic plexi (GP)
    atrial fibrillation and surgical ablation, 645, 646*f*, 659–664, 661*f*, 663*f*
    mapping and ablation, 337, 425
general endotracheal anesthesia (GETA), 436
GETA. *See* general endotracheal anesthesia
giant cell myocarditis, 881

H

HARMONY trial, 948
HCM. *See* hypertrophic cardiomyopathy
HD Mesh Ablator catheter, 332
heart block and conduction disturbances, surgical ablation and, 686
heart disease
    See also pediatric electrophysiology procedures, patients with congenital heart disease
    electrocardiographic findings of ventricular tachycardia with structural, 14, 14*f*
    mapping triggers of PMVT/VF in amyloid, 400, 603
    mapping triggers of PMVT/VF in ischemic, 397–400, 399*f*, 602–603, 602*f*
heart failure, monitoring of patients with, 156–157, 815–819, 816*f*, 817*f*, 818*f*
Heart Rhythm Society (HRS), 731, 732*t*–733*t*, 734, 735, 741, 747, 759, 825, 891, 908
hematomas
    groin, 970, 972
    postoperative, 711, 756–757
hemopericardium, 596
hemothorax, 758–759
heparin infusion, 466, 693, 706
HFJV. *See* high-frequency jet ventilation
HIFU. *See* high-intensity focused ultrasound
high-frequency jet ventilation (HFJV), 436
    apnea, physiology of, 445
    breath stacking and auto-PEEP, 442
    CO_2 elimination and monitoring, 445
    complications, 447
    devices and types of, 441
    entrainment of gas, 443

hemodynamic effects, 444–445
humidification, 444
monitoring airway pressure, 442–443, 443*f*
open versus semiclosed systems, 443–444, 443*f*, 444*f*
pulmonary vein isolation, 441, 445–447
reasons for using, 439, 441
ventilator settings, 447
high-intensity focused ultrasound (HIFU), 624, 624*f*
high right atrium (HRA) catheters, 6–8, 8*f*, 9*f*
His bundle
    anatomy, 23, 38, 38*f*, 192, 193*f*
    damage to, 12–13, 53
His position catheters, 6, 8*f*, 9*f*
His-Purkinje arborization, 391–392
HOBIPACE. *See* Homburg Biventricular Pacing Evaluation
Homburg Biventricular Pacing Evaluation (HOBIPACE) trial, 901
HRA. *See* high right atrium
HRS. *See* Heart Rhythm Society
hybrid operating rooms
    costs, 131
    equipment, 130*t*
    example of, 131–132, 132*f*
    imaging equipment, 130
    for lead extraction, 826
    management of, 131
    operating table, 128, 130*f*
    periprocedural evaluation and care, 132
    personnel and educational requirements for, 131
    quality measures, 131
    radiation safety, 128
    room design, 128, 129*f*
    wireless technologies, 130
hybrid procedures/therapy
    antiarrhythmic drug combinations, 944–945, 944*f*, 945*f*
    antiarrhythmic drugs and atrial pacing, 950–951, 950*f*
    antiarrhythmic drugs and catheter ablation, 948–950, 949*t*
    arrhythmogenic right ventricular cardiomyopathy, 991
    atrial antitachycardia pacing and antiarrhythmic drugs, 984–986, 985*f*
    atrial fibrillation, antiarrhythmic drugs and, 973–974, 974*f*, 975*f*
    atrial fibrillation, catheter ablation and, 968–972, 969*f*, 970*f*, 971*f*
    atrial fibrillation, catheter ablation and antiarrhythmic drugs, 975–977, 976*f*
    atrial fibrillation, catheter ablation versus antiarrhythmic drugs, 972–973
    atrial fibrillation, impact of advances in mechanisms of, 945–946, 946*t*–947*t*
    atrial fibrillation, types of, 947–948, 948*t*
    atrial fibrillation, with heart failure, 961–962
    atrial fibrillation, without bradycardias, 962
    benefits of, 943–944
    Brugada syndrome, 990
    catecholaminergic polymorphic ventricular tachycardia, 991
    dual-site atrial pacing with catheter ablation and antiarrhythmic drugs,

958–963, 959f, 960t, 960f, 961f, 962f, 963f
electrical storm/incessant ventricular tachycardia, 988–989, 992–993, 992f
future roles of, 963t
implantable cardioverter-defibrillators and antiarrhythmic drugs, 982–986, 983t, 985f, 986f
implantable cardioverter-defibrillators and catheter ablation, 986–990
long QT syndrome, 990–991
multisite atrial pacing, 951–958, 951f, 952f, 955f, 957f, 958f
types of, 127–128, 128t
ventricular arrhythmias, 981–993
hypertrophic cardiomyopathy (HCM)
electrocardiographic findings, 21, 22f
implantable cardioverter-defibrillators, 873, 880, 912–913
indications for pacemaker implantation, 902, 903f
magnetic resonance imaging, 123
myocardial fibrosis, 572
risk factors for sudden cardiac death, 913t

I

IAVAs. *See* idiopathic annular ventricular arrhythmias
ibutilide, atrial fibrillation ablation and, 261–262
ICDs. *See* implantable cardioverter-defibrillators
ICE. *See* intracardiac echocardiography
IDCM. *See* idiopathic dilated cardiomyopathy
idiopathic annular ventricular arrhythmias (IAVAs)
anatomy, 379
diagnosis and management, 379
electrocardiograms, 379–383, 380f, 381f, 382f
mitral annulus, 380–381, 380f, 381f
para-Hisian region, 381–382
prognosis and follow-up, 383
tricuspid annulus, 380, 380f, 381f
idiopathic automatic junctional tachycardia, 844
idiopathic dilated cardiomyopathy (IDCM), 571, 580–581
idiopathic ventricular arrhythmias (IVAs)
catheter ablation, 355, 356f
classification, 355, 356t
epicardial ventricular arrhythmias, 383–386, 384f
idiopathic annular ventricular arrhythmias, 379–383, 380f, 381f, 382f
left fascicular ventricular tachycardias, 367–376, 368f, 369f, 370f, 371f, 372f, 373f, 375f
outflow tract ventricular tachycardias, 11–13, 12f, 13f, 111, 112f, 357–367, 357f, 358f, 359f, 360f, 361f, 362f, 364f, 366f, 553–566
papillary muscle arrhythmias, 376–379, 376f, 377f, 378f
idiopathic ventricular tachycardia
See also fascicular ventricular tachycardia
endocavitary structures, 566

originating from the mitral annulus, 566–567
IEAPs. *See* industry employed allied professionals
IHM. *See* implantable hemodynamic monitoring
IHR. *See* intrinsic heart rate
IJV. *See* internal jugular vein
ILRs. *See* implantable loop recorders
imaging
See also computed tomography; echocardiography; intracardiac echocardiography; magnetic resonance imaging; radiography; transesophageal/transthoracic echocardiography (3D)
clinical applications, 106–113
during electrophysiology procedures, 6
future applications for integration techniques, 114
importance of, 97
integrating 3D mapping systems, 101–105, 102f, 103f, 105f, 106f
registration, technical aspects of, 102–103, 102f, 103f
registration errors, minimizing, 104–105
Tissue Doppler, 719, 719f
virtual, 671
Immediate Risk Stratification Improves Survival (IRIS) trial, 909t, 911, 912, 915, 916
implantable and heart failure devices. *See* cardiovascular/cardiac implantable electronic devices (CIEDs)
implantable cardioverter-defibrillators (ICDs)
See also cardiovascular/cardiac implantable electronic devices; cardiac rhythm management devices; devices; implantation techniques; leads
antiarrhythmic drugs with, 982–986, 983t, 985f, 986f
battery technology, 141–142
catheter ablation and, 986–990
clinical cardiac training requirements, 870, 870t
comorbidities and other variables on the outcome of, 915–916
guidelines for, 907–908
indications for, 75–79, 908
limitations of current, 141, 982
magnetic resonance imaging and, 121–122, 122f, 123f, 139–140, 145–146
pacing devices, programming and physiologic stimulation, 143–144, 144f
recommendations for, in structural heart disease, 872t
shocks, 141, 981–982, 987–988, 989–990
subcutaneous, 142, 142f
sudden cardiac death and primary prevention, 877, 878t, 879t, 910–912
sudden cardiac death and secondary prevention, 871, 908, 910
trials, 871, 872t, 877–885, 908, 909t, 915–916
implantable cardioverter-defibrillators, applications
arrhythmogenic right ventricular cardiomyopathy, 991
arrhythmogenic right ventricular dysplasia/cardiomyopathy, 873, 880–881, 913

Brugada syndrome, 882–883, 883t, 913–914, 990
catecholaminergic polymorphic ventricular tachycardia, 883, 883t, 991
coronary artery disease, 871–873, 874, 877–879
electrical storm/incessant ventricular tachycardia, 988–989, 992–993, 992f
hypertrophic cardiomyopathy, 873, 880, 912–913, 913t
long QT syndrome, 882, 882f, 914–915, 990–991
nonischemic dilated cardiomyopathy, 873, 874, 879–880
pediatric and congenital heart patients, 883–884, 884t
structural heart disease, 871, 873–874, 874t
implantable hemodynamic monitoring (IHM) systems, 815–817, 816f
implantable loop recorders (ILRs), 814–815, 814f
implantation techniques
See also lead extraction; leads
anesthesia for, 278, 455–456, 695
atrial lead placement, 699
closure, 702, 702f
complications, 711–715, 715t, 726–727
defibrillation threshold testing, 700–702, 701t
device failure, 712
incision, 695
infections, 710, 712–713, 757, 757f
lead dislodgement, 711–712
lead explantation, 713
lead measurements, 699–700, 700f
lead tie-down and pulse generator placement, 700
lead tunneling, 710
left ventricular, 135–136, 139, 720–721, 723, 723f, 774–775, 774f
for pectoral implants, 708–710, 709f, 710f
postoperative care, 702–703, 711–715, 715t
preoperative planning, 693–694, 705–707
pulse generator pocket, 695, 700, 719, 710f
right ventricular lead placement, 697, 698f, 699
room set-up, 694–695, 706
surgical site preparation, 706–708, 707f, 708f
venous access, 695–697, 696f, 697f, 706–710, 707f, 708f, 709f, 710f
inappropriate sinus tachycardia (IST), 285–286
catheter ablation, 476–477, 476f
diagnosis of, 679
surgical ablation, 680–683, 681t, 681f, 682f, 683t
treatment options, 679–680
industry employed allied professionals (IEAPs), 739–740
infections
as indication for lead extraction, 824–825, 825f
postoperative, 710, 712–713, 757, 757f
inferior vena cava (IVC), 180, 181, 283, 283f, 324, 508, 511, 512, 513, 514
informed consent, for electrophysiology procedures, 3, 55, 457

interatrial dyssynchrony, 718, 718f
inter-electrode spacing, 25
internal jugular vein (IJV), as an access site, 5
interventricular dyssynchrony, 718–719, 718f
intra-atrial dyssynchrony, 718, 718f
intracardiac echocardiography (ICE)
    baseline image acquisition using, 85–86, 85f, 86f
    catheter ablation for atrial fibrillation and, 89, 89f
    catheter ablation for ventricular tachycardia and, 90–93, 90f–93f
    catheters, 83, 84f, 84t, 85
    compared to transesophageal echocardiography, 86–87, 88
    coronary sinus lead placement and, 88
    currently available technologies, 83, 84f, 84t, 85, 112
    focal atrial tachycardias and, 322
    image integration techniques, 112
    indications for, 75–79
    left atrial appendage occlusion and, 88, 88f
    left atrial appendage thrombus and, 86–87
    for outflow tract arrhythmia, 560–561
    role of, 35, 36–37, 66–69
    three-dimensional imaging with, 93–94, 530, 531f
    transseptal catheterization and, 87, 87f, 88f
Intracardiac Echocardiography Guided Cardioversion Helps Interventional Procedures (ICE-CHIP) study, 86–87, 120, 120
intraoperative mapping
    activation maps, 47, 48f, 420
    atrial fibrillation and, 51–52, 52f, 422–425, 423f, 424f, 425f
    atrial tachycardias and, 51, 422
    atrioventricular bypass tracts and, 47, 48f, 49f
    atrioventricular conduction system, identifying normal, 52–53
    coordinate system, 46, 46f
    electrodes for, 417–419, 418f, 419f
    future perspectives, 428
    limitations of, 53
    potential distribution mapping, 421
    preparation for, 46
    process, 45–46, 46f
    signal processing and analysis, 419–420
    tools, 47f
    use of, 45, 417
    ventricular tachycardias and, 49–51, 49f, 50f, 51f, 425–427, 426f, 427f, 428f
    voltage mapping, 420–421
    Wolff–Parkinson–White syndrome and, 47, 52, 421–422, 421f
intrathoracic impedance monitoring, 817–819, 817f, 818f
intraventricular conduction delay (IVCD), 718
intraventricular dyssynchrony, 718–719, 718f
intrinsic heart rate (IHR), calculating, 286–287
IRIS. *See* Immediate Risk Stratification Improves Survival
ischemic cardiomyopathy
    ablation outcomes, 578

ablation techniques and endpoints, 572–573, 577–578
    anatomic and electrophysiologic substrate, 571
    electrocardiograms analysis, 574, 576
    entrainment mapping, 573–574, 573t, 574t, 575f
    imaging substrate, 123
    late potential mapping, 576
    localizing conducting channels, 576–577
    pace mapping during sinus rhythm, 576, 576f
    radiofrequency techniques, 577–578
    substrate mapping, 573t, 574
    unmappable, troubleshooting, 574t
    ventricular tachycardia in, 123, 571–584
isoflurane, 275f, 276, 438, 456, 457
isoproterenol, 3, 8, 9, 56, 56t
    atrial fibrillation ablation and, 261, 333
    for Brugada syndrome, 990
    for tachycardia ablation, 260
ISSUE3 trial, 899
IST. *See* inappropriate sinus tachycardia
ivabradine, 284
IVAs. *See* idiopathic ventricular arrhythmias
IVC. *See* inferior vena cava
IVCD. *See* intraventricular conduction delay

J

J-wave syndromes, electrocardiographic findings, 20

K

ketamine, 271f, 273–274, 279t, 437t, 438

L

LAA. *See* left atrial appendage
Larmor frequency, 99–100
laryngeal mask airway (LMA), 436, 446, 453, 454f
laser ablation, 227–228, 228f, 543–546, 544f, 545f, 546t
    advantages and disadvantages, 858t
laser balloon device, 544, 544f, 545f, 546t
lead extraction
    complication rates, 826–828, 826t, 827f
    complications of, 173, 173t, 182, 714–715, 715t, 831, 831t
    definitions, need for uniform, 173
    echocardiography prior to, 829, 829f
    failure of, 183
    femoral tools, 179, 179f
    foreign-body response, 171, 172f
    indications, 174, 175t, 823–825, 824f, 825f
    lead abandonment versus, 174, 174f
    locking stylets, 176–177, 177f
    operating site, 826
    pericardial tamponade, 831
    postprocedure care, 182–183
    powered sheaths, 178, 178f, 179f

    preoperative planning, 174, 176, 713–714, 828, 828t
    reimplantation following, 182
    risk profiles, 825
    safety issues, 831–833, 832f, 833f
    success rates, 171, 172f
    surgical approach, 181, 831, 831t
    techniques, 179–182, 180f, 181f, 714
    telescoping sheaths, 177, 177f
    temporary pacing, 829
    tools/equipment, 176–179, 177f, 178f, 179f
    training experience, 173–174, 825–826
    vascular tears, 831
    vegetations, 829–830, 830f
    venoplasty, 181–182
leads
    See also implantation techniques; lead extraction
    atrial placement, 699
    Biotronik, 138, 138f, 139f
    biventricular, 720
    Boston Scientific, 138, 138f
    changes in, 135, 136
    coronary sinus, 831–832
    dislodgement, 711–712, 726–727, 757–758, 758f
    endocardial, 142–143
    explantation, 713
    infections, 710, 712–713, 757, 757f, 824–825, 825f
    left ventricular, 135–136, 139, 720–721, 723, 723f, 724–727, 725f, 772, 774–775, 774f
    malfunctions, 135, 712, 715, 824
    measurements, 699–700, 700f
    Medtronic Attain, 137, 137f, 138f
    Medtronic Revo MRI SureScan Pacing System, 139–140
    Medtronic Sprint Fidelis, 143, 712, 714, 824, 832, 832f
    perforation, 758
    right ventricular placement, 697, 698f, 699
    St. Jude Medical CPS Direct ST Slittable Outer Guide Catheter, 136, 136f
    St. Jude Medical Quartet LV pacing, 136, 137f, 137t
    St. Jude Medical Riata, 143, 712, 712f, 715, 824, 832, 833f
    subcutaneous ICDs and, 142, 142f
    tie-down, 700
    tunneling, 710
left atrial appendage (LAA)
    function and size, echocardiography, 66, 67
    surgical ablation, 645, 649, 650f, 671, 926
    3D echocardiography, 72–75, 73f, 74f, 75f
    thrombus and intracardiac echocardiography, 86–87
left atrial appendage (LAA) occlusion
    devices and implantation techniques, 166–167, 166f, 167f
    imaging, 169
    indications, 165
    intracardiac echocardiography, 88, 88f
    safety and success rates, 167–169, 168f
left atrial lesion set, 653–657, 655f
left atrioventricular junction, anatomy, 197
left atrium, anatomy, 194–195, 195f

left fascicular ventricular tachycardias (LFVTs)
    anatomy, 367–368, 368f, 369f–370f
    diagnosis and management, 368, 371f
    electrocardiograms, 371, 371f, 372f, 373–375, 373f, 375f
    prognosis and follow-up, 375–376
left inferior pulmonary vein (LIPV) electrophysiological techniques, 331
    mapping, 85f, 89f, 90f
left superior pulmonary vein (LSPV), mapping, 85f, 89f, 320
left ventricle
    anatomy, 200–202, 201f, 202f
    noncompaction of, 881
left ventricular diastolic function, echocardiography, 69
left ventricular dyssynchrony, 77–79, 78f, 79f, 719–720, 719f
left ventricular ejection fraction (LVEF), 71, 75–79, 76f
left ventricular endocardial pacing, 143–144, 775–776
left ventricular leads, 135–136, 139, 720–721, 723, 723f, 724–727, 725f, 772, 774–775, 774f
left ventricular outflow tract (LVOT)
    anatomy, 554–555, 554f, 555f
    electrocardiographic findings, 12–13, 12f, 13f, 554f, 556–557
    intracardiac echocardiography, 560–561
    location of intracardiac catheters, 557, 558f, 559–560, 559f, 560f
    mapping, 561–564, 561f
left ventricular pacing leads, 139
legal issues, remote monitoring and, 158–159
Lenègre's disease, 293
Levs disease, 293
LEXICON trial, 825, 827
LFVTs. See left fascicular ventricular tachycardias
lidocaine, 268–270, 269f, 276, 277, 695
linear catheter ablation
    atrial fibrillation, 519–524, 521f, 522f, 523f
    atrial linear ablation, 523
    in CPVA, 520–522, 521f, 522f
    endocardial coronary sinus ablation, 522
    endocardial septum ablation, 522, 523f
    epicardial coronary sinus ablation, 523, 523f
    future of, 524
    left atrial ablation, 523
    posterior and mitral isthmus lines, 522, 522f
    PV disconnection, 521, 521f, 522f
    right atrium ablation, 523
LIPV. See left inferior pulmonary vein
LMA. See laryngeal mask airway
long QT syndrome
    adrenaline/procainamide infusion worksheet, 255t–256t
    channelopathies and associated proteins and channels, 250t
    description of, 249–252
    electrocardiograms, 250f, 251–252
    hybrid procedures/therapy, 990–991
    implantable cardioverter-defibrillators for, 882, 882f, 914–915, 990–991
    pacing, 885, 885t, 902
    pharmacological provocation for diagnosis of channelopathies, 252t
    polymorphic ventricular tachycardia and ventricular fibrillation in, 395–396, 396f, 601, 882, 882t
lorazepam, 272, 436
LSPV. See left superior pulmonary vein
Lumos-T Safely Reduces Routine Office Device Follow-up (TRUST), 153, 154, 155–156, 160
LVEF. See left ventricular ejection fraction
LVOT. See left ventricular outflow tract

M

macroreentrant arrhythmias, 45
macroreentrant atrial tachycardias, 51
    after catheter or surgical ablation, 515
    catheter ablation, 324
    characteristics, 315
    diagnosis and mapping, 322–324, 323f
    mapping strategies, 505–506, 506f, 507f
    pathophysiology, 316
MADIT I and II. See Multicenter Automatic Defibrillator Implantation Trials I and II
magnetic resonance angiography (MRA), 121
magnetic resonance imaging (MRI), 65, 71, 75
    advantages and disadvantages of, 101, 121
    clinical applications, 106–113, 123–124
    electromechanic interference, 145–146
    image modalities, 100
    imaging process, 99–100, 120–121, 121f
    implantable cardioverter-defibrillators and, 121–122, 122f, 123f, 139–140, 145–146
    registration with electroanatomic mapping systems, 103–105, 105f, 106f
    scar identification, 770–771
    3D mapping systems with, 101, 530
Mallampati classification, 434, 435f, 452–453
mapping techniques
    See also electroanatomic mapping; entrainment mapping; intraoperative mapping
    atrial fibrillation and focal and map-guided ablation, 527–537, 528f, 529f, 531f, 532f, 533f, 535f, 536f, 537f, 538f
    atrioventricular node and, 296
    basket, 562
    catheter rigs, 23–25, 23f, 24f, 25f, 25t
    endocardial, 49, 49f, 427
    epicardial, 24, 24f, 25f, 49, 50, 352, 427, 428f, 559f, 564, 579–580, 579f, 580f, 589–596, 611
    multielectrode, 562
    noncontact, 352
    pace, 30, 350–351, 350f, 562–563, 576, 576f
    point-to-point, 562
    recording systems and techniques, 25–26
    return-cycle, 426, 427f
    substrate, 30
    supraventricular tachycardias and, 26–27, 26t, 27f, 28f, 28t, 29, 29t, 30f
    3D mapping systems, 101–108, 102f, 103f, 105f, 106f, 107f, 337–338, 338f, 339f, 340f, 341f
    transseptal, transaortic, and epicardial approaches, 24, 24f, 25f
    ventricular tachycardia and, 30–31, 31f, 31t, 345–352, 561–564, 561f
marcaine, 695
MAVERIC. See Midlands Trial of Empirical Amiodarone versus Electrophysiology-guided Interventions and Implantable Cardioverter-defibrillators
MDPs. See mid-diastolic potentials
Medtronic, 222
    Arctic Front, 547–548, 547f
    Attain leads and deliver system, 137, 137f, 138f
    Cardioblate BP2 Irrigated RF Surgical Ablation System, 237
    Cardioblate LP System, 237
    Cardioblate Standard Ablation Pen, 236
    Cardioblate XL Surgical Ablation Pen, 236
    CareLink Network, 150–151
    Cryo, 234
    cryoconsole, 223, 224f
    Paceart data management, 743, 745f
    Reveal, 814, 814f
    Revo MRI SureScan Pacing System, 139–140
    SarFix, 832
    Sprint Fidelis, 143, 712, 715, 824, 832, 832f
Medtronic/Ablation Frontiers, Pulmonary Vein Ablation Catheter, 215
mepivacaine, 269
metformin, 694
methacholine, 333
methohexital, 272, 279t
mexiletine, 944
micropuncture kits, 5
microwave ablation, 230, 230f
    advantages and disadvantages, 858t
midazolam, 4, 270–271, 271f, 276, 277, 279t, 436, 437t, 456, 457
mid-diastolic potentials (MDPs), 31
MidHeft trial, 817
Midlands Trial of Empirical Amiodarone versus Electrophysiology-guided Interventions and Implantable Cardioverter-defibrillators (MAVERIC) study, 910
MILOS. See Multicenter Longitudinal Observational Study
MIRACLE trials 769t
mitral annulus, 566–567
mitral-aortic continuity, 358, 358f
mitral isthmus
    linear lesions, 854–855, 856f
    line of block, 513–514, 514f
    posterior and lines, 522, 522f
mitral isthmus ventricular tachycardia, 14, 14f
mitral valve damage, 614
MOde Selection Trial (MOST), 811–812, 898, 950
monitoring devices
    See also cardiovascular/cardiac implantable electronic devices, remote monitoring and; remote navigation
    anticoagulation, 810–812, 811f, 812f, 813f
    for atrial arrhythmias, 803–813, 805f, 806f, 807f, 808f, 809f, 810f, 811f, 812f, 813f

event, 814
for heart failure, 815–819, 816f, 817f, 818f
for heart rate variability, 818
implantable loop recorders, 814–815, 814f
intrathoracic impedance, 817–819, 817f, 818f
pressure monitoring systems, 815–817, 816f
remote, 762, 813, 818
for syncope, 813–815
Monsoon Universal Jet Ventilator, 441, 442, 444, 447
morphine, 274, 279t
MOST. *See* MOde Selection Trial
MRA. *See* magnetic resonance angiography
MRI. *See* magnetic resonance imaging
MUGA. *See* multiple uptake gated acquisition
Multicenter Automatic Defibrillator Implantation (MADIT) trials
    CRT trial, 718, 721, 768, 769t, 771, 776, 901, 911
    RIT study, 762, 912
    Trials I and II, 161, 762, 872t, 877, 879, 909t, 910, 911, 912, 915, 916, 936, 981, 982, 983, 992
Multicenter Longitudinal Observational Study (MILOS), 911
Multicenter THERMOCOOL Ventricular Tachycardia Ablation Trial, 611, 875, 987, 988
Multicenter Unsustained Tachycardia Trial (MUSTT), 877, 879, 909t, 910, 911
multiple uptake gated acquisition (MUGA) scans, 71, 75
muscle relaxants, 275, 446
muscular dystrophies, 293
Mustard procedure, 51, 410t, 411, 412
MUSTIC trial, 769t
MUSTT. *See* Multicenter Unsustained Tachycardia Trial

N

naloxone, 279t, 456
nasal cannulae, 436
Nd-YAG (neodymium-doped yttrium-aluminum-garnet), 227, 543, 544
nContact, VisiTrax, 236
neonatal lupus, 292–293
neurocardiogenic syncope, 899, 902t, 903t
neuromyopathies, 293
NICM. *See* nonischemic cardiomyopathy
NIDCM. *See* nonischemic dilated cardiomyopathy
Niobe catheter system, 213, 214f, 533
nitrous oxide, 276
noncompaction of left ventricle, 881
nonischemic cardiomyopathy (NICM)
    See also type of
    ablation techniques and endpoints, 572–573
    anatomic and electrophysiologic substrate, 571
    catheter ablation for, 580–582
    endpoints, 578
    epicardial mapping, 579–580, 579f, 580f
    imaging, 123
    indications for implantable cardioverter-defibrillators, 76–77
    mapping triggers of PMVT/VF in dilated, 401, 401f, 604
    septal substrates, 582–583
    ventricular tachycardia ablation outcomes, 876
    ventricular tachycardia in, 123, 124f, 571–584
nonischemic dilated cardiomyopathy (NIDCM)
    heart failure in, 879–880
    implantable cardioverter-defibrillators trials, 873, 879–880
North American Society of Pacing and Electrophysiology, 908

O

obstructive sleep apnea (OSA), 435, 446, 452, 693, 899
OEDIPE. *See* One Day Pacemaker Implantation Program with Home-monitoring
OFISSER trial, 818
One Day Pacemaker Implantation Program with Home-monitoring (OEDIPE), 153–154
opioids, 274–275, 436–437, 456
OPTIC study, 984
OSA. *See* obstructive sleep apnea
OT-VT. *See* outflow tract ventricular tachycardias
outflow tract ventricular tachycardia (OT-VT), 111, 112f
    anatomy, 357–358, 357f, 358f, 554–555, 554f, 555f
    cardiac conduction system damage, 567–568
    diagnosis and management, 358–367, 359f
    electrocardiograms, 11–13, 12f, 13f, 360–361, 360f, 361t, 554f, 556–557
    intermediate morphology, 365–367, 366f
    intracardiac echocardiography, 560–561
    left side morphology, 367
    location of intracardiac catheters, 557, 558f, 559–560, 559f, 560f
    mapping, 561–564, 561f
    myocardial sleeves extensions, 555
    prognosis and follow-up, 367
    right side morphology, 362–365, 362f, 364f
oval fossa, anatomy, 191, 196–197, 197f

P

pacemakers/pacing
    See also cardiac rhythm management devices; devices; implantation techniques
    antiarrhythmic drugs and, 976
    atrial, 29, 29t, 720–722, 721f, 722f, 950–958, 950f, 951f, 952f, 955f, 957f, 958f, 958–963, 959f, 960t, 960f, 961f, 962f, 963f
    atrial antitachycardia, 984–986, 985f
    atrioventricular junction ablation and, 467, 977
    biventricular, 772, 776, 776f, 777f, 810, 810f, 811f, 885, 900, 901
    for bradycardias, 892–895, 894f, 897–899
    cardiac resynchronization therapy, 900–902, 902t, 903t
    confirming mechanisms of tachycardia, 27, 28t
    development of, 891, 897
    devices, programming and physiologic stimulation, 143–144, 144f
    dual-chamber, 897–899
    for falls in the elderly, 899–900, 900t
    indications for, 891–892, 902t, 903t
    left ventricular endocardial, 143–144, 775–776
    limitations of current, 141
    mapping, 30, 350–351, 350f, 562–563, 576, 576f
    mode selection, 897–899
    for neurocardiogenic syncope, 899, 902t, 903t
    for obstructive sleep apnea, 899
    prevention of ventricular arrhythmias, 884–885, 885t
    right ventricular, 901
    for sinus node dysfunction, 895–897, 896f, 897f, 902t, 903t
    for tachycardias, 902–903, 902f, 903f
    ventricular, 29, 29t
PAF. *See* paroxysmal atrial fibrillation
PainFREE trials, 985
pain management, 460
pancuronium, 275
papillary muscle (PapM) arrhythmias
    anatomy, 376–377, 376f
    diagnosis and management, 377
    electrocardiograms, 377–378, 377f, 378f
    prognosis and follow-up, 378–379
PapM. *See* papillary muscle
paroxysmal atrial fibrillation (PAF), 921, 926
paroxysmal supraventricular tachycardias (PSVTs)
    ablation sites, mapping criteria to identify, 309, 311–312, 311f
    categories, 299t
    catheter ablation, 840–841
    diagnosis of, from surface electrocardiogram, 300–302, 301f, 302f
    drug testing, 312
    electrophysiological study and mapping, 302–309, 303f–310f
    narrow QRS complexes, 300–301, 301f
    preexcited QRS complexes, 301–302, 302f
    regular wide, 301
    other names for, 299
PARTITA trial, 583
PATH-CHF-II trial, 721, 769t
patient care agreement, 735, 738f
patient history, needed for electrophysiology procedures, 3–4
patients
    discharging, 741, 742f, 754, 756
    education, 744, 746, 747f
    responsibilities of, 735, 735t, 738f
PEA. *See* peak endocardial acceleration

peak endocardial acceleration (PEA), measuring, 818
PECA. *See* percutaneous epicardial catheter ablation
pediatric electrophysiology procedures
    access issues, 58, 58*f*, 59*f*
    anesthesia/sedation, 56, 56*t*, 409–410, 457
    biophysical issues, 60–61
    developmental and psychosocial issues, 55
    diagnoses and types of arrhythmias, 56–57
    equipment, 59–60, 60*f*
    indications and complications, 57
    laboratory setting, 55–56
pediatric electrophysiology procedures, mapping and ablation techniques
    catheter techniques and patient size, 408–409, 408*f*
    cryoablation, 409
    cryomapping, 408–409
    patient safety, 405–406
    patient size, 406–407, 407*t*
    radiation exposure, 408
pediatric electrophysiology procedures and patients with congenital heart disease
    anesthesia/sedation, 409–410
    electroanatomic mapping systems, 410
    general concepts, 409
    implantable cardioverter-defibrillators, 883–884, 884*t*
    navigation and visualization technology, 410
    rhythm disturbances: atrial, 411–414, 412*f*
    rhythm disturbances: ventricular tachycardia, 414–415
    types of defects, 409*t*
    voltage mapping, 410–411
percutaneous epicardial catheter ablation (PECA), 667
percutaneous left atrial appendage occlusion. *See* left atrial appendage (LAA) occlusion
Percutaneous Left Atrial Appendage Transcatheter Occlusion (PLAATO), 166, 167, 166*f*, 168*f*
pericardial effusions, 79, 80*f*
pericardial tamponade, 831
permanent junctional reciprocating tachycardia (PJRT), 843
PET. *See* positron emission tomography
phenylephrine, 456
phrenic nerve palsy (PNP)/injury, 549–550, 612, 671, 688
phrenic nerve stimulation, 726
physicians
    educational requirements, 735, 739
    reimbursement, 748–749, 749*t*–750*t*
PJRT. *See* permanent junctional reciprocating tachycardia
PLAATO. *See* Percutaneous Left Atrial Appendage Transcatheter Occlusion
PLEXUS trial, 827
PMVT/VF. *See* polymorphic ventricular tachycardia and ventricular fibrillation
pneumothorax, 711, 758–759
PNP. *See* phrenic nerve palsy

polymorphic ventricular tachycardia and ventricular fibrillation (PMVT/VF)
    catheter ablation, 882, 882*t*
    in early repolarization syndrome, 396–397, 397*f*, 601
    His-Purkinje arborization, role of, 391–392
    idiopathic, 394–395, 395*f*, 599–600, 600*f*, 882
    initiation and maintenance of, 391–392
    in long QT and Brugada syndromes, 395–396, 396*f*, 601, 601*f*, 882–883
    mapping, invasive, 392–397, 393*f*, 394*f*, 395*f*, 396*f*, 397*f*
    mapping triggers of, in amyloid heart disease, 400, 603
    mapping triggers of, idiopathic, 599–600, 600*f*
    mapping triggers of, in ischemic heart disease, 397–400, 399*f*, 602–603, 602*f*
    mapping triggers of, in nonischemic dilated cardiomyopathy, 401, 401*f*, 604
positron emission tomography/computed tomography (PET/CT), 108–109, 109*f*
postoperative care. *See* cardiac rhythm management devices
post-pacing interval (PPI), 27, 27*f*, 31
postural orthostatic tachycardia syndrome (POTS), 286, 482
potential distribution mapping, 421
POTS. *See* postural orthostatic tachycardia syndrome
povidone-iodine, 459–460
PPI. *See* post-pacing interval
Predictors of Response to Cardiac Resynchronization Therapy (PROSPECT) study, 69, 71, 78, 719, 769
PREFER. *See* Prospective Randomized Evaluation of a New Fabric Attenuation Device in Endovascular Interventional Radiology
PRELUDE. *See* PRogrammed ELectrical stimUlation preDictive valuE
premature ventricular complexes (PVCs)
    ablation, 886, 886*t*
    pacing maneuvers, 29, 29*t*
    ventricular fibrillation and, 20–21, 21*f*
PREPARE. *See* Primary Prevention Parameters Evaluation
pressure monitoring systems, 815–817, 816*f*
primary electrical disorders, 882–883
Primary Prevention Parameters Evaluation (PREPARE), 762
procainamide, 56*t*
    adrenaline and, infusion worksheet, 254, 255*t*–256*t*
PRogrammed ELectrical stimUlation preDictive valuE (PRELUDE), 913–914
propafenone, 944, 944*f*
propofol, 4, 271*f*, 272–273, 276, 277, 279*t*, 437, 437*t*, 439, 446, 456, 457
PROSPECT. *See* Predictors of Response to Cardiac Resynchronization Therapy
Prospective Randomized Evaluation of a New Fabric Attenuation Device in Endovascular Interventional Radiology (PREFER), 153, 154, 813
provocative drug testing, 9
PSVTs, *See* paroxysmal supraventricular tachycardias

Pulmonary Vein Ablation Catheter (PVAC), 215
pulmonary vein isolation (PVI)
    circumferential antral, 530, 531*f*, 532*f*, 533*f*
    cryoballoon for, 548, 548*f*
    electrogram-guided antral, 530, 531*f*, 532*f*, 533, 536*f*, 537*f*, 538*f*
    high-frequency jet ventilation and, 441, 445–447
    safety issues, 853
    segmental, 529–530
    surgical ablation, 643–651, 654–655
pulmonary veins (PVs)
    anatomy, 195
    electrical isolation of, 852–853, 853*f*
    endpoints and limitations, 534
    linear catheter ablation and disconnection, 521, 521*f*, 522*f*
    stenosis, 550, 612, 670, 687, 853, 970–971, 972
pulmonary vein triggers
    atrial fibrillation and focal and map-guided ablation, 527–537, 528*f*, 529*f*, 531*f*, 532*f*, 533*f*, 535*f*, 536*f*, 537*f*, 538*f*
    catheter ablation, 851–852
    ectopy, recognizing, 527–529, 528*f*, 529*f*
    non-, 534
pulse generator pocket, 695, 700, 710, 710*f*
PVAC. *See* Pulmonary Vein Ablation Catheter
PVCs. *See* premature ventricular complexes
PVI. *See* pulmonary vein isolation
PVs. *See* pulmonary veins

Q

Quality of Recovery score, 460
QUIDAM study, 990
quinidine, 944, 990

R

RAAFT. *See* Radiofrequency Ablation for Atrial Fibrillation Trial
radiation exposure
    computed tomography and, 99
    electrophysiology procedures and, 5–6
    pediatric patients and, 408–409
    reducing, 671
radiation safety, 41, 42*f*, 128
radiofrequency
    See also catheter ablation
    advantages and disadvantages, 858*t*
    biophysics of, 205–207, 206*f*, 207*f*
    bipolar, 237–238, 237*f*, 583, 623, 623*f*, 630, 644, 644*f*
    catheter impedance and determining lesion status, 209
    catheter improvements, 209–212, 210*f*, 211*f*
    coagulum (char) formation, 208, 208*f*
    conductive heating, 206
    contact force, 212–213, 213*f*, 214*f*
    cryoballoon compared with, 549
    duty-cycled phased energy, 215
    ischemic cardiomyopathy and, 577–578

laser ablations compared with, 545–546, 546t
lesion size, determinants of, 207
in pediatric patients, 405–408
resistive heating, 205
steam popping, 209
surgical ablation, 623, 623f
thermal latency, 206–207, 207f
unipolar, 235–236, 236f
Radiofrequency Ablation for Atrial Fibrillation Trial (RAAFT), 948–949, 973
radiography
complications and use of, 784, 785f, 786f
device recognition, 791–792, 791f, 792t–793t, 793f
leads, coils, and patches, 793–794, 794f, 795f
postimplantation use, 783, 784f, 787f, 788f, 789–791
postimplant lead assessment, 785–787, 785f, 786f, 789f, 790f, 791f
preprocedural assessment, 797–798, 797f, 798f
troubleshooting with, 795–796, 795f, 796f, 797f
uses for, 783
RAFT. See Resynchronization-Defibrillation for Ambulatory Heart Failure Trial
ranolazine, 944, 948
RASTA trial, 949
recalls and safety alerts, 743–744, 744t, 746f
recording systems, for electrophysiology procedures, 6
REDUCEhf. See Reducing Events in Patients with Chronic Heart Failure
Reducing Events in Patients with Chronic Heart Failure (REDUCEhf) trial, 816
REFORM. See Remote Follow-up for ICD-Therapy in Patients Meeting MADIT II Criteria
reimbursement, 748–749, 749t–750t
remifentanil, 279t, 437, 439, 446
remifentanyl, 271f, 275
Remote Follow-up for ICD-Therapy in Patients Meeting MADIT II Criteria (REFORM), 153, 161
remote monitoring, 762, 813, 818
See also cardiovascular/cardiac implantable electronic devices, remote monitoring and; monitoring devices
remote navigation
atrial fibrillation and, 533, 859, 859f
goals of, 241
magnetic, 243–245, 243f, 244f
robotic, 241–243, 242f, 245, 533
repolarization abnormalities, 20, 21f
respiratory inductance plethysmography (RIP), 442, 443f
RESPONSE-HF trial, 779
Resynchronization-Defibrillation for Ambulatory Heart Failure Trial (RAFT), 769t, 901, 911
RethinQ trial, 720
return-cycle mapping, 426, 427f
revascularization, 932–933
REVERSE trial, 768, 769t, 900
Riata lead, 143, 712, 712f, 715, 824, 832, 833f
right atrium, anatomy, 190, 190f
right ventricle, anatomy, 199–200, 199f, 200f
right ventricular apex (RVA) catheters, 6, 8, 9f

right ventricular lead placement, 697, 698f, 699
right ventricular outflow tract (RVOT)
anatomy, 554–555, 554f, 555f
electrocardiographic findings, 11–13, 12f, 13f, 554f, 556–557
intracardiac echocardiography, 560–561
location of intracardiac catheters, 557, 558f, 559–560, 559f, 560f
mapping, 561–564, 561f
right ventricular pacing, 901
RIP. See respiratory inductance plethysmography
rivaroxaban, 706
rocuronium, 275, 277
Roentgen, W., 6
ropivacaine, 269, 270
RVA. See right ventricular apex
RVOT. See right ventricular outflow tract

S

SACT. See sinoatrial conduction time
SAFE. See Septal Pacing for Atrial Fibrillation Suppression Evaluation
SAFE PACE trial, 899–900
safety alerts, 743–744, 744t, 746f
SAFS. See Surgical Atrial Fibrillation Suppression
sarcoid cardiomyopathy, 881
sarcoidosis, 124, 572, 582, 582f
SAVE PACE study, 951
SCD. See sudden cardiac death
SCD-HeFT. See Sudden Cardiac Death in Heart Failure Trial
SCIP. See Surgical Care Improvement Project
sedation. See anesthesia/sedation
sedative-hypnotics, 437–438
Seldinger, S. I., 5
Seldinger technique, 5
Senning procedure, 51, 410t, 411, 412
Sensei Robotic Catheter System, 213, 214f, 533, 859
SensorMedics High-Frequency Oscillator, 441
Septal Pacing for Atrial Fibrillation Suppression Evaluation (SAFE) study, 950, 955
septal substrates, 582–583
SERF. See Synergistic Effects of Risk Factors for Sudden Cardiac Death
sevoflurane, 275f, 276, 438, 456, 457
SHIELD. See Shock Inhibition Evaluation with Azimilide
shock
implantable cardioverter-defibrillators, 141, 981–982, 987–988, 989–990
postoperative, 756, 762
Shock Inhibition Evaluation with Azimilide (SHIELD) trial, 984, 992
sick sinus syndrome (SSS), 284–285, 284f, 285f, 898
signal filtration, 25
sinoatrial conduction time (SACT), 7, 287
sinus nodal reentrant tachycardia, 477, 844
sinus node
anatomy, 52, 191, 192f, 283–284, 283f, 475
autonomic testing, 286–287
catheter ablation, 475

damage to, 52
electroanatomic mapping, 287–289, 288f, 289f
electrophysiology of, 284
indications for evaluating, 286
reentry, 844
sinus node dysfunction (SND)
See also inappropriate sinus tachycardia
clinical presentation, 896
electrocardiogram manifestations of, 895–896, 896f
etiology and pathophysiology, 896
pacemaker indications for, 896–897, 897f, 902t, 903t
sick sinus syndrome, 284–285, 284f, 285f, 898
sinus node recovery time (SNRT), 7, 287
sinus tachycardia (ST)
electrocardiographic findings, 14–16, 15f, 16f
inappropriate, 285–286, 476–477, 477f, 679–683, 681t, 681f, 682f, 683t
skin infections, implants and, 713, 757
skin preparation and sterilization, 459–460, 694, 707
SMART-AV. See Smart Delay Determined AV Optimization
Smart Delay Determined AV Optimization (SMART-AV) trial, 778
SMASH-VT. See Substrate Mapping and Ablation in Sinus Rhythm to Halt Ventricular Tachycardia
SND. See sinus node dysfunction
SNRT. See sinus node recovery time
Society of Thoracic Surgeons, 908
sotalol, 702, 944, 944f, 974f, 984
spatial frequency, 100
Speckle Tracking Assisted Resynchronization Therapy for Electrode Region (STARTER), 772
Sprint Fidelis, 143, 712, 715, 824, 832, 832f
SSS. See sick sinus syndrome
ST. See sinus tachycardia
STARTER. See Speckle Tracking Assisted Resynchronization Therapy for Electrode Region
Stereotaxis Magnetic Navigation System, 533, 859
sternotomy approach, surgical, 621
STICH trial, 936
St. Jude Medical
Confirm, 814
CPS Direct ST Slittable Outer Guide Catheter, 136, 136f
EnGuide, 410, 415
EnSite NavX, 104, 337, 338f, 410, 530, 855
EnSite Velocity Cardiac Mapping System, 35, 39–40, 39f, 40f, 41f, 104, 105
EnSite Versimo, 102
Merlin.net Patient Care System, 152
Quartet LV pacing, 136, 137f, 137t
Riata, 143, 712, 712f, 715, 824, 832, 833f
STOP AF. See Sustained Treatment of Paroxysmal Atrial Fibrillation
STRATUM VT trial, 584
structural heart disease
evaluation and testing, 871, 873–874, 874t

role of ventricular tachycardia and
ablation in, 14–16, 14f, 15f, 345–352,
874–875, 875t
Substrate Mapping and Ablation in Sinus
Rhythm to Halt Ventricular Tachycardia
(SMASH-VT), 578, 611, 876, 989
subxiphoid approach, surgical, 620, 621f
succinylcholine, 275
sudden cardiac death (SCD)
congenital heart disease, 884
defined, 907
implantable cardioverter-defibrillator
trials for prevention of, 871, 872t
primary prevention of, 877, 878t, 879t,
910–912
secondary prevention of, 871, 908, 910
Sudden Cardiac Death in Heart Failure Trial
(SCD-HeFT), 762, 872t, 877, 879, 909t,
910, 911, 912, 915, 916, 982
sufentanil, 279t
supraventricular tachycardias (SVTs)
See also paroxysmal supraventricular
tachycardias
mapping and, 26–27, 26t, 27f, 28f, 28t,
29, 29t, 30f
pacing maneuvers, 27, 28t, 29, 29t
in pediatric patients, 56
surgical ablation
atrial flutter, 926
complications, 669–675, 685–688
energy sources, 621–622
hybrid surgical/catheter ablation, 927
inappropriate sinus tachycardia, 679–683,
681t, 681f, 682f, 683t
left anterior thoracotomy approach,
620–621
left atrial appendage, 645, 649, 650f, 671,
926
paroxysmal atrial fibrillation, 921, 926
pericardioscopy, midline, 925, 925f
sternotomy approach, 621, 924–925
subxiphoid approach, 620, 621f
thoracoscopic approach, 621, 622f, 925
ventricular tachycardia with hybrid
endocardial and epicardial approaches,
619–626, 620f, 621f, 622f, 623f, 624f,
626f
surgical ablation, for atrial fibrillation
See also radiofrequency
anatomic issues, 234
bipolar radiofrequency energy, 237–238,
237f, 583, 644, 644f
Cox-Maze IV procedure, 629–633, 629f,
630f, 631f, 632f, 653–654
cryoablation, 234–235, 234f
cryosurgical Cox-Maze procedure,
635–640, 636f, 637f, 637t, 638f, 638t,
639f
development of, 976–977, 976f
energy sources, 924
extended left atrial lesion set, 653–657,
655f
ganglionic ablation, 645, 646f, 659–664,
661f, 663f
hybrid procedures, 667–675, 672f, 673f,
674f
indications for, 921
lesion patterns, 922–924, 922f, 923f, 924f
patient-specific recommendations,
925–926

patients with prior nodal balation and
pacemaker, 927
requirements for, 233
results, 922t
stand-alone, 926
surgical approaches, 924–925
unipolar radiofrequency energy, 235–236,
236f
with left antral pulmonary vein isolation,
ganglionic plexi ablation and excision
of left atrial appendage, 643–651,
644f, 645t, 646f, 646t, 647f, 648f, 649f,
650f
surgical ablation, for ventrical tachycardia
cryoablation, 622–623, 623f
current techniques and results, 931, 932f
endocardial resection and cryoablation,
933–934, 933f, 934t, 935f
energy sources, 621–622
high-intensity focused ultrasound, 624,
624f
history of, 929
hybrid, 624–625, 626f
indications for, 936–937
ischemic, 930
left anterior thoracotomy approach,
620–621
nonischemic, 930–931
radiofrequency, 623, 623f
rationale for, 619–620, 620f
revascularization, 932–933
sternotomy approach, 621
subxiphoid approach, 620, 621f
surgical ventricular restoration, 935–936
thoracoscopic approach, 621, 622f
Surgical Atrial Fibrillation Suppression
(SAFS) study, 976
Surgical Care Improvement Project (SCIP),
457
surgical scar, 124
surgical ventricular restoration (SVR),
935–936
SurgiFrost CryoSurgical probe, 623f
Sustained Treatment of Paroxysmal Atrial
Fibrillation (STOP AF), 549
SVR. See surgical ventricular restoration
SVTs. See supraventricular tachycardias
SYNBIAPACE study, 956
syncope, monitoring for, 813–815
Synergistic Effects of Risk Factors for Sudden
Cardiac Death (SERF) study, 915
SYNPACE. See Vasovagal Syncope and Pacing
systemic inflammatory diseases, 293

T

tachycardia cycle length (TCL), 505, 506,
507f, 515
tachycardias, indications for pacemaker
implantation, 902–903, 902f, 903f
TactiCath catheter, 213
tamponade, 611, 670, 831, 970, 972
TARGET. See Targeted Left Ventricular
Lead Placement to Guide Cardiac
Resynchronization Therapy
Targeted Left Ventricular Lead Placement to
Guide Cardiac Resynchronization Therapy
(TARGET) study, 772

TCL. See tachycardia cycle length
TDI. See Tissue Doppler Imaging
TEE. See transesophageal echocardiography
terminal crest, anatomy, 190, 190f
tetralogy of Fallot, 51, 199, 293, 413, 414–415,
427
Thebesian valve, anatomy, 190f, 191
thiopental, 271f, 272, 279t
thoracoscopic approach, surgical, 621, 622f
thoracotomy approach, surgical left anterior,
620–621
three-dimensional imaging with intracardiac
echocardiography, 93–94
three-dimensional mapping systems
atrial fibrillation and, 106–108, 107f,
337–338, 338f, 339f, 340f, 341, 341f
clinical applications, 106–113
integrating, 101–105, 102f, 103f, 105f,
106f
three-dimensional rotational angiography
(3DRA), 112–113, 113t, 114f
three-dimensional transesophageal
echocardiography. See transesophageal/
transthoracic echocardiography (3D)
thromboembolism, 613, 670
Tissue Doppler Imaging (TDI), 719, 719f
torsades de pointes, 249, 251, 262, 392, 607,
610, 840, 893, 895, 902, 931, 973, 974, 974f
transaortic mapping, 24
transesophageal echocardiography (TEE), 572
compared to intracardiac
echocardiography, 86–87, 88
complications, 459
role of, 66, 67–68, 71, 72f
transesophageal/transthoracic echocardiography (3D)
left atrial appendage, 72–75, 73f, 74f, 75f
left ventricular dyssynchrony, 77–79,
78f, 79f
left ventricular ejection fraction, 71,
75–76, 76f
nonischemic cardiomyopathies, 76–77
overview of, 71–72
pericardial effusions, 79, 80f
role of, 66, 67–68, 71, 72f
transseptal catheterization (TSC), intracardiac
echocardiography and, 87, 87f, 88f
transseptal mapping, 24, 24f
transthoracic echocardiography (2D), 71, 72
transvenous lead extraction. See lead extraction
TRENDS study, 812
triangle of Koch, 15, 18f, 53, 192, 193f, 200,
289, 290f, 296, 478, 478f
trifascicular block, 895
TRUST (Lumos-T Safely Reduces Routine
Office Device Follow-up), 153, 154,
155–156, 160
TSC. See transseptal catheterization
TTE. See transesophageal/transthoracic
echocardiography (3D); transthoracic
echocardiography (2D)
Twiddler's syndrome, 710
two-dimensional transthoracic
echocardiography. See transthoracic
echocardiography (2D)

U

UKPACE. *See* United Kingdom Pacing and Cardiovascular Events
ultrasound ablation, 228–230, 229*f*
   advantages and disadvantages, 858*t*
ULV. *See* upper limit of vulnerability
United Kingdom Pacing and Cardiovascular Events (UKPACE) trial, 897–898
upper limit of vulnerability (ULV) testing, 702

V

VA. *See* ventriculoatrial
valve annuli. *See* idiopathic annular ventricular arrhythmias
VANISH. *See* Ventricular Tachycardia Ablation vs. Enhanced Drug Therapy in Structural Heart Disease
vascular access, for electrophysiology procedures, 5
vascular complications, 614
vascular tears, 831
Vasovagal Pacemaker Study II (VPS-II), 899
Vasovagal Syncope and Pacing (SYNPACE) trial, 899
venoplasty, 181–182
venous access, implantation techniques, 695–697, 696*f*, 697*f*, 706–710, 707*f*, 708*f*, 709*f*, 710*f*
ventricles, anatomy, 198–202, 199*f*, 200*f*, 201*f*, 202*f*
ventricular dyssynchrony (inter and intra), 718–719, 718*f*
ventricular fibrillation (VF)
   clinical and animal studies on triggers, 604–605
   hybrid procedures/therapy, 981–993
   mapping of Purkinje triggers and postablation monitoring, 599
   pacing and prevention of, 884–885, 885*t*
   polymorphic ventricular tachycardia and, 391–402, 393*f*, 394*f*, 395*f*, 396*f*, 397*f*, 399*f*, 401*f*, 599–604, 881–882
   premature ventricular complexes and, 20–21, 21*f*
ventricular pacing maneuvers, 29, 29*t*
ventricular tachyarrhythmias (VTAs)
   See also ventricular tachycardias (VTs)
   biventricular pacemakers in preventing, 885
   catheter ablation training requirements, 870–871, 871*t*
   classification of recommendations, 869, 869*f*, 870*t*
   clinical cardiac electrophysiology training requirements, 870, 870*t*
   clinical characteristics, morphologies and outcomes, 868*t*
   hybrid procedures/therapy, 981–993

ventricular tachyarrhythmias, interventional strategies
   arrhythmogenic right ventricular dysplasia/cardiomyopathy, 873
   coronary artery disease, 871–873, 874
   hypertrophic cardiomyopathy, 873
   nonischemic dilated cardiomyopathy, 873, 874
   in patients with normal hearts, 885–886
   structural heart disease, 871, 873–874, 874*t*
Ventricular Tachycardia Ablation in Coronary Disease (VTACH) trial, 989
Ventricular Tachycardia Ablation Versus Enhanced Drug Therapy in Structural Heart Disease (VANISH) trial, 583, 988
ventricular tachycardias (VTs)
   See also surgical ablation, for ventricular tachycardia
   ablation complications, 567–568
   ablation outcomes, in patients with prior myocardial infarction, 875–877
   Belhassen's, 13, 13*f*, 367
   bundle branch reentrant, 21, 21*f*, 876
   catecholaminergic polymorphic, 257, 258*f*, 883, 883*t*, 991
   catheter ablation and intracardiac echocardiography for, 90–93, 90*f*–93*f*
   catheter ablation clinical trials, 583–584
   classification of recommendations, 869, 869*f*, 870*t*
   clinical characteristics, morphologies and outcomes, 868*t*
   complications, 610–611
   computed tomography, magnetic resonance imaging, and 3D mapping systems for, 108–110, 109*f*, 110*f*, 123, 124*t*
   cryoablation, 622–623, 623*f*, 933–934, 933*f*, 934*t*, 935*f*
   echocardiography, 68
   electrical storm/incessant, 988–989, 992–993, 992*f*
   electrocardiograms, surface, 345–346, 346*f*
   endocavitary structures, 566
   epicardial mapping, 24, 24*f*, 25*f*, 50, 352, 427, 428*f*, 559*f*, 564, 579–580, 579*f*, 580*f*, 589–596, 589*f*, 590*f*, 590*t*, 591*f*, 592*f*, 593*f*, 594*f*, 595*f*
   fascicular, 13, 13*f*, 564–566
   focal, intraoperative mapping, 50–51, 50*f*, 51*f*
   hybrid procedures/therapy, 981–993
   implantable cardioverter-defibrillators electrograms, 346–347, 347*f*
   interfascicular reentry, 566
   ischemic and nonischemic cardiomyopathies, 571–584, 930–931
   left fascicular, 367–376, 368*f*, 369*f*, 370*f*, 371*f*, 372*f*, 373*f*, 375*f*

   magnetic navigation, 245
   mapping, 30–31, 31*f*, 31*t*, 561–564, 561*f*, 573–574, 573*t*, 574*f*, 575*f*
   mapping of, in acquired heart disease, 345–349, 349*f*
   mapping, intraoperative, 49–51, 49*f*, 50*f*, 51*f*, 425–427, 426*f*, 427*f*, 428*f*
   mitral annulus, 566–567
   mitral isthmus, 14, 14*f*
   noninvasive imaging, 346, 347*f*
   outflow tract, 11–13, 12*f*, 13*f*, 111, 112*f*, 357–367, 357*f*, 358*f*, 359*f*, 360*f*, 361*t*, 362*f*, 364*f*, 366*f*, 553–566
   in pediatric patients with congenital heart disease, 414–415
   polymorphic, 391–402, 393*f*, 394*f*, 395*f*, 396*f*, 397*f*, 399*f*, 401*f*, 599–604, 881–882
   reentrant, initiating, 348
   with structural heart disease, 14, 14*f*, 345–352, 873–875, 874*t*, 875*t*
   unmappable, 350–352, 350*f*, 351*f*
ventriculoatrial (VA) interval, 27, 28*t*
Venturi effect, 443
VF. *See* ventricular fibrillation
voltage mapping, 410–411, 420–421
VPS-II. *See* Vasovagal Pacemaker Study II
VTACH. *See* Ventricular Tachycardia Ablation in Coronary Disease
VTAs. *See* ventricular tachyarrhythmias
VTs. *See* ventricular tachycardias

W

Waldo, A., 26
warfarin, 74, 90, 91, 165, 168, 169, 579, 592, 613, 633, 637, 644, 686
   implantation techniques and, 693, 706
Watchman LAA Closure Technology, 165, 167, 167*f*, 168
Wenckebach, 8, 8*f*, 143, 295
Wolff–Parkinson–White syndrome, 6, 379, 619, 842
   electrocardiographic findings, 16–17, 17*f*, 18*f*
   mapping, intraoperative, 47, 52, 421–422, 421*f*
   in pediatric patients, 57
Wolf Lumitip dissector with GlidePath Transfer Guide, 648–649, 648*f*
Wolf technique, 643, 645, 645*t*, 647, 650, 651

X

x-rays, 6
   See also radiography